CLINICAL
RESPIRATORY
MEDICINE

CLINICAL RESPIRATORY MEDICINE

FOURTH EDITION

Stephen G. Spiro, BSc, MD, FRCP

Professor of Respiratory Medicine, Honorary Consultant Physician, Department of Cancer Medicine, University College London Hospitals, National Health Service Foundation Trust; Honorary Consultant Physician, The Royal Brompton Hospital, London, United Kingdom

Gerard A. Silvestri, MD, MS

Professor of Medicine, Medical University of South Carolina, Charleston, South Carolina

Alvar Agustí, MD, PhD, FRCPE

Professor, Senior Consultant and Director, Thorax Institute, Hospital Clinic, University of Barcelona, Barcelona, Spain; Scientific Director, CIBER Enfermedades Respiratorias, Fundacio D'Investigacio Sanitaria Illes Balears, Mallorca, Spain

ELSEVIER
SAUNDERS

1600 John F. Kennedy Boulevard
Suite 1800
Philadelphia, PA 19103-2899

Notices

Knowledge and best practice in this field are constantly changing. As new research and experience broaden our understanding, changes in research methods, professional practices, or medical treatment may become necessary.

Practitioners and researchers must always rely on their own experience and knowledge in evaluating and using any information, methods, compounds, or experiments described herein. In using such information or methods they should be mindful of their own safety and the safety of others, including parties for whom they have a professional responsibility.

With respect to any drug or pharmaceutical products identified, readers are advised to check the most current information provided (i) on procedures featured or (ii) by the manufacturer of each product to be administered, to verify the recommended dose or formula, the method and duration of administration, and contraindications. It is the responsibility of practitioners, relying on their own experience and knowledge of their patients, to make diagnoses, to determine dosages and the best treatment for each individual patient, and to take all appropriate safety precautions.

To the fullest extent of the law, neither the Publisher nor the authors, contributors, or editors, assume any liability for any injury and/or damage to persons or property as a matter of products liability, negligence or otherwise, or from any use or operation of any methods, products, instructions, or ideas contained in the material herein.

Content Strategist: Pamela Hetherington
Senior Content Development Specialist: Anne Snyder
Publishing Services Manager: Patricia Tannian
Senior Project Manager: Sarah Wunderly
Design Direction: Louis Forgione

Printed in China

Last digit is the print number: 9 8 7 6 5 4 3 2 1

DEDICATION

To my parents, Ludwig and Anna, who supported me in my earlier years and taught me the importance of education and knowledge. To Alison, who always gave me the time to work and enjoy my career while she cared for the family and engaged in her own profession.
STEPHEN SPIRO

For my father, who taught me to aspire to greatness in my career while never forgetting where I came from and those who truly matter—my family. For my mother, who passed along a love of reading and the gift of memory. For my children, Nate and Mia, who are already better people than I could ever have hoped. Most of all, for my wife, Joanne, whose love and support are the glue that holds it all together.
GERARD SILVESTRI

To my wife Gemma, daughters Belén and Inés, and son Alvaro, the best family any man could think of.
ALVAR AGUSTÍ

CONTRIBUTORS

Asia A. Ahmed, MBBS, MRCP, FRCR
*Senior Specialist Registrar in Radiology, Department of Imaging,
University College London Hospital National Health Service
Foundation Trust, London, United Kingdom*
Percutaneous Biopsy Procedures: Techniques and Indications

Richard K. Albert, MD
*Chief of Medicine, Denver Health; Professor of Medicine,
University of Colorado, Aurora, Colorado*
Chest Pain

Mark S. Allen, MD
*Professor of Surgery, Chair, Division of General Thoracic
Surgery, Mayo Clinic, Rochester, Minnesota*
Diagnostic Thoracic Surgical Procedures

Douglas Arenberg, MD
*Associate Professor, Division of Pulmonary and Critical
Care Medicine, University of Michigan Medical Center,
Ann Arbor, Michigan*
Lung Cancer: Treatment

Phil Bearfield, MB, ChB, FRCA, EDIC, FFICM
*Consultant Intensivist, Royal Free Hospital, London,
United Kingdom*
Hemodynamic Monitoring in Critical Illness

Thomas Benfield, MD, DMSc
*Associate Professor, Department of Infectious Diseases,
University of Copenhagen, Hvidovre University Hospital,
Hvidovre, Denmark*
Noninfectious Conditions in Patients with Human
Immunodeficiency Virus Infection

Ilya Berim, MD
*Fellow, Pulmonary and Critical Care Medicine, School of
Medicine and Biomedical Sciences, University at Buffalo,
The State University of New York, Buffalo, New York*
Community-Acquired Pneumonia

Kathryn G. Bird, MD
Occupational Physician, Concentra, Golden, Colorado
Toxic Inhalational Lung Injury

Surinder S. Birring, MD, MRCP
*Honorary Senior Lecturer Division of Asthma, Allergy and
Lung Biology, King's College London; Consultant Physician,
Department of Respiratory Medicine, King's College Hospital,
London, United Kingdom*
Cough

Lukas Brander, MD
*Department of Intensive Care Medicine, Inselspital, Bern
University Hospital, University of Bern, Bern, Switzerland*
Invasive Mechanical Ventilation

Jeremy S. Brown, MBBS, PhD, FRCP
*Reader, Centre for Respiratory Research, University College
London, London, United Kingdom*
Pneumonia in the Non–HIV-Infected Immunocompromised
Patient

Kevin K. Brown, MD
*Professor and Vice Chairman, Department of Medicine, Division
of Pulmonary and Critical Care Medicine, National Jewish
Health, University of Colorado, Aurora, Colorado*
Idiopathic Pulmonary Fibrosis and Other Interstitial
Lung Diseases

Todd M. Bull, MD
*Associate Professor, Pulmonary Sciences and Critical Care
Medicine; Director, Pulmonary Vascular Center, University of
Colorado, Aurora, Colorado*
Pulmonary Embolism

Felip Burgos, MSc, RPFT, RN
*Servei de Pneumologia i Allèrgia Respiratòria, ICT,
Departament de Medicina, Institut D'Investigacions
Biomèdiques August Pi i Sunyer, Hospital Clínic,
Universitat de Barcelona, Barcelona, Spain*
Exercise Testing

Peter M.A. Calverley, MB, ChB, FRCP, FRCPE
*Professor of Respiratory Medicine, Institute of Ageing and
Chronic Disease, University of Liverpool; Consultant Physician,
Clinical Sciences Centre, University Hospital Aintree, Liverpool,
United Kingdom*
Bronchodilators

Philippe Camus, MD
*Professor, Division of Pulmonary and Critical Care, Centre
Hospitalier Universitaire de Dijon, Hôpital du Bocage,
Université de Bourgogne, Dijon, France*
Drug-Induced and Iatrogenic Respiratory Diseases

Paolo Carbonara, MD
*Physician, Division of Respiratory and Critical Care Medicine,
Sant'Orsola-Malpighi Hospital, University of Bologna,
Bologna, Italy*
Noninvasive Mechanical Ventilation

William Graham Carlos III, MD
*Assistant Professor of Clinical Medicine, Indiana University
School of Medicine, Indianapolis, Indiana*
Nonbacterial Infectious Pneumonia

Stephen D. Cassivi, MD, MSc, FRCSC
Associate Professor of Surgery, Division of General Thoracic Surgery; Director of Lung Transplantation, Mayo Clinic, Rochester, Minnesota
Chest Tube Insertion and Management
Diagnostic Thoracic Surgical Procedures

Rodrigo Cavallazzi, MD
Assistant Professor of Medicine, Assistant Director, Intensive Care Services, University of Louisville Health Sciences Center, Louisville, Kentucky
Pulmonary Complications of Hematopoietic Stem Cell Transplantation

Bartolome R. Celli, MD
Professor of Medicine, Harvard Medical School, Brigham and Women's Hospital, Boston, Massachusetts
Treatment of the Stable Patient with Chronic Obstructive Pulmonary Disease

William Y.C. Chang, MBMCh, MA(Oxon)
Research Fellow, Division of Therapeutics and Molecular Medicine, University of Nottingham, Nottingham, United Kingdom
Rare Diffuse Interstitial Lung Diseases

Chung-Wai Chow, MD, PhD
Assistant Professor, Division of Respirology, Department of Medicine, University of Toronto; Staff Respirologist, Division of Respirology, Multiorgan Transplant Unit, University Health Network, Toronto, Ontario, Canada
Pulmonary Host Defenses

Andrew M. Churg, MD, FRCP(C)
Professor of Pathology, University of British Columbia; Pathologist, Vancouver General Hospital, Vancouver, Canada
Macro and Micro Structure of the Lung

Jean-François Cordier, MD
Professor of Respiratory Medicine, Claude Bernard Lyon 1 University; Head of Department of Respiratory Medicine, Reference Center for Rare Pulmonary Diseases, Louis Pradel University Hospital, Lyon, France
Eosinophilic Lung Disease
Organizing Pneumonia

Borja G. Cosio, MD, PhD, MCP
Consultant, Department of Respiratory Medicine, Hospital Universitario Son Espases, Palma de Mallorca, Spain
Asthma: Epidemiology, Pathophysiology, and Risk Factors

Vincent Cottin, MD, PhD
Professor of Respiratory Medicine, Claude Bernard Lyon 1 University; Department of Respiratory Medicine, Reference Center for Rare Pulmonary Diseases, Louis Pradel University Hospital, Lyon, France
Eosinophilic Lung Disease
Organizing Pneumonia

Bruce H. Culver, MD
Associate Professor of Medicine, Division of Pulmonary and Critical Care Medicine, University of Washington School of Medicine, Seattle, Washington
Respiratory Mechanics
Pulmonary Circulation
Pulmonary Function Testing

Charles L. Daley, MD
Professor and Chief, Division of Mycobacterial and Respiratory Infections, National Jewish Health; Professor, Division of Pulmonary and Critical Care Medicine and Infectious Diseases, University of Colorado, Aurora, Colorado
Tuberculosis and Nontuberculous Mycobacterial Infections

Helen E. Davies, MD, MRCP
Consultant in Respiratory Medicine, University Hospital of Wales, Cardiff, United Kingdom
Pleural Effusion, Empyema, and Pneumothorax

Chadrick E. Denlinger, MD
Assistant Professor, Medical University of South Carolina, Charleston, South Carolina
Diagnostic Thoracic Surgical Procedures

Christophe Deroose, MD, PhD
Assistant Professor, Catholic University; Deputy Clinical Head, Positron Emission Tomography Centre, Department of Nuclear Medicine, University Hospital Gasthuisberg, Leuven, Belgium
Positron Emission Tomography Imaging

Claude Deschamps, MD
Professor of Surgery, Division of General Thoracic Surgery; Chair, Department of Surgery, Mayo Clinic, Rochester, Minnesota
Chest Tube Insertion and Management

Christophe Dooms, MD, PhD
Assistant Professor of Internal Medicine, Catholic University; Deputy Clinical Head, Pulmonology, University Hospital Gasthuisberg, Leuven, Belgium
Positron Emission Tomography Imaging

Gregory P. Downey, MD
Professor and Executive Vice President, Academic Affairs, Division of Pulmonary and Critical Care Medicine, Departments of Medicine and Pediatrics, National Jewish Health; Professor, Department of Medicine, Integrated Department of Immunology, University of Colorado, Aurora, Colorado
Pulmonary Host Defenses

Miquel Ferrer, MD, PhD
Assistant Professor of Medicine, University of Barcelona; Senior Consultant, Respiratory Intensive Care Unit, Thorax Institute, Hospital Clinic, Barcelona, Spain
Nosocomial Respiratory Infections

Rodney J. Folz, MD, PhD
*Professor of Medicine, Biochemistry, and Molecular Biology;
Chief, Pulmonary, Critical Care, and Sleep Disorders Medicine;
Director; Adult Cystic Fibrosis Program; Distinguished
University Scholar, University of Louisville Health Sciences
Center, Louisville, Kentucky*
Pulmonary Complications of Hematopoietic Stem
Cell Transplantation

Edward R. Garrity, Jr., MD, MBA
*Professor of Medicine, Section of Pulmonary and Critical Care
Medicine, University of Chicago, Chicago, Illinois*
Lung Transplantation

Alex H. Gifford, MD
*Assistant Professor of Medicine, Dartmouth Medical School,
Hanover, New Hampshire*
Dyspnea

Robb W. Glenny, MD
*Professor of Medicine, Physiology, and Biophysics; Head,
Division of Pulmonary and Critical Care Medicine, University
of Washington, Seattle, Washington*
Pulmonary Circulation

Kelsey Gray, MD, MS
*Fellow, Pulmonary and Critical Care Medicine, University of
Colorado, Aurora, Colorado*
Extrinsic Allergic Alveolitis

Ruth H. Green, MBChB, MSc, MD, FRCP
*Consultant Respiratory Physician and Honorary Senior Lecturer,
Institute for Lung Health, Glenfield Hospital, University
Hospitals of Leicester National Health Service Foundation Trust,
Leicester, United Kingdom*
Diagnosis and Management of Asthma in Adults

Michael P. Gruber, MD
*Assistant Clinical Professor, University of Colorado, Aurora,
Colorado*
Pulmonary Embolism

J.C. Grutters, MD, PhD
*Professor, Department of Pulmonology, Center of Interstitial Lung
Diseases, St. Antonius Hospital, Nieuwegein, The Netherlands;
Division of Heart and Lungs, University Medical
Center Utrecht, Utrecht, The Netherlands*
Connective Tissue Diseases

Andrew R. Haas, MD, PhD
*Assistant Professor of Medicine, Perelman School of Medicine;
Director of Clinical Operations, Section of Interventional
Pulmonology and Thoracic Oncology, Pulmonary, Allergy, and
Critical Care Division, University of Pennsylvania Medical
Center, Philadelphia, Pennsylvania*
Bronchoscopy

Chadi A. Hage, MD
*Assistant Professor of Medicine, Indiana University; Staff
Physician, Roudebush VA Medical Center, Indianapolis, Indiana*
Nonbacterial Infectious Pneumonia

Pranabashis Haldar, MD, MRCP
*Senior Lecturer, Department of Respiratory Medicine, Institute
for Lung Health, Glenfield Hospital, University Hospitals of
Leicester National Health Service Foundation Trust, Leicester,
United Kingdom*
Diagnosis and Management of Asthma in Adults

David M. Hansell, MD, FRCP, FRCR
*Professor of Thoracic Imaging, National Heart and Lung
Institute, Imperial College School of Medicine; Consultant
Radiologist, Royal Brompton and Harefield National Health
Service Foundation Trust, London, United Kingdom*
Imaging Techniques

Nicholas Hart, BSc, PhD, MRCP, FFICM
*Clinical Research Consultant, Respiratory and Critical Care
Medicine, National Institute of Health Research, Comprehensive
Biomedical Research Centre, King's College London; Clinical
and Academic Director, Lane Fox Respiratory Unit, St. Thomas'
Hospital, Guy's and St. Thomas' National Health Service
Foundation Trust, London, United Kingdom*
Diseases of the Thoracic Cage and Respiratory Muscles

Felix J.F. Herth, MD, PhD, FCCP
*Professor of Medicine, Chairman and Head, Department of
Pneumology and Critical Care Medicine, Thoraxklinik,
University of Heidelberg, Heidelberg, Germany*
Endobronchial and Endoesophageal Ultrasound Techniques

Kristin B. Highland, MD, MSCR
*Associate Professor of Medicine, Division of Pulmonary, Critical
Care, Allergy, and Sleep Medicine, Medical University of South
Carolina, Charleston, South Carolina*
Pulmonary Hypertension

Andre Holmes, MD
*Senior Pulmonary Fellow, Division of Pulmonary, Critical Care,
Allergy, and Sleep Medicine, Medical University of South
Carolina, Charleston, South Carolina*
Pulmonary Hypertension

John R. Hurst, PhD, FRCP
*Senior Lecturer, Academic Unit of Respiratory Medicine,
University College London Medical School, London,
United Kingdom*
Management of Exacerbations in Chronic Obstructive
Pulmonary Disease

Michael C. Iannuzzi, MD, MBA
*Edward C. Reifenstein Professor and Chair, Department of
Medicine, State University of New York, Upstate Medical
University, Syracuse, New York*
Sarcoidosis

Ferrán Barbé Illa, MD
*Respiratory Department, Hospital University Arnau
de Vilanova, University of Lleida, Lleida; CIBERES,
Madrid, Spain*
Obstructive Sleep Apnea: Epidemiology, Risk Factors,
and Pathophysiology

Cyrielle Jardin, MD
Pulmonary Medicine Fellow, Service de Pneumologie et Immuno-allergologie, Centre de Competence des Maladies Pulmonaires Rares, Hôpital Albert Calmette, CHRU at Universite de Lille 2, Lille, France
Silicosis and Coal Worker's Pneumoconiosis

Simon R. Johnson, MBBS, DM, FRCP
Professor of Respiratory Medicine, Division of Therapeutics and Molecular Medicine, University of Nottingham and National Centre for Lymphangioleiomyomatosis, Nottingham, United Kingdom
Rare Diffuse Interstitial Lung Diseases

Robert M. Kacmarek, RRT, PhD
Professor, Department of Anesthesia, Harvard University; Director, Department of Respiratory Care, Massachusetts General Hospital; Boston, Massachusetts
Acute Respiratory Distress Syndrome

Harsha H. Kariyawasam, MBBS, MRCP, BSc, PhD
Consultant Physician, Department of Allergy and Medical Rhinology, Royal National Throat, Nose and Ear Hospital, London, United Kingdom
Upper Airway Disease: Rhinitis and Rhinosinusitis

Joel D. Kaufman, MD, MPH
Professor, Departments of Medicine, Environmental and Occupational Health Sciences, and Epidemiology, University of Washington, Seattle, Washington
Air Pollution

John W. Kreit, MD
Professor of Medicine and Anesthesiology and Director of Fellowship Training Programs, Division of Pulmonary, Allergy, and Critical Medicine, University of Pittsburgh School of Medicine, Pittsburgh, Pennsylvania
Hemoptysis

Michael J. Krowka, MD
Professor of Medicine, Division of Pulmonary and Critical Care Medicine, Mayo Clinic, Rochester, Minnesota
Hepatic and Biliary Disease

Mark Lambert, FRCA, BA(Hons), MBBS
Specialist Registrar in Anaesthesia, Royal Free Hospital, London, United Kingdom
Hemodynamic Monitoring in Critical Illness

J.-W.J. Lammers, MD, PhD
Professor, Division of Heart and Lungs, Department of Respiratory Medicine, University Medical Center Utrecht, Utrecht, The Netherlands
Connective Tissue Diseases

Stephen E. Lapinsky, MB BCh, MSc, FRCPC
Professor of Medicine, University of Toronto; Site Director, Intensive Care Unit, Mount Sinai Hospital, Toronto, Canada
Pregnancy

Y.C. Gary Lee, MBChB, PhD, FCCP, FRACP
Winthrop Professor of Respiratory Medicine, The University of Western Australia; Consultant and Director of Pleural Services, Respiratory Department, Sir Charles Gairdner Hospital; Head, Pleural Disease Unit, Lung Institute of Western Australia, Perth, Australia
Pleural Effusion, Empyema, and Pneumothorax

Gianluigi Li Bassi, MD
Researcher, Institut D'Investigacions Biomèdiques August Pi i Sunyer; Attending Physician, Respiratory Critical Care Unit, Thorax Institute, Hospital Clinic, Barcelona, Spain
Nosocomial Respiratory Infections

Marc C.I. Lipman, MC, FRCP
Senior Lecturer and Consultant Physician, Centre for Respiratory Medicine, Royal Free Hospital, University College London, London, United Kingdom
Pulmonary Infections in Patients with Human Immunodeficiency Virus Disease

David A. Lomas, PhD, ScD, FRCP, FMedSci
Professor, Department of Medicine, University of Cambridge, Cambridge Institute for Medical Research, Cambridge, United Kingdom
Basic Aspects of Cellular and Molecular Biology

William MacNee, MBChB, MC(Hons), FRCP(Glas), FRCP(Edin)
Professor, The Edinburgh Lung and the Environment Group Initiative Colt Research Laboratories, Medical Research Council Centre for Inflammation Research, Queen's Medical Research Institute, University of Edinburgh, Edinburgh, Scotland, United Kingdom
Chronic Obstructive Pulmonary Disease: Epidemiology, Pathophysiology, and Clinical Evaluation

Donald A. Mahler, MD
Professor of Medicine, Dartmouth Medical School; Director, Pulmonary Function and Cardiopulmonary Exercise Laboratories, Dartmouth-Hitchcock Medical Center, Lebanon, New Hampshire
Dyspnea

Jean-Luc Malo, MD
Professor, Université de Montréal, Hôpital du Sacré-Coeur de Montréal, Montreal, Canada
Occupational Asthma

Stefan J. Marciniak, MA, FRCP, PhD
Medical Research Council Senior Clinical Fellow, Cambridge Institute for Medical Research, University of Cambridge; Honorary Consultant Physician, Addenbrooke's Hospital National Health Service Foundation Trust, Cambridge, United Kingdom
Basic Aspects of Cellular and Molecular Biology

José M. Marin, MD, PhD
Hospital Universitario Miguel Servet, Aragon Institute of Health Sciences, Zaragoza, Spain
Obstructive Sleep Apnea: Clinical Features, Diagnosis, and Treatment

Miguel Ángel Martínez-García, MD
Respiratory Department, Polytechnic and University Hospital, Valencia, Spain
Obstructive Sleep Apnea: Epidemiology, Risk Factors, and Pathophysiology

Peter Mazzone, MD, MPH, FCCP
Director, Lung Cancer Program, Cleveland Clinic Respiratory Institute, Cleveland, Ohio
Preoperative Pulmonary Evaluation

Alan McGlennan, BSc, MBBS, FRCA
Consultant Anaesthetist, Royal Free Hospital, London, United Kingdom
Airway Management in the Intensive Care Unit

Pamela J. McShane, MD
Assistant Professor of Medicine, Section of Pulmonary and Critical Care Medicine, University of Chicago, Chicago, Illinois
Lung Transplantation

Tarek Meniawy, MBBS, FRACP
Medical Oncology Fellow, Department of Medical Oncology, Sir Charles Gairdner Hospital; Research Fellow, University of Western Australia School of Medicine and Pharmacology and National Centre for Asbestos Related Diseases, Nedlands, Australia
Malignant Pleural Mesothelioma

David E. Midthun, MD
Professor of Medicine, Mayo Clinic, Rochester, Minnesota
Benign Lung Tumors

Robert F. Miller, MBBS, FRCP, CBiol, FSB
Professor and Reader in Clinical Infection; Honorary Consultant Physician, Camden Provider Services, University College London, London, United Kingdom
Pulmonary Infections in Patients with Human Immunodeficiency Virus Disease

Theo J. Moraes, MD, PhD
Assistant Professor, Department of Pediatrics, University of Toronto; Pediatric Respirologist, Division of Respirology, Department of Pediatrics, The Hospital for Sick Children, Toronto, Canada
Pulmonary Host Defenses

Alison Morris, MD, MS
Associate Professor of Medicine, Immunology, and Clinical and Translational Research, Department of Medicine, University of Pittsburgh School of Medicine, Pittsburgh, Pennsylvania
Pulmonary Infections in Patients with Human Immunodeficiency Virus Disease

Gimbada B. Mwenge, MD
Center for Sleep Medicine, Cliniques Universitaires Saint-Luc, Université Catholique de Louvain, Brussels, Belgium
Obesity Hypoventilation Syndrome

Stefano Nava, MD
Director, Division of Respiratory and Critical Care Medicine, Sant'Orsola-Malpighi Hospital, Bologna, Italy
Noninvasive Mechanical Ventilation

Lee S. Newman, MD, MA
Professor, Department of Environmental and Occupational Health, Colorado School of Public Health, Department of Medicine, School of Medicine, University of Colorado, Aurora, Colorado
Asbestosis
Toxic Inhalational Lung Injury

Aynur Okcay, MD
Cardiopulmonary Research Fellow, Mayo Clinic, Rochester, Minnesota
Hepatic and Biliary Disease

Simon P.G. Padley, BSc, MBBS, FRCP, FRCR
Reader in Radiology, Imperial College School of Medicine; Consultant Radiologist, Chelsea and Westminster Hospital National Health Service Foundation Trust, Royal Brompton Hospital and Harefield National Health Service Foundation Trust, London, United Kingdom
Imaging Techniques

Ganapathi Iyer Parameswaran, MBBS
Research Assistant Professor, Department of Medicine, University at Buffalo, State University of New York; Physician, Division of Infectious Diseases, VA Western New York Healthcare System, Buffalo, New York
Viral Pneumonia

Nicholas J. Pastis, MD
Assistant Professor of Medicine, Division of Pulmonary and Critical Care Medicine, Medical University of South Carolina, Charleston, South Carolina
Chest Tube Insertion and Management

Manju Paul, MD
Fellow, Division of Pulmonary and Critical Care Medicine, Department of Medicine, State University of New York Upstate Medical University, Syracuse, New York
Sarcoidosis

Ian D. Pavord, DM, FRCP
Consultant Physician and Honorary Professor of Medicine, Institute for Lung Health, Glenfield Hospital, University Hospitals of Leicester National Health Service Foundation Trust, Leicester, United Kingdom
Cough
Diagnosis and Management of Asthma in Adults

Hilary Petersen, MPAS, PA-C
Physician Assistant, Lung Cancer Program, Cleveland Clinic Respiratory Institute, Cleveland, Ohio
Preoperative Pulmonary Evaluation

Michael I. Polkey, PhD, FRCP
Professor of Respiratory Medicine, National Institute for Health Research, Respiratory Biomedical Research Unit, Royal Brompton and Harefield National Health Service Foundation Trust, National Heart and Lung Institute, Imperial College London, London, United Kingdom
Diseases of the Thoracic Cage and Respiratory Muscles

Jennifer Quint, MBBS, MRCP, PhD
*Doctor, London School of Hygiene and Tropical Medicine,
University College London, National Health Service Foundation
Trust, London, United Kingdom*
Pneumonia in the Non–HIV-Infected Immunocompromised
Patient

Klaus F. Rabe, MD, PhD
*Professor of Medicine, Department of Internal Medicine,
Christian-Albrechts University, Kiel, Germany; Medical
Director, Grosshansdorf Clinic, Grosshansdorf, Germany*
Antiinflammatory Drugs

Michelle Ramsay, BSc, MRCP
*Clinical Research Fellow in Respiratory Physiology, Department
of Asthma, Allergy, and Respiratory Science, Division of Asthma
and Lung Biology, King's College London; Lane Fox Respiratory
Unit, St. Thomas' Hospital, Guy's and St. Thomas' National
Health Service Foundation Trust, London, United Kingdom*
Diseases of the Thoracic Cage and Respiratory Muscles

Felix Ratjen, MD, PhD, FRCPC
*Professor, Department of Pediatrics, University of Toronto; Head,
Division of Respiratory Medicine, H.E. Sellers Chair in Cystic
Fibrosis, Hospital for Sick Children, Toronto, Canada*
Cystic Fibrosis

M. Katayoon Rezaei, MD
*Assistant Professor of Pathology, The George Washington
University Medical Center, Washington, DC*
Lung Cancer: Epidemiology, Surgical Pathology,
and Molecular Biology

Seppo T. Rinne, MD, PhD
*Senior Pulmonary Fellow, University of Washington, Seattle,
Washington*
Air Pollution

Bruce W.S. Robinson, MBBS, MD, FRACP, FRCP, DTM&H, FCCP
*Professor of Medicine, University of Western Australia School of
Medicine and Pharmacology; Consultant Respiratory Physician,
Department of Respiratory Medicine; Sir Charles Gairdner
Hospital; Director, National Centre for Asbestos Related
Diseases, Nedlands, Australia*
Malignant Pleural Mesothelioma

Josep Roca, MD
*Servei de Pneumologia i Allèrgia Respiratòria, ICT, Departament
de Medicina, Institut D'Investigacions Biomèdiques August Pi i
Sunyer, Hospital Clínic, Universitat de Barcelona, Barcelona,
Spain*
Exercise Testing

Daniel Rodenstein, MD, PhD
*Professor, Pneumology Department and Center for Sleep
Medicine, Cliniques Universitaires Saint-Luc, Université
Catholique de Louvain, Brussels, Belgium*
Obesity Hypoventilation Syndrome

Jaime Rodríguez Rosado, MD
*Pulmonologist, Department of Respiratory Medicine, Hospital
Universitario Son Espases, Palma de Mallorca, Spain*
Asthma: Epidemiology, Pathophysiology, and Risk Factors

Melissa L. Rosado-de-Christenson, MD, FACR
*Clinical Professor of Radiology, University of Missouri–Kansas
City; Section Chief, Thoracic Radiology, Department of
Radiology, Saint Luke's Hospital of Kansas City, Kansas City,
Missouri*
Disorders of the Mediastinum

Cecile Rose, MD, MPH
*Professor of Medicine, University of Colorado, Aurora;
Occupational Medicine Program Director, National Jewish
Health, Denver, Colorado*
Extrinsic Allergic Alveolitis

Federico Fiorentino Rossi, MD
*Pulmonologist, Department of Respiratory Medicine, Hospital
Universitario Son Espases, Palma de Mallorca, Spain*
Asthma: Epidemiology, Pathophysiology, and Risk Factors

Luis G. Ruiz, MD
*Pulmonologist, Kaiser Permanente Mid Atlantic Medical Group,
Washington, DC*
Lung Transplantation

Glenis K. Scadding, MA, MD, FRCP
*Honorary Consultant Physician, Department of Allergy and
Medical Rhinology, Royal National Throat, Nose and Ear
Hospital, London, United Kingdom*
Upper Airway Disease: Rhinitis and Rhinosinusitis

Frank Schneider, MD
*Assistant Professor of Pathology, Department of Pathology,
University of Pittsburgh Medical Center, Pittsburgh,
Pennsylvania*
Inflammatory Bowel Disease

Arnold M. Schwartz, MD, Phd
*Professor of Pathology and Surgery, The George Washington
University Medical Center, Washington, DC*
Lung Cancer: Epidemiology, Surgical Pathology,
and Molecular Biology

Amen Sergew, MD
*Instructor, Division of Pulmonary and Critical Care Medicine,
National Jewish Health, University of Colorado, Aurora,
Colorado*
Idiopathic Pulmonary Fibrosis and Other Interstitial
Lung Diseases

Sanjay Sethi, MD, FACP
*Division Chief, Pulmonary, Critical Care, and Sleep Medicine,
University at Buffalo, The State University of New York; Staff
Physician, Pulmonary, Critical Care, and Sleep Medicine, VA
Western New York Healthcare System, Buffalo, New York*
Community-Acquired Pneumonia
Viral Pneumonia

Penny J. Shaw, MBBS, MRCP, DMRD, FRCR
*Consultant Radiologist, Department of Imaging, University
College London Hospital National Health Service Foundation
Trust, London, United Kingdom*
Percutaneous Biopsy Procedures: Techniques and Indications

Anita K. Simonds, MD, FRCP
Professor, NIHR Respiratory Disease Biomedical Research Unit, Royal Brompton and Harefield National Health Service Foundation Trust, London, United Kingdom
Scoliosis and Kyphoscoliosis

Arthur S. Slutsky, MD, PhD
Professor of Medicine, Surgery, and Biomedical Engineering, University of Toronto; Director, Interdepartmental Division of Critical Care Medicine, Department of Critical Care Medicine, St. Michael's Hospital, Keenan Research Center, Li Ka Shing Knowledge Institute of St. Michael's Hospital, Toronto, Canada
Invasive Mechanical Ventilation

Ulrich Specks, MD
Professor of Medicine, Mayo Clinic College of Medicine, Division of Pulmonary and Critical Care Medicine, Mayo Clinic, Rochester, Minnesota
Pulmonary Vasculitis and Hemorrhage

Jonathan R. Spiro, MBBS, BSc, MD, MRCP
Specialist Registrar in Cardiology, University Hospitals Birmingham, The New Queen Elizabeth Hospital, Birmingham, United Kingdom
Echocardiography in Respiratory Medicine

Michael Spiro, MBBS, BSc, FRCA
Specialist Registrar in Anaesthesia and Critical Care Medicine, Royal Free Hospital, London, United Kingdom
Airway Management in the Intensive Care Unit

Stephen G. Spiro, BSc, MD, FRCP
Professor of Respiratory Medicine, Honorary Consultant Physician, Department of Cancer Medicine, University College London Hospitals, National Health Service Foundation Trust; Honorary Consultant Physician, Royal Brompton Hospital, London, United Kingdom
Chest Pain

Richard P. Steeds, MA, MC, FRCP
Honorary Lecturer, University of Birmingham; Consultant Cardiologist with Special Interest in Imaging, University Hospitals Birmingham, The New Queen Elizabeth Hospital, Birmingham, United Kingdom
Echocardiography in Respiratory Medicine

Daniel H. Sterman, MD
Assistant Professor of Medicine, Perelman School of Medicine; Chief, Section of Interventional Pulmonology and Thoracic Oncology, Pulmonary, Allergy, and Critical Care Division; Co-Director, PENN Mesothelioma and Pleural Program, Hospital of the University of Pennsylvania, Philadelphia, Pennsylvania
Bronchoscopy

Kaylan E. Stinson, MSPH
Senior Professional Researcher, Colorado School of Public Health, University of Colorado, Aurora, Colorado
Asbestosis

Robert Stockley, MD, DSc, FRCP
Professor, Department of Lung Function and Sleep, The New Queen Elizabeth Hospital, Birmingham, United Kingdom
Bronchiectasis

Diane C. Strollo, MD, FACR
Associate Professor of Radiology, Thoracic Radiology, University of Pittsburgh Medical Center, Pittsburgh, Pennsylvania
Disorders of the Mediastinum

Demet S. Sulemanji, MD
Instructor, Department of Anesthesia, Harvard University; Research Coordinator, Department of Respiratory Care, Massachusetts General Hospital, Boston, Massachusetts
Acute Respiratory Distress Syndrome

Lynn Tanoue, MD
Professor of Medicine, Section of Pulmonary and Critical Care Medicine; Vice-Chair for Clinical Affairs, Department of Internal Medicine, Yale School of Medicine, New Haven, Connecticut
Lung Cancer: Clinical Evaluation and Staging

Magali N. Taylor, BSc, MBBS, FRCR
Consultant Radiologist with Thoracic Subspecialty Interest, Department of Imaging, University College London Hospital National Health Service Foundation Trust, London, United Kingdom
Percutaneous Biopsy Procedures: Techniques and Indications

Antoni Torres, MD, PhD
Professor of Medicine, University of Barcelona; Director, Respiratory Intensive Care Unit, Thorax Institute, Hospital Clinic, Barcelona, Spain
Nosocomial Respiratory Infections

Elizabeth Tullis, MD, FRCP
Associate Professor of Medicine, Department of Respirology, University of Toronto; Head, Division of Respirology; Director, Adult Cystic Fibrosis Program, St. Michael's Hospital, Toronto, Canada
Cystic Fibrosis

Anil Vachani, MD
Assistant Professor of Medicine, Pulmonary, Allergy, and Critical Care Division, Perelman School of Medicine; Attending Physician, Philadelphia VA Medical Center, Philadelphia, Pennsylvania
Bronchoscopy

Olivier Vandenplas, MD, PhD
Professor of Medicine, CHU Mont-Godinne, Université Catholique de Louvain, Yvoir, Belgium
Occupational Asthma

Johan Vansteenkiste, MD, PhD
Professor of Internal Medicine, Catholic University; Deputy Clinical Head Pulmonology, University Hospital Gasthuisberg, Leuven, Belgium
Positron Emission Tomography Imaging

Theodoros Vassilakopoulos, MD, PhD
Associate Professor, Department of Critical Care and Pulmonary Services, University of Athens Medical School, Evangelismos Hospital, Athens, Greece
Control of Ventilation and Respiratory Muscles

Kristen L. Veraldi, MD, PhD, FCCP
Assistant Professor of Medicine, University of Pittsburgh School of Medicine, Division of Pulmonary, Allergy, and Critical Care Medicine, The Dorothy P. and Richard P. Simmons Center for Interstitial Lung Disease, University of Pittsburgh Medical Center, Pittsburgh, Pennsylvania
Inflammatory Bowel Disease

Jesús Villar, MD, PhD, FCCM
Chief, Group 29, CIBER de Enfermedades Respiratorias, Instituto de Salud Carlos III, Madrid, Spain; Director, Research Unit, Hospital Universitario Dr. Negrin, Las Palmas de Gran Canaria, Spain; Adjunct Scientist, Keenan Research Center, Li Ka Shing Knowledge Institute, St. Michael's Hospital, Toronto, Canada
Acute Respiratory Distress Syndrome

Peter D. Wagner, MD
Distinguished Professor of Medicine and Bioengineering, University of California–San Diego, La Jolla, California
Gas Exchange

Benoit Wallaert, MD
Professor of Medicine, Service de Pneumologie et Immuno-allergologie, Centre de Competence des Maladies Pulmonaires Rares, Hôpital Albert Calmette, CHRU at Universite de Lille 2, Lille, France
Silicosis and Coal Worker's Pneumoconiosis

Nicholas Walter, MD, MS
Instructor, Division of Pulmonary Sciences and Critical Care Medicine, University of Colorado, Aurora, Colorado
Tuberculosis and Nontuberculous Mycobacterial Infections

Jadwiga A. Wedzicha, MD, FRCP
Professor of Respiratory Medicine, Academic Unit of Respiratory Medicine, University College London Medical School, Royal Free Campus, London, United Kingdom
Management of Exacerbations in Chronic Obstructive Pulmonary Disease

Athol Wells, MBChB, MD, FRCP, FRCR
Professor of Respiratory Medicine, The Royal Brompton Hospital, Imperial College, London, United Kingdom
Approach to Diagnosis of Diffuse Lung Disease

Deborah Whitters, MBChB, MRCP(UK)
Clinical Research Fellow, Department of Lung Function and Sleep, The New Queen Elizabeth Hospital, Birmingham, United Kingdom
Bronchiectasis

Mark A. Woodhead, BSc, DM, FRCP
Clinical Professor of Respiratory Medicine, University of Manchester; Consultant in General and Respiratory Medicine, Department of Respiratory Medicine, Manchester Royal Infirmary, Manchester, United Kingdom
Approach to the Diagnosis of Pulmonary Infection

Joanne L. Wright, MD, FRCP(C)
Professor of Pathology, University of British Columbia; Pathologist, St. Paul's Hospital, Vancouver, Canada
Macro and Micro Structure of the Lung

John M. Wrightson, MB, BChir, MA, MRCP
Research Fellow in Pleural Diseases, Oxford Centre for Respiratory Medicine, Oxford University Hospitals National Health Service Trust; National Institute for Health Research, Oxford Biomedical Research Centre, Clinical Training Fellow, University of Oxford, Oxford, United Kingdom
Pleural Effusion, Empyema, and Pneumothorax

PREFACE

We have been very encouraged by the success of the previous editions of *Clinical Respiratory Medicine*, and we are proud to publish the fourth edition. Although the contents have changed considerably with each edition, we still hold to the principle of providing a book that teaches both the basics of respiratory medicine and the details of individual diseases.

When we set out in 1999, our idea was to bring the global respiratory medicine community together within a single publication. We aimed to use the extraordinary advances in computer graphics and publishing to combine detailed presentations of lung structure and physiology with clinical material. In this fourth edition we extended this philosophy to include videos of most practical procedures to help explain how these investigations are performed.

This edition has seen the departure of co-editors Professors James Jett and Richard Albert, and we welcome the "new blood" and ideas from Professors Alvar Agusti and Gerard Silvestri, both preeminent in the respiratory medicine field. They helped enormously in giving the book a new look. We changed more than 30% of authors to ensure the material in this edition is current. The chapters with the same author as in the previous edition have been rewritten and updated. Also, each chapter includes five multiple-choice questions to aid the learning process. We are fortunate to include many of the most world-renowned writers in their respective fields, who have contributed willingly and on time, and we are most grateful to them for their kindness and commitment.

The senior editor has always felt the importance of pulmonary physiology in understanding lung function and the disease processes that occur. Therefore we make no apology for strengthening this part of the book, with superb chapters from the leaders in their specialty areas. Entirely new chapters are included on lung structure, echocardiography, obesity and its effects, and benign tumors, as well as a much expanded section on lung cancer.

The format of the book has remained essentially unchanged, with the first 300 or so pages focusing on physiology, host defenses, techniques and indications (much improved with videos), and principles of respiratory care. This is followed by detailed, disease-focused chapters. The book has never been intended as an exhaustive source of references, but summary reading lists are provided for each topic.

The fourth edition remains directed at trainees in respiratory medicine, physicians practicing general medicine, respiratory therapists, and all respiratory medicine clinicians. Once again, we have been well supported by Elsevier and in particular by Anne Snyder, who has kept the project on schedule and worked so efficiently on our behalf. Her guidance and always prompt advice are greatly appreciated.

We have enjoyed preparing this text as a teaching tool for the profession and hope *Clinical Respiratory Medicine* maintains its place among the leading respiratory texts. Enjoy it.

Stephen G. Spiro
Gerard A. Silvestri
Alvar Agusti

CONTENTS

Video Contents   **xxi**

Section 1
NORMAL STRUCTURE AND FUNCTION

1. **Macro and Micro Structure of the Lung**   **1**
   Joanne L. Wright and Andrew M. Churg

2. **Basic Aspects of Cellular and Molecular Biology**   **7**
   Stefan J. Marciniak and David A. Lomas

3. **Respiratory Mechanics**   **19**
   Bruce H. Culver

4. **Pulmonary Circulation**   **29**
   Bruce H. Culver and Robb W. Glenny

5. **Gas Exchange**   **37**
   Peter D. Wagner

6. **Control of Ventilation and Respiratory Muscles**   **50**
   Theodoros Vassilakopoulos

Section 2
DIAGNOSTIC TECHNIQUES

7. **Imaging Techniques**   **63**
   Simon P.G. Padley and David M. Hansell

8. **Positron Emission Tomography Imaging**   **122**
   Johan Vansteenkiste, Christophe Dooms, and Christophe Deroose

9. **Pulmonary Function Testing**   **133**
   Bruce H. Culver

10. **Exercise Testing**   **143**
    Josep Roca and Felip Burgos

11. **Bronchoscopy**   **154**
    Anil Vachani, Andrew R. Haas, and Daniel H. Sterman

12. **Endobronchial and Endoesophageal Ultrasound Techniques**   **174**
    Felix J.F. Herth

13. **Percutaneous Biopsy Procedures: Techniques and Indications**   **180**
    Asia A. Ahmed, Magali N. Taylor, and Penny J. Shaw

14. **Echocardiography in Respiratory Medicine**   **193**
    Jonathan R. Spiro and Richard P. Steeds

Section 3
RESPIRATORY PHARMACOLOGY

15. **Bronchodilators**   **202**
    Peter M.A. Calverley

16. **Antiinflammatory Drugs**   **213**
    Klaus F. Rabe

17. **Drug-Induced and Iatrogenic Respiratory Diseases**   **221**
    Philippe Camus

Section 4
AN APPROACH TO RESPIRATORY SYMPTOMS

18. **Cough**   **242**
    Surinder S. Birring and Ian D. Pavord

19. **Dyspnea**   **250**
    Alex H. Gifford and Donald A. Mahler

20. **Hemoptysis**   **261**
    John W. Kreit

21. **Chest Pain**   **267**
    Richard K. Albert and Stephen G. Spiro

Section 5
INFECTIOUS DISEASES

22. **Pulmonary Host Defenses**   **275**
    Theo J. Moraes, Chung-Wai Chow, and Gregory P. Downey

23. **Approach to the Diagnosis of Pulmonary Infection**   **288**
    Mark A. Woodhead

24. **Community-Acquired Pneumonia**   **296**
    Ilya Berim and Sanjay Sethi

25. **Viral Pneumonia**   **309**
    Ganapathi Iyer Parameswaran and Sanjay Sethi

26. **Nonbacterial Infectious Pneumonia**   **315**
    William Graham Carlos III and Chadi A. Hage

27. **Nosocomial Respiratory Infections**   **322**
    Gianluigi Li Bassi, Miquel Ferrer, and Antoni Torres

28. **Pneumonia in the Non–HIV-Infected Immunocompromised Patient** 330
Jennifer Quint and Jeremy S. Brown

29. **Pulmonary Infections in Patients with Human Immunodeficiency Virus Disease** 346
Robert F. Miller, Marc C.I. Lipman, and Alison Morris

30. **Noninfectious Conditions in Patients with Human Immunodeficiency Virus Infection** 374
Thomas Benfield

31. **Tuberculosis and Nontuberculous Mycobacterial Infections** 383
Nicholas Walter and Charles L. Daley

Section 6
CRITICAL CARE RESPIRATORY MEDICINE

32. **Invasive Mechanical Ventilation** 406
Lukas Brander and Arthur S. Slutsky

33. **Noninvasive Mechanical Ventilation** 431
Paolo Carbonara and Stefano Nava

34. **Airway Management in the Intensive Care Unit** 437
Michael Spiro and Alan McGlennan

35. **Hemodynamic Monitoring in Critical Illness** 445
Mark Lambert and Phil Bearfield

36. **Acute Respiratory Distress Syndrome** 454
Jesús Villar, Demet S. Sulemanji, and Robert M. Kacmarek

Section 7
AIRWAY DISEASES

37. **Upper Airway Disease: Rhinitis and Rhinosinusitis** 471
Glenis K. Scadding and Harsha H. Kariyawasam

38. **Asthma: Epidemiology, Pathophysiology, and Risk Factors** 487
Borja G. Cosio, Jaime Rodríguez Rosado, and Federico Fiorentino Rossi

39. **Diagnosis and Management of Asthma in Adults** 501
Ian D. Pavord, Ruth H. Green, and Pranabashis Haldar

40. **Occupational Asthma** 521
Olivier Vandenplas and Jean-Luc Malo

41. **Chronic Obstructive Pulmonary Disease: Epidemiology, Pathophysiology, and Clinical Evaluation** 531
William MacNee

42. **Treatment of the Stable Patient with Chronic Obstructive Pulmonary Disease** 553
Bartolome R. Celli

43. **Management of Exacerbations in Chronic Obstructive Pulmonary Disease** 562
John R. Hurst and Jadwiga A. Wedzicha

44. **Cystic Fibrosis** 568
Felix Ratjen and Elizabeth Tullis

45. **Bronchiectasis** 580
Deborah Whitters and Robert Stockley

Section 8
PARENCHYMAL LUNG DISEASES

46. **Approach to Diagnosis of Diffuse Lung Disease** 588
Athol Wells

47. **Idiopathic Pulmonary Fibrosis and Other Interstitial Lung Diseases** 599
Amen Sergew and Kevin K. Brown

48. **Sarcoidosis** 607
Manju Paul and Michael C. Iannuzzi

49. **Eosinophilic Lung Disease** 620
Vincent Cottin and Jean-François Cordier

50. **Organizing Pneumonia** 629
Vincent Cottin and Jean-François Cordier

51. **Silicosis and Coal Worker's Pneumoconiosis** 637
Cyrielle Jardin and Benoit Wallaert

52. **Asbestosis** 645
Lee S. Newman and Kaylan E. Stinson

53. **Connective Tissue Diseases** 653
J.C. Grutters and J.-W.J. Lammers

54. **Rare Diffuse Interstitial Lung Diseases** 667
Simon R. Johnson and William Y.C. Chang

55. **Extrinsic Allergic Alveolitis** 676
Kelsey Gray and Cecile Rose

56. **Toxic Inhalational Lung Injury** 682
Lee S. Newman and Kathryn G. Bird

Section 9
PULMONARY VASCULAR DISORDERS, VASCULITIDES, AND HEMORRHAGE

57. **Pulmonary Embolism** 690
Michael P. Gruber and Todd M. Bull

58. **Pulmonary Hypertension** 710
Kristin B. Highland and Andre Holmes

59. **Pulmonary Vasculitis and Hemorrhage** 722
Ulrich Specks

Section 10
SLEEP-DISORDERED BREATHING

60. **Obstructive Sleep Apnea: Epidemiology, Risk Factors, and Pathophysiology** 731
Ferrán Barbé Illa and Miguel Ángel Martínez-García

61. Obstructive Sleep Apnea: Clinical Features, Diagnosis, and Treatment   **741**
José M. Marin

62. Obesity Hypoventilation Syndrome   **749**
Gimbada B. Mwenge and Daniel Rodenstein

Section 11
CHEST WALL DISORDERS

63. Scoliosis and Kyphoscoliosis   **756**
Anita K. Simonds

64. Diseases of the Thoracic Cage and Respiratory Muscles   **763**
Michelle Ramsay, Michael I. Polkey, and Nicholas Hart

Section 12
LUNG TUMORS

65. Lung Cancer: Epidemiology, Surgical Pathology, and Molecular Biology   **776**
Arnold M. Schwartz and M. Katayoon Rezaei

66. Lung Cancer: Clinical Evaluation and Staging   **788**
Lynn Tanoue

67. Lung Cancer: Treatment   **801**
Douglas Arenberg

68. Benign Lung Tumors   **810**
David E. Midthun

Section 13
DISORDERS OF THE PLEURA AND MEDIASTINUM

69. Pleural Effusion, Empyema, and Pneumothorax   **818**
John M. Wrightson, Helen E. Davies, and Y.C. Gary Lee

70. Malignant Pleural Mesothelioma   **837**
Tarek Meniawy and Bruce W.S. Robinson

71. Disorders of the Mediastinum   **846**
Diane C. Strollo and Melissa L. Rosado-de-Christenson

Section 14
THORACIC SURGERY

72. Chest Tube Insertion and Management   **862**
Stephen D. Cassivi, Claude Deschamps, and Nicholas J. Pastis

73. Preoperative Pulmonary Evaluation   **869**
Hilary Petersen and Peter Mazzone

74. Diagnostic Thoracic Surgical Procedures   **876**
Chadrick E. Denlinger, Stephen D. Cassivi, and Mark S. Allen

75. Lung Transplantation   **882**
Pamela J. McShane, Luis G. Ruiz, and Edward R. Garrity, Jr.

Section 15
SPECIAL CLINICAL CONDITIONS

76. Pregnancy   **904**
Stephen E. Lapinsky

77. Pulmonary Complications of Hematopoietic Stem Cell Transplantation   **912**
Rodrigo Cavallazzi and Rodney J. Folz

78. Hepatic and Biliary Disease   **920**
Aynur Okcay and Michael J. Krowka

79. Inflammatory Bowel Disease   **927**
Frank Schneider and Kristen L. Veraldi

80. Air Pollution   **937**
Seppo T. Rinne and Joel D. Kaufman

VIDEO CONTENTS

14. Echocardiography in Respiratory Medicine
1. The Parasternal Long-Axis View
2. The Parasternal Short-Axis View
3. The Apical Four-Chamber View
4. The Subcostal View
5. The Tilted Parasternal Long-Axis View
6. The Right Ventricular Outflow Tract, Pulmonary Valve, and Pulmonary Artery
7. Flattening of the Interventricular Septum
8. Tricuspid Regurgitation
9. The Inferior Vena Cava
10. Dilated Right Ventricle
11. Modified Apical Four-Chamber View of a Dilated Right Heart
12. Subcostal View of a Dilated Right Heart
13. Parasternal Long-Axis View of a Pericardial Effusion
14. Apical Four-Chamber View of a Large Pericardial Effusion
15. Apical Four-Chamber View of a Pericardial Effusion
16. Infiltrative Cardiomyopathy

34. Airway Management in the Intensive Care Unit
1. Conventional Direct Laryngoscopy Using a Macintosh Blade
2. Laryngoscopy Using the AP Advance as a Direct Laryngoscope
3. Indirect Laryngoscopy Using the AP Advance as a Video Laryngoscope.
4. Indirect Laryngoscopy Using the AP Advance Video Laryngoscope with the Difficult Intubation Blade

61. Obstructive Sleep Apnea: Clinical Features, Diagnosis, and Treatment
An Adult with Obstructive Sleep Apnea
A Young Man with Obstructive Sleep Apnea

68. Benign Lung Tumors
Respiratory Papillomatosis
Endobronchial Hamartoma
Endobronchial Hamartoma Removal

Chapter 1

Macro and Micro Structure of the Lung*

Joanne L. Wright • Andrew M. Churg

LUNG DEVELOPMENT

The emergence of a normal, functioning respiratory system requires simultaneous development of the conducting airway system and the vascular system. Of interest, the mechanisms that drive this process also hold true for other branched-structure organ systems, such as the kidney and breast. Lung development, beginning with organogenesis, is divided into several stages, as indicated in **Table 1-1.** However, considerable overlap of the signaling cascades between the various stages is recognized.

The earliest stage of lung development is known as the *embryonic* stage—that of organogenesis—and continues to approximately week 7. The primary lung buds arise from the ventral wall of the anterior foregut at approximately day 28. The trachea develops independently as a foregut tube anterior to the lung buds. Although it initially also includes the esophagus, the tube subsequently separates into two parts, with the ventral aspect forming the trachea, which then connects to the lung buds. The lung bud–tracheal domain is characterized by expression of Nkx2-1 (also called Titf1 [thyroid transcription factor 1]). Signal proteins from the mesenchyme, including bone morphogenetic proteins (BMPs), Noggin, fibroblast growth factors (FGFs), and Wnts, influence patterning, and deficiencies in some of these proteins result in failure of foregut separation with or without abnormal differentiation of epithelium and mesenchyma. Retinoic acid also plays an important role in lung morphogenesis during primary bud formation. Canonical Wnt signaling appears to be important in the regulation of cell proliferation and differentiation and also plays a role in lung branching. Beta-catenin phosphorylation is an integral portion of this pathway, with subsequent translocation to the cell nucleus and activation of T cell factor/lymphoid enhancer factor (TCF/LEF) target genes. Epigenetic changes, including methylation of DNA or histones, may influence developmental processes.

Vasculogenesis is initiated at the same time as that for development of the foregut bud. The vascular endothelial growth factor (VEGF) signaling cascade is integral to lung development and is necessary for endothelial proliferation and continued maintenance of the maturing vessels. The VEGF signaling event may be downstream from the *Fgf* signaling pathway.

The *pseudoglandular* stage generally is considered to encompass weeks 5 to 17, during which the lung has the appearance of a tubular gland. Continuing development of the lung buds is dependent on expression of FGF10 in the mesoderm and FGF receptor 2 (FGF2) in the endoderm. Branching is controlled by expression of Br1 (Branchless), a ligand of FGF, in small clusters of endodermal and mesodermal cells. Patterning genes determine the position of the clusters. The signaling network involved in this stage is complex, with feedback loops that significantly influence the morphogenetic signals.

In the *canalicular* stage (weeks 16 to 26) and extending into the saccular stage (weeks 24 to 38), the endoderm differentiates to form type I and II epithelial cells, and the air-blood barrier forms as capillaries remodel and become applied to the type I cells. The *saccular* stage is characterized by formation of saccules, the precursors of the alveoli. Matrix proteins assemble into a scaffold configuration at this time and also act as a reservoir for growth proteins such as transforming growth factor-β (TGF-β). Multiple signaling pathways are involved, with the *Fgf* pathway appearing to have a critical role in alveolar development.

The *postnatal* stage is characterized by rapid alveolarization and microvascular maturation, with an approximate 20-fold multiplication of surface area and an increase from approximately 50 million to 300 million alveoli. New alveoli arise from septa containing a double capillary network, or new septa are formed from mature septa, with induced formation of capillary network. Myofibroblasts and collagen and elastic fibers appear to be necessary for continued septation, and platelet-derived growth factor (PDGF) is necessary in this process, whereas VEGF is necessary for capillary maturation and maintenance.

NORMAL LUNG ANATOMY

The lungs can move freely within the thorax, attached normally only at the hila. The lungs are covered by a serosal membrane known as the visceral pleura. This membrane is then reflected as the parietal pleura over the hilum to cover the mediastinum, chest wall, and diaphragm. The serosal space is a theoretic space between the two pleural layers; normally, only a thin layer of pleural fluid separates the two layers. The pleura itself is formed as a layer of mesothelial cells supported by an elastic fiber network, which in turn is supported by a loose fibroconnective tissue layer. Mesothelial cells are characterized by their long microvilli.

As shown in **Table 1-2** and **Figure 1-1,** *A* to *D,* the lungs are asymmetrically paired. The right lung is divided by major and minor fissures into three lobes: the upper, lower, and middle lobes. By contrast, the left lung has a single fissure dividing it into upper (superior) and lower (inferior) lobes. In the left lung, the homologue of the right lung's middle lobe is the *lingula,* made up of the anterior and inferior portions of the upper lobe. In some persons there may be an incomplete fissure separating the lingula from the upper lobe. Bronchopulmonary segments are subunits of the lobes that derive from

---

*Additional content for this chapter can be found on Expert Consult.

Table 1-1   Stages of Lung Development

Stage	Time	Growth Characteristics	Important Genes/Growth Factors
Embryonic	4-7 weeks	• Beginning organogenesis • Development of major airways	Nkx2-1, BMPs, FGFs, Wnts, retinoic acid, VEGF
Fetal pseudoglandular	5-17 weeks	• Bronchial tree formation • Beginning of parenchyma differentiation	FGFs, Wnt, PDGF, BMP
Fetal canalicular	16-26 weeks	• Conducting airways • Epithelial differentiation	Wnts, FGFs, TGF-β
Fetal saccular	24 weeks–term	• Air space expansion • Beginning alveolarization	VEGF, PDGF
Postnatal	Term–early childhood	• Remodeling with continued septation and alveolarization • Maturation of capillary bed	PDGF, VEGF

BMP, bone morphogenetic protein; *FGFs*, fibroblast growth factors; *PDGF*, platelet-derived growth factor; *TGF-β*, transforming growth factor-β; *VEGF*, vascular endothelial growth factor.

Table 1-2   Segments of Lung

Right Lung	Left Lung
Upper Lobe	*Upper Lobe*
1. Apical	1, 2. Apical-posterior
2. Posterior	
3. Anterior	3. Anterior
Middle Lobe	*Lingula*
4. Lateral	4. Superior
5. Medial	5. Inferior
Lower Lobe	*Lower Lobe*
6. Superior	6. Superior
7. Medial basal	
8. Anterior basal	8. Anterior basal
9. Lateral basal	9. Lateral basal
10. Posterior basal	10. Posterior basal

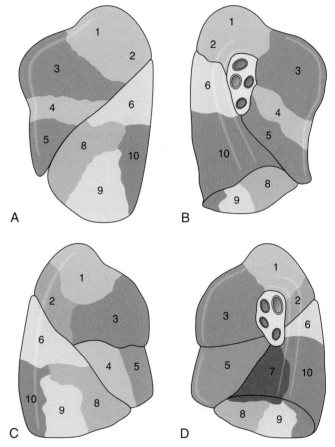

Figure 1-1   Lobes for left (**A** and **B**) and right (**C** and **D**) lungs. The numbered segments are identified in Table 1-2.

the first generation of bronchi below the lobar bronchi. These also are asymmetric between lungs; Table 1-1 shows the nomenclature.

The next-smallest unit of the lung below the gross level of definition is the *pulmonary lobule*, also known as the secondary lobule of Miller. On the pleural surface, the secondary lobule is outlined by connective septa and has a roughly polygonal shape, measuring between 1 and 2 cm in diameter. Examination of the cut surface of lung again shows the interlobular septa demarcating the edges of the lobule (**Figures 1-2 and 1-e1**); these are best seen in the periphery, because interlobular septa are less well developed in the center of the lungs. Lobules also can be identified on microscopic examination (**Figures 1-e2 and 1-e3**). Each lobule contains three to five acini, which are the basic units of gas exchange. An *acinus* is defined as the lung parenchyma that derives from a single terminal membranous bronchiole and includes three successive generations of respiratory bronchioles and their subtending alveolar ducts, alveolar saccules, and alveoli. The terminal bronchioles branch near the center of the lobules, and their acini abut the interlobular septa. This relationship allows assessment of alterations

in the lung parenchyma in terms of its location within the lung lobule (centrilobular, panlobular, paraseptal).

AIRWAYS

The bronchial system generally is divided into conducting and respiratory airways. The conducting airways extend from the trachea to the membranous bronchioles, and the architecture changes as the airways decrease in size. The trachea has a membranous posterior aspect composed of transverse smooth muscle bundles that together make up the trachealis muscle,

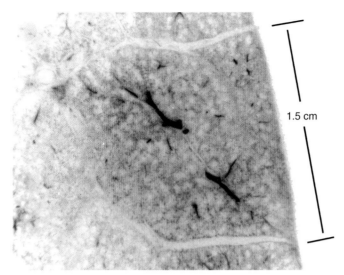

Figure 1-2   Gross specimen of a secondary lobule of Miller, identified as the lung parenchyma surrounded by venous septa, or pleura and venous septa.   *(Photo obtained from Gough section.)*

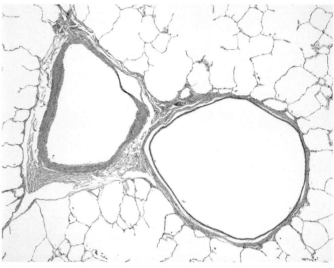

Figure 1-4   Membranous bronchiole with adjacent pulmonary artery. The diameters of the airway and the artery are roughly similar.

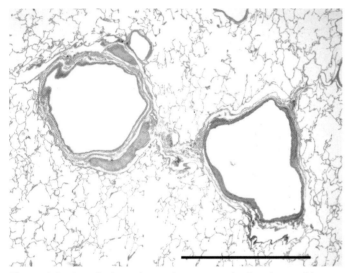

Figure 1-3   A cartilaginous intrapulmonary conducting airway with adjacent pulmonary artery. Of note, the diameters of airway and artery are similar. *Bar* indicates 2 mm.

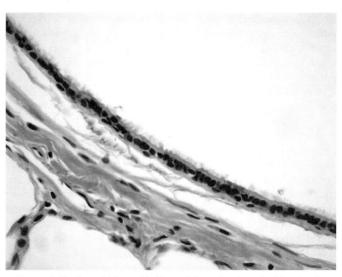

Figure 1-5   Bronchiolar epithelium with predominantly ciliated cells.

with protective cartilaginous rings on the anterior aspect (**Figure 1-e4**). In the *cartilaginous* bronchi, the cartilage plates enclose but do not completely surround the airway, and the muscle fibers wind around the airway in a spiral. These airways are surrounded by loose connective tissue, which contains the bronchial arteries, venous trunks, lymphatics, and nerves (**Figures 1-3** and **1-e5**). In the upper airways, the epithelium is predominantly ciliated, with a modest number of goblet cells. The cells are supported by a thin basement membrane. The bronchial mucous glands lie deep to the epithelium, with the mucous gland pits emptying onto the surface of the airway (**Figure 1-e6**). The glands contain both serous and mucous cells, with myoepithelial cells, all enclosed within the basal lamina of the glands (**Figure 1-e7**).

The noncartilaginous conducting airways extend from approximately generation 5 to generation 14 and are termed membranous bronchioles (**Figure 1-4**). The more proximal airways have a ciliated cell predominance (**Figure 1-5**), whereas the more distal airways acquire increasing numbers of non-ciliated bronchiolar (Clara) cells until they account for

approximately 11% of the total epithelial cell numbers in the terminal membranous bronchioles. Each bronchiole has a complete fibromuscular wall, with the muscle arranged in a tight spiral. An inconspicuous compartment located between the basement membrane and the muscle layer contains a few collagen fibers and longitudinally oriented elastic fibers. The bronchioles have an adventitial sheath into which adjacent alveoli insert.

The respiratory bronchioles have an incomplete fibromuscular wall, because they are partially alveolarized (**Figure 1-6**); the degree of alveolarization increases in each generation. The muscle bundles continue down the walls of the alveolar ducts, which are airways with completely alveolate walls, and end at the alveolar saccule entrance rings (**Figure 1-e8**).

AIRWAY EPITHELIAL CELLS

Mucin-secreting cells are differentiated toward goblet cells and are characterized by a bulging apex distended by secretory vacuoles.

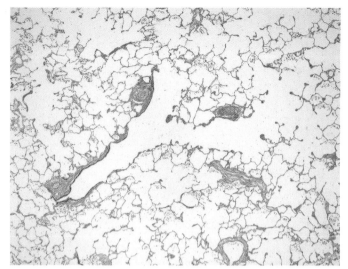

Figure 1-6 Terminal membranous bronchiole bifurcating into two respiratory bronchioles, which in turn have subtending alveolar ducts, saccules, and alveoli.

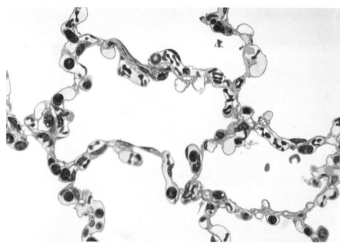

Figure 1-7 Plastic section showing the components of an alveolus.

The *ciliated cells* arise from differentiation of the basal and nonciliated cells; they are columnar in type and attach to the basal lamina. The cilia are complex structures with dynein arms, nexin links, and radial spokes, all configured to utilize adenosine triphosphatase to control cilial beat.

Clara cells are nonciliated secretory cells that produce Clara cell secretory protein, some of the surfactant apoproteins, and antileukoproteinase and are a rich source of oxidases.

Neuroendocrine cells are known by several different names: *Feyrter cells* and *Kulchitsky cells* are more modern terms, but *amine precursor uptake and decarboxylation (APUD) cells* and *"small granular" cells* are found in earlier literature. The cells are roughly flask-shaped, with an apical protrusion found between the columnar cells extending to the airway surface. They express immunohistochemical neural markers such as chromogranin and synaptophysin, in addition to peptide hormones such as substance P, calcitonin, and gastrin-releasing peptide.

ALVEOLUS

The alveolus is the main gas exchange area of the lung and is composed of a thin epithelial layer supported by its basement membrane, a capillary endothelium supported by its own basement membrane, and the interstitium between the two basement membranes (**Figures 1-7** and **1-e9**). Where the two basement membranes are fused, the alveolus is optimized for gas exchange; this region is known as the "thin" portion of the blood-air barrier. In the "thick" portion, by contrast, the basement membranes are separate, and there are fibroblasts, collagen and elastin fibers, and contractile interstitial cells (myofibroblasts, pericytes, and smooth muscle cells).

The alveolus is penetrated by openings known as the pores of Kohn (**Figure 1-8**). These appear early in postnatal life and increase in number with age. A majority of the pores are filled by alveolar lining fluid, but their geometry is affected by lung volumes. They may be important in collateral ventilation or may represent an acquired degenerative lesion.

Alveolar Epithelial Cells

Most of the alveolar surface is covered by simple squamous cells known as type I pneumocytes (**Figure 1-9**). These cells have a small nucleus with highly branched cytoplasmic

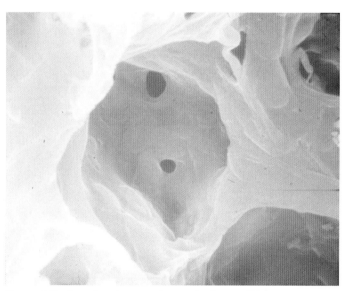

Figure 1-8 Scanning electron micrograph of pore of Kohn. *(Courtesy Dr. William Thurlbeck.)*

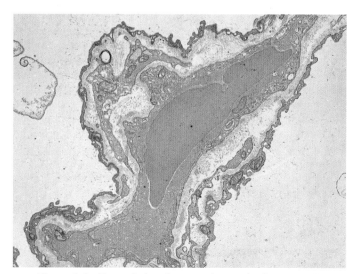

Figure 1-9 Transmission electron micrograph of a type I cell.

processes covering 4000 to 5000 μm^2. The cytoplasm contains sparse organelles. Type I cells form by mitotic division and transformation of type II cells. The normal ratio of type I to type II cells is 1:2.

Type II epithelial cells have a granular appearance and, in humans, are noted to protrude into the alveolar space (**Figure 1-10**). They have abundant mitochondria, endoplasmic reticulum, and a large Golgi apparatus, in addition to conspicuous secretory granules, called lamellar bodies, which are composed of surfactant. Surfactant is approximately 90% lipid in nature, the major portion of which is phosphatidylcholine; surfactant apoproteins A, B, C, and D make up the remainder.

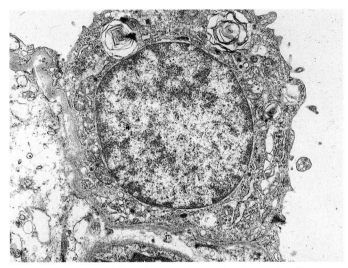

Figure 1-10 Transmission electron micrograph of a type II cell. Lamellar granules are evident within the cytoplasm.

VASCULAR SYSTEM

The main pulmonary artery splits into its two main branches within the mediastinum and beneath the aortic arch. The right pulmonary artery passes beneath the aortic arch and enters the lung anterior to the main bronchus. The left pulmonary artery travels above the main bronchus, passes over the superior lobar bronchus, and can then be identified posterior to the bronchus. The pulmonary arteries branch in company with the bronchi (see Figures 1-3 and 1-4) and can be identified down to the level of the tertiary respiratory bronchioles–alveolar ducts where they are small and poorly muscularized (see Figure 1-6). These precapillary vessels feed into the alveolar-capillary network, which consists of a gridlike mesh (**Figure 1-11**). The capillaries empty into the pulmonary veins, which travel a path independent of the bronchi, at the periphery of the acinus. When the interlobular septa are well formed, the veins lie within the septal fibrous tissue. At the hilus of each lung, the two pulmonary veins independently enter into the left atrium.

The bronchial blood supply is through the systemic circulation, arising from the aorta or the intercostal, internal mammary, or subclavian arteries. In gross specimens, the bronchial arteries can be identified in the connective tissue of the bronchial wall. Venous blood from the central bronchial circulation flows through bronchial veins and empties into the azygos and hemiazygos veins; that from the peripheral bronchi enters into the pulmonary venous system.

LYMPHATIC SYSTEM

The lymphatic vessels run in the visceral pleura as a superficial network of channels and are present in the fibroconnective tissue of the interlobular septa and the bronchovascular bundles, where they form a deep plexus. These vessels have valves to direct the flow toward the lung hilus. Lymph travels to the

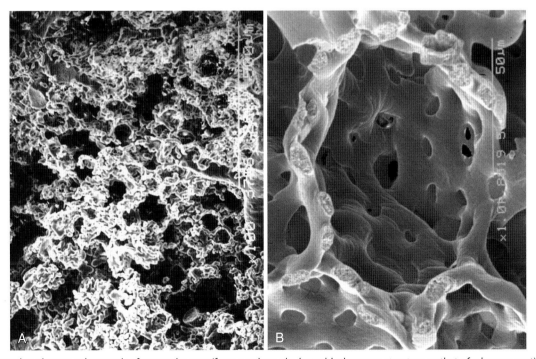

Figure 1-11 Scanning electron micrograph of a vascular cast (from a guinea pig, but with the same structure as that of a human cast). **A,** Low-power magnification showing three-dimensional relationship of alveoli. **B,** High-power magnification showing ringlike structure of alveolar capillaries.

tracheal bifurcation (node 7 in lymph node mapping systems in current use) and along the trachea to the right and left mediastinal nodes (t4R and 4L nodes, followed by 2R and 2L nodes); the lymph nodes function to filter the lymphatic fluid. The right lymphatic channel empties into the right subclavian vein, whereas lymph from the left flows into the thoracic duct and then into the left subclavian vein.

SUGGESTED READINGS

Burri PH: Structural aspects of postnatal lung development—alveolar formation and growth, *Biol Neonate* 89:313–322, 2006.

Cardoso WV, Kotton DN: Specification and patterning of the respiratory system (July 16, 2008), *StemBook*, Cambridge, Mass, Harvard Stem Cell Institute (serial online): http://www.stembook.org, accessed March 5, 2011.

Lauweryns JM: The blood and lymphatic microcirculation of the lung, *Pathol Annu* 6:365–415, 1971.

Morrisey EE, Hogan BL: Preparing for the first breath: genetic and cellular mechanisms in lung development, *Dev Cell* 18:8–23, 2010.

Ochs M, Weibel ER: Functional design of the human lung for gas exchange. In Fishman AP, Elias J, Fishman J, et al, editors: *Fishman's pulmonary diseases and disorders*, ed 4, New York, 2008, McGraw-Hill, pp 23–70.

Parent RA: *Comparative biology of the normal lung*, Ann Arbor, Mich, 1992, CRC Press.

Pinkerton KE, Green FH: Normal aging of the lung. In Harding R, Pinkerton KE, Plopper CG, editors: *The lung: development, aging, and the environment*, New York, 2004, Academic Press, pp 213–233.

Plopper CG, Hill LH, Mariassy AT: Ultrastructure of the nonciliated bronchiolar epithelial (Clara) cell of mammalian lung. III. A study of man with comparison of 15 mammalian species, *Exp Lung Res* 1:171–180, 1980.

Plopper CG, George J, Mariassy A, et al: Species differences in airway cell distribution and morphology. In Crapo JD, Miller FJ, editors: *Extrapolation of dosimetric relationships for inhaled particles and gases*, New York, 1989, Academic Press, pp 19–34.

Chapter 2

Basic Aspects of Cellular and Molecular Biology

Stefan J. Marciniak • David A. Lomas

The 20th century saw pulmonary medicine blossom with scientific advances. Although physiology remains at the core of this specialty, pulmonologist investigators are now at the leading edge of research in cell and molecular biology. These laboratory-based disciplines provide tools to study lung disease both in entire populations and at the level of individual proteins. Molecular biology encompasses both genetics and structural biology, which underpin cell biology, from which physiology emerges. Genetics helps to identify the alleles of genes that increase the risk of disease; structural and cell biology then aim to provide the mechanism. It is through an understanding of disease mechanisms that this century will see its major clinical breakthroughs. A working knowledge of these disciplines is therefore essential for today's pulmonologist.

MOLECULAR BIOLOGY

THE GENETIC BASIS OF LUNG DISEASE

Genetic factors play an important role in diseases that affect the airways (asthma, chronic obstructive pulmonary disease [COPD], cystic fibrosis, primary ciliary dyskinesia), parenchyma (pulmonary fibrosis, Birt-Hogg-Dubé syndrome, tuberous sclerosis), and vasculature (hereditary hemorrhagic telangiectasia) of the lung (**Table 2-1**). Such conditions include simple monogenic disorders such as Kartagener syndrome and α_1-antitrypsin deficiency, in which mutations of critical genes are sufficient to induce well-defined disease phenotypes. By contrast, many other disease processes affecting the lung are complex genetic traits in which inheritance subtly affects pathogenesis. This group of entities includes COPD, asthma, and idiopathic pulmonary fibrosis. Extending current understanding of the genetic basis of pulmonary conditions will be essential to provide new insights into their underlying pathophysiology, to make predictions about outcome, and to develop novel therapeutic strategies.

Identification of single-gene defects in families that show the same phenotype is now relatively straightforward, owing to completion of the human genome project and improvements in DNA sequencing. Consequently, the past 20 years have seen rapid progress in elucidation of the genetic basis of disease. This rate of progress can be appreciated by a consideration of the many years required to identify the gene associated with cystic fibrosis. Dorothy Hansine Andersen first defined the condition in 1938 when she described cystic fibrosis of the pancreas in association with lung and intestinal disease. Only later was it recognized to be a recessive condition. The sweat test that is used to diagnose the condition was developed after the detection of abnormal sweat electrolytes by Paul di Sant' Agnese in 1952. The search for the cystic fibrosis gene started in the early 1980s, and the gene was localized to chromosome 7 in 1985 through recognition of linkage with the highly polymorphic gene paraoxonase in many populations. This achievement was followed by the identification of additional markers more closely linked to the cystic fibrosis locus, MET and D7S8, allowing prenatal diagnosis of the disorder and eventually leading directly to the mapping of the causative gene in 1989 by teams headed by Lap-Chi Tsui, Francis Collins, and Jack Riordan. This gene was called the cystic fibrosis transmembrane conductance regulator (*CFTR*), and now more than 1000 different mutations have been identified that cause cystic fibrosis.

By contrast, today, what had once taken many groups a decade to complete can be undertaken in a single laboratory in days. For example, modern exome sequencing enables all 180,000 exons encoded by the human genome to be characterized in an individual patient or an entire kindred. Although the exome equates to only 1% of the genome, or about 30 megabases, it is thought to contain 85% of the mutations responsible for mendelian disorders. This technology, for example, was recently used to identify the causative gene of Miller syndrome, a rare disorder that manifests with cleft palate, absent digits, and ocular anomalies. The entire exomes of four persons so affected were sequenced, allowing mutations to be identified in the causative gene encoding dihydroorotate dehydrogenase (*DHODH*).

The major challenges now are therefore no longer the single-gene disorders but complex genetic diseases such as cancer, COPD, asthma, and interstitial lung disease. These diseases are the result of interactions between multiple genes and environmental factors. Consequently, the diseases cluster within families but do not show a clear pattern of inheritance.

SINGLE-GENE DISORDERS AND RESPIRATORY DISEASE

Many single-gene disorders have been linked with respiratory disease (see Table 2-1). They are perhaps best typified by the autosomal recessive condition α_1-antitrypsin deficiency. This condition shows a clear genotype-phenotype correlation with current understanding of the molecular basis providing new insights into the pathogenesis of disease. α_1-Antitrypsin is the archetypal member of the serine proteinase inhibitor

Table 2-1   Examples of Genetic Factors That Underlie Lung Disease

Condition	Inheritance	Gene(s) Associated With Disease	Chromosomal Location	Affected Protein(s)
Respiratory distress syndrome	Multifactorial	SFTPA1	10q22.2-q23.1	Surfactant protein A
		SFTPB	2p12-p11.2	Surfactant protein B
		SFTPC	8p21	Surfactant protein C
Primary ciliary dyskinesia (CILD1-13)	Autosomal recessive	CILD1 (DNAI1)	9p21-p13	Dynein intermediate chain 1, axonemal
		CILD2 (?)	19q13.3	?
		CILD3 (DNAH5)	5p	Dynein heavy chain 5, axonemal
		CILD4 (?)	15q13	?
		CILD5 (?)	16p12	?
		CILD6 (TXNDC3)	7p14.1	Thioredoxin domain containing 3
		CILD7 (DNAH11)	7p21	Dynein heavy chain 11, axonemal
		CILD8 (?)	15q24-q25	?
		CILD9 (DNAI2)	17q25	Dynein intermediate chain 2, axonemal
		CILD10 (KTU)	14q21.3	Kintoun
		CILD11 (RSP4A)	6q22	Radial spoke head 4 A
		CILD12 (RSPH9)	6p21	Radial spoke head 9
		CILD13 (LRRC50)	16q24.1	Leucine-rich repeat containing 50
Asthma	Multifactorial	ADAM-33	20p13	A disintegrin and metalloproteinase domain 33
		CHI3L1	1q32.1	Chitinase 3-like 1
		DPP10	2q12.3-q14.2	Dipeptidyl peptidase X
		HLA-G	6p21.3	Histocompatibility antigen class I G
		ORMDL3	17q21.1	Orosomucoid 1-like protein 3
		GSDMB	17q21	Gasdermin B
Interstitial lung disease	Multifactorial	TERT	5p15.33	Telomerase reverse transcriptase
		TERC	3q21-q28	Telomerase RNA component
		SFPA1	10q22.2-q23.1	Surfactant protein A1
		SFTPA2	10q22-q23	Surfactant protein A2
		SFTPC	8p21	Surfactant protein C
Cystic fibrosis	Autosomal recessive	CFTR	7q31.2	Cystic fibrosis conductance regulator
α_1-Antitrypsin deficiency	Autosomal recessive	SERPINA1	14q32.1	α_1-Antitrypsin
Pneumothorax and emphysema secondary to Marfan syndrome	Autosomal dominant	FBN1	15q21.1	Fibrillin
Emphysema secondary to Menkes disease	X-linked recessive	ATP7A	Xq12-q13	Copper-transporting ATPase
COPD	Single-gene defect	ELN	7q11.2	Elastin
Emphysema secondary to cutis laxa	Autosomal recessive	FBLN4	11q13	Fibulins
		FBLN5	14q32.1	
COPD	Multifactorial	SERPINE2	2q33-q35	Thrombin protease inhibitor
		MMP12	11q22.2-q22.3	Matrix metalloproteinase-12
		CHRNA-3/5	2q24-q32	α-Nicotinic acetyl choline receptor
		HHIP	4q28-q32	Hedgehog-interacting protein
		FAM13A	4q22.1	Family with sequence similarity, member A

Table 2-1   Examples of Genetic Factors That Underlie Lung Disease—cont'd

Condition	Inheritance	Gene(s) Associated With Disease	Chromosomal Location	Affected Protein(s)
Hyper-IgE (Job's syndrome)	Autosomal dominant	STAT3	17q21	Signal transducer and activator of transcription 3
Familial pneumothorax (Birt-Hogg-Dubé syndrome)	Autosomal dominant	FLCN	17p11.2	Folliculin
Tuberous sclerosis with pulmonary cysts/ lymphangioleiomyomatosis	Autosomal dominant	TSC1	9q34	Hamartin
		TSC2	16p13.3	Tuberin
Hereditary hemorrhagic telangiectasia (Osler-Weber-Rendu syndrome)	Autosomal dominant	HHT1	9q34.1	Endoglin
		ALK1	12q11-q14	Activin receptor–like kinase-1
Primary pulmonary hypertension	Autosomal dominant	BMPR2	2q33	Bone morphogenetic protein receptor type II
		ALK1	12q11-q14	Activin receptor–like kinase-1

("serpin") superfamily. It is synthesized in the liver and secreted into the plasma, where it is the most abundant circulating proteinase inhibitor. Most people of North European descent carry the normal M allele, but 1 in 25 carries the Z variant (Glu342Lys), which results in plasma α_1-antitrypsin levels in the homozygote that are 10% to 15% of the normal M allele. The Z mutation causes the accumulation of α_1-antitrypsin in the rough endoplasmic reticulum of the liver, predisposing the homozygote to the development of juvenile hepatitis, cirrhosis, and hepatocellular carcinoma. The greatly reduced circulating levels of α_1-antitrypsin are unable to protect the lungs against proteolytic damage by neutrophil elastase, predisposing the Z homozygote to the development of early-onset emphysema.

The structure of α_1-antitrypsin is based on a dominant β-pleated sheet A and nine α-helices (**Figure 2-1**). This scaffold supports an exposed mobile reactive loop that presents a peptide sequence as a pseudosubstrate for the target proteinase. After docking, the proteinase is inactivated by a mousetrap-type action that swings it from the top to the bottom of the serpin in association with the insertion of an extra strand into β-sheet A (see Figure 2-1). This six-stranded protein bound to its target enzyme is then recognized by hepatic receptors and cleared from the circulation. The structure of α_1-antitrypsin is central to its role as an effective antiproteinase but also renders it liable to undergo conformational change in association with disease. The Z mutation is at residue P_{17} (17 residues proximal to the key P_1 amino acid that defines the inhibitory specificity of α_1-antitrypsin) at the head of a strand of β-sheet A and the base of the mobile reactive loop (see Figure 2-1). The mutation opens β-sheet A, thereby favoring the insertion of the reactive loop of a second α_1-antitrypsin molecule to form a dimer (see Figure 2-1). This dimer can then extend to form polymers that tangle in the endoplasmic reticulum of the liver to form the inclusion bodies resulting in liver disease. Support for this pathomechanism comes from the demonstration that Z α_1-antitrypsin formed chains of polymers when incubated under physiologic conditions. The rate was accelerated by raising the temperature to 41° C and could be blocked by peptides that compete with the loop for annealing to β-sheet A. The role of polymerization in vivo was clarified by the finding of

α_1-antitrypsin polymers in inclusion bodies from the livers of Z α_1-antitrypsin homozygotes (see Figure 2-1).

Although many α_1-antitrypsin deficiency variants have been described, only three other mutants of α_1-antitrypsin have similarly been associated with plasma deficiency and hepatic inclusions: α_1-antitrypsin Siiyama (Ser53Phe), α_1-antitrypsin Mmalton (Phe52 deleted), and α_1-antitrypsin King's (His334Asp). All of these mutants lie in the shutter domain that controls opening of β-sheet A. They destabilize the molecule to allow the formation of loop-sheet polymers in vivo. Further investigations have shown that polymerization also underlies the mild plasma deficiency of the S (Glu264Val) and I (Arg39Cys) variants of α_1-antitrypsin. The point mutations that are responsible for these variants have less effect on β-sheet A than does the Z variant. Thus, the associated rate of polymer formation is much slower than that for Z α_1-antitrypsin, which results in less retention of protein within hepatocytes, milder plasma deficiency, and the lack of a clinical phenotype. However, if a mild, slowly polymerizing I or S variant of α_1-antitrypsin is inherited with a rapidly polymerizing Z variant, then the two can interact to form heteropolymers within hepatocytes. These polymers underlie the inclusions that cause cirrhosis.

Emphysema associated with α_1-antitrypsin deficiency results from lack of protection against proteolytic attack in the lungs associated with reduced levels of circulating proteinase inhibitor. This is particularly the case with individuals who smoke tobacco. The Z α_1-antitrypsin that does escape from the liver into the circulation is less efficient in protecting the tissues from enzyme damage and, like M α_1-antitrypsin, may be inactivated by oxidation of the P1 methionine residue. The demonstration that Z α_1-antitrypsin can undergo a spontaneous conformational transition in association with liver disease raised the possibility that this might also occur within the lung. Indeed, polymers have been detected in bronchoalveolar lavage fluid in patients with Z α_1-antitrypsin deficiency. This observation may have important implications for the pathogenesis of disease, because polymerization obscures the reactive loop of α_1-antitrypsin, rendering the protein inactive as an inhibitor of proteolytic enzymes. Thus, the spontaneous polymerization of α_1-antitrypsin within the lung will exacerbate the already reduced antiproteinase screen, thereby increasing the

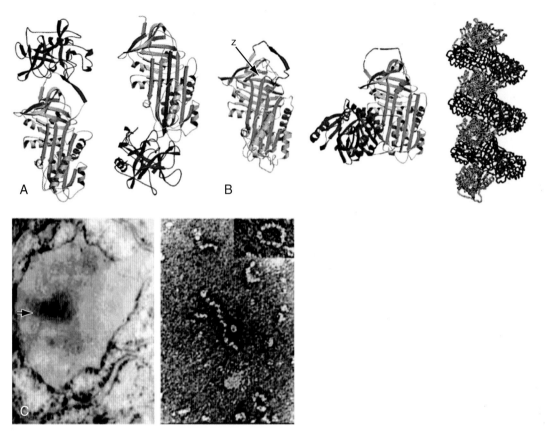

Figure 2-1 The molecular basis of α_1-antitrypsin deficiency. α_1-Antitrypsin may be considered to act by a mousetrap mechanism. **A,** After docking (*left*), the target proteinase (*gray*) is inactivated by movement from the upper to the lower pole of the protein (*right*). This is associated with insertion of the reactive loop (*red*) as an extra strand into β-sheet A (*green*). The mousetrap mechanism may be triggered spontaneously by point mutations in association with disease. The Z mutation (Glu342Lys) of α_1-antitrypsin is at the head of a strand of β-sheet A (*green*) and the base of the reactive loop. **B,** Mutations in this region can destabilize β-sheet A to allow the insertion of a reactive loop of a second molecule (*middle*). This dimer then extends to form long chains of polymers (*right*). Each molecule of α_1-antitrypsin in the polymer is shown in a different color. It is these polymers that tangle in the endoplasmic reticulum to cause inclusions resulting in liver disease. **C,** An inclusion body (*arrow*) from the liver of a patient with α_1-antitrypsin deficiency (*left*). The inclusions are composed of chains of molecules of α_1-antitrypsin (*right*). *(Modified from Gooptu B, Lomas DA: Conformational pathology of the serpins—themes, variations and therapeutic strategies, Annu Rev Biochem 78:147–176, 2009.)*

susceptibility of the tissues to proteolytic attack and increasing the rate of progression of emphysema. Finally, the α_1-antitrypsin polymers themselves are inflammatory for neutrophils, which will also increase the proteolytic load in the lung. Recent data suggest that cigarette smoke can induce the intrapulmonary polymerization of Z α_1-antitrypsin, thereby exacerbating the lung damage associated with smoking.

GENE HUNTING FOR COMPLEX GENETIC DISEASES AND ITS PITFALLS: COPD AND ASTHMA

One approach to looking for genes associated with complex genetic disorders is by means of an *association study*, which analyzes genetic variation between cases and controls (i.e., without disease) matched for various factors. The genetic variation commonly used in such studies is the single-nucleotide polymorphism (SNP) (DNA sequence variation) found approximately every 300 base pairs across the genome. These studies have been undertaken in patients with COPD matched with control subjects who do not have COPD but who are the same age and have the same smoking history and the same ethnic background. The early studies typically were small (100 to 150 cases plus controls) and often were confounded by failure to match carefully cases and controls. To increase the likelihood of finding a disease-associated gene, such studies frequently included SNPs in multiple genes in the same cohort. However, such *multiple comparisons* can result in false-positive results. With study of sufficient numbers of genes, purely by chance a variant will arise that erroneously appears to be associated with the disease being studied. Careful statistical analysis is necessary to avoid this problem.

The analysis was made more complex in COPD by the inherent complexity of the disease phenotype—a heterogeneous mix of airway disease and emphysema. Indeed, larger family-based studies have shown the independent clustering of the airway disease and emphysema components of COPD within families. This finding suggests that different genetic factors predispose to each of these components of the phenotype. The only way to overcome the inherent variation in COPD is to focus on groups of patients with well-characterized disease components or to undertake studies with large sample sizes and then to replicate any positive findings in other cohorts. This is now the case with candidate gene studies, and good evidence has emerged to show that heterozygosity for α_1-antitrypsin deficiency (phenotype PiMZ) and polymorphisms in genes involved in oxidative stress—those encoding microsomal epoxide hydrolase (*EPHX1*), glutathione *S*-transferase (*GST-P1* and *GST-M1*), heme oxygenase (*HMOX1*), and superoxide dismutase 3 (*SOD3*)—are associated with an increased risk of COPD (**Figure 2-2**). More recently, a minor

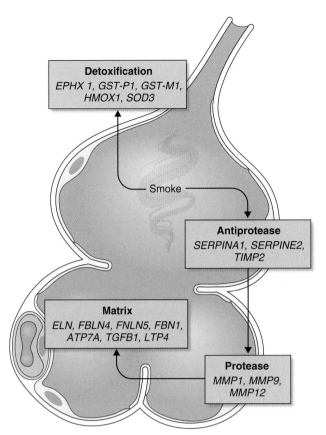

Figure 2-2 Genes implicated in chronic obstructive pulmonary disease (COPD). When smoke enters the alveolus, many of its constituent compounds are absorbed. Some of these are detoxified by an array of enzymes; those that escape detoxification cause local damage and inflammation. The influx and activation of inflammatory cells lead to the liberation of proteases that attack the extracellular matrix, primarily elastin. The effect of these proteases is attenuated by endogenous antiprotease activities, whereas growth factor signals are thought to modulate the repair and remodeling of the extracellular matrix.

allele of an SNP in the matrix metalloprotease-12 gene (*MMP12*) has been shown to protect against COPD in adult smokers.

The limitation of association studies using a *candidate gene approach* is that they are by definition restricted to pathways already recognized to be associated with the disease—in the case of COPD, the proteinase-antiproteinase balance, the oxidative stress pathway, and the integrity of the extracellular matrix (see later). Consequently, this approach lacks the capacity to identify unanticipated players and is thus restricted to *hypothesis testing*, rather than *hypothesis generation.*

In recent years, the collection of large cohorts of patients combined with technologic advances has allowed unbiased *genome-wide association studies* of many patients with lung disease. It is currently possible to use microarrays to assay up to a million different SNPs in the genome in the same patient. The variation in SNPs is then compared between cases and controls. The largest study was undertaken in a cohort from Bergen, Norway, and then replicated in the International COPD Genetics Network, the National Emphysema Treatment Trial with controls from the Normative Ageing study, and then finally in the Boston Early Onset COPD cohort. Top hits from this analysis were SNPs in the α-nicotinic acetylcholine receptor *CHRNA-3/5* and the hedgehog-interacting protein *HHIP*. The first of these (rs8034919) in the α-nicotinic acetylcholine

receptor also was identified in three genome-wide association studies of lung cancer and also is thought to be important in peripheral vascular disease and nicotine addiction. It is possible that this SNP functions as a marker for an addiction gene. People who carry this SNP may require more cigarettes to satisfy nicotine addiction, may inhale more deeply, and may find it more difficult to withdraw from cigarette smoking. If this hypothesis is correct, the disease-associated allele of this gene would account for 12% of the population risk for COPD.

In interpreting any association study, it is important to consider two important caveats. First, many genetic associations studies report false-positive findings owing to a failure to appreciate the *prior probability* of an association and the *power* of the study to detect a meaningful effect. When the prior probability of an association is low, that is to say when there is little functional or epidemiological data to support an association, the numbers of subjects required to guard against a false-positive result increases. Consequently, the identification of a genetic association in a single study must always be treated with caution. Clearly, in the case of the α-nicotinic acetylcholine receptor, it is possible to construct very plausible models for its potential role in COPD, so the prior probability is not low. Moreover, those studies in which it was identified were well powered. The second caveat, however, relates to the phenomenon of *linkage disequilibrium*. The combination of more than one genetic variant or *allele* is called a *haplotype*. Some haplotypes occur in the population more often than one would expect by random association of alleles. This can be caused by, but is not restricted to, the inheritance of blocks of adjacent genes on a chromosome. Clearly, nearby genes are less likely to be separated by recombination during gametogenesis than are more distantly spaced genes. Each population of humans has its own characteristic set of common haplotypes. In this light, a disease-associated SNP can more accurately be viewed as a marker of the haplotype that is associated with the disease under study and the causative gene must be identified within that group. Indeed, in the case of disease-associated SNPs in the α-nicotinic acetylcholine receptor, there does appear to be linkage disequilibrium with SNPs in the iron-responsive element binding protein 2 IREB2. This was identified from expression analysis in lung tissue from persons with COPD and then confirmed in three separate COPD cohorts. IREB2 is localized to the human epithelial cell surface and may play a role in protecting against epithelial damage from oxidative stress.

It is, of course, possible that a haplotype identified in large genome-wide association studies may contain multiple disease-associated genes, so each one needs individual validation. Indeed, many diseases appear to involve the interaction of multiple disease-associated alleles, each with relatively small contributions when studied individually. The chances of identifying an allele that imparts a small *relative risk* for developing a disease are improved both by increasing the numbers of cases studied (increased *power*) and by carefully selecting cases of the same phenotype. With diseases such as COPD that are likely to represent the final common pathway of many forms of lung damage, this consideration is particularly important.

The analysis of still larger numbers of patients with COPD has identified a disease-associated SNP in *FAM13A*. The role of this gene in disease is unclear, but expression has been associated with hypoxia. *FAM13A* also has been associated with lung function in a second independent study. A detailed analysis of these genes in well-characterized cohorts showed that SNPs in the α-nicotinic acetylcholine receptor are associated with smoking intensity, airflow obstruction, and emphysema, and SNPs in the hedgehog-interacting protein are associated with systemic features of COPD (low body mass index) and exacerbations, whereas SNPs in *FAM13A* are associated with airflow obstruction.

Familial clustering of asthma has also been recognized for many years, and comparisons between monozygotic and dizygotic twins suggest that 70% of asthma-related population variance is accounted for by genetic factors. Classical positional cloning using linkage analysis of large families has identified several candidates, including *ADAM33*, *CHI3L1*, *DPP10*, and *HLA-G*, and more recently, asthma-specific genome-wide association studies have identified further disease-associated loci (see Table 2-1). The first of these was in the long arm of chromosome 17 and found to contain two genes, *ORMDL3* and *GSDMB*, whose expression levels are altered in asthmatic persons. The pathways implicated by such studies can now be tested to determine what role they play in disease pathogenesis.

CELL BIOLOGY

INTRACELLULAR SIGNALS

Oxidative Stress

Cigarette smoke contains 10^{17} free radicals per puff, including superoxide ions, hydrogen peroxide, hydroxyl radicals, nitric oxides, peroxynitrite, and semiquinone. Migrating neutrophils also can release superoxide radicals in response to inflammatory stimuli, including pathogens and smoke. Alveolar macrophages from the lungs of smokers are more activated compared with controls and release more reactive oxygen species (ROS) in vitro. These toxic products can all modify proteins, lipids, and DNA during oxidative stress. Oxidized proteins can be found in lung tissue and their level increases with worsening lung disease. This damage leads directly to cell death and emphysema. When ROS react with phospholipids in the cell membrane (*lipid peroxidation*), they generate products such as F_2 isoprostanes and malondialdehyde that can trigger intracellular signaling pathways. For example, isoprostanes cause muscle constriction and induce cell growth by way of prostaglandin receptors. Other diffusible peroxides act as chemoattractants, thereby contributing to inflammation.

Normally, homeostatic mechanisms maintain the reducing environment of the cytoplasm. Glutathione (GSH) is an abundant sulfhydryl chemical that exists in the cytosol predominantly in its reduced form (GSH), with only 1% in the oxidized disulfide-bonded form (GSSG). The cell maintains the ratio of GSH to GSSG strongly in favor of the reduced form by reducing GSSG to GSH, or by excreting GSSG. However, during the adaptive response to oxidative stress, de novo synthesis of GSH also is important. Alterations in GSH metabolism have been shown to affect the sensitivity of cells to oxidative damage. For example, ROS can induce signaling by a number of stress pathways including c-Jun N-terminal kinase (JNK), extracellular signaling kinase, and p38 kinase. These are linked to signaling cascades that ultimately regulate gene transcription.

Oxidative stress is an important activator of nuclear factor κB (NFκB). This proinflammatory transcription factor is held in the cytosol in unstressed cells through binding to its inhibitor, IκB. When cell surface receptors are activated, they can trigger an IκB kinase (IKK) that phosphorylates IκB, targeting it for degradation. NFκB is thus released to migrate to the nucleus, where it transactivates genes involved in many pathways, including the inflammatory response. The precise mechanism whereby NFκB is activated by oxidative stress is not fully understood but may involve the direct activation of IKK by ROS.

ROS also modulate gene transcription by modifying chromatin, so-called *epigenetic regulation*. Chromatin structure determines the access of transcription factors to target sequences within the promoters of genes and is subject to regulation. Posttranslational modification of histones can alter DNA coiling around them. For example, the relative activities of histone acetyltransferases (HATs) and histone deacetylases (HDACs) profoundly alter histone function and consequently gene transcription. Cigarette smoke and oxidative stress can enhance histone acetylation by impairing HDAC activity resulting in altered gene expression.

A number of genes have been studied that might plausibly modify the cells' responses to cigarette smoke and ROS. These include genes involved in detoxification of toxins and genes involved in neutralization of ROS. Many toxins in cigarette smoke are subject to first-pass metabolism in the liver, and one of the enzymes involved in this is microsomal epoxide hydrolase (encoded by *EPHX1*) localized to 1q42.1, which has been studied intensely in the context of COPD (see Figure 2-2). Several *EPHX1* SNPs have been described that affect its activity. One of these leads to a 40% loss of in vitro activity (Tyr113His, the "slow" allele), whereas another increases activity by 25% (His139Arg, the "fast" allele). A recent systematic metaanalysis found homozygosity for the "slow" (Tyr113His) allele to be *protective* against COPD (odds ratio, 0.5). Analysis of the National Emphysema Treatment Trial (NETT) dataset has suggested a role for *EPHX1* polymorphism in both severity of COPD and the distribution of emphysematous changes. In addition to EPHX1, glutathione S-transferase (GST) comprises a large family of enzymes capable of catalyzing the conjugation of GSH to noxious compounds. The GSTs are highly polymorphic, and SNPs in *GSTP1* have been associated with COPD, the distribution of emphysema, and more rapid decline in lung function. The null mutation of *GSTM1* (localized to 1p13.1) also has been associated with COPD.

Several other proteins can loosely be considered as having antioxidant activity and thus protective against ROS. Heme oxygenase catalyzes the first step in heme degradation. Heme oxygenase 1 (encoded by *HMOX1*, localized to 22q13.1) is the inducible isoform that can be upregulated by a wide range of stresses. Bile pigments generated by heme cleavage are believed to have antioxidant properties; thus, HMOX-1 induction is protective during cellular oxidant injury, and overexpression of HMOX-1 in lung tissue protects against hyperoxia. The *HMOX1* gene 5′-flanking region contains stretches of GC repeats that are highly polymorphic in length. A higher proportion of long repeats that are associated with impaired promoter activity has been observed in patients with COPD and increased severity of disease. By contrast, superoxide dismutase (SOD) directly catalyzes the conversion of superoxide to oxygen and hydrogen peroxide. The extracellular isoform (encoded by *SOD3*, localized to 4p15) is abundant in lung parenchyma, and in the cross-sectional Copenhagen Heart Study, the R213G allele that results in higher plasma levels was associated with significantly less severe COPD in smokers.

Oxidative stress also is important in the pathogenesis of emphysema associated with α₁-antitrypsin deficiency. Free radicals released from neutrophils or cigarettes can oxidize the key P1 methionine at residue 358, which is central to the inhibitory activity of α_1-antitrypsin. This change results in a 2000-fold reduction in the association rate constant with neutrophil elastase. A reduction in the intrapulmonary concentration of α_1-antitrypsin in persons with α_1-antitrypsin deficiency means that fewer free radicals are required to have a significant impact on the inactivation of α_1-antitrypsin. In addition to Met358, methionines at positions 226, 242, and 351 and the cysteine residue at 232 in α_1-antitrypsin are similarly available for oxidation. These molecules may be considered to function as a sump to "mop up" free radicals, thereby reducing their toxicity. However, persons with α_1-antitrypsin deficiency have fewer molecules to bind free radicals. Moreover, polymer formation masks two of the four methionines, thereby further reducing the capacity of α_1-antitrypsin to detoxify these toxic species. Thus, α_1-antitrypsin from persons with Z α_1-antitrypsin deficiency is more prone to oxidative damage and less able to protect the tissues from oxidative stress as a result of both local deficiency and polymer formation.

Endoplasmic Reticulum Stress

The early steps in the biogenesis of secreted and membrane proteins occur in the lumen of the endoplasmic reticulum, where resident proteins that make up the endoplasmic reticulum machinery assist in their folding, maturation, and complex assembly (**Figure 2-3**). Variation in the load of endoplasmic reticulum client proteins and in the function of its protein-folding machinery can lead to an imbalance between the two that is referred to as *endoplasmic reticulum stress*. This imbalance triggers a cellular response, mediated by signaling pathways that restore balance between the protein-folding environment in the organelle by increasing the expression of genes that enhance most aspects of endoplasmic reticulum

function and by transiently repressing the biosynthesis of new client proteins. This response has been termed the *unfolded protein response* (UPR) and is mediated by three signaling molecules, PERK, IRE1, and ATF6, located in the endoplasmic reticulum membrane (see Figure 2-3). It is now clear that the UPR plays a role in many human diseases, including many that affect the lung.

Cigarette smoke can directly induce endoplasmic reticulum stress in cells. When cultured airway epithelial cells are treated with cigarette smoke extracts, they activate the UPR. Similar responses have been observed in vivo in the lungs of cigarette smoke–exposed mice and even in the lungs of human smokers. Overexpression of the endoplasmic reticulum chaperones BiP in cultured bronchial epithelial cells protects them from smoke-induced apoptosis, supporting a role for endoplasmic reticulum stress in cigarette cytotoxicity. Precisely how smoke induces endoplasmic reticulum stress remains to be determined, but the protective effects of coadministered N-acetylcysteine or GSH suggest that oxidation of an unknown target is likely to be important.

The existence of IRE1β, a lung- and gut-specific IRE1 isoform, suggests that endoplasmic reticulum stress has important consequences for mucosal tissues. IRE1 signals through splicing the messenger RNA (mRNA) for the transcription factor XBP-1, which transactivates many UPR genes but it is not clear why airways and bowel require a tissue-specific IRE1 isoform. A clue may come from the *XBP1*-mutant mouse, which exhibits impaired mucosal defense against *Listeria monocytogenes* and has poorly bactericidal gut secretions. These observations suggest that the IRE1-XBP1 pathway may play an important role in host-pathogen interactions at epithelial surfaces. Endoplasmic reticulum stress can itself affect the acquired

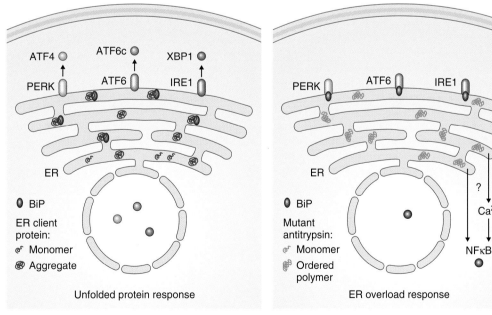

Figure 2-3 Unfolded protein response and endoplasmic reticulum (ER) overload response. *Unfolded protein response* (UPR): In the resting endoplasmic reticulum, the chaperone BiP holds the stress-signaling molecules PERK, IRE1, and ATF6 inactive. When proteins misfold in the endoplasmic reticulum, they sequester BiP (*purple*). This enables PERK, IRE1, and ATF6 to become active and signal to the cytosol. PERK phosphorylates a cytosolic translation initiation factor eIF2α, thereby halting most protein synthesis. In parallel, the translation of a subset of proteins increases. These include the transcription factor ATF4, which transactivates genes of the integrated stress response (ISR). When IRE1 is activated, it splices out an intron from the messenger RNA (mRNA) encoding the transcription factor XBP1. This causes a frameshift in the mRNA, accompanied by the translation of an activated form of XBP1, which can transactivate UPR genes. When ATF6 is released from BiP, it migrates initially to the Golgi apparatus, where it is cleaved by proteases to release a soluble fragment, ATF6c. This migrates to the nucleus, where it transactivates UPR genes. *Endoplasmic reticulum overload response* (EOR): When excess folded proteins accumulate in the endoplasmic reticulum, they cause calcium-dependent activation of nuclear factor κB (NFκB) through a poorly understood mechanism.

immune response. It is clear that the IRE1-XBP-1 pathway is crucial for differentiation programs that require expansion of the endoplasmic reticulum—for example, during the differentiation of B lymphocytes into plasma cells. This requirement can be explained by the regulation of many lipid synthetic genes by XBP-1. In addition, XBP-1–dependent processes appear to be responsible for heightened inflammatory signaling in inflamed airway epithelium. When forced to express active XBP-1, bronchial epithelial cells show elevated bradykinin-induced IL-8 release.

One of the disease-causing mutations of the surfactant protein C gene *SFTPC* is a deletion of exon 4. This change generates a protein that fails to exit the endoplasmic reticulum and induces endoplasmic reticulum stress. When expressed transiently in cultured cells, this mutant of SFTPC accumulates as large ubiquitinated inclusions and inhibits normal proteasome function, ultimately killing the cell. When cell lines that stably express this mutant are infected with respiratory syncytial virus, the cells accumulate high levels of mutant protein, activate the UPR, and show increased toxicity compared with wild type SFTPC–expressing cells. Of interest, evidence of UPR activation has been seen in a majority of cases of interstitial lung disease, both with and without SFTPC mutations. This finding may suggest an even greater role for endoplasmic reticulum stress in idiopathic pulmonary fibrosis. Very recently, it was shown that endoplasmic reticulum stress caused by a variety of insults, including mutant SFPC, can induce *epithelial to mesenchyme transition* (EMT). This is the process by which epithelia can transdifferentiate into cells of a more fibroblast-like phenotype. This mechanism has been suggested to contribute to pulmonary fibrosis and would explain why treatment strategies for idiopathic pulmonary fibrosis involving antiinflammatory drugs have been less than entirely successful. It may instead prove more beneficial to prevent EMT by ameliorating endoplasmic reticulum stress.

Cystic fibrosis is caused by *CFTR* mutations that impede protein folding. High levels of $\Delta F508$ CFTR expression, but not of wild type protein, induce a UPR in cultured cells. However, rather than CFTR expression affecting endoplasmic reticulum stress, the clinically relevant relationship may be the converse. Recent data have suggested endoplasmic reticulum stress affects CFTR expression. In cells treated with agents that induce the UPR, levels of mature CFTR protein are markedly diminished. This involves a selective reduction of genomic CFTR expression; an effect that is not seen with recombinantly expressed CFTR or with endogenous control genes. Repression of the CFTR promoter is achieved both by selective recruitment of ATF6 and by epigenetic changes, including altered DNA methylation and histone deacetylation. This is especially unfortunate, because mucopurulent secretions from patients with cystic fibrosis are sufficient to induce endoplasmic reticulum stress in human bronchial epithelial cells, suggesting that chronic airway sepsis may actually contribute to further impairment of CFTR expression in those cases in which milder mutations allow some of the protein to reach the cell surface. This effect of endoplasmic reticulum stress on CFTR also may explain previous studies that have identified impaired CFTR expression and function in the upper airway of smokers who do not have the disease. This finding had been attributed to oxidant effects alone but now might be explained equally well as a response to smoke-induced endoplasmic reticulum stress. Whether this effect contributes to the pathologic lung changes associated with smoking is unclear, but if it does so, it would provide a novel therapeutic target.

Hypoxia is a far more common cause of protein misfolding than these single-gene disorders. The endoplasmic reticulum requires large amounts of energy to function, so it is one of the first organelles to malfunction when energy supplies are disrupted. This effect can follow nutrient deprivation or hypoxia and appears to play a role in tissue survival during ischemia. Cancers provide a good example of this mechanism. Tumors frequently outgrow their blood supply, so their cores become hypoxic. It has been found that tumors from animals with defective endoplasmic reticulum stress signaling fail to grow well, and most lung cancers show evidence of UPR activation. Consequently, modulation of endoplasmic reticulum stress may offer a target for treating thoracic malignancies. Attempts to identify antimesothelioma therapies found that proteasome inhibition with bortezomib could cause cell cycle arrest and death of cultured mesothelioma lines. The mechanism is not certain, but because bortezomib induces the UPR in several cancer models, endoplasmic reticulum stress may plausibly be involved. In some cancers, bortezomib appears to target hypoxic cells preferentially, perhaps because of their basal endoplasmic reticulum stress.

Endoplasmic Reticulum Overload

Remarkably, when $Z \alpha_1$-antitrypsin polymerizes within the endoplasmic reticulum of its cell of synthesis, it fails to induce a strong UPR. Instead, the predominant signaling response appears to be activation of NFκB through a poorly understood mechanism that has variously been termed the *endoplasmic reticulum overload response* or the *ordered polymer response* (Figure 2-3). In the liver, this ultimately can lead to cirrhosis. $Z \alpha_1$-antitrypsin appears also to be synthesized locally in the lung by some cell types, including bronchial and alveolar epithelial cells and macrophages. These too are likely to activate NFκB signaling cascades that would increase the production of inflammatory mediators and further amplify neutrophil recruitment and tissue damage. Chronic activation of NFκB would accelerate apoptosis within alveolar cells and thus contribute to the pathogenesis of emphysema. Because this effect would occur in all alveolar cells, it provides another explanation for the panlobular distribution of emphysema that characterizes α_1-antitrypsin deficiency. Although $Z \alpha_1$-antitrypsin serves as an excellent model disease to study endoplasmic reticulum overload, it is likely that more common diseases such as some viral infections involve this form of signaling.

MAINTENANCE OF THE EXTRACELLULAR MATRIX

As in all tissues, cells of the lung communicate with one another through direct contact and by way of released diffusible and matrix molecules. This communication network is important during the inflammatory response but also is required for the maintenance of normal lung architecture. The extracellular matrix comprises a complex network of scaffolding proteins, principally elastin and collagen. The elastin filaments form from tropoelastin monomers that self-assemble into aggregates and then fuse with microfilaments. Multiple covalent cross-links between the lysines in neighboring filaments provide stability. Cutis laxa is a family of autosomal dominant, X-linked, and recessive human diseases characterized by excessively slack connective tissues. Several families with the milder autosomal dominant form show early-onset pulmonary pathology including emphysema, particularly if inherited with the Z allele of α_1-antitrypsin. Mutations have been identified within the *ELN* (elastin) gene that cause mild cutis laxa and early-onset COPD

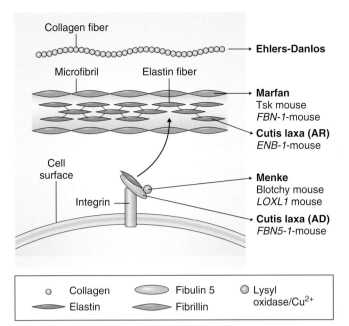

Figure 2-4   Extracellular matrix structure. The extracellular matrix of the lung is composed primarily of collagen and elastin fibers. Large fibrils of collagen assemble within the endoplasmic reticulum and traverse the Golgi apparatus, ultimately to be secreted. Elastin filaments form in association with microfilaments and integrin-anchored fibulin 5. *AD*, autosomal dominant; *AR*, autosomal recessive.

(see Table 2-1). The *ELN* gene maps to 7q11.23 in humans, but because chromosome 7 has not been identified in linkage analysis as a site associated with COPD, it is likely that *ELN* mutations are a rare cause of this disease.

Elastin fibers bind other proteins, including fibulins, which in turn bind multiple extracellular matrix components and the basement membrane (**Figure 2-4**). The fibulins are a family of six proteins, at least two of which (those encoded by *FBLN4*, mapped to 11q13, and *FBLN5*, on 14q32.1) are mutated in severe autosomal recessive forms of cutis laxa and whose phenotype often includes early-onset emphysema. Both pathogenic mutations are located within an epidermal growth factor–like domain of each protein, suggesting these are critical for fibulins to maintain the integrity of the extracellular matrix within the lung. Of interest, analogous mutations in fibrillin, which bares homology to the fibulins, cause Marfan syndrome. Moreover, mutations of fibrillin (encoded by *FBN1*, localized to 15q21.1) have been described in neonatal Marfan syndrome with very-early-onset emphysema.

Menkes disease, characterized by abnormal hair and specific dysmorphic features, is caused by mutations in an intracellular copper transporter (encoded by *ATP7A*, localized to Xq13.3). The clinical features are due to defective connective tissue synthesis believed to be the result of dysfunction of lysyl oxidase. This copper-dependent enzyme is required for proper cross-linking of both collagen and elastin fibers. A recent case report described a child with Menkes disease and severe bilateral panlobular emphysema who died at only 14 months of age. Gene sequencing revealed a splice-site mutation in *ATP7A*, suggesting that proper extracellular matrix cross-linking is vital for stability of the lung parenchyma.

In contrast with animal models of COPD, mutations in collagen have not been identified in humans. This difference does not appear to be due to an incompatibility of mutated collagen with survival, because numerous collagen mutations have been

described that cause other human diseases. Instead, it may reflect a more important role for elastin integrity in emphysema in humans than in mice.

Noxious stimuli such as cigarette smoke that cause lung inflammation help establish chemotactic gradients of interleukin-8 (IL-8) and leukotriene B_4 (LTB$_4$) that encourage macrophages and neutrophils to migrate from capillaries into the small airways and alveoli. Neutrophils initially are concentrated in the centrilobular regions of the lung parenchyma where they release serine and cathepsin proteinases. These enzymes damage and degrade elastin and other structural proteins, thereby causing disease. The degraded elastin fragments themselves act as chemoattractants that recruit additional inflammatory cells. A direct correlation has been noted between the numbers of neutrophils within the interstitium and the severity of emphysema.

REPAIR

The lung comprises more than 40 specialized cell types, each with its own individual functions and distribution. Of importance, only a subset of these possesses replication potential. Those that can divide must serve as a stem cell population for the other, terminally differentiated cell types. Regeneration of the lung is a source of much debate. It appears that in humans, the primary regenerative capacity of airway epithelia comes from resident precursor cells. Limited colonization of the airway by exogenous precursors has been described in humans. For example, male epithelial cells have been identified in the lungs of women who have just given birth to a male infant, and chimerism of the bronchial epithelium has been detected in bone marrow recipients. Conversely, limited numbers of recipient-derived cells have also been detected in engrafted transplant lungs. In the absence of lung damage, however, such engraftment of non–lung-derived cells appears to be a rare event.

Alveoli are composed of capillaries and lymphatics encased in a thin epithelial layer. More than 90% of the alveolar surface is composed of *type I pneumocytes* (**Figure 2-5**). These are terminally differentiated, large flat squamous epithelial cells that possess a relatively simple ultrastructure. Their function is to allow gaseous exchange between the alveolar gas and the bloodstream; consequently, they require little more than a nucleus and cell membrane with a few mitochondria and a limited secretory pathway. They are unable to replicate and are susceptible to noxious insults from inhaled toxins such as cigarette smoke and therefore must be replenished by the major stem cell found within the alveolus, which is the *type II pneumocyte*. These are small cuboidal cells located predominantly at the alveolar septal junctions. Although contributing little surface area to the lung, they are abundant, making up half of the alveolar cells by number. Tight gap junctions separate their polarized apical and basolateral domains, enabling selective secretion toward their apical surface, readily identified by its many microvilli.

Type II pneumocytes have two primary functions: to secrete surfactant and to act as the sole stem cell of the alveolus. Surfactant is a complex mixture of phospholipids (mainly dipalmitoylphosphatidylcholine and phosphatidylglycerol) and surfactant proteins A to D (encoded by *SFTPA*, *SFTPB*, *SFTPC*, and *SFTPD*, respectively). Intracellular surfactant inclusions, or multilamellar bodies, give these cells their granular appearance. After exocytosis at the apical surface, these spheroid lamellar bodies form a membrane lattice called *tubular myelin* that plays

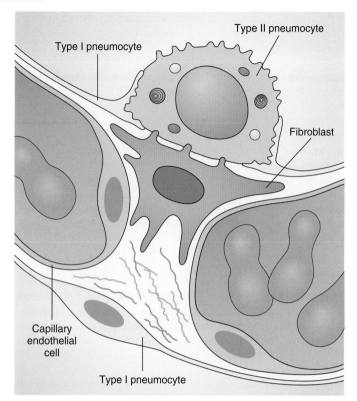

Figure 2-5   Pneumocytes. Alveoli are composed primarily of type I and type II pneumocytes. Type I pneumocytes are thin, terminally differentiated nonsecretory cells that make up 90% of the alveolar surface area. Type II pneumocytes contain lamellar bodies composed of surfactant proteins and lipids. After injury, these cells can divide and give rise to type I pneumocytes.

an important role in reducing the surface tension of the alveolar lining fluid and in host defense. Surfactant proteins A and D are members of the hydrophilic collectin family that have a carboxyl-terminal (C-terminal) lectin domain able to bind and opsonize many inhaled pathogens. In addition, they also have direct toxicity against gram-negative organisms. By contrast, surfactant proteins B and C both are small hydrophobic proteins that interact with surfactant lipids.

Because type II cells first appear in significant numbers after 24 weeks of gestation, prematurely newborn are impaired in surfactant production, which can lead to the development of respiratory distress syndrome, the most common cause of respiratory death in infants in the Western world. Those children who survive are at increased risk for respiratory disability as a result of bronchopulmonary dysplasia. Fortunately, the deficit can now be corrected by instilling surfactant into the trachea. But despite a marked improvement in survival as a result of this therapy, a significant minority (5% to 25%) nevertheless develop long-term complications. Family studies have shown clustering of disease, which suggests a genetic susceptibility to respiratory distress in infancy. The most likely causes of this susceptibility are mutations in the surfactant protein genes and some extrapulmonary gene products (such as granulocyte-macrophage colony-stimulating factor and its receptor). Mutations in the hydrophobic *SFTPB* and *SFTPC* are clearly linked to neonatal respiratory disease. The substitution of GAA for C in codon 121 in *SFTPB* gene underlies 60% of hereditary deficiency of surfactant protein B. This substitution results in a truncated protein, a lack of protein on immunohistochemical

staining of lung tissue, and a *loss-of-function* phenotype, in which the homozygote experiences onset of respiratory distress within the first 12 to 24 hours of life and death by 1 to 6 months of age. A total of 27 mutations have now been described in the *SFTPB* gene, some of which have a milder effect on the production of surfactant protein B, with a later onset of respiratory failure. One family also has been described with a splice site mutation in intron 4 of the *SFTPC* gene. Infants with this mutation do not suffer neonatal respiratory distress but instead develop interstitial lung disease in the first year of life with an autosomal dominant pattern of inheritance. Furthermore, mutations within the genes encoding granulocyte-macrophage colony-stimulating factor or its receptor cause pulmonary alveolar proteinosis in children, a condition characterized by the overproduction of surfactant.

Idiopathic pulmonary fibrosis is a progressive interstitial lung disease characterized by inflammation and fibrosis of the alveolar walls. Although most cases of pulmonary fibrosis are sporadic, some rare familial cases have been described. In a number of early-onset familial cases of idiopathic pulmonary fibrosis, causative mutations have been identified in the *SFTPC* gene. This encodes a large transmembrane pro-protein that is proteolytically processed to the mature small surfactant C protein. As discussed earlier, one of its disease-causing mutants, characterized by a deletion of exon 4, misfolds to induce endoplasmic reticulum stress.

When type I cells are injured, type II cells can proliferate and differentiate into the larger type I cells. In bronchi, *intermediate and basal cells* form the pool of progenitor cells, whereas in terminal bronchioles, the *Clara cell* plays this role. These latter cells are highly metabolically active and serve to detoxify many inhaled chemicals by way of their cytochrome P-450 monooxygenase system in their smooth endoplasmic reticulum. They are able to multiply and differentiate into both ciliated and nonciliated bronchial epithelial cells. This response involves first dedifferentiation and then loss of their secretory granules and smooth endoplasmic reticulum, followed by reentry into the cell cycle. However, not all Clara cells behave identically. A variant that shows resistance to naphthalene, a toxin that targets the cytochrome P-450 isoenzyme found in Clara cells, may represent the main progenitor subtype and has been called either the *toxin-resistant variant Clara cell* or the *bronchiolar stem cell.*

Cells have been identified at the junction between terminal bronchioles and the alveoli that express markers of both Clara cells and type II pneumocytes. These have been named *bronchoalveolar stem cells* (BASCs), because when isolated and grown in vitro, they have been shown to be capable of self-renewal. At least in culture, they can differentiate into cells that express markers of bronchial epithelium, alveolar type I or type II cells. The identity of the progenitor cells of the interstitium, smooth muscle, and endothelium remains unclear. In adults, transdifferentiation of one cell type to another may be important. In disease, many examples of epithelial to mesenchymal transition have been described.

There is growing interest in the potential of stem cell technology in the treatment of lung disease. In young mice, the administration of retinoic acid derivatives can induce lung regeneration, presumably from endogenous stem cells; whether such regeneration can be induced in adult humans, however, is not clear. Instead, it may be possible to deliver exogenous stem cells to the lung. Among the potential sources for such cells, the most controversial are embryonic stem cells. When grown in vitro, these cells can be made to develop toward a type II pneumocyte–like phenotype expressing surfactant proteins that contain lamellar bodies or to form pseudoglandular structures. However, there are currently no clinical data to support their use. By contrast, mesenchymal stem cells derived from bone marrow or cord blood have been more extensively studied. In mouse models of acute lung injury and lung fibrosis, mesenchymal stem cells have yielded promising results. Moreover, in a clinical trial administering human mesenchymal stem cells to patients after acute myocardial infarction, an increase in forced expiratory volume in 1 second (FEV_1) was reported. Further trials designed specifically to test the effectiveness of such therapies in well-defined human lung disease are now required.

The major hurdle in administering exogenous cells is the potential for immune reaction and rejection. If the patient's own cells can be used, this problem can be circumvented. In one recent case involving a 10-year-old boy with congenital tracheal stenosis, a segment of trachea was grown ex vivo on a collagen scaffold from stem cells derived from his bone marrow. This was subsequently implanted to correct the stenosis. Modern technologies now enable progenitor cells to be generated from adult peripheral tissues. Induced pluripotent stem cells (iPS cells) can be derived by expressing stem cell transcriptional regulators such as SOX-2 and Oct-3 in adult cells such as skin fibroblasts. The resulting dedifferentiated cells have the potential to differentiate into many other tissues—hence their pluripotency. This technology has been used to generate hepatocyte-like cells from the skin of patients with α_1-antitrypsin deficiency. Ultimately, when such iPS cells are reprogrammed to correct the genetic defect, it is hoped that they will provide a source of autologous tissue to replace damaged or malfunctioning organs.

PITFALLS AND CONTROVERSIES

NATURE OF THE α_1-ANTITRYPSIN POLYMER

Although the "loop-sheet" model of polymerization described earlier has long been accepted as the mechanism of the retention of Z α_1-antitrypsin within cells, the field was recently revitalized by a new model for polymerization. This model was based on the finding that another serpin molecule, antithrombin, could be re-folded in vitro to form dimers linked by the swapping of a large hairpin structure rather than by the single strand of the reactive center loop. This "domain swap" model initially garnered significant support and led to revival of the molecular mechanism of α_1-antitrypsin deficiency. An important consequence of this renewed interest was the development of a novel monoclonal antibody called 2C1, which specifically recognizes α_1-antitrypsin polymers generated by heating the purified protein. This development was significant because up to that point, heating rather than refolding after chemical denaturation had been the source of most serpin polymers studied in vitro. The crucial observation that 2C1 also recognizes polymers formed within the livers of affected patients, while showing no reactivity against polymers formed by refolding in vitro, strongly supports the original loop-sheet hypothesis. However, this renewed bout of interest in serpin polymerization, while having been prompted most likely by an in vitro antithrombin artifact, has left researchers with an excellent new monoclonal antibody that will be of great use in the study (and perhaps future diagnosis) of this disease. This field remains ripe for future discoveries, and it is unlikely that the last word on serpin polymerization has yet been written.

ALVEOLAR REGENERATION IN RESPONSE TO RETINOIC ACID

In 1997 it was shown that retinoic acid could induce alveolar regeneration in rats. This observation suggested a possible future therapy for emphysema in humans. However, subsequent studies that have attempted to replicate these findings have met with mixed results, some positive and others not. This inconsistency may reflect strain-specific differences, because it has been noted that the successful studies were restricted to certain strains of mice and rats. Recent observations have demonstrated that it is not responsiveness or lack thereof to retinoic acid per se that is strain-specific, but instead that each strain differs in its sensitivity to the agent. What is not clear is if the effects can be recapitulated in animals other than rodents. A single study in humans has so far failed to show clinical improvement in indices of emphysema, although that study has been criticized for methodologic flaws including lack of power. Larger-scale, well-controlled studies are necessary to settle this important controversy.

STEM CELL BIOLOGY

As discussed earlier, the potential for regeneration of lung tissue from a stem cell pool is a research subject of considerable interest, with ongoing controversy surrounding the origins of these cells. Indeed, opinion remains split on whether to call these "stem cells," "progenitor cells," or even "reparative cells." Clearly, endogenous pulmonary cells are responsible for recovery of the lung from many insults, but it has not been established how these could be used therapeutically unless mechanisms can be found to augment their function. The use of iPS, bone marrow–derived, or even embryonic stem cells remains a controversial area but holds the potential to revolutionize therapy for emphysema.

AUTOPHAGY VERSUS ENDOPLASMIC RETICULUM–ASSOCIATED DEGRADATION IN α_1-ANTITRYPSIN DEFICIENCY

In many diseases, the accumulation of aberrant proteins in the endoplasmic reticulum directly contributes to the pathogenesis of disease, be these misfolded surfactant proteins or polymers of α_1-antitrypsin. It is a goal of several laboratories to devise ways of helping the cell dispose of these retained proteins, but a useful therapy remains elusive. For some time, it was thought that polymers within the endoplasmic reticulum were too large to be degraded by the classical endoplasmic reticulum–associated degradation (ERAD) pathway and so an alternative disposal mechanism must be involved. Indeed, a number of reports described the activation of autophagy by retained serpin polymers. Autophagy is the process by which intracellular components are engulfed by double-membraned structures called autophagosomes that ultimately "digest" their contents in what translates literally as "self-eating." However, it appears that the disposal of polymerogenic serpins shows significant cell type differences, and most in fact are degraded primarily by ERAD, with autophagy playing a secondary role. This area requires further study. An exciting recent report has described how the use of a commonly prescribed drug, carbamazepine, can stimulate both the ERAD and autophagy of polymerized α_1-antitrypsin and result in the resolution of liver disease in transgenic Z α_1-antitrypsin mice. The doses required currently are far higher than those that can safely be employed in humans, so further clinical trials are needed.

THE CANDIDATE GENE APPROACH

When hunting for a disease-associated mutation or polymorphism, it is essential to maintain a high degree of skepticism and statistical rigor. The involvement of a biologic statistician at an early stage of the study design is therefore essential. The attempt to link tumor necrosis factor (TNF)-α variants with the pathogenesis of COPD illustrates this pitfall well. The involvement of TNF-α was biologically plausible, because the levels of this multifunctional cytokine are elevated in bronchoalveolar lavage fluid, induced sputum samples, and lung biopsy specimens from patients with COPD. Moreover, well-studied promoter polymorphisms had been shown to alter expression levels and were linked with other inflammatory conditions. It was the observation of an association (with a staggering odds ratio of over 10) between a specific allele of TNF-α and "bronchitis" in Taiwanese men that ignited interest in this gene in COPD. That study was difficult to interpret, however, because a third of the men involved were "never smokers" and thus were unlikely to suffer from COPD. More than 10 subsequent studies have found little evidence that TNF-α polymorphisms are associated with, or modify the progression of, COPD. Although tempting as it may be to restrict study to a "favorite gene," it is far more fruitful to look first in an unbiased fashion for associations and only then to focus on individual genes or pathways.

FUTURE DIRECTIONS

The first human genome took a global effort of 13 years to complete. Today, genomes can be sequenced in a single laboratory in less than a week. Before very long, sequencing studies will be affordable for most research groups and may potentially even enter clinical practice, truly revolutionizing medicine. Such genomic elucidation will determine far more than whether a few disease-causing mutations are present; it will make possible individually tailored treatments like never before.

Pharmacogenetics will identify the most effective therapies and avoid the worse complications. In clinical practice, experienced prognostication and risk stratification will inform the hard decisions that both patient and physician need to make. In parallel, structural and cell biologists will continue to tease apart the components that make pneumocytes work and, more important, allow them to fail. These advances can be expected to lead to a new understanding of pathology and to provide signposts to new treatments. This century promises to be one in which all physicians can look forward to an exciting role as clinician scientists.

SUGGESTED READINGS

Barnes KC: Genetic studies of the etiology of asthma, *Proc Am Thorac Soc* 8:143–148, 2011.

Gooptu B, Lomas DA: Conformational pathology of the serpins—themes, variations and therapeutic strategies, *Annu Rev Biochem* 78:147–176, 2009.

Marciniak SJ, Lomas DA: α₁-Antitrypsin deficiency and autophagy, *N Engl J Med* 363:1863–1864, 2010.

Marciniak SJ, Lomas DA: What can naturally occurring mutations tell us about the pathogenesis of COPD? *Thorax* 64: 359–364, 2009.

Marciniak SJ, Ron D: The unfolded protein response in lung disease, *Proc Am Thorac Soc* 7:356–362, 2010.

Miranda E, Pérez J, Ekeowa UI, et al: A novel monoclonal antibody to characterize pathogenic polymers in liver disease associated with α₁-antitrypsin deficiency, *Hepatology* 52:1078–1088, 2010.

Online Mendelian Inheritance in Man (OMIM) (website): http://www.ncbi.nlm.nih.gov/omim; accessed March 5, 2011.

Pearson H: Human genetics: one gene, twenty years, *Nature* 460:164–169, 2009.

Pillai SG, Ge D, Zhu G, et al: A genome-wide association study in chronic obstructive pulmonary disease (COPD): identification of two major susceptibility loci, *PLoS Genet* 5:e1000421, 2009.

Stinchcombe SV, Maden M: Retinoic acid–induced alveolar regeneration: critical differences in strain sensitivity, *Am J Respir Cell Mol Biol* 38:185–191, 2008.

Chapter **3**
Respiratory Mechanics
Bruce H. Culver

INTRODUCTION

This chapter describes the physical properties of the lungs and chest wall involved in the cyclic processes of ventilation supporting the metabolic needs of the body. The contribution of respiratory muscles to these processes is reviewed here; their function is described more fully in Chapter 6. Clinical measurements of some of these mechanical properties are an important part of pulmonary function testing, as discussed in Chapter 9.

STRUCTURE OF THE THORAX AND LUNGS

THORAX

The bony thorax protects the lungs, heart, and great vessels but also allows the lungs to change volume from a minimum of 1.5 to 2.0 L to a maximum of 6 to 8 L. This large expansion is made possible by the articulation of the ribs with the spine and the sternum, the arrangement of the muscles, and the motion of the diaphragm. The ribs articulate with the transverse processes of the thoracic vertebrae and have flexible cartilaginous connections with the sternum. The ribs angle down, both from back to front and from midline to side, so that as they elevate, both the anteroposterior and the transverse dimensions of the thorax increase (**Figure 3-1**). The external intercostal muscles that angle down from posterior to anterior (**Figure 3-2**) are well situated to elevate the ribs. With deep inspiratory efforts, the first and second ribs are elevated and stabilized by the accessory muscles of respiration in the neck. If the upper extremities are fixed, the pectoralis muscles also can act to raise the ribs (e.g., leaning onto a chair back or against a wall when out of breath). Expiration normally is passive, driven by the elastic recoil of the lung, but can be assisted by the internal intercostal muscles. Forced expiration or a cough requires the abdominal muscles to force the diaphragm upward.

The diaphragm is dome-shaped in its relaxed position and can be pulled flatter by muscle contraction. The diaphragm most often is described as fixed at the periphery so that its action pulls down the center of the dome, lengthening the lungs. However, if it is fixed centrally by the pressure of the abdominal contents, the peripheral attachments will lift the ribs, which swing outward when elevated, increasing the transverse diameter of the chest. In addition, the increase in abdominal pressure associated with descent of the diaphragm acts on the lower ribs in the so-called *zone of apposition* to impart an outward force. The actual action of the diaphragm is a combination of these mechanisms in a proportion that varies with position and abdominal wall tension.

The intercostal muscles are innervated from the thoracic spine at their own level, and the abdominal muscles are innervated from lower thoracic and lumbar level, but the diaphragm is served by the phrenic nerves, which originate at the cervical level (C3 to C5). Thus, the diaphragm remains functional in patients who have spinal injuries below the midcervical level. The long course of each phrenic nerve along the mediastinum, however, makes it vulnerable to both transient and permanent interruptions by disease, injury, or surgery. Occasionally, local irritation of a phrenic nerve leads to intractable singultus (i.e., hiccups). The respiratory muscles are more fully discussed in Chapter 6.

PLEURAL SPACE

The lungs are covered by a thin visceral pleura, which is invaginated into the lobar fissures. The inner aspect of each hemithorax, including the top of the diaphragm and the mediastinal surface, is lined with the parietal pleura, which joins the visceral pleura on each side at the lung hilum. The pleural space extends deeply into the posterior and lateral costophrenic recesses and is a potential space, normally containing only a few milliliters of fluid to serve a lubricating function.

The inspiratory force of the chest wall and diaphragm is transmitted to the lung by creation of a more negative pressure in this potential space. In pathologic states, pleural effusions may form and necessarily make the lung volume smaller by occupying part of the intrathoracic space. Penetration of the chest wall or rupture of the lung surface can allow air to enter the pleural space, creating a pneumothorax.

AIRWAYS

The upper respiratory passages (nasal cavities and pharynx) conduct, warm, and moisten air as it moves into the lungs. The respiratory system develops as an offshoot from the digestive system and, like the digestive system, has an absorptive function. The entire system is continuously exposed to particulate and infective agents and accordingly is protected by a well-developed lymphoid barrier and, more superficially, a mucous barrier. The upper respiratory passages contain the olfactory areas and also conduct and help shape the sounds that produce speech.

The larynx opens off the lowest part of the pharynx. During swallowing, the larynx is closed off from both the pharynx above and the esophagus posteriorly by the epiglottis. The trachea begins at the lower border of the cricoid cartilage of the larynx, at the level of the sixth cervical vertebra. The lumen of the trachea is held open by incomplete, C-shaped

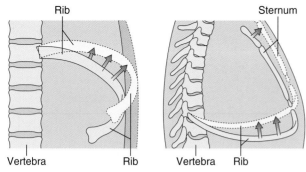

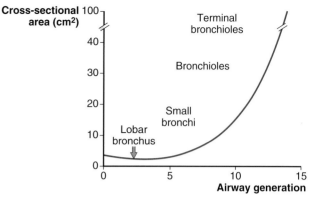

Figure 3-1 Frontal (*left*) and lateral (*right*) views of thorax movement. With rib elevation, both the transverse and anteroposterior dimensions increase.

Figure 3-3 Total cross-sectional area of the airways. The aggregate luminal area increases greatly from approximately 2.5 cm² in the trachea and major airways to more than 100 cm² at the level of the terminal bronchioles. (*Modified from Culver BH, editor:* The respiratory system, *Seattle, University of Washington Publication Services, 2006; data from Weibel ER:* Morphometry of the human lung, *New York, Springer-Verlag, 1963.*)

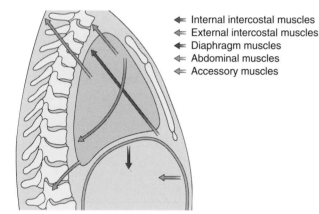

- ← Internal intercostal muscles
- ← External intercostal muscles
- ← Diaphragm muscles
- ← Abdominal muscles
- ← Accessory muscles

Figure 3-2 Action of the major respiratory muscle groups—intercostals, accessories, diaphragm, and abdominals.

cartilaginous rings. The posterior membranous portion contains smooth muscle. When the intrathoracic pressure exceeds the intraluminal pressure, as during a cough, the membranous portion becomes invaginated, the ends of the rings may overlap, and the lumen is greatly narrowed. Smooth muscle contraction narrows the lumen but increases its rigidity. With deep inspiration, the trachea enlarges and lengthens. The trachea bifurcates into the main bronchi, which become in turn lobar, segmental, and then subsegmental bronchi, and end in bronchioles, which lack cartilage and are approximately 1 mm in diameter. Beyond these are the respiratory bronchioles, alveolar ducts, sacs, and alveoli, which make up the respiratory zone in which gas exchange and other functions take place.

The intraparenchymal bronchi are invested with overlapping helical bands of smooth muscle wound in clockwise and counterclockwise fashion. The amount of smooth muscle increases proportionately in the smaller bronchioles to occupy approximately 20% of the wall thickness. Elastic fibers are present at every level of the respiratory system and become a rich component of the connective tissue in the smaller bronchi and bronchioles. They stretch when the lungs are expanded in inspiration, and their recoil helps to return the lungs to their end-exhalation volume. Although the smooth muscle stops at the portals of the respiratory zone, elastin and collagen contribute to the alveolar wall and form an irregular, wide-meshed net of delicate, interlacing fibers.

The number of airway generations required to reach the respiratory zone varies with pathway length, so that areas near the hilum may be reached in 15 generations, whereas those in the periphery may require 25 generations. Although the size of individual airways becomes smaller, the number of

airways approximately doubles with each new generation, so that the total cross-sectional area of the combined air path increases. This is especially so in the smaller bronchi and bronchioles, where the "daughters" of each division are only slightly smaller than the "parent." The rapidly increasing total cross-sectional area of small airways, shown diagrammatically in **Figure 3-3**, means that their contribution to airflow resistance in the lungs is small. Thus, diseases that affect these peripheral airways may be functionally silent until they reach an advanced state.

There is further dramatic expansion in the gas-exchanging respiratory zone as the airways terminate in an estimated 480 million alveoli with a surface area of 130 m².

INTERDEPENDENCE IN THE LUNG

Because the lung parenchyma is made up of interconnected alveolar walls, interstitial tissues, and fibers, any local distortion must be opposed by the surrounding tissue. That is, if a small zone of alveoli within a lobe begins to collapse, the surrounding tissue is stretched and thus tends to pull the alveoli back open. This property, termed *structural interdependence*, in concert with surfactant and the presence of collateral air pathways, helps to prevent alveolar collapse, even when small bronchioles become plugged. When collapsed areas of lung cannot expand despite distention of the surrounding alveoli, lung injury may develop as a result of extremely large stretching forces that are generated at the interface. These forces contribute to the ventilator-induced lung injury seen with mechanical ventilation at high tidal volumes and the more overt barotrauma that may result when high levels of end-expiratory pressure are applied. Because the bronchi and blood vessels travel through, and have attachments to, the lung parenchyma, they too are affected by the surrounding tissue. As the lung expands, the caliber of these channels also increases, and at low lung volumes, airway closure may occur.

RESPIRATORY MECHANICS

The properties of the lung and chest that affect and effect the movement of air into and out of the lungs are central to understanding both normal and abnormal lung function.

LUNG VOLUMES

The total gas-containing capacity of the lungs can be divided into a series of "volumes," as shown in **Figure 3-4**, which, in combination, give lung "capacities." The largest amount of air that can be held in the lungs at full inspiration is the total lung capacity (TLC). After a complete forced exhalation, the lungs are not empty but contain a residual volume (RV). The difference between TLC and RV—that is, the greatest volume of air that can be inhaled or exhaled—is the vital capacity (VC). The vital capacity can be affected by factors that either limit expansion of the lung (restrictive processes) or limit lung emptying (airflow obstruction).

A normal breath has a tidal volume (VT) that is only a small portion of the vital capacity (approximately 10%), and even during strenuous exercise, VT increases to only 50% to 60% of VC. Increases in VT occur by extending into the inspiratory reserve and expiratory reserve volumes as shown in Figure 3-4. At the end of a relaxed tidal exhalation, the lungs and chest wall return to a resting position, which normally is approximately 50% of TLC. The volume contained in the lungs at this end-tidal position is the functional residual capacity (FRC), and the volume that can be inhaled from this point is the inspiratory capacity (IC).

THE LUNG-CHEST WALL SYSTEM

To understand the process of normal breathing, special maneuvers such as coughing, and the effects of positive-pressure ventilators requires knowledge of the mechanical properties of the thorax. Three primary forces are involved:

- Elastic recoil properties of the lung
- Elastic recoil properties of the chest wall
- Muscular efforts of chest wall, diaphragm, and abdomen

In combination, these forces result in changes in lung (and thorax) volume, in alveolar pressure (PA), and in intrapleural pressure (Ppl).

VOLUMES OF ELASTIC STRUCTURES

The recoil tendency of a spring can be expressed in terms of its unstressed or resting length and its length-tension relationship. Similarly, for expandable volumetric structures, the relevant properties are the unstressed volume and the relationship between volume and the transmural pressure required to achieve that volume (**Figure 3-5**). By convention, transmural pressures are expressed as the difference between the pressure inside and the pressure outside the structure (Pin − Pout). It is convenient to think of this as the *distending pressure* required to achieve a certain volume. In addition, this distending pressure also represents the *recoil pressure*, or the tendency of the structure to return to its unstressed volume (where transmural pressure is zero). A positive recoil pressure indicates a tendency

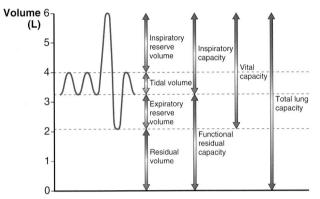

Figure 3-4 The normal spirogram and subdivisions of lung volume. By convention, *volume* is used to describe the smallest subdivisions that do not overlap (residual volume, expiratory reserve volume, tidal volume, and inspiratory reserve volume), and *capacity* is used to describe combinations of these volumes (functional residual capacity, inspiratory capacity, vital capacity, and total lung capacity). *(From Pulmonary terms and symbols: a report of the ACCP-ATS Joint Committee on Pulmonary Nomenclature, Chest 67:583–593, 1975.)*

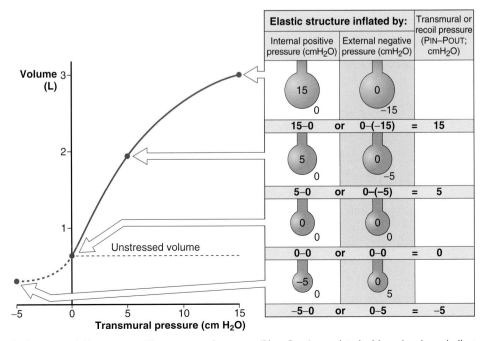

Figure 3-5 Elastic recoil of an expandable structure. The transmural pressure (Pin − Pout) associated with each volume indicates the tendency to return to the unstressed volume. Positive pressure and negative pressure inflation are equivalent.

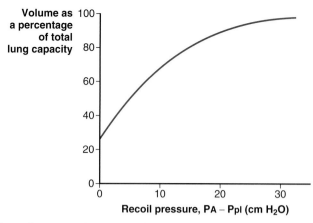

Figure 3-6 Normal pressure-volume curve of the lung. The elastic recoil pressure of the lung was obtained during a very slow expiration from total lung capacity (the curve on inspiration is somewhat different). *P*A, alveolar pressure; *Ppl*, intrapleural pressure. *(Modified from Culver BH, editor: The respiratory system, Seattle, University of Washington Publication Services, 2006.)*

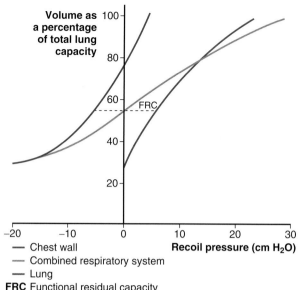

Figure 3-7 Pressure-volume curves of the combined thoracic system. The relaxed chest wall has a relatively high unstressed volume. The recoil of the combined respiratory system is the sum of the recoil of the chest wall plus that of the lung. *(Modified from Culver BH, editor: The respiratory system, Seattle, University of Washington Publication Services, 2006; data from Rahn H, Otis AB, Chadwich LE, Fenn WO: The pressure-volume diagram of the thorax and lung, Am J Physiol 146:161–178, 1946.)*

to become smaller. A structure distorted to a volume below its unstressed volume has a negative recoil pressure, which indicates its tendency to become larger.

ELASTIC PROPERTIES OF THE LUNG

The lungs are elastic structures with a tendency to recoil to a small "unstressed volume" (usually slightly less than RV). To maintain any lung volume larger than this unstressed volume requires a force that distends the lungs; this force is the difference between the alveolar pressure (PA) and the pressure surrounding the lungs, the intrapleural pressure (Ppl). The elastic properties of the lungs and their tendency to recoil are represented by a plot of the relationship between lung volume and transmural pressure (**Figure 3-6**). Such graphs apply to an excised lung being inflated by a pump, an in vivo lung inflated by a ventilator, or the more physiologic normal lung inflated by expanding the chest (to create a more negative pleural pressure). In each case, the curve of volume versus the transpulmonary pressure difference (PA – Ppl) is the same.

The slope of this pressure-volume curve represents the compliance of the lungs (CL), as represented by Equation 1.

$$C_L = \Delta V/\Delta P \qquad (1)$$

The CL varies with volume, decreasing as the lungs near the limit of their distensibility at TLC. Usually, CL is measured just above FRC in the tidal breathing range. Because it normally is expressed in absolute volume units (e.g., L/cm H_2O), CL is strongly dependent on the lung size. A single lung, for example, undergoes only half the volume change that would result from the same pressure change in two lungs. A small child's normal CL is considerably lower than that of an adult. For this reason, CL often is divided by lung volume to give the volume-independent *specific compliance*.

ELASTIC PROPERTIES OF THE CHEST WALL

The chest wall has elastic properties that can be expressed in the same way as for those of the lung (**Figure 3-7**). The chest wall differs from many common elastic structures in that its unstressed volume (where recoil pressure = 0) normally is quite high. When expanded above its unstressed volume, it recoils

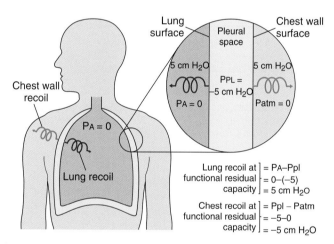

Figure 3-8 Balance of pressures and forces at functional residual capacity. The opposing recoils of lung and chest wall create a negative intrapleural pressure. *(Modified from Culver BH, editor: The respiratory system, Seattle, University of Washington Publication Services, 2006.)*

inward, but if the chest wall is "distorted" to a smaller volume, its tendency is to recoil outward. Recoil pressure for the relaxed chest wall is Ppl – Patm, or simply Ppl, because Patm is taken to be zero (**Figure 3-8; Table 3-1**). The compliance of the chest wall is similar to that of the lungs in the midvolume range; of note, however, at TLC, the chest wall remains as distensible as it is at FRC. At low thoracic volumes, the chest wall compliance becomes very low, resisting further exhalation, and this is the mechanism determining residual volume in children and young adults. By middle age, losses in the elasticity of the tissue attachments supporting small airways cause airway closure to be the mechanism limiting further active exhalation.

Table 3-1	Recoil Pressures of the Lungs, Chest Wall, and Respiratory System, Measured as the Transmural Pressure Difference*
Locus of Measurement	**Pressure Components**
Lungs	Alveolar pressure (PA) – pleural pressure (Ppl)
Chest wall	Ppl – atmospheric pressure (Patm), or simply Ppl
Respiratory system	(PA – Ppl) + (Ppl – Patm) = PA – Patm

*For example, pressure inside minus pressure outside.

LUNG AND CHEST WALL: THE RESPIRATORY SYSTEM

In the intact thorax, the lungs and chest wall must move together. The muscular effort required to inspire a volume of air, or the pressure that must be developed by a ventilator to achieve the same volume change, is determined by the pressure-volume curve of the combined respiratory system, shown by the red line in Figure 3-7. The lungs and chest wall normally contain the same volume of air, so that only points at the same horizontal level in Figure 3-7 can coexist. Because both the lungs and the chest wall are expanded together, the distending pressure for the respiratory system is the sum of the distending pressures required by the lungs and chest wall. The transmural pressure for the respiratory system is PA – Patm (see Table 3-1). Figure 3-7 shows that a greater pressure change is required to add volume to the respiratory system than to either of its components alone, and thus the compliance of the respiratory system is lower than that of either lungs or chest wall at the same volume. This may at first seem paradoxical, because the tendency of the chest wall to expand might be thought to help lung expansion; however, as the system volume is increased, the outward recoil of the chest wall decreases, and this force must be replaced by additional work.

The third mechanical factor, muscle force, is not considered in Figure 3-7. Thus, the pressure difference across the lung, which has no muscle, can always be taken from its curve, but the pressure across the chest wall (and diaphragm) may reflect muscle tension and is described by this curve only during complete relaxation. Similarly, the curve for the respiratory system shows the pressure that would be measured by a manometer held tightly in the mouth after the subject has inhaled or exhaled to a particular volume and then relaxed all muscle effort.

At the resting end-tidal position of the respiratory system (FRC), no active muscular forces are applied, and PA = Patm (distending pressure = 0). The lung is distended above its low unstressed volume, and the chest wall is held below its relatively high unstressed volume. The relaxed FRC is the volume at which the opposing tendencies of the lungs to recoil inward and the chest wall to recoil outward are evenly balanced. Any change in the unstressed volume or the compliance of either lungs or chest wall results in a new FRC. For example, obesity reduces the unstressed volume of the chest wall and thus also reduces the FRC (and expiratory reserve volume) (see Chapter 62). Emphysema increases both compliance and unstressed volume of the lung, which results in a higher FRC and a "shift to the left" of the respiratory system pressure-volume curve.

The opposing forces of lung and chest wall create a subatmospheric (negative) pressure in the intrapleural space at the FRC (see Figure 3-8). Because the lungs and chest wall are not directly linked, it is actually the intrapleural pressure that opposes lung recoil and chest wall recoil. Thus, at a relaxed

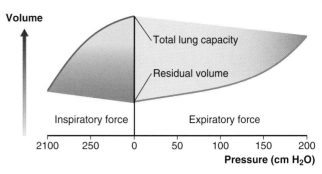

Figure 3-9 Maximum inspiratory and expiratory forces. The normal maximum force generated by inspiratory muscles is greatest at low lung volume, and the expiratory force is greatest at high lung volume. *(Modified from Culver BH, editor: The respiratory system, Seattle, University of Washington Publication Services, 2006.)*

FRC, it must have the same magnitude as each of these recoil forces. The average pleural pressure normally is approximately –5 cm H$_2$O at FRC.

EVENTS OF THE RESPIRATORY CYCLE

Inspiration is an active process. Contraction of the inspiratory muscles (primarily the intercostals and the diaphragm) tends to expand the thorax, which creates a more negative intrapleural pressure. This change increases the distending pressure applied to the lung, and the subsequent expansion causes the alveolar pressure to become negative with respect to the atmosphere, drawing air into the lungs. This process continues until the lung volume increases to a point at which its recoil pressure is increased to balance the combined muscular and elastic forces of the chest wall. At this point, alveolar pressure becomes zero, and the inspiratory flow stops, because a pressure gradient no longer exists along the airways.

During normal breathing, *expiration* is a passive process. The inspiratory muscles relax, and the balance of forces shifts so that lung recoil predominates. The alveolar pressure becomes positive, and the air moves from alveoli through the airways to the outside atmosphere until FRC conditions are reached, with the forces again balanced and the alveolar pressure zero. Of note, with a typical small VT, the chest wall volume remains below its unstressed volume, with a small outward recoil force, and pleural pressure can be negative throughout the cycle. During active expiration, this process can be assisted by contraction of the expiratory muscles (intercostal and abdominal wall muscles), which makes pleural pressure positive.

RESPIRATORY MUSCLE EFFORT

The maximum inspiratory and expiratory pressures measure the maximal efforts of the respiratory muscles (**Figure 3-9**). That is, with an inhalational effort against a closed pressure manometer, the maximum negative pressure that can be generated at the mouth is approximately 100 cm H$_2$O at a low lung volume. At TLC, no negative pressure can be generated, so no more air can be drawn into the chest. Maximum expiratory pressures are somewhat greater, measuring 150 to 200 cm H$_2$O at high lung volume, and fall to zero at RV.

SURFACE TENSION

At the surface of a liquid, the intermolecular forces are not balanced by the more widely spaced molecules of the gas phase, which creates a surface tension. The surface tension of the air-liquid interface that lines the alveoli contributes an important part of the elastic properties of the lung shown by the pressure-volume curve. If a lung is filled with liquid, surface forces are abolished, and the resultant pressure-volume curve (**Figure 3-10**) reflects only the tissue properties of the lung. This liquid-filled curve is shifted to the left, indicating that the lung can be distended with much less pressure. The air-filled lung, in addition to requiring greater pressures, demonstrates marked hysteresis; that is, the pressure-volume curve during inflation is different from that during deflation.

The air-filled deflation curve approaches the liquid-filled curve at low lung volume, indicating that the pressure from surface tension becomes small at this volume. Given no other parameters, however, the prediction would be that pressure from surface forces should *increase* as alveoli become smaller. Laplace's law relates the pressure within a sphere to wall tension (T) and radius (r), P = 2T/r, whereas for a cylinder, P = T/r. If the surface tension remains constant as "r" decreases (smaller alveoli or airway), the pressure from the surface tension should rise. This situation is avoided in the lung by the presence of a unique

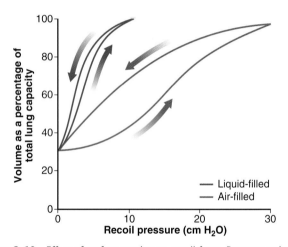

Figure 3-10 Effect of surface tension on recoil force. Pressure-volume curves obtained on inflation and deflation of a normal air-filled lung and the same lung when filled with saline. The horizontal difference between the curves reflects the effect of surface tension, which is greater on inspiration than expiration and abolished when the lung is liquid filled. *(Modified from Culver BH, editor: The respiratory system, Seattle, University of Washington Publication Services, 2006; data from Bachofen H, Hildebrandt J, Bachofen M: Pressure-volume curves of air- and liquid-filled excised lungs—surface tension in situ, J Appl Physiol 29:422–431, 1970.)*

Figure 3-11 Pulmonary surfactant at the air-liquid interface in an alveolus. The nonpolar fatty acid chains project into the alveolar gas phase, whereas the hydrophilic polar end lies within the surface of the liquid phase or may be able to bond directly to the epithelium. The close arrangement of the molecules facilitates their surface tension–lowering properties. The fluid hypophase tends to fill alveolar corners and surface irregularities.

surface-lining material, surfactant, which not only reduces surface tension but does so in a volume-dependent manner. As lung volume and surface area decrease, the lining layer compresses, and surface tension decreases until it is nearly abolished at RV. This property has important beneficial consequences in the lung, including the following:

- The work needed to expand the lungs is greatly reduced.
- Stability of alveoli and terminal airways is maintained. (If pressure increased within an alveolus as it became smaller, the alveolus would tend to empty into interconnected, larger alveoli with lower pressure.)
- Inwardly directed forces of surface tension in the "corners" of alveoli act to draw fluid from the capillaries and interstitium into the alveoli, so lowering surface tension helps prevent alveolar edema (discussed in Chapter 4).

Pulmonary surfactant is produced in alveolar type II cells in the form of lamellar bodies, appears in the alveolar lining liquid as tubular myelin, and then spreads as a monolayer at the air-liquid interface. The major component, and the component that is primarily responsible for the surface tension–lowering effects, is dipalmitoyl phosphatidylcholine (DPPC). DPPC has a nonpolar end, made up of two saturated fatty acid chains, and a polar end that tends to have a positive charge. At the air-liquid interface, the molecules orient with the hydrophilic polar end in the liquid and the fatty acid chains projecting into the air (**Figure 3-11**). Both ends have similar cross-sectional area allowing them to pack closely together. The molecules may also adsorb directly to the epithelial surface, which tends to have a negative charge, in areas where a liquid subphase is absent.

FLOW RESISTANCE

Airflow between the atmosphere and alveolar gas depends on the driving pressure (i.e., alveolar – atmospheric) and the airway resistance, as shown in Equation 2.

$$\text{Flow} = \dot{V} = \frac{\Delta P}{R} = \frac{\text{Patm} - \text{P}_A}{\text{Raw}} \qquad (2)$$

Airflow resistance (Raw) is affected by the following factors:

- Viscosity of air
- Length of airways (Raw is directly proportional to length)
- Caliber of airways (Raw is proportional to $1/r^4$)

Thus, a doubling of length doubles resistance, but a halving of caliber causes a 16-fold increase in resistance. Factors affecting airway caliber include the following:

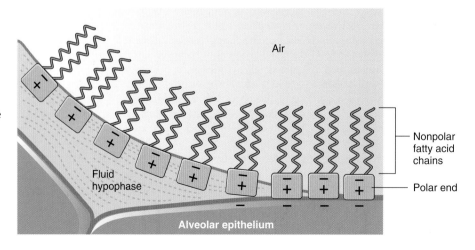

- Position of the airway in the bronchial tree
- Lung volume
- Bronchial muscle tone
- Mucous secretions
- Pressure across the airway wall

All of these factors are similar during both inspiration and expiration, except the last. During inspiration, the intrathoracic pressure that surrounds the airways is more negative than the intraluminal pressure, so airways tend to be distended (**Figure 3-12**). During passive exhalation, the magnitude of the airway distending force is lower, so airflow resistance is somewhat higher. With active expiratory efforts, the pleural pressure becomes positive, and with the addition of lung recoil, the pressure in the alveoli is even higher. However, the intraluminal pressure decreases progressively in airways mouthward of the alveoli, reflecting both frictional losses and a decrease in lateral pressure through the Bernoulli effect, because the decreasing cross-sectional area of the composite airway requires a marked increase in velocity of air movement (convective acceleration). Because their cartilaginous structure is incomplete, airways are compressed under such forces, and calculated resistance is much higher.

Maximum airflow rates are evaluated by having the subject take a full inspiration to TLC and blow the air out as forcefully and completely (to RV) as possible. With use of a spirometer, this forced vital capacity (FVC) is recorded as an expiratory spirogram (volume versus time), or if the flow rate is directly measured, the same information can be recorded as a maximum expiratory flow versus volume curve (**Figure 3-13**). A remarkable feature of this maneuver is that the maximum flow rate for any volume, except the higher lung volumes near the beginning of the exhalation, is achieved with submaximal effort and cannot be exceeded with further effort. This flow limitation, or "effort independence," is demonstrated in **Figure 3-14** and is a consequence of the dynamic compression noted previously. The mechanism of this flow limitation is related to the rate of propagation of a pressure wave through a compliant tube, but the result can be understood with a simpler conceptual model of dynamic compression. Because this compression begins just beyond the point at which intraairway pressure falls to equal pleural pressure, the effective pressure driving flow from the alveoli to this point becomes PA – Ppl (i.e., in Figure 3-12, for forced expiration, 30 – 20 = 10 cm H₂O). This is the same as the elastic recoil pressure of the lung and is a function of lung volume, not effort. If, in the example of Figure 3-12, a greater expiratory effort is made and the pleural pressure is raised to 40 cm H₂O at the same lung volume, the alveolar pressure becomes 50 cm H₂O and the effective driving pressure = (50 – 40) = 10 cm H₂O, so the resultant flow rate remains unchanged.

This mechanism may have its major physiologic significance in normal persons during a cough. Although overall airflow rate (L/second) out of the lungs is not increased by the high pleural pressure generated, the airflow velocity (m/second) through the narrowed major airways is greatly increased, which aids in the removal of secretions and foreign material.

WORK OF BREATHING

The muscle effort required to raise lung volume above the FRC during inspiration is a form of work. Part of this is the *elastic* work used to stretch the tissues and the surface lining of the lung, whereas another part is the *frictional* work required to

Inspiration
Active diaphragm and chest wall muscles

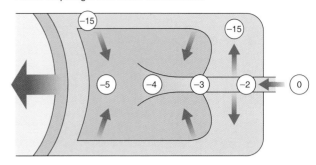

Passive expiration
Partially relaxed muscles

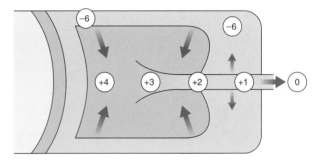

Forced expiration
Active abdominal and chest wall muscles

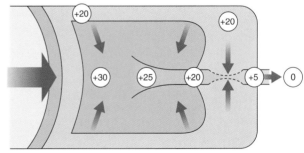

Figure 3-12 Dynamic compression. Comparison of intrathoracic and intraluminal pressures during inspiration, passive expiration, and forced expiration. In each case, the lung volume is the same, with a recoil pressure of 10 cm H₂O. During *inspiration*, the intrathoracic airways tend to be distended, which lowers airway resistance. In *passive expiration*, although intrapleural pressure may remain slightly negative, a positive alveolar pressure is generated by lung elastic recoil. Central airways are less distended than during inspiration. In *forced expiration*, high intrapleural pressure, plus lung recoil, creates a large, positive alveolar pressure to drive flow but also compresses central airways. Flow is limited once dynamic compression begins downstream from the point where intraluminal pressure falls below pleural pressure (the so-called equal pressure point). Further effort increases alveolar driving pressure but also increases compression. Airway resistance becomes high and varies with the degree of effort.

overcome airflow resistance in the airways. The elastic work stored in stretched fibers on inspiration then provides the energy needed to push air out on the subsequent passive exhalation. With active expiratory efforts, additional muscle work is done on expiration as well.

The elastic and frictional components of respiratory work are affected differently by lung volume. At low lung volume,

Expiratory spirogram

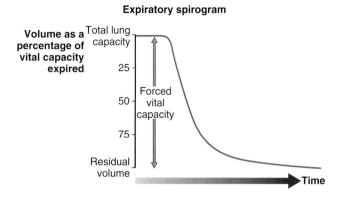

Flow–volume curve

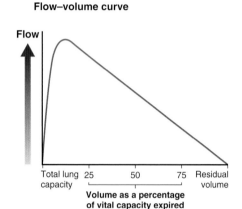

Figure 3-13 Forced vital capacity maneuver. This common breathing test can be displayed as an expiratory spirogram or as a flow-volume curve. Volume axes show percentage of vital capacity expired. *(Modified from Culver BH, editor: The respiratory system, Seattle, University of Washington Publication Services, 2006.)*

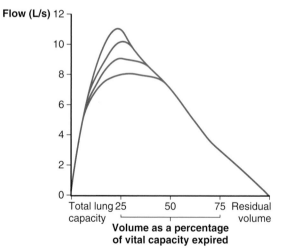

Figure 3-14 Effort-independent flow. The *top curve* represents a maximum expiratory effort, and the *lower curves* show the flow that results from progressively less effort. At lower lung volumes, the maximum flow rate is relatively independent of effort. *(Modified from Bates DV, Macklem PT, Christie RV: Respiratory function in disease, ed 2, Philadelphia, WB Saunders, 1971, pp 10–95.)*

airways are narrower, and resistance (and thus frictional work) increases rapidly (R is proportional to $1/r^4$). At higher lung volumes, the airways are larger, but muscles must do more elastic work to keep the lungs stretched. The relaxed FRC is the volume at which the static recoil forces of the lung and chest wall are balanced, but **Figure 3-15** shows that FRC also

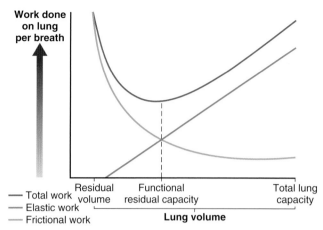

Figure 3-15 Work of breathing. The combined work of lung and chest wall expansion (elastic) and airflow resistance (frictional) is normally lowest near functional residual capacity. *(Modified from Culver BH, editor: The respiratory system, Seattle, University of Washington Publication Services, 2006.)*

is the volume at which work of breathing is least. If either the elastic or frictional contributions to work of breathing change, FRC may change rapidly or chronically.

The narrowed airways in obstructive disease increase frictional work and the volume at which work is the least increases. The accompanying shift of the tidal breathing range to a higher volume may occur quite suddenly in an asthma attack or may develop slowly with chronic obstructive disease. When airflow rates increase, frictional work becomes relatively more important, so that patients who have obstructive disease may shift to a higher end-expiratory volume during exercise or voluntary hyperventilation.

Restrictive disease processes reduce lung compliance (CL). Accordingly, the force the muscles must generate to stretch the lung increases. The elastic work required to breathe at any lung volume is higher, and this shifts the volume for least work lower. Increased CL, as with emphysema, has the opposite effect. Figure 3-7 shows that the static forces predict the same changes in FRC (greater lung recoil results in lower FRC volume and vice versa).

Normally, the energy consumed by breathing is very small. In metabolic terms, less than 1 mL/minute of oxygen consumption is required for each liter per minute of ventilation, or only a few percent of total body oxygen consumption at rest. Derangements of respiratory mechanics may increase the work of breathing significantly, contributing to the common symptom of dyspnea. With severe airflow obstruction, the energy cost of breathing becomes much higher. Increases in respiratory frequency associated with activity may cause COPD patients to shift their tidal ventilation to a higher end-expiratory lung volume whereby the increased airway caliber allows the tidal breath to be exhaled within the shorter expiratory time available. This dynamic hyperinflation places the inspiratory muscles at further mechanical disadvantage and is a major contributor to exertional dyspnea and exercise limitation. If the expiratory time does not allow the alveolar pressure to fully equilibrate to atmospheric pressure, then the residual positive end-expiratory alveolar pressure (termed auto-PEEP) must be overcome by additional inspiratory effort before inspiratory airflow can begin. The same phenomenon also is seen during mechanical ventilation of patients with airflow obstruction and may have hemodynamic consequences, as well as impairing their ability to initiate breaths.

DISTRIBUTION OF VENTILATION

The incoming air of each tidal breath is not distributed evenly to all alveoli in the lung. Pleural pressure is not the same throughout the chest but has a vertical gradient of several centimeters of water because of the effects of gravity, the configuration of the chest and diaphragm, the presence of the heart and mediastinal structures, and the need for the lung to fit within the thorax irrespective of the shape of either the lung or the thorax. At FRC measured with the patient in the upright position, -5 cm H_2O is an average value at chest midlevel; near the apices, however, the pressure outside the lung might be -8 cm H_2O, whereas near the bases it might be only -2 cm H_2O. Because alveoli throughout the lung seem to have similar maximum volume and pressure–volume relationships, and because alveolar pressure is everywhere the same, those alveoli near the top of the lung are held at larger volume (distending pressure of 8 cm H_2O) than those near the bottom (distending pressure of 2 cm H_2O). This places the lower alveoli on a steeper (more compliant) portion of their pressure-volume curve. In addition, the proximity of the basal alveoli to the motion of the diaphragm exposes them to a greater increase in distending pressure with inspiration. These two factors combine to give the lower portion of the normal lung a relatively greater proportion of the tidal ventilation than that distributed to the apices.

A second consequence of the higher (i.e., less negative) pleural pressure in the basal portions of the lung is that the distending pressure of the small airways also is less. At low lung volume, airways may close, and the dependent portions of the lung reach this "closing volume" first, whereas higher portions of the lung are still partially distended. Thus, in a patient who breathes at very low lung volumes, near residual volume (e.g., with obesity), basal airway closure may occur, with consequent poor ventilation of the lung bases.

In summary, respiratory units in the basal portion of the lung contain less gas but receive more ventilation so long as they remain open. However, they are more susceptible to airway closure and loss of ventilation at low lung volume.

SUMMARY

The mechanical properties of the lungs and chest wall are described by the interactions of volume and pressure within the thorax, and by flows and resistance during dynamic changes in lung volume. Alterations in these properties underlie many respiratory diseases and contribute to their associated symptoms. Measurement of these properties is important in elucidation of the pathophysiology of lung diseases and in diagnosis and monitoring of disease in the pulmonary function laboratory (see Chapter 9), and the increasing sophistication of modern ventilators makes an understanding of thoracic mechanics essential in the intensive care unit (see Chapter 32).

CONTROVERSIES AND PITFALLS

The principles of lung mechanics discussed in this chapter have been well established for the past 40 to 60 years, but their application in some clinical situations is less clear-cut. Inadequate understanding of lung–chest wall pressure relationships underlies the occasionally heard bedside comment that increasing positive end-expiratory pressure (PEEP) to improve hypoxemia in a mechanically ventilated patient with acute lung injury (ALI) will not affect hemodynamics "because the lungs are stiff and no added pressure will be transmitted to the pleural space." It is true that low lung compliance will result in a lesser expansion of lung volume for any increase in alveolar pressure, with less increase in average intrapleural pressure than in a normal chest. If there is an improvement in oxygenation, however, the likely mechanism is recruitment of alveoli with an increase in end-expiratory lung volume, and this necessitates that the chest wall also must be expanded along its passive pressure-volume curve (see Figure 3-7). Because this relationship has a positive slope throughout, any increase in thoracic volume must be accompanied by at least some increase in intrapleural pressure, with its potential for a hemodynamic effect.

Since the recognition that mechanical ventilation may cause or contribute to lung injury, an ongoing issue has been the optimal tidal volume and pressures to avoid this complication. It was demonstrated in animal work many years ago that ventilation with a high tidal volume, generated by an inspiratory pressure of 40 cm H_2O, was injurious, but that this injury was greatly mitigated by a modest level of PEEP. Accordingly, in addition to concerns for the limits of lung expansion, subsequent work has focused on the stresses associated with cyclic closing and reopening of small peripheral airspaces.

It has been demonstrated that the use of a tidal volume of 6 mL/kg is associated with lower mortality in acute lung injury–acute respiratory distress syndrome (ALI-ARDS) than that with a volume of 12 mL/kg, but the relative contributions of tidal volume, end-inspiratory pressure, and PEEP remain controversial. Although it is likely to be the change in, or maximal extent of, tissue stretch due to lung volume expansion, that is the injurious force, the best bedside indicator of that force may be the airway pressure, because even a small tidal volume may overexpand the more compliant regions of an injured lung. Some clinicians feel that tidal volume reduction may be unnecessary if end-inspiratory pressure is maintained below 30 cm H_2O, but the 6 mL/kg tidal volume strategy was similarly beneficial at all levels of initial end-inspiratory pressure.

With the wide acceptance of "lung-protective ventilation," some consideration has emerged for extending this approach to patients at risk for ALI, or even to all ventilated patients. There does appear to be a trend in this direction, with initial tidal volumes of 8 to 10 mL/kg increasingly common, and those of 10 to 12 mL/kg less so. It is difficult to know how best to prevent ventilator-induced lung injury without better understanding of its cause. Potential mechanisms include tissue failure from high stresses during lung expansion, which are magnified at the junction of atelectatic lung and adjacent expandable tissue, as well as cytokine release associated with the deformations of repetitive cycling.

SUGGESTED READINGS

Faffe DS, Zin WA: Lung parenchymal mechanics in health and disease, *Physiol Rev* 89:759–775, 2009.

Gibson GJ: Lung volumes and elasticity. In Hughes JM, Pride NB, editors: *Lung function tests: physiologic principles and clinical applications*, London, 1999, WB Saunders, pp 45–56.

Hager DN, Krishnan JA, Hayden DL, Brower RG: Tidal volume reduction in patients with acute lung injury when plateau pressures are not high, *Am J Respir Crit Care Med* 172:1241–1245, 2005.

Heil M, Hazel AL, Smith JA: The mechanics of airway closure, *Respir Physiol Neurobiol* 163:214–221, 2008.

Hubmayer RD: Straining to make mechanical ventilation safe and simple, *Am J Respir Crit Care Med* 183:1289–1290, 2011.

Hills BA: Surface-active phospholipids: a Pandora's box of clinical applications. Part I: the lung and air spaces, *Int Med J* 32:170–178, 2002.

Loring SH, Garcia-Jacques M, Malhotra A: Pulmonary characteristics in COPD and mechanisms of increased work of breathing, *J Appl Physiol* 107:309–314, 2009.

Lucangelo U, Bernabe F, Blanch L: Lung mechanics at the bedside: make it simple, *Curr Opin Crit Care* 13:64–72, 2007.

O'Donnell DE, Laveneziana P: Dyspnea and activity limitation in COPD: mechanical factors, *COPD* 4:225–236, 2007.

Pride NB: Airflow resistance. In Hughes JM, Pride NB, editors: *Lung function tests: physiologic principles and clinical applications*, London, 1999, WB Saunders, pp 27–44.

Ratnovsky A, Elad D, Halpern E: Mechanics of respiratory muscles, *Respir Physiol Neurobiol* 168:82–89, 2008.

Schurch S, Bachofen H, Possmeyer F: Alveolar lining layer: functions, composition, structures. In Hlastala MP, Robertson HT, editors: *Lung biology in health and disease, vol 121: complexity in structure and function of the lung*, New York, 1998, Marcel Dekker, pp 35–98.

Weibel ER: What makes a good lung? The morphometric basis of lung function, *Swiss Med Wkly* 139:375–386, 2009.

Chapter **4**
Pulmonary Circulation
Bruce H. Culver • Robb W. Glenny

The lungs are served by two circulations—the pulmonary circulation, which accommodates the entire cardiac output from the right side of the heart through a low-pressure circulation, and the bronchial circulation, which arises from branches of the aorta with systemic pressure and usually carries less than 1% of the cardiac output.

CIRCULATORY STRUCTURE

PULMONARY CIRCULATION

The pulmonary arteries lie near and branch in unison with the airways in the bronchovascular bundle. They are much thinner than systemic arteries and have proportionately more elastic tissue in their walls. The walls of the arterioles, with a diameter less than 100 μm, are so thin relative to those of their systemic counterparts that fluid and gas can move across them. Within the gas-exchanging zone, the arterioles give rise to a network of pulmonary capillaries in the alveolar walls that is continuous throughout the lungs. They are so numerous that, when distended, blood flows almost as an unbroken sheet between the air spaces (**Figure 4-1**). "Sheet flow" reduces vascular resistance and optimizes gas exchange by creating a very large surface area, estimated at over 100 m^2. When the transmural pressure difference between the inside and outside of the vessels is low, many of the capillary segments are closed, but flow switches among segments frequently as some open and others close. Nonflowing segments are rapidly recruited into the pulmonary vascular bed as needed to accommodate increased flow and may be further distended by an increase in transmural pressure. Both recruitment and distention of the pulmonary capillary bed reduce resistance to blood flow and help to maintain a low pressure in the face of increased blood flow. This low pressure allows the capillary-alveolar membrane to be very thin (approximately 1 μm), facilitating diffusion of respiratory gases between blood and alveoli. A red cell that follows a capillary path from the pulmonary artery to a vein may cross several alveoli, with the average transit time through the vessels engaged in gas exchange calculated to be approximately 0.75 second. The capillaries unite to form larger alveolar microvessels, which become venules and then veins that run between the lobules toward the hila, where upper and lower pulmonary veins from each lung empty into the left atrium.

BRONCHIAL CIRCULATION

The bronchial arteries arise directly from the aorta or from intercostal arteries to supply the walls of the trachea and bronchi and also to nourish the major pulmonary vessels, nerves, interstitium, and pleura. Extensive small-vessel anastomoses occur between these (systemic) vessels and both the precapillary and postcapillary pulmonary vasculature. The bronchial veins from the larger airways and hilar region drain through the systemic veins (particularly the azygos system) into the right atrium. However, bronchial flow to the intrapulmonary structures connects to the pulmonary circulation and drains through the pulmonary veins into the left atrium. This small aliquot of desaturated blood contributes to the normal (2% to 5%) right-to-left shunt, which may increase when the bronchial circulation hypertrophies to supply inflammatory or neoplastic lesions. The bronchial circulation has a role in the regulation of temperature and humidity in the airways and supplies the fluid for secretion through the airway mucosa.

LYMPHATIC CIRCULATION

Pulmonary lymphatics are not found in alveolar walls but originate in interstitial spaces at the level of the respiratory bronchioles and at the pleural surface, then follow the bronchovascular bundles to the hila. The lymph flows through the right lymphatic duct and the thoracic duct into the right and left brachiocephalic veins. The total flow from the lungs is quite low under normal conditions (less than 0.5 mL/minute in experimental animals) but can increase many-fold with pulmonary edema. The lymphatics have valves to prevent backflow and can generate sufficient pressures to maintain flow when systemic venous pressure is as high as 20 cm H_2O.

CIRCULATORY PHYSIOLOGY

The pulmonary circulation conducts the entire cardiac output with a remarkably low driving pressure from the pulmonary artery (mean Ppa of 15 to 20 mm Hg) to the left atrium (Pla of 7 to 12 mm Hg). As in the airways, the branching pattern of vessels leads to an increase in total cross-sectional area as the alveolar vessels are approached, but unlike in the airways, this increase is not associated with a decrease in resistance. Total cross-sectional area increases at a branching point if the number of daughter branches (*n*) is greater than the ratio of the parent to daughter radii squared, (a/b)^2, but resistance decreases only if *n* is greater than (a/b)^4. The latter case occurs in the peripheral airways but not in the vessels, so although small peripheral airways contribute little to normal airflow resistance, pulmonary microvessels make up a substantial portion of vascular resistance. Efforts to partition the pressure drop longitudinally suggest that approximately 20% to 30% is in the arterial portion (including arterioles), 40% to 60% in the microvascular portion, and the remainder in the veins. With increases in flow,

Resting   **Engorged**

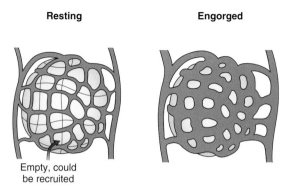

Empty, could
be recruited

Figure 4-1 Alveolar capillaries. The normal cardiac output requires only a portion of the sheet of capillaries; any remaining vessels can be recruited when cardiac output rises during exercise. *(Modified with permission from Butler J: The circulation of the lung. In Culver BH, editor: The respiratory system, Seattle, 2006, University of Washington Publication Services, p 8.2.)*

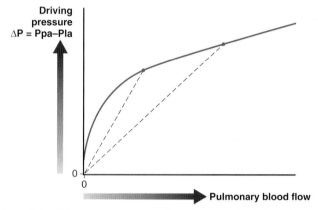

Figure 4-2 Driving pressure across the pulmonary circulation. Mean pulmonary artery pressure (Ppa) minus mean left atrial pressure (Pla) increases nonlinearly with cardiac output. Resistance, represented by the slope from the origin to any point on the line, decreases with increased pulmonary blood flow, which reflects recruitment and distention of vessels.

recruitment occurs mainly at the level of microvascular vessels, so their relative contribution to resistance becomes less.

The pulmonary circulation is a network of segmental resistors that share common upstream (i.e., Ppa) and downstream (i.e., Pla) pressures. Flow is distributed to the various segments in proportion to the reciprocal of the total serial resistance through any segment. The benefit of having the highest resistance at the microvascular level is that the control of blood flow distribution can occur at a finer level, allowing active mechanisms of flow regulation (see further on) to adjust blood flow to relatively small lung regions.

The pulmonary vascular resistance, PVR, is calculated as transvascular driving pressure, ΔP (mean upstream Ppa minus mean downstream Pla), divided by the flow: PVR = $\Delta P/Q$. The calculated resistance must be interpreted in the context of flow, because the relationship of driving pressure to flow usually is not linear and its plotted curve does not pass through zero. As shown in **Figure 4-2**, pulmonary vascular resistance decreases as flow and pressure increase with the attendant recruitment and distention of vessels.

The resistance to flow through a vessel increases with its length, with the viscosity of the fluid, and, most important, with the inverse of the radius to the fourth power. In addition

Low lung volume   **High lung volume**

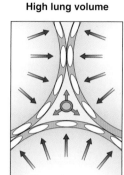

Figure 4-3 Lung volume affects alveolar and extraalveolar vessels differently. At high lung volumes, alveolar microvessels are stretched and compressed as vascular pressures fall relative to alveolar pressure. Extraalveolar vessels, however, tend to be expanded as the pressure surrounding them decreases. *(Modified with permission from Butler J: The circulation of the lung. In Culver BH, editor: The respiratory system, Seattle, 2006, University of Washington Publication Services, p 8.4.)*

to muscle activity in the wall, the caliber of a distensible vessel depends passively on the transmural pressure difference between intravascular and extravascular pressures. This mechanism is particularly important in the lungs, where the vessels are embedded in expandable parenchyma. It is convenient to consider separately the effect of lung expansion on the extraalveolar arterial and venous vessels, which differs from the effect on the microvessels of the alveolar zone. With lung volume increase, extraalveolar vessels are distended as the pressure is lowered in the expanding perivascular space around them (**Figure 4-3**), and they are elongated as the lung expands.

By contrast, the alveolar microvessels in the alveolar walls are elongated but partially collapsed by lung inflation, because the alveolar pressure that surrounds them tends to increase relative to the intravascular pressure. This effect is easy to recognize with positive-pressure ventilation, but it also occurs with spontaneous inspiration, because intravascular pressures fall relative to atmospheric and alveolar pressure. The sheets of capillaries in the alveolar walls are protected from the full compressive force of the alveolar pressure by the surface tension of the fluid that lines curved portions of the alveolar surface. Microvessels in the "corners" where alveolar walls meet are more fully protected from compression by the sharper curvature of the surface film and perhaps by local distending forces, analogous to the situation with extraalveolar vessels (**Figure 4-4**). The pulmonary vascular resistance is the sum of that through alveolar and extraalveolar vessels and thus has a complex relationship with lung volume. It is lowest at approximately the normal resting lung volume (functional residual capacity) but increases at higher and lower volumes.

BLOOD FLOW DISTRIBUTION

Both vascular geometry and gravity influence the distribution of blood flow within the lung. If the upright lung is viewed as a stacked series of slices, a vertical gradient occurs in which the average flow per slice rises progressively down the lung, consistent with the influence of gravity. Within each slice, however, a marked variability of blood flow is found among regions, with high-flow areas distributed dorsally. The tendency of blood flow to be higher in dorsal and basal regions is largely preserved even when the gravitational direction is reversed, which indicates

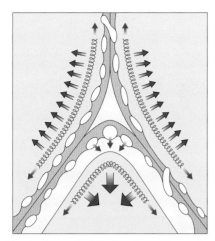

Figure 4-4 Alveolar "corner" at the junction of three alveolar walls. Surface tension (depicted by "springs") holds vessels open, particularly in corners, and promotes fluid transudation by lowering the pressure around vessels. *(Modified with permission from Butler J: The circulation of the lung. In Culver BH, editor: The respiratory system, Seattle, 2006, University of Washington Publication Services, p 8.5.)*

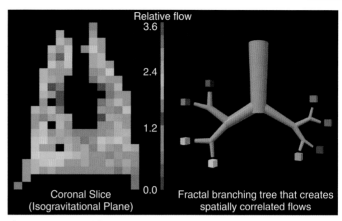

Figure 4-6 Blood flow distribution. The *left half* of the figure shows an isogravitational coronal plane of a canine lung divided into cubes of tissue 1.2 cm on a side. The color scale shows the relative blood flow, indicated by the number of flow-directed microspheres trapped in each cube. Note that low flow (*blue*) cubes tend to cluster together, as do high flow (*yellow-red*) cubes. The *right half* shows how the geometry of shared, more proximal vessel segments can account for this spatial correlation further downstream.

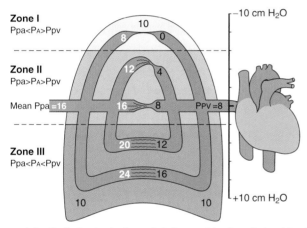

Figure 4-5 Perfusion in the lungs is influenced by the relationship of pulmonary arterial and venous pressures (Ppa and Ppv) to alveolar pressure (PA). In this example, the alveolar pressure is 10 cm H_2O, as might be found in a patient who receives positive-pressure ventilation. *(Modified with permission from Culver BH: Hemodynamic monitoring: physiologic problems in interpretation. In Fallat RJ, Luce JM, editors: Cardiopulmonary critical care, Edinburgh, 1988, Churchill Livingstone.)*

that anatomic branching patterns are a major determinant of flow distribution.

The gravitational effect has been conceptualized by dividing the lung into four zones, one above another, on the basis of the relationship of vascular and alveolar pressures (**Figure 4-5**). Intravascular pressures are higher at the bottom of the lung than at the top by an amount equal to a vertical hydrostatic column as high as the lung. Near the lung apex, *zone I*, the pressure in the alveoli (PA) exceeds that in both the pulmonary arteries (Ppa) and pulmonary vein (Ppv) and collapses the alveolar vessels, except those in the alveolar corners, which remain patent and allow some flow to continue. Below this, in *zone II*, Ppa exceeds PA, but PA is greater than Ppv, so flow depends on the pressure difference between Ppa and PA. The vessels remain open but are critically narrowed at the downstream end, where venous pressure is lower than alveolar pressure. This condition creates independence of flow from the downstream venous pressure, analogous to a waterfall in which

a stream that flows over a precipice is unaffected by a rising level in the pool below until it rises above the level of the lip. In the middle to lower portion of the lung, *zone III*, both Ppa and Ppv exceed PA, the vessels are distended, and blood flow is the highest. *Zone IV* is restricted to a small area in the most dependent region, where flow diminishes. It has been postulated that this reduction is the result of increased vascular resistance secondary to low lung volume or perivascular edema in this area.

Although the gravitational effect expressed in the vertical zone concept contributes to the average increase in flow down the lung, it does not explain the observed large variability in flow within an isogravitational slice, which implies that other anatomic or vasoregulatory factors are important at this level. More recent studies have determined that the heterogeneous distribution of blood flow within horizontal (isogravitational) planes is due to asymmetric branching geometries (and hence resistances) of the vascular tree. Because the vascular tree is largely a dichotomous branching structure, differences in resistances between daughter branches cause flow to be distributed unevenly between the branches. With differences in resistances occurring at every bifurcation in the vascular tree, blood flow becomes progressively more heterogeneous, resulting in a broad distribution of flows at the terminal branches. Owing to the shared heritage up the vascular tree, neighboring lung regions have similar magnitudes of flow, with high-flow regions near other high-flow regions and low-flow regions neighboring other low-flow regions. Hence, the spatial distribution of pulmonary blood flow is not random but rather exhibits a clear pattern of high and low flows (**Figure 4-6**). Studies have demonstrated that the pattern of perfusion distribution is very stable over time and with growth, and that the pattern is genetically determined. These insights provide a new perspective on blood flow distribution in the lung. The traditional model of vertically stacked zones needs to be replaced by one in which the multiple zones can exist within horizontal planes. In addition, the large degree of heterogeneity within isogravitational planes suggests that mechanisms other than gravity must be responsible for the tight matching between regional ventilation and blood flow.

REGULATION OF PULMONARY BLOOD FLOW

Besides their responses to passive mechanisms (anatomy, gravity, lung volume, alveolar pressure), the pulmonary vessels exhibit vasomotor activity regulated by both neural and non-neural factors. Motor efferents from three autonomic networks are in anatomic proximity to the vasculature: sympathetic, parasympathetic, and nonadrenergic noncholinergic fibers. The *sympathetic* efferents have a vasoconstrictor effect, whereas *parasympathetic* stimulation dilates constricted vessels. Although acetylcholine is a potent pulmonary vasodilator, there is little cholinergic innervation of the pulmonary resistance vessels. The *nonadrenergic noncholinergic* system is inhibitory, constantly releasing small vasodilatory peptides at the ganglia and postganglionic ends of its unique network. This vasodilator function is augmented with exercise.

Pulmonary arteries demonstrate an intrinsically low tone as they remain relaxed when isolated from the lung. This state reflects a balance between effects of endothelium-derived vasoconstrictor and vasodilator substances. Although their relative roles are yet to be clarified, many vasoactive peptides are found in the lung. Those exerting vasoconstrictor activity on the pulmonary circulation include angiotensin II, arginine vasopressin, endothelin 1, peptide tyrosine Y, and substance P. Vasodilatory peptides include adrenomedullin, atrial natriuretic peptide, calcitonin gene–related peptide, endothelin 3, somatostatin, and vasoactive intestinal peptide.

Nitric oxide is produced in endothelial cells in the pulmonary circulation and elsewhere and is now recognized as an important mediator of vasodilatation. The oxidation of a nitrogen from L-arginine is catalyzed by nitric oxide synthase, present in both a constitutive form and a form that is inducible by products of inflammation. Nitric oxide activates guanylate cyclase, which increases cyclic guanosine monophosphate (cGMP) within vascular smooth muscle cells. This in turn reduces intracellular Ca^{++} by several mechanisms, leading to vascular relaxation. Nitric oxide also is abundantly produced in the nasal sinuses, providing an intriguing mechanism whereby inhaled nitric oxide may enhance blood flow to the best-ventilated areas of lung.

Although the role of nasal nitric oxide in ventilation-perfusion matching is still speculative, the role of alveolar hypoxia in vasoregulation has been recognized for more than 50 years, but the mechanisms involved are still uncertain. Pulmonary arterioles constrict when the P_{O_2} in the alveoli they serve falls, and additional vasoconstriction results if alveolar P_{CO_2} rises (**Figure 4-7**). Thus, when ventilation is decreased by an obstructed airway or other injury, local hypoxic pulmonary vasoregulation decreases blood flow to the affected region, which tends to restore the local ventilation-perfusion ratio ($\dot{V}/\dot{Q}$) toward normal and thereby improve the P_{O_2} of the blood flowing through that area. The diverted blood flow can be directed to better-ventilated regions, which further contributes to an improvement in overall matching. This hypoxic vasoconstriction seems to be a response to a low P_{O_2} in the air spaces, rather than in the intraluminal blood, which normally is desaturated in these prealveolar vessels. The effector cell is thought to be pulmonary artery smooth muscle located at the entrance to the acinus, and the sensor may be the oxygen-consuming mitochondria within these cells. Several candidate signaling pathways to generate the increase in intracellular calcium necessary for muscle contraction are under investigation.

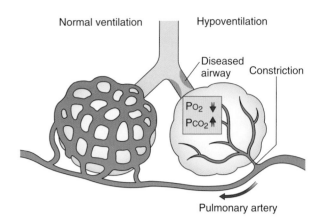

Figure 4-7 Hypoxic vasoconstriction reduces blood flow to poorly ventilated areas. This adaptation improves ventilation-perfusion matching and oxygenation but, if generalized, contributes to pulmonary hypertension. *(Modified with permission from Butler J: The circulation of the lung. In Culver BH, editor: The respiratory system, Seattle, 2006, University of Washington Publication Services, p 8.7.)*

Considerable individual variability is found in the hypoxic vasoconstrictor response, and it may be diminished by vasodilating drugs. Diversion of blood flow is most effective in atelectatic areas of lung, in which hypoxic vasoconstriction is unopposed by the radial traction of surrounding expanded lung tissue. A reciprocal reflex in the airways also contributes to better matching: Small airways constrict when intraluminal P_{CO_2} falls and dilate when it rises. Hypoxic vasoconstriction is a helpful, adaptive response to local or regional lung abnormalities, but when alveolar hypoxia is generalized (e.g., hypoventilation or altitude), the increased resistance can lead to pulmonary hypertension.

NONRESPIRATORY FUNCTIONS OF THE PULMONARY CIRCULATION

FILTERING

Aggregates of blood elements and emboli of various types (e.g., fat, air, particulate matter) carried in the systemic venous return are continually filtered out, dissolved, or engulfed by the cells of the pulmonary capillary bed. This process provides vital protection for the cerebral, coronary, and other systemic vascular beds and is a benefit of the entire cardiac output from the right side of the heart passing through the lungs. Emboli that bypass the pulmonary circulation through anatomic shunts are called "paradoxical emboli" and are the most common cause of strokes in young persons. Larger emboli have the potential to cause ischemia in affected regions of the pulmonary vascular bed, but this may be countered in part by limited perfusion from the bronchial circulation through bronchopulmonary anastomoses and by exposure to oxygenated pulmonary venous blood that backflows into the occluded region during tidal lung volume changes. Thus, ischemic damage to the alveoli is prevented while a thrombus is lysed and the pulmonary flow restored.

Large numbers of white cells, mainly polymorphonuclear leukocytes, are sequestered in the small vessels of the pulmonary bed. The numbers of leukocytes sequestered in the lung increases markedly if the pulmonary endothelium expresses ligands that cause these cells to adhere and then traverse the vascular wall into the interstitial and alveolar spaces. Many reticuloendothelial cells are found in the lung, and some evidence suggests that the vascular endothelial cell itself can be phagocytic when stimulated.

MODIFICATION OF MEDIATORS

Some mediators in the blood that have regulatory functions throughout the body are secreted, taken up, or inactivated through specific receptors and enzyme systems in the pulmonary endothelial cells. Best-known is angiotensin-converting enzyme, which converts inactive angiotensin 1 into the systemic vasoconstrictor angiotensin 2. Histamine, bradykinin, serotonin, and acetylcholine are largely inactivated by the pulmonary endothelium in one pass through the lungs.

COAGULATION

When local injury is present, pulmonary endothelial cells can be a source of thromboplastin and tissue plasminogen activator. Despite vascular stasis and closure of vessels when flow decreases, clots do not form in pulmonary vessels because of the structure of the endothelial surface and because the secretion of anticlotting substances bathes the surface and prevents the adherence of platelets and cells. Nitric oxide, produced by the pulmonary endothelium, is a potent inhibitor of platelet aggregation. Embolic thrombi are dissolved remarkably quickly by local thrombolytic secretions.

FLUID EXCHANGE IN THE PULMONARY CIRCULATION

The fluid flux across the pulmonary vascular endothelium is influenced by the same pressure relationship as in the systemic capillaries, summarized in the modified Starling equation presented in **Table 4-1**. The hydrostatic pressure in the pulmonary microvessels (Pmv) exceeds the interstitial hydrostatic pressure outside the microvessels, i.e., the perimicrovascular pressure (Ppmv). This effect favors filtration. The interstitial tissue fluid protein osmotic pressure is approximately two thirds that in the vessel; thus, the net osmotic force is absorptive and inward. The components of this equation make it convenient to categorize abnormal fluid flux into the lung into two broad types: *hydrostatic* edema, when the primary abnormality is an increase in Pmv minus Ppmv, and *permeability* edema, when endothelial injury increases fluid conductivity across the membrane (incorporated into the permeability factor) and decreases the osmotic reflection coefficient and osmotic gradient. The terms *cardiogenic* and *noncardiogenic* also are commonly used for these two mechanisms of edema formation.

Table 4-1	Modified Starling Equation

$$F = K_f [(Pmv - Ppmv) - \sigma(pv - pt)]$$

Symbol	Description
F	Net fluid flux out of vessels
K_f	Permeability factor (constant)
σ	Reflection coefficient for oncotic agents
Pmv	Pressure in microvessels
Ppmv	Perimicrovascular pressure
pv	Osmotic pressure in vessels
pt	Osmotic pressure of tissues

Fluid flux is sensitive to small intravascular or perivascular pressure changes. Intravascular pressure rises may originate downstream (as with a failing left ventricle) or may follow overall vascular volume increments (as in overhydration) or displacement of blood from the systemic to the pulmonary vessels. The pulmonary capillary endothelium is much less permeable than that of systemic capillaries, and the interstitial space around alveolar microvessels is tightly restricted by the collagen network between the alveolar walls, forming an inexpansible space, so leakage at this site is limited. The extraalveolar arterioles and venules, which are not so confined and are more permeable, appear to constitute an additional important site of fluid leakage and reabsorption in the lungs.

Surface tension in the fluid film that lines the alveoli opposes alveolar pressure and tends to lower the interstitial pressure around pulmonary microvessels, particularly in corner areas (see Figure 4-4). An increase in surface tension may contribute to edema when surfactant is lost in an injured lung. Interstitial pressure around the extraalveolar vessels is close to intrathoracic (pleural) pressure and falls as the lungs are distended, which favors relatively more leakage from them at high rather than low lung volumes (see Figure 4-3).

INTERSTITIAL EDEMA

Several factors tend to keep the lung from becoming edematous. Normally, a net outflow of fluid from the upstream arterioles and capillaries is reabsorbed into the downstream capillaries and venules, where the intravascular pressure is lower. Fluid leakage causes local perivascular pressures to rise, particularly in the restricted space between the alveolar walls, which reduces the outward fluid flux. It also may compress the vessels, thereby reducing the total surface available for leakage. Because the fluid that leaks through intact endothelium is largely protein-free, it dilutes and washes out the interstitial protein. This alteration reduces the perivascular osmotic pressure of tissues and thus increases the inward osmotic pressure difference and reduces the local fluid leak. If excess leakage does occur, the fluid moves from the alveolar walls, where it could interfere with gas exchange, into the low-pressure interstitial zones around the bronchovascular bundles, where it forms relatively innocuous venous, arterial, and peribronchial cuffs. This fluid may be absorbed in part by the rich bronchial vascular network and by the many lymphatics in the adventitia of the airways and vessels. Edema fluid also may reach the pleural space, where it is absorbed by the pleural lymphatic and blood vessels. Finally, experimental data suggest that all the blood perfusing the capillaries in alveolar walls must first pass through capillaries located in alveolar corners and that the negative interstitial pressure surrounding these corner capillaries is critically dependent on alveolar surface tension. When surface tension is eliminated by alveolar flooding, interstitial pressure around these vessels increases, thus serving to compress the corner vessels and diminish flow through the capillaries in the alveolar wall of these flooded alveoli. This mechanism provides for much more precise control of perfusion, virtually on an alveolus-to-alveolus basis, compared with the effects of alveolar hypoxia, which are directed to much more proximal vessels.

When the capillary endothelium is injured, locally or through the effect of circulating mediators, the vascular permeability to fluids and solutes is increased; consequently, even a modest outward pressure gradient causes a large fluid leak. The ability to retain large molecules is lost, protein-rich plasma leaks out, and the osmotic pressure in tissues approaches that in vessels, so that the osmotic force opposing intravascular hydrostatic pressure is lost. This high-permeability or "leaky capillary" edema can be a fulminant process that leads to severe abnormalities in gas exchange.

ALVEOLAR EDEMA

The epithelial cells that line the air spaces have tight junctions along their apical surface, so this membrane normally is even less permeable than the endothelial membrane, protecting alveolar spaces as interstitial edema increases. After total lung water has increased by approximately 50%, the edema fluid appears in the alveoli. A structural failure, at the epithelial cell junctions or elsewhere, is suspected, because there is no protein gradient between interstitial and alveolar edema fluid. Fluid initially is seen only in the corners of the alveoli, where surface tension causes the pressure below the curved fluid film to be lowest. As more fluid accumulates, the alveoli rapidly become completely filled, again because of surface tension effects. As alveoli fill, the radius of the curvature of the meniscus of the fluid becomes shorter, and the effect of surface tension becomes greater (Laplace's law), which pulls fluid in more strongly (**Figure 4-8**). Thus, the sequence of edema development progresses from the perimicrovascular interstitium to peribronchovascular "sump" to patchy alveolar flooding.

Fluid and ions normally exchange across the bronchial and alveolar epithelial surfaces to regulate the character of the mucous blanket and maintain the subphase film beneath the surfactant that lines the alveoli. Alveolar edema can be cleared by an active process of sodium reabsorption with water following osmotic transport. The type II epithelial cells take in sodium through channels on their apical surface and move it by active Na^+,K^+-ATPase pumping on the basolateral surfaces into the interstitium. The type I cells seem to have similar, though less prominent, apparatus and, because they cover about 90% of the alveolar surface, might have a significant role. Fluid removal also may occur in distal airways, where epithelial and Clara cells actively transport sodium. These active mechanisms also are crucial in the initial clearance of fetal lung fluid at birth. In experimental models, fluid clearance from air spaces is enhanced by β_2-agonists and blocked by antagonists such as propranolol.

HIGH-ALTITUDE PULMONARY EDEMA

Some persons traveling or climbing to high altitudes develop pulmonary edema that may be severe and life-threatening. The

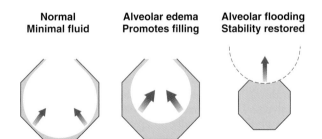

Normal   **Alveolar edema**   **Alveolar flooding**
Minimal fluid   **Promotes filling**   **Stability restored**

Figure 4-8 Alveoli tend to fill with fluid in an "all-or-none" fashion. In the normal alveolus, a small amount of fluid rounds off the corners. Alveolar edema decreases the radius, which increases the inward force of surface tension and pulls in more fluid. When the alveolus is filled, the radius of the surface increases, so stability is regained. *(Modified with permission from Butler J: The circulation of the lung. In Culver BH, editor: The respiratory system, Seattle, 2006, University of Washington Publication Services, p 8.11.)*

mechanisms are becoming better understood and seem to involve both hydrostatic and permeability factors. The underlying abnormality in people who are susceptible to high-altitude pulmonary edema (HAPE) and who are subject to repeated episodes with repeated exposures is an exaggerated elevation of pulmonary artery pressure in response to hypoxia. Susceptible persons may experience only slight elevations in Ppa at rest or during routine activities when breathing air at sea level but demonstrate a greater increase in response to exercise than that observed in control subjects. In response to a hypoxic challenge, HAPE-susceptible subjects experience a rise in Ppa that is three- to four-fold higher than that in control subjects. At altitude, typically greater than 3000 m above sea level, Ppa in susceptible persons would be expected to rise rapidly in response to alveolar hypoxia and to increase further with the exertion that is common to mountaineering activities. Symptomatic edema develops after 24 hours up to a few days later but rarely arises after 5 days at altitude. The few hemodynamic measurements made under these circumstances have shown marked elevation of pulmonary artery systolic pressure, as high as 80 to 100 mm Hg, but usually normal or only modestly elevated pulmonary artery occlusion pressure. Thus, although high hydrostatic forces are involved, this is not a typical cardiogenic mechanism, with elevation of left atrial pressure reflected into the pulmonary microvasculature. The site of hypoxic vasoconstriction is in small pulmonary arteries and arterioles, although some venoconstriction also occurs, which could contribute to a pressure increase at the capillary level. It has been hypothesized that a heterogeneous distribution of the increased pulmonary vascular resistance might divert relatively high blood flow to low-resistance arterioles, thereby increasing local microvascular pressure sufficiently to cause the patchy edema pattern typically seen on lung radiographs of patients with HAPE. Because some persons with a similarly exaggerated hypoxic vasoconstrictor response do not develop edema, it is suggested that a defect in alveolar epithelial fluid clearance also may contribute to HAPE.

Of interest, bronchoalveolar lavage fluid obtained from climbers on Mt. McKinley and elsewhere with symptomatic HAPE has shown high levels of protein, which is consistent with increased vascular permeability, and red cells, suggesting further loss of barrier function. Because granulocytes and inflammatory markers are seen in only modest quantities and tend to appear later in the course, the underlying mechanism is believed to be a noninflammatory permeability change. This may be explained by the stretching of pores under hydrostatic forces or, in more severe cases, by overt capillary stress failure with endothelial, epithelial, and basement membrane disruption, as described in experiments in rabbit lungs subjected to high intravascular pressure. Although the cellular mechanisms responsible for the exaggerated pulmonary vascular response are yet to be explained, a plausible sequence of events leading to pulmonary edema in HAPE-susceptible persons has now emerged, and pulmonary vasodilators have been shown to be protective.

RESPIRATORY-CIRCULATORY INTERACTIONS

SPONTANEOUS BREATHING

The phasic changes of intrathoracic pressure and lung volume of the respiratory cycle alter the preload and afterload of the right and left sides of the heart, which interact to vary cardiac output and blood pressure with the respiratory cycle. The changes are modest during normal tidal breathing, when intrathoracic pressure swings are small, but can be more notable in pathologic states. During inhalation, the decrease in intrathoracic pressure enhances systemic venous return to the chest. The right atrium and ventricle fill, and right heart output to the pulmonary vessels increases as the alveoli fill with air. Lung expansion dilates the extraalveolar pulmonary arterial vessels, which reduces their resistance and helps to accommodate the increased flow. Ppa stays almost constant relative to alveolar pressure. The increase in right ventricular volume tends to stiffen or compress the left ventricle within the common pericardium, but the surge of pulmonary flow reaches the left heart after two or three beats, so that systemic output and blood pressure begin to rise in late inspiration or early expiration. This preload effect normally is dominant, but the inspiratory drop in intrathoracic pressure also can add effective afterload to the left ventricle. When the pressure surrounding the heart is lower, the myocardium would have to generate a greater transmural pressure difference to maintain the same stroke volume and systemic arterial pressure. Accordingly, systemic blood pressure falls a few millimeters of mercury coincident with inspiration and rises a few millimeters of mercury during exhalation. Depending on the respiratory rate, this direct pressure effect may be enhanced or countered by the arrival at the left ventricle of the inspiratory surge of venous return.

When intrathoracic pressure swings are exaggerated, as occurs during an asthma attack or an exacerbation of chronic obstructive pulmonary disease, the inspiratory drop in blood pressure can be 20 to 30 mm Hg, creating the clinical observation of pulsus paradoxus. Of interest, such markedly negative inspiratory pressures do not generate a proportionate increase in systemic venous return because of a flow-limiting, or waterfall, mechanism in the central veins. When the intraluminal pressure falls in these intrathoracic veins, the vessels collapse at the point where they are first exposed to atmospheric pressure, in the neck, axilla, and abdomen, and their flow becomes independent of the increasingly negative downstream right atrial pressure.

When the pericardial space is limited (e.g., pericardial effusion, constrictive pericarditis, enlarged heart), the interaction between the two ventricles is more prominent. Inspiratory filling of the right side of the heart limits the diastolic expansion of the left side of the heart. This ventricular interaction contributes to an inspiratory decrease in systemic outflow and blood pressure and allows both to increase when the right side of the heart is less full during expiration.

POSITIVE-PRESSURE VENTILATION

When patients are mechanically ventilated with positive inspiratory pressure, the same mechanisms seen in spontaneous breathing are involved, but the pressure effects shift phase in the tidal cycle. For example, the pressure outside the left ventricle rises during inspiration, so the same contraction yields a higher blood pressure early in the inspiratory phase. This increase may be augmented by blood pushed out of the capillaries by the positive alveolar pressure (see Figure 4-3). During late inspiration or early expiration, the blood pressure decreases as the effect of an inspiratory decrease in venous return to the right heart reaches the left side. If the expiratory phase is long enough, the blood pressure will begin to rise, reflecting enhanced venous return to the right heart earlier in expiration.

In addition to the cyclic changes, overall effects on cardiac output are seen when spontaneous breathing is replaced by positive-pressure ventilation, particularly when positive end-expiratory pressure (PEEP) is added. The mean airway pressure and the mean intrathoracic pressure both are high, and the latter is reflected in the pressure outside the right heart. This in turn causes the right atrial pressure to be higher, which may decrease the pressure difference driving venous flow from the systemic capacitance vessels. In addition, the increase in lung volume may partially compress the inferior vena cava as it runs through the lung just above the diaphragm, thereby increasing resistance to venous return. A resultant decrease in cardiac output typically is seen, accompanied by a decrease in right atrial transmural pressure and a decrease in right ventricular end-diastolic volume, particularly if intravascular volume is low. This effect may be opposed by a rise in abdominal pressure as thoracic volume increases and by increased venous tone to help restore the driving pressure for venous return.

When an increase in end-expiratory lung volume is recruited by PEEP, the chest wall also must be passively expanded, and its pressure-volume relationship (see Chapter 3, Figure 3-7) would predict at least a modest increase in pleural pressure. As shown by direct measurement with suitable flat devices, however, when the lungs are distended with PEEP, the pressure in the cardiac fossa may rise more than that measured by an esophageal balloon, and the pressure in the pericardium may be still higher. Bedside measurements of a decreased cardiac output accompanied by a higher pulmonary arterial occlusion pressure may suggest a decrease in cardiac function or contractility, but when accurate measurements of juxtacardiac pressure or left ventricular end-diastolic volume are made, the ventricle is seen to be operating at a lower preload on the same function curve. The same phenomenon may be seen when patients with severe airflow obstruction develop dynamic hyperinflation with an associated increase in cardiac fossa pressure.

High levels of PEEP and of end-inspiratory alveolar pressure compress alveolar septal capillaries, outweighing any distention of extraalveolar vessels with the lung volume increase, and thus increase pulmonary vascular resistance and right ventricular afterload. If this effect becomes dominant, a decrease in cardiac output may be associated with an increase in right ventricular end-diastolic volume.

The increase in juxtacardiac pressure with PEEP decreases the stroke work the left ventricle must do to maintain any given systemic blood pressure, thus effectively decreasing left ventricular afterload. In most circumstances, the preload effect previously described dominates, but a failing ventricle is quite sensitive to afterload, and this effect becomes more important in patients with severe heart disease. In such patients, the benefit of continuous positive airway pressure (CPAP) may be more hemodynamic than ventilatory.

CONTROVERSIES AND PITFALLS

The "classic" three- (or four-) zone model of lung blood flow distribution with its emphasis on gravitational effects has evolved to a more complete understanding of this distribution, as discussed earlier in this chapter. No real controversy clouds the accuracy of either the earlier data or more recent work, but the role of gravity has been so extensively taught that some misconceptions persist. Studies measuring blood flow with radioactive tags and relatively large counters placed over the upper, middle, and lower thorax clearly demonstrated a vertical gradient of flow increasing toward the base. The effect of alveolar and intravascular pressures on blood flow, with the latter decreasing with vertical height due to gravitational hydrostatic force, provided a plausible explanation for this finding. More recent data measuring regional flow by various techniques confirm this vertical gradient in upright lungs, but studies of inverted lungs do not show the reversal expected of a gravitational effect, and studies in zero or increased gravity show less-than-expected redistribution of regional flow. With the development of techniques to measure regional flow on increasingly smaller anatomic scales, wide variation in local blood flow is observed within an isogravitational plane, whereas flow in a specific region remains consistent despite different gravitational states. These data indicate that the distribution of blood flow is dominated by the arrangement of serial vascular resistances, due to anatomic development and largely under genetic control, with a relatively small superimposed effect of gravity. The influences of alveolar and intravascular pressures described in the zone model remain important but should not be tied to a stacked vertical alignment, because the physiology of different zones may coexist at the same height in the lung. The measurement techniques used to measure flow on a small anatomic scale require subsequent lung excision and destructive sampling, so they have been applied only to animals, including primates; whatever controversy remains, therefore, is related to the less-substantiated proof in human lungs and continuing debate over the relative importance of vascular structure and hydrostatic gradients in determining regional blood flow.

Failure to appreciate this newer description of blood flow distribution in the lung can lead to misunderstanding of clinical events. For example, considerable interest has emerged in the improved oxygenation that commonly occurs with prone positioning in acute lung injury. The gravitational model would suggest that the improved ventilation-perfusion distribution could be attributed to a shift in perfusion, but available data show that it is predominantly the ventilation that shifts to better match the maintained higher perfusion of the dorsal-caudal regions of lung.

SUGGESTED READINGS

Circulatory Structure

Butler J, editor: *The bronchial circulation*, vol 57 of Lenfant C, editor: *Lung biology in health and disease*, New York, 1992, Marcel Dekker.

Culver BH, Butler J: Mechanical influences on the pulmonary circulation, *Annu Rev Physiol* 42:187–198, 1980.

Paredi P, Barnes PJ: The airway vasculature: recent advances and clinical implications, *Thorax* 64:444–450, 2009.

Weibel ER: What makes a good lung? The morphometric basis of lung function, *Swiss Med Wkly* 139:375–386, 2009.

Blood Flow Regulation and Distribution

Baumgartner WA Jr, Jaryszak EM, Peterson AJ, et al: Heterogeneous capillary recruitment among adjoining alveoli, *J Appl Physiol* 95:469–476, 2003.

Glenny RW: Determinants of regional ventilation and blood flow in the lung, *Intensive Care Med* 35:1833–1842, 2009.

Glenny RW, Bernard S, Robertson HT, Hlastala MP: Gravity is an important but secondary determinant of regional pulmonary blood flow in upright primates, *J Appl Physiol* 86:623–632, 1999.

Glenny RW, Robertson HT: Regional differences in the lung: a changing perspective on blood flow distribution. In Hlastala MP, Robertson HT, editors: *Complexity in structure and function of the lung*, vol 121 of Lenfant C, editor: *Lung biology in health and disease*, New York, 1998, Marcel Dekker, pp 461–481.

Prisk GK, Yamada K, Henderson AC, et al: Pulmonary perfusion in the prone and supine postures in the normal human lung, *J Appl Physiol* 103:883–894, 2007.

Sommer N, Dietrich A, Schermuly RT, et al: Regulation of hypoxic pulmonary vasoconstriction: basic mechanisms, *Eur Respir J* 32:1639–1651, 2008.

Fluid Exchange

Bhattacharya J: Physiological basis of pulmonary edema. In Matthay M, Ingbar D, editors: *Pulmonary edema*, vol 116 of Lenfant C, editor: *Lung biology in health and disease*, New York, 1998, Marcel Dekker.

Effros RM, Parker JC: Pulmonary vascular heterogeneity and the Starling hypothesis, *Microvasc Res* 78:71–77, 2009.

Matthay M, Folkesson HG, Clerici C: Lung epithelial fluid transport and the resolution of pulmonary edema, *Physiol Rev* 82:569–600, 2002.

Ware LB, Matthay MA: Clinical practice. Acute pulmonary edema, *N Engl J Med* 353:2788–2796, 2005.

High-Altitude Pulmonary Edema

Bartsch P, Mairbaurl H, Maggiorini M, Swenson E: Physiological aspects of high-altitude pulmonary edema, *J Appl Physiol* 98:1101–1110, 2005.

Scherrer U, Rexhaj E, Jayet PY, et al: New insights in the pathogenesis of high-altitude pulmonary edema, *Prog Cardiovasc Dis* 52:485–492, 2010.

Respiratory-Circulatory Interactions

Feihl F, Broccard AF: Interactions between respiration and systemic hemodynamics. Part 1: basic concepts, *Intensive Care Med* 35:45–54, 2009.

Marini JJ, Culver BH, Butler J: Mechanical effects of lung distension with positive pressure on cardiac function, *Am Rev Respir Dis* 124:382–386, 1981.

Tyberg JV, Grant DA, Kingma I, et al: Effects of positive intrathoracic pressure on pulmonary and systemic hemodynamics, *Respir Physiol* 119:163–171, 2000.

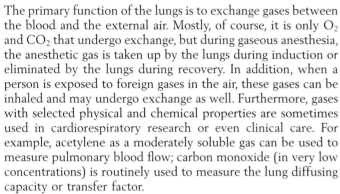

Chapter **5**

Gas Exchange

Peter D. Wagner

The primary function of the lungs is to exchange gases between the blood and the external air. Mostly, of course, it is only O_2 and CO_2 that undergo exchange, but during gaseous anesthesia, the anesthetic gas is taken up by the lungs during induction or eliminated by the lungs during recovery. In addition, when a person is exposed to foreign gases in the air, these gases can be inhaled and may undergo exchange as well. Furthermore, gases with selected physical and chemical properties are sometimes used in cardiorespiratory research or even clinical care. For example, acetylene as a moderately soluble gas can be used to measure pulmonary blood flow; carbon monoxide (in very low concentrations) is routinely used to measure the lung diffusing capacity or transfer factor.

Fortunately, all such gases behave in accordance with the same basic physical principles underlying gas transport and exchange—mass conservation—explained in some detail further on. Although different gases appear to behave differently, this reflects their different physicochemical properties related to how they are transported in blood, and not differences in conforming to the mass conservation principles of exchange. Moreover, gas uptake from air into blood obeys the same rules as for gas elimination from the blood to the air. Thus, the topic of gas exchange can be treated as a general process applicable to all gases, whether taken up or eliminated. Subsequent applications can be made for individual gases in accord with their blood transport properties. In this chapter, the focus is primarily on the respiratory gases O_2 and, to a lesser extent, CO_2.

THE BASIS OF GAS EXCHANGE: VENTILATION, DIFFUSION, AND PERFUSION

The lungs conduct gas exchange through three interacting processes: ventilation, diffusion, and perfusion (or blood flow). Ventilation brings O_2 from the air to the alveoli (and simultaneously eliminates CO_2, transferred from the blood, to the air). Diffusion is the process by which O_2 in the alveoli passes across the alveolar wall into the pulmonary capillary. Perfusion moves the blood through the pulmonary circulation and allows continuously flowing red cells to take on O_2. Ventilation and perfusion are mostly convective processes that require energy expenditure by the organism. Ventilation is an alternating, bidirectional process of inspiration and expiration, while perfusion is unidirectional from right ventricle to left atrium. Inspiration is accomplished by the respiratory muscles (diaphragm and external intercostal muscles mostly), which on contraction expand the thoracic cage, thus reducing the intrapleural pressure around the lungs, resulting in passive lung expansion. Expiration generally is passive and occurs as the respiratory

muscles relax and allow the elastic recoil of the lung to expel air. Diffusion is passive and does not require the organism to expend energy. It simply reflects random molecular motion that over time tends to equalize molecular concentrations in space.

RELATIONSHIPS BETWEEN LUNG STRUCTURE AND FUNCTION

The evolutionary "decision" to conduct gas exchange by passive diffusion (rather than by energy-requiring active transport) was a profound one that dictated the basic structure of the lungs. The laws of diffusion show that diffusive mass transfer rates are directly proportional to the surface area available for diffusion and are inversely proportional to the distance the molecule must diffuse. The fundamental unit of structure in the lung is the alveolus, small and roughly spherical in shape, with an average radius of 150 micrometers (μm). There are about 300 million alveoli in the human lung. Each is supplied with air that must pass through the branching bronchial tree (conducting airways). The wall of each alveolus, shared by adjacent alveoli, is packed with capillaries. The tissue separating alveolar gas from the blood in the capillaries consists of the capillary endothelium, interstitial matrix, alveolar epithelium, and a thin layer of fluid. The entire wall is less than 0.5 μm in thickness.

These dimensions imply a total alveolar surface area of about 80 m^2, yet a gas volume of only 4 L (small enough to fit within the chest cavity). Thus, the actual lung can conduct diffusive exchange efficiently because of the large surface area and small diffusion distance. By contrast, if the lungs consisted of just a single large sphere of the same 4-L volume, its surface area would be only $\frac{1}{8}$ m^2 (640-fold less). Moreover, if the same mass of 0.5-μm-thick alveolar wall tissue covering all 300 million alveoli were spread around this one sphere, its thickness would be over 300 μm, also about 600 times greater than in the actual lung. Because diffusion rates depend on the ratio of area to thickness, the real lung is about 640 × 600, or 400,000 times better at diffusive transport than would be a single sphere of the same volume and mass. The message is that by dividing up the lung into a very large number of very small structures, diffusion becomes a feasible and energy-efficient method of gas exchange, circumventing the need for active transport.

This picture of the lungs is similar in some ways to a bunch of grapes in which each grape is an alveolus, the skin is the alveolar wall (containing the capillaries) and the pulp inside is the alveolar air space. The stalks connecting each grape to its cluster depict the conducting airways and blood vessels. A major shortcoming to the grape analogy, however, is that each grape in a bunch is physically detached from all others in the bunch. However, all alveoli are connected, sharing common alveolar walls, much like the cells of a honeycomb. This connectivity means that the alveoli are mechanically interdependent—they pull on each other, forming a self-stabilizing three-dimensional network.

CHALLENGES TO LUNG FUNCTION CAUSED BY ITS STRUCTURE

Lung structure may be optimized for diffusion, but it results in several potentially life-threatening challenges:

Inequality of ventilation and blood flow: Because the lungs are ventilated through a single main airway (trachea), yet air must reach all 300 million alveoli, there must be a substantial branching airway system. Indeed, some 23 orders of largely dichotomous branching are recognized, resulting in a very large number of very small airways arranged in parallel with each other—much like tree branches emanating and serially dividing from a single trunk. It is impossible to imagine that inhaled air can be distributed homogeneously to all 300 million alveoli, and nonuniform ventilation distribution is well known to occur. Similarly, blood flow reaches the lungs from the main pulmonary artery by a corresponding branching system, and it also is known that perfusion is nonuniform. Nonuniform distribution of ventilation and blood flow are important for gas exchange efficiency as will be shown later.

Wasted ventilation (dead space): The first 17 or so generations of the airways are conducting airways—plumbing whose walls are unable to perform any gas exchange. Their total volume is about 150 mL. This means that with every single breath, 150 mL of inhaled air never reaches the alveoli yet must be moved by muscle contraction. Normally, each breath is about 500 mL in total volume, so about 30% of each breath represents wasted effort. This is not important in health, but in some lung diseases, the effort of breathing is so high that this wasted ventilation, called *dead space*, leads to insufficient ventilation of fresh gas to the alveoli.

Alveolar collapse: A very large number of very small collapsible structures is potentially physically unstable, due to surface tension forces. The laws of physics show that the pressure inside a soap bubble caused by surface tension is inversely proportional to the bubble radius. To the extent that the soap bubble analogy applies to the alveoli, which simply are not all exactly equal in size, surface tension forces will therefore tend to empty small alveoli into larger alveoli. Unchecked, this progression would lead to massive alveolar collapse with loss of gas exchange surface area and could prove fatal. In fact, the neonatal respiratory distress syndrome is considered to represent an example of just this phenomenon. The body has solved this problem by generating, in normal full-term newborns, a surfactant that lines each alveolus. It reduces surface tension by about an order of magnitude, greatly mitigating the risk of alveolar collapse. What also helps prevent collapse is the aforementioned interdependence whereby adjacent alveoli share common alveolar walls, creating a mesh or network that is inherently self-stabilizing.

Particle deposition: An array of about 20 orders of dichotomous branching leads to a very large (2^{20} in this case) number of small peripheral airways. Although individually each is very small, there are so many of them that their total cross-sectional area becomes very large. With this arrangement, the forward velocity of the air in each small airway is reduced as air is inhaled, which in turn increases the chance that an inhaled dust (or other) particle will settle out and deposit on the small airway wall (compared with larger, more proximal airways, in which the velocity of air flow is much greater). If such a particle is physically, chemically, or biologically dangerous, disease may result, often starting in those small peripheral airways—as is the case for emphysema caused by inhalation of tobacco smoke.

Airway obstruction by mucus: Although the airways have developed a sophisticated particle clearance mechanism using mucociliary transport, the mucus that traps the particles may itself occlude small airways, impairing distal ventilation of the alveoli.

Capillary stress failure: The pulmonary microcirculation is at risk from the inherent structure of the lungs. With capillaries poorly supported in very thin alveolar walls (good for diffusion), they risk rupture into the alveolar space when intravascular pressures rise even modestly. Such alveolar hemorrhage occurs in several conditions, and especially in racehorses, whose lungs are relatively small, leading to high vascular pressures, which in this setting can be fatal.

Pulmonary hypertension: Because all of the cardiac output has to pass through the lungs (compare the systemic circulation, for which flow is divided among all of the body's other tissues and organs), the potential for high vascular pressures is considerable. The twin processes of capillary distention and recruitment mitigate increases in pressure when perfusion is increased, as in exercise.

In sum, many life-threatening challenges may be associated with a lung built for diffusion, affecting the airways, alveoli, and blood vessels. In the normal lung, defenses against them are satisfactory, but in lung disease, they often are inadequate, with sometimes fatal outcomes.

GAS EXCHANGE IN THE HOMOGENEOUS LUNG: VENTILATION, DIFFUSION, AND PERFUSION

Because gas exchange obeys mass conservation rules and occurs by passive diffusion, the exchange of gases can be understood and predicted quite accurately in a quantitative sense. In fact, quantitative discussion is essential to understanding of not just the principles but also the clinically very important differences in behavior of O_2, CO_2, and other gases. It is best to start with a perfectly homogeneous lung—one in which every alveolus is assumed to be identical and to receive an equal share of both ventilation and blood flow. Although an obvious oversimplification, this assumption allows the establishment of the basic principles, which can then be readily applied to lungs in which differences in ventilation and blood flow exist among alveoli.

Ventilation

For ventilation, *mass conservation* means that the amount of O_2 diffusing into the pulmonary capillary blood from the alveolar gas in a given period (say, 1 minute—i.e., $\dot{V}O_2$) can be expressed as the difference between how much O_2 was inhaled and how much was exhaled (over that minute). This relation holds because inhaled O_2 has only two fates—diffusing into the blood or being exhaled. The amount inhaled is the product of minute ventilation and the concentration of O_2 in inhaled air; the amount exhaled is the product of minute ventilation and the concentration of O_2 in the exhaled gas. Because O_2 concentration is constantly changing during the course of an exhalation, it is appropriate to use the mean concentration over exhalation. Minute ventilation is the product of the volume of each breath (L/breath) and the frequency of breathing (breaths/minute). Although the volumes inhaled and exhaled might be expected to be the same (or the lungs would either blow up or collapse), exhaled volume usually is 1% less than that inhaled because the amount of O_2 absorbed into the blood is a little more than the amount of CO_2 eliminated from the blood. This small difference can be neglected in most circumstances, as is the case in the following discussion. The mass conservation equation that then describes O_2 uptake as a function of ventilation is

$$\dot{V}_{O_2} = \dot{V}_E \times F_{IO_2} - \dot{V}_E \times F_{EO_2} \tag{1}$$

where $\dot{V}_{O_2}$ is the volume of O_2 taken up into the blood per minute, and $\dot{V}_E$ is the minute ventilation, both expressed in L/minute. F_{IO_2} and F_{EO_2} are, respectively, the inhaled and exhaled mean O_2 fractional concentrations. $\dot{V}_E$ commonly is about 7 L/minute. Because about 21 of every 100 molecules in air are O_2 molecules (the rest being mostly nitrogen), F_{IO_2} is 0.21. F_{EO_2} at rest is about 0.17; this difference shows that $\dot{V}_{O_2}$ is about 0.3 L/minute. Because the conducting airways that feed the alveoli do not exchange O_2 or CO_2, it has become conventional to subtract the volume of gas left in the conducting airways each breath—the so-called *anatomic dead space*—from the total breath volume before multiplying by respiratory frequency to calculate ventilation, resulting in a variable known as *alveolar ventilation* ($\dot{V}_A$). Equation 1 then becomes

$$\dot{V}_{O_2} = \dot{V}_A \times F_{IO_2} - \dot{V}_A \times F_{AO_2} \tag{2}$$

where F_{AO_2} is now the mean alveolar O_2 concentration. F_{AO_2} is higher than F_{EO_2} because the latter combines the inhaled air from the dead space with the alveolar gas, which is lower because of O_2 transfer into the blood.

The tendency is to use partial pressure (P_{IO_2}, inhaled; P_{AO_2}, alveolar) rather than fractional concentration (F_{IO_2}, F_{AO_2}) in describing these relationships: From Dalton's law of partial pressure, $P_{O_2} = F_{O_2} \times$ (barometric pressure − water vapor pressure). Allowing for proper units, Equation 2 can then be rewritten as

$$\dot{V}_{O_2} = 1.159 \times \dot{V}_A \times (P_{IO_2} - P_{AO_2}) \tag{3}$$

$\dot{V}_{O_2}$ is now expressed in mL/minute, $\dot{V}_A$ in L/minute, and P in mm Hg.

$\dot{V}_{O_2}$ is the whole-body metabolic rate and as such is dictated by the body tissues, not the lungs. Because P_{IO_2} is a constant, Equation 2 can be used to demonstrate the dependence of alveolar P_{O_2} on alveolar ventilation for a given value of $\dot{V}_{O_2}$ (**Figure 5-1**). The same concepts apply to CO_2, for which it is simpler, because CO_2 is essentially absent from inhaled air. The corresponding equation is

$$\dot{V}_{CO_2} = 1.159 \times \dot{V}_A \times P_{ACO_2} \tag{4}$$

How ventilation affects P_{ACO_2} also is shown in Figure 5-1. It is evident that a relatively small reduction in ventilation will reduce P_{AO_2} and increase P_{ACO_2}—both substantially.

Dividing Equation 4 by Equation 3 gives

$$\dot{V}_{CO_2}/\dot{V}_{O_2} = R = P_{ACO_2}/(P_{IO_2} - P_{AO_2}) \tag{5}$$

which can be rearranged into what is called the *alveolar gas equation*:

$$P_{AO_2} = P_{IO_2} - P_{ACO_2}/R \tag{6}$$

This equation, which relates alveolar P_{O_2} to alveolar P_{CO_2} for a given respiratory exchange ratio R, is very useful at the bedside, as discussed later on.

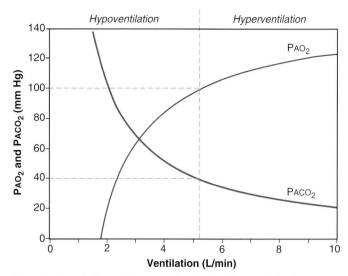

Figure 5-1 Relationship between alveolar P_{O_2}/P_{CO_2} and alveolar ventilation when metabolic rate is held constant. *Dashed lines* indicate normal ventilation, P_{O_2} and P_{CO_2}. Note that as ventilation is reduced, even moderately, P_{O_2} falls sharply and P_{CO_2} rises similarly.

Diffusion

The laws of diffusion dictate that the rate at which a gas diffuses between two points is the product of the diffusion coefficient for the gas and the partial pressure difference between the two points. In the lungs, the diffusion coefficient, measured as the diffusing capacity, is determined by surface area and distance of the diffusion pathway (see earlier). When a red cell leaves the pulmonary arteries and enters the pulmonary capillary, it arrives with a reduced level of O_2, because the tissues visited by that red cell took O_2 from the red cell for the tissue's metabolic needs. The P_{O_2} in the red cell in this blood commonly is about 40 mm Hg. Alveolar P_{O_2}, on the other hand, usually is about 100 mm Hg. The large P_{O_2} difference ("driving gradient") of 60 mm Hg leads to rapid diffusion of O_2 from the alveolar gas into the capillary blood. Consequently, however, the blood P_{O_2} increases, reducing the driving gradient, and O_2 diffusion slows down as the red cell progresses along the lung capillary network. With modeling of this process, again using mass conservation principles, P_{O_2} is seen to rise approximately exponentially as the red cell moves along the lung capillary until P_{O_2} in the red cell has reached the alveolar value, indicating that diffusion equilibration has occurred. This process is shown in **Figure 5-2**. Note that for O_2, equilibration occurred in about 0.25 second. On average, each red cell takes about 0.75 second to move through the alveolar capillary system, so that diffusion equilibration is complete already a third of the way along the capillary, and thus well before its end. As might be expected, during exercise, time available for a red cell to pick up O_2 in the lung is reduced, because blood flow rate is increased, and at very high exercise intensity, there may not be sufficient time for P_{O_2} in the red cell to reach the alveolar value. Accordingly, P_{O_2} in the systemic arterial blood will be lower than that in the alveolus—a situation referred to as hypoxemia caused by diffusion limitation. This effect is seen commonly in exceptional athletes exercising heavily at sea level, and in all subjects exercising at altitude.

While CO_2 moves from blood to gas, the principle is the same as for O_2. Here, the red cell enters the alveolar capillary

Figure 5-2   A, Rate of rise in gas partial pressure along the capillary. Inert gases equilibrate very rapidly, and O_2 more slowly, but CO fails to equilibrate. **B,** Rate of fall in CO_2 partial pressure along the capillary. CO_2 equilibrates about twice as rapidly as does O_2.

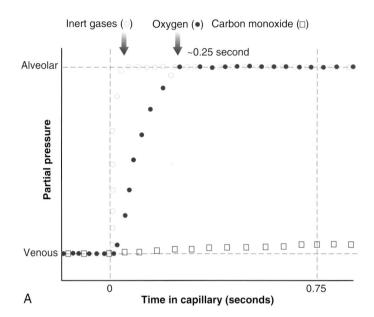

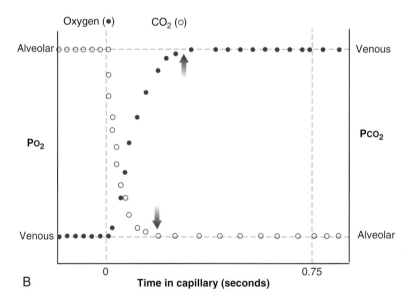

with a high PCO_2 (because of addition of waste CO_2 from tissues visited by the red cell), whereas alveolar PCO_2 is lower. Thus, diffusion will move CO_2 from red cell to alveolar gas, and red cell PCO_2 will fall toward the alveolar value in mirror image to the rise in PO_2 described earlier (see Figure 5-2). The speed of equilibration for CO_2 is about twice that for O_2, so it takes about half the time to reach equilibration. In practice, CO_2 is never diffusion-limited. Gases carried in blood only in physical solution (i.e., inert and anesthetic gases) equilibrate even faster—about 10 times as quickly as for O_2 (see Figure 5-2). This rule holds true for gases of any solubility.

In the remainder of this chapter, diffusion equilibration is assumed to be complete for all gases discussed. What this means is that the alveolar (A) and end-of-the-capillary (ec) PO_2 values are the same for any one gas. Thus, for O_2, $PAO_2 = PecO_2$.

Perfusion

From the preceding, it is clear that O_2 brought to the alveoli by ventilation then diffuses into the flowing blood in lung capillaries. O_2 uptake into the blood can be described using mass conservation principles, just as for ventilation. Thus, the amount

of O_2 taken up into the flowing blood per minute ($\dot{V}O_2$) is the amount of O_2 in the blood leaving the lungs each minute heading for the left atrium, minus the amount that had entered the lungs in the pulmonary arterial blood. These amounts are the product of the concentration of O_2 in each site and the blood flow rate. If $CecO_2$ is the concentration of O_2 in the end-capillary blood, CvO_2 is the concentration of O_2 in the capillary blood as it enters the lung capillaries, and $\dot{Q}$ is the blood flow rate through the lungs, mass conservation gives

$$\dot{V}O_2 = \dot{Q} \times CecO_2 - \dot{Q} \times CvO_2 \qquad (7)$$

Because O_2 concentration in end-capillary blood is virtually unchanged between the end of the capillary and the systemic arterial circulation, end-capillary O_2 concentration can be replaced with arterial CaO_2, giving

$$\dot{V}O_2 = \dot{Q} \times (CaO_2 - CvO_2) \qquad (8)$$

This relationship is known as the *Fick principle*. For CO_2, the corresponding equation is

$$\dot{V}CO_2 = \dot{Q} \times (CvCO_2 - CaCO_2) \qquad (9)$$

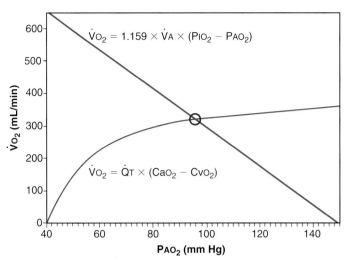

Figure 5-3 The two mass conservation equations for calculating O_2 transfer rate ($\dot{V}O_2$): one as a function of ventilation ($\dot{V}A$, *straight line*) and the other based on blood flow ($\dot{Q}T$, *curved line*), as alveolar PO_2 (PAO_2) varies. Inspired and mixed venous O_2 levels are held constant, as are $\dot{V}A$ and $\dot{Q}T$. The point of intersection (*open circle*) is the only combination of $\dot{V}O_2$ and PAO_2 for which mass of O_2 is conserved and indicates the PAO_2 that must exist for the given values of $\dot{V}A$ and $\dot{Q}T$.

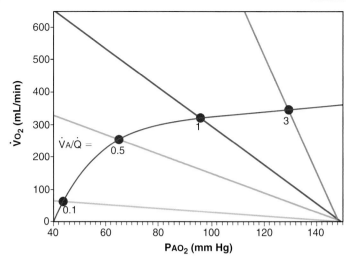

Figure 5-4 Same analysis as in Figure 5-3, with the *four straight lines* reflecting four values of ventilation, $\dot{V}A$, but only one value of blood flow, $\dot{Q}T$ (and thus yielding four values of their ratio, $\dot{V}A/\dot{Q}$). PAO_2 increases with $\dot{V}A/\dot{Q}$, as shown by the *four filled circles*.

GAS EXCHANGE

Focusing on O_2, Equations 3 and 8 should now be considered together. They both embody mass conservation but express it differently, with Equation 3 reflecting alveolar loss of O_2 into blood and Equation 8, red cell gain of O_2 into blood. **Figure 5-3** shows how, for given constant values of $\dot{V}A$ and $\dot{Q}$, and for designated values of inspired PO_2 (PIO_2) and inflowing pulmonary arterial O_2 concentration (CvO_2), $\dot{V}O_2$ would have to vary with alveolar PO_2 (to satisfy both these equations) when determined by each of the two equations independently. Because each molecule of O_2 that leaves the alveolus by crossing the blood gas barrier appears in the capillary blood, the $\dot{V}O_2$ calculated from the two equations must be the same—again, conservation of mass. Thus, only a single value of PAO_2 can exist—that at the point of intersection of the two relationships in Figure 5-3. If the calculations in Figure 5-3 were repeated for different values of $\dot{V}A$, and thus $\dot{V}A/\dot{Q}$ (in this example, keeping $\dot{Q}$ the same), the lines and their point of intersection would change as in **Figure 5-4**. This figure shows that alveolar PO_2 (x axis) and the amount of O_2 that can be taken up ($\dot{V}O_2$, y axis) both depend on $\dot{V}A$ and $\dot{Q}$. Commonly, Equations 3 and 8 are combined, because $\dot{V}O_2$ must be the same when calculated from either equation. This yields the ventilation-perfusion equation:

$$\dot{V}O_2 = 1.159 \times \dot{V}A \times (PIO_2 - PAO_2) = \dot{Q} \times (CaO_2 - CvO_2)$$

or

$$\dot{V}A/\dot{Q} = 0.863 \, (CaO_2 - CvO_2)/(PIO_2 - PAO_2) \qquad (10)$$

and the equivalent for CO_2:

$$\dot{V}A/\dot{Q} = 0.863 \, (CvCO_2 - CaO_2)/PACO_2 \qquad (11)$$

These equations say that it is the *ratio* of $\dot{V}A$ to $\dot{Q}$ that determines the alveolar PO_2 and PCO_2 in any region of the lungs.

Figure 5-5 shows how alveolar PO_2 and PCO_2 vary with $\dot{V}A/\dot{Q}$ when inspired PO_2 is that of room air and the pulmonary arterial (mixed venous) PO_2 is normal (i.e., 40 mm Hg).

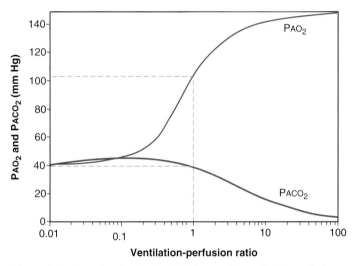

Figure 5-5 How alveolar PO_2 (and PCO_2) vary with ventilation-perfusion ratio ($\dot{V}A/\dot{Q}$), based on the analysis of Figures 5-3 and 5-4. *Dashed lines* show normal values for a $\dot{V}A/\dot{Q}$ of 1. Normal conditions are assumed: inspired $PO_2 = 150$ mm Hg, $PCO_2 = 0$ mm Hg, mixed venous $PO_2 = 40$ mm Hg, $PCO_2 = 45$ mm Hg. PAO_2 and $PACO_2$ approach mixed venous values as $\dot{V}A/\dot{Q}$ approaches zero and inspired values as $\dot{V}A/\dot{Q}$ approaches infinity.

Important conclusions to be drawn from this figure are that as $\dot{V}A/\dot{Q}$ falls, PO_2 falls, approaching the mixed venous value at low $\dot{V}A/\dot{Q}$ values, and conversely, PCO_2 rises. Also, as $\dot{V}A/\dot{Q}$ rises, PO_2 approaches the inspired value, while PCO_2 falls. The dashed lines show that at the normal value for the $\dot{V}A/\dot{Q}$ ratio of about 1, PO_2 is about 100 mm Hg, and PCO_2 is about 40 mm Hg.

Although the behavior of the two gases is qualitatively similar (even if opposite in direction), their quantitative behaviors are different. Most of the variance in PO_2 occurs over the $\dot{V}A/\dot{Q}$ range 0.3 to 3, whereas for CO_2, most of its change is seen in the $\dot{V}A/\dot{Q}$ range 2 to 20, almost a decade higher. The gases obey the very same conservation of mass rules in their exchange, so their quantitative differences are due to differences in their transport properties in blood.

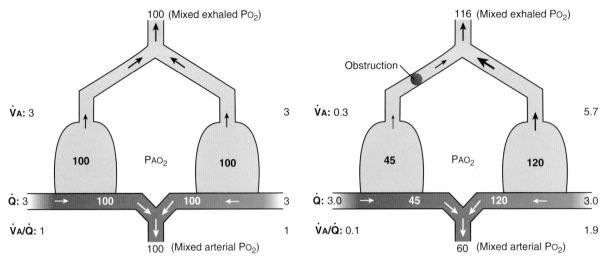

Figure 5-6   A two-compartment representation of ventilation-perfusion distribution showing how maldistribution interferes with gas exchange. **Left,** The homogeneous example in which each compartment having the same $\dot{V}A/\dot{Q}$ also must have the same PAO_2. When exhaled air and end-capillary blood from the two compartments mix, the mixed exhaled gas and mixed arterial blood have the same PO_2. **Right,** Effects of altered distribution of ventilation due to airway obstruction on the left side, reducing ventilation and thus $\dot{V}A/\dot{Q}$ each 10-fold. Mixed exhaled PO_2 is higher and mixed arterial PO_2 is lower than in the homogeneous case, and total O_2 uptake is reduced—all as total ventilation and total blood flow are held constant.

VENTILATION-PERFUSION INEQUALITY AND GAS EXCHANGE

The preceding analysis accounts for gas exchange in the intact, homogeneous lung, in which a single value is taken for $\dot{V}A/\dot{Q}$ (equal to the ratio of total alveolar ventilation to total pulmonary blood flow). In real life, not all alveoli enjoy the same $\dot{V}A$ to $\dot{Q}$ ratio. In fact, even in healthy young humans there is about a 10-fold difference between the lowest and highest values, from a low of about 0.3 to a high of about 3. This difference is due to both gravitational influences (higher $\dot{V}A/\dot{Q}$ in non-dependent than in dependent regions) and nongravitational factors such as variation in length and diameter of airways and blood vessels. Alveoli with different $\dot{V}A/\dot{Q}$ ratios are connected in parallel: Mixed venous blood reaches them all, and then the end-capillary blood from each flows into the pulmonary veins, much like tributaries joining a river. In lung diseases, variation in $\dot{V}A/\dot{Q}$ (also called $\dot{V}A/\dot{Q}$ inequality) can be extreme and even fatal. Thus, it is essential to consider how such inequality affects the ability of the lungs to take up O_2 and eliminate CO_2.

This analysis can be done by comparing a homogeneous lung to one with the simplest degree of inequality—a lung imagined to have two "alveoli" of different $\dot{V}A/\dot{Q}$ ratios. This schema is illustrated in **Figure 5-6.** In the left panel, the homogeneous case, with a total ventilation of 6 L/minute and a total blood flow also of 6 L/minute, both equally divided between two identical "alveoli," PO_2 and PCO_2 values can be read off Figure 5-5 for the resulting $\dot{V}A/\dot{Q}$ ratio of 1.0. In the case of inequality, the example in the right panel shows the effect of severe but incomplete airway obstruction, causing 90% reduction in ventilation of the left "alveolus," with corresponding redistribution of ventilation to the right "alveolus" (that is, total ventilation and blood flow are assumed to be unaltered by the airway obstruction). The PO_2 values are again read from Figure 5-5 and are now 45 and 120 mm Hg, respectively. As the two "alveoli" exhale, their gas streams mix in proportion to the relative gas flow rates, resulting in a mixed exhaled PO_2 of 116 mm Hg. Similarly, the blood leaving each "alveolus" has the same PO_2 as in the respective alveolar gas, as shown, and these two blood streams mix again in proportion to their blood flows. Here the

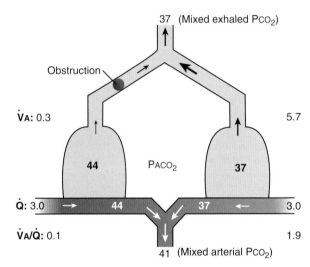

Figure 5-7   Corresponding calculations for CO_2 in the same model as in Figure 5-6, *right*. CO_2 output is impaired, whereas arterial PCO_2 is increased and exhaled PCO_2 is decreased, although the changes are less than for O_2.

computation is performed using the concentrations, not partial pressures, and when this is done, the mixed arterial PO_2 is reduced to only 60 mm Hg.

Thus, what this simple calculation shows is that when the $\dot{V}A/\dot{Q}$ ratio is not everywhere the same, gas exchange suffers: Arterial PO_2 falls, and the amount of O_2 taken up by the whole lung also falls (which can be deduced from the *increase* in mixed exhaled PO_2, which means that because more O_2 was exhaled, less O_2 was transferred into the blood).

The same occurs for PCO_2, but in the opposite direction: $\dot{V}A/\dot{Q}$ inequality increases arterial PCO_2, reduces mixed exhaled PCO_2, and thus also reduces the amount of CO_2 eliminated. **Figure 5-7** shows the values for CO_2 for the same case as in Figure 5-6. What is seen, however, is a quantitatively larger negative effect on O_2 than on CO_2, in terms of both the arterial partial pressures and total amounts of gas transferred.

That O_2 is more affected than CO_2 in this instance reflects the nature of the example: The obstructed "alveolus" has a very low $\dot{V}A/\dot{Q}$ ratio. With modeling of exactly the same problem but this time reducing blood flow in one "alveolus" by 90%, rather than reducing ventilation as in Figures 5-6 and 5-7, $\dot{V}A/\dot{Q}$ inequality would still be present and both gases would be affected, but because the abnormal "alveolus" has a high and not low $\dot{V}A/\dot{Q}$ ratio, the quantitative effects are different: CO_2 is affected more than is O_2.

This result points out that the effects of $\dot{V}A/\dot{Q}$ inequality are always to impair gas exchange for all gases, but the degree to which any one gas is affected depends on the exact pattern of distribution of ventilation and blood flow. The basic reason why O_2 and CO_2 are differently affected in any given pattern is found in the differences in their dissociation curves in blood. That for O_2 is quite nonlinear; that for CO_2 is almost linear and also is much steeper. In sum, O_2 is affected more when low $\dot{V}A/\dot{Q}$ regions dominate; CO_2 is more affected when high $\dot{V}A/\dot{Q}$ regions dominate.

SHUNT

Shunt refers to blood that crosses from the right to the left side of the heart without encountering any alveolar gas. This pathophysiologic entity can be due to ventricular or atrial septal defects and other intracardiac anomalies, or to lung lesions such as complete airway obstruction, atelectasis, pneumothorax, pulmonary edema, pneumonic consolidation, and large arteriovenous intrapulmonary vascular malformations. Referring back to Figure 5-6, which illustrates partial airway obstruction, a shunt could be modeled by assigning zero ventilation to the left "alveolus" and all the ventilation to the right side. The effects would be slightly more severe than those illustrated for partial obstruction, but the point is that a shunt can be thought of as an extreme of $\dot{V}A/\dot{Q}$ inequality: a region with $\dot{V}A/\dot{Q} = 0$, because ventilation is absent.

There is, however, a special feature of shunt that merits discussion: response to inhalation of 100% O_2. When $\dot{V}A/\dot{Q}$ inequality is present, and 100% O_2 is inhaled, all alveolar nitrogen that had been present in the lungs of a subject breathing room air will eventually wash out, and the only gases in the alveoli will be O_2 and CO_2. PO_2 in all alveoli will be above about 600 mm Hg, no matter what the $\dot{V}A/\dot{Q}$ ratio is for each alveolus. Accordingly, on 100% O_2, a lung with $\dot{V}A/\dot{Q}$ inequality will exchange O_2 normally. In the presence of shunt, however, the shunted blood is never exposed to 100% O_2, and its PO_2 remains low (at PO_2 in the inflowing pulmonary arterial blood). This, using the same principles as in Figure 5-6, causes the mixed arterial PO_2 to be abnormally low even as 100% O_2 is inhaled.

THE FOUR CAUSES OF HYPOXEMIA

As characterized in the preceding discussion, arterial hypoxemia (defined as a subnormal value of arterial PO_2) has four different causes:

1. Hypoventilation (see Figure 5-1)
2. Diffusion limitation (not illustrated but discussed earlier)
3. $\dot{V}A/\dot{Q}$ inequality (see Figure 5-6)
4. Shunt, as discussed previously

The alveolar gas equation derived earlier (Equation 6) is useful in separating hypoxemia from these various insults: For hypoventilation alone, the equation predicts exactly how much arterial PO_2 will fall for any given increase in arterial PCO_2, because the alveolar PO_2 and the arterial PO_2 remain equal. However, as shown in Figure 5-6, for $\dot{V}A/\dot{Q}$ inequality, the exhaled alveolar PO_2 increases while the arterial PO_2 falls. Equation 6 is used to compute alveolar PO_2 by inserting arterial PCO_2 into the equation, and when this is done and the arterial PO_2 is subtracted from it, one has what is called the alveolar-arterial PO_2 difference $PO_2(A-a)$. The typical patterns of arterial PO_2, PCO_2, and $PO_2(A-a)$ are illustrated in **Table 5-1** for each cause of hypoxemia, together with the response to 100% O_2 breathing mentioned earlier. In Table 5-1, it is specifically assumed that the body has not reacted to the hypoxemia by any of the compensatory mechanisms normally available to it, as discussed next. In life, such compensatory reactions are the rule, unless special circumstances such as trauma, heart disease, or narcotic overdose also are present.

COMPENSATORY MECHANISMS

When hypoxemia develops for any reason, three principal compensatory mechanisms are invoked:

1. *Greater O_2 extraction from blood by the tissues.* When arterial PO_2 falls, the initial response of the body is to extract more O_2 from the flowing blood. In this way, $\dot{V}O_2$ can be restored passively, both rapidly and effectively. It does result in a lower PO_2 in the venous blood returning to the lungs, which may further impair arterial oxygenation, thereby worsening the hypoxemia, but metabolism is protected. The same occurs in reverse for CO_2: More CO_2 is added to the tissue venous blood, raising the CO_2 level in the blood reaching the lungs. If ventilation remains unchanged, arterial PCO_2 must rise as a result.
2. *Hyperventilation.* Within seconds of the emergence of hypoxemia, chemoreceptors are stimulated, and reflex increase in ventilation occurs. This response usually is very effective in reducing an elevated arterial PCO_2 to normal but often is less

Table 5-1	Effects of Different Causes of Hypoxemia on Gas Exchange			
Cause of Hypoxemia	**Arterial PO_2**	**Arterial PCO_2**	**$PO_2(A-a)$**	**Arterial PO_2 on 100% O_2**
Hypoventilation	Reduced	Increased	Normal	Normal
Diffusion limitation	Reduced	Normal	Increased	Normal
$\dot{V}A/\dot{Q}$ inequality	Reduced	Increased	Increased	Normal
Shunt	Reduced	Normal	Increased	Reduced

$PO_2(A-a)$, alveolar-arterial PO_2 difference; PCO_2, partial pressure of carbon dioxide; PO_2, partial pressure of oxygen; $\dot{V}A/\dot{Q}$, alveolar ventilation-perfusion ratio.

effective in restoring arterial P_{O_2}. Indeed, in an attempt to normalize P_{O_2}, ventilation commonly is increased to the point of causing arterial hypocapnia despite gas exchange abnormalities that in themselves impair CO_2 exchange. Hyperventilation is not especially effective in restoring arterial P_{O_2} in conditions associated with very low $\dot{V}_A/\dot{Q}$ ratios, such as asthma, pneumonia, and acute lung injury. It is much more effective in diseases in which high $\dot{V}_A/\dot{Q}$ ratios are the principal pulmonary abnormality—especially pulmonary thromboembolic disease.

3. *Increased cardiac output.* The sympathetic stimulation resulting from hypoxemia and other factors in many lung diseases may result in tachycardia and an elevated cardiac output. The increased output allows less fractional extraction of O_2 in the tissues, which has the effect of increasing the P_{O_2} of the venous blood returning to the heart, which in turn elevates and partly restores arterial P_{O_2}. This clinical situation commonly is seen in asthmatic patients during acute episodes, especially when β-sympathetic agonists have been taken in large doses, but is unusual in chronic, stable disease states.

These mechanisms act to restore the mass flow of O_2 and CO_2 across the lungs, returning $\dot{V}_{O_2}$ and $\dot{V}_{CO_2}$ to levels necessary to sustain tissue metabolism. Failure to invoke these mechanisms leads to tissue death and can be fatal.

CLINICAL ASSESSMENT OF GAS EXCHANGE BASED ON PHYSIOLOGIC PRINCIPLES

The entire preceding discussion has provided a physiologic basis for clinical tools to assess pulmonary gas exchange. All of these tools are based on measurement of P_{O_2} and P_{CO_2} in an arterial blood sample. Because measuring the entire distribution of ventilation and of blood flow is complex and time-consuming, several simplified methods of gas exchange analysis have been proposed.

Alveolar-Arterial P_{O_2} Difference: $P_{O_2}(A-a)$

As noted earlier, Equation 6, derived previously, is called the *alveolar gas equation.*

$$P_{AO_2} = P_{IO_2} - P_{ACO_2}/R$$

If an arterial blood gas sample is taken, arterial P_{O_2} (P_{aO_2}) and arterial P_{CO_2} (P_{aCO_2}) are available. P_{aO_2} as measured can then be subtracted from P_{AO_2} as calculated from Equation 6, to get $P_{O_2}(A-a)$:

$$P_{O_2}(A-a) = P_{AO_2} - P_{aO_2} = P_{IO_2} - P_{aCO_2}/R - P_{aO_2} \quad (12)$$

In a perfect lung, $P_{O_2}(A-a)$ would be zero. In a normal lung in a young, healthy subject, $P_{O_2}(A-a)$ is about 4 to 10 mm Hg. It can increase to as much as 60 mm Hg in severe lung disease.

Shunt: $\dot{Q}s/\dot{Q}t$

Even if the lung is complex in disease, it can always be modeled as consisting of two "compartments": one normal and one completely unventilated (i.e., in which all the blood flow is shunted). As described previously, shunted blood takes on no O_2, so that the blood leaving has the same low O_2 level as that entering in the mixed venous blood. The objective is to calculate that fraction of the cardiac output ($\dot{Q}s/\dot{Q}t$) necessary to flow through the "shunt" compartment to explain the measured arterial P_{O_2}. This calculation is done using the shunt equation, as follows:

$$C_{aO_2} \times \dot{Q}t = \dot{Q}s \times C_{vO_2} + (\dot{Q}t - \dot{Q}s) \times C_{ecO_2} \quad (13)$$

This is a *conservation of mass* or *mixing* equation that states that the arterial O_2 concentration (C_{aO_2}) is the blood flow–weighted average of the concentrations of O_2 coming from the shunt ($\dot{Q}s$, shunt flow; C_{vO_2}, mixed venous O_2 concentration) and the normal compartment ($\dot{Q}t - \dot{Q}s$, nonshunt blood flow; C_{ecO_2}, end-capillary O_2 concentration). $\dot{Q}t$ is total blood flow, or cardiac output. Equation 13 can be rearranged as follows:

$$\dot{Q}s/\dot{Q}t = (C_{ecO_2} - C_{aO_2})/(C_{ecO_2} - C_{vO_2}) \quad (14)$$

This is called the *shunt equation.* To use it, C_{ecO_2} is calculated using the oxygen-hemoglobin dissociation curve, and the P_{AO_2} as calculated from Equation 6; C_{aO_2} is determined from an arterial blood gas sample, and C_{vO_2} is either assumed or measured from a mixed venous blood sample. If C_{vO_2} is assumed to have a specific value, the calculated value of shunt fraction ($\dot{Q}s/\dot{Q}t$) is only as accurate as the assumed value of C_{vO_2}.

If data for this equation were collected with the patient breathing 100% O_2, a true value of shunt would be found. Recall that, as explained previously, when the subject is breathing 100% O_2, even low $\dot{V}_A/\dot{Q}$ alveoli have very high P_{AO_2} values, exceeding 600 mm Hg, and thus would not contribute to a discernible reduction in C_{aO_2}, because the alveolar blood is fully O_2-saturated. If, however, the data came from a patient breathing less than 100% O_2, the value for $\dot{Q}s/\dot{Q}t$ would in general be larger, because when less than pure O_2 is breathed, areas of low ventilation-perfusion ratio contribute numerically to what appears as $\dot{Q}s/\dot{Q}t$, because they show less than full O_2 saturation of hemoglobin.

Physiologic Dead Space: Vd/Vt

In a conceptual mirror-image formulation, total dead space can be calculated as another parameter of abnormal gas exchange. Conventionally, CO_2 has been used as the marker gas for this, not O_2. The basis is again conservation of mass, and the concept makes use of another two-compartment model. This time, while one compartment remains normal, the other is given an infinitely high ratio of $\dot{V}_A/\dot{Q}$—that is, it is ventilated ($\dot{V}_A > 0$) but unperfused ($\dot{Q} = 0$). No gas exchange occurs because there is no blood flow. This compartment therefore wastes any ventilation it gets. Its alveolar P_{CO_2} is thus that of inspired gas, namely, zero. The objective is to explain the P_{CO_2} in mixed exhaled gas (P_{ECO_2}) as a ventilation-weighted average of the P_{CO_2} coming from each compartment—alveolar P_{CO_2} (P_{ACO_2}) from the normal compartment and zero from the dead space compartment. The mass conservation equation parallels that for shunt, as follows:

$$P_{ECO_2} \times Vt \times f = P_{ACO_2} \times (Vt - Vd) \times f + 0 \times Vd \times f \quad (15)$$

Here f is respiratory frequency, Vd is the volume of air inhaled per breath by the unperfused compartment, and Vt is total inhaled volume of air per breath. Rearranging this equation gives

$$Vd/Vt = (P_{ACO_2} - P_{ECO_2})/P_{ACO_2} \quad (16)$$

Usually, alveolar P_{CO_2} (P_{ACO_2}) is replaced by arterial P_{CO_2} (P_{aCO_2}) from an arterial blood sample, to arrive at

$$Vd/Vt = (P_{aCO_2} - P_{ECO_2})/P_{aCO_2} \quad (17)$$

This dead space equation needs as input arterial P_{CO_2} as well as P_{CO_2} measured in mixed exhaled gas.

The foregoing discussion makes it clear that taking an arterial blood sample is critical for estimating all three parameters of gas exchange. For accurate results, an arterial blood sample is not sufficient. Mixed exhaled gas is required to determine R ($\dot{V}_{CO_2}/\dot{V}_{O_2}$) in Equation 12 and for measuring mixed exhaled P_{CO_2} (P_{ECO_2}) as used in Equation 17. Moreover, Equation 14 requires an estimate of mixed venous O_2 concentration.

ACID-BASE RELATIONSHIPS

For the body to function, hydrogen ion concentration must be kept within narrow limits. Expressed as pH (negative log of [H^+] in moles per liter), normal acidity in circulating blood is 7.40 (40 nanomoles of free H^+ per liter). About the lowest pH that can be survived is 6.8; what is the highest survivable value is unclear (probably about 7.9). A pH of 6.8 corresponds to about 160 nmol/L, whereas a pH of 7.9 corresponds to 13 nmol/L.

It is not surprising that the body has several mechanisms available to maintain pH within this very narrow range. There are in essence three homeostatic mechanisms that together work toward keeping pH normal. The first is chemical buffering by weak acids or bases. The second is renal excretion or retention of H^+, and the third is the process of ventilation.

BUFFERING

When blood is examined, several weak acids and bases are present in solution in plasma, red cells, or both. The major concept here is that they are all in chemical equilibrium with the existing [H^+]. Should the concentration of H^+ ions (i.e., protons) increase for any reason (that is, should *acidosis* develop), positively charged protons can react with the negatively charged ionic form of the weak acid to form the combined, nonionic species. In this way, protons are removed from solution, thus raising the pH back toward normal. This sequence is evident when the chemical equation for this process is displayed:

$$H^+ + A^- \rightarrow HA \qquad (18)$$

The ionic form of the weak acid A (i.e., A^-) combines with a proton (H^+) to form the associated nonionic form HA, thus reducing free [H^+] and thereby raising pH.

Should the opposite condition exist—a reduction in free [H^+] (known as *alkalosis*), the reaction shown in Equation 18 can run from right to left, thereby increasing H^+ ion levels and lowering pH back toward normal.

Important buffers in blood include plasma proteins, especially albumin, phosphate ions, and, inside the red cell, hemoglobin. These buffers form the body's first line of defense against an alteration in pH. They are immediately available and work instantly. Once deployed, however, they can be of little further use until new molecules are synthesized. Thus, they are of limited long-term value for modulating acid-base disturbances and have limited quantitative effect.

THE KIDNEYS

The kidneys can retain or excrete H^+ and bicarbonate ions (HCO_3^-) to preserve their levels in the blood and thus play a major role in controlling pH changes arising from acid-base disturbances. The details of renal function are beyond the scope of this discussion, and further information is available in any of several texts on the subject.

Two important aspects of the renal contribution to acid-base disturbances are as follows: First, the kidneys are slow to react noticeably to an alteration in pH. Somewhat akin to a freight train starting from a dead stop, renal action may begin as soon as pH is changed, but it takes hours to "get up to speed" and affect pH. Second, just as normal kidneys can play a major homeostatic role in restoring pH toward normal, when renal disease develops, the ability to excrete a normally acid urine may be compromised, resulting in accumulation of H^+ ions, with consequent development of acidosis. The kidneys can therefore be a cause of acidosis when they themselves are abnormal, owing to failure of H^+-excreting mechanisms that are invoked to deal with excess H^+ in normal kidneys.

THE LUNGS

Just as the kidneys can counteract either an acidosis or an alkalosis, the lungs have the ability to do likewise. The lungs contribute to regulation of blood pH through changes in P_{CO_2} brought about by changes in ventilation. In sum, an increase in [H^+] in the blood stimulates both central (ventral medullary) and peripheral (carotid body) chemoreceptors, which send neural signals to the respiratory control areas of the brain, which in turn direct the respiratory muscles to produce an increase in ventilation, thereby decreasing P_{CO_2} (refer to Equation 4). A decrease in [H^+] does the opposite. This effect is achieved through the buffering principle, as described, with carbonic acid (H_2CO_3) as the weak acid, as follows. The reaction is greatly accelerated by carbonic anhydrase:

$$H^+ + HCO_3^- \rightarrow H_2CO_3 \rightarrow H_2O + CO_2 \qquad (19)$$

Thus, if acidosis develops, the entire reaction proceeds rightward, removing H^+ ions, raising pH, and producing more CO_2 that can (usually) be easily eliminated by a (usually) modest increase in ventilation. Conversely, should alkalosis develop, the reaction proceeds leftward, liberating H^+ ions to restore pH. The source of the CO_2 necessary to "feed" this backward reaction is a reduction in ventilation. In sum, changes in ventilation affect changes in P_{CO_2}, which then cause the chemical reaction in Equation 19 to proceed rightward when there is acidosis (increased ventilation and lowering P_{CO_2}) or leftward when there is alkalosis (lowering ventilation and raising P_{CO_2}).

By writing the equilibrium version of Equation 19, the concentrations of H^+, HCO_3^-, and CO_2 can be related as follows:

$$K = [H^+] \times [HCO_3^-]/[CO_2] \qquad (20)$$

or

$$K = [H^+] \times [HCO_3^-]/[0.03 \times P_{CO_2}] \qquad (21)$$

where 0.03 is the solubility of CO_2 in plasma (water) in mmoles per liter per mm Hg unit. Taking logarithms of equation 21 and rearranging K and [H^+] gives:

$$-\log[H^+] = -\log K + \log([HCO_3^-]/[0.03 \times P_{CO_2}]) \qquad (22)$$

or

$$pH = pK + \log([HCO_3^-]/[0.03 \times P_{CO_2}]) \qquad (23)$$

where pK is the negative logarithm of the equilibrium constant for the reaction in Equation 19 and equals 6.1. This equation is known as the *Henderson-Hasselbalch equation* and is widely used in describing acid-base disturbances. As can be seen, it relates pH to [HCO_3^-] and P_{CO_2}.

Because this equation contains three variables, their relationship should be expressed in three dimensions, which is difficult. Several ways of working with the equation to surmount this problem have been devised, and they are in essence graphical.

Henderson-Hasselbalch equation:

$$pH = pK + \log\left(\frac{[HCO_3^-]}{0.03 \times Pco_2}\right)$$

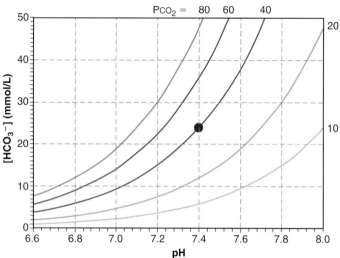

Figure 5-8   The Davenport diagram: Representation of the Henderson-Hasselbalch equation relating pH, [HCO$_3^-$], and Pco$_2$. Each *curved line* shows the unique relationship between [HCO$_3^-$] and pH for each single value of Pco$_2$ shown on the graph. The *filled circle* is the point corresponding to normal arterial blood.

Perhaps the most intuitive and widely used is the *Davenport diagram*, which plots [HCO$_3^-$] on the ordinate and pH on the abscissa and uses isopleths of Pco$_2$ to allow consideration of variation in that variable. For example, if Pco$_2$ is held constant at its normal value of 40 mm Hg, the equation simplifies to

$$pH = 6.1 + \log([HCO_3^-]/[0.03 \times 40]) \qquad (24)$$

In this way, the value of [HCO$_3^-$] for any given pH can be calculated, forming a single line on which each point satisfies Equation 24 for the same value of Pco$_2$—in this example, 40 mm Hg. **Figure 5-8** shows this line on a Davenport diagram for a Pco$_2$ of 40 mm Hg and also for several other fixed Pco$_2$ values, as indicated. This set of Pco$_2$ isopleths then forms the framework for considering acid-base relationships, both normal and abnormal. The value in normal arterial blood is shown in this figure by the solid circle located at Pco$_2$ of 40 mm Hg, pH of 7.40, and [HCO$_3^-$] of 24 mmol/L.

Figure 5-9 plots as a series of solid circles the relationship between pH and [HCO$_3^-$] when the same *normal* blood sample is exposed to and equilibrated with gases of different Pco$_2$ values (one at a time), after which pH and [HCO$_3^-$] are measured. From Equation 23, the Henderson-Hasselbalch equation, it is evident that as the applied Pco$_2$ is raised above normal, pH must fall to below normal, and as Pco$_2$ falls below normal, pH rises above normal, as shown. The pH/[HCO$_3^-$] relationship turns out to be almost straight, as the figure indicates. The steeper the line, the less is the change in pH for a given Pco$_2$. That is, the steeper the line, the more effectively [H$^+$] is kept from changing. Because these results pertain to a single blood sample in vitro, no renal intervention is possible, and the line can be said to represent the buffering ability of the blood sample. Indeed, it is called the *blood buffer line*. The higher the plasma and red cell buffer levels, the steeper will be the buffer line.

Henderson-Hasselbalch equation:

$$pH = pK + \log\left(\frac{[HCO_3^-]}{0.03 \times Pco_2}\right)$$

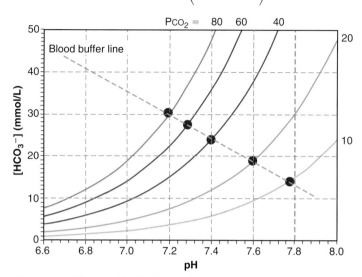

Figure 5-9   The blood buffer line on the Davenport diagram. It is the line relating pH to [HCO$_3^-$] as Pco$_2$ is varied in a given blood sample. See text for details.

Respiratory acidosis
Henderson-Hasselbalch equation:

$$pH = pK + \log\left(\frac{[HCO_3^-]}{0.03 \times Pco_2}\right)$$

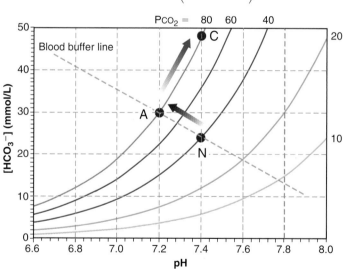

Figure 5-10   The Davenport diagram for respiratory acidosis. An acute increase in Pco$_2$ moves blood pH from the normal position (N) to point A—that is, movement up the normal blood buffer line. Over several hours to days, renal compensation slowly restores pH through HCO$_3^-$ retention, moving blood to point C.

Use of the Davenport diagram to describe acid-base disturbances is illustrated in **Figures 5-10** through **5-13**. Each figure depicts the consequences of one of the four possible types of acid-base disturbance—respiratory acidosis, respiratory alkalosis, metabolic acidosis, and metabolic alkalosis. In each, the CO$_2$ isopleths and normal blood buffer line are shown, along with the normal point, N. These diagrams often are very useful at

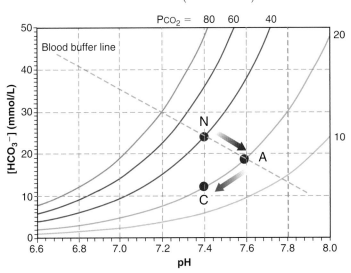

Respiratory alkalosis
Henderson-Hasselbalch equation:

$$pH = pK + \log\left(\frac{[HCO_3^-]}{0.03 \times P_{CO_2}}\right)$$

Figure 5-11 The Davenport diagram for respiratory alkalosis. An acute decrease in P_{CO_2} moves blood pH from the normal position (N) to point A—that is, down the normal blood buffer line. Over several hours to days, renal compensation slowly restores pH through HCO_3^- excretion, moving blood to point C.

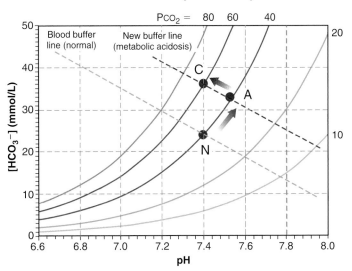

Metabolic alkalosis
Henderson-Hasselbalch equation:

$$pH = pK + \log\left(\frac{[HCO_3^-]}{0.03 \times P_{CO_2}}\right)$$

Figure 5-13 The Davenport diagram for metabolic alkalosis. An acute decrease in $[H^+]$ moves blood pH from the normal position (N) to point A—that is, up the line for normal P_{CO_2}. Over seconds to minutes, ventilatory compensation quickly restores pH through hypoventilation, thereby increasing P_{CO_2}, and moving blood to point C.

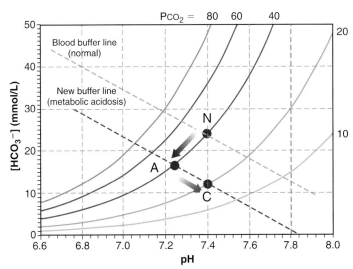

Metabolic acidosis
Henderson-Hasselbalch equation:

$$pH = pK + \log\left(\frac{[HCO_3^-]}{0.03 \times P_{CO_2}}\right)$$

Figure 5-12 The Davenport diagram for metabolic acidosis. An acute increase in $[H^+]$ moves blood pH from the normal position (N) to point A—that is, down the line for normal P_{CO_2}. Over seconds to minutes, ventilatory compensation quickly restores pH through hyperventilation, thereby reducing P_{CO_2}, and moving blood to point C.

ventilation to keep P_{CO_2} normal at 40 mm Hg for the given rate of metabolic production of CO_2. It is the necessary consequence of mass conservation as expressed in Equation 4. From the Henderson-Hasselbalch equation, a rise in P_{CO_2} due to insufficient ventilation causes a fall in pH. When changes in ventilation or metabolic rate occur rapidly (minutes), the movement of P_{CO_2} is along the blood buffer line (from N to A in the particular example in Figure 5-10), because the kidneys have not had time to affect pH. This early situation is called *acute* respiratory acidosis. How far up the buffer line the value moves will depend on the degree to which ventilation is insufficient to maintain P_{CO_2}. In the example of Figure 5-10, the point has moved from the $P_{CO_2} = 40$ mm Hg isopleth to the $P_{CO_2} = 80$ mm Hg isopleth. Using Equation 4, it becomes evident that doubling P_{CO_2} from 40 to 80 mm Hg must have happened because either ventilation was, for some reason, cut in half while maintaining metabolic rate or metabolic rate doubled while ventilation did not change (or a combination of these two). If the acute respiratory acidosis is not treated but persists, the kidneys will start to retain HCO_3^-, excreting acid until after a day or so, the pH, from Equation 23, is (almost) restored to normal (point C in Figure 5-10). The situation is now termed *compensated* respiratory acidosis. As can be seen from Figure 5-10 and the Henderson-Hasselbalch equation, doubling $[HCO_3^-]$ will return the ratio of $[HCO_3^-]$ to P_{CO_2} to normal, and therefore also restore pH to 7.40. In real life, renal compensation (as this process is called) is rarely complete, and so as long as P_{CO_2} remains elevated (in this example, at 80 mm Hg), the point labeled C will be at a lower pH and lower $[HCO_3^-]$ than depicted but must still lie on the isopleth for $P_{CO_2} = 80$ mm Hg.

Common clinical causes of respiratory acidosis are central nervous respiratory depression from drugs, brain injury, phrenic nerve damage, neuromuscular diseases, chest wall trauma, and

the bedside because they allow the caregiver to visually assess, diagnose, understand, and quantify the sometimes complex acid-base states encountered in clinical practice.

Figure 5-10 presents a Davenport diagram for *respiratory acidosis*. As the name implies, it is the result of insufficient lung diseases causing ventilation-perfusion inequality such as chronic obstructive pulmonary disease (COPD).

Figure 5-11 depicts the mechanism of *respiratory alkalosis*, which is the exact mirror image of respiratory acidosis as just described. It occurs when ventilation is increased in relation to metabolic rate, lowering both P_{CO_2} and lowering [HCO_3^-], and increasing pH. Acute (point A, no renal compensation due to short duration) and fully renally compensated (C) points are indicated along with the normal (N) values. Again, complete compensation usually is not seen, so that point C is a little above and to the right of where it is shown in Figure 5-11 (but still on the same isopleth for CO_2).

A common cause of respiratory alkalosis is hyperventilation, either in intact awake persons, usually due to anxiety, or in ventilated patients, as in the ICU or during anesthesia. Additional causes are high-altitude exposure, leading to hypoxic stimulation of respiration, and lung diseases such as asthma, COPD, and interstitial pulmonary fibrosis, as evidenced by a P_{CO_2} lower than normal.

Figure 5-12 depicts the third type of acid-base disturbance, called *metabolic acidosis*. In contrast with respiratory acidosis (in which the high P_{CO_2} was the primary disturbance, which then led to a lower pH), metabolic acidosis achieves a low pH through generation of protons from some metabolic or external source. Referring to the Henderson-Hasselbalch equation, addition of protons must reduce [HCO_3^-] as they combine with HCO_3^- to produce H_2CO_3. Although the chemoreceptors will react to the low pH rapidly (seconds), thus raising ventilation, it is useful to depict what would happen before that compensatory action takes place. In Figure 5-12, point A represents acute respiratory acidosis without change in ventilation (or, therefore, in P_{CO_2}). The more severe the disturbance, the further down and to the left will be point A, but before ventilatory compensation, it must lie on the normal P_{CO_2} = 40 isopleth. Point C shows normalization of pH, achieved by hyperventilation, which lowers P_{CO_2} and allows pH to be restored. This is called respiratory compensation and usually is also incomplete.

In contrast with respiratory acidosis, the data point (A) lies well off (i.e., below) the normal blood buffer line, even before compensation, as Figure 5-12 shows. The vertical drop between the two essentially parallel buffer lines (in this instance, about 11 units) is termed the *base deficit*. It signifies how much base must be added to the blood to fully compensate for the acidosis and restore pH—in this case, 11 mmol of base/L of blood.

Common causes of metabolic acidosis include lactic acidosis (as with exercise or in multiple organ failure) and diabetic ketoacidosis.

Finally, Figure 5-13 depicts the mirror image of metabolic acidosis: *metabolic alkalosis*. The acute response is an increase in pH and [HCO_3^-], from point N to A. Depression of ventilation may ensue, causing P_{CO_2} to rise and pH to normalize. This is a much weaker response than the converse (i.e., hyperventilation in acidosis), but if it occurs, normalization to point C results if compensation is complete.

Common causes of metabolic alkalosis are overdosing on (alkaline) antacid medications, persistent vomiting (of acid gastric fluid) secondary to a duodenal obstruction such as a scar from a previous ulcerative lesion or from cancer, and continuing use of some diuretics.

An important observation with this depiction of acid-base disturbances is that the Davenport diagrams for respiratory acidosis and metabolic alkalosis look similar after compensation—normal pH, high [HCO_3^-], and high P_{CO_2}. In principle, then,

it is impossible to tell by which pathway the patient arrived at the compensated state, and therefore which abnormality was primary and which was the secondary, compensating process. The patient profiles usually are very different, however, and in practice, confusion is uncommon. Exactly the same issue arises for respiratory alkalosis and metabolic acidosis, and again, the clinical situations usually are very different.

CONTROVERSIES AND PITFALLS

The subject of pulmonary gas exchange is well established and is grounded in the fundamental and irrefutable principle of mass conservation. Accordingly, few real controversies remain among researchers who study the topic. Where pitfalls arise is in clinical application of the methods used to assess gas exchange.

Some pitfalls are methodologic, especially the well-known difficulty in accurately measuring arterial P_{O_2} in patients breathing 100% O_2. Here, essentially all errors cause the value provided by the laboratory to be erroneously low. To minimize this effect, samples should be completely free of air bubbles, immediately placed on ice, and measured within a few minutes. Although this admonition should be respected for all blood samples, it is especially key when F_{IO_2} is high.

Other pitfalls are conceptual. Clinicians understandably desire to simplify gas exchange tests by assuming values for key variables that are hard to measure. Important here is the respiratory exchange ratio (R), which is necessary in calculation of the alveolar-arterial P_{O_2} difference ($P_{O_2}(A-a)$; see Equation 12). Uncertainty in R can cause substantial errors in $P_{O_2}(A-a)$. Furthermore, with its basis in mass conservation principles, appropriate use of this equation is limited to the steady state. If the patient's gas exchange condition is not in a steady state but rather actively in flux, $P_{O_2}(A-a)$ is likely to be uninterpretable.

Similarly, the shunt equation (Equation 14) requires knowledge of mixed venous (i.e., pulmonary arterial) O_2 concentration, C_{VO_2}. Without a direct measurement of this entity using a pulmonary arterial catheter, the value of C_{VO_2} must be assumed, and especially in critically ill patients, this is problematic, causing potentially large errors in calculated shunt. However, using the Fick principle (see Equation 8), C_{VO_2} can be calculated if $\dot{V}_{O_2}$ (oxygen uptake), $\dot{Q}$ (cardiac output), and C_{aO_2} (arterial oxygen concentration) all are measured, considerably improving the reliability of the calculated shunt value.

SUGGESTED READINGS

Davenport HW: *The ABC of acid-base chemistry: the elements of physiological blood-gas chemistry for medical students and physicians*, Chicago, 1974, University of Chicago Press.

Kelman GR: Computer program for the production of O_2-CO_2 diagrams, *Respir Physiol* 4:260–269, 1968.

Olszowka AJ, Farhi LE: A digital computer program for constructing ventilation-perfusion lines, *J Appl Physiol* 26:141–146, 1969.

Rahn H: A concept of mean alveolar air and the ventilation-blood flow relationships during pulmonary gas exchange, *Am J Physiol* 158:21–30, 1949.

Rahn H, Fenn WO: *A graphical analysis of the respiratory gas exchange*, Washington, DC, 1955, American Physiological Society.

Riley RL, Cournand A: "Ideal" alveolar air and the analysis of ventilation-perfusion relationships in the lungs, *J Appl Physiol* 1:825–847, 1949.

Weibel ER: *Morphometry of the human lung*, Heidelberg, 1963, Springer.

Weibel ER, Gil J: Structure-function relationships at the alveolar level. In West JB, editor: *Bioengineering aspects of the lung*, New York, 1977, Marcel Dekker, pp 2–81.

West JB: Causes and compensations for hypoxemia and hypercapnia, *Comp Physiol* 1:1541–1553, 2011.

West JB: *Respiratory physiology: the essentials*, ed 8, Baltimore, 2008, Williams & Wilkins.

West JB: Ventilation-perfusion inequality and overall gas exchange in computer models of the lung, *Respir Physiol* 7:88–110, 1969.

West JB: *Ventilation/bloodflow and gas exchange*, ed 5, Philadelphia, 1990, Lippincott.

Chapter **6**

Control of Ventilation and Respiratory Muscles

Theodoros Vassilakopoulos

The respiratory muscles are the only muscles, along with the heart, that must work continuously, although intermittently, to sustain life. They have to repetitively move a rather complex elastic structure, the thorax, to achieve the entry of air into the lungs and thence effect gas exchange. The presence of multiple muscle groups in this system mandates that these muscles interact properly to perform their task despite their differences in anatomic location, geometric orientation, and motor innervation. They also should be able to adapt to a variety of working conditions and respond to many different chemical and neural stimuli.

This chapter describes some aspects of respiratory muscle function that are relevant to current understanding of the way these muscles accomplish the action of breathing and how their function is controlled by the respiratory centers located in the central nervous system.

THE RESPIRATORY CENTERS

Early studies of the neural control of breathing involved the section and ablation of various brain stem structures. From these studies emerged the classical description of the neural control of breathing that required centers in the medulla for the rhythmic generation of ventilatory drive plus additional areas in the pons (traditionally known as the pneumotaxic and apneustic centers) that modulated and regulated the basic rhythm. Nowadays, the very complex and inadequately explored and understood respiratory center structure and function can be summarized as follows (**Figure 6-1**):

- Primary centers responsible for the generation of respiratory rhythm are located in the medulla. Within the medulla, there are two bilateral aggregations of neurons having respiratory related activity.
  - The *dorsal respiratory group* (DRG) neurons are primarily inspiratory (firing on inspiration) and are located in the nucleus tractus solitarius (NTS). These neurons project contralaterally to the phrenic and intercostal motor neurons in the spinal cord and provide the primary stimulus for respiration. In addition, this region is the recipient of important afferent stimuli, most notably from peripheral and central chemoreceptors and from receptors in the lung. Many connections are present between the dorsal and ventral groups of neurons.
  - The *ventral respiratory group* (VRG) consists of a long column of respiratory neurons, some of which are

inspiratory (firing on inspiration) and some of which are expiratory (firng on expiration). It contains the nucleus ambiguus, which contains primarily inspiratory neurons that project to the larynx, pharynx, and tongue. Stimulation of these neurons causes dilation of the upper airways, which minimizes airway resistance during inspiration. The VRG connects polysynaptically, with inspiratory motor neurons in the thorax at T1 to T12 that transmit the drive to external intercostal muscles, and polysynaptically, with expiratory motor neurons in the thorax and abdomen that supply expiratory muscles such as the internal intercostal and abdominal muscles.

- An area of the ventrolateral medulla next to the nucleus ambiguus, the pre-Bötzinger complex, is hypothesized to be a critical site for respiratory rhythmogenesis. Current theory proposes that a group of pacemaker neurons depolarize, fire, and repolarize in a rhythmic fashion. This endogenous oscillatory activity can be modulated by afferent inputs, generating an efferent output that is translated into the respiratory drive. Apart from the pre-Bötzinger complex principally involved in controlling inspiratory motor activity, the retrotrapezoid-parafacial respiratory group (RTN/pFRG) appears to play at least a modulatory role and may be a conditional oscillator that controls active expiration.

- An additional mechanism is voluntary control of the respiratory muscles, signals for which originate in the motor cortex and pass directly to the spinal motor neurons by way of the corticospinal tracts. The medullary respiratory control center is bypassed. The voluntary control competes with automatic control at the level of the spinal motor neuron.

AFFERENT INPUTS TO THE RESPIRATORY CENTERS

The respiratory controller receives information from a variety of sources. Some of these involve the relatively straightforward chemoreceptor signals that provide closed-loop information on the gas exchange functions of the lung. These signals arise mainly from the central and peripheral chemoreceptors that mediate the response to hypoxia, hypercapnia, and acidemia. In addition, at any given time, many other inputs from the upper airways, the lung, the respiratory muscles, and the thoracic cage may be important in determining ventilatory drive (**Figure 6-2**). The states of cortical arousal, sleep, and emotion play important roles in the level of ventilation and the response to other stimuli.

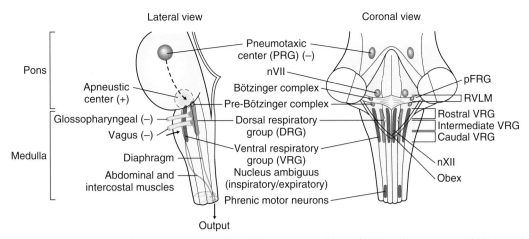

Figure 6-1 The respiratory centers. *nVII,* nucleus of cranial nerve VII; *pFRG,* retrotrapezoid-parafacial respiratory group; *RVLM,* rostral ventrolateral medulla.

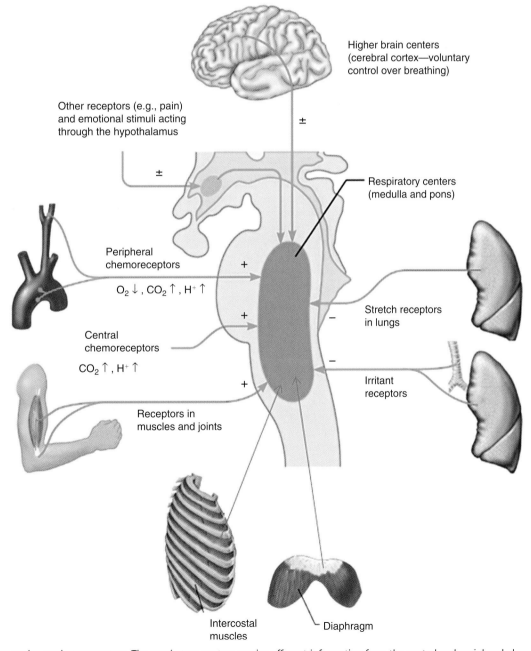

Figure 6-2 Input to the respiratory centers. The respiratory centers receive afferent information from the central and peripheral chemoreceptors, and from various receptors located in the respiratory system and other parts of the body, and input from higher brain centers.

CENTRAL CHEMORECEPTORS

Central chemoreception involves neurons (and glial cells) at many sites within the hindbrain, including, but not limited to, the retrotrapezoid nucleus (glutaminergic neurons), the medullary raphe (serotoninergic neurons), the locus ceruleus (noradrenergic neurons), the nucleus tractus solitarius, the lateral hypothalamus (orexin neurons), and the caudal ventrolateral medulla. Central chemoreception also has an important nonadditive interaction with afferent information arising at the peripheral chemoreceptors (carotid body). The exact role of each area and its relative importance may vary depending on the condition (e.g., sleep versus wakefulness) and is currently not definitely established. The central chemoreceptors respond to either local increases in CO_2 or decreases in pH. However, because the chemoreceptors are located on the brain side of the blood-brain barrier and H^+ ions do not readily cross this barrier, the central chemoreceptors are much more sensitive to increases in $PaCO_2$ than to decreases in blood pH. The central chemoreceptors are not sensitive to blood PO_2.

PERIPHERAL CHEMORECEPTORS

The peripheral chemoreceptors include the carotid bodies and the aortic bodies. The carotid bodies are much more important than the aortic bodies in humans. The peripheral chemoreceptors are sensitive to both hypoxia and hypercapnia or acidosis. The site of chemoreception in the carotid body is the type I glomus cells; the type II cells play more of a supporting role, similar to that of glial cells. The hypoxic response causes a sharp increase in firing rate of the carotid sinus nerve when the PaO_2 is lowered below 60 mm Hg. Signal transduction involves the depolarization of the type I cells (by closing a potassium channel that normally is open at resting membrane potential). After the transduction in the type I cells, the signal is transmitted to the carotid sinus nerve endings. Rather than there being a single neurotransmitter, multiple inhibitory and excitatory neurochemicals function both as classical neurotransmitters and also as neuromodulators. Dopamine is abundant in type I cells but seems to be an inhibitory neurotransmitter. Adenosine triphosphate (ATP), by contrast, functions as the primary excitatory neurotransmitter, perhaps coreleased with acetylcholine.

The Hypercapnic Ventilatory Response

CO_2 is the most important factor in the control of ventilation under normal circumstances. The $PaCO_2$ is held very close to 40 mm Hg, during the course of daily activity with periods of rest and exercise. During sleep, it may vary a little more. Increasing $PaCO_2$ acts through a negative feedback loop to increase alveolar ventilation.

Both the central and peripheral chemoreceptors respond to hypercapnia. The carotid body provides about 20% to 30% of the total hypercapnic response. This response is fast, with a time constant of 10 to 30 seconds. The central chemoreceptor response accounts for about 70% to 80% of the total hypercapnic response but is slower, with a time constant in the range of 60 to 150 seconds. This slow central response requires 5 to 6 minutes of hypercapnia to reach steady-state ventilation. Steady-state ventilation has an apparently linear relationship to increasing $PaCO_2$ (normal values for the hypercapnic ventilatory response slope range between 1 and 2 L/minute/mm Hg of PCO_2). Hypoxia augments the hypercapnic response by shifting the CO_2 response curve to the left and increasing its slope. A number of factors can influence the response to CO_2 (e.g., drugs, sleep-wakefulness).

The Hypoxic Ventilatory Response

The hypoxic ventilatory response is due almost solely to the carotid bodies. Very little ventilatory response occurs until the arterial oxygen is lowered below 60 mm Hg, and then there is a sharp increase, just as in the firing rate of the carotid sinus nerve. Hypercapnia greatly augments the hypoxic response. Hypoxia and hypercapnia interact at the level of the carotid body, and their combination is an extremely powerful stimulus to ventilation.

UPPER AND LOWER RESPIRATORY TRACT RECEPTORS

Important receptors in the lung and the upper respiratory tract provide afferent information to the respiratory centers. This information is used in normal ventilation as well as to initiate maneuvers such as sneezing and coughing that need to override the gas exchanging role of the ventilatory system.

Reflexes from all along the respiratory tract provide information to the respiratory centers that will modify or sometimes even block the respiratory drive. Many of the reflexes of the airway are involved in protection, either through trying to clear the airway of foreign material through sneezing or coughing, or in preventing aspiration by closing the larynx during the swallowing of emesis. *Irritant receptors* are found in the nose and upper airways. They are triggered by nonspecific irritants, and their stimulation leads to reflex apnea. Pharyngeal reflexes are important in maintaining a patent airway. During inspiration, the pressure in the airway is negative, and because no intrinsic structures are present to hold the pharyngeal airway open (as with the tracheal cartilages), muscle tone must provide the counterforces to maintain an open airway. Receptors in the pharynx sense this negative pressure and signal the need for increased drive to the upper airway muscles during inspiration. In obstructive sleep apnea, this reflex may not be sufficient to overcome the forces that collapse the airway during inspiration.

Reflexes in the lower airway (tracheobronchial tree) also are involved in both shaping the ventilatory pattern and protecting the airway. *Rapidly adapting pulmonary stretch receptors* are so named because during constant stimulation they initially fire very rapidly but then soon decrease their firing rate. These receptors are located between airway epithelial cells and are found in abundance throughout the carina and at subsequent bronchial bifurcations. These locales are where contaminants in the inspired air (particles) are most likely to impact because of their mass. They are stimulated by irritant gases, histamine, and rapid or extreme lung inflation. They mediate reflex cough, bronchoconstriction, and hyperpnea. The *slowly adapting pulmonary stretch receptors* are located in airway smooth muscle and carry impulses in the vagus nerve by way of large myelinated fibers. They are activated by high lung volume or bronchoconstriction and mediate the Hering-Breuer reflex (early termination of inspiration, which in humans becomes active at an inspired volume of about 1 to 1.5 L). The *J receptors*, whose impulses are carried in small unmyelinated C fibers of the vagus nerve, have been so called because the nerve endings are found near ("juxta") the alveolus in the walls of pulmonary capillaries or interstitium. They respond to mechanical deformation (e.g., pulmonary edema). Activation of these receptors causes rapid, shallow breathing and dyspnea.

RESPIRATORY MUSCLE–THORACIC CAGE RECEPTORS

Receptors in the respiratory muscles themselves also are very important: tendon organs that sense changes in tension, muscle spindles that sense changes in muscle length, and unmyelinated small afferent fibers that sense metabolic-inflammatory products. These somatic receptors provide information on the length-tension relationship of the respiratory muscles and make essential contributions to control the work of breathing and respiratory loads. In addition to somatic receptors located in the intercostal muscles, rib joints, accessory muscles, and tendons, the output of receptors in other parts of the body, including skeletal muscles, can influence the respiratory pattern. At the onset of exercise, an increase in ventilation occurs that precedes the increase in PCO_2 that would be required for chemoreceptor signals. It is believed that the observed increase in ventilation is mediated by other mechanisms. For example, passively moving the limbs causes an increase in ventilation. The aforementioned somatic receptors presumably account for these observations. The control of ventilation during exercise and with changes in metabolic rate also involves afferent information from temperature and nociceptive receptors.

THE EFFERENT LIMB: THE RESPIRATORY MUSCLES

FUNCTIONAL ANATOMY

The Intercostal Muscles

The intercostal muscles are two thin layers of muscle fibers occupying each of the intercostal spaces. They are termed external and internal because of their surface relations, the external being superficial to the internal. The muscle fibers of the two layers run at approximately right angles to each other. The *external intercostals* extend from the tubercles of the ribs dorsally to the costochondral junctions ventrally, and their fibers are oriented obliquely, downward, and forward, from the rib above to the rib below. The *internal intercostals* begin posteriorly as the posterior intercostal membrane on the inner aspect of the external intercostal muscles. From approximately the angle of the rib, the internal intercostal muscles run obliquely, upward, and forward from the superior border of the rib and costal cartilage below to the floor of the subcostal groove of the rib and the edge of the costal cartilage above,

ending at the sternocostal junctions. All of the intercostal muscles are innervated by the intercostal nerves.

The external intercostal muscles have an inspiratory action on the rib cage, whereas the internal intercostal muscles are expiratory. An illustrative clinical example of the "isolated" inspiratory action of the intercostal muscles is offered by *bilateral diaphragmatic paralysis*. In patients with this deficit, inspiration is accomplished solely by the rib cage muscles. As a result, the rib cage expands during inspiration, and the pleural pressure falls. Because the diaphragm is flaccid and no transdiaphragmatic pressure can be developed, the fall in pleural pressure is transmitted to the abdomen, causing an equal fall in the abdominal pressure. Hence, the abdomen moves paradoxically inward during inspiration, opposing the inflation of the lung (**Figure 6-3**). This paradoxical motion is the cardinal sign of diaphragmatic paralysis on clinical examination and is invariably present in the supine posture, during which the abdominal muscles usually remain relaxed during the entire respiratory cycle. However, this sign may be absent in the erect posture.

The Diaphragm

The floor of the thoracic cavity is closed by a thin musculotendinous sheet, the diaphragm—the most important inspiratory muscle, accounting for approximately 70% of minute ventilation in normal subjects. The diaphragm is anatomically unique among the skeletal muscles in that its fibers radiate from a central tendinous structure (the central tendon) to insert peripherally into skeletal structures. The muscle of the diaphragm has two main components as defined at its point of origin: the crural (vertebral) part and the costal (sternocostal) part. The *crural* part arises from the crura (strong, tapering tendons attached vertically to the anterolateral aspects of the bodies and intervertebral disks of the first three lumbar vertebrae on the right and two on the left) and the three aponeurotic arcuate ligaments. The *costal* part of the diaphragm arises from the xiphoid process and the lower end of the sternum and the costal cartilages of the lower six ribs. These costal fibers run cranially so that they are directly apposed to the inner aspect of lower rib cage, creating a *zone of apposition*.

The shape of the relaxed diaphragm at the end of a normal expiration (at functional residual capacity [FRC]) is that of two domes joined by a "saddle" that runs from the sternum to the

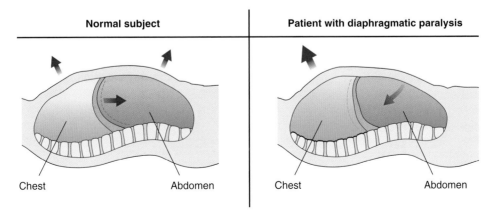

Normal subject	Patient with diaphragmatic paralysis
Chest Abdomen	Chest Abdomen

Figure 6-3 Schematic demonstration of normal abdominal and rib cage movement (*left panel*) and the paradoxical abdominal motion of isolated diaphragmatic paralysis (*right panel*). The diaphragm at resting end expiration is shown as a *solid line* and after inspiration as a *dashed line*. In the normal subject, the diaphragm moves caudally, and in the patient with diaphragmatic paralysis, the diaphragm moves in a cephalic direction. The anterior abdominal wall moves inward instead of outward.

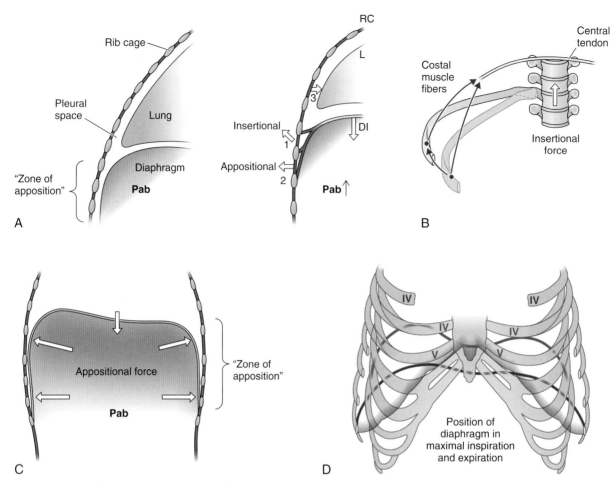

Figure 6-4 Actions of the diaphragm. **A,** Zone of apposition and summary of diaphragmatic actions. When the diaphragm contracts, a caudally oriented force is being applied on the central tendon, and the dome of the diaphragm descends (DI). Furthermore, the costal diaphragmatic fibers apply a cranially oriented force to the upper margins of the lower six ribs that has the effect of lifting and rotating them outward (insertional force, *arrow 1*). The zone of apposition makes the lower rib cage part of the abdomen, and the changes in pressure in the pleural recess between the apposed diaphragm and the rib cage are almost equal to the changes in abdominal pressure *(Pab)*. Pressure in this pleural recess rises rather than falls during inspiration because of diaphragmatic descent, and the rise in abdominal pressure is transmitted through the apposed diaphragm to expand the lower rib cage *(arrow 2)*. All of these effects result in expansion of the lower rib cage. Within the upper rib cage, isolated contraction of the diaphragm causes a decrease in the anteroposterior diameter, and this expiratory action is caused primarily by the fall in pleural pressure *(arrow 3)*. **B,** Insertional force; **C,** appositional force; **D,** shape of the diaphragm and the bony thorax at maximum inspiration and expiration.

anterior surface of the spinal column (**Figure 6-4**). The motor innervation of the diaphragm is from the phrenic nerves, which also provide a proprioceptive supply to the muscle. When tension develops within the diaphragmatic muscle fibers, a caudally oriented force is applied on the central tendon, and the dome of the diaphragm descends; this descent has two effects. First, it expands the thoracic cavity along its craniocaudal axis, and consequently the pleural pressure falls. Second, it produces a caudal displacement of the abdominal visceral contents and an increase in the abdominal pressure, which in turn results in an outward motion of the ventral abdominal wall and the lower rib cage (appositional force). Thus, when the diaphragm contracts, a cranially oriented force is being applied by the costal diaphragmatic fibers to the upper margins of the lower six ribs that has the effect of lifting and rotating them outward (insertional force) (see Figure 6-4). The actions mediated by the changes in pleural and abdominal pressures are more complex. Viewed as the only muscle acting on the rib cage, the diaphragm has two opposing effects when it contracts: On the upper rib cage, it causes a decrease in the anteroposterior diameter, and this expiratory action results primarily from the fall in pleural pressure (see Figure 6-4). On the lower rib cage, it causes an expansion. In fact, this is the pattern of chest wall motion observed in *tetraplegic patients* with transection injury at the fifth cervical segment of the spinal cord or below, who have complete paralysis of the inspiratory muscles except for the diaphragm. This inspiratory action on the lower rib cage is caused by the concomitant action of two different forces, the "insertional" force already described and the "appositional" force.

The Sternocleidomastoids

The sternocleidomastoids arise from the mastoid process and descend to the ventral surface of the manubrium sterni and the medial third of the clavicle. Their neural supply is from the accessory nerve. The action of the sternocleidomastoids is to displace the sternum cranially during inspiration, to expand the upper rib cage more in its anteroposterior diameter than in its transverse one, and to decrease the transverse diameter of the lower rib cage. In normal subjects breathing at rest, however, the sternocleidomastoids are inactive, being recruited only when the inspiratory muscle pump is abnormally loaded or when ventilation increases substantially. Therefore, they should be considered to be accessory muscles of inspiration.

The Scalenes

The scalenes are composed of three muscle bundles that run from the transverse processes of the lower five cervical vertebrae to the upper surface of the first two ribs. They receive their neural supply mainly from the lower five cervical segments. Their action is to increase (slightly) the anteroposterior diameter of the upper rib cage. Although initially regarded as accessory muscles of inspiration, they are invariably active during inspiration. In fact, seated normal subjects cannot breathe without contracting the scalenes even when they reduce the required inspiratory effort by reducing tidal volume. Therefore, scalenes in humans are primary muscles of inspiration, and their contraction is an important determinant of the expansion of the upper rib cage during breathing.

The Abdominal Muscles

The abdominal muscles with respiratory activity are those constituting the ventrolateral wall of the abdomen (i.e., the rectus abdominis ventrally and the external oblique, internal oblique, and transversus abdominis laterally). They are innervated by the lower six thoracic nerves and the first lumbar nerve. As they contract, they pull the abdominal wall inward, thus increasing the intraabdominal pressure. This in turn causes the diaphragm to move cranially into the thoracic cavity, increasing the pleural pressure and decreasing lung volume. Thus, their action is expiratory. Expiration usually is a passive process but can become active when minute ventilation has to be increased (e.g., during exercise) or during respiratory distress. Expiratory muscle action also is essential during cough.

PHYSIOLOGY: THE ABILITY TO BREATHE: THE LOAD-CAPACITY BALANCE

For a person to take a spontaneous breath, the inspiratory muscles must generate sufficient force to overcome the elastance of the lungs and chest wall (lung and chest wall elastic loads), as well as the airway and tissue resistance (resistive load). This effort requires an adequate output of the centers controlling the muscles, anatomic and functional nerve integrity, unimpaired neuromuscular transmission, an intact chest wall, and adequate muscle strength. The mechanisms involved can be schematically represented by considering the ability to take a breath as a balance between inspiratory load and neuromuscular competence (**Figure 6-5**). Under normal conditions, this system is polarized in favor of neuromuscular competence (i.e., there are reserves that permit considerable increases in load). For spontaneous breathing, however, the inspiratory muscles should be able to sustain the aforementioned load over time as well as adjusting the minute ventilation to afford adequate gas exchange. The ability of the respiratory muscles to sustain this load without the onset of fatigue is called endurance and is determined by the balance between energy supply and energy demand (**Figure 6-6**).

Energy supply depends on the inspiratory muscle blood flow, the blood substrate (fuel) concentration and arterial oxygen content, the muscle's ability to extract and use energy sources, and the muscle's energy stores. Under normal circumstances, energy supply is adequate to meet the demand, and a large recruitable reserve exists (see Figure 6-6). Energy demand increases proportionally with the mean pressure developed by the inspiratory muscles per breath (P_I), expressed as a fraction of maximum pressure that the respiratory muscles can voluntarily develop ($P_I/P_{I_{max}}$), the minute ventilation ($\dot{V}_E$), the inspiratory duty cycle (T_I/T_{TOT}), and the mean inspiratory flow rate

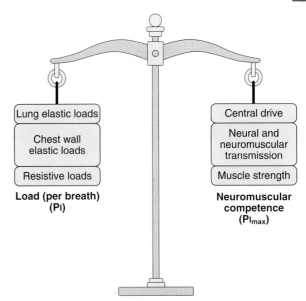

Figure 6-5 Balance between inspiratory load and neuromuscular competence. The ability to take a spontaneous breath is determined by the balance between the load imposed on the respiratory system (pressure developed by the inspiratory muscles, P_I) and the neuromuscular competence of the ventilatory pump (maximum inspiratory pressure; $P_{I_{max}}$). Normally, this balance weighs in favor of competence, permitting significant increases in load. However, if the competence is, for whatever reason, reduced below a critical point (e.g., drug overdose, myasthenia gravis), the balance may then weigh in favor of load, rendering the ventilatory pump insufficient to inflate the lungs and chest wall. *(Modified from Vassilakopoulos T, Roussos C: Neuromuscular respiratory failure. In Slutsky A, Takala R, Torres R, editors: Clinical critical care medicine, St. Louis, 2006, Mosby.)*

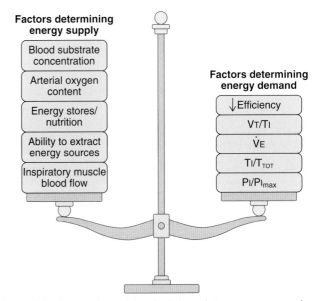

Figure 6-6 Factors determining the balance between energy supply and energy demand in maintaining neurorespiratory capacity. Respiratory muscle endurance is determined by the adequacy of energy for ventilatory needs. Normally, the supply is adequate to meet the demand, and a large reserve exists. Whenever this balance weighs in favor of demand, the respiratory muscles ultimately become fatigued, leading to inability to sustain spontaneous breathing. $P_I/P_{I_{max}}$, inspiratory pressure–maximum inspiratory pressure ratio; T_I/T_{TOT}, duty cycle (ratio of fraction of inspiration to total breathing cycle duration); $\dot{V}_E$, minute ventilation; V_T/T_I, mean inspiratory flow (tidal volume–inspiratory time ratio). *(Modified from Vassilakopoulos T, Roussos C: Neuromuscular respiratory failure. In Slutsky A, Takala R, Torres R, editors: Clinical critical care medicine, St. Louis, 2006, Mosby.)*

(V_T/T_I) and is inversely related to the efficiency of the muscles. Fatigue develops when the mean rate of energy demands exceeds the mean rate of energy supply (i.e., when the balance is polarized in favor of demands).

The product of T_I/T_{TOT} and the mean transdiaphragmatic pressure expressed as a fraction of maximal transdiaphragmatic pressure (Pdi/Pdi_{max}) defines a useful "tension-time index" (TTIdi) that is related to the endurance time (i.e., the time that the diaphragm can sustain the load imposed on it). Whenever TTIdi is smaller than the critical value of 0.15, the load can be sustained indefinitely, but when TTIdi exceeds the critical zone of 0.15 to 0.18, the load can be sustained for only a limited period—in other words, the endurance time. This variable was found to be inversely related to TTIdi. The TTI concept is assumed to be applicable not only to the diaphragm but also to the respiratory muscles as a whole:

$$TTI = P_I/P_{I_{max}} \times T_I/T_{TOT}$$

Because endurance is determined by the balance between energy supply and demand, TTI of the inspiratory muscles has to be in accordance with the energy balance view. In fact, as Figure 6-6 demonstrates, $P_I/P_{I_{max}}$ and T_I/T_{TOT}, which constitute the TTI, are among the determinants of energy demand; an increase in either that will increase the TTI value also will increase the demand. But what determines the ratio $P_I/P_{I_{max}}$? The numerator, the mean inspiratory pressure developed per breath, is determined by the elastic and resistive loads imposed on the inspiratory muscles. The denominator, the maximum inspiratory pressure, is determined by the neuromuscular competence (i.e., the maximum inspiratory muscle activation that can be voluntarily achieved). It follows, then, that the value of $P_I/P_{I_{max}}$ is determined by the balance between load and competence (see Figure 6-5). But $P_I/P_{I_{max}}$ also is one of the determinants of energy demand (see Figure 6-6); therefore, the two balances (i.e., between load and competence and between energy supply and demand) are in essence linked, creating a single system (**Figure 6-7**). Schematically, when the central hinge of the system moves upward or is at least at the horizontal level, spontaneous ventilation can be sustained indefinitely

(see Figure 6-7). The ability of a subject to breathe spontaneously depends on the fine interplay of many different factors. Normally, this interplay moves the central hinge far upward and creates a great ventilatory reserve for the healthy person. When the central hinge of the system, for whatever reason, moves downward, spontaneous ventilation cannot be sustained, and ventilatory failure ensues.

HYPERINFLATION

Hyperinflation (frequently observed in obstructive airway diseases) compromises the force-generating capacity of the diaphragm for a variety of reasons: First, the respiratory muscles, like other skeletal muscles, obey the length-tension relationship. At any given level of activation, changes in muscle fiber length alter tension development. This is because the force-tension developed by a muscle depends on the interaction between actin and myosin fibrils (i.e., the number of myosin heads attaching and thus pulling the actin fibrils closer within each sarcomere). The optimal fiber length (Lo) for which tension is maximal is the length at which all myosin heads attach and pull the actin fibrils. Below this length (as with hyperinflation, which shortens the diaphragm), actin-myosin interaction becomes suboptimal, and tension development declines. Second, as lung volume increases, the zone of apposition of the diaphragm decreases in size, and a larger fraction of the rib cage becomes exposed to pleural pressure. Hence, the diaphragm's inspiratory action on the rib cage diminishes. When lung volume approaches total lung capacity, the zone of apposition all but disappears (**Figure 6-8**), and the diaphragmatic muscle fibers become oriented horizontally internally (see Figure 6-8). The insertional force of the diaphragm is then expiratory, rather than inspiratory, in direction. This observation explains the inspiratory decrease in the transverse diameter of the lower rib cage in subjects with emphysema and severe hyperinflation (Hoover's sign). Third, the resultant flattening of the diaphragm increases its radius of curvature (Rdi) and, according to Laplace's law, $Pdi = 2Tdi/Rdi$, diminishes its pressure-generating capacity (Pdi) for the same tension development (Tdi).

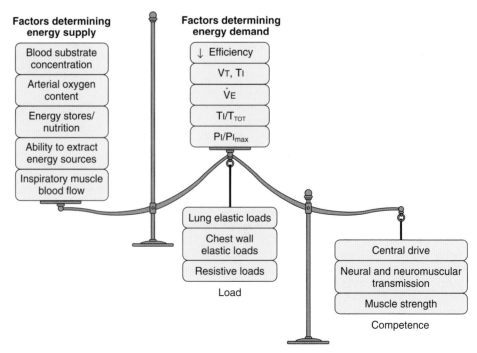

Figure 6-7 Factors determining the two aspects of balance in the system maintaining neurorespiratory capacity: (1) load and competence and (2) energy supply and demand. The relationship between these system components is depicted schematically. The $P_I/P_{I_{max}}$, one of the determinants of energy demand (see Figure 6-6), is replaced by its equivalent: the balance between load and neuromuscular competence (see Figure 6-5). In fact, this correlation is the reason the two balances are linked. When the central hinge of the system moves upward or is at least at the horizontal level, a balance exists between ventilatory needs and neurorespiratory capacity, and spontaneous ventilation can be sustained. In healthy persons, the hinge moves far upward, creating a large reserve. For abbreviations, see legends to Figures 6-5 and 6-6. *(Modified from Vassilakopoulos T, Roussos C: Neuromuscular respiratory failure. In Slutsky A, Takala R, Torres R, editors:* Clinical critical care medicine, *St. Louis, 2006, Mosby.)*

Factors determining energy supply

- Blood substrate concentration
- Arterial oxygen content
- Energy stores/ nutrition
- Ability to extract energy sources
- Inspiratory muscle blood flow

Factors determining energy demand

- ↓ Efficiency
- V_T, T_I
- $\dot{V}_E$
- T_I/T_{TOT}
- $P_I/P_{I_{max}}$

Lung elastic loads
Chest wall elastic loads
Resistive loads

Load

Central drive
Neural and neuromuscular transmission
Muscle strength

Competence

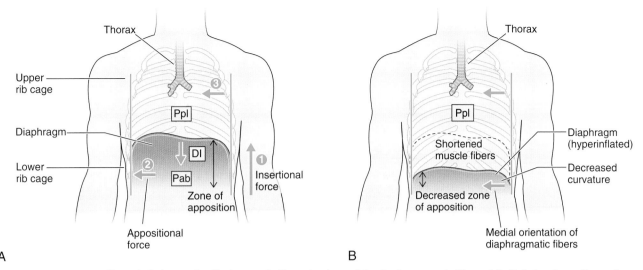

Figure 6-8 Consequences of hyperinflation on the diaphragm. **A,** Normal actions of the diaphragm, as in Figure 6-2. **B,** Deleterious effects of hyperinflation on the diaphragm. *DI*, diaphragmatic force; *Pab*, abdominal pressure; *Ppl*, pleural pressure.

RESPIRATORY MUSCLE RESPONSES TO CHANGES IN LOAD

ACUTE RESPONSES TO INCREASED LOAD

Respiratory Muscle Fatigue

Fatigue is defined as the loss of capacity to develop force and/or velocity in response to a load that is reversible by rest. Fatigue should be distinguished from weakness, in which reduced force generation is fixed and not reversed by rest, although the presence of weakness may itself predispose a muscle to fatigue. The site and mechanisms of fatigue remain controversial. Theoretically, the site of fatigue may be located at any link in the long chain of events involved in voluntary muscle contraction leading from the brain to the contractile machinery. A widely used convention is to classify fatigue as central fatigue, peripheral high-frequency fatigue, or peripheral low-frequency fatigue.

Central fatigue is present when a maximal voluntary contraction generates less force than does maximal electrical stimulation. If maximal electrical stimulation superimposed on a maximal voluntary contraction can potentiate the force generated by a muscle, a component of central fatigue exists. This procedure applied to the diaphragm consists of the *twitch occlusion test*, which may separate central from peripheral fatigue. This test examines the transdiaphragmatic pressure (Pdi) response to bilateral phrenic nerve stimulation superimposed on graded voluntary contractions of the diaphragm. Normally, the amplitude of the Pdi twitches in response to phrenic nerve stimulation decreases as the voluntary Pdi increases. During Pdi_{max}, no superimposed twitches can be detected. When central diaphragmatic fatigue is present, superimposed twitches can be demonstrated. A number of experiments have suggested that a form of central diaphragmatic "fatigue" may develop during respiratory loading such that, at the limits of diaphragmatic endurance, a significant portion of the reduction in force production is due to failure of the central nervous system to completely activate the diaphragm. Central fatigue may be caused by a reduction in the number of motor units that can be recruited by the motor drive or by a decrease in motor unit discharge rates, or both. The observed decreased central firing rate during fatigue may in fact be a beneficial

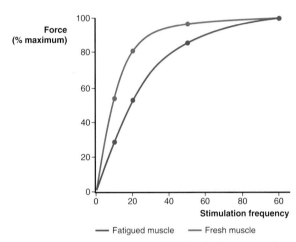

Figure 6-9 Force-frequency relationship of in vivo human respiratory muscles. The force-frequency curve for fresh muscle is shown in *red*, and that for muscle after a fatiguing task is shown in *blue*; a disproportionate force loss at low stimulation frequencies is evident. *(Modified from Moxham J, Wiles CM, Newham D, Edwards RH: Contractile function and fatigue of the respiratory muscles in man, Ciba Found Symp 82:197–212, 1981.)*

adaptive response preventing the muscle's self-destruction by excessive activation.

Peripheral fatigue refers to failure at the neuromuscular junction or distal to this structure and is present when muscle force output falls in response to direct electrical stimulation. This type of fatigue may occur as a consequence of failure of impulse propagation across the neuromuscular junction, the sarcolemma or the T tubules (transmission fatigue), impaired excitation-contraction coupling, or failure of the contractile apparatus of the muscle fibers. Peripheral fatigue can be further classified into high- and low-frequency types on the basis of the shape of the muscle force-frequency curve (**Figure 6-9**). High-frequency fatigue results in depression of the forces generated by a muscle in response to high-frequency electrical stimulation (50 to 100 Hz), whereas low-frequency fatigue results in depression of force generation in response to low-frequency stimuli (1 to 20 Hz). *High-frequency fatigue* (see Figure 6-9) is attributed to transmission fatigue. Teleologically, transmission block could be beneficial in some instances by protecting the muscle against excessive depletion of its ATP stores. Normal subjects breathing against high-intensity inspiratory resistive loads develop high-frequency fatigue, which resolves very quickly after cessation of the strenuous diaphragmatic contractions.

When the loss of force is not accompanied by a parallel decline in the electrical activity, impaired excitation-contraction coupling is thought to be responsible. This type of fatigue is characterized by a selective loss of force at low frequencies of stimulation (see Figure 6-9) despite maintenance of the force generated at high frequencies of stimulation, indicating that the contractile proteins continue to generate force so long as sufficient calcium is released by the sarcoplasmic reticulum. This *low-frequency fatigue* is characteristically long-lasting, with recovery occurring over several hours. Low-frequency fatigue occurs during high-force contractions and is less likely to develop when the forces generated are smaller, even if these are maintained for longer time periods, thereby achieving the same total work. As previously stated, fatigue develops when the mean rate of energy demands exceeds the mean rate of energy supply to the muscle (see Figure 6-6), resulting in depletion of muscle energy stores, acidosis from lactate accumulation, and excessive production of oxygen-derived free radicals. The exact interplay of all of these factors is not yet identified. Low-frequency fatigue occurs in the diaphragm of experimental animals during cardiogenic or septic shock, and in the diaphragm and sternocleidomastoid of normal subjects after breathing against very high inspiratory resistance or after sustaining maximum voluntary ventilation (for 2 minutes) (**Figure 6-10**). The clinical relevance of respiratory muscle fatigue is difficult to ascertain, because performing the measurements that are required for fatigue detection is problematic in situations in which fatigue is likely to be present (such as during acute hypercapnic respiratory failure).

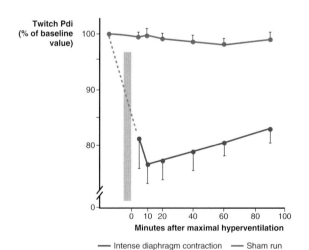

Figure 6-10 Low-frequency fatigue of the diaphragm in normal subjects. The mean twitch tension (i.e., twitch transdiaphragmatic pressure [Pdi]) is shown before and at intervals up to 90 minutes after intense diaphragmatic contraction (in this case, a 2-minute period of maximal normocapnic hyperventilation) in nine healthy adults (*blue symbols*). Data after a sham ("normal breathing") run in the same subjects are shown in *red*. A significant decline in twitch Pdi is observed that has only partially recovered at 90 minutes, which confirms the presence of low-frequency diaphragmatic fatigue. (*Data from Hamnegård CH, Wragg SD, Kyroussis D, et al: Diaphragm fatigue following maximal ventilation in man, Eur Respir J 9:241-247, 1996.*)

INFLAMMATION AND INJURY

Strenuous diaphragmatic contractions (induced by resistive breathing, which accompanies many disease states such as chronic obstructive pulmonary disease [COPD] and asthma) initiate an inflammatory response consisting of elevation of plasma cytokines and recruitment and activation of white blood cell subpopulations. These cytokines are produced within the diaphragm secondary to the increased muscle activation. Strenuous resistive breathing results in diaphragmatic ultrastructural injury (such as sarcomere disruption, necrotic fibers, flocculent degeneration, and influx of inflammatory cells) in both animals and humans. The mechanisms involved are not definitively established but may involve intradiaphragmatic cytokine induction, adhesion molecule upregulation, calpain activation, and reactive oxygen species formation. Cytokines also are essential in orchestrating muscle recovery after injury by enhancing proteolytic removal of damaged proteins and cells (through recruitment and activation of phagocytes) and by activating satellite cells. Satellite cells are quiescent cells of embryonic origin that reside in the muscle and are transformed into myocytes when the muscle becomes injured, to replace damaged myocytes.

CHRONIC RESPONSES TO INCREASED LOAD

Plasticity and Adaptation

The respiratory muscles are plastic organs that respond with structural and functional changes or adaptations to chronic changes in the load they are facing and thus in their activity.

COPD is the paradigm of a disease characterized by chronically increased respiratory muscle load. A major adaptation of the respiratory muscles is fiber type transformation. The myosin heavy chain component of the myosin molecule constitutes the basis for the classification of muscle fibers as either type I or type II (**Figure 6-11**). Myosin heavy chain exists in various isoforms, which in increasing order of maximum shortening velocity are myosin heavy chain (MHC) I, IIa, and IIb, the last type being the fastest (see Figure 6-11). The diaphragm in healthy humans is composed of approximately 50% type I fatigue-resistant fibers, 25% type IIa, and 25% type IIb. Muscles can modify their overall MHC phenotype in two ways: (1) preferential atrophy or hypertrophy of fibers containing a specific MHC isoform and (2) actual transformation from one fiber type to another. In COPD, a transformation of type II to type I fibers occurs, resulting in a great predominance of type I fatigue-resistant fibers. This altered makeup increases the resistance of the diaphragm to fatigue development but at the same time compromises the force-generating capacity, because type I fibers can generate less force than type II fibers can.

Adaptation is not restricted to only fiber type transformation. In an animal model of COPD (in emphysematous hamsters), the number and the length of sarcomeres decrease, resulting in a leftward shift of the length-tension curve, so that the muscle adapts to the shorter operating length induced by hyperinflation. These alterations may help restore the mechanical advantage of the diaphragm in chronically hyperinflated states. In humans, this adaptation seems to occur by sarcomere length shortening.

Respiratory Muscle Response to Inactivity: Unloading

Respiratory muscles adapt not only when they function against increased load but also when they become inactive, as happens

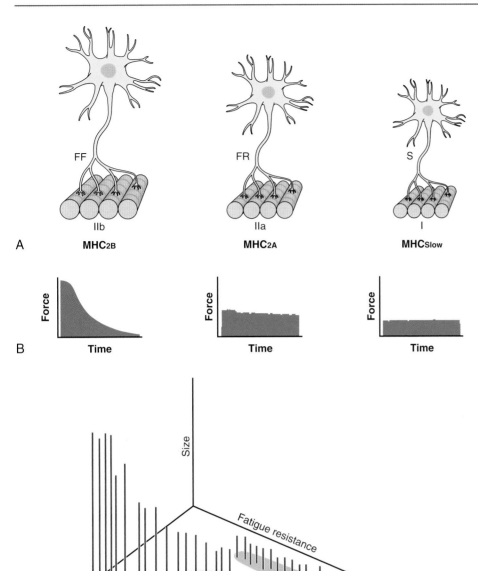

Figure 6-11 Properties of skeletal muscle fiber types. Different fiber types in the diaphragm muscle are distinguished by size, myosin heavy chain content, contractile characteristics (force and speed of contraction), and fatigue resistance (type S, slow; type FR, fast-twitch, fatigue-resistant; and type FF motor units, fast-twitch, fatigable—types I, IIa, and IIb, respectively), as well as myosin heavy chain (MHC) isoform expression (MHCSlow, MHC2A, and MHC2B). **A,** Size; **B,** force; **C,** size-speed of contraction-fatigue resistance. *(Modified from Mantilla CB, Sieck GS: Mechanisms underlying motor unit plasticity in the respiratory system,* J Appl Physiol *94:1230-1241, 2003; and Jones DA: Skeletal muscle physiology. In Roussos C, editor:* The thorax, *ed 2, New York, 1995, Marcel Dekker, pp 3-32.)*

during denervation or when a mechanical ventilator takes over their role as force generator to create the driving pressure permitting airflow into the lungs. Inactivity and unloading of the diaphragm associated with mechanical ventilation are harmful, resulting in decreased diaphragmatic force-generating capacity, diaphragmatic atrophy, and diaphragmatic injury. This combination of effects has been designated *ventilator-induced diaphragmatic dysfunction* (VIDD). The mechanisms are not fully explained, but muscle atrophy, oxidative stress, structural injury, and muscle fiber remodeling contribute to a variable extent in the development of VIDD.

TESTING RESPIRATORY MUSCLE FUNCTION

Muscles have two functions: to develop force and to shorten. In the respiratory system, *force* usually is estimated as pressure and *shortening* as lung volume change.

VITAL CAPACITY

Vital capacity (VC) is easily measured with spirometry; decreases in VC point to respiratory muscle weakness. The VC averages approximately 50 mL/kg in normal adults. VC changes are not specific, however, and decreases may result from both inspiratory and expiratory muscle weakness and may be associated with restrictive lung and chest wall diseases. A marked fall (of greater than 30%) in VC in the supine compared with that in the erect posture (which in the normal person is 5% to 10%) is associated with severe bilateral diaphragmatic weakness.

MAXIMAL STATIC MOUTH PRESSURES

Measurement of the maximum static inspiratory (PI_{max}) or expiratory (PE_{max}) pressure that a subject can generate at the mouth is a simple way to estimate inspiratory and expiratory

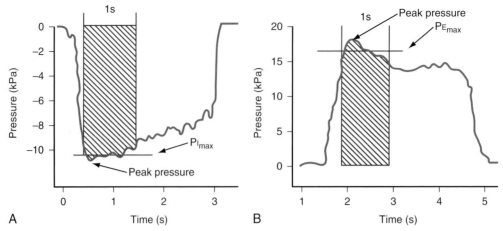

Figure 6-12 Maximum inspiratory-expiratory pressures. **A,** Pressure tracing from a subject performing a maximal inspiratory maneuver (PI_{max}). A peak pressure is seen, and the 1-second average is determined by calculating the *shaded area*. **B,** Typical pressure tracing from a subject performing a maximal expiratory maneuver (PE_{max}). *(Modified from American Thoracic Society/European Respiratory Society: ATS/ERS statement on respiratory muscle testing, Am J Respir Crit Care Med 166:518-624, 2002.)*

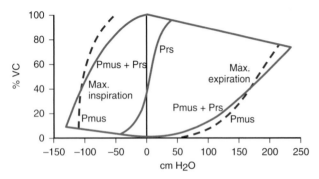

Figure 6-13 Relationship of muscle and respiratory pressures at different lung volumes. *Vertical axis* represents lung volume as a percentage of vital capacity (% VC). *Horizontal axis* represents alveolar pressure in cm H_2O. The *broken lines* indicate the pressure contributed by the muscles. *Pmus,* pressure developed by the respiratory muscles; *Prs,* pressure of the respiratory system. *(Modified from Agostoni E, Mead J: Statics of the respiratory system. In Fenn WO, Rahn H, editors: Handbook of physiology: respiration, vol 1, section 3, Washington, DC, 1964, American Physiological Society, pp 387-409.)*

muscle strength. These pressures are measured at the side port of a mouthpiece that is occluded at the distal end. A small leak is incorporated to prevent glottic closure and buccal muscle use during inspiratory or expiratory maneuvers. The pressure must be maintained for at least 1.5 seconds, so that the maximum pressure sustained for 1 second can be recorded (**Figure 6-12**). The pressure measured during these maneuvers (Pmo) reflects the pressure developed by the respiratory muscles (Pmus), plus the passive elastic recoil pressure of the respiratory system including the lung and chest wall (Prs) (**Figure 6-13**). At FRC, Prs is 0, so Pmo represents Pmus. However, at residual volume (RV), where PI_{max} usually is measured, Prs may be as much as 30 cm H_2O and thus makes a significant contribution to PI_{max} of up to 30% (or more if Pmus is decreased). Similarly, PE_{max} is measured at total lung capacity (TLC), where Prs can be up to 40 cm H_2O. Clinical measures and normal values of PI_{max} and PE_{max} do not conventionally subtract the elastic recoil of the respiratory system. Normal values are available for adults, children, and elderly persons. The tests are easy to perform and well tolerated, yet they are associated with significant between- and within-subject variability, as well as learning effect.

Nevertheless, a PI_{max} of −80 cm H_2O usually excludes clinically important inspiratory muscle weakness.

TRANSDIAPHRAGMATIC PRESSURE

When inspiratory muscle weakness is confirmed, the next diagnostic step is to unravel whether the underlying problem is diaphragmatic weakness, because the diaphragm is the most important inspiratory muscle. This determination is accomplished by the measurement of maximum transdiaphragmatic pressure (Pdi_{max}). Pdi_{max} is the difference between gastric pressure (reflecting abdominal pressure) and esophageal pressure (reflecting intrapleural pressure) on a maximal inspiratory effort after the insertion of appropriate balloon catheters in the stomach and the esophagus, respectively.

SNIFF PRESSURES

A *sniff* is a short, sharp voluntary inspiratory maneuver performed through one or both unoccluded nostrils. It achieves rapid, fully coordinated recruitment of the diaphragm and other inspiratory muscles. The nose acts as a Starling resistor, so nasal flow is low and largely independent of the driving pressure that is the esophageal pressure. Pdi measured during a sniff (sniff Pdi) reflects diaphragm strength, and Pes reflects the integrated pressure of the inspiratory muscles on the lungs (sniff Pes) (**Figure 6-14**). Pressures measured in the mouth, nasopharynx, or one nostril give a clinically useful approximation of esophageal pressure during sniffs without the need to insert esophageal balloons, especially in the absence of significant obstructive airway disease.

The nasal sniff pressure is the easiest measurement for the subject. Pressure is measured by wedging a catheter in one nostril by use of foam, rubber bungs, or dental impression molding (**Figure 6-15**). The subject sniffs through the contralateral unobstructed nostril. A wide range of normal values has been documented, reflecting the variability in normal muscle strength from person to person. In clinical practice, Pdi,sn_{max} values greater than 100 cm H_2O in males and 80 cm H_2O in females are unlikely to be associated with clinically significant diaphragm weakness. Values of maximal sniff esophageal or nasal pressure greater than 70 cm H_2O (in males) or 60 cm

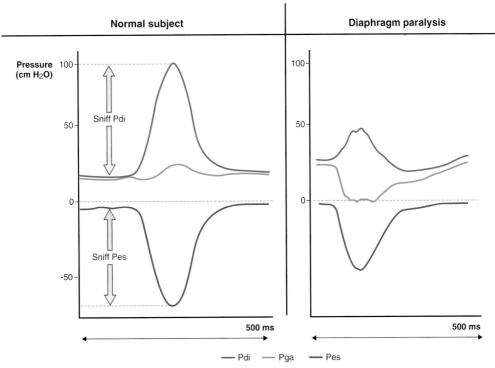

Figure 6-14   Examples of the sniff maneuver. *Left panel* shows a recording from a healthy subject. Note that the esophageal (pleural) pressure change is subatmospheric, whereas the intraabdominal pressure becomes more positive. Measurement conventions for the sniff esophageal (sniff Pes) and sniff transdiaphragmatic (sniff Pdi) pressures are illustrated. The *right panel* shows a recording from a patient with bilateral diaphragmatic paralysis. Note that there is now a negative pressure change in the abdominal compartment, because the diaphragm fails to prevent pressure transmission from the thorax.

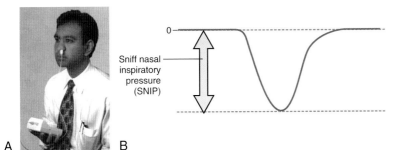

Figure 6-15   The sniff maneuver. A nasal bung and an adapted pressure meter are used for this test. **A,** Measurement setup. The meter returns a numerical value that represents the amplitude of the pressure swing between atmospheric (0) pressure and the nadir. **B,** The tracing produced. The meter returns a numerical value that is the amplitude of the pressure swing between atmospheric (0) pressure and the nadir.

H_2O (in females) also are unlikely to be associated with significant inspiratory muscle weakness.

ELECTROPHYSIOLOGIC TESTING

Electrophysiologic testing helps in determining whether weakness is due to muscle, nerve, or neuromuscular transmission impairment. This determination requires the measurement of Pdi in response to bilateral supramaximal phrenic nerve electrical or magnetic stimulation, with concurrent recording of the elicited electromyogram (EMG) at the diaphragm—the compound muscle action potential (CMAP)—with either surface or esophageal electrodes (**Figure 6-16**).

If the phrenic nerve is stimulated, the diaphragm contracts. Each contraction is called a twitch. If the stimulus is intense enough, all phrenic fibers are activated synchronously, giving reproducible results. The intensity of the twitch increases with the frequency of stimulation. If multiple impulses stimulate the phrenic nerve, the contractions summate to cause a tetanic contraction. Thus, if both phrenic nerves are stimulated with various frequencies (1, 10, 20, 50, and 100 Hz) at the same lung volume with closed airway (to prevent entry of air with consequent changes in lung volume and initial length of the diaphragm), the isometric *force-frequency curve* of the diaphragm is obtained (see Figure 6-9). Stimulation of the phrenic nerve with high frequencies is technically difficult to achieve (because of displacement of the stimulating electrode by local contraction of the scalene muscles and movement of the arm and shoulder due to activation of the brachial plexus). Therefore, the transdiaphragmatic pressure developed in response to single supramaximal phrenic nerve stimulation at 1 Hz, called the *twitch Pdi*, is commonly measured. Although technically demanding, this approach has the great advantage of being independent of patient effort or motivation. The twitch Pdi also allows for the measurement of *phrenic nerve conduction time*, or *phrenic latency* (i.e., the time between the onset of the stimulus and the onset of CMAP [M wave] on the diaphragmatic EMG tracing) (see Figure 6-16, *B*). A prolonged conduction time suggests nerve involvement.

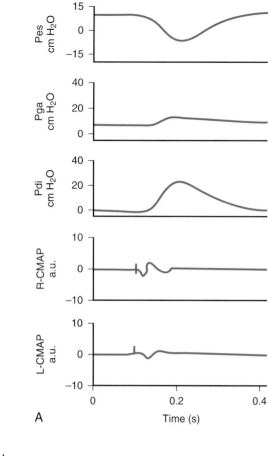

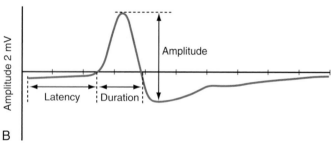

Figure 6-16 Electrophysiologic testing: The "twitch Pdi." **A,** The twitch transdiaphragmatic pressure (Pdi) after magnetic or electrical stimulation. **B,** A detailed (enlarged) view of a compound muscle action potential (M wave), in which the latency (time from stimulus to muscle depolarization), the duration, and the amplitude of the electromyogram are evident. *a.u.,* arbitrary units; *L-CMAP,* left compound motor action potential; *Pes,* esophageal pressure; *Pga,* gastric pressure; *R-CMAP,* right compound motor action potential. *(Modified from Vassilakopoulos T, Roussos C: Neuromuscular respiratory failure. In Slutsky A, Takala R, Torres R, editors: Clinical critical care medicine, St. Louis, 2006, Mosby.)*

CONTROVERSIES AND PITFALLS

- The actual mechanisms of respiratory rhythmogenesis have not been definitively established. When the pre-Bötzinger complex was discovered, it was hypothesized to be the sole generator of respiratory rhythm. Subsequent work suggested the presence of a second respiratory rhythm generator, located rostral to the pre-Bötzinger complex in the region of the retrotrapezoid nucleus–parafacial respiratory group (RTN/pFRG) and functioning primarily as a conditional oscillator for generating expiratory motor output; this model is the core of the "two-oscillator" hypothesis. The existence

of a second respiratory oscillator is still controversial, and whether it persists into adulthood also is still debated (although with waning intensity).

- Still to be determined within the framework of respiratory rhythm generation is whether single pacemaker neurons in the pre-Bötzinger complex generate the respiratory rhythm or whether the pre-Bötzinger complex network functions as a self-organized group pacemaker, wherein individual pacemaker neurons can be embedded but are not essential for emergent network rhythms that depend on connectivity and synaptically activated burst-generating currents. So-called emergent systems are widespread in biology. They consist of autonomous agents that interact according to simple rules and produce meaningful population-level behaviors. When these behaviors are rhythmic, the underlying network always incorporates two essential features: positive feedback, which serves to coordinate individual elements and promote the formation of a collective temporal pattern, and negative feedback, which can temporarily halt or reverse the assembly process fueled by positive feedback. These processes, by their nature, alternate. The rhythms are called *emergent* because individual agents interact in accordance with simple rules, but none possesses a blueprint for the collective behavior that results.

- The clinical relevance of respiratory muscle fatigue is controversial. Physicians usually institute noninvasive or invasive mechanical ventilation in patients presenting with conditions in which the load the respiratory muscles are facing is fatiguing, because clinical signs of severe respiratory distress (such as tachypnea, accessory muscle use, and diaphoresis) develop before respiratory muscle fatigue is established. Furthermore, the objective diagnosis of respiratory muscle fatigue is impractical in the clinical arena (such as the emergency department), because the required electrophysiologic testing is time-consuming and technically demanding, which makes it hard to implement in acutely dyspneic patients with respiratory distress.

- With most volitional tests of respiratory muscle function, a significant learning effect is characteristic. Thus, repeat testing is required before the diagnosis of respiratory muscle weakness is established, especially in elderly persons or in patients for whom cooperation may be difficult.

SUGGESTED READINGS

American Thoracic Society/European Respiratory Society: ATS/ERS statement on respiratory muscle testing, *Am J Respir Crit Care Med* 166:518–624, 2002.

Mantilla CB, Sieck GS: Invited review: mechanisms underlying motor unit plasticity in the respiratory system, *J Appl Physiol* 94:1230–1241, 2003.

Roussos C, Zakynthinos S: Fatigue of the respiratory muscles, *Intensive Care Med* 22:134–155, 1996.

Vassilakopoulos T: Ventilator-induced diaphragmatic dysfunction: the clinical relevance of animal models, *Intensive Care Med* 34:7–16, 2008.

Vassilakopoulos T, Roussos C: Neuromuscular respiratory failure. In Slutsky A, Takala R, Torres R, editors: *Clinical critical care medicine,* St. Louis, 2006, Mosby, pp 275–282.

Vassilakopoulos T, Roussos C, Zakynthinos S: The immune response to resistive breathing, *Eur Respir J* 24:1033–1043, 2004.

Vassilakopoulos T, Zakynthinos S, Roussos C: Respiratory muscles and weaning failure, *Eur Respir J* 9:2383–2400, 1996.

Vassilakopoulos T, Zakynthinos S, Roussos C: Muscle function: basic concepts. In Marini JJ, Slutsky A, editors: *Physiologic basis of ventilator support,* New York, 1998, Marcel Dekker, pp 103–152.

Chapter **7**
Imaging Techniques
Simon P.G. Padley • David M. Hansell

Today, clinicians have two main imaging techniques at their disposal for the investigation of patients with chest disease—plain radiography, which produces a projectional image, and computed tomography (CT), which provides a cross-sectional view. Other techniques, such as magnetic resonance imaging (MRI), radionuclide scanning, and ultrasonography, can provide valuable additional information but are rarely performed without previous chest radiography or CT. Because imaging is an integral part of the practice of respiratory medicine, an understanding of the strengths and weaknesses of these various techniques is vital. The advent of high-resolution and spiral (helical) CT techniques has lent further precision to the clinical investigation of suspected chest disease, but the use of such sophisticated tests should not be indiscriminate; accurate interpretation of the chest radiograph remains the mainstay of thoracic imaging.

PLAIN CHEST RADIOGRAPHY

TECHNICAL CONSIDERATIONS

The views of the chest most frequently performed are the erect posteroanterior and lateral projections, taken with the patient's breath held at total lung capacity. On a frontal (posteroanterior) chest radiograph, just under half of the lung is free from overlying structures, such as the ribs or diaphragm. Many technical factors determine how well the lungs are demonstrated. The characteristics of current digital imaging systems make it possible to adjust the final image and optimize exposure of the least and most dense parts of the chest in a single are image.

Because the coefficients of x-ray absorption for bone and for soft tissue approach one another at high kilovoltage, the skeletal structures do not obscure the lungs on a higher-kilovoltage radiograph to the same degree as on low-kilovoltage radiographs. The high-kilovoltage radiograph thus demonstrates much more of the lung. Improved penetration of the mediastinum also allows some of the central airways to be seen. Although high-kilovoltage radiographs are preferable for routine examinations of the lungs and mediastinum, low-kilovoltage radiographs provide good detail of unobscured lung because of the improved contrast between lung vessels and surrounding lung. Furthermore, dense lesions—for example, calcified pleural plaques—are particularly well demonstrated on low-kilovoltage films.

The past decade has seen a major change in plain film radiography with the development of digital imaging systems, which are now ubiquitous in modern radiology departments. Digital chest radiography, yielding images either stored on a phosphor plate and then digitally scanned or captured directly onto a detector plate, has been combined with computer-based picture archiving and communications systems (PACSs) for distribution of images around the hospital or over wider networks. The much wider latitude of digital systems also allows the image to be "postprocessed" to provide optimum visualization of the relevant structures

The frontal (posteroanterior) (**Figure 7-1**) and lateral (**Figure 7-2**) projections are sufficient for most purposes in chest radiography. Other radiographic views are less frequently required, but they should not be overlooked because they may solve a particular problem quickly and cheaply. The lateral *decubitus* view is not, as its name implies, a lateral view. It is a frontal view taken with use of a horizontal beam and the patient in a side-lying position. Its main purpose is to demonstrate the movement of fluid in the pleural space (**Figure 7-3**). An adaptation of this view is the "lateral shoot-through" sometimes used in bed-bound patients: A lateral radiograph of the supine patient is taken to show an anterior pneumothorax behind the sternum (not always visible on a frontal chest radiograph) (**Figure 7-4**). If a pleural effusion is not loculated, it gravitates, to some extent, to the dependent part of the pleural cavity. Thus, in a decubitus patient, the fluid will layer between the chest wall and the lung edge. This view also may be useful for demonstrating a small pneumothorax, because the visceral pleural edge of the lung falls away from the chest walls in the nondependent hemithorax.

For the *lordotic* view, now rarely performed, the x-ray beam is angled 15 degrees cranially, either by positioning the patient upright and directing the beam up or by leaving the beam horizontal and leaning the patient backward. On this view, the lung apices are demonstrated free from the superimposed clavicle and first rib. It may be useful to differentiate pulmonary shadows from incidental calcification of the costochondral junctions (**Figure 7-5**).

PORTABLE CHEST RADIOGRAPHY

Portable or mobile chest radiography has the obvious advantage that the examination can be carried out without moving the patient from the ward. However, the portable radiograph has disadvantages. Use of the shorter-focus film distance results in undesirable magnification, and most portable machines are unable to deliver the power required for high-kilovoltage techniques. Furthermore, the maximum current is limited so that longer exposure times are needed, which potentially increases blurring of the image. Portable lateral radiographs are even less likely to be successful because of the extremely long exposure times required to obtain adequate penetration.

Patient positioning for portable radiography is difficult, and the resultant radiographs often are suboptimal. Even with use of the so-called erect position, in which the patient sits up, the chest is rarely as vertical as it is in a standing patient. Because many patients are unable to move to the radiography department for a formal radiograph, any method of improving the quality of a portable chest radiograph, such as digital radiography, represents a significant advance.

DIGITAL CHEST RADIOGRAPHY

The most widely employed systems use conventional radiographic equipment but use a reusable photostimulatable plate instead of conventional film. The reusable phosphor plate is housed in a cassette and stores some of the energy of the incident x ray as a latent image. On scanning the plate with a laser beam, the stored energy is emitted as light that is detected by a photomultiplier and converted into a digital signal. The digital information is then manipulated, displayed, and stored in whatever format is desired. The phosphor plate can be reused once the latent image has been erased by exposure to light. Most currently available computed radiography systems produce a

digital radiograph with a resolution of more than 10 line pairs per millimeter. The fundamental requirement to segment the image into a finite number of pixels has resulted in much work to determine the relationship between pixel size, which affects spatial resolution, and the detectability of focal abnormalities. Although it might seem desirable to aim for an image composed of pixels of the smallest possible size, an inverse relationship occurs between pixel size and the cost and speed of data handling. Thus, pixel size is ultimately a compromise between image quality and ease of data processing and storage.

An unequivocal advantage of digital computed radiography over conventional film radiography is the linear

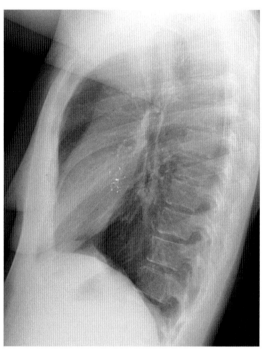

Figure 7-2 Standard lateral chest radiograph. The dorsal spine vertebral bodies are of progressively lower density toward the diaphragm. The metallic density over the cardiac silhouette is an atrial septal defect closure device.

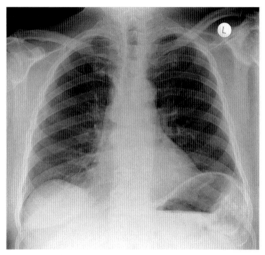

Figure 7-1 A standard digital posteroanterior radiograph demonstrating the wide latitude that can be routinely achieved. This image provides good detail of both lung and mediastinal anatomy.

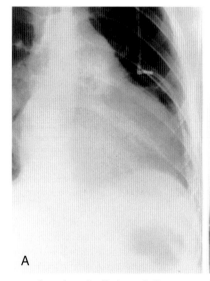

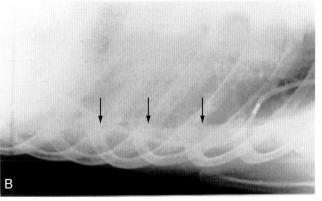

Figure 7-3 Demonstration of small effusions. **A,** Posteroanterior chest radiograph obtained in a patient with a ventriculoperitoneal shunt. More soft tissue than usual is present between the gastric air bubble and the base of the lung because of a subpulmonic effusion. **B,** Decubitus view shows redistribution of fluid to the dependent part of the chest (*arrows*).

photoluminescence-dose response, which is much greater than that of conventional film. This extremely wide latitude coupled with the facility for image processing produces diagnostic images over a wide range of exposures.

Observer performance studies have shown that computed radiography is just as useful as conventional film radiography for virtually any relevant application. However, postprocessing of the digital image has to be used to match the digital radiograph to the specific task. Enhancement of the image for one purpose often degrades it for another but is easily achieved in most PACS reporting systems.

COMPUTED TOMOGRAPHY

The same basic principles that allow film radiography apply with CT—namely, the absorption of x rays by tissues that contain constituents of different atomic number. By use of multiple projections and computed calculations of radiographic

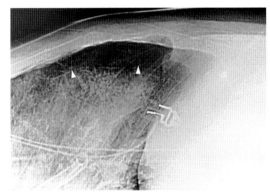

Figure 7-4   Lateral shoot-through digital radiograph of the chest obtained in a patient in the intensive care unit. The anterior pneumothorax (*arrowheads* indicate the visceral pleural edge) was not obvious on the anteroposterior portable radiograph.

density, slight differences in x-ray absorption are displayed as a cross-sectional image. The components of a CT scanner include an x-ray tube that rotates around the patient and an array of x-ray detectors opposite the tube, together contained within the gantry. The patient lies on the examination couch, which moves the patient through the aperture of the CT gantry. The data acquired are then processed by the CT computer, resulting in the final images as displayed on the CT monitor.

An impressive and rapid improvement in CT hardware capability has occurred over the past decade. Most particularly, the advent of multiple-channel CT scanners has resulted in the ability to acquire simultaneous helical datasets. An accompanying increase in gantry rotation speed coupled with the reduction in the size of the individual detectors has resulted in the ability to acquire extremely detailed images in very short scan times. On the current "top specification" scanners from the major manufacturers, up to 320 channels are available, each with a detector size of as small as 0.5 mm. The entire thorax can now be scanned at submillimeter resolution in 1 to 2 seconds. Thus, spiral (also known as volume or helical) scanning entails continuous scanning and table movement into the CT gantry (**Figure 7-6**). The information is reconstructed into axial sections, perpendicular to the long axis of the patient, identical to conventional CT sections.

Temporal resolution has been further improved, because data reconstruction algorithms now allow CT images to be generated after a partial rotation of the gantry. Thus, temporal resolution of as little as 65 msec is now possible, enabling modern multichannel CT scanners to acquire cardiac gated images that effectively freeze cardiac motion. This capability in turn can be applied to allow detailed analysis of coronary artery and cardiac anatomy.

The analysis of what is frequently hundreds of individual images that are produced as the result of a single CT examination is undertaken on dedicated CT or PACS workstations. Postprocessing of these thin sections also allows the production

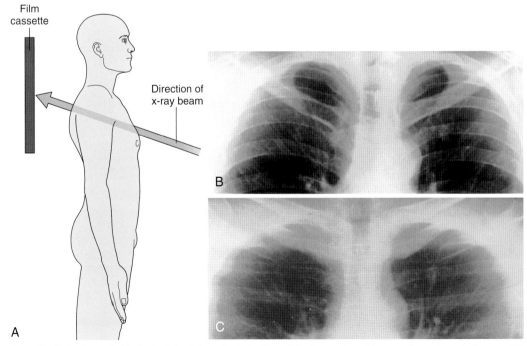

Figure 7-5   The value of lordotic views. **A,** Method of obtaining a lordotic view of the lung apices: The x-ray beam is angled upward. **B,** Selected area from a standard posteroanterior view of the upper lung zones in a patient who presented with hemoptysis, with a suggestion of a small opacity projected over the anterior end of the left first rib. **C,** A lordotic view confirms that the small opacity is intrapulmonary (rather than calcified costochondral cartilage).

of multiplanar reformats (MPRs), maximum and minimum intensity projections (MIPs and MinIPs), and angiographic images. Skeletal structures can be automatically removed, or surface-rendered images that mimic appearances familiar to the bronchoscopist can be produced with a few mouse clicks. These images are visually pleasing and allow an exquisite appreciation of anatomy. They also have a role in the planning of interventional procedures, including transbronchial needle biopsy and endoluminal stent insertion (**Figure 7-7**).

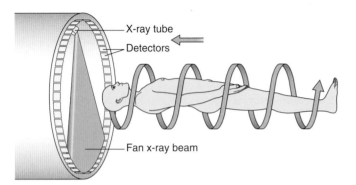

Figure 7-6 The principle of spiral (helical) computed tomography. The patient moves into the scanner with the x-ray tube continuously rotating and the detectors acquiring information. The rapidity of data acquisition allows a complete examination of the thorax to be performed in a single breath-hold.

TECHNICAL CONSIDERATIONS

The CT image is composed of a matrix of picture elements (*pixels*). A fixed number of pixels make up the matrix, so the size of each pixel varies according to the diameter of the circle to be scanned. A typical matrix in a modern CT system would be 512 by 512 pixels. The smaller the image field of view, the smaller the area represented by a pixel and the higher the spatial resolution of the image. In practical terms, the field of view size is adjusted to the size of the area of interest, usually the chest diameter.

Often, marked differences can be seen in the "look" of the images obtained on the various models of CT scanners. Such differences are largely the result of specific features of the software reconstruction algorithms used to smooth the image, to a greater or lesser extent, by averaging the density of neighboring pixels. The lung is a high-contrast environment, so less smoothing is needed than in other parts of the body. Higher-spatial-resolution algorithms (which make image "noise"—a granular appearance—more conspicuous) generally are more desirable for lung work.

SECTION THICKNESS

Although a CT section is viewed as a two-dimensional image, it has a third dimension of depth. The depth, or section thickness, is determined by a combination of factors, depending on

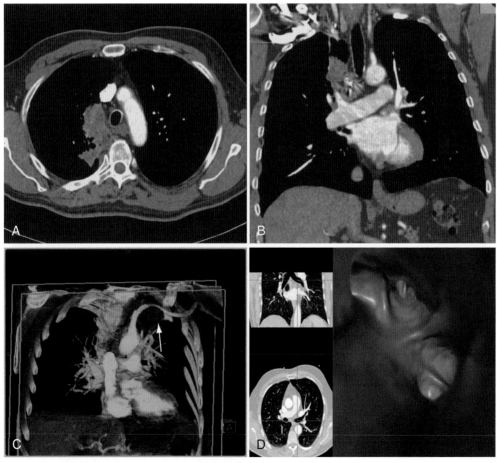

Figure 7-7 Dataset from a multidetector computed tomography study. **A,** This axial image demonstrates a bronchogenic carcinoma in a right paratracheal position. **B,** A reformatted image derived from the same data demonstrates the same abnormality in the coronal plane without loss of resolution. **C,** A coronal volume-rendered image obtained in a different patient demonstrates a left superior sulcus tumor encasing the left subclavian artery (*arrow*). **D,** Virtual bronchoscopy image from a normal subject.

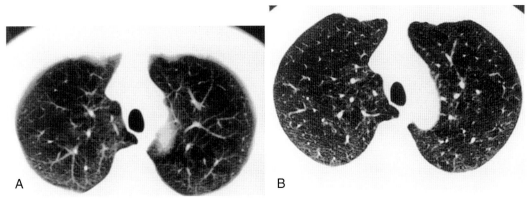

Figure 7-8 The partial volume effect on computed tomography (CT) scan appearance. **A,** This 10-mm CT section shows a poorly defined opacity, adjacent to the left superior mediastinum, apparently within the lung. **B,** The 1.5-mm section through the same region reveals that the appearance in **A** results from a partial volume effect—that is, the aortic arch is partially included in the 10-mm-thick sections.

the exact parameters utilized, including focal spot size, thickness of the individual detector elements, and width of the x-ray beam collimation. Because a section has a predetermined thickness, each pixel has a volume and this three-dimensional element is referred to as a *voxel*. The computer calculates the average radiographic density of tissue within each voxel, and the final CT image consists of a representation of the numerous voxels (not individually visible without magnification) in the section. The single attenuation value of a voxel represents the average of the attenuation values of all of the various structures within the voxel. The thicker the section, the greater the chance that different structures will be included within the voxel and the greater the signal averaging that occurs. This is known as the *partial volume effect*; the easiest way to reduce this effect is to use thinner sections (**Figure 7-8**).

When the entire chest is examined, contiguous thin sections are reconstructed for analysis. If the study is undertaken on a multichannel system, the dataset may be reconstructed at thinner intervals predetermined by the thickness of the detector rows, and these thinner sections may be used for reporting or multiplanar reconstructions. Thinner sections also are used to study fine detail and complex areas of anatomy, such as the aortopulmonary window and subcarinal regions. Another specific example for which narrow sections may be useful is to display differential densities (which would otherwise be lost because of the partial volume effect) of the small foci of fat or calcium that are sometimes seen within a hamartoma.

If exposure factors are otherwise kept the same, the total patient radiation dose varies very little between different multichannel systems. Of note, however, a striking difference in the radiation dose to the patient is associated with use of contiguous sections versus interspaced fine sections. Thus, the effective dose to the patient with interspaced fine sections (e.g., 1 or 2 mm) every 10 mm, such as used for high-resolution CT of the lung parenchyma, is 5 to 10 times less than that imposed by single-channel or multichannel spiral CT of the entire chest volume. The disadvantage of interspaced sections is the inability to view the data in any plane, but for the purposes of assessment of the lung interstitium, this added refinement usually is not of sufficient added diagnostic value to warrant the increased radiation burden. This consideration is especially important in the relatively younger patient.

WINDOW SETTINGS

The average density of each voxel is measured in Hounsfield units (H); these units have been arbitrarily chosen so that zero is water density and –1000 is air density. The span of Hounsfield units reflecting density in the thorax is wider than in any other part of the body, ranging from that for aerated lung (approximately –800 H) to that for ribs (+700 H). Two variables are used that allow the operator to select the range of densities to be viewed—window width and window center (or level).

The *window width* determines the number of Hounsfield units to be displayed. Any densities greater than the upper limit of the window width are displayed as white, and any below the limit of the window are displayed as black. Between these two limits, the densities are displayed in shades of gray. The median density of the window chosen is the *window center* or level; this center can be moved higher or lower as desired, thus moving the window up or down through the range. The narrower the window width, the greater the contrast discrimination within the window. No single window setting can depict the wide range of densities encountered in the chest on a single image. For this reason, at least two sets of images are required to demonstrate the lung parenchyma and soft tissues of the mediastinum, respectively (**Figure 7-9**). Standard window widths and centers for thoracic CT vary between departments, but generally for the soft tissues of the mediastinum, a window width of 400 to 600 H and a center of +30 H is appropriate. For the lungs, a wide window of 1500 H and a center of approximately –500 H are usually satisfactory. For bones, the widest possible window setting at a center of +30 H is best.

Window settings have a profound influence on the size and conspicuity of normal and abnormal structures. Nonetheless, it is impossible to prescribe precise window settings because of the element of observer preference and also differences between machines. The most accurate representation of an object seems to be achieved if the value of the window level is halfway between the density of the structure to be measured and the density of the surrounding tissue. For example, the diameter of a pulmonary nodule, measured on soft tissue settings appropriate for the mediastinum, will be grossly underestimated. When inappropriate window settings are used, imaging of smaller structures (e.g., peripheral pulmonary vessels) will be affected proportionately much more than that of larger structures.

INTRAVENOUS CONTRAST ENHANCEMENT

Intravenous contrast enhancement is needed only in specific instances, because of the high contrast on CT between vessels and surrounding air in the lung and between vessels and surrounding fat within the mediastinum. One such instance is to

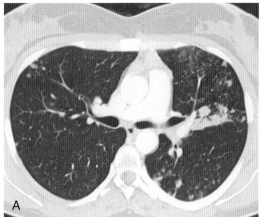 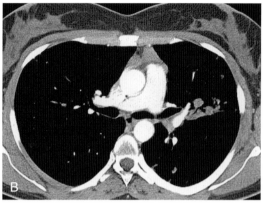

Figure 7-9   The effect of window settings on computed tomography scan appearance. A 5-mm-thick computed tomography section is displayed on different window settings. **A,** On lung windows (center, 500 H; width, 1500 H), nodules in the lungs and pulmonary vessels are clearly visible. **B,** On soft tissue windows (center, 35 H; width, 400 H), the contrast-enhanced vessels in the mediastinum and the soft tissue structures are delineated, but the lung detail is lost.

aid the distinction between hilar vessels and a soft tissue mass. The exact timing of the injection of contrast material depends most on the time the CT scanner takes to scan the thorax. With multichannel CT scanners, the circulation time specific for the patient becomes an important factor.

Contrast medium rapidly diffuses out of the vascular space into the extravascular space, so that opacification of the vasculature after a bolus injection with a "power injector" quickly declines, and structures such as lymph nodes steadily increase in density over time. Such dynamics result in a point at which a solid structure may have exactly the same density as an adjacent vessel. The timing and duration of the contrast medium infusion must therefore be taken into account in interpreting images obtained in a contrast-enhanced CT study. Rapid scanning protocols with automated injectors tend to improve contrast enhancement of vascular structures at the expense of enhancement of solid lesions because of the rapidity of scanning. With spiral CT, it is possible to achieve good opacification of all of the thoracic vascular structures by using small volumes of contrast material. Optimal contrast enhancement is a prerequisite for the diagnosis of pulmonary embolism or aortic and great vessel abnormalities. To achieve optimal contrast enhancement, many CT systems now use an automated triggering system. Thus, in examining the pulmonary arteries, a low-dose repeating scan will monitor the density in the pulmonary outflow tract once every second. When a predetermined density threshold is reached as a result of the arrival of intravenous contrast, the preplanned examination is triggered. The couch rapidly moves the patient from the monitoring position to the start position, a prerecorded breath-hold instruction is given to the patient over a loudspeaker, and the data acquisition commences. The acquisition is timed to correspond with appropriate enhancement of anatomic structures if contrast has been administered.

For examining inflammatory lesions, such as the reaction around an empyema, it may be necessary to delay scanning by 30 seconds, to allow contrast to diffuse into the extravascular space. For examining the liver and adrenals in evaluation of a patient with suspected lung cancer, the optimal phase of contrast enhancement to maximize the conspicuity of hepatic metastases is during the portal venous phase of contrast enhancement, and this occurs 60 to 80 seconds after contrast injection.

HIGH-RESOLUTION COMPUTED TOMOGRAPHY

TECHNICAL CONSIDERATIONS

Over the past two decades, the development of high-resolution computed tomography (HRCT) has had great impact on the approach to the imaging of diffuse interstitial lung disease and bronchiectasis. Images of the lung produced by HRCT correlate closely with the macroscopic appearance of pathologic specimens, so in the context of diffuse lung disease, HRCT represents a substantial improvement over chest radiography. Three factors associated with significantly improved spatial resolution of CT—hence the designation "high-resolution"—are narrow beam collimation, use of a high-spatial-frequency reconstruction algorithm, and a small field of view.

Narrow collimation of the x-ray beam reduces volume averaging within the section and so increases spatial resolution compared with standard 10-mm collimation. For routine HRCT scanning, 1.50-mm beam collimation generally is regarded as optimal. Narrow collimation has a marked effect on the appearance of the lungs, notably the vessels and bronchi—the branching vascular pattern seen particularly in the midzones on standard 10-mm sections has a more nodular appearance with narrow sections, because shorter segments of the obliquely running vessels are included in the section. In addition, parenchymal details become more clearly visualized (**Figure 7-10**).

In HRCT lung imaging, a high-spatial-frequency algorithm is used to take advantage of the inherently high-contrast environment of the lung. The high-spatial-frequency algorithm (also known as the edge-enhancing, sharp, or formerly "bone" algorithm) reduces image smoothing and makes structures visibly sharper but at the same time makes image noise more obvious (see Figure 7-10).

Several artifacts are consistently identified on HRCT images, but they do not usually degrade the diagnostic content of the images. Nevertheless, it is useful to be able to recognize the more common ones. Probably the most frequently encountered is a streaking appearance, which arises from patient motion. Cardiac motion sometimes causes movement of the adjacent lung with consequent degradation of image quality. Some CT scanners are able to eliminate this artifact by triggering the acquisition of the slice from the electrocardiogram (ECG) tracing so that the data are collected during diastole, when

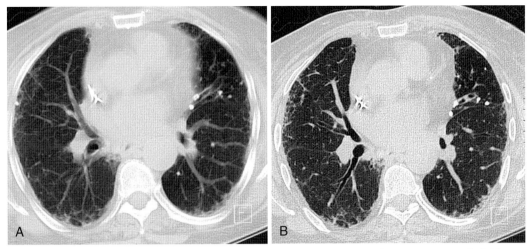

Figure 7-10   The effect of computed tomography (CT) section thickness and edge enhancement on image appearance. **A,** A 10-mm-thick section reconstructed with edge enhancement from a multidetector CT (MDCT) dataset. **B,** A 1.5-mm-thick section with high edge enhancement from the same dataset, typical of a high-resolution CT (HRCT) lung image from a volume acquisition.

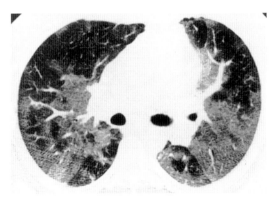

Figure 7-11   High-resolution computed tomography image demonstrating artifact caused by aliasing and quantum mottleing. Detail is obscured in the posterior parts of the lungs. The patchy parenchymal opacification results from desquamative interstitial pneumonitis.

cardiac motion is minimized. To optimize this technique, the scanner must have a short rotation time and also be capable of formatting a CT image from data from a partial rotation. This reduces the data acquisition time window to as little as 360 msec.

The size of the patient has a direct effect on the quality of the lung image—the larger the patient, the more conspicuous the noise, which is seen as granular streaks because of increased x-ray absorption by the patient. This artifact is particularly evident in the posterior lung adjacent to the vertebral column. The phenomenon of aliasing results in a fine, streaklike pattern radiating from sharp, high-contrast interfaces. The severity of the aliasing artifact is related to the geometry of the CT scanner, and, unlike quantum mottle, aliasing is independent of the radiation dose. These artifacts are exaggerated by the non-smoothing, high spatial-resolution reconstruction algorithm but do not mimic normal anatomic structures and are rarely severe enough to obscure important detail in the lung parenchyma (**Figure 7-11**).

The degree to which HRCT samples the lung depends primarily on the spacing between the thin sections. An HRCT examination also may vary in terms of the number of sections, the position of the patient, the phase in which respiration is suspended, the window settings at which the images are displayed, and the manipulation of the image by postprocessing.

No single protocol can be recommended to cover every eventuality. However, the simplest protocol entails 1.5-mm collimation sections at 20-mm intervals from apex to lung bases. Any given scanning protocol may need to be modified—a patient referred with unexplained hemoptysis ideally is scanned with contiguous standard sections through the major airways (to show a small endobronchial abnormality) and interspaced narrow sections through the remainder of the lungs (to identify bronchiectasis).

When early interstitial disease is suspected, for example, in asbestos-exposed persons in whom the chest radiograph is normal in appearance, HRCT scans often are performed with the patient in the prone position, to prevent any confusion with the increased opacification seen in the dependent posterior basal segments in many normal subjects scanned in the usual supine position. The increased density seen in the posterior dependent lung with supine positioning disappears in normal persons when the scan is repeated at the same level with prone positioning. No advantage is gained by scanning a patient in the prone position if no obvious diffuse lung disease is found on a contemporary chest radiograph.

A limited number of scans taken at end expiration can reveal evidence of air trapping caused by small airway disease, which may not be detectable on routine inspiratory scans. Areas of air trapping range from a single secondary pulmonary lobule to a cluster of lobules that give a patchwork appearance of low attenuation areas adjacent to higher attenuation, normal lung parenchyma (**Figure 7-12**).

Alterations of the window settings of HRCT images sometimes make detection of parenchymal abnormalities impossible when there is a subtle increase or decrease in attenuation of the lung parenchyma. Uniformity of window settings from patient to patient aids consistent interpretation of the lung images. In general, a window level of −500 to −800 HU and a width of between 900 and 1500 HU are usually satisfactory. Modification of the window settings for particular tasks is often desirable; for example, in looking for pleuroparenchymal abnormalities in asbestos-exposed patients, a wider window of up to 2000 HU may be useful. Conversely, a narrower window of approximately 600 HU may emphasize the subtle density differences that characterize emphysema and small airway disease.

The relatively high radiation dose to the patient inherent in all CT scanning needs to be appreciated. The radiation burden

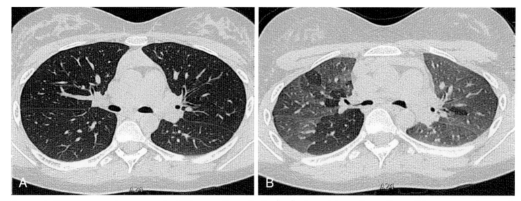

Figure 7-12 **A,** High-resolution computed tomography (CT) scan through the lower lung lobes of a patient with severe asthma. The inspiratory image through the upper zones is normal. **B,** A high-resolution CT image at end expiration emphasizes the regional air trapping due to small airways obstruction.

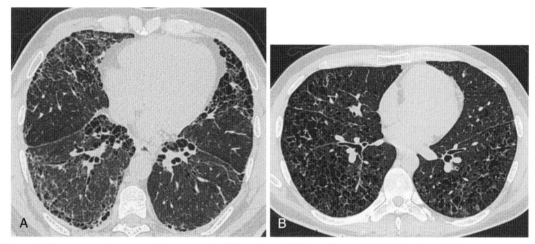

Figure 7-13 High-resolution computed tomography patterns in diffuse interstitial lung disease. **A,** Subpleural reticular pattern typical of established fibrosing alveolitis. **B,** Multiple irregularly shaped cystic spaces within the lungs in a young patient with preserved lung volumes. Images through the lung bases were more normal. This high-resolution computed tomography pattern and distribution combination is virtually pathognomonic for Langerhans cell histiocytosis.

to the patient is considerably less with HRCT than with conventional CT scanning. It has been estimated that the mean radiation dose delivered to the skin with HRCT by use of 1.5-mm sections at 20-mm intervals is 6% that of conventional 10-mm contiguous scanning protocols. A further method of reducing the radiation burden to the patient is to decrease the milliamperage; it is possible to reduce the milliamperage by up to 10-fold and still obtain comparably diagnostic images. Although continuous refinement in CT technology is reducing the radiation burden to patients, CT still delivers a relatively high radiation dose to patients, so this imaging modality must not be used indiscriminately.

CLINICAL APPLICATIONS OF HIGH-RESOLUTION COMPUTED TOMOGRAPHY

Increasingly, HRCT is used to confirm or refute the impression of an abnormality seen on a chest radiograph. It may also be used to achieve a histospecific diagnosis in some patients who have obvious, but nonspecific, radiographic abnormalities.

It probably is impossible to determine the frequency with which HRCT will show significant parenchymal abnormalities when the chest radiograph appears normal. Studies of individual diseases show that HRCT demonstrates abnormalities despite normal chest radiographs in 29% of patients with

systemic sclerosis and in up to 30% of those with asbestosis. For hypersensitivity pneumonitis, the proportion may be even higher. As indicated by the average sensitivity results of several studies, HRCT seems to have a sensitivity of approximately 94%, compared with 80% for chest radiography; this increased sensitivity does not seem to be achieved at the expense of decreased specificity.

In patients with clinical and lung function evidence of diffuse lung disease, HRCT is now central in the diagnostic workup, with clinical performance greatly exceeding that of plain chest radiography and may obviate the need for lung biopsy. In the original study that compared the diagnostic accuracy of chest radiography and CT in the prediction of specific histologic diagnosis in patients with diffuse lung disease, Mathieson and associates showed that three observers could make a confident diagnosis in 23% of cases on the basis of chest radiographs and in 49% of cases with use of CT; the correct diagnosis was made in 77% and 93% of these readings, respectively (**Figure 7-13**).

A number of subsequent early HRCT studies acted as the forerunners of a large body of work that has established HRCT as a cornerstone in the assessment of patients suspected of having diffuse lung disease but for whom the clinical features and appearance on the chest radiograph do not allow a confident diagnosis to be made. A number of diffuse lung diseases

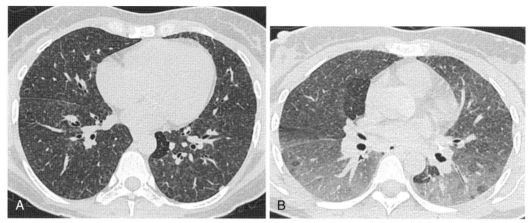

Figure 7-14   High-resolution computed tomography scans of the chest in a patient with subacute hypersensitivity pneumonitis. **A,** Widespread nodular and ground glass patterns. **B,** The areas of decreased attenuation evident posteriorly are made more obvious on this scan obtained at end expiration.

can have a "diagnostic" appearance on HRCT when findings are interpreted by experienced chest radiologists; such diseases include fibrosing alveolitis, sarcoidosis, Langerhans cell histiocytosis, lymphangioleiomyomatosis, pneumoconiosis, and hypersensitivity pneumonitis (**Figure 7-14**). An intriguing observation is that the ability of HRCT to allow observers to provide correct histospecific diagnoses seems to be maintained in advanced end-stage disease.

However, HRCT is sometimes used indiscriminately for patients in whom the high certainty of diagnosis from clinical and radiographic findings does not justify the extra cost and radiation burden. No evidence shows that an HRCT examination adds anything of diagnostic value for a patient who has progressive shortness of breath, finger clubbing, crackles at the lung bases, and the typical radiographic pattern and lung function profile of fibrosing alveolitis. Nevertheless, the ability of HRCT to characterize disease, and often to deliver a definite and correct diagnosis in patients with nonspecific radiographic shadowing, frequently is helpful.

Much interest has been shown in defining the role of HRCT in staging disease activity, particularly for fibrosing alveolitis, in which cellular histology indicates disease activity and is used to predict both responses to treatment and prognosis. As shown by more recent evidence, a predominance of ground glass opacification in fibrosing alveolitis predicts a good response to treatment and increased actuarial survival compared with patients with a more reticular pattern, which denotes established fibrosis. Similar observations about the potential reversibility of disease can be made with use of HRCT in patients who have sarcoidosis, in whom a ground glass or a nodular pattern predominates. In other conditions, the identification of ground glass opacification on HRCT, although nonspecific, almost invariably indicates a potentially reversible disease—for example, extrinsic allergic alveolitis, diffuse pulmonary hemorrhage, and *Pneumocystis jiroveci* pneumonia (**Box 7-1**). An important exception is bronchoalveolar cell carcinoma, in which areas of ground glass opacification that merge into areas of frank consolidation or a more nodular pattern may be seen. Another caveat applies with the situation in which fine, intralobular fibrosis is seen on HRCT as widespread ground glass opacification; in this rare occurrence, evidence of traction bronchiectasis usually is present within the areas of ground-glass opacification.

The ability of CT to discriminate among various patterns of disease has clarified the basis for the sometimes complex mixed

---

Box 7-1	**Causes of Ground Glass Opacification**

Pneumocystis jiroveci or cytomegalovirus pneumonia
Acute respiratory distress syndrome–acute interstitial pneumonia
Hypersensitivity pneumonitis—subacute
Desquamative interstitial pneumonitis
Pulmonary edema
Idiopathic pulmonary hemorrhage
Bronchioloalveolar cell carcinoma
Alveolar proteinosis
Lymphocytic interstitial pneumonia
Respiratory bronchiolitis-interstitial lung disease

---

obstructive and restrictive functional deficits found in some diffuse lung diseases. A good example is hypersensitivity pneumonitis, in which both interstitial and small airway disease coexist; patterns caused by these different pathologic processes can be readily appreciated on HRCT. The extent of the various HRCT patterns correlates with the expected functional indices of restriction and obstruction, respectively. Other conditions in which CT is able to tease out the morphologic abnormalities responsible for complex functional deficits include fibrosing alveolitis with coexisting emphysema and sarcoidosis associated with a combination of interstitial fibrosis and small airway obstruction by peribronchiolar granulomata.

In patients for whom lung biopsy is deemed necessary, HRCT may be invaluable to indicate which type of biopsy procedure is likely to be successful in obtaining diagnostic material. The broad distinction between peripheral disease versus central and bronchocentric disease is easily made on HRCT. Thus, disease with a subpleural distribution, such as fibrosing alveolitis, is most unlikely to be sampled by transbronchial biopsy, whereas diseases with a bronchocentric distribution on HRCT, such as sarcoidosis and lymphangitis carcinomatosa, are consistently accessible to transbronchial biopsy. In patients for whom an open or thoracoscopic lung biopsy is contemplated, HRCT assists in determining the optimal biopsy site. Pathologic examination of a lung biopsy specimen can still justifiably be regarded as the final arbiter of the presence or absence of subtle interstitial lung disease. Because HRCT images provide a kind of "in vivo big picture," many lung pathologists now combine the imaging and pathologic information before assigning a final diagnosis, and in many centers, the benefits of a team approach to the diagnosis of diffuse lung disease are recognized. The indications for HRCT

Box 7-2   **Indications for High-Resolution Computed Tomography of the Lungs**

■ To narrow the differential diagnosis or to make a histospecific diagnosis in patients with obvious but nonspecific radiographic abnormalities
■ To detect diffuse lung disease in patients with normal or equivocal radiographic findings
■ To elucidate unexpected pulmonary function test results
■ To investigate the underlying problem in patients presenting with hemoptysis
■ To evaluate disease reversibility, particularly in patients who have fibrosing alveolitis
■ To guide the type and site of lung biopsy

that have been developed over the past 20 years are summarized in **Box 7-2**.

MAGNETIC RESONANCE IMAGING

Plain radiography, CT, ultrasound imaging, contrast angiography, and isotope scanning constitute the mainstays of thoracic disease imaging. Although magnetic resonance imaging (MRI) has developed a role complementary to these techniques, it generally is considered a problem-solving tool rather than a technique of first choice.

MRI entails placing the subject in a very strong magnetic field (typically 0.2 to 1.5 tesla) and then irradiating the area under examination with pulses of radiowaves. Anatomic MRI depends on the presence of water within tissue to produce the signal required for interpretation. Protons within this water exist within different local atomic environments and, consequently, have different properties. These differences, measured as magnetic resonance, can be exploited by sequence manipulation to generate differences in contrast between tissues in the final image. Thus, the frequency of the radiofrequency pulse transmitted into the patient is carefully selected so that it causes hydrogen protons within water to be disturbed from the orientation that they have assumed as a result of being placed inside the powerful magnetic field within the bore of the magnet. After the transient disturbance caused by the radiofrequency pulse, these protons, which are acting akin to small bar magnets, relax back into their original resting position. As they do this, they release energy as a further pulse of radio waves, which are detected by the receiver coils located in the wall of the bore of the magnetic coil or, more commonly, in a variety of receiver coils placed more directly around the area under investigation. These coils frequently are known by the body part they have been designed to examine—thus, a knee, head, neck, or body coil is placed appropriately at the start of the examination. In the case of thoracic imaging, the body coil usually consists of a pair of coil mats placed in front of and behind the patient.

Historically, the main strengths of MRI are the high intrinsic soft tissue contrast generated, the lack of artifact from bone, the absence of exposure to ionizing radiation, and the ability to produce images in any chosen plane. The major weaknesses of MRI in the thorax have, until recently, been its susceptibility to image degradation secondary to respiratory and cardiac motion, as well as the relatively long times required to perform an examination. In general, the quality of MR images is related to the field strength of the scanner and the peak power and

speed of the amplifiers that generate the interrogating radiofrequency pulses.

For thoracic imaging, ECG-triggering facilities, whereby the acquisition of imaging data can be coordinated with the cardiac cycle to reduce flow artifact, are essential. Various methods of compensation for respiratory motion have been developed. Some approaches use external devices such as respiratory bellows, which detect movement of the chest wall, with data collection occurring when motion is at its least. Other methods are essentially software developments that compensate for respiratory disruption of magnetic spins. Most of these techniques have been superseded on modern scanners by the ability to acquire images of the thorax with use of breath-hold techniques.

MEDIASTINAL AND CHEST WALL IMAGING

The most common indications for the use of MRI in respiratory disease are for investigation of neoplastic disease, most commonly bronchogenic carcinoma. In addition to the primary disease, secondary complications such as cerebral secondaries, spinal metastases, and retroperitoneal fibrosis all lend themselves to evaluation by MRI. MRI also permits assessment for invasion of mediastinal structures such as the major airways, heart and great vessels, chest wall, and diaphragm and allows differentiation among different forms of soft tissue, fluid, hemorrhage, local hematoma formation, and aneurysms (**Figures 7-15 and 7-16**). With modern multichannel CT techniques, MRI now holds relatively little advantage over CT in assessing chest wall invasion, except with superior sulcus tumors. However, MRI does provide superb anatomic detail without subjecting the patient to radiation exposure—an important consideration in the pediatric age group, in which a number of follow-up studies may be required (**Figure 7-17**). The disadvantage of MRI in the very young child is the necessity for general anesthesia in many cases.

LUNG PARENCHYMAL IMAGING

Use of magnetic resonance techniques for imaging the lungs has been limited by a number of significant technical challenges. First, the lungs are constantly moving because of respiratory and cardiac motion. Second, they have a low water content relative to other biologic tissues, so they have a low proton density and return relatively little signal. Third, because of the multiple interfaces between air and soft tissue, innumerable small disturbances arise in the magnetic field. This loss of homogeneity at air-tissue interfaces results in a phenomenon known as magnetic susceptibility artifact, further reducing signal and increasing noise. Thus, on standard sequences, normal lung exhibits little signal and often is obliterated by artifact. Attempts to tackle this problem are showing increasing promise—for example, in the area of suppurative lung disease in younger patients.

VENTILATION STUDIES

Another area of intense interest has been the use of polarized gases (helium 3 and xenon 129) to show pulmonary ventilation. With this technique, a process of heating and irradiating with polarized light produces polarized gases. The gases (which have a short half-life) are inhaled and imaged using optimized sequences. The use of dual-frequency probes allows gas and proton images to be acquired and registered, enabling function and anatomy to be correlated.

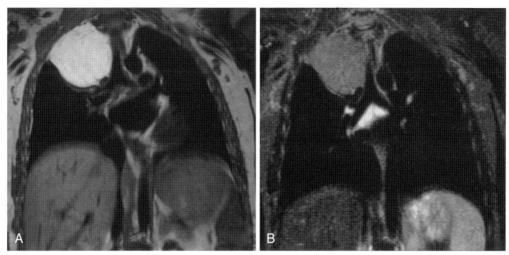

Figure 7-15 Magnetic resonance imaging of a right upper zone lung mass in an 11-year-old boy. **A,** A coronal T1-weighted sequence demonstrates a high-signal-intensity apical mass. **B,** With the addition of fat saturation, reducing the signal returned from fat, the signal intensity in the mass falls significantly. This imaging feature confirms the fatty nature of the mass, which was a large pleural lipoma.

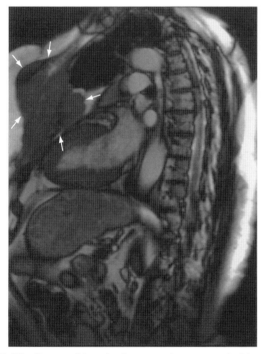

Figure 7-16 Chest wall invasion by tumor demonstrated with magnetic resonance imaging. Oblique sagittal T2-weighted image through the long axis of the left ventricle demonstrates an adjacent chest wall mass (*arrows*) extending through the interior chest wall into the overlying breast tissue. This was due to recurrent breast carcinoma.

MAGNETIC RESONANCE ANGIOGRAPHY

Magnetic resonance also can be used to demonstrate vascular anatomy by differential visualization of flowing blood and stationary tissue; this may be achieved with or without intravenous MRI contrast agents. Generally, the use of contrast increases the signal returned from blood, increases the signal-to-noise ratio, and allows acquisition times to be shorter. This modality, known as magnetic resonance angiography (MRA), can be used to look at venous or arterial flow, together or separately (see Figure 7-17).

The contrast agents used in MRI generally and MRA in particular are based almost exclusively on gadolinium chelates.

Most such agents are sequestered in the extracellular spaces; they cause shortening of the T1 relaxation time and thus increase the signal from the enhanced tissue on T1-weighted sequences. The distribution of these agents is very similar to that of the iodinated contrast agents used routinely in CT.

PULMONARY EMBOLI AND INFARCTION

At present, MRI is not routinely used in patients with suspected pulmonary embolism and infarction, but it has been the subject of much research: In a number of published series, breath-hold pulmonary MRA has been found to show fifth-order pulmonary vessels and to permit diagnosis of emboli to the segmental level. Presence of smaller pulmonary emboli can be inferred by lack of segmental and subsegmental perfusion. Three-dimensional MRA datasets can be acquired and displayed on workstations as moving projections to demonstrate areas of deficient perfusion.

VASCULAR MALFORMATIONS AND CONGENITAL ANOMALIES

Increasing evidence suggests that MRI can clearly define a number of vascular and developmental anomalies of the lungs by combining anatomic and flow studies. Such anomalies include the scimitar syndrome, hypogenetic lung syndrome, pulmonary artery agenesis, bronchopulmonary sequestration, and vascular malformations (see Figure 7-17).

CARDIOVASCULAR IMAGING

MRI is now a key technique for imaging the heart and great vessels and is widely used for the assessment of cardiac anatomy and function. Rapid and accurate assessment of wall motion, determination of ejection fraction, and stress testing for reversible ischemia, hibernating myocardium, and valvular disease are now routine. The ultimate challenge—namely, accurate imaging of the coronary arteries—is under intense investigation, although this application has not yet reached routine practice. Nevertheless, MRI is now able to provide comprehensive noninvasive cardiac assessment that is likely to challenge more established techniques such as nuclear medicine and echocardiography.

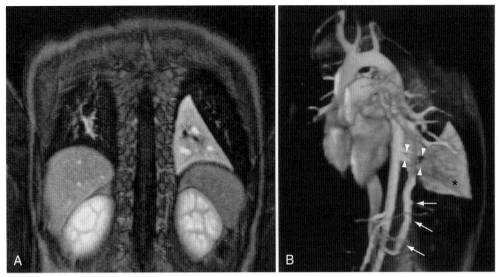

Figure 7-17 Extralobar pulmonary sequestration. **A,** A coronal contrast-enhanced breath-hold image demonstrates the avidly enhancing pulmonary sequestration at the left lung base. Note the clear plane between the triangular sequestrated segment and the diaphragm and underlying spleen. **B,** Volume-rendered angiographic image demonstrating the same triangular sequestrated segment *(asterisk)* with two supplying branches from the aorta *(arrowheads)* and complex venous drainage. The largest vein drains subdiaphragmatically *(arrows)* into the left renal vein.

PULMONARY ANGIOGRAPHY

Pulmonary angiography is used to investigate pulmonary circulation when other, less invasive, methods have failed to provide the requisite information. The most frequent indication is for suspected pulmonary embolism, often after ventilation-perfusion scanning. In the acute assessment of pulmonary embolism, the angiogram is undertaken within 24 hours of clinical presentation. However, a delay of 48 to 72 hours should not preclude the use of pulmonary angiography, although the diagnostic yield progressively declines because of fragmentation of thrombi over time, especially if anticoagulation has been instituted.

Pulmonary angiography is now rarely used. Apart from the relative expense and invasive nature of angiography, it is perceived to have a high complication rate (although this is not supported by the published evidence), so it has been largely replaced by CT.

The technique of pulmonary angiography involves fluoroscopically directed insertion of a guidewire followed by a modified pigtail catheter into the right and then the left main pulmonary arteries in turn, with injection of a nonionic contrast administered at an appropriate flow rate. At least two views per side are required, with additional oblique or magnification views as necessary. Catheter access usually is through the femoral vein, with use of the internal jugular and subclavian veins as possible alternatives. Most departments undertake angiography with digital subtraction vascular equipment **(Figure 7-18)**. Problems with misregistration artifact, inherent in digital subtraction systems and caused by respiratory or cardiac cycle phase differences between the mask image and the contrast image, usually can be overcome. Crossing the tricuspid valve may induce an arrhythmia that usually is transient. Therefore, electrocardiogram (ECG) monitoring is mandatory, and the use of prophylactic antiarrhythmic agents or temporary pacing-wire insertion is common practice in some centers. Right-sided heart catheter pressure measurements and gas analysis also may be undertaken.

When a pulmonary embolus is present, it most frequently is situated in the posterior segments of the lower lobe. Thrombi

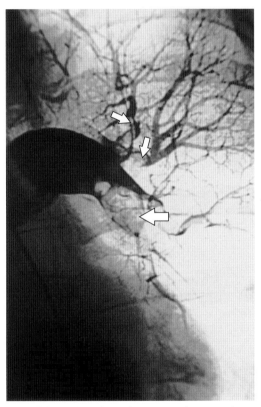

Figure 7-18 Digital subtraction pulmonary angiogram. A large thrombus causes a filling defect within the contrast in the artery of the left lower lobe *(large arrow)*. Smaller thrombi are present within the proximal branches to the upper lobe *(small arrows)*.

beyond the segmental vessel level are detected less reliably than more central thrombi. However, the significance of thrombi confined to subsegmental vessels is unclear. The typical angiographic findings with pulmonary embolism are those of vascular cutoff or, when vascular occlusion is not complete, an intraluminal filling defect with contrast passing around and beyond the clot. Indirect signs of embolism include areas of relatively delayed or reduced perfusion, late filling of the venous circulation, and vessel tortuosity. When the angiogram is performed to investigate suspected chronic thromboembolic disease, vascular changes to look for include local stenosis or thin webs, luminal ectasia, and irregularities of the normal tapering pattern.

BRONCHIAL ARTERY EMBOLIZATION

Bronchial artery embolization usually is performed to treat massive hemoptysis in patients who are unsuitable candidates for surgical management. The most common causes of bronchial artery hypertrophy and consequent hemorrhage are suppurative lung diseases (particularly bronchiectasis) and fibrocavitary disease that involves mycetomas. Less common causes of hemorrhage from the bronchial circulation include bronchial carcinoma, chronic pulmonary abscess, and congenital cyanotic heart disease. No absolute contraindications to bronchial artery embolization are known, although the patient should be hemodynamically stable and able to cooperate.

The most common anatomic arrangement on bronchial arteriography is that of one main right bronchial artery arising from a common intercostobronchial trunk, which comes off the thoracic aorta at approximately the level of T5, and two left bronchial arteries arising more inferiorly. However, bronchial arteries may arise from the thyrocervical trunk, the internal mammary artery, the costocervical trunk, the subclavian artery, a lower intercostal artery, or the inferior phrenic artery or even the abdominal aorta. The right intercostal bronchial trunk takes off from the aorta at an acute upward angle, whereas the left bronchial arteries leave the aorta at more-or-less right angles, and special catheters have been designed to facilitate selective catheterization. Superselective catheterization of the bronchial circulation allows precise delivery of embolic material, thereby preventing spillover into the aorta or inadvertent embolization of the spinal artery.

Fiberoptic bronchoscopy often is advocated before bronchial artery embolization to establish the site of hemorrhage. However, a large-volume hemoptysis almost invariably results in vigorous coughing, thereby spreading blood throughout the bronchial tree, which makes localization impossible. CT angiography also is a useful preliminary investigation, delineating bronchial artery anatomy, guiding intervention, and sometimes localizing the lobe or segment from which the bleeding originates. Few criteria exist to determine which angiographically demonstrated bronchial arteries should be embolized. Guidelines are particularly relevant when several bronchial arteries have been identified and the site of hemorrhage is not obvious from previous thoracic imaging. Embolization is directed at the vessels considered most likely to be the source of hemorrhage (**Figure 7-19**). Bronchial arteries of diameter greater than 3 mm may be considered to be pathologically enlarged. In patients with diffuse, suppurative lung disease, most commonly cystic fibrosis, attempts are made to embolize all significantly enlarged bronchial arteries bilaterally. If no abnormal bronchial arteries are identified, a systematic search is made for aberrant bronchial arteries. When a patient continues to experience hemoptysis after embolization, all suspicious systemic arteries should be examined for a source of bleeding, and it may be necessary to angiographically investigate the pulmonary circulation for a source of bleeding.

A variety of embolic materials have been used for the embolization of bronchial arteries, ranging from spheres of polyvinyl alcohol in a variety of sizes to small pieces of surgical gel (Gelfoam). Although coils lodged proximally in the bronchial artery have been used, they can prevent subsequent catheterization.

After bronchial artery embolization, many patients experience transient fever and chest pain. Some patients cough up a small amount of blood, which possibly arises from limited infarction of the bronchial mucosa. Serious complications after bronchial artery embolization are rare, the most serious being transverse myelitis, probably caused by contrast toxicity rather than inadvertent embolization. Inadvertent spillover of embolization material into the thoracic aorta may cause distant ischemia in the legs or abdominal organs.

The aim of bronchial artery embolization is the immediate control of life-threatening hemoptysis, which is achieved in more than 75% of patients. Failures usually result from nonidentification of significant bronchial arteries and an inability to maintain the catheter position to allow subsequent embolization. Up to 20% of patients rebleed within 6 months of an initially successful bronchial artery embolization. The reasons cited for recurrent hemorrhage are recanalization of previously embolized vessels, incomplete initial embolization, and hypertrophy of small bronchial arteries not initially embolized.

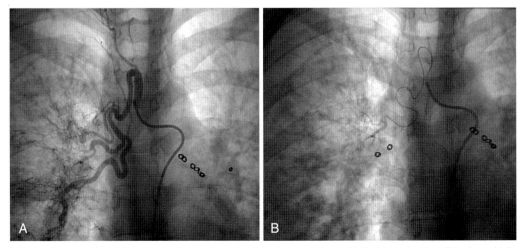

Figure 7-19 Bronchial arteriogram obtained in a patient who presented with hemoptysis. **A,** Marked hypertrophy of the bronchial artery to the right upper zone is evident. These changes were caused by cystic fibrosis. Previous embolization coils are seen over the right upper lobe. **B,** After embolization with a combination of small coils and particles, no further flow into these branches occurs.

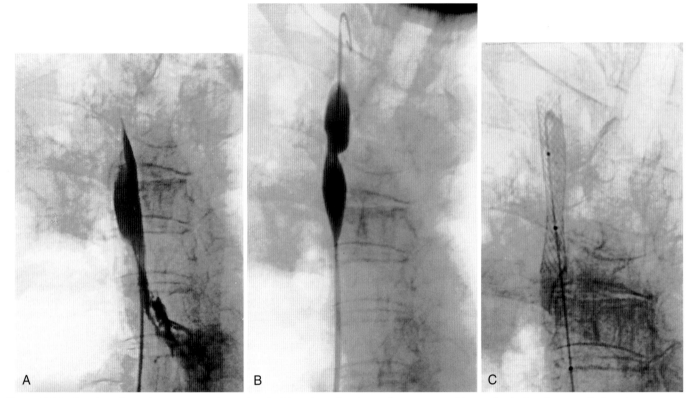

Figure 7-20 Stenting of superior vena cava obstruction. In this patient, the obstruction was caused by mediastinal malignancy. **A,** Superior venacavagram showing a tight stricture in the midportion of the superior vena cava. **B,** Balloon dilation of the stricture. **C,** Placement of a mesh-wire stent in the now-patent superior vena cava.

However, bronchial artery embolization usually can be satisfactorily repeated in patients who rebleed.

SUPERIOR VENA CAVA STENTING

Superior vena cava obstruction (SVCO) is characterized by facial and upper limb swelling, headache, and shortness of breath and usually is caused by advanced mediastinal malignancy. Conventional palliative treatment relies on radiotherapy, chemotherapy, and sometimes surgery. Radiotherapy usually produces an initial improvement, although subsequent recurrence of symptoms is frequent. Balloon angioplasty for treatment of both benign and malignant causes of SVCO has been reported, but not surprisingly, symptoms are liable to recur soon after angioplasty alone.

The percutaneous placement of metallic stents for the treatment of SVCO has several attractions. With increasing experience, reliable and successful palliation of SVCO has been reported with use of various stent designs. A superior venacavagram is necessary to identify the length of the stenosis and its site in relation to the confluence of the brachiocephalic veins and the right atrium. Identification of intraluminal thrombus or tumor may require thrombolysis before stent insertion, or the use of a covered stent. After balloon dilatation of the superior vena cava stricture, the stent is positioned across the stricture, and a postplacement venacavagram is performed to confirm free flow of blood into the right atrium (**Figure 7-20**). Subsequent to angioplasty and stent placement, relief of SVCO symptoms usually is rapid and dramatic. Recurrence of symptoms may be caused by venous thrombosis or tumor progression. Although rupture of the superior vena cava at the time of angioplasty is a risk, this complication seems to be extremely rare, possibly because of the tamponade provided by surrounding tumor or postirradiation fibrosis.

The role of intravascular stents in the management of nonmalignant SVCO has not yet been defined. Patients who have SVCO caused by benign fibrosing mediastinitis have been treated successfully, although occlusion of the stent secondary to the progression of the mediastinal fibrosis or with endothelial proliferation may occur.

NORMAL RADIOGRAPHIC ANATOMY

MEDIASTINUM AND HILAR STRUCTURES

The mediastinum is delineated by the lungs on either side, the thoracic inlet above, the diaphragm below, and the vertebral column posteriorly. In the context of radiographic anatomy, the various structures that make up the mediastinum are superimposed on each other, so they cannot be separately identified on a two-dimensional chest radiograph; for this reason, the normal anatomy of the individual components of the mediastinum is considered in more detail in the later section on CT of the mediastinum. Nevertheless, because a chest radiograph usually is the first imaging investigation, it is necessary to appreciate the normal appearances of the mediastinum and the considerable possible variations resulting from the patient's body habitus and age.

The mediastinum is conventionally divided into superior, anterior, middle, and posterior compartments (**Figure 7-21**). The practical benefit of use of these arbitrary divisions is that specific mediastinal pathologies show a definite predilection for individual compartments (e.g., a superior mediastinal mass most frequently is caused by intrathoracic extension of the

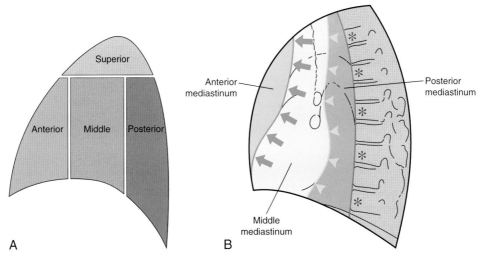

Figure 7-21 The mediastinal compartmental divisions. **A,** Arbitrary division of the mediastinum into superior, anterior, middle, and posterior compartments. **B,** An alternative scheme omits the superior mediastinal compartment. The area posterior to the sternum and anterior to the heart and great vessels *(blue arrows)* defines the anterior mediastinum in both cases. Likewise, a line placed along the posterior aspect of the trachea and heart *(yellow arrowheads)* distinguishes the middle from the posterior mediastinum, which is bounded posteriorly by the vertebra *(red asterisks)*.

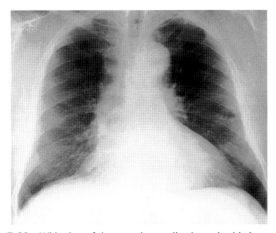

Figure 7-22 Widening of the superior mediastinum in this image is caused by abundance of mediastinal fat. In addition, bilateral cardiophrenic fat pads are present.

thyroid gland; a middle mediastinal mass usually results from enlarged lymph nodes). However, localization of a mass within one of these compartments does not normally allow a specific diagnosis to be made, and neither do the arbitrary boundaries preclude disease from involving more than one compartment.

Only the outline of the mediastinum and the air-containing trachea and bronchi (and sometimes esophagus) is clearly seen on a normal posteroanterior chest radiograph. On a chest radiograph, the right brachiocephalic vein and superior vena cava form the right superior mediastinal border. This border usually is vertical and straight (in contrast with the situation in which right paratracheal lymphadenopathy is present, when the right superior mediastinal border tends to be undulate), and it becomes less distinct as it reaches the thoracic inlet. The right side of the superior mediastinum can appear to be considerably widened in patients who have an abundance of mediastinal fat (**Figure 7-22**); such persons often have prominent cardiophrenic fat pads. The mediastinal border to the left of the trachea above the aortic arch is the result of summation of the left carotid and left subclavian arteries, together with the left brachiocephalic and jugular veins. The left cardiac border

consists of the left atrial appendage, which merges inferiorly with the left ventricle. The silhouette of the heart should always be sharply outlined. Any blurring of the border results from loss of immediately adjacent aerated lung, usually by collapse or consolidation.

The density of the heart shadow to the left and right of the vertebral column should be identical—any difference indicates pathology (e.g., an area of consolidation or a mass in a lower lobe). On a well-penetrated film, a density with a convex lateral border frequently is seen through the right heart border—this apparent mass is caused by the confluence of the right pulmonary veins as they enter the left atrium and is of no clinical significance.

The trachea and main bronchi should be visible through the upper and middle mediastinum. The trachea is rarely straight and often is to the right of the midline at its midpoint. In older persons, the trachea may be markedly displaced by a dilated aortic arch below. In approximately 60% of normal subjects, the right wall of the trachea (the right paratracheal stripe) can be identified as a line of uniform thickness (less than 4 mm in width); when visible, it excludes the presence of any adjacent space-occupying lesion, most usually lymphadenopathy. The angle between the left and right main bronchi, which forms the carina, usually is somewhat less than 80 degrees. Splaying of the carina is a relatively crude sign of subcarinal disease, in the form of either a massive subcarinal lymphadenopathy or a markedly enlarged left atrium. A more sensitive sign of subcarinal disease is obscuration of the upper part of the azygoesophageal line, which usually is visible in its entirety on a chest radiograph with good penetration (**Figure 7-23**). The origins of the lobar bronchi, when they are projected over the mediastinal shadow, usually can be identified, but segmental bronchi within the lungs generally are not seen on plain radiography.

The normal hilar shadows on a chest radiograph represent the summation of the pulmonary arteries and veins, with little contribution from the overlying bronchial walls or lymph nodes of normal size. The hila are of approximately the same size, and the left hilum normally lies between 0.5 and 1.5 cm above the level of the right hilum. The size and shape of the hila show remarkable variation in normal persons, making subtle abnormalities difficult to identify.

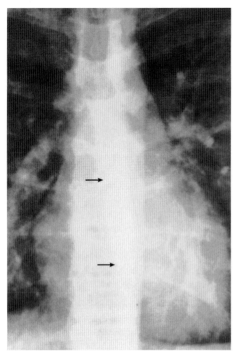

Figure 7-23 Chest radiograph made using the advanced multiple beam equalization radiography (AMBER) system. The normal azygoesophageal line is demonstrated (*arrows*).

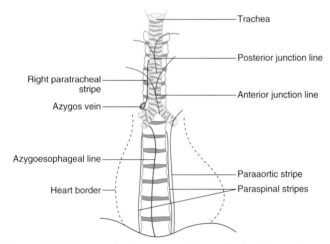

Figure 7-24 Diagram showing some of the mediastinal lines and stripes frequently seen on a frontal chest radiograph.

PULMONARY FISSURES, VESSELS, AND BRONCHI

The two lungs are separated by the four layers of pleura behind and in front of the mediastinum. The resultant posterior and anterior junction lines often are visible on frontal chest radiographs as nearly vertical stripes, the posterior junction line lying higher than the anterior (**Figure 7-24**). Because these junction lines are not invariably seen (their visibility is largely dependent on whether the pleural reflections are tangential to the x-ray beam), their presence or absence is not usually of significance.

The lobes of lung are surrounded by visceral pleura—the major (or oblique) fissure separates the upper and lower lobes of the left lung. The major (or oblique) fissure and the minor (horizontal or transverse) fissure separate the upper, middle, and lower lobes of the right lung. In the absence of abnormality, the minor fissure is visible in more than half of posteroanterior

chest radiographs. In normal persons, the minor fissure is slightly bowed upward and runs horizontally; any deviation from this configuration usually is caused by loss of volume of a lobe. The major fissures are not visible on a frontal radiograph and are inconsistently identifiable on lateral radiographs. Inability to detect a fissure usually reflects that the fissure is not exactly in the line of the x-ray beam. Occasionally, however, fissures may be incompletely developed—a point familiar to thoracic surgeons, who sometimes encounter difficulty in performing a lobectomy because of incomplete cleavage between lobes. Accessory fissures are occasionally seen; for example, in the left lung a minor fissure can be present, which separates the lingula from the remainder of the upper lobe.

All of the branching structures seen within normal lungs on a chest radiograph represent pulmonary arteries or veins. The pulmonary veins may sometimes be differentiated from the pulmonary arteries—the superior pulmonary veins have a distinctly vertical course. Often, however, it is impossible to differentiate arteries from veins in the lung periphery. On a chest radiograph taken in the erect position, a gradual increase in the diameter of the vessels is seen, at equidistant points from the hilum, traveling from lung apex to base; this gravity-dependent effect disappears if the patient is supine or in cardiac failure.

The lobes of the lung are divided into segments, each of which is supplied by its own segmental pulmonary artery and accompanying bronchus. The walls of the segmental bronchi are rarely seen on the chest radiograph, except when lying parallel with the x-ray beam, in which case they are seen end on as ring shadows measuring up to 8 mm in diameter. The most frequently identified segmental airways are the anterior segmental bronchi of the upper lobes.

DIAPHRAGM AND THORACIC CAGE

The interface between aerated lung and the hemidiaphragms is sharp, and the highest point of each dome normally is medial to the midclavicular line. The right dome of the diaphragm is higher than the left by up to 2 cm in the erect position, unless the left dome is elevated by air in the stomach. Laterally, the hemidiaphragm forms an acute angle with the chest wall. Filling in or blunting of these costophrenic angles usually represents pleural disease, either pleural thickening or an effusion. In elderly persons, localized humps on the dome of the diaphragm, particularly posteriorly (and therefore most obvious on a lateral radiograph), are common and represent minor weaknesses or defects of the diaphragm. Interposition of the colon in front of the right lobe of the liver is a frequently seen normal variant (so-called Chilaiditi syndrome).

Apparent pleural thickening along the lateral chest wall in the middle zones is a frequent observation in obese patients; it is caused by subpleural fat bulging inward. Deformities of the thoracic cage may cause distortion of the normal mediastinum and so simulate disease. One of the most common deformities is pectus excavatum, which, by compressing the heart between the depressed sternum and vertebral column, causes displacement of the apparently enlarged heart to the left and blurring of the right heart border (**Figure 7-25**). A similar appearance may arise with an unusually straight thoracic spine, referred to as *straight back syndrome*.

ANATOMY OF THE LATERAL CHEST RADIOGRAPH

Consistent viewing of lateral chest radiographs in the same orientation, whether a right or a left lateral projection, improves

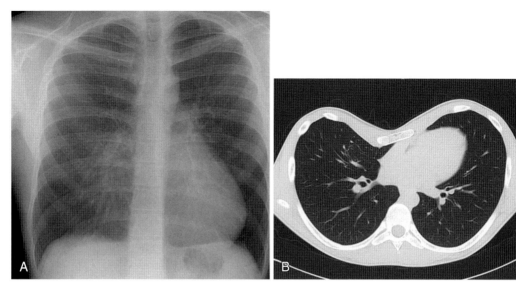

Figure 7-25 A, Chest radiograph, posteroanterior view, obtained in a patient with marked pectus excavatum. The blurring of the right heart border and the apparent increase in heart size are a direct consequence of a depressed sternum. Note the 7 configuration of the ribs. **B,** Computed tomography scan shows the sternal depression.

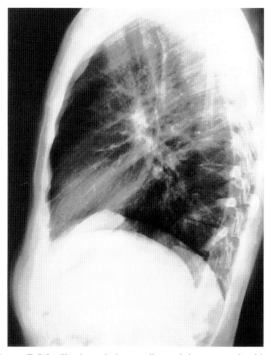

Figure 7-26 The lateral chest radiograph in a normal subject.

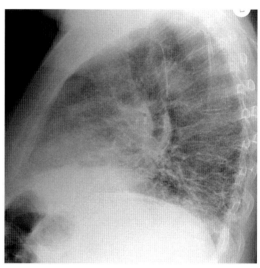

Figure 7-27 Loss of the normal increase in transradiancy toward the lower part of the dorsal spine in a patient with interstitial lung disease.

the ability to detect deviations from normal. In the lateral view, the trachea is angled slightly posteriorly as it runs toward the carina, and its posterior wall is always visible as a fine stripe (**Figure 7-26**). The posterior walls of the right main bronchus and the right intermediate bronchus are outlined by air and also are seen as a continuous stripe on the lateral radiograph. The overlying scapulae are invariably seen running almost vertically in the upper part of the lateral radiograph (and may be misinterpreted as intrathoracic structures). Further confusing shadows are formed by the soft tissues of the outstretched arms, which project over the upper mediastinum. The carina is not visible as such on the lateral radiograph, and the two transradiancies projected over the lower trachea represent the right main bronchus (superiorly) and the left main bronchus (inferiorly).

Overlying structures on a lateral radiograph obscure most of the lung. In normal persons, the unobscured lung in the retrosternal and retrocardiac regions should be of the same transradiancy. Furthermore, as the eye travels down the spine, a gradual increase in transradiancy should be apparent. The loss of this phenomenon suggests the presence of disease in the posterior-basal segments of the lower lobes (e.g., fibrosing alveolitis) (**Figure 7-27**).

The two major fissures are seen as diagonal lines, of a hair's breadth, that run from the upper dorsal spine to the anterior surface of the diaphragm. Care must be taken not to confuse the obliquely running rib edges with fissures. The minor fissure extends horizontally from the middle right major fissure. It is often not possible to differentiate the right from the left major fissures with confidence. Similarly, although the two hemidiaphragms may be identified individually (especially if the gastric bubble is visible under the left dome of the diaphragm), differentiation between the right and the left hemidiaphragm is often impossible. A useful sign is the relative heights of the two

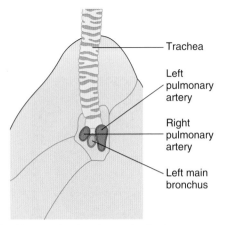

Figure 7-28 Diagram showing the proximal pulmonary arteries seen on a lateral chest radiograph.

Table 7-1	**Causes of Consolidation**
Common	**Rare**
Infection	Allergic lung diseases
Infarction	Connective tissue diseases
Cardiogenic pulmonary edema	Drug reactions
Noncardiogenic pulmonary edema	Hemorrhage
Acute respiratory distress syndrome	Lymphoma
Neurogenic edema	Radiation injury
Drug-induced edema	Amyloid
Miscellaneous	Eosinophilic lung disease
Sarcoid	
Alveolar proteinosis	

domes—the dome farther from the film normally appears higher because of magnification.

The summation of both hilar on the lateral radiograph generates a complex shadow. However, one general point is useful in the interpretation of this difficult area—the right pulmonary artery lies anterior to the trachea and right main bronchus, whereas the left pulmonary artery arches over the left main bronchus so that a large part of it lies posterior to the major bronchi (**Figure 7-28**). A bandlike opacity often is seen along the lower third of the anterior chest wall behind the sternum. It represents a normal density and occurs because less aerated lung is in contact with the chest wall, because the space is occupied by the heart; it should not be confused with pleural disease.

POINTS IN THE INTERPRETATION OF A CHEST RADIOGRAPH

Even when an obvious radiographic abnormality is present, use of a systematic method of reviewing the chest radiograph is essential. With increasing experience, appreciation of deviation from normal appearances becomes rapid, which leads quickly to a directed search for related abnormalities. Before interpretation of a chest radiograph, it is vital to establish whether any previous radiographs are available for comparison—the sequence and pattern of change often are as important as the identification of a radiographic abnormality. Information gained from preceding radiographs, particularly the lack of serial change, often prevents needless further investigation.

A check that the radiograph is of satisfactory quality includes an estimation of the adequacy of radiographic exposure, depth of inspiration, and position of the patient. The intervertebral disk spaces of the entire dorsal spine should be visible on a correctly exposed chest radiograph, and the midpoint of the right hemidiaphragm lies at the level of the anterior end of the sixth rib if the (normal) subject has taken in a satisfactory breath. The medial ends of the clavicles should be equidistant from the spinous processes of the cervical vertebral bodies.

The order in which the various parts of a chest radiograph are examined is unimportant. A suggested sequence is to start with a check of the position of the trachea, the mediastinal contour (which should be sharply outlined in its entirety), and then the position, outline, and density of the hilar shadows. The certain identification of a hilar abnormality often requires comparison with a previous radiograph; any suspicion of a hilar abnormality necessitates the retrieval of any previous chest

radiographs. At least as important as an abnormal contour for detecting a mass at the hilum is a discrepancy in density between the two sides—both hilar shadows, at equivalent points, should be of equal density, and a mass at the hilum (or an intrapulmonary mass projected over the hilum) is evident as an increased density of the affected hilum. For a questionably abnormal hilum, the lateral radiograph sometimes is helpful in clarifying the situation, provided that the normal anatomy is kept in mind (i.e., most of the right pulmonary artery lies anterior to the trachea and the bulk of the left pulmonary artery lies behind the trachea). Thus, a suspected right hilar mass on a frontal radiograph that appears to be behind the trachea on a lateral view is unlikely to represent a prominent right pulmonary artery and is therefore most likely to be an abnormal mass (the converse rule applies to a suspicious left hilum).

The lungs may then be examined in terms of their size, the relative transradiancy of each zone, and the position of the horizontal fissure. Pulmonary vessels are seen as far out as the outer third of the lung, and the number of vessels should be roughly symmetric on the two sides. Next, the position and clarity of the hemidiaphragms should be noted, followed by an assessment of the ribs and soft tissues of the chest wall. Before a chest radiograph can be regarded as normal, close inspection of areas that are poorly demonstrated, or that contain structures sometimes misinterpreted, is indicated. Such areas include the central mediastinum (where even a large mass may be invisible on the posteroanterior view), the lungs behind the diaphragm and heart, the lung apices (often obscured by the overlying clavicles and ribs), and the lung and pleura just inside the chest wall.

RADIOGRAPHIC SIGNS

Consolidation

Consolidation, also referred to as air space shadowing, is caused by opacification of the air-containing spaces of the lung. The causes of consolidation are numerous (**Table 7-1**) and include almost any pathologic process that results in the filling of the normal alveolar spaces and small airways. The responsible material is almost invariably of fluid density, and usually the volume of the displacing fluid equals the volume of air displaced. This normally results in no net change in size of the lobar anatomy. Typically, it is not possible to tell from the radiologic appearances what has caused the air space filling, especially in the absence of a clinical history. The possible exception to this generalization is with air space shadowing resulting from cardiogenic alveolar edema, when associated signs of congestive cardiac failure are found. In analyzing an area of pulmonary opacification, the presence of a number of radiologic characteristics allows the confident characterization of air space shadowing.

Typically, the shadowing is ill-defined, except when it directly abuts a pleural surface (including the interlobar fissures), in which case it is sharply demarcated (**Figure 7-29**). Although consolidation respects lobar boundaries, there are no such barriers to spread into adjacent lung segments, which are frequently contiguously involved. Thus, an area of consolidation within a single lobe often enlarges in an irregular manner, and a discrete, well-defined opacity (so-called round pneumonia) is the exception and not the rule (**Figure 7-30**).

The vascular markings within an area of consolidation usually become obscured, because the contrast between the air-containing lung and the soft tissue density vascular markings is lost. By contrast, the bronchi, which usually are too thin-walled to be differentiated from the surrounding lung parenchyma, become apparent in negative contrast to the air space opacification, to produce the true hallmark of consolidation, the air bronchogram (**Figure 7-31**). A relatively uncommon but very suggestive radiologic sign of consolidation is the acinar shadow, in which an individual secondary pulmonary lobule becomes opacified but remains surrounded by normally aerated lung. The resultant soft tissue density nodule usually is on the periphery of a more confluent area of consolidation and normally measures 0.5 to 1 cm in diameter. These acinar opacities most commonly are seen in association with mycobacterial and varicella-zoster pneumonias but can occur with any other cause of consolidation (**Figure 7-32**). Occasionally, an acinus is left normally aerated but surrounded by opacified air spaces; this radiologic sign has been termed the *air alveologram*. When consolidation is not fully developed and has caused only partial filling of the air spaces, the resultant radiographic appearance is ground glass opacification (**Figure 7-33**). Again, a wide range of possible causes has been documented, and in addition to causes of consolidation, this pattern may result from interstitial lung infiltration.

When an area of consolidation undergoes necrosis, because of either infection or infarction, liquefaction may result, and if

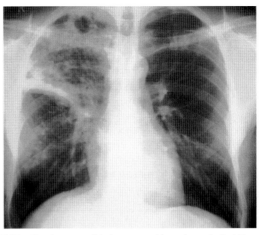

Figure 7-29 Patchy consolidation caused by tuberculosis. Where this area of involvement abuts the horizontal fissure, the inferior surface of the consolidation is sharply defined.

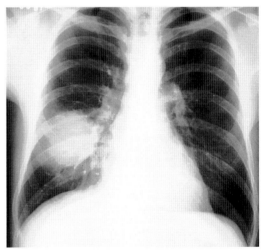

Figure 7-30 Well-defined, rounded opacity in the right middle lung zone, which fades out peripherally. This "round pneumonia" was caused by pneumococcal infection.

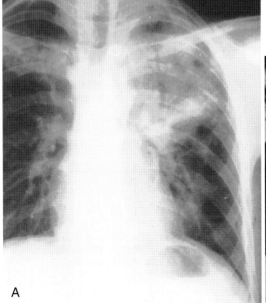

A

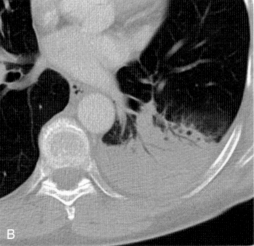

B

Figure 7-31 Air bronchogram in consolidation. **A,** Plain radiograph of the left upper zone in a patient with tuberculosis shows an air bronchogram. **B,** Computed tomography scan through the left lower lobe in a different patient demonstrates an area of segmental pneumonia.

either a gas-forming organism or communication with the bronchial tree is present, an air-fluid level may develop in addition to cavity formation (**Figure 7-34**). Consolidation frequently produces a silhouette sign, as described by Felson and Felson. Although this radiographic sign may be seen in association with a wide number of intrapulmonary pathologic processes, it is the relatively transitory nature of many forms of consolidation that best demonstrates the features of this finding. The original description stated that when an intrathoracic lesion touched a border of the heart, aorta, or diaphragm, it obliterated that border on the radiograph. Furthermore, a small area of consolidation may obliterate a normal air–soft tissue interface as effectively as a large area. This contingency is demonstrated well by the obliteration of the right heart border by subtle middle lobe consolidation that might otherwise be overlooked.

Understanding the significance of the silhouette sign allows the observer to localize an area of consolidation or other pulmonary opacity. Only if an area of consolidation lies in direct contact with a normal structure is the silhouette of that structure lost. If an area of consolidation and a normal structure–lung interface merely lie along the same x-ray path, they are superimposed on the radiograph but do not demonstrate the silhouette sign. Thus, lingular consolidation is likely to obscure the heart border, but left lower lobe consolidation usually does not (**Figures 7-35 through 7-37**). Several potential causes for a falsely positive silhouette sign are recognized. Some relatively common anatomic variants that result in a reduced anteroposterior diameter of the thorax, such as pectus excavatum or straight back syndrome, cause loss of the right heart border as the depressed sternum distorts the normal anatomy (see Figure 7-25). Occasionally, a scoliosis, usually concave to the left and often of relatively trivial clinical significance, causes the right heart border to be projected over the spine. It is only when the heart border is projected over the right lung that the silhouette sign can be elicited. Underexposed radiographs may appear to demonstrate the silhouette sign, so it is imperative that the technical quality of the radiograph be taken into account.

Collapse

Partial or complete volume loss in a lung or lobe is referred to as *collapse* or *atelectasis*. The two terms are essentially interchangeable, and both imply a diminished volume of air in the lung with associated reduction of lung volume. Any of several different mechanisms may be responsible for lung or lobar collapse.

Relaxation or Passive Collapse

The lung retracts toward its hilum when air or an abnormal amount of fluid accumulates in the pleural space.

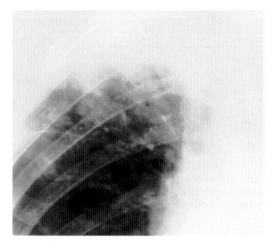

Figure 7-32 Acinar opacities seen at the periphery of confluent right upper lobe consolidation in a patient with tuberculosis. Note the elevation of the horizontal fissure.

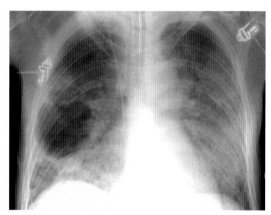

Figure 7-34 Large right lower lobe cavity in a patient with widespread pneumonic consolidation. In this radiograph obtained with the patient supine, an air-fluid level is not evident.

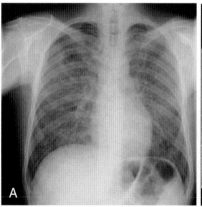 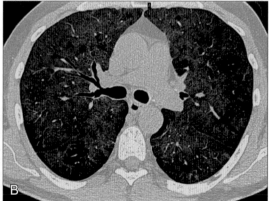 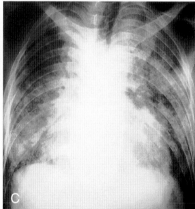

Figure 7-33 Ground glass opacification in the middle and lower zones associated with *Pneumocystis jiroveci* pneumonia. **A,** Chest radiograph shows perihilar poorly defined, increased (ground glass) density. The patient was a young man who was seropositive for human immunodeficiency virus (HIV) infection. **B,** High-resolution computed tomography image from the same patient demonstrates variable lung attenuation with markedly black airways highlighted by the ground glass patchy infiltrate. **C,** Diffuse and severe ground glass and air space infiltrate is seen on a chest radiograph obtained in a different patient with *P. jiroveci* pneumonia. (**A,** Courtesy Dr. M. Taylor.)

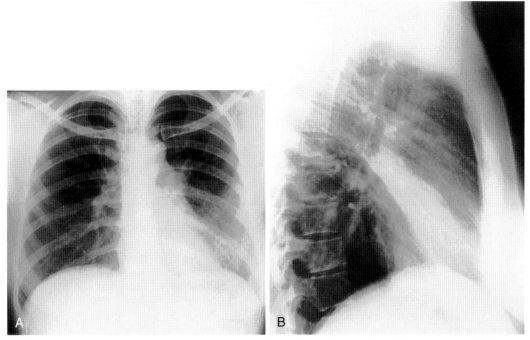

Figure 7-35   Radiographic appearance of lingular consolidation. **A,** Loss of the left heart border with a diffuse pulmonary infiltrate in the left middle and lower zones. The outer aspect of the left diaphragm is preserved. **B,** Lateral view in the same patient as in **A,** showing consolidation within the lingula, delineated posteriorly by the major fissure.

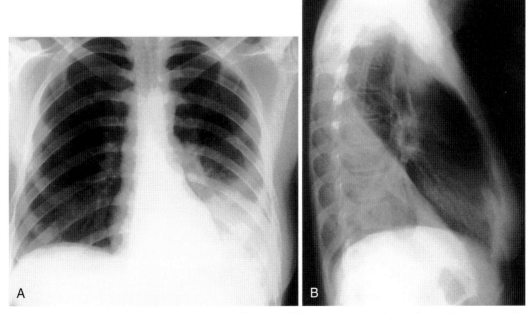

Figure 7-36   Middle and lower zone consolidation in the left lower lobe. **A,** On this posteroanterior view, radiographic features include preservation of the left heart border with loss of the left hemidiaphragm silouette. **B,** Lateral view shows the consolidation in the lower lobe delineated anteriorly by the major fissure.

Cicatrization Collapse

The normal expansion of the lung, to contact the parietal pleura, depends on a balance between outward forces in the chest wall and opposite elastic forces in the lung. If the lung is abnormally stiff, this balance is disturbed, lung compliance is decreased, and the volume of the affected lung is reduced. Perhaps the best example of this phenomenon is volume loss associated with pulmonary fibrosis.

Adhesive Collapse

In the normal lung, the forces that govern surface tension become more pronounced as the surface area of the air space is reduced. Hence, the collapse of smaller airways and alveoli tends to occur at lower lung volumes—a tendency that is offset by surfactant, which reduces the surface tension of the fluid that lines the alveoli. This reduction usually is sufficient to overcome the tendency to collapse in the normal lung. However,

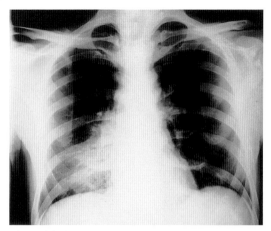

Figure 7-37 Right lower lobe consolidation. The right heart border is clearly defined. Because the consolidation is not complete, the hemidiaphragm has not been effaced.

if the mechanism is disturbed, as in respiratory distress syndrome, collapse of the alveoli occurs, and typically the larger airways remain patent.

Reabsorption Collapse

In acute bronchial obstruction, gases in the alveoli are steadily taken up by the blood in the pulmonary capillaries and are not replenished, leading to alveolar collapse. The degree of collapse may be counteracted by collateral air drift if the obstruction is distal to the main bronchus and also by infection and accumulation of secretions. If the obstruction becomes chronic, subsequent reabsorption of intraalveolar secretions and exudate may result in complete collapse—the usual mechanism of collapse seen in carcinoma of the bronchus. When the cause of collapse is a proximal obstructing mass, the S sign of Golden may be apparent. This sign refers to the S shape made by the relevant fissure as the distal part of a lobe collapses, but the proximal part of a lobe maintains its bulk because of the presence of a tumor.

Radiographic Signs of Lobar Collapse

The radiographic appearance in pulmonary collapse depends on a number of factors, including the mechanism of collapse, the extent of collapse, the presence or absence of consolidation in the affected lung, and the preexisting state of the pleura. This last factor includes the presence of underlying pleural tethering or thickening and the presence of pleural fluid. Preexisting lung disease, such as fibrosis and pleural adhesions, may alter the expected displacement of anatomic landmarks in lung collapse. An air bronchogram is rare in reabsorption collapse but is usual in passive and adhesive collapse and may be seen in cicatrization collapse if fibrosis is particularly dense.

Signs of collapse may be direct or indirect. *Indirect* signs are the result of compensatory changes that occur as a consequence of the volume loss. The *direct* signs of collapse include displacement of interlobar fissures, loss of aeration, and vascular and bronchial signs. Indirect signs include elevation of the hemidiaphragm, mediastinal displacement, hilar displacement, compensatory hyperinflation, and crowding of the ribs. There tends to be a reciprocal relationship between the individual compensatory signs of collapse, so with mediastinal shift to the side of collapse, significant diaphragmatic elevation is unlikely. For example, in lower lobe collapse, if hemidiaphragmatic elevation is marked, hilar depression is less marked.

Displacement of Interlobar Fissures Displacement of interlobar fissures is the most reliable sign, and the degree of displacement depends on the extent of collapse.

Loss of Aeration The increased density of a collapsed area of lung may not become apparent until collapse is almost complete. However, if the collapsed lung is adjacent to the mediastinum or diaphragm, the presence of the silhouette sign may indicate loss of aeration.

Vascular and Bronchial Signs If a lobe is partially collapsed, crowding of its vessels may be visible; also, if an air bronchogram is seen, the bronchi may appear to be crowded together.

Elevation of the Hemidiaphragm Elevation of the hemidiaphragm may be seen in lower lobe collapse but is uncommon in collapse of the other lobes.

Mediastinal Displacement In upper lobe collapse, the trachea often is displaced toward the affected side; in lower lobe collapse, the heart may be displaced to the same site.

Hilar Displacement The hilum may be elevated in upper lobe collapse and depressed in lower lobe collapse.

Compensatory Hyperinflation The remaining normal lung may become hyperinflated and thus may appear more transradiant, with the vessels more widely spaced than in the corresponding area of the contralateral lung. With considerable collapse of a lung, compensatory hyperinflation of the contralateral lung may occur, with herniation of lung across the midline.

Crowding of the Ribs On the side of the collapse, common radiographic features include narrowing of the intercostal spaces with crowding together of the ribs, which reflects the diminished overall volume of the affected hemithorax.

Complete Lung Collapse

With complete collapse of an entire lung (in the absence of an accompanying pneumothorax, large pleural effusion, or extensive consolidation), complete opacification of that hemithorax is seen, with displacement of the mediastinum to the affected side and elevation of the hemidiaphragm. Compensatory hyperinflation of the contralateral lung occurs, often with herniation across the midline. Herniation most often is in the retrosternal space, anterior to the ascending aorta, but may occur posterior to the heart (**Figure 7-38**).

Individual Lobar Collapse

The descriptions that follow apply to collapse of individual lobes, uncomplicated by preexisting pulmonary or pleural disease. The alterations in the positions of the fissures, mediastinal structures, and diaphragms are shown in **Figures 7-39** to **7-43**.

Right Upper Lobe Collapse As the right upper lobe collapses (see Figure 7-39), the horizontal fissure rotates around the hilum and the lateral end moves upward and medially toward the superior mediastinum. The anterior end moves upward, toward the apex. The upper half of the oblique fissure moves anteriorly. The two fissures become concave superiorly. In severe collapse, the lobe may be flattened against the superior mediastinum and may obscure the upper pole of the hilum. The hilum is elevated, and its lower pole may be prominent. Deviation of the trachea to the right is usual, and compensatory hyperinflation of the right middle and lower lobes may be apparent.

Middle Lobe Collapse In right middle lobe collapse (see Figure 7-40), the horizontal fissure and lower half of the oblique fissure move toward each other, a feature best seen on the lateral projection. Because the horizontal fissure tends to be more mobile, it usually shows greater displacement. On the frontal (anteroposterior) radiograph, changes associated with middle lobe collapse may be subtle, because the horizontal fissure may not be visible, and increased opacity does not become apparent until collapse is almost complete. Critical analysis of the radiograph sometimes reveals obscuration of the right heart border as the only clue. The lordotic anteroposterior projection is rarely required but may be used to bring the displaced fissure into the line of the x-ray beam and occasionally may elegantly demonstrate middle lobe collapse. Because the volume of this lobe is relatively small, indirect signs of volume loss are rarely obvious.

Left Lower Lobe Collapse In left lower lobe collapse (see Figure 7-41), the normal oblique fissures extend from the level of the fourth thoracic vertebra posteriorly to the diaphragm, close to the sternum anteriorly. The position of these fissures on the lateral projection is the best index of lower lobe volumes. When a lower lobe collapses, the oblique fissure moves posteriorly but maintains its normal slope. In addition to posterior movement, the collapsing lower lobe causes medial displacement of the oblique fissure, which may become visible in places on the frontal projection.

Right Lower Lobe Collapse Right lower lobe collapse (see Figure 7-42) causes partial depression of the horizontal fissure, which may be apparent on the frontal projection. Increased opacity of a collapsed lower lobe is usually visible on the frontal projection also. A completely collapsed lower lobe may be so small that it flattens and merges with the mediastinum to produce a thin, wedge-shaped shadow. In left lower lobe collapse, the heart may obscure this opacity, and a penetrated view may be required to demonstrate it. Mediastinal structures and parts of the diaphragm adjacent to the nonaerated lobe are obscured. When significant lower lobe collapse occurs, especially when the collapsed lobe is so small as to be invisible as a separate opacity, confirmatory evidence usually is apparent from close inspection of the relevant hilum. This area typically is depressed and rotated medially, with loss of the normal hilar vascular structures, which is made all the more obvious if a previous film is available for comparison. In addition, indirect signs of collapse, such as upper lobe hyperinflation, are present. Diaphragmatic elevation is unusual.

Lingula Collapse The lingula often is involved in collapse of the left upper lobe, but occasionally it may collapse individually, in which case the radiographic features are similar to those of middle lobe collapse. With absence of a horizontal fissure on the left, however, anterior displacement of the lower half of the oblique fissure and increased opacity anterior to it become important signs. On the frontal projection, the left heart border becomes obscured.

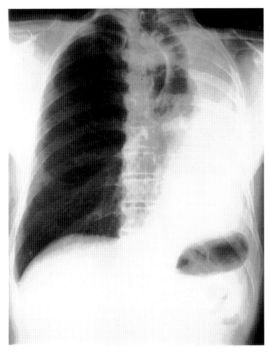

Figure 7-38 Collapse of the left lung. A proximal obstructing tumor is evident within the left main bronchus, with complete collapse of the left lung and a mediastinal shift to the left.

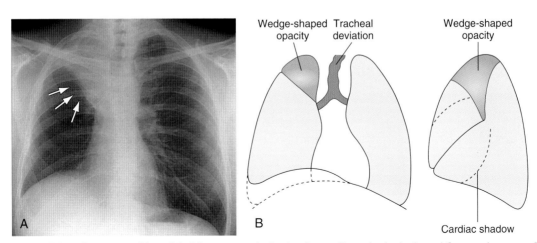

Wedge-shaped opacity   Tracheal deviation   Wedge-shaped opacity

A   B   Cardiac shadow

Figure 7-39 Right upper lobe collapse caused by a right hilum tumor. **A,** On the chest radiograph, the horizontal fissure takes on an S configuration, known as the S sign of Golden (*arrows*). **B,** Line diagram of pathoanatomic changes: *left,* frontal view; *right,* lateral view.

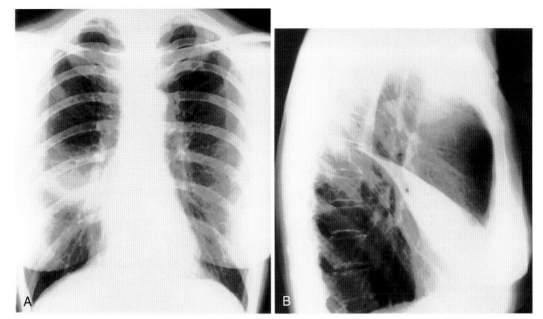

Figure 7-40 Middle lobe collapse. **A,** Loss of the right heart border is seen on the anteroposterior radiograph. **B,** A well-defined wedge-shaped opacity on the lateral radiograph is delineated by the horizontal and oblique fissures.

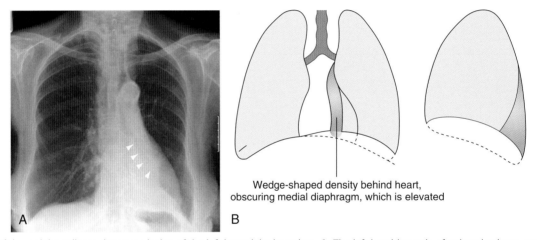

Wedge-shaped density behind heart, obscuring medial diaphragm, which is elevated

Figure 7-41 Left lower lobe collapse due to occlusion of the left lower lobe bronchus. **A,** The left hemithorax is of reduced volume, and there is loss of the normal silhouette of the left lower lobe pulmonary artery. The left lower lobe has contracted behind the cardiac silhouette (*arrowheads*). **B,** Line diagram of pathoanatomic changes: *left,* frontal view; *right,* lateral view.

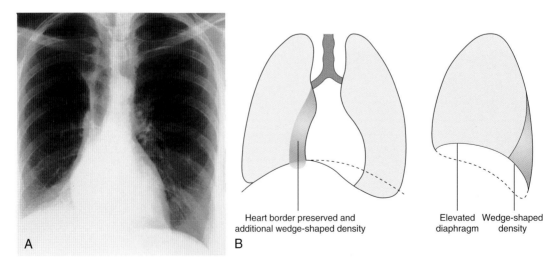

Heart border preserved and additional wedge-shaped density

Elevated diaphragm   Wedge-shaped density

Figure 7-42 Right lower lobe collapse in a patient with asthma. **A,** Radiographic features include preservation of the right heart border with reduction in volume of the right hemithorax and shift of the trachea to the right side. **B,** Line diagram of pathoanatomic changes: *left,* frontal view; *right,* lateral view.

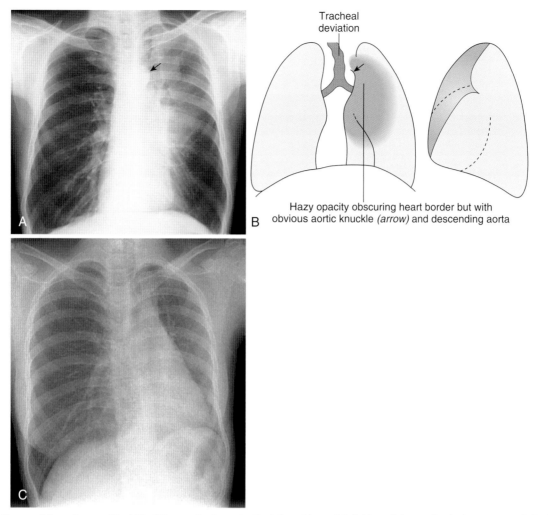

Figure 7-43 Left upper lobe collapse with shift of the mediastinum to the left and loss of definition of the mediastinal structures. **A,** In this patient, a large tumor *(arrow)* is causing left upper lobe and lingula collapse. The opacification fades out more inferiorly. **B,** Line diagram of pathoanatomic changes: *left,* frontal view; *right,* lateral view. **C,** In another patient, very tight left upper lobe collapse was due to a small tumor. The appearances are different, but volume loss is marked in both instances.

Left Upper Lobe Collapse The pattern of upper lobe collapse is different in the two lungs. Left upper lobe collapse (see Figure 7-43) is apparent on the lateral projection as anterior displacement of the entire oblique fissure, which becomes oriented almost parallel to the anterior chest wall. With increasing collapse, the upper lobe retracts posteriorly and loses contact with the anterior chest wall. With complete collapse, the left upper lobe may lose contact with the chest wall and diaphragm and retract medially against the mediastinum. On a lateral film, therefore, left upper lobe collapse is seen as an elongated opacity that extends from the apex and reaches, or almost reaches, the diaphragm; it is anterior to the hilum and is bounded by the displaced oblique fissure posteriorly and by the hyperinflated lower lobe.

A collapsed left upper lobe does not produce a sharp outline on the frontal view. An ill-defined, hazy opacity is present in the upper, middle, and sometimes lower zones, the opacity being densest near the hilum. Pulmonary vessels in the hyperinflated lower lobe usually are visible through the haze. The aortic knuckle typically is obscured, unless the upper lobe has collapsed anterior to it, in which case hyperexpansion of the lower lobe apical segment may occur, separating the collapsed upper lobe from the mediastinal silhouette and aortic knuckle. This separation produces an unusual-looking but characteristic medial crescent of lucency termed the Luftsichel sign. If the lingula is involved, the left heart border is obscured. The hilum often is elevated, and the trachea is deviated to the left.

Combined Lobar Collapses

Right Lower and Middle Lobe Collapse Because the right lower and middle lobes take their origin from the bronchus intermedius, an extensive lesion involving those sites may cause combined collapse. The radiographic appearance is similar to that in right lower lobe collapse (**Figure 7-44**), except that the horizontal fissure is not apparent, and the opacification reaches the lateral chest wall on the frontal view and similarly extends to the anterior chest wall on the lateral view.

Right Upper and Middle Lobe Collapse Combined collapse of the right upper and middle lobes is unusual because of the distance between the origins of their bronchi; it generally can be taken to imply the presence of more than one lesion. This combination produces appearances almost identical to those of left upper lobe collapse (**Figure 7-45**). On occasion, isolated right upper lobe collapse also produces appearances that are identical to those with left upper lobe collapse.

Rounded Atelectasis Rounded atelectasis is an unusual form of pulmonary collapse that may be misdiagnosed as a pulmonary tumor. The plain film will show an opacity that may

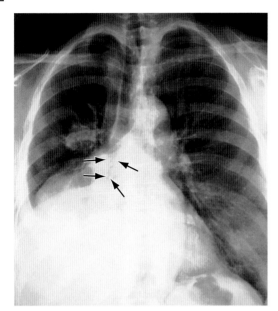

Figure 7-44   Right middle and lower lobe collapse caused by an obstructing lesion in the bronchus intermedius. A bronchial cutoff sign is visible (*arrows*). A separate pulmonary mass is present in the right upper lobe.

be several centimeters in diameter, frequently with ill-defined edges. Rounded atelectasis is always pleura-based and associated with pleural thickening. Vascular shadows may radiate from part of the opacity, said to resemble a comet's tail (**Figure 7-46**). The appearance is caused by peripheral lung tissue folding in on itself. Rounded atelectasis usually is related to previous asbestos exposure but also may be secondary to any exudative pleural effusion. It is not of any other pathologic significance, although when present often raises the question of a malignancy. The CT appearance usually is sufficiently diagnostic to allow differentiation from other pulmonary masses.

Unilateral Increased Transradiancy
The most common causes of increased unilateral transradiancy are technical factors, such as patient rotation, poor beam centering, or an offset grid. Usually, hypertransradiancy caused by technical factors can be identified by comparison of the soft tissues around the shoulder girdle and particularly over the axillae. Nevertheless, a number of pathologic causes of unilateral increased transradiancy are recognized.

Chest Wall   A hemithorax may appear of increased transradiancy (blacker) if the x rays are less attenuated because of a reduction in the amount of overlying soft tissue. The most common cause for this appearance is a mastectomy. Rarely, the same phenomenon may be seen in patients who have congenital unilateral absence of pectoral muscles in Poland syndrome (**Figure 7-47**). This defect may be accompanied by associated skeletal abnormalities in the ipsilateral ribs but may be recognized by loss of the normal axillary skin fold.

Reduced Vascularity   Interruption or significant reduction in the blood supply to one lung, either congenital or acquired, has increased transradiancy (**Figure 7-48**).

Lung Hyperexpansion   If a lung is overexpanded because of either air trapping secondary to the presence of a foreign body or asymmetric emphysema, that hemithorax may demonstrate increased transradiancy. When the entire lung is affected, the

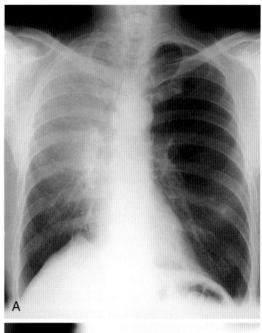

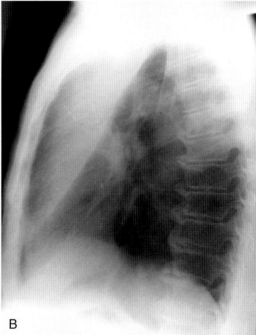

Figure 7-45   Occasionally, the combination of right middle and upper lobe collapse mimics left upper lobe and lingular collapse on the chest radiograph. Both posteroanterior (**A**) and lateral (**B**) views demonstrate changes similar to those seen on the opposite side. The major fissure shifts anteriorly and extends from the lung apex to the anterior costophrenic recess.

hemithorax usually is relatively larger than the opposite side. However, the same phenomenon may occur with compensatory emphysema due to collapse or removal of an ipsilateral lobe. In this instance, the transradiant hemithorax may be of normal volume, and the presence of the increased transradiancy should prompt a search for other evidence of collapse or previous surgery.

A relatively increased transradiancy of one hemithorax with no obvious cause suggests the possibility of a generalized increase in radiopacity of the opposite side (for example, the posterior layering of a pleural effusion in a supine patient) (**Figure 7-49**).

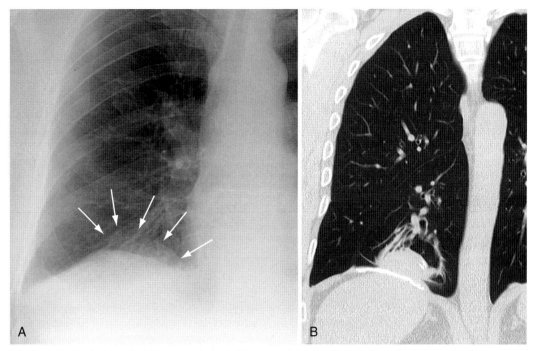

Figure 7-46 Rounded atelectasis. **A,** A poorly defined opacity is visible on the frontal radiograph (*arrows*). **B,** Coronal reformatted image from computed tomography scan reveals the characteristic pleurally based mass with radiating bronchovascular strands.

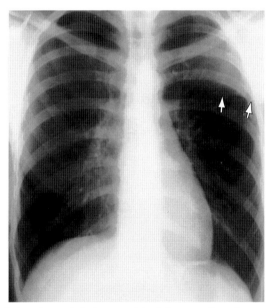

Figure 7-47 Congenital absence of the left pectoralis major muscle in Poland syndrome. In this patient, the muscle deficit was an incidental finding on a chest radiograph. Note the alteration in the left axillary skin fold compared with the right (*arrows*).

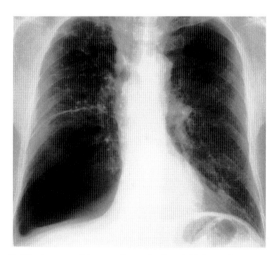

Figure 7-48 Increased transradiancy in the right lower lung zone. A large emphysematous bulla occupies the lower half of the right lung, and the apical changes are in keeping with previous tuberculosis.

The Pulmonary Mass

The finding of a solitary pulmonary nodule on the chest radiograph requires careful analysis, because the diagnostic possibilities are numerous. Once a pulmonary mass has been identified, the observer must decide first, if the lesion is genuine and second, whether the lesion is truly intrapulmonary. The possibility of a cutaneous lesion should not be overlooked, especially if only a part of the nodule is well defined. If doubt remains, repeat radiographs are obtained, with a lateral view and, if relevant, use of nipple markers. What appears at first glance to represent a solitary pulmonary mass may, on closer inspection, actually represent the most obvious of a number of pulmonary nodules. The radiology of multiple pulmonary nodules is discussed later.

When a pulmonary mass is clearly defined around its entire circumference and is projected over the lung on frontal and lateral projections, the mass is truly intrapulmonary (**Figure 7-50**). If a surface is in contact with another soft tissue structure, however, the possibility of an extrapulmonary mass projecting into the lung must be considered. Analysis of the breadth of the base of the lesion, the angle made with the adjacent structure, and the presence of bone destruction often allows the observer to differentiate an extrapulmonary mass that extends into the adjacent lung from an intrapulmonary mass that has grown to contact the mediastinum, diaphragm, or chest wall.

The analysis of a solitary pulmonary mass relies on a number of radiologic and clinical factors. The latter include patient age, geographic and ethnic origins, smoking history, and medical history. The likelihood that a pulmonary nodule represents a malignancy in a young nonsmoker who comes from an area in which histoplasmosis is endemic clearly is different from that for an elderly patient with a lifetime history of smoking.

Radiographic features of a pulmonary nodule that should be analyzed include size, density, margins, vascular markings, and growth rate.

Size
Generally, the likelihood of malignancy is greater with increasing size, although the opposite argument is not reliable.

Density
Most pulmonary masses are of soft tissue density. However, careful inspection must be made for the presence of calcification, because certain patterns of calcification are typical of benign lesions that may be safely observed rather than resected (**Figure 7-51**). A completely or centrally calcified nodule is diagnostic of a tuberculoma or histoplasmoma. Often, CT is required to confirm this pattern of calcification. Likewise, concentric rings of calcification are typical of healed histoplasmosis infection. Popcorn calcification, within the matrix of a

pulmonary nodule, is highly suggestive of a hamartoma (**Figure 7-52**). Other forms of calcification do not reliably indicate whether a nodule is benign or malignant, and dystrophic calcification within a pulmonary malignancy is relatively common.

Margins
Perfectly smooth, round lesions are likely to be benign. This is not a completely reliable rule, however, because some primary lung malignancies and secondary deposits, particularly from soft tissue sarcomas, may be perfectly spherical. By contrast, lobulated or spiculated masses are much more likely to represent malignancy.

Vascular Markings
A rare, benign, but important cause of a pulmonary nodule is an arteriovenous malformation. The diagnosis may be suggested on the plain radiograph if a prominent feeding artery or draining vein is identified.

Growth Rate
Review of previous radiographs, when available, may establish whether a lesion is static or increasing in size. It is usual practice to express the growth of a pulmonary tumor in terms of the time taken for it to double in volume, which equates to an increase in diameter of 25%, assuming that the tumor is roughly spherical, as is usually the case. Tumors with a doubling time of less than 30 days or more than 2 years are very unlikely to result from malignancy. Often, however, no previous films are available, so the use of growth rate as a diagnostic aid is limited. Modern CT allows small pulmonary lesions to be followed over increasing intervals to confirm lack of growth. This is facilitated by the use of automated software that allows volumetric information to be derived from the CT dataset (**Figure 7-53**).

ENHANCEMENT CHARACTERISTICS

By the same token, it has been shown that failure of enhancement of a small lung mass after administration of a bolus of intravenous radiographic contrast also is a strong indicator of a benign histologic type and may strengthen the case for an observational approach to a small (1 to 3 cm) lung nodule in the low-risk patient.

When a solitary lung mass is evident on the chest radiograph, and no features suggest whether it is of benign etiology or a

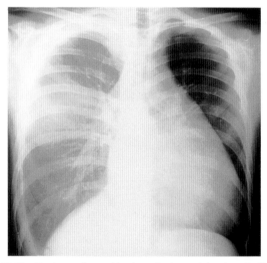

Figure 7-49   Supine radiographic view of a large right pleural effusion. The generalized increase in radiopacity of the right side is caused by posterior layering of a pleural effusion.

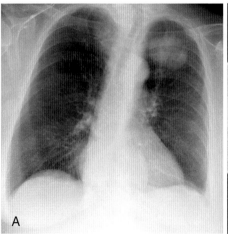
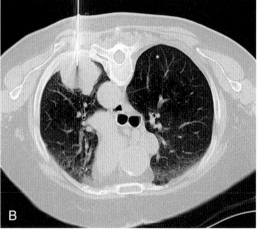

Figure 7-50   A rounded pulmonary mass. **A,** Posteroanterior chest radiograph obtained in a patient with a well-defined left upper lobe pulmonary mass. The entire circumference is visualized on the film, which shows minimal contact of the lesion with adjacent structures. **B,** Image obtained at computed tomography–guided needle biopsy demonstrates that the mass is largely surrounded by aerated lung.

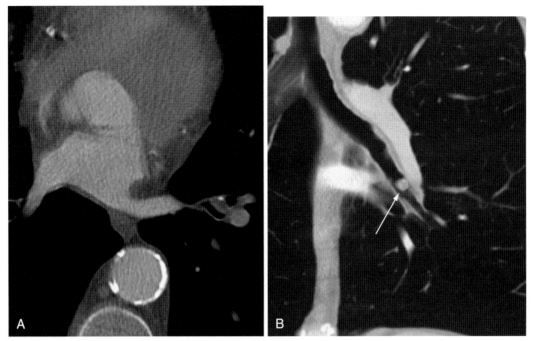

Figure 7-51 Fat and calcium density in a small endobronchial mass seen on computed tomography. A small lesion in the left lower lobe bronchus is evident on both axial (**A**) and coronal (**B**) reformatted images. This density (*arrow* in **B**) confirms that the lesion is a hamartoma.

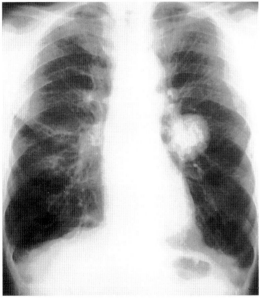

Figure 7-52 Pulmonary mass calcification. Posteroanterior chest radiograph shows a mass that projects over the left hilum. This is smoothly marginated and contains central popcorn calcification; it is unusually large but otherwise is a typical pulmonary hamartoma.

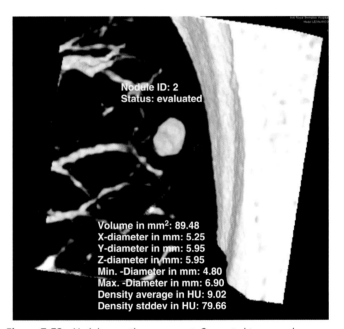

Nodule ID: 2
Status: evaluated

Volume in mm^2: 89.48
X-diameter in mm: 5.25
Y-diameter in mm: 5.95
Z-diameter in mm: 5.95
Min. -Diameter in mm: 4.80
Max. -Diameter in mm: 6.90
Density average in HU: 9.02
Density stddev in HU: 79.66

Figure 7-53 Nodule growth assessment. Computed tomography workstation volumetric assessment allows accurate follow-up imaging of small pulmonary nodules to detect interval growth.

malignant lesion, it should be assumed to be a primary lung carcinoma until proven otherwise. In the assessment of a potential lung primary tumor, certain guidelines may be helpful.

Approximately half of primary lung carcinomas arise centrally in a proximal or segmental bronchus and as a result manifest as a hilar mass.

Because carcinoma of the bronchus arises in the bronchial mucosa, the tumor is likely to grow into the bronchial lumen and around the bronchus. As the bronchial lumen narrows, the distal lung may become consolidated and lose volume. Depending on the site of the tumor, a malignant solitary lung mass may

be associated with lobar or segmental collapse (**Figure 7-54**) or even collapse of an entire lung (see Figure 7-38).

Peripheral tumors usually appear as solitary nodules or masses, but no features on plain films reliably differentiate a benign from a malignant pulmonary nodule. As described previously, malignant tumors often are larger, poorly defined, spiculated, or lobulated. Satellite opacities around a mass are more commonly seen with benign lesions, notably granulomatous diseases (see Figure 7-32). At least 5% of bronchial carcinomas cavitate as a consequence of central necrosis or abscess formation; the resultant cavity typically is thick-walled with an irregular inner margin (**Figure 7-55**). Peripheral tumors may invade the ribs or spine directly. Bone destruction must be specifically looked for and, when present, almost invariably indicates malignancy (**Figure 7-56**).

MULTIPLE PULMONARY NODULES

The differential diagnosis of multiple pulmonary nodules is wide in scope (**Box 7-3**), but analysis of the chest radiograph and a review of the clinical status of the patient will rapidly narrow the number of possibilities. Many of the radiographic features used in the analysis of the solitary pulmonary nodule can be used to advantage in the assessment of multiple lesions.

Radiographically, multiple nodules are described in terms of size, number, distribution, density, definition, cavitation, speed of growth (if serial films are available), and accompanying pleural, mediastinal, or skeletal abnormalities. Further important clinical clues may come from the clinical status of the patient. Specifically, evidence of infection, systemic illness, and previous malignancy is sought (**Figures 7-57** to **7-60**). Miliary nodules are a particular form of nodular shadowing. The term

miliary derives from the resemblance in size and shape of the nodules to millet seeds, being round, well defined, and 2 to 3 mm in diameter. Although the description usually is associated with tuberculosis, this pattern of nodular infiltrate also may be due to histoplasmosis, organic and inorganic dust diseases, sarcoid, or metastases.

DIFFUSE SHADOWING

Many diseases cause diffuse lung shadowing on chest radiography. Careful analysis is required to correctly determine the nature of the abnormality and narrow the differential diagnosis. Appearances on the chest radiograph can be misleading, and the pattern of disease demonstrated at histopathologic examination or HRCT may differ considerably from the pattern of abnormality suggested by the chest radiograph. The summation of multiple small linear opacities on the chest radiograph may produce the appearance of multiple small nodules. Likewise, the superimposition of multiple small nodules may produce a granular or ground glass pattern. A variety of descriptive terms

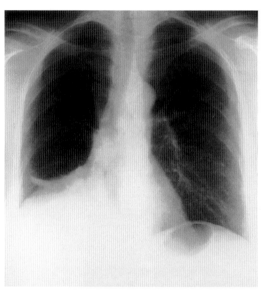

Figure 7-54 Right lower and partial middle lobe collapse secondary to a proximal bronchogenic carcinoma.

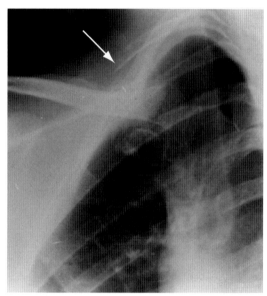

Figure 7-56 Oblique view of the right apex demonstrating bone destruction within the first rib (*arrow*). The patient has peripheral bronchogenic carcinoma.

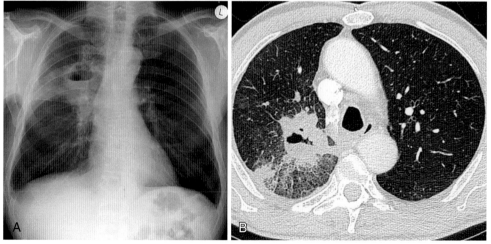

Figure 7-55 A right upper lobe bronchogenic carcinoma with central necrosis and cavitation. On the chest radiograph (**A**) and computed tomography scan (**B**), the cavity wall is seen to be thick and irregular.

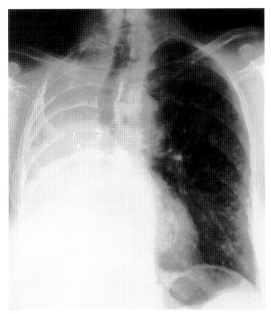

Figure 7-57 Chest radiograph of a patient who had a previous right pneumonectomy for adenocarcinoma. Multiple pulmonary nodules, due to metastases, are now evident within the remaining lung.

| Box 7-3 | **Causes of Acquired Pulmonary Nodules** |

Neoplastic
Benign
    Hamartomas
    Papillomatosis
    Bronchogenic cysts
Malignant
    Metastases
    Lymphoma
    Multifocal tumor
    Kaposi sarcoma
    Bronchoalveolar cell carcinoma

Inflammatory
Infectious
    Viral infections—chickenpox and measles
    Granulomatous infections
    Multiple embolic abscesses
    Round pneumonias
    Parasites—hydatid cysts, paragonimiasis
Noninfectious
    Caplan syndrome and rheumatoid nodules
    Wegener's granulomatosis
    Sarcoidosis

Other
Progressive massive fibrosis
Amyloid
Infarcts
Bronchial impaction

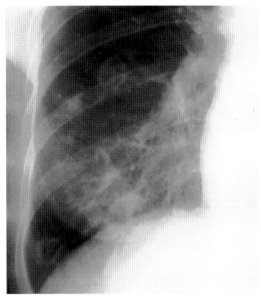

Figure 7-58 Magnified view of the right lower zone. The multiple pulmonary nodules are cavitating in this case of multiple staphylococcal abscesses in an intravenous drug abuser.

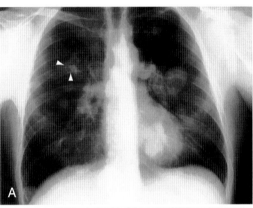

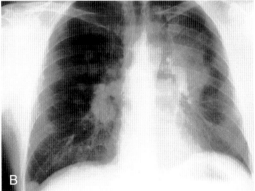

Figure 7-59 Multiple pulmonary nodules. **A,** On the initial chest radiograph, multiple pulmonary nodules are smoothly defined and of variable size; some are cavitating (*arrowheads*). **B,** Subsequent radiograph obtained within a few days of the initial film. The left perihilar nodules are no longer visible because they lie within the now collapsed left upper lobe. The patient proved to have multiple metastases from soft tissue sarcoma.

are used in the analysis of a chest radiograph in this context, and frequently appearances are classified as being either interstitial or air space. A number of processes are capable of producing both patterns, however, so such classification may lead to erroneous narrowing of the differential diagnosis at an early stage of analysis. Thus, it is preferable to analyze the pattern in purely descriptive terms, such as reticular or nodular shadowing, to avoid this pitfall.

Reticular Shadowing

Reticular or linear shadowing (**Figure 7-61**) is made up of multiple, short, irregular linear densities, usually randomly oriented and often overlapping to produce a netlike pattern. When profuse, they may summate to form ring shadows or

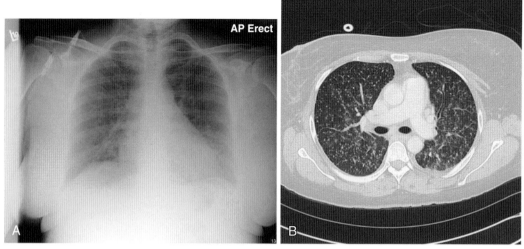

Figure 7-60   Miliary tuberculosis. **A,** Anteroposterior erect chest radiograph demonstrating innumerable 2- to 3-mm soft nodules. **B,** Computed tomography scan showing discrete miliary nodules.

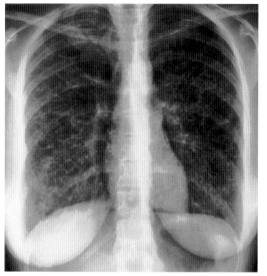

Figure 7-61   Extensive reticular infiltrate in lungs of normal volume. The patient had Langerhans cell histiocytosis.

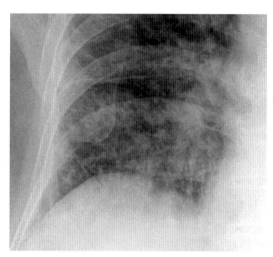

Figure 7-62   Kerley B lines in a patient with heart failure. Of note, the reticular opacities are oriented at right angles to the pleural surface.

sometimes a nodular pattern. Occasionally, the linear shadows may be oriented at right angles to the pleural surface, so-called Kerley B lines (**Figure 7-62**)—a feature that indicates thickening of the interlobular septa. When the linear opacities are extremely profuse or coarse, the impression of a ring or honeycomb pattern is typical.

Nodular Opacities

Nodules may be well or poorly defined and of varying density, ranging from soft tissue to calcific (**Figure 7-63**). They may be discrete or coalescent, with areas of confluence producing consolidation. When the nodules are greater than a few millimeters in diameter, the differential diagnosis changes. Larger discrete nodules were discussed previously.

Reticulonodular Shadowing

Often, it is impossible to confidently assign a pattern of diffuse shadowing to one of the two previously described categories, because they overlap. The reticulonodular pattern probably is the most common form of diffuse lung shadowing.

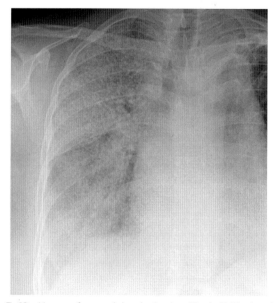

Figure 7-63   Very profuse nodular shadowing. The individual nodules are of high density. The patient had alveolar microlithiasis.

Ground Glass Shadowing

Ground glass shadowing (see Figure 7-33) refers to a generalized increase in density of the lung, which may be diffuse or patchy but most commonly is bilateral and in a middle and lower zone or perihilar location. The underlying vascular branching pattern is not totally obscured as it is in consolidation, but the vessels become less distinct; likewise, the hila and hemidiaphragms may appear less sharp. This subtle abnormality is considerably easier to appreciate with the benefit of a previous normal film for comparison.

In addition to determining the radiographic pattern of diffuse abnormality, a number of other features must be sought, including whether the distribution of disease is central or peripheral, in the upper, middle, or lower zone, and whether distortion of the lung architecture is present. Additional important features include signs of cardiac failure or fluid overload, such as increased heart size, equalization of upper and lower lobe vein size, and pleural effusions. Hilar or mediastinal enlargement caused by lymph node or vascular enlargement also should be specifically sought. In addition, the bones and soft tissues of the chest wall may provide important clues, such as evidence of previous breast surgery or an erosive arthritis. The accuracy of radiographic analysis is reduced in the absence of appropriate clinical information. For example, ascertaining whether the patient is well, acutely or chronically unwell, of normal immune status, or immunocompromised can dramatically narrow a wide range of possibilities in the radiologic differential diagnosis.

AIRWAY DISEASE

Plain tomography has been replaced by CT as the investigation of choice for the examination of airway abnormalities.

Tracheal Narrowing

Tracheal narrowing may be caused by an extrinsic mass, mediastinal fibrosis, or an intrinsic abnormality of the tracheal wall. Chronic inflammatory causes include fibrosing mediastinitis, sarcoidosis, chronic relapsing polychondritis, infection (**Figure 7-64**), and Wegener's granulomatosis. Primary tumors of the trachea are rare. Benign tumors manifest as small, well-defined, intraluminal nodules that are difficult or impossible to visualize on the chest radiograph. Malignant tumors of the trachea tend to occur close to the carina (**Figure 7-65**), although they may be quite extensive and cause a long stricture. Tracheal wall thickening and tracheal luminal narrowing can be detected on the plain chest radiograph, especially when specifically sought, but are best appreciated on CT (**Figure 7-66**). The right lateral

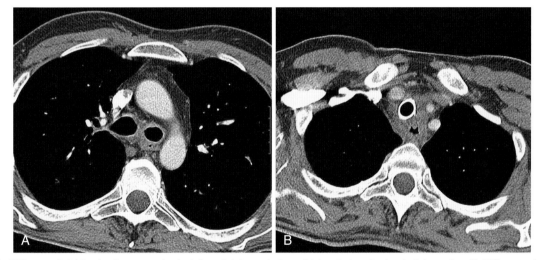

Figure 7-64 **A,** Diffuse wall thickening is present in the left and right main bronchi, just below the level of the carina. **B,** Diffuse tracheal wall thickening is evident at the high level, where a silicone stent is in place.

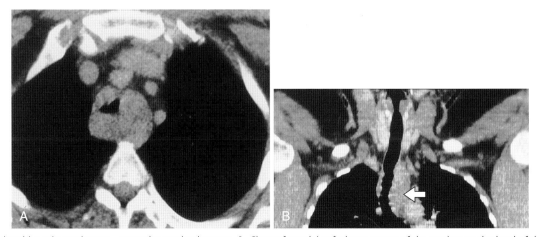

Figure 7-65 Adenoid cystic carcinoma—extensive tracheal tumor. **A,** Circumferential soft tissue tumor of the trachea at the level of the great vessels. **B,** Coronal reformatted image showing extensive tracheal wall thickening measuring, on the left, almost 2 cm (*arrow*).

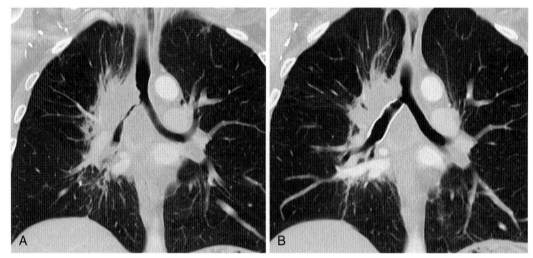

Figure 7-66   Coronal reformatted images from computed tomography scan of the chest. **A,** An extensive mediastinal lymph node mass is the cause of tracheal narrowing. **B,** After stent insertion, airway caliber is restored.

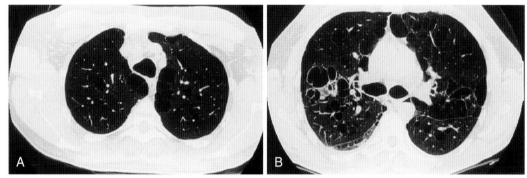

Figure 7-67   Tracheobronchomegaly. Computed tomography scans showing diffuse moderate dilatation of the trachea and main bronchi in association with cystic bronchiectasis: **A,** At the level of the trachea. **B,** At the level of the carina.

wall of the trachea (the right paratracheal stripe) above the level of the azygos vein, typically is a 2-mm-thick soft tissue stripe, and tracheal wall thickening can be detected on the plain radiograph if this portion of the airway is involved.

Tracheal Widening

The normal dimensions of the trachea have been assessed by use of a variety of techniques, most recently CT. The trachea becomes slightly larger with increasing age. On CT scanning, the maximal coronal diameter of the trachea is 23 mm in a man and 20 mm in a woman. Dilatation of the trachea is rare and may result from a generalized defect of connective tissue.

Mounier-Kuhn syndrome is the condition that causes the most dramatic tracheal dilatation (**Figure 7-67**). It is extremely rare and was first described in 1932. On the plain radiograph, shift of the right paratracheal stripe to the right often is the only sign of tracheal widening, and because the trachea frequently is not central in location, tracheal widening can be recognized only if the left wall of the trachea also is identified. The Mounier-Kuhn syndrome is underreported because it may go undiagnosed—clinical signs and symptoms are similar to those of chronic bronchitis, COPD, or bronchiectasis. Other features include marked dilatation of the trachea and major bronchi associated with repeated respiratory infections and copious sputum production. CT scans demonstrate tracheo-bronchial dilatation; some will often reveal parenchymal scarring secondary to chronic infection. Bronchoscopy demonstrates

dilated central airways with thickened walls. Dilatation results in ineffective mucociliary expectoration, and the subsequent chronic inflammation contributes to the cycle of infection and continued inflammation, leading to bronchiectasis and recurrent pneumonia and the development of emphysema.

Histopathologic inspection reveals loss of cartilage and muscle within the airway walls associated with dilatation and saccular diverticulosis. There may be associated connective tissue diseases such as Ehlers-Danlos syndrome in adults and cutis laxa in children. Airways usually return to normal caliber at the fourth or fifth bronchial generation. In some cases, the disease may be acquired, because a complete absence of symptoms until the third or fourth decade of life has been described.

The chest radiograph often is reported to be normal even when extensive disease is evident on CT. Management options are limited, because the central airway involvement prevents extensive surgical intervention. Postural drainage and antibiotic therapy are necessary, in parallel with other forms of bronchiectasis. In some reported cases, bronchoscopy was used to clear secretions, tracheostomy has been necessary, and transplantation has been attempted.

Another unusual form of airway dilatation was described by Williams and Campbell. All patients presented in early childhood with symptoms of cough and wheezing and recurrent pulmonary infections. On examination, the chest was barrel-shaped, and inspiratory and expiratory wheezes and clubbing were noted. In this original cohort, plain radiography and

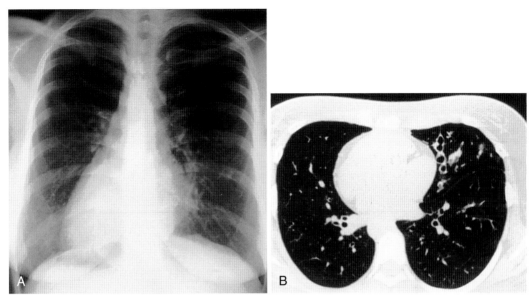

Figure 7-68 Bronchiectasis. **A,** The chest radiograph of a patient with primary ciliary dyskinesia. Dextrocardia is obvious. Some questionable bronchial wall thickening adjacent to the left heart border is obscured. **B,** The changes of bronchiectasis are much more convincingly demonstrated on high-resolution computed tomography.

bronchography demonstrated thin-walled cystic bronchiectasis and ballooning of more peripheral airways on inspiration with collapse on expiration. Inspiratory and expiratory CT images have proved useful in the diagnosis of this syndrome in more recent reports.

Bronchiectasis

The chest radiograph is relatively insensitive for the detection of bronchiectasis, and in most series, a significant proportion of plain radiographs obtained in patients with clinical bronchiectasis are judged to be normal (**Figure 7-68**). The use of HRCT is discussed later on; this modality is now the investigation of choice for bronchiectasis. Abnormalities present on the chest radiograph are as follows.

Bronchial wall thickening is evident as parallel, linear opacities radiating from the hilum, with lack of the normal convergence more peripherally. Ring shadows occur when the dilated airway is seen end on, may be thick- or thin-walled, and may contain secretions that produce an air-fluid level. Bronchiectatic airways that become plugged with secretions may produce tubular, soft tissue density opacities radiating from the hilum, more commonly in the lower lobes.

Distortion of the lobar anatomy with volume loss and crowding together of bronchovascular structures may be an associated finding. However, patients who have cystic fibrosis, also characterized by bronchiectasis, may have significant air trapping, which results in overexpansion. Even severe bronchiectasis may be invisible within a completely collapsed lobe.

Cylindrical (or tubular) bronchiectasis produces a dilated bronchus with parallel walls, in varicose bronchiectasis the walls are irregular, and in saccular (or cystic) bronchiectasis the airways terminate as round cysts. In an individual patient, presence of more than one pattern is typical. Bronchiectasis usually involves the peripheral bronchi more severely than the central bronchi. Although it has long been held that in allergic bronchopulmonary aspergillosis, this pattern may be reversed, overall the distribution and morphology demonstrated by CT give no more than a clue to the underlying etiology.

MEDIASTINAL ABNORMALITIES

The normal radiographic anatomy of the mediastinum was discussed earlier in this chapter. When a mediastinal abnormality is present on the posteroanterior radiograph, a lateral view should be obtained to aid anatomic localization. Today, the imaging of mediastinal masses depends heavily on CT scanning, which is discussed elsewhere. However, a familiarity with normal anatomy is required to detect mediastinal masses that at first appear as a subtle distortion of the normal mediastinal contours. A considerable volume of mediastinal tumor or lymph node enlargement may be present despite a normal appearance on the chest radiograph.

The most common cause of mediastinal enlargement visible on the chest radiograph in children is the normal thymus, which may enlarge and contract in certain disease states but typically remains relatively prominent, especially on CT scans, until puberty (**Figure 7-69**). Lymphadenopathy, tumor, hiatal hernia, and vascular abnormalities account for most mediastinal masses seen in adults.

Mediastinal Lymphadenopathy

Lymph nodes are present in all compartments of the mediastinum but are visible on the chest radiograph only when they are calcified or enlarged. Causes of mediastinal nodal enlargement are discussed elsewhere. The chest radiograph is a relatively insensitive indicator of lymphadenopathy. Enlargement of right paratracheal nodes is identified more easily than that of left paratracheal nodes, aortic-pulmonary nodes, and subcarinal lymphadenopathies (**Figure 7-70**). Barium swallow is a simple method of identifying some cases of subcarinal lymphadenopathy, but CT is the most comprehensive and accurate method of assessing mediastinal nodes.

Abnormalities of the Thoracic Aorta

The thoracic aorta arises in the middle mediastinum and then arches through the anterior, middle, and posterior mediastinal compartments. The greater vessels arise from the aortic arch in the superior mediastinum (**Figure 7-71**). Dilatation or tortuosity of the aortic arch or its branches may cause widening of the

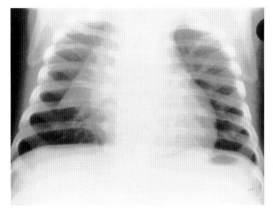

Figure 7-69 A prominent but normal thymic silhouette in an infant. Note the characteristic sail shape of the thymus as it projects over the right lung and the typically slightly lobulated contour as it conforms to the overlying ribs.

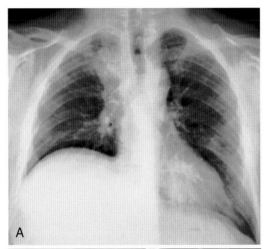

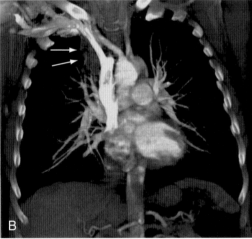

Figure 7-70 Right paratracheal lymph node enlargement caused by bronchogenic carcinoma. **A,** A right phrenic nerve palsy results in elevation of the right hemidiaphragm. **B,** Coronal volume-rendered slab image from a multidetector computed tomography machine obtained in a different patient. As in **A,** right paratracheal lymph node enlargement (*arrows*) abuts but does not distort the right brachiocephalic vein and superior vena cava.

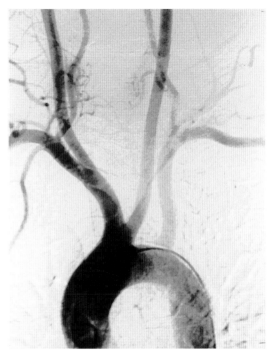

Figure 7-71 Digital subtraction arch aortogram. Two vessels can be seen arising from the arch—a common variant of the normal three-vessel anatomy. The image was obtained with the patient in a 30-degree left anterior oblique position.

mediastinal shadow. So-called unfolding of the aorta is a common chest radiographic finding in elderly or hypertensive patients. Aneurysm of the aorta most often results from atherosclerosis (**Figure 7-72**). Cystic medial necrosis (Marfan syndrome), infection (mycotic aneurysm), syphilitic aortitis, and a history of trauma are less common causes. Most aortic aneurysms are asymptomatic and manifest as mediastinal opacities on the radiograph, sometimes with curvilinear calcification visible in the wall. Aneurysms of the ascending aorta are best appreciated on the lateral radiograph as a filling in of the retrosternal window. Aneurysms of the arch and descending aorta frequently are evident on the frontal radiograph, but a lateral view often is required for more accurate localization, and cross-sectional imaging may be warranted to confirm that the mediastinal abnormality in question is of vascular origin.

In the acutely injured patient, traumatic aortic rupture may be suspected from the appearance on the chest radiograph, and confirmation of injury usually requires angiography (**Figure 7-73**). When the chest radiographic findings are equivocal, however, in concert with a degree of trauma less than that usually associated with aortic injury, a spiral CT scan may be performed in the stable patient to exclude a mediastinal hematoma. If any doubt remains, the patient should proceed to angiography. If the aortic injury remains undetected and the patient survives, an aneurysm secondary to the trauma may develop subsequently. Such lesions almost always are confined to the junction of the aortic arch and descending aorta. Aortic abnormalities may produce remodeling due to chronic pressure in adjacent skeletal structures.

Aneurysm of the ascending aorta may be associated with erosion of the posterior surface of the sternum, and descending aortic aneurysms may cause scalloping of the spine. Tortuosity of the innominate artery is a common cause of widening of the superior mediastinum in elderly persons. Right-sided aortic arch (**Figure 7-74**) and pseudocoarctation of the aorta are two anomalies that may alter the appearance of the mediastinum, suggestive of a mass.

Abnormalities of the Esophagus

Abnormalities of the esophagus are relatively common. They include infection and inflammation, trauma and perforation,

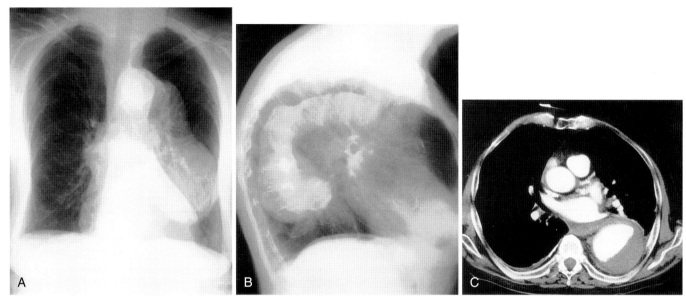

Figure 7-72 Thoracic aortic aneurysm. **A,** On the posteroanterior radiographic view, marked dilatation and tortuosity of the descending thoracic aorta are present. Of note, the left heart border is still evident, indicating the abnormality is likely to lie in the posterior thorax. **B,** Lateral view in the same patient demonstrates that the aneurysm involves the posterior arch and descending thoracic aorta. Note calcification within the ascending aorta. **C,** Computed tomography scan demonstrating extensive mural thrombus.

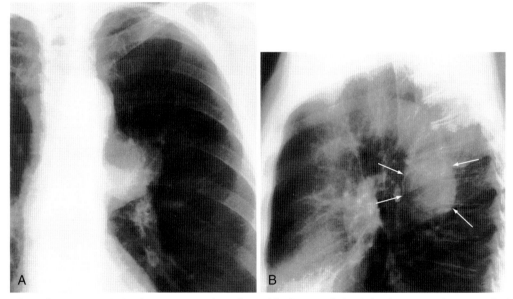

Figure 7-73 Traumatic aortic aneurysm. **A,** On the posteroanterior radiographic view, a soft tissue density mass projects over the left hilum. Of note, the left lower lobe artery is still visible through this mass, indicating that it is separate from the hilum. The medial surface blends smoothly with the mediastinal structures, indicating that it is likely to be extrapulmonary. **B,** The lateral view confirms presence of an aneurysm secondary to previous trauma at the typical site, the junction of the posterior arch and descending thoracic aorta (*arrows*).

and benign and malignant neoplastic processes. Esophageal abnormalities may be associated with diseases that also involve the lungs. Such conditions are best exemplified by achalasia of the cardia (**Figure 7-75**) or systemic sclerosis (**Figure 7-76**), in which esophageal motility disorders resulting in significant dilatation and reflux may be encountered in conjunction with pulmonary fibrosis and the sequelae of recurrent aspiration.

Dilatation of Central Veins

The superior vena cava and the azygos vein may dilate because of increased pressure, increased flow, obstruction, or congenital abnormality. Increased flow in the superior vena cava is seen with supracardiac, total, anomalous pulmonary venous drainage

(**Figure 7-77**), and in the azygos vein, with congenital absence of the inferior vena cava. Rarely, aneurysmal dilatation of the superior mediastinal veins produces an abnormal mediastinal silhouette. Likewise, obstruction of the superior vena cava may cause dilatation of the great veins in the superior mediastinum, which results in widening of the mediastinal contour. However, the clinical features are likely to be obvious by the time radiographic abnormalities become significant.

Other Mediastinal Abnormalities

Pneumomediastinum or *mediastinal emphysema* is the presence of air between the tissue planes of the mediastinum. This condition may be secondary to interstitial pulmonary emphysema

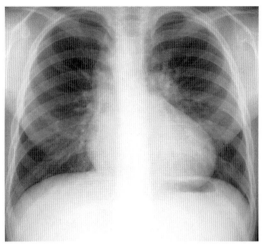

Figure 7-74 Tetralogy of Fallot. A right-sided aortic arch can be seen, in addition to elevation of the ventricular apex secondary to developing ventricular hypertrophy. Note the relatively oligemic lungs.

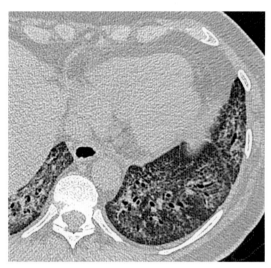

Figure 7-76 Systemic sclerosis with esophageal involvement. HRCT scan shows a coarse bibasal reticular infiltrate with marked traction bronchiectasis. In addition, the esophagus is moderately dilated and contains an air-fluid level.

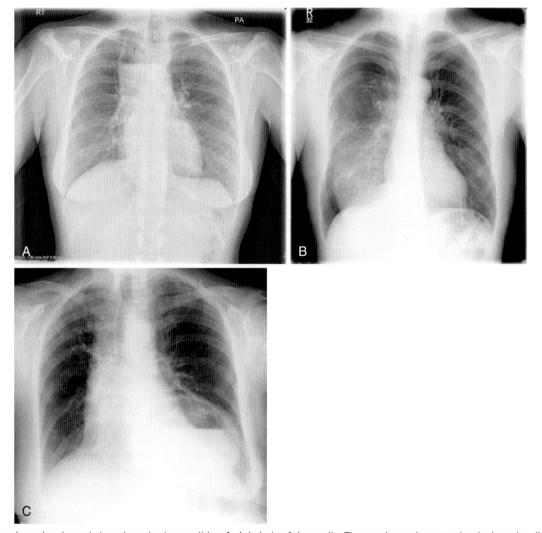

Figure 7-75 Esophageal and gastric intrathoracic abnormalities. **A,** Achalasia of the cardia. The esophagus is empty, but its lateral walls are seen running up the mediastinum. **B,** Chest radiograph obtained in a patient who had a gastric pull-up subsequent to esophagectomy. The wall of the stomach is seen near the right chest wall margin. The stomach contains solid matter in its lower part and mainly air in its upper part. The missing rib was resected for the necessary surgery. **C,** Large hiatal hernia with fluid level more or less overlying the heart. No stomach bubble is seen on the chest film obtained in the conventional site, and the left hemidiaphragm is poorly demarcated. (*B* and *C* Courtesy of Dr. M. Taylor.)

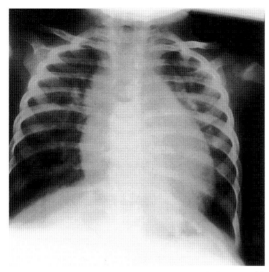

Figure 7-77 Total anomalous pulmonary venous drainage. Widening of the superior mediastinum on the chest radiograph is caused by dilatation of the superior vena cava.

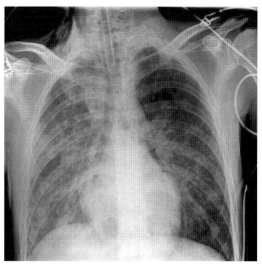

Figure 7-78 Pneumomediastinum. Air separates the tissue planes within the mediastinum and extends into the soft tissues of the neck and chest. A left-sided intercostal drain is in situ. *(Courtesy Dr. M. Taylor.)*

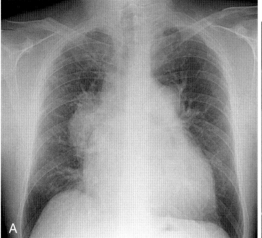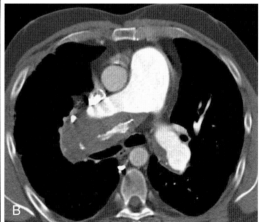

Figure 7-79 Recurrent pulmonary emboli resulting in marked dilatation of the proximal pulmonary arteries. **A,** The cardiac silhouette is enlarged. **B,** Computed tomography angiogram demonstrating contrast and clot in the pulmonary arteries.

(most often caused by mechanical ventilation); to perforation of the esophagus, trachea, or a bronchus; or to a penetrating chest injury. Chest radiography may show vertical, translucent streaks in the mediastinum, which represent the soft tissue planes separated by air (**Figure 7-78**). The air may extend up into the neck and over the chest wall (causing subcutaneous emphysema) and also over the diaphragm. The mediastinal pleura may be displaced laterally and then become visible as a thin stripe alongside the mediastinum.

Acute mediastinitis typically is caused by perforation of the esophagus, pharynx, or trachea, and a chest radiograph usually shows widening of the mediastinum. A pneumomediastinum often is apparent, and air-fluid levels may be visible in the mediastinum. Chronic or fibrosing mediastinitis usually manifests as SVCO. Mediastinal hemorrhage may occur from venous or arterial bleeding. The mediastinum appears widened, and blood may be seen to track over the lung apices. It is obviously imperative to identify a life-threatening cause such as aortic rupture.

HILAR ABNORMALITIES

Having identified a hilar abnormality, the observer must differentiate between a vascular and a nonvascular cause. Vascular prominence often is bilateral and accompanied by enlargement of the main pulmonary artery (**Figure 7-79**). Although the hila are large, they are of relatively normal density, and it usually is possible to trace the pulmonary artery branches in continuity from the adjacent lung to their point of convergence with the interlobar arteries, known as the *hilar convergence sign*. By comparison, enlargement caused by lymph nodes or hilar tumor generally produces a lobulated hilar contour, with discernible lateral or inferior borders. Frequently, the normal hilar point is obliterated, and on the left, the aortopulmonary angle is filled in (**Figure 7-80**).

Occasionally, a pulmonary lesion is superimposed directly on the hilum on the frontal radiograph, which produces a spuriously large or dense hilum. The true position of the abnormality is revealed on the lateral radiograph (see Figure 7-72). A further pitfall arises when the vessels to the lingula or, more

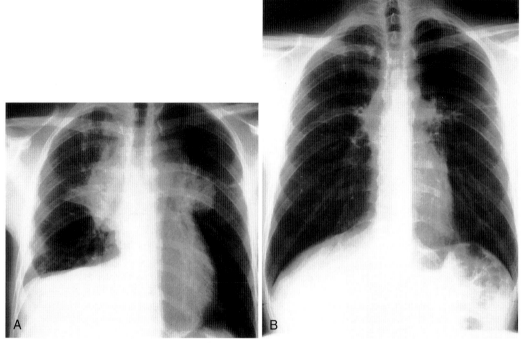

Figure 7-80   Non-Hodgkin lymphoma. **A,** Bilateral hilar lymph node enlargement, with obliteration of the normal aortopulmonary angle and subcarinal nodes. A right-sided pleural effusion is present. **B,** Residual abnormality after chemotherapy.

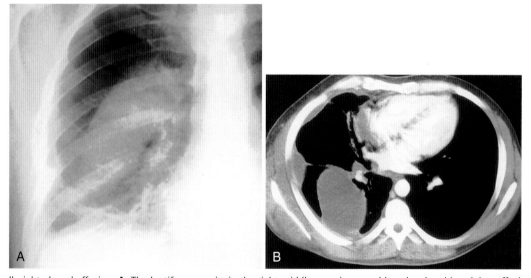

Figure 7-81   Small, right pleural effusion. **A,** The lentiform opacity in the right middle zone is caused by a loculated interlobar effusion. **B,** Computed tomography scan on mediastinal settings demonstrating the position of the loculated fluid within the oblique fissure.

commonly, the right middle lobe are superimposed on the lower part of the hilar shadow, particularly when the film is taken anteroposteriorly, in a lordotic projection, or with a poor inspiratory effort. A lateral radiograph usually confirms the vascular nature of the shadowing.

PLEURAL DISEASE

Pleural Fluid

The most dependent recess of the pleural space is the posterior costophrenic angle, which is where a small effusion tends to collect. As little as 100 to 200 mL of fluid accumulated in this recess can be seen above the dome of the diaphragm on the frontal view. Even smaller effusions may be seen on a lateral radiograph, and it is possible to identify effusions of only a few

milliliters by use of decubitus radiographic views made with a horizontal beam, ultrasound imaging, or CT. Eventually, the costophrenic angle on the frontal view fills in, and with increasing fluid a homogeneous opacity spreads upward, obscuring the lung base (**Figure 7-81**). The fluid usually demonstrates a concave upper edge, higher laterally than medially, and obscures the diaphragm. Fluid may track into the fissures. A massive effusion may cause complete opacification of a hemithorax with passive atelectasis. The space-occupying effect of the effusion may push the mediastinum toward the opposite side, especially when the lung does not collapse significantly (**Figure 7-82**).

Lamellar effusions are shallow collections between the lung surface and the visceral pleura, sometimes sparing the costophrenic angle. Subpulmonary effusions accumulate between

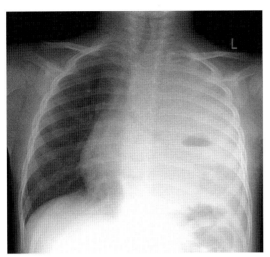

Figure 7-82 Large left pleural effusion. The patient presented with an acute empyema resulting from a lung abscess (note the air-fluid level). The mediastinal shift to the right is due to the space-occupying effects of the fluid.

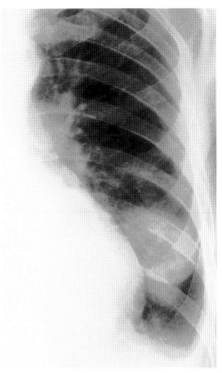

Figure 7-83 Small, left basal pleural effusion. The opacity in the left middle zone is caused by fluid loculated in the oblique fissure.

the diaphragm and undersurface of a lung, mimicking elevation of the hemidiaphragm. Usually, the contour to the top of such an effusion differs from the normal diaphragmatic contour, the apparent apex being more lateral than usual. Also, some blunting of the costophrenic angle or tracking of fluid into fissures may be visible. On the left side, increased distance between the gastric air bubble and lung base may be apparent. A subpulmonary effusion may be confirmed by ultrasound imaging. However, because the fluid is free to shift within the pleural cavity with changes in patient position, a decubitus film may be needed for confirmation.

Encapsulated or encysted fluid may be difficult to differentiate from an extrapleural opacity, parenchymal lung disease, or mediastinal mass. Of note, however, an encysted effusion often is associated with free pleural fluid or other pleural shadowing and may extend into a fissure (see Figure 7-81). Loculated effusions tend to have comparatively little depth but considerable width, rather like a biconvex lens. Their appearance, therefore, depends on whether they are viewed end on, in profile, or obliquely. Extrapleural opacities tend to have a much sharper outline, with tapered, sometimes concave edges where they meet the chest wall. Peripheral, pleurally based lung lesions may show an air bronchogram, which differentiates them from true pleural disease. The differentiation between pleural thickening or mass and loculated pleural fluid may be difficult on plain films; CT and ultrasound imaging are particularly useful in this context.

Fluid may become loculated in the interlobar fissures and most frequently is seen in heart failure. Fluid that collects in the horizontal fissure produces a lenticular, oval, or round shadow, with well-demarcated edges. Loculated fluid in an oblique fissure may be poorly defined on a frontal radiograph, but a lateral film usually is diagnostic, because the fissure is seen tangentially and the typical lenticular configuration of the effusion is demonstrated. Loculated interlobar effusions can appear rounded on two views and may disappear rapidly. Hence, they are sometimes known as pulmonary pseudotumors (**Figure 7-83**). With subsequent episodes of heart failure, they may return at the same site.

Diagnosis of an empyema usually requires thoracentesis. Nevertheless, the diagnosis may be suspected radiographically by the spontaneous appearance on a plain film of an air-fluid level in a pleural effusion, because this feature usually equates with loculation and communication with the tracheobronchial tree or the presence of a gas-forming organism. Loculation is best demonstrated with ultrasound imaging.

Pneumothorax

A small pneumothorax is easily overlooked, and in an erect patient, the air usually collects at the apex. The lung retracts toward the hilum, and on a frontal chest film, the sharp white line of the visceral pleura is visible, separated from the chest wall by the radiolucent pleural space, which is devoid of lung markings. This appearance should not be confused with that of a skin fold (**Figure 7-84**). The lung usually remains aerated, although perfusion is reduced in proportion to ventilation, so the radiodensity of the partially collapsed lung remains relatively normal. A closed pneumothorax is easier to see on an expiratory film, although expiratory radiographs are not routinely required to detect clinically significant pneumothoraces. A lateral decubitus film made with the affected side uppermost occasionally is helpful, because the pleural air can be seen along the lateral chest wall. This view is particularly useful in infants, because small pneumothoraces are difficult to see on supine anteroposterior films, because the air tends to collect anteriorly and medially.

A large pneumothorax may lead to complete relaxation and retraction of the lung, with some mediastinal shift toward the normal side (**Figure 7-85**). Because it constitutes a medical emergency, tension pneumothorax often is treated before a chest radiograph is obtained. However, if a radiograph is taken in this situation, it shows marked displacement of the mediastinum (**Figure 7-86**). Radiographically, the lung may be squashed against the mediastinum or herniate across the midline, and the ipsilateral hemidiaphragm may be depressed.

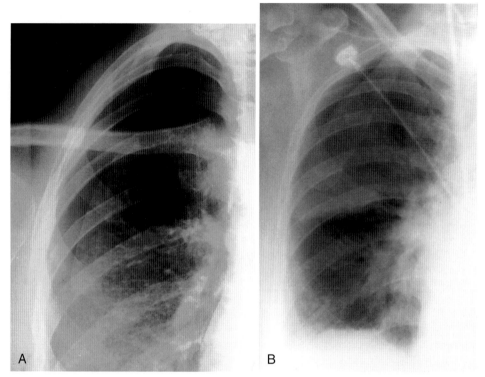

Figure 7-84   Shallow right pneumothorax. **A,** A discrete pleural white line is seen. Peripheral to this line, lung markings are absent. **B,** In this skin fold, although a change in density parallels the chest wall, no discrete pleural line is present, and lung markings are seen to extend beyond the apparent lung edge. This appearance is caused by a superficial fold of skin produced by the x-ray cassette.

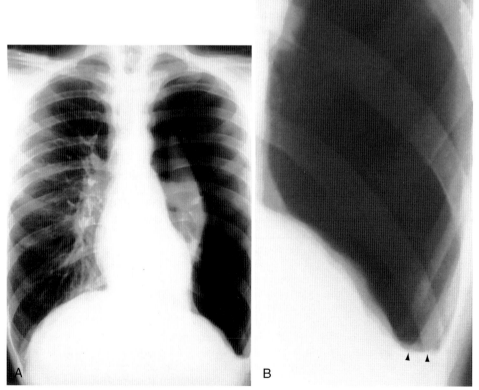

Figure 7-85   Left-sided pneumothorax. **A,** Complete collapse of the left lung, which is retracted to the left hilum. **B,** Magnified view of the left lower zone demonstrates the "short" air-fluid level commonly seen in a costophrenic angle when a pneumothorax is present (*arrowheads*).

Complications of Pneumothorax

Pleural adhesions may limit the distribution of a pneumothorax and result in a loculated or encysted pneumothorax. The usual appearance is an ovoid air collection adjacent to the chest wall, which may be radiographically indistinguishable from a thin-walled, subpleural pulmonary cyst or bulla. Pleural adhesions occasionally are seen as line shadows that stretch between the two pleural layers; they prevent relaxation of the underlying lung. Rupture of an adhesion may produce a hemopneumothorax. Collapse or consolidation of a lobe or lung in association with a pneumothorax is important because it may delay reexpansion of the lung.

Because the normal pleural space contains a small volume of fluid, blunting of the costophrenic angle by a "short" fluid level commonly is seen on radiographs of a pneumothorax (see Figure 7-85). In a small pneumothorax, this fluid level may be the most obvious radiologic sign. A higher fluid level usually signifies a complication and represents exudate, pus, or blood, depending on the etiology of the pneumothorax (**Figure 7-87**).

The usual radiographic appearance of a hydropneumothorax is that of a pneumothorax containing a horizontal fluid level that separates opaque fluid below from lucent air above. A hydrothorax or pyopneumothorax may arise as a result of a bronchopleural fistula (an abnormal communication between the bronchial tree and the pleural space). This may be a complication of surgery but also may occur as a complication of a subpleural lung tumor (**Figure 7-88**).

Pleural Thickening

Blunting of a costophrenic angle is a common observation and usually is caused by localized pleural thickening secondary to previous pleuritis. In the asymptomatic patient and in the absence of other radiologic abnormalities, it is of no significance other than that it may simulate a pleural effusion. When relevant, the possibility of pleural fluid may have to be excluded by other techniques. Localized pleural thickening that extends into the inferior end of an oblique fissure may produce so-called tenting of the diaphragm and is of similar significance, although a similar appearance may result from scarring caused by previous pulmonary infection or infarction.

Bilateral apical pleural thickening is common, usually symmetric in distribution, and more frequent in elderly patients and does not necessarily indicate previous tuberculosis. The

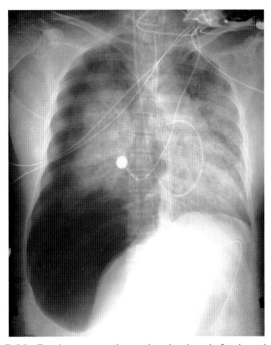

Figure 7-86 Tension pneumothorax that developed after insertion of a Swan-Ganz catheter. Note the shift of the mediastinum toward the left and reversal of the normal contour of the right hemidiaphragm.

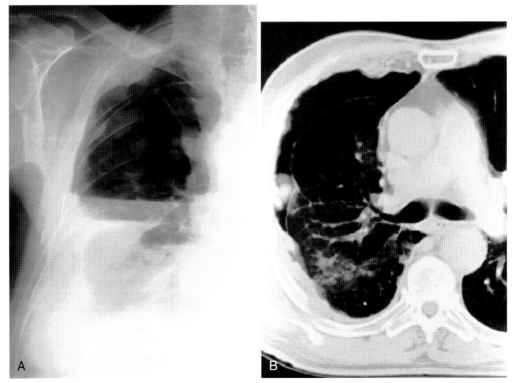

Figure 7-87 Hydropneumothorax in a patient with a mesothelioma. **A,** Chest radiograph shows normal thickness of the visceral pleura, but with lobulated soft tissue shadowing caused by tumor within the parietal pleura. **B,** Computed tomography scan demonstrates the lobulated pleural tumor.

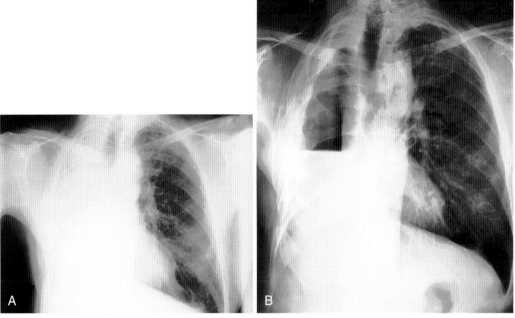

Figure 7-88 Pneumonectomy: appearances and complications. **A,** Chest radiograph showing the normal appearances after a right pneumonectomy. **B,** Spontaneous development of an air-fluid level, caused by a bronchopleural fistula from local recurrence.

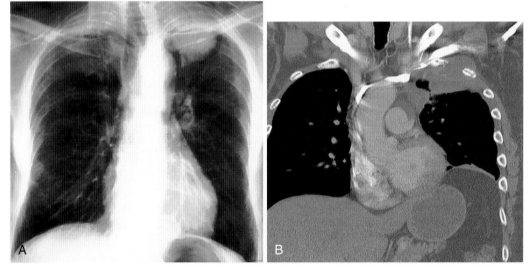

Figure 7-89 Apical abnormalities. **A,** Benign apical pleural thickening is visible (*right*); a Pancoast tumor also is present (*left*). **B,** Coronal reformatted image from a computed tomography scan from another patient who also had an apical tumor.

etiology is uncertain, but in some affected persons, the "caps" represent extrapleural fat that has descended because of scarring and consequent retraction of the upper lobes. By contrast, asymmetric or unilateral apical pleural thickening may be highly significant, especially if associated with pain. Asymmetric apical pleural shadowing may represent a Pancoast tumor, and bone destruction should be specifically sought (**Figure 7-89**).

More extensive unilateral pleural thickening usually is the result of a previous thoracotomy or an exudative pleural effusion. A simple transudate typically resolves completely, but empyema and hemothorax are more likely to resolve with residual pleural fibrosis. The thickened pleura may calcify (**Figure 7-90**), and the entire lung may become surrounded by fibrotic pleura, which may be as much as a few centimeters thick (**Figure 7-91**). Bilateral (parietal) pleural plaques are a common manifestation of asbestos exposure, and occasionally more diffuse, visceral pleural thickening is seen.

Pleural Calcification

In general, pleural calcification has the same causes as for pleural thickening. Unilateral pleural calcification is therefore likely to be the result of previous empyema or hemothorax, and bilateral calcification occurs after asbestos exposure (**Figure 7-92**). Pleural calcification may be discovered in a patient who was not aware of previous chest disease.

The calcification associated with previous pleurisy, empyema, or hemothorax occurs in the visceral pleura (**Figure 7-93**); associated pleural thickening is almost always present and separates the calcium from the ribs. The calcium may be in a continuous sheet or in discrete plaques, which usually produce dense, coarse, irregular shadows, often sharply demarcated

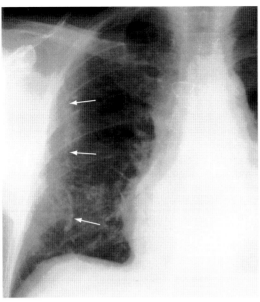

Figure 7-90 Previous thoracotomy (note sternotomy sutures) for mitral valve replacement. Pleural calcification is seen on the right side (*arrows*).

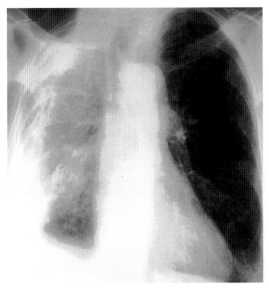

Figure 7-91 Previous tuberculosis. Extensive right-sided pleural thickening and calcification, with reduction in volume of the right hemithorax, are evident.

laterally. When a plaque is viewed end on, it may be less well defined, mimicking a pulmonary infiltrate.

Pleural Masses

Primary tumors of the pleura are rare. Benign tumors of the pleura include pleural fibroma and lipoma (**Figure 7-94**). The most common malignant disease of the pleura is metastatic, usually adenocarcinoma from the bronchus or breast (**Figure 7-95**). Malignant mesothelioma typically is associated with previous asbestos exposure.

COMPUTED TOMOGRAPHY

ANATOMY OF THE MEDIASTINUM

The soft tissue contrast provided by CT, as well as its cross-sectional nature, makes the diagnostic information available from CT far superior to that provided by two-dimensional

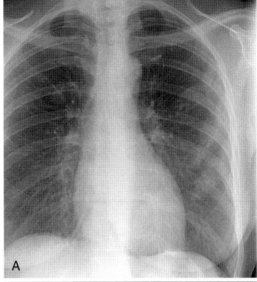

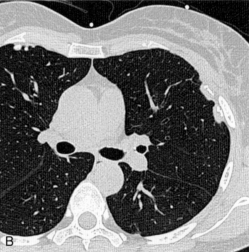

Figure 7-92 Calcified pleural thickening secondary to asbestos exposure. The subtle plaques seen on the chest radiograph (**A**) are better demonstrated on the computed tomography scan (**B**).

radiography. Modern CT scanners can acquire a volume of imaging information that includes the whole of the mediastinum within the time of a single breath-hold. This three-dimensional dataset can then be displayed as continuous or overlapping axial slices, free from breathing movement artifact. Usually, a collimation and slice width of between 5 and 10 mm is used, and it is usual, but not always essential, to give intravenous contrast. The normal mediastinal anatomy is demonstrated in **Figures 7-96** to **7-101**.

Great Vessels

The great vessels constitute the most familiar anatomic landmarks within the mediastinum. Knowledge of the relationship of these vessels to other mediastinal components allows accurate description of the location of pathology and has important implications for planning the approach to either an open operation or mediastinoscopy. The most common branching pattern of the aortic arch is for three arteries to arise from the upper arch—the right innominate, left common carotid, and left subclavian (see Figure 7-96). However, many variations to this basic anatomy exist (see Figures 7-71, 7-74, and 7-77). The transverse portion of the aortic arch is the most readily recognizable vascular structure within the mediastinum (see Figure 7-97). The great veins lie anterior to the arterial structures. The left brachiocephalic vein is situated above and anterior to the aortic arch and aortic branches, although its position is variable. The right brachiocephalic vein descends more directly in the anterior right mediastinum to merge with its counterpart to form the superior vena cava. Because CT contrast is given from one arm, one brachiocephalic vein is heavily opacified, whereas the other remains of soft tissue density.

The pulmonary outflow tract ascends, usually outlined by fat within the pericardium, to divide adjacent and just posterior to the ascending aorta. The main pulmonary artery diameter typically is equal to or less than that of the ascending aorta as measured on CT. When the pulmonary artery diameter exceeds the aortic diameter, underlying pulmonary hypertension is likely. The right pulmonary artery swings dorsally and to the right, behind the ascending aorta and the superior vena cava and anterior to the right main bronchus (see Figure 7-99). After giving a branch to the upper lobe, it descends posterolaterally to the bronchus intermedius. The left pulmonary artery follows a shorter course and arches up and over the left main bronchus.

Hilar anatomy is well demonstrated on contrast-enhanced CT, especially when vascular structures are traced sequentially over contiguous images. Knowledge of normal anatomy enables differentiation of vascular structures from normal or enlarged mediastinal lymph nodes, even on unenhanced scans; however, if there is any cause for doubt, intravenous contrast always clarifies the situation (see Figure 7-101).

Airways

The trachea descends through the thoracic inlet, where reduction in caliber may occur, and usually appears rounded on scans obtained in full inspiration. If scans are obtained during expiration, the membranous posterior wall of the trachea is seen to bow forward into the tracheal lumen. The wall of the trachea is only 2 mm thick, and any intramural thickening is well demonstrated on CT. Modern scanners also allow reformatting of

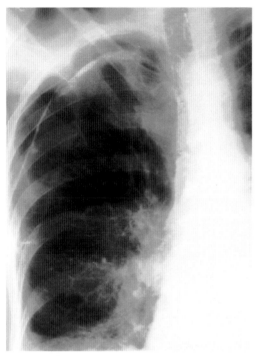

Figure 7-93 Previous sternotomy resulting in pleural thickening and calcification. A small pneumothorax is visible. Of note, the pleural thickening is associated with the visceral pleura.

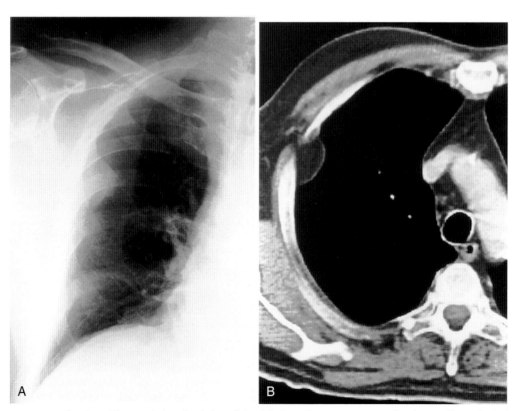

Figure 7-94 The appearances of a pleural lipoma. **A,** Localized view of the right lung from a posteroanterior chest radiograph. A pleurally based opacity is present in the right middle zone, well defined medially but fading out laterally. **B,** Computed tomography scan of the same lesion. The opacity was due to a pleural lipoma. Note the identical signal attenuation with this mass and the subcutaneous fat.

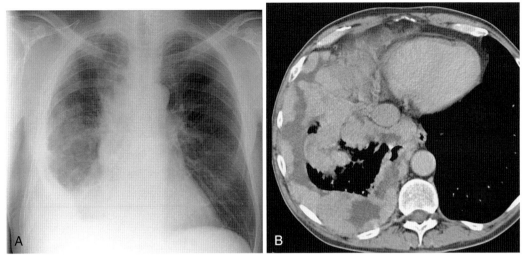

Figure 7-95 Malignant pleural involvement from metastatic adenocarcinoma. **A,** Appearance on chest radiograph. **B,** Computed tomography after contrast enhancement shows a lobulated rind of pleural thickening extending from the right apex down to the right diaphragm, which appears elevated. The overall volume of the right hemithorax is reduced.

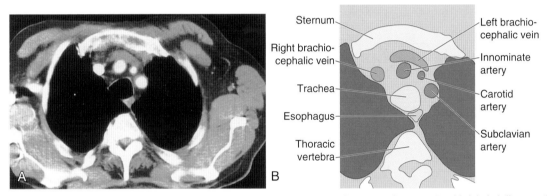

Figure 7-96 Mediastinal anatomy at the level of the great vessels: computed tomography scan (**A**) with labeled diagram (**B**).

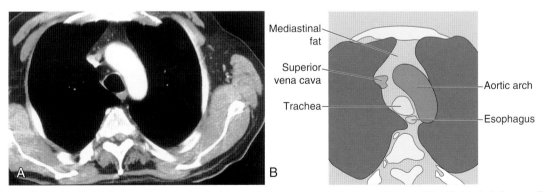

Figure 7-97 Mediastinal anatomy at the level of the aortic arch: computed tomography scan (**A**) with labeled diagram (**B**).

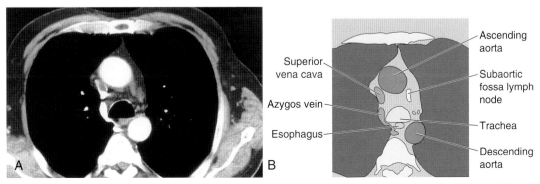

Figure 7-98 Mediastinal anatomy at the level of the subaortic fossa: computed tomography scan (**A**) with labeled diagram (**B**).

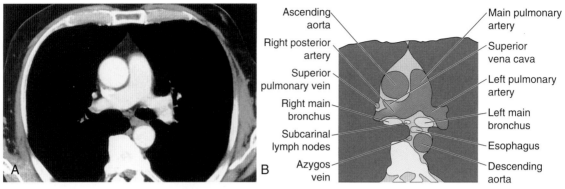

Figure 7-99 Mediastinal anatomy through the division of the main pulmonary artery: computed tomography scan (**A**) with labeled diagram (**B**).

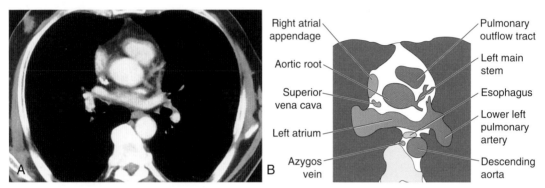

Figure 7-100 Mediastinal anatomy through the aortic root: computed tomography scan (**A**) with labeled diagram (**B**).

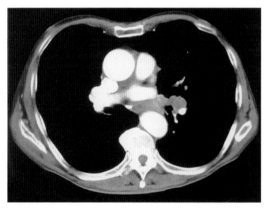

Figure 7-101 Contrast-enhanced computed tomography scan showing left hilar lymph node enlargement with extension of abnormal tissue anterior to the descending aorta.

the data in sagittal or coronal planes, thus allowing more elegant demonstration of tracheal abnormalities. The anatomy of the bronchial tree can be traced from the tracheal carina out into the lungs, at least to the segmental level, with excellent correlation between CT and bronchoscopic findings. Furthermore, the three-dimensional dataset acquired on modern spiral scanners can be manipulated to provide a computer simulation of the bronchoscopic appearances (see Figure 7-7, *D*).

Thymus

The thymus, in the normal state, is not visible on the chest radiograph of the adult patient, but the thymic remnant frequently is evident on CT. The thymus decreases in size after puberty. It lies in the anterior mediastinum, just in front of the root of the aorta; it is bilobed, with the left lobe usually being the larger. Generally, the thymus is assessed by examining the contours of the gland, which should be concave, and the thickness of the individual lobes. In childhood, the thymus is of soft tissue density on CT scanning, but after puberty, it starts to involute, and the gland undergoes atrophy and fatty replacement. Traces of thymic tissue within the anterior mediastinal fat frequently are identifiable on CT in young adults.

Thyroid

Usually, the thyroid is confined to the neck, but mediastinal extension frequently occurs with thyroid enlargement (see further on). Typically, the thyroid lies on either side of the extrathoracic trachea and is bounded laterally by the carotid artery and internal jugular vein. On contrast enhancement, normal thyroid tissue enhances avidly; it usually is of relatively high attenuation on unenhanced scans because of its relatively high iodine content.

Esophagus

The esophagus often is completely collapsed on CT scanning and is thus inconspicuous, but it is easily identified if it contains air or contrast. Initially, the esophagus lies directly posterior to the trachea; below the bifurcation, it usually deviates slightly to the left and lies adjacent to the aorta. The esophageal wall typically is only 2 to 3 mm in thickness.

Lymph Nodes

Numerous lymph nodes occur within the mediastinum, usually less than 1 cm in long axis and discrete; they may not be visible on CT scanning. Previous granulomatous disease may result in extensive mediastinal lymph node calcification, which reveals the true extent of normal mediastinal lymph node distribution (**Figure 7-102**). An extensive chain of lymph nodes also accompanies the internal mammary vessels bilaterally. Additional nodes are present in the intercostal chain adjacent to the heads

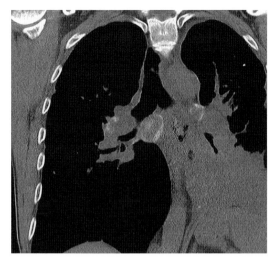

Figure 7-102 Unenhanced computed tomography scan through the thorax showing faint eggshell calcification in mediastinal lymph nodes secondary to previous granulomatous disease.

of the ribs in a posterior, paraspinal position and alongside the esophagus and descending thoracic aorta. These merge with the retrocrural lymph node chain and the paraaortic nodes in the abdomen.

Pericardium

The pericardial membrane is composed of visceral and parietal layers and surrounds the heart. The visceral layer is separated from the myocardium by a variable amount of epicardial fat. The parietal layer is variably fused with the mediastinal pleura. Where they are separate, mediastinal fat may accumulate (such as in the epiphrenic fat pad). Fluid within the pericardial sac may be evident on the chest radiograph, CT scan, or ultrasound image.

COMPUTED TOMOGRAPHIC EVALUATION OF MEDIASTINAL MASSES

Most patients who have a mediastinal mass present with symptoms from the local compressive or invasive effects of the mediastinal mass, but in a surprising number, the mass is discovered on a chest radiograph taken for an unrelated cause. Generally, the PA and lateral chest radiographs enable localization of the mass to one of the compartments of the mediastinum, which refines the differential diagnosis. However, current practice is for patients who present with a mediastinal mass to undergo a contrast-enhanced CT scan or sometimes MRI.

The differential diagnosis of a mediastinal mass is wide in scope. Masses can arise from any of the normal structures in the mediastinum, as well as from metastatic disease from a distant primary tumor. In addition, mediastinal abscesses also may manifest as a mass. The diagnosis is considerably narrowed by CT, which enables the organ of origin of the mass to be assessed, defines the attenuation and enhancement characteristics, and detects evidence of invasion of adjacent structures. It is usual to classify mediastinal masses according to the anatomic portion of the mediastinum from which they appear to arise (**Figure 7-103**).

Superior Mediastinal Masses

Thyroid

An enlarged thyroid may extend inferiorly into the superior mediastinum and may be large enough to reach into the middle

Solid masses

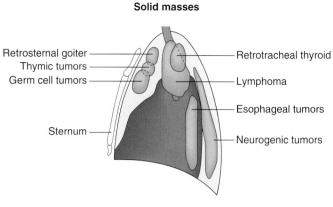

Cystic masses

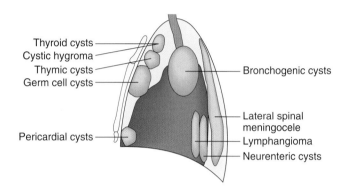

Fat density masses

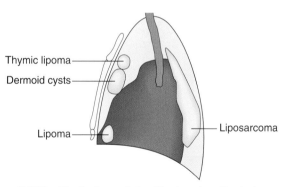

Figure 7-103 Distribution and classification of mediastinal masses depending on density derived from computed tomography scan.

mediastinum. However, this picture rarely presents a diagnostic problem, because the mass is obviously continuous with the cervical thyroid tissue and enhances avidly after intravenous contrast. Frequently, the enlarged gland contains low-density cysts and areas of calcification, particularly within cyst walls. Large thyroid masses may cause tracheal deviation or narrowing and may enlarge acutely with hemorrhage into the gland (**Figure 7-104**). Although the thyroid originates anterior to the trachea, extension to the right and even posterior to the trachea within the upper mediastinum may be observed.

Lymphatic Malformations

Lymphatic malformations are rare and may arise in the superior mediastinum. The most common of these is the cystic hygroma, which usually manifests in infants as a cervical mass with an extensive intrathoracic component. Although these lesions are considered benign, complete resection is difficult to

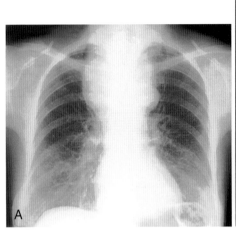
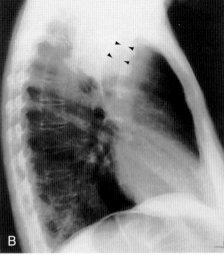
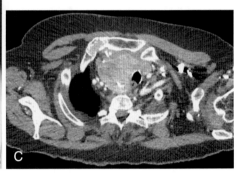

Figure 7-104 Retrosternal thyroid mass. **A,** Posteroanterior chest radiograph shows a large superior mediastinal mass mainly to the right of the trachea. **B,** The lateral view demonstrates an extension behind the trachea, which is narrowed in its anteroposterior dimension (*arrowheads*). **C,** The thyroid frequently extends into a retrotracheal position in the upper mediastinum, as demonstrated on this computed tomography scan from a different patient.

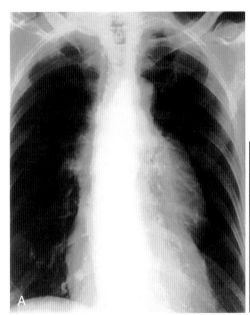
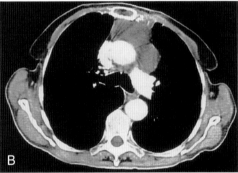

Figure 7-105 Thymic cyst. **A,** Anteroposterior chest radiograph shows mediastinal widening. **B,** Contrast-enhanced computed tomography scan confirms an anterior mediastinal abnormality of fluid density.

accomplish because of their tendency to spread around normal structures.

Anterior Mediastinal Masses

Most anterior mediastinal masses arise from the thymus, thyroid (see earlier), germ cell tumors, and enlarged lymph nodes.

Thymus

The normal thymus involutes after puberty but may show reactive enlargement in certain disease states or after chemotherapy. Intrinsic neoplasia of the thymus, however, is a relatively common cause of an anterior mediastinal mass in adult life. Causes of thymic neoplasia include thymoma, thymic carcinoma, thymic cysts (**Figure 7-105**), thymic lipoma, thymic carcinoid, and thymic lymphoma. With CT, fat or fluid

elements may be identified within a thymic mass, and invasion of adjacent structures can be shown. With the exception of thymolipoma and thymic cysts, histopathologic examination usually is required for definitive diagnosis.

Teratomas and Germ Cell Tumors

Teratomas and germ cell tumors originate from primitive stem cell rests. It is useful to separate these neoplasms into benign and malignant forms—the former is the benign cystic teratoma (synonymous with dermoid cyst). Benign cystic teratomas (**Figure 7-106**) may contain differentiated elements and consequently may display a variety of densities on CT, ranging from fat to calcified tissue, and even that of teeth. The malignant teratomas comprise a variety of tumors that usually arise in the testes—namely, seminomas, teratocarcinoma, embryonal

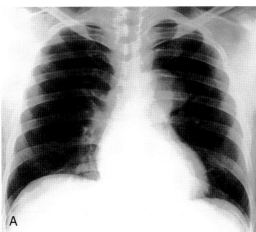
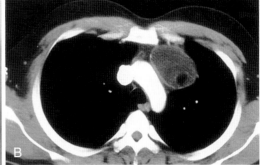

Figure 7-106 Cystic teratoma. **A,** Posteroanterior, erect chest radiograph demonstrates a mass arising from the mediastinum. Note that the posterior aortic arch and descending aorta are still visualized, which indicates an anterior position. **B,** Computed tomography scan shows fluid and fat elements within an anterior mediastinal mass.

carcinoma, yolk sac tumors, and choriocarcinoma. Some mediastinal germ cell tumors may be secondary to a primary tumor arising within the gonads. Malignant germ cell tumors usually are found in young men, secrete tumor markers, and are chemosensitive.

Lymph Node Enlargement

Lymph node enlargement is a common cause of an anterior mediastinal mass, although many processes that involve lymph nodes cause generalized mediastinal nodal enlargement. These processes may be infective (such as tuberculosis or histoplasmosis), neoplastic, reactive, or of unknown etiology (such as sarcoidosis).

Lymphoma

Hodgkin disease and, to a lesser extent, non-Hodgkin lymphoma and lymphatic leukemia frequently involve the mediastinum, especially the paratracheal, tracheobronchial, and anterior mediastinal nodes. The lymph node enlargement typically is asymmetric.

Middle Mediastinal Masses

Middle mediastinal masses most frequently are malignant, usually from metastatic nodal enlargement. The presence of enlarged nodes, however, is not an accurate predictor of malignancy, because reactive enlargement also is common. The classification of mediastinal lymph node enlargement is discussed under staging of lung cancer.

Some important developmental middle mediastinal masses are recognized. These lesions frequently are identified as an incidental abnormality in adult life, although they may manifest earlier if complications supervene. Bronchogenic cysts may arise anywhere along the course of the trachea but usually are found close to a carina. On the chest radiograph they appear as well-defined, round masses that may, on rare occasion, calcify. On CT scans they may appear as either cystic or solid masses. MRI may be diagnostic.

Posterior Mediastinal Masses

The posterior mediastinum contains neural elements, which give rise to a range of benign and malignant neural tumors. These may attain considerable size by the time of clinical presentation, and modeling abnormalities may occur in the

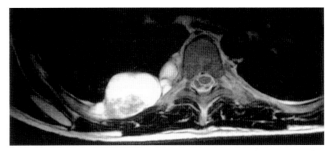

Figure 7-107 Paraganglionoma in an adult: appearance on magnetic resonance imaging. A right paraspinal T2-weighted high-signal-intensity lobulated mass is present. There is no extension into the soft tissues of the chest wall or through the neural foramina into the spinal canal.

adjacent ribs and spine, which provide a clue to their chronicity. On CT scanning, they typically are paraspinal in location and of soft tissue density, with patchy calcification. Also, CT may show the typical dumbbell extension of a neurofibroma, from an extraspinal position through an intervertebral foramen. In the assessment of neurogenic tumors, MRI has a distinct advantage over CT in that it can definitively confirm or exclude tumor extension into the spinal canal (**Figure 7-107**).

The esophagus lies in the posterior mediastinum. Esophageal carcinoma usually manifests with dysphagia or weight loss, without presence of a mass on the chest radiograph. CT usually is reserved for the staging of esophageal malignancy, in addition to the assessment of local tumor bulk. Benign esophageal lesions may reach a considerable size before the onset of symptoms, so at initial detection on the plain radiograph, the mass may be quite large. Such tumors include fibroma, leiomyoma, and lipomas.

Neuroenteric cysts are rare congenital masses that occur in the posterior mediastinum, usually inseparable from the esophagus, and sometimes within the esophageal wall. If a vertebral or neural canal abnormality is present, these are known as neuroenteric cysts, but if not, they are termed esophageal duplication cysts. Posterior mediastinal masses may arise directly from the spinal column and may represent primary or secondary tumors, infective processes, or sequelae of trauma or degeneration.

INTERPRETATION OF HIGH-RESOLUTION COMPUTED TOMOGRAPHY SCANS OF THE LUNGS

APPEARANCE OF NORMAL LUNG ANATOMY

Accurate interpretation of HRCT scans of the lung requires an understanding of the normal appearance of the bronchi, blood vessels, and the secondary pulmonary lobule. The close correspondence between gross pathologic specimen appearance and HRCT features enables the use of anatomic terms to describe the patterns of lung disease depicted by HRCT.

Throughout the lung, the bronchi and pulmonary arteries run together and taper slightly as they travel radially; this anatomic feature is easiest to appreciate in the bronchovascular bundles that run within and parallel to the plane of HRCT section. At any given point, the diameter of the bronchus is the same as its accompanying pulmonary artery. The bronchovascular bundle is surrounded by connective tissue from the hilum to the bronchioles in the lung periphery. The concept of connected components making up the lung interstitium is useful for the understanding of HRCT findings in interstitial lung disease—the peripheral interstitium around the surface of the lung beneath the visceral pleura extends into the lung to surround the secondary pulmonary lobules. Within the lobules, a finer network of septal, connective tissue fibers supports the alveoli. The "axial" fibers form a sheath around the bronchovascular bundles. Thus, the connective tissue stroma of these three separate components is in continuity, forming a fibrous skeleton for the lungs.

In normal persons, HRCT shows a clear and definite interface between the bronchovascular bundle and surrounding lung. Any thickening of the connective tissue interstitium results in apparent bronchial wall thickening and blurring of this interface. The size of the smallest subsegmental bronchi visible on HRCT scans is determined by the thickness of the bronchial wall, rather than by the bronchial diameter. In general, bronchi with a diameter less than 3 mm and walls less than 300 mm thick are not consistently identifiable on HRCT scans. Airways reach this critical size at approximately 2 to 3 cm from the pleural surface. The secondary pulmonary lobule is the smallest anatomic unit of the lung that is surrounded by a connective tissue septum (**Figure 7-108**). Within the septa lie lymphatic vessels and venules. The lobule contains between 5 and 12 acini, which each measure approximately 6 to 10 mm in diameter. Each lobule is approximately 2 cm in diameter and polyhedral in shape and often resembles a truncated cone. In the lung periphery, the bases of the cone-shaped lobules lie on a visceral pleural surface. In the central parts of the lung, the interlobular septa and thus the lobules are less well developed. The centrilobular bronchiole and accompanying pulmonary artery enter through the apex of the lobule.

The interlobular septa measure approximately 100 µm in thickness. The lower limit of resolution with HRCT is approximately 200 µm, so normal septa are infrequently identified on HRCT scans. The few interlobular septa that are visible in normal persons are seen as straight lines 1 to 2 cm in length that terminate at a visceral pleural surface. Sometimes several septa that join end to end are seen as a nonbranching, linear structure, which can measure up to 4 cm in length; these are most frequent at the lung bases, just above the diaphragmatic surface.

The secondary pulmonary lobule is supplied by a centrilobular artery and bronchiole that are approximately 1 mm in diameter as they enter the lobule. In the normal state, the core structures, effectively the 500-µm-diameter centrilobular artery, are visible as dots 1 cm deep to the pleural surface. On standard window settings, the lung parenchyma is of almost homogeneous low density, marginally greater than that of air.

Patterns of Parenchymal Disease

Vague terms traditionally used in the lexicon of plain chest radiography can be replaced by precise descriptions derived from an understanding of HRCT anatomy. Abnormal patterns on HRCT scans that represent pulmonary disease usually can be categorized into one of four patterns: reticular and linear opacities, nodular opacities, increased lung density, and cystic air spaces with areas of decreased lung density.

Although each of these patterns generally has a corresponding pattern on chest radiography, they are seen with much greater clarity on cross-sectional HRCT images, and the precise distribution of disease can be more readily appreciated. Increasing conformity is emerging in the terminology used to describe the HRCT abnormalities of diffuse infiltrative lung diseases.

Reticular Pattern

A reticular pattern on HRCT scans always indicates significant pathology. A reticular pattern caused by thickening of interlobular septa is a cardinal sign of many interstitial lung diseases. Numerous interlobular septa that join up to form an obvious network indicate an extensive interstitial abnormality caused by infiltration with fibrosis, abnormal cells, or fluid (e.g., fibrosing alveolitis, lymphangitis carcinomatosa, or pulmonary edema, respectively). Interlobular septal thickening that results from fibrosing alveolitis often is associated with intralobular, interstitial thickening (beyond the resolution of HRCT) and a coarse reticular pattern that contains cystic air spaces and produces the honeycomb pattern of destroyed lung. Thickening of the interlobular septa may be smooth or irregular, but this distinction is not always obvious. Irregular septal thickening is a feature of lymphangitic spread of tumor, whereas pulmonary edema and alveolar proteinosis cause smooth thickening. Sarcoidosis is typified by some nodular septal thickening, although widespread septal thickening is not characteristic of this condition.

Because the various parts of the lung interstitium are in continuity, widespread interstitial disease that causes interlobular septal thickening also results in bronchovascular interstitial thickening (e.g., by lymphangitis carcinomatosa). The bronchovascular thickening seen on HRCT is equivalent to the peribronchial "cuffing" seen around bronchi in end-on views on chest radiography. The HRCT finding of peribronchovascular thickening in isolation must be interpreted with caution, because it may be seen in reversible pure airway disease, for example, asthma. With thickening of the subsegmental and segmental bronchovascular bundles caused by lymphangitis

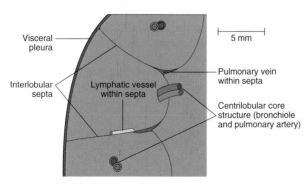

Visceral pleura

Interlobular septa

Lymphatic vessel within septa

5 mm

Pulmonary vein within septa

Centrilobular core structure (bronchiole and pulmonary artery)

Figure 7-108 Anatomy of the secondary pulmonary lobule.

carcinomatosa, for example, the interface between the thickened bronchial wall and surrounding lung sometimes has a "feathery" appearance (**Figure 7-109**).

The coarseness of the network that makes up the reticular pattern on HRCT is determined by the level at which the interstitial thickening is most severe. Thickening of the intralobular septa results in a very fine reticular pattern on HRCT, visible only on an optimal HRCT scan. Some of the very delicate linear structures that make up such a fine reticular pattern

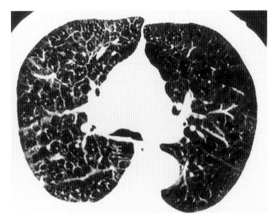

Figure 7-109 High-resolution computed tomography scan showing generalized, irregular thickening of the interlobular septa in the right lung. The patient had lymphangitis carcinomatosa.

are so small as to be below the resolution limits of HRCT, even with the narrowest collimation. The result is an amorphous increase in lung density ("ground glass" opacification) (see further on) caused by volume averaging within the section.

Extensive pulmonary fibrosis causes complete destruction of the architecture of the secondary pulmonary lobules, which results in a coarse reticular pattern made up of irregular, linear opacities. The reticular pattern of end-stage fibrotic or honeycomb lung mirrors the appearance on chest radiographs and is characterized by cystic spaces that measure a few millimeters to several centimeters across and are surrounded by discernible walls (**Figure 7-110**). Paradoxically, thickened interlobular septa are not an obvious feature of advanced fibrosing alveolitis, probably because of the severe disturbance of the normal lung architecture. The distortion that accompanies interstitial fibrosis may result in irregular dilatation of the segmental and subsegmental bronchi without honeycomb change, a phenomenon termed *traction bronchiectasis* (see Figure 7-110).

Nodular Pattern

A nodular pattern on HRCT consists of innumerable, small, discrete opacities that range in diameter from 1 to 10 mm and is a feature of both interstitial and air space diseases. The location of nodules in relation to the lobules and bronchovascular bundles, as well as their density, clarity of outline, and uniformity of size, may indicate whether the nodules lie predominantly within the interstitium or air spaces. Because most

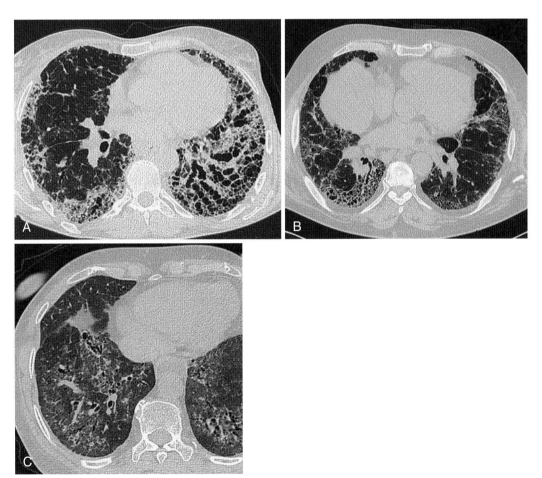

Figure 7-110 High-resolution computed tomography in fibrosing alveolitis. **A,** In the first patient, coarse cystic spaces are visible throughout the lung bases. **B,** In a second patient, finer fibrotic changes are seen. Traction bronchiectasis is evident in both cases, which is a typical feature of the usual interstitial pneumonitis (UIP) pattern. **C,** In a third patient, the much more marked ground glass changes are characteristic of nonspecific interstitial pneumonia (NSIP) pattern.

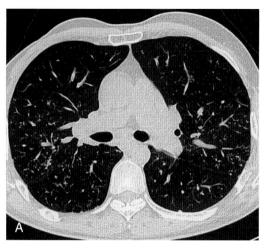

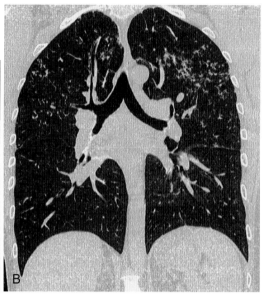

Figure 7-111 High-resolution computed tomography imaging of the lungs in a patient with sarcoidosis. **A,** Parenchymal nodularity together with thickening and beading of the bronchovascular bundles is typical of sarcoidosis. **B,** Coronal reformatted image through the lungs of the same patient demonstrates the middle and upper zone predominance of disease.

diffuse lung pathoses have both interstitial and air space components, this distinction does not always aid in the diagnosis. Whether pulmonary nodules can be detected on CT depends on their size, profusion, and density and on the scanning technique. Narrow-collimation HRCT clearly is superior to conventional CT for the detection of micronodular disease because it is associated with less partial volume effect, which can average out the attenuation of tiny nodules. A further refinement is the use of maximum-intensity projection images obtained with spiral CT to detect extremely subtle micronodular disease. Nodules within the lung interstitium are seen in the interlobular septa, subpleural regions (particularly in relation to the fissures), and in a peribronchovascular distribution. Nodular thickening of the bronchovascular interstitium results in an irregular interface between the margins of the bronchovascular bundles and the surrounding lung parenchyma. These features are most pronounced in cases of sarcoidosis, in which coalescent, perilymphatic granulomas cause a beaded appearance of the thickened bronchovascular bundles. The bronchovascular distribution of nodules, in conjunction with a perihilar concentration of disease, is virtually pathognomonic for sarcoidosis **(Figure 7-111)**.

The nodular pattern seen in coal worker's pneumoconiosis and silicosis generally is more uniform in distribution. Centrilobular nodules may be more numerous in the upper zone and in subpleural regions, but overall they tend to be more evenly spread throughout the lung parenchyma than those seen in sarcoidosis.

When the air spaces are filled, or partially filled, with exudate, individual acini may become visible as poorly defined nodules approximately 8 mm in diameter. Acinar nodules may merge with areas of ground glass opacification and sometimes are seen around the periphery of areas of dense parenchymal consolidation **(Figure 7-112)**. Such nodules usually are centrilobular, although this localization may be difficult to appreciate if the nodules are very profuse. Conditions in which this nonspecific pattern is seen include organizing pneumonia, hypersensitivity pneumonitis **(Figure 7-113)**, endobronchial spread of tuberculosis, idiopathic pulmonary hemorrhage, and some cases of bronchoalveolar cell carcinoma.

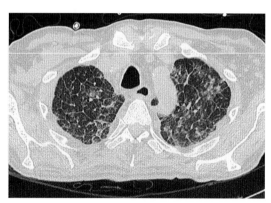

Figure 7-112 Poorly defined acinar nodules. Generalized ground glass density and interlobular septal thickening also are evident. The patient had cardiogenic pulmonary edema.

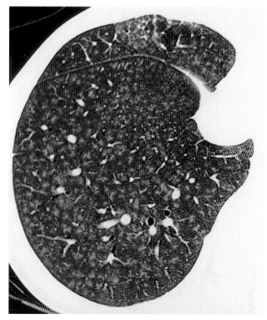

Figure 7-113 High-resolution computed tomography scan showing poorly defined nodular opacities merging with ground glass opacification. The patient had subacute hypersensitivity pneumonitis.

Increased Lung Density

An amorphous increase in lung density on HRCT often is described as a ground glass opacification appearance (**Figure 7-114**). Unlike the equivalent abnormality on chest radiography, in which the pulmonary vessels often are indistinct, a ground glass pattern on HRCT does not obscure the pulmonary vasculature. In cases in which the presence of a ground glass pattern is equivocal, HRCT often is useful to compare the density of the lung parenchyma with air in the bronchi—in the normal state, the difference in density is marginal. Although this HRCT abnormality usually is easily recognizable, particularly when it is interspersed with areas of normal lung parenchyma, subtle degrees of increased parenchymal opacification may not be obvious. It is important to recognize that a normal increase in parenchymal density, indistinguishable from a generalized opacification caused by infiltrative lung disease, results in a ground glass pattern in patients who breath-hold at end expiration.

On a pathologic level, the changes responsible for ground glass opacification are complex and include partial filling of the air spaces and thickening of the interstitium, or a combination of the two (**Figure 7-115**). Conditions that are characterized by these pathologic changes and result in the nonspecific pattern of ground glass opacification include fibrosing alveolitis in the active cellular phase, *Pneumocystis* pneumonia, subacute hypersensitivity pneumonitis, sarcoidosis, drug-induced lung damage, diffuse pulmonary hemorrhage, and acute lung injury. The amorphous ground glass density seen on HRCT in these conditions usually represents a potentially reversible process. However, mild thickening of the intralobular interstitium by irreversible fibrosis may rarely produce a ground glass appearance in fibrosing alveolitis. Furthermore, ground glass opacification may be seen in areas of bronchoalveolar cell carcinoma, usually in conjunction with patches of denser, consolidated lung (**Figure 7-116**).

A pitfall in identifying a ground glass pattern on HRCT occurs when regional differences in pulmonary perfusion are present—regional alterations in pulmonary blood flow, caused by thromboembolism, for example, may result in striking differences in lung density (**Figure 7-117**). The density difference between the underperfused lung and normal lung may give the appearance of a ground glass density in normal (but relatively overperfused) lung parenchyma. These areas of different density have often been termed mosaic oligemia. A similar appearance is seen in patients who have patchy air trapping caused by small airway disease, such as in an obliterative bronchiolitis: The relatively transradiant areas of underventilated and thus underperfused lung make the normal lung parenchyma appear more than usually dense and thus simulate a ground glass infiltrate. This potential pitfall often can be recognized for what it is by the relative paucity of vessels in the underventilated parts of the lungs caused by hypoxic

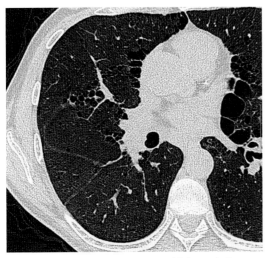

Figure 7-114 Ground glass appearance on high-resolution computed tomography. Extensive ground glass opacification in a patient with desquamative interstitial pneumonitis. Note that the vessels are visible within the areas of ground glass opacification.

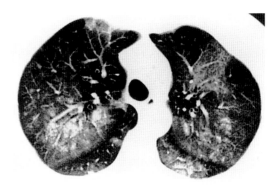

Figure 7-116 Patchy areas of ground glass opacification in a patient with biopsy-proven bronchoalveolar cell carcinoma.

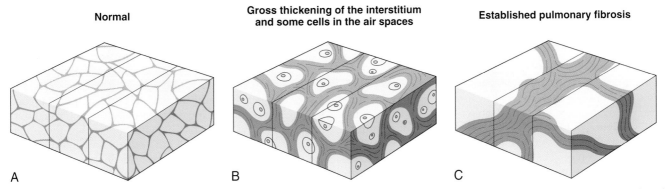

Normal

Gross thickening of the interstitium and some cells in the air spaces

Established pulmonary fibrosis

A   B   C

Figure 7-115 Normal and diseased lung voxels. **A,** In the normal state, most of the volume of these voxels is made up of air. **B,** Gross thickening of the interstitium and some cells within the air spaces causes displacement of air and a corresponding increase in density within the voxels—this produces ground glass opacification on a high-resolution computed tomography image. **C,** In established pulmonary fibrosis, the strands of fibrotic lung occupy much of the volume of individual voxels, which is reflected in their density; pulmonary fibrosis thus has a reticular pattern on high-resolution computed tomography.

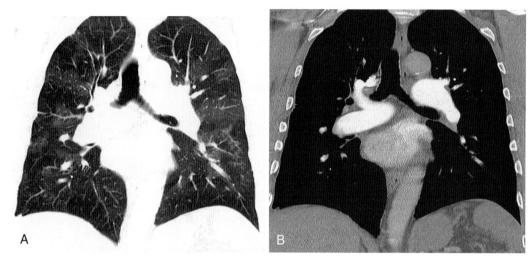

Figure 7-117 Coronal reformatted images from MDCT dataset. Uneven density of the lung parenchyma caused by perfusion inhomogeneity. The patient had chronic thromboembolism. **A,** Coronal reformatted image using lung window settings demonstrates the mosaic attenuation pattern. **B,** On mediastinal window settings, the large central pulmonary arteries are evident.

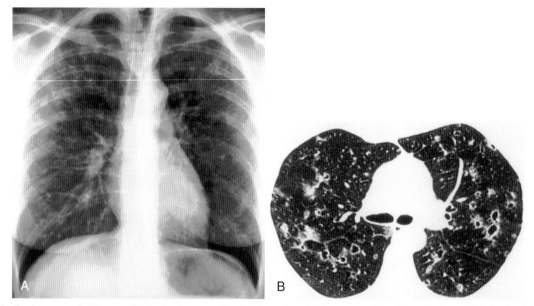

Figure 7-118 Cystic air spaces. **A,** Nonspecific shadowing on a chest radiograph, with the suggestion of a cavitating nodule in the right upper zone. **B,** High-resolution computed tomography scan through the upper lobes reveals multiple curious-shaped, cavitating lesions, typical of Langerhans cell histiocytosis.

vasoconstriction. The vessels in the relatively normal lung of higher density are engorged because of shunting of blood to these regions (see Figure 7-117).

Cystic Air Spaces

The term *cystic air space* describes a clearly defined, air-containing space that has a definable wall 1 to 3 mm thick. Many conditions are characterized by a profusion of cystic air spaces, which may not be recognizable as such on chest radiography (**Figure 7-118**), whereas the size and distribution of these cysts on HRCT may suggest the diagnosis.

The destruction of alveolar walls that characterizes emphysema produces areas of low attenuation on HRCT, which often merge imperceptibly with normal lung (**Figure 7-119**). In patients who have predominantly centrilobular emphysema, circular areas of lung destruction may resemble cysts; however, the centrilobular core usually is visible as a dotlike structure in the center of the apparent cyst. Although bullae of varying sizes

are clearly seen on HRCT in patients who have emphysema, usually a background permeative, destructive parenchyma prevents confusion with other conditions in which cystic air spaces are a prominent feature.

Cystic air spaces as the dominant abnormality are seen in only a few conditions, which include lymphangioleiomyomatosis, Langerhans cell histiocytosis, end-stage fibrosing alveolitis, and postinfective pneumatoceles. In lymphangioleiomyomatosis, the cysts usually are uniformly scattered throughout the lungs, with normal lung parenchyma intervening; the individual cysts rarely are larger than 4 cm in diameter (**Figure 7-120**). As the disease progresses, the larger cystic air spaces coalesce; the circumferential, well-defined walls of the cysts become disrupted; and the HRCT pattern in advanced lymphangioleiomyomatosis, and indeed in Langerhans cell histiocytosis, may be practically indistinguishable from that in severe centrilobular emphysema. Distinction of the delicate, "lacelike" reticular pattern of lymphangioleiomyomatosis on HRCT from that of

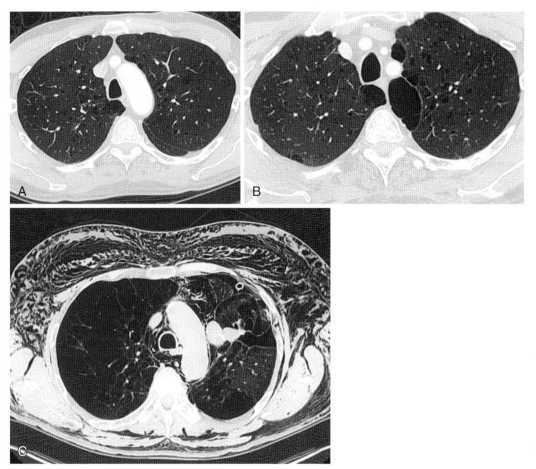

Figure 7-119 High-resolution computed tomography in centrilobular versus other forms of emphysema. **A,** Centrilobular emphysema. Note the permeative destruction of the lung parenchyma with scattered centrilobular lucent areas. **B,** Paraseptal emphysema. The disease is concentrated in the subpleural lung. **C,** Panacinar emphysema. Large swathes of completely destroyed lung are evident, with almost no vascular or soft tissue structures demonstrated within.

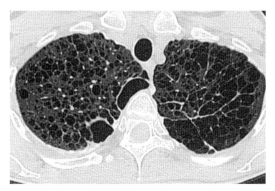

Figure 7-120 High-resolution computed tomography in advanced lymphangioleiomyomatosis. Note the coalescence of cystic air spaces, which resembles that in severe centrilobular emphysema.

end-stage fibrosing alveolitis usually is possible, because the cystic air spaces in a fibrotic honeycomb lung are smaller and have thicker walls. Furthermore, the tendency for fibrosing alveolitis to have a peripheral distribution, even in its end stage, usually is still obvious in the upper zones.

Similar, confluent cystic air spaces that give a delicate pattern on HRCT are seen in images obtained in patients who have advanced Langerhans cell histiocytosis. Earlier in the disease, however, a nodular component is present, and some of the nodules cavitate. The combination of cavitating nodules, some of which have curious shapes (e.g., cloverleaf shape), and cystic

air spaces with a predominantly upper zone distribution is virtually pathognomonic for this diagnosis (see Figure 7-118). Serial HRCT scans show the natural history of nodules, which cavitate, become cystic air spaces, and, in end-stage disease, coalesce. In a few cases, these pathologic changes may resolve, with the lung parenchyma reverting to a normal appearance. Some of the cavitating nodules in Langerhans cell histiocytosis superficially resemble bronchiectatic airways, but a lack of continuity between these lesions will be observed on adjacent sections, and the segmental bronchi, when they can be identified, do not have any of the HRCT features of bronchiectasis.

DISEASES OF THE AIRWAYS

Now that bronchography is rarely performed, the imaging modality of choice to diagnose bronchiectasis is HRCT. *Bronchiectasis* is defined as damage to the bronchial wall that results in irreversible dilatation of the bronchi, whatever the cause. Thus, the main feature of bronchiectasis on HRCT is dilatation of the bronchi with or without bronchial wall thickening. Criteria for the HRCT identification of abnormally dilated bronchi depend on the orientation of the bronchi in relation to the plane of the HRCT section (**Figure 7-121**).

Vertically oriented bronchi are seen in transverse section, so reference can be made to the accompanying pulmonary artery, which in normal persons is of approximately the same caliber; any dilatation of the bronchus results in the so-called signet ring sign (**Figure 7-122**). Although this generally constitutes reliable evidence of abnormal bronchial dilatation, care must be taken in comparing the diameter of the bronchi and adjacent pulmonary arteries just below the division of the lower lobe bronchus. At this level, pairs of segmental and sometimes subsegmental bronchi converge, and the resulting fusion of the two bronchi may give the spurious impression of an abnormally dilated bronchus. Bronchi that have a more horizontal course on CT scans, particularly the anterior segmental bronchi of the upper lobes and the segmental bronchi of the lingula and right middle lobe, are demonstrated along their length, and abnormal dilatation is seen as nontapering parallel walls or even flaring of the bronchi as they course distally (**Figure 7-123**). In more severe cases of bronchiectasis, the bronchi are obviously dilated and have a varicose or cystic appearance.

Bronchial wall thickening is a frequent but not invariable feature of bronchiectasis. The definition of what constitutes abnormal bronchial wall thickening remains contentious, particularly because mild degrees of wall thickening are seen in normal subjects, asymptomatic smokers, asthmatic individuals,

and patients affected by an acute, lower respiratory tract, viral infection. In brief, no robust and reproducible criterion for the identification of abnormal bronchial wall thickening has been identified, so bronchial wall thickening remains a subjective sign with an attendant high variation in observer interpretation. However, it is the presence of peribronchial thickening that renders the smaller peripheral airways visible on HRCT. Although there is no exact level beyond which visualization of the bronchi can be regarded as abnormal on HRCT, normal bronchi should not be visible within 2 to 3 cm of the pleural surface. Large elliptical and circular opacities, which represent secretion-filled, dilated bronchi, constitute a sign of gross bronchiectasis and are almost invariably seen in the presence of other obviously dilated bronchi, some of which may contain air-fluid levels (**Figure 7-124**). When mucous plugging of the smaller airways occurs, minute branching structures or dots in the lung periphery may be identifiable. In some cases, plugging of the numerous centrilobular bronchioles gives a curious nodular appearance to the lungs (**Figure 7-125**).

Supplementary HRCT evidence of bronchiectasis includes crowding of the affected bronchi, with obvious volume loss of the lobe as shown by the position of the major fissures. In many lobes affected by bronchiectasis, areas of decreased attenuation of the lung parenchyma adjacent to the abnormal airways can

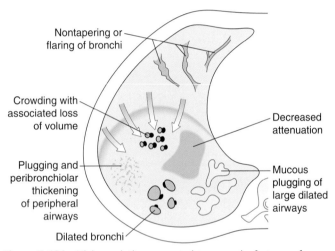

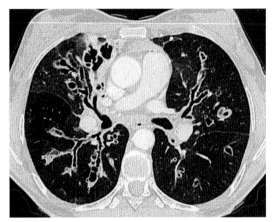

Figure 7-121 High-resolution computed tomography features of bronchiectasis: nontapering or flaring of bronchi lying within the plane of section; "signet ring" sign of dilated bronchi running perpendicular to the plane of computed tomography section; mucous plugging of large, dilated airways; plugging and peribronchiolar thickening of small peripheral airways; crowding with associated loss of volume (see position of oblique fissure); and areas of decreased attenuation, which reflect associated small airway disease.

Figure 7-123 High-resolution computed tomography scan obtained in a patient with cystic fibrosis. Nontapering and flaring of the bronchiectatic airways are evident in the apical segment of the right lower lobe. In addition, mosaic perfusion is present, reflecting associated small airway disease.

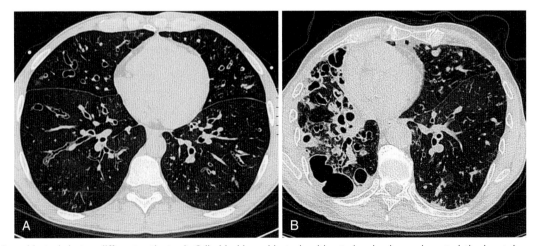

Figure 7-122 Bronchiectasis in two different patients. **A,** Cylindrical bronchiectasis without plugging has a characteristic signet ring appearance. **B,** With more severe disease, some airway plugging is seen in the tip of the lingula.

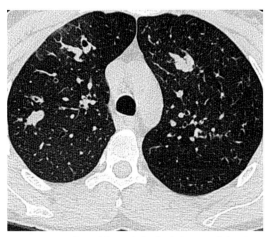

Figure 7-124 Severe bronchiectasis in the left upper lobe. Some bronchi are filled with secretions, which results in multiple tubular and elliptical opacities. The patient had allergic bronchopulmonary aspergillosis.

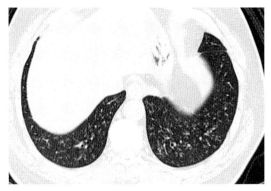

Figure 7-125 Numerous small irregular opacities in the left lower lobe representing plugged bronchioles. The patient had panbronchiolitis.

be identified; this pattern of mosaic attenuation is thought to reflect accompanying small airway disease, and the extent of the pattern correlates well with functional evidence of airflow obstruction, particularly indices of small airway dysfunction.

A positive diagnosis of bronchiectasis on HRCT is straightforward in patients who have moderate and severe disease. In some situations, however, subtle signs of bronchiectasis may be obscured by technical artifacts. Conversely, the HRCT appearance of bronchiectasis may be mimicked by other lung pathoses. Some of the causes of false-negative and false-positive diagnoses of bronchiectasis are listed in **Table 7-2**.

Interest in the ability of HRCT to detect small airway disease is increasing. In the exudative form of bronchiolar disease (typified by Japanese panbronchiolitis), HRCT directly shows the

Table 7-2	Causes of False-Positive and False-Negative Diagnosis of Bronchiectasis on High-Resolution Computed Tomography
False-Negative Factors	**False-Positive Factors**
Inappropriately thick computed tomography section	Cardiac pulsation causing "double vessels"
Movement artifact obscuring lung detail	Confluence of subsegmental bronchi leading to spurious impression of bronchiectasis, at a single level (particularly in the lower lobes)
Focal, inconspicuous, thin-walled bronchiectasis	Cavitating nodules mimicking bronchiectasis (e.g., Langerhans cell histiocytosis)
Masking of bronchiectatic airways by surrounding fibrosis	Reversible dilatation of bronchi with acute pneumonic consolidation

plugged small airways as small, irregularly branching opacities. The HRCT signs of constrictive obliterative bronchiolitis (e.g., in patients with rheumatoid arthritis or postviral obliterative bronchiolitis) are indirect—areas of decreased attenuation occur within which the vessels are of reduced caliber (but not distorted, in contrast with emphysema). The areas of decreased attenuation may merge with those of more normal lung or may have sharply demarcated, "geographic" boundaries (mosaic attenuation pattern). The density differences that characterize constrictive obliterative bronchiolitis may be extremely subtle, but because they represent areas of reduced ventilation with consequent air trapping, they may be dramatically emphasized on scans performed at end expiration. Most patients affected by small airway disease ill exhibit some bronchiectatic changes on HRCT, which tend to be more severe in those who have immunologically mediated obliterative bronchiolitis.

SUGGESTED READINGS

Hansell DM, Lynch DA, McAdams HP, Bankier AA: *Imaging of diseases of the chest*, St. Louis, 2010, Mosby.

Webb R, Higgins C: *Thoracic imaging*, Philadelphia, 2010, Lippincott Williams & Wilkins.

Muller N, Silva C: *Imaging of the chest*, Philadelphia, 2008, Saunders.

de Lacey G, Simon Morley S, Berman L, editors: *The chest X-ray: a survival guide*, London, 2008, Saunders.

Collins J, Stern EJ, editors: *Chest radiology: the essentials*, Philadelphia, 2007, Lippincott Williams & Wilkins.

Brant WE, Helms CA: *Fundamentals of diagnostic radiology*, Philadelphia, 2007, Lippincott Williams & Wilkins.

McLoud TC, Boiselle PM: *Thoracic radiology: the requisites*, St. Louis, 2009, Mosby.

Chapter **8**
Positron Emission Tomography Imaging

Johan Vansteenkiste • Christophe Dooms • Christophe Deroose

Conventional imaging relies on differences in the *structure* of tissues, measured by differences in density, as in chest radiography and computed tomography (CT); surface reflectivity, as in ultrasonography; or chemical environment, as in magnetic resonance imaging (MRI). With the exquisite anatomic detail they provide, these modalities play a crucial role in the evaluation of many respiratory diseases. Nonetheless, assessment of structural differences often does not lead to a definitive diagnosis; in such instances, invasive tests with tissue sampling also are needed.

Positron emission tomography (PET) brought a revolutionary and novel aspect to imaging: It allows accurate, noninvasive measurement of *metabolism* of tissues, a valuable complement to the structural information provided on conventional imaging. This combined information allows better distinction between malignant and benign tissues and also can be used in monitoring of disease by the study of metabolic alterations, which can be different from or even precede the anatomic changes.

USE OF POSITRON EMISSION TOMOGRAPHY IN RESPIRATORY MEDICINE

PET with ^{18}F-fluorodeoxyglucose (FDG) tagging is a noninvasive imaging technique with high sensitivity for detection of both oncologic and nononcologic disorders in respiratory medicine. It has been suggested that FDG-PET might be useful in several diseases associated with FDG uptake based on inflammatory mechanisms, such as granulomatous diseases (e.g., sarcoidosis) or other proliferative inflammatory disorders (e.g., idiopathic pulmonary fibrosis, posttransplantation lymphoproliferative disorders).

Classical forms of sarcoidosis with intrathoracic nodal and/or pulmonary disease are in general assessed by combining clinical examination, pulmonary function and laboratory tests, and a CT scan of the chest. The extent and activity of the disease can be more accurately assessed by FDG-PET–CT than by gallium 67 single photon emission CT (^{67}Ga-SPECT) scintigraphy. FDG-PET–CT in sarcoidosis is better at identifying occult sites of extrathoracic disease and has a superior spatial and contrast resolution, as well as better interobserver agreement, compared with ^{67}Ga-SPECT. FDG-PET–CT currently is undergoing further evaluation of its clinical utility to monitor disease activity during treatment of interstitial pulmonary diseases such as sarcoidosis and idiopathic pulmonary fibrosis.

Posttransplantation lymphoproliferative disorder (PTLD) is a serious complication occurring after solid organ or bone marrow transplantation. The incidence of PTLD in lung transplant recipients is 5%. In this disorder, FDG-PET–CT allows more accurate evaluation of disease extent, with better follow-up after treatment, than that achievable with conventional CT imaging.

The most common application of FDG-PET is in investigation of respiratory malignancies. The indications for PET in this setting are listed in **Box 8-1**.

PRINCIPLES OF POSITRON EMISSION TOMOGRAPHY IMAGING

POSITRON EMISSION TOMOGRAPHY CAMERAS

A PET camera produces three-dimensional images that represent the distribution of radioactivity in the body. Any molecule that can be labeled with a positron-emitting radioisotope can be used to generate PET images (more than 400 PET tracers are listed in the NIH Molecular Imaging and Contrast Agent Database [MICAD], available at www.ncbi.nlm.nih.gov/books/NBK5330/).

The spatial resolution of older PET cameras was 6 mm or higher; for contemporary PET cameras, this is around 4 mm. Lesions with a diameter up to twice that resolution can be characterized with virtually no size-related (partial volume effect) underestimation of the tracer uptake, whereas for smaller lesions, the tracer uptake will gradually be underestimated as the size becomes smaller. In practice, lesions larger than 8 to 10 mm will be well characterized, whereas smaller ones, other than strongly FDG-avid lesions, cannot be accurately depicted.

The main difference between standard radionuclide imaging with gamma cameras and imaging with dedicated PET cameras is that the latter type of camera has a full ring of several thousands of scintillation detectors and does not need lead collimators—which absorb more than 99% of the emitted photons—to generate the image, resulting in higher sensitivity to radioactivity and higher spatial resolution.

Historically, PET cameras were "stand-alone" machines, either dedicated PET cameras or specially designed gamma cameras with which dual-head gamma camera coincidence imaging was performed. To overcome the lack of anatomic information of PET imaging, this type of camera has been replaced by hybrid systems in which a dedicated PET camera is combined with an anatomic tomograph—mostly with a computed tomography (CT) camera but sometimes a magnetic resonance imaging (MRI) camera. These fusion PET-CT cameras are considered the new standard ("stand-alone" PET cameras are not manufactured anymore), whereas PET-MRI is an emerging technology. The use of hybrid PET-CT cameras offers three main advantages: (1) attenuation correction (AC), which is needed to correct the image for the fact that some of the

Diagnosis of Single Pulmonary Nodules or Masses
Differentiation of malignant versus benign nodules
   Reduce the need of unwanted invasive procedures
   Reduce cost
   Aid in decision algorithms in screening studies
False-negative results
   Small or ground glass opacity tumors
   Low-metabolism tumors (carcinoid, bronchioloalveolar
     carcinoma)
False-positive results
   Inflammatory respiratory disorders

Mediastinal Lymph Node Staging
High negative predictive value for lymph node metastasis
   Reduction in number of invasive tests, without loss of accuracy
   Reduction in cost
   Better guidance of invasive procedures
False-negative results
   Low FDG uptake in primary tumor
   Centrally located tumors
   Major hilar lymph node involvement
False-positive results
   Inflammatory lymph nodes

Extrathoracic Staging
Significant complement to conventional imaging
   Detection of unexpected metastasis
   Characterization of equivocal lesions
False-negative results
   Low FDG uptake in primary tumor
   Small metastatic deposits
False-positive results
   Inflammatory/benign: always confirm single suspect lesion
   Second primary tumor

Innovative Indications
Selective use in lung cancer screening
Assessment of pleural mesothelioma
Diagnosis of recurrence after radical therapy
Prognosis and assessment of therapy
   Prognostic information
   Early response evaluation during chemotherapy
   Restaging after induction treatment
Radiotherapy planning
Response prediction in molecular therapy

FDG, ^{18}F-fluorodeoxyglucose.

photons coming from radioactive decay are absorbed by the body, can be performed with the CT dataset, resulting in significant time reduction (approximately 10 minutes gained per patient); (2) increased accuracy of the exact position of the lesion and morphologic characterization of the underlying correlate, reducing equivocal findings; and (3) significantly increased confidence in reported findings. Typical scan times for modern PET-CT are in the 6- to 20-minute range for a skull-to-thigh image (i.e., whole-body scan). The data reported in this chapter derive from either dedicated PET or PET-CT applications.

The advent of PET-CT has resulted in two different strategies: so-called *low-dose CT*, which is used only for AC and localization, and "one-stop shopping" *high-dose, contrast-enhanced diagnostic CT* together with PET. It has been demonstrated that the use of oral or intravenous contrast agents does

not induce clinically significant changes in the PET images. The combination of contrast-enhanced CT with PET changes tumor-node-metastasis (TNM) staging in 8% of patients and is nowadays mandatory for applications such as radiation therapy planning. The drawback is an increase in radiation dose, with low-dose techniques adding about 3 mSv to the approximately 8 mSv from the radiopharmaceutical, whereas contrast-enhanced CT adds some 10 to 20 mSv.

METABOLIC TRACERS

For cancer imaging, 2-^{18}F-fluoro-2-deoxy-D-glucose (FDG), described in 1978, is by far the most commonly used metabolic tracer. The usefulness of this tracer relates to the increased cellular uptake of glucose (due to an increased expression of glucose transporter proteins) and a much higher rate of glycolysis in cancer cells. FDG, a glucose analogue in which the oxygen molecule in position 2 is replaced by a positron-emitting fluorine 18 atom, undergoes the same uptake as for glucose but is metabolically trapped and accumulated in the neoplastic cell after phosphorylation by hexokinase.

INTERPRETATION OF POSITRON EMISSION TOMOGRAPHY IMAGES

GENERAL PRINCIPLES

If the aim of the FDG-PET study is just to stage the patient's cancer, visual analysis of non-AC images (i.e., "hot spots" with higher-than-background activity not caused by physiologic processes are positive for tumor) probably is just as good as AC images, as has been pointed out by different prospective studies, both for the discrimination of nodules and for the evaluation of mediastinal involvement. Non-AC images should be examined to detect small lung lesions, because they are better visualized, owing to higher contrast, than are AC images.

THE NORMAL FDG-PET IMAGE

High physiologic FDG uptake occurs in brain, kidney, and urinary tract (urinary excretion) and can be present in the heart. Particularly in the brain, this interferes with lesion detection. A low degree of physiologic uptake of FDG has been noted in thoracic structures, including the lung, the heart, the aorta and large arteries, esophagus, thymus, trachea, thoracic muscles, bone marrow, and joints and soft tissues. This low background tracer activity builds the image contour.

FALSE-POSITIVE RESULTS

FDG uptake is not tumor-specific and may be observed in all active tissues with high glucose metabolism, in particular, those in which inflammation is present. Therefore, a finding of clinically relevant FDG uptake, especially if isolated and decisive for patient management, requires confirmation. The differentiation between metastasis and a benign or inflammatory lesion, or even an unrelated second malignancy, should be made by means of other tests or tissue diagnosis.

The major causes of false-positive results (**Box 8-2**) in chest pathology are infectious, inflammatory, and granulomatous disorders. Iatrogenic procedures, such as thoracocentesis, placement of a chest tube, percutaneous needle biopsy, mediastinoscopy, thoracoscopy, and talc pleurodesis, also may give false-positive results.

Box 8-2   Causes of False-Positive and False-Negative Results on Positron Emission Tomography

False-Positive Findings
Infection/Inflammation
(Postobstructive) pneumonia/abscess
Mycobacterial or fungal infection
Granulomatous disorders (sarcoidosis, Wegener granulomatosis)
Chronic nonspecific lymphadenitis
(Rheumatoid) arthritis
Occupational exposure (anthracosilicosis)
Bronchiectasis
Organizing pneumonia
Reflux esophagitis

Iatrogenic Causes
Invasive procedure (puncture, biopsy)
Talc pleurodesis
Radiation esophagitis and pneumonitis
Bone marrow expansion post chemotherapy
Colony-stimulating factors
Thymic hyperplasia post chemotherapy
FDG embolism

Benign Mass Lesions
Salivary gland adenoma (Warthin tumor)
Thyroid adenoma
Adrenal adenoma
Colorectal dysplastic polyps

Focal Physiologic FDG Uptake
Gastrointestinal tract
Muscle activity
Brown fat
Unilateral vocal cord activity
Atherosclerotic plaques

False-Negative Results
Lesion-Dependent
Small-sized lesion
Bronchioloalveolar carcinoma
Carcinoid tumors
Ground glass opacity neoplasms

Technique-Dependent
Hyperglycemia
Paravenous FDG injection
Increased time between injection and scanning

FDG, ^{18}F-fluorodeoxyglucose.

FALSE-NEGATIVE RESULTS

False-negative results are less common and may be due to lesion-dependent or technical factors (see Box 8-2). A critical mass of metabolically active malignant cells is required for PET detection. Interpretation thus is a critical process with tumors exhibiting decreased FDG uptake such as small, very well-differentiated adenocarcinoma, bronchioloalveolar carcinoma, or carcinoid tumors. FDG-avid lesions smaller than 5 mm may be false-negative as a consequence of the limitations in spatial resolution and partial volume effect. In the lower lung fields, the detection limit may even go down to 10 mm, owing to additional respiratory motion. CT-based AC can cause artifacts in the event of misregistration between the CT and the PET data, which can lead to occultation of liver metastasis on the AC images.

Factors related to technique are paravenous FDG injection and high baseline glucose serum levels. Blood glucose levels should be checked, and it is advised to proceed only if the glucose level is within an acceptable range before tracer injection (typically 60 to approximately 180 mg/dL). Although diabetic patients often were excluded in the prospective studies, FDG uptake probably is not significantly influenced in these patients if the blood glucose levels are under reasonable control.

POSITRON EMISSION TOMOGRAPHY IN DIAGNOSIS

The value of FDG-PET in differentiating benign from malignant lung lesions (**Figure 8-1**) has been studied in many prospective studies and documented in different metaanalyses. In these series, in which a *standardized uptake value* (SUV) cutoff of 2.5 often was used to suggest malignancy, a sensitivity of about 90% to 95% (range, 83% to 100%), a specificity of about 80% (range, 52% to 100%), and an accuracy of about 90% (range, 86% to 100%) were reported. Differences in the results can be explained mainly by the prevalence of malignancy in the study population, which is the result of the varying epidemiology of solitary pulmonary nodules (SPNs) in different areas of the world (e.g., regions with more tuberculosis or histoplasmosis), and by the inclusion criteria of the different series (e.g., a lower sensitivity can be expected in series with smaller nodules). The causes for false-negative and false-positive findings in SPNs are listed in Box 8-2.

Studies listed in the metaanalyses included only solid nodules of at least 1 cm in diameter. Therefore, use of a threshold SUV above 2.5 is questionable for smaller or ground glass lesions. In mostly Japanese series with smaller or faint lesions, use of the 2.5 threshold missed malignancy in a quarter of the cancerous lesions. Many of these could, however, be diagnosed on the basis of weak FDG uptake on visual analysis (corresponding to an SUV of about 1.5).

FDG-PET should be used in relation to other clinical (age, smoking history) and radiologic (spiculation) factors determining the likelihood of malignancy. In clinical decision algorithms, FDG-PET will mostly add information for SPNs with an intermediate probability of malignancy. It is important to be aware of possibilities and limitations (see Box 8-2). Strong data point to use of FDG-PET for characterization of solid pulmonary nodules larger than 2 cm in diameter. Sensitivity is around 95%, negative predictive value (NPV) is very high, malignancy can be excluded correctly in the vast majority of cases, and unnecessary invasive procedures can be avoided. In order to minimize the chance of missing malignancy in smaller or faint SPNs, any lesion with FDG uptake resulting in higher-than-background activity should be considered suspect, and the overall use of the "magic" SUV threshold of 2.5 should be abandoned.

Finally, specificity and positive predictive value (PPV) are suboptimal, and clinicians should be aware that a false-positive scan is possible in the conditions listed in Box 8-2, which should be evaluated by appropriate tests. In case of doubt, lesions with increased FDG uptake should be considered to be malignant until proven otherwise and should be managed accordingly.

POSITRON EMISSION TOMOGRAPHY IN STAGING

TUMOR-NODE-METASTASIS STATUS

On the basis of extension of the primary tumor (T), spread to locoregional lymph nodes (N), and presence of distant metastasis (M), patients with lung cancer can be grouped according to different disease stages. Stage is the most important factor in prognosis and choice of treatment. Therefore, reliable

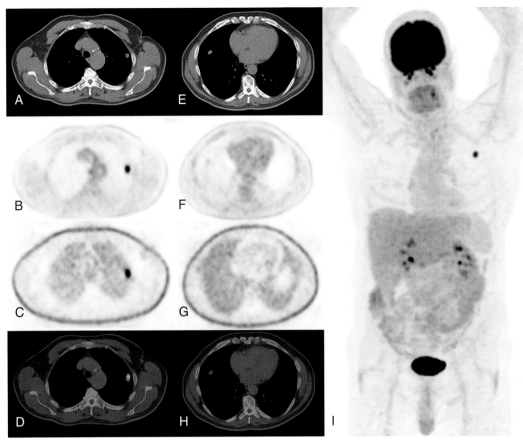

Figure 8-1 ^{18}F-fluorodeoxyglucose (FDG) positron emission tomography–computed tomography (PET–CT) for investigation of coin lesions. Patient with focal nodular lesion in right lung on chest radiograph (*not shown*). CT showed two coin lesions 13 mm in diameter, one in the right middle lobe and one in the left upper lobe. **A,** CT image of left lung coin lesion. **B,** Intense focal FDG uptake (SUV$_{max}$ = 11.3) at the site of the lesion on transverse attenuation coefficient (AC) images. **C,** Transverse non-AC image also demonstrates intense FDG uptake. **D,** Fusion image shows colocalization of PET signal and coin lesion. **E,** CT image of right lung lesion. **F,** A transverse AC PET image shows only faint uptake (SUV$_{max}$ = 1.2) at the site of the lesion, less intense than the blood pool activity seen in the mediastinum. **G,** A transverse non-AC image shows no increased uptake at all. **H,** Fusion image shows lack of uptake in the lesion. **I,** Maximum intensity projection PET image showing FDG-uptake in the left lung lesion only. At resection, the lesion on the left was found to be a well-differentiated primary lung adenocarcinoma. The lesion in the right lung was regarded as postinfectious scarring and did not change during further years of follow-up. *SUV,* standardized uptake value.

noninvasive methods for accurate staging are very important. CT scan, endoscopic techniques, and surgical staging procedures are key staging tools, but addition of FDG-PET to these conventional methods has been shown to improve the staging process substantially, by distinguishing patients who are candidates for radical approaches such as surgical resection or intense multimodality treatments from those who are not.

For the *T factor*, the detailed images of modern multislice CT allow evaluation of the relationship of the tumor to the fissures (which may determine the type of resection), to mediastinal structures, or to the pleura and chest wall. The integrated FDG-PET–CT images (**Figure 8-2**) may allow more precise evaluation of chest wall and mediastinal infiltration or correct differentiation between tumor and peritumoral inflammation or atelectasis.

FDG-PET–CT has been used to assess pleural disease with variable results, because small pleural deposits can be missed on PET-CT, owing to their low tumor load or partial volume effect, whereas false-positive results have been documented in patients with inflammatory pleural lesions. If pleural abnormalities determine the chance for radical treatment, often histopathologic verification with cytologic analysis or thoracoscopic biopsy is needed.

For the *N factor*, the addition of FDG-PET to CT results in more accurate lymph node staging than CT alone, with an overall sensitivity of 80% to 90% and a specificity of 85% to 95% in metaanalyses.

On the one hand, the absence of mediastinal lymph node disease on FDG-PET–CT has a high NPV, so that invasive lymph node staging tests can be omitted, and the patient can proceed to straightforward surgical resection. Restrictions on this NPV apply in case of insufficient FDG uptake in the primary tumor, central location of the tumor, or presence of important hilar nodal disease that may obscure coexisting N2 disease on PET images.

On the other hand, the combination of FDG-PET and CT illustrates the location of suspect lymph nodes, thereby helping to direct tissue sampling procedures such as endobronchial ultrasound–guided transbronchial needle aspiration or cervical mediastinoscopy. Because false-positive results are possible with lymph node imaging (under the conditions listed in Box 8-2), histopathologic proof of lymph node involvement should be sought in most patients with imaging-positive mediastinal nodes on FDG-PET, except those with obvious bulky nodes on imaging (**Figure 8-3**).

For the *M factor*, FDG-PET added to CT is almost uniformly superior to CT alone, except in brain imaging, for which sensitivity is unacceptably low owing to the high glucose uptake in normal surrounding brain tissue. CT and, even better, MRI remain the methods of choice for brain imaging.

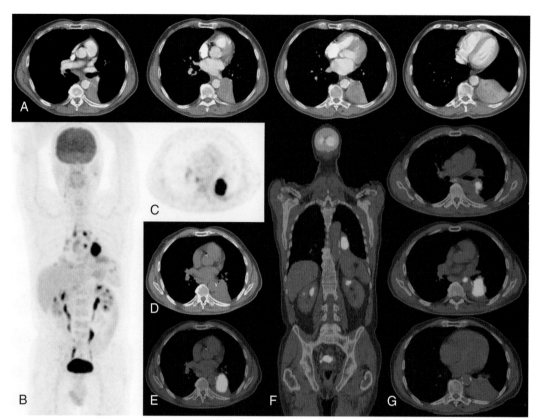

Figure 8-2 ^{18}F-fluorodeoxyglucose positron emission tomography–computed tomography (FDG-PET–CT) aids in the determination of T stage. Patient with adenocarcinoma of the left lower lobe. **A,** CT images show densification of the left lower lobe due to a solid lesion with accompanying retro-obstructive atelectasis, without clear delineation between tumor and benign parenchyma. **B,** Coronal image of the FDG-PET–CT shows a large rounded hypermetabolic lesion in the left lower lobe with smaller foci of intense activity in the mediastinum medial and cranial to the tumor, corresponding to lymph nodes. **C,** Transverse PET image showing a nicely delineated rounded tumor mass, allowing appropriate size determination (47 mm, or T2a). **D,** Corresponding low-dose CT image. **E,** Corresponding fusion image. **F,** Coronal image showing limited size of tumor compared with the atelectatic region. **G,** Consecutive fusion images allowing determination of involved and spared tissue, which are of high value in radiation therapy planning.

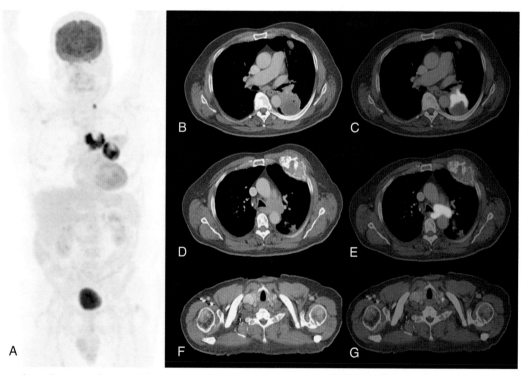

Figure 8-3 ^{18}F-fluorodeoxyglucose positron emission tomography–computed tomography (FDG-PET–CT) in the determination of nodal (N) stage. Patient with a squamous cell carcinoma of the left lower lobe. **A,** Coronal image shows hypermetabolic tumor in left lower lobe with a hypometabolic area at the cranial part indicating necrosis, hypermetabolic bulky mediastinal nodes, and focal increased uptake in the left supraclavicular region. **B,** CT image of primary tumor. **C,** Fusion image of primary tumor. **D,** CT image of bulky enlarged subaortic nodes and calcified rib lesion. **E,** Fusion image demonstrates hypermetabolic nodes and absence of metabolic activity in the rib. **F,** Nonenlarged supraclavicular lymph node behind the jugular vein. **G,** Focal intense FDG uptake in this node (SUV$_{max}$ = 12.2) is indicative of N3 involvement. The benign nature of the rib lesion was confirmed through biopsy, and the malignant nature of the supraclavicular node, by fine needle aspiration. *SUV,* standardized uptake value.

For bone metastases, FDG-PET is more accurate than technetium 99m–tagged medronate disodium (formerly methylene diphosphonate) (^{99m}Tc-MDP) bone scan: Sensitivity is at least as good (90% to 95%), and specificity is far better (95%, versus 60% for bone scan). Limitations are the restricted area of imaging for PET (only from the head to just below the pelvis) and possibility of a false-negative result with osteoblastic lesions (rare in lung cancer). For adrenal gland metastases, FDG-PET has a high sensitivity for detection of such disease, so an equivocal-appearing lesion on CT without FDG uptake usually will not be metastatic. FDG-PET also can be of help for investigation of hepatic lesions that remain indeterminate by conventional studies. PET also may reveal metastases in sites that escape attention on conventional staging (e.g., soft tissue lesions, retroperitoneal lymph nodes, barely palpable supraclavicular nodes, painless bone lesions). Exclusion of malignancy requires caution in case of smaller lesions (less than 1 cm in diameter) (see Box 8-2). In this respect, the small contralateral lung nodule(s)—a common finding in the era of spiral multislice CT—often still requires invasive sampling, such as by thoracoscopy.

INFLUENCE ON TREATMENT CHOICES

FDG-PET has a significantly complementary role to that of CT for two reasons: First, PET may detect unexpected lymph node or distant organ metastatic spread (**Figure 8-4**). After a negative result on conventional staging, unknown metastases are found on PET-CT in 5% to 20% of the patients, in increasing numbers from clinical stage I to III tumors. Second, FDG-PET is able to determine the nature of some equivocal lesions on conventional imaging. Consequently, PET induces a change of stage in 27% to 62% of patients with non–small cell lung carcinoma (NSCLC), in general more upstaging than downstaging, related mainly to the detection of unexpected distant lesions (**Table 8-1**). Such findings lead to a change in management in 25% up

Table 8-1	Impact of Positron Emission Tomography on Stage Designation and Patient Management in Non-Small Cell Lung Carcinoma		
Study	**N**	**Change of Stage**	**Change in Management**
Lewis et al., 1994	34	NR	41%
Bury et al., 1997	109	34%	25%
Saunders et al., 1999	97	27%	37%
Pieterman et al., 2000	102	62%	NR
Hicks et al., 2001	153	43%	35%
Schmucking et al., 2003	63	NR	52%
Hoekstra et al., 2003	57	30%	19%

NR, not reported.

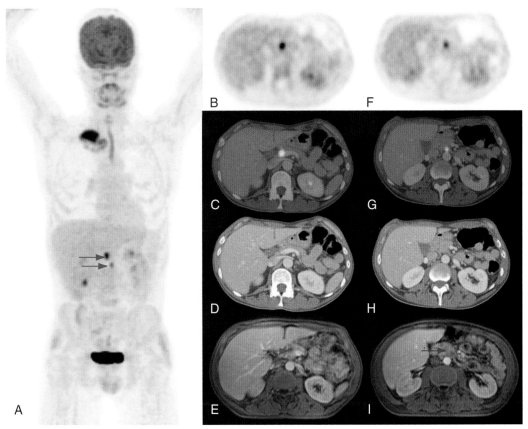

Figure 8-4 ^{18}F-fluorodeoxyglucose positron emission tomography–computed tomography (FDG-PET–CT) may detect unsuspected metastases. Patient with large cell carcinoma of the right upper lobe assessed with FDG-PET–CT after concurrent chemotherapy and radiotherapy. **A,** Coronal image shows a persistent, intensely hypermetabolic mass in the right upper lung. Pronounced linear FDG uptake in the esophagus corresponded to treatment-induced inflammation. Two additional foci project on the midline of the epigastrium *(arrows)*. **B,** Transverse PET image of the cranial epigastric lesion. **C,** Fusion image shows an intra- or juxtapancreatic location, highly suspicious for metastasis. **D,** Corresponding CT image shows no significant lesion. **E,** Hypointense focal intrapancreatic lesion on a subsequent contrast-enhanced T1-weighted MRI study, compatible with metastasis *(arrow)*. **F-I,** Similar findings in the caudal lesion. Echoendoscopy-directed fine needle aspiration confirmed metastasis. *MRI*, magnetic resonance imaging.

to 52% of the patients. Documented changes have involved both treatment intent (curative versus palliative) and choice of treatment modalities (chemotherapy versus radiotherapy, radical radiotherapy versus surgery).

No problem arises in interpretation when whole-body FDG-PET shows multisite metastases, but presence and character of an isolated suspect lesion that determines radical treatment intent should always be verified by other tests or tissue sampling, because of the ever-present risk of false-positive lesions (see Box 8-2) or a second primary tumor. In one large retrospective series, solitary extrathoracic lesions were documented in approximately 20% of the patients. About half of these were metastatic; the other half were not related to lung cancer, as either inflammatory or other benign lesions, or were second primary tumors (**Figure 8-5**).

Before the advent of integrated FDG-PET–CT, it remained unclear if PET alone could *replace* conventional imaging. One randomized study compared staging with upfront FDG-PET alone (i.e., directly after first presentation) versus

guideline-based CT imaging in 465 patients. Patients with FDG-avid, noncentrally located tumors without signs of mediastinal or distant spread on PET proceeded directly to surgical resection. Frequency of noninvasive tests to reach a clinical TNM diagnosis was about the same in both treatment groups, but that of invasive tests (i.e., mainly mediastinoscopy) was significantly reduced with PET. With the contemporary use of integrated FDG-PET–CT, this question has become an academic one.

The effect of *adding* FDG-PET or FDG-PET–CT was investigated in several randomized controlled trials (**Table 8-2**). Two earlier trials that looked at the addition of PET alone reported seemingly contradictory results. Clear differences in trial design probably accounted for this finding. In the Dutch trial, the end point "futile thoracotomy" was clearly defined (benign disease, explorative thoracotomy, pathologic stage IIIA-N2/IIIB, or postoperative relapse or death within 12 months), whereas in the Australian study, there were no benign lesions, surgery was considered to be of use in some patients with stage IIIA-N2

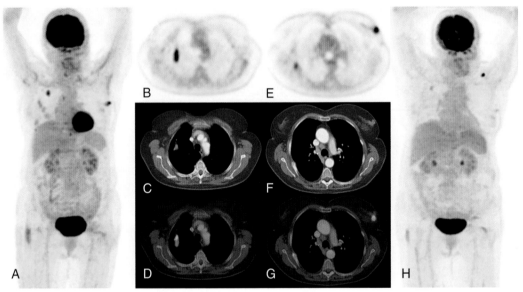

Figure 8-5 ^{18}F-fluorodeoxyglucose positron emission tomography–computed tomography (FDG-PET–CT) detects synchronous tumors, as in this patient with adenocarcinoma in the right upper lobe. **A,** Coronal image shows focal intense uptake in the right upper lobe as well as in the left breast. Moderately increased uptake is apparent in a right paratracheal lymph node. Note multifocal, moderately increased uptake in the right ribs (secondary to inflammation due to recent fractures) and next to the right trochanter femoris (enthesopathy). **B,** Transverse PET image shows the intensely FDG-avid lung lesion, compatible with the known malignancy. **C,** CT image of lung lesion. **D,** Fusion image. **E,** Transverse PET image of the intensely FDG-avid focal lesion in the left breast, highly suspicious for malignancy. **F,** CT shows an enhancing solid lesion at the site of FDG uptake. **G,** Fusion image of breast lesion that proved to be an invasive ductal adenocarcinoma. **H,** Coronal image after induction chemotherapy for the pulmonary adenocarcinoma and antihormonal therapy for the breast lesion. Note the strong decrease in uptake in both primary tumors, indicating a partial metabolic response. The intense focus in the left supraclavicular region is an artifact due to tracer retention in the patient's Portacath.

Table 8-2   **Effects on Outcome With Addition of FDG-PET or FDG-PET-CT to Clinical Assessment**

Study	N	Population	Study Question	Comparison	Outcome	Findings
Van Tinteren et al., 2002	188	Proven/suspected resectable NSCLC	Reduction in "futile thoracotomies"?	CS → surgery	Yes	Futile thoracotomy 41% vs. 21% (P = .003)
Viney et al., 2004	184	Proven stage I-II NSCLC	Impact on "decision to operate"?	CS → surgery CS + PET → surgery	No	No difference in avoided thoracotomies (P = .20)
Fischer et al., 2009	189	Proven/suspected resectable NSCLC	Reduction in "futile thoracotomies"?	CS → surgery PET-CT → surgery	Yes	Futile thoracotomy 52% vs. 35% (P = .05)
Maziak et al., 2009	337	Proven stage I-IIIA NSCLC	Improvement in correct upstaging?	CS PET-CT	Yes	Correctly upstaged pts 7% vs. 14% (P = .05)

CS, conventional staging; *CT,* computed tomography; *FDG,* ^{18}F-fluorodeoxyglucose; *NSCLC,* non-small cell lung carcinoma; *PET,* positron emission tomography.

disease, and no strict follow-up terms were predefined. The Australian trial focused on patients with clinical stage I and II disease only, where less additional benefit of PET was demonstrated in previous nonrandomized accuracy studies. The later trials used FDG-PET–CT imaging in addition to standard workup. The study by Fischer and colleagues largely reproduced the Dutch experience, with a significant reduction in futile thoracotomies. However, the number of nonfutile thoracotomies and the overall survival rate were similar in both treatment groups. Finally, the study reported by Maziak and associates mainly looked at correct upstaging and met this primary end point. Even in this study, which was the largest, no significant survival difference at 3 years was noted. This apparent lack of improvement was attributed by the investigators to the fact that larger patient numbers may be needed, and to the fact that some patients did not have their planned surgery.

The overall evidence thus points at significantly more accurate TNM staging with PET-CT compared with conventional imaging alone. This improved accuracy leads to more appropriate treatment policies, such as the avoidance of futile surgery in more patients than when only conventional imaging is used. In nonrandomized settings, this also has been reported to lead to other treatment adaptations—for example, a change between radical and palliative intent of radiotherapy, or adaptations in the radiation fields. Although all of this evidence certainly leads to true benefits such as stage migration and better patient management, it remains unknown if survival of individual patients has improved since the introduction of FDG-PET.

SURVIVAL

Indeed, several FDG-PET staging studies clearly demonstrated stage migration. The possible effects of stage migration may account in part for improvements in survival of patients treated for both early- and advanced-stage disease, widely referred to as the "Will Rogers phenomenon." Examples are the prospective multicenter trials on the use of FDG-PET in patients with stage III NSCLC, in which upstaging was confirmed in about 25% to 30% of the patients, and in which overall survival was significantly longer ($P = .006$) in patients whose disease was staged by PET than in those who did not undergo PET. The aforementioned randomized controlled trials were underpowered to evaluate the potential real survival benefit brought by PET.

FDG-PET also has been shown to predict the prognosis for patients with NSCLC. A recent systematic review and meta-analysis including retrospective studies demonstrated that the SUV, a semiquantitative measure of FDG uptake, for the primary tumor at diagnosis may predict outcome in NSCLC, especially at earlier stages. These studies almost consistently found a better overall survival among patients with a metabolic activity lower than the threshold SUV value, calculated from either the most discriminative log-rank SUV value or the median SUV. However, although SUV may be a way to assess prognosis, no true cutoff point has been recognized as suitable for broad clinical use. Rather, a continuous SUV spectrum of a gradually worsening prognosis might be a more realistic concept. Baseline SUV, incorporated as a continuous variable in a Cox proportional hazards model, showed a 7% increase in hazard of death after a one-unit increase in SUV in patients with resected stage I to III NSCLC and a 6% increase in hazard of death after a one-unit increase in SUV in patients with inoperable NSCLC treated with radiotherapy.

HEALTH ECONOMICS

Today's respiratory oncologists aim for the best-quality health care for the patient, but in acknowledgment of the need for financial prudence. The major cost of modern oncology practice, however, does not lie in the baseline diagnostic process but is attributable to the delivery of expensive treatments and the morbidity related to possible side effects. Therefore, application of economic modeling in the use of FDG-PET has to be based on both diagnostic and therapeutic aspects of health care expenditure within the day-to-day clinical setting.

In a recent overview of all economic evaluations on FDG-PET in oncology performed between 2005 and 2010, the strongest evidence for cost-effective use of PET alone was for the staging of NSCLC. Studies suggested that PET for staging of NSCLC may benefit patients in terms of a (slight) increase in life expectancy and may benefit the health care system in terms of cost savings resulting from the number of invasive procedures avoided. Since the introduction of PET-CT technology into clinical medicine in 2001, only a few additional studies in respiratory oncology have evaluated the cost-effectiveness of this integrated scanning method. Taking into account the superior accuracy of FDG-PET–CT over that of PET alone in lung cancer staging, the health economic impact in terms of cost-effectiveness probably can be extended to PET-CT. Furthermore, FDG-PET is cost-effective for characterizing and diagnosing solitary pulmonary nodules and constitutes the most cost-effective strategy for assessment of nodules of low to moderate pretest probability of malignancy on CT.

OTHER INDICATIONS FOR POSITRON EMISSION TOMOGRAPHY

Small Cell Lung Cancer

Small cell lung cancer (SCLC) typically shows very high FDG accumulation. In a systematic analysis of seven studies, FDG-PET or PET-CT provides more accurate staging of SCLC, mainly based on high sensitivity rates ranging from 92% to 100%. In one study, involved nodes were detected in 14% of patients in whom results on CT were negative. This increased lesion detection resulted in stage migration in a median of 13% of patients, 9% (0 to 33%) upstaged from limited stage (LS) to extensive stage (ES), and 4% (0 to 17%) downstaged from ES to LS. The data on the use of FDG-PET in the management of SCLC are less robust than for NSCLC, because the emphasis on systemic and radiation therapy provides less histologic data to serve as gold standard. Furthermore, most studies were rather small (mean $n = 40$) and retrospective in nature. Detection of brain metastases also is poor, so additional specific brain imaging with conventional methods is still mandatory. Nevertheless, the use of FDG-PET information is associated with considerable changes in patient management, ranging from 27% to 47% across studies. The use of FDG-PET–CT resulted in changes to the three-dimensional conformal radiation therapy plan in 58% of patients, mainly by decreasing the target volume (in case of atelectasis) or by detecting unsuspected nodal or pulmonary foci.

Mesothelioma

Integrated FDG-PET–CT imaging is playing an increasing role in the assessment of suspected or known malignant pleural mesothelioma (MPM) (**Figure 8-6**). PET-CT is useful in the correct differentiation of malignant (mainly MPM) from benign pleural diseases in asbestos-related CT findings, with an overall

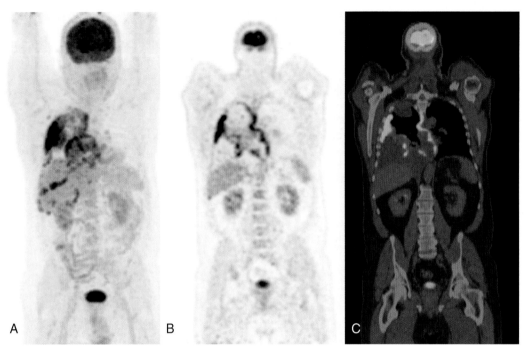

Figure 8-6 ^{18}F-fluorodeoxyglucose positron emission tomography–computed tomography (FDG-PET–CT) for evaluation of a patient with right-sided epithelioid pleural mesothelioma. Pleuroscopy with talc pleurodesis was performed before the PET scan. **A,** Coronal image showing diffuse and irregular area of intense FDG uptake in the right hemithorax, mainly in the apical part but with also demonstrating multiple foci in the costodiaphragmatic sinus. **B,** Coronal PET image showing hypermetabolic activity in the lateral and medial right pleura. **C,** Fusion images show areas of pleural effusion without increased FDG uptake.

accuracy greater than 90% and a high NPV of more than 90%. PET-CT is significantly more accurate in baseline TNM staging in patients who are appropriate candidates for multimodality therapy based on spiral CT findings alone. Although PET-CT does not provide additional information about the primary tumor beyond that supplied by CT alone, it identifies a higher number of metastatic mediastinal lymph nodes and/or unknown distant metastatic disease in up to two thirds of patients, with a significant clinical impact on treatment planning. Early evidence also suggests that PET-CT may have a role in evaluating response to therapy in MPM. This is an interesting possibility, because the assessment of response in patients with MPM according to standard response criteria on CT is far from simple. More work to define response criteria for MPM on FDG-PET is needed. Furthermore, a prospective study in patients with nonsarcomatoid malignant pleural mesothelioma observed that baseline total glycolytic volume on PET was more predictive of survival than CT-assessed TNM stage on multivariate analysis. These observations of prognostic capability still require prospective validation.

Therapy Assessment

FDG uptake in tumors is related to (1) the number of viable cancer cells, (2) their metabolic activity and proliferation capacity, and (3) the presence of inflammatory cells. In many clinical settings, the metabolic changes caused by cancer therapy precede the morphologic changes. This discrimination of viable from nonviable tumor is the basis for the use of FDG-PET for the determination of response to therapy.

Restaging of locally advanced lung cancer after neoadjuvant or induction therapy has been extensively studied (**Table 8-3**). In the restaging of mediastinal lymph nodes, FDG-PET added to CT was more accurate than CT alone but with more moderate results than when used for baseline nodal staging (sensitivity of 50% to 80% and specificity of 60% to 90%). Later studies

using integrated PET-CT found better sensitivity (up to 77%) with an increase in specificity (up to 92%). Mediastinal restaging with PET-CT thus reaches an accuracy level of some clinical value but is especially useful in directing additional tissue sampling techniques such as endobronchial ultrasound-guided transbronchial needle aspiration (EBUS-TBNA), esophageal ultrasound–guided fine needle aspiration (EUS-FNA), or mediastinoscopy, which usually need to be added to certify the nodal status.

The findings on outcome prediction in this setting are even more interesting. The classic prognostic parameters for surgery in these patients are obtained from the resection specimen—(1) downstaging of mediastinal nodes and (2) the pathologic response in the primary tumor. Outcomes are poorly predicted by the evolving clinical or CT imaging characteristics during therapy. In the prospective studies, both the residual FDG uptake in the primary tumor after induction and the change in FDG uptake in comparison of pre- and postinduction values had strong power to predict outcome after combined-modality treatment. With the advent of endoscopic baseline mediastinal staging (EBUS-TBNA and EUS-FNA) to confirm N2 or N3 disease, the postinduction assessment can be based on primary tumor response information on (serial comparison of) FDG-PET and lymph node assessment by a first mediastinoscopy after induction therapy. In one model, the combination of lymph node involvement and primary tumor response on FDG-PET could discriminate patients with a good prognosis (defined as a 5-year survival rate of 62%) from those with a poor prognosis (survival rate of only 6%; hazard ratio, 0.18) in a cohort of patients with surgical multimodality treatment.

Targeted therapies are advancing at a rapid pace in the treatment of NSCLC, and conceptually FDG-PET might be of great interest in the assessment of these cytostatic rather than cytotoxic drugs. Two recent independent studies have shown that early FDG-PET can predict progression-free and overall

Table 8-3 Results of PET and Integrated PET-CT in Restaging After Induction Treatment for Locally Advanced Non-Small Cell Lung Carcinoma

Study	N	Stage	CTRT	Imaging	Sensitivity	Specificity
Vansteenkiste et al., 2001	31	IIIA-N2	0	PET + CT (visual corr.)	71%	88%
Akhurst et al., 2002	56	I-III	29%	PET + CT (visual corr.)	67%	61%
Ryu et al., 2002	26	III	100%	PET + CT (visual corr.)	58%	93%
Cerfolio et al., 2003	34	IB-IIIA	21%	PET + CT (visual corr.)	71%	77%
Hellwig et al., 2004	37	III	70%	PET + CT (visual corr.)	50%	88%
Port et al., 2004	25	I-IIIA	0	PET + CT (visual corr.)	20%	71%
Hoekstra et al., 2005	25	IIIA-N2	0	PET + CT (visual corr.)	50%	71%
Yamamoto et al., 2006	26	III	100%	PET + CT (visual corr.)	88%	89%
Eschmann et al., 2007	70	III	100%	PET + CT (visual corr.)	77%	68%
Cerfolio et al., 2006	93	IIIA-N2	100%	Integrated PET-CT	62%	88%
Pottgen et al., 2006	37	IIIA/B	100%	Integrated PET-CT	73%	89%
De Leyn et al., 2006	30	IIIA-N2	0	Integrated PET-CT	77%	92%

CT, computed tomography; CTRT, % patients with chemoradiotherapy; PET, positron emission tomography.

survival in patients treated with erlotinib, even in the absence of a Response Evaluation Criteria in Solid Tumors (RECIST) response.

For patients managed with the newer locoregional treatment strategy of radiofrequency ablation, FDG-PET may potentially be useful in the assessment of the therapeutic success and prediction of prognosis. This specific setting, however, necessitates a careful pattern analysis next to semiquantitative determination of the glucose metabolism, because there can be a strong and persisting inflammatory response.

For all settings in which FDG-PET scans at different time points are to be compared, it is crucial to perform the PET procedure according to a consistent methodology, including interval from last therapy, patient preparation, camera setting, reconstruction parameters, and image analysis. Recommendations on this very crucial point of standardization in a multicenter setting have been published recently.

Radiotherapy Planning

Just as careful TNM staging is important to select patients who are candidates for surgical options, the accurate delineation of target volumes for radiotherapy is crucial to avoid geographic treatment misses leading to treatment failures.

It has been shown in many radiotherapy planning studies that use of FDG-PET or FDG-PET–CT influences the target volumes. The PET-based volume delineations were in general smaller than those with CT alone, mainly to permit potentially more precise nodal irradiation. This approach allowed for radiation dose escalation to the tumor in a substantial number of patients. Prospective clinical trials using PET-CT–based selective nodal irradiation reported isolated nodal failures in less than 5% of patients treated with (chemo)radiotherapy. This rate is lower than the 13% rate of false-negative PET results in CT-positive lymph nodes in a metaanalysis, which might be explained by the incidental irradiation of lymph nodes adjacent to the planning target volume. Because of the possibility of false-positive lymph nodes on PET, invasive nodal staging using endosonography or mediastinoscopy may be warranted, if the nodes concerned would have a major impact on the radiation treatment field. The clinical gain with PET-based delineation of the primary tumor compared with CT-based delineation is in general smaller, except in situations with postobstructive atelectasis.

In recent studies, automated PET-CT delineation also reduced the interobserver variability in treatment planning compared with that for CT alone. Furthermore, FDG-PET also may have a role in monitoring treatment during the course of radiotherapy. PET may identify radioresistant areas within the primary tumor before and during treatment, with high accuracy. Work is in progress on how to use this information to plan higher radiation doses to these areas, for improved outcomes.

FUTURE INNOVATION

Evolution in PET is largely driven by advances in camera technology (hardware and software) and by the development of new tracers. Spatial resolution improvement is driven by size reduction of the crystal detectors and by novel reconstruction algorithms that take into account the point spread function of the camera. A resolution of approximately 2 mm probably will be the limit, because the two photons emitted during positron annihilation do not travel at exactly 180 degrees ("noncolinearity"). Time-of-flight (TOF) PET uses the time difference between two crystals that detect an incoming photon to reduce these photons' origin from a line (as is classically done) to a short segment of this line. This reconstruction method results in improved signal-to-noise ratio, allowing faster acquisition times or tracer dose reduction.

Another feature that could improve the quality of the images, especially in respiratory medicine, is respiratory gating of PET acquisition. Because of respiratory motion, the volume of a lung lesion is "smeared out" and thus overestimated, while the FDG intensity is underestimated, especially in the lower lung fields. Synchronization of the acquisition of the PET emission images with respiratory motion is now available and being clinically evaluated, with exact quantification of tracer uptake and radiotherapy planning as the most promising fields. Reconstruction algorithms are being developed that incorporate anatomic information from either CT or MRI to obtain higher-resolution images with sharper edges, allowing better volume delineation in radiotherapy planning.

The other major driver of innovation in PET is new tracer development. Although FDG imaging allows highly accurate tumor detection and characterization, FDG uptake in inflammatory tissues remains a major limitation. Development of novel tracers offering a similar sensitivity with higher specificity is ongoing, but until now, no molecule has outperformed FDG in respiratory oncology. Molecular imaging of key molecules and cellular processes could, however, play an important role in noninvasive tumor characterization. Many crucial cellular processes can be studied, such as proliferation, angiogenesis, and expression of different receptor types. PET imaging with 3'-deoxy-3'-^{18}F-fluorothymidine (^{18}F-FLT) allows noninvasive assessment of proliferation and offers theoretical advantages in determination of response to cytostatic therapies. A whole range of PET tracers have been developed to image angiogenesis, the most intensively studied based on ligands for the dividing endothelial cell marker integrin $\alpha v\beta 3$. These tracers are being evaluated mainly in the context of prediction or assessment of response to antiangiogenic therapies. Tumor characterization based on receptor expression can be performed by PET imaging with binding of radiolabeled peptides to the somatostatin receptor (mainly types 2, 3, and 5), thereby allowing diagnosis and staging of carcinoid tumors. PET also is studied to assess the presence of pharmaceutical targets in tumor tissue. One example is 1-(2'-deoxy-2'-fluoroarabinofuranosyl) cytosine (FAC), a substrate for deoxycytidine kinase, the enzyme responsible for the conversion of gemcitabine from a prodrug to its active form. Selection of patients based on genetic mutations will become increasingly common, and novel PET tracers are being developed that allow detection of specific mutations, such as ^{18}F-PEG6-IPQA, a radiotracer with increased selectivity and irreversible binding to the active mutant L858R EGFR kinase (which is sensitive to gefitinib) but not to wild type or T790M-mutated EGFR kinase.

Many other tracers are being developed, and their clinical testing is eagerly awaited to help in the selection of patients for targeted therapies. The fact that PET imaging, with use of FDG or other, more specific molecular tracers, is being incorporated in some of the pivotal clinical trials establishing novel therapies will help to generate needed evidence for use of this modality in clinical decision making.

SUGGESTED READINGS

Boellaard R, O'Doherty MJ, Weber WA, et al: FDG PET and PET/CT: EANM procedure guidelines for tumour PET imaging: version 1.0, *Eur J Nucl Med Mol Imaging* 37:662–671, 2010.

De Cabanyes-Candela S, Detterbeck FC: A systematic review of restaging after induction therapy for stage IIIA lung cancer: prediction of pathologic stage, *J Thorac Oncol* 5:389–398, 2010.

Dooms C, Verbeken E, Stroobants S, et al: Prognostic stratification of stage IIIA-N2 non-small cell lung cancer after induction chemotherapy: a model based on the combination of morphometric-pathologic response in mediastinal nodes and primary tumour response on serial 18-fluoro-2-deoxy-glucose positron emission tomography, *J Clin Oncol* 26:1128–1134, 2008.

Fischer B, Lassen U, Mortensen J, et al: Preoperative staging of lung cancer with combined PET-CT, *N Engl J Med* 361:32–39, 2009.

Hicks J: Role of ^{18}F-FDG in assessment of response in non-small cell lung cancer, *J Nucl Med* 50(Suppl 1):31S–42S, 2009.

Mavi A, Lakhani P, Zhuang H, et al: Fluorodeoxyglucose-PET in characterizing solitary pulmonary nodules, assessing pleural diseases, and the initial staging, restaging, therapy planning, and monitoring response of lung cancer, *Radiol Clin North Am* 43:1–21, 2005.

Thomson D, Hulse P, Lorigan P, Faivre-Finn C: The role of positron emission tomography in management of small cell lung cancer, *Lung Cancer* 73:121–126, 2011.

Van Baardwijk A, Baumert BG, Bosmans G, et al: The current status of FDG-PET in tumour volume definition in radiotherapy treatment planning, *Cancer Treat Rev* 32:245–260, 2006.

Vansteenkiste J, Fischer BM, Dooms C, Mortensen J: Positron-emission tomography in prognostic and therapeutic assessment of lung cancer: systematic review, *Lancet Oncol* 5:531–540, 2004.

Vansteenkiste J, Dooms C: Positron emission tomography in nonsmall cell lung cancer, *Curr Opin Oncol* 19:78–83, 2007.

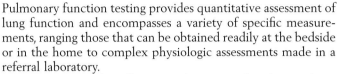

Chapter **9**
Pulmonary Function Testing

Bruce H. Culver

Pulmonary function testing provides quantitative assessment of lung function and encompasses a variety of specific measurements, ranging those that can be obtained readily at the bedside or in the home to complex physiologic assessments made in a referral laboratory.

Spirometry in the office is used to screen for abnormalities of airflow or lung volume, to test bronchodilator responsiveness, and for interval assessments in patients who have asthma or chronic obstructive pulmonary disease (COPD). Screening spirometry has been recommended for middle-aged smokers and former smokers to identify airflow obstruction at an earlier stage than that typical for persons presenting with dyspnea. Although COPD often is suspected from smoking history and symptoms, the diagnosis rests on the demonstration of airflow obstruction from spirometry testing, and current measures of clinical quality require that such testing be done. COPD has now become the third leading cause of death (in U.S. statistics) yet frequently is diagnosed late in the course as it becomes disabling. Up to one half of the persons with this condition may remain undiagnosed, because the most common early symptoms, cough and exertional dyspnea, often are attributed to other causes.

Testing in the pulmonary function laboratory allows further classification and quantification of lung disease by adding data from the measurement of lung volumes and assessment of gas exchange through measurement of diffusing capacity and arterial blood gases, and from tests of gas distribution. Special testing is available for prethoracotomy evaluation, assessment of upper airway obstruction, bronchoprovocation challenge testing, and cardiopulmonary exercise response (discussed in Chapter 10). Although even comprehensive lung function testing may not provide a specific diagnosis, the pattern of physiologic derangements guides further assessment, and demonstration of the severity of impairment aids in prognosis.

Guidelines for pulmonary function equipment specifications, procedural techniques, and interpretation of results were most recently published in 2005 by a joint panel of the American Thoracic Society (ATS) and the European Respiratory Society (ERS). The multipart series of statements are included in the "Suggested Readings" listing, and the recommendations presented in this chapter are consistent with these guidelines.

SPIROMETRY

THE FORCED EXPIRATORY VOLUME MANEUVER

Assessments of vital capacity (VC), or forced vital capacity (FVC) and airflow are based on the forced expiratory volume maneuver, in which the subject inhales maximally to total lung

capacity (TLC) and then exhales forcefully and completely to residual volume (RV). The expiratory flow rate at any point during this maneuver is determined by the driving pressure for airflow and the airway resistance. During a forceful exhalation, the intrathoracic pressure that surrounds the central airways exceeds the intraluminal pressure, causing dynamic compression of the airway (see Chapter 3, Figure 3-12). As a result, the effective driving pressure becomes the difference between alveolar pressure and the pleural pressure that compresses airways. This pressure difference ($P_A - P_{pl}$) is equivalent to the elastic recoil pressure of the lung tissue. Thus, even during a forceful effort, the intrinsic elastic properties of the lung are a major determinant of airflow. Airway resistance upstream from the point of compression is determined primarily by airway caliber, which varies directly with lung volume. Throughout exhalation from TLC, both recoil pressure and airway caliber progressively decrease, so that airflow rates, after an early peak, also progressively decrease. Although the peak expiratory flow rate varies with the rapidity and forcefulness of the expiratory effort, once dynamic compression begins, the flow rate during the middle to later portions of the maneuver is limited and independent of further effort beyond the threshold needed to begin compression. These flows also are independent of added resistance downstream from the point of flow limitation. This physiologic arrangement aids in making the basic measurements of spirometry quite reproducible on repeated efforts.

To obtain a satisfactory spirometric tracing, the preceding inspiration must be maximal and the forced expiratory volume maneuver must be continued to cessation of flow or, when emptying is slowed, for at least 6 to10 seconds. The resultant information commonly is displayed in one of two formats. The traditional *spirogram* (**Figure 9-1**) plots volume versus time, with flow rate indicated by the steepness of the plot. The orientation of the axes varies with equipment, with time moving to the right and exhaled volume plotted either up or down. In the *flow-volume display* (**Figure 9-2**), the instantaneous flow rate is measured continuously and directly plotted on the vertical axis with volume on the horizontal axis. Time is not shown on this plot but may be indicated by tick marks. With this display, the reproducibility of successive efforts and some patterns of abnormality may be more easily seen. It is important to recognize that both the traditional spirogram and the expiratory flow-volume display are obtained from the same maneuver but emphasize different aspects of the information thus obtained.

EXPIRATORY FLOW MEASUREMENTS

Basic measurements from the forced expiratory volume maneuver include FVC, the forced expiratory volume in 1 second

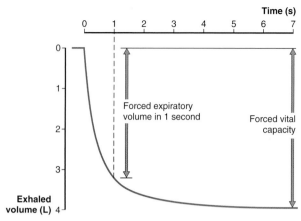

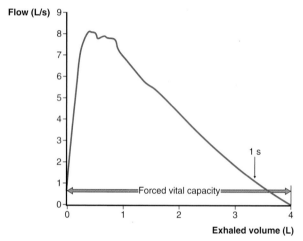

Figure 9-1 Normal forced expiratory spirogram plotted as exhaled volume versus time. The forced expiratory volume at 1 second (FEV_1) and forced vital capacity (FVC) are indicated by *arrows*. In this example, FEV_1 = 3.35 L, FVC = 4 L, and FEV_1/FVC = 0.84.   *(Modified from Culver BH: Pulmonary function testing. In Kelly WN, editor:* Textbook of internal medicine, *Philadelphia, 1988, JB Lippincott.)*

Figure 9-2 Normal expiratory flow-volume curve. The same forced expiratory volume maneuver shown in Figure 9-1 is plotted here as a flow-volume curve. The airflow rate reaches a peak early in the exhalation and then decreases progressively until flow ceases at residual volume. *(Modified from Culver BH: Pulmonary function testing. In Kelly WN, editor:* Textbook of internal medicine, *Philadelphia, 1988, JB Lippincott.)*

(FEV_1), and the ratio of FEV_1 to FVC. The FVC or total volume exhaled is equivalent in normal subjects to a so-called *slow VC*, obtained with a complete but not forceful exhalation. Patients who have advanced obstructive airway disease often manifest exaggerated dynamic compression (narrowing airways with forceful efforts), so that the FVC is smaller than the slow VC. A reduction in VC reflects either a reduction in TLC, an increase in RV, or a combination of both. The FEV_1 is readily obtained from the volume-time spirogram by observing the volume exhaled in the first 1 second of effort. This measurement cannot be seen on the flow-volume display but can be calculated by the microprocessors in the equipment that use this display. Determination of FEV_1/FVC is easily performed using simple equipment; this ratio provides the best index of airflow limitation. When the slow VC also is available, and if it is larger, this may be substituted for FVC, thereby increasing the sensitivity of the ratio for detection of obstruction. This ratio is commonly expressed as a percentage and sometimes is referred to as the "percent FEV_1"; however, this terminology may cause confusion, because the FEV_1 itself is commonly expressed as a percentage of its predicted value. Misunderstanding is lessened if the ratio is reported and discussed as a decimal (e.g., 0.82).

An additional flow measurement widely reported from the spirogram is the average forced expiratory flow rate between 25% and 75% of the exhaled VC (FEF_{25-75}), formerly referred to as the maximum midexpiratory flow rate. This measurement shows wider variability than that typical for FEV_1 or FEV_1/FVC, both within and between individual subjects. When this variability is appropriately accounted for, FEF_{25-75} is not more sensitive than FEV_1/FVC for the detection of airflow limitation. Numerous other flow measurements can be obtained from the forced expiratory volume maneuver, but they are highly interdependent with those already described and add little new information. The $FEV_{0.5}$ may be used to assess the initiation of effort but adds little diagnostic information in adults. In young children, the $FEV_{0.5}$ or $FEV_{0.75}$ can be a useful index of flow, because children may fully empty their lungs within the first second.

Because it may be difficult for some subjects to consistently maintain the forced expiratory maneuver to full exhalation, which may take 10 to 15 seconds when airflow obstruction is present, the forced expiratory volume in 6 seconds (FEV_6) may be taken as a surrogate for FVC and used to calculate an FEV_1-to-FEV_6 ratio, which can be compared with appropriate reference values.

The peak expiratory flow rate achieved during the FVC maneuver cannot be accurately calculated from a spirogram display but is readily seen on the flow-volume display and can be calculated by microprocessors. It can show considerable effort-to-effort variability, even when FEV_1 and FVC measurements are nearly identical. A peak flow measurement also can be obtained with simple handheld devices, which are useful for interval follow-up evaluation and for home management of patients who have reactive airway disease but are less accurate and less sensitive than spirometry for screening. Whereas spirographic flow measurements are obtained over a time interval or volume interval, measurements from the flow-volume display or current microprocessors can be reported at specific lung volumes. Maximum flow rates at 50% and 75% of exhaled volume are commonly reported, but nomenclature varies, and the latter may be designated as the flow rate at 25% of remaining VC. Routine use of these measurements is not recommended.

The maximum voluntary ventilation (MVV) is measurable on some office spirometers but is primarily a laboratory measurement. The subject is instructed to breathe deeply and rapidly, typically at 60 to 70 breaths per minute, and the total volume of ventilation over a 12- to 15-second period is extrapolated to liters per minute. Historically, this was the initial dynamic test for obstructive disease; however, it has been supplanted by the forced expiratory maneuver for the diagnosis of airflow limitation. The MVV currently is used as a global assessment of ventilatory capacity in the evaluation of dyspnea, in the interpretation of exercise limitation, in disability assessment, in some preoperative testing, and to evaluate neuromuscular disease of the chest wall and diaphragm.

REVERSIBILITY

The usefulness of spirometry in the office or laboratory often is enhanced by the assessment of bronchodilator response. Spirometry is repeated after the administration of an inhaled bronchodilator, waiting 15 minutes after a beta agonist or 30 minutes after ipratropium bromide. An increase of more than 12% in the FEV_1 represents a significant response in a patient who has near-normal baseline spirometry results. With more severe obstructive disease, the magnitude of improvement also should be at least 200 mL to differentiate the pharmacologic response from test-to-test variability. FVC often improves in parallel with FEV_1. An improvement in FVC by more than 12% and 200 mL, in the absence of a significant change in FEV_1, may reflect either an improvement in flow rates after the first second or simply a longer duration of effort.

Although determination of the FEV_1/FVC ratio is the most useful test for the diagnosis of airflow limitation, the value may remain the same or even decrease after administration of a bronchodilator, depending on the relative change in its two components, so this ratio is not a useful index of reversibility. Because of its large intraindividual variability, FEF_{25-75} must show an increase of 30% to 40% to represent a significant bronchodilator effect. Occasionally, this parameter changes little or even decreases despite a clear improvement in FEV_1 or, particularly, FVC. This apparent paradox occurs because the bronchodilator has allowed exhalation to continue to a lower RV, so that the 25% to 75% increment is now measured at a lower lung volume, with consequent lower flow rates.

REFERENCE EQUATIONS AND LIMITS OF NORMALITY

Unlike many laboratory tests, lung function parameters vary greatly with body size and age, so the expected values must be determined on an individual basis. Numerous prediction equations have been derived from spirometric surveys of normal reference populations. Currently accepted studies exclude all smokers as well as persons who have any thoracic or cardiopulmonary disease. Most studies have found that lung function parameters can be predicted on the basis of gender, age, and height, and that the addition of other body size measurements does not improve the accuracy of the equations. The prediction equations give the midpoint of the normal range, which is unfortunately wide for most spirometry measurements.

The lower limit of normal (LLN) must be established from the variability among individual subjects who have the same prediction parameters. The limits of the normal range are chosen to exclude 5% of a normal population; that is, 5% will be misclassified as having disease. In screening a generally healthy population for a rare disease, a borderline-low result is more likely to reflect this misclassification than to represent true identification of disease. However, when spirometry is done for persons at risk for lung disease, or with suggestive symptoms, the probability that a borderline result reflects a true abnormality is much higher. For the spirometry measurements, only low values are considered of concern, so the LLN is set at the 5th percentile of the reference sample. Because the distribution of values in the reference population is adequately symmetric above and below the mean, the 5th percentile LLN often is taken as the predicted value minus 1.645 times the standard error of the estimate (SEE) of the regression equation. The predicted value and the LLN both are readily calculated from the reference data programmed into the spirometry equipment, and both should be reported for comparison against the actual measured value.

Spirometry reference data from a large, systematic survey of the U.S. population (the Third National Health and Nutrition Examination Survey [NHANES III]) are recommended for use in North America. Equations are provided for Caucasians, African Americans, and Mexican Americans ranging in age from 8 to 80 years. No single reference source currently is recommended for use in Europe, but an international effort is under way to merge the NHANES data with those for many reference populations from throughout Europe and elsewhere, to generate a new, widely applicable reference dataset.

The use of a percentage of the predicted value as a lower limit is convenient but less accurate than the 5th percentile, because it causes the normal range to vary with the magnitude of the predicted value, whereas the true variance is similar around small and large values. A lower limit value equal to 80% of the predicted value has been widely used in spirometric interpretation. Although this is a reasonable approximation of the LLN for FEV_1 and FVC at the midrange of age and height, it creates an overly broad normal range for younger, taller persons (in whom the true LLN is approximately 82% to 83%), and it is overly sensitive for older or smaller subjects (in whom the LLN may be as low as 73% to 75%). An 80% lower limit is quite inappropriate for FEF_{25-75}, because the normal range extends to 65% of the predicted value in the young and below 50% of predicted in older persons. The normal value for FEV_1/FVC varies little with height but does decline progressively with age (e.g., from 0.87 at age 20 to 0.77 at age 70 in females, and from 0.84 to 0.74 in males). The LNN is approximately 0.10 below the predicted ratio. Because the ratio often is expressed as a percentage, reporting this value as a percent of the predicted value is potentially confusing.

INTERPRETATION OF SPIROMETRIC ABNORMALITIES

Obstructive Impairment

A decrease in airflow is the hallmark of the obstructive diseases; this physiologic diagnosis rests primarily on the demonstration of an FEV_1/FVC (or FEV_1/VC) value below the age-appropriate LLN. When the FEV_1/FVC value is low, even persons with an FEV_1 itself as high as 100% of the predicted value (and, necessarily, with a high-normal FVC) are considered to have mild airflow obstruction, which has been shown to be associated with increased morbidity over time. Typically, FVC is normal early in the course of airflow obstruction but is reduced in more severe disease as the RV is increased because of trapped air. The severity of obstructive impairment is best quantified by the decrement in FEV_1 as a percent of predicted, because progressive loss of FVC with advanced severity and air trapping limits the reduction in FEV_1/FVC. Varying recommendations for categories of severity have been made by different groups, although an apparent consensus suggests that an FEV_1 below 50% of the predicted value reflects a "severe" impairment. A simple schema that represents a compromise between one included in the ATS-ERS guidelines and that used in the Global Initiative for Chronic Obstructive Lung Disease (GOLD) guidelines is shown in **Table 9-1**.

Restrictive Impairment

A restrictive defect is defined by a reduction in TLC, but restriction in lung volume can be suspected from spirometry findings when the FVC is below the LLN and FEV_1 is similarly reduced, so that FEV_1/FVC is normal or high. In such cases, some persons will be found to have a normal TLC (see later under "Nonspecific Pattern"), but if the FVC is reduced below 60%, then the likelihood of true restriction is 80%. A decrement in FVC secondary to the increased RV of obstruction should not be classified as a restrictive defect, because TLC would then be normal to large. When both FVC and FEV_1/FVC are decreased, the presence and magnitude of any

Table 9-1	**Suggested Categories of Ventilatory Impairment** Based on FEV_1 expressed as a percent of the predicted value. Applicable to obstructive, restrictive, or mixed impairments after diagnosis of airflow obstruction by FEV_1/FVC and/or restriction by TLC.

Degree of Impairment	% Pred FEV_1
Mild	70-100%
Moderate	50-69%
Severe	30-49%
Very severe	<30%

concomitant restrictive impairment can be determined only by an assessment of TLC. Even when TLC is measured, the ATS-ERS guidelines recommend that the severity of a restrictive (or mixed) impairment be based on the reduction in FEV_1, because that correlates with exercise limitation and morbidity.

Mixed Impairment

The problem is clearly obstructive when the FEV_1/FVC ratio is low with a normal FVC, and restriction can be suspected when FEV_1/FVC is normal with a low FVC, with increased confidence when the FVC is more markedly reduced; however, other combinations leave uncertainty when only spirometry findings are available. A low ratio with a low FVC may reflect the air trapping of obstructive disease or a mixed pattern with both obstructive and restrictive components. When FEV_1/FVC is reduced to 0.55 (55%) or lower, a low FVC is most likely due to air trapping, because lung volume measurements show a normal TLC in more than 90% of cases. Conversely, when the ratio is only mildly reduced but the FVC is quite low, the likelihood of a mixed disorder is increased. When both FEV_1/FVC and FVC are low, and lung volume measurement is not available, it may be more helpful to note the overall "ventilatory impairment" indicated by the loss of FEV_1, than to try to separately assess the components.

LUNG VOLUMES

Spirometry can measure only those subdivisions of lung volume contained within the VC range (see Chapter 3, Figure 3-4). Measurement of TLC or FRC requires a method of measuring the gas that remains in the lungs at RV. Typically, the gas volume contained in the lungs at FRC is measured, with TLC and RV determined by adding or subtracting the appropriate increments from an accompanying spirogram. The methods used most widely to measure lung volumes include helium dilution, nitrogen washout, and body plethysmography. Also, TLC can be quite accurately determined from calculations based on planimetry of posteroanterior and lateral chest radiographs or from CT scans, using one of several geometric models.

MEASUREMENT BY HELIUM DILUTION

A spirometer is prepared that contains a known volume and concentration of an inert gas, typically 10% helium (**Figure 9-3**). While the subject breathes through a mouthpiece with nose clipped, a valve is turned at end-tidal exhalation to connect the airway to this closed system. As normal tidal breathing continues over the course of a few minutes, the gas in the

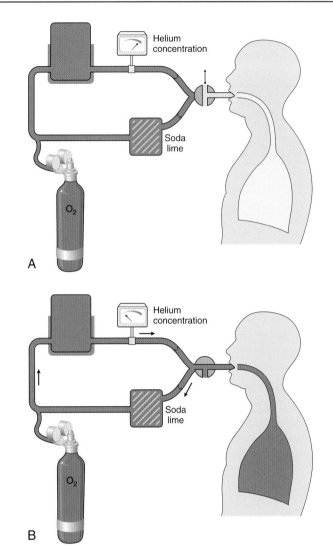

Figure 9-3 Lung volume measurement by helium dilution. **A,** The spirometer and circuit are prepared with a known gas volume and concentration of helium. **B,** The subject breathes through the circuit, as CO_2 is absorbed and O_2 consumption is replaced, until a new, lower helium concentration is established. The unknown lung volume added to the circuit when the valve was turned is calculated from the dilution of the initial helium concentration: $[He]_{initial} \times Vol_1 = [He]_{final} \times (Vol_1 + FRC)$.

subject's lung equilibrates with gas in the spirometer, and the helium concentration, which is continuously monitored, falls to a new, lower, steady-state level. Carbon dioxide is removed from the closed system by soda lime absorption, and a low flow of oxygen is added to compensate for the subject's ongoing oxygen consumption by keeping the mixing chamber or spirometer volume constant. The ratio of the initial to the final concentration of helium allows calculation of the unknown volume (FRC) added to the system. A continuous tracing of the spirogram, including a maximum inspiratory and expiratory effort, allows calculation of the subdivisions of lung volume, and correction for any offset from the relaxed FRC at the moment the valve was opened to start the test.

MEASUREMENT BY NITROGEN WASHOUT

The nitrogen washout technique also is based on the principle of conservation of mass of an inert gas—in this case, the nitrogen normally resident within the lungs. The subject breathes on a

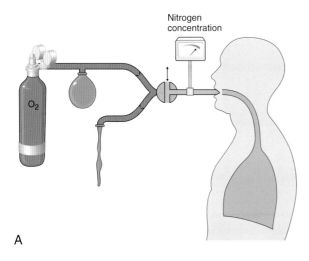

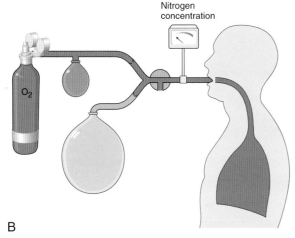

Figure 9-4 Lung volume measurement by nitrogen washout. **A,** Before the test, as the subject breathes air, the nitrogen concentration in the lungs is 80%, and the collection system is flushed free of nitrogen. **B,** The subject inhales 100% O_2 and exhales into the collection bag until the exhaled N_2 concentration approaches zero. The total volume of the bag and its final N_2 concentration are measured, and the unknown initial lung volume (including valve and mouthpiece dead space) is calculated: $[N_2]_{bag} \times Vol_{bag} = 0.80 \times FRC$.

mouthpiece that, at the end of a relaxed tidal exhalation, is connected to an inspiratory source of 100% oxygen (**Figure 9-4**), while the subsequent exhaled gas is directed by one-way valves into a collection bag, previously flushed with oxygen so that it contains no nitrogen. The resident nitrogen is washed out of the lungs progressively and monitored with continuous analysis at the mouthpiece. When the exhaled nitrogen concentration falls below 2%, the test is terminated, and the volume of nitrogen collected is measured. The FRC can be calculated on the basis that this nitrogen volume represents 80% of the lung gas contained at the beginning of the test. Instead of the collection bag, current microprocessors use a calculation based on instantaneous, breath-by-breath measurement of exhaled volume times nitrogen concentration. Washout can be completed in 3 to 4 minutes in normal subjects but may require longer than 15 minutes with severe obstructive airway disease, so that the gas volume in slowly exchanging spaces can be measured.

MEASUREMENT BY BODY PLETHYSMOGRAPHY

The volume of gas within the thorax, whether in communication with airways or not, can be measured by the technique of

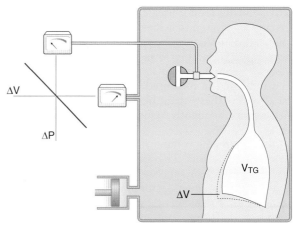

Figure 9-5 Lung volume measurement by body plethysmography. See text for description of the procedure. As the subject makes panting efforts against a closed airway shutter valve, the product of pressure and thoracic gas volume (V_{TG}) stays constant (Boyle's law). Thus, $P_B \times V_{TG} = (P_B - \Delta P) \times (V_{TG} + \Delta V)$. Solving for V_{TG} yields: $V_{TG} = P_B (\Delta V / \Delta P) - \Delta V$. Because ΔV is very small relative to V_{TG}, it is ignored, so $V_{TG} = P_B (\Delta V / \Delta P)$. ΔP is directly obtained from the airway pressure transducer, and ΔV is obtained from the pressure change in the plethysmograph, after calibration by cycling a known volume with a piston pump. V_{TG} is obtained from the slope of this relationship plotted during the panting maneuver.

body plethysmography, based on the physical principles of gas compression described by Boyle's law. The subject sits within a fully enclosed rigid box and breathes through a mouthpiece connected through a shutter to the internal volume of the box (**Figure 9-5**). Sensitive manometers monitor the pressure at the airway and inside the chamber. The apparatus is calibrated with the subject in place, so that the volume addition required within the chamber to raise the chamber pressure by 1 cm H_2O is known. At the end of a tidal exhalation, the airway shutter is closed, and the subject is asked to make panting efforts with the glottis open. An effort to expand the chest decompresses intrathoracic gas and reciprocally compresses that in the chamber; the opposite occurs during an expiratory effort.

Under conditions of constant temperature, which is well maintained by the high blood flow through the lungs, the product of airway pressure and lung gas volume is a constant. The slope of the relationship between the change in airway pressure and the change in thoracic volume, which can be calculated continuously or plotted on an oscilloscope, is inversely related to the intrathoracic volume. Because this technique is sensitive to gas volume not in free communication with the airways, such as that in bullae or even a pneumothorax, the measurement often is called "thoracic gas volume," which may exceed the FRC measured by gas dilution techniques. Advantages of this method, besides its inclusion of "trapped" gas, are that several measurements can be repeated rapidly, and that airway resistance can be measured with the same apparatus when panting is continued with the shutter open.

INTERPRETATION OF LUNG VOLUME ABNORMALITIES

Inspiration is limited at TLC when the maximum inspiratory force that can be applied by the chest muscles and diaphragm is opposed equally by the increasing recoil force of the lungs as they are distended to higher volumes. TLC is limited primarily by the elastic properties of the lungs, because variations in muscle strength have only a small effect on total chest expansion until weakness becomes quite marked. Parenchymal restrictive diseases reduce lung compliance, so greater distending pressure is required to achieve any volume change, and the maximum volume that can be achieved (TLC) is reduced. The displacement of intrathoracic gas volume by effusions, edema, intravascular volume, and inflammatory cells also can contribute to a reduction in measured lung gas volumes. Except for pleural effusions, these quantities are relatively small and outweighed by the frequently associated changes in lung elastic properties.

The minimum lung volume, or RV, is determined by a combination of two factors. The smallest volume to which the expiratory muscles can squeeze the chest wall and raise the diaphragm is the dominant factor in youth. By middle age, with the normal loss of tissue elastic recoil forces, the lung volume at which small airways close and trap remaining gas behind them increases and becomes the dominant factor in determining RV.

Restrictive Lung Diseases

Restrictive lung impairment is defined by a decrease in TLC below its lower limit of normal. In most parenchymal infiltrative processes, this is accompanied by parallel decrements in FRC, RV, and VC. The reduction in FRC reflects a shift in the balance of lung and chest wall recoil forces (see Chapter 3, Figure 3-7) and the reduction in RV occurs as increased tissue recoil delays airway closure. However, some patients with clear interstitial lung disease by radiologic evaluation or biopsy maintain lung volumes within the normal range. Obesity causes true restriction only when extreme but affects lung volumes in a pattern that differs from that of parenchymal lung diseases. The primary effect is on the relaxed end-expiratory volume or FRC, because the large abdomen and heavy chest wall reduce the outward recoil of the thoracic cage, which allows the inward recoil of the lung parenchyma to reduce FRC. RV is determined by airway closure, however, and is therefore less affected, and the TLC achievable using maximum inspiratory force is only minimally reduced until obesity becomes extreme (body mass index [BMI] greater than 40). Thus, the typical spirogram in even moderate obesity shows an end-expiratory volume (FRC) that approaches RV (i.e., the expiratory reserve volume is markedly reduced), but with a relatively large inspiratory capacity and a near-normal TLC and VC.

Obstructive Diseases

Airflow obstructive processes lead to airway closure that limits exhalation at higher lung volume because of the combined effects on luminal caliber of airway inflammation and loss of tissue recoil. These changes result in a progressive increase in RV (**Figure 9-6**), as increasing amounts of gas are trapped behind closed airways. Affected patients breathe at an increased FRC because of the combined effects of a decrease in lung recoil force from emphysema and the need to increase luminal caliber to minimize the resistive work of air flow. The TLC is normal to high, which again reflects the loss of lung recoil forces. Because RV increases to a greater extent than that seen in TLC, the VC decreases with severe airway obstruction.

Mixed Obstruction and Restriction

Obtaining lung volume measurement allows further characterization of the underlying problem in patients with both a low FEV_1/FVC and a low FVC. If the TLC is below the LLN, then they have restriction in addition to the obstructive abnormality, or a so-called mixed disorder. In such cases, the decrement in

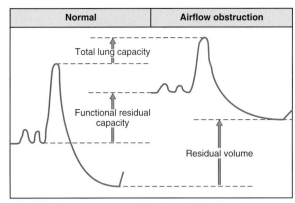

Figure 9-6   Severe airflow obstruction is associated with an increase in residual volume. Prolonged expiratory airflow may continue until the subsequent inhalation, and alveolar gas is trapped behind narrowed and closed airways. The functional residual capacity at which tidal breathing occurs also is increased, and total lung capacity may be high as well. (*Modified from Culver BH: Pulmonary function testing. In Kelly WN, editor: Textbook of internal medicine, Philadelphia, 1988, JB Lippincott.*)

FEV_1 will reflect the contributions of both conditions, so it should not be attributed entirely to obstruction. For example, a patient with an FEV_1/FVC ratio of 0.65, a TLC of 60% predicted, and an FEV_1 of 45% predicted certainly has a "severe ventilatory impairment" but probably does not have severe airflow obstruction. It has been recently suggested that the severity of the obstructive component can be more appropriately attributed if the % predicted FEV_1 is divided by the % predicted TLC. Separate quantification of the components often is difficult, however, and clinical estimation of the overall severity of the combined impairment may be more important, because this is what affects the patient.

Nonspecific Pattern

Some persons with reduction in both FVC and FEV_1 and with a normal ratio of FEV_1 to FVC will be found on lung volume testing to have a TLC within normal limits. Thus, they do not meet the definition for either obstruction or restriction, yet the low FEV_1 indicates some degree of impairment. The associated increase in RV may reflect early airway closure of uncertain cause. This so-called nonspecific pattern may be seen with obesity. Repeat studies over several years show that in most such cases, the same pattern is retained, with differentiation to either an obstructive or a restrictive pattern observed less frequently. The decrement in FEV_1 can be characterized as a mild ventilatory impairment of uncertain cause.

DIFFUSING CAPACITY

PRINCIPLES AND TECHNIQUE

The diffusing capacity (DL), also called transfer factor, is a measure of the capacity to transfer gas from alveolar spaces into the alveolar capillary blood. This process occurs by passive diffusion and is a function of the pressure difference that drives gas, the surface area over which exchange takes place, and the resistive properties to gas movement through the membrane and into chemical combination with the blood. The units are milliliters per minute per millimeter of mercury of driving pressure (mL/minute/mm Hg). (In SI units, 1 mole/minute/kPa = 2.896 mL/minute/mm Hg.) Carbon monoxide is used for the clinical test of diffusing capacity (DLCO), because its extreme avidity for hemoglobin allows the back pressure to diffusion to be considered negligible.

In the widely used single-breath method, the subject exhales to RV and then takes a VC inhalation of the test gas, which contains a low level of carbon monoxide (0.3%) and an inert gas not taken up in the blood (e.g., 10% helium). After breath-holding at full inspiration for 8 to 10 seconds, the subject exhales quickly. The initial portion of the expirate, which includes anatomic dead space, is discarded, and a sample of the subsequent alveolar gas is collected or measured by a rapidly responding sensor. The reduction in helium concentration in the alveolar sample allows calculation of the alveolar volume at TLC into which carbon monoxide was distributed, and of the initial carbon monoxide concentration after its dilution by the resident RV. The final concentration of carbon monoxide measured in the exhaled alveolar sample is applied in calculating the volume of carbon monoxide transferred out of alveoli and also allows a calculation, for which an exponential decline is assumed, of the mean carbon monoxide driving pressure during breath-holding. An effective residence time is calculated from the breath-hold period plus a portion of the time of inspiration and sample collection.

A significant problem with the diffusing capacity measurement is that numerous variations in the handling of small correction factors (for gas conditions, apparatus dead space, timing measurement, and so on) can cumulatively cause the calculated value to vary substantially among laboratories. Typically, two measurements are done and the results are averaged. Although reproducibility within a laboratory can be quite acceptable (±2.5 mL/minute/mm Hg), the accuracy of comparisons between laboratories or to reference data is much less consistent, as reflected by published predicted values that vary by 20% or more. It is essential that each laboratory choose prediction equations that are appropriate to the nuances of its equipment and technique.

INTERPRETATION OF DIFFUSION ABNORMALITIES

Although diffusion often is thought of as a function of alveolar membrane thickness, the dominant factor is usually the capillary blood volume, which influences both the surface area available for exchange and the volume of blood and hemoglobin available to accept carbon monoxide. The influence of hemoglobin concentration, [Hb], can be accounted for by theoretical or empirical correction factors. The velocity of blood flow is not important, because carbon monoxide is taken up even by stagnant blood (or extravasated blood in the case of pulmonary hemorrhage), but the recruitment of additional capillary segments during high flow conditions such as exercise or with congenital left-to-right shunt increases the measured diffusing capacity.

Many laboratories also report the diffusing capacity as a ratio of such capacity to the alveolar volume (DL/VA). This also is called the transfer coefficient (K_{CO}). The implication is that loss of lung volume secondary to mechanical abnormalities is accompanied by a parallel loss of diffusion capacity. This, however, is not the case with a voluntary limitation of inspiration, in which capillaries remain perfused and DL/VA rises, or with pneumonectomy, in which capillaries are recruited in the remaining lung and DL/VA is again high. Diffusing capacity is commonly reduced in parenchymal inflammatory diseases, primarily because of the loss of available capillaries. The most common pattern in diseases such as sarcoidosis and interstitial fibrosis is for DL to be reduced and DL/VA to be slightly low

or "normal," because volume also is lost. Both DL and DL/VA are low with the loss of capillary surface area and blood volume in emphysema and in diseases that are primarily vascular, such as vasculitis, recurrent emboli, and pulmonary hypertension. Clinical interpretation of diffusion abnormality should be based primarily on the DL, not on the DL/VA, with small correction factors available for [Hb] and the lower oxygen levels of altitude.

TESTS OF GAS DISTRIBUTION

Abnormalities of spirometry and airflow rate reflect overall narrowing of airways, but most lung diseases affect airways heterogeneously, which leads to abnormalities of gas distribution that may be more sensitive indicators of early airway disease.

CLOSING VOLUME

As lung volume decreases, the smaller, intraparenchymal airways decrease in caliber until they close at low lung volume and ventilation to or from alveoli beyond them ceases. Because there is a vertical gradient in the pleural pressure that surrounds the lungs, the lung tissue is less distended in dependent regions than at higher levels in the thorax. In late exhalation, dependent airways close (i.e., these areas reach their regional RV), whereas air continues to flow from the upper portions of the lung until they too close, and overall RV is reached. The beginning of this wave of ascending airway closure can be detected by physiologic tests and is termed *closing volume*. Closing volume usually is expressed as a percentage of VC. That is, a closing volume of 20% means that airway closure can be detected during a slow exhalation when 20% of the VC remains before RV is attained (**Figure 9-7**). Alternatively, when RV is measured, this can be added to closing volume, and the sum, termed *closing capacity*, is expressed as a percentage of TLC.

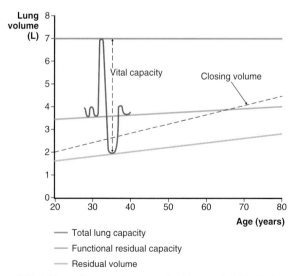

— Total lung capacity

— Functional residual capacity

— Residual volume

Figure 9-7 Effects of age on the normal spirogram. Residual volume progressively increases, with an associated small reduction in vital capacity. The functional residual capacity (FRC) increases slightly, but the closing volume, at which dependent airways cease to ventilate, increases more steeply and exceeds the normal FRC in older ages. *(Modified from Culver BH, Butler J: Alterations in pulmonary function. In Andres R, Bierman E, Hazzard W, editors:* Principles of geriatric medicine, *New York, 1985, McGraw-Hill.)*

Both of these measures have been used as tests of early airway dysfunction in the natural history of COPD. Abnormalities can be detected in a high percentage of smokers, but the prognostic usefulness is limited, because this group includes many who do not go on to develop progressive airflow limitation. On an individual patient basis, the closing volume is most helpful in its relationship to the lung volume at which tidal breathing occurs. When airway closure occurs at a volume below FRC, the airways are open throughout the lungs during tidal breathing, but when airway closure occurs above FRC, the affected alveoli are underventilated. Because the dependent regions are well perfused, premature airway closure creates a low ventilation-perfusion region, which contributes to hypoxemia. This abnormality occurs when the closing volume is increased by normal aging or COPD, and by the effect of peribronchial edema in left ventricular failure. Similar consequences are observed when FRC is reduced by recumbent posture or by obesity.

ARTERIAL BLOOD GAS MEASUREMENT

Measurement of pH, P_{CO_2}, and P_{O_2} in arterial blood is commonly included in the complete pulmonary function assessment of patients suspected to have significant lung disease. The pH and P_{CO_2} are directly measured, and the accompanying bicarbonate concentration is calculated from the Henderson-Hasselbalch equation. (The value of this "calculated" blood gas component must not be discounted; it is every bit as accurate as the pH and P_{CO_2} measurements from which it is derived.)

An increase in arterial P_{CO_2} means that alveolar ventilation is low relative to carbon dioxide production. This may be because total ventilation is low, the effective alveolar ventilation is reduced by excessive wasted ventilation, or the carbon dioxide production level has increased without a concomitant increase in ventilation. The matching of ventilation to metabolic need is a function of both mechanical capabilities and ventilatory drive. Most patients who suffer hypercapnia have severe mechanical impairments, but those who also have relatively low drive are more likely to retain carbon dioxide. Patients who have an FEV_1 greater than 1 L rarely retain carbon dioxide unless lack of drive is a major factor. Despite the airflow obstruction present during an acute asthmatic attack, multiple stimuli tend to increase drive and ventilation. However, when obstruction becomes extreme, again with an FEV_1 in the realm of 1 L or less for an adult, the development of acute hypercapnia is likely. Most parenchymal restrictive diseases tend to be associated with mild hyperventilation, presumably from mechanical stimuli to the respiratory centers, until the functional abnormalities become very severe.

The normal P_{CO_2} remains in a narrow range, around 40 mm Hg, throughout life, but the normal P_{O_2} diminishes progressively with age. This decline is more marked when P_{O_2} is measured with the subject in the supine position and in both cases reflects the progressive increase in closing volume with age (see Figure 9-7). Abnormal reductions in P_{O_2} are caused by hypoventilation, as reflected (but not caused) by an increase in P_{CO_2}, or result from the combined effects of pulmonary blood flow to poorly ventilated areas (low ventilation-perfusion ratio [$\dot{V}/\dot{Q}$]) and right-to-left shunting. Diffusion abnormalities, unless extremely severe, rarely contribute to a low P_{O_2} in patients at rest. The low P_{O_2} commonly seen in patients who have diffusion abnormalities reflects the concomitant presence of ventilation-perfusion abnormalities associated with their

disease. Diffusion limitation may make a small contribution to a reduction in P_{O_2} observed during exercise, but again, the major component is a worsened effect of the ventilation-perfusion abnormalities.

SPECIAL TESTING

UPPER AIRWAY OBSTRUCTION

Obstruction in the central airways (e.g., tracheal tumor or stenosis) affects the expiratory flow-volume relationship in a different way than does the more common peripheral airway obstruction of COPD. The latter has its predominant effect late in expiration, with slowing of terminal flow rates, so that peak flow tends to be relatively maintained while the remaining flow-volume curve becomes progressively convex toward the horizontal axis (**Figure 9-8**). Central obstructions have their primary effect early, which results in a truncated, flat-topped flow-volume curve (**Figure 9-9**), reflecting a steady effort against a constant resistance. In the latter portion of the expiration, the decreasing lung volume and airway caliber shift the site of major resistance to the more peripheral airways, so that the latter portion of the flow-volume curve is normal.

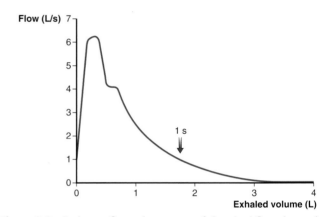

Figure 9-8 Expiratory flow-volume curve of chronic airflow obstruction. Airflow rates are markedly reduced at mid- to lower lung volumes, with a curve that is convex to the horizontal axis. In this example, just under 50% of the vital capacity has been exhaled in 1 second. (*Modified from Culver BH: Pulmonary function testing. In Kelly WN, editor:* Textbook of internal medicine, *Philadelphia, 1988, JB Lippincott.*)

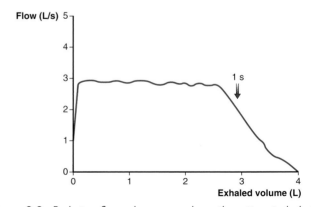

Figure 9-9 Expiratory flow-volume curve shows the pattern typical of central airway obstruction. Peak flow is markedly truncated, but the flow rates at low lung volume are unaffected. Despite the dramatic effect on the flow-volume curve, the ratio of FEV_1 to FVC is only modestly affected, with a value of 0.71 in this example. (*Modified from Culver BH: Pulmonary function testing. In Kelly WN, editor:* Textbook of internal medicine, *Philadelphia, 1988, JB Lippincott.*)

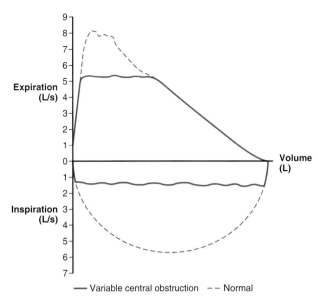

Figure 9-10 Flow-volume loop showing both forced expiratory and inspiratory airflows. The expiratory peak flow is somewhat truncated, consistent with a mild central obstruction during exhalation; inspiratory flow is markedly reduced from that for the normal curve. This pattern is typical of a flexible, extrathoracic obstruction, such as that secondary to paralysis of the vocal cords. *(Modified from Culver BH: Pulmonary function testing. In Kelly WN, editor:* Textbook of internal medicine, *Philadelphia, 1988, JB Lippincott.)*

When a central obstruction is in the extrathoracic airway and has some flexibility (e.g., vocal cord paralysis), its effect is much greater during inspiratory flow than expiratory flow. The negative intraluminal pressure generated during inspiration narrows the airway, which exacerbates the obstruction, whereas during expiration, the positive airway pressure below the site of obstruction tends to distend the airway, which reduces the abnormality. These lesions are assessed by recording on the flow-volume display the maximum effort inspiratory flow curve, as well as that during expiration, to complete a flow-volume "loop." The normal inspiratory flow pattern has a semicircular shape with peak inspiratory flow at midvolume that consistently exceeds midvolume expiratory flow (**Figure 9-10**).

BRONCHOPROVOCATION TESTING

Patients who have suspected reactive airway disease frequently demonstrate normal spirometry values when asymptomatic. When the diagnosis is unclear, provocation testing may be performed in an attempt to explain symptoms or predict future risks. A common clinical provocation of asthma is the airway mucosal cooling and drying effect of exercise hyperpnea or cold air inhalation. Provocation testing with *exercise* can utilize free running, treadmill running, or bicycle pedaling, with the relative yield of abnormal tests in that order. To provide a sufficient ventilatory stimulus, exercise level is increased over 2 to 3 minutes to 70% to 90% of maximal capability, as estimated from heart rate, and then sustained for an additional 4 to 6 minutes. Spirometric testing is done before exercise and repeated after exercise, with the most marked decrease in flow rates noted at 5 to 10 minutes after exercise. A reduction in FEV_1 of 10% is considered significant, because normal subjects typically show a small increase shortly after exercise. *Cold air challenge*, in which spirometric testing is done before and after isocapneic hyperventilation of air that has been dehumidified

and cooled to 4° C, is less widely available as a provocation maneuver.

Methacholine responsiveness is a nonspecific indicator of airway reactivity. Starting with a single inhalation at a very low concentration, patients are tested after progressively increasing inhaled doses until either a predetermined maximum dose has been achieved or the FEV_1 has been observed to fall by 20%. Normal subjects do not respond to the maximum dose, whereas patients with asthma usually respond to very low to intermediate doses. A negative response at the maximum dose in a patient suspected to have asthma and recently symptomatic makes that diagnosis very unlikely, but positive responses are less specific. Persons who have a family history of asthma or hay fever symptoms may show intermediate responses, as may patients with COPD or cystic fibrosis, as well as some normal persons in the recovery period after viral respiratory infections.

Whereas methacholine directly stimulates smooth muscle contraction, indirect stimuli such as exercise or the recently developed mannitol challenge test act through changes in mucosal osmolarity and release of endogenous mediators. These stimuli are more specific for asthma and more responsive to variations in airway inflammation, but they tend to be less sensitive than methacholine challenge.

In selected circumstances, provocation testing may be carried out with suspected specific allergens or occupational exposures. Dose preparation needs to be very careful, to avoid an excessive and dangerous response. Studies may be designed to mimic the circumstances of the patient's clinical or occupational exposure. Testing may need to be continued for several hours to identify a late-phase reaction.

SUGGESTED READINGS

American Thoracic Society–European Respiratory Society Task Force Guidelines for Lung Function Testing
Brusasco V, Crapo R, Viegi G, series editors: ATS/ERS task force: standardisation of lung function testing, *Eur Respir J* 26, 2005.

MacIntyre N, Crapo RO, Viegi G, et al: Standardisation of the single-breath determination of carbon monoxide uptake in the lung, *Eur Respir J* 26:720–735, 2005.

Miller MR, Crapo R, Hankinson J, et al: General considerations for lung function testing, *Eur Respir J* 26:153–161, 2005.

Miller MR, Hankinson J, Brusasco F, et al: Standardisation of spirometry, *Eur Respir J* 26:319–338, 2005.

Pellegrino R, Viegi G, Brusasco F, et al: Interpretative strategies for lung function tests, *Eur Respir J* 26:948–968, 2005.

Wanger J, Clausen JL, Coates A, et al: Standardisation of the measurement of lung volumes, *Eur Respir J* 26:511–522, 2005.

General
American Thoracic Society: Guidelines for methacholine and exercise challenge testing—1999, *Am J Resp Crit Care Med* 161:309–329, 2001.

Anderson SD: Indirect challenge tests: airway hyperresponsiveness in asthma: its measurement and clinical significance, *Chest* 138:25S–30S, 2010.

Crapo RO, Jensen RL, Wanger JS: Single-breath carbon monoxide diffusing capacity, *Clin Chest Med* 22:637–649, 2001.

Ferguson GT, Enright PL, Buist AS, Higgins MW: Office spirometry for lung health assessment in adults, *Chest* 117:1146–1161, 2000.

Gardner ZS, Ruppel GL, Kaminsky DA: Grading the severity of obstruction in mixed obstructive-restrictive lung disease, *Chest* 140:598–603, 2011.

Hankinson JL, Odencratz JR, Fedan KB: Spirometric reference values from a sample of the general US population, *Am J Resp Crit Care Med* 159:179–187, 1999.

Hayes D Jr, Kraman SS: The physiologic basis of spirometry, *Respir Care* 54:1717–1726, 2009.

Hughes JMB, Pride NB: *Lung function tests: physiologic principles and clinical applications*, London, 1999, WB Saunders.

Iyer VN, Schroeder DR, Parker KO, et al: The "non-specific" pulmonary function test: longitudinal follow up and outcomes, *Chest* 2010.

Jones RL, Nzekwu MM: The effects of body mass index on lung volumes, *Chest* 130:827–833, 2006.

Stanojevic S, Wade A, Stocks J, et al: Reference ranges for spirometry across all ages, *Am J Respir Crit Care Med* 177:253–260, 2008.

Vandevoorde J, Verbanck S, Schuermans D, et al: Forced vital capacity and forced expiratory volume in six seconds as predictors of reduced total lung capacity, *Eur Respir J* 31:391–395, 2008.

Chapter **10**
Exercise Testing

Josep Roca • Felip Burgos

Clinical exercise testing is widely accepted as an important component of the clinical assessment of patients with chronic respiratory illness, because impaired exercise capacity in these patients shows significant associations with health-related quality of life and with relevant clinical outcomes such as hospitalization rates and survival.

Impaired exercise capacity can be defined by the inability of the subject to sustain a required work rate long enough for the successful completion of a given task that could be achieved by a healthy person. Limitation of oxygen transport from the atmosphere to the cell is the most common cause of exercise limitation in chronic respiratory disease, but altered oxygen utilization due to abnormally low mitochondrial oxidative potential also can be a contributing factor in patients with advanced disease (**Figure 10-1**).

Clinical manifestations of limited exercise capacity are breathlessness, perception of limb fatigue, or even, in some conditions, frank pain. Abnormally low exercise capacity is the hallmark of a range of cardiovascular, respiratory, and other systemic diseases, of which congestive heart failure and chronic obstructive pulmonary disease (COPD) are the most prominent. However, the causes of a reduced exercise capacity are many, ranging from physical unfitness and obesity to muscle and neurologic diseases, anemia, and locomotor disorders.

Several studies have shown that the functional reserve (i.e., aerobic capacity) of patients with COPD and interstitial lung disease is not accurately predicted from resting lung function indices. In this scenario, cardiopulmonary exercise testing (CPET) constitutes a proper tool to assess both magnitude and mechanisms of impaired exercise capacity. CPET also can provide indices of the functional reserve of the different systems (pulmonary, cardiovascular, skeletal muscle) involved in the exercise response, with implications for factors contributing to the limitation of oxygen uptake at peak exercise. Moreover, CPET also is useful for establishing the profiles and adequacy of the system responses at submaximal exercise.

The chapter describes the laboratory exercise protocols more commonly used for clinical purposes, but it also covers simple exercise tests of increasing clinical usefulness that are extensively used outside the laboratory with well-defined purposes.

CLINICAL INDICATIONS FOR EXERCISE TESTING

The various clinical indications for CPET can be divided into three principal groups: assessment of functional reserve (aerobic capacity), identification of predominant factors limiting exercise capacity, and, last but not least, diagnostic purposes. Of note, adequate identification of the clinical problem requiring exercise testing should be considered a necessary prelude to CPET, as should an appropriate preassessment of the patient by (1) medical history, (2) physical examination, (3) chest radiograph, (4) resting pulmonary function testing, and (5) electrocardiogram (ECG). The clinical problem that prompts CPET and the specific aims of such testing (e.g., assessment of aerobic capacity, analysis of pulmonary gas exchange during exercise) determine both the type of exercise protocol to be used and the variables to be considered in the interpretation of the findings.

Assessment of aerobic capacity and identification of potential limiting factors constitute the most important indications for CPET. These goals are particularly important in evaluating dyspnea but also for assessing the degree of functional impairment in patients with chronic diseases. Appropriate use of CPET allows the investigator (1) to quantify the degree of functional limitation and to discriminate among causes of impairment of exercise capacity, (2) to differentiate between dyspnea of cardiac or pulmonary origin when respiratory and cardiac diseases coexist, and (3) to analyze unexplained dyspnea when initial pulmonary function testing does not provide conclusive results. CPET also is useful to assess the effects of pharmacologic interventions.

An important area for CPET is preoperative assessment in certain conditions—for example, for planned major abdominal surgery in elderly patients. Also, CPET is indicated before lung cancer resection and lung volume reduction surgery, either to confirm the patient's fitness to survive the procedure, if this is in question, or to ensure that postoperative respiratory function will be adequate. Information on predicted postoperative lung function can help to modulate the amount of lung parenchyma to be removed and determines the type of perioperative strategy needed to prevent complications. Pulmonary function tests performed in the resting state are considered adequate to evaluate low-risk patients (FEV_1 greater than 2 L and D_{LCO} within the reference limits), but CPET plays a pivotal role in the evaluation of patients at high risk.

CPET should always play a central role in assessing candidates for a rehabilitation program and in the subsequent modulation of the exercise prescription.

Assessment of impairment-disability also constitutes a major indication for CPET. It is now well accepted that CPET provides different and relevant information, compared with resting cardiopulmonary measurements, in impairment-disability evaluation and therefore constitutes a key tool in this area.

Finally, CPET plays a role in the diagnosis of a range of disease conditions, namely: exercise-induced asthma, cardiac ischemia, foramen ovale patency with development of right-to-left shunt during exercise, and McArdle syndrome.

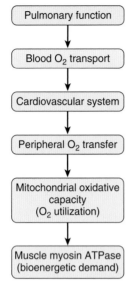

Figure 10-1   Major elements of the O_2 transport–O_2 utilization pathway. Integrated effects of all steps involved to move oxygen from air to mitochondria are essential to determine maximum capacity of the system. In disease, nonuniformity of ventilation-perfusion ratios in the lung, altered response of the cardiovascular system to exercise, and/or mismatching of metabolism-perfusion ratios in the peripheral tissues may be of considerable importance in determining cell oxygenation. Moreover, in patients with advanced chronic obstructive pulmonary disease (COPD), impaired oxygen utilization due to altered mitochondrial oxidative capacity has been demonstrated.

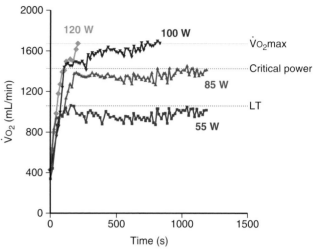

Figure 10-2   Response of oxygen uptake to four different constant-work-rate exercise tests carried out using a cycle ergometer in a healthy subject. From moderate to heavy exercise: *Green*, 55 watts, corresponding to a work rate moderately above the lactate threshold (LT), approximately 58% of $\dot{V}O_2$max, indicates the transition from moderate to intense exercise; *dark blue*, 85 watts, indicates the critical power (approximately 88% $\dot{V}O_2$max) corresponding to the highest level of sustainable exercise; *red*, 100 watts, indicates nonsustainable exercise above the critical power; and *light blue*, 120 watts, supramaximal nonsustainable exercise intensity. Of note, the two last exercise intensities, 100 and 120 watts, generate identical oxygen uptake that, by definition, corresponds to maximal O_2 uptake, $\dot{V}O_2$max.

EXERCISE INTENSITY AND ENERGY REQUIREMENTS

Availability of oxygen to all body tissues and cells is essential for survival. During steady-state conditions, oxygen consumption ($\dot{V}O_2$) matches the turnover of adenosine triphosphate (ATP), the high-energy phosphate needed to fulfill the bioenergetic requirements of the cells. ATP is efficiently generated by oxidative phosphorylation into the mitochondria. Within the inner mitochondrial matrix, pyruvate is converted to acetyl coenzyme A (CoA) and metabolized aerobically by way of the tricarboxylic acid cycle to yield water and carbon dioxide (CO_2) as residual products to be subsequently eliminated.

Alternative pathways of energy production not requiring oxygen constitute rapid but only transient solutions to fulfill the bioenergetic requirements. That is, anaerobic reduction of pyruvate to lactic acid in the cytosol is inefficient in terms of ATP production. Moreover, increased lactate levels provoke a marked fall in intracellular pH that may alter mitochondrial function. Likewise, skeletal muscle contains high levels of phosphocreatine (PCr) compared to other tissues, but the breakdown of muscle PCr stores can supply cellular needs of ATP for only a few seconds of strenuous contractions. Compared with glycolysis, aerobic metabolism requires longer to become activated. Energy utilization during exercise may require higher ATP turnover than the synthesis from aerobic pathways in the muscles allows. This phenomenon causes an "oxygen debt" that must be repaid after exercise. Aerobic metabolism, in turn, is more efficient in terms of ATP production and it enables the cell to utilize stored lipid as fuel via fatty acid metabolism. Consequently, the integrity of the different pathways governing cellular O_2 transport–O_2 utilization is a pivotal determinant of exercise capacity in both health and disease (see Figure 10-1).

In the progression from mild to high-intensity exercise, four conceptual steps that are important to a proper understanding of exercise testing can be identified:

Lactate threshold (LT), or anaerobic threshold, is the threshold $\dot{V}O_2$ for arterial lactate concentration increase. The LT should be considered to partition moderate from heavy-intensity exercise, and it corresponds to a transitional exercise intensity that triggers a series of physiologic responses associated with increased lactate production that stress ventilation, pulmonary gas exchange, and acid-base regulation. Of note, the LT is highly task-specific. It occurs at an appreciably lower $\dot{V}O_2$ for arm exercise than for leg exercise and typically is lower for cycle ergometry than for treadmill exercise, reflecting the magnitude of muscle mass over which the work is distributed. A wide range of techniques have been advocated for estimation of LT, including both direct measurements and indirect estimation, as described next.

Critical power is the highest sustainable level of $\dot{V}O_2$ and usually is at an intensity below the maximal $\dot{V}O_2$ for an individual subject and at an intensity of exercise that can still generate a plateau in $\dot{V}O_2$ (**Figure 10-2**). Heavier exercise intensities, well beyond LT, are not sustainable and may peak at $\dot{V}O_2$max (see Figure 10-2). During moderate intensity submaximal exercise, the components of the O_2 transport pathway can provide adequate O_2 flux between the air and the mitochondria. Mitochondrial oxidative capacity will not have been reached, symptoms usually are tolerable, and muscle fatigue has not occurred, or at least may be insufficient to impair performance appreciably. Although the concept of critical power is relevant for understanding the exercise response, it is not assessed in clinical exercise testing, because no normal ranges for submaximal exercise comparable between laboratories or diseases have been established.

Maximal exercise ($\dot{V}O_2$max) corresponds to maximal aerobic capacity, as displayed in Figure 10-2. At this point, maximal oxygen transport capacity and/or maximal mitochondrial oxidative potential have been reached. The subject cannot increase $\dot{V}O_2$ when work rate is increased or the highest tolerated work rate is sustained for a period of time. Often, $\dot{V}O_2$max can only be clearly identified in fit subjects that can sustain high levels of exercise for a few minutes. Extreme motivation is needed to reach true $\dot{V}O_2$max, and it is, in general, an unsuitable and unsafe test for patient populations.

Peak exercise ($\dot{V}O_2$peak) occurs when maximal work rate has been limited by severe symptoms at a level that does not require maximal O_2 transport or maximal oxidative capacity. Under these conditions, a plateau in O_2 ($\dot{V}O_2$max) has not been reached, and the appropriate designation is *peak* rather than *maximal* $\dot{V}O_2$. Symptom-limited exercise testing is common in the clinical setting, and this approach does not preclude adequate interpretation of the test results.

Because the catabolic capacity of the myosin ATPase is such that it outstrips by far the capacity of the respiratory system to deliver energy aerobically, exercise tolerance ($\dot{V}O_2$max) is determined by the capacity of the O_2 transport–O_2 utilization system, rather than by the muscle's contractile machinery (see Figure 10-1).

Two physiologic muscle properties—muscle strength and muscle fatigability—may modulate functional performance of the patient in daily life activities as well as during clinical exercise testing. *Muscle strength* is defined as the force generated by a muscle. It is determined by the number and type of motor units recruited. *Muscle fatigue* has been defined as a loss of contractile functions (force, velocity, power, or work) that is caused by prolonged exercise and is reversible by rest. Factors involved in muscle fatigue are complex, consisting mainly of contractile machinery, muscle respiratory capacity, and redox status of the muscle.

RESPONSES TO EXERCISE IN HEALTH AND DISEASE

As the patient with lung disease exercises harder, O_2 consumption, CO_2 production, ventilation, and cardiac output all increase to fulfill increased muscle bioenergetic requirements, as they do in the normal subject, but submaximal exercise response is abnormal and peak levels attained are lower, and increasingly so with increasing severity of the disease.

PULMONARY RESPONSE TO EXERCISE IN HEALTHY HUMANS

Ventilation and cardiac output markedly increase during exercise to match O_2 transport with augmented cellular O_2 requirements. Because ventilation increases to a relatively higher extent than pulmonary blood flow, the ratio of total alveolar ventilation to blood flow (overall $\dot{V}A/\dot{Q}$ ratio) rises rather substantially. At moderate levels of exercise, the dispersion of the $\dot{V}A/\dot{Q}$ distributions does not change, but the $\dot{V}A/\dot{Q}$ ratios as the mean of both ventilation and perfusion distributions increase markedly owing to the higher overall $\dot{V}A/\dot{Q}$ ratio. Consequently, the efficiency of the lung as an O_2 and CO_2 exchanger improves at these exercise levels. Mixed venous PO_2 falls dramatically during exercise because the relative increase in $\dot{V}O_2$ is considerably greater than that of cardiac output, and

mixed venous PCO_2 levels rise equally remarkably. Arterial PO_2 levels generally remain unchanged until extremely high levels of exercise are undertaken. Arterial PCO_2 levels also are relatively stable until the appearance of high blood lactate levels generates acidosis with even more ventilation and a corresponding fall in PCO_2 levels. The alveolar-arterial O_2 gradient, $PO_2(A-a)$, progressively increases with the level of exercise, reaching values of 20 mm Hg close to maximal exercise ($\dot{V}O_2$ peak) in average subjects and even greater—up to 40 mm Hg or more—in some elite athletes. Such an increase in $PO_2(A-a)$ indicates inefficiency of pulmonary gas exchange during heavy exercise that is even more apparent in other animal species. It has been shown that the increase in the $PO_2(A-a)$ during exercise is due in part to ventilation-perfusion mismatching, but it is mostly explained by alveolar–end-capillary O_2 diffusion limitation. Experimental studies suggest that development of subclinical pulmonary edema may explain the deterioration of pulmonary gas exchange during heavy exercise in elite athletes.

PULMONARY RESPONSE TO EXERCISE IN LUNG DISEASE

In patients with COPD, resting levels of minute ventilation ($\dot{V}E$) are abnormally high but, during exercise, the slope between $\dot{V}E$ and work rate is normal. For a given level of $\dot{V}E$ during exercise, tidal volume (VT) tends to be lower and respiratory rate (f) higher in patients than in healthy subjects. Moreover, the O_2 cost of breathing per unit ventilation is higher in persons with COPD than in healthy subjects. Impaired respiratory mechanics requires more effort to move a given volume of air. Peak exercise VT is strongly related to vital capacity in these patients, in whom two strategies are adopted during exercise to increase $\dot{V}E$: First, end-expiratory lung volume (EELV) increases, allowing higher maximum expiratory flow rates. This dynamic hyperinflation does not occur in normal persons, who show a fall in EELV during exercise (**Figure 10-3**).

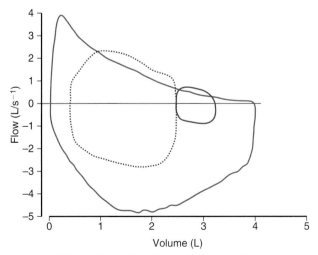

Figure 10-3 The resting maximal flow-volume curve from a patient with chronic obstructive pulmonary disease is represented by the *blue solid line*. The *solid smallest green loop* corresponds to tidal volume at rest, and the *dashed red curve* indicates tidal volume at maximal exercise. During exercise, end-inspiratory and end-expiratory lung volumes are increased (dynamic hyperinflation), and expiratory flow limitation is seen over most of expiration.   *(From Roca J, Rabinovich R: Clinical exercise testing. In Gosselink R, Stam H, editors: Lung function testing, Eur Resp Mon 31:146-165, 2005.)*

Second, inspiratory flow rate increases, so that inspiratory time decreases and more time is available for expiration.

Impaired respiratory mechanics (i.e., dynamic hyperinflation) seems to play a major role limiting exercise tolerance in these patients. During exercise in COPD, a balance is struck between the need for ventilation and the high cost of the work of breathing. The most common end result is a small rise in arterial PCO_2 and similar fall in PaO_2. However, unless pulmonary CO transfer capacity ($DLCO$) is severely impaired (less than 50% predicted value), PaO_2 does not fall during exercise, and may even increase in some subjects. Studies using the multiple inert gas elimination technique in COPD show that ventilation-perfusion mismatch usually is unchanged from that at rest, that shunts do not develop, and that diffusion limitation also does not occur. This is the case even when COPD is severe. In milder disease, there is evidence that small improvements in $\dot{V}A/\dot{Q}$ relationships may occur on exercise, providing a partial reason for improvement in arterial PO_2. It is not infrequently observed, however, that when the patient with COPD is encouraged to maximal effort, sudden hypoxemia and hypercapnia can develop just before the patient quits exercising.

In a variety of chronic respiratory disorders such as interstitial lung disease (ILD) and pulmonary vascular disease (PVD), abnormally high resting levels of $\dot{V}E$ and normal slope between $\dot{V}E$ and work rate during exercise are commonly observed but not dynamic hyperinflation, as seen in patients with COPD. In these patients, end-expiratory lung volume does not change significantly during exercise. Oxygen cost of breathing per unit ventilation is increased in patients with ILD because the increased elastic recoil requires more inspiratory muscle activity. They show a strong linear relationship between peak exercise VT and vital capacity, suggesting that differences in peak VT are due mainly to abnormal respiratory mechanics. During exercise, patients with ILD generally show typical and substantial blood gas changes, even at moderate effort. Although arterial PCO_2 generally is unaffected, PaO_2 falls in almost all patients, sometimes severely, as does mixed venous PO_2. It is this profound degree of arterial hypoxemia (and not respiratory mechanics) that mostly limits exercise tolerance in ILD. Worsening of ventilation-perfusion mismatching and shunt does not play a relevant role in exercise-induced hypoxemia seen in these patients. Therefore, the blood gas changes on exercise are mostly the consequence of (1) insufficient increase of alveolar ventilation relative to the rise in $\dot{V}O_2$ and $\dot{V}CO_2$ and (2) secondary effects from the fall in mixed venous PO_2 causing a fall in arterial PO_2. Also, O_2 diffusion limitation is seen in most patients with ILD during exercise, further adding to the hypoxemia. The presence of O_2 diffusion limitation in these patients, despite the relatively low cardiac output at peak exercise (less than 10 L/min) probably is related to the combination of (1) an abnormally low mixed venous PO_2, (2) a short capillary transit time, and (3) some increased interstitial resistance for the diffusion of O_2 from the alveolar gas to the capillary blood caused by the large collagen deposits there.

Exercise-induced hypoxemia in patients with ILD is found to be due largely to the fall in venous PO_2, because there is no systematic change in $\dot{V}A/\dot{Q}$ relationships, nor does diffusion limitation develop.

HEMODYNAMIC RESPONSES TO EXERCISE IN HEALTH AND DISEASE

In healthy subjects, cardiac output ($\dot{Q}T$) shows a linear increase in relation to O_2 uptake during exercise. Likewise, both stroke volume and heart rate also increase as $\dot{V}O_2$ rises. In well-trained subjects, up to a five-fold increase (approximately 25 L/min) in $\dot{Q}T$ at peak exercise can be seen. Systolic pulmonary pressure increases during exercise, but pulmonary vascular resistance falls because of vascular recruitment of underperfused areas of the pulmonary vascular bed. At systemic levels, systolic pressure increases, but not diastolic pressure. It is of note, however, that elite athletes at peak exercise show a potent sympathetic vasoconstriction at systemic level inducing massive redistribution of cardiac output, which ensures preferential perfusion to active skeletal muscle (due to local exercise-induced vasodilator effects) while preserving blood flow and O_2 delivery to essential organs such as the brain. During high-intensity exercise in COPD, restriction of intercostal muscle perfusion with preservation of quadriceps blood flow, along with attainment of a plateau in cardiac output, indicates the inability of the cardiovascular system to satisfy the energy demands of both the locomotor and respiratory muscles. In affected patients, the increase in thoracic and abdominal pressures due to dynamic hyperinflation and activity of abdominal expiratory muscles seems to preclude adequate increase in cardiac output during intense exercise.

In chronic respiratory diseases, pulmonary vascular abnormalities are present well before overt heart failure occurs. There is pulmonary hypertension often even evident at rest, and usually during exercise. The increase in pressure per unit increase in cardiac output is some three times greater in these patients than in the normal subjects.

In contrast with normal subjects, in whom pulmonary vascular resistance normally falls during exercise owing to a combination of vascular recruitment and distention in the lungs, in those with COPD, vascular resistance remains constant or may even rise. The vascular destruction or obstruction that occurs in these diseases, together with some vascular distortion and hypoxic vasoconstriction, are the reasons underlying these physiologic abnormalities. Eventually, as the diseases progress, the right heart will hypertrophy and ultimately fail, and clinically significant cor pulmonale will develop. Despite the two- to three-fold increase in vascular resistance and high pulmonary artery pressures, it is remarkable that even in advanced lung disease, the heart can pump essentially normally as a function of filling pressure.

At peak exercise, systemic O_2 delivery is clearly below normal predicted levels. Although the obvious culprit is impaired pulmonary function, it is not always through a reduction in SaO_2 that systemic O_2 delivery is reduced, because despite $\dot{V}A/\dot{Q}$ inequality and reduced effective alveolar ventilation, hypoxemia may not necessarily provoke a marked fall in arterial O_2 content. It is accepted that cardiac output at peak exercise is always well below normal levels. However, in COPD as in the absence of disease, cardiac output increases linearly in relation to oxygen uptake, because work rate increases during incremental exercise such that cardiac output at a given submaximal O_2 uptake is close to the expected normal value. Of note, however, the rise in cardiac output during exercise usually is achieved through a higher heart rate and lower stroke volume than in healthy subjects.

Because total ventilation, cardiac output, and exercise intensity remain closely coupled in COPD as in health, the inability to increase ventilation appears to be the principal governor of the O_2 transport process: A low ceiling on ventilation means a low ceiling on cardiac output and thus on systemic O_2 delivery. However, the mechanisms that couple ventilation to cardiac output during exercise are still not well understood. It has been proposed that the large pleural pressure swings observed during exercise can be paramount in constraint of left ventricular function, thus limiting both peak cardiac output and exercise tolerance in severe COPD. It also is accepted that abdominal expiratory muscles can play a role in limiting increases of cardiac output during exercise, as indicated previously. The coupling between whole-body O_2 uptake and cardiac output during exercise implies that the O_2 difference between arterial and mixed venous blood and the fractional O_2 extraction are normal or near normal. The cardiac response to exercise in patients with ILD is similar to the description for persons with COPD. By contrast, patients with PVD show a different cardiac response to exercise. Certainly, at peak exercise, cardiac output is lower. More important, however, the slope of the relationship between $\dot{V}O_2$ and cardiac output appears different. This observation suggests that for any given degree of exercise (i.e., $\dot{V}O_2$), cardiac output in patients with PVD does not increase as much as in control subjects or patients with COPD or ILD. This abnormal behavior is likely to be related to the increased afterload of the right ventricle. As expected, patients with PVD have, at rest, pulmonary artery hypertension and increased pulmonary vascular resistance. Compared with patients with COPD and ILD, patients with PVD show much worse hemodynamic responses. During exercise, pulmonary artery pressure increases in direct proportion to the increase in cardiac output and reaches extremely high values. This effect highlights the lack of pulmonary vascular reserve. In fact, the pathologically elevated pulmonary vascular resistance seen at rest does not change substantially during exercise.

MUSCLE O_2 UTILIZATION IN HEALTH AND DISEASE

It has been reported that well-trained men show O_2 supply dependency of maximum O_2 uptake, indicating that mitochondrial capacity does not constitute the rate-limiting factor for maximum exercise performance. By contrast, data from healthy sedentary subjects strongly suggest that muscle mitochondrial function is a limiting step for maximum O_2 uptake in sedentary persons. A recent study including direct measurements of cell PO_2 saturation during exercise with different levels of FIO_2 further indicates that sedentary subjects do not show O_2 supply dependency of $\dot{V}O_2max$. The plasticity of skeletal muscles during high-intensity physical training programs fully accounts for the differences alluded to between athletes and sedentary subjects. The scenario is far more complex in patients with COPD. Femoral blood flow ($\dot{Q}leg$) measurements in patients with moderate to severe airflow limitation have shown, as for cardiac output, a marked reduction in peak $\dot{Q}leg$. However, leg blood flow (and leg O_2 delivery) at a given submaximal whole-body O_2 uptake is above normal, which may indicate increased peripheral muscle O_2 demand. Moreover, poor muscle capillary networks in these patients seem to suggest that low peripheral O_2 diffusion capacity also may contribute to exercise-induced cell hypoxia, even in the absence of arterial hypoxemia. Increased lactate production is responsible for the fall in muscle pH, which in turn may play a role determining exercise intolerance in these patients. Premature lactic acidosis during exercise in COPD has been associated with reduced oxidative enzyme concentrations in the lower limb muscles that can be at least partly reversed by physical training.

Several studies exercising different muscle groups in heterogeneous groups of patients with COPD have consistently shown lower cellular bioenergetic status (^{31}P-nuclear magnetic resonance spectroscopy) and lower pH than in healthy sedentary

control subjects at equivalent levels of exercise. Some evidence suggests that muscle deconditioning plays an underlying role in the disturbances of skeletal muscle bioenergetics in COPD. Recent evidence indicates that intrinsic skeletal muscle dysfunction may be present in COPD, as well as in other chronic disorders such as congestive heart failure. Abnormal redox status plays a central role in precipitating muscle mass wasting, particularly in susceptible subsets of patients with COPD.

It is accepted that the level of exercise tolerance is set by the integrity of each of the functions involved in the O_2 transport–O_2 utilization system, as well as by proper interactions among all of the aforementioned physiologic responses. Complex integrative pathways both at whole body level and at cellular level have been identified. Because not only intracellular pH but also cell PO_2 has been shown to modulate mitochondrial function, O_2 transport (cell PO_2) and O_2 utilization (mitochondrial capacity) cannot be analyzed as separate systems.

Also of major interest are the events surrounding peak or maximal $\dot{V}O_2$ and the physiologic basis of why peak or maximal $\dot{V}O_2$ is reduced, as it almost always is in disease. Of note in this regard, the amount of $\dot{V}O_2$ achieved by a given patient not only is set by the intrinsic characteristics of the system but also depends on several other factors that modulate the physiologic response of the whole body, such as (1) environmental conditions (e.g., altitude above sea level, FIO_2); (2) amount of exercising muscle mass (e.g., with cycling, walking, or localized quadriceps exercise); and (3) type of exercise protocol (e.g., incremental, endurance test, 6-minute walking test, shuttle test).

CLINICAL EXERCISE PROTOCOLS

The goal of CPET protocols is to stress the organ systems involved in the exercise response in a controlled manner. For this reason, the testing generally involves exercising large muscle groups, usually the lower extremity muscles. A key requirement is that the exercise stimulus must be quantifiable in terms of external work and power performed. Clinical exercise protocols are grouped into those carried out in the laboratory and simple exercise testing. As indicated earlier, the first step is proper identification of the clinical question to be answered through CPET, such that the appropriate protocol and corresponding measurements can be properly chosen.

INCREMENTAL EXERCISE IN THE LABORATORY

The appropriateness of the integrated systemic responses is best studied using incremental exercise testing either as a ramp function or as small work-rate increments of short duration. This approach provides a smooth incremental stress to the subjects, so that the entire range of exercise intensities can be spanned in a short period of time.

CPET has been classically built around the rapid ramp-incremental exercise test (performed on a cycle ergometer or motorized treadmill), breath-by-breath monitoring of cardiopulmonary variables (e.g., O_2 uptake, CO_2 output, ventilation, heart rate), and formulation of graphical clusters of response profiles that optimize estimation of key parameters such as $\dot{V}O_2$ peak and the lactate threshold and the characterization of pertinent response profiles (e.g., heart rate–$\dot{V}O_2$, oxygen pulse–$\dot{V}O_2$, $\dot{V}E$-$\dot{V}CO_2$). This approach provides a convenient way of (1) determining whether the magnitude and pattern of response of particular variables is normal with respect to other variables or to work rate, (2) establishing a subject's limiting or maximum attainable value for physiologic variables of interest, and (3) establishing exercise intensity domains, such as the transition between moderate and heavy-intensity exercise.

For incremental exercise testing, electronically braked cycle ergometry with constant pedaling frequency, of 60 revolutions per minute (rpm) is recommended. Equivalent results are obtained when work rate is increased either continuously (ramp test) or by a uniform amount each minute (1-minute incremental test) until the patient is limited by symptoms (i.e., the person cannot cycle faster than 40 rpm) or is not able to continue safely. The increment size should be set according to the clinical characteristics of the patient in order to obtain approximately 10 minutes of exercise. This may represent incremental rates of 10 to 20 watts per minute in a healthy sedentary subject or less in a patient with COPD. Data to be acquired in a test lasting less than 20 minutes from start to finish should include (1) measurements at rest, (2) 3 minutes of unloaded exercise, (3) incremental exercise (approximately 10 minutes), and (4) 2 minutes of recovery, at least. Standard noninvasive CPET carried out with the subject breathing room air ($FIO_2 = 0.21$) involves acquisition of breath-by-breath expired O_2 and CO_2 concentrations (FEO_2 and $FECO_2$, respectively), work rate, expired airflow, heart rate, and systemic arterial pressure as primary variables. ECG and pulse oximetry tracings should be continuously monitored during the test. It is useful to establish a sense of the patient's exercise-related perceptions during the exercise test and at the point of discontinuation of exercise. Such perceptions should encompass exertion, dyspnea, chest pain, and skeletal muscle effort, with quantification achieved by means of standardized rating procedures (e.g., Borg visual analogue scale).

Proper evaluation of pulmonary gas exchange in patients with lung disease requires assessment of arterial blood gases (**Figure 10-4**). In such cases, arterial cannulation (preferably of the radial or brachial artery) is needed to obtain partial pressures of respiratory gases (PaO_2 and $PaCO_2$) and to determine $PO_2(A-a)$. This also provides information on acid-base status (pH, $PaCO_2$ and base excess) and allows continuous monitoring of systemic arterial blood pressure during the test. However, although "arterialized venous blood" (e.g., from the dorsum of the heated hand or vasodilated ear lobe) gives good values for PCO_2 and pH, it is not appropriate for PO_2. Furthermore, arterial respiratory blood gas values estimated using expired O_2 and CO_2 profiles or with "transcutaneous" electrodes and pulse oximetry should not be used as indices of arterial PO_2 and PCO_2 during exercise. It is important to recognize that arterial blood sampling immediately after exercise does not provide an adequate assessment of blood gas values at peak exercise. However, although pulse oximetry does not indicate arterial PO_2, it does provide valuable information on oxyhemoglobin saturation during exercise.

If the ergometer used in the CPET is a motor-driven treadmill, then the *Balke protocol* is considered the most appropriate for its simplicity. The speed of the treadmill is kept constant (3 to 3.5 mph) during the protocol while the slope is progressively increased (by 1% to 2% each minute). Of note, $\dot{V}O_2$peak assessed using treadmill usually is 10% to 15% higher than measurements obtained with a cycle ergometer, owing to a higher exercising muscle mass with the treadmill. Moreover, the assessment of the relationship between oxygen uptake and external work rate is more accurately done with use of a cycle ergometer than a treadmill.

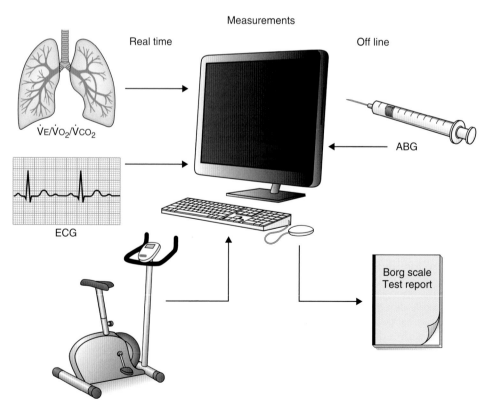

Figure 10-4 Measurements done during a standard incremental cardiopulmonary exercise protocol in the laboratory; see text for further explanation. *ABG,* arterial blood gas [analysis]; *ECG,* electrocardiogram; $\dot{V}_{CO_2}$, carbon dioxide production; $\dot{V}_E$, minute ventilation; $\dot{V}_{O_2}$, oxygen uptake.

CONSTANT-WORK-RATE EXERCISE IN THE LABORATORY

Constant-work-rate protocols can result in steady-state responses when work rate is below the critical power (usually up to 60% of maximal). By contrast, a constant work rate of high intensity for the individual subject typically results in continually changing values in most variables of interest. Consequently, attainment of, or failure to attain, a steady-state $\dot{V}O_2$ during a constant-load test can be used to determine if a particular task is sustainable by the patient.

In the clinical setting, high-intensity constant-work-rate exercise (at approximately 75% of $\dot{V}O_2$peak) to exhaustion is a highly reproducible test to assess the effects of an intervention (e.g., bronchodilators, vasodilators, rehabilitation). Moreover, endurance time (time to exhaustion) properly reflects aerobic potential. Alternatively, the use of a high-intensity constant work rate to assess exercise-induced asthma has traditionally been used in the clinical setting, but it might be progressively substituted by a bronchial challenge with mannitol.

During a constant-work-rate protocol, the period of dynamic adjustment (time constant) to a constant-work-rate test provides information regarding the dynamic behavior of lung function, hemodynamics, and tissue O_2 utilization. To date, however, virtually no information is available on the confidence limits, reproducibility, and predictive value of the derived parameters in patient populations. In summary, incremental exercise testing with a cycle ergometer constitutes the standard exercise protocol in the laboratory to assess aerobic capacity and to explore limiting factors. In specific cases in which the effects of an intervention are to be explored, high-intensity, sustainable, constant-work-rate exercise using a cycle ergometer is the protocol of choice. Of note, simple exercise testing outside the laboratory is *not* an acceptable alternative choice to exercise testing in the laboratory; rather, it should be considered a complementary option that constitutes a useful expansion of the potential of clinical exercise testing.

SIMPLE EXERCISE TESTING OUTSIDE THE LABORATORY

Although incremental cycling protocols are designed to facilitate the assessment of the relationship between O_2 uptake and work rate throughout the test, timed-walking tests have important limitations in this regard. The three most important factors determining energy requirements during timed-walking tests are walking speed, ergonomics of the walking, and body weight. Because body weight remains unchanged, the other two factors modulate intrasubject variability of energy requirements during the test. Proportionality between $\dot{V}O_2$ and walking speed supports the contention that walking speed is a key determinant of work rate, together with body weight. The study displayed in **Figure 10-5** demonstrates that physiologic responses during

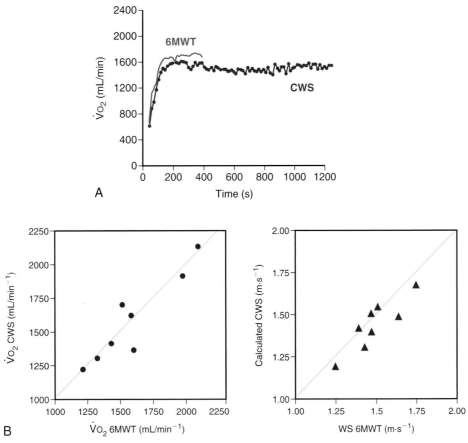

Figure 10-5 Equivalence of oxygen uptake responses for the 6-minute walking test (6MWT) and critical power in patients with chronic obstructive pulmonary disease (COPD). **A,** The upper graph indicates the $\dot{V}O_2$ response in a representative patient during 6MWT, in *blue*, and during timed-walking speed at the critical power (critical walking speed [CWS]), in *red*. **B,** Individual relationships between $\dot{V}O_2$ during CWS (y-axis) and $\dot{V}O_2$ during 6MWT (x-axis) (*r* = .93, *P* < .001) (*left*) and between CWS and walking speed (WS) during 6MWT (*r* = .90, *P* < .01) (*right*). Similar relationships were observed for heart rate and minute ventilation. $\dot{V}O_2$, oxygen uptake. *(From Casas A, Vilaro J, Rabinovich R, et al: Encouraged 6-min walking test indicates maximum sustainable exercise in COPD patients,* Chest *128:55–61, 2005.)*

the 6-minute walking test (6MWT) in patients with moderate to severe COPD are equivalent to those seen in persons walking at critical power (to achieve critical walking speed [CWS]), which corresponded to approximately 90% of maximum $\dot{V}O_2$ in the patients studied. The study seems to indicate that patients with moderate to severe COPD set their walking speed during the test to achieve critical O_2 uptake. The level of $\dot{V}O_2$ achieved at CWS may indicate the integrated response of the systems involved in O_2 transport–O_2 utilization that ultimately determine the highest sustainable level of exercise. These results may constitute the underlying explanation for the high prognostic value of the 6MWT, which, together with its simplicity, applicability, and acceptable reproducibility, prompts its recommendation as the most suitable choice for conventional clinical assessment in COPD, as part of the multidimensional evaluation of disease severity. At present, 6MWT is recognized to add prognostic information useful to the staging of patients with COPD, primary pulmonary hypertension, and congestive heart failure. Results of timed walking tests (e.g., 6MWT) are sensitive to changes after interventions such as inhaled bronchodilators, volume reduction surgery, and pulmonary rehabilitation.

Figure 10-6 and **Table 10-1** compare the physiologic responses with three simple exercise protocols (stair climbing test, incremental shuttle test, and 6MWT) and incremental cycling exercise using a cycle ergometer, all of them carried out by patients with moderate to severe COPD. It is clearly shown that approximately 80% of $\dot{V}O_2$peak was already achieved within the first minute of encouraged stair climbing.

Incremental cycling exercise and incremental shuttle test showed similar $\dot{V}O_2$ profiles (see Figure 10-6 and Table 10-1). At peak exercise, however, incremental cycling showed higher CO_2 output and higher respiratory exchange ratio than with the incremental shuttle test. Likewise, symptom scores also were higher during cycling exercise than for incremental shuttle test. The differences between these two tests could be explained by higher blood lactate levels, hence ventilatory requirements, during incremental cycling compared with timed-walking tests. In the study, $\dot{V}O_2$peak during incremental cycling was similar to $\dot{V}O_2$ at peak incremental shuttle (see Table 10-1), despite the fact that the amount of exercising muscle mass during cycling exercise is significantly smaller than in timed-walking tests and the characteristics of the exercise are different. As described earlier, patient's $\dot{V}O_2$max was observed at exhaustion in most of the exercise protocols carried out in Figure 10-5, irrespective of the amount of exercising muscle mass. A potential explanation for this finding is that the ceiling of whole-body $\dot{V}O_2$ in patients with COPD is defined mainly by the degree of pulmonary impairment and not by the amount of exercising muscle mass.

In summary, despite its well-recognized limitations, simple exercise testing (i.e., with the 6MWT) constitutes a complementary option to laboratory exercise testing in the clinical assessment of patients with chronic respiratory conditions.

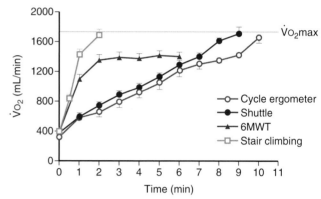

Figure 10-6 Comparison of mean O_2 uptake profiles for eight patients with moderate to severe chronic obstructive pulmonary disease (COPD) during four different clinical exercise protocols (mean ± SEM): incremental cycling (*open circles*), incremental shuttle (*solid circles*), 6MWT-90 (*solid triangles*), and stair climbing (*open squares*). See text for further explanation. *SEM,* standard error of the mean. *(From Casas A, Vilaro J, Rabinovich R, et al: Encouraged 6-min walking test indicates maximum sustainable exercise in COPD patients, Chest 128:55–61, 2005.)*

Table 10-1	Comparison Among Clinical Exercise Protocols									
Test Variable	**Stair Climbing (peak)**			**Incremental Cycling (peak)**			**Incremental Shuttle (peak)**			**6MWT-90 (last 3 min)**	
Time to exhaustion (s)	88	±	37	546	±	95	465	±	54	—	
$\dot{V}E$ (L/min)	57.7	±	14.1	56.0	±	8.3	48.2	±	10.0	44.2	± 10.0*†
$\dot{V}O_2$ (mL/min)	1693	±	256	1661	±	180	1651	±	243	1429	± 227*†
$\dot{V}CO_2$ (mL/min)	1749	±	359	1687	±	151	1473	±	273‡	1273	± 220*†
RER	1.03	±	0.12	1.02	±	0.06	0.89	±	0.09‡§	0.89	± 0.05*†
Heart rate (beats/min)	131	±	18	133	±	15	130	±	14	128	± 13
Sao₂ (%)	91%	±	5%	91%	±	4%	91%	±	2%	90%	± 5%
Borg scale score—dyspnea	8 [3-10]			7 [3-9]			5 [1-9]‡§			4 [1-7]*†	
Borg scale score—leg fatigue	5 [3-8]			6 [3-8]			4 [1-5]‡			4 [1-7]*	

Results expressed as means ± SD except for Borg's scores that are expressed as mean and range.
*6MWT-90 vs incremental cycling: $\dot{V}O_2$ ($p < 0.01$); $\dot{V}CO_2$ ($p < 0.01$); $\dot{V}E$ ($p < 0.01$); Dyspnea ($p < 0.01$); Leg ($p < 0.05$)
†6MWT-90 vs stairs climbing: $\dot{V}O_2$ ($p < 0.005$); $\dot{V}CO_2$ ($p < 0.01$); $\dot{V}E$ ($p < 0.01$); Dyspnea ($p < 0.05$)
‡Incremental shuttle vs incremental cycling: $\dot{V}CO_2$ ($p < 0.01$); RER ($p < 0.01$); Dyspnea ($p < 0.05$); Leg ($p < 0.05$)
§Shuttle vs stair climbing: RER ($p < 0.05$); Dyspnea ($p < 0.05$)
6MWT-90, 6-minute walking test on a 90-meter course; *RER,* respiratory exchange ratio; *Sao₂,* blood oxygen saturation; *$\dot{V}CO_2$,* carbon dioxide production; *$\dot{V}E$,* minute ventilation; *$\dot{V}O_2$,* oxygen uptake.

TESTING PROCEDURES

Cardiopulmonary exercise testing should be conducted only by adequately trained personnel with a basic knowledge of exercise physiology. Technicians familiar with normal and abnormal responses during exercise and trained in cardiopulmonary resuscitation (CPR) should be present throughout the test. CPET should be performed under the supervision of a physician who is appropriately trained to conduct exercise tests and in advanced CPR. The degree of subject supervision needed during the test can be determined by the clinical status of the subject being tested and the type of exercise protocol. Although presence of the physician during the test is preferable, if this is not possible, a physician must be readily available to respond as needed. Additional roles for the physician are in the evaluation of the patient immediately before the test and in the interpretation of the results.

PATIENT PREPARATION

At the time of scheduling, the patient should be instructed to adhere to the usual medical regimen; he or she should not eat for at least 2 hours before the test, avoid cigarette smoking and caffeine, and dress appropriately for the exercise test. A brief history (with detailed inquiries about the medications) and physical examination should be done to rule out contraindications to testing. Results of recent resting-state pulmonary function tests—as a minimum, forced spirometry—should be available for patients in whom pulmonary disease is suspected.

On the patient's arrival at the CPET laboratory, a detailed explanation of the testing procedure and equipment should be provided, outlining risks and potential complications as described further on. The patient needs to become familiar with the equipment. If the treadmill is used, time is provided for several practice trials of starting and stopping until the patient feels confident. If the cycle ergometer is used, the seat height is adjusted so that the subject's legs are almost completely extended when the pedals are at the lowest point and the cycling rhythm is practiced.

Before the test, the ECG electrodes are carefully placed and secured after preparing the skin to ensure good recordings (if necessary, the area of the electrode placement can be shaved). A sphygmomanometer cuff is placed on the upper arm. The mouth piece and nose clip are then tried and the position adjusted until a comfortable position has been established. The patient is informed that it is acceptable to swallow with the mouth piece in place and that any unexpected difficulty should be signaled by a "thumb down" gesture. The patient is advised to point to the site of discomfort if chest or leg pain is experienced.

During the test, the patient is encouraged to carry on with a regular pedaling cadence (60 cycles/minute). Monitoring for symptoms and degree of discomfort is performed periodically (in accordance with the safety precautions described next). Good communication with the patient throughout the whole procedure increases the subject's confidence and promotes good effort. During recovery, the patient is told to continue to pedal, without external work load (or walk at a slow pace on the treadmill), for at least 2 minutes, to prevent fainting and to accelerate lactate removal. At the point of discontinuation of exercise, after the patient has removed the mouthpiece, the physician should ascertain the symptoms (type and intensity graded on the Borg scale) that prompted the patient to stop exercise. If the test does not provide adequate diagnostic information because of premature termination or inadequate cooperation of the patient, it should be repeated after a rest period of 30 to 45 minutes.

Although CPET may be considered to be a safe procedure, risks and complications have been reported. Good clinical judgment should be paramount in defining indications and contraindications for exercise testing. Cardiac (bradyarrhythmias, ventricular tachycardia, myocardial infarction, heart failure, hypotension, and shock) and noncardiac (musculoskeletal trauma, severe fatigue, dizziness, fainting, body aches) complications of CPET have been reported. Consequently, during the test, laboratory personnel should be alert to any abnormal event. The indications to stop the test must be clearly established and known by all persons involved in testing. These indications include symptoms and signs such as acute chest pain, sudden pallor, loss of coordination, mental confusion, extreme dyspnea, ECG changes including depression of the ST segment by more than 0.1 mV (values are less specific in female patients) and T wave inversion, sustained ventricular tachycardia, and fall in systolic blood pressure either below the resting value or about 20 mm Hg below its highest value during exercise testing. Relative indications to stop the test are occurrence of polymorphic and/or frequent premature ventricular beats and hypertension (blood pressure above 250 mm Hg systolic and above 130 mm Hg diastolic).

If the exercise test has been stopped for one of the aforementioned reasons, the patient should be monitored in the CPET laboratory until symptoms or ECG changes have completely cleared. Admission to the hospital for longer observation or more often for complementary investigation will be necessary in very rare cases. If necessary, intensive care can be administered on site. Full CPR equipment should be available in the CPET laboratory.

INTERPRETATION STRATEGIES

For the greatest diagnostic potential and impact on the clinical decision-making process, exercise testing should rely not on the utility of any one individual measurement, although some are obviously more important than others, but rather on their integrated use. Identification of a cluster of responses characteristic of different diseases often is useful. The major portion of the interpretation strategy is focused on CPET results generated during maximal, symptom-limited, incremental exercise testing. This is currently the most popular albeit not the exclusive protocol in use. **Figure 10-7** displays data obtained in a normal subject performing cycle ergometry, for which the ergometer used an "assist" to provide an actual zero-watt work rate at "unloaded" pedaling. The four plots labeled *A* to *D* on this figure depict, in addition to the peak $\dot{V}O_2$, the variables commonly used to provide an indirect estimation of the lactate threshold. That is, they allow identification of the O_2 uptake at the transition between moderate to heavy-intensity exercise. Plot *E*—O_2 uptake versus work rate—reflects the exercise efficiency and the limits of exercise tolerance of the subject. Plot *F*—ventilation versus CO_2 output—and plot *H*—tidal volume versus ventilation—characterize aspects of the ventilatory response during submaximal and maximal exercise. Some investigators, however, find the relationship between $\dot{V}E$ and $\dot{V}O_2$ during such tests to be useful. Finally, plot *G*—heart rate (and O_2 pulse) versus O_2 uptake—is informative with respect to the characteristics of the hemodynamic response to exercise. The next step is to choose adequate reference values to establish patterns of normal or abnormal response.

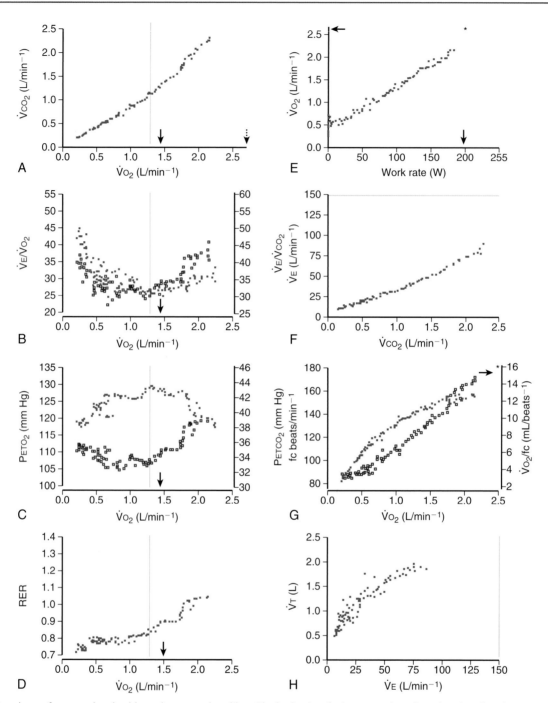

Figure 10-7   Exercise performance in a healthy sedentary male subject. The basic plots for interpretation of results of cardiopulmonary exercise testing are depicted. In **A** to **D**, in addition to peak oxygen uptake ($\dot{V}_{O_2}$), the variables commonly used to indirectly estimate lactate threshold (LT) are given. That is, the $\dot{V}_{O_2}$ at which the transition from moderate- to high-intensity exercise occurs is identified (*vertical dashed line*). The expected LT for a healthy subject (55% of predicted $\dot{V}_{O_2}$peak) is indicated in **A** to **D** by a *small arrow with a solid shaft*. Predicted $\dot{V}_{O_2}$peak is indicated in **A** by a *small arrow with a dashed shaft*. In **E**, $\dot{V}_{O_2}$ versus work rate reflects the exercise efficiency and limits of exercise tolerance of the subject, with the expected peak exercise performance represented by the *asterisk*. **F** and **H** indicate minute ventilation ($\dot{V}_E$) versus carbon dioxide uptake ($\dot{V}_{CO_2}$) and tidal volume ($\dot{V}_T$) versus $\dot{V}_E$, respectively; these two plots describe the characteristics of the ventilatory response during submaximal and peak exercise. Finally, **G** presents characteristics of the hemodynamic response to exercise, with estimated peak heart rate represented by the *asterisk* and predicted peak O_2 pulse by the *arrow*. P_{ETO_2}, end-tidal pressure of oxygen; P_{ETCO_2}, end-tidal pressure of carbon dioxide; *RER*, respiratory exchange ratio.   *(From Roca J, Rabinovich R: Clinical exercise testing. In Gosselink R, Stam H, editors: Lung function testing, Eur Resp Mon 31:146–165, 2005.)*

SUMMARY

The chapter provides an overview of the clinical use of exercise testing in patients with chronic pulmonary disease. The roles and complementary benefits of both laboratory testing and simple exercise protocols are analyzed, with emphasis on the pivotal role of the O_2 transport–O_2 utilization system in determining maximum O_2 uptake in an integrative manner. Also described are the systemic responses to exercise in healthy subjects, both athletes and sedentary persons, and in patients with common pulmonary diseases. Finally, basic principles of exercise testing and interpretation of the results are reviewed.

SUGGESTED READINGS

American Thoracic Society; American College of Chest Physicians: ATS/ACCP statement on cardiopulmonary exercise testing, *Am J Respir Crit Care Med* 167:211–277, 2003.

Casas A, Vilaro J, Rabinovich R, et al: Encouraged six minute walking test indicates maximum sustainable exercise in COPD patients, *Chest* 128:55–61, 2005.

Celli BR, Cote CG, Marin JM, et al: The body-mass index, airflow obstruction, dyspnea, and exercise capacity index in chronic obstructive pulmonary disease, *N Engl J Med* 350:1005–1012, 2004.

Fletcher GF, Balady GJ, Amsterdam EA, et al: Exercise standards for testing and training. AHA Statement, *Circulation* 104:1694–1740, 2001.

Nici L, Donner CL, Wouters E, et al: ATS/ERS statement on pulmonary rehabilitation, *Am J Respir Crit Care Med* 173:1390–1413, 2006.

Palange P, Ward S, Carlsen KH, et al: Recommendations on the use of exercise testing in the clinical practice, *Eur Respir J* 29:185–209, 2007.

Palange P, Ward S, Whipp BJ: Clinical exercise testing, *Breathe* 3:159–163, 2006.

Roca J, Rabinovich R: Clinical exercise testing. In Gosselink R, Stam H, editors: Lung function testing, *Eur Resp Mon* 31:146–165, 2005.

Ward S, Palange P, editors: *Clinical exercise testing*, European Respiratory Society Monograph 40, vol 12, Sheffield, UK, 2007, European Respiratory Society Journals Ltd, pp viii–ix.

Wasserman K, Hansen JE, Sue DY, et al. *Principles of exercise testing and interpretation*, ed 4, Philadelphia, 2005, Lippincott Williams & Wilkins.

Chapter **11**

Bronchoscopy

Anil Vachani • Andrew R. Haas • Daniel H. Sterman

The first bronchoscopy was performed by Gustav Killian in 1897. Technologic advances during the next century facilitated development of bronchoscopy as a pivotal diagnostic and therapeutic tool in pulmonary medicine. Although a number of bronchoesophagologists contributed to refinement of the technique based on the use of a rigid instrument, the advent of flexible fiberoptic bronchoscopy, pioneered by Shigeto Ikeda in 1967, opened new horizons to clinicians. At the end of the 1980s, the development of videobronchoscopy brought significant improvements in imaging quality and data storage. Subsequently, several other bronchoscopic applications have been developed for both diagnostic and therapeutic purposes.

This chapter presents an overview of bronchoscopy and related techniques. After a general discussion of bronchoscopy and associated instrumentation, applications of the technique and patient preparation are considered, and safety factors, contraindications, and complications of bronchoscopy are reviewed. Finally, specific indications for diagnostic and therapeutic bronchoscopy are discussed.

TYPES OF BRONCHOSCOPY AND GENERAL INSTRUMENTATION

RIGID BRONCHOSCOPY

The initial bronchoscope, developed by Killian and further optimized by Chevalier Jackson, was a rigid metal tube that permitted either spontaneous or mechanical ventilation. Over the decades, rigid bronchoscopes of various lengths and sizes that are adaptable for diverse applications in children and adults have become available. Although the flexible bronchoscope has to a large extent replaced the rigid scope for most diagnostic and some therapeutic indications, rigid bronchoscopy still has vital therapeutic applications.

Both rigid and flexible modern systems are equipped with optic capabilities for airway observation alone. With the rigid scope, various types of telescopic rods, equipped with circumferential illumination, permit direct and magnified visualization (**Figure 11-1**). Specially designed telescopes allow viewing not only directly forward but also at oblique and lateral angles. Various diagnostic and therapeutic instruments can be inserted through the rigid scope while the patient remains ventilated. Rigid bronchoscopy allows a number of therapies such as laser photoresection, endobronchial stents, balloon dilation, electrocautery, argon beam coagulation, and cryotherapy to be performed safely and effectively. Perhaps most important, a rigid scope can be used to "core out" large bulky airway tumors and to dilate central airway strictures and areas of stenosis very effectively and efficiently. In addition, the rigid bronchoscope

also can be used for the passage of a flexible scope, which may be necessary for dealing with tortuous airways or distal lesions.

FLEXIBLE BRONCHOSCOPY

The flexible scope is used in most bronchoscopic procedures. Although initial flexible bronchoscopes used fiberoptic systems, most such instruments now use a charge-coupled device (CCD) camera at the tip that allows transmission of digital images to a monitor. The main advantages of flexible scopes include their ease of manipulation and greater flexibility, allowing a more complete tracheobronchial tree evaluation than with rigid bronchoscopy, and a less challenging path to expertise, permitting more rapid acquisition of skills (favorable learning curve), for use of these devices (**Figure 11-2**).

Flexible scopes vary in size, ranging from ultrathin devices allowing for endoscopy in infants and neonates to larger, adult-sized therapeutic scopes. The working channel of the bronchoscope can be used for aspiration of secretions and to accommodate various diagnostic or therapeutic accessories. Four main diagnostic tools have been developed for use during bronchoscopy in order to obtain diagnostic material: bronchoalveolar lavage (BAL), brushings, forceps biopsy, and needle aspiration (**Figure 11-3**). Since the inception of bronchoscopy more than 100 years ago, these diagnostic modalities have been hampered by limited ability to ensure direct localization of pulmonary nodules, masses, infiltrates, or lymph nodes. However, recent technologic developments in navigational technology and endoscopic ultrasound imaging have improved the ability to localize these lesions, to obtain diagnostic tissue, and to prevent unnecessary surgical intervention. The use of endobronchial ultrasound probes is discussed in Chapter 12.

Biopsy forceps are available in various sizes and may have smooth or serrated edges. In some models, a small central needle is present between the cups for anchoring and stabilization. Smooth cup edges also may reduce tissue trauma and the concomitant bleeding risk. Lesions not accessible to direct forceps biopsy can be approached with a bronchial brush. This device consists of a rigid central wire surrounded by bristles of various size and shape. Repeated brush movement against the adjacent tissue produces minor trauma but enables collection of cellular specimens for cytologic or microbiologic analysis. Uncontaminated specimens from the lower respiratory tract can be collected with a brush protected by an additional sheath and tip. Needles of various sizes can be used to obtain both cytologic and histologic material from transbronchial lesions (e.g., lymph nodes, mediastinal masses) or from endobronchial and submucosal lesions.

PATIENT PREPARATION AND MONITORING DURING BRONCHOSCOPY

All patients undergoing bronchoscopy should undergo a complete prebronchoscopy evaluation, including a medical history, physical examination, and chest imaging (**Box 11-1**). Although routine laboratory tests are not required, each evaluation should be individualized on the basis of patients' underlying conditions and the diagnostic and therapeutic procedures planned.

Most flexible bronchoscopy procedures are performed after patient sedation with any of a variety of pharmacologic agents. Most frequently, a combination of a short-acting benzodiazepine (e.g., midazolam) and a narcotic agent (e.g., fentanyl) are used for bronchoscopic sedation. Local anesthesia of the upper airway, larynx, and tracheobronchial tree is achieved with inhaled or bronchoscopically instilled lidocaine. Although rigid bronchoscopy initially was performed with use of minimal

anesthesia and later with the patient under general anesthesia, the recent trend has been to perform the procedure with patients either breathing spontaneously or ventilated with a jet ventilator, often under total intravenous anesthesia (TIVA) with agents such as propofol and remifentanil. With appropriate monitoring, good oxygenation and adequate ventilation can be ensured.

Success of bronchoscopy, whether diagnostic or therapeutic, depends in large part on proper preparation of the patient, including relief of anxiety, muscle relaxation, cough suppression, and adequate anesthesia. Time spent in achieving these goals will be justified in reducing the complication risk and in increasing the ease of procedural performance.

TECHNIQUE

The flexible bronchoscope usually is inserted nasally, orally, or through an endotracheal tube or a tracheotomy stoma. When necessary, it also can be inserted through a rigid bronchoscope. The nasal route often is preferred because the nasal passage

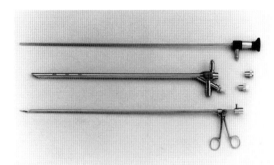

Figure 11-1 A typical rigid bronchoscope (*middle*) with Hopkins rod rigid telescope (*top*) and optical biopsy forceps (*bottom*). *(Courtesy John Beamis, MD.)*

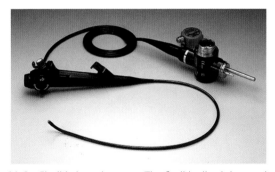

Figure 11-2 Flexible bronchoscope. The flexible distal tip permits easy maneuverability in all lobar and segmental bronchi. *(Courtesy Olympus Corporation of the Americas, Center Valley, Pennsylvania.)*

Box 11-1   Prebronchoscopy Checklist

1. Is there an appropriate indication for bronchoscopy?
2. Has there been a previous bronchoscopy?
3. If the answer to the preceding question is yes, were there any problems or complications?
4. Does the patient (and close relative[s] if patient is unable to communicate) fully understand the goals, risks, and complications of bronchoscopy?
5. Does the patient's medical history (allergy to medications or topical anesthesia) and present clinical condition pose special problems or predispose to complications?
6. Are all the appropriate tests completed and the results available?
7. Are the premedications appropriate and the dosages correct?
8. Does the patient require special consideration before bronchoscopy (e.g., corticosteroids for asthma, insulin for diabetes mellitus, or prophylaxis against endocarditis) or during bronchoscopy (e.g., supplemental oxygen, extra sedation)?
9. Is the plan for postbronchoscopy care appropriate?
10. Are all the appropriate instruments and personnel available to assist during the procedure and to handle the potential complications?

Modified from Prakash UBS, Cortese DA, Stubbs SE: Technical solutions to common problems in bronchoscopy. In Prakash UBS, editor: *Bronchoscopy*, New York, Raven, 1994.

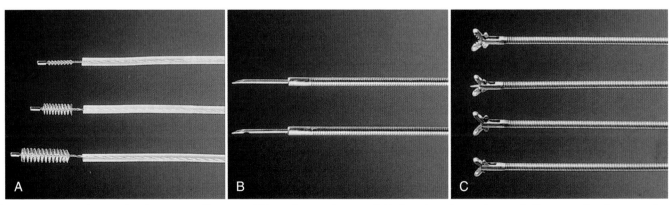

Figure 11-3 Bronchoscopy brushes (**A**), needles (**B**), and biopsy forceps (**C**) are available in various sizes and types. **B,** Biopsy needles shown are the standard 21 G aspiration needle *(top)*, and needle with side port *(bottom)*, allowing for cell collection from the side and tip of the needle. **C,** Biopsy forceps shown *(top to bottom)* are alligator-jaw, alligator-jaw with needle, elongated, and standard cup forceps. *(Courtesy Olympus Corporation of the Americas, Center Valley, Pennsylvania.)*

often provides some resistance against the scope and allows for somewhat better control during airway inspection. When the oral route is used, a "bite block" should be inserted to prevent the patient from biting and damaging the scope. Supplemental oxygen should be administered to prevent hypoxemia, which is fairly common during bronchoscopy, particularly in patients with underlying lung disease.

The bronchoscopic evaluation should begin with a thorough examination of the upper airway, as well as assessment of the integrity and function of the larynx. The vocal cords should be examined for any abnormalities, such as polyps or tumors, and evaluated for paralysis during phonation.

Once the upper airway inspection is completed, a systematic evaluation of the lower respiratory tract should be performed, beginning with an evaluation of the trachea and then all segmental bronchi. Airway integrity should be assessed including thorough evaluation of the mucosal and delineation of carinal size and shape for any abnormalities with special attention paid to changes in dynamic airway caliber during either relaxed breathing or forced expiration and coughing.

It is important to distinguish among normal anatomy, anatomic variations without clinical significance, and frankly pathologic conditions. These considerations have important implications regarding potential diagnostic and therapeutic approaches. For example, an abnormal branching of a bronchus may be of no clinical significance. On the other hand, such an abnormality could explain frequent infections caused by impaired ventilation and drainage of the affected area. Bronchoscopy is particularly useful in documenting posttraumatic or postsurgical changes in bronchial integrity, such as bronchial rupture, tracheoesophageal or bronchopleural fistulas, or anastomotic complications after reconstructive or lung transplantation surgery. Similarly, bronchoscopy can be used to document tracheal injuries occurring in critically ill patients after prolonged intubation or tracheostomy. Although tracheal injuries have decreased in incidence over the past decade, tracheal stenosis, tracheomalacia, and tracheoinnominate artery fistula are still clinically important complications that must be considered and identified. Complications specific to the use of percutaneous tracheotomy include protrusion of ruptured cartilage into the tracheal lumen and extraluminal tracheostomy tube placement.

A thorough evaluation of the mucosal surface is an important part of the bronchoscopic examination. The most common abnormality is a change in mucosal coloration, with prominent hypervascular areas seen in patients with chronic bronchitis. The presence of granulation tissue can be due to reaction to a foreign body. Inflammatory mucosal reactions, although not very characteristic, should raise the possibility of mycobacterial infection, nonspecific viral and nonviral infections, and other granulomatous diseases, such as sarcoidosis (**Figure 11-4**). Mucosal ulcerations are more characteristic of Wegener granulomatosis or malignancy. Loss of the usual mucosal luster and presence of a roughened surface may be early signs of an infiltrative or neoplastic process.

The trachea and bronchi are surrounded by mediastinal and parenchymal structures. Developmental or pathologic changes in these organs may be noted during bronchoscopic evaluation. An enlarged goiter or thymus can compress upper airways, resulting in airflow obstruction. Lymphadenopathy may produce structural changes, including widening of the main carina caused by subcarinal involvement, and compression of other bronchi—as, for example, in the right middle lobe syndrome. Peribronchial calcified lymph nodes may erode through

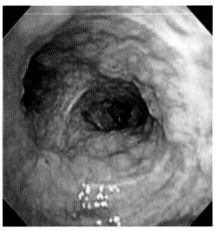

Figure 11-4 Endobronchial sarcoidosis. Bronchoscopy demonstrates edematous airways with a "cobblestone" appearance, often seen in endobronchial sarcoidosis. *(Courtesy Meeta Prasad, MD.)*

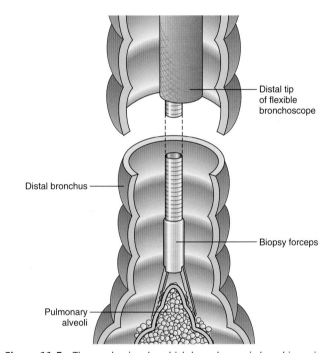

Figure 11-5 The mechanism by which bronchoscopic lung biopsy is obtained. The biopsy forceps pinches off the lung tissue located between two branches of terminal bronchi.

the bronchial wall, resulting in broncholith formation. Such lesions are potential sources of obstruction, infection, or hemoptysis.

After the bronchoscopic inspection of the airways and surrounding structures has been performed, appropriate samplings should be obtained from the abnormalities identified. Aspirated secretions can be sent for microbiology cultures to determine the offending organism in cases of infection or suspected infection. Endobronchial lesions can be sampled with cytology brushes, biopsy forceps, or needles. Bronchoscopic lung biopsy can be performed for either focal abnormalities or diffuse lung diseases (**Figure 11-5**). For small or focal lesions, fluoroscopy helps guide peripheral forceps placement and improves the diagnostic yield of biopsies for focal lesions. The use of fluoroscopy also may obviate the need for routine chest radiography after transbronchoscopic lung biopsy. In the case of diffuse lung disease, such as sarcoidosis, use of

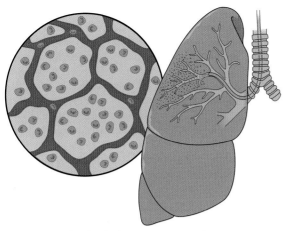

Figure 11-6 Bronchoalveolar lavage (BAL) is performed by wedging the tip of the flexible bronchoscope in the segmental bronchus leading to the parenchymal abnormalities detected by imaging techniques. Normal saline, 100 to 150 mL, in aliquots of 10 to 50 mL, is instilled through the bronchoscope channel and suctioned back into a container for analysis.

fluoroscopy has *not* been demonstrated to improve the diagnostic yield of transbronchial biopsies. Fluoroscopy is useful, however, in providing information regarding the proximity of the forceps to the pleura and in more rapidly establishing the diagnosis of complications (e.g., pneumothorax). Transbronchoscopic needle aspiration (TBNA) and biopsy (TBNB) permit sampling of peribronchial lymph nodes. These transbronchial approaches provide cost-effective diagnostic modalities with less risk and a lower complication rate than with mediastinoscopy (see Chapter 17).

Bronchoalveolar lavage (BAL) is a useful and generally well-tolerated bronchoscopic sampling technique (**Figure 11-6**). BAL is safe, even in critically ill patients, when biopsy or brushing methods are not recommended because of bleeding risk. Normal saline solution, devoid of any bacteriostatic material, is instilled into distal air spaces through the "wedged" flexible scope and then aspirated through the instrument's suction channel or from a sterile trap. The fluid collected can be analyzed for gross appearance to detect possible alveolar hemorrhage. The fluid also may be subjected to a variety of tests, depending on the clinical circumstances: microbiologic testing, specific cytologic analysis and cell count, immunologic parameters, presence of various biochemical mediators related to pathologic processes, tissue markers, polymerase chain reaction (PCR) assay, electron microscopy, flow cytometry, and DNA probes. The diagnostic yield of BAL very much depends on specific patient characteristics, the underlying pathologic process, and technical factors.

INDICATIONS FOR DIAGNOSTIC BRONCHOSCOPY

Many potential indications have been recognized for both diagnostic and therapeutic bronchoscopy, many of which are listed in **Boxes 11-2** and **11-3**. The most common reason for bronchoscopy remains the evaluation of a lung mass or nodule. Other major indications include investigation of pulmonary infiltrates, evaluation of opportunistic infections in immunocompromised persons, investigation of hemoptysis, assessment for suspected foreign body, and treatment of airway complications related to neoplasms in the tracheobronchial tree. Some of these indications are discussed next.

Box 11-2 Indications for Diagnostic Bronchoscopy

Cough
Hemoptysis
Wheeze and stridor
Abnormal chest radiograph
Pulmonary infections
Diffuse interstitial lung disease
Intrathoracic lymphadenopathy or mass
Bronchogenic carcinoma
Metastatic carcinoma
Esophageal and mediastinal tumors
Foreign body in the tracheobronchial tree
Tracheobronchial strictures and stenoses
Airway burns
Thoracic trauma
Vocal cord paralysis
Bronchopleural fistula
Tracheoesophageal fistula
Assessment of endotracheal tube placement or complications
Assessment of airway anastomosis

Box 11-3 Indications for Therapeutic Bronchoscopy

Hemoptysis
Atelectasis
Foreign body removal
Neoplasms of the tracheobronchial tree
    Bronchoscopic removal
    Laser therapy
    Argon plasma coagulation
    Brachytherapy
    Stent placement
Strictures and stenoses
    Bronchoscopic dilation
    Laser therapy
    Balloon dilation
    Stent replacement
Lung lavage (pulmonary alveolar proteinosis)
Bronchoscopic drainage
    Lung abscess
    Mediastinal or bronchogenic cysts
Thoracic trauma
Endotracheal tube placement

CHRONIC COUGH

Chronic cough remains one of the most common reasons for patients to seek medical attention. Although flexible bronchoscopy frequently is used in the evaluation of chronic cough, its role has not been clearly defined, particularly in patients without other indications for the procedure. The routine use of bronchoscopy for investigation of chronic cough has a diagnostic yield of less than 5%. When chronic cough is associated with localizing signs and symptoms, such as hemoptysis, a focal wheeze, or abnormalities on an imaging study, a specific diagnosis by bronchoscopy is much more likely. In nonsmokers with normal findings on chest imaging, the most likely causes of cough are asthma, gastroesophageal reflux disease, and rhinitis. Bronchoscopy can be considered if these etiologic entities have been effectively ruled out by a combination of empirical treatment and diagnostic testing, including the use of spirometry, bronchoprovocation tests, sinus imaging, and esophageal pH probes.

HEMOPTYSIS

Hemoptysis is a common clinical sign and one of the most frequent indications for bronchoscopic evaluation. The most common causes of scant hemoptysis include chronic bronchitis, tuberculosis, and bronchiectasis, whereas massive hemoptysis, usually defined as bleeding greater than 200 mL in a 24-hour period, most often is due to tuberculous cavities, lung cancer, mycetomas, or lung abscess (see Chapter 24). Bronchoscopy can be of help in localizing the site and cause of bleeding. Although the timing of the procedure should be dictated by clinical circumstances, studies have shown that early bronchoscopy (within 48 hours) is more likely to demonstrate active bleeding and allow for the determination of the bleeding site. Chest imaging, with either chest radiograph or computed tomography (CT) scan, can assist in bleeding site localization and, in stable patients without massive hemoptysis, should precede bronchoscopy. In patients with a normal appearance on the chest film, the prevalence of malignancy is approximately 5%, which in most cases is visible by CT scan. The yield of bronchoscopy in patients with normal findings on CT scan is extremely low, and a conservative approach consisting of observation and serial imaging should be considered. Beyond its role as a diagnostic tool, bronchoscopy often can be used to perform various therapeutic procedures in patients experiencing hemoptysis (see further on).

PULMONARY INFECTIONS

Bronchoscopy is a useful technique in the diagnosis of pulmonary infections, allowing for the collection of respiratory samples for evaluation with special stains and culture. Respiratory samples can be collected by one or more techniques, including bronchial washing, BAL, protected specimen brushing (PSB), bronchoscopic lung biopsy, and TBNA (Table 11-1).

Bronchoscopy is not indicated for the diagnosis of community-acquired pneumonia, which is currently treated empirically with appropriate antibiotic therapy. Bronchoscopy is likely to be useful in cases of nonresolving pneumonia, ventilator-associated pneumonia (VAP), or new infiltrates in immunocompromised patients. Nonresolving pneumonia is defined as lack of improvement or worsening of symptoms despite a minimum of 10 days of antibiotic therapy or failure of radiographic abnormalities to resolve after 2 to 3 months. The causes of nonresolving pneumonia are myriad and include inadequate antibiotic therapy, resistant or highly virulent organisms, impaired host defenses, obstructing endobronchial lesions, or a noninfectious cause. Although controversial, bronchoscopy should be considered in these patients.

Ventilator-Associated Pneumonia

Ventilator-associated pneumonia is defined as a pneumonia occurring more than 48 hours after intubation and initiation of mechanical ventilation. Intubated patients are at increased risk for pneumonia because of the impairment in mucociliary clearance caused by the endotracheal tube. These patients also are often on broad-spectrum antibiotics and therefore are at greater risk for infections with resistant organisms. Recent guidelines support the use of either a quantitative or semiquantitative strategy (e.g., tracheal aspirates) in the diagnosis of VAP. Two quantitative bronchoscopic methods that are particularly useful are BAL and PSB. The threshold for VAP diagnosis with PSB is 10^3 colony-forming units (CFU) per milliliter. PSB seems to have higher specificity than sensitivity for the presence of VAP—a positive result greatly increases the likelihood that pneumonia is present. For quantitative BAL, a threshold of 10^4 or 10^5 CFU/mL is used for VAP diagnosis. The detection of VAP by quantitative BAL culture has a sensitivity of 40% to 90% and a specificity of 45% to 100%. Because a larger proportion of lung parenchyma is sampled with BAL, this may be a better method than PSB for VAP diagnosis. Techniques

Table 11-1 Bronchoscopic Techniques and Applications in Respiratory Infections

Technique	Clinical Applications
Bronchoscopy—visualization	Assessment of mucosal, intraluminal, and extraluminal pathology Evaluation of endobronchial tuberculosis, mycoses, viral vesicles (in AIDS) Evaluation of invasive tracheobronchial aspergillosis, candidiasis, and other conditions Follow-up evaluation of endobronchial disease (e.g., tuberculosis)
Bronchial washing	Culture for identification of mycobacteria, fungi, and viruses and *Pneumocystis* smears
Bronchoalveolar lavage	Culture for identification of all organisms, especially mycobacteria, fungi, cytomegalovirus and other viruses and *Pneumocystis* smears
Protected specimen brushing	Culture for aerobic and anaerobic bacteria
Nonprotected bronchial brushing	Stains and culture for identification of mycobacteria, fungi, *Pneumocystis*, and viruses
Endobronchial biopsy	Mucosal lesions caused by mycobacteria, fungi, protozoa Removal of obstructing lesions responsible for infection (e.g., tumor, foreign body) Drainage of lung abscess; piecemeal removal of mycetomas (aspergillomas, other fungus balls)
Bronchoscopic needle aspiration	Stains and culture of extrabronchial lymph node specimens for identification of mycobacteria and fungi Drainage of bronchogenic cyst and instillation of sclerosing agent
Bronchoscopic lung biopsy	Stains and culture for identification of all organisms, especially *Pneumocystis jiroveci*, mycobacteria, and fungi Detection of parasitic lung infections
Rigid or flexible bronchoscopy—therapeutic intervention	Insertion of tracheobronchial prosthesis (stent) to overcome airway obstruction caused by intrinsic stenosis (posttuberculosis or fungal) or extrinsic compression caused by mediastinal fibrosis due to histoplasmosis

incorporating molecular testing in addition to microbiologic cultures are currently being evaluated.

Mycobacterial Infections

In cases in which pulmonary tuberculosis is suspected, the initial diagnostic evaluation should consist of serial examination of sputum for the presence of acid-fast bacilli (AFB) in stained smears. Ideally, induced sputum samples should be obtained. If sputum study results are negative and tuberculosis is still suspected, bronchoscopy with BAL and biopsy should be performed. Both induced sputum collection and bronchoscopy should be performed with appropriate infection control precautions to minimize the risk of nosocomial transmission. A bronchoscopy may cause the patient to produce sputum for several days afterwards; these specimens also should be collected and analyzed, if possible. The utility of bronchoscopy varies widely in the literature, with reported diagnostic yields of 50% to 95%. The yield in patients with miliary tuberculosis, in whom sputum smears frequently are negative, is approximately 70%. Bronchoscopy also is useful in tuberculosis manifesting as an endobronchial lesion or with mediastinal and hilar adenopathy, in which case diagnostic tissue can be obtained with TBNA (**Figure 11-7**). The yield of diagnostic procedures, including bronchoscopy, can be expected to improve as newer interferon release assays and nucleic acid amplification techniques are incorporated into everyday practice (see Chapter 31).

Infections in Immunocompromised Patients

Pulmonary infection in immunocompromised patients is a frequent complication and represents an important contributor to mortality. Such infections are increasingly common, reflecting the expanding use of aggressive chemotherapeutic regimens and the ever-increasing number of solid organ and hematopoietic stem cell transplantations. The differential diagnosis of pulmonary infiltrates is broad in scope; however, most cases are caused by infectious agents, including bacterial, fungal, viral, and mycobacterial pathogens. Bronchoscopy is the most commonly used diagnostic procedure in these patients and should be performed as early as possible, because a delay in diagnosis of longer than 5 days has been shown to significantly increase mortality among these patients.

The sensitivity of bronchoscopy varies, depending on the immunocompromised population studied and the specific etiologic disorder. In non–human immunodeficiency virus (HIV)-infected patients, the yield of BAL for *Pneumocystis jiroveci* is

approximately 80%, compared with a greater than 95% yield observed in HIV-seropositive patients. This difference is due to the much lower organism load present in non–HIV-seropositive subjects. Although empirical therapy often is initiated in patients suspected of having *P. jiroveci* infection, bronchoscopy should be performed in most cases to confirm the diagnosis. Bronchoscopic lung biopsy may increase the diagnostic yield of BAL for diagnosis of *P. jiroveci* infection, particularly in the non–HIV-infected population. Bronchoscopy also has a high diagnostic yield for cytomegalovirus (CMV); however, because CMV cultures from BAL are not specific, the diagnosis of CMV pneumonia should be limited to patients with pathologic evidence of CMV infection demonstrated by the presence of CMV inclusion bodies on BAL or biopsy. Although bronchoscopy also is useful for the diagnosis of aspergillosis—the sensitivity is approximately 50%—the disease often is peripheral and patchy and thus is not easily diagnosed by BAL or bronchoscopic biopsy. Overall, in immunocompromised patients with infiltrates, bronchoscopy is successful in establishing the diagnosis in as many as 80% of cases.

Human Immunodeficiency Virus Syndrome

The introduction of highly active antiretroviral therapy (HAART) led to a sharp decline in the incidence of opportunistic infections in HIV-infected patients. Nevertheless, infectious complications remain one of the most common indications for bronchoscopy in this population. *Pneumocystis* pneumonia remains the most frequent serious opportunistic infection in HIV-seropositive patients. Bronchoscopy with BAL remains the preferred diagnostic procedure for this disease, although in select centers, the use of sputum induction has had a relatively high diagnostic yield and may avoid the need for bronchoscopy. As previously mentioned, bronchoscopic lung biopsy may increase the diagnostic yield of BAL. Empirical therapy often is initiated in patients with suspected *Pneumocystis* infection; such therapy can impair the diagnostic yield of BAL if the procedure is not performed within 24 hours. In patients receiving pentamidine prophylaxis, the diagnostic yield is decreased unless the upper lobes are sampled. Several PCR assays have been tested on BAL fluid, induced sputum, and oral wash specimens; these generally have been more sensitive but less specific than traditional microbiologic methods.

Bronchoscopy also plays an important diagnostic role in HIV-positive patients with infections caused by mycobacteria, including tuberculosis, atypical bacterial pneumonias, and various fungal infections. Kaposi sarcoma, caused by human herpesvirus type 8 (HHV8), can manifest with violaceous endobronchial plaques that typically occur at airway bifurcations; pulmonary parenchymal involvement is characterized by lymphangitic infiltration of tumor, leading to the development of nodules and masses.

BRONCHOGENIC CARCINOMA

Diagnosis

Bronchoscopy most commonly is performed in the evaluation of patients with suspected lung cancer. It remains the most commonly used modality for the diagnosis of bronchogenic carcinoma and plays an important role in staging of the disease as well. Centrally located lesions generally can be approached using flexible bronchoscopy with minimal risk. Bronchogenic carcinoma of the central airways can manifest as exophytic mass lesions with partial or total bronchial lumen occlusion, as peribronchial tumors with extrinsic compression of the airway,

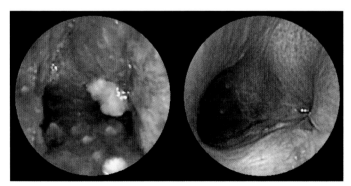

Figure 11-7 Endobronchial tuberculosis involving distal trachea and main bronchi. Image on the *left* was obtained before chemotherapy; the posttherapy appearance is shown in image on the *right*. Endobronchial tuberculosis is commonly mistaken for bronchogenic carcinoma.

as submucosal tumor infiltration, or as some combination of these entities. The mucosal abnormalities seen with peribronchial tumors or with submucosal infiltration often are subtle—the airways should be examined closely for characteristic changes such as erythema, loss of bronchial markings, and nodularity of the mucosal surface.

Central lesions usually are sampled with a combination of bronchial washes, bronchial brushings, and endobronchial biopsies. The yield of endobronchial biopsy is highest for exophytic lesions, with a diagnostic yield of approximately 80%. Attempts should be made to obtain the biopsy specimens from areas of the lesion that seem viable. Endobronchial needle aspiration (EBNA) to obtain a "core" biopsy from centrally located tumors should be considered, particularly if the lesion appears necrotic. For submucosal lesions, EBNA can be performed by inserting the needle into the submucosal plane at an oblique angle, and in patients with peribronchial disease causing extrinsic compression, the needle should be passed through the bronchial wall into the lesion. For all of these indications, EBNA has been shown to increase the diagnostic yield of conventional sampling methods.

Peripheral lesions usually are sampled with a combination of bronchial wash, brushes, transbronchial biopsy, and TBNA. The diagnostic yield of bronchoscopy for peripheral lesions depends on a number of factors, including lesion size, the distance of the lesion from the central airways, and the relationship between the lesion and bronchus. The yield of bronchoscopy for lesions smaller than 3 cm varies, ranging from 14% to 50%, compared with a diagnostic yield of 46% to 80% when the lesion is larger than 3 cm. The presence of a bronchus sign on chest CT predicts a much higher yield of bronchoscopy for peripheral lung lesions. In these cases, fluoroscopic guidance should be used to ensure proper positioning of the diagnostic accessory (**Figure 11-8**).

Several newer methods have been developed for the evaluation of peripheral lung lesions, including endobronchial ultrasound (EBUS) imaging (see Chapter 12) and navigational bronchoscopy. The first U.S. Food and Drug Administration (FDA)-approved navigational system, the Electromagnetic Navigation Bronchoscopy (EMN) system (InReach System, SuperDimension, Inc., Minneapolis, Minnesota), uses an electromagnetic board to generate a magnetic field around the patient, a magnetic sensor probe, an extended working channel, and three-dimensional integration of CT scan reconstruction and flexible bronchoscope position (**Figure 11-9**). In essence, this navigational system works on the same triangulation principle as for a global positioning system and allows the bronchoscopist to direct the flexible scope through the airways to the target. Several studies have demonstrated EMN diagnostic sensitivity to range between 67% and 74%, independent of lesion size. Studies also show improved diagnostic yield with the combination of EMN with mini-ultrasound probes for sampling of small peripheral lesions. Beyond standard diagnostic utilization, novel navigational applications have been demonstrated in targeted therapeutic delivery, such as EMN-guided stereotactic radiosurgery fiducial placement or implantation of radiotherapy monitoring devices.

Several new navigational bronchoscopy systems have recently been introduced (LungPoint System, Broncus Technologies, Mountain View, California; SPiN Drive System, Veran Medical Technologies, St. Louis, Missouri; Bf-NAVI, Cybernet Systems, Tokyo, Japan). With LungPoint and Bf-NAVI, virtual bronchoscopic images are displayed adjacent to the actual procedural video, allowing an electronic pathway to be overlaid onto the endoscopic image. An image of the target lesion can be overlaid on the virtual bronchoscopy and actual video images for localization during biopsy.

Navigational bronchoscopy systems may be limited in general application by their high capital cost and training necessary for optimal utilization. These newer navigational technologies have not yet been rigorously evaluated but appear to offer improvements in diagnostic yield beyond that attainable with standard approaches. The lack of randomized, comparative studies with this technology raises concerns about its role relative to traditional or ultrasound-guided approaches.

Staging

Bronchoscopy is an important modality for establishing lung cancer stage. In patients with potentially resectable tumors, a thorough airway examination helps confirm the absence of a

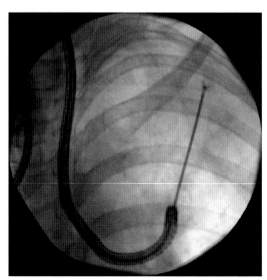

Figure 11-8   Bronchoscopic lung biopsy with fluoroscopic guidance. Fluoroscopy assists in the placement of the diagnostic accessory for investigation of small or focal lesions and improves the diagnostic yield.

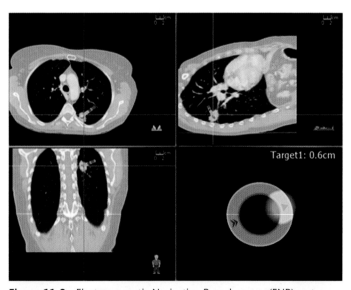

Figure 11-9   Electromagnetic Navigation Bronchoscopy (ENB) system: Representative images obtained at bronchoscopy performed using electromagnetic guidance. The parenchymal lesion is visible in sagittal, coronal, and axial views.   *(Courtesy SuperDimension, Inc., Minneapolis, Minnesota.)*

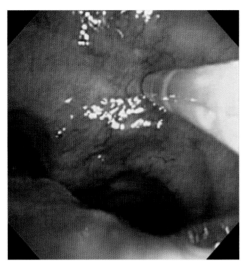

Figure 11-10 Transbronchial needle aspiration (TBNA) of a precarinal lymph node.

concomitant, radiographically occult lesion. For lesions that involve the central airways, it is important to document the extent of disease and the degree of involvement of "mainstem" bronchi and main carina.

TBNA has emerged as a valuable tool for the investigation of enlarged or metabolically active mediastinal lymph nodes (**Figure 11-10**). The procedure is particularly useful for evaluation of patients who are marginal or poor surgical candidates; in these patients, more invasive approaches, such as mediastinoscopy or mediastinotomy, may be obviated. TBNA has proved particularly useful with the use of *rapid onsite evaluation* (ROSE), whereby a cytopathologist working in or near the bronchoscopy suite can evaluate obtained specimens in real time (see Chapter 14).

Several precautions should be observed during the performance of TBNA to minimize the risk of false-positive results. The bronchoscope should be introduced into the bronchial tree without suction, and TBNA should be performed before distal airway inspection and before any other sampling procedures. N3 nodes should be sampled first, followed by N2 and N1 nodes.

Because of a relatively high false-negative rate (approximately 25%), a negative result with standard TBNA should prompt consideration of more invasive staging methods (i.e., mediastinoscopy). A positive result on TBNA is more likely with significant adenopathy on CT scanning, endoscopically visible tumors, subcarinal lymph nodes larger than 2 cm in diameter, or an abnormal-appearing carina. The use of image guidance with TBNA, such as ENB or EBUS, is promising and may provide higher diagnostic yields. This is particularly true of EBUS-TBNA.

Molecular and Immunohistochemical Assessment

In the past several years, the advent of targeted agents has improved survival rates in both recurrent and metastatic non–small cell lung cancer (NSCLC). It is increasingly apparent that both histologic analysis and molecular typing will be necessary to determine appropriate therapy for patients with NSCLC. For example, patients with activating mutations in the endothelial growth factor receptor (*EGFR*) gene are more likely to respond to EGFR inhibitors, whereas tumors with *EML4-ALK* translocations have recently been shown to improve with crizotinib therapy. Because a majority of patients

with NSCLC are diagnosed by bronchoscopy with either transbronchial biopsy or cytology specimens, mutation testing often is limited by insufficient material. In addition to molecular typing, advanced histologic analysis is increasingly important, because the choice of specific cytotoxic agents now relies on distinguishing among the various NSCLC histologic subtypes. For example, pemetrexed appears to have preferential activity in adenocarcinoma over that in squamous cell or large cell carcinoma. These considerations require careful attention to sampling technique: adequate tissue must be obtained at diagnostic flexible bronchoscopy for subtype classification and molecular testing.

DIFFUSE LUNG DISEASES

A wide range of acute and chronic pulmonary disorders are capable of causing diffuse interstitial lung diseases with more than 150 distinct clinical entities. These processes include infection, neoplasm, pulmonary edema, alveolar hemorrhage, alveolar proteinosis, occupational lung diseases, drug-induced disease, and various types of interstitial lung disease. In general, patients with diffuse lung disease should undergo high-resolution CT (HRCT) scanning, which helps to narrow the differential diagnosis and in some cases is virtually diagnostic of certain disorders. In many cases, it is still necessary to obtain samples for cytologic and histologic evaluation to confirm a specific diagnosis and to help exclude other possible disorders.

The most common bronchoscopic procedures used to help establish the diagnosis in diffuse lung disease are BAL and bronchoscopic lung biopsy. The findings on HRCT can be used to determine the best location for BAL or lung biopsy. In truly diffuse disease, the right middle lobe and the lingula are the best locations for BAL; with these sites, ease of access and good fluid retrieval are typical. BAL should be performed using a total of 100 to 200 mL of saline instilled in multiple aliquots. It is important to obtain a reasonable sampling of the alveolar spaces for the necessary cellular analysis.

Certain findings on BAL can be suggestive or virtually diagnostic of a number of interstitial lung diseases (**Table 11-2**). It is important that the BAL findings be correlated with the clinical and HRCT findings. For example, specific characteristics of the freshly retrieved lavage fluid can support the diagnosis of alveolar hemorrhage, pulmonary alveolar proteinosis, microlithiasis, or lipid aspiration. In patients with suspected eosinophilic pneumonia, a high eosinophil count is diagnostic, and in cases of pulmonary Langerhans cell histiocytosis, BAL flow cytometry should be performed to evaluate for CD1at cells.

In a number of disorders, BAL findings may be suggestive, but additional diagnostic procedures probably will be required. Such diseases include sarcoidosis, hypersensitivity pneumonitis, and organizing pneumonia. Bronchoscopic lung biopsy should be considered in situations in which the diagnosis has not been established by HRCT and BAL. In many situations, bronchoscopic lung biopsy can establish the diagnosis and avoid the need for surgical lung biopsy (**Box 11-4**). For example, with pulmonary sarcoidosis, the diagnosis usually is established by a combination of BAL and biopsy findings. The BAL can be used to exclude the presence of tuberculosis and fungal infections and can demonstrate the characteristic high CD4$^+$/CD8$^+$ ratio seen in sarcoidosis, whereas bronchoscopic biopsy specimens may demonstrate the classic finding of noncaseating granulomas. In general, bronchoscopic biopsy should be performed in several affected areas, and at least five or six specimens should

Table 11-2 Bronchoalveolar Lavage (BAL) in Diffuse Interstitial Disease

Disorder	BAL Fluid Findings
Pulmonary hemorrhage	Progressive increase in RBCs with sequential aliquots; hemosiderin-laden macrophages
Pulmonary alveolar proteinosis (PAP)	Grossly cloudy, milky appearance; positive PAS stain
Eosinophilic pneumonia	Eosinophilia >25%
Sarcoidosis	CD4$^+$/CD8$^+$ ratio >3.5
Pulmonary Langerhans cell histiocytosis	CD1at cells >5%
Hypersensitivity pneumonitis	Lymphocytosis; decreased CD4$^+$/CD8$^+$ ratio
Lipid pneumonia	Oily material that layers above aqueous phase
RBILD/DIP	Brown macrophages

DIP, diffuse interstitial pneumonia; *PAS*, periodic acid–Schiff; *RBCs*, red blood cells; *RBILD*, respiratory bronchiolitis–associated interstitial lung disease.

Box 11-4 Pulmonary Disease in Which Bronchoscopic Lung Biopsy Provides High Diagnostic Yield

Sarcoidosis
Hypersensitivity pneumonitis
Pulmonary Langerhans cell histiocytosis
Pulmonary alveolar proteinosis
Lymphangitic metastasis
Diffuse pulmonary lymphoma
Diffuse alveolar cell carcinoma
Pneumocystis jiroveci infection
Mycobacterial infection
Mycoses
Cytomegalovirus infection
Pneumoconioses
Lung transplant rejection

be taken. The sensitivity for diagnosis of sarcoidosis is only approximately 60% to 70%, and many patients require further invasive testing, such as surgical lung biopsy. Recently, the use of EBUS-TBNA has been extended to the diagnosis of sarcoidosis, especially in patients with mediastinal and hilar adenopathy. The addition of TBNA to transbronchial biopsy can provide the diagnosis in more than 85% of sarcoidosis cases.

Bronchoscopy has a limited role in the diagnosis of idiopathic pulmonary fibrosis (IPF). A nonspecific increase in levels of neutrophils, eosinophils, and, less commonly, lymphocytes has been documented in BAL fluid. Bronchoscopic biopsy is limited by the small size of the specimen obtained and the lack of histologic preservation because of mechanical crushing of the tissue. In the cases in which the diagnosis of IPF is probable or definite on the basis of clinical and HRCT criteria, bronchoscopy (and surgical lung biopsy) is not required. In situations in which the HRCT findings are "nondiagnostic," bronchoscopy should be considered to evaluate for the presence of other potential etiologic disorders. If the specific diagnosis cannot be established on the basis of BAL and bronchoscopic biopsy findings, surgical lung biopsy should be considered.

SAFETY FACTORS IN BRONCHOSCOPY

Bronchoscopy is a specialized procedure that requires extensive training. Familiarity with both the physiology and anatomy of the airways and other intrathoracic structures is essential. As with any other procedure, analysis of each patient's risk-benefit ratio will help reduce the complication rate. Mild sedation, muscular relaxation, and anterograde amnesia increase patient cooperation and permit quicker and less traumatic procedures. During and shortly after the procedure, appropriate monitoring of hemodynamic parameters (heart rate, rhythm, and blood pressure), oxygenation, and ventilation all contribute to the safety of bronchoscopy. Last but not least, knowledge and proper application of safety standards and maintenance procedures will decrease bronchoscopy cost.

In general, bronchoscopy is a safe and well-tolerated procedure, with few absolute contraindications. Of note, bronchoscopy should not be performed in patients with severe refractory hypoxemia, unstable cardiac disease, or life-threatening arrhythmias. Bronchoscopic lung biopsy should be performed with caution in patients with moderate to severe pulmonary hypertension or refractory coagulopathy.

COMPLICATIONS OF BRONCHOSCOPY

Complications generally are due to inappropriate patient preparation before bronchoscopy, effects of local or general anesthesia, and manipulation of various instruments. Appropriate training and experience of the bronchoscopist and supporting team are crucial to limiting the complication rate.

ANESTHESIA AND RELATED BLOOD GAS ABNORMALITIES

The major complications of diagnostic bronchoscopy include respiratory depression, hypoventilation, hypotension, and syncope. Risk is significantly increased among elderly persons and in patients with serious concomitant illnesses, including cardiovascular disease, chronic pulmonary disease, renal and hepatic dysfunction, seizures, and altered mental status. In patients with underlying organ dysfunction, doses of sedative agents and topical anesthetics should be adjusted as appropriate. Conscious sedation techniques using short-acting benzodiazepines (e.g., midazolam) offer significant anterograde amnesia but less muscle relaxation and have reduced the incidence of potentially dangerous hypotension and respiratory depression.

Inadequate topical anesthesia potentiates coughing, gagging, and patient discomfort and increases the risk of injury during bronchoscopy. However, topical anesthetics such as lidocaine, the most frequently used agent, are absorbed systemically through the respiratory mucosa, increasing the risk of cardiac or central nervous system toxicity. These complications are more likely to occur in patients with underlying low cardiac output, hepatic dysfunction, and oropharyngeal candidiasis. Another, less frequent complication of excessive lidocaine use is methemoglobinemia and tissue hypoxia.

Introduction of the bronchoscope frequently results in a decrease in oxygenation and in hypoventilation with demonstrable increases in $PaCO_2$. In patients with underlying chronic lung disease, severe hypoxemia may occur, triggering life-threatening cardiac arrhythmias. All patients should, therefore, be monitored continuously (electrocardiogram, blood pressure, O_2 saturation, and, if indicated, expiratory CO_2 concentration) from initiation of topical anesthesia through recovery from conscious sedation. Use of supplemental oxygen during the procedure should be routine.

FEVER AND INFECTION

A variety of pulmonary procedures, including bronchoscopy, have been reported to cause transient bacteremia. However, data demonstrating a link between bronchoscopy and increased risk of infective endocarditis are lacking. For patients at high risk for this condition (e.g., those with prosthetic valves, history of previous endocarditis, or congenital heart disease), the American Heart Association does not recommend the use of prophylactic antibiotics before bronchoscopy unless the procedure involves incision of the respiratory tract mucosa. Antibiotic prophylaxis should be considered, however, in high-risk patients who are undergoing a procedure to treat an active infection, such as drainage of an abscess.

Transient fever after bronchoscopy is fairly common and generally does not require any therapy. However, persistent fever in the setting of progressive radiographic infiltrates necessitates antibiotic therapy. The incidence of fever is increased in elderly persons, in patients with underlying chronic pulmonary disease or documented endobronchial obstruction, and in those undergoing bronchoscopic interventions for malignancy. The incidence of fever and extension of pulmonary infiltrates increase with the volume of BAL fluid and the total number of pulmonary segments lavaged. The incidence of postbronchoscopic infection is higher in immunocompromised persons and in patients with chronic suppurative lung disease, such as cystic fibrosis.

PNEUMOTHORAX

Pneumothorax after transbronchial biopsy occurs in approximately 4% of cases, even when the procedure is done under fluoroscopic guidance (**Figure 11-11**). The impact of fluoroscopy on the incidence of pneumothorax remains controversial. Uncontrolled studies have not found a difference in the incidence of pneumothorax after transbronchial biopsy when performed with and without fluoroscopy.

The incidence of pneumothorax is increased, however, in immunocompromised persons. This probably is due to the increased risk of pneumothorax associated with *Pneumocystis*

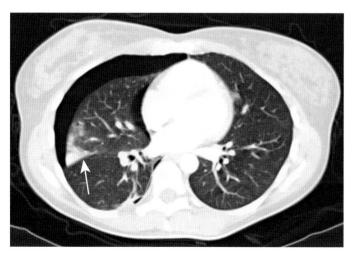

Figure 11-11 Computed tomography (CT) image demonstrating a pneumothorax of the right lung that developed after transbronchial lung biopsy. An area of focal hemorrhage in the lateral right upper lobe (*white arrow*) as a result of biopsy also can be seen.

infection. The risk also is elevated in mechanically ventilated patients, with peripheral lung biopsy, and in the presence of bullous lung disease. The risk of pneumothorax does not seem to be related to the size of the bronchoscopic biopsy forceps. In case of a significant pneumothorax, a chest tube should be inserted immediately to avoid oxygen desaturation and/or pathophysiologic changes in oxygen tension.

HEMORRHAGE

One of the most frequently reported complications related to bronchoscopy is hemorrhage. Patients with uremia or with underlying bleeding disorders, especially those caused by platelet dysfunction or thrombocytopenia, have an increased risk of bleeding during bronchoscopy. Bronchoscopic lung biopsy should not be performed if the platelet count is less than 50,000/μL, and aggressive interventional procedures (laser therapy, bronchoplasty, or stent placement) probably are safe only with platelet counts greater than 75,000/μL. Manipulation of the bronchoscope, mechanical trauma, vigorous suctioning, endobronchial brushing and biopsy may result in bleeding during bronchoscopy. In one large series, the overall rate of bleeding after transbronchial biopsy was 4.7%, although the risk of severe bleeding (defined as the need for a bronchus blocker, application of fibrin, critical care admission, or blood transfusion) was less than 1%. Hemorrhage also can occur with inadvertent perforation of pulmonary vessels during transbronchial needle aspiration or biopsy.

SPECIAL BRONCHOSCOPIC TECHNIQUES

ULTRATHIN BRONCHOSCOPY

Bronchoscopes with small external diameters (less than 3 mm), otherwise known as ultrathin bronchoscopes, were developed to deal with specific clinical situations, such as performing bronchoscopy in pediatric patients, investigating peripheral lung lesions, and evaluating tracheobronchial stenoses. The external diameter of traditional bronchoscopes generally is 5 to 6 mm, and these devices cannot easily examine beyond fourth- to fifth-order bronchi in adults. The use of ultrathin bronchoscopes with small working channels allowing for BAL and the use of a cytology brush have demonstrated promise in the diagnosis of peripheral lung lesions. The newest generations of ultrathin scopes have larger channels that can accommodate forceps and larger cytology brushes.

VIRTUAL BRONCHOSCOPY

Virtual bronchoscopy (VBS) is a novel radiographic reconstruction technique that exploits the versatility of helical (spiral) CT by transforming axial CT data into simulated three-dimensional intraluminal views of the airways. This form of perspective rendering has benefited enormously from continued advances in computing technology and currently is capable of providing images that in many ways mimic those obtained during conventional bronchoscopy (**Figure 11-12**). Although VBS has yet to find its place in routine clinical practice, it has nonetheless proved useful in the evaluation and management of a wide range of pulmonary diseases and conditions involving the tracheobronchial tree, including bronchogenic carcinoma, benign airway stenoses, tracheobronchomalacia, lung transplantation, and bronchiectasis. With this technique, which provides the bronchoscopist with a "virtual camera" inside the patient's tracheobronchial tree, images and perspectives can be obtained and procedures can be planned before conventional bronchoscopy is undertaken. Specific advantages include examination of airways distal to a completely occluded bronchus, retroflexion of the bronchoscope, and en face views. Current limitations of VBS include its inability to adequately characterize mucosal abnormalities, identify subtle submucosal disease, or visualize small endobronchial lesions. Obviously, however, VBS can never completely replace conventional bronchoscopy because it does not allow biopsy or therapeutic intervention.

AUTOFLUORESCENCE AND NARROW BAND IMAGING

The development of *autofluorescence bronchoscopy* (AFB) has improved the detection of dysplasia, carcinoma in situ, and invasive carcinoma of the central airways. AFB systems rely on the principle that infiltrating tumors disturb the fluorescence characteristics of normal tissue. Fluorophores, substances responsible for fluorescence, are variously concentrated within organs and may change according to prevailing conditions. When the bronchial tree is illuminated with blue light (442 nm in wavelength), subepithelial fluorophores within normal tissues emit light with a higher fluorescence intensity than that observed for pre-neoplastic or neoplastic lesions, especially in the green light emission spectrum. Reasons for the weaker green fluorescence in dysplasia, carcinoma in situ, and

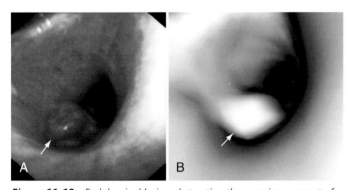

Figure 11-12 Endoluminal lesion obstructing the superior segment of the left lower lobe in a patient with metastatic melanoma. The images of this lesion (*arrow*) were obtained by flexible bronchoscopy (*top left*, **A**) and by virtual bronchoscopy (*top middle*, **B**). *(From Finkelstein SE, Schrump DS, Nguyen DM: Comparative evaluation of super high-resolution CT scan and virtual bronchoscopy for the detection of tracheobronchial malignancies, Chest 124:1834-1840, 2003.)*

microinvasive carcinoma include epithelial thickening, tumor hyperemia, and reduced fluorophore concentrations. Thus, the intensity of the emitted light is weaker, and observed light shifts to the red spectrum.

Several recent studies have evaluated the utility of AFB as a screening tool for dysplasia or carcinoma of the central airways in comparison with *white light bronchoscopy* (WLB). These studies have included patients at high risk for such pathology (e.g., those with a history of asbestos exposure, smokers), with known or suspected lung cancer, and after surgical resection for lung tumors. Although the sensitivity for detecting high-grade dysplasia or carcinoma in situ was increased two- to six-fold on average, AFB has limited specificity. Furthermore, no accepted algorithm has emerged for management of the lesions identified by AFB, and the question of whether screening bronchoscopy improves cancer survival remains unanswered. An additional important consideration is the significant interobserver variability documented among AFB endoscopists and histopathologists.

Narrow band imaging (NBI) uses a unique filter to select light wavelengths that preferentially are absorbed by hemoglobin, thereby permitting superior microvasculature detection. Because angiogenesis preferentially occurs in dysplastic and neoplastic lesions, NBI may identify early dysplastic lesions better than WLB or AFB. Studies suggest similar sensitivity between AFB and NBI, but improved NBI specificity for detecting abnormal lesions. Although current clinical applications for AFB and NBI in the general pulmonary population are limited, they may play an important role in future risk stratification, prognostication, and chemoprevention trials in high-risk patients.

OPTICAL COHERENCE TOMOGRAPHY

Optical coherence tomography (OCT) is the optical ultrasound analogue whereby near-infrared light transit time and reflection are used rather than sound waves and provides a macroscopic optical cross-sectional view of hollow organs. By using light instead of sound waves, OCT overcomes two major ultrasound limitations in the lung: (1) the inability to image through air and (2) poor spatial resolution. OCT resolution is between 4 and 20 nm, which is approximately 25 times higher than that of other modalities. In the airway, dysplastic, invasive cancer, or inflammatory changes appear to have unique OCT image patterns (**Figure 11-13**). The ability of OCT to provide

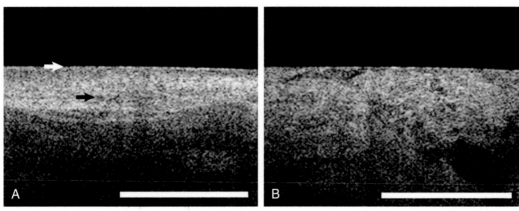

Figure 11-13 Optical coherence tomography images of bronchial mucosa in a patient with small cell carcinoma. **A,** Normal bronchial mucosa in uninvolved area of lung. Layers of epithelium (*white arrow*) and lamina propria (*black arrow*) can be seen. **B,** Within the tumor area, loss of identifiable microstructures is evident. The scale bars are 1 mm. *(From Ross RG, Kinawewitz GT, Fung KM, et al: Optical coherence tomography as an adjunct to flexible bronchoscopy in the diagnosis of lung cancer: a pilot study, Chest 138:984-988, 2010.)*

an "optical biopsy" with information about microinvasive airway lesion evolution, airway wall remodeling in obstructive lung diseases, or interstitium alterations in idiopathic interstitial pneumonia (IIP) without the risk of tissue biopsy could provide a valuable bronchoscopic tool. Such data may provide diagnostic information, but more important, longitudinal evaluation in an individual patient may allow therapeutic tailoring in the future.

FIBERED CONFOCAL FLUORESCENCE MICROSCOPY

Fibered confocal fluorescence microscopy (FCFM) is a modification of confocal microscopy that allows imaging of thin-section biologic specimens by replacing the microscope's objective with a flexible fiberoptic miniprobe that can be introduced through a flexible bronchoscope. This technology does not rely on light reflectance, as in OCT, but rather is based on cellular and tissue autofluorescence on laser excitation. The predominant source of airway wall autofluorescence is the subepithelial elastin fibers, and alterations in this elastin network can be detected in microinvasive and invasive proximal airway lesions. FCFM can image alveolar and acinar elastin fiber alterations and alveolar macrophage accumulation in patients who smoke, compared with nonsmoking patients. Therefore, although available data are limited, this technology may have evolving applications in diagnosis and monitoring of therapeutic interventions in a variety of parenchymal lung diseases, including obstructive lung diseases, sarcoidosis, IIP, and microinvasive malignant lesions.

THERAPEUTIC BRONCHOSCOPY TECHNIQUES

Since the introduction of bronchoscopy, the technique has been used not only for observation and diagnostic purposes but also for treatment of airway disorders.

RIGID BRONCHOSCOPIC DEBULKING OR BALLOON DILATATION

The ideal tool for rapid reestablishment of airway patency in endoluminal obstruction is the rigid bronchoscope. Rigid bronchoscopes have beveled tips, which are ideal for "coring through" large airway tumors and for dilating strictures, and they have large internal diameters, which facilitates débridement of tumors, evacuation of clots, simultaneous insertion of multiple instruments, and concomitant ventilation. Despite advances in other adjunctive endoscopic techniques, rigid bronchoscopic recanalization remains the treatment of choice for life-threatening tracheobronchial obstruction.

Balloon dilation has become an attractive alternative to dissection with a blunt rigid bronchoscope in less urgent cases of obstruction caused by malignant tumors and benign strictures. High-pressure balloons of various lengths and diameters commonly were used in the past. There are now balloons designed specifically for tracheobronchial use that are expandable to specific diameters by application of defined positive pressure. These are inserted through the bronchoscope working channel under direct vision or fluoroscopic guidance. The balloon, filled with saline or radiopaque contrast media, is inflated at the site of interest until the desired diameter is attained. This technique often is used in combination with bronchoscopic thermal treatments (laser, argon plasma coagulation, electrocautery) and tracheobronchial stent placement for the treatment of airway stenosis (**Figure 11-14**).

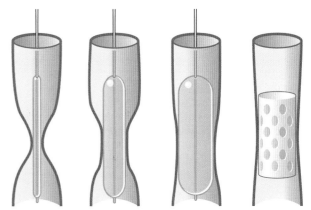

Figure 11-14 Diagrammatic representation of bronchoscopic balloon dilatation of tracheal stenosis. This procedure can be accomplished using a flexible or rigid bronchoscope with graduated dilating balloons. After optimal dilatation, a silicone stent (*far right*), placed using a rigid bronchoscope, relieves airway obstruction.

Balloon bronchoplasty also has been used successfully to treat other disorders, including endobronchial tuberculosis, fibrosing mediastinitis, and strictures associated with lung transplantation or prolonged intubation. It is less successful when used alone to treat stenosis accompanied by extrinsic airway compression and generally is not beneficial in patients with tracheobronchomalacia.

Complications of balloon dilation of airway lesions include bronchospasm, chest pain, mucosal laceration, airway perforation, bleeding, postprocedure airway edema, pneumothorax, and pneumomediastinum.

ENDOBRONCHIAL LASER THERAPY

Perhaps the most widely known technique in therapeutic bronchoscopy is laser photocoagulation or photoablation. Lasers produce a beam of monochromatic, coherent light that can induce tissue vaporization, coagulation, hemostasis, and necrosis. Although primarily useful in the ablation of endoluminal malignant tumors, bronchoscopic laser therapy also is beneficial for the treatment of other tracheobronchial disorders, including inflammatory strictures, obstructive granulation tissue, amyloidosis, and benign tumors such as hamartomas and lipomas.

Since the initial report of endobronchial laser ablation of an obstructive neoplasm by Laforet in 1976, several types of lasers have become available for the management of tracheobronchial obstruction. The carbon dioxide (CO_2) laser, used primarily by otolaryngologists, allows shallow penetration of tissue (to a depth of 0.1 to 0.5 mm) and highly precise cutting, but it has minimal hemostatic properties and traditionally was used through a rigid bronchoscope or with suspension laryngoscopy. More recently developed technology has facilitated the delivery of CO_2 laser energy by means of unique reflective fiberoptic probes allowing applications with flexible laryngoscopy and bronchoscopy. The CO_2 laser, with its fine control of tissue ablation, is ideal for the management of laryngeal lesions (e.g., webs, vocal cord nodules). For therapeutic bronchoscopy, neodymium:yttrium-aluminum-garnet (Nd:YAG) laser ablation is most commonly used and provides deeper tissue penetration (to a depth of 3 to 5 mm), superior coagulation, and improved hemostasis, but with less cutting precision. Nd:YAG laser procedures can be performed through a rigid or flexible bronchoscope. Success rates and complications directly related to laser therapy are not different when the procedure is performed through a rigid bronchoscope with the patient under general anesthesia or through a flexible bronchoscope with use of topical anesthesia and conscious sedation.

Nd:YAG laser photoablation therapy has demonstrated a single-modality recanalization rate greater than 90% for endobronchial obstruction of large central airways but is less successful for management of peripheral lesions or with associated extrinsic airway compression. Laser therapy may improve the chances of successful weaning from mechanical ventilation in patients with advanced endoluminal lung cancer presenting in respiratory failure. In addition, photocoagulation with an Nd:YAG laser is an invaluable treatment for patients with airway obstruction caused by benign endoluminal tumors.

Although endobronchial laser therapy generally is safe and well tolerated, it may be complicated by cardiac arrhythmias, airway perforation, pneumothorax, hemorrhage, hypoxemia, or endobronchial fire (ignition of the bronchoscope or endotracheal tube). The use of a laser in the tracheobronchial tree requires careful consideration of the anatomic location and configuration of the lesion. If the lesion is in close proximity to the esophagus or the pulmonary artery, endobronchial laser therapy carries a risk of fistula formation. Laser therapy in a patient with tracheobronchial narrowing caused by extrinsic compression may result in airway perforation. In rare cases, pulmonary edema or fatal pulmonary venous gas embolism has been reported. Patients with standard silicone endotracheal tubes or silicone tracheobronchial stents and those who require high concentrations of supplemental oxygen are at increased risk for endobronchial fire. Fortunately, the overall risk is less than 0.1%. The overall rate of mortality associated with endoscopic laser therapy is quite low, not exceeding 0.3% to 0.5% in several large series.

ENDOBRONCHIAL CRYOTHERAPY AND ELECTROCAUTERY

Cryotherapy and electrocautery are cost-effective alternatives to laser therapy for the management of tracheobronchial obstruction. The depth of penetration and resulting injury are, however, much more difficult to control. As with the Nd:YAG laser, both electrocautery and cryotherapy can be administered through a rigid or flexible bronchoscope. The effects of electrocautery on tissue are similar to those of Nd:YAG laser, with tissue destruction induced by coagulative necrosis. *Argon plasma coagulation* (APC) is similar to electrocautery except that it uses argon gas to conduct the electrical current, rather than a contact probe. APC has a depth of penetration of only 1 to 3 mm and is therefore more suitable for the treatment of superficial and spreading lesions. In contrast with cautery or APC, cryotherapy probes induce tissue necrosis through hypothermic cellular crystallization and microthrombosis. Specially designed cryoprobes are inserted through the bronchoscope until they contact the target tissue. Through the probe in the bronchoscopy working channel, liquid nitrous oxide or liquid nitrogen is introduced through a small orifice under pressure, resulting in rapid cooling with creation of an "ice ball" (approximate temperature of −20° C) at the probe tip. This freezing effect is maintained for approximately 20 seconds; the area is then allowed to thaw. Cryotherapy treatment of an endobronchial lesion requires several freeze-thaw cycles.

Cryotherapy and electrocautery have been used successfully to relieve airway obstruction caused by benign tracheobronchial tumors, polyps, and granulation tissue. These techniques—cryotherapy in particular—may be superior to lasers for distal lesions because of the lower risk of airway perforation. Similarly, carcinoma in situ and mucosal dysplasia may be adequately treated with cryotherapy or electrocautery alone, although multiple treatments may be required for optimal results. Cryotherapy is effective in the removal of certain foreign bodies that can be frozen to the probe and extracted. Of interest, cryotherapy can very effectively freeze endobronchial blood clots and mucous plugs to the probe, which can be easily extracted from the airway.

Endobronchial cryotherapy generally is not effective for management of paucicellular lesions that are relatively impervious to freezing, such as fibrotic stenoses, cartilaginous or bony lesions, and lipomas. Furthermore, endobronchial cryotherapy, unlike either laser therapy or electrocautery, is inefficient in achieving rapid relief of symptomatic airway obstruction. The most common serious complication of both electrocautery and cryotherapy is bleeding secondary to disruption of endobronchial tumor without full coagulation of distal tissue and tumor vessels. The estimated incidence of clinically significant bleeding in patients treated with electrocautery is 2.5%.

ENDOBRONCHIAL BRACHYTHERAPY

Brachytherapy is the local treatment of tumors with radiation delivered internally through implanted radioactive seeds or in a circumferential fashion with inserted wires. This technique ensures the delivery of a maximal therapeutic radiation dose to the tumor with a minimal effect on normal surrounding tissues. Endobronchial brachytherapy involves the bronchoscopic insertion of a thin, hollow "afterloading" catheter through or parallel to a malignant obstruction under fluoroscopic guidance. A radioactive implant is then inserted into the catheter and left in position for a predetermined period (2 to 40 hours, depending on the dose rate).

In 1922, Yankauer described the use of rigid bronchoscopic brachytherapy for the palliation of airway obstruction caused by malignant tumors. Modern techniques, including the use of flexible bronchoscopes, polyethylene afterloading catheters, and iridium 192 implants, were first described in 1983. Since the development of techniques involving high dose-rate delivery in the 1980s, endobronchial brachytherapy has become an option for outpatient treatment of peribronchial tumors.

Relief of airway obstruction is the primary goal of endobronchial brachytherapy, although curative treatment may be attempted in conjunction with external beam irradiation in selected patients. For rapid and sustained airway recanalization in malignant airway obstruction, brachytherapy generally is used as an adjunct to thermal tumor ablation, endobronchial stent placement, or conventional external beam irradiation. Brachytherapy is safest and most effective for management of central airway lesions, although in one study, small peripheral tumors proved to be more responsive than bulkier central tumors. Among patients with malignant airway obstruction, rates of recanalization range from 60% to 90%, with decreased dyspnea, cessation of hemoptysis, and relief of cough in most cases. Endobronchial brachytherapy may require multiple treatments to be effective.

Serious complications of brachytherapy include massive hemoptysis and fistula formation secondary to necrosis of the airway wall and adjacent vascular structures. Because of the risk of fatal hemorrhage, every effort should be made to rule out central vascular involvement of the tumor before brachytherapy administration. The reported incidence of serious complications varies widely, with rates as low as zero to 10% in some of the largest studies and as high as 30% to 40% in smaller studies.

PHOTODYNAMIC THERAPY

Photodynamic therapy (PDT) currently is approved by the FDA for malignant airway obstruction palliation and as an alternative to surgery in select patients with minimally invasive central lung cancer. PDT works on the principle that certain compounds, such as hematoporphyrin derivatives (Photofrin) or aminolevulinic acid (ALA), function as photosensitizing agents, rendering malignant cells susceptible to damage from monochromatic light. Tumor necrosis occurs as a result of cellular destruction through the generation of oxygen free radicals or by ischemic necrosis mediated by vascular occlusion resulting from thromboxane A_2 release. The selective effect of PDT on malignant cells is thought to be due to the greater uptake and retention of photosensitizing agents in neoplastic cells compared with normal cells—with the exception of cells of the reticuloendothelial system, particularly those in the skin. This relative tumor selectivity effect seems to be most pronounced within 24 to 48 hours after photosensitizing agent infusion. For this reason, bronchoscopic treatment of target lesions often is performed 1 or 2 days after agent administration. In view of the delayed onset of PDT action, it is not useful in patients with acute respiratory distress from malignant airway obstruction. Follow-up "toilet" bronchoscopies are required to debride necrotic tissue.

Ideal candidates for PDT include patients with airway obstruction caused by malignant endobronchial masses with minimal extrinsic airway compression, and patients with minimally invasive tumors of the central airways. Although surgical resection remains the treatment of choice for early lung cancer, some patients refuse surgery or have tumors that are deemed inoperable because of high surgical risk. In such cases, PDT may represent an appropriate alternative. Response rates are highest in patients with small tumors and minimal depth of penetration. In patients with bulky tumors, endobronchial PDT may substantially reduce the obstruction, with objective increases in spirometric measurements and subjective improvements in dyspnea and the quality of life. Metastatic tumors also have been treated successfully with PDT. Complications include increased skin photosensitivity and hemoptysis resulting from extensive tumor necrosis. Cutaneous photosensitivity, similar to that seen with sunburn, occurs in up to 20% of patients in various reported series and can be obviated by adequate sunlight precautions. Sensitivity to sunlight after photosensitizer administration can persist for 6 weeks or longer.

TRACHEOBRONCHIAL STENTING

The medical term *stent* refers to any device designed to maintain the integrity of hollow tubular structures, such as the coronary arteries and the esophagus. Anecdotal reports of attempts to implant stents in the tracheobronchial tree date back to 1915. The Montgomery T tube, designed in the 1960s, was the first reliable, dedicated airway stent. However, stent implantation in the lower trachea and bronchi did not become standard medical practice until Dumon's 1990 report on the safety and ease of placement of a dedicated airway stent made of silicone.

Two main types of endobronchial stents are in use today: tube stents made of silicone and self-expandable metallic stents (SEMSs). Silicone stents are placed by rigid bronchoscopy with the patient under general anesthesia. Silicone stents are relatively inexpensive (in the range of $400 to $500 USD) compared with SEMSs ($1800 to $2000 USD). Bifurcated silicone stents also are available for the palliation of distal tracheal and main carinal lesions. These stents have been effectively used in the management of carinal compression associated with malignant tumors, tracheoesophageal fistulas, and tracheobronchomalacia. Custom silicone stents can be designed by the treating bronchoscopist to deal with unique anatomic problems such as stump-related bronchopleural fistula after pneumonectomy. In one large single-center series, the complications of silicone stents included a 5% migration rate, a 10% incidence of granulation tissue formation, and a 27% incidence of partial stent occlusion by inspissated secretions.

Unlike silicone stents, SEMSs can be placed with flexible bronchoscopy, are less likely to migrate, and are more likely to preserve normal mucociliary clearance. However, if metal stents are misplaced in the airway, rigid bronchoscopy often is required for their removal. In addition, mucosal inflammation and the granulation tissue formation are common with uncovered SEMSs and at the proximal and distal ends of covered SEMSs, and repeated endoscopic intervention may be required to restore airway patency. For all these reasons, SEMSs have an FDA warning against their utilization in *benign* airway stenosis, unless all other treatment options, including silicone stenting, have been obviated. One exception to this rule is the development of dehiscence of the bronchial anastomosis in lung transplantation. In this setting, temporary uncovered SEMS insertion across the dehiscence has been used to induce focal granulation tissue formation, which promotes dehiscence closure.

Endobronchial stents have a critical role in multimodality endoscopic approaches to both benign and malignant airway obstruction. Airway obstruction caused by locally advanced bronchogenic carcinoma can be treated with a combination of thermal tumor ablation and stent implantation to regain and to preserve airway lumen diameter by preventing tumor ingrowth (**Figure 11-15**). Stent placement also can be used to maintain airway patency after endobronchial brachytherapy or can be combined with laser therapy and balloon dilation in the endoscopic management of benign fibrotic strictures. Most large studies of endobronchial stent placement have demonstrated impressive efficacy. Dumon and colleagues reported excellent clinical outcomes and few complications with silicone stent use in patients with malignant airway obstruction but a lower success rate among patients with tracheal stenosis caused by other disorders. Success rates, with "success" broadly defined as symptomatic relief, have ranged in limited studies between 78% and 98%, although none of the early trials used objective measures such as the Lung Cancer Symptom Score (LCSS) to determine efficacy. In two small studies in patients who were intubated because of respiratory failure secondary to unresectable tracheobronchial and mediastinal disease, stent placement facilitated extubation in most patients.

The benefits of stent placement seem to persist in patients who survive for a period of several months or years after stent implantation. Long-term follow-up data, however, are derived from patients with benign disease, because the mean follow-up period in patients with malignant airway obstruction does not usually exceed 3 to 4 months, because of limited underlying disease survival. Some investigators have reported poor long-term results with the use of metal stents in patients with fibroinflammatory stenosis caused by nonmalignant disorders. In addition, there have been case reports of massive hemorrhage associated with the use of stents in patients with extrinsic

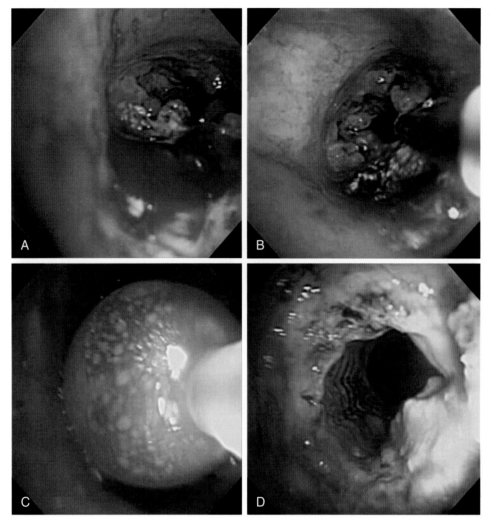

Figure 11-15 **A,** Endoluminal tumor with extrinsic compression treated with a combination of modalities: bronchoscopic laser therapy (**B**), balloon bronchoplasty (**C**), and stent placement (**D**).

compression attributable to aneurysmal dilatation or congenital aortic malformations.

INDICATIONS FOR THERAPEUTIC BRONCHOSCOPY

Therapeutic bronchoscopy most commonly is performed for aspiration of retained secretions and mucous plugs and for the treatment of airway obstruction. The indications for therapeutic bronchoscopy are listed in Box 11-3; many of these are discussed next.

ENDOLUMINAL AIRWAY OBSTRUCTION

Endoluminal obstruction of the tracheobronchial tree may result from various benign and malignant processes. The most common cause of endobronchial obstruction is advanced bronchogenic carcinoma. In patients with inoperable central airway tumors, restoration of airway patency may provide palliation and may even prolong life, particularly in the case of impending respiratory failure or postobstructive pneumonia.

Signs and symptoms of central malignant airway obstruction vary but often include progressive dyspnea and functional limitation, wheezing, cough, stridor, hoarseness, hemoptysis, and chest pain. A careful pretreatment evaluation should be performed to distinguish symptoms attributable to focal tracheobronchial lesions from those related to underlying obstructive lung disease or parenchymal lung disease, or both. A mild obstruction, for example, may contribute only marginally to the dyspnea experienced by a patient with concomitant severe chronic obstructive pulmonary disease (COPD). Although pulmonary function testing and thoracic imaging techniques such as chest CT may be useful in the evaluation of a patient with suspected malignant airway obstruction, bronchoscopy, either rigid or flexible, remains the diagnostic and therapeutic "gold standard." Increasingly, however, three-dimensional reconstruction CT imaging—so-called virtual bronchoscopy—is being applied as a reliable noninvasive method of assessing the nature and extent of malignant airway obstruction to allow preprocedural intervention planning.

The bronchoscopic approach to management of malignant airway obstruction depends on the lesion location, the presence or absence of associated extrinsic compression, and the degree of clinical urgency (**Table 11-3**). Rigid bronchoscopic debulking with adjunctive thermal ablation is recommended when airway recanalization must be performed on an emergency basis. If endobronchial obstruction is accompanied by marked extrinsic compression, stent placement may be beneficial (**Figure 11-16**).

The complexity of a lesion is equally important in determining the best approach to resection. Benign tracheal webs often are managed by laser or electrocautery-mediated resection

Table 11-3 Bronchoscopic Therapies

Therapy	Type of Lesion Therapy	Type of Bronchoscope	Rapidity of Positive Result	Repeatability
Mechanical débridement	Endoluminal or submucosal	Rigid or flexible (rigid preferable)	++++	+
Laser	Endoluminal	Rigid or flexible (rigid preferable)	++++	++++
Argon plasma	Endoluminal	Rigid or flexible	++++	++++
Brachytherapy	Endoluminal or submucosal	Flexible	+	+
Cryotherapy	Endoluminal	Rigid or flexible	++	+++
Balloon dilation	Endoluminal or submucosal with extraluminal compression	Rigid or flexible (rigid preferable)	++++	++++
Photodynamic therapy	Endoluminal	Flexible	++	+++
Electrocautery	Endoluminal	Rigid or flexible	+++	++++
Stent	Endoluminal with extraluminal compression	Rigid or flexible (Dumon stent requires rigid bronchoscope; Wall stents and Gianturco stents require fluoroscopy)	++++	+++

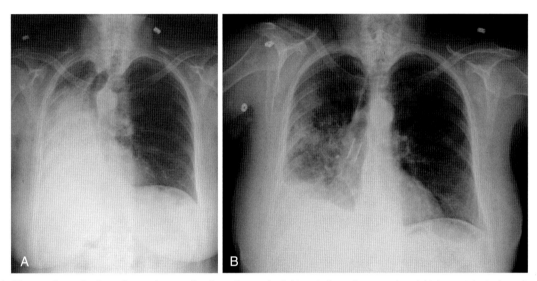

Figure 11-16 **A,** Chest radiograph of an obstructing small cell carcinoma in right main bronchus, causing right lung atelectasis and mediastinal shift. **B,** Radiographic appearance after rigid bronchoscopic debulking of the lesion and placement of a Dumon silicone stent. *(**A** and **B,** Courtesy Colin Gillespie, MD.)*

alone, whereas complex fibrotic strictures may warrant the combination of rigid bronchoscopic or balloon dilation, thermal incision, and stent placement. For focal tracheal stenosis in patients at low risk for complications, surgical resection with primary reanastomosis should remain the treatment of choice.

EXTRINSIC AIRWAY COMPRESSION

Extrinsic airway compression usually results from malignant involvement of structures adjacent to the central airways, such as mediastinal lymph nodes or the esophagus, but it may be associated with a benign process, such as fibrosing mediastinitis, tuberculosis, aneurysmal dilatation of the aorta, or sarcoidosis. The clinical signs and symptoms of extrinsic airway compression often mimic those of endobronchial obstruction. The diagnosis is established on the basis of bronchoscopic detection of marked airway narrowing in the absence of an endoluminal mass.

Therapeutic options in the management of extrinsic airway compression are limited. Ablative endoscopic approaches such as laser therapy, cryotherapy, PDT, and electrocautery are contraindicated because of the lack of demonstrable benefit and risk of airway perforation. Although some patients with malignant disease may benefit from endobronchial brachytherapy, tracheobronchial stent placement is the palliative treatment of choice for patients with symptomatic extrinsic airway compression.

TRACHEOBRONCHOMALACIA

Diffuse or focal tracheobronchomalacia is perhaps the most challenging disorder encountered by the therapeutic bronchoscopist. *Cartilaginous* tracheobronchomalacia, as seen in patients with relapsing polychondritis, reflects a loss of the structural integrity of the trachea and/or main bronchi secondary to airway cartilaginous ring destruction. *Membranous,* or *crescentic,* tracheobronchomalacia, also known as excessive dynamic airway collapse (EDAC), is manifested by displacement of the posterior membrane toward the anterior tracheal wall during exhalation as a result of trachea and main bronchus posterior membrane laxity and usually is seen in patients with

Figure 11-17 A, Tracheal buckling. In a patient presenting with dyspnea, cough, and stridor, bronchoscopic examination revealed localized upper tracheal buckling on hyperflexion of the neck. Symptoms cleared after three tracheal rings were resected. Histopathologic analysis showed localized tracheomalacia. **B,** "Saber sheath trachea." Fixed reduction in coronal diameter with concomitant increase in sagittal diameter of the trachea results in the classic bronchoscopic appearance of this lesion.

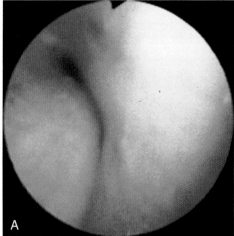
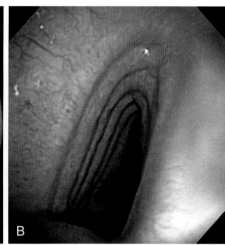

long-standing COPD. Focal tracheobronchomalacia may be a complication of long-standing intubation or an anastomotic complication after lung transplantation.

Tracheobronchomalacia is best diagnosed on the basis of findings on flexible bronchoscopy, performed with the patient breathing spontaneously (**Figure 11-17,** *A*), although dynamic CT scanning, with images obtained on inspiration and expiration, often is helpful. Tracheobronchomalacia should be distinguished from a *saber sheath trachea*, which is characterized by a fixed reduction of the transverse diameter of the intrathoracic portion of the trachea, in the presence of accentuation of the sagittal diameter (see Figure 11-17, *B*).

The endoscopic treatment of choice for patients with diffuse tracheobronchomalacia is the insertion of a standard or bifurcated silicone tracheobronchial stent. This intervention is more likely to be successful in patients with the cartilaginous type of tracheobronchomalacia than in those with the membranous type. Patients with membranous tracheobronchomalacia may benefit from a trial of silicone stent placement. For those who benefit in terms of decreased respiratory symptoms and improved pulmonary function, surgical plication or buttressing of the posterior membrane, or both, can be performed, often with good results and with facilitation of stent removal. For many patients with focal tracheomalacia, particularly from postintubation injury, surgical resection with primary reanastomosis is the best therapeutic option. An alternative treatment for selected patients with diffuse tracheobronchomalacia is the "pneumatic stent" provided by noninvasive ventilatory techniques such as continuous positive airway pressure.

CONTROL OF HEMOPTYSIS

In cases of hemoptysis, bronchoscopy may be of value not only for diagnosis but frequently for emergency management of endobronchial bleeding (**Box 11-5**). Because of difficulties with visualization, instruments with large and maximally effective suction channels should be used. Rigid bronchoscopy generally is preferred with massive bleeding and when the need to remove large clots is anticipated.

When continuous suctioning of blood fails to clear the airways, other means can be used. An iced saline solution can be instilled along with vasoactive drugs, such as epinephrine, to induce vasoconstriction. The bronchoscope itself can occlude the lumen of the bronchus from which the bleeding originates. The same effect, perhaps with better local control, can be

---

Box 11-5 Measures and Agents for Bronchoscopic Control of Hemoptysis

- Repeated suctioning (to keep open the airways)
- Iced saline irrigation
- Vasoactive drugs (epinephrine, vasopressin analogues)
- Bronchoscopic tamponade
- Balloon tamponade
- Tamponade with gauze or surgical gel (Gelfoam)
- Thrombin or fibrinogen instillation
- Laser coagulation
- Argon plasma coagulator
- Electrocautery
- Cryotherapy*
- Bronchoscopic brachytherapy†
- Isolation of bronchial tree (e.g., double-lumen endotracheal tube)

*Not suitable for management of massive hemoptysis.
†Not suitable for management of massive hemoptysis or for acute control of hemoptysis.

---

achieved with bronchoscopic balloon catheters (**Figure 11-18**). Specially designed catheters have been developed for introduction through the working channel of the flexible bronchoscope, several permitting subsequent removal of the scope while the tamponading balloon remains in place, as well as the potential for suctioning beyond the balloon for clearance of blood from distal airways. Another effective method for control of visible sources of bleeding, particularly from endobronchial neoplasms, is Nd:YAG laser photocoagulation.

Recent reports have demonstrated the benefit of endobronchial packing, accomplished using either flexible or rigid bronchoscopy, with oxidized regenerated cellulose (Surgicel), which functions in multiple capacities, including local tamponade and isolation at the segmental or subsegmental bleeding site, absorption of blood, and promotion of endobronchial clot formation by induction of fibrin polymerization. This procedure may obviate the need for bronchial artery embolization or other, more invasive procedures.

REMOVAL OF FOREIGN BODIES

Foreign body aspiration is more likely to occur in children than in adults, with most occurring in children younger than 3 years. In children the obstruction most often involves a mainstem

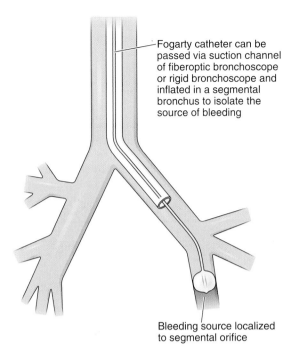

Fogarty catheter can be passed via suction channel of fiberoptic bronchoscope or rigid bronchoscope and inflated in a segmental bronchus to isolate the source of bleeding

Bleeding source localized to segmental orifice

Figure 11-18 Placement of a Fogarty balloon catheter under bronchoscopic guidance to control massive hemorrhage from a segmental or lobar bronchus. *(From Lordan JL, Gascoigne A, Corris PA: The pulmonary physician in critical care: illustrative case 7: assessment and management of massive hemoptysis, Thorax 58:814-819, 2003.)*

bronchus, whereas in adults most foreign bodies are wedged distally, most commonly in the right lower lobe. Before the development of bronchoscopy, most foreign body aspirations resulted in high morbidity and mortality, commonly from postobstructive pneumonia. Until the introduction of the flexible bronchoscope, all foreign body removals were accomplished with rigid bronchoscopy. Even at present, the rigid bronchoscope remains the tool of choice for the removal of foreign bodies, especially in children. The advantage of the rigid instrument resides in its larger access channel, permitting use of larger and more adaptable retrieval tools and ability to simultaneously provide and maintain ventilation. In adults, flexible bronchoscopy is the most common initial diagnostic tool for foreign body aspiration and allows for successful foreign body removal in most cases.

Various types of instruments have been developed for use with bronchoscopy for the removal of foreign bodies, including grasping forceps, balloon catheters, retrieval baskets, snares, and magnetic extractors. The instrument choice depends on the specifics of the type of foreign body and its location in the tracheobronchial tree. Grasping forceps may be helpful in the retrieval of hard objects with an irregular surface. Smooth objects or organic material (e.g., nuts, food particles) may require the use of expandable baskets or a combination of balloon catheters, suction devices, and grasping forceps. Fogarty balloon catheters frequently are used to dislodge a foreign body and bring it proximally into the trachea before its removal with other instruments.

Special attention should be paid to the period after removal of the foreign body, because serious complications can occur. Patients should be observed closely for any signs of hemoptysis, subcutaneous emphysema, or subglottic edema. Trauma inflicted during the extraction or forceful manipulation of instruments greatly accentuates the risk of postoperative complications, particularly if oversized instruments are used or if the bronchoscopy procedure is prolonged.

ASPIRATION OF SECRETIONS

According to a survey of bronchoscopists in the United States, removal of retained secretions is cited as a leading indication for therapeutic bronchoscopy. Bronchoscopic secretion aspiration may be indicated in patients presenting with respiratory muscle weakness (e.g., because of underlying neuromuscular disease or the postoperative state) or disorders leading to recurrent aspiration of food or excessive upper airway secretions. In critically ill or mechanically ventilated patients, removal of secretions and mucous plugs usually can be rapidly achieved through the flexible bronchoscope. A flexible scope with a large-diameter suction channel should be chosen for this procedure. The nature of the retained material—its consistency and viscosity—may dictate frequent bronchoscopy procedures to relieve segmental or lobar atelectasis because of inspissated mucous plugs. Underlying pulmonary diseases, such as bronchiectasis, may aggravate the airway secretion retention. Bronchoscopic secretion aspiration should not be considered "routine" in the postoperative period or in other conditions in which good chest physiotherapy and maintenance of adequate pulmonary toilet could be more effective.

Two specific disorders are worth highlighting in the context of therapeutic bronchoscopy: pulmonary alveolar proteinosis (PAP) and allergic bronchopulmonary aspergillosis (ABPA). In PAP, BAL has been used for therapeutic clearance of alveolar material, although the standard approach is whole-lung lavage that uses double-lumen endotracheal tube intubation. In ABPA, lavage with saline solution may be insufficient to remove tenacious impactions (described as "plastic bronchitis"). In these circumstances, use of bronchoscopic forceps or snare may prove helpful.

CLOSURE OF BRONCHIAL FISTULAS

Prolonged air leaks are a common problem associated with primary or secondary pneumothorax and are the most frequent complication after pulmonary resection, with the highest rate after lung volume reduction surgery (LVRS). The current management for prolonged air leaks usually includes prolonged chest tube drainage with Heimlich valve, attempts at surgical repair, and/or blood patch and pleurodesis.

Either flexible or rigid bronchoscopy can be a useful intervention in confirming suspected bronchopleural fistulas or alveolopleural fistulas and in specifying their precise location. The most common approach is to perform selective airway occlusion with a balloon catheter while observing the chest tube air leak rate or volume. Depending on the fistula location and the size, bronchoscopic procedures can be attempted with the goal of occlusion and sealing the bronchopleural fistulas. Small bronchial openings in an otherwise normal bronchus after thoracic surgery respond much better, with a higher rate of success of bronchoscopic sealing. It is much more difficult to achieve good obliteration of a fistula if it is infected or is due to an underlying malignancy. Many different techniques for permanent closure have been used, including introduction of bronchial mucosal irritants (e.g., silver nitrate), with the object of stimulating reactive granulation tissue formation. Several potentially useful agents have been described, including surgical gel (Gelfoam), autologous blood patch, cryoprecipitate, and thrombin injection to create fibrin clot. In addition, laser photocoagulation surrounding small, proximal bronchopleural fistulas has been reported to be beneficial. Recent case series suggest that the placement of one-way endobronchial valves leads to complete or partial resolution in the large majority of patients with prolonged air leaks from diverse causes.

BRONCHOSCOPIC TREATMENTS FOR COMMON "BENIGN" LUNG DISEASES

One of the major advances in therapeutic bronchoscopic use over the past decade has been the development of experimental bronchoscopic interventions for highly prevalent lung diseases such as asthma and emphysema.

BRONCHOSCOPIC TREATMENTS FOR EMPHYSEMA

The risks associated with LVRS, in which diseased portions of emphysematous lung are resected through median sternotomy or with use of videothoracoscopy, including a perioperative mortality of 5% or greater, as well as substantial perioperative morbidity, have spurred the development of minimally invasive approaches for dyspnea palliation in patients with emphysema. The bronchoscopic lung volume reduction (BLVR) approaches evaluated have used a range of different techniques, including airway occlusion with silicone plugs (i.e., Endobronchial Watanabe Spigot [EWS]); insertion of one-way bronchial valves; and creation of artificial noncompressible communications ("bypass tracts") between cartilaginous airways and emphysematous parenchyma. Endobronchial valves are designed to limit ventilation to the most severely emphysematous regions of lung and reduce dynamic hyperinflation. When placed correctly, the valves allow one-way flow of secretions and air out of the occluded pulmonary segment. The major advantage of the bronchial valve approach for emphysema palliation is the potential for reversibility—the valves generally are removable with minimal risk to the patient. The bane of the pulmonologist attempting to use bronchial valves in the treatment of emphysema is collateral ventilation, which inhibits induction of atelectasis, thereby preventing successful lung volume reduction. Results from the first randomized study of endobronchial valves, a double-blinded sham-controlled multicenter trial of the Zephyr endobronchial valve, demonstrated modest increases in forced expiratory ventilation in 1 second (FEV_1) and 6-minute walk distance at 6 months, but unfortunately with an increased rate of complications, including COPD exacerbations and hemoptysis.

The results from the randomized study of Airway Bypass also did not demonstrate statistically significant improvements in the primary end points of forced vital capacity (FVC) and dyspnea score. Studies evaluating the use of other novel endobronchial approaches are ongoing. These include the placement of airway implants (e.g., Nitinol coils); intrabronchial injection of steam to induce tissue necrosis resulting in loss of lung tissue, volume, and ventilation; and biologic restructuring of emphysematous lung parenchyma to induce tissue fibrosis, atelectasis, and contraction, with consequent lung volume reduction. The latter approach was inspired by numerous case reports of "medical" lung volume reduction, in which patients with heterogeneous emphysema achieved significant clinical and physiologic improvements in lung function after receiving external beam radiation therapy for an upper lobe non–small cell carcinoma or after developing infection or inflammation in an upper lobe bulla resulting in fibrosis and contraction of the bullous lung tissue after resolution of the infectious or inflammatory process. One of the major downsides of the biologic approach to lung volume reduction is the permanent destruction of lung tissue, with no option for reversibility in the event of worsening lung function.

BRONCHIAL THERMOPLASTY

Chronic asthma is a major cause of morbidity and death and also a major contributor to rapidly rising health care costs. Bronchial thermoplasty (BT) is a new bronchoscopic procedure that delivers controlled thermal energy to the bronchial wall of conducting airways, with the intent to inhibit airway smooth muscle contractile function. This offers the potential to attenuate bronchoconstriction occurring during asthma exacerbations. BT is performed by use of a single-use radiofrequency device that delivers thermal energy to the bronchial wall during an outpatient bronchoscopic procedure. Three separate procedures are performed in order to treat all accessible upper and lower lobe airways, ranging from 3 to 10 mm in diameter. The initial randomized, multicenter Airway Intervention with Radiofrequency (AIR) trial in patients with moderate to severe disease demonstrated decreased asthma exacerbations in the group undergoing BT compared with those patients treated with standard medical treatment alone. This was followed by a randomized, sham-controlled multicenter trial (AIR2) demonstrating significant improvement in the primary end point, asthma-related quality of life. Although an increase was noted in early posttreatment asthma exacerbations requiring emergency department visits and hospitalizations, the long-term follow-up data showed decreased asthma-related health care utilization for patients undergoing BT as opposed to the sham procedure. On the basis of these data, BT should be considered for patients with severe asthma that is not well controlled by medication therapy. Studies are ongoing to collect additional safety data and to assess the durability of the BT treatment effect.

COMPLICATIONS OF THERAPEUTIC BRONCHOSCOPIC TECHNIQUES

The advent of interventional bronchoscopy has resulted in complications not ordinarily seen with diagnostic bronchoscopy. Inappropriate use of lasers has resulted in endobronchial burns and bronchial perforations associated with catastrophic bleeding, pneumomediastinum, or pneumothorax. Endobronchial edema and mucosal sloughing also may occur as a result of laser thermal effects.

As noted previously, the use of airway stents is associated with several complications. Stents may not be properly adapted to the diameter of the airway, resulting in either incomplete stent deployment or stent migration, possibly engendering life-threatening airway obstruction. The presence of an endoprosthesis in the airway may predispose the patient to difficulties with secretion clearance and accumulation of inspissated mucus. Placement of SEMSs may be followed by severe local airway reactions, with consequent formation of granulation tissue, hemorrhage, or bronchial perforation.

SUMMARY

Technologic advances in bronchoscopy continue to improve the pulmonologist's ability to perform minimally invasive, accurate evaluations of the tracheobronchial tree and to implement an ever-increasing array of diagnostic, therapeutic, and palliative interventions. The role of both diagnostic and therapeutic bronchoscopy will continue to evolve as further improvements are made in bronchoscopes, accessory equipment, and imaging technologies. Therapeutic bronchoscopy may soon be used to provide treatment for conditions that traditionally have been treated with surgery. The major challenge in the adoption of the many new bronchoscopic techniques into routine clinical practice is the need for well-designed studies to delineate the appropriate use of these interventions and to better define their limitations.

SUGGESTED READINGS

Beamis JF Jr, Mathur PN, Mehta AC, editors: *Interventional pulmonary medicine*, New York, 2004, Marcel Dekker.

Bolliger CT, Mathur PN, Beamis JF, et al: ERS/ATS statement on interventional pulmonology. European Respiratory Society/American Thoracic Society, *Eur Respir J* 19:356–373, 2002.

Cox G, Thomson NC, Rubin AS, et al: AIR Trial Study Group: Asthma control during the year after bronchial thermoplasty, *N Engl J Med* 356:1327–1337, 2007.

Ernst A, Silvestri GA, Johnstone D: ACCP Interventional/Diagnostic Procedures Network Steering Committee: Interventional pulmonary procedures. Guidelines from the American College of Chest Physicians, *Chest* 123:1693–1717, 2003.

Mehta AC, Prakash US, Garland R, et al: 2005 American College of Chest Physicians and American Association for Bronchology Consensus Statement: prevention of flexible bronchoscopy-associated infection, *Chest* 128:1742–1755, 2005.

Seijo LM, Sterman DH: Medical progress: interventional pulmonology, *N Engl J Med* 344:740–749, 2001.

Simoff MJ, Sterman DH, Ernst A, editors: *Thoracic endoscopy: advances in interventional pulmonology*, Malden, Mass, 2006, Blackwell.

Wang KP, Mehta AC, Turner JF Jr, editors: *Flexible bronchoscopy*, Malden, Mass, 2004, Blackwell.

Chapter **12**

Endobronchial and Endoesophageal Ultrasound Techniques

Felix J.F. Herth

Lung cancer is still the leading cause of cancer deaths worldwide, with an overall 5-year survival rate of 10% to 15%. Mediastinal lymph node sampling in lung cancer is important for adequate staging to determine appropriate treatment, as well as for predicting outcome. Adequate staging of lung cancer also is important in order to improve research into lung cancer, both for accurate comparison of data and for quality control.

Mediastinal lymph node staging can be performed preoperatively by radiologic imaging, endoscopically, or surgically. CT scanning, magnetic resonance imaging (MRI), positron emission tomography (PET), and integrated PET-CT are useful noninvasive imaging techniques for staging of lung cancer; however, they are not sufficiently sensitive or specific to determine mediastinal lymph node involvement. CT scanning usually is the initial method for staging of mediastinal nodes. Only lymph nodes with a short-axis diameter greater than 1 cm (with or without positive findings on PET-CT or other PET study) usually are considered to be suspicious for malignant involvement by radiologic criteria set forth in national and international guidelines. Nevertheless, in view of the high false-positive rate for CT and PET-CT, neither of which provides a tissue diagnosis, it is important to obtain lymph node tissue to determine operability.

Mediastinoscopy with nodal biopsy has been the "gold standard" for mediastinal staging for many years and has a sensitivity of 90% to 95% for detection of metastases in this region. Only certain lymph node stations—2, 4, and anterior 7—are accessible by this approach, in which access to the posterior and inferior mediastinum is limited, typically necessitating extending the procedure to cervical mediastinoscopy or thoracoscopy. However, it is essentially a surgical approach requiring general anesthesia and occasionally hospitalization. Endoscopic techniques provide a minimally invasive alternative to surgical staging. Accordingly, the past few years have seen the development of a number of less invasive staging modalities, including endobronchial ultrasound (EBUS) and endoesophageal ultrasound (EUS) techniques.

TRANSBRONCHIAL NEEDLE ASPIRATION

Merely a curiosity at its inception, flexible bronchoscopy has emerged as an essential diagnostic and therapeutic modality in the management of a variety of lung diseases. The addition of transbronchial needle aspiration (TBNA) not only improved bronchoscopy's diagnostic yield but further extended the role of this modality in the evaluation of mediastinal disease, and in the diagnosis and staging of bronchogenic carcinoma. The first description of sampling mediastinal lymph nodes through the tracheal carina using a rigid bronchoscope was by Schieppati. In 1978, Wang and associates demonstrated that it was feasible to sample paratracheal nodes using TBNA. Subsequent publications highlighted the use of the technique in the diagnosis of endobronchial (**Figure 12-1**) and peripheral lesions and the ability of TBNA to provide a diagnosis even in the absence of endobronchial disease.

The diagnostic yield of TBNA in the assessment of hilar-mediastinal lymph node involvement in lung cancer varies greatly in published series, with reported rates ranging from 15% to 85%. Recently, a metaanalysis assessing TBNA for mediastinal staging in non–small cell lung cancer demonstrated that TBNA is highly specific for the identification of mediastinal metastases, with sensitivity depending heavily on the study population under investigation. In studies that included patient populations with a prevalence of mediastinal metastases of 34%, sensitivity was only 39%, whereas in a population with a prevalence of 81%, sensitivity for detection of metastases was 78%.

Nevertheless, even after more than 50 years since the advent of TBNA, the technique is still underused. The main reasons for the limited use of TBNA have been lack of needle monitoring, difficulties in performing the procedure, and a belief, despite good evidence to the contrary, that TBNA is not useful.

ENDOBRONCHIAL ULTRASOUND TECHNIQUE

The integration of ultrasound technology and flexible fiberoptic bronchoscopy enables imaging of lymph nodes, lesions, and vessels located beyond the tracheobronchial mucosa. Developed in 2002, the EBUS bronchoscope looks similar to a normal bronchovideoscope (**Figure 12-2**) but is 6.9 mm wide and has a 2-mm instrument channel and a 30-degree side viewing optic. Furthermore, a curved linear array ultrasound transducer sits on the distal end and can be used either with direct contact to the mucosal surface or with an inflatable balloon that can be attached at the tip. This setup produces a conventional endoscopic picture side by side with the ultrasound view. Ultrasound scanning is performed at a frequency of 7.5 to 12 MHz, with tissue penetration of 20 to 50 mm. An ultrasound processor generates the ultrasound image.

EBUS allows the bronchoscopist to visualize airway structures as well as surrounding processes. It is useful for staging advanced cancer, especially as it relates to intramural or nodal

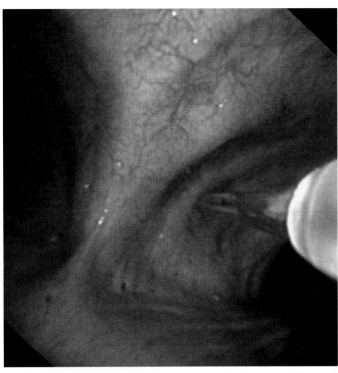

Figure 12-1   Classical transbronchial needle aspiration (TBNA) biopsy of the lymph node.

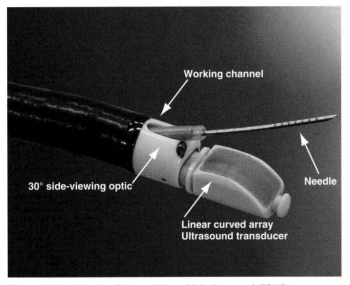

Figure 12-2   The tip of the endobronchial ultrasound (EBUS) scope. The transbronchial needle aspiration (TBNA) needle is already inserted.

Working channel

30° side-viewing optic

Linear curved array Ultrasound transducer

Needle

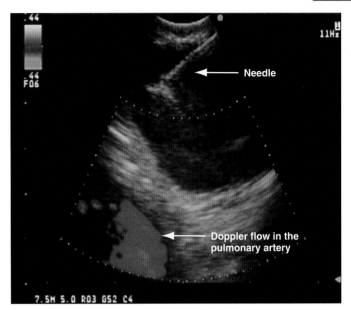

Figure 12-3   Endobronchial ultrasound–transbronchial needle aspiration (EBUS-TBNA) of a lymph node in position 4R.

Needle

Doppler flow in the pulmonary artery

spread. EBUS can identify N1, N2, and N3 nodes without the need for surgical intervention and can hence decrease the need for expensive surgery.

Procedure

The actual TBNA is performed using direct transducer contact with the wall of the trachea or bronchus. When a lesion is outlined, a 21 or 22 gauge needle can be advanced through the working channel, and lymph nodes can be punctured under real-time ultrasound visualization. The needle is encased in an internal sheath in order to avoid contamination during biopsy. At the same time, color Doppler can be used to identify surrounding vascular structures. Once the target lymph node or mass has been clearly identified with EBUS, the needle is

inserted under real-time ultrasound guidance and then placed within the lesion (**Figures 12-3** and **12-4**). Suction is applied with a syringe, and the needle is moved back and forth to achieve multiple punctures. The stylet of the needle is left in place on the first puncture to minimize bronchial cell contamination; once the needle tip is inside the target tissue, the stylet is removed. We stab the target 10 to 15 times without suction and apply suction only for the last two or three stabbing motions. Before retraction of the needle into the needle sheath, suction must be removed to minimize sample loss into the syringe. The specimen is then air-flushed onto a slide, and the needle is flushed with heparin-saline solution to avoid clotting; the same procedure is repeated three times at every lymph node station.

Lymph node stations that can be reached using EBUS are the highest mediastinal (station 1), the upper paratracheal (2L and 2R), the lower paratracheal (4R and 4L), the subcarinal (station 7), the hilar (station 10) nodes, as well as the interlobar (station 11) and lobar (station 12) nodes. The highest-staging node (e.g., an N3 contralateral mediastinal lymph node before an N2, an ipsilateral mediastinal lymph node before an N1 hilar lymph node) should be biopsied first; otherwise, the needle needs to be changed each time.

Lymph nodes at a size of 5 mm and upwards can be successfully sampled and have to date shown excellent diagnostic yield. The number of mediastinal lymph node stations to sample depends on the purpose of the examination.

Every attempt should be made to sample nodes at these sites, even if size and ultrasonographic features are normal. At our institution, we routinely sample mediastinal lymph nodes that are 5 mm or larger in short-axis diameter.

The learning curve for EBUS-TBNA has been evaluated: performance of at least 10 procedures is necessary in order to achieve excellent sensitivity and diagnostic accuracy, although that number may be higher, depending on operator skill level.

Results

In recently published metaanalysis, EBUS-TBNA has been shown to have a high pooled sensitivity of 93% and specificity of 100%. Multiple publications have shown that even in

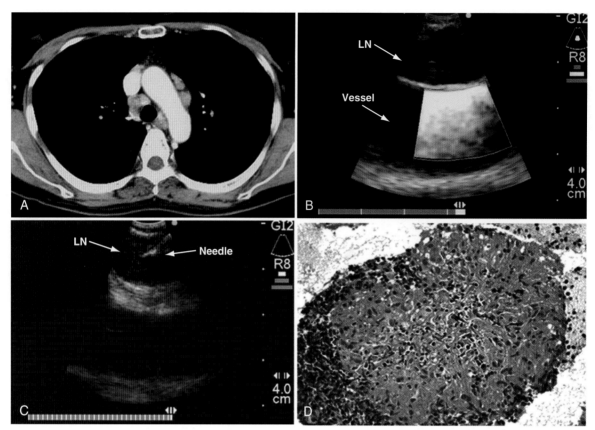

Figure 12-4 **A,** Enlarged lymph node in the upper mediastinum in position 4r. **B,** The vessels are readily seen on the power Doppler image. **C,** Real-time ultrasound image of the aspiration biopsy procedure. **D,** The histopathologic pattern was consistent with a diagnosis of sarcoidosis. *LN*, lymph node.

patients with lymph nodes less than 1 cm in diameter (which had been termed N0 by CT criteria), with the use of EBUS-TBNA, a large percentage could still be shown to have N2 or N3 disease (in some cases, despite a negative result on PET-CT).

Numerous studies have looked at the use of EBUS-TBNA for biomarkers and tumor genetics in lung cancer. In a recent published trial, endothelial growth factor receptor (EGFR) gene analysis of the EBUS-TBNA sample was feasible in 26 of 36 patients (72.2%) with lymph node metastasis. Somatic mutations of the *EGFR* gene were detected in tissue obtained through EBUS-TBNA in 2 of 20 patients (10%) with metastatic lung adenocarcinoma. Complications such as bleeding or infection are very rare and have been reported only as case reports.

EBUS-TBNA also has been shown to have utility in diagnosis of other pulmonary diseases besides lung cancer. In patients with clinically suspected lymphoma, the reported diagnostic sensitivity is 70% to 80%. If more tissue specimens are needed for histologic analysis, it is even possible to insert a 1.15-mm mini-forceps through the EBUS scope and past the airway wall via a needle puncture, to obtain forceps biopsy specimens of mediastinal lymph nodes under real-time ultrasound guidance.

Different prospective studies have assessed the usefulness of EBUS-TBNA in evaluation of patients with suspected sarcoidosis. EBUS-TBNA has been reported to have a diagnostic yield of 85% to 93%, which increases with the number of passes performed. In one study in which a cytopathologist performed on-site evaluations, the diagnostic yield was greater than 80% at five passes and did not increase further after seven passes. In a recently published randomized controlled trial, EBUS-TBNA

provided a diagnostic yield superior to that with conventional TBNA (83% versus 54%). In patients with suspected sarcoidosis, EUS-FNA has a similar diagnostic yield of 82% to 86%. The choice between the two diagnostic methods is therefore based on the location and accessibility of the enlarged lymph nodes and on the expertise of the operator.

ENDOESOPHAGEAL ULTRASOUND TECHNIQUE

Gastroenterologists have been using the endoesophageal ultrasound (EUS) technique for many years in the investigation of esophageal and pancreatic malignancies. Mediastinal EUS-guided fine needle aspiration (FNA) was first used in the early 1990s and subsequently has become a popular method to diagnose a variety of intraabdominal and intrathoracic masses, including mediastinal lesions. EUS-FNA has been shown to be useful in biopsying mediastinal lesions, even in patients in whom a previous conventional technique was nondiagnostic, and may be more cost-effective as an initial staging procedure in patients with non–small cell lung cancer (NSCLC) than classical techniques.

Procedure

The linear EUS bronchoscope has the same basic architecture as that of the EBUS scope and uses a scanner frequency of between 5 and 10 MHz. The penetrating ultrasound depth can be up to 8 cm. Needles used for biopsy are 19 or 21 gauge, again equipped with a stylet. The procedure usually is performed on an outpatient basis and takes approximately 30 minutes. As with EBUS, the puncture of lymph nodes is performed under real-time ultrasound guidance (**Figure 12-5**).

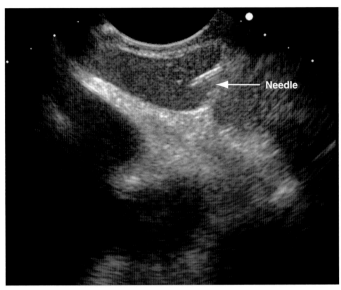

Figure 12-5 Endoesophageal ultrasound–guided fine needle aspiration (EUS-FNA) of an enlarged node in station 7.

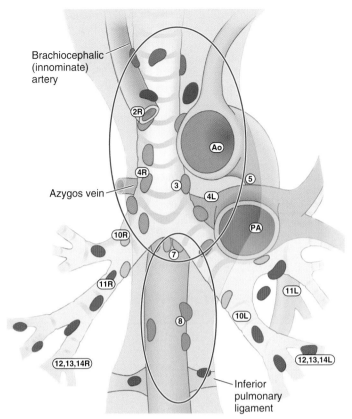

Figure 12-6 Region of access for endobronchial needle aspiration (*blue-outlined oval*) and for endoesophageal needle aspiration (*red-outlined oval*). *Ao,* aorta; *PA,* pulmonary artery.

However, EUS-FNA has limited access, because only lymph node stations 2L, 4L, 7, 8, and 9 are accessible through a transesophageal approach. Lymph node station 5 is not routinely accessible by EUS, and transvascular FNA may be required to sample this tissue.

Results

EUS is especially useful in staging of the posterior mediastinum. The left adrenal can be reached and identified in 97% of cases. It has a characteristic "seagull" shape on ultrasound images and is particularly well visualized in cases of metastatic enlargement. Furthermore, the left lobe of the liver also can be reached. The hilar and precarinal lymph nodes cannot be reached.

The procedure carries only a very small risk of mediastinitis or bleeding. Unless cysts are punctured antibiotics do not need to be administered routinely.

EUS is more accurate and has a higher predictive value than either PET scan or CT for assessment of posterior mediastinal lymph nodes.

Multiple publications and a metaanalysis of data on EUS-FNA have shown high sensitivity and specificity. Even in cases in which mediastinal lymph node enlargement is not seen on CT, EUS-FNA has been able to demonstrate metastases in 25% of patients with lung cancer.

For both techniques, however, it is important to recognize that the negative predictive value (NPV) is limited. Therefore, if samples do not contain tumor cells, follow-up evaluation with a more definitive procedure such as mediastinoscopy with biopsy or video-assisted thoracoscopic surgery (VATS) is indicated.

COMBINING ENDOBRONCHIAL AND ENDOESOPHAGEAL ULTRASOUND TECHNIQUES

For tissue sampling of mediastinal lymph nodes after conventional TBNA, our own preference is for minimally invasive methods such as EBUS-TBNA and EUS-FNA over more invasive procedures such as mediastinoscopy and VATS. EUS-FNA and EBUS-TBNA have been shown to avoid the need for mediastinoscopy to a large extent (**Figure 12-6**). EBUS-TBNA

and EUS-FNA have a complementary reach in analyzing mediastinal nodes: EBUS has access to the paratracheal, subcarinal, and hilar regions, and EUS, to the lower mediastinum and aortopulmonary window.

Increasingly, EUS-FNA and EBUS-TBNA are thought of as complementary rather than competitive procedures. In principle, the combined access to mediastinal, hilar, and periesophageal disease affords the most complete staging possible.

As shown above, EUS and EBUS provide access to different areas of the mediastinum. In combining techniques, most lymph node stations as well as the left adrenal gland can be reached (apart from stations 5 and 6). In six recent series, the accuracy of EUS-FNA and EBUS-TBNA used in combination for the diagnosis of mediastinal cancer was 95%. With use of the EBUS scope for concurrent endobronchial and endoesophageal sampling in the same patient, the sensitivity for cancer detection combining the results with both modes of access can be as high as 96% (sensitivity of 89% for EUS and 91% for EBUS); specificity, 100%; and NPV value, 96% (NPV for EUS alone of 82% and for EBUS alone, 92%).

In a recently published trial, the hypothesis of the current guidelines recommending minimally invasive endosonography followed by surgical staging (if no nodal metastases are found by endosonography) as an alternative to immediate surgical staging was proved in a randomized design. Patients were randomly assigned to undergo either surgical staging alone (the surgical staging group, representing the current standard of care) or endosonography (combined EUS-FNA and EBUS-TBNA) followed by surgical staging if no nodal metastases were found at endosonography (the endosonography group, representing a novel alternative staging strategy). A total of 241 patients were enrolled in the trial. Nodal metastases were found in 41 patients by surgical staging and in 56 patients by endosonography, and in 62 patients by endosonography followed by surgical staging. These findings corresponded to sensitivity of 79% (versus 85%) and 94%. Thoracotomy was unnecessary in 21 patients in the mediastinoscopy group, versus 9 in the endosonography group (P = .02). The complication rates were similar in both groups, although a majority of complications in the endosonography group were due to the addition of surgery. The investigators concluded that among patients with NSCLC, a staging strategy combining endosonography and surgical staging versus surgical staging alone resulted in greater sensitivity for detection of mediastinal nodal metastases without unnecessary thoracotomies.

A reasonable approach, therefore, is to begin the staging evaluation with EBUS or EUS. If the result is positive, the staging process is complete. If it is negative, a strategy of surgical staging followed by immediate surgery is recommended.

RESTAGING PATIENTS WITH LUNG CANCER AFTER CHEMOTHERAPY

Patients with N2 disease (stage IIIA) considered unresectable at diagnosis may nevertheless become candidates for surgical resection if chemotherapy or chemoradiation therapy can lead to successful downstaging. Documentation of downstaging (complete histopathologic response in N2 lymph nodes) is essential for such potentially curative resection. Imaging procedures (CT and PET-CT) are helpful in this regard but show unacceptably high rates of false-positive and false-negative results, and a tissue diagnosis is required to guide management. EUS-FNA or EBUS-TBNA, or both, can be performed depending on the location of the lymph nodes initially involved. Usually the mediastinal N2 lymph node that initially was proved to be positive should be rebiopsied using the same techniques. Mediastinoscopy, which is technically difficult as a consequence of fibrosis, especially after radiation therapy, usually is reserved for cases in which analysis of samples obtained by endoscopic needling techniques fails to show malignancy. Compared with initial mediastinoscopy, repeat mediastinoscopy is associated with lower sensitivity and diagnostic accuracy. With all other diagnostic techniques, restaging sensitivity and accuracy are lower than for the initial procedure as a result of the effects of chemotherapy and irradiation on tissues with ensuing fibrosis, as well as tumor shrinkage, necrosis, and cystic degeneration. In a study of 124 patients with NSCLC who had undergone induction chemotherapy, restaging by EBUS-TBNA found persistent nodal metastases in 89 patients (72%); however, 28 of the 35 patients with negative results on EBUS were found to have residual N2 disease at surgery. Therefore, the NPV of EBUS-TBNA in restaging was only 20%.

In a recent published trial, a total of 61 patients underwent restaging EBUS-TBNA. EBUS-TBNA revealed metastatic lymph node involvement in 30% of patients. In 43 patients with negative or uncertain results on EBUS-TBNA, metastatic disease remaining in nodes was diagnosed in nine patients, in seven in stations accessible for EBUS-TBNA, and in two stations not accessible for EBUS-TBNA. The false-negative results of biopsies were found only in small nodes. Moreover, all positive N2 nodes diagnosed by surgery contained only small metastatic deposits. Reported values for diagnostic sensitivity, specificity, accuracy, positive predictive value (PPV), and NPV of the restaging EBUS-TBNA were 67%, 86%, 80%, 91%, and 78%, respectively.

The value of EUS-FNA in restaging of the mediastinum also was evaluated in other trials. The numbers of patients included in these trials are limited in comparison with the EBUS trials, but all series showed an NPV above 90%.

As mentioned before, the adequate restaging technique remains a matter of debate, because comparison of the different techniques is still problematic. Endoscopic techniques are safe and minimally invasive and produce accurate results in comparison with surgical data from repeat mediastinoscopy. However, if results on needle aspiration are negative, surgical restaging is required for adequate assessment of the mediastinum.

CONCLUSIONS AND OUTLOOK

Overall, EBUS and EUS are safe and effective techniques for staging of mediastinal disease. The novel diagnostic modalities of EBUS-guided TBNA and transesophageal ultrasound–guided FNA allow ultrasound-controlled mediastinal tissue sampling. These techniques are minimally invasive, avoiding many of the risks associated with invasive staging procedures.

At present, the main limitation with TBNA is the current restriction of its use to EBUS and EUS, which are performed predominantly at major clinical centers and hence only in selected patients. Training of physicians and surgeons remains the issue, and performance of an adequate numbers of procedures per year is required in order to maintain competency. Reimbursement remains an issue in some countries, as well as actual implementation and incorporation into cancer guidelines within hospitals. Increasingly, both techniques are being used in hospitals across the world, with consequent improvement in diagnostic yield. Use of combined EBUS and EUS, as the first ultrasound techniques for detection of metastases to the mediastinum, has been termed "complete endo-echo staging."

Beyond doubt, implementation of these techniques can be expected to drastically alter lung cancer staging algorithms in the near future. Thanks to its minimally invasive approach, safety record, accuracy, and diagnostic reach, complete ambulatory endoscopic staging of lung cancer may be the way of the future.

SUGGESTED READINGS

Annema JT, van Meerbeeck JP, Rintoul RC, et al: Mediastinoscopy vs endosonography for mediastinal nodal staging of lung cancer: a randomized trial, *JAMA* 304:2245–2252, 2010.

Gu P, Zhao YZ, Jiang LY, et al: Endobronchial ultrasound-guided transbronchial needle aspiration for staging of lung cancer: a systematic review and meta-analysis, *Eur J Cancer* 45:1389–1396, 2009.

Herth FJ: Mediastinal staging—the role of endobronchial and endo-oesophageal sonographic guided needle aspiration, *Lung Cancer* 45(Suppl 2):S63–S67, 2004.

Herth FJ, Eberhardt R, Krasnik M, Ernst A: Endobronchial ultrasound-guided transbronchial needle aspiration of lymph nodes in the radiologically and positron emission tomography-normal mediastinum in patients with lung cancer, *Chest* 133:887–891, 2008.

Herth FJ, Krasnik M, Kahn N, et al: Combined endoesophageal-endobronchial ultrasound-guided, fine-needle aspiration of mediastinal lymph nodes through a single bronchoscope in 150 patients with suspected lung cancer, *Chest* 138:790–794, 2010.

Holty JE, Kuschner WG, Gould MK: Accuracy of transbronchial needle aspiration for mediastinal staging of non-small cell lung cancer: a meta-analysis, *Thorax* 60:949–955, 2005.

Hwangbo B, Lee GK, Lee HS, et al: Transbronchial and transesophageal fine-needle aspiration using an ultrasound bronchoscope in mediastinal staging of potentially operable lung cancer, *Chest* 138: 795–802, 2010.

Micames CG, McCrory DC, Pavey DA, et al: Endoscopic ultrasound-guided fine-needle aspiration for non-small cell lung cancer staging: a systematic review and metaanalysis, *Chest* 131:539–548, 2007.

Silvestri GA, Gould MK, Margolis ML, et al: Noninvasive staging of non-small cell lung cancer: ACCP evidence-based clinical practice guidelines (2nd edition), *Chest* 132:178S–201S, 2007.

Varadarajulu S, Eloubeidi M: Can endoscopic ultrasonography-guided fine-needle aspiration predict response to chemoradiation in non-small cell lung cancer? A pilot study, *Respiration* 73:213–220, 2006.

Vilmann P, Herth F, Krasnik M: State of the art lecture: mediastinal EUS, *Endoscopy* 38(Suppl 1):S84–S87, 2006.

Wang KP, Terry P, Marsh B: Bronchoscopic needle aspiration biopsy of paratracheal tumors, *Am Rev Respir Dis* 118:17–21, 1978.

Yasufuku K, Chiyo M, Sekine Y, et al: Real-time endobronchial ultrasound-guided transbronchial needle aspiration of mediastinal and hilar lymph nodes, *Chest* 126:122–128, 2004.

Chapter 13

Percutaneous Biopsy Procedures: Techniques and Indications

Asia A. Ahmed • Magali N. Taylor • Penny J. Shaw

This chapter describes the techniques and equipment available to obtain diagnostic samples from intrathoracic and selected extrathoracic lesions by the percutaneous route. The common lesions sampled and their locations are listed in **Figure 13-1**. The most frequent methods of sampling intrathoracic lesions, depending on their site, are summarized in **Figure 13-2**. The techniques and indications are different from those required to diagnose more diffuse intrapulmonary disease. The latter, which includes conditions such as idiopathic pulmonary fibrosis, requires a transbronchial lung biopsy or an open lung biopsy through a mini-thoracotomy or video-assisted thoracoscopy (VATS) procedure.

Imaging plays an important role in detecting and confirming the site of lesions and in evaluating their size and the quality of the surrounding tissues. Imaging is also used to assess the extent of pathology and the presence of other diseases. The radiologist determines whether lesions are amenable to percutaneous sampling, selects the optimum target for biopsy (often with the aid of positron emission tomography [PET] imaging), and decides which imaging modality is best suited to guide intervention. The choice and size of needle depend on the site, size, and solidity of the lesion, as well as the operator's personal preference. Cores of tissue are invariably obtained, in keeping with requirements for immunohistochemistry analysis, and, increasingly, to assess for the presence of mutations to assist targeted therapy in lung cancer.

METHODS OF TISSUE SAMPLING

Imaging Techniques

Several factors are considered in selecting the most appropriate imaging modality to guide percutaneous tissue sampling. These include the site, size, and depth of the lesion; its proximity to the pleura and neurovascular structures; and performance status of the patient.

Ultrasound

Ultrasound techniques are ideal for imaging superficial lesions including lymph nodes, the pleura, chest wall lesions, and the liver. Certain characteristics, such as the normal fatty hila of lymph nodes, are better depicted on ultrasound examination. Other advantages include easy access, real-time needle visibility leading to reduced time of procedure, and absence of radiation exposure. High-resolution transducers allow access to technically difficult areas, such as the supraclavicular fossae, and

patients can be placed in different positions to optimize access. Mobile lesions can be secured by applying gentle pressure with the probe, and if the lesion is close to major vessels, local anesthetic can be introduced to create space around the lesion. Color Doppler imaging is useful to assess lesion vascularity as well as the surrounding structures.

The use of ultrasound imaging becomes limited when lesions lie deep to the skin surface, because resolution decreases and visibility becomes poor. Imaging through air (e.g., the lungs) and bone is inadequate.

Computed Tomography

Computed tomography (CT) offers better contrast resolution between tissues of differing density. Pulmonary and mediastinal lesions, which are often partly surrounded by air, are better depicted. Deeper structures are clearly visualized, and detailed vascular anatomy is obtained with or without contrast enhancement. CT with multiplanar reconstruction provides a panoramic view of any lesion—in particular, its relationship to key structures, including the heart and great vessels. In the lung, CT allows accurate targeting of small lesions and tracking of mobile lesions located close to the diaphragm.

Unlike ultrasonography, CT does involve radiation exposure to the patient. It is of limited use in sampling central parenchymal and nodal disease, because biopsy in this region is associated with greater risks and complications; however, it remains useful for biopsy of mediastinal masses and pulmonary lesions.

Integrated Positron Emission Tomography–Computed Tomography

Positron emission tomography (PET) has an established role in the detection and staging of neoplastic diseases. In lung cancer it provides information on the primary lesion, early nodal involvement, and distant metastases. The positron-emitting agent most frequently used is ^{18}F-fluorodeoxyglucose (FDG). This tracer accumulates at sites of increased glycolysis (e.g., tumor cells), and this activity is then detected by the PET camera. The intensity of activity is displayed on a color scale, and a quantitative assessment is made by measuring the *standardized uptake value* (SUV).

CT combined with PET allows accurate anatomic localization of FDG-avid foci. This technique is particularly useful in isolating active foci surrounded by benign changes, such as within thickened pleura, or in separating tumor from collapse, allowing greater precision in positioning the biopsy needle (**Figure 13-3**).

The sensitivity of PET is limited by the size of the lesion. Small lesions (usually less than 1 cm) may not accumulate sufficient FDG to be detected on PET imaging, leading to false-negative results. The latter can also occur in tumors with relatively low metabolic activity such as carcinoids and alveolar cell cancers.

Inflammatory conditions such as bacterial pneumonias, abscesses, tuberculosis, and active sarcoidosis are associated with increased granulocytic activity. Such activity promotes increased uptake of FDG, potentially giving rise to false-positive results.

Needles

The two main modes of sampling are fine needle aspiration (FNA) for cytologic study and core biopsy for histopathologic

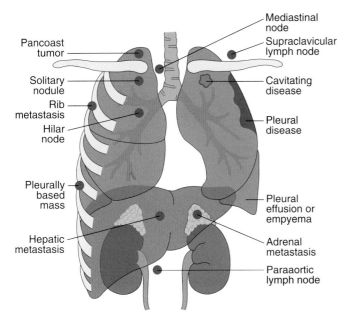

Figure 13-1 Common sites for biopsy.

examination. Both methods retrieve samples that are suitable for culture. Although the sensitivity of FNA is improved by having a cytologist present to ensure that an adequate sample is obtained, the diagnostic yield in benign disease remains low (20% to 50%) compared with that for core biopsy (70%) (Greif et al., 1999). In malignant disease, the techniques are analogous, with a sensitivity of 90% to 95% (Klein et al., 1996). The clinical requirement for cores of tissue for immunohistochemical analysis has led to a reduction in the use of FNA, and when feasible, cores are always obtained.

FNA involves inserting a fine needle into a lesion and carefully moving the tip to and fro within the tissue, to obtain an aspirate. Gentle suction can be applied by attaching a 5-mL syringe to the needle hub. A variety of fine needles are available, including the Westcott, Chiba, Franseen, and Rotex needles, which range in size from 20 to 23 gauge. Larger-gauge needles are smaller in caliber and less rigid in design, which can limit their use. The Westcott needle has the advantage of having a trough close to the needle tip, which captures small cores of tissue in approximately 50% of cases. The main use of FNA is to obtain nodal aspirates.

Core biopsy specimens are obtained using cutting needles, which are larger in diameter (14 to 18 gauge) and are available in different lengths (6-, 9-, and 15-cm lengths are commonly used). These needles are more sturdy, allowing greater control in placement. Cutting needles are typically mounted on a spring-loaded mechanism. Older designs such as the Bard Biopty biopsy system, when triggered, simultaneously fire an inner notched stylet and an outer cutting cannula. The handle of the Bard system is bulky but reusable (**Figure 13-4**). Newer, lighter designs include the Cook Quickcore and Bauer Temno devices, which allow the inner notched stylet to be advanced and secured within the lesion before the cutting cannula is activated. The throw can be increased from 1 to 2 cm to obtain better core samples (**Figure 13-5**). The Cook device seems to have a slightly sharper needle tip, which in practice can be advanced through tougher tissues.

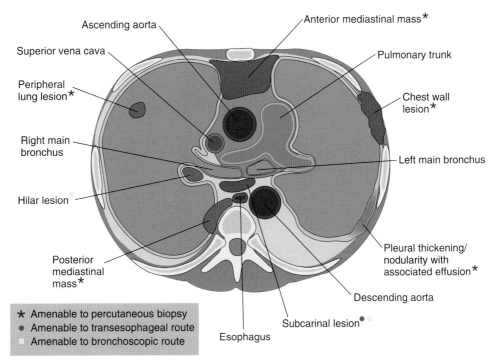

★ Amenable to percutaneous biopsy
● Amenable to transesophageal route
▫ Amenable to bronchoscopic route

Figure 13-2 Common routes for biopsy according to site.

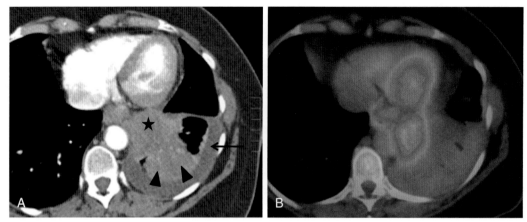

Figure 13-3 Differentiating central tumor from distal lung collapse. **A,** The computed tomography (CT) scan shows central low-density tumor in the left lower lobe (*star*) with distal collapse (*arrowheads*), but differentiation is subtle. A small pleural effusion (*arrow*) is evident. **B,** CT–positron emission tomography (PET) study demarcates the FDG-avid tumor from the area of distal collapse. Note normal physiologic left ventricular avidity. *FDG,* ¹⁸F-2-fluorodeoxyglucose.

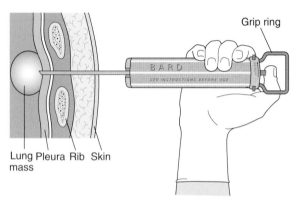

Figure 13-4 The Bard Biopty biopsy system. The needle is introduced at a point on the thorax so that the tip reaches the area in which biopsy will be performed.

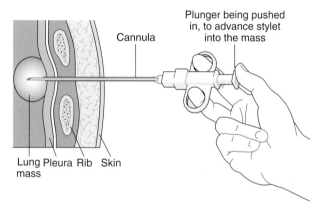

Figure 13-5 The Bauer Temno biopsy instrument. The cutting needle is positioned within the lesion to be biopsied by pushing the plunger. The advantages include that the instrument is lightweight and requires use of only one hand, and that it is easy to use under computed tomography or ultrasound guidance.

Historically, it was believed that use of larger cutting needles carried higher complication rates than those associated with fine needles. A 2002 study of practice based in the United Kingdom analyzed data from 5444 lung biopsy and FNA procedures and found no difference between the two methods, a conclusion supported by other studies (Richardson et al., 2002).

With transpulmonary biopsy, the risk of pneumothorax is more closely related to the number of pleural passes. The introduction of a coaxial system has transformed lung biopsies. A single pleural pass is made with a thin-walled introducer needle (usually 16 gauge). A smaller cutting needle (usually 18 gauge with a 1- or 2-cm throw) is inserted through the introducer and multiple cores are taken without repuncturing the pleura. The process is quicker, simpler, and safer than attempting multiple pleural passes, leading to a reduction in the complication rate with an improved diagnostic yield (**Figure 13-6**).

PERCUTANEOUS BIOPSY OF INTRAPULMONARY LESIONS

Indications

The role of percutaneous lung biopsy in diagnosing malignant disease is well established, with a sensitivity of 90% to 95%. Its main application is in patients with inoperable lung cancer, when sputum cytology and bronchoscopy are nondiagnostic, to provide a means of establishing cell type before chemotherapy

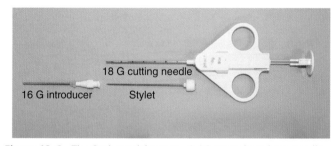

Figure 13-6 The Cook coaxial system. A 16-gauge introducer needle, together with its stylet and 18-gauge inner cutting needle, is shown.

and radiotherapy. In the past, both FNA and core biopsy have been comparable in diagnosing and distinguishing small cell lung cancer (SCLC) from non-SCLC (NSCLC), providing oncologists with sufficient information to make choices regarding appropriate chemotherapy regimens. New targeted chemotherapy and biologic agents (e.g., the epidermal growth factor receptor [EGFR] inhibitor drugs) have proven prognostic benefit with particular histologic subtypes. This has meant that core sampling is essential to allow routine performance of detailed tissue analysis. FNA can be adequate to differentiate between subtypes of NCSLC, but it remains less accurate overall than core biopsy. The latter allows sufficient material to

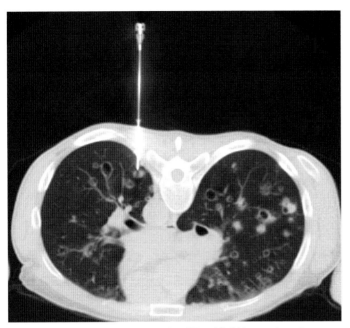

Figure 13-7 Computed tomography (CT)-guided biopsy of a pulmonary nodule using a coaxial system. The patient is in the prone position. Multiple cystic and solid pulmonary nodules in a patient with a history of lymphoma. The diagnosis was Langerhans cell histiocytosis.

Table 13-1	Contraindications to Needle Biopsy
Type of Contraindication	**Comment**
Relative	Inability of patient to cooperate: uncontrollable cough, inability to lie prone or supine
	Poor lung function/chronic obstructive pulmonary disease (FEV$_1$ <40% of predicted normal or multiple bullae)
	Pneumonectomy
	Bleeding disorder
	Pulmonary hypertension
	Pulmonary fibrosis
	Small nodules (<5 mm in diameter)
	Hydatid disease (associated with risk of anaphylactic reaction)
Absolute	Arteriovenous malformation with high pulmonary artery pressure

FEV$_1$, forced expiratory volume in 1 second.

be obtained for both accurate histologic subtyping and molecular testing (e.g., to determine EGFR mutation status) (Barnes et al., 2010).

Biopsy also is widely used to exclude lung metastases in patients with potentially operable lung tumors, and in those with extrathoracic malignancies (**Figure 13-7**).

With solitary pulmonary lesions, core biopsy remains the prudent approach for confirming benign disease. The combined use of CT guidance and the coaxial biopsy system, which allows multiple cores to be taken safely, has improved the diagnostic accuracy of this technique in both benign and malignant disease. If malignancy is strongly suspected, it may be best to avoid biopsy and proceed straight to surgery.

Transthoracic biopsy and FNA also have a role in the diagnosis of non-neoplastic disease. Both techniques are increasingly being used to obtain samples for identification of microorganisms, particularly in immunocompromised patients with consolidation and masses. All samples are routinely sent to both histology (or cytology) and microbiology. Communication with the referring clinician is essential. In cases in which infection is suspected, the first sample should be sent to microbiology should the procedure need to be unexpectedly abandoned. The converse is true in suspected cases of malignancy where the first sample is sent to histology. The working diagnosis may also influence the choice of needle size.

Contraindications

The contraindications to percutaneous lung biopsy are largely relative and are summarized in **Table 13-1**. In general, patients need to be able to cooperate, including lying still in the desired position, resisting excessive coughing, and controlling breathing. In patients with very poor lung function, biopsy of a lesion is still possible, provided that the lesion is peripheral and a carefully considered route is identified (usually with CT) that does not traverse lung parenchyma. In performing the biopsy, care is taken to avoid creating a pneumothorax, which could be life-threatening. Before the procedure, a coagulation screen

is performed according to local protocol, and bleeding diatheses are corrected, when appropriate, to keep within safe guidelines. Biopsy of parenchymal hydatid lesions has been documented, but an increased and probably unacceptable risk of anaphylactic reaction has been documented in patients with such lesions.

Method

Pulmonary lesions are usually sampled under CT guidance using cutting needles rather than fine needles. The coaxial technique is preferred because it allows multiple consecutive cores to be obtained without delay, helping to improve diagnostic accuracy while minimizing risk. The number of biopsy specimens varies, but in practice, two to five samples are required (fewer if the patient is at high risk of complications). The aim is to obtain a diagnosis without compromising patient safety.

Peripheral lesions located away from fissures and large vessels are ideally targeted, to minimize complications of pneumothorax and hemorrhage. When possible, the approach should cover the shortest distance from the skin surface to the lesion, using a route that allows the patient to be positioned comfortably for a period of at least 30 minutes. The latter consideration is important, because patients are often elderly or frail and breathless at rest.

In lesions obscured by atelectasis, intravenous contrast can be administered to localize abnormal tissue from collapsed lung. PET-CT is useful in identifying avid foci in these cases. If the lesion is cavitating or exhibits central necrosis, the biopsy must be taken from the periphery of the lesion.

Procedure

Preparation

Percutaneous biopsy procedures are arranged as short-stay cases, with the expectation that patients will return home the same day, after a period of observation.

Before the appointment, all patients must have a complete blood count (CBC), and the international normalized ratio (INR) must be checked and corrected when appropriate, to reduce the risk of bleeding. A platelet count greater than 150 × 10^9/L and an INR of 1.4 or less are acceptable lower and upper limits, respectively. Antiplatelet agents (e.g., aspirin, clopidogrel) should be withheld for several days preceding intervention (5 days for aspirin, 7 to 10 days for clopidogrel).

Percutaneous lung biopsy requires that the patient fast beforehand. On the day of the procedure, the patient is admitted to the programmed investigation unit (PIU), where a baseline set of observations are recorded (including heart rate, blood pressure, and oxygen saturation).

The radiologist performing the procedure explains the process, enquires about relevant allergies, and after addressing any queries, obtains written informed consent, documenting potential complications, which occur at a rate greater than 1%. The patient is informed that several samples may need to be taken. Sedation is rarely required but can be used in anxious patients. For administration of such agents, intravenous access is established, and cardiorespiratory monitoring is required. Audio aids (e.g., iPods) are invaluable in relaxing younger patients and adults who are restless.

Practical Aspects

The patient is positioned supine or prone, depending on the anteroposterior location of the lesion. Pillows are used to elevate one side of the chest if necessary, and the arms are positioned to optimize access, avoiding elevation above the head, which typically causes shoulder discomfort in elderly persons.

Radiopaque surface skin markers are placed 0.5 to 1.0 cm apart over the region of interest, and a limited CT scan covering the area is performed with the patient in gentle respiration (**Figure 13-8**). Once the target lesion is identified, the safest percutaneous route to the lesion is mapped along the axial and sagittal axes, using the CT slice number and surface markers, respectively, as a guide. A cross is drawn on the patient's skin to mark the corresponding entry site and a sterile field is created. Lidocaine 1% (10 to 15 mL) or 2% (5 mL) is infiltrated down to the pleura, with care taken not to puncture the visceral pleura or lung. The patient is warned that it is not always possible to anesthetize the pleura fully, because of the risk of pneumothorax from the anesthetic needle.

With use of the coaxial system, the introducer needle is advanced first, through a small skin incision. Because formal breathing instructions can be confusing to the patient, the respiratory phase is judged from movements of the chest wall. A slight "give" is felt when the pleura is breached, and this thrust should be performed with a smooth, firm motion to avoid shearing the pleura, thereby increasing the chance of a pneumothorax. The progression of the needle toward the lesion and the final position of its tip are intermittently checked by repeating the initial scan as required. One-centimeter markers visable along the length of the introducer needle are a useful guide when advancing the needle. Accurate placement of the needle tip is essential and may take time with small and mobile lesions.

Once the introducer needle is optimally positioned, the central stylet is removed and a finger placed over the hub to prevent air embolism. The cutting needle is then inserted through the lumen of the introducer, and multiple cores are taken, with replacement of the stylet between biopsy maneuvers. The tip of the cutting needle can be angled differently with each thrust, to obtain a representative sample—a technique that is particularly useful when tumors show histologic heterogeneity. Saline (2 to 3 mL) can be injected and aspirated through the introducer needle to obtain microorganisms, when indicated.

Once sufficient samples are obtained safely, the introducer needle is removed in a single swift motion during expiration, and a postbiopsy scan is performed if a pneumothorax is suspected.

Specimen Handling

Specimens should be handled appropriately and sent to the laboratory promptly. Aspirated material is smeared onto slides, with some fixed in alcohol and the rest air-dried, and sent for cytologic studies. A saline wash of the needle is taken for microbiologic analysis. Cores of tissue are placed in formalin for histopathologic examination and in saline for microbiologic studies. Advanced cytologic procedures such as flow cytometry for lymphoma, estrogen receptor status assay for metastatic breast cancer, and immunohistochemistry staining for malignancies are additional useful tests.

Patient Aftercare

After lung biopsy, the patient is monitored in the hospital setting for 4 to 5 hours. A biopsy side–down position should be maintained whenever possible, and excessive talking, laughing, and coughing should be avoided to reduce the risk of pneumothorax. Hourly observations are recorded, and a chest radiograph is taken at 1 and 4 hours after biopsy, to identify any pneumothorax and to monitor its size. If a pneumothorax is detected, high-flow oxygen (10 L/minute) is given, because it improves the rate of reabsorption by up to four-fold. Patients with a small, stable pneumothorax who are otherwise clinically well can still be discharged home safely, provided that they are able to return without delay if signs or symptoms develop.

Complications

A risk-benefit analysis should always be made before any procedure, particularly in high-risk groups (**Table 13-2**).

The most common complication after lung biopsy is pneumothorax (**Figure 13-9**). Most pneumothoraces are small (less than 2 cm on chest film) and are managed conservatively. Those requiring intervention usually are detected early: 88% immediately after biopsy and the remainder after 1 hour. A delayed presentation is rare. Intervention can involve aspiration by way of a three-way tap or drainage through a one-way (Heimlich) valve; drainage is performed at a frequency of 0 to 17%. Positioning the patient with the puncture site dependent can reduce the pneumothorax rate and should be considered

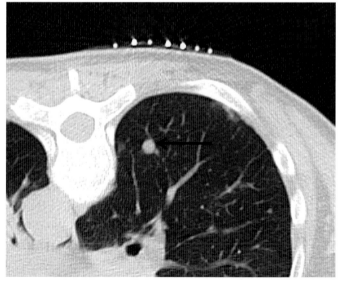

Figure 13-8 Computed tomography (CT)-guided biopsy of a right lower lobe nodule (*arrow*). Surface grid markers, together with slice position, are used to determine the site of needle insertion.

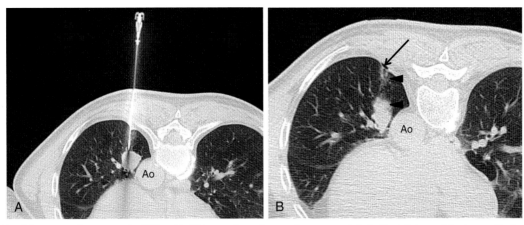

Figure 13-9 **A,** Coaxial computed tomography (CT)-guided biopsy of a solitary pulmonary nodule in the left lower lobe in a patient with a history of colonic carcinoma. The needle is angled away from the aorta (Ao). **B,** After biopsy, a tiny pneumothorax (*arrow*) can be seen, along with the needle tract and perilesional hemorrhage (*arrowheads*). The diagnosis was carcinoid.

Table 13-2	Complications of Needle Biopsy
Category	**Complication/Cause**
Early complications	Pneumothorax: 5-50% Hemoptysis: 5-10% Hemorrhage: 10-40% Air embolism: rare
Late complications	Tumor seeding: extremely rare Empyema Bronchopleural fistula
Increased risk of pneumothorax	*Common associations*: • Chronic obstructive pulmonary disease or bullae • Uncontrollable coughing during the procedure • A small central lesion *Less common associations*: • Multiple pleural passes during procedure • Passage of instrumentation across fissure during procedure • Prolonged procedure

in patients at high risk. Surprisingly, use of a cutting needle does not increase the incidence of pneumothorax over that with fine needle aspiration, the pneumothorax rate being in the range of 3% to 42%. Tension pneumothorax is rare but may be seen in patients with emphysema. It develops within minutes and constitutes a medical emergency.

Minor perilesional hemorrhage is common (see Figure 13-9); however, actual hemoptysis occurs in only 4% to 5% of biopsy procedures (Richardson et al., 2002) and is more common in patients with pulmonary hypertension. It often follows a bout of coughing and can be extremely frightening for the patient. Supportive measures are initiated with the patient positioned biopsy side down. Treatment is rarely required, because spontaneous recovery is rapid. Massive hemoptysis rarely occurs and can be fatal.

Although rare, a systemic arterial air embolism is a serious and increasingly recognized complication of interventional lung procedures, and its effects can be clinically subtle (Hiraki et al., 2007). It occurs when air enters into the pulmonary venous circulation, is pumped through the left side of the heart, and subsequently enters the cerebral and coronary arteries, which become occluded. Air may enter the pulmonary veins by two

main processes. It can be drawn in from the atmosphere, through the introducer needle on deep inspiration, when the hub is temporarily exposed in between biopsies. Entry of air through this route is avoided by promptly covering the hub with the thumb each time the cutting needle or stylet is withdrawn, and by asking the patient to hold the breath during the process. Alternatively, air can enter the pulmonary veins through the airways along the needle tract during a bout of coughing. To prevent this from occurring, needles should be removed during uncontrollable coughing. Rapid diagnosis and treatment of a pulmonary venous air embolism are essential. The patient should be placed in the right lateral decubitus position, and 100% oxygen should be administered while awaiting transfer to a hyperbaric oxygen chamber if available. A CT scan of the head and chest should be performed to confirm the diagnosis.

Reported mortality rates for transpulmonary biopsy range from 0.07% to 0.15% (Richardson et al., 2002; Tomiyama et al., 2006). Death may result from cardiac arrest, systemic arterial air embolism, tension pneumothorax, or hemorrhage.

Pitfalls and Controversies

In malignant disease, percutaneous sampling of pulmonary lesions carries a high sensitivity with use of the coaxial system, even if the nodules are small. This has reduced the need to recall patients for repeat biopsies, because the sensitivity for detection of malignancy has risen to 90% to 95%.

In benign disease, FNA has a relatively poor diagnostic yield. Sensitivity is improved by obtaining multiple cores using a cutting needle and the coaxial system, a technique that has been used in the diagnosis of cryptogenic organizing pneumonia, Wegener granulomatosis, and some infections.

Diagnostic difficulties still arise with lesions exhibiting a high level of fibrosis—for example, metastatic breast carcinoma and Hodgkin disease. Excess mucus production as in bronchoalveolar carcinoma also can interfere with establishing the diagnosis.

Biopsy of a solitary mass with suspected malignancy that is potentially operable remains controversial, because the lesion is likely to need removal. In any case, the advantages of biopsy are that the patient and the surgeon are better informed, and that the operation time is shortened by avoiding the need for frozen sections.

There remain four indications for biopsy of a noncalcified solitary pulmonary nodule: First, if benign disease is suspected, biopsy may obviate the need for surgery; second, in a lung

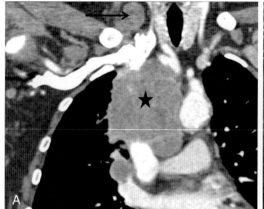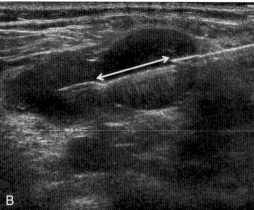

Figure 13-10 **A,** Coronal computed tomography (CT) image showing a large right paratracheal lymph node mass (*star*) and right supraclavicular lymphadenopathy (*arrow*). **B,** Ultrasound-guided biopsy of the supraclavicular lymphadenopathy in the same patient. Two adjacent nodes have been targeted, allowing for a longer, 2-cm sample to be taken. The recess of the biopsy needle is seen (*double arrow*) before triggering of the cutting mechanism. The diagnosis was small cell lung cancer.

cancer patient who is a poor operative candidate, it may be necessary to obtain tissue to optimize treatment with nonsurgical therapies (radiotherapy with curative intent); third, in a patient with an extrathoracic malignancy where a metastasis is suspected; fourth, a fully informed patient may wish to confirm the diagnosis of cancer, even if the suspicion of cancer is high, before proceeding to surgery.

ULTRASOUND-GUIDED BIOPSY: GENERAL PRINCIPLES

Preparation

Ultrasound-guided sampling of superficial lesions usually requires no fasting or formal hospital admission, and observations are recorded only if the patient history includes clinical concerns. Hematologic indices are checked and optimized beforehand, and antiplatelet therapy is withheld, in accordance with protocols for CT-guided procedures.

Practical Aspects

The site of the lesion or tissue usually determines the optimal positioning of the patient. For example, nontargeted pleural biopsy requires that the patient sit upright, facing away from the radiologist, with the arms folded to spread apart the shoulder blades. Supraclavicular node sampling, on the other hand, is performed with the patient supine, with the shoulders raised on a pillow, allowing the neck to be slightly hyperextended. Time spent ensuring that both patient and radiologist are comfortable helps ensure a quick procedure, avoiding unwanted "shuffling."

With targeted biopsy procedures, the ultrasound probe (curvilinear or linear) is adjusted until the lesion can be seen along its greatest length. Once this is achieved, the probe is held secure, and a line is drawn on the patient's skin to mark the orientation of the probe, which is then removed. The skin entry site is prepared, and a cryogesic (ethyl chloride) freezing spray can be applied to numb the skin, particularly in young patients.

Under sterile conditions, the probe is reapplied to the skin (using the marker as a guide to positioning), and local anesthetic (up to 10 mL of 1% lidocaine) is infiltrated down to the lesion using a 21 gauge (green) needle. Deep to the skin, the needle is kept in view by advancing it directly in line with the transducer. The angle between the needle and the skin is adjusted depending on the depth of the lesion. Administering

local anesthetic reduces discomfort for the patient, creates a passage to the lesion, and also gives the radiologist an idea of how to angle the larger biopsy needle.

Depending on the size of the lesion, a cutting needle with a 1- or 2-cm throw is selected. Adjacent lymph nodes can be lined up and sampled simultaneously, enabling the 2-cm throw to be used more often, which is preferable, because it provides a better specimen (**Figure 13-10**). After a small skin incision is made, the biopsy needle is introduced and carefully observed as it is advanced toward and into the lesion. With the tip of the needle secured well within the lesion (which often requires a firm nudge to pierce its capsule or wall), the whole apparatus can be flattened out, so that the inner stylet can be advanced through but not out of the lesion. Once the stylet is optimally positioned, the biopsy specimen is taken by pushing the trigger, after the patient is warned to expect a clicking sound. The needle is then swiftly withdrawn, and pressure is applied to the skin to control any bleeding; the process is repeated as appropriate after the first sample is retrieved.

Aftercare

After an uncomplicated superficial biopsy procedure, the patient can be discharged home after a brief period of observation, if clinical stability is maintained. Advice is given on necessary precautions and signs and symptoms necessitating urgent medical attention. High-risk patient groups (e.g., elderly persons and those with an underlying coagulopathy) and high-risk procedures (e.g., targeted liver biopsy, as discussed later on), are the exceptions and require closer observation or an overnight stay.

PERCUTANEOUS SAMPLING OF EXTRAPULMONARY INTRATHORACIC TISSUES

MEDIASTINAL NODES AND MASSES

Method

Depending on the location, mediastinal lesions can be accessed endoscopically (by the transbronchial or transesophageal route), surgically with VATS or through an anterior mediastinotomy, or percutaneously under image guidance, if a safe route that avoids traversing the lung is available.

CT is preferred to ultrasound imaging to guide percutaneous mediastinal biopsy, because it helps to map a direct route

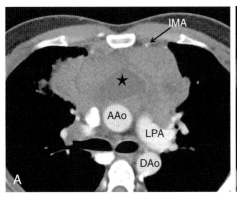
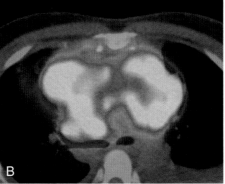
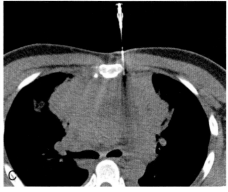

Figure 13-11 A, Contrast-enhanced computed tomography (CT) scan shows a large anterior mediastinal mass with central low-density necrosis (*star*). **B,** Integrated CT–positron emission tomography (PET) study shows FDG avidity within the mass, with a central photopenic area corresponding to the necrosis on CT scan. **C,** CT=guided biopsy. The approach is medial to the left internal mammary artery and targets the non-necrotic portion of the tumor. *AAo,* ascending aorta; *DAo,* descending aorta; *FDG,* ^{18}F-fluorodeoxyglucose; *IMA,* internal mammary artery; *LPA,* left main pulmonary artery.

through the chest wall to the mass, which avoids puncturing lung or vessels (particularly the internal mammary vessels). Contrast-enhanced CT and color Doppler ultrasound techniques are essential tools for assessing vascularity.

With large mediastinal masses abutting the chest wall, a biopsy route that avoids the lung parenchyma is readily available (**Figure 13-11**). With smaller lesions, a safer route may be achieved with use of a transpleural approach through an existing effusion or pneumothorax. Saline can be injected into the pleural space where there is no effusion, or directly into the mediastinum, providing an extrapleural route. Placing the patient in the lateral decubitus position to shift the mediastinum also can help to create an extrapulmonary route. These alternative approaches are associated with reduced incidence of complications.

Core biopsy specimens are necessary to diagnose primary mediastinal tumors (e.g., lymphomas, thymomas). Multiple cores for immunohistochemistry studies are required to differentiate lymphoma from other lesions and can be obtained using the coaxial needle technique.

Limitations and Complications

Breathing can cause small lesions to move out of the biopsy plane and, with use of the extrapleural route, can result in inadvertent introduction of the biopsy needle into the lung or pleura. With biopsy of anterior mediastinal lesions, damage to the internal mammary vessels can result in serious hemorrhage. When feasible, a parasternal approach is adopted, with use of CT guidance to minimize this risk. With biopsy of posterior mediastinal lesions, a paravertebral route can occasionally cause injury to the paravertebral and intercostal neurovascular structures, and the azygous vein.

MEDIASTINAL COLLECTIONS

Mediastinal abscess secondary to esophageal rupture is a life-threatening condition associated with high mortality. Percutaneous aspiration or drainage is considered a useful alternative to surgery, particularly in patients unfit for a general anesthetic procedure.

Method

Mediastinal drainage is performed under CT guidance using a Seldinger technique. After administration of a local anesthetic, a 17 or 18 gauge, long puncture needle is advanced into the collection, often under gentle suction applied with a syringe.

This technique allows aspiration of the contents when the fluid collection is breached and also helps to confirm the position of the needle tip. The syringe is removed, and a guidewire is fed through the needle into the fluid collection. With the guidewire held firmly at the entry site, the needle is withdrawn and a tract is dilated over the guidewire. The drain then replaces the dilator, and the guidewire is withdrawn. Usually size 10 or 12 French (10F or 12F) drains are used, depending on the viscosity of the fluid.

HILAR LESIONS

Percutaneous CT-guided biopsy of hilar lymph nodes and masses has been performed, but the technique is limited by the depth of the location, proximity to major vessels, and the associated risks of pneumothorax and hemorrhage. Endobronchial ultrasound (EBUS) has largely replaced CT-guided biopsy for this indication, providing better access to the central thoracic structures and a safer route for sampling hilar and mediastinal tissues.

PLEURAL AND CHEST WALL DISEASE

Non-targeted pleural biopsy often is performed to diagnose benign conditions such as pleural tuberculosis. Targeted pleural and chest wall biopsies usually are undertaken to exclude malignant disease, which may be suggested by focal FDG avidity detected on PET imaging. Cores of tissue are essential in differentiating mesothelioma from metastatic adenocarcinoma.

Method for Non-targeted Pleural Biopsy

If no discrete pleural mass is present, or there is simply diffuse pleural thickening, a non-targeted ultrasound-guided biopsy is performed. This procedure can be undertaken only if sufficient pleural fluid is present. A suitable biopsy site is identified on ultrasound imaging, and the depth from the skin to the parietal pleura is measured. Local anesthetic is administered down to the pleural space until fluid is aspirated. The depth of the anesthetic needle at this point also gives an estimate of the distance from the skin to the parietal pleura. Guided by these measurements, the tip of the biopsy needle is positioned proximal to the parietal pleura, so that when the stylet is advanced, the notch traverses the width of the pleura to enter the pleural space. The core obtained should therefore contain the full thickness of the pleura and some pleural fluid.

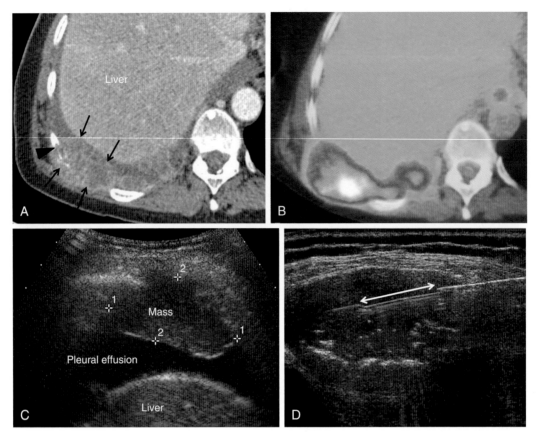

Figure 13-12 A, Contrast-enhanced computed tomography (CT) scan shows a heterogeneous pleural mass (*arrows*) that is invading the chest wall and destroying the adjacent rib (*arrowhead*). A small pleural effusion is evident. **B,** CT–positron emission tomography (PET) study was performed for staging and shows that the mass is FDG-avid. **C,** Ultrasound image demonstrates the mass (*cursor* at *1, 2*). **D,** Ultrasound-guided biopsy, with the recess of the needle advanced through the tumor (*double arrow*). The diagnosis was metastatic adenocarcinoma. *FDG,* ¹⁸F-fluorodeoxyglucose.

Method for Targeted Pleural and Chest Wall Biopsies

Targeted pleural and chest wall biopsies are indicated to sample a discrete mass and are usually performed under ultrasound guidance (**Figure 13-12**). If visualization is difficult with use of ultrasound imaging, or if the lesion is small, with insufficient pleural fluid, biopsy is performed under CT guidance. The optimum route is one that runs along the main axis of the pathologic process (i.e., an oblique tract), allowing more of the lesion to be sampled with less risk of pneumothorax (**Figure 13-13**).

Several cores (at least three) are taken, and if the pleura is not particularly thickened, multiple passes may be required. Radiologists favor the 18 gauge Cook Quickcore or Temno cutting device. The coaxial system can be used for pleural biopsy procedures performed under CT guidance. Samples are sent for microbiologic and histologic examination. If the pleural lesion is large and the patient remains asymptomatic after biopsy, no chest radiograph is required before discharge.

Diagnostic Yield

Imaging-guided pleural biopsy using a cutting needle has a sensitivity of 88%, specificity of 100%, and an overall accuracy of 91% for detection of malignant disease.

PERCUTANEOUS SAMPLING OF EXTRATHORACIC LESIONS

During staging of thoracic malignancies, lesions may be identified in the liver, adrenal glands, lymph nodes or bones. If

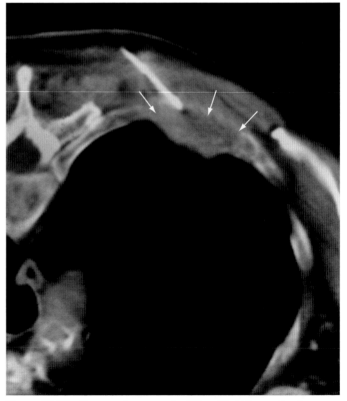

Figure 13-13 Computed tomography (CT)-guided biopsy of a rib metastasis (*arrows*). The diagnosis was non–small cell carcinoma.

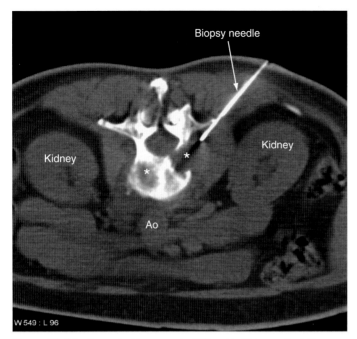

Figure 13-14 Computed tomography (CT)-guided biopsy of a lytic vertebral lesion (*star*). *Ao*, aorta.

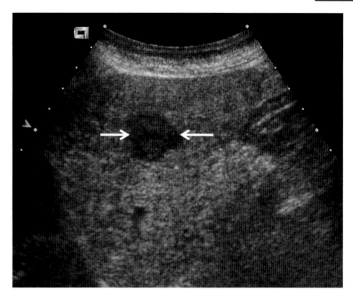

Figure 13-15 Ultrasound image showing a hypoechoic liver metastasis (*arrows*), which can be targeted for biopsy.

appearances suggest metastases (e.g., increased FDG avidity on PET imaging), it is essential to perform a biopsy to confirm inoperability (**Figure 13-14**). If multiple sites are involved, several factors are considered in deciding which tissue to sample—for example, the extent of the disease, the likelihood of obtaining a diagnostic sample safely, and how accessible the site is with a minimally invasive approach.

LIVER

Method

Hepatic lesions usually are biopsied under ultrasound guidance, where they are easily imaged and rapidly sampled (**Figure 13-15**). Owing to the risk of bleeding and the potential need for intervention, preoperative preparation of the patient includes fasting for 6 hours before the procedure.

Ultrasound scanning is performed with the patient supine, with the right arm elevated to allow access to the right upper quadrant. The liver is scanned with a curvilinear probe, and the optimum target is identified. Metastatic deposits can be well- or ill-defined and will vary in size, number, echogenicity, and echotexture, but most often they are solid and hypoechoic relative to the surrounding parenchyma. The lesion that can be reached by the shortest intraparenchymal route while avoiding the gallbladder and the hepatic and portal vessels (which are highlighted on color Doppler) is selected for sampling.

With strict adherence to aseptic technique, local anesthetic is infiltrated down to the liver capsule, which has a rich neurovascular supply. The tip of the anesthetic needle is kept in full view to avoid breaching the capsule, because this can increase the risk of bleeding. A small skin incision is then made, and a larger cutting needle is introduced (usually 18 gauge); radiologists at our institution favor the traditional Bard Biopty biopsy system, which obtains a 1-cm core. The biopsy sample is taken with the patient in arrested respiration to limit movement. If insufficient tissue is obtained with a single core, the biopsy can be repeated. However, careful risk-benefit analysis should be made, owing to the increased risk of hemorrhage

associated with multiple passes (Grant et al., 1999). In practice, no more than two cores are usually taken. Although multiple cores are avoided, the coaxial system can still be useful, as hemostatic agents (such as Gelfoam sponge) can be inserted down the introducer needle as it is withdrawn, helping to control bleeding along the biopsy tract.

Aftercare

Post biopsy, patients are observed for at least 6 hours. Blood pressure and pulse are recorded at gradually increasing intervals to observe for signs of early bleeding, and analgesia is prescribed if pain develops. Patients can remain supine or lie right side down, with no evidence to support a particular position.

A study of more than 9000 liver biopsies showed that the risk of hemorrhage not only is related to the number of passes made but also is closely associated with the presence of malignancy and the age of the patient (McGill et al., 1990). Given these risk factors, in the context of malignant liver disease, patients undergoing targeted biopsy usually are admitted overnight for careful observation.

A retrospective study of 68,276 percutaneous liver biopsy procedures (performed over a decade) demonstrated that the majority of complications occur early on (61% in the first 2 hours), with most detected within a day (96% within 24 hours). Death was uncommon (with 9 deaths reported per 100,000 procedures) but occurred in patients with either underlying malignant disease or cirrhosis and was due to intraperitoneal hemorrhage, with signs of bleeding seen within 6 hours (Piccininio et al., 1986). After 24 hours, if clinical status remains stable and pain has subsided, the patient can be discharged home with advice to return if any delayed symptoms are experienced.

ADRENAL GLANDS

Biopsy of adrenal lesions is usually performed under CT guidance (**Figure 13-16**). It may be necessary to traverse the pulmonary or hepatic parenchyma to enter the adrenal mass. If the mass is on the side opposite the primary lung carcinoma, the pulmonary parenchymal route should be avoided, because a pneumothorax could delay surgery or result in significant

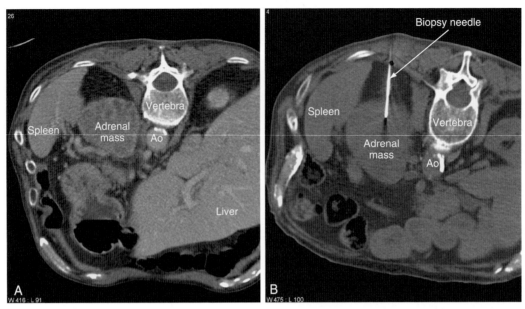

Figure 13-16   A, Contrast-enhanced computed tomography (CT) scan shows a large adrenal mass lateral to the vertebral body and aorta (Ao). **B,** CT-guided biopsy with the patient in the prone position. The needle tip is in the mass. The diagnosis was metastatic lung cancer.

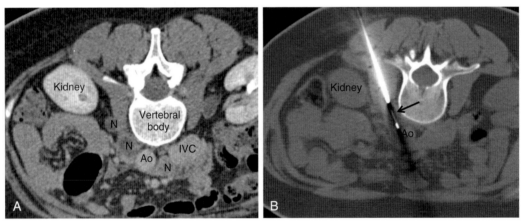

Figure 13-17   A, Contrast computed tomography (CT) scan shows necrotic retroperitoneal lymph nodes (N). *Ao,* aorta; *IVC,* inferior vena cava. **B,** Coaxial CT-guided biopsy. The patient is prone, and the outer needle has been advanced through the left psoas muscle. The inner cutting needle also has been advanced, the recess of which can be seen within the lymph node *(arrow).*

respiratory compromise. A coaxial system is invaluable, allowing several aspirates or cores to be obtained with a single pass of the introducer needle.

LYMPH NODES

Biopsy of enlarged lymph nodes (greater than 1 cm in short axis) often provides diagnostic tissue when it is difficult to obtain from the primary lung lesion and also aids staging. Smaller, subcentimeter nodes can be targeted if increased FDG activity on PET imaging suggests early metastatic involvement.

The supraclavicular regions, axillae, and retroperitoneum are the usual sites of lymphadenopathy in primary diseases of the lung. In lung cancer, detecting supraclavicular lymph node metastases is crucial, because it constitutes a contraindication to surgery (stage IIIB).

Ultrasound imaging is commonly used to identify and sample abnormal nodes. Nearly a third of patients with lung cancer have nonpalpable supraclavicular nodal metastases, detectable on ultrasound-guided FNA. This frequency increases

to almost 50% in patients who have mediastinal nodal metastases. The advantage of ultrasound imaging is that it allows accurate assessment of nodal size and can identify pathologic features (e.g., rounded morphology, loss of echogenic hilum, peripheral vascularity) that are not detectable clinically.

Superficial nodes, including supraclavicular and axillary, are amenable to ultrasound-guided biopsy, which is a simple and safe procedure. Biopsy of retroperitoneal masses (including lymph nodes) requires CT guidance (**Figure 13-17**). Core biopsy is preferable to FNA. A 16 or 18 gauge cutting needle is used, depending on the site.

BONE LESIONS

The presence of bone metastases confirms stage IV lung cancer. Lesions are typically osteolytic and common sites for metastasis include the spine, ribs, and pelvic bones. The indications for bone biopsy are variable but typically include a suspicious bone lesion (usually detected on CT, PET-CT, or bone scan) in a patient with potentially curable disease. A bone biopsy is considered to complete the staging process, if no other tissue amenable to sampling (e.g., a lymph node) is available. If the bone lesion is superficial (e.g., a rib metastasis), biopsy can be performed under ultrasound guidance. CT guidance is preferred if the lesion lies deep and is close to major neurovascular structures.

PLEURAL DRAINAGE

Indications and Contraindications

Common causes of exudative effusions are malignancy and empyemas. In patients with a community-acquired pneumonia, 40% develop a parapneumonic effusion. Most cases resolve spontaneously, but the effusion can progress to form an empyema. Early and rapid drainage of an empyema is essential to prevent fibrin deposition, which potentially leads to pleural fibrosis and possibly a restrictive defect. An esophageal rupture or endobronchial lesion should be considered in a patient with an empyema without an obvious predisposing cause.

A pleural effusion can be tapped for diagnostic purposes, and a pleural biopsy performed at the same time if indicated. A pleural effusion can be drained for therapeutic purposes if it is large and the patient is symptomatic (usually with a malignant effusion), if it is infected or is an empyema (if the glucose is low, or the pH is less than 7.2), or if a hemothorax is present (usually after trauma). A bleeding disorder is a relative contraindication to pleural drainage, predisposing to hematoma formation.

Technique

Ultrasound imaging is the easiest and quickest way to confirm the presence and volume of pleural fluid and also demonstrates the presence of echogenic material, septa, and multiple locules, which may require multiple drainage tubes (**Figure 13-18**).

CT has an advantage in evaluating any underlying lung or mediastinal pathology. In empyemas, the pleurae characteristically are smooth and diffusely thickened and enhance after intravenous contrast injection.

Procedure

A large effusion can be drained without image guidance, but smaller or multiloculated effusions are better drained by the radiologist. For this procedure, the seated patient leans forward, "hugging" a pillow against the chest to bring the arms forward and clear the scapulae from the back. A small stool placed under the feet makes the patient feel more comfortable, and the optimum skin position is marked, just above a rib to avoid the intercostal vessels and nerves. A sterile technique with local anesthetic is used. The size of the drainage catheter varies, ranging between small pigtail catheters and large catheters for empyemas.

The depth of the effusion can be judged by both ultrasound imaging and with use of the local anesthetic needle. The catheter can be positioned by means of a Seldinger technique or with a single-step procedure. The latter is often used and involves advancing the catheter with its central stylet into the pleural space. A slight "give" is felt when the pleura is breached, and at this point the catheter is advanced into the effusion while the central stylet is simultaneously withdrawn. The catheter is connected rapidly to a drainage bag and a three-way tap. Samples for cytologic, microbiologic, and biochemical analysis are taken. If drainage is for a short time (24 to 48 hours), use of a bag will normally suffice. If drainage is required for a longer duration (normal with empyemas) or if the effusion is large—presumably because of active fluid production, the drainage bag is replaced by an underwater drainage system.

If aspiration is undertaken, no more than 1.5 L of fluid should be removed at any one time because of the risk of reexpansion pulmonary edema. Larger catheters can be used, but smaller catheters usually are adequate and more comfortable. The catheters should be securely fastened to the skin, and regular saline irrigation should be performed to maintain patency (20 mL of saline every 4 to 6 hours). In some patients, intrapleural fibrinolytics (e.g., streptokinase) given early may improve drainage but are not routinely used, because use of such agents has not been found to reduce long-term mortality or complication rates and may be associated with adverse reactions.

Complications

Complications are few, provided that no bleeding disorder is present. Pneumothorax occurs in less than 5% of cases. Puncture of other viscera can be avoided by inserting the catheter under ultrasound guidance and with blunt dissection through the chest wall to avoid traumatizing the catheter. Pain may occur at the site of insertion, but this is minimized by inserting the catheter laterally for patient comfort. Reactions to streptokinase are much fewer when the purified form is used but previously have included anaphylaxis and bleeding, both intrapleurally and systemically, with larger doses.

Pitfalls and Controversies

The routine use of intrapleural streptokinase has still not been widely adopted because of the expense and the complications associated with the use of the less purified form and the occasional occurrence of large hemorrhages. Its efficacy in the overall management of empyemas remains uncertain.

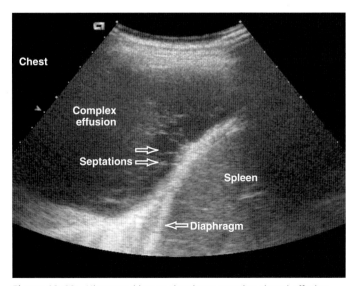

Figure 13-18 Ultrasound image showing a complex pleural effusion with multiple septations.

SUGGESTED READINGS

Adams RF, Gleeson FV: Percutaneous image-guided cutting-needle biopsy of the pleura in the presence of a suspected malignant effusion, *Radiology* 219:510–514, 2001.

Arakawa H, Nakajima Y, Kurihara Y, et al: CT-guided transthoracic needle biopsy: a comparison between automated biopsy gun and fine needle aspiration, *Clin Radiol* 51:503–506, 1996.

Barnes D, Souza C, Entwisle J: The role of percutaneous biopsy in the evolving diagnosis and treatment of lung cancer, *Clin Radiol* 65:951–952, 2010.

Fultz PJ, Harrow AR, Elvey SP, et al: Sonographically guided biopsy of supraclavicular lymph nodes: a simple alternative to lung biopsy and other more invasive procedures, *AJR Am J Roentgenol* 180:1403–1409, 2003.

Gould MK, Fletcher J, Iannettoni MD, et al: Evaluation of patients with pulmonary nodules: when is it lung cancer? ACCP evidence-based clinical practice guidelines (2nd edition), *Chest* 132(3 Suppl):108S–130S, 2007.

Grant A, Neuberger J: Guidelines on the use of liver biopsy in clinical practice, *Gut* 45:IV1–IV11, 1999.

Greif J, Marmor S, Schwarz Y, et al: Percutaneous core needle biopsy versus fine needle aspiration in diagnosing benign lung lesions, *Acta Cytol* 43:756–760, 1999.

Gupta S, Seaberg K, Wallace MJ, et al: Imaging-guided percutaneous biopsy of mediastinal lesions: different approaches and anatomic considerations, *Radiographics* 25:763–786, 2005.

Hare SS, Gupta A, Goncalves AT, et al: Systemic arterial air embolism after percutaneous lung biopsy, *Clin Radiol* 66:589–596, 2011.

Henry M, Arnold T, Harvey J: BTS guidelines for management of spontaneous pneumothorax, *Thorax* 58:ii39, 2003.

Hiraki T, Fujiwara H, Sakurai J, et al: Nonfatal systemic air embolism complicating percutaneous CT-guided transthoracic needle biopsy: four cases from a single institution, *Chest* 132:684–690, 2007.

Klein JS, Salomon G, Stewart EA: Transthoracic needle biopsy with a coaxially placed 20-gauge automated cutting needle: results in 122 patients, *Radiology* 198:715–720, 1996.

Lacasse Y, Wong E, Guyatt G, Cook D: Transthoracic needle aspiration biopsy for the diagnosis of localised pulmonary lesions: a meta-analysis, *Thorax* 54:884–893, 1999.

Lucidarme O, Howarth N, Finet J-F, Grenier PA: Intrapulmonary lesions: percutaneous automated biopsy with a detachable, 18-gauge, co-axial cutting needle, *Radiology* 207:759–765, 1998.

McGill DB, Rakela J, Zinsmeister AR, et al: A 21-year experience with major haemorrhage after percutaneous liver biopsy, *Gastroenterology* 99:1396–1400, 1990.

Piccininio F, Sagnelli E, Pasquale G, et al: Complications following percutaneous liver biopsy, *J Hepatol* 2:165–173, 1986.

Richardson CM, Pointon KS, Manhire AR, Macfarlane JT: Percutaneous lung biopsies: a survey of UK practice based on 5444 biopsies, *Br J Radiol* 75:731–735, 2002.

Tokuda Y, Matsushima D, Stein GH, Miyagi S: Intrapleural fibrinolytic agents for empyema and complicated parapneumonic effusions: a meta-analysis, *Chest* 129:783–790, 2006.

Tomiyama N, Yasuhara Y, Nakajima Y, et al: CT-guided needle biopsy of lung lesions: a survey of severe complications based on 9783 biopsies in Japan, *Eur J Radiol* 59:60–64, 2006.

Westcott JL, Rao N, Colley DP: Transthoracic needle biopsy of small pulmonary nodules, *Radiology* 202:97–103, 1997.

Chapter **14**
Echocardiography in Respiratory Medicine
Jonathan R. Spiro • Richard P. Steeds

The role of echocardiography within clinical medicine has grown dramatically over recent decades, for several reasons. First, the progressive increase in use of echocardiography has mirrored a decline in clinical examination skills previously required for cardiorespiratory diagnosis. Second, it generally is recognized that the clinical diagnosis of many common cardiac conditions such as pericardial effusion, early ventricular dysfunction, and silent valvular disease is a challenge for even the most experienced clinician, yet such conditions can be rapidly diagnosed by echocardiography. Third, early etiologic diagnosis leads to rapid institution of an appropriate management plan, as evidenced by the fact that the frequency of cardiorespiratory misdiagnosis in unselected patients who died while hospitalized has halved over the past 20 years, in parallel with the increasing use of echocardiography. The combination of sophisticated technology, powerful computing, and improved operator ability has, however, translated to the production of large amounts of data, often highly complex in nature, which can be difficult to interpret. Consequently, training in performing and interpreting an echocardiogram has become significantly more rigorous.

Owing to the inherent interrelationship of the cardiovascular and respiratory systems, important clinical and prognostic information may be obtained from echocardiographic evaluation of patients with acute and chronic respiratory disease. Advantages of the technique include wide availability, portability, low cost, and provision of high-quality diagnostic imaging without the use of ionizing radiation. Despite many favorable characteristics, echocardiography has important limitations. Accuracy of data is reliant on the availability of a high-quality acoustic window, which often may be limited in respiratory disease, when hyperexpansion of lungs or the use of ventilatory support may limit ultrasound transmission. In such circumstances, echocardiography is technically challenging. This chapter provides an overview of the important components of the echocardiographic examination, including techniques, views, and structurally based measurements, in evaluation for specific respiratory disease states. The information thus obtained may assist or influence decisions regarding diagnosis, management, and prognosis.

ECHOCARDIOGRAPHIC PLANES AND RIGHT-SIDED HEART STRUCTURES

The right ventricle (RV) is located anterior to the left ventricle (LV) and is positioned just behind the sternum. When viewed anteriorly, the right ventricular cavity appears triangular in shape; however, it takes a crescentic shape in cross section. This anatomic orientation means that no single acoustic window allows visualization of the whole of the RV, so multiple transducer positions must be used. Standard echocardiography of the right side of the heart includes use of the parasternal (long-axis, right ventricular inflow, short-axis) (see Videos 1 and 2), apical (four-chamber) (see Video 3) and (modified four-chamber), and subcostal acoustic windows (see Video 4), generating a report that includes a qualitative description of right-sided heart anatomy and function, with at least one measurement of right atrial and right ventricular size, and a quantitative assessment of right ventricular function (**Table 14-1**). The venous inflow to the right side of the heart comprises the coronary sinus, superior vena cava, and inferior vena cava. The venous inflow is easily visualized from the parasternal acoustic window, in the right ventricular inflow view (**Figure 14-1**, *A*, and Video 5) and from the parasternal acoustic window, in the right ventricular inflow view (see Figure 14-1, *B*, and Video 4). The right atrium, tricuspid valve, and RV (inlet, free wall, apex, and infundibulum) are seen from the parasternal short axis (see Figure 14-1, *C*) and modified apical four-chamber views (see Figure 14-1, *D*). The tricuspid valve comprises septal, anterosuperior, and posterior leaflets, attached by chordae tendineae to papillary muscles located within the septum and lateral walls of the RV. Unlike with the aortic and mitral valves, it is not possible to see all three leaflets of the tricuspid valve from any single two-dimensional view—the septal and anterosuperior leaflets are seen in the apical four-chamber view, with the posterior and anterosuperior leaflets seen in the right ventricular inflow view. The pulmonary valve consists of three cusps without subvalvular apparatus and, along with the main pulmonary artery and proximal branch pulmonary arteries, is best seen on the parasternal short axis (see Figure 14-1, *C*, and Video 6) and rotated subcostal views. Normal ranges for right ventricular and right atrial size have been derived from normal healthy populations. An important point in this context is that these measures are not indexed to body surface area, so reported values may lose discriminatory power in assessment of these structures at either end of the normal distribution curve for size.

ASSESSMENT OF RIGHT VENTRICULAR FUNCTION BY ECHOCARDIOGRAPHY

The orientation of the myocardial fibers within the right ventricular wall is different from that within the LV, leading to three definable modes of contraction. First, the right ventricular contraction is sequential and peristaltic, from inlet to infundibulum, and results in *longitudinal shortening*, which is the main driver behind right ventricular stroke volume. Second, the right ventricular free wall is observed to move inwards toward the interventricular septum (IVS), contributing to stroke volume through a bellows-like effect. Third, twist or torsion of the RV is less important than in the LV but arises

Table 14-1 Normal Limits for Recommended Measurements of Right-Sided Heart Structure and Function

Variable	Abnormal	Illustrated in:
Chamber Dimensions		
RV subcostal wall thickness	>0.5 cm	Figure 14-1, B
RVOT PLAX proximal diameter	>3.3 cm	Figure 14-1, C
RV basal diameter (RVD1)	>4.2 cm	Figure 14-1, D
RA major diameter	>5.3 cm	Figure 14-1, D
RA minor diameter	>4.4 cm	Figure 14-1, D
Systolic Function		
Tricuspid annular plane systolic excursion (TAPSE)	<1.6 cm	Figure 14-2, A
Peak lateral TV annular velocity, S'	<10 cm/s	Figure 14-2, B
Myocardial performance index (MPI) Pulsed-wave Doppler imaging Tissue Doppler imaging	>0.40 >0.55	Figure 14-2, C
Fractional area change (FAC)	<35%	Figure 14-2, D
Diastolic Function		
E/A	<0.8 or >2.1	Figure 14-3, A
E/E'	>6	

A, velocity of active ventricular filling (see Figure 14-3, A); E, velocity of passive right ventricular filling (see Figure 14-3, A); E', a tissue Doppler measurement of the motion of the lateral tricuspid valve annulus during early diastole (see Figure 14-2, B); PLAX, parasternal long axis; RV, right ventricle; RVOT, right ventricular outflow tract; RA, right atrium; TV, tricuspid valve.
Data from Rudski L, Lai W, Afilalo J, et al: Guidelines for the echocardiographic assessment of the right heart in adults: a report from the American Society of Echocardiography, *J Am Soc Echocardiogr* 23:685–713, 2010.

predominantly from contraction against the insertion points of the RV into the septum. Although longitudinal (rather than radial) shortening is most important, the IVS contributes between 20% to 40% of right ventricular stroke volume. Echocardiographic evaluation of right ventricular function is complicated, because volumetric assessment of the RV (using end-diastolic and end-systolic volumes to calculate an ejection fraction) cannot be performed without advanced three-dimensional techniques. Visual assessment of right ventricular function may provide an initial qualitative evaluation of the function of the right side of the heart but suffers from inter-study variability of up to 15%; however, one or more of the following quantitative measurements should be incorporated.

TRICUSPID ANNULAR PLANE SYSTOLIC EXCURSION

Tricuspid annular plane systolic excursion (TAPSE) is measured using M-mode echocardiography in the apical four-chamber view to generate an image that illustrates the systolic longitudinal displacement of the lateral tricuspid annulus toward the apex (**Figure 14-2, A**). Because the septal attachment of the tricuspid annulus is relatively fixed, the major component of longitudinal systolic motion occurs at this point. The greater the displacement, the better is right ventricular function—a value less than 16 mm is considered abnormal. TAPSE correlates closely with right ventricular ejection fraction (RVEF) measured by radionuclide angiography, the "gold standard" modality for assessment of right ventricular function. TAPSE is simple to perform, with reproducible results, and is

less dependent on optimal image quality than other measurements. It does not require complex calculations (the result obtained may be multiplied by 3.2 to give a value for RVEF, if desired) and can predict likelihood of death among patients with pulmonary arterial hypertension (PAH). However, TAPSE makes the assumption that displacement of a single segment represents function of the entire RV, which does not apply in the presence of regional dysfunction, particularly that affecting the septum. TAPSE is afterload dependent and falls with increasing severity of PAH.

PEAK SYSTOLIC VELOCITY OF LATERAL TRICUSPID ANNULUS DISPLACEMENT

Tissue Doppler imaging (TDI) can be used to measure the velocity of longitudinal displacement of the lateral tricuspid valve annulus during systole (S') (see Figure 14-2, B). S' values correlate closely with radionuclide angiography findings, and population-based validation studies indicate that a value less than 10 cm/s is abnormal. The data share the disadvantage of TAPSE in assuming that the velocity of a single wall region reflects the entire function of the complex three-dimensional shape of RV. Velocities are measured using Doppler imaging and therefore can underestimate function if measured off-angle by more than 20 degrees.

Myocardial Performance Index

The right ventricular myocardial performance index (MPI), also known as the Tei index, is the ratio of isovolumetric relaxation time (IVRT) plus isovolumetric contraction time (IVCT) to ventricular ejection time (see Figure 14-2, C). This index gives an accurate, global estimate of both systolic and diastolic right ventricular function. It avoids the need to use the geometric assumptions that are required for volumetric measurement of global right ventricular function, because MPI is based on time intervals from either blood pool Doppler (right ventricular outflow tract [RVOT] and tricuspid valve inflow) or tissue Doppler (lateral tricuspid valve annulus) measurements. A value greater than 0.4 is abnormal for blood pool Doppler, and a value greater than 0.55 is abnormal for tissue Doppler. Advantages of this technique include high reproducibility and the fact that it is relatively unaffected by variation in heart rate. The MPI can be falsely low under conditions of raised right atrial pressure, which may decrease the IVRT.

Fractional Area Change

Fractional area change (FAC) is obtained by tracing the endocardial border of the right ventricle in systole and diastole in the apical four-chamber view (see Figure 14-2, D). The percent FAC is then calculated using the formula (end-diastolic area − end-systolic area/end-diastolic area) × 100%, with a value below 35% considered abnormal. This method correlates closely with magnetic resonance imaging (MRI) assessment of right ventricular function, and reduced FAC is an independent predictor of adverse outcome after pulmonary embolism. The main practical disadvantage arises in defining contours in highly trabeculated RVs.

Three-Dimensional Volume Estimation

Three-dimensional volume estimation of right ventricular function correlates closely with radionuclide angiography and with MRI estimates of right ventricular function. It delivers accurate and reproducible measurements, but at present, the methodology is complicated and time-consuming, and the

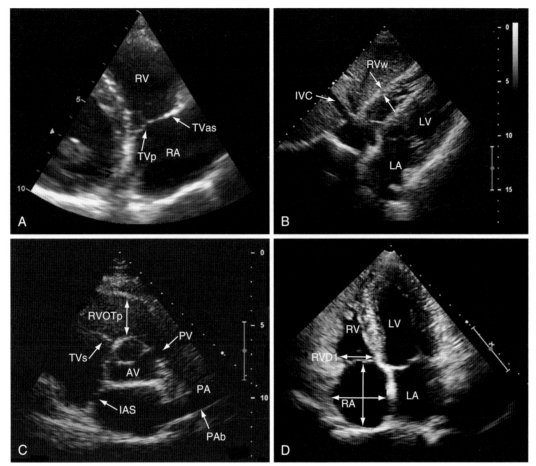

Figure 14-1   Echocardiographic views. **A,** Tilted right ventricular inflow view; **B,** subcostal view; **C,** parasternal short axis view; **D,** apical four-chamber view. *AV,* aortic valve; *IAS,* interatrial septum; *IVC,* inferior vena cava; *LA,* left atrium; *LV,* left ventricle; *PA,* pulmonary artery; *PAb,* pulmonary artery bifurcation; *PV,* pulmonary valve; *RA,* right atrium; *RV,* right ventricle; *RVD1,* right ventricular basal diameter; *RVOTp,* right ventricular outflow tract proximal diameter; *RVw,* site of measurement of right ventricular wall thickness; *TV,* anterosuperior (*TVas*), posterior (*TVp*), and tricuspid valve with septal (*TVs*) leaflets.

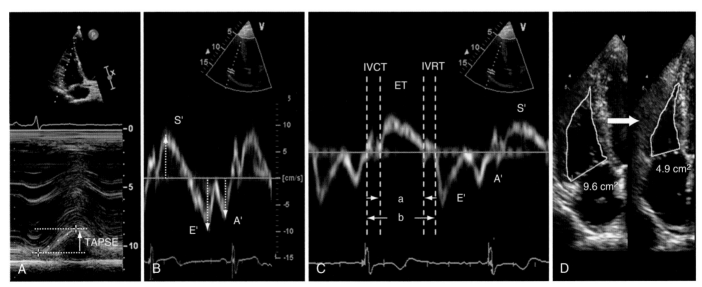

Figure 14-2   Assessment of right ventricular systolic function by various modalities: **A,** tricuspid annular plane systolic excursion (TAPSE); **B,** S′ wave measurement by tissue Doppler imaging; **C,** myocardial performance index (MPI), or Tei index, calculated as isovolumetric relaxation time (IVRT) plus isovolumetric contraction time (IVCT) divided by ventricular ejection time (ET), or $a/b - a$; **D,** fractional area change (FAC)—here, from 9.6 cm^2 to 4.9 cm^2 = 49%. E/E′ is calculated as follows: peak velocity of pulsed-wave Doppler E wave (measured at the tips of the tricuspid valve; see Figure 14-3, *A*) divided by peak velocity of the E′ wave (measured using tissue Doppler imaging at the lateral tricuspid valve annulus).

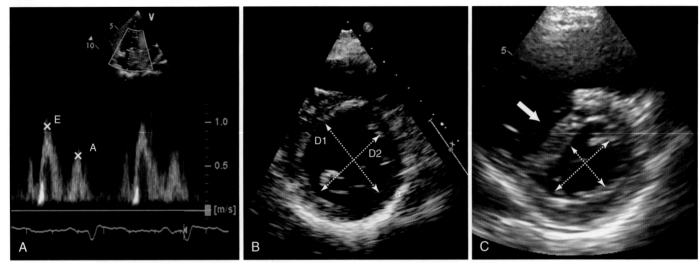

Figure 14-3 A, Pulsed-wave Doppler assessment of tricuspid valve inflow from the apical four-chamber view. E wave velocity reflects passive ventricular filling, whereas A wave velocity represents ventricular filling secondary to atrial systole. **B** and **C,** Flattening of the interventricular septum (*arrow*). *D1,* minor axis dimension perpendicular to and bisecting septum; *D2,* minor axis dimension parallel to the septum. Eccentricity index (EI) is calculated as *D2/D1.* Normal EI value is 1.0; EI greater than 1.0 at end-diastole is indicative of volume overload of right ventricle, whereas EI greater than 1.0 at end-systole is indicative of pressure overload.

equipment not widely available. The lower limit of normal is 44%, lower than that for the LV.

RIGHT VENTRICULAR DIASTOLIC FUNCTION

Diastolic function, which reflects the relaxation and filling of the RV, can be a useful early marker predicting deterioration in right ventricular function and may be of prognostic utility in patients with a number of acute and chronic respiratory conditions, although further data are needed. The parameters used for assessment of right ventricular diastolic function are essentially the same as those used in left ventricular diastolic assessment, including pulsed-wave Doppler-derived transtricuspid E/A ratio, tissue Doppler–derived E/E' ratio, IVRT, and right atrial size (**Figure 14-3,** *A*). IVRT is a tissue Doppler measurement of the time taken for the right ventricle to relax, which is made at the basal right ventricular free wall. This relaxation period occurs after pulmonary valve closure (end of the S' wave) and before tricuspid valve opening (beginning of the E' wave) (see Figure 14-2, *C*). A prolonged IVRT (longer than 75 ms) may represent impaired myocardial relaxation and can be highly suggestive of PAH. Diastolic measurements should be acquired in end-expiration, and interpretation of the results should take account of the age of the patient (see Table 14-1). One additional important finding is the presence of late antegrade flow measured by pulsed-wave Doppler midway between the pulmonary valve leaflets and the pulmonary artery bifurcation, which is a sign of restrictive right ventricular filling and is associated with a poor prognosis.

HEMODYNAMIC ASSESSMENT OF THE RIGHT SIDE OF THE HEART BY ECHOCARDIOGRAPHY

In health, the right side of the heart ejects blood into a low-resistance, highly distensible pulmonary vascular bed. The RV is thin-walled and more compliant than the LV (so it adapts well to increases in volume) but demonstrates heightened sensitivity to change in afterload (so it adapts poorly to increases in pulmonary vascular resistance). The LV and RV interact with one another during systole, and this ventricular

interdependence is mediated mainly by the motion of the IVS. Both changes in volume (preload) or pressure (afterload) within the right side of the heart will have an impact on the motion of the IVS. Under normal conditions, the higher intracavity pressure in the LV, as compared with that in the RV, helps to maintain a circular shape of the LV when imaged in cross section (see Video 2). Pressure loading of the RV results in a "flattening" of the IVS during systole, creating a more D-shaped left ventricular cavity. Volume loading of the RV results in a "flattening" of the IVS during diastole (see Figure 14-3, *B* and C; see also Video 7). This is an important marker of loading conditions within the RV, which can be measured by calculating the "eccentricity index" of the LV in the parasternal short-axis view (i.e., the ratio of the anterior-posterior dimension to septal-lateral dimension of the left ventricular cavity).

A number of direct parameters can be used for hemodynamic assessment of the right ventricular and pulmonary circulations, the most common being measurement of right ventricular systolic pressure (RVSP) estimated from the velocity of the jet of the tricuspid regurgitation (**Figure 14-4,** *A* and *B*, and Video 8). Using the simplified Bernoulli equation,

$$RVSP = 4v^2 + \text{Right atrial pressure}$$

where v = maximal velocity of the jet of tricuspid regurgitation (in m/s) and right atrial pressure is estimated from resting inferior vena cava diameter taking into account the degree of inspiratory collapse (see Figure 14-4, *C*, and Video 9). In the absence of a gradient across the pulmonary valve or RVOT, RVSP equals the *systolic* pulmonary artery pressure (PAP). Care must be taken to ensure that this measurement is made with an adequate Doppler signal; if the signal is not clear, it can be improved with the injection of an agitated mixture of blood, saline, and air for contrast. The measurement should be made several times, and the highest velocity obtained used in calculation. A normal value for a peak tricuspid regurgitation signal is less than 2.6 m/s (equivalent to a pressure of 27 mm Hg + right atrial pressure), but this value increases with age and with increasing body mass index. This method may underestimate RVSP when severe tricuspid regurgitation is present.

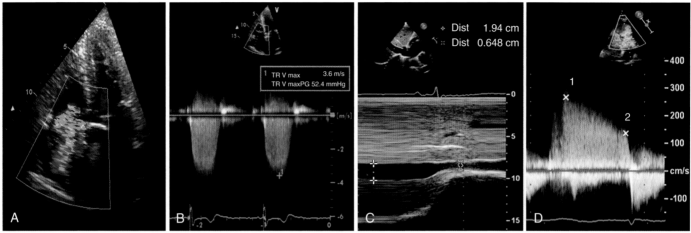

Figure 14-4 Hemodynamic measurements in echocardiography. **A,** Color flow Doppler imaging demonstrating tricuspid regurgitation (TR), with blood being ejected back into the right atrium. **B,** Continuous-wave Doppler interrogation of the regurgitant jet. Point *1* denotes peak jet velocity, which measures 3.6 m/s in this example. **C,** M-mode assessment of the inferior vena cava (IVC) from the subcostal acoustic window. The IVC can be seen to collapse with short sharp inspiration, decreasing in size from 1.94 cm to 0.648 cm in this example. Right atrial pressure can be estimated by assessing the diameter of the IVC at rest and then recording the change in size in response to inspiration: normal IVC diameter (i.e., less than 1.5 cm) with full collapse, 0 to 5 mm Hg; IVC diameter 1.5 to 2.5 cm with greater than 50% collapse, 5 to 10 mm Hg; IVC diameter 1.5 to 2.5 cm with less than 50% collapse, 10 to 15 mm Hg; IVC diameter greater than 2.5 with less than 50% collapse, 15 to 20 mm Hg; and IVC diameter greater than 2.5 cm with no change, 20 mm Hg or greater. **D,** Echocardiographic determination of diastolic and mean pulmonary artery pressure (PAP) by continuous-wave Doppler assessment of the signal generated by pulmonary regurgitation (PR). Point *1* indicates the maximal velocity of the jet of pulmonary regurgitation at the beginning of diastole. Mean PAP can be calculated as 4 × (early pulmonary regurgitation jet velocity)² + estimated right atrial pressure. Point *2* indicates the pulmonary regurgitant jet velocity at end-diastole, with diastolic PAP calculated as 4 × (end pulmonary regurgitant jet velocity)² + estimated right atrial pressure.

The simplified Bernoulli equation also can be used to estimate diastolic PAP from the end-diastolic velocity of the pulmonary regurgitant jet: diastolic PAP = $4v^2$ + right atrial pressure (see Figure 14-4, *D*), where v = terminal velocity of the regurgitant jet (in m/s). Mean PAP can then be calculated using a standard formula: mean PAP = 1/3 systolic PAP + 2/3 diastolic PAP. It also can be estimated directly from the early peak of the regurgitant jet velocity: mean PAP = $4v^2$ (v = early maximal velocity of the regurgitant jet [in m/s]) plus right atrial pressure (see Figure 14-4, *D*). Echocardiography also can deliver measurements of pulmonary vascular resistance, pulmonary capillary wedge pressure, and pulmonary capacitance, although these are not in routine use. These measurements provide important insights into right ventricular and pulmonary hemodynamic status, although any conclusions should be based not only on a single hemodynamic parameter, such as jet velocity in tricuspid regurgitation, but also in the context of a full assessment of right ventricular and right atrial size, shape, and function.

Right ventricular adaptation to disease is complex and depends on many factors. The most important factors appear to be the type and severity of myocardial stress, the time course of the disease (acute or chronic), and the time of onset of the disease process (young age or adult years). The remodeling of the right side of the heart produces classic anatomic and hemodynamic characteristics that are used by echocardiographers to diagnose and assess prognosis in specific disease states, as discussed next.

ECHOCARDIOGRAPHY IN EVALUATION OF SPECIFIC DISEASE STATES

PULMONARY ARTERIAL HYPERTENSION

PAH is a hemodynamic and pathophysiologic condition defined as an increased mean PAP of 25 mm Hg or more at rest, as assessed invasively at right-sided heart catheterization. The evaluation process in a patient with suspected PAH requires a number of investigations, but echocardiography should always be performed. The primary rationale is to provide an estimate of PAP, although the echocardiographic study most often measures the systolic and not the mean pressure, and this method is no longer recommended for screening patients with mild PAH.

The principal technique used to estimate PAP from Doppler ultrasound measurement of the maximal velocity of the tricuspid regurgitation jet consists of application of the simplified Bernoulli equation and addition of estimated right atrial pressure, as discussed previously. Historically, Doppler echocardiography has been considered to correlate well with direct (invasive) measurements of PAP; more recent studies, however, have brought this relationship into question. Indeed, in a study of 163 patients recruited to the National Emphysema Treatment Trial, who were assessed by both Doppler echocardiography and right-sided heart catheterization, echocardiographic estimates of PAP correlated weakly with invasive measurements, with investigators reporting poor sensitivity (60%), specificity (74%), and positive (68%) and negative (67%) predictive values for Doppler imaging. Poor image quality was common and was thought to be a major factor in the relative inaccuracy of PAP estimation in this study. However, these findings were replicated in a more recent study of 65 patients with PAH secondary to a variety of conditions, in which Doppler imaging and right-sided heart catheterization were performed "simultaneously" (within 1 hour). Once again, Doppler echocardiography continued to provide inaccurate estimates of PAH. The accuracy of the measurement can be limited not only by poor image quality but also by extremes of jet velocity or character, observed as trivial, severe, or eccentric, resulting in an incomplete regurgitation signal. Estimation of right atrial pressure from inferior vena cava dimensions and collapsibility may contribute to this inaccuracy, because correct identification of right atrial pressure, within a range of 5 mm Hg, may be achievable in only about half of all cases. Accuracy of this estimation can be improved by an assessment of hepatic vein flow, because increasing right atrial pressure is associated with a relative decline in systolic forward hepatic vein flow relative to atrial reversal. In summary, although a strong correlation is recognized between jet velocity in tricuspid regurgitation and pressure gradient, Doppler echocardiography may not be accurate in the individual patient to assess systolic PAP. An alternative approach to the use of a Doppler-derived pressure gradient is simply to measure the jet velocity in tricuspid regurgitation and compare this against values from the normal population. This approach has the disadvantage that the value does not directly link to the accepted pressure-derived definition of PAH; use of velocity alone, however, does avoid the cumulative error that arises in calculating pressure.

Attention should always be paid to other echocardiographic features that may reinforce the suspicion of PAH. These include dilatation of the RV and right atrium (see Videos 10 to 12), the presence of right ventricular hypertrophy (greater than 5 mm in cross section) measured from the subcostal acoustic window, early systolic flattening of the IVS, and dilatation of the pulmonary artery. The sensitivity of such findings is likely to be low, as they are late pathologic consequences of PAH. Other indirect measures resulting from high afterload in the pulmonary circulation are useful and include prolongation of the right ventricular IVRT (greater than 75 ms) and shortening of the acceleration time of right ventricular ejection into the pulmonary artery (less than 105 ms). High afterload also results in a fall in longitudinal contraction within the RV, resulting in a negative correlation with S' wave velocity on TDI (less than 12 cm/s) and TAPSE (less than 18 mm). Finally, the degree of PAH correlates with an increase in the velocity of the jet of pulmonary regurgitation, measured on pulsed Doppler in the parasternal short-axis view.

Echocardiography can not only be helpful as a screening tool in patients with suspected PAH but can also provide useful prognostic information. Multivariable analysis of various echocardiographic parameters has demonstrated prognostic utility for (1) the presence of pericardial effusion (hazard ratio, [HR], 2.08 [95% CI = 1.12 to 3.86; $P = .017$]), (2) indexed right atrial area (HR, 1.33 [95% CI = 1.06 to 1.66; $P = .012$]), (3) left ventricular eccentricity index greater than 1.7 (HR, 1.45 [95% CI = 1.12 to 1.86; $P = .004$]), (4) right ventricular systolic function as determined by FAC, (5) right ventricular tissue Doppler, (6) right ventricular MPI, and (7) TAPSE less than 15 mm (HR, 2.74 [95% CI = 1.11 to 6.77; $P = .022$]).

Furthermore, echocardiography also may provide information regarding the cause of PAH—for example, significant left-sided heart disease, which may include left ventricular or valvular dysfunction. Echocardiography is vital in the exclusion of significant congenital heart disease and in the identification of systemic to pulmonary shunts. Detection of high pulmonary blood flow on Doppler interrogation of the RVOT or two-dimensional detection of an enlarged right heart chamber in the absence of a clear shunt on transthoracic echocardiography (TTE) should precipitate a more intensive examination using transesophageal echocardiography (TEE). This modality not only provides a closer inspection of the atrial septum but also ensures that a sinus venosus–type septal defect can be excluded (which cannot be seen on TTE) and that anomalous pulmonary venous drainage is not present. The latter defects are of particular importance to distinguish from atrial septal defects, because these are not amenable to percutaneous closure. The

accuracy of both TTE and TEE can be improved by the use of an agitated mixture of saline, air, and blood contrast, which also can be used to identify intrapulmonary shunts in patients with portal vein and pulmonary artery (porto-pulmonary) hypertension.

Thus, echocardiography is an integral part of the diagnostic algorithm for investigation of suspected PAH and may provide quantitative data useful for the assessment of prognosis in patients with proven disease.

ACUTE RIGHT-SIDED HEART FAILURE

Acute right ventricular dysfunction may occur as a consequence of various disease processes, which include ischemic heart disease, myocarditis, and pulmonary embolism. Among patients presenting with suspected acute pulmonary embolism, neither TTE nor TEE have sufficient sensitivity to be used as the primary imaging modality for diagnosis but may provide useful supportive data and can identify those persons at high risk for adverse outcomes. Typically, the abrupt vascular obstruction sets up a cascade of adverse hemodynamic effects that not only exert strain on the RV but also may impair left ventricular function and coronary artery perfusion (**Figure 14-5**).

Although echocardiography may be normal in up to 50% of patients with confirmed pulmonary embolism, sensitivity is increased with increasing hemodynamic compromise from the event. Typical echocardiographic findings include dilatation of the RV with reduced thickening of the free wall, flattening of the IVS in systole, dilatation of the right atrium due to elevated right ventricular end-diastolic pressure, paradoxical atrial septal motion due to high right atrial pressure, which also is associated with dilatation of the inferior vena cava, and loss of respiratory variation. Hemodynamic measurements altered by acute pulmonary embolism include increased jet velocity in tricuspid regurgitation (more than 2.7 m/s) and reduction in TAPSE and S', together with shortened RVOT acceleration time. Rarely, thrombus may be seen in the right side of the heart or pulmonary artery. The McConnell sign, consisting of hypokinesis of

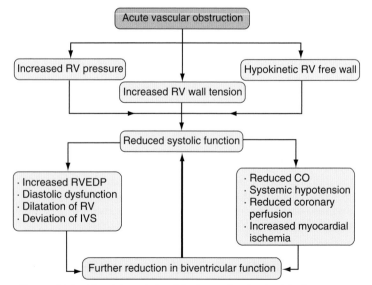

Figure 14-5 The vicious circle of detrimental pathophysiologic events that may occur in the setting of acute vascular obstruction, such as with acute pulmonary embolism. *CO,* cardiac output; *IVS,* interventricular septum; *RV,* right ventricle; *RVEDP,* right ventricular end-diastolic pressure.

the mid–free wall in the presence of normal apical wall motion, is reported to be 77% sensitive and 94% specific for acute pulmonary embolism.

In the setting of acute pulmonary embolism, the presence of right ventricular dysfunction and/or elevated PAP has been shown to predict poor outcome. Consequently, using echocardiography early in the assessment of patients with acute hemodynamic instability may assist with rapid detection of these high-risk features and may identify a cohort of subjects who may benefit from more aggressive management, perhaps involving the use of thrombolysis. An important point in this context is that these changes occur in patients with acute pulmonary embolism who have no preexisting thromboembolism or PAH, in which case the effect of chronic pressure overload on the RV modifies the appearance of the right side of the heart.

CHRONIC RIGHT-SIDED HEART FAILURE (COR PULMONALE)

The most common cause of chronic right-sided heart failure is chronic left ventricular failure (LVF). Both in LVF and in chronic lung disease, such as chronic interstitial disease, chronic obstructive pulmonary disease (COPD), or chronic thromboembolic disease, the pulmonary vasculature gradually remodels over time from a low- to a high-pressure system. This insidious transformation exerts an impact on the function and architecture of the RV as it attempts to maintain stroke volume and is characterized by right ventricular hypertrophy (RVH). This hypertrophy is not similar to that seen in the physiologically trained or athletic heart but involves other processes that include myocardial fibrosis, inflammation, and myocyte apoptosis and necrosis. The RV in general responds better to chronic volume than to pressure overload, which leads to a more pronounced increase in the density of myocardial connective tissue observed at histologic examination. Initially on visual inspection, right ventricular systolic function appears to be maintained, although a reduction in systolic contraction is preceded by impaired right ventricular diastolic function and by changes in myocardial strain. *Strain* is an echocardiographic measure of myocardial deformation in thickening or shortening that is independent of myocardial velocity and translational cardiac motion. Ultimately, however, the effect of the continued pressure overload on the hypertrophied right ventricular myocardium predisposes the patient toward full decompensation in function, which is reflected in right ventricular dilatation, thinning of the right ventricular free wall, and fall in right ventricular systolic function.

Right ventricular function is a strong and independent predictor of mortality in LVF. Progressive reduction in right ventricular FAC is associated with worse outcomes in patients with heart failure after myocardial infarction, independent of severity of reduction in left ventricular ejection fraction. Other independent right-sided indices of adverse outcome in patients with LVF include reductions in right ventricular MPI and TDI S′. Adverse prognosis in RVH, secondary to chronic lung disease and in the absence of LVF, is similarly predicted by reductions in TAPSE and TDI S′, but increased right ventricular dilatation assessed by right ventricular end-diastolic volume index is an additional predictor of death.

PERICARDIAL EFFUSION AND TAMPONADE

The pericardium consists of a monolayer of mesothelial cells that directly overlie the epicardial fat (visceral layer) and reflects back upon itself to form a second (parietal) layer. In health, the pericardium contains a small volume (15 to 35 mL) of plasma ultrafiltrate, which acts as a lubricant. Under physiologic conditions of low stress, the pericardium is elastic, but under higher stress, it has the tensile strength of rubber and becomes stiff and resistant to stretch. This transition in mechanical properties occurs close to the upper limit of normal pericardial volume. As the pericardial reserve volume is exceeded, pressure within the pericardium increases rapidly. This rise in pressure is dependent not only on the volume but also on the rate of accumulation, which explains why large pericardial effusions may cause no hemodynamic compromise if they have developed slowly, whereas very small volumes can cause hemodynamic collapse if the ultrafiltrate accumulated rapidly. Under conditions in which pericardial pressure rises, the mechanical properties of the pericardium become an important determinant of right atrial and right ventricular filling, and cardiac function may be adversely affected, with loss of normal ventricular interdependence.

Pericardial effusion is detected easily by TTE and is distinguished from pleural fluid by its presence anterior to the descending aorta in the parasternal long-axis view (**Figure 14-6** and Video 13). Pericardial fluid almost never overlaps the left atrium and usually collects behind the right atrium and then the RV and extends to the lateral wall of the LV. This localization obviously depends on patient position, but the effusion can be a focal process with a localized accumulation of fluid—for example, after cardiothoracic surgery. Assessing the size of a pericardial effusion is important for prognostication: The larger the collection, the worse the outcome. The presence of even a small pericardial effusion, however, is a marker for increased risk of death.

Although cardiac tamponade remains a clinical diagnosis, certain echocardiographic features are often used to confirm the presence of a hemodynamically significant pericardial collection. As the pericardial pressure increases, the first effect is for ventricular interdependence to be exaggerated—this means that respiratory variation in tricuspid valve inflow measured at the tips of the valve on pulsed-wave Doppler imaging is exaggerated at the expense of mitral valve inflow. On inspiration, for example, tricuspid valve inflow velocity and volume increase, whereas mitral valve inflow velocity and volume decrease. As pressure rises further and diastolic filling of the heart is impaired, the chambers of the heart start to "collapse" in order of intracavity pressure—first the right atrium, then the RV, and subsequently the left atrium (see Videos 14 and 15; see also Video 13). Abnormal posterior motion of the anterior right ventricular free wall during diastole seen in the parasternal long-axis view should prompt urgent review, with consideration of pericardiocentesis. TTE can then play a vital role in guiding percutaneous needle aspiration, or drain insertion, which may rapidly alleviate symptoms. Echocardiography-guided aspiration has a high procedural success rate and carries a risk of major complications of only 1% to 2%.

PERICARDIAL CONSTRICTION

The pericardium can be affected by a variety of inflammatory, infective, or neoplastic insults that may trigger a healing process characterized by granulation and scar tissue formation, promoting fibrosis sufficient to obliterate the pericardial space. Under such conditions, the pericardium becomes a firm and poorly compliant structure that can encase, or "constrict," the heart, leading to impairment of ventricular diastolic filling.

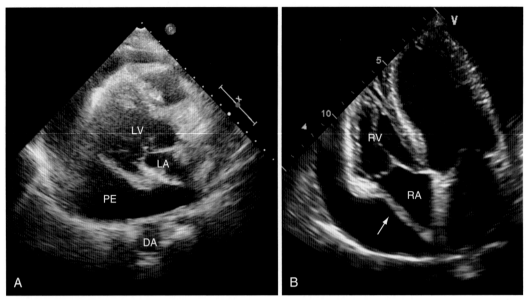

Figure 14-6 A large pericardial effusion, viewed from the parasternal long-axis (PLAX) (**A**) and apical four-chamber (**B**) acoustic windows. In **A**, the effusion can be seen to lie anterior to the descending thoracic aorta (DA), thereby differentiating it from a left-sided pleural effusion, which usually is seen to extend posteriorly to the descending aorta. In this example, the effusion extends alongside the left atrium (LA), which is unusual. In **B**, the right atrium (RA) is seen to collapse during diastole *(arrow)*, which may be a feature of significantly increased intrapericardial pressure and may be an early sign of tamponade.

Historically, tuberculous pericarditis was the most common cause of pericardial constriction; today, however, the most common causes include healing after cardiac surgery, neoplastic pericarditis, mediastinal irradiation, chronic uremia, inflammation associated with pulmonary asbestosis, and recurrent pericarditis secondary to connective tissue disorders.

It can be difficult to differentiate between pericardial constriction and a restrictive cardiomyopathy, because both manifest with signs and symptoms suggestive of right ventricular failure and a restrictive filling pattern on pulsed-wave Doppler, assessed at the tips of the mitral and tricuspid valves. Early diastolic filling is rapid, owing to raised intraatrial pressure, which is seen as an elevated E wave velocity. However, intraventricular pressure rises abruptly, as a consequence of the lack of either pericardial or myocardial compliance (from pericardial constriction or restrictive cardiomyopathy, respectively), so that by mid-diastole, rapid cessation of passive filling is seen, corresponding to a shortened E wave deceleration time (less than 150 ms). Owing to high interventricular pressure, atrial systole does not contribute as much as normal to ventricular filling, so the A wave velocity is reduced, resulting in an E/A ratio greater than 2. Although these echocardiographic features are shared by the two conditions, clinical distinction is vital, because the treatment of choice for pericardial constriction is pericardiectomy, which carries a high risk and is of no benefit in restrictive cardiomyopathy.

RESTRICTIVE CARDIOMYOPATHY SECONDARY TO CHRONIC RESPIRATORY DISEASE

Cardiomyopathies (CMs) are a group of conditions characterized by abnormalities of the myocardium. CMs are broadly divided into three main functional categories: dilated, hypertrophic, and restrictive. Among patients with certain respiratory diseases, such as sarcoid or hypereosinophilic (Löffler) syndrome, cardiac involvement caused by infiltration of the myocardium may give rise to a restrictive cardiomyopathy. The hallmark of a restrictive cardiomyopathy is a stiff and poorly compliant myocardium that limits diastolic filling, resulting in elevated end diastolic pressures and the characteristic echo features as described. The diagnosis of cardiac involvement in patients with established respiratory disease often is difficult, but TTE is an important first step. On two-dimensional echocardiography, the left ventricular cavity size is often normal or reduced, in contrast with left ventricular wall thickness, which may be normal or increased—the presence of concentric LVH in the absence of a history of systemic hypertension should prompt further investigation (see Video 16). Being compliant chambers, both the left and right atria are considered "barometers" of ventricular filling pressure. This means that biatrial enlargement is often present in restrictive cardiomyopathy as a result of increased biventricular filling pressures. The RV may be hypertrophied and ultimately dilated, in the presence of elevated pulmonary artery pressure. Right-sided heart failure is a final common pathway, often as a sequel to chronic PAH driven by the underlying respiratory disorder.

Echocardiographic features that support a diagnosis of pericardial constriction, rather than restrictive cardiomyopathy, may include the presence of an echodense or thickened pericardium (often, however, it may appear normal), normal chamber size, normal wall thickness, and preservation of systolic function. Other data in support of pericardial constriction include the finding of a normal early annular myocardial relaxation velocity on TDI, exaggeration of the usual variation in tricuspid and mitral valve inflow observed during respiration, and reversal of the normal annular early relaxation velocities measured by TDI (a higher E′ velocity is found in the septum compared to the lateral annulus). Conversely, in restrictive cardiomyopathy early annular myocardial relaxation may be reduced (E′ is less than 7 cm/s), variation in tricuspid and mitral inflow is within normal range, and annular early relaxation velocities are higher laterally than in the septum (lateral E′

higher than septal E′). Finally, paradoxical motion of the IVS is observed in pericardial constriction and not in restriction and represents an exaggeration of the normal physiologic ventricular interdependency secondary to the equalization of intraventricular pressures after encasement of the heart within the noncompliant diseased pericardium, with increased right ventricular filling on inspiration (shift of the IVS toward the LV) and increased left ventricular filling on expiration (movement of the IVS toward the RV).

CONCLUSIONS

Traditionally, the right side of the heart has often been ignored relative to the LV, but right ventricular function is well recognized to play a vital role in determining clinical outcome in both acute and chronic respiratory disease. Careful qualitative and quantitative examination of the right side of the heart with echocardiography can provide valuable data to assist in diagnosis, guiding treatment, and establishing prognosis in patients with cardiorespiratory disease. Echocardiography provides this information cheaply and at no risk to the patient. Those clinicians limiting their understanding of echocardiography to the reading of report conclusions may be limiting the care that they are providing to their patients. When interpreting echocardiographic reports, however, clinicians should pay particular attention to the quality of the data presented to them, because acquisition of good-quality images can be challenging, especially in patients with respiratory disease.

Acknowledgments
With thanks to Jenny Green, Echocardiographer, University Hospitals Birmingham, The New Queen Elizabeth Hospital Birmingham, and Kam Rai, Lead Echocardiographer, University Hospitals Coventry and Warwickshire NHS Trust, United Kingdom.

SUGGESTED READINGS

Arcasoy S, Christie J, Ferrari V, et al: Echocardiographic assessment of pulmonary hypertension in patients with advanced lung disease, *Am J Respir Crit Care Med* 167:735–740, 2003.

Forfia P, Fisher M, Mathai S, et al: Tricuspid annular displacement predicts survival in pulmonary hypertension, *Am J Respir Crit Care Med* 174:1034–1041, 2006.

Guidelines for the diagnosis and treatment of pulmonary hypertension. The Task Force for the Diagnosis and Treatment of Pulmonary Hypertension of the European Society of Cardiology and the European Respiratory Society, endorsed by the International Society of Heart and Lung Transplantation, *Eur Heart J* 30:2493–2537, 2009.

Haddad F, Doyle R, Murphy D, et al: Right ventricular function in cardiovascular disease, part II: pathophysiology, clinical importance, and management of right ventricular failure, *Circulation* 117:1717–1731, 2008.

Haddad F, Hunt S, Rosenthal D, et al: Right ventricular function in cardiovascular disease, part I: anatomy, physiology, aging, and functional assessment of the right ventricle, *Circulation* 117:1436–1448, 2008.

McConnell M, Solomon S, Rayan M, et al: Regional right ventricular dysfunction detected by echocardiography in acute pulmonary embolism, *Am J Cardiol* 78:469–473, 1996.

McQuillan B, Picard M, Leavitt M, et al: Clinical correlates and reference intervals for pulmonary artery systolic pressure among echocardiographically normal subjects, *Circulation* 104:2797–2802, 2001.

Milan A, Magnino C, Veglio F: Echocardiographic indexes for the non-invasive evaluation of pulmonary hemodynamics, *J Am Soc Echocardiogr* 23:225–239, 2010.

Rudski L, Lai W, Afilalo J, et al: Guidelines for the echocardiographic assessment of the right heart in adults: a report from the American Society of Echocardiography, *J Am Soc Echocardiogr* 23:685–713, 2010.

Vieillard-Baron A, Page B, Augarde R, et al: Acute cor pulmonale in massive pulmonary embolism: incidence, echocardiographic pattern, clinical implications and recovery rate, *Intensive Care Med* 27:1481–1486, 2001.

Chapter **15**
Bronchodilators
Peter M.A. Calverley

Bronchodilator drugs are among the most widely used respiratory medicines, and substantial developments, particularly in duration of action, have increased their effectiveness in recent years. Essentially these drugs act to increase airway caliber and permit faster and more effective lung emptying. The concept of bronchodilatation has evolved as well, and the designation "bronchodilator" is now largely synonymous with any drug that acts relatively rapidly to cause relaxation of airway smooth muscle.

Breathlessness and wheezing are cardinal symptoms of many respiratory diseases, and from the 19th century it was recognized that smoking cigarettes made from the leaves of the plant *Atropa belladonna* lessened the symptoms of asthma. This therapy was largely superseded when epinephrine (adrenaline) was purified in the early 20th century. Subsequently, synthetic analogues of epinephrine were developed, as was atropine, the first synthetic antimuscarinic agent. Both atropine and epinephrine could be added to organ baths containing airway smooth muscle, and their potency in relieving or preventing induced smooth muscle contraction could be measured. These developments led to the current understanding of the control of airway smooth muscle, as shown in **Figure 15-1**. Changes in airway smooth muscle length translate into changes in airway caliber—an especially important issue when airway diameter is reduced, as in chronic obstructive pulmonary disease (COPD) (**Figure 15-2**). In clinical practice, this aspect of pulmonary function is assessed indirectly as an increase in the forced expiratory volume in 1 second (FEV_1) after drug administration. When a bronchodilator is given orally, the time to onset of action (i.e., improvement in lung function) is prolonged, reflecting the absorption and circulation of the drug; this time can be considerably shortened when treatment is administered by inhalation. Of note, not all drugs that increase FEV_1 do so by changing airway smooth muscle activity; for example, antiinflammatory agents can reduce the mucosal thickening and thickening of the airway wall, thereby leading to improvements in FEV_1. These processes take some time to develop, however, because agents such as corticosteroids have both nuclear and extranuclear effects on protein synthesis, which reduce the number of proinflammatory messenger molecules. Hence, for practical purposes, bronchodilators can be considered as those drugs with a proven direct effect on airway smooth muscle and a relatively rapid onset of effect (minutes to several hours) in clinical circumstances in which some measure of airway resistance is the marker for effectiveness.

This chapter presents an overview of the principal classes of bronchodilator drugs, including their mechanisms of action and specific indications. As background for these considerations, it is useful first to examine why these drugs should be so useful in respiratory disease, and to identify those settings in which they should be deployed.

PHYSIOLOGIC BASIS FOR BRONCHODILATOR ACTION

Under resting conditions in healthy people, the work of breathing performed by the respiratory muscles is relatively small. Inspiration is an active process, and sufficient flow has to be generated by overcoming respiratory resistive, elastive, and frictional loads to ensure adequate alveolar ventilation. Expiration is passive and ends when the expiratory recoil pressure of the lungs and the chest wall are balanced. There is little expiratory flow resistance within the bronchial tree, and expiratory flow limitation (no increase in flow despite increasing expiratory driving pressure) is detected only during the last part of the maximum forced expiration (**Figure 15-3**, *top*). Ventilation increases during exercise but not to the point at which flow limitation significantly limits performance.

Airway resistance is influenced significantly by the caliber of the bronchial tree (see Figure 15-2). In health, most of the resistance lies in the region of the larynx, with less than 20% coming from the periphery of the lung. The evidence points to resting airway smooth muscle tone that decreases physiologically during exercise to reduce the resistive work required when ventilation has to increase. Bronchodilator drugs abolish this smooth muscle tone in both healthy persons and patients with disease. In healthy people, the increase in FEV_1 after administration of a β-agonist is between 50 and 120 mL, a value similar to that in patients with COPD, whose baseline FEV_1 usually is much lower. By contrast, in patients with asthma, in which airway smooth muscle bulk is greater and resting muscle tone may be increased by indirect reflex mechanisms, the response to bronchodilator drugs is more dramatic, and substantial increases in lung function occur after the acute administration of a bronchodilator. The improvement in lung emptying that results from bronchodilation has important effects on the operating lung volume and hence on the work of breathing.

In general, wheezing reflects areas of local flow limitation within the airway. Expiratory flow limitation can occur in the absence of audible wheeze and contributes to the slow emptying of the lungs and the higher lung volumes that lead to breathlessness and chest tightness in obstructive lung disease. Expiratory flow limitation may be abolished completely after a bronchodilator drug in asthma (see Figure 15-3), although asthmatic symptoms often will recur when the effects of the bronchodilator wear off (see further on). In COPD, the absolute change in lung function is much smaller than in asthma,

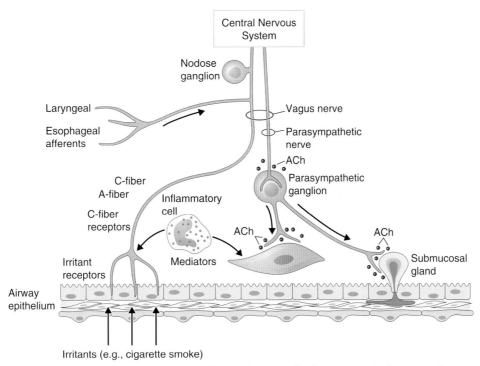

Figure 15-1 Control of airway smooth muscle in humans. Preganglionic and postganglionic parasympathetic nerves release acetylcholine (ACh) and can be activated by airway and extrapulmonary afferent nerves. There is no direct sympathetic innervation to the airways. Mediators released from inflammatory cells directly activate airway smooth muscle cells, as well as acting through a cholinergic reflex. This may explain why antimuscarinics are less effective than β_2-agonists as bronchodilators in asthma, because the latter drugs counteract the effect of all bronchoconstrictors.   *(From Barnes PJ: β_2-Agonists, anticholinergics, and other nonsteroid drugs. In Albert RK, editor:* Clinical respiratory medicine, *ed 3, Philadelphia, Mosby, 2008.)*

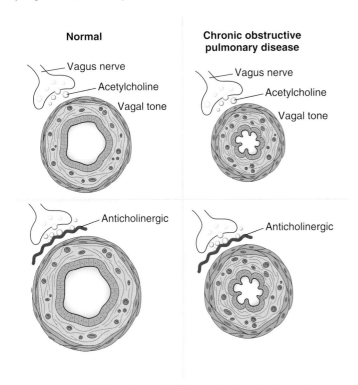

Figure 15-2 Cholinergic control of airways in chronic obstructive pulmonary disease (COPD). The normal airway has a certain degree of vagal cholinergic tone caused by tonic release of acetylcholine, which is blocked by muscarinic antagonists. This effect may be exaggerated in patients who have COPD, because of fixed narrowing of the airways as a result of geometric factors. The absolute increase in forced expiratory volume in 1 second (FEV$_1$) after administration of these agents is similar to that seen in healthy smokers, but the relative change is much greater, reflecting the lower initial airway diameter.   *(From Barnes PJ: β_2-agonists, anticholinergics, and other nonsteroid drugs. In Albert RK, editor:* Clinical respiratory medicine, *ed 3, Philadelphia, Mosby, 2008.)*

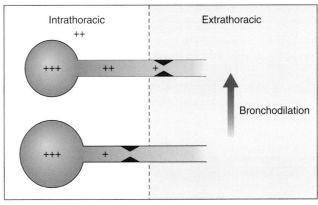

Figure 15-3 Expiratory flow limitation in health and disease. *Top,* The pressure change within and outside the airway in health. Intraluminal driving pressure producing expiratory flow declines owing to frictional resistance. The *opposing triangles* mark the point at which pressures within and outside the airway are equal (choke point) when expiratory flow limitation is present. This occurs outside of the thorax in healthy people (*dotted line*) and only during a maximum forced expiration. *Bottom,* The resistive pressure drop is greater, the choke point is more proximal in the airway, and expiratory flow limitation occurs within the thorax and can be present in tidal breathing. The bronchodilator moves the choke point distally and thus may abolish resting flow limitation altogether or allow more lung emptying to occur before onset of flow limitation.

and flow limitation often persists, particularly in severe disease, although to a less severe degree. These subtle changes in lung mechanics, however, can produce clinically relevant changes in operating lung volumes, particularly in the end-expiratory lung volume, which is significantly elevated in many patients with COPD and constitutes is a good guide to the degree of exercise impairment experienced by affected persons. A further effect of bronchodilator drugs is to increase the threshold at which symptoms are induced. This increased threshold is important in the prevention of exercise-induced asthma and also in the reduction of symptoms produced more predictably by exercise, as occurs when patients with COPD undertake certain daily activities. This ability to increase baseline lung function and reduce the impact of external stimuli on the airways is likely to be important in explaining why bronchodilator drugs are associated with fewer exacerbations of airways disease when given in effective doses over the long term.

A different situation obtains in patients with restrictive lung function secondary to diffuse pulmonary fibrosis or chest wall disorders, in which the work of breathing is increased because of the greatly increased elastic load on the inspiratory muscles and the airways are largely spared from involvement. In such patients, bronchodilator drugs will have little effect on breathlessness, and their use is associated with unwanted side effects, rather than clinical benefit. Thus, bronchodilators are indicated only for the relief of symptoms that are caused by obstructive lung disease and not when a restrictive disorder is the dominant clinical problem.

PHARMACOLOGIC BASIS OF BRONCHODILATOR ACTION

Although by definition the focus of action of bronchodilator drugs is the airway smooth muscle, a number of other secondary or incidental effects occur that can be clinically useful. The balance of these nonbronchodilator effects differs significantly between the two main classes of bronchodilator drugs.

β-AGONISTS

Based on the classical work of Ahlquist in defining different subtypes of adrenoreceptors, a range of relatively specific β-agonist agents were developed. Because β_2-receptors are almost the only subtype expressed on human airway smooth muscle, it makes sense to use highly selective β-agonists and there is no place for nonselective agents in clinical practice today. The chemical structures of the principal β-agonists are shown in **Figure 15-4**.

β_2-Agonists produce bronchodilatation by directly stimulating β_2-receptors in airway smooth muscle, which leads to relaxation. This can be demonstrated in vitro by the relaxant effect of β-agonists on human bronchi and small airways—an effect confirmed in humans by a rapid decrease in airway resistance after administration of drug by inhalation. β-Receptors have been demonstrated in airway smooth muscle by direct receptor-binding techniques, and autoradiographic studies indicate that β-receptors are localized to smooth muscle of all airways from the trachea to the terminal bronchioles, although a wide distribution within the lungs as a whole, including the alveoli, is characteristic.

The β-receptor is a seven transmembrane–spanning G protein. Binding of the β_2-agonist to the disulfide bonds on the extracellular surface leads to activation of adenylate cyclase and a consequent increase in intracellular cyclic adenosine-3′,

5′-monophosphate (cAMP). This leads in turn to activation of a specific kinase (protein kinase A) that phosphorylates several target proteins within the cell, resulting in several specific effects:

- A fall in the intracellular calcium ion (Ca^{2+}) concentration by active removal of Ca^{2+} from the cell into intracellular stores
- Inhibition of phosphoinositide hydrolysis
- Direct inhibition of myosin light chain kinase
- Opening of large-conductance, calcium-activated potassium channels (K_{Ca}) that repolarize the smooth muscle cell and may stimulate the sequestration of Ca^{2+} into intracellular stores
- β_2-Agonists act as functional antagonists and reverse bronchoconstriction, irrespective of the contractile agent. This is an important property, because multiple bronchoconstrictor mediators (inflammatory mediators and neurotransmitters) are released in asthma.

β_2-Agonists may have other effects on airways, and β_2-receptors are localized to several different airway cells. Thus, additional effects may include the following:

- Inhibition of mediator release from mast cells and other inflammatory cells
- Inhibitory effects on neutrophil migration and activation
- Reduction and prevention of microvascular leakage and, consequently, development of bronchial mucosal edema after exposure to mediators such as histamine and leukotrienes
- Increased mucus secretion from submucosal glands and ion transport across airway epithelium (effects that may enhance mucociliary clearance, thereby reversing the defect in clearance found in asthma)
- Reduction in neurotransmitter release from airway cholinergic nerves, thus reducing cholinergic reflex bronchoconstriction
- Inhibition of the release of bronchoconstrictor and inflammatory peptides, such as substance P, from sensory nerves

How relevant any of these effects are to the observed clinical effects in disease is hard to determine. They may be more important in preventing bronchoconstriction from other stimuli in asthmatic patients than in directly influencing airway dimensions. The immediate impact on airway smooth muscle remains the most important of these various mechanisms, as illustrated in **Figure 15-5**. Recognized polymorphisms of the β-receptor show variable responses to agonist drugs in vitro. Translation of these observations into clinically noticeable differences in response in the clinical setting has been difficult, however, and at present these observations remain primarily of academic interest.

Antiinflammatory Effects of β_2-Agonists

The inhibitory effects of β-agonists on the release of mast cell mediators and on microvascular leakage can be considered to be antiinflammatory effects, although this term is not well defined. Nonetheless, available data suggest that β-agonists may modify acute inflammation. How well sustained such actions are remains unclear. To date, β-agonists have not been shown to modify chronic inflammation, but whether this reflects their basic pharmacology or is simply a result of a limited duration of action is less clear. The advent of very long-acting agents (see below) may resolve this point if any investigators have the courage to test this application in asthmatic patients without a

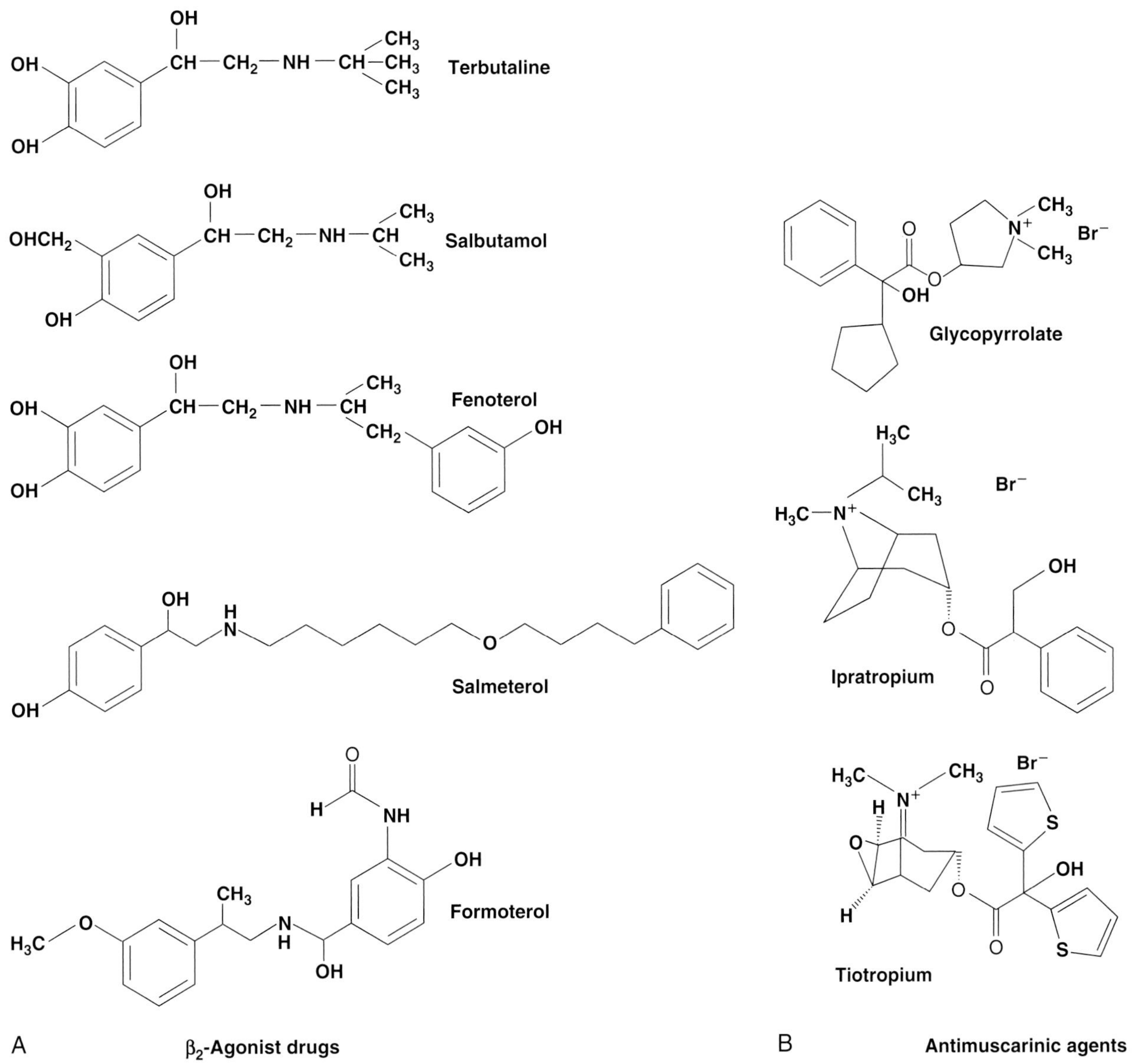

Terbutaline

Salbutamol

Fenoterol

Glycopyrrolate

Ipratropium

Salmeterol

Formoterol

Tiotropium

A   β₂-Agonist drugs

B   Antimuscarinic agents

Figure 15-4   Chemical structures of commonly used bronchodilator drugs. **A,** β₂-Agonists. **B,** Antimuscarinic drugs.

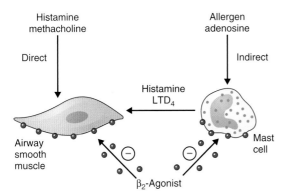

Figure 15-5   Direct and indirect bronchodilator effects of β₂-agonists. These agents stimulate β₂-receptors throughout the bronchial tree but cause bronchodilatation directly by means of activation of β₂-receptors on airway smooth muscle and also indirectly by inhibition of mediator release from mast cells. The latter mechanism is more likely to operate in allergic asthmatic patients, but its relative significance is unknown. *LTD₄,* leukotriene D₄. *(From Barnes PJ: β₂-Agonists, anticholinergics, and other nonsteroid drugs. In Albert RK, editor: Clinical respiratory medicine, ed 3, Philadelphia, Mosby, 2008.)*

background of other antiinflammatory treatment. Bronchial biopsy specimens in asthmatic patients who regularly take β-agonists show no significant reduction in the number of or activation in inflammatory cells in the airways, in contrast with suppression of inflammation that occurs with inhaled corticosteroids.

ANTIMUSCARINIC AGENTS

Antimuscarinic agents are specific antagonists of muscarinic receptors and inhibit cholinergic nerve–induced bronchoconstriction. Muscarinic receptors bind to acetylcholine released after stimulation of the parasympathetic nerves. These nerves innervate the bronchi and small airways of the human bronchial tree but do not extend to the respiratory bronchioles and alveoli. The receptor has seven membrane-spanning loops, the third of which shows considerable heterogeneity—explaining the existence of several different functional variants. Many of these receptors (M_1 to M_3) occur in different sites and with rather different functions, as shown in **Figure 15-6.**

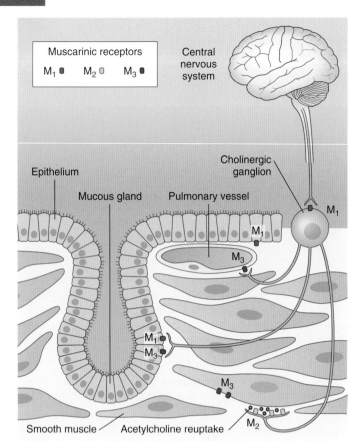

Figure 15-6 Distribution of muscarinic receptors in the lung. Note that different receptors have different roles, so their blockade will have different effects. M_1 receptors on the ganglia in the airway wall seem to regulate overall bronchomotor tone. M_2 receptors are involved in the autoregulation of acetylcholine reuptake from the synaptic cleft. M_3 receptors are postsynaptic on airway and pulmonary vascular smooth muscle, and their blockade leads to smooth muscle relaxation.

A small degree of resting bronchomotor tone is caused by tonic cholinergic nerve impulses, which release acetylcholine in the vicinity of airway smooth muscle, and cholinergic reflex bronchoconstriction may be initiated by irritants, cold air, or stress. Although anticholinergics offer some protection against acute challenge by sulfur dioxide, inert dusts, cold air, and emotional factors, they are less effective against antigen challenge, exercise, and fog. This is not surprising, because anticholinergic drugs only inhibit reflex cholinergic bronchoconstriction and have no significant blocking effect on the direct effects of inflammatory mediators, such as histamine and leukotrienes, on bronchial smooth muscle. Furthermore, cholinergic antagonists probably have little or no effect on mast cells, microvascular leak, or the chronic inflammatory response. For these reasons, in patients who have asthma, anticholinergics are less effective as bronchodilators than β_2-agonists. In COPD the drugs appear to be more equivalent, although differences in their duration of action are as likely to explain their relative benefit as are fundamental pharmacologic differences.

β_2-AGONISTS: CLINICAL CONSIDERATIONS

Although historically, nonselective adrenaline derivatives such as isoprenaline were used to treat airway disease, cardioselective β_2-agonists are now recognized as being the safest and most effective compounds in this class. The most widely prescribed drug at present is salbutamol (albuterol in the United States), although the closely related compound terbutaline is popular in some parts of Europe. Fenoterol, a more potent β_2-agonist, was widely used in the 1980s, although it was associated with an increased risk of asthma death in New Zealand. Whether this association was causal or coincidental remains a subject of heated debate, which still affects current attitudes toward drugs in this class today. Although oral β-agonists were popular for many years, their slow onset of action and significant side effect profile have led to a decline in their use, and the inhaled route is now preferred, because the effects develop more rapidly and the total dose of drug given is smaller. In general, drugs such as salbutamol and terbutaline are considered short-acting β-agonists (SABAs), to distinguish them from long-acting agents such as salmeterol and formoterol (LABAs), which also are given by inhalation. Once-daily long-acting β-agonists, such as indacaterol and vilanterol, have been developed recently and, in the case of indacaterol, are now licensed for use in certain medical conditions. Intravenous treatment with β-agonist initially was used for emergency care and is still offered to some people in intensive care units; however, this regimen has declined in popularity, and higher doses of these drugs are now given principally by nebulization. The doses, duration of action, and formulations of the most widely used agents are presented in **Table 15-1**.

The relationship between increases in dose of β_2-agonists and the spirometric response in health and disease is at best a shallow one. This is most easily seen in people with asthma, in whom changes in FEV_1 after administration of these drugs are more dramatic and hence can be defined more reliably. A similar situation, however, applies in patients with COPD. The increase in adverse events is more clearly dose-related, thereby limiting the amount of drug that can be given.

In general, SABA drugs have a duration of action (assessed by a measurable difference in FEV_1 compared with that after administration of placebo) of 4 to 6 hours (**Figure 15-7**). Although the changes in lung function are statistically significant compared with either baseline or placebo, these effects really are very modest and often below the threshold of a clinically important difference, which for operational purposes is set at around 100 mL from baseline. Some evidence points to a much shorter period of protection against nonspecific challenges (e.g., to methacholine) than the total duration of effect measured in this way. By contrast, long-acting inhaled agents produce more substantial bronchodilation for at least 12 hours relative to their baseline value, and again, the duration of protraction against agonist challenges is much longer (see Figure 15-7). Salmeterol and formoterol are given twice-daily to maintain a bronchodilator effect over the 24-hour day. Salmeterol has a relatively slower onset of action, whereas formoterol, which is a full agonist, induces bronchodilation at a rate similar to that seen with salbutamol. This difference is important only when treatment is given on a maintenance basis, but the fast onset of action of formoterol allows it to be used as a rescue therapy; this has led to the "single inhaler" approach to asthma management. Newer data derived from patients with COPD managed with indacaterol and vilanterol show that these drugs have a rapid onset of action that lasts throughout the day after a single dose.

Although consideration has been given to the possibility of tachyphylaxis with β_2-agonists, it has been difficult to establish that this occurs in clinical settings. Some data suggest that it may happen to a minor degree with formoterol, but this does not seem to lead to any clinically important difference, and

Table 15-1   Formulations and Typical Doses of Medications for Treatment of Chronic Obstructive Pulmonary Disease*

Drug	Inhaler Dose (µg)	Solution for Nebulizer (mg/mL)	Oral	Vials for Injection (mg)	Duration of Action (hours)
β₂-Agonists					
Short-Acting					
Fenoterol	100-200 (MDI)	1	0.05% (syrup)		4-6
Levalbuterol	45-90 (MDI)	0.21, 0.42			6-8
Salbutamol (albuterol)	100, 200 (MDI, DPI)	5	5 mg (tablet), 0.024% (syrup)	0.1, 0.5	4-6
Terbutaline	400, 500 (DPI)		2.5 mg, 5 mg (tablet)		4-6
Long-Acting					
Formoterol	4.5-12 (MDI, DPI)	0.01†			12+
Arformoterol		0.0075			12+
Indacaterol	150-300 (DPI)				24
Salmeterol	25-50 (MDI, DPI)				12+
Anticholinergics					
Short-Acting					
Ipratropium bromide	20, 40 (MDI)	0.25-0.5			6-8
Oxitropium bromide	100 (MDI)	1.5			7-9
Long-Acting					
Tiotropium	18 (DPI), 5 (SMI)				24+
Combination Short-Acting β₂-Agonists Plus Anticholinergic‡					
Fenoterol/ipratropium	200/80 (MDI)	1.25/0.5			6-8
Salbutamol/ipratropium	75/15 (MDI)	0.75/0.5			6-8
Methylxanthines					
Aminophylline			200-600 mg (tablet)	240	Variable, up to 24
Theophylline (SR)			100-600 mg (tablet)		Variable, up to 24
Combination Long-Acting β₂-Agonists Plus Corticosteroids‡					
Formoterol/budesonide	4.5/160, 9/320 (DPI)				
Salmeterol/fluticasone	50/100, 250, 500 (DPI) 25/50, 125, 250 (MDI)				

DPI, dry powder inhaler; *MDI*, metered dose inhaler; *SMI*, soft mist inhaler.
*Not all formulations are available in all countries; in some countries, other formulations may be available.
†Formoterol nebulized solution is based on the unit dose vial containing 20 µg in a volume of 2.0 mL.
‡In one inhaler.

there is certainly no waning of the bronchodilator and clinically relevant actions of any of these drugs when tested in clinical trials. By contrast, an oral agent, viozan, which was developed because of its combination of β₂ and dopaminergic agonist effects, is associated with dramatic tachyphylaxis after several months of use and was never taken forward. Hence, this can be a problem when β-agonists are delivered in certain ways, but it does not seem to be an issue when the inhaled route is adopted.

SIDE EFFECTS

The principal side effects associated with β₂-agonists are shown in **Table 15-2**. Although these are less evident with inhaled than oral therapy, they still occur, especially when recommended doses are exceeded, as happens in patients with poorly controlled disease with use of β₂-agonist rescue therapy. The metabolic effects associated with these drugs do show tachyphylaxis, which helps explain why reports of hypokalemia after acute administration of the drugs have not been confirmed during larger clinical trials in which the drugs are given repeatedly. Also reported, however, is a variable susceptibility to tachycardia and tremor, which can be very troublesome, particularly in elderly patients. Sleep disturbance and anxiety appear to be nonspecific effects of higher doses of inhaled β-agonists, although the mechanisms leading to such problems remain unclear.

Recently, most concern has been focused on the risk of death associated with these drugs. This problem is confined to patients with asthma, rather than those with COPD, for which large, appropriately powered clinical trials have shown a reduction rather than an increase in all-cause and cardiac-related mortality rates. Equivalent prospective control data on asthma are lacking, and the concerns associated with the use of long-acting

Figure 15-7   Schematic time course of inhaled bronchodilator action. This usually is expressed in terms of the change in forced expiratory volume in 1 second (FEV_1) from baseline and here is normalized as a percentage of maximum achieved in the disease under treatment. Graph segment *A* reflects changes in the first 2 hours after inhalation. *Red line* plots data for short-acting β-agonist (SABA); *blue line* represents formoterol or indacaterol; *purple line* represents salmeterol or long-acting muscarinic antagonist (LAMA). Graph segment *B* depicts action from 4 to 12 hours. Of note, the SABA has already passed its peak effect (*orange line*). The *purple line* reflects indacaterol and tiotropium dose profile, whereas the *red line* reflects both salmeterol and formoterol time courses. Graph segment *C* extends duration to 24 hours and represents the effect of tiotropium and indacaterol.

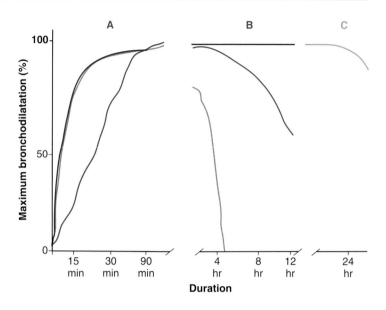

Table 15-2   Side Effects of Bronchodilator Drugs

| Drug Class | Side Effect(s)* | | |
	Minor	Troublesome	Major
β₂-Agonists	Muscle tremor Tachycardia Palpitations Metabolic (increase in free fatty acids, pyruvate)[†] Hypokalemia[†] Worsening of hypoxemia due to ventilation-perfusion mismatch[†]		Perceived increase in risk of death (see text for discussion)
Antimuscarinics	Dry mouth Prostatism Blurred vision		Apparent increase in risk of death with soft mist formulation—disputed (see text for discussion)
Theophyllines	Diuresis	Headache Nausea Vomiting Gastric discomfort Behavioral disturbance (?)	Cardiac arrhythmias, including ventricular tachycardia Grand mal epileptic convulsions

*Minor: side effects unlikely to modify treatment use, often decreasing over time; usually dose-dependent. *Troublesome*: side effects severe enough to lead to treatment discontinuation. *Major*: side effects severe enough to be life-threatening.
[†]Usually a first-dose effect in subjects previously naive to the drug. Patient often shows tachyphylaxis in the first weeks of treatment.

inhaled β-agonists have come both from earlier concerns about SABA use and from observational studies mainly conducted after the drugs have been licensed. The most important of these was a large observational trial of the use of salmeterol in asthmatic persons in the United States. This study found an apparent increased risk of death among African American asthmatic patients, many of whom were using these drugs for monotherapy, rather than in combination with inhaled corticosteroids. This observation has led to somewhat conflicting opinions across the Atlantic about the risks of β₂-agonist treatment. European clinicians, who have always been enthusiastic advocates of inhaled corticosteroids as a primary treatment for asthma, have been reassured by safety data about β₂-agonists, provided that they are used in combination with inhaled corticosteroids, while U.S. physicians remain concerned about the class effects of these drugs. Large monitoring studies are being conducted on the use of fixed combinations of these treatments

in a single inhaler in U.S. asthmatics, with the goal of resolution of the concerns that still cling to use of this group of drugs.

ANTIMUSCARINIC AGENTS: CLINICAL CONSIDERATIONS

Antimuscarinic drugs (which also are called anticholinergic agents almost interchangeably, adding an element of confusion to any consideration of this topic) have been developed exclusively for use by the inhaled route. This limited approach reflects the significant side effect profile associated with systemically available drugs such as atropine, which produce a range of pharmacologically predictable adverse events including tachycardia, dry mouth, blurred vision, constipation, and prostatism. The pharmacologic manipulation of the atropine molecule by the addition of an ammonium residue greatly reduces the ability of the drug to cross lipid membranes and hence limits the action of the agent to the airways, rather than allowing systemic absorption. By far the most widely used agent in the past has been ipratropium, which is a short-acting muscarinic antagonist (SAMA) whose duration of effects measured by FEV_1 change is similar to and in general slightly greater than that for SABA drugs (see Figure 15-7). The development of tiotropium, an effective long-acting once-daily inhaled muscarinic antagonist (LAMA), has greatly reduced the use of ipratropium, and newer agents in this class also are being developed. Details of the dose, duration of action, and formulation of these drugs are presented in Table 15-1.

Inhaled antimuscarinic drugs are relatively nonspecific antagonists that block the uptake of acetylcholine at all three clinically relevant muscarinic receptor sites. The main benefit is the result of blockade at the M_3 receptors, but to some extent, blocking the M_2 receptors is a disadvantage because this reduces the reuptake of acetylcholine from the synaptic cleft and antagonizes the blockade of these receptors by the drug. It has been argued that this effect is less important with drugs like tiotropium, but in fact the relative kinetics of receptor occupancy, although longer with tiotropium than with ipratropium, are the same, so any specific advantage for this LAMA, beyond its extended duration of action as a bronchodilator, is unlikely. As with the β-agonists, there is a relatively shallow dose-response relationship with antimuscarinic drugs. These agents do protect against specific agonist challenge, such as with methacholine, and this protective effect has been demonstrated in asthmatic subjects. However, the efficacy of receptor antagonism appears to be less than that seen with agonist drugs, at least in asthma (see earlier), so the major portion of the data on antimuscarinic agents has come from patients with COPD. In this context, high doses of ipratropium (250 to 500 μg administered by nebulizer) have been shown to be more effective in improving lung function (as assessed by changes in FEV_1 and inspiratory capacity) than lower doses of ipratropium (40 μg). Although these differences appear to be small, they may be relevant, particularly when patients have difficulty using inhaled devices and when they are experiencing an acute exacerbation of disease. This explains the popularity of nebulized anticholinergic drugs for use in management of acute exacerbations of airways disease (see later).

As with β-agonists, the duration of effect of SAMA drugs is relatively brief, certainly compared with once-daily agents like tiotropium. And even when ipratropium is taken on a four-times-daily regimen, its clinical effectiveness is significantly less in patients with COPD than once-daily tiotropium, which is associated with better health status, fewer exacerbations, and better-maintained morning lung function. As a result, within the context of COPD, LAMA drug regimens are now the preferred form of maintenance bronchodilator therapy. Other agents in this class are currently being developed, such as glycopyrrolate and aclidinium bromide. The latter drug was believed to have a full 24-hour action, but clinical trials have suggested that it is likely to be more effective if used as a twice-daily inhaled drug. In general, little evidence of tachyphylaxis has been accrued for any of the antimuscarinic agents.

SIDE EFFECT PROFILE

The adverse events associated with inhaled antimuscarinic drugs follow those that would be anticipated with use of systemic available agents like atropine. The incidence of these side effects is much lower, however, although dry mouth is a frequent but not necessarily persistent reported change. This alteration reflects a direct local effect on salivary gland secretion, seen with all agents in this class but seldom sufficient to lead to discontinuation of treatment. When ipratropium is given in a wet nebulizer, it is possible, if a face mask is used, for some of the drug to enter the eye, and cases in which acute glaucoma was precipitated in this fashion have been reported. This is a rare problem, however, and does not seem to result in patients who take the drug by inhalation without the risk of direct contamination. As noted already, it is possible to administer high doses of ipratropium to increase the clinical benefit in certain circumstances, but there is less confidence that this is the case with tiotropium and related agents, so the stated dose of tiotropium (18 μg once daily) should not be exceeded.

As with β-agonists, cardiac events have been associated with the use of inhaled anticholinergic drugs. This risk is predominantly an issue for patients with COPD and was observed initially with ipratropium in the first Lung Health Study, a 5-year trial examining the effects of regular bronchodilator therapy and smoking cessation on the natural history of early COPD. A post hoc analysis of these data suggested a higher frequency of cardiac events in patients who received ipratropium. Although this finding fell short of statistical significance, it has contributed significantly to subsequent metaanalyses of data with these agents. Concerns about the use of long-acting drugs such as tiotropium have been raised, but the data from the large, 4-year randomized control Long-Term Impacts on Function with Tiotropium (UPLIFT) trial were very reassuring, with fewer, if any, cardiac events in patients who receive tiotropium. More recently, again based on metaanalysis, concern has emerged that the route of delivery may potentially influence the risk of death associated with tiotropium. Patients who receive tiotropium as a soft mist in the Respimat device demonstrated a 50% greater risk of dying during the clinical trials than in those who received this drug by Handihaler. The absolute number of events was small, however, and follow-up studies to the end of the trial, to determine mortality status, did not include all patients. A larger prospective, appropriately conducted study is under way to resolve these issues. It is difficult at present to see why a change in the delivery system should have such an apparently dramatic effect on mortality rates. The overall impression, however, is that these drugs are clinically safe and valuable, particularly in the context of COPD.

THEOPHYLLINE

Theophylline drugs have been used for many years in the treatment of airway disease. These drugs were developed after the original observation that xanthine-containing preparations such as coffee and tea had some mild bronchodilator action. Because this group of agents was in use before current drug licensing processes were developed, they have not been subjected to the same rigorous safety and efficacy evaluation required for newer drugs. Direct comparison of theophylline with those inhaled agents already described provides a fairly clear picture of their relative efficacy. Theophylline is the typical example of this class, although it has been modified as aminophylline for intravenous use. These drugs have complex pharmacologic effects, including inhibition of a range of phosphodiesterase enzymes with a rise in intracellular cAMP as a result, as well as adenosine antagonism and a range of potentially antiinflammatory actions. In terms of bronchodilatation, these seem to be associated mainly with antagonism of the phosphodiesterase-3 (PDE3) receptor. This is not necessarily a very potent way to produce

Table 15-3 Factors Affecting Theophylline Metabolism in Chronic Obstructive Pulmonary Disease (COPD)*

Increased	Decreased
Cigarette smoking++	Arterial hypoxemia (<45 mm Hg)++
Anticonvulsant drugs	Respiratory acidosis+
Rifampicin	Congestive cardiac failure+
	Liver cirrhosis
	Erythromycin++
	Ciprofloxacin (NOT ofloxacin)
	Cimetidine (NOT ranitidine)
	Viral infections
	Old age+

*Factors posing particular problems in COPD are indicated by superscript plus signs, the number depending on the likely hazards.

Table 15-4 Technique for Use of Metered Dose Inhalers in Obstructive Lung Disease

Ideal Method	Difficulties Observed/Reported in Clinical Use
1. Remove cap.	Occasionally forgotten
2. Shake inhaler.	Occasionally forgotten
3. Hold inhaler upright.	Often forgotten
4. Tilt head back 10-55 degrees.	Often forgotten
5. Hold inhaler in front of open mouth.	Confusion about this step is common
6. Begin to inspire and activate inhaler.	Coordination problems
7. Breathe in slowly and deeply.	Difficult if lungs are hyperinflated already
8. Breath-hold for 10-15 seconds.	Breath-hold time reduced
9. Breath out slowly through the nose.	Harder with high respiratory rate
10. Use one puff at a time—wait 3-5 minutes between puffs.	Frequent use of multiple puffs in a single inspiration

bronchodilatation, and these agents are less effective, both in vitro and in vivo, than other, alternative medications.

Theophyllines can be used only by the oral or intravenous route and, for reasons that remain somewhat unclear, appear to be entirely ineffective when given by inhalation. This limitation is unfortunate, because these drugs have a significant adverse event profile, as summarized in **Table 15-3**. The most dramatic problems are those associated with the unanticipated onset of ventricular tachycardia and of grand mal epileptic convulsions. However, a number of other troublesome side effects are typical of this group and probably are mediated by PDE4 inhibition—namely, headache, nausea, insomnia, vomiting, diarrhea, and poor appetite. These effects occur frequently with theophyllines and are dose-related. Unfortunately, the pharmacokinetics of this class of agents is rather variable, and their absorption is influenced by food and the way in which the drug is presented. Although slow-release preparations have been developed, their use increases the cost of what would otherwise be relatively inexpensive medication. It has been suggested, but not conclusively established, that introducing these drugs in low doses with gradual buildup subsequently is associated with lower incidence of unpleasant adverse events. Nonetheless, it also is a requirement that theophylline levels be monitored to ensure that the patient is not exposed to undue risks of toxicity.

More recently, interesting experimental data have suggested that these agents when given at lower dose have an antiinflammatory effect, and a mechanism has been suggested to explain why this might be important in patients who are smokers, because it would overcome antagonism directly created by the effects of inhaled corticosteroids. This experimental data need to be translated into a clinical setting to ensure that the magnitude of benefit is worth the hazard associated with taking even low doses of these drugs. In most clinical guidelines, theophyllines are now regarded as drugs to be tried in patients where other therapies have not been effective, so their overall use has declined significantly in the past decade.

DRUG DELIVERY

As noted earlier, the most effective bronchodilator drugs are delivered by the inhaled route, which minimizes the dose to the patient while increasing the directly available concentration of the drug at the desired site of action within the airways. Inhalation therapy is more complex than oral treatment,

however, and in some settings and cultures, barriers to its uptake remain. As noted in Table 15-1, short-acting inhaled bronchodilators are available both as metered dose inhalers and in dry powder devices. Long-acting inhaled β-agonists also are available in both these forms, but at present tiotropium, the most widely used LAMA drug, is available only as a dry powder. No standardization of inhalation devices used to deliver these drugs has been attempted, but the general requirements for effective inhaler use have been codified and are presented in **Table 15-4**. An assessment of the effectiveness of the patient's inhaler technique is one of the most important components of the clinical review on follow-up visits. The ability to use inhalers properly is not related to educational status or age and seems to be somewhat unpredictable. The use of spacer devices can improve the percentage of drug delivered and often can sidestep problems with incoordination. A variety of such devices are available for use with metered dose inhalers. Spacers can be helpful when the need to limit side effects due to inhaled corticosteroids is a primary consideration but also can increase the effectiveness of bronchodilator delivery if the drug is reaching the airway, rather than being swallowed and metabolized. Breath-activated inhalers help some patients who find it hard to coordinate inspiration and device actuation, and often a change to a different delivery system (e.g., switching to a dry powder formulation from a metered dose inhaler) can improve matters significantly. Wet nebulization formulations of both SABA and SAMA drugs are available, but their potential for greater effect reflects the much higher doses given, rather than improvement in the deposition of the drug. These systems are operator-independent and thus well suited for use by distressed patients experiencing exacerbations of symptoms. How much of this acute benefit derives from the drug and how much from the cooling effects on the face of the mist in which it is delivered remain to be quantified.

USE OF BRONCHODILATOR DRUGS IN CLINICAL PRACTICE

The uses of bronchodilators in specific diseases are considered elsewhere in this book. This section presents a brief overview of the main clinical indications for this group of agents at present.

AID TO DIAGNOSIS

Bronchodilator reversibility testing is still widely performed in many laboratories. The principle is simple: Lung function, normally assessed as the FEV_1, is measured before and at an appropriate interval after the inhalation of a bronchodilator. Any change greater than that expected by chance would represent a *positive response*, which has been defined operationally as a change greater than 12% of the baseline which also exceeds 200 mLs. This information can be helpful as an adjunct to other diagnostic and clinical assessments but unfortunately cannot be relied on by itself as a guaranteed way of defining specific diseases. In asthma, it is the within- and between-day variability in lung function that is more important than the acute response to a drug, although a return to normal lung function after a bronchodilator test on a day when lung function is impaired constitutes strong evidence for this diagnosis. If the patient is tested when lung function is close to normal, however, the bronchodilator test result may be negative, but the diagnosis will still be asthma. Similarly, in COPD, many patients show responses to drugs on some occasions but not others. This inconsistency reflects the categorical nature of the response criteria and the fact that even in COPD, some physiologic variation in day-to-day lung function is typical. In general, the likelihood of a response falls as the baseline lung function worsens, along with the degree of clinical emphysemas. If more than one drug is used, then the chance of a positive response increases, so testing the combination of a β-agonist and an anticholinergic will produce a prevalence of disease different from that observed with use of a β-agonist alone. The latter drug has the advantage that only 15 minutes is required before the patient can be retested, explaining its popularity in many laboratories.

MANAGEMENT OF STABLE DISEASE

Use of inhaled short-acting β-agonists is a valuable way of relieving acute symptoms, and the rapid onset of action of these agents is much appreciated in both patients with asthma and those with COPD. Short-acting bronchodilator treatment with any class of these drugs is not appropriate for the management of these diseases, however, and long-acting inhaled drugs are preferred. An important distinction emerges regarding how these drugs are used in combination with other agents: Fixed-dose drug combinations of inhaled corticosteroids and long-acting β-agonists in a single inhaler have been available for some years and have proved to be very effective in the management of both asthma and COPD. In the context of asthma management, inhaled corticosteroids should always be the first line of treatment before the addition of a long-acting β-agonist to improve asthma control. LABA treatment should not be used as monotherapy for this condition. In COPD, it is clear that long-acting β-agonists and especially long-acting antimuscarinic drugs can be safely used and are very effective in disease management. Here the decision to add a combination inhaler is guided more by symptom severity and complications, as

indicated in recent treatment guidelines. As noted, the use of oral theophyllines remains a third-line therapy in both the major obstructive lung diseases. Data on the use of bronchodilators in conditions such as bronchiectasis are much more limited, and although these drugs are widely prescribed in this context, their use is based largely on extrapolation from pharmacologic management of clinical entities such as asthma and COPD, for which much more information is available.

MANAGEMENT OF ACUTE EXACERBATIONS OF DISEASE

High doses of nebulized bronchodilators, often as combinations of SABAs and SAMAs, are the mainstay of management of acute asthma and exacerbations of COPD that necessitate hospitalization. These drugs also are given to patients who require invasive ventilation, although in this context the β-agonist may be given intravenously. Intravenous therapy is not appropriate with antimuscarinic drugs but has been widely used to deliver aminophylline for both asthma exacerbations and acute COPD for many years. Evidence from metaanalysis of existing clinical trials shows no benefit in either setting from the use of aminophylline and is associated with a considerable risk of toxicity, especially when the patient has been receiving theophyllines as part of the regular medication regimen before intravenous therapy begins. Accordingly, intravenous aminophylline is no longer recommended in patients who can use appropriate nebulized short-acting bronchodilator drugs.

CONTROVERSIES AND PITFALLS WITH BRONCHODILATOR DRUGS

Despite the well-described pharmacologic properties and abundant clinical trial data on the use of bronchodilator drugs, some areas of controversy remain. It is now accepted that inhaled β₂-agonists produce greater degrees of bronchodilatation than those achievable with antimuscarinic agents in the treatment of asthma. This observation probably reflects the additional pharmacologic properties of these drugs as discussed, plus the potential advantages of an agonist over an antagonist agent in inducing smooth muscle relaxation. By contrast, antimuscarinic drugs such as ipratropium and tiotropium have been thought, on balance, to be more effective than inhaled β₂-agonists. As noted, however, this view is now being challenged with the advent of drugs such as indacaterol and oldanterol, which have a truly 24-hour duration of action and, in terms of lung function, appear to be as effective as antimuscarinic drugs in the management of COPD. Almost all available data on the action of bronchodilator drugs in lung disease come from studies in COPD and asthma, and these drugs commonly are used to help airflow obstruction in other settings, such as those of bronchiectasis and obliterative bronchiolitis. Whether these agents have equivalent effects in different disease states remains unclear, although it seems unlikely that their use will be prohibited on these grounds. Most of the data on bronchodilators come from trials of efficacy that established that the treatment is beneficial but have not necessarily studied how effective such treatment is in a "real-world" clinical setting. Here, many other factors come into play, such as adherence to treatment and patient choice, as well as perception and information, and optimizing these aspects of care is as likely to be important as any minor differences in the pharmacology of the agents selected. Finally, a much-needed look at these issues could be realized with good studies of the use of theophylline in stable lung disease on a background of other existing modern treatments. Implementation of such studies would be particularly problematic in the context of bronchial asthma, for which inhaled corticosteroids are seen as first-line therapy but would seem to be possible in COPD, a condition that affects many people, particularly those in the developing economies, who cannot afford more expensive combination treatment.

Concerns about safety of bronchodilator drugs have been present for many years since the first asthma epidemics were associated with excess use of nonspecific adrenergic stimulants such as isoprenaline and the subsequent problems associated with the use of fenoterol. These issues have not been helped by the sometimes overoptimistic promotion of new bronchodilator drugs by their advocates, including the manufacturers. The issues of β_2-agonists and asthma safety have already been considered, but it is unlikely that a clear-cut response to these concerns can be obtained until the large 6-month safety trials being conducted by the U.S. Food and Drug Administration (FDA) have been completed. Inevitably, some clinicians and patients will remain suspicious of the ultimate benefit of these agents in this context. Similar concerns about the cardiovascular safety of antimuscarinic drugs have been raised, although in general it has been possible to offer good clinical trial data that these risks have been exaggerated. The latest concerns, based on a metaanalysis of registration studies for the soft mist form of tiotropium, also have suggested a significant increase in the risk of death for patients who use this agent. A very large prospective clinical trial is now under way that should resolve this issue as well. Nonetheless, the requirement for large numbers of people who have to be studied to exclude a potential risk serves as a brake on development of new drugs in these classes.

Despite the foregoing concerns, bronchodilator drugs remain relatively safe and easy to administer. The pitfalls in their use are practical. In particular, failure to check that the patient is using the inhaler properly remains an issue with both metered dose and dry powder inhalers. Although new devices have been developed, adherence to treatment in a "real-world" setting is likely to be lower than in clinical trials. Use of "reliever" treatment is clearly preferred over maintenance therapy in patient-delivered management of many diseases, and this inclination is a particular concern in patients with asthma, in whom additional use of reliever therapy is a marker for poor asthma control. Understanding the reasons for such patient behaviors is key to effective bronchodilator use. Drugs such as theophyllines are no longer in widespread use, but patients on maintenance treatment, who often are suffering from COPD, are at serious risk for major complications if intravenous aminophylline is added to a regimen associated with already high theophylline levels. In view of the minimal evidence for efficacy of intravenous preparations, these agents are best avoided in the interest of patient safety.

THE FUTURE OF BRONCHODILATOR THERAPY

Although other mechanisms including potassium channel blockade have been explored, the risk of toxicity or lack of clinical effect with alternative approaches has meant that bronchodilator treatment is still focused on the manipulation of the adrenergic and cholinergic systems recognized more than a century ago. In practice, an easier approach has been to modify the duration of drug action rather than its potency, so new treatments are likely to be given once daily. The resulting consistent bronchodilation over the 24-hour day is a particular benefit in patients with COPD and other conditions associated with persistent airflow obstruction, as was seen when

tiotropium became available. Indacaterol is the first inhaled once-daily long-acting β-agonist and has been licensed in Europe for treatment of COPD. It produces improvement in lung function comparable with that seen with tiotropium, and more studies are awaited to establish whether it is equivalent to or more effective than this agent. Vilanterol and oldanterol appear to have similar properties when given by inhalation, and clinical data have been presented in abstract, although these drugs are yet to be licensed. Like formoterol, both drugs have a relatively rapid onset of action; the importance of this property when the drug is used as for maintenance therapy remains unclear, however. New LAMA drugs are being developed, and an old agent, glycopyrrolate, has been revived and repackaged as an effective once-daily anticholinergic bronchodilator.

Combining drugs of different classes may potentially achieve greater effect for a given level of adverse effects associated with each agent. This approach proved popular in the 1990s, when the combination of salbutamol and ipratropium was widely used by patients with COPD, and the concept is now being revisited with different combinations of once-daily LAMA and SABA agents. Similarly, new inhaler regimens of once-daily LABA (and potentially LAMA) drugs plus an inhaled corticosteroid are being developed as successors to the single inhaler combinations noted previously. Although the combination of all three agents in a single inhaler is being considered, complex technical issues remain to be solved regarding the simultaneous administration of consistent doses of three chemically different agents.

The limiting factor for dual-agent bronchodilator drugs, and also for new LABA combinations in general, is the concern of the FDA that such treatment might be given to patients with asthma even if that is not the labeled indication. Reflecting FDA concerns already noted that treatment with LABA drugs in patients with asthma may be dangerous, as well as the possible cardiovascular risk associated with anticholinergic agents, large (comprising approximately 11,500 patients) and hence expensive clinical trials are now a regulatory requirement to ensure the safety of such drugs. This requirement can be expected to impede the development of new treatment formulations; accordingly, the agents already discussed in detail are likely to remain the mainstay of clinical management for some time to come.

SUGGESTED READINGS

Albert P, Calverley PM: Drugs (including oxygen) in severe COPD, *Eur Respir J* 31:1114–1124, 2008.

Baker WL, Baker EL, Coleman CI: Pharmacologic treatments for chronic obstructive pulmonary disease: a mixed-treatment comparison meta-analysis, *Pharmacotherapy* 29:891–905, 2009.

Calverley PM: COPD: what is the unmet need? *Br J Pharmacol* 155(4):487–493, 2008.

Cazzola M, Celli B, Dahl R, Rennard S, editors: *Therapeutic strategies in COPD*, Oxford, 2005, Clinical Publishing.

Cazzola M, Matera MG: Emerging inhaled bronchodilators: an update, *Eur Respir J* 34:757–769, 2009.

Cazzola M, Segreti A, Matera MG: Novel bronchodilators in asthma, *Curr Opin Pulm Med* 16:6–12, 2010.

Global Initiative for Asthma: *Global strategy for asthma management and prevention* (website), NHLBI/WHO Workshop Report: www.ginasthma.com; accessed May 2011.

Global Initiative for Chronic Obstructive Lung Disease (GOLD): *Global strategy for the diagnosis, management and prevention of COPD* (website): www.goldcopd.org/guidelines-global-strategy-for-diagnosis-management.html; accessed May 2011.

Chapter **16**
Antiinflammatory Drugs

Klaus F. Rabe

Asthma and chronic obstructive pulmonary disease (COPD) are both inflammatory diseases. The nature of the inflammatory cascade is complex but different in each disease, asthma involving eosinophils and COPD and severe asthma involving neutrophils, among other inflammatory cell types. Therefore, asthma and COPD should be treated differently. Corticosteroids (also known as glucocorticoids or simply steroids), and particularly inhaled corticosteroids, constitute the most effective treatment for persistent asthma and are recommended as first-line agents in both adults and children. This group of drugs improves quality of life and lung function, by relieving symptoms, combating airway hyperresponsiveness, reducing inflammation, and limiting exacerbations. They are less effective at reducing COPD-specific inflammation and are not recommended until the disease has progressed to more advanced stages. Oral and systemic steroids are of benefit in treating COPD exacerbations, although their use is limited by side effects.

Bronchodilators, alone or in combination with an inhaled steroid, are the mainstay of COPD therapy, although a significant number of patients continue to suffer exacerbations while using these drugs. Only recently has a new class of antiinflammatory drug, the phosphodiesterase-4 (PDE4) inhibitors, been proved effective for the treatment of COPD, and at present only one drug in this class, roflumilast, has been approved for clinical use.

This chapter reviews these two classes of antiinflammatory drugs, highlighting their mode of action, clinical efficacy, and possible side effects. Some of the most commonly used systemic and inhaled corticosteroids are compared, with particular attention to dosing equivalence.

CORTICOSTEROIDS

Corticosteroids have been the cornerstone of treatment for various inflammatory diseases affecting any and all body systems and structures for more than 60 years. They were first applied to the treatment of inflammatory diseases of the lungs in 1949. The development of inhaled corticosteroids has revolutionized the treatment of asthma, providing local antiinflammatory properties while minimizing the side effects that limit the use of oral and systemic steroids.

PHARMACODYNAMICS

Cellular, Tissue, and Systemic Effects

The primary therapeutic effect of corticosteroids in respiratory disease results from reducing the number of inflammatory cells in the airways, such as eosinophils, T lymphocytes, mast cells, and dendritic cells. Corticosteroids inhibit the recruitment of inflammatory cells by reducing chemotaxis and adhesion, phagocytosis, and respiratory burst activity, as well as the production of inflammatory mediators such as cytokines and eicosanoids. Corticosteroids also have lytic effects on circulating lymphocytes and induce neutrophilia through decreased adhesion and demargination of polymorphonuclear cells. In particular, airway endothelia are thought to be a major target for the antiinflammatory properties of inhaled steroids in asthma.

In COPD, however, even high-dose inhaled corticosteroids have little effect on airway inflammation, although they are effective when combined with a long-acting β_2-agonist (LABA) (**Figure 16-1**).

MOLECULAR MECHANISMS

The primary effect of corticosteroids appears to be at the genetic level, activating transcription of antiinflammatory genes and repressing proinflammatory genes. They act primarily by binding to intracellular glucocorticoid receptors, which in turn regulate gene expression through glucocorticoid response elements (GREs) (**Figure 16-2**). Once inside the nucleus, glucocorticoid receptors dimerize and bind to GREs in the promoter regions of steroid-responsive genes, altering gene transcription and initiating a cascade of antiinflammatory effects downstream. Mediators affected by corticosteroids include cytokines, adhesion molecules, and chemokines. Nuclear glucocorticoid receptor monomers also interact with transcription factors such as nuclear factor (NF)-κB, to suppress expression of a number of proinflammatory genes. Corticosteroids can also decrease protein synthesis by decreasing messenger RNA (mRNA) stability.

Recent work has focused on the role of corticosteroids in regulating gene expression through effects on histone acetylation and chromatin compaction. Inflammatory signals cause chromatin unwinding by histone acetyltransferase activity. Corticosteroids can directly inhibit histone acetyltransferases and recruit histone deacetylases (HDACs) to their site of action, seemingly independent of glucocorticoid receptor binding to GREs. Corticosteroids interact with specific HDACs (such as HDAC2) that target specific histone proteins (e.g., histone H$_4$), regulating expression of particular regions of the genome. The net effect is to decrease histone acetylation, promoting chromatin compaction and downregulation of inflammatory gene expression (**Figure 16-3**).

SYNERGY WITH BRONCHODILATORS

Inhaled corticosteroids and β_2-agonists appear to work in synergy: The steroids upregulate β_2-adrenoreceptors and

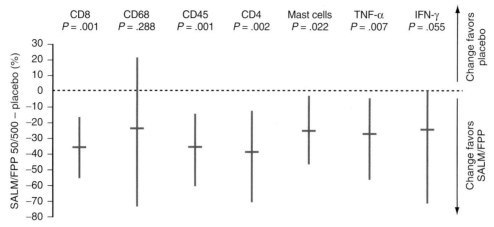

Figure 16-1 Inhaled corticosteroids and long-acting β-agonists reduce airway inflammation in chronic obstructive pulmonary disease (COPD). This figure demonstrates the reduction in inflammatory cells and cytokines in endobronchial biopsy specimens after 12 weeks of treatment with combination therapy, compared with placebo. *IFN-γ*, interferon-γ; *SALM/FPP*, salmeterol/fluticasone propionate; *TFN-α*, transforming growth factor-α. (*From Barnes NC, Qiu Y, Pavord ID, et al: Antiinflammatory effects of salmeterol/fluticasone propionate in chronic obstructive lung disease, Am J Respir Crit Care Med 173:736-743, 2006.*)

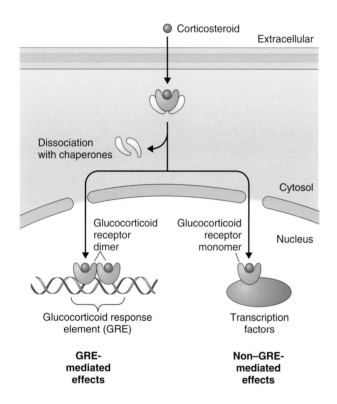

Figure 16-2 Molecular mechanisms of corticosteroid action. Corticosteroids diffuse readily across the cell membrane, where they bind glucocorticoid receptors. Corticosteroid binding causes dissociation of chaperone proteins (such as heat shock protein 90), thereby allowing translocation of the glucocorticoid receptor to the nucleus. Once in the nucleus, the glucocorticoid receptor can dimerize and bind to glucocorticoid response elements (GREs), or it can bind to other transcription factors (such as activator protein 1 and nuclear factor-κB) as a monomer. (*From McGhan RM: Corticosteroids. In Albert RK, Spiro SG, Jett JR, editors: Clinical respiratory medicine, ed 3, Philadelphia, Mosby, 2008, p 484.*)

prevent tachyphylaxis in response to β$_2$-agonists, while β$_2$-agonists increase translocation of glucocorticoid receptors from the cytoplasm to their site of action in the nucleus. As might be expected, then, these two important drug classes have an additive effect when given in combination, which may explain the greater efficacy of fixed-dose combinations in COPD compared with that achieved with inhaled steroid monotherapy.

STEROID RESISTANCE

Resistance to corticosteroids is problematic, because high doses are associated with side effects. Several mechanisms of steroid resistance have been described. Inactivating mutations in the glucocorticoid receptor occur in rare cases; these patients typically suffer no side effects of corticosteroid treatment. More commonly, steroid resistance is acquired during the course of inflammatory diseases and may, in fact, be induced selectively in inflamed tissues through the action of inflammatory cytokines. Alternative splicing of the glucocorticoid receptor may result in accumulation of β-glucocorticoid receptors that do not bind steroids, and may decrease the activity of steroid-bound α-glucocorticoid receptors through formation of heterodimers and through competitive binding to GREs. Additional mechanisms may include phosphorylation of glucocorticoid receptors that alters their pharmacologic activity and acquired HDAC deficiency, resulting in decreased steroid-induced chromatin compaction.

PHARMACOKINETICS

Systemic

The route of administration for systemic steroids depends, to some degree, on the indication. Very high doses of corticosteroids given for acute conditions generally require parenteral administration. When the prescribed steroid dose can be achieved by oral administration (e.g., prednisone, 1 mg/kg daily), there is no clear benefit to parenteral therapy. The pharmacologic activity of systemic steroids depends on both the pharmacokinetic and pharmacodynamic properties of the drug. Dosing equivalence is based on the biologic activity of a given dose, as measured by antiinflammatory activity and sodium-retaining activity.

Oral steroids are readily absorbed by the gastrointestinal tract. The degree of first-pass hepatic elimination varies, with oral bioavailability ranging from 60% to 90%. Cortisone and prednisone are prodrugs and require hydroxylation in the liver for activation. After absorption, steroids are bound to proteins such as albumin and circulate systemically. The rate-limiting

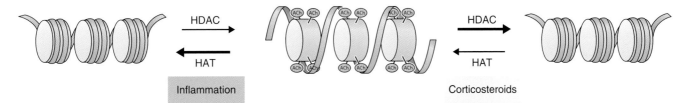

Figure 16-3 Effects of inflammation and corticosteroids on chromatin compaction. Inflammation promotes acetylation of histones by increasing histone acetyltransferase (HAT) activity; in addition, histone deacetylase (HDAC) activity is decreased in inflammatory lung diseases including asthma and chronic obstructive pulmonary disease (COPD). Corticosteroids promote chromatin compaction and silencing of gene transcription by inhibiting HAT activity and by increasing HDAC activity. *ACh,* acetylcholine.   *(From McGhan RM: Corticosteroids. In Albert RK, Spiro SG, Jett JR, editors:* Clinical respiratory medicine, *ed 3, Philadelphia, Mosby, 2008, p 485.)*

Table 16-1	Receptor Affinity and Pharmacokinetic Properties of Inhaled Corticosteroids					
Corticosteroid	Relative Receptor Affinity*	Half-Life (hr)	Oral Bioavailability (%)	Protein Binding (%)	Lipid Conjugation	Prodrug
Beclomethasone[†]	0.5/13	0.1/2.7	15/26	87/NA		Yes
Budesonide	9.4	2-3	11	88	Yes	
Flunisolide	1.8	1.6	21	80		
Fluticasone	18	4-14	<1	90		
Triamcinolone	3.6	1.5	23	71	Yes	
Mometasone	2200	4.5	<1	NA		
Ciclesonide[†]	0.1/12	0.4/3.6-5.1	<1/<1	99/99	Yes	Yes

NA, not available.
*Affinity relative to dexamethasone.
[†]Values are given for prodrug/active compound.
From McGhan RM: Corticosteroids. In Albert RK, Spiro SG, Jett JR, editors: *Clinical respiratory medicine*, ed 3, Philadelphia, Mosby, 2008, p 486.

step in the elimination of a steroid drug is reduction and conjugation in the liver, although the final fate of these water-soluble metabolic end products is excretion in the urine. The metabolism of parenteral steroids is similar, except without first-pass elimination.

Inhaled

Between 10% and 60% of a dose of inhaled corticosteroid (ICS) is deposited in the lung, where it is absorbed into the systemic circulation and cleared through the liver. The remainder of the dose is deposited in the oropharynx, which can lead to local side effects. Any of the dose that is swallowed undergoes absorption into the portal circulation and undergoes first-pass elimination, as for oral steroids.

A number of methods have been developed for delivering inhaled steroids, including use of metered dose inhalers (MDIs), dry powder inhalers, and, less commonly, nebulizers. Historically, the propellants used in MDIs were chlorofluorocarbons, but recognition of the environmental impact of these agents led to the development of hydrofluoroalkanes as the propellant. All of these methods of delivery vary with respect to the particle size generated and velocity of delivered drug, resulting in small differences in equivalent dosing but similar efficiency of drug delivery.

The pharmacokinetic characteristics of inhaled steroidal agents are more complex than those of systemic steroids. These drugs have undergone extensive development to improve activity in the lungs while decreasing systemic activity. An "ideal" inhalational agent of this class would have a small particle size (to allow access to small airways of the lung), low oral bioavailability, long residence in the lung (through slow absorption and/or lipid conjugation), delivery of a lung-activated prodrug,

high receptor affinity, and high binding to proteins in circulating blood. **Table 16-1** reviews many of these properties for seven available ICSs.

Direct comparison of the pharmacologic activity of various inhaled agents is difficult but nevertheless important, because management of airway diseases requires the ability to titrate the potency of delivered drug to achieve the desired clinical effect. The National Asthma Education and Prevention Program (NAEPP) Expert Panel Report, the Global Initiative for Asthma (GINA), and the Global Strategy for Asthma Management and Prevention have integrated a large amount of clinical and pharmacokinetic data to classify equivalent doses of a variety of different ICSs (**Table 16-2**). In general, a dose-response relationship without increased systemic effects is typical in the low to medium dose range.

SIDE EFFECTS

Generally, side effects are more common with systemic steroids than with inhaled agents (**Table 16-3**). Tolerability can be improved further by reducing dosage or treatment duration where possible, and with improvements in formulation as described above. Long-term use of systemic steroids can be associated with weight gain, increased susceptibility to infection secondary to immunosuppression, growth retardation in children, and osteoporosis. All forms of corticosteroids can hinder growth in children, although growth retardation associated with inhaled steroids is transient and of no long-term significance. The Childhood Asthma Management Program study monitored growth in 1041 children treated with budesonide, nedocromil, or placebo for 4 to 6 years and found a 1.1-cm lag in height gained in patients taking budesonide

Table 16-2   Adult Dosing for Inhaled Corticosteroids*

Corticosteroid	Delivery	Dose Per Actuation (μg)	Low Dose (μg)	Medium Dose (μg)	High Dose (μg)
Beclomethasone	CFC	42 or 84	168-504	504-840	>840
	HFA	40 or 80	80-240	240-480	>480
Budesonide	DPI	200	200-600	600-1200	>1200
Flunisolide	MDI	250	500-1000	1000-2000	>2000
Fluticasone	MDI	44, 110, 220	88-264	264-660	>660
	DPI	50, 100, 250	100-300	300-600	>600
Triamcinolone	MDI	100	400-1000	1000-2000	>2000
Mometasone	MDI	220	220-440	440-660	>660
Ciclesonide	MDI	80,160	80-160	160-320	>320

*For dosing in children, see package insert for each drug.
Modified from the NAEPP Expert Panel Report and the GINA Global Strategy for Asthma Management and Prevention. Available at www.ginasthma.org. Accessed December 2011.

compared with placebo. This lag was experienced primarily during the first year of the study.

Corticosteroids adversely affect bone health, with osteoporosis, osteoporotic fractures, and avascular osteonecrosis being relatively common and severe toxicities resulting from systemic administration. The incidence of osteoporosis seems to be related to daily use, prolonged duration of use, and significant cumulative lifetime dose, and this complication has been seen with doses as low as 5 to 7.5 mg/day of prednisone.

Adrenal insufficiency is a well-described consequence of systemic corticosteroid use. The risk seems minimal with inhaled steroidal agents. Although suppression of morning cortisol levels does occur in response to these agents, the risk of clinically apparent adrenal insufficiency is small (although supported by published case reports).

Systemic corticosteroids are potent immunosuppressors, particularly when prescribed in higher doses and for prolonged periods of time. Courses of 2 to 8 weeks of systemic steroids used to treat acute exacerbations of COPD do not seem to be associated with increased rates of infection. Chronic corticosteroid use is recognized to carry a risk for *Pseudomonas* and *Pneumocystis* infections, tuberculosis, and herpes zoster.

Side effects of inhaled steroidal agents are mostly associated with deposition of the drug in the oropharynx, such as oral candidiasis (thrush) and dysphonia, although the incidence of these events can be reduced by rinsing the mouth after taking the drug. Inhaled formulations have been associated with decreased bone mineral density in at least one randomized controlled trial. Inhaled steroids initially were not thought to increase the risk of lung infections, but more recently, the TORCH (Towards a Revolution in COPD Health) trial found an increased frequency of pneumonia among patients receiving inhaled steroids (fluticasone propionate, with or without salmeterol), possibly a result of localized immunosuppression in the lungs.

PREVENTION AND MANAGEMENT OF CORTICOSTEROID TOXICITY

To reduce side effects associated with inhaled corticosteroid use, patients should be educated on proper inhaler technique and on washing out the mouth after use, and those who use MDIs should be given a spacer to add to their device. Symptoms associated with use of an MDI sometimes may be reduced or eliminated by a switch to a dry powder inhaler. Children who use a nebulizer for steroid delivery should wash the face after using the medication.

In patients on pharmacologic doses of systemic steroids, periodic ophthalmologic examination can detect the development of cataracts and glaucoma, which may respond to reduction in dose or, if the steroid dose cannot be reduced, other treatments. The role of ophthalmologic assessment in patients on inhaled steroidal agents is less clear, but these patients should certainly be referred for evaluation of any ophthalmologic symptoms and for routine, age-appropriate care.

Screening for and management of cardiovascular risk factors, including hypertension, hyperglycemia, and hyperlipidemia, also are warranted in patients receiving chronic systemic steroids.

Patients receiving chronic systemic or inhaled steroid therapy should have routine bone mineral density measurements (particularly in high-risk groups), and they should be encouraged to perform weight-bearing exercise and to take calcium and vitamin D supplements (in the absence of any contraindications). Hormone replacement, bisphosphonates, calcitonin, and hydrochlorothiazide (HCTZ) can be considered in patients with established osteoporosis.

Avoidance of nonsteroidal antiinflammatory drugs (NSAIDs) is appropriate in patients receiving systemic steroids. Vigilance for psychiatric symptoms is prudent; if such symptoms are present, the patient can be managed by reducing the dose of steroid and/or by pharmacotherapy targeting the psychiatric symptoms.

Patients receiving chronic steroid therapy should be alerted to the increased risk of infection and should be encouraged to seek prompt evaluation at the earliest sign of infection. If possible, any vaccinations that are appropriate should be administered before therapy starts. If long-term administration of moderate to high doses of systemic corticosteroids is anticipated, prophylaxis for *Pneumocystis* pneumonia may be appropriate.

Patients receiving chronic systemic steroid therapy should be alerted to the symptoms of adrenal insufficiency and should be encouraged not to skip doses.

PHOSPHODIESTERASE 4 INHIBITORS

PDE4 is one of 11 PDEs in the phosphodiesterase enzyme superfamily. It is expressed in many cell types, notably in inflammatory cells such as neutrophils, and in airway smooth muscle cells, where it regulates inflammation by means of the

Table 16-3 Adverse Effects of Inhaled and Systemic Corticosteroids

System/Structure	Inhaled	Systemic	Prevention
Upper airway	Thrush	Thrush	Wash out mouth after using inhaled steroids
	Dysphonia		Use a spacer device
Musculoskeletal	Growth delay	Decreased adult height	Follow bone mineral density
	Decreased bone mineral density	Osteoporosis	Calcium/vitamin D
	Possible increase in fractures	Fractures	Bisphosphonates
		Avascular osteonecrosis	Weight-bearing exercise
		Myopathy	HCTZ
HPA axis	Suppression of cortisol secretion	Adrenal insufficiency well described	Avoid abrupt discontinuation of chronic steroids
	Case reports of clinical adrenal insufficiency		Stress dosing when appropriate
Ocular	Possible increase in posterior subcapsular cataracts, glaucoma	Posterior subcapsular cataracts Glaucoma	Serial ophthalmologic examination
Skin and soft tissues	Ecchymosis	Ecchymosis	Face washing after use of nebulized drug in children
	Atrophy	Atrophy Acne Impaired wound healing Striae Buffalo hump Moon facies Weight gain	
Immunologic	Increased pneumonias	Increased infection	Tuberculosis screening and prophylaxis when appropriate
		Opportunistic infection	*Pneumocystis* prophylaxis
Central nervous system	Case reports of psychiatric disturbance	Euphoria Depression Psychosis Memory loss Hypomania Sleep disturbance	
Gastrointestinal	None	Gastrointestinal bleeding in conjunction with NSAIDs Visceral perforation Steatohepatitis	Avoid NSAIDs
Cardiovascular	None	Increased cardiovascular events Hypertension Hyperlipidemia Hyperglycemia	Treat modifiable risk factors (high lipids, blood pressure, glucose)

HCTZ, hydrochlorothiazide; *HPA*, hypothalamic-pituitary-adrenal; *NSAIDs*, nonsteroidal antiinflammatory drugs.
From McGhan RM: Corticosteroids. In Albert RK, Spiro SG, Jett JR, editors: *Clinical respiratory medicine*, ed 3, Philadelphia, Mosby, 2008, p 488.

second messenger cyclic adenosine monophosphate (cAMP). PDE4 was identified as a potential target for antiinflammatory therapies many years ago, and several PDE4 inhibitors have been developed specifically as treatments for respiratory disease. Most of these agents have failed in clinical testing owing to a high incidence of gastrointestinal side effects, although compounds with greater substrate potency and specificity have increased efficacy at low doses (**Table 16-4**).

Theophylline is a weak and nonspecific inhibitor of several PDE isoforms, often incorrectly considered to be a PDE4 inhibitor. It is associated with severe side effects, and its use in treating respiratory disease is becoming less common.

The focus of the remainder of this section is on roflumilast, the only PDE4 inhibitor approved to treat COPD (granted approval by the European Medicines Agency in 2010).

PHARMACODYNAMICS

Molecular Mechanisms

Roflumilast and other PDE4 inhibitors bind directly to PDE4 to block its activity, thereby reducing inflammation (**Figure 16-4**). PDE4 is expressed in many cells involved in the inflammatory response that underlies COPD.

Table 16-4 Relative Potency and Suggested Dosage of Selected Phosphodiesterase 4 (PDE4) Inhibitors and Theophylline for Chronic Obstructive Pulmonary Disease

	PDE4 Inhibition: IC$_{50}$ (nM)*	Dosage
Roflumilast	0.8	0.5 mg once daily
Cilomilast	120	15 mg twice daily
Rolipram	1100	—
Theophylline	>10,000	100-600 mg daily

*Potency expressed as half-maximal inhibition concentration for PDE4 activity. Modified from Wang D, Cui X: Evaluation of PDE4 inhibition for COPD, *Int J COPD* 1:373-379, 2006.

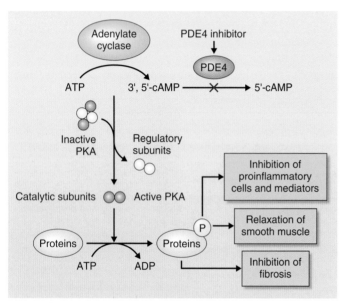

Figure 16-4 Molecular pathways affected by inhibition of phosphodiesterase 4 (PDE4). PDE4 inhibitors block the activity of PDE4, causing accumulation of cyclic adenosine monophosphate (cAMP) and downstream increase in protein kinase A (PKA) activation. This in turn leads to protein phosphorylation (P), resulting in an overall antiinflammatory effect. Although increased cAMP levels generally are associated with smooth muscle relaxation, this is not a characteristic of roflumilast. *ADP*, adenosine diphosphate; *ATP*, adenosine triphosphate. *(Modified from Rabe KF: Roflumilast for the treatment of chronic obstructive pulmonary disease,* Expert Rev Respir Med *4:543–555, 2010.)*

Cellular, Tissue, and Systemic Effects

PDE4 inhibitors work over many weeks to reduce the inflammation associated with COPD. Studies in animals have provided evidence that roflumilast can reduce smoke-induced inflammatory responses, remodeling in the airways and pulmonary vasculature, and oxidative stress. In a 4-week crossover study in patients with COPD, roflumilast significantly reduced the number of inflammatory cells and mediators in induced sputum samples. This finding correlated with improved lung function in the same patients, supporting an antiinflammatory basis for the clinical actions of the drug.

Synergy With Bronchodilators

PDE4 inhibitors have no immediate bronchodilatory effects but work over time to target chronic inflammation. Because bronchodilators work through a different mechanism of action,

PDE4 inhibitors can offer additional clinical benefit when added to regimens of these drugs, such as reducing exacerbation rates even further. In fact, roflumilast currently is licensed only for add-on therapy to bronchodilators.

PHARMACOKINETICS

In humans, roflumilast is rapidly converted to roflumilast *N*-oxide, which is responsible for most therapeutic effects. It has a long half-life, which allows once-daily dosing, and is taken orally at the optimal dose of 500 µg. In clinical studies, the main benefit of this drug in patients with COPD was found to be reduction in the frequency of moderate to severe COPD exacerbations.

Phase III clinical testing has shown that roflumilast is most effective in a subpopulation of patients with COPD who are at increased risk for COPD exacerbations. The target subgroup includes patients with severe COPD (i.e., with a postbronchodilator forced expiratory volume in 1 second [FEV$_1$] less than 50%), symptoms of chronic bronchitis (which is linked to an increased risk of exacerbations), and a history of more than one exacerbation in the past year. These patients are most likely to suffer from repeated exacerbations (the "frequent exacerbator" phenotype) and therefore benefit the most from the clinical effects of roflumilast—that is, in reducing exacerbation frequency. Clinical studies have shown that roflumilast significantly improves lung function and reduces exacerbations when added to most COPD maintenance therapy regimens—including a LABA, a long-acting muscarinic antagonist (LAMA), or inhaled steroid—in this patient subgroup as described (**Figure 16-5**).

SIDE EFFECTS

All PDE4 inhibitors have been associated with gastrointestinal side effects such as nausea and diarrhea. Roflumilast is clinically effective at a relatively low dose (compared with other PDE4 inhibitors), thereby minimizing the risk of side effects. In 1-year phase III clinical studies, the incidence of side effects was 67% with roflumilast and 62% with placebo, although study discontinuations were more often associated with roflumilast (14%) than with placebo (11%). Diarrhea, headache, and weight loss appear to be the most limiting side effects associated with roflumilast, although in most cases, these appear to resolve with continued use of the drug. Further investigation has shown that the weight reduction associated with roflumilast was due mostly to loss of fat mass rather than fat-free body mass, and additional metabolic effects of this systemic drug are the subject of ongoing investigations.

PIPELINE PRODUCTS

A number of new inhaled steroid formulations are in development, either as monotherapy for COPD and asthma or in combination with bronchodilators. Since the approval of roflumilast, several PDE4 inhibitors have been investigated in clinical development, including oglemilast (which failed to meet clinical efficacy end point in midstage clinical testing) and tetomilast (currently in phase II testing). Inhaled formulations of PDE4 inhibitors have been investigated, showing promising efficacy in mild asthma, but with no proven efficacy in COPD to date.

At present, of the 17 antiinflammatory drugs in the pipeline for COPD treatment, none represents a new molecule or class of drug. Eleven of the 17 pipeline products are in phase III

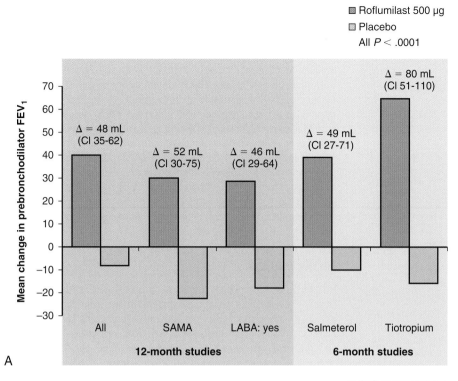

Roflumilast 500 μg
Placebo
All P < .0001

Figure 16-5 Clinical effects of roflumilast on lung function (**A**) and exacerbation rate (**B**). Both 12- and 6-month studies were performed in patients with chronic obstructive pulmonary disease (COPD), chronic bronchitis (not required in the salmeterol study), and at least one exacerbation in the past year. Patients were allowed to take long-acting β_2-agonists (LABAs) or short-acting muscarinic antagonists (SAMAs) as concomitant medications in the 12-month studies; all patients were taking salmeterol or tiotropium in the 6-month studies. Effects of roflumilast were observed on top of effects of concomitant medications. The 6-month studies were not powered to detect differences in exacerbation rate. *Indicates post hoc analyses. *CI*, confidence interval; *FEV₁*, forced expiratory volume in 1 second. *(Modified from Rabe KF: Update on roflumilast, a phosphodiesterase 4 inhibitor for the treatment of chronic obstructive pulmonary disease,* Br J Pharmacol *163:53–67, 2011.)*

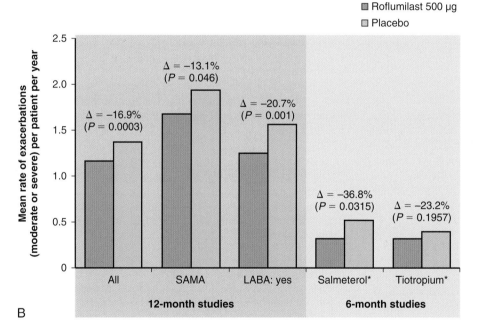

Roflumilast 500 μg
Placebo

testing, 3 are in phase II testing, and 3 are in phase I testing. Intracellular signaling proteins that have been researched as antiinflammatory agents for use in other diseases are now being investigated for treatment of COPD, including inhibitors of mitogen-activated protein (MAP) kinases (particularly p38), phosphatidylinositol 3 (PI3) kinase, and matrix metalloproteinases (MMPs). Many clinical trials with asthma treatments are ongoing, focusing on increasing the specificity for the targeted protein and identifying specific "responder populations" likely to experience the most clinical benefits. Monoclonal antibodies to various cytokines and cytokine receptors, notably the interleukins IL-5 and IL-17, currently are in phase II/III testing for asthma, with promising results.

In addition, stem cell therapy is an emerging area of research on treatment of respiratory disease. **Figure 16-6** depicts novel molecular targets for COPD and asthma drugs.

CONTROVERSIES AND PITFALLS

Tolerability issues associated with systemic steroid use are well known and not specific to respiratory disease. Although inhaled steroidal agents are accepted as highly beneficial for asthma treatment, their role in the management of COPD remains unclear. It is known that the inflammatory pathways underlying asthma and COPD are different, and this may underlie the relative resistance to inhaled steroids in COPD. CD8+

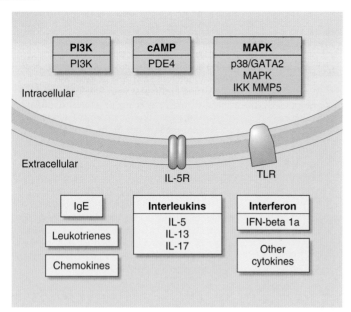

Figure 16-6 Novel targets for antiinflammatory treatments for chronic obstructive pulmonary disease (COPD) and asthma. Several components of inflammatory intracellular signaling pathways (including MAPK, PI3K, and cAMP-dependent pathways) are novel targets for respiratory drug development. *IFN-beta*, interferon-beta; *IgE*, immunoglobulin E; *IKK*, inhibitor of kappa B (IKK) kinase; *IL-5R*, interleukin-5 receptor; *PDE4*, phosphodiesterase 4; *PI3K*, phosphatidylinositol 3-kinase; *MAPK*, mitogen-activated protein kinase; *MMP5*, matrix metalloproteinase 5; *TLR*, toll-like receptor. (*Data from the National Institutes of Health–sponsored database of clinical trials www.clinicaltrials.gov; and from Gross NJ: The COPD pipeline x, COPD 8:244–247, 2011.*)

lymphocytes and neutrophils appear to drive COPD-specific inflammation; airway biopsy studies have shown that an inhaled steroid–LABA combination reduces the number of airway CD8+ cells to a greater degree than does an inhaled steroid alone. Another mechanism that could underlie resistance to inhaled steroids in COPD is the inactivation of nuclear translocation of glucocorticoid receptors and reduced activity of HDAC2, by both cigarette smoke and oxidative stress. These mechanisms both can lower the ability of inhaled corticosteroids to inhibit inflammatory gene expression.

The combination of inhaled steroid–LABA appears to have synergistic effects in COPD, as highlighted by trials such as the large TORCH study, in which a combination of a LABA and the inhaled steroidal agent fluticasone had a greater effect on exacerbations than that observed with the individual components alone. However, TORCH failed to show any significant effect of a LABA–inhaled steroid combination on long-term mortality, and a metaanalysis of inhaled steroid use in 13,000 patients with COPD reported no positive effect on FEV$_1$ decline or mortality, although a 25% reduction in exacerbations was noted. Additionally, the TORCH and INSPIRE (Investigating New Standards for Prophylaxis in Reducing Exacerbations) studies showed a small increase in episodes of nonfatal pneumonia in fluticasone-treated patients, which requires further study to confirm the exact nature of this relationship. However, the increased risk of pneumonia, which probably is associated with all types of inhaled steroids, should be balanced by the large reduction in exacerbations that these drugs can provide.

Development of alternative therapies therefore remains a priority in COPD management. The recent approval of roflumilast as the first antiinflammatory agent targeting COPD-specific inflammation has been a major advance, although the incidence of gastrointestinal side effects has been a concern with use of this drug. Much of this concern stems from the history of PDE4 inhibitor development—rolipram was associated with a high incidence of gastrointestinal side effects, and cilomilast was associated with nausea and vomiting. These compounds have lower potency than roflumilast, however, and have poor tolerability at the relatively high concentrations required for efficacy. Roflumilast is a potent and highly specific inhibitor of PDE4. The most limiting side effect of this agent is diarrhea, which resolves after a few weeks of treatment, and the long-term benefits on exacerbations appear to outweigh tolerability issues.

CONCLUSION

Inhaled corticosteroid regimens remain the most effective therapy for asthma, with innovations in formulation and delivery improving the efficacy of these agents and reducing side effects. Inhaled corticosteroids are less effective for treating COPD, and bronchodilators continue to be the mainstay of therapy for this disease. PDE4 inhibition is the only new approach to treating COPD in many years. Roflumilast currently is licensed as an agent for add-on treatment for a specific subpopulation of patients with COPD, in which its main benefit is reducing exacerbations.

Acknowledgments
This chapter was based in part on Chapter 37 on corticosteroids, by Ryan McGhan, in the third edition of this book. Sarah Nelson provided editorial assistance with preparation of the chapter.

SUGGESTED READINGS

Allen DB, Bielory L, Derendorf H, et al: Inhaled corticosteroids: past lessons and future issues, *J Allergy Clin Immunol* 112:S1–40, 2003.

Barnes PJ: Glucocorticosteroids: current and future directions, *Br J Pharmacol* 163:29–43, 2011.

Calverley PM, Rabe KF, Goehring UM, et al: Roflumilast in symptomatic chronic obstructive pulmonary disease: two randomized clinical trials, *Lancet* 374:685–694, 2009.

Derendorf H, Nave R, Drollman A, et al: Relevance of pharmacokinetics and pharmacodynamics of inhaled corticosteroids to asthma, *Eur Respir J* 28:1042–1050, 2006.

Fabbri LM, Calverley PM, Izquierdo-Alonso JL, et al: Roflumilast in moderate-to-severe chronic obstructive pulmonary disease treated with longacting bronchodilators: two randomized clinical trials, *Lancet* 374:695–703, 2009.

Hatzelmann A, Morcillo EJ, Lungarella G, et al: The preclinical pharmacology of roflumilast—a selective oral phosphodiesterase 4 inhibitor in development for chronic obstructive pulmonary disease, *Pulm Pharmacol Ther* 23:235–256, 2010.

Leung DY, Bloom JW: Update on glucocorticoid action and resistance, *J Allergy Clin Immunol* 111:3–22, 2003.

Rabe KF: Roflumilast for the treatment of chronic obstructive pulmonary disease, *Expert Rev Respir Med* 4:543–555, 2010.

Rodrigo GJ: Rapid effects of inhaled corticosteroids in acute asthma: an evidence-based evaluation, *Chest* 130:1301–1311, 2006.

Sin DD, Man SF: Corticosteroids and adrenoceptor agonists: the compl[e]ments for combination therapy in chronic airways diseases, *Eur J Pharmacol* 533:28–35, 2006.

Chapter **17**

Drug-Induced and Iatrogenic Respiratory Diseases

Philippe Camus

For both many older and newer therapeutic agents, the risk-benefit ratio is clearly in favor of treatment of many neoplastic conditions, rheumatoid arthritis, systemic or pulmonary hypertension, and cardiac dysrhythmias. In a small fraction of patients exposed to drugs taken at normal dosage to treat these conditions, adverse respiratory effects may develop. It is the duty of practitioners in oncology, cardiology, rheumatology, primary care, emergency medicine, pathology, and respiratory medicine to be cognizant of drug-induced respiratory diseases.

Recognition that a respiratory problem has been caused by the administration of a drug or a combination of drugs is of primary importance in the clinical setting. Patients may be spared unnecessary invasive evaluation including lung biopsy and/or empirical corticosteroid therapy for an alternative condition pending the results of a dechallenge-challenge test, which can be diagnostic. Further damage usually can be prevented if use of the offending agent is stopped early. Measures should be taken so that the underlying illness for which the drug was given is managed appropriately using other medications and so that the patient is not unduly reexposed to the culprit agent. In each individual case, careful exclusion of another cause is warranted, and considerations in the differential diagnosis will vary with the clinical presentation, pattern of respiratory injury, specific drug, and underlying illness.

An ever-increasing number of therapeutic drugs ($n = 455$), hormones, and investigational compounds have been associated with severe adverse respiratory reactions in adults, children, health care professionals, and persons who work in the drug industry or otherwise handle drugs, as well as in companion animals, horses, and cattle. A periodically updated online list of causal drugs is maintained on the Pneumotox website (www.pneumotox.com), sponsored by the GEPPI (Groupe d'Etudes de la Pathologie Pulmonaire Iatrogène) investigators. Agents of recent interest or concern are listed in **Table 17-1**. Adverse effects of drugs such as amiodarone, antineoplastic chemotherapy agents, nitrofurantoin, or nonsteroidal anti-inflammatory drugs (NSAIDs) are still commonly observed. Owing to their less trendy nature, however, the number of publications dealing with these medications represents an underestimate of the true incidence. With the recently renewed interest in nitrofurantoin for use as a urinary antiseptic agent, a resurgence of new cases of nitrofurantoin lung may potentially be expected. The same holds true for thalidomide. The clinical problem of drug overdose, although capable of producing severe pulmonary edema, is beyond the scope of drug-induced lung disease in this chapter.

Some presentations of drug-induced respiratory disease (DIRD) are distinctive clinically, radiologically, or histopathologically, and in such cases the evidence points almost unequivocally to the drug itself as the cause. Drug-induced anaphylaxis, angioedema, bronchospasm, noncardiac pulmonary edema (NCPE), diffuse alveolar hemorrhage (DAH), amiodarone-induced pulmonary toxicity, exogenous lipoid pneumonia, and the rare diffuse pattern of pulmonary calcification are classic examples of conditions highly suggestive of drug-induced injury.

A few drugs produce gender-specific adverse respiratory reactions because they are reserved for treating diseases that are more prevalent in or specific to one or the other gender (e.g., nilutamide and amiodarone in men, trastuzumab and nitrofurantoin in women). Still other drugs capable of causing lung damage, such as gold salts, penicillamine, or methyldopa, have been supplanted by novel agents and are falling out of favor. In addition, certain drugs—including aminorex, benfluorex, fenfluramine, dexfenfluramine, hexamethonium, L-tryptophan, and mecamylamine—have been recalled from the pharmaceutical lineup for the reason of respiratory or other adverse effects. Rare sporadic cases of adverse reactions from these agents are still being reported.

One of the greatest challenges in determining drug toxicity in suspected cases is that most patients are taking multiple medications to treat complex underlying conditions, and more than one drug may be capable of causing respiratory damage. Diagnosing drug-induced disease in this situation can be problematic, particularly if the underlying disease also manifests with interstitial lung disease (ILD) or is associated with opportunistic pulmonary infections. For instance, patients with rheumatoid arthritis may receive methotrexate or leflunomide in addition to an anti–tumor necrosis factor (TNF) agent; cardiac patients may receive anticoagulants, antiplatelets, and amiodarone; and patients with neoplastic conditions typically are exposed to several drugs, including chemotherapy agents, all capable of causing lung damage.

In addition to the usual over-the-counter and prescription drugs, numerous agents including whole blood, platelets, plasma concentrates, parenteral nutrition solutions, substances of abuse (e.g., cocaine, heroin, morphine, marijuana, propofol, anesthetic gases), herbal preparations (e.g., *Sauropus*), drug excipients (e.g., crospovidone, talc, cornstarch, lipids, sesame oil) present in therapeutic drugs, adulterants used in street drugs (e.g., brodifacoum, levamisole), illegally used chemicals such as fluid silicone or paraquat, and external or internal radiation therapy

Table 17-1   Drugs/Drug Families Recently Implicated as Agents of Respiratory Injury

Drug Family	Underlying Condition	Drug(s)	Pattern(s) of Respiratory Injury
TNF-α receptor inhibitors	Rheumatoid arthritis	Infliximab, etanercept, adalimumab	Infusion reactions, anaphylaxis Accelerated ILD ILD with granulomas Opportunistic pulmonary infections
		Leflunomide	ILD
		Tacrolimus	ILD
ACE inhibitors	LVF, systemic hypertension	Captopril, enalapril, lisinopril	Angioedema
EGFR TKIs	Non–small cell lung cancer	Gefitinib, erlotinib, ?cetuximab	ILD-DAD
Antineoplastic chemotherapy	Colorectal cancer	Oxaliplatin plus 5-FU and leucovorin (FOLFOX), irinotecan plus 5-FU and leucovorin (FOLFIRI)	ILD, DAD, BOOP
Multitargeted TKIs	Chronic myelogenous leukemia	Imatinib Dasatinib	ILD, pleural effusion Lymphocyte-rich or chylous pleural effusion
Anti-CD20 Mo-Ab	Malignant lymphoma	Rituximab	ILD, BOOP, DAH, ARDS
Platelet glycoprotein IIB-IIIA receptor inhibitors	Coronary heart disease	Abciximab, clopidogrel, eptifibatide, ticlopidine	Alveolar hemorrhage
Mo-Ab	Asthma	Omalizumab	Anaphylaxis
Leukotriene receptor antagonists	Asthma	Montelukast, pranlukast, zafirlukast	Churg-Strauss vasculitis
Antithyroid drugs	Hyperthyroidism	Propylthiouracil	ANCA-positive systemic vasculitis
mTOR receptor inhibitors	Transplantation	Everolimus, sirolimus, temsirolimus	ILD, DAH, BOOP, pulmonary vasculitis
HMG-CoA reductase inhibitors	Hypercholesterolemia	Statins	ILD, BOOP, ARDS
Opiates	Illicit drug use/abuse	Cocaine and adulterants thereof	ILD, vasculitis, DAH

ACE, angiotensin-converting enzyme; *ANCA*, antineutrophil cytoplasmic antibody; *ARDS*, acute respiratory distress syndrome; *BOOP*, bronchiolitis obliterans organizing pneumonia; *DAD*, diffuse alveolar damage; *DAH*, diffuse alveolar hemorrhage; *EGFR*, epidermal growth factor receptor; *5-FU*, 5-fluorouracil; *HMG-CoA*, hydroxymethylglutaryl coenzyme A; *ILD*, interstitial lung disease; *LVF*, left ventricular failure; *Mo-Ab*, monoclonal antibody; *mTOR*, mammalian target of rapamycin; *TKI*, tyrosine kinase inhibitors; *TNF-α*, tumor necrosis factor-α.

may injure the respiratory system by similar pharmacologic-cytopathic mechanisms.

Virtually any route of administration of drugs may be associated with increased risk for DIRD. The oral, parenteral (intramuscular, intravenous), inhaled, dermal, and topical routes are cited most often. Drugs instilled into the pleural space, coronary artery, hepatic artery, urinary bladder, uterine cavity, myometrium, subcutaneous fat, or vertebral body, or given intrathecally or aspirated into the bronchial tree, also can cause respiratory injury.

With reference to respiratory disease, the term *iatrogenic* encompasses pulmonary damage from medical or surgical procedures such as liposuction, chest tube placement, coronary artery bypass graft, and insertion of pacemaker leads or central venous line, as well as retained foreign bodies (also known as gossypibomas), all of which may cause potentially serious respiratory compromise.

Interstitial-infiltrative lung disease (i.e., ILD) is the most common clinical-imaging-pathologic pattern of respiratory involvement from drugs, accounting for about two thirds of all cases of DIRD. Conversely, drugs account for about 3% of all ILD cases. The relative preponderance of ILD must not overshadow other, less common DIRD patterns such as involvement of the upper or lower airways, pleural membrane, pericardium, heart, heart valves, pulmonary circulation, mediastinum, respiratory muscles and nerves, central respiratory

oscillator, and hemoglobin, which may have detrimental clinical consequences.

DIRD may be detected at a subclinical stage on imaging or bronchoalveolar lavage (BAL) fluid analysis, or it can be clinically evident and serious, requiring prompt recognition, immediate drug withdrawal, and emergent management aimed at securing airway patency, restoring gas exchange, and correcting hemoglobin dysfunction. DIRD presentations that portend particular severity (**Table 17-2**) include drug-induced anaphylaxis, angioedema, and bronchospasm, which may cause acute airway obstruction; NCPE; diffuse alveolar damage (DAD); DAH; extensive ILD, including eosinophilic pneumonia; opportunistic infections including *Pneumocystis* and viral pneumonias; massive pleural effusion; methemoglobinemia; neuromuscular failure; and multiorgan dysfunction. Drug-induced and iatrogenic events that occur intraoperatively, including drug-induced explosive coughing, curare- or latex-induced anaphylaxis, opiate-induced pulmonary edema, transfusion-related acute lung injury (TRALI), protamine-induced acute pulmonary hypertension, or negative-pressure pulmonary edema, raise difficult diagnostic and management issues. Awareness and emergent management are essential; however, some DIRDs are not survivable (see Table 17-2).

Several drugs within certain pharmacologic classes—curares, opiates, angiotensin-converting enzyme (ACE) inhibitors, β-adrenergic receptor blockers, antidepressants, appetite

Table 17-2 Life-Threatening Drug-Induced Respiratory Conditions Requiring Emergent Management

Injury Pattern	Prototypical Causal Drugs	Time to Onset	Life-Threatening Pathomechanism(s)
Acute upper airway obstruction	ACE inhibitor–induced angioedema	Minutes	Throat closure, airway obstruction, shock
	Drug/biologic-induced anaphylaxis	Minutes	Airway obstruction, shock, pulmonary edema
Catastrophic bronchospasm	Beta blockers, NSAIDs (including aspirin)	Minutes	Locked airway, acute hypercapnic respiratory failure, hypoxic brain damage
Noncardiac pulmonary edema	Antineoplastic chemotherapy agents, chlorothiazide, aspirin	Typically minutes to a few hours	ARDS, ARF, hypoxemia
Diffuse alveolar damage	Antineoplastic chemotherapy agents, amiodarone	Hours to weeks	ARDS, ARF *Later:* pulmonary fibrosis
Diffuse alveolar hemorrhage	Anticoagulants, antiplatelet agents	Days	ARDS, ARF, diffuse clotting in airways
	Cocaine, propylthiouracil	Weeks to months	Pneumorenal syndrome, extrapulmonary involvement
Acute cellular interstitial lung disease	Methotrexate	Weeks to years	ARF
Amiodarone-induced pulmonary toxicity	Amiodarone	Weeks to years	ARF *Later:* pulmonary fibrosis
Acute eosinophilic pneumonia	Minocycline, tobacco smoke	Days to months	ARF
Acute radiation-induced lung injury	Radiation therapy	Weeks	ARF
Opportunistic infection	Corticosteroids, biologics	Weeks to months	ARF
Massive pleural effusion/hemothorax	Dantrolene, lupus-inducing drugs, anticoagulants	Weeks to months	Compression of heart, lung and venous return
Catastrophic pulmonary hypertension	Protamine	Minutes	Acute RHF, hypoxemia
Methemoglobinemia	Benzocaine, dapsone, oxidizing chemicals	Hours to days	Tissue hypoxia, pulmonary edema, brain damage
Neuromuscular failure	Aminosides, curares, dantrolene	Hours to days	ARF
Multiorgan dysfunction syndrome	Drugs that induce DRESS syndrome	Weeks to months	Multiorgan failure

ACE, angiotensin-converting enzyme; *ARDS*, acute respiratory distress syndrome; *ARF*, acute renal failure; *DAD*, diffuse alveolar damage; *DRESS*, drug rash, eosinophilia, and systemic symptoms; *NSAIDs*, nonsteroidal antiinflammatory drugs; *RHF*, right[-sided] heart failure.

suppressants (anorectics), anticonvulsants, antineoplastic chemotherapy agents, ergots and ergolines, leukotriene receptor antagonists (LTRAs), mTOR (*mammalian target of rapamycin*) inhibitors, NSAIDs, and statins—may cause similar kinds of DIRD, suggesting a common pharmacologic cytopathic mechanism (**Table 17-3**). Furthermore, patients who exhibit an adverse reaction from one drug are at risk for cross-reaction if challenged with another drug of the same family. In the case of anticonvulsants, relatives of patients with the syndrome of drug rash, eosinophilia, and systemic symptoms (DRESS) may be at risk for development of a similar complication with exposure to this class of medications.

Certain antineoplastic agents may cause acute or subacute lung injury when used in a single-drug regimen (e.g., azathioprine, bleomycin, busulfan, chlorambucil, cyclophosphamide, dasatinib, imatinib, methotrexate, nitrosoureas). Typically, however, these agents are given as part of a multiagent regimen, so that it is difficult to discern which drug caused the reaction, unless pulmonary toxicity is observed to occur only after addition of a specific drug to an otherwise nonpneumotoxic regimen. Toxicity in this latter setting has been documented for bleomycin, gemcitabine, methotrexate, radiation therapy, and

rituximab. Combinations of certain chemotherapy agents, such as gemcitabine and bleomycin, or of drugs and radiation therapy may be particularly toxic, dramatically increasing the incidence of severe pulmonary toxicity. Oxygen also synergizes the pulmonary toxicity of chemotherapy agents, amiodarone, and radiation therapy. Radiation therapy may synergize chemotherapy-induced lung damage, causing augmented toxicity or rebound pneumonitis in the previously treated patient. Several antineoplastic agents of the newer generation—erlotinib, gefitinib, imatinib, dasatinib, everolimus, trastuzumab, temozolomide, temsirolimus, thalidomide, lenalidomide, omalidomide, and topotecan—may cause acute pneumonitis, DAD, pulmonary fibrosis, organizing pneumonia (the preferred designation for bronchiolitis obliterans organizing pneumonia [BOOP]), infusion reactions, bronchospasm, anaphylaxis, capillary leak, methemoglobinemia, and pulmonary hemorrhage. In addition to subacute and acute presentations, antineoplastic agents may cause subtle insidious pneumonitis or fibrosis particularly in children, typically noted years after completion of therapy, in the form of indolent or progressive restrictive lung dysfunction. In a few such patients, lung transplantation may be necessary.

Table 17-3   Specific Agents/Drug Families Implicated in Drug-Related Respiratory Disease

Drug Family	Specific Agent(s)	Frequency of Adverse Effects	Pattern(s) of Respiratory Damage	Comments
Abused drugs	Heroin, cocaine, crack, marijuana	++++	Airway burns	Suggestive of exposure to crack cocaine
			Severe bronchospasm	Suggestive of exposure to insufflated heroin
			Acute NCPE	Suggestive of heroin overdose
			DAH	Suggestive of exposure to cocaine
			Pneumothorax	May follow injection of drug in central vein
			Systemic vasculitis	Suggests exposure to drugs tainted with levamisole
ACE inhibitors	Captopril, enalapril	++++	Cough	Chronic, annoying cough; remits with drug avoidance
		+++	Angioedema	Drug etiology often missed
		++	Rare PIE	Rare
Anorectic agents	Aminorex, fenfluramine	+++	Pulmonary hypertension	Can be irreversible/progressive Drugs are recalled
Antibiotics	Minocycline, sulfasalazine, penicillin	+++	Anaphylaxis	Can cause ARF
			PIE	Can cause ARF
Anticonvulsants	Carbamazepine, phenytoin, lamotrigine	++++	DRESS	Cutaneous rash, deep organ involvement ± PIE
Anticoagulants: oral	Warfarin	++	Bland DAH	Risk increases in parallel with the INR
		++	Laryngeal, tongue, tracheal hematoma	May cause acute upper airway obstruction
		+	Pulmonary calcium deposits	Unusual
Anticoagulants: intravenous	Heparin, streptokinase, urokinase, alteplase	++	Bland DAH	
		++	Hemothorax	Can cause compression and circulatory failure
Antidepressants	Sertraline, venlafaxine	++	Eosinophilic pneumonia, DRESS	May cause respiratory failure
Antithyroid drugs	Propylthiouracil	+++	Vasculitis, capillaritis, DAH	Demonstrable pulmonary capillaritis; in some cases perinuclear or cytoplasmic ANCA detectable at high titers Renal involvement possible
β-Agonists (parenteral tocolytics)	Salbutamol, terbutaline, isoxuprine	+++	NCPE	Usually transient and benign
Beta blockers	Most β-blocking drugs	+++	Acute bronchospasm	Can be fatal
		++	Lupus syndrome	Pleural/pleuropericardial effusion and a positive ANA test result
		+	ILD/BOOP	Rare
Biologics	Anti-TNF agents, rituximab, omalizumab	++	Anaphylaxis	
		++	Acute ILD	More common with rituximab or infliximab
		++	Pulmonary granulomas	More common with etanercept
		++	Lupus syndrome	Serositis and a positive ANA test result and ds-DNA
Blood, blood products	Whole blood, platelets, FFP	++++	TRALI/NCPE	Early onset Diuretics detrimental
Curares	Pancuronium, tubocurarine	+++	Anaphylaxis	
		++++	Respiratory muscle palsy	

Table 17-3 Specific Agents/Drug Families Implicated in Drug-Related Respiratory Disease—cont'd

Drug Family	Specific Agent(s)	Frequency of Adverse Effects	Pattern(s) of Respiratory Damage	Comments
Cytotoxic agents	Busulfan, bleomycin, cyclophosphamide	+++	Transient pulmonary infiltrates	Caution, as rechallenge may cause full-blown NCPE/ARDS
	Gemcitabine, nitrosoureas, taxanes	++++	NCPE, DAH	May lead to an ARDS picture
			Later: pleuropulmonary fibrosis	Improvement may follow corticosteroid therapy
	Oxaliplatin	++	Anaphylaxis	Can be fatal Skin tests useful in diagnosis
DMARDs	NSAIDs	+++	Acute asthma, PIE	Class effect
	Methotrexate	++++	Acute cellular ILD	Must be separated from *Pneumocystis jiroveci* pneumonia
	Leflunomide	++	Cellular ILD	Described mostly in Japanese patients with RA
	Tacrolimus	+	ILD	Described in Japanese patients with RA
	Biologics			See biologics
Ergots	Bromocriptine, cabergoline	++++	Pleural effusion	Resolves with drug discontinuance
	Ergotamine, dihydroergotamine, methysergide	++++	Pleural thickening	Decreases with drug discontinuance
	Nicergoline, pergolide	+++	Acquired valvular heart disease	Reversal of changes possible with drug discontinuance
Interferon alfa/beta		+++	Cellular or granulomatous ILD	Clinical improvement with drug discontinuance/corticosteroid therapy
			BOOP	Reversal of changes with drug discontinuance/corticosteroid therapy
			Sarcoidosis-like reaction	Subsides with drug discontinuance/corticosteroid therapy
Leukotriene receptor antagonists	Montelukast, pranlukast, zafirlukast	++	Churg-Strauss syndrome	Strong suspicion for a causal relationship
Lipids: aspirated/inhaled	Paraffin	++++	Exogenous lipoid pneumonia	Lipid droplets present in sputum, BAL fluid, and alveoli
Lipids: infused	Parenteral nutrition, drug excipient	++	Fat embolism syndrome	May also cause DAH
mTOR inhibitors	Everolimus, sirolimus, temsirolimus	+++	Cellular ILD, BOOP, DAH	Dose-related Abates with reduced dosage or discontinuance
NSAIDs, including aspirin	ASA, ibuprofen, indomethacin	+++	Catastrophic bronchospasm	Can be fatal
	Naproxen, piroxicam	++	PIE	Remits with avoidance, relapses on rechallenge
	Aspirin	+++	NCPE	Anion gap, metabolic acidosis, elevated blood salicylate
Platelet glycoprotein IIb-IIIA inhibitors	Abciximab, clopidogrel, eptifibatide	++	DAH	More common in smokers and in presence of LVF
	Ticlodipine, tirofiban			DAH generally not associated with low platelet counts
Radiation—therapeutic				
Lung		++++	Radiation-induced lung injury	Localizes along the radiation beam
		+++	Stereotactic irradiation	Whorled appearance May be tracer-avid on PET scan

Continued

Table 17-3 Specific Agents/Drug Families Implicated in Drug-Related Respiratory Disease—cont'd

Drug Family	Specific Agent(s)	Frequency of Adverse Effects	Pattern(s) of Respiratory Damage	Comments
Mediastinum		++	Mediastinal fibrosis	
Trachea		++	Tracheal disruption	
Endobronchial		++	Airway damage	Dehiscence, fatal hemoptysis
Breast		+++	BOOP	Corticosteroids may be indicated
Liver		++	ARDS	^{131}I (radioiodine)
Statins	Fluvastatin, pravastatin, simvastatin	+++	Cellular ILD	Ground glass shadowing on HRCT scan
			BOOP	Fixed or migratory alveolar opacities Statin myopathy may be present
TKI inhibitors	Erlotinib, gefitinib	+++	DAD/ALI	Difficult to separate from disease progression or from an infection Previous ILD may increase risk
	Imatinib	++	Cellular ILD	
	Dasatinib	++	Pleural exudate, chylous effusion	
TNF-α antibody agents	Etanercept, infliximab, adalimumab	+++	Accelerated ILD	May mimic an infection or exacerbation of underlying rheumatoid lung
			Pulmonary granulomatosis	May mimic sarcoidosis
			Opportunistic infections including TB	Pretherapy evaluation for latent TB indicated using TST and IGRA

ACE, angiotensin-converting enzyme; *ALI*, acute lung injury; *ANA*, antinuclear antibody; *ANCA*, antineutrophil cytoplasmic antibody; *ARDS*, acute respiratory distress syndrome; *ARF*, acute renal failure; *ASA*, acetylsalicylic acid; *BAL*, bronchoalveolar lavage; *BOOP*, bronchiolitis obliterans organizing pneumonia; *DAD*, diffuse alveolar damage; *DAH*, diffuse alveolar hemorrhage; *DMARDs*, disease-modifying antirheumatic drugs; *DRESS*, drug rash, eosinophilia, and systemic symptoms [syndrome]; *ds-DNA*, double-stranded DNA; *FFP*, fresh frozen plasma; *HRCT*, high-resolution computed tomography; *IGRA*, interferon-gamma release assay; *ILD*, interstitial lung disease; *INR*, international normalized ratio; *mTOR*, mammalian target of rapamycin; *PET*, positron emission tomography; *RA*, rheumatoid arthritis; *TB*, tuberculosis; *TKI*, tyrosine kinase inhibitor; *TNF-α*, tumor necrosis factor-α; *TST*, tuberculosis skin test.

INCIDENCE AND RISK EVALUATION

The incidence of DIRD varies with the specific drug or agent. Amiodarone, antineoplastic drugs (bleomycin, cyclophosphamide, gefitinib, methotrexate, nitrosoureas), nitrofurantoin, disease-modifying antirheumatic drugs (DMARDs) (leflunomide, methotrexate, anti-TNF agents), NSAIDs, mTOR inhibitors, and radiation therapy are associated with the highest reported rates of DIRD. The true incidence is modulated by the number of patients receiving the drug. Although the incidence rate for mTOR inhibitor–induced ILD has been reported as up to 36%, the actual number of patients with the disease is low, because this class of medications is given mainly to patients with selected malignancies and to recipients of solid organ transplants. By contrast, the incidence rate of amiodarone pulmonary toxicity is 1% to 2%, but the number of affected patients is greater, because the drug is widely used to treat various forms of arrhythmias. Incidence of DIRD increases with age, in parallel with exposure to drugs.

Mechanisms and risk factors for DIRD have been deduced from studies in animals and in humans and in many cases have been matched with specific agents, as follows:

Pharmacokinetics and sequestration of the drug—amiodarone, desethyl-amiodarone, bleomycin, mTOR inhibitors

Albumin levels—methotrexate

Metabolic activation of drug in lung cells—paraquat and possibly nitrofurantoin

Cumulated drug dosage—amiodarone, bleomycin, nitrosoureas

Sequential exposure to the drug, an important consideration when retreatment is being considered—bleomycin, nitrosoureas

Combinations of pneumotoxic drugs—gemcitabine plus bleomycin, gemcitabine or other chemotherapy agent plus radiation therapy to the chest

Volume of irradiated lung

Cytochrome P-450 variant allele carrier status—oral anticoagulants, cocaine, and possibly other drugs

Impurities formed during drug synthesis—"peak E" contaminant of L-tryptophan

Extremes of age—amiodarone or bleomycin in older people, nitrosoureas in younger persons

History of smoking—amiodarone, bleomycin

Gender—amiodarone in male patients, bischloroethyl nitrosourea (BCNU) in female patients

Renal failure—bleomycin, amiodarone

Preexisting lung disease—amiodarone, DMARDs including methotrexate, leflunomide, anti-TNF agents, gefitinib

Atopy—minocycline, NSAIDs, drugs causing hypersensitivity or anaphylaxis

Ethnicity—enhanced risk for development of ACE inhibitor–induced angioedema in dark-skinned people, and of ILD in association with use of gefitinib, bortezomib, leflunomide, and tacrolimus in persons of Japanese ancestry

Unfortunately, DIRDs often occur unexpectedly in predisposed persons and generally are not amenable to early detection with use of serial lung function tests, including diffusing capacity, although this parameter often decreases substantially concomitant with the administration of chemotherapeutic drugs without necessarily indicating clinical toxicity, or by imaging. Nevertheless, an appreciation of the aforementioned risk factors by physicians who prescribe those drugs is essential, particularly the dose-limiting toxicity of bleomycin and nitrosoureas, the hazard of bleomycin combined with gemcitabine, the 6- to 12-month time window for onset of amiodarone pulmonary toxicity, and the risk associated with use of excessive concentrations of oxygen in patients who have received chemotherapeutic agents, or amiodarone which may lead to acute deterioration of subclinical pneumonitis.

DIAGNOSING DRUG-INDUCED RESPIRATORY DISEASE

Diagnosing DIRD accurately is essential with regard to decisions to discontinue or continue the presumptively offending agent, because inappropriate drug withdrawal may have a negative impact on outcome, and because rechallenge may lead to fatal relapse. Issues regarding the diagnosis of DIRD and the corresponding differential diagnosis differ according to the underlying illness and specific clinical context (**Table 17-4**). Particularly difficult issues arise in patients with solid tumors, hematologic malignancies, or rheumatoid arthritis and in recipients of bone marrow or hematopoietic stem cell transplants, who are immunosuppressed under the combined influence of the underlying condition and the drugs (including corticosteroid therapy) and the radiation used to treat it.

Although the expression of bacterial and fungal pulmonary infections on imaging studies often is distinctive, viral and *Pneumocystis* pneumonias resemble drug-induced ILD, with no clinical or radiographic discriminator to separate these two entities. Therefore, meticulous examination of BAL and other body fluids is indicated. Further complicating the issue, recipients of hematopoietic stem cell transplants may develop diffuse nonspecific pulmonary complications unrelated to drugs, such as acute pulmonary edema, DAH, the periengraftment respiratory distress syndrome, and idiopathic pneumonia syndrome, leading to substantial diagnostic confusion. Drug-induced ILD also is difficult to diagnose in patients with rheumatoid arthritis and in those with certain other systemic conditions, for several reasons: such patients often receive more than one DMARD (e.g., NSAID, methotrexate, an anti-TNF drug, cyclophosphamide, or rituximab) each having the potential to cause lung damage. In addition, the underlying rheumatic or systemic condition itself may manifest with progressive ILD. Furthermore, opportunistic infections can occur as a consequence of the underlying disease and/or therapy with corticosteroids and anti-TNF agents. Similarly, ILD in cardiac patients who are taking amiodarone raises complex issues, because amiodarone-induced pulmonary toxicity must be reliably and noninvasively separated from heart failure and from any incidental ILD.

The evidence base for respiratory disease as being drug-induced is wide-ranging, because the literature on DIRD consists mostly of case reports and is subject to reporting bias. There is a paucity of epidemiologic studies showing a convincing association of exposure to a drug and occurrence of pulmonary events. Investigating a case of possible DIRD requires a high degree of awareness, careful exclusion of conditions that DIRD can resemble (e.g., *Pneumocystis* or viral pneumonia with use of BAL), cessation of administration of the suspected agent (underlying disease permitting), and discussion of whether corticosteroid therapy is indicated, bearing in mind that corticosteroid therapy itself may complicate evaluation of the effect of drug withdrawal on signs and symptoms (drug withdrawal may be without an effect in patients with explosive or severe presentations). Evidence indicating that a respiratory reaction is drug-induced consists of the following: (1) the likelihood of exposure to a compatible drug, particularly if given as a solo agent, (2) previous conclusive reports of reactions to the drug, (3) pattern of involvement compatible with the specific drug, (4) compatible temporal relationship of exposure and onset and progression of symptoms, best demonstrated in patients who experience an acute reaction such as acute bronchospasm, anaphylaxis, angioedema, or pulmonary edema; (5) abatement of signs and symptoms after cessation of drug administration; (6) supportive findings on BAL fluid and histopathologic analysis; (7) lack of an alternative diagnosis after meticulous investigation using BAL and, in selected cases, lung biopsy; and (8) relapse of signs and symptoms on rechallenge, a potentially hazardous test. **Box 17-1** summarizes these diagnostic criteria and presents a useful approach to diagnosis and management of DIRD.

The Naranjo scale is well known for grading the evidence. Case histories are heterogeneous in the literature and rarely include all criteria. Patients may give a history of periods on and off the drug, and it is important to correlate timing of these with onset, fading, and recurrence of respiratory signs and symptoms. Although drugs are an important consideration in the differential diagnosis for ILD, video-assisted surgical lung biopsy (VATS) is rarely performed owing to its relative invasiveness and associated risks. The transbronchial approach is a valuable alternative, although the limited size of the sample obtainable with this technique confers a lesser degree of diagnostic certainty than that achieved with the open approach. Although the possibility of drug-induced ILD sometimes is raised by the pathologist on the basis of typical changes in the tissue, lung biopsy usually can be avoided, because lung tissue changes may lack specificity for the drug. Important exceptions include *amiodarone pulmonary toxicity*, which demonstrates features of dyslipoidosis; *chemotherapy lung*, characterized by DAD and an abundance of reactive epithelial cells; *lung injury from illicit drugs*, in which presence of carbonaceous deposits or drug excipient within and around the pulmonary vasculature is typical; *exogenous lipoid pneumonia*, in which oil is seen lying free in the alveoli and in the tissue; and *fluid silicone embolism*, associated with distinctive nonstainable vacuoles.

In most other instances, histopathologic examination discloses changes that are consistent with, rather than diagnostic for, the drug etiology. However, the lung biopsy has an important diagnostic role in that it may confidently exclude other potential etiologic disorders, including infection, if appropriate stains and molecular techniques are applied to the specimen.

PATTERNS OF DRUG-INDUCED RESPIRATORY DISEASE

More than 60 discrete clinical-imaging-pathologic patterns of DIRD have been identified. The most common presentation is

Table 17-4   Diagnosis and Differential Diagnosis of Drug-Induced Respiratory Disease

Setting/ Specialty	Prototypical Causal Drugs	Clinical Pattern of Involvement	Main Competing Diagnosis
Emergency department	ACE inhibitors, AA2R	Acute upper airway obstruction	Epiglottitis
	Drugs that cause NCPE, ALI, ARDS, DAH, ILD, PIE, BOOP	Diffuse pulmonary infiltrates with or without ARF	Infection, LVF
	Drugs that cause anaphylaxis	Shock, acute airway obstruction	Sudden severe asthma
	Anticoagulants, antiplatelet agents	DAH Hemothorax	DAH of other causes Spontaneous hemothorax, trauma
Oncology: solid tumors	Chemotherapy agents including TKIs (gefitinib, erlotinib)	NCPE, DAD, DAH, anaphylaxis, pulmonary fibrosis	NCPE, DAD, DAH of other causes, including opportunistic pulmonary infection, ILD due to other drugs, TRALI, overload pulmonary edema
	mTOR inhibitors G-CSF, GM-CSF Blood and fractions	ILD, BOOP, DAH Ranges from pulmonary infiltrates to NCPE TRALI	ILD, BOOP, DAH of other causes NCPE of other causes Overload pulmonary edema
Oncology: hematologic malignancies	Chemotherapy agents including TKIs and imatinib	NCPE, DAD, DAH, anaphylaxis, pulmonary fibrosis	NCPE, DAD, ILD, DAH of other causes, including opportunistic pulmonary infections
	ATRA	ATRA syndrome ILD, pleural effusion	NCPE, ARDS, DAH of other causes
	Imatinib	Pleural effusion, chylous effusion	Underlying disease
	Dasatinib	Pleural effusion, chylous effusion	Underlying disease
	Thalidomide, lenalidomide, pomalidomide	ILD	ILD of other causes
Rheumatology	Corticosteroids	Opportunistic infections including *Pneumocystis* pneumonia	Drug-induced ILD
	Methotrexate	Acute methotrexate pneumonitis	Opportunistic pulmonary infection
	Leflunomide	Subacute ILD	Rheumatoid lung, ILD of other causes
	Anti-TNF agents	Accelerated ILD, opportunistic infection including tuberculosis, autoimmune phenomena	Idiopathic ILD
Cardiology	Amiodarone	Insidious or acute ILD	Left ventricular failure, pulmonary edema
	β-Adrenergic receptor blockers	Acute bronchospasm	"Cardiac asthma"
	ACE inhibitors	Coughing	Coincidental lung disease
Dermatology	Minocycline	Pulmonary infiltrates and eosinophilia	PIE of other causes
	Acitretin	Acute ILD	Underlying disease
Endocrinology	Propylthiouracil	Diffuse alveolar hemorrhage, pneumorenal syndrome	ANCA-associated vasculitis (Wegener granulocytosis/microscopic polyangiitis)
Anesthesia	Curares Opiates	Neuromuscular failure—anaphylaxis	Other causes of intraoperative anaphylaxis
	Propofol	NCPE Acute explosive coughing	Overload pulmonary edema, TRALI
Neurology	Anticonvulsants Ergots	DRESS Pleural effusion/thickening	Other causes of pleural effusion

AA2R, Angiotensin 2 receptor inhibitors, *ACE*, angiotensin-converting enzyme; *ANCA*, antineutrophil cytoplasmic antibody; *ARDS*, acute respiratory distress syndrome; *ATRA*, all-*trans* retinoic acid; *BOOP*, bronchiolitis obliterans organizing pneumonia; *DAD*, diffuse alveolar damage; *DAH*, diffuse alveolar hemorrhage; *DRESS*, drug rash, eosinophilia, and systemic symptoms [syndrome]; *G-CSF, GM-CSF*, granulocyte/granulocyte-macrophage colony-stimulating factor; *ILD*, interstitial lung disease; *LVF*, left ventricular failure; *mTOR*, mammalian target of rapamycin; *NCPE*, noncardiac pulmonary edema; *TKIs*, tyrosine kinase inhibitors; *PIE*, pulmonary infiltrates and eosinophilia; *TNF-α*, tumor necrosis factor-α; *TRALI*, transfusion-related acute lung injury.

one of diffuse or focal pulmonary infiltrates, with or without hypoxemia. This pattern often is referred to as ILD, although histopathologic evidence is rarely available to confirm the diagnosis. Under the influence of cultural differences throughout the world, a given clinical imaging pattern may be named using various descriptor English terms. A recent trend is to ascribe a specific "pathologic diagnosis" to a given pattern on high-resolution computed tomography (HRCT). This should be done with caution, however, because correlation of these two diagnostic modalities can be suboptimal. Drugs can elicit virtually any pattern of naturally occurring ILD, which as noted is a clinical, radiologic, and histopathologic mimic of numerous

Box 17-1 Approach to Diagnosis and Management of Drug-Induced Respiratory Disease

Diagnostic Criteria
- Confirmed exposure to an eligible drug
- Confirmatory literature data
- Pattern of reaction appropriate for the drug
- Appropriate latency period and timing of onset of respiratory symptoms relative to taking the drug
- Supportive BAL and histopathologic findings
- Resolution of symptoms after dechallenge
- Exclusion of any other cause including other drugs
- Relapse after rechallenge, if performed

Checklist for Fine-Tuning Diagnosis and Management
In patients with compatible clinical presentation or supportive imaging or histopathologic findings (summarized on the Pneumotox website):

1. Depending on level of consciousness and presence or level of respiratory distress, take history of exposure to drugs, occupational/environmental agents, chemicals, and toxic substances. Confirm drug history from relatives, friends, or pharmacist when needed.
2. Evaluate risks associated with discontinuance of drug for underlying condition. Substitute when appropriate.
3. Arrange for timely evaluation of drug and metabolites in blood and/or urine (e.g., opiates, amiodarone, aspirin, mTOR inhibitors) and a urine drug screen.
4. List patterns of respiratory involvement attributable to an underlying disease if present. Match with pattern of involvement from the drug or drugs under consideration. Check for overlapping features.
5. Check complete blood count, CD4+ count, autoimmunity (ANA, ANCA), and HIV serostatus whenever appropriate.
6. Retrieve earlier, pretreatment, and baseline imaging studies, respiratory physiology reports, laboratory data, and autoantibody assay results.
7. List exposure to any drug (even if remote), blood transfusion, blood products, radiation therapy, concealed exposure to illicit drugs, substances of abuse, and chemicals used to synthesize drugs in the household.
8. List possible risk factors related to dosing or blood levels (see text).
9. Examine timing of exposure—discontinuation versus latency period, onset, peak, and resolution of pulmonary symptoms and signs on imaging studies.
10. Match clinical presentation, imaging data, and findings on BAL, laboratory testing, ANA and ANCA assays, and histopathologic analysis (if available) with the drug under study. Contribution of KL-6 glycoprotein assay and in vitro tests is limited.
11. Examine other diagnostic possibilities including *Pneumocystis* and viral pneumonia and pulmonary involvement from the underlying disease.
12. Check laboratory findings for involvement of organs other than the lung.
13. If patient has been exposed to more than one drug, assess causality for each specific drug.
14. Examine whether adverse reaction may result from the known pharmacologic effect of the drug
15. Determine pharmacogenetic trait when appropriate.
16. Evaluate whether corticosteroid therapy is indicated in addition to drug withdrawal (as indicated by clinical severity).
17. Schedule follow-up assessment for signs/symptoms and imaging and laboratory abnormalities after drug withdrawal, to confirm positive dechallenge.
18. Ensure proper communication with any health professional so that the patient is not inadvertently rechallenged with the drug.
19. Discuss whether deliberate rechallenge is indicated (reserved for vital drugs for which no substitute is available). This procedure is performed using low doses in a hospital setting close to an ICU. Tolerance can be induced for a limited number of drugs.
20. Report to national/federal drug safety monitoring authorities; plan publication of findings.

ANA, antinuclear antibody; *ANCA*, antineutrophil cytoplasmic antibody; *BAL*, bronchoalveolar lavage; *HIV*, human immunodeficiency virus; *ICU*, intensive care unit; *mTOR*, mammalian target of rapamycin.

entities: nonspecific cellular or fibrotic nonspecific interstitial pneumonia (NSIP), eosinophilic pneumonia, BOOP, desquamative interstitial pneumonia (DIP), ILD with a granulomatous component, interstitial pulmonary fibrosis, or pulmonary alveolar proteinosis. Drugs also may cause NCPE, DAD, and DAH.

Other patterns of respiratory involvement include angioedema, bronchospasm, pleural effusion with or without the lupus syndrome, pulmonary vasculopathy with or without pulmonary arterial hypertension, neuromuscular failure, and methemoglobinemia. Although DIRD generally occurs in isolation, concomitant involvement of the liver has been reported with nitrofurantoin, nilutamide, and amiodarone.

DIRD may at times manifest as a systemic condition with extrapulmonary and pulmonary involvement. Systemic presentations include the drug-induced lupus syndrome, antineutrophil cytoplasmic antibody (ANCA)-positive vasculitis with DAH, and the Churg-Strauss syndrome. In these conditions, involvement of the skin, kidney, heart, and lung occurs in a manner similar to that seen in the idiopathic conditions. The DRESS syndrome includes a distinctive cutaneous rash and involvement of the liver, kidney, central nervous system, fever, and blood eosinophilia; in a fraction of affected patients, pneumonitis is present. Propythiouracil and anticonvulsants epitomize the culprit agents for drug-induced ANCA–related vasculitis and DRESS, respectively (**Table 17-5**).

PARENCHYMAL PATTERNS

ILD is the most common pattern of DIRD and sometimes is assigned as a "definitive" diagnosis, although lung biopsy is rarely used to confirm this. Severity ranges from the asymptomatic state or mild changes on imaging, to the gas exchange characteristics of acute lung injury (ALI) or adult respiratory distress syndrome (ARDS). If performed, lung biopsy can reveal almost any form of ILD or interstitial and alveolar lung disease including NSIP (the most common reaction), eosinophilic pneumonia, BOOP, DAD, and DAH. Of importance, these patterns may overlap in different areas of a given lung biopsy. The potential for harm versus possible gain with transbronchial or surgical lung biopsy should be weighed in each individual patient, inasmuch as the biopsied tissue may show only nonspecific changes. A state of immunosuppression, severe hypoxemia, and rapidly deteriorating lung function all are contraindications to undertaking an invasive diagnostic procedure.

Nonspecific Interstitial Pneumonia: Cellular Interstitial Pneumonitis

On histopathologic examination, the pattern of NSIP consists of interstitial inflammation with expansion of alveolar septa by a mild to moderate mononuclear cell infiltrate, occasional eosinophils, and interstitial edema. Among the well over 100 drugs that may cause this condition, β-blocking drugs, amiodarone, flecainide, fludarabine, gold salts, imatinib, lenalidomide,

Table 17-5 Systemic Drug-Induced Reactions With Possible Pulmonary Involvement

Systemic Condition	Protypical Drugs(s) or Family	Presentation	Potential for Severity
Lupus syndrome	Lupus-inducing drugs	Pleural/pleuropericardial effusion arthralgias, neutropenia	–
ANCA-positive vasculitis	Propylthiouracil	DAH ± renal failure; pneumorenal syndrome	+++
Churg-Strauss syndrome	Leukotriene receptor antagonists	Eosinophilia, pulmonary infiltrates, mononeuritis multiplex	+
DRESS or anticonvulsant syndrome	Anticonvulsants (e.g., phenytoin), minocycline	Eosinophilia, pneumonitis, hepatitis	+++
Polymyositis	Statins	Diffuse ILD/BOOP and myopathy	+++
Systemic inflammatory response	Aspirin	Temperature disturbances, hyperventilation, tachycardia, leukocytosis or leukopenia, NCPE, acid-base disturbances	++

ANCA, antineutrophil cytoplasmic antibody; *BOOP*, bronchiolitis obliterans organizing pneumonia; *DAH*, diffuse alveolar hemorrhage; *DRESS*, drug rash, eosinophilia, and systemic symptoms [syndrome]; *ILD*, interstitial lung disease; *NCPE*, noncardiac pulmonary edema.

methotrexate, mTOR inhibitors, nilutamide, nitrofurantoin, propylthiouracil, statins, sulfasalazine, thalidomide and its congeners, tocainide, and venlafaxine are cited most often (see under categories Ia and Ib on the Pneumotox website). Methotrexate pneumonitis in rheumatoid arthritis seems to typify acute drug-induced NSIP. Collection of evidence for drug relatedness can be done using the approach set forth in Box 17-1.

Onset of signs and symptoms can be insidious or rapid, with a dry cough, dyspnea, fever, fatigue, and malaise (**Figure 17-1**). In patients who develop this complication with methotrexate and particularly if the drug is continued, the disease may accelerate without notice, causing further shadowing and progressive respiratory failure. The chest radiograph exhibits areas of ground glass attenuation, confluence, or consolidation, which often predominate in the bases, where such changes may extend rather than migrate. In more advanced cases, findings include areas of consolidation with air bronchograms and generalized volume loss, which can be marked. In early or mild cases, HRCT discloses a discrete and diffuse haze, ground glass shadowing, or mosaic attenuation, which may resemble hypersensitivity pneumonitis in appearance. Other signs on imaging include disseminated or diffuse inter- and/or intralobular septal thickening or "crazy paving"; in severe cases, an associated pleural exudate can be present. The BAL fluid typically reveals a CD8+-dominant lymphocytosis, except with bacillus Calmette-Guérin (BCG)-induced pneumonitis, and sometimes an associated increase in neutrophils and/or a modest increase in eosinophil counts. The results of BAL fluid analysis are influenced by timing of the test in the course of the disease and whether the patient has received corticosteroids. BAL has an important exclusionary role: It is used to rule out a coincidental or drug-induced infection, the main competing diagnosis in drug-induced ILD. Particularly important is the use of the most recent nucleic acid–targeted molecular techniques to diagnose *Pneumocystis jiroveci* infection, as opposed to colonization, and viral infections. Nevertheless, BAL is not 100% sensitive for detection of infection. If lung biopsy is performed, the specimen will show uniform expansion of the interstitium by edema and a chronic, inflammatory cellular mononuclear infiltrate composed of lymphocytes and occasional plasma cells. Eosinophils and interstitial fibrosis are inconspicuous. Occasionally scarce and loosely formed granulomas and giant cells may be evident in methotrexate- and sirolimus-induced ILD. Special stains and in situ hybridization studies in the tissue must be used to reliably rule out an infection, which drug-induced ILD can closely resemble.

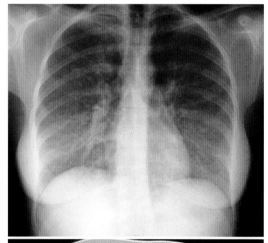
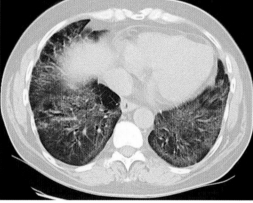

Figure 17-1 Methotrexate lung. Changes include presence of fine interstitial infiltrates in the context of dyspnea, dry cough, and fever. Clinical improvement followed discontinuance of the drug. Although not used in this particular case, corticosteroids are indicated in patients with severe presentations, after an infection has been carefully ruled out. Drug-induced cellular interstitial pneumonitis may manifest with bilateral opacification and transient acute respiratory failure; a list of drugs that may cause this pattern is available on the Pneumotox website, under categories Ia and Ib (www.pneumotox.com).

Outcome with this form of drug-induced ILD is good, with dissipation of signs and symptoms after drug discontinuance. Corticosteroid therapy is reserved for severe presentations or cases in which the disease progresses despite cessation of the drug. Dose and duration of treatment with corticosteroids are adjusted to clinical response; the usual regimen generally is for

2 to 12 weeks, using tapered dosages. The recent trend of administration of methylprednisolone in 1-g boluses has no proven efficacy as compared with conventional dosages. Pneumonitis associated with use of mTOR inhibitors may respond to simple dose reduction. Rechallenge for the purpose of an academic diagnosis is not recommended, because of the risk of life-threatening relapse or death, which would be difficult to justify from a medical-legal standpoint. Reexposure can be contemplated only if use of the specific agent is vital and no substitute drug is available, with administration of small initial doses in a hospital setting. Adequate communication among the patient, primary care provider, specialists, and pharmacist must be established to ensure that the patient is not rechallenged with the drug. Pulmonary fibrosis developing after resolution of this condition is exceedingly rare.

Amiodarone Pulmonary Toxicity

Amiodarone is an antiarrhythmic drug that is widely used to treat supraventricular and ventricular arrhythmias. Amiodarone is an amphiphilic drug, which, like most amphilics, sequesters in tissues, notably the lung, where it causes coarsely foamy changes in resident cells and macrophages of the lung—the so-called amiodarone effect. Such changes are found in the BAL fluid in most asymptomatic nontoxic patients on this medication and do not imply or predict the development of pulmonary toxicity. Amiodarone-induced pulmonary toxicity is a distinctive and potentially devastating pulmonary reaction to the drug and its metabolite. It may affect up to 2% to 5% of patients on the medication, manifesting as new-onset pulmonary infiltrates, and carries a mortality rate of about 10%. Advanced age and a history of ILD may increase the patient's risk for development of this condition. Amiodarone pulmonary toxicity typically develops in older men 6 to 12 months into treatment, which corresponds to an accumulated intake of 100 to 150 g of amiodarone, although a few cases emerged within a few days and a few others after several years. Serial monitoring of imaging and pulmonary function tests (PFTs), even if repeated frequently, generally is not capable of detecting the development of this complication early enough, because changes in PFT variables may develop abruptly. However, a pretherapy chest radiograph and lung function testing are advisable. Most cases of amiodarone pulmonary toxicity take the form of cough, breathlessness, malaise, and moderate fever, with slow and insidious onset over weeks or months. On imaging studies, disseminated, asymmetric parenchymal involvement is present and, in a few cases, pulmonary infiltrates. The liver may exhibit increased attenuation from the iodine in the amiodarone molecule. Other supportive features include a decline of 15% or greater in total lung capacity and vital capacity, or more than 20% from baseline for diffusing capacity. BAL fluid examination discloses foamy-appearing macrophages, with an inconsistent increase in lymphocytes and/or neutrophils. Amiodarone pulmonary toxicity must be distinguished from left ventricular failure using a combination of amino-terminal (N-terminal) pro-B-type natriuretic peptide (NT-pro-BNP) assay and appropriate imaging studies, particularly HRCT, heart ultrasound evaluation, cardiac catheterization, and re-imaging after a few days of induced diuresis.

The various clinical imaging patterns of amiodarone pulmonary toxicity (**Figure 17-2**) include asymmetric pulmonary infiltrates abutting a thickened pleura, segmental or lobar consolidation, a pattern undistinguishable from that of interstitial pulmonary fibrosis, DAH, multiple ill-defined nodules that may exhibit avid uptake on a fluorodeoxyglucose positron emission

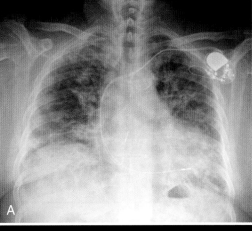

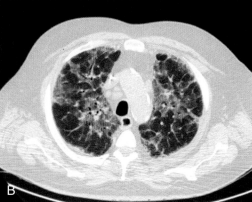

Figure 17-2 Amiodarone pulmonary toxicity (APT). **A,** The chest radiograph shows scattered infiltrates and volume loss. The presence of a pacemaker is a clue to the diagnosis of APT. **B,** Lobular filling is evident on the high-resolution computed tomography (HRCT) scan. Pulmonary involvement in APT is diverse and can be asymmetric or localize in the apices. Other, less common APT patterns include inter/intralobular septal thickening, lobar consolidation, areas of pleural thickening, zonal high attenuation due to the high iodine content of amiodarone, nodules, and masses.

tomography (FDG-PET) scan, pleuropericardial effusion, masses with a center of decreased attenuation, or white lungs and an ARDS picture, particularly after thoracic surgery. Thoracic surgery should be considered a triggering factor for serious amiodarone pulmonary toxicity. Histopathologic analysis, if performed, discloses a pattern of NSIP with foamy-appearing or vacuolated alveolar macrophages, giving the lung a desquamative interstitial pneumonia appearance, foamy changes in pneumocytes and endothelial cells, BOOP, acute fibrinous organizing pneumonia (AFOP), lymphocytic agents, and sterile suppurative masses. Eosinophilic pneumonia, DAD, DAH, and pulmonary fibrosis are less common manifestations of amiodarone pulmonary toxicity, and foam cells may accompany these changes, depending on the interval from cessation of amiodarone administration. A noninvasive approach, as opposed to the more invasive biopsy and its attendant risk of complications, is recommended, inasmuch as a risk-benefit evaluation is not available. Accordingly, causality is more often inferred rather than proved.

The most important aspect of recommended therapy for amiodarone-induced pulmonary toxicity is curtailing exposure to the drug. Corticosteroids are given if drug discontinuance fails to provide demonstrable benefit and in severe cases are quite efficacious. Because of concern about a flare of toxicity-related symptoms while corticosteroids are tapered, a slow diminution of steroid dose is indicated, and corticosteroids typically are given for at least 6 months. Prolonged treatment with corticosteroids requires that patients be regularly monitored for the possible development of steroid-induced adverse effects, including amyotrophy, osteopenia, and opportunistic infections.

Pulmonary Infiltrates and Eosinophilia: Eosinophilic Pneumonia

Eosinophilic pneumonia is a not uncommon complication of pharmaceutical exposures, with more than 80 distinct drugs and substances including substances of abuse recognized as potentially causative agents. Eosinophilic pneumonia can be divided into several clinically distinct entities, which may have overlapping features:

- Patients with methotrexate or nitrofurantoin lung may exhibit mild to moderate peripheral eosinophilia without displaying significant or predominant eosinophilia in BAL fluid or in tissue. Such cases do not strictly meet the definition for eosinophilic pneumonia.
- Eosinophilic pneumonia, when pulmonary infiltrates and peripheral blood and BAL fluid eosinophilia coexist, is an elective complication of treatment with drug families such as ACE inhibitors, antibiotics (minocycline, sulfa drugs, daptomycin), antidepressants (venlafaxine, sertraline), and NSAIDs. Occasional cases have been reported with the administration of bleomycin, cocaine, heroin, fludarabine, and leukotriene receptor antagonists, but eosinophilic pneumonia is not the primary pattern of pulmonary reaction with these latter drugs. Fever and a skin rash can be present at onset of the condition. On the chest radiograph and HRCT scan (**Figure 17-3**), pulmonary infiltrates may predominate in the upper lung fields and can be accentuated in the subpleural regions of the lung bilaterally, but this finding is not universal. Eosinophilic pneumonia can be diffuse or migratory and at times may be difficult to separate from other drug-induced ILD on imaging. Blood eosinophil counts can be normal, whereas BAL fluid eosinophils are more specifically increased up to 50% of the total score or more, obviating the need for the lung biopsy. The diagnosis of drug-induced eosinophilic pneumonia rests on the combination of exposure to a compatible drug, consistent temporal relationship, compatible imaging findings, and a confirmatory blood and/or BAL fluid cell count that decreases on drug discontinuance. A lung biopsy was performed in approximately 6% of all cases reported in the literature. Findings included eosinophil-rich interstitial inflammation and, in some cases, a relative abundance of eosinophils perivascularly. Occasional patients present with overlapping imaging features of eosinophilic *and* organizing pneumonia, with migratory opacities and histopathologic evidence of luminal fibrosis. Extrapulmonary signs and symptoms in patients with eosinophilic pneumonia should raise suspicion for the Churg-Strauss syndrome (see further on). Other causes and contexts for eosinophilic pneumonia including parasitic infestation must be carefully excluded. Outcome of this condition is good if the causal drug is withheld. Corticosteroid therapy is indicated in severe cases. Rechallenge has been safely used to confirm the diagnosis and typically results in the early return of fever and blood eosinophilia in a few hours, which is sufficient to confirm the diagnosis, and of the full-blown picture in a few days.
- Acute eosinophilic pneumonia (AEP) is a grave illness manifesting with fever, cough, dyspnea, dense pulmonary

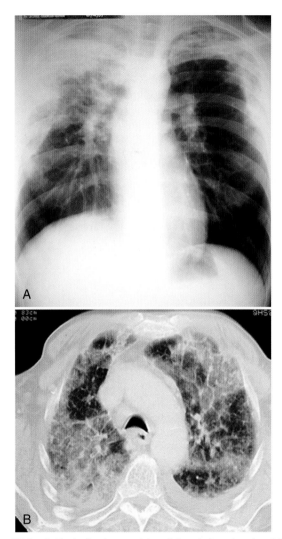

Figure 17-3 A, Typically, the opacities of drug-induced eosinophilic pneumonia (caused by minocycline in this case) localize in the apices subpleurally, as seen on this chest radiograph, although they may be more diffuse. **B,** On high-resolution computed tomography (HRCT) scan, lobular ground glass shadowing, interlobular septal thickening, and pleural effusion may be present. See under category Ic on the Pneumotox website (www.pneumotox.com).

infiltrates, blood, and/or BAL fluid eosinophilia and respiratory failure requiring mechanical ventilation. HRCT shows scattered or more diffuse areas of so-called crazy paving, with areas of consolidation and air bronchograms in more advanced cases. A bilateral pleural effusion may be present at the peak of the disease course. Extreme BAL fluid eosinophilia is the rule, but peripheral eosinophilia is not present in every case. Even though AEP can occur in patients exposed to a compatible drug, not all AEP cases are drug-related, because rechallenge with the drug may not lead to relapse in every patient. The list of causal drugs and substances overlaps with that for eosinophilic pneumonia and includes chloroquine, daptomycin, minocycline, venlafaxine, L-tryptophan (a now-recalled dietary supplement), cocaine, heroin, cannabis, and tobacco use with recent onset of smoking. Drug-induced AEP may represent the upper end of the severity spectrum of eosinophilic pneumonia. Early discontinuation of the offending drug and corticosteroid therapy are indicated.

- Exposure to minocycline, allopurinol, mexiletine, tricyclic antidepressants, anticonvulsants, ibuprofen, and a few other drugs may induce a systemic reaction characterized by prominent and extensive cutaneous rash, pharyngitis, and involvement of the liver, kidney, heart, and central nervous system; in about 15% to 20% of patients, pulmonary infiltrates or eosinophilic pneumonia also is present. The syndrome is known as *DRESS* (drug rash, eosinophilia, and systemic symptoms) or the *anticonvulsant syndrome*, because cases may follow the administration of carbamazepine, phenobarbital, phenytoin, or lamotrigine. DRESS may occur in 1 of 1000 to 10,000 patients receiving these medications. DRESS seems to be poorly recognized, and delay time to diagnosis often is described as "too long," although early recognition is essential. Reactivation of human herpesvirus type 6 or 7 (HHV6, HHV7) or Epstein-Barr virus (EBV) infection may play a causative role by expanding a pool of activated CD8$^+$ T lymphocytes directed against *Herpesvirus* sequences. Drug withdrawal and corticosteroid therapy are indicated. Although outcomes are considered as good, myocardial involvement may adversely affect prognosis.
- Still other patients, mostly asthmatics, develop the Churg-Strauss syndrome during the course of drug therapy. Most cases (more than 90%) occurred in association with LTRAs, and a minority with a few other drugs. Recent case reports have described the onset of Churg-Strauss syndrome in connection with treatment with omalizumab. With LTRA, a few Churg-Strauss cases developed after the other antiasthma drugs were tapered, suggesting that the disease was suppressed by the non-LTRA antiasthma drugs and had been masked until these were omitted. The current view, however, is in favor of an independent and statistically significant causal relationship of LTRA administration and the development of the syndrome.

Infiltrative Lung Disease with a Granulomatous Component

Drugs causing granulomatous ILD include BCG therapy, interferon alfa or beta, methotrexate, sirolimus, and etanercept. On imaging studies, this condition manifests with diffuse interstitial micronodular or linear infiltrates with or without concomitant hilar or mediastinal lymphadenopathy. In some patients, an abundance of CD4$^+$ or CD8$^+$ lymphocytes in the BAL fluid is seen, whereas in others, lymphocyte numbers are normal. Treatment with interferons and etanercept may induce a clinical-imaging and pathologic picture similar to that in sarcoidosis, sometimes with the typical extrathoracic and laboratory features of the naturally occurring disease. Not all cases of sarcoidosis-like disease in hepatitis C virus infection are related to interferon, however, because in about a quarter of the patients with the association, no antiviral agent was being given at the time of diagnosis. The diagnosis of granulomatous inflammation can be confirmed by transbronchial or open lung biopsy, although biopsy of extrapulmonary sites, preferably the skin, is a desirable means of noninvasively establishing the diagnosis. The granulomas in methotrexate pulmonary toxicity are loosely formed, as opposed to those seen with interferons. Recent evidence suggests that treatment with anti-TNF agents in rheumatoid arthritis, mainly etanercept, may be associated with the development of lymphohistiocytic pulmonary infiltrates and non-necrotizing granulomas showing negative results on cultures and special stains for microorganisms. A blunted response to a yet-to-be identified microorganism, a *forme fruste* of rheumatoid lung nodules, and an authentic pulmonary reaction to etanercept are among the possibilities. With a finding of pulmonary granulomatosis in a patient who is on anti-TNF therapy, it is crucially important to rule out pulmonary tuberculosis using sputum stains and cultures and interferon gamma release assay, even if findings on pretherapy evaluation for latent tuberculosis were negative, because anti-TNF agents predispose to the development of this complication. It also is important that patients on anti-TNF agents be tested for antinuclear and anti–double-stranded DNA (anti-ds-DNA) antibodies, because *drug-induced lupus syndrome* appears to be a common complication of treatments with anti-TNF agents. A few patients have developed both a sarcoid-like reaction and drug-associated lupus with anti-TNF antibody therapy. Drug discontinuance and corticosteroid therapy are associated with improvement in nearly all cases. In published reports, symptomatic patients with granulomatous ILD due to BCG administration were given antituberculosis drugs prophylactically.

Organizing Pneumonia

Organizing pneumonia, or BOOP (see under category Id on the Pneumotox website), is a distinctive but nonspecific pulmonary reaction to several infectious and noninfectious insults including inhalation injury, aspiration, drugs, and radiation therapy. BOOP also can occur in recipients of hematopoietic stem cell transplants and in patients with systemic diseases such as rheumatoid arthritis, lupus erythematosus, inflammatory myopathies, temporal arteritis, and ulcerative colitis. BOOP can also occur idiopathically in patients not exposed to drugs. Thus, the multiplicity of underlying causes or contexts for BOOP makes drug causality assessment in BOOP cases difficult. Reasonable evidence suggests that amiodarone, bleomycin, beta blockers, interferon alfa or beta, nitrofurantoin, rituximab, statins, trastuzumab, and radiation therapy to the breast all may cause BOOP. Regardless of the inciting agent, clinical manifestations will include fever, dyspnea, crackles, and sometimes chest pain. Imaging studies will show focal areas of alveolar consolidation, which can migrate, wander, or levitate on chest films taken serially (**Figure 17-4**). Less common presentations include lung nodules or masses containing air bronchograms or diffuse shadowing and acute respiratory failure. On histopathologic examination (although lung biopsy is rarely performed in typical cases), buds of young connective tissue are seen to populate the distal air spaces, which become solid, and widespread florid interstitial inflammation is typical.

In general, BOOP responds well to drug withdrawal and corticosteroid therapy. Unlike idiopathic BOOP, the drug-related condition may relapse, because corticosteroids are still given at elevated dosages if the culprit drug is inappropriately continued—a clue to the diagnosis of drug-induced BOOP. Statin-induced BOOP can be associated with myalgias and a concomitant increase in creatine kinase levels, indicating statin myopathy. In isolated reports, some patients developed a picture of polymyositis thought to be triggered by statin administration. In a few cases, the recently recognized pattern of AFOP was noted as a possible adverse pulmonary reaction to amiodarone or statins. AFOP shares pathologic features with both BOOP and DAD, and it is characterized by diffuse shadowing on imaging studies and by the gas exchange abnormalities of ALI. Outcome in patients with AFOP is distinctly not as good as in those with BOOP. Some BOOP or AFOP cases diagnosed on histopathologic examination may represent the resolving phase of ALI and DAD (see further on).

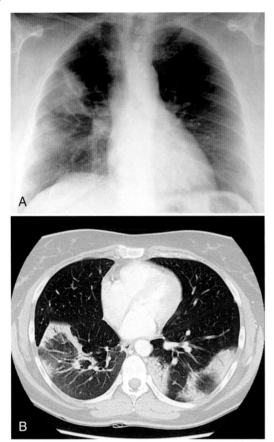

Figure 17-4 Probable organizing pneumonia that developed during treatment with a statin drug. **A** and **B,** Areas of alveolar consolidation and air bronchograms "wandered" from one to another area of the lung on serial chest films, until the drug was eventually withdrawn. See under category Id on the Pneumotox website (www.pneumotox.com). Severe bronchiolitis obliterans organizing pneumonia (BOOP) may overlap with acute fibrinous organizing pneumonia (AFOP).

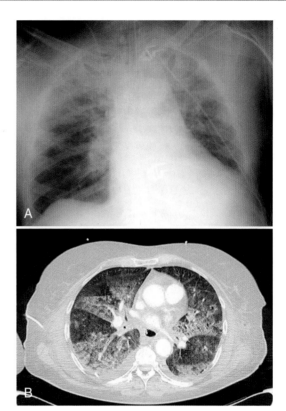

Figure 17-5 Acute noncardiac pulmonary edema (NCPE) after administration of chemotherapeutic drugs in the treatment of solid malignancy. **A** and **B,** Imaging discloses gravity-dependent alveolar opacities, ground glass, interlobular septal thickening, areas of consolidation and moderate pleural effusion. Drug-induced NCPE typically occurs shortly after the administration of chemotherapy or nonchemotherapeutic drugs, or after blood transfusion–related acute lung injury (TRALI). Mechanical ventilation may be necessary in patients with acute respiratory failure. Vigorous inspiration against a closed airway may cause barotrauma and precipitate negative-pressure pulmonary edema. See under category II on the Pneumotox website (www.pneumotox.com).

Acute Pulmonary Edema

Acute pulmonary edema can complicate deliberate or accidental ingestion of large quantities of several drugs and appears to be a nonspecific effect of drug overdose. True drug-induced NCPE is defined by the simultaneous presence of bilateral infiltrates of sudden or rapid onset and severe hypoxemia in a patient with normal pulmonary capillary wedge pressure and absence of changes on heart ultrasound imaging who is receiving a compatible drug at normal dosage, and in whom other causes for NCPE are excluded. The abrupt onset of signs and symptoms after exposure and rapid disappearance on stopping the drug characterize this condition, as opposed to ILD, which runs a more protracted course. Histopathologic confirmation is rarely available, so most cases are suspected rather than proved. In acute, florid cases that came to autopsy after therapy with cytosine arabinoside, methotrexate, gemcitabine, or heroin, alveolar spaces were found to be filled with acellular proteinaceous fluid or fibrin, or there were diffusely distributed hyaline membranes of DAD, a condition with overlapping features, depending on the time frame for diagnosis. Interstitial inflammation is inconspicuous or modest. Interlobular septa may be grossly enlarged by fluid (**Figure 17-5**).

The mechanisms for NCPE include loss of endothelial cell integrity with consequent extravascular plasma leakage. This is confirmed by the high edema fluid–to–plasma protein ratio. Clinically, NCPE is heralded by the sudden onset of

dyspnea and pulmonary opacities sometimes within less than 1 minute after oral, parenteral, or topical administration of a compatible drug, such as epinephrine, all-*trans* retinoic acid (ATRA), arsenic trioxide (As_2O_3), aspirin, hydrochlorothiazide, interleukin-2, nafazoline, narcotics (opiates), propofol, tocolytic agents, antineoplastic chemotherapy (gemcitabine, methotrexate, taxanes), blood and blood products (as in TRALI), or radiocontrast media. In severe cases of NCPE, particularly in drug abusers, a plume of pink frothy sputum is noted at the mouth or in ventilator tubing. Imaging studies disclose the rapid onset of diffuse haze or ground glass shadowing with thickened septal lines and pleural effusion. Typically, there is no cardiomegaly or pedicle enlargement. Notable signs and symptoms include low blood pressure concomitant with the onset of pulmonary infiltrates indicating extravascular fluid loss. In patients with low blood pressure, diuretics are likely to further aggravate the hemodynamic condition and are contraindicated. Epinephrine-induced pulmonary edema can be of the vasoconstrictive type, with marked and transient hypertension concomitant with the onset of pulmonary edema. Hydrochlorothiazide produces a so-called allergic pulmonary edema, characterized by accumulation of pulmonary infiltrates shortly after administration of as little as one tablet of the drug. It may take more than one episode of inadvertent challenge with hydrochlorothiazide before the drug is eventually recognized as a causative agent. Salicylate-induced pulmonary edema can occur in acute and chronic aspirin users, especially in elderly patients with impaired renal function and consequent high plasma drug levels. Patients may present with fever and an impaired level of consciousness, making it difficult to obtain a reliable drug history. Anion gap and metabolic acidosis are characteristic biologic features of salicylate-induced NCPE. Monitoring of drug levels in blood is advised early after hospital admission to confirm the diagnosis, and 30 mg/dL is considered the threshold above which toxicity is likely to occur. Treatment of salicylate-induced pulmonary edema includes serum and urine alkalinization, with hemodialysis reserved for cases with pulmonary edema and other organ damage. Outcomes generally are good if administration of the offending agent is stopped promptly and appropriate supportive care including mechanical ventilation is given. A few cases progress to pulmonary failure or ARDS. The effect of corticosteroid therapy is unclear, but these drugs often are given empirically. The development of pulmonary edema in relation to cardiac dysfunction occasionally has been reported with the administration of doxorubicin and trastuzumab.

Diffuse Alveolar Damage: Chemotherapy Lung

DAD is a pathologic diagnosis that corresponds clinically to acute interstitial pneumonia and the gas exchange characteristics of ALI or ARDS. The condition runs a subacute or acute clinical course and may complicate therapy with numerous antineoplastic agents, particularly when such drugs are given in the form of a multiagent regimen at high dosages, or in conjunction with oxygen and radiation therapy, each of which may cause DAD on its own. Patients treated for solid tumors and hematologic malignancies are at risk for this condition, dubbed "chemotherapy lung" (see under category II on the Pneumotox website). Drugs reported to cause DAD include antineoplastic antibiotics (bleomycin, mitomycin C), alkylating agents (busulfan, cyclophosphamide, chlorambucil, melphalan), antimetabolites (aracytine, azathioprine, gemcitabine, fludarabine, 6-mercaptopurine, methotrexate), nitrosamines (BCNU, chloroethyl-cyclohexyl nitrosourea [CCNU], and novel nitrosoureas), oxaliplatin, podophyllotoxins (etoposide), bortezomib, docetaxel, etoposide, paclitaxel, erlotinib, gefitinib, cetuximab, irinotecan, granulocyte-monocyte colony-stimulating factors (GM-CSFs), and a few nonchemotherapeutic drugs such as amiodarone, carbamazepine, everolimus, opiates, nitrofurantoin, rituximab, salicylate, sertraline, sirolimus, statins, and ticlopidine, as well as blood and blood products used in transfusion. Features of DAD may overlap with those of NCPE, with transition from benign pulmonary infiltrates to noncardiac pulmonary edema or DAD in some patients with inappropriately continued exposure to the causal drug. DAD manifests with cough, dyspnea, disseminated or diffuse haze, ground glass shadowing that may progress to widespread consolidation, lung volume loss, and hypoxemia. HRCT imaging displays linear interlobular and/or intralobular opacities; ground glass attenuation and, on occasion, moderate bilateral pleural effusions are present. Although no study has specifically addressed the contribution of BAL to confirmation of drug-induced DAD, reported series that included a few patients diagnosed with drug-induced DAD showed increased neutrophil counts in their BAL samples; in severe cases, hemosiderin-laden macrophages and bizarre type II cells also were present. It is critical to monitor patients on sequential chemotherapy for the development of subclinical pulmonary infiltrates on imaging studies, because this finding may indicate early NCPE and reflect

impending DAD on continued exposure to the drug. PFTs also are often performed serially, and caution is required in the asymptomatic patient when the diffusing capacity for carbon monoxide falls by more than 30% or 40%. A confirmatory lung biopsy is rarely requested, because the procedure often is deemed to have an unacceptable attrition rate, as measured against a modest diagnostic output. On histopathologic examination, depending on stage of the illness, findings may include interstitial edema, alveolar fibrin, hyaline membranes, various stages of resolving or organizing alveolar damage, and an increased prominence of alveolar lining cells, which is a marker of epithelial cell injury. Although DAD certainly is a distinctive pattern of pulmonary involvement, histopathologic analysis is not capable of separating drug-induced from idiopathic DAD, or to pinpoint its cause. DAD has been observed in the setting of infection, after hematopoietic stem cell transplantation (HSCT) or solid organ transplantation, and with exacerbations of preexisting pulmonary fibrosis; in about a fifth of the cases, no cause is found. Thus, drug causality assessment is a difficult task, unless the results of workup for infection are negative and a straightforward drug exposure–symptom relationship is recognized. Empirical corticosteroids often are given, but the results of this form of therapy are unpredictable. Patients treated early in the course of DAD may respond, whereas others may experience progression to an ARDS picture despite high-dose corticosteroids. The overall mortality rate for iatrogenic DAD is 45%.

Diffuse Alveolar Hemorrhage

DAH is a diffuse and synchronous bleeding from the pulmonary capillaries to the alveolar spaces causing shortness of breath, hypoxemia, anemia, and accumulation of pulmonary infiltrates. Before the diagnosis of drug-induced DAH is considered, exposure to inhaled hydrocarbons or cocaine, ingestion of the super-warfarin brodifacoum rodenticide, or subcutaneous injection of fluid silicone should be ruled out, because any of these may cause severe pulmonary bleeding. Bleeding after accidental or deliberate ingestion of brodifacoum can be especially difficult to treat, because the compound has a very long half-life. From 11% to 18% of DAH cases are considered to be due to drugs. On imaging studies, hazy or ground glass opacities of alveolar filling may assume a butterfly or batwing configuration or have a more diffuse appearance, and on HRCT, scattered, loosely demarcated areas of increased attenuation may be seen.

DAH requires emergent management, because clotting may take place in the distal air spaces or major airways, causing respiratory failure or airway blockage. Hemoptysis occurs in less than a third of the patients, even though significant anemia may be present. An increase in the diffusing capacity for carbon monoxide suggesting free hemoglobin in air spaces is an insensitive finding, because it was noted in a quarter of all reported cases of DAH. A hemorrhagic BAL fluid return is the key diagnostic feature in DAH, and most cases are undiagnosed clinically before the test. A progressively bloody return is noted on serial BAL fluid aliquots. Iron-laden macrophages are revealed by Prussian blue staining, and a correlative increase in the Golde score is seen on microscopy. Drug causality assessment necessitates careful exclusion of other causes, because DAH can occur as a manifestation of cytomegalovirus (CMV) pneumonitis, *Strongyloides stercoralis* infestation, coagulation disturbances, thrombocytopenia, or left ventricular dysfunction, or on a background of lupus, ANCA-related vasculitis, or HSCT, or idiopathically. DAH may be an isolated finding (so-called bland DAH), or it may occur in association with features of extrapulmonary involvement such as microscopic hematuria, renal failure, or microscopic vasculitis in the skin. Indications for and benefits of lung biopsy in DAH constitute a matter of debate, because BAL is the key contributor to definitive diagnosis in the presence of compatible imaging. The finding of capillaritis in the form of invasion and permeation of the capillary walls by neutrophils, along with red cells in alveolar spaces, may not change the treatment approach substantially, and the attendant risks are not negligible.

DAH is the main predictable adverse effect of heparin, thrombolytic agents, oral anticoagulants, and a newer class of antiplatelet agents, the glycoprotein IIb-IIIa inhibitors (abciximab, clopidogrel, eptifibatide, ticlopidine, tirofiban). With the last group of drugs, left ventricular dysfunction and smoking are additional risk factors. Platelet counts generally are within the normal range. In the case of DAH and oral anticoagulants, although a high INR is associated with increased risk of bleeding, coagulation studies can be in the normal therapeutic range at the time of clinical onset of DAH. DAH is an occasional adverse effect of amiodarone, ATRA, nitrofurantoin, rituximab, sirolimus, and chemotherapy drugs. Rarely, DAH is secondary to thrombocytopenia occurring with use of abciximab or quinidine.

Distinctive drug-induced DAH contexts have recently attracted attention:

- Antithyroid drugs, mainly propylthiouracil (PTU) and, less often, benzylthiouracil, carbimazole, or methimazole, may induce perinuclear ANCA, with or without clinically demonstrable vasculitis. These antibodies more often exhibit an anti-myeloperoxidase (anti-MPO), antilactoferrin, or antileukocyte elastase staining pattern and, less often, anticathepsin or antiazurocidin reactivity. ANCAs are unusual in untreated Graves' disease and are strongly associated with exposure to antithyroid drugs, and titers are found to be higher than in naturally occurring ANCA vasculitis, which should attract clinical attention. An anti-PR3 specificity similar to that in naturally occurring ANCA-related vasculitis (Wegener) is an unusual finding. Rare patients have exhibited dual anti-MPO and PR3 ANCA specificity. About 25% of patients with PTU-induced ANCA disease present with pulmonary involvement, and pulmonary capillaritis is found in about 20% of those with PTU-related DAH who undergo a lung biopsy. Renal involvement of various stages is a finding in approximately 75% of the patients, ranging from microscopic hematuria to necrotizing and/or crescentic glomerulonephritis. Patients may present with violaceous skin changes related to vasculitis in the skin on the ears or limbs. A few patients will require induction therapy with corticosteroids, cyclophosphamide, and plasma exchange in a manner similar to that for idiopathic DAH or pneumorenal syndromes. Terminal renal failure is reported in about 5%, and death occurs in approximately 15% of the patients, with respiratory death due to uncontrollable DAH. Recognition of the drug-induced disorder as opposed to an idiopathic etiology is important, because all manifestations of the disease including elevation of ANCA titers are likely to fade on discontinuance of PTU. About a third of the patients with Graves' disease who receive PTU, but not those unexposed to the drug, also demonstrate development of ANCA. Monitoring and follow-up but not drug discontinuance are indicated in asymptomatic cases, because only a fraction of the patients who develop ANCA with exposure to PTU will develop overt vasculitis. Only a few cases of ANCA-related or mixed ANCA and ANA-related autoimmune disease have occurred with the use of penicillamine and hydralazine.
- Inhalation of cocaine may be followed in a few days by acute episodes of hemorrhage, and evidence for DAH is a common finding at autopsy in drug addicts. Although anti-basement membrane–related DAH (Goodpasture syndrome) was once considered an idiopathic condition, 9 of 10 patients in a recent study were smokers, and a history of illicit inhaled drug use (cocaine, cannabis, heroin) was elicited in up to a third of the patients. Thus, Goodpasture syndrome may be a form of inhalational lung injury.
- Although not a real drug, fluid silicone is used subcutaneously in cosmetic surgery to augment breast size in women or to feminize body shape in transsexual persons. Fluid silicone can gain access to the venous circulation, potentially causing severe lung injury, DAH, ARDS, and neurologic death. The *silicone embolism syndrome* shares several clinical and imaging features with the fat embolism syndrome: It may develop over a few hours to 2 weeks, typically in a woman or a transsexual person with a history of illegal subcutaneous injections of fluid silicone. Clinical presentation is with any combination of fever, dyspnea, cough, chest pain, hypoxemia, hemoptysis, alveolar hemorrhage, petechiae, and altered consciousness. Imaging findings are remarkably similar across cases and series and include dense, predominantly basilar subpleural shadowing and air bronchograms. On HRCT, these features may resemble those of eosinophilic pneumonia. Specific attention to the breast is required, because breast tissue may show signs of recent subcutaneous injection of silicone on HRCT. Silicone can be found in BAL fluid macrophages, which contain large, pleomorphic, cytoplasmic inclusions, on a background of neutrophils and/or hemorrhage. On histopathologic examination, nonstainable interstitial vacuoles of fluid silicone conform to the shape of pulmonary capillaries, and a foreign body reaction is diagnostic of this condition. The outcome with silicone embolism syndrome is good, except in patients with very early onset of symptoms after the procedure or in those with a neurologic presentation, which is thought to result from transmigration of silicone through the lung or via an atrial septal defect to the brain. Such patients sustain a high mortality.

The management of DAH includes drug therapy withdrawal, supportive care, and, depending on the clinical context, vitamin K, fresh frozen plasma, platelet transfusion, pulmonary lavage with iced saline, activated recombinant factor VII, or corticosteroids. Immunosuppressant regimens or plasma exchange procedures are reserved for refractory or drug-induced DAH in a manner similar to that for DAH or pneumorenal syndrome occurring idiopathically.

Pulmonary Fibrosis

Diagnosing the cause for pulmonary fibrosis in a patient with a history of exposure to drugs is nearly always problematic, in view of the commonness of idiopathic pulmonary fibrosis. Clubbing of the fingers and honeycombing are less common in drug-induced than in idiopathic pulmonary fibrosis. Drug-induced and iatrogenic pulmonary fibrosis can occur as a late complication of antineoplastic combination chemotherapy using bleomycin, busulfan, chlorambucil, cyclophosphamide, melphalan, mitomycin C, or nitrosoureas (BCNU, CCNU). Estimates indicate a 3% to 4% prevalence of clinically detectable pulmonary fibrosis in long-term survivors of Hodgkin disease, and figures are higher if patients with subclinical restrictive lung function are included. The delayed pulmonary toxicity syndrome in hematopoietic stem cell transplant recipients may correspond to radiation- and chemotherapy-induced pulmonary fibrosis. Pulmonary fibrosis may follow an episode of early drug-induced lung injury; it also seems to arise de novo.

Drug-induced pulmonary fibrosis manifests with dyspnea, cough, crackles, and weight loss. Imaging studies disclose predominantly basilar linear or streaky opacities and volume loss. HRCT reveals coarse reticular thickening along with traction bronchiectasis. Histopathologic examination demonstrates mutilating interstitial fibrosis with sparse inflammation. The late changes of nitrosourea- and cyclophosphamide-induced pulmonary fibrosis may have a predilection for the apices. The late changes of cyclophosphamide-induced disease include pleural thickening, which adds to the restrictive lung dysfunction. The thickened pleura is paradoxically liable to spontaneous pneumothorax, which appears to be difficult to treat. Evidence for nonchemotherapy drugs as agents of pulmonary fibrosis is tenuous. Amiodarone has been reported to cause lung fibrosis either after an episode of classic unresolved pulmonary toxicity or unexpectedly during or after the end of therapy with the drug. An association with nitrofurantoin, occasionally with a positive result on ANA testing that reverses on cessation of therapy with the drug, also has been described. Recently, sudden deterioration of previously diagnosed "rheumatoid lung" has been seen in association with administration of various anti-TNF agents. Curtailing exposure to the suspected agent is indicated in all cases of fibrosis thought to be induced or aggravated by a drug. Improvement is inconsistent, as is the response to corticosteroid therapy. Lung transplantation must be considered and has been successfully implemented in a few patients.

Radiation-Induced Injury

The extent, location, and likelihood of radiation-induced changes depend on radiation dose, associated chemotherapy, portals, and irradiation technique. Sporadic radiation pneumonitis typically occurs in the first few months after delivery of therapy. Late radiation-induced lung fibrosis predominates in the mediastinum in patients with lymphoma who received Y-shaped irradiation fields and in the irradiated lung in patients who received oblique radiation therapy for the treatment of lung cancer. This process takes the form of a limited, whorled or convoluted area of fibrosis developing after stereotactic body radiation therapy, or it can be diffuse when occurring after whole-lung or total-body irradiation.

AIRWAY INVOLVEMENT

Upper Airway Obstruction

Angioedema, the most serious upper airway complication of drugs, occurs more often as a complication of ACE inhibitors than with any other drugs, and ACE inhibitors may account for two thirds of all angioedema cases. An underdiagnosed clinical entity, angioedema is poorly identified as drug-induced, and the long delay until diagnosis, during which exposure to the drug continues despite repeated episodes of edema, puts the patient at risk for development of an asphyxiating episode of airway blockage. Incidence of drug-induced angioedema is on the rise, and ACE inhibitor–induced angioedema is seen more often, and in the United States, a disproportionately greater (fourfold) frequency of this disorder has been documented among African Americans or Afro-Caribbeans than among whites. Incidence is greater with enalapril or lisinopril than with

captopril. Angioedema tends to occur more frequently in the first few weeks of treatment in dark-skinned people, whereas in whites, angioedema can occur months and up to a few years into treatment. About a quarter of affected patients give a history of previous spontaneously resolving episodes, which failed to be recognized as drug-induced. ACE inhibitor–induced angioedema develops unexpectedly or after manipulation of the airway. It manifests with nonspecific signs and symptoms of sore throat, drooling of saliva, dysphagia, and pruritus, followed by the rapid development of edema of the lips, floor of the mouth, and/or larynx.

Drug-induced angioedema can be classified as type 1, edema limited to the face; type 2, involvement of the floor of the mouth, base of tongue, and uvula; and type 3, involvement of the oropharyngeal, glottic, and supraglottic regions and, rarely, the thoracic trachea. Patients with type 2 and type 3 edema are more liable to experience breathing difficulties and to require admission to an intensive care unit (ICU), or to need intubation. It is crucially important to identify and secure the airway early, using fiberoptic bronchoscopy, because if the edema progresses, complete airway obliteration can occur. Identification of the airway may prove impossible, and emergent tracheostomy may be required. Overall, 40% of patients with angioedema require ICU admission, and mechanical ventilation is indicated in about 10%. Outcome is good with supportive care. Patients need to remain hospitalized for an average of 2 days, because rebound edema has been reported. Autopsy series of asphyxiating ACE inhibitor angioedema point to the need for careful identification and management of this condition.

A similar pattern of acute upper airway obstruction may develop with anaphylaxis. Anaphylaxis is an explosive reaction that may follow the administration of drugs, notably antibiotics or radiocontrast media. Signs and symptoms of the condition include wheezing, bronchospasm, airway obliteration, cramping, cardiovascular collapse, shock, loss of consciousness, seizures, and pulmonary edema. Although outcome is good in most instances, a fraction of affected patients may die from the condition. Drugs and foodstuffs account for most cases of fatal anaphylaxis, with anesthetic agents and antibiotics making up a majority of causal drugs. Time to cardiac or respiratory arrest generally is within 5 minutes of ingestion. Distinction between an asthma attack and anaphylaxis is not made in every patient. Although a fraction of the patients initially are resuscitated, secondary death from hypoxic brain damage may occur. Although epinephrine is administered in most patients, it rarely is given early enough before the arrest.

Less common causes of large airway obstruction include laryngeal hematoma and bleeding around the trachea in patients chronically exposed to oral anticoagulants.

Acute Bronchospasm

Bronchospasm can closely follow exposure to oral or parenteral drugs, with acetylsalicylate, β-blocking agents, analgesics, NSAIDs, antibiotics, and cardiovascular drugs accounting for three fourths of the cases and miscellaneous drugs including corticosteroids accounting for the remainder. About 10% to 15% of cases of acute asthma necessitating ICU admission may be secondary to drugs. Asthma, atopy, and a history of drug allergy are risk factors. A stream of an inhaled drug also can cause bronchospasm.

Although acute bronchospasm may develop with no warning sign or symptom in a subject free from antecedent asthma, most of the time it occurs in patients who have underlying asthma and/or chronic obstructive airway disease. Many of the aforementioned drugs are contraindicated or should be used with caution in patients with asthma or chronic obstructive pulmonary disease (COPD), although novel selective beta blockers may have a favorable risk-benefit ratio in terms of mortality in established COPD.

Aspirin sensitivity and intolerance to NSAIDs do not usually result from acquired sensitization but are intrinsic to the patient, who may exhibit the Widal or Samter triad of recalcitrant sinusitis or nasal polyps and intermittent watery nasal discharge, difficult-to-treat asthma, and intolerance to NSAIDs, including aspirin. Nasal symptoms and severe bronchospasm are precipitated by inadvertent exposure to an NSAID within minutes to a few hours after ingestion of the drug. Although avoidance of any NSAID, including aspirin, is recommended, desensitization using incremental dosages has been successful in patients who need to be treated with these drugs. Continued exposure is required for maintenance of the state of tolerance; otherwise, the drug hypersensitivity will return in a few days. Desensitization also can be undertaken in patients with antibiotic hypersensitivity.

Bronchospasm from beta blockers may be catastrophic and difficult to treat, because the state of beta blockade may blunt the response to β_2-agonists used to reverse the bronchospasm.

A hypersensitivity reaction with pruritus and bronchospasm can occur in patients receiving vinca alkaloids, taxanes, or the novel biologics rituximab, infliximab, etanercept, and cetuximab. The reaction can be quenched or ameliorated in most cases by reducing the perfusion rate and premedicating patients with antihistamines and corticosteroids.

In the recent past, inhaled or insufflated heroin was recognized as a cause for acute bronchospasm necessitating emergency intubation. It is nowadays good clinical practice to raise this possibility in the evaluation of adults presenting with acute asthma attacks, using the urine drug screen performed at the time of admission to identify presumptive cocaine and heroin users.

Solitary Cough

ACE inhibitors can cause a chronic annoying cough in up to 30% of patients taking one of these drugs. Incidence is higher in patients of Asian ancestry. The cough develops for no identifiable reasons and occurs in women more frequently than in men, usually after 1 to 2 months of treatment but occasionally later. All ACE inhibitors can induce chronic cough, although the incidence rate differs among different ACE inhibitors. The direct angiotensin receptor II antagonists appear to induce cough less often. Patients with preexisting asthma are not at increased risk, and no relation of ACE inhibitor cough with ACE inhibitor angioedema has been documented. Of importance, careful pulmonary evaluation is necessary, because the cough that develops during therapy with an ACE inhibitor may reveal lung cancer or other pleuropulmonary conditions.

The exact cause for ACE inhibitor cough is unclear, although the bradykinin catabolic pathway may be involved. Drug discontinuance results in improvement within a few days or weeks, but relapse will follow rechallenge with the drug, another ACE inhibitor, or, rarely, an angiotensin II antagonist. No treatment has proved effective in controlling the cough.

Anesthetic agents such as propofol, fentanyl, and isoflurane can induce violent coughing on induction in the perioperative setting.

Isolated cough can occur during chronic treatment with methotrexate without necessarily indicating impending methotrexate pneumonitis. BAL fluid shows a modest increase in lymphocytes. The cough may abate despite continuation of the drug.

Circumstantial evidence relates chronic cough to the administration of interferon, paroxetine, sirolimus, and topiramate. Generally, a drug holiday is indicated in any patient who complains of chronic, otherwise unexplained coughing during the drug exposure period.

Obliterative Bronchiolitis

The rapid development of obliterative bronchiolitis is a rare complication of therapy with gold or penicillamine in patients with rheumatoid arthritis. Evidence for this association is not strong, because bronchiolitis obliterans is a recognized complication of rheumatoid arthritis. Due to the advent of more efficacious drugs, these drugs have fallen out of favor.

The condition also has been reported in recipients of bone marrow or stem cell transplants, in whom it may represent a form of graft-versus-host reaction, and in recipients of lung transplants.

Patients with obliterative bronchiolitis experience increasing dyspnea and cough. Physical examination findings may be normal, or overinflation squeaks may be auscultated over the lung bases. The chest radiographs may show hyperinflation, and the expiratory HRCT scan may disclose a mosaic pattern, probably related to disseminated air trapping. Histopathologic examination reveals subacute or chronic bronchiolitis and/or *bronchiolitis fibrosa obliterans*.

PLEURAL PATTERNS

Iatrogenic pleural involvement can take the form of unilateral (without predilection for either side) or bilateral, subacute or chronic, free-flowing lymphocyte-rich or eosinophilic exudates (from dantrolene, ergots, or hydralazine or after coronary artery bypass graft surgery), serositis with pleuropericardial inflammatory effusion or constriction (from dantrolene, dasatinib, ergots, or drugs that induce the lupus syndrome), pleural bleeding (from oral anticoagulants, heparin, antiplatelets, or alteplase), pneumothorax (in patients receiving chemotherapy or mTOR inhibitors for the treatment of pulmonary metastases), chylous effusion (from dasatinib), pleural thickening (from ergots), or acute chest pain (from bleomycin or methotrexate or with drug-induced lupus) (**Figure 17-6**). Drug withdrawal generally is followed by resolution of the effusion. Clinically, pleural disease develops in isolation, concomitant with pericardial involvement or with systemic symptoms and a positive antinuclear antibody test result, which is suggestive of drug-induced lupus. Anti-TNF agents are notable for an increased propensity for causing anti–ds-DNA antibodies similar to that in naturally occurring lupus. Patients may be asymptomatic or present with dyspnea, restrictive lung function, chest pain, compression of the contralateral lung, respiratory distress, anemia, pericardial tamponade, or pericardial constriction. Patients with massive effusion, especially if bilateral or hemorrhagic, or with tension pneumothorax need expeditious therapeutic intervention.

A serous or, less often, serosanguineous pleural exudate may accompany the florid phase of amiodarone, methotrexate, and nitrofurantoin pneumonitis in up to 30%, 10%, and 16% of the cases, respectively. Pleural effusion can develop as a manifestation of fluid retention, capillary leak, and hyperpermeability during treatment with interleukin-2, GM-CSF, cytosine arabinoside, dasatinib, gemcitabine, ATRA, glitazones, gonadotropins, or imatinib. By contrast, pleural effusion is rare in drug-induced pulmonary edema.

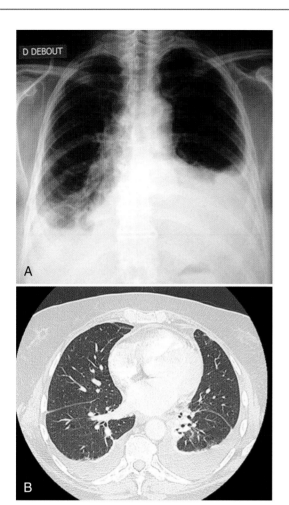

Figure 17-6 Eosinophilic or lymphocytic pleural effusion is visible on chest radiograph **(A)** and/or HRCT **(B)**. The free-flowing effusion is usually an exudate, or pleural thickening may develop during treatments with ergots, dantrolene, or dasatinib, and after chest radiation therapy. In a few cases, pleural effusion and chest pain are the expression of drug-induced lupus, which is diagnosed by the presence of circulating antinuclear and/or anti-DNA antibodies in a patient exposed to a compatible lupus inducer including anti-TNF agents. See under category V on the Pneumotox website (www.pneumotox.com).

The novel orally available multitargeted tyrosine kinase inhibitors imatinib and dasatinib can produce lymphocyte-rich pleural effusions in up to about a third of patients suffering with leukemia who take the drug, and effusions can be chylous in patients on dasatinib. Chylothorax is a rare iatrogenic complication of radiation therapy and coronary artery bypass graft surgery.

Chronic therapy with ergots (e.g., bromocriptine, cabergoline, ergotamine, methysergide, nicergoline) can be complicated by bilateral pleural effusion and thickening, resulting in so-called fibrothorax, manifesting with marked lung restriction and chronic respiratory insufficiency. Previous exposure to asbestos is an additional risk factor. Patients complain of dyspnea, pleuritic chest pain, or a dull sensation in the chest, or they may present with systemic symptoms and congestive heart failure. Muffled breath sounds and a friction rub synchronous with breathing are evident on auscultation, and the noise has been compared by nautically versed patients to that of a mooring rope on a gunwale. Ergot-induced pleural changes develop insidiously over months. Imaging reveals diffuse pleural thickening, areas of folded lung or rounded atelectasis, and loculated or free pleural fluid, but no pleural plaques. These changes are

best seen on HRCT, which also may provide evidence of pericardial thickening or pericardial effusion. Restriction, hypoxemia, and sometimes hypercapnia are seen as measures of abnormal pulmonary physiology. ANA assay results are negative. Drug withdrawal is followed by slow and often incomplete resolution of the pleural changes, leaving residual pleural thickening and a restrictive lung function defect. Heart ultrasound examination is advised, because ergots may produce valvular heart disease.

PULMONARY VASCULOPATHY

Pulmonary vasculopathy is a well-documented adverse effect of various drugs. Also included in this category are DAD and the silicone embolism syndrome, described earlier.

A few drugs are associated with an increased specific risk for venous thromboembolism and pulmonary embolism. Important examples are thalidomide, intravenous immunoglobulins, GM-CSF, and antipsychotic agents.

Several amphetamine-like anorectic agents (aminorex, benfluorex, fenfluramine, dexfenfluramine) can produce pulmonary arterial hypertension, and this is one reason why these drugs were recalled in the past. These drugs also can induce valvular heart disease. Illicit amphetamines also may produce pulmonary hypertension in abusers.

Severe pulmonary hypertension, usually progressive, is a recognized complication of intravenous injection of crushed pharmaceutical tablets by drug abusers. Micronodular infiltrates can be present on imaging studies. Examination of lung tissue discloses foreign body reaction around pulmonary arterioles, with drug additives such as talc, cornstarch, microcrystalline cellulose, and crospovidone discernible within granulomas with use of polarized light and appropriate staining.

Lipiodol-laden acrylate used to treat brain arteriovenous fistulas may spill, with consequent access to the distal pulmonary circulation, causing chest pain and transient opacities on the chest radiograph. Similarly, methacrylate cement used in vertebroplasty procedures also may enter the pulmonary circulation, causing formation of micro- or massive pulmonary emboli of radiopaque cement, which may be evident on contrast unenhanced computed tomography (CT) scans.

Pulmonary venoocclusive disease is characterized by occlusion of pulmonary venules, causing interstitial opacities, subclinical hemorrhage, and pulmonary hypertension. The usual presenting manifestation is dyspnea of insidious onset. Chest radiographs may show Kerley B lines in the absence of left ventricular enlargement. Venoocclusive disease has been reported to occur in the aftermath of chemotherapy with cytotoxic agents or radiation therapy for malignant lymphoma or solid tumors, and after bone marrow, stem cell, or cord blood transplantation. Evidence for a causal relationship is not strong.

MEDIASTINAL PATTERNS

Long-term corticosteroid therapy can lead to mediastinal lipomatosis—a radiographic curiosity in most patients and a cause for cough or mediastinal hemorrhage in a few.

Patients with drug-induced granulomatosis resulting from administration of interferons, etanercept, or infliximab, or patients with the DRESS or anticonvulsant syndrome may present with mediastinal lymphadenopathy.

Oral anticoagulants may on occasion be associated with formation of a mediastinal hematoma, which may compress the trachea, causing respiratory distress.

Drugs and enteral nutrition may desiccate in the esophagus, leading to bezoar formation. Bezoars may protrude anteriorly, causing tracheal narrowing and respiratory discomfort. Esophagoscopy with fragmentation and lavage of the condensed material is indicated to rectify the problem.

METHEMOGLOBINEMIA

Oxidizing agents, dapsone, benzocaine, inhaled "poppers" (alkyl nitrites), nitrates, and nitric oxide may convert hemoglobin from its normal ferrous (Fe^{2+}) to the oxidized ferric (Fe^{3+}) state. Methemoglobin is a poor oxygen carrier, and its bluish chocolate-brown color confers a slate-gray, cyanotic appearance to the skin and also results in interference with pulse oximetry, unless the oximeter has a four-wavelength emitter. Newborns are at risk for this disorder owing to their immature reductase system. Patients with methemoglobinemia present with dyspnea, oxygen-resistant cyanosis, and a normal measured PaO_2. Pulse oximetry gives oxygen saturation values in the 60% to 80% range. Measured arterial blood oxygen content is subnormal. The diagnosis is confirmed by actual measurement of methemoglobin. Normal levels are less than 1% to 2%. Levels greater than 50% are life threatening and can be associated with neurologic symptoms and pulmonary edema, which can be life-threatening. Oxygen therapy is indicated. Methylene blue is the therapeutic agent of choice, should drug withdrawal not suffice to correct the problem.

CONTROVERSIES AND PITFALLS

In any patient with new, otherwise unexplained respiratory signs and symptoms, the possibility of a drug reaction (whatever the route of administration) must be sought. Early recognition, careful exclusion of an infection, and drug withdrawal are paramount and may be lifesaving.

Although a few drugs are associated with a distinctive pattern of reaction, most produce nonspecific changes. The clue to diagnosis is development of such changes in conjunction with exposure to the drug, with abatement on withdrawal of the agent. Exposure to abused drugs must be looked for carefully.

The diagnosis of drug-induced respiratory involvement is more often suspected or probable, rather than definite or proved. A lung biopsy may not resolve the issue, and a risk-versus-benefit analysis in terms of diagnosis input and/or exclusion of other causes often is not available. Rechallenge, although providing strong evidence for causality if followed by relapse, is hazardous. It is possible, however, to induce a state of tolerance in hypersensitive patients by rechallenging them with small incremental doses of such drugs as antibiotics or NSAIDs.

Drug-induced involvement may mimic the pulmonary and extrapulmonary features of idiopathic autoimmune conditions such as the lupus syndrome, ANCA-related vasculitis, Churg-Strauss syndrome, antiglomerular basement membrane antibody–related disease, and myositis. Antithyroid drugs, statins, and anti-TNF antibody therapy are under scrutiny at this time. It is important to test patients receiving such agents for autoantibodies, which may be found in high titers, and to relate drug discontinuance with abatement of signs and symptoms, imaging abnormalities, and autoantibodies.

Novel biologic agents when given to patients with systemic conditions capable of involving the lung may be temporally associated with lung injury that is difficult to separate from underlying disease-related pulmonary involvement. Also, anti-TNF blockers increase the likelihood of infection, and excluding an opportunistic infection is vital. Whether biologics cause acute progression or exacerbation of incipient pulmonary involvement from the underlying systemic condition is unclear as yet.

BAL is a powerful test for excluding infection. The finding of a lymphocyte- or eosinophil-rich BAL fluid supports but does not prove a drug etiology. Foamy macrophages point to the diagnosis of amiodarone-associated pulmonary toxicity. The merit of a lung biopsy versus a more conservative approach is not established in the management of this drug toxicity. Amiodarone pulmonary toxicity may be associated with some degree of interstitial cardiac pulmonary edema. The two conditions must be separated with use of measurements of NT-pro-BNP and diuresis.

Evaluation of respiratory physiology and a baseline chest radiograph (against which any further change can be compared) are indicated before initiation of treatment with amiodarone, DMARDs, or a chemotherapy regimen, particularly if bleomycin is to be given. Serial follow-up chest radiographs are indicated in patients exposed to amiodarone and in those receiving bleomycin. Serial respiratory physiology testing is indicated in patients on bleomycin, although a drop in carbon monoxide diffusing capacity does not equate to toxicity in all patients.

The following *risk reduction strategies* are recommended:

- Maintain cognizance of all aspects of drug-induced respiratory disease.
- Use recommended dosages of drugs.
- Adjust dosages if renal failure is present.
- Consult Pneumotox website if needed.
- Relate exposure to drug to onset and nature of signs and symptoms.
- Discontinue the suspected drug and substitute with another active agent.
- Use corticosteroids sparingly, and taper them slowly.

Preventive treatment with corticosteroids is rarely indicated.

Acknowledgment
This chapter is presented in memory of Dorothy A. White, MD.

SUGGESTED READINGS

Afessa B, Abdulai RM, Kremers WK, et al: Risk factors and outcome of pulmonary complications after autologous hematopoietic stem cell transplant (HSCT), *Chest* 141:442–450, 2012.

Barclay JA, Ziemba SE, Ibrahim RB: Dapsone-induced methemoglobinemia: a primer for clinicians, *Ann Pharmacother* 49:1103–1115, 2011.

Beasley MB: The pathologist's approach to acute lung injury, *Arch Pathol Lab Med* 134:719–727, 2010.

Briasoulis E, Pavlidis N: Noncardiogenic pulmonary edema: an unusual and serious complication of anticancer therapy, *Oncologist* 6:153–161, 2001.

Camus P, Colby TV, Rosenow EC: Amiodarone pulmonary toxicity. In Camus P, Rosenow EC, editors: *Drug-induced and iatrogenic lung disease*, London, 2010, Oxford University Press, Chapter 23.

Camus P, Rosenow EC, editors: *Drug-induced and iatrogenic lung disease*, London, 2010, Hodder Arnold, p 344.

Erasmus JJ, McAdams HP, Rossi SE: High-resolution CT of drug-induced lung disease, *Radiol Clin North Am* 40:61–72, 2002.

Foucher P, Camus P, GEPPI (Groupe d'Etudes de la Pathologie Pulmonaire Iatrogène): Pneumotox Online: *The drug-induced lung diseases*, 1997 (website): http://www.pneumotox.com (last update May 28, 2011); accessed on June 20, 2011.

Goldblatt M, Huggins JT, Doelken P, et al: Dasatinib-induced pleural effusions: a lymphatic network disorder? *Am J Med Sci* 338:414–417, 2009.

Hagan IG, Burney K: Radiology of recreational drug abuse, *Radiographics* 27:919–940, 2007.

Hamblin MJ, Horton MR: Rheumatoid arthritis-associated interstitial lung disease: diagnostic dilemma, *Pulm Med* 2011:1–12, 2011.

Khasnis AA, Calabrese LH: Tumor necrosis factor inhibitors and lung disease: a paradox of efficacy and risk, *Semin Arthritis Rheum* 40:147–163, 2010.

Lara AR, Schwarz MI: Diffuse alveolar hemorrhage, *Chest* 137:1164–1171, 2010.

Larici AR, Del Ciello A, Maggi F, et al: Lung abnormalities at multi-modality imaging after radiation therapy for non-small cell lung cancer, *Radiographics* 31:771–789, 2011.

Larsen BT, Vaszar LT, Colby TV, et al: Lymphoid hyperplasia and eosinophilic pneumonia as histologic manifestations of amiodarone-induced lung toxicity, *Am J Surg Pathol* 2012 Feb 2. [Epub ahead of print.]

Ledingham J, Wilkinson C, Deighton C: British Thoracic Society (BTS) recommendations for assessing risk and managing tuberculosis in patients due to start anti-TNF-α treatments, *Rheumatology (Oxford)* 44:1205–1206, 2005.

Leslie KO: My approach to interstitial lung disease using clinical, radiological and histopathological patterns, *J Clin Pathol* 62:387–401, 2009.

Levine M, Brooks DE, Truitt CA, et al: Toxicology in the ICU: part 1: general overview and approach to treatment, *Chest* 140:795–806, 2011.

Popovsky MA: Pulmonary consequences of transfusion: TRALI and TACO, *Transf Apheresis Sci* 34:243–244, 2006.

Restrepo CS, Carrillo JA, Martinez S, et al: Pulmonary complications from cocaine and cocaine-based substances: imaging manifestations, *Radiographics* 27:941–956, 2007.

Rossi SE, Erasmus JJ, McAdams P, et al: Pulmonary drug toxicity: radiologic and pathologic manifestations, *Radiographics* 5:1245–1259, 2000.

Ruangchira-Urai R, Colby TV, Klein J, et al: Nodular amiodarone lung disease, *Am J Surg Pathol* 32:1654–1660, 2008.

Vahid B, Marik PE: Pulmonary complications of novel antineoplastic agents for solid tumors, *Chest* 133:528–538, 2008.

Wu R, Li R: Propylthiouracil-induced autoimmune syndromes: 11 case report, *Rheumatol Int* 2010 Dec 7. [Epub ahead of print]

Yousem SA, Dacic S: Pulmonary lymphohistiocytic reactions temporally related to etanercept therapy, *Mod Pathol* 18:651–655, 2005.

Chapter **18**

Cough

Surinder S. Birring • Ian D. Pavord

COUGH IN HEALTH AND DISEASE

Cough is an important defense mechanism that clears the airways of secretions and prevents entry of foreign bodies and irritants to the lower respiratory tract. It is a universal experience in health but also a nonspecific presenting feature of most respiratory conditions and a number of nonrespiratory conditions. Acute cough is one of the most common presenting symptoms in the patient population encountered by the general practitioner. In most cases, cough results from viral and bacterial upper respiratory tract infection, is a self-limiting problem, and does not require further evaluation, but a small proportion of patients will have persistent cough that necessitates specialist opinion.

Chronic cough is arbitrarily defined as presence of cough for longer than 8 weeks. It affects 3% to 10% of the general population and is responsible for between 10% and 20% of respiratory outpatient referrals. Chronic cough with significant sputum production (i.e., more than a tablespoonful per day) is likely to be due to intrapulmonary disease such as chronic bronchitis or bronchiectasis. A chronic dry or minimally productive cough may be related to extrapulmonary factors; the cough is likely to be the result of abnormal sensitization of the cough reflex secondary to the effects of local inflammation on sensory nerve endings or an intrinsic abnormality of airway nerves. Most patients complain of an abnormal sensation in the laryngeal area such as a tickle in the throat (laryngeal paresthesia). Chronic cough often is perceived as a trivial annoyance but can be a disabling problem responsible for impairment of quality of life and associated with distressing symptoms such as musculoskeletal chest pains, syncope, incontinence, disturbed sleep, and social embarrassment.

The key to successful management is establishing a clear diagnosis and applying effective treatment for long enough to reset the activity of cough receptors at a more physiologic level. Important pitfalls include atypical presentations, the presence of multiple pathologic conditions, and inadequate therapy of the underlying disorder. Further difficulty arises from the fact that evidence for the efficacy of specific therapies in chronic cough is largely based on expert opinion or uncontrolled trials, as well as the paucity of randomized controlled trials with well-validated outcome measures to guide the clinician. Nevertheless, a systematic approach based on the so-called *anatomic diagnostic protocol*, which focuses on disease processes within the anatomic distribution of vagal afferent nerves, seems to be successful, and various studies have reported a high rate of treatment success even in tertiary referral populations. The general consensus is that in most cases of chronic cough in patients with no other respiratory symptoms or signs and normal findings on spirometry and chest radiography, the underlying cause is asthma, eosinophilic bronchitis, gastro-esophageal reflux, or rhinitis, or a combination of these. Many of these conditions can be recognized clinically, and successful diagnosis and management often are possible without recourse to expensive or invasive investigations.

This chapter focuses primarily on isolated chronic cough, because it is a common condition not dealt with elsewhere in this book. In addition, an isolated chronic cough often is a difficult diagnostic problem for both primary and secondary care physicians. This category of cough is thought to involve a primary abnormality of the cough reflex leading to a heightened response to known tussive stimuli.

THE COUGH REFLEX

Cough is a reflex that occurs when afferent nerve receptors are stimulated by inhaled, aspirated, or endogenous substances. The most sensitive sites for initiating cough are the larynx, the carina, and the points of bronchial branching. Cough receptors also are present in extrapulmonary structures, including the esophagus, diaphragm, and stomach. A broad group of rapidly adapting "irritant" receptors (RARs) found in the larynx and tracheobronchial tree can be stimulated by a wide range of stimuli, including cigarette smoke, ammonia, ether vapor, acid and alkaline solutions, hypotonic and hypertonic saline, and mechanical stimulation by direct contact, mucus, or dust; all such stimuli can provoke cough. Another closely related fiber is the slowly adapting stretch receptor (SAR), which terminates inspiration and initiates expiration when the lungs are at an adequate level of inflation. SARs also may influence cough. C-fiber receptors, which have thin, nonmyelinated vagal afferent fibers, are found in the laryngeal, bronchial, and alveolar walls. They are relatively insensitive to mechanical stimulation and lung inflation but are exquisitely sensitive to chemicals such as bradykinin, capsaicin, prostaglandins, and acid pH. Stimuli that are known to cause cough in human subjects such as capsaicin, bradykinin, and citric acid activate C-fiber afferents, particularly those located in the bronchi. Afferent nerve fibers pass to a central cough receptor in the medulla, triggering a forced expiratory maneuver against a closed glottis, followed by glottal opening and high-velocity expiration (**Figure 18-1**).

DIFFERENTIAL DIAGNOSIS OF COUGH

The causes of cough can be conveniently divided into acute and chronic (**Box 18-1** and **Table 18-1**). An *acute* cough is arbitrarily defined as a cough of less than 3 weeks' duration. Infectious and allergic conditions are by far the most common

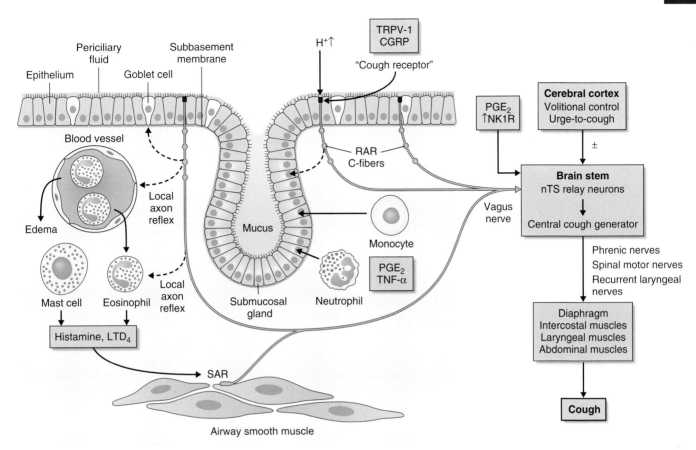

Figure 18-1 Representative scheme of afferent and efferent pathways that regulate cough, and of the pathophysiology of the enhanced cough reflex. Laryngeal and pulmonary receptors, such as rapidly adapting receptors (RARs), C-fibers, and slowly adapting fibers (SARs), and putative cough receptors provide input to the brain stem medullary central cough generator through the intermediary of the relay neurons in the nucleus tractus solitarius (nTS). The central cough generator then decides and coordinates the efferent output to the muscles that causes the cough effort. Also present is an efferent output to airway smooth muscle and mucosal glands (*not shown*). The cerebral cortex may control the motor output of cough volitionally or influence the "urge-to-cough" sensation. Potential factors involved in the enhancement of the cough reflex both in the upper airways and at the brain stem level are illustrated. Inflammatory responses with expression of mediators, neuropeptides, and vanilloid receptors (e.g., TRPV1) may influence the cough response and brain stem modulation of the afferent pathways. *CGRP*, calcitonin gene–related peptide; *LTD₄*, leukotriene D$_4$; *PGE₂*, prostaglandin E$_2$; *TNF-α*, tumor necrosis factor-α; *TRPV1*, transient receptor potential cation channel subfamily V member 1 [i.e., vanilloid receptor 1 or capsaicin receptor].

Box 18-1	Common Causes of Acute Cough

Upper respiratory tract infections
Acute sinusitis
Allergic rhinitis
Asthma

---

etiologic disorders. Most acute coughs related to viral upper respiratory tract infection resolve by 3 weeks, but a small proportion become persistent and require further evaluation.

Most pulmonary conditions implicated in causing chronic cough, such as chronic obstructive pulmonary disease, lung cancer, an inhaled foreign body, pulmonary tuberculosis, sarcoidosis, idiopathic pulmonary fibrosis, and heart failure, will be obvious on clinical assessment, spirometry, and chest radiography. Assessment and management of these conditions are dealt with elsewhere in this book. Thus, a majority of patients referred for investigation of chronic cough are nonsmokers with normal findings on physical examination and chest radiography. Most present with a nonproductive or minimally productive cough, and 60% to 75% are female. A recognized tendency is for cough to manifest initially around the time of menopause. The most common conditions implicated in aggravating or causing chronic cough in these patients are listed in Table 18-1.

Table 18-1 Common Conditions Implicated in Causing Chronic Cough

Diagnosis	Approximate Incidence (%)
Rhinitis	25-30
Asthma/eosinophilic bronchitis	20-25
Gastroesophageal reflux	15-20
Post-viral infection cough	5-10
Chronic bronchitis	5-10
Bronchiectasis	5-10
ACE inhibitor–induced cough	5-10
Unexplained	5-20

ACE, angiotensin-converting enzyme.

CLINICAL ASSESSMENT

An initial assessment of a patient with chronic cough is directed at finding a specific cause, assessing severity, and initiating trials of treatment. A careful history and physical examination are paramount in the evaluation of a patient with chronic cough (**Table 18-2**). Details of the factors surrounding the onset of

Table 18-2 Initial Evaluation of the Patient with Chronic Cough

Evaluation Component	Assessment Factors
History	Cough: onset, duration, character, triggers, laryngeal paresthesia Sputum: volume, character Smoking, occupation Upper respiratory tract infection Drug history (ACE inhibitors) Asthma: breathlessness, wheeze, nocturnal symptoms, atopy Gastroesophageal reflux: reflux-associated symptoms Rhinitis: postnasal drip, sinusitis, throat clearing, nasal congestion Adverse quality of life: musculoskeletal chest pains, incontinence, syncope, social embarrassment, anxiety, disturbed sleep Snoring
Examination	Clubbing External nasal: polyps External ears: excessive wax Oropharyngeal: signs of postnasal drip, tonsillar enlargement Chest: signs of airflow obstruction, crackles
Investigations	Chest radiograph Spirometry ± bronchodilator reversibility Serial peak expiratory flow Complete blood count and eosinophil differential cell count
Optional investigations	Bronchoprovocation challenge test, induced sputum, allergen skin tests Exhaled nitric oxide test Sinus radiography/sinus CT study 24-hour esophageal pH and manometry Chest CT/bronchoscopy in selected patients
Treatment for identified causes	Directed at cause(s)

ACE, angiotensin-converting enzyme; *CT*, computed tomography.

cough and associated symptoms and a careful assessment of the upper airways and the respiratory system are particularly important. Basic initial investigations should include up-to-date chest radiography, spirometry, and tests of bronchodilator reversibility, if appropriate. An abrupt onset of coughing while eating or chewing should raise the possibility of an inhaled foreign body, and the onset of cough shortly after introduction of angiotensin-converting enzyme (ACE) inhibitor therapy suggests ACE inhibitor associated cough. The presence of significant quantities of sputum, hemoptysis, systemic symptoms, prominent breathlessness, wheeze, or abnormal physical signs increases the probability of intrinsic lung disease and should trigger appropriate investigations, which may include a CT scan of the chest and bronchoscopy even in the absence of suggestive findings with more simple investigations. The onset of cough with symptoms suggesting an upper or lower respiratory tract infection raises the possibility of a postinfectious cough; prominent whoops, a very troublesome nocturnal cough, and cough associated with vomiting all are associated with pertussis, a condition that is increasingly recognized in both school-age children and adults. Otherwise, little evidence is available to suggest that information on the timing, nature, complications,

and potential aggravating factors is predictive of the underlying cause of the cough.

Findings on history and physical examination often are unremarkable, in which case the patient evaluation should focus on the recognition of corticosteroid-responsive conditions (i.e., asthma and eosinophilic bronchitis) and extrapulmonary factors that may be aggravating the cough, such as rhinitis and gastroesophageal reflux. One approach to the assessment of patients with chronic cough is outlined in **Figure 18-2**. The emphasis is on early recognition of corticosteroid-responsive cough, which can be detected easily in most cases with appropriate investigations or treatment trials. By contrast, the management of patients with nonasthmatic cough can be complex, time-consuming, and expensive, often with disappointing response to specific therapy. Far from clear, however, is whether extrapulmonary factors implicated in the pathogenesis of cough are aggravating a preexisting tendency or represent the underlying cause. Several factors point to the former, including the tendency for nonasthmatic chronic cough to affect middle-aged women and the frequent clinical observation that interventions against potential causes of chronic cough often help, but rarely cure the cough. It is best to have no preconceptions about the underlying causative factors in nonasthmatic cough and to view extrapulmonary factors such as rhinitis and gastroesophageal reflux as potential aggravating factors rather than as causes of the problem. This model has the advantage of providing a basis for the incomplete response to the treatment of these conditions seen in many patients; it also should stimulate research into the cause and treatment of the underlying heightened cough reflex sensitivity.

A further difficulty in evaluating patients with nonasthmatic chronic cough is the poor correlation between the presence of symptoms or abnormalities on investigation of the potential aggravating factor and the success of treatment directed against that factor. Thus, the diagnosis is secured largely by demonstrating clinical improvement as indicated by decrease in frequency or severity of cough after a suitable trial of treatment. Spontaneous improvement is common, and multiple potential aggravating factors typically are present; these factors add another layer of complexity to the clinical encounter. Results of treatment trials are more easily interpreted when combined with attempts to assess cough severity objectively before and after treatment. Suitable methods for such assessment include use of a simple cough visual analogue (with scores of 0 to 100 mm) (**Figure 18-3**), cough-specific health-related quality of life questionnaires, and evaluation of cough reflex sensitivity. A 15-mm change in visual analogue score, a 2-point change in Leicester Cough Questionnaire quality of life score, and a 2–doubling dose change in C2 (concentration of capsaicin that causes 2 coughs) can be regarded as evidence of a significant response to treatment. The remainder of this section focuses on the evaluation of the commoner conditions implicated in causing chronic cough.

COUGH VARIANT ASTHMA/EOSINOPHILIC BRONCHITIS

Asthma is a condition characterized by airway hyperresponsiveness and inflammation that manifests with variable symptoms of cough, dyspnea, and wheeze. A subgroup of patients can present with an isolated chronic cough known as *cough variant asthma*. Heightened cough reflex sensitivity is a common finding in cough variant asthma but not in non–cough-predominant asthma. The airway inflammation in cough variant asthma is essentially similar to that seen in classic

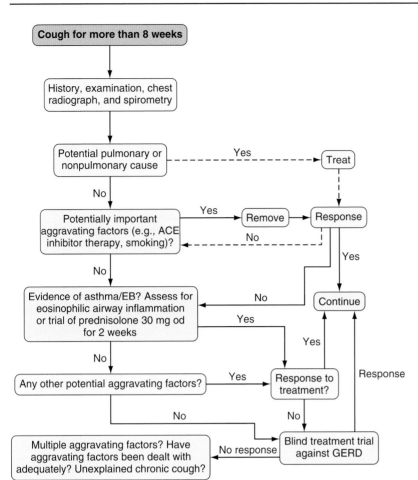

Figure 18-2   Diagnostic algorithm for investigation of chronic cough. *ACE,* angiotensin-converting enzyme; *EB,* eosinophilic bronchitis; *GERD,* gastroesophageal reflux disease.

Flowchart labels:

Cough for more than 8 weeks

History, examination, chest radiograph, and spirometry

Potential pulmonary or nonpulmonary cause — Yes → Treat

No

Potentially important aggravating factors (e.g., ACE inhibitor therapy, smoking)? — Yes → Remove → Response

No

Evidence of asthma/EB? Assess for eosinophilic airway inflammation or trial of prednisolone 30 mg od for 2 weeks

No

Any other potential aggravating factors? — Yes → Response to treatment?

No

Multiple aggravating factors? Have aggravating factors been dealt with adequately? Unexplained chronic cough? — No response → Blind treatment trial against GERD

Continue

asthma. The cough typically is dry or minimally productive; it may occur nocturnally, or after exercise or allergen and occupational exposure, although clinical clues often are lacking. The key to diagnosing asthma is demonstrating variable airflow obstruction. Serial peak flow recordings and spirometry with bronchodilator response are routine first-line investigations, but findings often are normal in cough variant asthma. Demonstration of airway hyperresponsiveness by bronchoprovocation testing is a more sensitive and specific index of variable airflow obstruction, and the hyperresponsiveness may be the only abnormality found. Blood or sputum eosinophilia, a raised exhaled nitric oxide concentration, the presence of atopy, and a positive result on allergen skin prick testing or allergen-specific IgE assay provide supportive evidence for the presence of asthma.

The diagnosis of so-called cough variant asthma usually is confirmed by observation of clinical improvement with therapy. Although originally described as manifesting with a bronchodilator-responsive cough, cough variant asthma is much more commonly associated with a corticosteroid-responsive cough, and inhaled corticosteroids are the mainstay of treatment. A blood eosinophil count above 0.4×10^9/L, a sputum eosinophil count more than 3%, and an exhaled nitric oxide concentration above 50 parts per billion (ppb) at an exhalation flow of 50 L/minute are strongly associated with a positive response to corticosteroid therapy in patients with cough. These tests are arguably more fruitful and clinically informative than tests of airway dysfunction. A 2-week trial of oral corticosteroids may be a useful alternative if these tests are unavailable.

Eosinophilic bronchitis is an increasingly recognized entity that presents with a corticosteroid responsive cough and is characterized by sputum eosinophilia (**Figure 18-4**), heightened cough reflex sensitivity, but no evidence of variable airflow obstruction or airway hyperresponsiveness. Most patients also have a raised exhaled nitric oxide concentration, and blood eosinophilia often is present. Studies suggest that eosinophilic bronchitis is responsible for 10% to 15% of cases of chronic cough. The airway inflammation is similar to that seen in asthma although available evidence indicates that differences in the pattern of airway dysfunction are due to differences in the site of mast cell localization within the airway, with infiltration of the epithelium occurring in eosinophilic bronchitis and infiltration of the airway wall smooth muscle occurring in asthma. Recognition of eosinophilic bronchitis is important, because like cough variant asthma, it responds well to inhaled corticosteroids. This is best achieved by assessing airway inflammation using induced sputum or exhaled nitric oxide; if these techniques are not available, a trial of corticosteroid therapy is indicated irrespective of the presence of airway hyperresponsiveness.

ANGIOTENSIN-CONVERTING ENZYME INHIBITOR-ASSOCIATED COUGH

ACE inhibitors increase cough reflex sensitivity and cough frequency in patients and healthy research volunteers. Around 8% of patients develop a persistent troublesome cough. This is a class effect that is not obviously dose-related. The cough often is triggered by a viral upper respiratory tract infection or an obvious environmental insult, but it persists long after these stimuli are removed. Thus, there may not be a close temporal relationship between starting treatment and the onset of cough. ACE inhibitor–associated cough occurs more commonly in

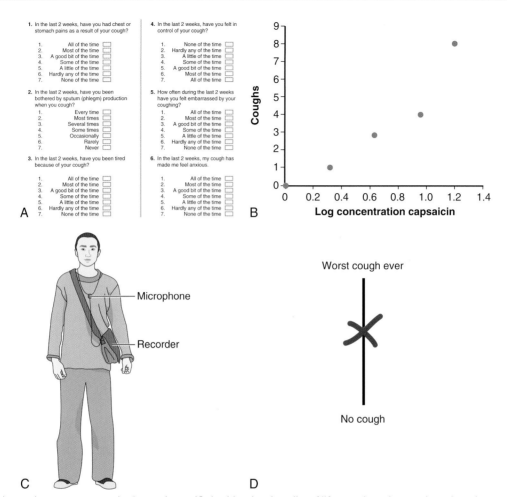

Figure 18-3 Cough severity assessment tools: **A,** cough-specific health-related quality of life questionnaires, such as the Leicester Cough Questionnaire; **B,** cough reflex sensitivity measurement; **C,** 24-hour ambulatory automated cough frequency monitoring; and **D,** 100-mm cough visual analogue scale.

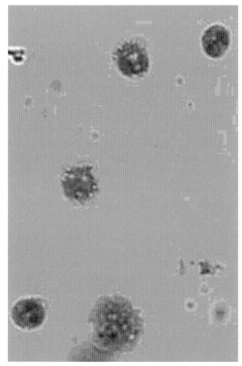

Figure 18-4 Sputum eosinophilia in eosinophilic bronchitis. Eosinophils are the cells with cytoplasmic granules stained *red*.

females and in patients of South East Asian ancestry. Excess cough is not seen with use of ACE receptor antagonists. Increased airway concentrations of antitussive mediators such as bradykinins and prostaglandins are thought to be responsible for heightened cough reflex sensitivity and increased cough in patients with ACE inhibitor cough. The cough usually resolves within 2 months of withdrawal. Persistence may suggest asthma, the onset of which has been linked to the use of ACE inhibitors.

COUGH DUE TO UPPER AIRWAY DISEASE

Rhinitis, often associated with sinusitis and postnasal drip, is one of the most common conditions implicated as an aggravating factor in chronic cough. Allergy and infection are common causes of rhinitis and are thought to result in cough by mechanical stimulation from a postnasal drip and extension of local inflammation to the pharyngeal and laryngeal area where the cough receptors are most concentrated. Patients may report nasal congestion, nasal discharge, and facial pain; they may be aware of a postnasal drip and the frequent need to clear the throat. Careful examination of upper airways may reveal a nasal quality to the voice, nasal polyps, sinus tenderness, and inflammation of the posterior pharyngeal wall, with evidence of draining secretions. Investigations for rhinitis include nasal endoscopy and radiography or CT scan of the sinuses, which may reveal mucosal thickening and fluid levels.

A causal link between upper airway inflammation and cough has not been clearly established. No evidence has established that upper airway symptoms are more common in patients with chronic cough than in control subjects, or that specific findings on investigations are predictive of successful resolution of cough developing after treatment directed against rhinitis, nor is there good-quality evidence from double blind studies that interventions against rhinitis are associated with a reduction in cough frequency in a general cough population. Thus, rhinitis may represent an epiphenomenon not directly causally linked to cough.

Other upper airway conditions including viral upper respiratory tract infection, chronic tonsillar enlargement, disease of the external auditory canal, obstructive sleep apnea, and chronic snoring have been associated with chronic cough, supporting the concept that structural and inflammatory conditions of the upper airway disease can aggravate coughing. Therefore, it seems reasonable to suppose that structural abnormalities and chronic inflammation of the upper airway are potential albeit unproven aggravating factors for chronic cough, and to offer appropriate treatment in patients with suggestive symptoms or clinical findings.

GASTROESOPHAGEAL REFLUX–ASSOCIATED COUGH

Signs and symptoms suggesting gastroesophageal reflux and abnormalities of esophageal function are common in patients with chronic cough, and effective treatment of gastroesophageal reflux has been associated with decreased frequency and severity of cough, supporting a causal association. Potential mechanisms include microaspiration of esophageal contents to the tracheobronchial tree and stimulation of a neural esophageal-tracheobronchial reflex. Gastroesophageal reflux is associated with the relaxation of the lower esophageal sphincter and often occurs during eating and talking and on waking; also of note, many patients with chronic cough report increased cough during these activities. The presence of symptoms such as heartburn, dysphagia, sore throat, globus, and dysphonia may not be a good guide to the success of antireflux treatment, because some evidence suggests that cough can be the sole clinical manifestation of gastroesophageal reflux in up to 75% of patients.

Many of the aforementioned problems with cough due to rhinitis also apply for cough associated with gastroesophageal reflux. Good evidence indicates that reflux symptoms and abnormalities of esophageal function occur more commonly in patients with cough than control subjects, but this is also the case for other airway diseases such as asthma and chronic obstructive pulmonary disease (COPD), so it is difficult to make a case for a specific link between cough and gastroesophageal reflux. Moreover, it has not been possible to identify particular features on investigation that are predictive of the success of treatment directed against gastroesophageal reflux, and randomized trials of acid suppression therapy in gastroesophageal reflux associated cough have been disappointing. Potentially the link between reflux and cough is more dependent on the volume of reflux than on acid reflux, and therapeutic strategies that reduce reflux volume by addressing gastro-esophageal sphincter function may be more effective. Another possibility, however, is that the occurrence of excess gastroesophageal reflux in cough is a function of coughing itself, or else a manifestation of a global abnormality of upper aerodigestive reflexes, with no direct causal link between one and the other. The current state of knowledge is such that a reasonable approach is to offer a trial of treatment with acid suppression therapy with a proton pump inhibitor and an alginate for 2 to 3 months in patients with otherwise unexplained cough even when there are no suggestive upper gastrointestinal symptoms. More work is needed before more invasive treatments with a potentially greater effect on the volume of reflux, such as Nissen fundoplication, can be recommended in patients with suspected gastroesophageal reflux–associated cough if the sole motive is to relieve cough.

OTHER CAUSES OF COUGH

Community surveys suggest that most coughs related to upper respiratory tract infections resolve within 3 weeks. In such instances, however, the cough can take several months to resolve in a small proportion of subjects. The infection in most cases remains unidentified, but respiratory viruses, *Mycoplasma pneumoniae*, *Chlamydia pneumoniae*, basidiomycetous fungi, and *Bordetella pertussis* have been implicated in adults. Chronic bronchitis is a common cause of cough in smokers and may occur in nonsmokers with dusty occupations or living in polluted environments. These patients typically have a productive morning cough. Other conditions reported to be associated with isolated chronic cough include Holmes-Adie syndrome, premature ventricular complexes, and familial peripheral neuropathy.

Diffuse panbronchiolitis is a well-recognized cause of corticosteroid-resistant adult-onset chronic productive cough in Japan and other parts of Southeast Asia. This is an important diagnosis to consider, because treatment with low-dose macrolide antibiotics is associated with a striking improvement that appears to be independent of the antimicrobial effects of these drugs. Patients with diffuse panbronchiolitis typically exhibit sinusitis and prominent small airway changes on imaging studies. Significant airflow obstruction and respiratory failure can occur. Whether less clinically overt cases occur in a general cough population is unclear, but this is certainly a possibility.

FURTHER INVESTIGATIONS

The use of fiberoptic bronchoscopy and high-resolution CT scanning should be reserved for evaluation of patients suspected of inhaling a foreign body; for those with suggestive symptoms, signs, or chest radiograph findings; and for patients with no objective evidence of more common causes of cough, because the investigations are invasive and expensive, with low diagnostic yield. Cough reflex sensitivity measurement has limited value in the validation of the presence of chronic cough in clinical practice because of the wide overlap of cough sensitivity between health and respiratory disease causing cough. Ambulatory cough monitors have the advantage of providing objective evidence of the presence and frequency of cough, but their routine use is hampered by automation difficulty of analysis of the recordings. Recent advances in recording devices and improved battery life have led to a renewed interest in cough monitor development, and they should be available for clinical use in the near future.

TREATMENT

Treatment directed at the specific cause of chronic cough is summarized in **Table 18-3**. With use of the anatomic diagnostic protocol, success rates of up to 95% in the management of chronic cough have been reported. The success rate goes down to 60% to 80% in specialist cough clinics, possibly owing to the

Table 18-3 Specific Therapy for Chronic Cough

Cause	Treatment
Rhinitis	Nasal corticosteroids Selected patients: topical ipratropium, topical decongestants, oral antihistamines, surgery
Asthma	Inhaled corticosteroids Leukotriene antagonists
Eosinophilic bronchitis	Inhaled corticosteroids, oral corticosteroids in selected cases
GER-associated cough	Self-help measures: weight loss, smoking cessation, reduce alcohol intake, elevate head of bed, avoid eating within 2 hours of bedtime Acid suppression: proton pump inhibitors Prokinetic agents: metoclopramide or domperidone in selected patients Surgery: laparoscopic fundoplication in selected patients
Chronic bronchitis	Smoking cessation
ACE cough	Drug withdrawal; substitution of alternative if appropriate
Post-viral infection cough	Observation
Bronchiectasis	Chest physiotherapy and postural drainage, antibiotics
Idiopathic chronic cough	Antitussives (dextromethorphan, codeine); nebulized lidocaine; speech and language therapy or physiotherapy

ACE, angiotensin-converting enzyme; *GER*, gastroesophageal reflux.

complexity of cases referred. Reassessment of the patient after treatment with exclusion of additional aggravating factors or causes forms an integral part of management for chronic cough. A common dilemma faced by physicians managing these patients is that the diagnosis of cough often depends on successful trials of treatment, which if unsuccessful leads to the difficult question of whether the underlying condition has not responded or is not responsible for the cough. In some situations, the use of objective tests to make a diagnosis and careful validation of the effect of therapy for the underlying condition should minimize this problem. Therapeutic interventions for common causes of chronic cough are discussed next.

COUGH VARIANT ASTHMA/EOSINOPHILIC BRONCHITIS

Cough due to asthma responds well to inhaled corticosteroids. A response typically occurs within 1 to 2 weeks of starting therapy and reaches a maximum after 8 to 10 weeks. Leukotriene antagonists also are helpful in cough variant asthma. The duration of asthma therapy remains unclear, but return of the cough on gradual withdrawal of therapy suggests the need for long-term therapy. Patients with cough variant asthma often have coexisting rhinitis or postnasal drip, and a complete response may not be seen until all potential aggravating factors are treated. Treatment of cough due to eosinophilic bronchitis is with inhaled corticosteroids. Rarely, oral corticosteroids are required to suppress eosinophilic airway inflammation and cough.

RHINITIS

Topical corticosteroids are the mainstay of treatment for cough due to rhinitis. Antihistamines, particularly first-generation agents, are frequently used. When nasal obstruction is prominent, initial additional treatment with topical decongestant sprays may be necessary, and antibiotics should be administered if infection is suspected. Topical ipratropium bromide often is helpful if rhinorrhea is prominent, and antihistamines are useful when sneeze and nasal itch are prominent and in cases with coexisting atopy. Surgical treatment may be necessary to correct obvious anatomic abnormalities.

GASTROESOPHAGEAL REFLUX-ASSOCIATED COUGH

Gastroesophageal reflux–associated cough is managed with self-help measures such as weight reduction, avoidance of tight clothing, elevation of headrest during sleep, reduced alcohol and tobacco intake, and drug therapy for acid suppression. Use of proton pump inhibitors is the most effective treatment for heartburn associated with gastroesophageal reflux, but the effect of these agents in cough thought to be associated with reflux has been mixed. Anecdotal evidence suggests that high-dose therapy for at least 3 months often is required before clinical improvement is seen. In patients who appear to respond to proton pump inhibitors, confirmation of a link between cough and gastroesophageal reflux may be sought by withdrawal and rechallenge. Prokinetic agents such as metoclopramide and domperidone may have a role in some cases. The role of antireflux surgery is unclear.

ANTITUSSIVE THERAPIES

Treatments directed against potential aggravating factors often do not achieve perfect results, and antitussive therapies that target the heightened cough reflex directly are needed as well. Codeine and the non-narcotic antitussive dextromethorphan have been demonstrated to have some effect on cough associated with upper respiratory tract infections, although the effect on cough frequency is small and of uncertain clinical relevance. The use of morphine and diamorphine has been restricted to patients with the severe cough of malignant disease, which often is associated with pain and distress. Lidocaine delivered by aerosol or nebulizer has been used to treat chronic cough, although good evidence of the efficacy and safety of this approach is lacking.

A recent study has shown clinical improvement in patients with chronic cough in a randomized placebo-controlled trial of a speech therapy intervention; similar benefits have been shown with an outpatient physiotherapy approach. The key components of these interventions are unclear, but an important component of the latter approach is training in voluntary cough suppression, suggesting that excess coughing may be partly due to the continuation of a vicious circle whereby coughing leads to airway trauma and activation of the cough reflex.

There are no other well-established antitussive agents, and the value of much of the existing work evaluating the pharmacologic manipulation of the cough reflex is limited, because it has been carried out in animal models that are poorly predictive of effects in humans. Moreover, those agents that have been investigated in humans have been tested against models of questionable relevance for the at-need population. Early evidence points to a role for drugs that modulate nerves, such as amitriptyline and gabapentin, but further investigation is necessary. More relevant basic science is needed, and there is an urgent need for better treatments and clinical trials.

UNEXPLAINED CHRONIC COUGH

Cough remains unexplained after extensive investigations and treatment trials in up to 40% of patients. These patients are predominantly middle-aged females with objective evidence of airway abnormalities, including increased cough reflex sensitivity and airway inflammation. Organ-specific autoimmune diseases are common, suggesting that the airway abnormalities may have an autoimmune basis.

Unexplained cough is responsible for considerable physical and psychological morbidity. Many patients with unexplained chronic cough are labeled with a diagnosis of psychogenic cough, although little evidence is available to support this view, and it is perhaps more likely that any abnormal illness behavior is secondary to the adverse impact of cough on psychosocial aspects of quality of life. In evaluating a patient with unexplained cough, it is important to recognize common pitfalls in managing chronic cough (**Box 18-2**). Therapy for idiopathic chronic cough is disappointing, and there is therefore a large unmet need for better antitussive treatment in these patients. Referral to a respiratory physiotherapist or speech therapist for cough management coaching may be of some help.

CONCLUSION

All pulmonary and many nonpulmonary conditions can manifest with cough. Most will be evident after a simple clinical assessment that includes a careful history, physical examination, plain chest radiography, and spirometry. Cough that remains unexplained after such an assessment is a common reason for referral to a specialist. Potential causes include asthma, eosinophilic bronchitis, rhinitis, and gastroesophageal reflux. Satisfactory outcomes can be achieved in a majority of patients with a management strategy that includes targeted investigations and carefully controlled treatment trials. Complete cure is not always possible, however, particularly in patients with cough thought to be due to extrapulmonary factors, and a significant minority of predominantly middle-aged women have unexplained chronic cough. Whether this reflects failure to identify important causes or represents inadequate treatment of established factors is unclear.

WEB RESOURCES

American College of Chest Physicians: http://chestjournal.chestpubs.org/content/129/1_suppl/1S.full (*cough guideline summary*).
British Thoracic Society: http://www.britthoracic.org.uk/Portals/0/Clinical%20Information/Cough/Guidelines/coughguidelines august06.pdf (*cough guidelines*).
International Society for the Study of Cough: http://www.issc.info.

SUGGESTED READINGS

Birring SS: Controversies in the evaluation and management of chronic cough, *Am J Respir Crit Care Med* 183:708–715, 2011.

Birring SS, Berry M, Brightling CE, Pavord ID: Eosinophilic bronchitis: clinical features, management and pathogenesis, *Am J Respir Med* 2:169–173, 2003.

Birring SS, Brightling CE, Symon FA, et al: Idiopathic chronic cough: association with organ specific autoimmune disease and bronchoalveolar lymphocytosis, *Thorax* 58:1066–1071, 2003.

Birring SS, Prudon B, Carr AJ, et al: Development of symptom specific health status measure for patients with chronic cough: Leicester Cough Questionnaire (LCQ), *Thorax* 58:339–343, 2003.

Chung KF, Pavord ID: Prevalence, pathogenesis and causes of chronic cough, *Lancet* 371:1364–1374, 2008.

Irwin RS, Baumann MH, Bolser DC, et al: Diagnosis and management of cough executive summary: ACCP evidence-based clinical practice guidelines, *Chest* 129(1 Suppl):1S–23S, 2006.

Irwin RS, Madison JM: The diagnosis and treatment of cough, *N Engl J Med* 343:1715–1721, 2000.

Morice AH, Fontana GA, Belvisi MG, et al: ERS guidelines on the assessment of cough, *Eur Respir J* 29:1256–1276, 2007.

Morice AH, McGarvey L, Pavord I, for the British Thoracic Society Cough Guideline Group: Recommendations for the management of cough in adults, *Thorax* 61(Suppl 1):i1–i24, 2006.

Pavord ID, Chung KF: Management of chronic cough, *Lancet* 371:1375–1384, 2008.

Chapter **19**
Dyspnea
Alex H. Gifford • Donald A. Mahler

WHAT IS DYSPNEA?

In healthy people, breathing is an unconscious activity that is regulated by automatic command by groups of neurons in the brain stem to control cyclic contraction and relaxation of the respiratory muscles. With a perturbation of this process, the affected person may experience breathing difficulty or discomfort. This sensation is considered a symptom and typically is referred to as *dyspnea*, which literally means "disordered breathing" (*dys-* + *-pnea*). In 1999, the American Thoracic Society defined dyspnea as "a subjective experience of breathing discomfort that consists of qualitatively distinct sensations that vary in intensity." Patients typically cite such discomfort when describing their symptoms: "I am short of breath." "I can't get enough air." "It's hard to breathe."

A majority of studies investigating dyspnea have focused on patients with chronic obstructive pulmonary disease (COPD), for two reasons: (1) COPD is the most prevalent respiratory disease, and (2) exertional breathlessness is the major symptom of this condition. Thus, the accumulated knowledge of clinical features of dyspnea and current understanding of the relevant mechanisms and qualities derive in large part from studies involving patients with COPD.

An interesting point is that dyspnea shares many features with pain. Both symptoms are complex neurophysiologic processes that are influenced by physiologic, psychologic, social, and environmental factors. These sensations function as warning signals of potential harm that usually lead the affected individual to reduce activities in order to minimize the complaint and/or to seek medical attention. Like pain, dyspnea can be perceived only by the affected person and has both sensory (how bad is it?) and affective (how does it feel?) components. Because both dyspnea and pain are under behavioral control, any emotional state may worsen these experiences to a degree that may be out of proportion to the magnitude of physiologic impairment. For example, high levels of anxiety and panic attacks are associated with increased breathlessness and more intense pain.

Dyspnea is an important problem in the elderly population, often with a major impact on quality of life. It is estimated that more than 30% of those 65 years of age or older without known cardiorespiratory disease report breathlessness with various activities of daily living, including walking on a level surface or up an incline. An analysis of 124 patients over 70 years of age who were randomly selected from a large family medicine practice revealed that up to 37% had moderate to severe dyspnea, and that dyspnea was associated with poor perceived health, more anxiety and depression, and impaired daily functioning. With any physical activity, including exercise, older people exhibit higher levels of ventilation than those typical for younger persons performing the same amount of physical work. Not clear, however, is whether this increased ventilatory demand in older people is a direct result of the aging process in the respiratory system (secondary to a decrease in lung elasticity, increase in chest wall stiffness, and decrease in respiratory muscle strength) or a consequence of sedentary life style, deconditioning, and possible weight gain, which frequently occur with advancing age in populations of developed countries.

Gender differences in the prevalence and severity of dyspnea among patients with COPD have been documented. For example, women are more likely to report severe dyspnea compared with men despite significantly fewer pack-years of smoking cigarettes and similar frequencies of coughing. In the National Emphysema Treatment Trial involving 1053 patients with severe COPD (emphysema phenotype), women reported greater dyspnea than that described by men when findings were controlled for lung function, age, pack-years of smoking, and proportion of the lung affected by emphysema. Whether this gender difference in dyspnea relates to physiologic differences (compared with men, women have smaller airway lumina, with disproportionately thicker airway walls) is uncertain.

MECHANISMS OF DYSPNEA

The neurophysiologic pathways that mediate the control of breathing (to supply oxygen, to eliminate carbon dioxide, and to maintain acid-base balance) also are relevant to the mechanisms of dyspnea (**Figure 19-1**). In simple terms, nerve fibers (sensory receptors) send electrical signals (afferent impulses) to the spinal cord, which in turn transmits these signals to the brain.

The brain interprets these signals as a sensation (dyspnea). Outgoing commands from the brain may then elicit an appropriate response—the affected person may stop the offending activity, for example, or may use a rescue inhaler in an attempt to relieve the breathing difficulty.

Presented next is an overview of the neurophysiology of dyspnea, with details of the important components of the relevant pathways.

SENSORY RECEPTORS

Activation of sensory receptors provides afferent information to several brain areas that are perceived as respiratory sensations. Blood gas abnormalities (hypoxemia and hypercapnia), mechanical respiratory loads (increased airway resistance and elastance), disturbances in airway epithelium (e.g., edema,

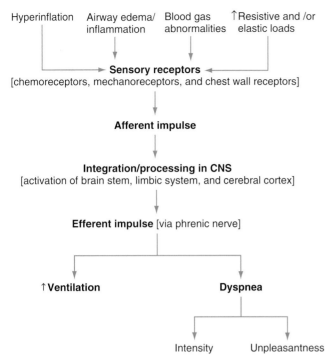

Figure 19-1 Neurophysiologic basis of dyspnea. *CNS*, central nervous system.

inflammation), and hyperinflation are stimuli that activate sensory receptors. For example, neurons in the carotid bodies (peripheral chemoreceptors) are more sensitive to arterial hypoxemia than are neurons in the aortic bodies, although both contribute to hypoxemic ventilatory responsiveness. Central chemoreceptors located in the ventral medulla respond to changes in bloodstream H^+-CO_2 equilibrium.

Mechanoreceptors are distributed throughout the lung and the chest wall. Parenchymal stretch receptors transmit information about airway caliber and lung volume to the somatosensory cortex through unmyelinated vagal nerve fibers. C-fibers relay information about airway irritation, which can be demonstrated using various chemical mediators. J-fibers are stimulated by interstitial pressure increases, especially pulmonary edema. The chest wall muscles are innervated by Golgi tendon organs and spindle fibers that project to anterior horn cells of spinal neurons. These structures transduce information on length-tension and spatial relationships to the somatosensory cortex.

AFFERENT IMPULSES

Afferent information from sensory receptors are transmitted to brain stem respiratory centers that automatically adjust breathing and also may project to higher brain areas for direct assessment of the status of various stimuli. Well-characterized examples include the following: The glossopharyngeal nerve transmits impulses for peripheral chemoreceptors; the vagus nerve transmits information for rapidly adapting, slowly adapting, and C-fiber lung mechanoreceptors; and cervical spinal nerves 3 to 5 (C3 to C5) transmit sensory information accrued by mechanoreceptors from the diaphragm.

Two different pathways have been proposed to process respiratory sensations to the cerebral cortex. One pathway reflects *discriminative processing*—that is, awareness of the spatial, temporal, and intensity components (e.g., how bad is it?). With activation of respiratory muscle receptors, afferent information is relayed into the brain stem medulla and is then

projected to the ventroposterior thalamus area; from here, projections ascend to the primary and secondary somatosensory cortex. These structures are thought to process the intensity component of dyspnea.

A second pathway reflects *affective processing* (e.g., how does it feel?). With activation of airway and lung receptors, afferent information is relayed by the vagal nerve to the brain stem medulla and is then projected to the amygdala and medial dorsal areas of the thalamus; from here, projections ascend to the insular and cingulate cortex. These structures are part of the limbic system, which forms the inner border of the cortex and contains rich interconnections among the cerebral cortex, thalamus, and brain stem, and are thought to process the affective component of dyspnea.

CENTRAL NERVOUS SYSTEM

The central nervous system integrates and processes the sensory information into a combined output carried by the phrenic nerve to the respiratory muscles. Neuroimaging studies demonstrate that the anterior cingulate cortex, amygdala, and thalamus are consistently activated in response to various respiratory perturbations. Activation of cortical neural processes appears to require a gating mechanism that can receive changes in respiratory afferent neural activity and distribute this sensory information to specific cortical areas for cognitive processing. It is believed that the thalamus and hippocampus are critical neural areas for the gating of respiratory sensory input to the cerebral cortex.

The experience of dyspnea is thought to result from a mismatch between incoming afferent information (from one or more activated sensory receptors) and the outgoing central respiratory motor activity.

NEUROMODULATION BY ENDOGENOUS OPIOIDS

Endogenous opioids and their receptors are expressed broadly throughout the peripheral and central nervous systems, as well as the respiratory system. Beta-endorphins are one of five groups of naturally occurring opioid peptides that modulate pain and dyspnea. In response to noxious and stressful stimuli, the pituitary gland releases beta-endorphins into the circulation, whereas the brain elaborates endogenous opioids into the cerebrospinal fluid.

Naloxone, an opioid antagonist that readily crosses the blood-brain barrier, has been used to uncover the putative effects of endogenous opioids on modulating dyspnea. Studies using methacholine-induced bronchoconstriction, high-intensity treadmill exercise, and inspiratory resistive breathing (as stimuli to provoke breathlessness) have shown that patients with asthma or COPD report higher ratings of dyspnea after receiving naloxone than after receiving normal saline. These observations support the role of endogenous opioids as neuromodulators of the perception of dyspnea.

THE LANGUAGE OF DYSPNEA

To help dyspneic patients describe their experience more accurately, questionnaires have been developed that allow for the selection of specific descriptors of breathlessness. It appears that the descriptors selected by patients relate in part to the underlying mechanisms contributing to dyspnea. For example, *chest tightness* is relatively specific to bronchoconstriction in patients with asthma but is not typically reported by patients

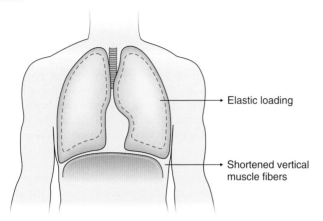

Figure 19-2 Mechanical consequences of dynamic hyperinflation.

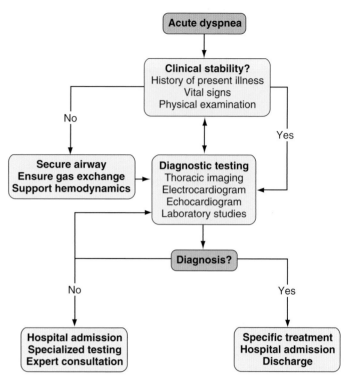

Figure 19-3 Initial evaluation of acute dyspnea.

with COPD. This perception of tightness presumably is due to activation of sensory receptors located in large airways and can be relieved with use of bronchodilator therapy.

The sense of respiratory *work* or *effort* commonly is reported by patients with various conditions including asthma, COPD, interstitial lung disease, and neuromuscular disease. The descriptor "work/effort" of breathing difficulty probably is related to activation of respiratory muscle afferents imposed by mechanical loads (airway narrowing → added resistance; parenchymal edema/infiltrates → added elastance) imposed by certain diseases as well as respiratory muscle weakness. For example, in patients with COPD, the lungs typically hyperinflate during the performance of physical tasks. This dynamic hyperinflation results in two major consequences that contribute to dyspnea: (1) an added elastic load and (2) functional weakening of the diaphragm by shortening of the vertical muscle fibers (**Figure 19-2**). Although patients with acute asthma initially may experience chest tightness, they typically report that the increased work or effort of breathing develops as airway narrowing progresses as a result of subsequent lung hyperinflation.

A perception of not being able to take in enough air has been described as *air hunger*, or "unsatisfied inspiration." This experience is not specific to any particular disease or stimulus. A consistent finding is that patients with various cardiorespiratory conditions generally report greater breathing difficulty during inspiration than with expiration. A clustering of reported sensations such as smothering, suffocating, and air hunger has been documented in patients with panic disorder and idiopathic hyperventilation syndrome who do not have any cardiopulmonary or neuromuscular disease. These findings are consistent with an increase in ventilatory drive.

The three qualities of dyspneic sensations, as described, do not explain all clinical features of breathlessness. Moreover, multiple pathways may combine to contribute to dyspnea in an individual patient. For example, in a patient with cardiogenic pulmonary edema, bilateral pleural effusions, cardiac cachexia, and arterial hypoxemia, dyspnea may be due to activation of carotid body neurons (hypoxemia), stretch receptors (interstitial edema), and Golgi tendon organs and spindle fibers (muscle weakness).

ACUTE DYSPNEA

INITIAL EVALUATION

The rapidity with which dyspnea develops is clinically important. Although a standard definition of acute dyspnea does not exist, potentially life-threatening cardiopulmonary processes often are heralded by unprecedented, severe dyspnea minutes to hours in duration. Whenever possible, details should be sought about the circumstances under which dyspnea began, whether it is associated with other symptoms, and how it has progressed. Knowledge of medications and comorbid conditions also is helpful. Dyspnea in the prehospital environment independently predicts a nearly seven-fold likelihood of hospital admission from the emergency department. Studies have shown that delays in seeking clinical attention for acute exacerbations of asthma, COPD, and congestive heart failure (CHF) are associated with a higher frequency of hospital admissions and worse outcomes.

With any clinical encounter, the focus of the initial assessment is on whether or not the patient is stable (**Figure 19-3**). If this evaluation reveals evidence of hemodynamic insult or lability, hypotension may need to be treated promptly with intravenous fluids, vasopressors, and/or vasodilators. Airway patency and adequacy may be threatened by a depressed level of consciousness, aspiration, or trauma. Endotracheal intubation may become necessary in such instances and when gas exchange derangements cannot be rectified by supplemental oxygen or noninvasive positive-pressure ventilation. Once these basic support elements are addressed, diagnostic testing can safely proceed.

DIFFERENTIAL DIAGNOSIS

One approach to the differential diagnosis for acute dyspnea is to consider how processes in certain anatomic regions contribute to this symptom (**Table 19-1**). Obstruction is the most common mechanism for dyspnea arising from upper airway problems. Stridor, a variably high-pitched, harsh inspiratory noise caused by turbulent airflow, often can be heard in the context of an aspirated foreign body and edema of the epiglottis and laryngeal soft tissues. Prompt evaluation and management of upper airway blockage are critical, because the airway is

Table 19-1 **Differential Diagnosis of Acute Dyspnea**

Anatomic Region/ Structure	Relevant Pathologic Process(es)	Related Signs/Symptoms	Physical Findings
Upper airway	Obstruction	Impaired phonation Cough Wheeze	Commonly child or infant Cyanosis Altered mental status Stridor
	Anaphylaxis/angioedema	Pruritus Flushing Throat/chest tightness Cough Nausea	Facial swelling Urticaria Stridor Hypotension Wheeze on auscultation
	Epiglottitis (E) Peritonsillar abscess (PTA) Retropharyngeal abscess (RPA)	Sore throat (E/PTA/RPA) Fever (E/PTA/RPA) Altered voice (E/PTA/RPA) Cervicalgia (RPA) Dysphagia (E/PTA/RPA)	Stridor (E) Drooling (E) Tripod posture (E) Fever (E/PTA/RPA) Uvula deviation (PTA) Trismus (PTA/RPA)
Lungs	Asthma exacerbation	Chest tightness Cough Wheeze	Wheeze on auscultation Prolonged expiratory phase Accessory muscle use
	COPD exacerbation	Increased cough frequency Wheeze Change in sputum production	Wheeze on auscultation Pursed-lip breathing Barrel chest Cyanosis
	Pulmonary embolism	Lateral chest pain Presyncope/syncope Palpitations Hemoptysis	Hypoxemia Hypotension Asymmetric extremity size
	Pneumonia	Cough ± sputum production Fever ± chills Pleurisy Hemoptysis	Altered mental status Rales on auscultation Sepsis
	Pneumothorax	Chest pain (anterior/superior) Anxiety	Tachypnea Hypotension Distant breath sounds
Heart	Congestive heart failure	Paroxysmal nocturnal dyspnea Orthopnea Weight gain Wheeze	Jugular venous distention Crackles on auscultation S3 gallop Lower extremity edema
	Acute coronary syndrome	Chest pain ± arm radiation Diaphoresis Nausea ± emesis	Hemodynamic instability S4 gallop Hypoxemia
Muscles	Acute idiopathic demyelinating polyneuropathy	Acral paresthesias Progressive global weakness Dysphagia	Autonomic dysregulation Symmetric weakness Areflexia
Other	Hyperventilation syndrome	Chest discomfort Complaint of "can't get enough air in"	Frequently normal findings on examination

endangered. Exacerbations of asthma and COPD typically are manifested as bronchospasm, wheeze, and cough. Sputum production is common to exacerbations of COPD associated with acute bronchitis and pneumonia, but its physical characteristics alone are not useful in predicting a causative pathogen. Pleuritic chest pain is sharp, incisive, breath-taking discomfort caused by irritation of the parietal pleural nerve supply along the thoracic cavity. This type of pain can accompany pulmonary embolism, pneumonia with or without pleural effusion, and pneumothorax.

In an acute coronary syndrome (ACS) or CHF, dyspnea is caused by pulmonary venous hypertension and interstitial fluid accumulation. Sudden dyspnea without chest discomfort is the presenting feature of myocardial infarction in 4% to 14% of events. Papillary muscle rupture with mitral valve incompetence, florid pulmonary edema, and shock complicates myocardial infarction in approximately 7% of affected patients. Neuromuscular diseases more commonly cause chronic, progressive dyspnea, but ventilatory failure can develop over just a few hours in acute idiopathic demyelinating polyneuropathy

(AIDP). Dyspnea is a frequent consequence of severe abdominal distention, such as that seen with bowel obstruction. The increased pressure of the abdominal cavity restricts diaphragm excursion, thereby decreasing functional residual capacity. Abdominal pain restricts ventilation as a consequence of muscle splinting, which also can cause atelectasis.

PHYSICAL EXAMINATION

Inspection of the patient in respiratory distress may be quite revealing. Stigmata of adrenergic excess commonly are present, including hypervigilance, diaphoresis, and tachycardia. The breathing pattern frequently is rapid and shallow, which foreshortens responses to clinical questioning. An exception is the deep and sometimes bradypneic pattern of Kussmaul respirations seen with severe metabolic acidosis, typical of diabetic ketoacidosis. Engagement of accessory inspiratory muscles (e.g., scalenes, intercostals, and sternocleidomastoids) often signals respiratory failure. This finding alone is associated with a nearly three-fold risk of death and a roughly doubled requirement for posthospital care in patients admitted through the emergency department for COPD exacerbation. Among adult asthmatics who were noted to use accessory breathing muscles at the time of hospitalization, percent-predicted FEV_1 values were lower than in patients who were not activating these muscles. Pursed-lip breathing (exhaling against partially occluded lips) can be seen in persons with airflow obstruction. In patients with moderate to severe COPD, pursed-lip breathing facilitates the recruitment of accessory muscles, decreases the electromyographic propensity for diaphragm fatigue, and improves tidal volume and arterial oxyhemoglobin saturation. Dyspnea observed in the context of altered mental status and cyanosis is worrisome, because taken together, these findings attest to profound gas exchange problems.

BIOMARKERS

Brain Natriuretic Peptides

Peripheral blood concentrations of brain-type natriuretic peptides (BNPs) commonly are used in emergency medicine to distinguish CHF from other causes of acute dyspnea. BNP is one of the natriuretic peptides released from cardiac myocytes with ventricular stretching and pressure overload. A prospective, multicenter study published in 2002 called the Breathing Not Properly trial evaluated the test characteristics and diagnostic accuracy of BNP for CHF in 1586 patients who presented for urgent evaluation of acute dyspnea. The clinical diagnosis of CHF was adjudicated by two cardiologists who were blinded to BNP results. At a cutoff value of 100 pg/mL, the diagnostic accuracy for CHF was 83%. Patients with BNP levels of 100 pg/mL or higher were nearly 30 times more likely than those with lower values to have CHF. Other clinical correlates of CHF, such as cephalization of pulmonary vessels on chest radiograph (odds ratio, 10.7), crackles on chest auscultation (odds ratio, 2.2), and jugular venous distention (odds ratio, 1.8), also were helpful.

A related natriuretic peptide called amino-terminal pro-BNP (NT-proBNP) also has been shown in the emergency department setting to strongly suggest CHF as the correct diagnosis for acute dyspnea. Nonetheless, elevated natriuretic peptide measurements do not independently secure a CHF diagnosis. Atrial arrhythmias, cardiomyopathies, regurgitant valvular disease, pulmonary arterial hypertension, obstructive sleep apnea, pulmonary embolism, and even sepsis can cause abnormal results on BNP assays. An echocardiogram can be beneficial when BNP levels return to within an indeterminate range.

Troponin Isoforms

Dyspnea is a common feature of ACS, affecting roughly 35% to 55% of patients. Although chest discomfort and diaphoresis are encountered more frequently, dyspnea alone can herald myocardial infarction, particularly in women. Troponin isoforms are cardiac myocyte proteins that leak into the circulation due to ischemic damage. Modern troponin assays are exquisitely sensitive such that positive results are obtained in many conditions other than ACS and MI. Patients are likely to experience dyspnea in a number of these conditions: aortic dissection, acute respiratory distress syndrome, pulmonary embolism, sepsis, and blunt chest trauma. Troponin elevation in the setting of nonmassive, symptomatic pulmonary embolism is associated with a four-fold increase in short-term mortality (i.e., risk of death in the immediate post–embolic event period). Unlike BNP and NT-proBNP, troponin isoforms are not sufficiently specific to distinguish cardiac from noncardiac causes of acute dyspnea in the emergency department setting.

D-Dimer

In the three largest investigations of diagnostic imaging modalities for acute pulmonary embolism, dyspnea as an isolated symptom was reported by only 22% to 46% of patients. Because dyspnea is not a completely reliable indicator of pulmonary embolism, which carries a mortality rate of about 30% without treatment, the aim of any workup is to confidently exclude this diagnosis. To this end, the D-dimer assay has found a place in the evaluation of acute dyspnea. D-dimer is a fibrin degradation product detectable in venous blood as a result of clot breakdown. Of utmost importance in clinical decision-making, the use of D-dimer results requires understanding that pretest probability and test characteristics of a given assay strongly influence diagnostic accuracy.

Prediction scores can help the clinician settle on a pretest probability of venous thromboembolism. The incidence of venous thromboembolism at 3 months is 1% or less when the clinical pretest suspicion is low and the D-dimer test result is normal (and anticoagulation therapy is withheld). When venous thromboembolism is more strongly suspected or D-dimer assay results are positive, more definitive testing using computed tomography (CT) pulmonary angiography should be considered.

THORACIC IMAGING

Chest Radiograph

Plain chest radiography is perhaps the most widely utilized imaging modality for the evaluation of acute dyspnea. Depending on patient stability and mobility, adequate views in anteroposterior or standing posteroanterior projections can be obtained using portable techniques. The chest radiograph complements the workup for an airway foreign body but has some limitations. Retrospective studies involving children have shown that the chest radiograph has a sensitivity of 73% to 85% and a specificity of 9% to 45% for foreign body, suggesting that direct visualization is warranted in most instances.

Certain technical caveats apply to the use of the chest radiograph to diagnose pneumothorax. The air collection appears as a lucent region between the chest wall and the line of the visceral pleura. This interface can be difficult to visualize in the supine patient, because air accumulates in subpulmonic regions. This pattern of localization causes the so-called deep sulcus sign. Chest radiography cannot be used to estimate the size of a pneumothorax, and there is no difference between expiratory and inspiratory views in terms of diagnostic yield.

The chest radiograph is insensitive for the diagnosis of pulmonary embolism. For example, a wedge-shaped peripheral opacity (Hampton's hump) and abrupt pulmonary arterial cut-off (Westermark's sign) were observed on the chest radiograph in only 22% and 14%, respectively, of pulmonary embolism cases confirmed by angiography.

Computed Tomography

Chest CT has become the most sensitive and specific chest imaging technique to evaluate acute dyspnea, especially when it is associated with pain or trauma. In the latter circumstance, CT elucidates pneumothorax, pulmonary contusion, and aortic injury very well. Sensitivity and specificity of CT pulmonary angiography (CTPA) for pulmonary embolism range from 57% to 100% and 78% to 100%, respectively, mostly because of technologic variability. A cross-sectional investigation of CTPA in 589 emergency department patients with suspected pulmonary embolism demonstrated a two-fold greater likelihood of discovering pulmonary nodules and lymphadenopathy than an embolism. A key implication of this finding is that using a CT scan for work up of acute dyspnea often begets further diagnostic studies. Nonetheless, CTPA may play a more important diagnostic role during COPD exacerbation because some data suggest that pulmonary embolism complicates up to 25% of hospitalized cases. Multidetector row CT scan is highly sensitive (95%) and specific (90%) for detection of obstructive coronary artery disease, but its utility in diagnosing acute myocardial infarction is not well defined.

TREATMENT

Further details on the treatment of acute dyspnea caused by the aforementioned processes are presented elsewhere in this book. Two interventions, oxygen therapy and noninvasive positive-pressure ventilation (NIPPV), merit a brief discussion here because of their application to several of these processes. **Table 19-2** presents a list of processes that cause acute dyspnea and their specific therapies.

Oxygen

Supplemental oxygen commonly is administered for acute dyspnea, regardless of hypoxemia, with perceived benefit. The mechanisms by which oxygen relieves dyspnea are surprisingly not well characterized. In a dose-dependent fashion, oxygen has been shown to relieve dyspnea and improve endurance in patients with COPD but without exercise-induced hypoxemia, potentially by slowing breathing rate and reducing dynamic lung hyperinflation. Similar physiologic effects may explain its utility during a COPD exacerbation. Alternatively, it could reduce dyspnea by rectifying oxygen debt of respiratory muscles already mechanically disadvantaged in COPD or by decreasing chemoreceptor output. Supplemental oxygen can overcome ventilation-perfusion mismatch, a process shared by other reasons for acute dyspnea such as CHF, pulmonary embolism, pneumonia, atelectasis, and asthma exacerbation.

Noninvasive Positive-Pressure Ventilation

NIPPV is a form of mechanical ventilation provided by mask or cannula that obviates the need for an invasive endotracheal

Table 19-2	Specific Therapies for Acute Dyspnea by Etiologic Condition
Etiologic Condition	**Therapeutic Intervention(s)/Agent(s)**
Aspirated foreign body	Endotracheal intubation Fiberoptic or rigid bronchoscopy with removal
Anaphylaxis/ angioedema	Antihistamines Subcutaneous epinephrine Systemic corticosteroids
Epiglottitis (E) Peritonsillar abscess (PTA) Retropharyngeal abscess (RPA)	Endotracheal intubation (PTA/RPA) Broad-spectrum antibiotics (PTA/RPA) Incision and drainage (PTA/RPA)
Asthma exacerbation	Supplemental oxygen Inhaled β_2-adrenergic agonists by nebulizer or MDI Systemic corticosteroids
COPD exacerbation	Supplemental oxygen Inhaled β_2-adrenergic agonists by nebulizer or MDI Inhaled anticholinergic agents by nebulizer or MDI Systemic corticosteroids Antibiotics for purulent sputum Noninvasive positive-pressure ventilation
Pulmonary embolism	Systemic anticoagulation Catheter-based thromboembolectomy
Pneumonia	Supplemental oxygen Antibiotics Airway clearance techniques Immunization
Pneumothorax	Thoracostomy tube placement Supplemental oxygen
Congestive heart failure	Supplemental oxygen Diuretics Systemic vasodilators Inotropic agents
Acute coronary syndrome	Percutaneous transluminal coronary angioplasty ± stent Antiplatelet agents Lipid-lowering therapies Diuretics
Acute idiopathic demyelinating polyneuropathy	Mechanical ventilatory support Intravenous immunoglobulin infusion Systemic corticosteroids
Hyperventilation syndrome	Anxiolytic medications Psychiatric evaluation

COPD, chronic obstructive pulmonary disease; *MDI,* metered dose inhaler.

airway. It has found particular utility in the management of acute ventilatory failure due to exacerbations of COPD and CHF. A bilevel airflow pattern can be established through the circuit such that inspiration is augmented by a higher pressure than that set during exhalation. NIPPV has been shown to help correct acute respiratory acidosis in COPD exacerbation, thereby avoiding the need for endotracheal intubation. Bilevel and continuous positive airway pressure delivered noninvasively can improve hypoxemia caused by cardiogenic pulmonary edema and atelectasis in the postoperative period. NIPPV is not appropriate for patients who are hemodynamically unstable, unable to protect their airway, and agitated to the point of not tolerating the apparatus.

CHRONIC DYSPNEA

Chronic dyspnea has been defined as lasting longer than 1 month. Prevalence statistics for chronic dyspnea vary by setting and population. In a cross-sectional survey from Australia, 8.9% of the nearly 5500 respondents acknowledged exertional breathlessness. Environmental tobacco smoke exposure independently increased the likelihood of dyspnea by a factor of 1.45 among 4197 Swiss never-smokers. In 2009, dyspnea was the most common symptom or reason for referral encountered by European hospital-based internists, constituting 19% of admissions. Chronic dyspnea accounts for 3% to 25% of general ambulatory practice visits and has a significant impact among the elderly.

Patients with chronic dyspnea can be disproportionately burdened with comorbid conditions. A 2006 telephone survey of 1003 patients with COPD, 61% of whom reported moderate or severe dyspnea, identified coexistent hypertension (55%), hypercholesterolemia (52%), depression (37%), cataracts (31%), and osteoporosis (28%). Retrospective and prospective data suggest that patients with COPD have a tendency to sustain falls. Idiopathic pulmonary fibrosis, a disease in which the vast majority of patients experience breathlessness, is associated with an excessive risk of cardiac ischemia, venous thromboembolism, and obstructive sleep apnea. From the U.S. Third National Health and Nutrition Examination Survey (NHANES III), researchers interested in asthma and obesity found that the proportion of subjects citing dyspnea during hill climbing rose as obesity worsened. The prevalence of airflow obstruction fell as body mass index increased, yet the most severely obese subjects were using bronchodilators more frequently. These observations led investigators to conclude that asthma may be overdiagnosed in severely obese patients.

DIFFERENTIAL DIAGNOSIS

Causes of chronic dyspnea are listed in **Table 19-3**. Conditions such as COPD and CHF (see Table 19-1) may have both acute and chronic phases. Relatively few studies have tried to identify those diseases that most commonly underlie chronic dyspnea in the outpatient setting. A prospective evaluation of 85 patients at a university-based pulmonary clinic showed that asthma (29%), COPD (14%), interstitial lung disease (14%), and cardiomyopathy (10%) explained two thirds of cases. Although the study investigators emphasized a rational diagnostic approach that incorporated the responses to disease-specific therapies, an average of 6.2 tests were conducted per patient, and no participants had pulmonary vascular disease or muscle weakness. Another investigation of 72 consecutive patients with chronic dyspnea and unrevealing history, physical examination, chest radiograph, and spirometry data found that 36% had pulmonary disease, 14% had cardiac disease, and 19% had primary hyperventilation. Only 3% had an extrathoracic reason for their breathlessness.

Dyspnea often affects patients without obvious heart or lung disease; therefore, the clinician must consider various etiologic conditions. Some of these processes, listed in Table 19-3, warrant further discussion, because dyspnea could be overlooked as a presenting symptom. Moderate to severe anemia can limit tissue oxygen delivery but does not lead to

oxyhemoglobin desaturation. Thus, the mechanism by which a low hemoglobin concentration provokes dyspnea probably is related to impaired muscle energetics and a compensatory increase in ventilation and cardiac output. Patients with many forms of advanced cancer indeed experience significant, albeit temporary, dyspnea relief from blood transfusions and erythropoietic growth factor support. Respiratory muscle weakness has been implicated as the cause of chronic dyspnea in patients with hypothyroidism and thyrotoxicosis, on the basis of responses to specific medical therapy. Limited data are available regarding the prevalence of dyspnea among patients with selected neuromuscular diseases. Roughly 40% of patients with amyotrophic lateral sclerosis, 23% of patients with postpoliomyelitis, and 12% of patients with multiple sclerosis complain of dyspnea. Both weight gain and a sedentary lifestyle are common causes of exertional dyspnea in those residing in developed countries.

MEDICAL HISTORY

Processes that cause chronic breathlessness are likely to have evolved to some extent before a patient presents for evaluation. Accordingly, it is incumbent on the clinician to ask about the ways in which the patient's dyspnea has changed. Questions might focus on how frequently dyspnea occurs, how long each episode lasts, how intense each episode is, and defining factors that both trigger and relieve it. Eliciting which activities of daily living provoke dyspnea can facilitate longitudinal assessment. This determination also sheds light on whether the patient is modifying behaviors as dyspnea worsens. Unless the clinician specifically asks about activities that the patient has stopped because of breathing difficulty, it can appear that breathlessness only modestly affects that patient's functional status. Perspectives on the patient's dyspnea from spouses, relatives, and friends frequently are useful and should be sought.

As discussed earlier, the correct diagnosis may be suggested by patient-selected descriptors of dyspnea, but it also can be substantiated by the presence or absence of associated symptoms. For example, asthmatic persons generally experience episodes of wheezing, chest tightness, and dyspnea with or without antecedent exposure to a discrete trigger such as an aeroallergen or cold air. A report of wheezing is nonspecific for asthma, however, because it can signify COPD, upper airway obstruction, or CHF. Many asthmatics also cough during bronchospasm periods, but asthma explains a chronic cough only about 25% of the time. The elderly asthmatic patient may describe exertional dyspnea and no other respiratory symptoms—a possible correlate of nonreversible airflow obstruction.

Paroxysmal nocturnal dyspnea and orthopnea may suggest CHF. A systematic review of studies investigating emergency department diagnosis of CHF found that a history of paroxysmal nocturnal dyspnea increased the pretest probability of CHF in the dyspneic patient by a factor of 2.6. Data from the Cardiovascular Health Study suggest that orthopnea and paroxysmal nocturnal dyspnea are relatively specific (87.5% and 89.8%, respectively) but somewhat insensitive (42.8% and 37.6%, respectively) indicators of CHF. Orthopnea also may be due to respiratory muscle weakness and abdominal "loading," as with ascites and obesity.

PHYSICAL EXAMINATION

A focused physical examination frequently yields sufficient clues about the origin of chronic breathlessness. The

Table 19-3 Differential Diagnosis of Chronic Dyspnea

Anatomy	Processes	Risk Factors
Upper airway	Vocal cord dysfunction	Head, neck, and lung cancer Neck surgery Head trauma Endotracheal intubation Viral infection Psychiatric disorder
	Subglottic stenosis	Endotracheal intubation ANCA-positive vasculitis
	Partially obstructing lesion(s)	Cancer Granulomatous inflammation
Thyroid	Thyrotoxicosis Hypothyroidism	Autoimmunity Viral infection
Blood	Anemia	Chemotherapy Chronic kidney disease Chronic gastrointestinal blood loss
Heart	Systolic heart failure Diastolic heart failure Pericardial disease Valvular disease Intracardiac shunt	Myocardial infarction Hypertension, obesity Pericarditis Mitral and aortic insufficiency Patent foramen ovale, ventricular septal defect
Lungs Airways	COPD	Tobacco abuse, α_1-antitrypsin deficiency
	Asthma	Atopy, genetic predisposition
	Cystic fibrosis	Heritable genetic defect
Parenchyma	Interstitial lung disease	Idiopathic interstitial pneumonia Pneumotoxic drug reaction Connective tissue disease
Vasculature	Pulmonary arterial hypertension	Idiopathic pulmonary arterial hypertension Chronic venous thromboembolism Vasculitis Obesity-hypoventilation syndrome
	Arteriovenous malformation	
Pleura	Pleural effusion	Systolic heart failure Cancer Infection Hepatic hydrothorax
Thorax	Kyphoscoliosis	Congenital Osteoporosis
Respiratory muscles	Mechanical loading	Morbid obesity Pregnancy
	Dyskinesia/dystonia Neurodegenerative disease	
Integrated	Deconditioning	Sedentary lifestyle Nutritional deficiency Obesity
Other	Hyperventilation syndrome	Anxiety

ANCA, antineutrophil cytoplasmic antibodies; *COPD,* chronic obstructive pulmonary disease.

investigation should begin with an appraisal of the patient's voice. Someone with "breathy" dysphonia whose voice tends to wane during prolonged speech could have vocal cord dysfunction. In the setting of chronic dyspnea, stridor most commonly is caused by the development of benign or malignant lesions or focal stenoses. The diagnostic utility of jugular venous pressure elevation for detection of decompensated CHF has been

extensively studied. The sensitivity and specificity of this finding for high pulmonary capillary occlusion pressure (i.e., pulmonary venous hypertension) are 70% and 79%, respectively. The jugular venous pressure can be difficult to measure in persons with an obese habitus and can be elevated as a consequence of pulmonary arterial hypertension, tricuspid regurgitation, pericardial constriction, or occlusion of the superior vena cava.

Examination of the neck also should involve palpation for thyroidomegaly and lymphadenopathy, because dyspnea can result from tracheal compression.

Inspection of the spine and thorax can provide a clear reason for why a patient experiences persistent dyspnea. Severe kyphosis reduces total lung capacity, limits alveolar ventilation, and eventually impairs gas exchange. The anteroposterior dimension of the thorax can be exaggerated in patients with COPD, but this adaptation to lung hyperinflation lacks sensitivity for this diagnosis. Central adiposity in the morbidly obese patient reduces functional residual capacity (FRC) and reserve volume, thereby increasing resistance to airflow and decreasing lung compliance. Collapse of small peripheral airways in the lung bases of obese patients can lead to ventilation-perfusion mismatch and breathlessness.

Crackles on lung auscultation can reflect several pathologic processes, all of which should be considered along with other aspects of the examination. The negative predictive value of crackles for interstitial lung disease and CHF has been reported as 98% and 89%, respectively, indicating that a majority of patients without crackles will not have these conditions. The sensitivity of crackles for CHF can be as low as 29%, even when echocardiography is used to affirm or refute presence of left ventricular dysfunction. In one study of 57 patients with pleural effusions, 49 of whom were dyspneic, dullness to percussion and decreased breath sounds were individually more suggestive of pleural fluid than crackles. Wheezes similarly are useful in diagnosing asthma and COPD, but their absence cannot exclude airflow obstruction. Emphysema is suggested by diminished breath sounds in the upper lung fields, sometimes associated with indistinct heart tones. The S3 gallop on heart auscultation is highly specific for elevated left ventricular end-diastolic pressure.

DIAGNOSTIC TESTING

Details from the history and physical examination should inform the selection of diagnostic tests that further refine decision-making. One approach involves categorizing these modalities according to their ability to investigate relevant anatomy and physiology (Table 19-4). Various guidelines on management of COPD recommend that the diagnosis be determined by a value of 70% or less for the ratio of postbronchodilator forced expiratory volume in 1 second (FEV_1) to forced vital capacity (FVC). However, the FEV_1/FVC ratio declines with aging, and the use of a "fixed" ratio may lead to overdiagnosis of COPD among patients older than 60 years of age. We concur with the American Thoracic Society–European Respiratory Society recommendation that airflow obstruction be diagnosed by a FEV_1/FVC value below the lower limit of normal for the specific patient.

A low FVC may be due to air trapping in a patient with airflow obstruction or may point to a restrictive lung process that can be confirmed by measurement of lung volumes. Analysis of the flow-volume loop can demonstrate evidence of upper airway obstruction (Figure 19-4). In cases of suspected asthma, a negative result on direct bronchoprovocation testing essentially rules out this diagnosis. However, false-positive results can be seen in normal persons as well as those with sarcoidosis or vocal cord dysfunction. Measurement of maximal inspiratory mouth pressure is sensitive for detection of respiratory muscle weakness.

Many cardiac causes of chronic breathlessness can be identified by echocardiography. In addition to quantifying left

Table 19-4 | **Diagnostic Testing for Chronic Dyspnea**

Test	Diagnostic Utility
Spirometry	Diagnose and quantify airflow obstruction and restriction
Flow-volume loop	Diagnose upper airway obstruction
Single-breath diffusion capacity for carbon monoxide (D_{LCO})	Reduced in emphysema, interstitial lung disease, and pulmonary hypertension Can be reduced in anemia Can be increased in alveolar hemorrhage, asthma
Lung volume determination	Confirms restrictive lung diseases
Bronchoprovocation testing	Diagnose airway hyperreactivity
Maximal inspiratory and expiratory mouth pressures	Evaluate neuromuscular weakness
Chest computed tomography	Interstitial lung disease Airway caliber well delineated; can identify endobronchial lesions Excellent characterization of pleural space and mediastinum
Echocardiography	Diagnose and quantify ventricular function Evaluate valvular incompetence, pericardium
Cardiopulmonary exercise testing	Diagnose cardiac dysfunction, ventilatory limitation, oxygen desaturation, deconditioning, psychogenic dyspnea
Complete blood count	Diagnose anemia

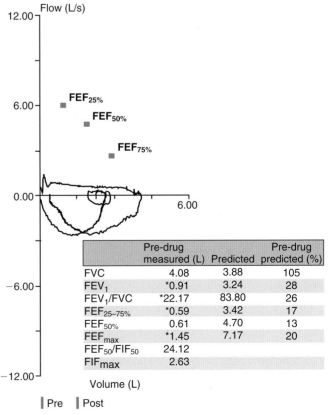

	Pre-drug measured (L)	Predicted	Pre-drug predicted (%)
FVC	4.08	3.88	105
FEV_1	*0.91	3.24	28
FEV_1/FVC	*22.17	83.80	26
$FEF_{25-75\%}$	*0.59	3.42	17
$FEF_{50\%}$	0.61	4.70	13
FEF_{max}	*1.45	7.17	20
FEF_{50}/FIF_{50}	24.12		
FIF_{max}	2.63		

| Pre | Post

Figure 19-4 Flow-volume loop and spirometry data for a patient with intrathoracic upper airway obstruction. Note plateau of expiratory flow.

Table 19-5 Cardiopulmonary Exercise Testing and Chronic Dyspnea

Measured Parameter	Deconditioning	Cardiac Process	Pulmonary Process
$V_{O_2}max$	↓	↓	↓
Anaerobic threshold (AT)	Normal	↓	↓ or normal
O_2 pulse (mL/beat)	Normal	↓	Normal
Heart rate reserve (normal ≤15%)	Normal	Normal	>15%
V_{O_2}/power slope (mL/min/W)	Normal	↓	Normal
Breathing reserve (normal ≥30%)	Normal	Normal	<30%
Sa_{O_2} (rest to exercise)	No change	No change	Possible ↓
Usual exercise-limiting symptom	Leg discomfort	Chest discomfort	Dyspnea

ventricular systolic function, this procedure provides information about peak systolic pulmonary artery pressure, pericardial structure, and valvular function. Intravenous administration of agitated saline solution coupled with echocardiography (i.e., contrast echocardiography) is more than 98% sensitive for detecting pulmonary arteriovenous malformations. In a study of nearly 18,000 patients without established coronary artery disease who were referred for radionuclide myocardial perfusion testing, evidence of inducible ischemia was similar for patients with self-reported dyspnea and for those with typical angina pectoris, prompting the investigators to conclude that a more systematic appraisal of dyspnea should occur at the time of stress testing referral.

The etiology of chronic dyspnea will sometimes remain elusive despite a careful history and physical examination and multiple diagnostic endeavors. Then, cardiopulmonary exercise testing should be considered to provoke the patient's dyspnea with comprehensive assessment of the oxygen transport system on an integrated level. Pulmonary gas exchange, cardiac function, and metabolic activity can be measured noninvasively (**Table 19-5**). Patients also are asked to rate dyspnea and leg discomfort throughout the exercise test. The results of cardiopulmonary exercise testing usually are able to distinguish cardiac dysfunction and ventilatory limitation but cannot always discriminate between cardiac disease and deconditioning.

TREATMENT

Disease-specific therapies generally are successful in mitigating chronic dyspnea, although this may not be the case with multiple concurrent processes or disease progression. Dyspnea is a prominent feature of CHF, yet most studies of various interventions for CHF consider death or utilization of health care resources as outcome metrics. Good-quality evidence supports exercise training to improve functional status in patients with CHF. Diuretics, inotropes, and vasodilators are mainstays of a management strategy of regulating volume status and controlling symptoms in CHF.

For patients with COPD, the combination of an inhaled corticosteroid and a long-acting β-agonist has been shown to improve lung function, relieve respiratory symptoms, and modestly reduce risk of death. Large trials of inhaled long-acting anticholinergic drugs also show a positive impact on dyspnea associated with COPD. Supplemental oxygen is indicated for patients with COPD who have resting hypoxemia, although its effect on mortality and symptoms in patients who display only exertional oxyhemoglobin desaturation is currently being investigated. Specific criteria to select patients with emphysema who could benefit from lung volume reduction surgery are well established. Pulmonary rehabilitation has been shown to have multiple benefits, including decreasing the severity of dyspnea, enhancing exercise tolerance, reducing the frequency of exacerbations, and improving quality of life. Interstitial lung disease is a broad category of infiltrative pulmonary disorders for which disease-modifying and symptom-relieving treatments are needed.

PALLIATION OF DYSPNEA

A recent consensus statement addresses management of dyspnea in advanced heart and lung disease. Its authors emphasize that dyspnea should be regularly assessed and documented, with a goal of determining whether this symptom is being adequately addressed. The statement affirms the potential for oxygen to palliate dyspnea in patients who are hypoxemic at rest or with modest physical activity. Recommended nonpharmacologic approaches to the management of dyspnea include pursed-lip breathing, relaxation, guided imagery, and NIPPV.

Systemic opioids are effective for palliating refractory dyspnea; the dose and frequency of opioid medications should account for altered pharmacokinetics due to liver or kidney disease. The consensus statement affirms that concerns about addiction or dependence should not curtail the effective palliation of dyspnea. Moreover, the principle of double effect provides an ethical basis for treating with a class of drugs that can hasten death by respiratory depression, so long as the primary intent is to relieve the disabling and distressing experience of dyspnea.

SUGGESTED READINGS

Davenport PW, Vovk A: Cortical and subcortical central neural pathways in respiratory sensations, *Respir Physiol Neurobiol* 167:72, 2009.

Gibson NS, Sohne M, Gerdes VE, et al: The importance of clinical probability assessment in interpreting a normal D-dimer in patients with suspected pulmonary embolism, *Chest* 134:789, 2008.

Horton R, Rocker G: Contemporary issues in refractory dyspnoea in advanced chronic obstructive pulmonary disease, *Curr Opin Support Palliat Care* 4:56, 2010.

Lansing RW, Gracely RH, Banzett RB: The multiple dimensions of dyspnea: review and hypotheses, *Respir Physiol Neurobiol* 167:53, 2009.

Mahler DA, Fierro-Carrion G, Baird JC: Evaluation of dyspnea in the elderly, *Clin Geriatr Med* 19:19, 2003.

Mahler DA, Selecky PA, Harrod CG, et al: American College of Chest Physicians consensus statement on the management of dyspnea in patients with advanced lung or heart disease, *Chest* 137:674, 2010.

Ohar JA, Sadeghnejad A, Meyers DA, et al: Do symptoms predict COPD in smokers? *Chest* 137:1345, 2010.

Pratter MR, Curley FJ, Dubois J, et al: Cause and evaluation of chronic dyspnea in a pulmonary disease clinic, *Arch Intern Med* 149:2277, 1989.

Von Leupoldt A, Dahme B: Cortical substrates for the perception of dyspnea, *Chest* 128:345, 2005.

Wang CS, FitzGerald JM, Schulzer M, et al: Does this dyspneic patient in the emergency department have congestive heart failure? *JAMA* 294:1944, 2005.

Chapter **20**

Hemoptysis

John W. Kreit

Hemoptysis is defined as the expectoration of blood that results from hemorrhage into the lower respiratory tract. It can be caused by a wide variety of disorders and constitutes a common reason for referral to a pulmonary specialist. The amount of blood expectorated can range from minimal streaking of the sputum to large volumes of pure blood and depends not only on the rate of bleeding but also on its location. For example, hemorrhage into the lung parenchyma or a distal airway may be accompanied by little or no hemoptysis, whereas even a relatively small amount of bleeding from a central airway may lead to a significant volume of expectorated blood.

Hemoptysis, by itself, does not usually lead to significant morbidity or death. Rather, it typically is important only as a sign of an underlying and often unrecognized disorder. Thus, hemoptysis is an extremely important symptom, and its cause must be determined by means of a thorough and orderly evaluation.

Massive hemoptysis is an uncommon but potentially life-threatening event, in that flooding of the airways and alveoli may quickly lead to respiratory failure. It requires rapid evaluation and emergent and specific therapy, so massive hemoptysis usually is considered to represent a distinct clinical entity and is discussed separately in a later section of this chapter.

DIFFERENTIAL DIAGNOSIS

A large number of disorders have been reported to cause hemoptysis, and the most important are listed in **Box 20-1**. Of these, bronchogenic carcinoma, bronchiectasis, bronchitis, and bacterial pneumonia are responsible for most cases. **Table 20-1** shows the relative frequency of disorders causing hemoptysis in major series published since 1980. The significant variability, especially in the frequency of bronchiectasis, bronchitis, and tuberculosis, probably reflects differences in the time of publication, the patient population studied, and the diagnostic tests and criteria used. **Figure 20-1** illustrates the percentage of patients with each diagnosis on the basis of pooled data from these studies.

NEOPLASMS

Malignancy is one of the most common causes of hemoptysis, and bronchogenic carcinoma accounts for most of these cases. In patients with hemoptysis, the tumor typically involves a central airway (i.e., a main, lobar, or segmental bronchus) and most commonly is a squamous cell carcinoma. Much less commonly, hemoptysis is caused by a peripherally located carcinoma or by other primary pulmonary neoplasms, such as carcinoid tumor or hamartoma. Extrathoracic malignancies,

especially melanoma and carcinoma of the breast, colon, and kidney, also may cause hemoptysis because of their propensity to metastasize to endobronchial locations in the tracheobronchial tree.

BRONCHIECTASIS

In studies published before the early 1960s, bronchiectasis often was the most common cause of hemoptysis and frequently accounted for 25% to 35% of cases. In the subsequent decades, this number dropped dramatically to less than 5%. Although this decline was correctly attributed to the greater availability and effectiveness of antibacterial and antituberculosis therapy, it probably was also caused by a marked decrease in the use of bronchography, the principal diagnostic modality of that era. Since the advent of high-resolution computed tomography (HRCT), bronchiectasis has been diagnosed with increasing frequency, and recent studies indicate that it remains a very important cause of hemoptysis.

ACUTE BRONCHITIS

Hemoptysis often is attributed to an acute infectious bronchitis on the basis of compatible clinical or bronchoscopic findings, and this is a common final diagnosis in most series. Although acute bronchitis undoubtedly may cause hemoptysis, the symptoms, signs, and bronchoscopic findings in this disorder are neither sensitive nor specific. In fact, several studies have demonstrated that the diagnosis of acute bronchitis often is made in patients with another source of bleeding. Thus, acute bronchitis must be considered to represent a diagnosis of exclusion, and great care must be taken to search for other causes of hemoptysis.

TUBERCULOSIS

Although tuberculosis remains relatively common in certain patient populations and geographic regions, successful methods of treatment and prevention have markedly reduced both its incidence and its importance as a cause of hemoptysis. Hemoptysis most commonly results from active disease, but it also may be caused by the sequelae of infection, particularly bronchiectasis, parenchymal cavitation, and mycetoma formation.

BACTERIAL PNEUMONIA

Hemoptysis may result from virtually any type of bacterial pneumonia but most often accompanies infection with *Streptococcus pneumoniae*. Other commonly implicated pathogens

Table 20-1 Causes of Hemoptysis in Published Series

Series	Santiago et al.	Johnston et al.	Hirshberg et al.	Fidan et al.	Tsoumakidou et al.
Year(s)	1974-1981	1977-1985	1980-1995	2000	2001-2003
Location	Los Angeles	Kansas City	Jerusalem	Istanbul	Crete
No. of cases	264	148	208	108	184
Neoplasms (%)	31	19	19	34	13
Bronchiectasis (%)	1	1	20	25	26
Bronchitis (%)	23	37	18	0	38
Pneumonia (%)	6	5	16	10	4
Tuberculosis (%)*	6	7	1	18	4
Cryptogenic (%)	22	3	8	0	10
Other (%)	11	26	18	13	5

Data from Santiago S, Tobaias J, Williams AJ: A reappraisal of the causes of hemoptysis, *Arch Intern Med* 151:2449-2451, 1991; Johnston H, Reisz G: Changing spectrum of hemoptysis, *Arch Intern Med* 149:1666-1668, 1989; Hirschberg B, Biran I, Glazer M, Kramer MR: Hemoptysis: etiology, evaluation, and outcome in a tertiary referral hospital, *Chest* 112:440-444, 1997; Fidan A, Ozdogan S, Oruc O, et al: Hemoptysis: a retrospective analysis of 108 cases, *Respir Med* 96:677-680, 2002; Tsoumakidou M, Chrysofakis G, Tsiligianni I, et al: A prospective analysis of 184 hemoptysis cases, *Respiration* 73:808-814, 2006.
*Active and inactive disease.

Box 20-1 Causes of Hemoptysis

Common (≥5% each)
Bronchogenic carcinoma
Bronchiectasis
Bronchitis
Bacterial pneumonia
Tuberculosis

Uncommon (1-4% each)
Pulmonary embolism
Left ventricular failure
Mycetoma
Nontuberculous mycobacterial infection
Traumatic or iatrogenic lung injury

Rare (<1% each)
Other primary lung neoplasms
Metastatic neoplasms
Nonbacterial pneumonia
Broncholithiasis
Foreign body aspiration
Mitral stenosis
Amyloidosis
Pulmonary arteriovenous malformation
Pulmonary artery aneurysm
Endometriosis
Pulmonary sequestration
Alveolar hemorrhage syndromes
   Goodpasture syndrome
   Wegener granulomatosis
   Microscopic polyarteritis
   Systemic lupus erythematosus

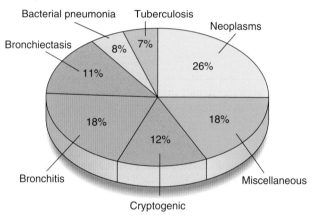

Figure 20-1 Final diagnosis in patients presenting with hemoptysis. The approximate percentage of cases attributed to each diagnosis is shown.

PATIENT EVALUATION

When the patient reports a history of expectorating blood, the first step must be to determine whether hemoptysis has actually occurred. That is, bleeding must be localized to the lower respiratory tract, and alternative sites, such as the nose, mouth, pharynx, larynx, and gastrointestinal tract, must be excluded. Few patients have difficulty distinguishing between vomiting and expectorating blood, although specific questions may be required to elicit a report of nausea and retching. Distinguishing between an upper and a lower airway source of bleeding occasionally is more difficult, although this usually can be accomplished by a directed history and physical examination. Patients with hemoptysis almost always report that the expectoration of blood follows an episode of coughing; in those with an upper airway source, it typically is preceded by a feeling of blood pooling in the mouth or the need to "clear the throat." A history of epistaxis also is an important indicator of upper airway hemorrhage. Routine examination of the nose, mouth, and pharynx is important to rule out an obvious site of bleeding. A thorough examination that includes rhinoscopy and laryngoscopy is indicated when an upper airway source cannot be reliably excluded.

include *Klebsiella pneumoniae, Staphylococcus aureus, Pseudomonas aeruginosa,* and anaerobic organisms.

CRYPTOGENIC HEMOPTYSIS

In almost all reported series, the cause of hemoptysis remains unknown in a significant percentage of patients. As shown in Table 20-1, the frequency of cryptogenic hemoptysis has varied widely, and this variability presumably is due to differences in diagnostic criteria and the extent of evaluation.

Table 20-2 Important Clinical Features in Patients with Hemoptysis

Category	Feature(s)	Disorder(s)
Historical	Cigarette smoking	Bronchogenic carcinoma
	Previously diagnosed malignancy	Metastatic malignancy
	Previously diagnosed pulmonary, cardiac, pulmonary vascular, or systemic disease	
	Recent chest trauma or procedure	Traumatic/iatrogenic lung injury
	Risk factors for aspiration	Lung abscess, foreign body aspiration
Symptom	Purulent-appearing sputum	Bronchiectasis, bronchitis, pneumonia, lung abscess
	Pleuritic pain	Pneumonia, pulmonary embolism
	Paroxysmal nocturnal dyspnea, orthopnea	Left ventricular failure, mitral stenosis
	Fever	Pneumonia, lung abscess
	Weight loss	Bronchogenic carcinoma, other malignancy, tuberculosis, lung abscess
Sign	Bronchial breath sounds, egophony	Pneumonia
	Localized decrease in breath sounds, localized wheezing	Bronchogenic carcinoma, broncholithiasis, foreign body
	Coarse crackles, rhonchi	Bronchiectasis, bronchitis
	Pleural rub	Pneumonia, pulmonary embolism
	S3 gallop	Left ventricular failure
	Diastolic murmur	Mitral stenosis

Table 20-3 Important Radiographic Findings in Patients with Hemoptysis

Radiographic Finding	Associated Disorder(s)
Nodule(s) or mass(es)	Bronchogenic carcinoma or other neoplasm, lung abscess, fungal infection, vasculitis
Atelectasis	Bronchogenic carcinoma or other endobronchial neoplasm, broncholithiasis, foreign body
Hilar/mediastinal adenopathy	Bronchogenic carcinoma or other neoplasm, mycobacterial or fungal infection, sarcoidosis
Dilated peripheral airways	Bronchiectasis
Air space consolidation	Pneumonia, alveolar hemorrhage, pulmonary contusion
Reticulonodular densities	Sarcoidosis, lymphangitic carcinoma
Cavity—single or multiple	Mycobacterial or fungal infection, mycetoma, lung abscess, bronchogenic carcinoma
Hilar/mediastinal calcification	Previous mycobacterial or fungal infection, broncholithiasis

INITIAL EVALUATION

Once hemoptysis has been confirmed, a search must be made for its cause. This process begins with an initial evaluation that consists of a complete history and physical examination and a chest radiograph.

Important symptoms, signs, and historical details that suggest one or more disorders are listed in **Table 20-2**. In some patients, such as those with pulmonary embolism, left ventricular failure, mitral stenosis, and traumatic or iatrogenic lung injury, the history and physical examination may provide the most important clues to the diagnosis.

As shown in **Table 20-3**, the chest radiograph also may yield important information about the underlying cause of hemoptysis. The chest film, however, is "localizing"—that is, it demonstrates a mass, cavity, infiltrate, lobar atelectasis, or other finding that is likely to be directly related to the cause of hemoptysis—in less than 40% of patients. In the remainder, the chest radiograph is either normal in appearance or demonstrates abnormal but nonspecific findings such as emphysema, interstitial fibrosis, minor atelectasis, or pleural thickening—a category referred to as "nonlocalizing." This radiographic classification has important diagnostic and prognostic implications. Malignancy is found in almost 40% of patients with hemoptysis associated with localizing findings on the chest radiograph.

On the other hand, cancer is diagnosed in only 6% to 10% of patients with normal-appearing or nonlocalizing chest radiographs.

ADDITIONAL TESTING

The history, physical examination, and plain chest radiography are essential to reduce the number of possible causes of hemoptysis, and findings often point toward specific disorders. This initial evaluation, however, yields a definitive diagnosis in only a small percentage of patients. In most cases, additional testing is required, which most commonly consists of computed tomography (CT) and fiberoptic bronchoscopy (FOB).

COMPUTED TOMOGRAPHY

Compared with conventional chest radiography, CT is clearly superior for imaging the peripheral and central airways, mediastinum, and lung parenchyma. Thus, it is not surprising that CT has been shown to be very useful in the evaluation of patients with hemoptysis. In the presence of a normal-appearing or nonlocalizing chest radiograph, CT reveals an unsuspected cause of hemoptysis, most commonly bronchiectasis, in approximately one third of patients (**Figure 20-2**). CT also may demonstrate an endobronchial lesion (**Figure 20-3**) or an unsuspected

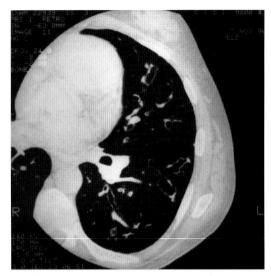

Figure 20-2 Computed tomography (CT) appearance of bronchiectasis. Dilated peripheral airways are clearly seen on this high-resolution CT image.

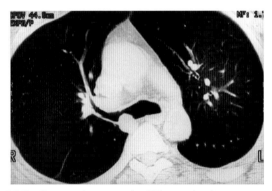

Figure 20-3 Computed tomography (CT) scan showing an endobronchial mass. The lesion, which proved to be a bronchogenic carcinoma, is clearly visible in the right main bronchus.

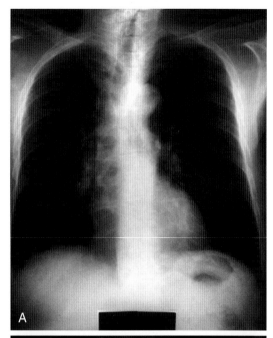

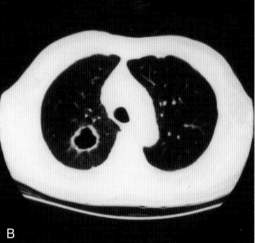

Figure 20-4 Chest radiograph and computed tomography (CT) scan obtained in a patient with a cavitary squamous cell carcinoma. **A,** The lesion cannot be seen on the chest radiograph but is clearly demonstrated on the CT scan, shown in **B.**

parenchymal mass, nodule, or cavity (**Figure 20-4**). CT also is useful in more than half of all patients whose chest radiograph is localizing, either by revealing a new source of hemoptysis or by providing additional information about a previously recognized abnormality.

FIBEROPTIC BRONCHOSCOPY

Since becoming widely available in the early 1970s, fiberoptic bronchoscopy (FOB) has been used almost routinely in the evaluation of patients with hemoptysis. By combining endoscopic examination with brushings, washings, endobronchial and transbronchial biopsy techniques, and transtracheal needle aspiration, FOB may be used both to identify the site of bleeding and to obtain a definitive diagnosis. FOB is most useful for diagnosing bronchogenic carcinoma and other endobronchial neoplasms (**Figure 20-5**); it is far less effective at detecting other causes of hemoptysis. The most common non-neoplastic diagnosis made by FOB is acute bronchitis, which is based on the presence of mucosal hyperemia and edema and purulent-appearing secretions. As previously discussed, however, these findings are nonspecific and often are unrelated to the actual cause of hemoptysis. When this diagnosis is excluded, a specific, non-neoplastic cause of hemoptysis is found by FOB in less than 10% of cases.

COMPUTED TOMOGRAPHY VERSUS BRONCHOSCOPY

Six studies have compared the sensitivity rates for CT and FOB for detection of bronchogenic carcinomas and other lung neoplasms in patients with hemoptysis. Five of these studies were published between 1990 and 1999 and used nonhelical, single-detector scanners. In most cases, images were acquired at 10-mm intervals, although additional sections usually were obtained through the central airways. A total of 296 patients were included in these studies, in whom the chest radiograph typically was either normal-appearing or nonlocalizing, and 83 were diagnosed with a pulmonary malignancy. CT demonstrated all but 1 tumor found by FOB and identified 12 cancers that were not detected by FOB.

Since that time, of course, a dramatic evolution has occurred in CT technology. The advent of continuous, helical scanning using multiple detectors has led to tremendous improvement in image quality and resolution. In a recently published retrospective comparison of FOB and CT in 270 patients with

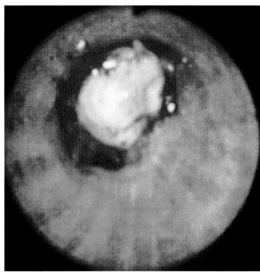

Figure 20-5 Bronchogenic carcinoma visualized through the fiberoptic bronchoscope. The tumor occludes the left upper lobe and is actively bleeding.

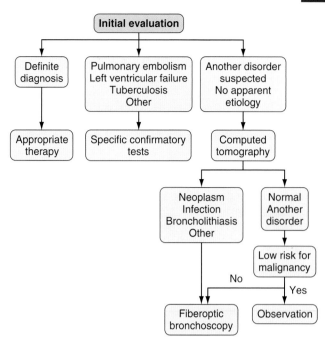

Figure 20-6 Diagnostic algorithm for patients presenting with hemoptysis.

hemoptysis and a normal-appearing chest radiograph, FOB and CT detected 14 and 25 of 26 lung malignancies, respectively. The 1 tumor missed by CT was found by FOB.

These studies clearly show that CT is much better than FOB at detecting and excluding malignancy. However, because CT can still miss small, endobronchial lesions and FOB can establish a definitive tissue diagnosis, both of these tests are recommended, to provide important complementary information in the evaluation of patients with hemoptysis.

Still more recent advances in CT technology have further improved imaging of the airways. Manipulation of CT data allows the creation of two-dimensional multiplanar images as well as three-dimensional internal views of the airways; the relevant technology often is referred to as "virtual bronchoscopy." Although these advancements would be expected to make CT an even more powerful tool, no studies have evaluated their efficacy in patients with hemoptysis.

DIAGNOSTIC ALGORITHM

A suggested approach to the patient with hemoptysis that is based on the preceding information is shown in **Figure 20-6**. If the initial evaluation yields a firm diagnosis, such as bacterial pneumonia or iatrogenic or traumatic lung injury, appropriate therapy is instituted. Alternatively, the initial evaluation may suggest a cause of hemoptysis that requires investigation using one or more specific tests. For example, an echocardiogram may confirm the presence of left ventricular failure or mitral stenosis, pulmonary embolism may be diagnosed by means of a CT angiogram, and sputum cultures may be diagnostic in patients with tuberculosis. In all other patients, CT is the most appropriate next step in the diagnostic evaluation. As discussed previously, CT often identifies an unsuspected cause of hemoptysis, even in patients whose chest radiograph is normal in appearance or nonlocalizing, and may provide important information in patients who already have a presumptive diagnosis. For example, in patients with suspected bronchogenic carcinoma, CT adds vital information for staging and also provides a "road map" for bronchoscopy by defining the exact location of a parenchymal mass and enlarged mediastinal lymph nodes.

If CT suggests a disorder that is amenable to bronchoscopic diagnosis, such as neoplasm or infection, FOB is performed next in the diagnostic evaluation. Additional studies such as mediastinoscopy or surgical lung biopsy may be required if FOB is nondiagnostic. When CT either yields normal findings or demonstrates another cause of hemoptysis, such as bronchiectasis, the role of FOB is less clearly defined. The absence of an endobronchial lesion on the CT scan is associated with a low risk of malignancy, and available data suggest that FOB may be safely omitted in never-smokers younger than 40 years. Because CT occasionally fails to detect small endobronchial lesions, however, FOB should be performed in all other patients.

MASSIVE HEMOPTYSIS

No generally accepted definition of *massive hemoptysis* has emerged, although the most commonly used criteria require the expectoration of between 200 and 600 mL of blood over 24 hours. Any definition based on the amount of expectorated blood is, of course, arbitrary, especially because the volume often is difficult to quantify.

From a clinical standpoint, it is more appropriate to define massive hemoptysis simply as bleeding that impairs ventilation and gas exchange. Because this effect depends not only on the volume of expectorated blood but also on the rate of bleeding, the ability of the patient to clear blood from the airways, and the extent and severity of any underlying lung disease, it is evident that the amount of bleeding needed to be considered "massive" will vary significantly from patient to patient.

Massive hemoptysis is relatively uncommon and occurs in fewer than 5% of patients with lower respiratory tract bleeding. Although any of the disorders listed in Box 20-1 may potentially give rise to life-threatening hemorrhage, massive hemoptysis most commonly is caused by bronchiectasis, bronchogenic carcinoma, mycetoma, lung abscess, and tuberculosis (active or inactive). Overall, the risk of death from massive hemoptysis is approximately 20%, although reported mortality rates vary widely, ranging between 0 and 75%.

The lungs have a dual blood supply. The pulmonary circulation has low pressure and resistance, carries the entire output of the right ventricle, and is responsible for the exchange of oxygen and carbon dioxide. The bronchial arteries are very small systemic arteries with high pressure and resistance. They usually arise from the aorta and normally contribute less than 1% of the blood flow entering the lung vasculature. The bronchial circulation provides oxygen and nutrients to the conducting airways, the pulmonary arteries and veins, the visceral pleura, and the esophagus. Chronic inflammatory disease or neoplasms within the lungs causes enlargement and proliferation of the bronchial arteries as well as recruitment of collateral vessels from extrapulmonary systemic arteries. These vessels tend to have thin walls and are more likely to rupture when exposed to systemic arterial pressure. Massive hemoptysis originates from a bronchial artery in about 90% of cases and from a nonbronchial systemic artery or a pulmonary artery in the remainder. Occasionally, bleeding comes from more than one type of artery.

Because of its associated morbidity and mortality, massive hemoptysis constitutes a respiratory emergency and necessitates rapid evaluation and therapy. Unlike in patients with small amounts of bleeding, in whom the emphasis is on determining the underlying cause, in patients with massive hemoptysis the goals are to maintain a patent airway and to localize and control the bleeding. Patients should be closely monitored in an intensive care unit, and intubation and mechanical ventilation are indicated if ventilation and gas exchange become sufficiently compromised.

Bronchoscopy should be performed immediately in an effort to identify the cause of bleeding or at least to localize the bleeding to a specific segment or lobe. Either rigid bronchoscopy or FOB may be used, depending largely on the clinical circumstances. Rigid bronchoscopy, with its large lumen, affords excellent airway control and suctioning capability, and is ideally suited to management of patients with very brisk bleeding. Disadvantages include poor visualization of the segmental and lobar bronchi and the need for general anesthesia. In most patients, FOB is the procedure of choice, because it can be performed rapidly and allows visualization of airways down to the subsegmental level. All patients with massive hemoptysis should be intubated before FOB. Implementation of this precaution optimizes airway control, allows effective suctioning should the rate of bleeding increase, and permits the bronchoscope to be easily removed and reinserted if the suction channel becomes occluded.

CT also is very effective in identifying both the cause and the site of bleeding in patients experiencing massive hemoptysis. In addition, CT angiography usually can provide images of the bronchial circulation that increase the ease and effectiveness of bronchial artery embolization (see later on) and identify patients who have a nonbronchial systemic arterial source of bleeding.

Localization of the bleeding site is important for two reasons. First, it provides a guide for embolization therapy to control ongoing hemorrhage (see further on). Second, in the setting of persistent, severe hemoptysis, it allows isolation of the bleeding site to prevent the spread of blood throughout the tracheobronchial tree. This potentially lifesaving intervention is performed by placing a bronchoscopically guided balloon catheter in a segmental or lobar airway. When bleeding can be localized only to one lung, a larger balloon may be inflated in a main bronchus, or the fiberoptic bronchoscope can be used to selectively intubate and ventilate the nonbleeding lung.

Once the bleeding site has been localized and a stable airway has been achieved, ongoing hemorrhage must be controlled. Guided by the results of bronchoscopy and CT angiography, bronchial or other intrathoracic arteries may be visualized by use of selective arteriography and occluded with embolized, nonabsorbable material. Arterial embolization is successful in rapidly controlling hemorrhage in 73% to 98% of attempted procedures. Emergent surgical resection is accompanied by a mortality rate that approaches 30% and usually is reserved for patients in whom arterial embolization is unsuccessful.

Once bleeding has resolved, either spontaneously or after embolization therapy, its cause, if not already identified, must be determined (see Figure 20-6). Specific treatment, such as antibacterial or antituberculosis therapy, often prevents further episodes of hemoptysis. When effective therapy is not available, recurrent and often life-threatening hemorrhage occurs with a frequency as high as 50%. Recurrent bleeding is especially likely in patients with bronchiectasis, a mycetoma, or pulmonary malignancy, and surgical resection should be considered in these cases. For patients who are not surgical candidates, repeat embolization therapy often is successful if bleeding recurs.

SUMMARY

Hemoptysis is a commonly encountered sign of extreme clinical importance in that it often signifies the presence of an underlying and sometimes unrecognized lung disease. Adherence to a thorough and orderly diagnostic approach to determine its cause is essential. Massive hemoptysis constitutes a life-threatening emergency, and therapy must focus on maintaining a patent airway and on identification and occlusion of the bleeding artery by means of selective arteriography and embolization.

SUGGESTED READINGS

Chun JY, Morgan R, Belli AM: Radiological management of hemoptysis: a comprehensive review of diagnostic imaging and bronchial arterial embolization, *Cardiovasc Intervent Radiol* 33:240–250, 2010.

Khalil A, Fartoukh M, Parrot A, et al: Impact of MDCT angiography on the management of patients with hemoptysis, *AJR Am J Roentgenol* 195:772–778, 2010.

Lee KS, Boiselle PM: Update on multidetector computed tomography imaging of the airways, *J Thorac Imaging* 25:112–124, 2010.

Thirumaran M, Sundar R, Sutcliffe IM, et al: Is investigation of patients with haemoptysis and normal chest radiograph justified? *Thorax* 64:854–856, 2009.

Tsoumakidou M, Chrysofakis G, Tsiligianni I, et al: A prospective analysis of 184 hemoptysis cases—diagnostic impact of chest x-ray, computed tomography, bronchoscopy, *Respiration* 73:808–814, 2006.

Chapter **21**
Chest Pain

Richard K. Albert • Stephen G. Spiro

Chest pain is a very common symptom, and its severity and etiology will depend, to a large extent, on the clinical circumstances in which it occurs. Chest pain is the most frequent new symptom reported by patients seen in outpatient clinics. Although it is an extremely nonspecific symptom (**Box 21-1**), it may be the presenting manifestation of a number of conditions, most of which will be relatively benign. Also, in many patients with such pain, a firm diagnosis may never be established. When chest pain is a presenting symptom in the emergency department setting, however, more serious, acute, and potentially life-threatening causes need to be considered. Accordingly, a complaint of chest pain requires thorough and careful investigation.

DIFFERENTIAL DIAGNOSIS

The pathophysiology of chest pain is understood for many but not all of the conditions with which it is associated. The most common form of chest pain is musculoskeletal pain. The causes of this form of chest pain are legion—in some instances involving an organic process, often due just to excessive coughing, as discussed later on. Of note, however, possible psychiatric or psychogenic reasons for chest pain need to be kept in mind. Cardiac disease is the most important cause of chest pain overall, so this entity is first in the overview of potential causes.

MYOCARDIAL ISCHEMIA

The chest pain associated with myocardial ischemia is attributed to an imbalance between myocardial oxygen (O_2) supply and demand. Most tissues can increase O_2 supply by increasing O_2 delivery, increasing O_2 extraction, or both. O_2 extraction by the myocardium is much greater than that occurring in other tissues, manifested by the O_2 content of coronary venous blood normally being much lower than that of blood coming from other muscles. Because the ability of the myocardium to increase O_2 extraction is limited, the primary mechanism by which the heart increases O_2 delivery in response to increased demands is to increase coronary blood flow.

Coronary blood flow is determined by the driving pressure (i.e., the aortic pressure minus the left ventricular end-diastolic pressure) and the resistance in the coronary arteries. Chest pain can therefore be caused by conditions that increase myocardial O_2 demand (e.g., hypertension, hyperthyroidism, exercise) in the setting of a limited ability to increase O_2 supply, decrease mean aortic pressure (e.g., aortic stenosis), decrease O_2 delivery (e.g., anemia, hypoxemia), or increase the downstream pressure for coronary arterial flow (e.g., aortic and mitral valve disease,

left or right ventricular hypertrophy, or dilatation). The importance of coronary arterial diameter is apparent in Poiseuille's law, which states that resistance is inversely related to the vessel radius taken to the fourth power, explaining why anything that might result in even a small change in coronary arterial diameter (e.g., coronary arterial spasm, thrombosis, atherosclerosis) can result in chest pain.

A wide range of disorders other than angina may be the cause of chest pain. These potential alternative diagnoses are summarized in **Box 21-2**.

PERICARDIAL PAIN

The visceral pericardium has no pain fibers, and the pain fibers in the parietal pericardium are localized to the caudal (i.e., diaphragmatic) region. This sparse, localized distribution of pericardial pain fibers may explain why most noninflammatory causes of pericardial effusions (e.g., myocardial infarction, uremia) are not associated with chest pain and why inflammatory problems may cause pain only when the inflammation spreads to the visceral pleura.

PULMONARY PAIN

The lung parenchyma and the visceral pleura are insensitive to most painful stimuli, and interference with stretch fibers tends to cause most intrapulmonary symptoms. Pain can arise from the parietal pleura, the major airways, the chest wall, the diaphragm, and the mediastinal structures. Inflammatory conditions affecting the lung periphery or the peripheral portions of either hemidiaphragm cause chest wall pain when the process extends to the parietal pleura and stimulates the intercostal nerves. Inflammation of the parietal pleura that lines the more central portions of the diaphragm stimulates the phrenic nerves, with the result that the pain is referred to the ipsilateral neck or shoulder. The augmentation of pulmonary pain during inhalation is attributable to the stretching of the inflamed pleura. Airway pain can be described as a burning pain, whereas mediastinal pain is a dull, central type of discomfort. For example, about 50% of patients with mediastinal metastatic disease describe this type of symptom.

PULMONARY EMBOLUS

Most cases of pulmonary embolism do not exhibit chest pain. If the embolism is big, chest tightness can be present, but most of the symptoms are related to circulatory disturbances. If pain is associated with acute pulmonary embolism, it is thought to result from distention of the central pulmonary artery or

Box 21-1 Causes of Chest Pain

Cardiac System
Myocardial infarction
Myocardial ischemia
   Angina pectoris
   Variant angina
   Syndrome X: microvascular angina in setting of non–insulin-
     dependent diabetes mellitus, dyslipidemia, and central
     obesity
   Myocarditis
Aortic dissection
Pericarditis (infections, Dressler syndrome)
Aortic stenosis
Syphilitic aortitis
Takayasu aortitis
Myocarditis
Hypertrophic cardiomyopathy

Pulmonary System
Pleurisy
Tracheobronchitis
Tumor
Pneumothorax
Pulmonary embolus (with or without infarction)
Pulmonary hypertension

Gastrointestinal System
Esophageal reflux
Esophageal dysmotility (e.g., spasm, achalasia, hyperactive lower
   sphincter)
Esophageal rupture
Peptic ulcer disease
Biliary colic
Pancreatitis
Splenic or hepatic flexure syndrome

Musculoskeletal Conditions
Costochondritis
Subacromial bursitis
Biceps, supraspinatus, or deltoid tendinitis
Shoulder or spinal arthritis
Intercostal muscle cramps
Hyperabduction or strain of the anterior scalene or rectus
   abdominis muscles
Fibromyalgia
Slipping rib syndrome (pain at the costochondral junction,
   generally affecting the eighth, ninth, or tenth rib; may be
   posttraumatic)
Rib fractures
Sternal marrow pain (with acute leukemia)

Neurologic Conditions
Neuritis-radiculitis (cervical compression, herpes zoster infection)
Brachial plexus involvement (cervical rib, spasm of the scalenus
   anterior, Pancoast tumors)

Others
Breast inflammation
Chest wall tumors
Mondor syndrome (thrombophlebitis of the superficial thoracic
   veins)
Diaphragm spasm
Mediastinal emphysema
Mediastinitis
Panic attacks
Hyperventilation syndrome

Box 21-2 Potential Causes of Chest Pain Other Than Angina

Cardiovascular
Aortic dissection; pericarditis

Pulmonary
Pulmonary embolism or infarction, pneumothorax, pneumonia,
   pleuritic pain

Gastroesophageal
Esophageal spasm and/or reflux, esophageal rupture, biliary
   inflammatory conditions, pancreatitis, peptic ulceration

Chest Wall
Costochondritis, fractured rib, rib/spinal metastases, herpes zoster,
   fibrositis, muscular strain

Pericardial
Inflammatory, neoplasia, post–myocardial infarction (Dressler
   syndrome), postirradiation, drug-induced, connective tissue
   disorders

Psychiatric
Anxiety disorders (panic, hyperventilation), depression, thought
   disorders and fixations

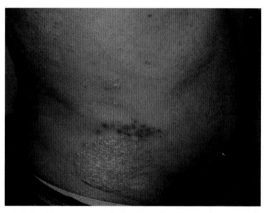

Figure 21-1 Herpes zoster infection affecting an intercostal nerve.

arteries. Pain occurring later in the illness is attributable to infarction of a peripheral segment of lung and occurs with concomitant inflammation of the adjacent pleura.

PULMONARY HYPERTENSION

The pain of chronic pulmonary hypertension is attributed to the disparity between right ventricular myocardial O_2 supply and demand, although vascular distention also may play a part.

MUSCULOSKELETAL PAIN

Costochondral and chondrosternal articulations are common sites of anterior and anterolateral chest pain. The articulations of the second, third, and fourth ribs are most commonly involved. When accompanied by swelling, redness, and heat, the condition is referred to as Tietze syndrome. Coughing or trauma can dislocate the costochondral junctions (most commonly those of ribs 10 to 12). The pain resulting from intercostal neuritis most frequently results from cervical osteoarthritis. Intercostal neuritis also is seen with herpes zoster infection, in which the onset of pain may precede the typical rash by 1 or 2 days (**Figure 21-1**). Thoracic roots most commonly are involved.

Subacromial bursitis, biceps or deltoid tendinitis, and arthritis of the shoulder can manifest as chest pain with extension to the shoulder and arm. The brachial plexus and subclavian artery can be compressed by a cervical rib, or by spasm of the scalenus anticus muscle. In the Pancoast syndrome (most commonly but not exclusively caused by bronchogenic carcinoma), invasion of the C8, T1, and T2 nerve roots by tumor may be the cause of considerable pain and other symptoms such as muscular weakness (**Figure 21-2**).

ESOPHAGEAL REFLUX OR DYSMOTILITY

The chest pain resulting from esophageal reflux or dysmotility (e.g., esophageal spasm, achalasia, hyperactive lower sphincter) results from acid irritation of the esophageal mucosa. Esophageal reflux or dysmotility accounts for the chest pain that

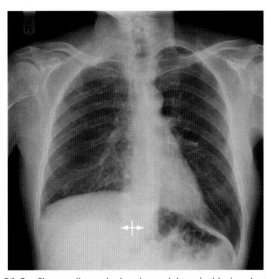

Figure 21-2   Chest radiograph showing a right apical lesion destroying the posterior parts of the first and second rib, with a soft tissue mass extending into the neck.

occurs in as many as 30% of patients with normal findings on a coronary arteriogram.

PATIENT EVALUATION

The approach to patients complaining of chest pain should focus initially on the potentially lethal causes of the symptom, especially in the emergency department or similar setting (**Figure 21-3**). Severe pain is more commonly associated with life-threatening causes, but any of these conditions may occur with minimal symptoms. Accordingly, patients frequently are treated as if the chest pain were life-threatening until these more serious conditions can be excluded by studies that yield more specific information than that obtainable at the time of the initial presentation.

CLINICAL PRESENTATION

If the pain is acute (and therefore generally of short duration) and the patient is hypotensive, myocardial infarction, pulmonary embolism, pericardial tamponade, dissecting aneurysm, and tension pneumothorax should be considered first (see Figure 21-3). Less commonly, this clinical syndrome can result from a ruptured esophagus, which not infrequently is missed because it is rare and the emergency physician may be reassured by normal findings on cardiac evaluation. In other patients, the approach is governed primarily by the findings on history and physical examination, which are interpreted on the basis of actual or estimated previous probabilities for each of the conditions listed in Box 21-1. For example, a middle-aged man with one or more risk factors for coronary artery disease (e.g., hypercholesterolemia, diabetes, hypertension, obesity, smoking) who experiences exertional chest pain typical for coronary artery disease that abates with rest has a greater than 90% probability of having myocardial ischemia as the cause of his symptoms. By contrast, a 20-year-old pregnant woman with a chest infection, cough, and localized chest pain is far more likely to have a spontaneous rib fracture.

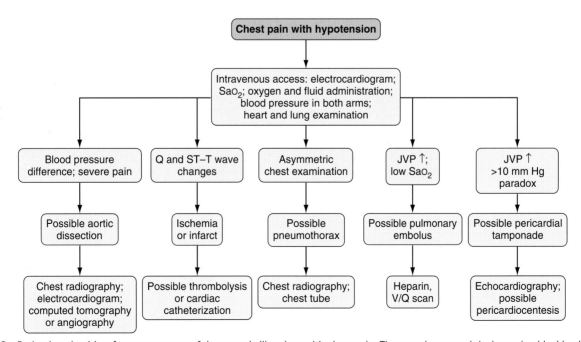

Figure 21-3   Evaluation algorithm for management of the severely ill patient with chest pain. Therapeutic approach is determined by blood pressure and findings on brief examination of the neck, chest, and head. *JVP*, jugular venous pressure; *SaO₂*, arterial oxygen pressure; *V/Q*, ventilation-perfusion.

HISTORY

The onset, duration, location, radiation pattern, character, and intensity of the pain should be ascertained, as should the factors that precipitate or diminish it. Unfortunately, both the sensitivity and specificity of the history are low for many of the conditions that must be considered in the differential diagnosis. For example, most episodes of electrocardiographically documented ischemia in patients with stable angina are asymptomatic. A history of cocaine, crack, or other stimulating drug use should be sought.

Cardiovascular Disorders

The pain of *myocardial ischemia* frequently is described as a dull pain accompanied by a sensation of tightness, pressure, squeezing, or heaviness in the chest. It characteristically radiates down the ulnar aspect of the left arm, but radiation to the neck or jaw also occurs. The pain develops gradually; occurs in association with exertion, emotional distress, or large meals; and abates within 2 to 10 minutes after the stressful activity is curtailed or within 5 minutes of administration of nitroglycerin.

The pain associated with *myocardial infarction* is of greater intensity and lasts longer. In addition, it can be associated with nausea (particularly with inferior infarctions), diaphoresis, hypotension, or arrhythmias and is not relieved by nitroglycerin.

Variant or *Prinzmetal angina* occurs in the early morning and at rest, rather than during stress, and results from coronary artery spasm. Patients with this type of angina frequently have other vasomotor symptoms such as migraine headaches or Raynaud phenomenon. Angina that occurs with a progressively lesser degree of exertion is considered unstable and is thought to be secondary to rupture of an atherosclerotic plaque with thrombin formation and coronary vasospasm.

Pericardial pain may be pleuritic in nature but more commonly is steady, worsens when the patient is recumbent or lying on the left side, and lessens when the patient sits up and leans forward. The pain often is centrally situated and radiates symmetrically to the upper portion of the trapezius muscles. The pain can be pleuritic if the adjacent parietal pleura is involved in the inflammatory process. Pericardial pain can radiate to the shoulder, neck, flank, or epigastrium. Because inflammatory causes are common, the history may include viral infection–type symptoms—myalgia, fever, and malaise. Similarly, in patients with known malignant disease, the main considerations in the differential diagnosis should be pericardial effusion and tamponade due to dissemination of an adenocarcinoma. Connective tissue disorders—rheumatoid arthritis, systemic lupus erythematosus, polymyositis, dermatomyositis, and scleroderma—also can be associated with pericardial pain.

The pain of a *dissecting aortic aneurysm* begins abruptly, becomes extremely severe within seconds or minutes, and radiates to the back, abdomen, neck, flank, and legs. It commonly is described as "tearing" and may be associated with an acute cerebrovascular event; a cold, pulseless extremity; and aortic insufficiency. Unusually large amounts of analgesic agents generally are needed to provide relief.

Pulmonary Inflammation and Chest Wall Problems

Many adjectives have been used by afflicted persons to describe the pain resulting from conditions that cause pulmonary inflammation or chest wall problems, but the pain is almost always pleuritic in nature in that it increases with forced

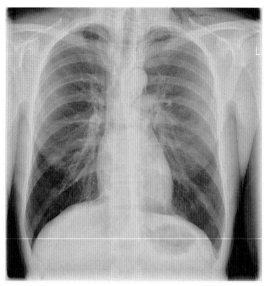

Figure 21-4   Chest radiograph obtained in patient with retrosternal pain of sudden onset. The image shows a pneumomediastinum, with air at the left heart border and around the aortic knuckle.

inhalation or exhalation (e.g., during coughing or sneezing), during spontaneous breathing, and when pressure is applied to the chest wall by bending or lying down. In response to the pleuritic or positional character of the pain, patients frequently limit their depth of inhalation and, accordingly, may complain of dyspnea, rather than or in addition to pain.

An abrupt onset suggests a rib fracture, pneumothorax, or pneumomediastinum (**Figure 21-4**). A more gradual onset over a few minutes or hours is seen with bacterial pneumonia and pulmonary emboli, and a gradual onset (e.g., days or weeks) is more compatible with chronic infections (e.g., tuberculosis, fungal infections) or tumor.

Patients with chronic obstructive pulmonary disease who experience an acute exacerbation of bronchitis frequently describe a burning type of chest pain that localizes to the substernal region. A similar symptom can occur in otherwise normal subjects in the setting of tracheobronchitis or during the hyperventilation that accompanies heavy exercise, particularly if the exercise is done in a cold environment.

In many instances, patients with costochondral pain or pain that results from muscle strains describe an episode of chest trauma or unusual upper extremity exercise (e.g., gardening, digging, scraping) that can result in an overuse syndrome. More commonly, no specific inciting event can be determined. The costosternal articulations are common "trigger sites" for the pain of fibromyalgia. Patients with this syndrome also have trigger sites in other locations (**Figure 21-5**). Musculoskeletal conditions generally are exacerbated by deep breathing and frequently are overlooked as causes of pleuritic or exercise-induced chest pain. The patient often can localize the painful area, where tenderness or muscular spasm may be elicited by palpation.

Intercostal neuritis commonly is described as being pleuritic. One potentially distinguishing characteristic is that patients may describe abrupt, electric shock–like sensations occurring in the same distribution as for the pleuritic pain.

Bursitis, Tendinitis, and Arthritis

Subacromial bursitis, biceps and deltoid tendinitis, and arthritis of the shoulder can manifest as chest pain with extension to

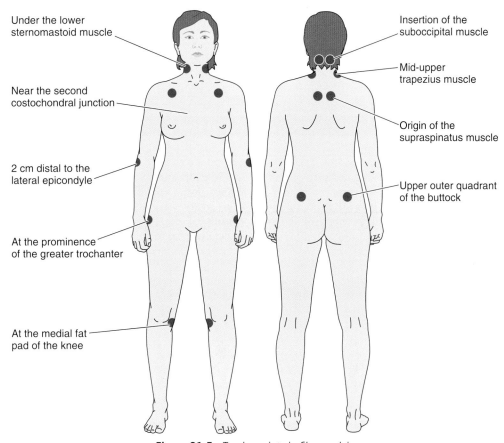

Under the lower
sternomastoid muscle

Near the second
costochondral junction

2 cm distal to the
lateral epicondyle

At the prominence
of the greater trochanter

At the medial fat
pad of the knee

Insertion of the
suboccipital muscle

Mid-upper
trapezius muscle

Origin of the
supraspinatus muscle

Upper outer quadrant
of the buttock

Figure 21-5 Tender points in fibromyalgia.

the shoulder and arm. In these conditions, the pain is worse with neck or shoulder movement but is not exercise-related.

Gastrointestinal Disorders

Like angina, the pain of esophageal reflux or dysmotility is located substernally; can radiate to the throat, neck, or left arm; and may be relieved by nitroglycerin. Unlike angina, however, the pain is rarely associated with exertion. Rather, it is exacerbated by bending, stooping, drinking alcohol, or lying supine and frequently is worse in the early morning, in association with acidic gastric secretions. Chest pain from esophageal reflux or spasm typically lasts for 1 hour or longer and may be relieved to a variable degree by sitting upright or by ingesting antacids or food. The history also may be positive for odynophagia, dysphagia, or regurgitation of undigested food.

Esophageal rupture is a life-threatening condition if not recognized rapidly and repaired. It can occur in otherwise healthy persons, in whom it may follow an episode of choking while swallowing, or violent or prolonged vomiting. It usually is accompanied by a distinct acute central episode of chest pain, sweating, and then hypotensive symptoms, with onset of pleuritic pain as gastric fluid leaks into the chest cavity. Dysphagia also may be pronounced. A CT scan with a contrast swallow can be diagnostic, showing air to have leaked into the mediastinum (**Figure 21-6**).

The pain associated with peptic ulcer disease, biliary colic, or pancreatitis generally begins 1 or 2 hours after eating. Pain associated with peptic ulcer disease may lessen or worsen with eating. The pain associated with biliary colic and pancreatitis frequently is accompanied by nausea and vomiting.

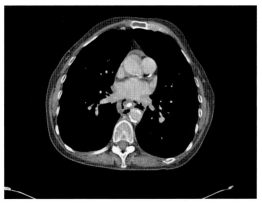

Figure 21-6 Computed tomography (CT) scan performed with contrast swallow shows the esophagus with air surrounding it in the mediastinum. This appearance is highly suggestive of esophageal rupture.

PSYCHIATRIC DISORDERS

Psychiatric disorders should always be considered only if physical explanations have been exhausted. Of note, however, chest pain is a well-recognized manifestation of anxiety, as, for example, in a patient with a near relative of emotional importance (i.e., with whom the patient identifies) who has suffered a heart attack. Depression can produce a myriad of physical symptoms, as can fixative ideology. It often can be most useful to ask the sufferer of chest pain about a particular anxiety regarding the cause of the pain, or if the person knows someone with a similar symptom.

PHYSICAL EXAMINATION

Although the physical examination may provide a number of clues, the findings may be entirely normal even when the pain results from a life-threatening condition. Shallow, more rapid respirations may suggest pleural inflammation or a musculoskeletal cause of pain. Cyanosis may suggest hypoxemia from a variety of pulmonary or cardiac problems. Xanthelasma and tuberous xanthomas suggest the presence of coronary disease. The onset of clubbing heralds intrapulmonary pathology, as may the finding of significant lymphadenopathy.

In addition to the standard vital signs, blood pressure should be measured in *both* upper extremities, because a disparity would suggest aortic dissection. Heart rate and rhythm abnormalities suggest acute ischemia or pulmonary embolism. Fever points away from musculoskeletal pain and suggests pneumonia, pulmonary embolus, pancreatitis, or biliary obstruction. Patients with myocardial infarction may be febrile, but the temperature rarely exceeds 38° C.

Elevated jugular venous pressure, abnormalities in the carotid upstroke, crackles, a pleural or pericardial rub, signs of parenchymal consolidation, gallop rhythms, paradoxical or fixed splitting or an increased intensity of the pulmonary component of the second heart sound, and cardiac murmurs have a high specificity for many of the cardiopulmonary disorders associated with chest pain. The sensitivity of these physical findings probably is low, however, because the physical examination may be entirely normal in patients with severe ischemia, pulmonary emboli, and many of the gastrointestinal causes of pain.

Attempts can be made to reproduce or exacerbate the pain by moving the patient's arms and shoulders and by thoroughly palpating the chest wall, particularly over the peristernal region and the costochondral junctions, as well as the subacromial bursae, the deltoid tendons, the shoulders, and the abdomen. Asking the patient to perform the maneuvers that produce the pain also can be helpful.

Intercostal neuritis frequently is associated with hyperalgesia or anesthesia over the distribution of affected intercostal nerves. Biliary colic and pancreatitis frequently are associated with right upper quadrant and midline abdominal tenderness, respectively. Clearly, it is vital not to miss important physical disease in the chest wall. Careful, gentle palpation with both hands over the skin, musculature, ribs, and vertebrae may identify tender areas that signify a serious problem (**Figure 21-7,** *A* and *B*).

DIAGNOSTIC TESTS

Patients without a previous diagnosis of coronary artery disease are not likely to have an acute myocardial infarction as the explanation for the acute onset of chest pain if the pain does not radiate to the neck, left shoulder, or arm and if the electrocardiogram and serial serum troponin levels are normal. Although the finding of flat or downsloping ST segment depression greater than 0.1 mV increases the likelihood that an episode of chest pain is caused by myocardial ischemia, the tracing may be normal at rest, between attacks, or even in the presence of active ischemia. Up to 80% of patients with coronary disease exhibit these ST segment changes during exercise, but such changes also may be found in up to 15% of patients with no evidence of disease at cardiac catheterization. Nonspecific ST-T wave changes have been documented in the setting of acute cholecystitis and esophageal spasm, as well as in other conditions for which chest pain is a presenting symptom (**Table 21-1**).

Chest radiographs should be obtained in all patients with chest pain unless a clear-cut musculoskeletal cause of the pain

Table 21-1	Electrocardiographic Findings in Conditions Manifesting with Chest Pain
Condition	**Electrocardiographic Finding(s)**
Acute cholecystitis	Inferior ST segment elevation
Pulmonary embolism	Inferior ST segment elevation
Dissecting aortic aneurysm	ST segment elevation ST segment depression
Pneumothorax	Poor R wave progression Acute QRS axis shift
Pericarditis	ST segment elevation (generally diffuse)
Myocarditis	ST segment elevation

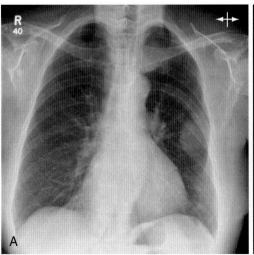
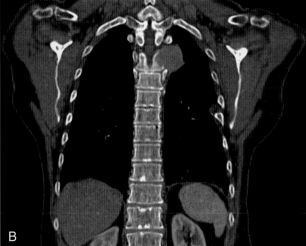

Figure 21-7 A, Chest radiography showing two soft tissue masses originating from bone. Clinical findings included tenderness on the left side of the chest and over the upper thoracic spine. **B,** Coronal computed tomography (CT) image showing the soft tissue mass invading and destroying a thoracic vertebra.

is evident on clinical evaluation. With myocardial ischemia or infarction, the chest radiograph may be entirely normal in appearance. Alternatively, it may reveal pulmonary edema, upper lobe vascular redistribution, valvular disease, or pericardial disease.

Chest radiographs may be normal-appearing in the setting of acute pulmonary emboli, although minor degrees of atelectasis, small effusions, or distention of the central pulmonary vessels may be seen. A small or an apical pneumothorax can be difficult to see, but if this lesion is suspected, a film exposed with the patient in full expiration will make it much larger and obvious. Careful radiographic review of all ribs should identify a fracture, most commonly located in the lower ribs if due to coughing. Local rib tenderness always warrants a chest radiograph (**Figure 21-8**). Anatomic anomalies such as a cervical rib, which may be the cause of root pain, should be looked for as appropriate. If pleuritic pain is associated with minor change, such as the obliteration of a costophrenic angle, obtaining a follow-up radiograph 24 hours later may show obvious development of the cause of chest pain. Pericardial causes of pain will become evident only if an effusion is gathering by causing the cardiac outline to enlarge; an effusion also may be a sign of malignant disease elsewhere within the chest, or of joint disease in connective tissue disorders.

A widened mediastinum or an apical effusion on films exposed with the patient in the supine position (**Figure 21-9**) suggests the possibility of a ruptured aortic aneurysm.

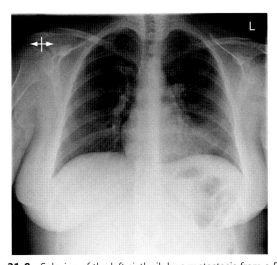

Figure 21-8 Splaying of the left sixth rib by a metastasis from a Ewing sarcoma manifesting as a soft tissue mass. The patient was a young man who presented with vague chest pain.

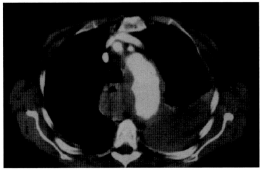

Figure 21-9 Aortic aneurysm. Chest computed tomography (CT) scan showing a dissecting aortic aneurysm.

A set of routine blood tests should be performed to identify abnormality of white cell count or renal or liver function an abnormality here may focus further investigations as appropriate. In addition, troponin T increases 4 to 12 hours after myocardial infarction and is a better predictor of acute infarction than creatine kinase–MB, because the latter increases in both infarction and ischemia. Troponin T can increase as a result of rhabdomyolysis in absence of ischemia, however. A normal result on D-dimer assay excludes pulmonary embolism for all practical purposes in all patients except those believed to be at high risk for this condition.

Computed tomography can be diagnostic for pulmonary embolism (especially when performed as a CT pulmonary angiogram), as well as for pneumothorax, esophageal rupture, pericardial disease, small pleural effusions, superior sulcus tumors, and mediastinal disease.

TREATMENT

Pharmacotherapy for patients with myocardial infarction or an acute coronary syndrome (e.g., patients with unstable angina or those with myocardial infarction but without non–ST segment elevation) includes aspirin, nitrates, β-adrenergic blockers, and low-molecular-weight heparin. Further details of management of these clinical entities are beyond the scope of this discussion.

The acute pericarditis that occurs in the setting of large myocardial infarctions generally responds to aspirin. Nonsteroidal antiinflammatory agents or corticosteroids may be contraindicated, because these agents slow the rate at which myocardial scar formation occurs and, therefore, may be associated with an increased frequency of myocardial rupture. The pain associated with Dressler syndrome (i.e., pericarditis developing 1 to 2 months after an infarction in association with fever, leukocytosis, and elevations of antimyocardial antibodies) is treated with nonsteroidal antiinflammatory agents. Systemic corticosteroids may be needed in more severe cases.

The pain associated with pulmonary inflammation may respond to nonsteroidal antiinflammatory agents, although opiates occasionally are needed. The pain associated with pneumothorax may be quickly replaced by that associated with the chest tube, and opiates may be required, to circumvent "guarding"-induced limitation of chest wall movement, with associated risk of respiratory infection.

In addition to elevating the head of the bed (or use of the reverse Trendelenburg position in markedly obese subjects), the pain associated with esophageal reflux also may be reduced by avoiding food or liquid intake before reclining, eliminating substances known to reduce the lower esophageal sphincter pressure (e.g., coffee, chocolate, alcohol, mint), and the use of antacids, calcium channel blockers, histamine H_2 receptor antagonists, metoclopramide, nitroglycerin, or proton pump inhibitors. Gastroplasty may be indicated in selected patients. Esophageal dysmotility has been treated with long-acting nitrates and calcium-channel blockers. Antacids, proton pump inhibitors, H_2 antagonists, sucralfate, and agents effective against *Helicobacter pylori* may be needed to eliminate the pain associated with peptic ulcer disease. The pain of pancreatitis generally requires narcotics. Meperidine is favored over other opiates, because it does not contract the sphincter of Oddi. Intractable pain is a common indication for surgical or invasive endoscopic approaches.

Patients with musculoskeletal pain can be treated with nonsteroidal antiinflammatory agents or the stretching exercises that are used in physical therapy. The chest pain associated with fibromyalgia may be relieved with use of amitriptyline. Most chest physicians see large numbers of patients with musculoskeletal pain, which can continue for months; an essential component of management of such patients is reassurance that the symptom is self-limiting and will go away over time. In some instances, a CT examination may be necessary to demonstrate the absence of a specific cause for the pain. Whiplash-associated pains within the chest and pain caused by seatbelts after road traffic accidents are common and can last for months; initial management should consist of reassurance, with regular analgesia only in the early days after the trauma. Long-term antiinflammatory medication is associated with its own problems, so physiotherapy, ultrasound, and graded exercise programs are very useful and important in this clinical scenario.

The pain associated with herpes zoster infections may be so severe as to require narcotics for control. Amitriptyline and fluphenazine also have been used, as have systemic corticosteroids.

SUGGESTED READINGS

Atar S, Barbagelata A, Birnbaum Y: Electrocardiographic diagnosis of ST-elevation myocardial infarction, *Cardiol Clin* 24:343–365, 2006.

Cayley WE Jr: Diagnosing the cause of chest pain, *Am Fam Physician* 72:2012–2021, 2005.

Eiseneman A: Troponin assays for the diagnosis of myocardial infarction and acute coronary syndrome: where do we stand? *Expert Rev Cardiovasc Ther* 4:509–514, 2006.

Fletcher GF, Mills WX, Taylor WC: Update on exercise stress testing, *Am Fam Physician* 74:1749–1754, 2006.

Fox M, Forgacs I: Unexplained (non-cardiac) chest pain, *Clin Med* 6:445–449, 2006.

Haro LH, Decker WW, Boie ET, Wright RS: Initial approach to the patient who has chest pain, *Cardiol Clin* 24:1–17, 2006.

Jones JH, Weir WB: Cocaine-induced chest pain, *Clin Lab Med* 26:127–146, 2006.

Schoepf UJ, Savino G, Lake DR, et al: The age of CT pulmonary angiography, *J Thorac Imaging* 20:273–279, 2005.

Tutuian R: Update in the diagnosis of gastroesophageal reflux disease, *J Gastrointest Liver Dis* 15:243–247, 2006.

Winters ME, Katzen SM: Identifying chest pain emergencies in the primary care setting, *Primary Care* 33:625–642, 2006.

Chapter **22**
Pulmonary Host Defenses
Theo J. Moraes • Chung-Wai Chow • Gregory P. Downey

The epithelial surface of the lung is continuously exposed to a variety of potentially pathogenic microorganisms, allergens, particulate pollutants, and other noxious agents. An intricate defense system has evolved over time to protect the lungs from these potentially harmful entities while preserving homeostasis and lung function (**Figure 22-1**). This system of defense mechanisms has two components: an innate (nonspecific) response and an adaptive or acquired (specific) response.

The *innate* immune response is evolutionarily conserved to provide immediate (occurring over seconds to minutes) host defense in a broad, nonspecific manner. Only vertebrates have an additional, *adaptive* immune system, which is directed at specific pathogens or molecules. Although the two systems work in concert to protect the host, each has several distinctive features. With rare exceptions, the innate component of the immune system depends on proteins and signaling pathways that exist in a fully functional form, does not require priming, and is not strengthened with subsequent exposures. By contrast, the adaptive immune response requires additional time (days to weeks) (see **Figures 22-2** and **22-3**) to ramp up to full capacity, is specific to the pathogen (and even to specific molecular determinants of the pathogen), and has memory to provide for stronger responses with subsequent attacks ("anamnestic response").

Together, these immune responses provide a formidable force to combat invading pathogenic microbes, as indicated by the rarity with which healthy humans succumb to lung infections. Specific components of the innate and adaptive host defense mechanisms are reviewed in this chapter.

STRUCTURAL DEFENSES

With a surface area in adults of 70 m^2, which comes into contact with roughly 10,000 L of air a day, the lung is confronted with constant threats from microbes. In addition to inhaled pathogens, high bacterial concentrations are present in oropharyngeal secretions (10^8/mL), and aspiration of these secretions also may pose a serious risk for invasive infection (aspiration pneumonia). Historically, the lung has been considered to be a sterile environment; recent developments in molecular analysis have provided evidence for the presence of a microbial flora of considerable diversity in the lung, which moreover is altered in disease states. Accordingly, the respiratory tract has developed a series of structural barriers that are designed both to minimize the number of pathogenic microbes entering the lungs and to hasten their clearance before an infection can be established (**Table 22-1**).

Particle size is an important factor determining the degree of penetration into the airways (**Table 22-2**). Very large particles are filtered by vibrissae (nasal hairs). Particles approximately 30 μm in diameter are removed in the nasal passages, where turbulent airflow results in prolonged air-mucosa contact, with subsequent particle impaction. Most particles between 10 and 30 μm in diameter also will be deposited on the turbinates and nasal septum, carina, or within the larger bronchi. The branching nature of the airways provides two additional mechanisms of protection: (1) the secondary, tertiary, and quaternary carinae force particles to embed in the airway mucosa, thereby preventing further penetration into the lung, and (2) reduced airflow with increased airway branching allows gravity to sediment most particles larger than 2 μm. Particles less than 0.2 to 0.5 μm across tend to stay suspended as aerosols and are exhaled. Much smaller particles (less than 0.1 μm) may be deposited as a result of brownian motion (bombardment with gas molecules).

Thus, only particles roughly between 2 and 0.2 μm in diameter will reach the alveoli. Unfortunately, most bacteria are from 0.5 to 2 μm in size and, when inhaled, may reach the terminal bronchioles, where they have the potential to establish an infection. Some exceptionally pathogenic bacteria require exceedingly small numbers (e.g., only 2 to 50 organisms) to establish infection.

In addition to particle size, other factors such as shape, charge, and state of hydration may influence the depth of penetration. For example, the grass heads of timothy grass, or *Alternaria*, can penetrate deeper into the lung than would be expected from their physical size.

NARES

The efficiency of the nose in filtering inspired air and trapping aerosolized particles has been highlighted by inhaled drug delivery studies that demonstrate better pulmonary drug deposition with mouth inhalers than with mask inhalers. Nasal congestion and increased mucus production also contribute to trapping of unwanted particles or microbes, preventing them from going further into the airways.

In addition to filtration, the nose functions to warm and humidify inspired air, thus protecting cells from physical stress and ensuring optimal performance of the mucociliary system. Olfaction also is protective, because sniffing allows potentially harmful gases to be detected before they contact the lower airways.

As noted previously, however, the upper respiratory tract may be a source of infection when aspiration of small amounts of upper airway secretions leads to compromise of the host pulmonary system. Microbial colonization is normal, and although potential pathogens can be isolated from the

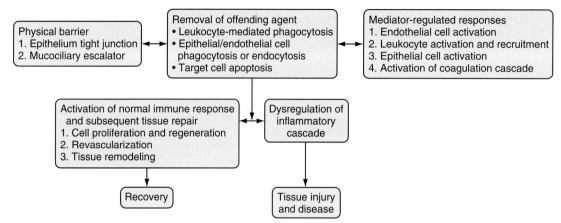

Figure 22-1 Pulmonary host defense. The pulmonary host defense system is composed of multiple components, including physical barriers such as the nose and mucous layer that lines the airways. Mechanisms also exist to remove offending microbial pathogens or noxious particles, either directly by phagocytosis or endocytosis or indirectly by mediator-regulated responses. Activation of the immune and inflammatory responses usually will facilitate resolution of the injury and clinical recovery of the patient. However, if these immune and inflammatory responses are excessive or unregulated, tissue injury and disease ensue.

Figure 22-2 Timeline of pulmonary host defense mechanisms—immediate, early (seconds to hours), and late (hours to days)—that serve to protect the lung.

Figure 22-3 Interactions among the different pulmonary host defense mechanisms—immediate, early, and late. These defense mechanisms augment the immune and inflammatory responses. *TLR*, Toll-like receptor.

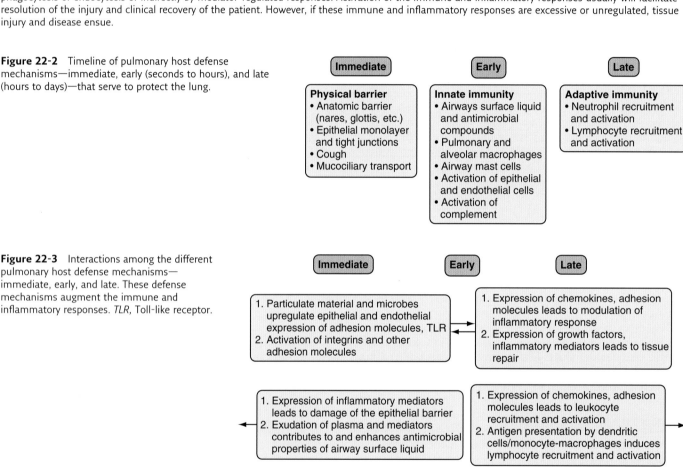

nasopharynx of healthy persons, under normal conditions, resident flora competitively inhibit the growth of pathogens.

COUGH/SNEEZE

Mechanical or chemical stimulation of receptors in the nose, larynx, or trachea or elsewhere in the respiratory tree may produce bronchoconstriction to prevent deeper penetration of irritants and also may trigger the cough or sneeze reflex to expel particles deposited in the airways (**Table 22-3**). The cough reflex aids mucociliary transport to remove trapped particles. Mucus usually is conveyed to the carina by the cilia and then expelled by coughing from this location. Disruption of the

cough reflex (e.g., in smokers or patients with vocal cord palsy or stroke) results in a predisposition to pneumonias.

GLOTTIS

The digestive tract and the respiratory tract share both an embryologic origin and an opening to the external world (the mouth). The glottis protects the lungs from potential contamination of the airways with digestive tract material. Nevertheless, small amounts of aspiration do occur from the nasopharynx and oropharynx or esophagus in healthy people, usually without pathologic consequences. Of importance, frequent aspiration or episodes of aspiration of large amounts of material, as is seen

Table 22-1 Structural Defenses of the Airway

Structure	Functions
Nose	Filters air Warms and humidifies air Sediments particles Olfaction Sneeze reflex
Glottis	Protects from gastrointestinal and nasopharyngeal contamination Cough reflex
Mucociliary escalator	Traps foreign particles Facilitates physical removal of particles
Epithelium	Barrier to microbes Mucociliary escalator Production of antimicrobial factors Cytokine production Adhesion molecule expression

Table 22-2 Effect of Particle Size on Penetration into Airways

Particle Size	Fate
>>>30 μm	Filtered by vibrissae
>30 μm	Nasopharyngeal impaction
10 to 30 μm	Nasopharyngeal, tracheal, and large bronchial impaction
2 to 10 μm	Sedimentation in airways
0.2 to 2 μm	Reach alveoli
0.2 to 0.5 μm	Exhaled
<0.2 μm	Exhaled or deposited (brownian motion)

Table 22-3 Phases of Cough/Sneeze

Component	Event(s)
1. Inspiratory phase	Deep inspiration, usually 1 to 2 times tidal volume
2. Compression phase	Begins with closure of the glottis and contraction of respiratory muscles, resulting in the generation of high intrathoracic pressure (up to 100 to 200 cm H_2O in adults)
3. Expressive phase	Glottal opening, with airflow at rates as high as 25,000 cm/sec (partly helped by compression of airway cross section)
4. Relaxation phase	Relaxation of respiratory muscles with temporary bronchodilatation

in persons with glottic dysfunction, can lead to bacterial pneumonia and chemical pneumonitis and possibly contribute to pulmonary fibrosis.

RESPIRATORY EPITHELIUM

The respiratory epithelium is a highly effective barrier to microbes. Conducting airways are lined with pseudostratified columnar epithelial cells that become cuboidal as the branches extend to the alveoli. Specialized structures termed tight junctions separate the epithelial monolayer into apical (luminal) and basolateral components that form an important barrier to the passive passage of molecules and microbes from the airway lumen or alveolar space.

In addition to this important physical barrier function, epithelial cells, including ciliated cells, goblet cells, serous cells, basal cells, and Clara cells, are integral to the normal function of the mucociliary escalator, the production of a variety of antimicrobial molecules, and the initiation and regulation of inflammatory responses (see Figure 22-4).

MUCOCILIARY ESCALATOR

The airway epithelium is lined from the trachea to the respiratory bronchioles by the airway surface liquid (ASL), a 5- to 25-μm-thick surface film the primary function of which is to trap and facilitate the physical removal of foreign particles, as well as to provide an environment conducive to the activity of antimicrobial molecules (Table 22-4).

ASL is a critical component of the mucociliary escalator and is the result of secretion by glands and serous cells and of plasma transudation (Table 22-5). The inner low-viscosity periciliary sol facilitates the coordinated beating action of the cilia that propels the outer viscous mucous blanket toward the glottis, thereby facilitating the removal of trapped pathogens or particles by expectoration or ingestion. The viscous mucus is composed of mucopolysaccharides, produced predominantly by submucous glands in the larger airways, with increasing contributions from goblet cells and Clara cells with successively larger airway generations.

Dysfunction of the ASL is seen in conditions such as asthma and chronic bronchitis, in which excessive mucus is produced, resulting in airway obstruction. In cystic fibrosis, defects in ion transport are thought to reduce ASL volume, thus increasing viscosity of the mucus. This altered environment impairs mucociliary clearance and predisposes the lungs to bacterial colonization, highlighting the importance of the antimicrobial function of normal ASL.

The cilia are the second key component of the mucociliary escalator and are present from the upper airways down to the terminal bronchioles. There are approximately 200 cilia per ciliated cell. Each of these protuberances is approximately 6 μm long and 0.2 μm in diameter. The cilia are arranged longitudinally to coordinate a beating activity of 500 to 1500 beats/minute, which serves to efficiently propel the mucous layer. Abnormal ciliary function may be related to primary ciliary dyskinesia (most frequently consequent to defects in the microtubule structure of the cilia) and predisposes the lungs in affected persons to development of pneumonia and bronchiectasis. In turn, bronchiectasis, whether associated with genetic causes such as cystic fibrosis or arising as an acquired condition such as sequelae of pulmonary infections, including pulmonary tuberculosis, can lead to localized ciliary dysfunction.

Although these structural components of the respiratory system are not formally considered to be part of the immune system, together they nonetheless constitute a vital and early component of the microbial defense systems of the lung.

SPECIFIC CELL RESPONSES

Diverse cell populations contribute to the host defense system of the lung. In addition to the cells of the respiratory

Table 22-4	Properties of the Mucociliary Escalator	
Structure	**Function(s)**	**Dysfunction in Disease**

• Present from trachea down to level of respiratory bronchioles
• 200 cilia per ciliated cell
• Each cilia: 6 μm long and 0.2 μm in diameter
• Thickness of layer: 5-25 μm
  • *Inner layer*: low-viscosity, periciliary solutes
  • *Outer layer*: viscous mucous blanket
	• Traps foreign particles and transports them up and out of respiratory tract
	Transport rate: small airways: 0.5-1 mm/min; large airways and nose: 5-20 mm/min
	• Production of antimicrobial compounds
		• *Smokers*: decreased number of ciliated cells, depressed ciliary functions
		• Bronchiectasis
		• Cystic fibrosis
		• Primary ciliary dyskinesia
		• Stents

Table 22-5	Properties of Airway Surface Liquid (ASL)	
Composition	**Function**	**Dysfunction in Disease**
Secretions from glands and goblet cells Plasma transudation	Antimicrobial properties due to low pH and secreted antimicrobial compounds	Cystic fibrosis Asthma COPD

COPD, chronic obstructive pulmonary disease.

Table 22-6	Cells Mediating Pulmonary Host Defense and the Inflammatory Response	
Timing	**Immune Cells**	**Nonimmune Cells**
Early phase	Monocyte-macrophages Eosinophils Mast cells Neutrophils Natural killer cells	Endothelial cells Epithelial cells
Late phase	Lymphocytes Dendritic cells	Endothelial cells Epithelial cells Fibroblasts Mesenchymal cells

epithelium, these include other structural cells of the lung, the pulmonary vascular endothelium and fibroblasts, resident leukocytes, and, at later stages of immune responses, recruited immune cells (**Table 22-6**), as reviewed next.

EPITHELIAL CELLS

The contribution of the respiratory epithelium is not limited to its roles as a structural barrier and facilitator of mucociliary clearance (**Box 22-1**). Respiratory epithelial cells actively participate in the regulation of inflammation and are capable of mounting an immune response by internalization of organisms and secretion of cytotoxic and antimicrobial peptides. Inhaled microbial pathogens including bacteria and viruses and other antigens can trigger activation of pathogen recognition receptors (such as Toll-like receptors [TLRs], discussed later in some detail under "Innate Immune Receptors") expressed by epithelial cells. Epithelial cells are induced by bacterial components, such as LPS, and by cytokines such as tumor necrosis factor (TNF)-α and interleukin-1β (IL-1β) to express various gene products (by the NFκB signaling pathway, discussed later on) that modulate the inflammatory response (**Figure 22-4**). Such inducers include the following:

- Cytokines such as TNF-α, IL-1β, and thymic stromal lymphopoietin (TSLP)
- Chemokines that include macrophage inflammatory protein (MIP)-2, CXC chemokines, monocyte chemoattractant protein (MCP)-1, IL-7, IL-8, IL-15
- Nitric oxide (NO) and reactive nitrogen species (ONOO⁻)
- Adhesion molecules such as β-integrins and intercellular adhesion molecule-1 (ICAM-1)
- TLRs such as TLR-2 and TLR-4
- TNF-α receptors, TNFR1 and TNFR2
- Growth factor receptors such as epidermal growth factor receptor (EGFR) and platelet-derived growth factor receptor (PDGFR)
- Plasminogen activator receptors

TSLP, also produced by fibroblasts, is thought to aid in the maturation of dendritic cells. Consequently, epithelial products

---

Box 22-1	Immunomodulatory Molecules Secreted by Airway Epithelial Cells

Inflammatory Mediators
Cytokines
Chemokines
Leukotrienes
Calprotectin

Chemotactic Mediators
LL-37/CAP-18
β-Defensins
Chemokines
Leukotrienes

Antimicrobial Substances
β-Defensins
LL-37/CAP-18
Lysozyme
Lactoferrin
Secretory leukocyte proteinase inhibitor (SLPI)
Elafin
Calprotectin
Phospholipase A2
Surfactant proteins SP-A, SP-D
Anionic peptides

CAP-18, cathelicidin antimicrobial protein-18.

---

lead to innate cell (neutrophil) recruitment to limit local infection. Epithelial products can promote dendritic cell maturation and thus induce an adaptive immune response (including memory T cells and neutralizing antibodies). In addition to these molecules, pulmonary epithelial cells also express a number of antimicrobial mediators that are unique to the lung. These include the surfactant proteins SP-A and SP-D (members of the collectin family) and the β-defensins, potent antimicrobial peptides (discussed later on).

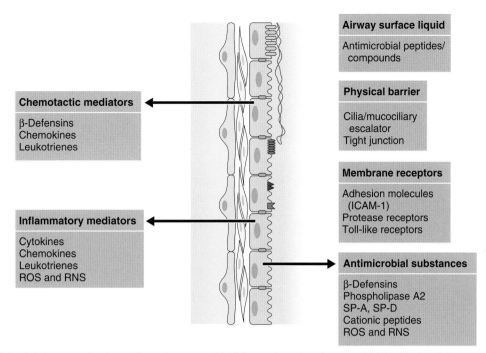

Figure 22-4 Epithelial cell defense mechanisms. The pulmonary epithelial monolayer functions as a highly effective defense system. The different mechanisms are illustrated, including the airway surface liquid that contains potent antimicrobial compounds, the mucous layer, junctions between the epithelial cells, and surface receptors expressed by the epithelial cells. *ICAM*, intracellular adhesion molecule; *RNS*, reactive nitrogen species; *ROS*, reactive oxygen species; *SP-A*, surfactant-associated protein A; *SP-D*, surfactant-associated protein D.

ENDOTHELIAL CELLS

Endothelial cells also play a pivotal role in the regulation of host defense and propagation of the inflammatory response. Like epithelial cells, endothelial cells also form tight junctions that separate the endothelial monolayer into apical and basal surfaces and prevent passive movement of particles and molecules. In addition to this physical barrier, activated endothelial cells modulate the expression of numerous proteins involved in different pathways that contribute to host defense. These include the following:

- Reactive nitrogen and oxygen species, including nitric oxide (NO•), peroxynitrite (ONOO⁻), superoxide (O₂⁻), and hydrogen peroxide (H₂O₂), which are cytotoxic to microorganisms and cells
- Inflammatory cytokines such as TNF-α, IL-1β, and IL-6, as well as chemokines such as IL-8, RANTES (*r*egulated on *a*ctivation, *n*ormal *T* cell–*e*xpressed and *s*ecreted), and MIP-1, which activate and recruit leukocytes
- Cytokine and chemokine receptors such as TNFR1 and IL-1R
- Adhesion molecules, including ICAM-1, ICAM-2, platelet endothelial cell adhesion molecule (PECAM), vascular cell adhesion molecule-1 (VCAM-1), E-selectin, and P-selectin, which have differential binding specificities for specific leukocyte populations
- Toll-like receptors (TLRs)
- Procoagulants and protease-activated receptors
- Proteases
- Leukotrienes and prostaglandins
- Growth factors such as vascular endothelial growth factor (VEGF) and transforming growth factor (TGF)-β
- Alterations in the surface adhesion molecules, cytoskeleton, and intercellular (junctional) proteins to allow for leukocyte adhesion transmigration and to regulate changes in vascular permeability

FIBROBLASTS

Although fibroblasts are classically viewed as structural cells and passive responders to exogenous influences, they are actually integral to the regulation of host defense. Fibroblasts synthesize extracellular matrix proteins, such as collagen and fibronectin, which are required to maintain the structural integrity of the lung during normal tissue turnover and tissue repair after infection and injury. They also express and secrete matrix-degrading proteases such as matrix metalloproteinases and cytokines such as IL-1, TNF, and TSLP, which play important roles in leukocyte recruitment and activation.

IMMUNE CELLS

Several leukocyte populations play distinct and vital roles in host defense in the lung and can be broadly classified as those that are normal residents of the lung (monocyte-macrophages, mast cells, dendritic cells) and those recruited in response to infection in injury (neutrophils and lymphocytes) (**Table 22-7**). Studies in animal models and in humans have demonstrated the increased risk of lung infection associated with defects in or absence of these cell types.

Monocyte-Macrophages

Macrophages (literally, "big eaters") are present within the interstitial tissues and alveolar spaces and on mucosal surfaces throughout the body. They function to provide

- Constant immune surveillance
- Orchestration of the immune response
- A bridge between the innate and adaptive arms of the immune system

Macrophages are derived from myeloid precursors in bone marrow, spleen, and fetal liver. Precursor cells termed *monocytes* leave the vascular space in response to chemokines or other

Table 22-7 Leukocyte Defense Mechanisms

Immune Cell	Primary Role(s)	Primary or Unique Inflammatory Mediators
Neutrophils	Killing and elimination of invading organisms	Reactive oxygen and nitrogen species Proteolytic enzymes and cationic proteins TNF-α, IL-1β, IL-6
Macrophages	Immune surveillance Killing and containment of invading microorganisms Removal of particulate matter Antigen presentation	TNF-α, IL-1β, IL-6 TGF-β ICAM-1 Reactive oxygen and nitrogen species
Mast cells	"Antennae" of immune response	Granule release (mediated via Fcϵ receptors) TLRs PAF, leukotrienes, and prostaglandins IL-1, IL-3, IL-4, IL-5, IL-6, IL-8, IL-10, IL-13, IL-16, TNF-α, VEGF, TGF-β, MIP-1α, MCP-1
Dendritic cells	Antigen presentation	TNF-α, IL-1β
Eosinophils	Allergic response Removal of parasites	Eosinophil-specific granules Cationic proteins Major basic protein Eosinophil peroxidase Eosinophil-derived neurotoxin Lipid mediators— leukotriene C$_4$ and PAF

ICAM-1, intercellular adhesion molecule-1; *IL-1*, interleukin-1 [etc.]; *MCP-1*, monocyte chemoattractant protein-1; *MIP-1*, macrophage inflammatory protein-1; *TGF-β*, transforming growth factor-β; *TNF-α*, tumor necrosis factor-α; *PAF*, platelet-activating factor; *TLRs*, Toll-like receptors; *VEGF*, vascular endothelial growth factor.

tissue-specific homing factors. The environment of the destination heavily influences the function of macrophages such that macrophages resident in different tissues display different patterns of function.

In response to infection or injury, the resident tissue macrophages can contribute to the innate immune response by phagocytosis, as well as expression of a variety of inflammatory and antimicrobial compounds, the pattern of which is differentially regulated by the microenvironment of the different tissues. Moreover, macrophages can function in antigen recognition, processing, and display to cells of the adaptive immune system (lymphocytes). Recent studies have determined that lung macrophages may be polarized along two lines, termed the M1 and M2 phenotypes, in response to specific cytokines and other mediators in their environment. The M1 phenotype, produced in response to exposure to microbial compounds (e.g., LPS) or interferon-γ, is a potent producer of reactive oxygen (O_2^-) and nitrogen (NO$^\bullet$) species and mediates

resistance against intracellular microbial parasites and tumors. By contrast, the M2 phenotype, produced in response to IL-4 and IL-13, participates in regulation of inflammatory and adaptive immune responses, scavenges debris, and promotes angiogenesis and tissue remodeling and repair.

Mast Cells

Mast cells are key elements in the innate immune system and have been termed the "antennae" of the immune response. Mast cells are located throughout the body in close proximity to epithelial surfaces, near blood vessels, nerves, and glands, placing them at strategic locations for detecting invading pathogens. In addition, mast cells express a number of receptors that allow them to recognize diverse stimuli.

In sensitized individuals, IgE is bound to Fcϵ receptors on the mast cell surface, and binding of antigen to surface-bound IgE results in mast cell activation. Thus, multiple stimuli (foreign antigens) may trigger the same class of receptor. However, there is specificity in this system as a result of multiple signal transduction pathways that are differentially activated on the basis of antigen size, receptor location, number, and subtype.

In addition, human mast cells also express TLRs: TLR-1, TLR-2, TLR-6, and TLR-4. TLRs are pattern recognition receptors that recognize specific molecular patterns of microorganisms. Expression of TLRs, in combination with other receptors, allows the mast cell to recognize many potential pathogens and mount a specific response. Of importance, mast cells are capable of releasing many immune modulating molecules that stimulate inflammation, and the adaptive immune response can polarize T cell subpopulations toward specific subtypes. Mast cell products include the following:

- Pre-formed mediators that are granule-associated (such as histamine)
- Mediators synthesized de novo (such as leukotriene C$_4$, platelet-activating factor, and prostaglandin D$_2$)
- A vast array of cytokines and chemokines, including IL-1, IL-3, IL-4, IL-5, IL-6, IL-8, IL-10, IL-13, IL-16, TNF-α, VEGF, TGF-β, MIP-1α, and MCP-1

In summary, the strategic location of mast cells in the body, their diversity of receptors, and cytokines indicate an important role for mast cells in regulating innate and adaptive immunity.

Dendritic Cells

Dendritic cells function as "conductors" of the immune response. These cells, resident within tissues, develop in vivo from hematopoietic precursor cells. Dendritic cells bind, internalize, and process antigens and then display them on their surface in the cleft of major histocompatibility complex (MHC I) or MHC II molecules. Activated dendritic cells then travel to local lymph nodes with processed antigen on their cell surface. These antigens are then "presented" to cells of the adaptive immune system (primarily lymphocytes). When a naive T lymphocyte recognizes an antigen-presenting dendritic cell with the requisite costimulatory signals, T lymphocyte differentiation usually occurs. A number of T helper (T$_H$) subsets have been described, including T$_H$1, T$_H$2, and T$_H$17 and regulatory T cells. These subsets are defined by cell surface markers, transcription factors expressed, and cytokines produced. Each subset is thought to be optimized for specific microbial challenges. Thus, T$_H$1 responses eliminate intracellular microorganisms, T$_H$2 responses eliminate parasites, and T$_H$17 responses eliminate conventional bacterial threats.

Recent studies have provided evidence for an increasing number of lung dendritic cell subsets identified and defined by their cell surface markers, cytokines produced, and functional attributes. Most of this work has been done in the murine models, although studies to define dendritic cell subsets in humans are being conducted. Further studies will reveal the relevance of various dendritic cell populations in host defense and lung pathology.

Eosinophils

Eosinophils (**Figure 22-5**) are considered to be effector cells of allergic responses and of parasite elimination. These bone marrow–derived cells contain four distinct granule cationic proteins: (1) major basic protein; (2) eosinophil peroxidase; (3) eosinophil cationic protein; and (4) eosinophil-derived neurotoxin.

During allergic inflammation, eosinophils release granule contents, as well as inflammatory mediators including lipid mediators such as leukotriene C_4 and platelet-activating factor, which may cause dysfunction and destruction of other cells.

Polymorphonuclear Neutrophils

The primary function of neutrophils in the innate immune response is to contain and kill invading microbial pathogens. Neutrophils merit particular mention in pulmonary host defense as the pulmonary microvascular endothelium preferentially recruits this leukocyte population in response to infection and inflammation (see **Figure 22-6**) by the expression of adhesion molecules and chemokines that target neutrophils. Recently it has been recognized that the T_H17 pathway involving the production of IL-17 and IL-23 can lead to neutrophil recruitment. Different stimuli including allergen sensitization, mast cell activation, various infections and TNF production, can promote a T_H17 response and thereby recruit neutrophils to the lung.

Neutrophils achieve their antimicrobial function through a series of rapid and coordinated responses that culminate in phagocytosis and destruction of the pathogens (**Figure 22-7**). Neutrophils have a potent antimicrobial arsenal that includes the following roles:

- Oxidants
- Powerful proteolytic enzymes (proteinases)
- Cationic peptides

Oxidants such as O_2^- and H_2O_2 are produced by a multi-component enzyme termed the phagocyte NADPH oxidase

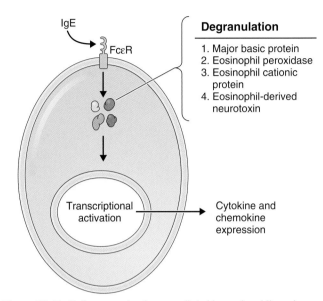

Figure 22-5 Defense mechanisms mediated by eosinophils and basophils. Immunoglobulin E (IgE)-mediated degranulation induces release of four distinct granule cationic proteins from eosinophils that can modulate the inflammatory response and display antihelminthic properties. Eosinophils and basophils also are capable of releasing cytokines and chemokines in a stimulus-specific manner.

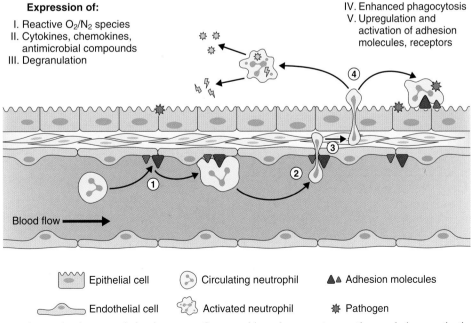

Figure 22-6 Leukocyte recruitment in airways and alveolar spaces. Contact with noxious agents or pathogens induces activation and enhanced expression of adhesion molecules on the apical surface of vascular endothelial cells (1) that facilitate leukocyte adhesion, recruitment, and activation; leukocytes then transmigrate across the endothelium, through the interstitial tissues, and across the epithelium and into the air space (2); leukocytes and the epithelial cells may become activated during these processes (3), leading to enhanced inflammatory cytokine and chemokine production (4).

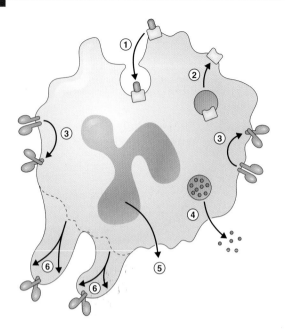

1. Receptor-mediated phagocytosis
2. Increased surface expression of adhesion molecules/receptors
3. Activation of integrins
4. Secretion of stored antimicrobial and inflammatory mediators
5. Increased production and expression of mediators
6. Migration to sites of infection or injury

Figure 22-7 Neutrophil-mediated defense mechanisms. Neutrophils play a central role in host defense of the lung through a variety of mechanisms (*1* to *6*), including their ability to phagocytose pathogens and, by oxidative and proteolytic mechanisms, kill the invading bacteria.

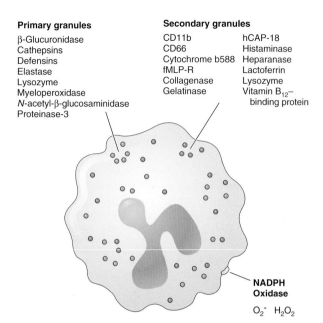

Primary granules	Secondary granules	
β-Glucuronidase	CD11b	hCAP-18
Cathepsins	CD66	Histaminase
Defensins	Cytochrome b588	Heparanase
Elastase	fMLP-R	Lactoferrin
Lysozyme	Collagenase	Lysozyme
Myeloperoxidase	Gelatinase	Vitamin B$_{12}$–
N-acetyl-β-glucosaminidase		binding protein
Proteinase-3		

NADPH Oxidase

O_2^- H_2O_2

Figure 22-8 Neutrophil-derived antimicrobial products. O_2^- and H_2O_2 are produced by a multicomponent enzyme, termed the phagocyte NADPH oxidase, which is expressed by neutrophils (PMNs) and macrophages. Leukocytes also contain unique secretory granules, the primary and secondary granules, which release potent proteolytic enzymes and cationic proteins that can digest a variety of microbial substrates. *fMLP-R*, fMet-Leu-Phe receptor; *hCAP-18*, human cathelicidin antimicrobial protein-18; *NADPH*, nicotinamide adenine dinucleotide phosphate (reduced); *PMNs*, polymorphonuclear neutrophils [leukocytes].

(NOX2). Granules within the cytoplasm of polymorphonuclear neutrophils (i.e., leukocytes) (PMNs) contain potent proteinases and cationic proteins that can digest a variety of microbial substrates. These compounds are released directly into the phagosome, compartmentalizing both the pathogen and the cytotoxic products (**Figure 22-8**). Conversely, neutrophil serine proteinases can be externalized in a weblike fashion together with nucleosomes to function as a trap for pathogens. These neutrophil extracellular traps (NETs) have been described in the vasculature and in the airways. NETs have an important antimicrobial function independent of phagocytosis by bringing and immobilizing microbial pathogens in close proximity to proteinases. NETs also provide a physical barrier to microbial spread. Of interest, some evidence suggests that eosinophils also produce NET-like structures in the lung.

ANTIMICROBIAL MOLECULES

Antimicrobial molecules (**Table 22-8**) are expressed by multiple cell types and play important roles in destruction and removal of pathogens. An overview of the important factors that have been shown to impede microbial growth and infection in the context of host defense of the lung is presented next.

ANTIMICROBIAL COMPONENTS IN THE AIRWAY SURFACE LIQUID

The acidic pH (6.4 to 7.3) of the ASL is inhibitory to microbial proliferation, as well as providing an optimal environment for the activity of the antimicrobial molecules found in the ASL. Important among these are lactoferrin and lysozymes.

Table 22-8 Antimicrobial Factors in Airway Surface Liquid

Factor	Role(s)/Function(s)
Lactoferrin	Binds iron Inhibits bacterial growth Enhances PMN function Modulates LPS activity
Lysozyme	Hydrolyzes peptidoglycan
Fibronectin	Binds to bacteria
Complement	Opsoninization Chemotactic Bacterial lysis
Immunoglobulins IgA and IgG	Opsoninization Complement activation
Defensins	Pore formation in microbial membranes Chemotactic Promotes cytokine production Stimulates dendritic cells
Cathelicidins	Modulates LPS Chemotactic Stimulates dendritic cells
Collectins	Binds carbohydrate domains of organisms, with reduced virulence and increased phagocytosis

LPS, lipopolysaccharide; *PMN*, polymorphonuclear neutrophil [leukocyte].

Lactoferrin

Lactoferrin is an iron-binding protein that is secreted by serous epithelial cells and neutrophils that competes with bacteria for iron, thereby inhibiting bacterial growth. Lactoferrin also possesses other antimicrobial properties, including the following:

- Enhancement of neutrophil functions—motility, adherence, and superoxide production
- Inhibition of biofilm formation by *Pseudomonas aeruginosa*
- The ability to injure bacterial membranes with resultant release of LPS
- Modulation of LPS activity by competitively binding LPS, thus preventing LPS-binding protein from binding and promoting an LPS-CD14 interaction, which would result in cell activation

Some evidence also suggests that lactoferrin can upregulate expression of various cytokine and growth factor genes such as IL-12 and IFN-β.

Lysozyme

Lysozyme is an enzyme produced by serous cells, macrophages, and PMNs that can hydrolyze peptidoglycan, a major component of gram-positive bacterial cell membranes, thus providing defense against infection by this type of bacteria. Lysozyme also aids in the defense against gram-negative bacteria and acts synergistically with lactoferrin, secretory leukoprotease inhibitor (SLPI), and LL-37 (an antimicrobial peptide) to provide multiple mechanisms for bacterial destruction and removal.

COMPLEMENT

Complement proteins are sequentially activated in a cascade encompassing three distinct pathways: (1) the classic antibody-antigen complex–dependent pathway, (2) the alternate pathway that is initiated by foreign or microbial products, and (3) a more recently identified pathway that is initiated by mannose-binding lectin (MBL), a member of the collectin family, and a related family of proteins called ficolins that are present in the lung. Complement proteins exude from plasma into airways in response to inflammation and are also produced by macrophages, type II pneumocytes, and fibroblasts. Specific complement components have important roles in host defense:

C5a: potent anaphylatoxin and chemoattractant that recruits neutrophils into the lung and enhances neutrophil-mediated microbial killing

C3a: another potent anaphylatoxin that also stimulates mucus production from goblet cells and enhanced LPS-induced synthesis of TNF and IL-1 by adherent phagocytes while decreasing synthesis in nonadherent cells

C5a-C9 complex: also known as the membrane attack complex (MAC), which creates pores in cell membranes, effectively killing bacteria

Multiple complement components can function as opsonins aiding phagocytosis of foreign particles (**Figure 22-9**). Of importance, hereditary deficiency of specific components of the complement pathway results in recurrent respiratory tract infections.

ANTIMICROBIAL PEPTIDES

A number of antimicrobial peptides are present in the airways. These can be classified conveniently into four groups on the basis of structural motifs: defensins, cathelicidins, histatins, and collectins.

DEFENSINS

Defensins are single-chain strongly cationic peptides that have a broad spectrum of antimicrobial activity against gram-positive

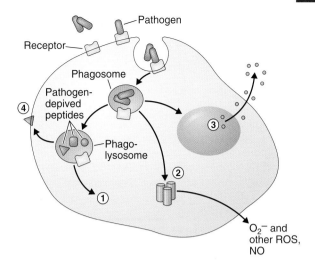

Figure 22-9 Immune defense mechanisms mediated by receptor-mediated phagocytosis and signaling. Internalization of pathogens or particulate matter induces multiple host defense mechanisms, including degradation of the offending agent (*1*), induction of the NADPH oxidase (neutrophils and macrophages) or iNOS (*2*), induction of chemokine and cytokine expression (*3*), and antigen presentation (particularly in dendritic cells and macrophages) (*4*). *iNOS*, inducible nitric oxide synthase; *NADPH*, nicotinamide adenine dinucleotide phosphate (reduced); *NO*, nitric oxide; *ROS*, reactive oxygen species.

bacteria, gram-negative bacteria, fungi, and viruses. They work synergistically with other host defense molecules such as lysozyme and lactoferrin. The antimicrobial activities of defensins include the ability to form pores in target membranes, to interfere with protein synthesis, and to directly damage DNA. Defensin activity is influenced by the salt concentration of the ASL, with higher concentrations decreasing their antimicrobial activity.

Defensins are defined by the presence of six cysteines and three intramolecular disulfide bridges and are classified into three different subgroups: α, β, and θ defensins. Only α and β defensins are of relevance in humans. The first four human α defensins (HD 1 to HD 4) are produced by neutrophils and are found in the airways, and the other two (HD 5 and HD 6) are found in the small intestine and female urogenital tract. Of the 28 human β defensins identified, 6 (HBDs 1 to 6) are expressed mainly by epithelial cells. HBDs 2 to 4 are inducible in response to a variety of stimuli, including bacterial and viral infection, IL-1, TNF, and LPS. The levels of HDs 1 to 4 are increased in inflammatory processes as a result of release by activated neutrophils.

In addition to their direct antimicrobial properties, defensins also contribute to host defense in other ways:

- Enhanced bacterial binding and killing and cytokine production by airway epithelial cells
- Chemotaxis for monocytes and immature dendritic cells
- Direct binding to CCR6 receptors on dendritic cells, thus linking the innate immune system to adaptive immunity (β-defensins)
- Promotion of phagocytosis in macrophages and neutrophils

- Downregulation of the inflammatory response by increasing SLPI release from airway epithelial cells, inhibiting the complement cascade, and reducing macrophage cytokine release and neutrophil oxidant production

CATHELICIDINS

The only human cathelicidin is LL-37, a peptide with a broad spectrum of antimicrobial activity that acts synergistically with lysozyme and lactoferrin. LL-37 is stored as a precursor, hCAP-18, in specific granules and also is secreted by mast cells and the respiratory epithelium. Other host defense activities of LL-37 include the following:

- Neutralization of LPS
- Chemotactic for neutrophils, eosinophils, mast cells, and T lymphocytes
- Direct interaction with dendritic cells to form T_H1 cells
- Mast cell degranulation
- Induction of cytokine and chemokine expression by epithelial cells and monocytes
- Induction of angiogenesis
- Induction of epithelial wound healing

HISTATINS

Histatins are a family of cationic histidine-rich peptides that are strongly antifungal and may have LPS-neutralizing properties. Histatins are present in saliva and play an important role in preventing oral infections. They have not been isolated from airway secretions.

COLLECTINS

The collectins, or collagenous C-type lectins, are a family of polypeptides that bind collagenous carbohydrates. Collectin proteins that play a role in pulmonary host defense include MBL and the surfactant proteins SP-A and SP-D. These molecules are secreted by the respiratory epithelium and are present in the airways. The collectins have broad antimicrobial activity against viruses, bacteria, and fungi by binding to conserved carbohydrate domains. In addition, collectins can bind organic antigens, apoptotic cells, nucleic acids, and host proteins. As discussed previously, MBL can activate the complement cascade and also has been shown to induce inflammatory mediator production from monocytes. The importance of these molecules is illustrated by the susceptibility of SP-A– and SP-D–deficient mice to various lung infections. In addition, some clinical studies suggest a link between severe pneumonia and reduced lung levels of SP-A or SP-D.

Together, these groups of antimicrobial molecules in the ASL function to destroy or inhibit microbes before they have a chance to proliferate and compromise the health of the host. If pathogens evade structural defenses and then survive the antimicrobial properties of the ASL, they can come into contact with host cell membranes, which allows for interaction with Toll-like receptors.

INNATE IMMUNE RECEPTORS

As highlighted earlier, the respiratory epithelium and other structural cells of the lung express innate immune receptors. These receptors function primarily as pattern recognition receptors to recognize conserved molecular patterns in

Table 22-9 Toll-Like Receptors (TLRs) and Their Ligands

Receptor	Reported Ligands
TLR-1	Heterodimerization with TLR-2, lipopeptides
TLR-2	Peptidoglycan and lipoteichoic acid (components of gram-positive bacteria) LPS Bacterial lipoproteins (components of *Borrelia burgdorferi*) Components of mycobacterial cell walls Mannuronic acid polymers (components of *Pseudomonas aeruginosa*) Glycosylphosphatidylinositol lipid (components of *Trypanosoma cruzi*) Phenol-soluble modulin (from *Staphylococcus epidermidis*) Soluble tuberculosis factor (19-kDa lipoprotein secreted by *Mycobacterium tuberculosis*) Whole bacteria (heat-killed *Listeria monocytogenes*)
TLR-3	dsRNA, polyinosinic:polycytidylic acid (poly I:C)
TLR-4	LPS Mannuronic acid polymers (components of *Pseudomonas aeruginosa*) RSV fusion protein Endogenous inflammation-related products (heat shock proteins HSP-60 and HSP90, fibronectin)
TLR-5	Flagellin
TLR-6	Heterodimerization with TLR-2, lipopeptides
TLR-7	ssRNA, antiviral compounds
TLR-8	ssRNA, antiviral compounds
TLR-9	Unmethylated CpG, bacterial DNA
TLR-10	?

CpG, cytosine-phosphate-guanine [DNA sequence]; *dsRNA*, double-stranded RNA; *LPS*, lipopolysaccharide; *RSV*, respiratory syncytial virus; *ssRNA*, single-stranded RNA.

microbial pathogens, called pathogen-associated molecular patterns (PAMPs), which are not normally found in the host (**Table 22-9**). This "pre-recognition" allows the host to respond to specific microbial products in the absence of an adaptive response; thus, the response does not require priming and is always present. Innate immune receptors include the membrane bound Toll-like receptors (TLRs) and additional cytosolic receptors. The 10 human TLRs share a protein structure characterized by an extracellular domain with a number of leucine-rich repeats (LRRs) and a cytoplasmic domain containing a Toll/IL1 receptor homology domain (TIR). They are highly expressed by leukocytes and in tissues in contact with the external environment, such as the lung. Cellular expression of TLRs is modulated by microbial stimuli. TLRs are found as homodimers with the exception of TLR-1 and TLR-6, which form heterodimers with TLR-2. TLR activation after binding of its cognate ligand triggers signal transduction pathways that ultimately lead to altered gene expression. The signaling pathway after recruitment of MyD88 is conserved for all TLRs (see **Figure 22-10**) with the exception of TLR-3, which utilizes TRIF. In addition, specific LPS chemotypes can activate TLR-4 in an MyD88-independent manner. Binding of MyD88 to the activated TLR leads to recruitment of IL-1 receptor–associated kinase (IRAK) and IRAK autophosphorylation. TNF receptor–

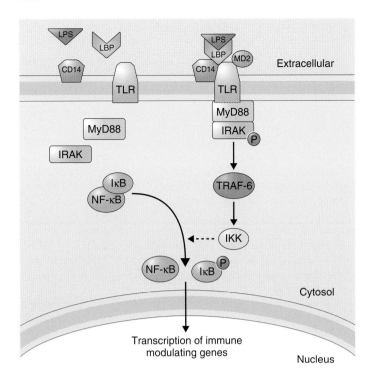

Figure 22-10 Toll-like receptor (TLR) signaling. The classical signaling pathway triggered by TLRs involves MyD88/IRAK (interleukin-1 receptor-associated kinase) and TRAF-6 (tumor necrosis factor [TNF] receptor-associated factor-6), leading to transcriptional regulation of immune and inflammatory genes. *IκB*, inhibitor of nuclear factor κB; *IKK*, IκB kinase; *LBP*, lipopolysaccharide-binding protein; *LPS*, lipopolysaccharide; *NFκB*, nuclear factor κB.

associated factor-6 (TRAF-6) links with this complex and activates IκB kinase (IKK). IKK phosphorylates IκB, leading to its dissociation from nuclear factor κB (NFκB). NFκB then translocates to the nucleus to activate gene transcription. Alternatively, TRIF leads to activation of IRF3 (interferon regulatory factor 3) that can translocate to the nucleus and lead to the transcription of interferon-α and -β. This pathway also activates NFκB.

Additional nonmembrane receptors enable cytosolic detection of microbial products. NOD1 and NOD2 (nucleotide-binding oligomerization domain proteins 1 and 2) are members of the NLR family of proteins (nucleotide-binding domain, leucine-rich repeat–containing) that recognize bacterial products and eventually lead to NFκB activation. NOD2 also may bind to single-stranded RNA and thus sense viruses. RNA viruses are recognized in the cytoplasm by retinoic acid–inducible gene (RIG)-I–like receptors (RLRs). These include RIG-1, MDA-5 (melanoma differentiation-associated gene-5), and LGP2 (laboratory of genetics and physiology-2). These proteins have a helicase domain and induce interferon production when activated. Double-stranded RNA (dsRNA) also can activate protein kinase R (PKR). PKR has an amino-terminal (N-terminal) RNA-binding domain and a carboxyl-terminal (C-terminal) kinase domain that is proapoptotic. PKR also can induce activation of other important molecules, including NFκB.

These innate immune receptors, whether on the membrane or in the cytosol, are critical for initiating an appropriate innate immune response to a microbial threat. In addition, strong evidence indicates that in the absence of appropriate TLR signaling, the adaptive immune response is impaired. The TLR response represents a "danger signal" and marks an associated antigen for an immune response. This signaling may be particularly relevant for the lung, which is constantly exposed to antigens yet must maintain a noninflamed environment in order to maximize gas exchange.

TOLL-LIKE RECEPTOR-2

Toll-like receptor-2 (TLR-2) is expressed on the surface of numerous cells and has a large number of reported ligands. These include components of gram-positive and gram-negative bacteria, mycobacteria, the protozoan parasite *Trypanosoma cruzi*, and zymosan, a yeast wall component. Additional ligands include secreted factors from *Staphylococcus epidermidis* and *Mycobacterium tuberculosis*, as well as whole bacteria (*Listeria monocytogenes*). TLR-2 does not recognize these PAMPs in isolation but rather forms heterodimers with TLR-6 and TLR-1, thus contributing to the diversity and specificity of TLR-2–mediated immune response.

TOLL-LIKE RECEPTOR-3

Toll-like receptor-3 (TLR-3) is activated by dsRNA), a marker of viral infection, and, through the activation of NF-κB, triggers the production of type I interferons. TLR-3 is found on plasma membranes, where it is believed to contact dsRNA after the lysis of infected cells and release of dsRNA into the extracellular milieu. Of note, additional evidence suggests that TLR-3 is found inside cells in vesicles associated with the endocytic pathway. TLR-3 is thought to have a more restricted pattern of expression but is found in dendritic cell populations.

TOLL-LIKE RECEPTOR-4

Toll-like receptor-4 (TLR-4) is the prototypical and most extensively studied of the TLRs. It recognizes lipopolysaccharide (LPS) (i.e., endotoxin), mannuronic acid polymers (components of *Pseudomonas aeruginosa*), and the F protein of the respiratory syncytial virus (RSV). Unlike the other TLRs, TLR4 also recognizes several endogenously derived molecules, including heat shock proteins HSP60 and HSP70 and fibronectin.

TOLL-LIKE RECEPTOR-5

Toll-like receptor-5 (TLR-5) recognizes a highly conserved cluster of 13 amino acid residues in flagellin, the structural component of flagella found in many pathogenic bacteria. This interaction triggers an innate immune response, resulting in cytokine production from leukocytes and dendritic cell activation and maturation.

TOLL-LIKE RECEPTOR-9

Toll-like receptor-9 (TLR-9) binds to unmethylated CpG (i.e., cytosine-phosphate-guanine sequence) elements in DNA and triggers a predominantly T_H1-weighted immune response. Unmethylated CpG dinucleotides are present at high frequencies in most bacterial genomes, whereas in the human genome, these dinucleotides are suppressed, methylated, and flanked by bases that are immune-neutralizing. TLR-9 is believed to be localized within endosomal compartments, thus facilitating its interaction with bacterial DNA.

OTHER TOLL-LIKE RECEPTORS

TLR-1 and TLR-6, as mentioned previously, interact with TLR-2 and function as a complex that recognizes a broad range of antigens. TLR-10 is related to TLR-1 and TLR-6, but its role remains to be clarified. TLR-7 and TLR-8 recognize single-stranded RNA.

INFLAMMATORY MEDIATORS

CYTOKINES

Cytokines (**Table 22-10**) are soluble, low-molecular-weight proteins that play important roles in host defense by regulating the inflammatory response and are expressed not only by leukocytes but also by endothelial cells, epithelial cells, and fibroblasts. Expression of cytokines is transcriptionally regulated, and secretion can be quickly enhanced after cell stimulation.

Signaling through cognate receptors, cytokines exert distinct responses in specific cell populations, stimulating some populations to activate, proliferate, and differentiate while having an inhibitory effect on other cell types. In this way, cytokines play a major role in regulating the intensity and duration of the inflammatory response. The cytokines that play important roles in inflammation, particularly in the early proinflammatory phase, include TNF-α, IL-1β, IL-6, and IL-10. Significant elevations of these cytokines are observed in generalized inflammatory states and particularly in gram-negative sepsis.

CHEMOKINES

Chemokines (**Table 22-11**) are 8- to 10-kDa glycoproteins that, although structurally related to cytokines, are distinct from them in their ability to bind and signal via G protein–coupled receptors. Chemokines are both chemotactic and cellular activating factors for leukocytes and can be classified into four groups on the basis of their amino acid structure. The two primary groups that play an important role in host defense are the CC chemokines (e.g., MCP-1, MIP-1α, and RANTES), which are chemotactic for monocytes, lymphocytes, basophils, and eosinophils and the CXC chemokines (e.g., IL-8, GRO-α [growth-related oncogene α], and ENA-78 [epithelial cell–derived neutrophil-activating peptide-78]), which act primarily on neutrophils.

The chemokine receptors are structurally related seven transmembrane–spanning proteins that transmit their signals through heterotrimeric G proteins. As with cytokines, the effect of chemokine activation results in diverse physiologic responses that are cell- and stimulus-specific. The binding specificity of individual chemokine receptors is determined by a region in the amino terminus of the protein. Some receptors

Table 22-10	Cytokines and Chemokines and Their Functions	
Cytokine	**Function**	**Other Clinical Roles**
TNF-α	Proinflammatory Neutrophil activation in ARDS	Proximate cytokine released in response to inflammatory stimulus
IL-1β	Proinflammatory Neutrophil activation in ARDS Upregulation of adhesion molecules on leukocytes, endothelium, and airway epithelium	One of first cytokines to be released in response to inflammatory stimulus
IL-6	Proinflammatory Leukocyte activation Promotes proliferation of myeloid progenitor cells Induces pyrexia Acute-phase reactant	Circulating levels are a marker of severity of ARDS of different causes
IL-10	Antiinflammatory Inhibits release of TNF-α, IL-1β, and IL-6 from monocyte-macrophages Stimulates the production of IL-1 receptor antagonist (IL-1RA) and soluble p75 TNF receptor	
GM-CSF	Alveolar macrophage function Lung host defense Surfactant homeostasis	Low circulating levels associated with poor prognosis in sepsis
PAF	Acts by way of receptors on platelets, leukocytes, and endothelial cells Increases vascular permeability Leukocyte recruitment Primes and triggers leukocyte secretion	
ICAM-1	Leukocyte recruitment and retention	Increased in inflammation
C5a	Product of classical and alternate complement cascade Potent anaphylatoxin and chemoattractant Acts via C5aR Can be both pro- and antiinflammatory	
Substance P	Neuropeptide that acts through its receptor NK1R Proinflammatory and associated with development of lung injury	

ARDS, acute respiratory distress syndrome; *GM-CSF*, granulocyte-macrophage colony-stimulating factor; *ICAM-1*, intercellular adhesion factor-1; *IL*, interleukin; *NK1R*, neurokinin 1 receptor; *TNF*, tumor necrosis factor; *PAF*, platelet-activating factor.

Table 22-11   **Chemokine Families**

Family	Member(s)	Function(s)
CXC	IL-8 MIP-2 GRO-α ENA-78 NAP-2	Chemotactic for and stimulatory to neutrophils
CC	MCP-1 MCP-2 MCP-3 RANTES MIP-1α MIP-1β	Chemotactic for and activation of: • monocytes • lymphocytes • eosinophils • basophils • mast cells
C	Lymphotactin	Attracts T cells
CXXXC	Fractalkine	Attracts T cells and monocytes Promotes adhesion

ENA-78, epithelial cell–derived neutrophil-activating peptide-78; *GRO-α*, growth-related oncogene; *IL-8*, interleukin-8; *MCP*, monocyte chemoattractant protein; *MIP*, macrophage inflammatory protein; *NAP-2*, neutrophil-activating protein-2.

are highly specific, whereas others bind multiple chemokines of both CC and CXC families. Differential regulation and expression of the chemokine receptor in different cell types play an important role in determining the biologic result of chemokine activation.

SUMMARY

It is apparent that the lung has multiple lines of defense against microbial pathogens and noxious environmental agents. These include physical barriers such as mucus and soluble factors such as antimicrobial peptides and proteins produced by epithelial cells, as well as leukocytes of the innate and adaptive immune systems. It is this combination of diversity and redundancy that enables the lung to thwart infection under most circumstances.

SUGGESTED READINGS

Gurish MF, Boyce JA: Mast cells: ontogeny, homing, and recruitment of a unique innate effector cell, *J Allergy Clin Immunol* 117:1285–1291, 2006.

Hiemstra PS: The role of epithelial beta-defensins and cathelicidins in host defense of the lung, *Exp Lung Res* 33:537–542, 2007.

Kuroki Y, Takahashi M, Nishitani C: Pulmonary collectins in innate immunity of the lung, *Cell Microbiol* 9:1871–1879, 2007.

Lambrecht BN: Lung dendritic cells: targets for therapy in allergic disease, *Curr Mol Med* 8:393–400, 2008.

Moraes TJ, Zurawska JH, Downey GP: Neutrophil granule contents in the pathogenesis of lung injury, *Curr Opin Hematol* 13:21–27, 2006.

Parker D, Prince A: Innate immunity in the respiratory epithelium, *Am J Respir Cell Mol Biol* 45:189–201, 2011.

Rohmann K, Tschernig T, Pabst R, et al: Innate immunity in the human lung: pathogen recognition and lung disease, *Cell Tissue Res* 343:167–174, 2011.

Chapter **23**
Approach to the Diagnosis of Pulmonary Infection

Mark A. Woodhead

The various clinical manifestations of respiratory tract disease are somewhat limited in scope and not specific to the causative disorder. The common signs and symptoms of cough, dyspnea, and chest pain and lung crackles or wheezes can be caused by infection but also by many other diseases. Accordingly, some detective work will be required to separate infection as a likely cause of illness from other possible etiologic conditions and then to identify the likely causative pathogen or pathogens and treat the infection.

Chapters 24 through 27 describe in detail aspects of pneumonia caused by specific pathogens. This chapter provides a framework from which to approach the individual patient in whom a pulmonary infection is likely. Assessment may begin by gathering specific information consisting of answers to the set of questions presented in **Box 23-1**. In this chapter, each of these questions is addressed in turn, although in clinical practice, the steps in this approach to the patient may be considered in parallel. Answers to the questions "Is it infection?" and "How severe is the illness?" are perhaps the most important.

THE APPROACH

IS IT INFECTION?

A careful history and physical examination are essential. No universally effective approach is recognized, however, and good clinical judgment often will be needed (**Table 23-1**). Typically, the patient with pulmonary infection will be pyretic and will have a cough characterized by purulent sputum. Rigors are even more specific to this disorder but occur only in more severe infections. An abrupt onset with pleuritic chest pain is a classical presentation in pneumonia but often is lacking. Wheeze may be present in airway infections, and focal chest signs are common in pneumonia. The more specific pneumonia signs of bronchial breathing, egophony, and whispering pectoriloquy are rare. Unfortunately, in real life, the presence of advancing age and immunosuppression can mean that infection is present despite the absence of any of these signs, and underlying lung disease may mean that some of them are present in the absence of infection.

For these reasons a confident diagnosis of pneumonia is difficult outside the hospital, where the cardinal feature of consolidation on the chest radiograph may be difficult to obtain. Even this feature may have other causes, but in the context of symptoms and signs suggesting infection, pneumonia is the likely diagnosis.

Very often the most important clinical considerations are whether an antibiotic should be prescribed (i.e., is this a bacterial infection?) and whether the patient should be admitted to the hospital. Historically, sputum purulence and the raised peripheral blood white cell count were considered to be suggestive of bacterial infection. Inflammatory markers such as C-reactive protein may be more specific and sensitive than the white cell count, and the hormokine procalcitonin may be an even more accurate marker of the presence or absence of bacterial infection. Available data are inconclusive, however, to allow recommendation of its routine use. The decision about hospital admission should be guided mainly by illness severity (see further on), but instability of comorbid diseases (e.g., diabetes mellitus) and social issues also are relevant to this decision.

Identification of a microorganism should be the best way to confirm infection, but this approach too has a number of limitations, most important of which is the insensitivity of available tests.

WHAT TYPE OF INFECTION IS IT?

Classification of Pulmonary Infections

The traditional anatomic classification of lung infection (e.g., upper respiratory, lower respiratory, pleural) forms a useful but far from perfect template on which to base a discussion of this topic. Although many infections are limited by anatomic boundaries (e.g., a lobar pneumonia), others do not fit easily into this classification schema (e.g., influenza virus infection).

The two main groups of acute adult pulmonary infections encountered in hospital practice are *acute exacerbations of chronic obstructive pulmonary disease* (COPD) (see Chapter 43) and *pneumonia* (Chapters 24 and 25). A chest radiograph is the key to separating these two, because it is the most sensitive screening method for detecting pulmonary consolidation (**Figure 23-1**, *A* and *B*). The presence of focal crackles is the most common feature of underlying consolidation. A pleural rub, or features of pleural effusion, may coexist. Other less common features include diarrhea, hypotension, and, in the elderly, mental confusion, hypothermia, and urinary incontinence. When pneumonia is suspected on clinical grounds and the chest radiograph is normal in appearance, a chest computed tomography (CT) scan may show changes in the lung parenchyma. However, other diseases may mimic pneumonia or be complicated by pneumonia (**Figures 23-2 to 23-4**).

It is important to identify the likely type of pneumonia according to the setting in which the infection was acquired

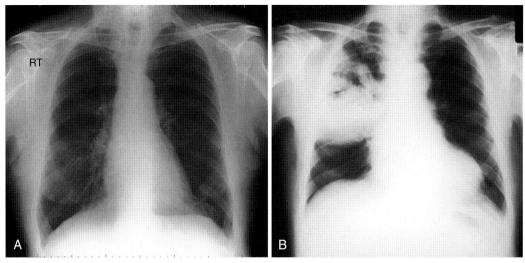

Figure 23-1 Chest radiographs obtained in two patients with underlying chronic obstructive pulmonary disease (COPD) who presented with cough, purulent sputum, and dyspnea. **A,** Uncomplicated COPD exacerbation with no lung consolidation. **B,** COPD exacerbation caused by pneumonia with right middle zone consolidation.

Box 23-1   Approach to the Patient with Suspected Pulmonary Infection

1. Is it infection?
2. What type of infection is it?
3. How severe is the illness?
4. What is the likely pathogen?
5. How is the causative pathogen best identified?
6. Is pathogen identification necessary?

Table 23-1   Features of Respiratory Infection and Alternative Causes

Feature	Pointer to Infection	Other Common Causes
Cough	Purulent sputum	Most other lung diseases
Temperature	Pyrexia Rigor	Bronchial carcinoma Pulmonary infarction
Sweats	"Drenching" and occurrence at night suggestive of tuberculosis	Septicemia Menopause
Chest signs	Features of consolidation	Bronchial carcinoma Any cause of alveolitis Pulmonary infarction
White cell count	Raised	Steroid therapy Bronchial carcinoma
C-reactive protein	Raised	Connective tissue disease
Chest radiographic appearance	Focal shadowing	Bronchial carcinoma Any cause of alveolitis Pulmonary infarction

---

Table 23-2   Classification of the Pneumonias According to Likely Origin and Immune Status

Pneumonia Group	Likely Pathogens
Community-acquired	Gram-positive bacteria *Mycoplasma, Chlamydia, Coxiella* Common viruses (e.g., influenza viruses)
Nosocomial, early	As for community-acquired pneumonias
Nosocomial, late	Gram-negative enterobacteria *Staphylococcus aureus* Antibiotic-resistant bacteria
Immunocompromised	Opportunistic organisms
Aspiration	Oropharyngeal anaerobic bacteria, chemical pneumonitis

diagnoses (e.g., bronchiectasis, pulmonary fibrosis, bronchial neoplasm); and, in some cases, guiding invasive investigation.

HOW SEVERE IS THE ILLNESS?

The severity of clinical illness guides decisions about the optimal setting in which to manage the patient—home versus hospital, general ward or intensive care unit (ICU)—and also may guide specific investigations and treatment strategies.

In the patient with an exacerbation of COPD, measures of respiratory distress (e.g., respiratory rate) and gas exchange are the best markers of illness severity.

Among patients with community-acquired pneumonia (CAP), those who die usually are severely ill at presentation, so the correct interpretation of presenting features is important. This information should be supplemented by the results of investigations as they emerge. Scoring systems have been developed as an aid to clinical judgment to assess CAP severity. The Pneumonia Severity Index (PSI) is a two-step severity score built from 20 clinical and laboratory features (**Figure 23-5**). It has been validated in a number of studies mainly as a tool for keeping low-risk patients out of the hospital. The simpler CURB-65 index also is well validated and is based on just five clinical features (**Figure 23-6**), whereas CRB-65, which may be used outside the hospital setting, is based on four. Comparisons

(**Table 23-2**). The spectrum of pathogens differs for the five pneumonia types—community-acquired, early, and late nosocomial; immunosuppression-related; and aspiration.

Other roles for plain chest radiography include assessing the extent of disease, for which it is especially useful; detecting complications (e.g., cavitation, abscess, pneumothorax, pleural effusion); identifying the lesions of additional or alternative of the scores confirm the slightly greater accuracy of the PSI but simpler application of CURB-65 and CRB-65. Use of these scoring systems is recommended in the most recent CAP management guidelines.

In nosocomial pneumonia as well as pneumonia in the immunocompromised patient, the importance of presenting features as opposed to features that develop during the course of the illness is less clearly defined than for patients who have CAP. Previous or inappropriate antibiotic therapy, renal failure, prolonged mechanical ventilation, coma, shock, and infection with *Pseudomonas aeruginosa, Acinetobacter* spp., and methicillin-resistant *Staphylococcus aureus* (MRSA) are additional markers for severe nosocomial pneumonia (**Box 23-2**).

High levels of lactate dehydrogenase that persist in peripheral blood, alveolar-arterial oxygen gradient greater than 30 mm Hg, and more than 5% neutrophils in bronchoalveolar lavage (BAL) fluid are markers for severe *Pneumocystis jiroveci* infection in patients with human immunodeficiency virus (HIV) infection.

WHAT IS THE LIKELY PATHOGEN?

A wide range of microbial pathogens can cause pulmonary infection. In most patients, the cause of the infection is never identified. In those in whom a pathogen is found, a delay always occurs between the time of clinical presentation and the availability of culture results. Because therapy should be started immediately, it is helpful to identify markers that may help to determine the cause of infection and hence to guide

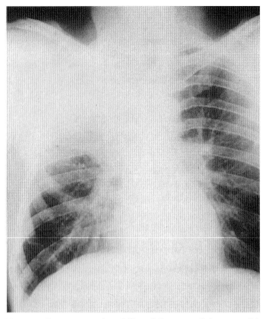

Figure 23-2 Pulmonary eosinophilia. Right upper lobe consolidation may mimic pneumonia, as in this case.

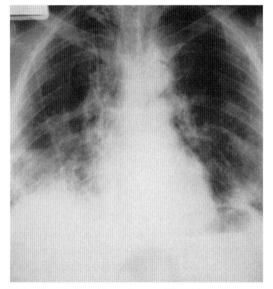

Figure 23-3 Drug-induced lung disease. Bilateral, patchy, predominantly basal consolidation was secondary to bleomycin administration.

Box 23-2 **Clinical Characteristics of Severe Nosocomial Pneumonia**

- Requirement for admission to the intensive care unit
- Respiratory failure (mechanical ventilation or the need for greater than 35% oxygen to maintain an artificial oxygen saturation above 90%)
- Rapid radiographic progression, multilobar pneumonia, or cavitating pneumonia
- Severe sepsis with hypotension and/or end-organ dysfunction:
  - Shock systolic blood pressure less than 90 mm Hg or diastolic blood pressure less than 60 mm Hg
  - Requirement for vasopressors for more than 4 hours
  - Urine output less than 20 mL/hour or total urine output less than 80 mL/hour in 4 hours (without other explanation)
  - Acute renal failure necessitating dialysis

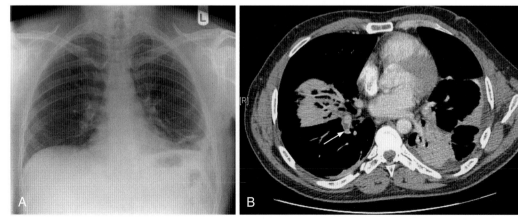

Figure 23-4 **A,** Appearance of left basal lung consolidation on chest radiograph. **B,** Contemporary computed tomography (CT) scan shows that consolidation is more extensive and is secondary to pulmonary embolism (*arrow*).

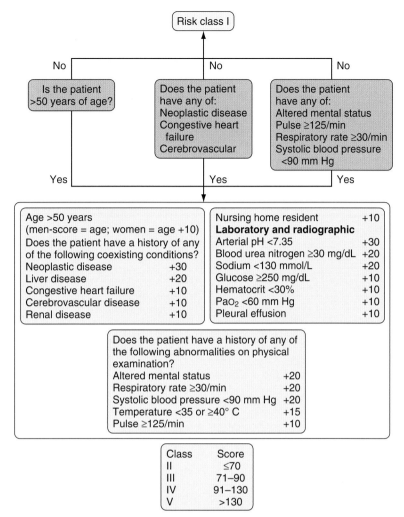

Figure 23-5 The Pneumonia Severity Index.

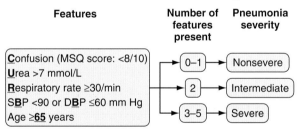

Figure 23-6 The CURB-65 score. *DBP*, diastolic blood pressure; *MSQ*, mental status questionnaire; *SBP*, systolic blood pressure.

decisions about therapy. Generally, information obtained at presentation may point to potential groups of pathogens, rather than to individual pathogens, because few features are pathogen-specific.

Airway infections often are of viral origin. When bacteria are present, *Haemophilus influenzae*, *Streptococcus pneumoniae*, and *Moraxella catarrhalis* are most frequently found, although such organisms may simply represent colonization, rather than being the responsible pathogens. These bacteria are important in bronchiectasis, in which *S. aureus* and *P. aeruginosa* also may be important. The latter two organisms are particularly important in patients with cystic fibrosis. In patients who suffer from bronchiectasis, knowledge of previous sputum culture results may be helpful (see Chapters 44 and 45).

The range of potentially treatable pathogens that may cause pneumonia is much more diverse. Classification of the pneumonia according to the immune status of the patient and the likely origin of the infection (see Table 23-2) is helpful. Risk factors for unusual exposures (e.g., birds for psittacosis, grazing animals for Q fever, or local ongoing outbreak, as with Q fever or Legionnaires' disease) and immunocompromise (e.g., unsuspected intravenous drug abuse or sexual contact for HIV infection risk) must always be sought in the history.

In CAP, the same pathogens usually are important regardless of age group, with *S. pneumoniae* the most frequent cause (see Table 23-2). The exception is that of a lower incidence of *Mycoplasma* infection in elderly persons. Gram-negative members of the family Enterobacteriaceae (e.g., *Escherichia coli*, *Proteus mirabilis*) may be a more frequent cause of pneumonias in some elderly nursing home populations, and MRSA is now being recognized as a community pathogen in this setting. Only varicella-zoster virus pneumonia has specific clinical features (i.e., the vesicular rash), but the presence of coincident skin or soft tissue infection may be a marker for the recently recognized community-associated MRSA pneumonia.

All of the pathogens encountered in the community setting can produce illnesses of variable severity, although *Legionella*, staphylococcal, and gram-negative enterobacterial infections are more commonly identified in severely ill patients (**Table 23-3**).

It may be helpful to retain the terms *atypical* and *typical* in the context of pneumonia to describe groups of pathogens

Table 23-3	Prediction of Microbial Etiology in Community-Acquired Pneumonia
Potential Agent of Community-Acquired Pneumonia	**Factor(s) With Higher Frequency of Association**
Streptococcus pneumoniae	Abrupt illness onset
Haemophilus influenzae	Preexisting lung disease
Staphylococcus aureus	Concurrent influenza epidemic Radiographic cavitation Severe illness Intravenous drug abuse
Legionella species	Recent foreign travel Concurrent epidemic Countries that border the Mediterranean
Mycoplasma pneumoniae	Age <65 years
Chlamydophila psittaci	Recent bird contact At-risk occupation
Coxiella burnetii	Animal contact (hoofed animals, cats, rabbits) At-risk occupation
Franciscella tularensis	Tick bites Rabbit contact
Brucella abortus	Cattle, sheep, goat, pig contact At-risk occupation (abattoirs, farming, veterinary work)
Gram-negative members of Enterobacteriaceae	Nursing home resident South Africa
Pseudomonas pseudomallei	Southeast Asia, northern Australia
Hantavirus pulmonary syndrome	Rodent contact
Mycobacterium tuberculosis, other mycobacteria	Nonindustrialized countries
Pneumocystis jiroveci	Risk factors for human immunodeficiency virus (HIV) infection Iatrogenic immune compromise

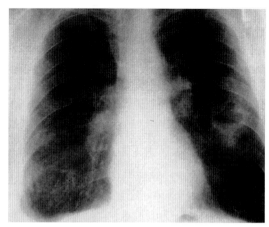

Figure 23-7 Cavitating pneumonia. Left midzone consolidation was caused by anaerobic infection.

allow an accurate prediction of the causative pathogen in nosocomial pneumonia; however, *P. aeruginosa* is less common in patients who have nosocomial pneumonia that developed outside the intensive care unit.

Bacterial antibiotic resistance is becoming increasingly important in both community-acquired and nosocomial pathogens. Patterns of resistance in community-acquired organisms usually are specific to the geographic region, whereas those in nosocomial organisms often are limited just to the treating institution. Knowledge of local resistance frequencies is therefore important in guideline-based empirical therapy.

The range of pathogens that cause pneumonia in the immunocompromised patient, in addition to routine bacterial and viral infections, also includes opportunistic organisms—those that usually are nonpathogenic in the immunocompetent host. Polymicrobial infections also occur more commonly in these patients. Prediction of likely pathogens is again imprecise, but attention should be paid to the nature and degree of the immunosuppression, time course of events, cytomegalovirus (CMV) status of donor and recipient, use of prophylactic therapies, and radiographic features (**Table 23-4**). Symptoms and signs, as in nosocomial pneumonia, are seldom helpful, although pancytopenia commonly accompanies CMV infections.

HOW CAN THE CAUSATIVE PATHOGEN BE IDENTIFIED?

Minimally Invasive Tests

Throat Swab Examination and Other Modalities

A throat swab may be used to identify some predominantly intracellular pathogens such as viruses (including influenza viruses), *Mycoplasma*, and *Chlamydophila*, by direct immunofluorescence (*Chlamydophila*, viruses) or cell culture. The yields are low and the methods often labor-intensive, which means that in adults, this approach usually is impractical, other than for research. In children, detection of respiratory syncytial virus by this method may be helpful. Increasingly, polymerase chain reaction (PCR) techniques are being used on such samples to detect organism-specific nucleotide sequences on throat swabs and other samples. Such tests are best for noncommensal organisms, for which significantly increased sensitivity over the older methods listed previously is found.

Sputum Examination

In many patients who have respiratory infection, sputum is easy to obtain. When such specimens are not available, sputum production may be induced by administration of nebulized

("atypical" referring to intracellular pathogens such as *Mycoplasma pneumoniae*, *Chlamydophila pneumoniae*, and *Coxiella burnetii*, and "typical" referring to conventional bacteria such as *S. pneumoniae* and *H. influenzae*), but recent studies have shown that a clinical distinction may not be helpful. *Legionella* pneumonia has been included in the "atypical" pneumonia group. In fact, the clinical features of this illness have much more in common with severe pneumococcal infection.

Radiographic features also usually do not help to differentiate among causative pathogens; however, cavitation occurs most commonly in staphylococcal, anaerobic (**Figure 23-7**), fungal, and tuberculous infections, and rarely with other pathogens.

It is helpful to distinguish nosocomial pneumonias that develop within the first 5 days of hospitalization from those that develop thereafter. *S. pneumoniae* and *H. influenzae* are not uncommon within the first 5 days, but are rarely found after 5 days, when *S. aureus* (both methicillin-sensitive and methicillin-resistant strains), *Acinetobacter* species, and *P. aeruginosa* are the most commonly seen. No specific clinical or laboratory features

Table 23-4	**Predicting Microbial Etiology in Pneumonia in Immunocompromised Patients**	
Feature	**Criteria**	**Organism**
Nature of immunosuppression	B cell dysfunction	Bacterial
	T cell dysfunction	Opportunist
	Neutropenia	Bacteria Fungi
Severity in HIV infection	CD4+ >200 cells/μL	Bacteria Tuberculosis
	CD4+ <200 cells/μL	*Pneumocystis jiroveci* pneumonia (PCP) Other opportunists
Time course of events	0-1 month after transplantation	Bacterial infection
	1-6 months after transplantation	Opportunist
Cytomegalovirus (CMV) status	CMV-positive donor to CMV-negative recipient	CMV
Prophylactic therapy	PCP prophylaxis	PCP less likely + atypical presentations
Radiology	Focal consolidation	Bacterial infection
	Nodule	Lung abscess Fungi
	Diffuse shadowing	PCP CMV

HIV, human immunodeficiency virus.

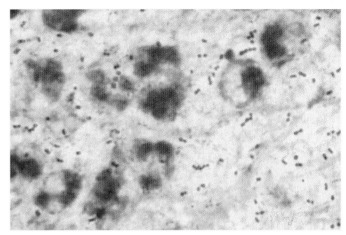

Figure 23-8 Sputum Gram stain. Gram-positive diplococci can be seen surrounded by degenerate neutrophils, which suggests pneumococcal infection.

hypertonic saline. This modality probably is of value only for the detection of *Mycobacterium tuberculosis* or of *Pneumocystis jiroveci* in immunocompromised patients. The value of examining sputum has been studied exhaustively, and its usefulness remains controversial. The main problem is that organisms identified in sputum may not be representative of what is happening in the lung. Second, bacteria may colonize the normally sterile airways when host defenses are compromised (e.g., by chronic bronchitis or intubation). The clinical illness may be attributed to these organisms when found in sputum even though another process (e.g., viral infection) is responsible.

Because some organisms are always pathogens (e.g., *Mycobacteria, Pneumocystis, Legionella*), their identification in sputum is always helpful. For other organisms, determination of the quality of the sputum sample is essential. Samples that contain 25 neutrophils and 10 or fewer squamous epithelial cells per high-power microscope field are considered to be representative of the lower respiratory tract. Other samples should be discarded, unless the pathogens listed previously are being sought.

Various tests can be performed on sputum; Gram stain and routine culture are the best known (**Figure 23-8**). Visualization of an organism on Gram stain is more specific than its identification by culture but is less sensitive. Culture is important for the identification of antibiotic-resistant strains. In a patient with CAP for which a predominant organism is identified within a purulent sputum sample, that organism usually is the cause of the pneumonia. Some organisms are identified in sputum only if appropriate stains are applied (e.g., with *Pneumocystis*) or if

culture is performed on specific media (as for *Legionella*, and some fungi).

Tracheal Aspiration

In nosocomial pneumonia, a tracheal aspirate can be obtained from the endotracheal tube. Even though the upper respiratory tract is bypassed, the frequency of colonization means that, as for sputum, microbiologic results from such a sample should be interpreted with caution. Culture results often are polymicrobial. Recent studies suggest that quantitative culture of tracheal aspirates may be as accurate as and less harmful than bronchoscopy in nosocomial pneumonia (see later under "Bronchoscopy").

Blood Culture

Blood culture is readily available and highly specific if positive. Its drawback is its relative insensitivity: Positive culture results are obtained in only 10% to 20% of hospitalized adult patients who have CAP. Its yield is even less in nosocomial pneumonia and very low in children with pneumonia.

Pleural Fluid/Tissue Sampling

When present, pleural fluid should be sampled, because the results are highly specific. Lymphocytosis suggests the possibility of tuberculosis. Pleural pH, as well as cell content, may help in the diagnosis of empyema. Pleural biopsy for histopathologic examination and culture may assist in the diagnosis of tuberculosis.

Urine Testing

Enzyme-linked immunosorbent assay (ELISA) testing of urine for *Legionella* antigen is now the most frequently performed test, yielding the most rapid results, for the diagnosis of *Legionella* infection. Minor drawbacks are that assay results are positive only in *Legionella pneumophila* serogroup I infection (more than 90% of cases of *Legionella* infection), that results may be negative if the assay is performed too early (antigen excretion begins on approximately day 3 of clinical illness), and that antigen excretion may persist for up to 1 year after the clinical illness. Urine antigen tests for *S. pneumoniae* probably are more sensitive and specific than is sputum examination, but their cost-effectiveness is uncertain.

Serologic Testing

In CAP, serologic studies may be the only method of diagnosis available for detection of *Mycoplasma*, *Chlamydia*, *Coxiella*, *Legionella*, and viral infections. This approach does not usually help in immunocompromised persons or in patients affected by nosocomial infections, unless *Legionella* is specifically suspected (e.g., during an ongoing epidemic). To establish such diagnoses, with certain exceptions, it is necessary to identify a four-fold rise in specific antibody titers to at least 1:128 between acute and convalescent samples. A single high titer of 1:256 is presumptive evidence of infection. The need to wait for the second sample limits the clinical value of this method, which is now being replaced in routine practice by PCR methodology.

Invasive Tests

Transtracheal Aspiration

Transtracheal aspiration performed by passing a catheter through the cricothyroid membrane was used quite frequently in the past. The associated risks of hemorrhage and subcutaneous emphysema, however, have rendered it rarely used today.

Bronchoscopy

Bronchoscopy allows direct sampling from the lungs, but because the bronchoscope passes through the nasopharynx and upper airway, it is important to use an approach that minimizes contamination. This technique is most useful for obtaining samples in patients who are not producing sputum. As other drawbacks, the procedure and the associated local anesthetic and sedation may further compromise the patient's already altered ventilatory status; transbronchial biopsy may cause hemorrhage or pneumothorax; and the bronchoscope itself may introduce infection. An advantage of BAL is that a wider area of the lung is sampled, but the risk of contamination is increased. Protected specimen brush (PSB) sampling may be more specific but is less sensitive, because only a small area is sampled. Bronchoscopy has been the most commonly used diagnostic technique in immunocompromised patients and those with nosocomial pneumonia; it is most strongly validated in the former.

The utility of bronchoscopic samples in the management of nosocomial pneumonia remains unclear; PSB sampling probably is better than BAL. Endotracheal aspirates may contain the same bacteria, and no outcome benefit has been conclusively shown. The technique cannot at present be recommended routinely.

In CAP, no evidence supports the routine addition of bronchoscopy to noninvasive sampling. It may be of value in the patient in whom initial therapy fails to produce improvement.

Percutaneous Fine Needle Aspiration

Percutaneous fine needle aspiration is performed by inserting a 22-gauge needle percutaneously into consolidated lung tissue through an 18-gauge needle placed in the chest wall. This technique carries a risk of pneumothorax and lung hemorrhage and cannot be recommended other than for research purposes in experienced hands.

Open Lung Biopsy

The value of open lung biopsy has not been systematically evaluated because of the potential risks. Anecdotally, it has helped to obtain a more definitive diagnosis in all three types of pneumonia when the patient has failed to respond to empirical therapy and when other tests have been unhelpful.

Other Techniques

Molecular biologic methods, especially polymerase chain reaction (PCR) techniques, are beginning to be used selectively for pathogen identification. Other roles of PCR analysis may be to detect multiple organisms at the same time in a single sample (so-called multiplex PCR assay) and to identify antibiotic resistance by detection of the specific gene defect that determines such resistance (e.g., rifampicin resistance in tuberculosis).

Interest also has emerged in "near-patient" tests that rely on antigen or nucleic acid detection, usually with a colorimetric marker. These tests enable a microbiologic diagnosis at the bedside, both in and outside the hospital. None are yet in routine use.

Is It Necessary to Identify the Causative Pathogen?

In some patients, it may be inappropriate to seek the causative pathogen because such investigation is impractical or is not cost-effective, or the potential risk to the patient outweighs any benefit. Within the community, 95% or more of respiratory infections are managed empirically without an attempt to identify the pathogen. In this setting, microbiologic investigations may be needed only when the patient fails to respond to initial therapy.

Microbiologic investigations on hospitalized patients are routine. However, in prospective studies of CAP in which intensive investigation is undertaken, pathogens are detected only in approximately 25% to 50% of patients, and the impact on treatment is small. Outcome benefit for bronchoscopic investigations in nosocomial pneumonia remains controversial. The reasons for the poor yield are multiple and relate to previous antibiotic therapy, inadequate sample collection, transport delays, and the use of insensitive laboratory methods that often depend on the presence of intact and viable organisms for a positive result. This situation may change with the advent of newer microbiologic methods, but because empirical, broad-spectrum antibiotics are easy to give and patients who are not severely ill usually recover, it can be argued that airway infections or CAP microbiologic investigations should be limited (or not performed at all) in the mildly ill and used extensively only in the severely ill patient. In nosocomial pneumonia and immunocompromise-related pneumonia, microbial investigation may be more important, because it often is necessary to differentiate infective from noninfective pathology. Possible approaches in CAP, nosocomial pneumonia, and the immunocompromise-related pneumonia are shown in **Figures 23-9**, **23-10**, and **23-11**, respectively.

CONTROVERSIES AND PITFALLS

CONTROVERSIES

- Pneumonia cannot be diagnosed without a chest radiograph.
- The distinction between typical and atypical pneumonias is clinically accurate and useful.
- Routine sputum examination is useful in CAP.
- Bronchoscopic sampling is useful in nosocomial pneumonia.

PITFALLS

- The symptoms and physical signs of respiratory infection are shared with other respiratory tract diseases.
- The elderly, the very young, and the immunosuppressed may not manifest typical features of respiratory infection.

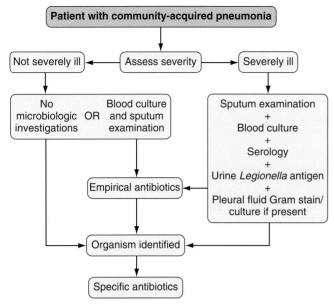

Figure 23-9 Diagnostic approach to the patient who has community-acquired pneumonia: Suggested algorithm to guide microbial investigation.

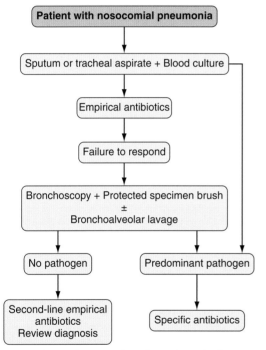

Figure 23-10 Diagnostic approach to the patient who has nosocomial pneumonia: Suggested algorithm to guide microbial investigation.

- Bacteria present in respiratory secretions may be commensal rather than pathogenic.
- Pneumococcal respiratory infections usually may still be treated by antibiotics to which a bacterium is resistant in vitro if appropriate doses are used.

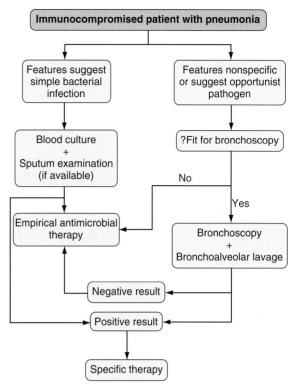

Figure 23-11 Diagnostic approach to pneumonia in an immunocompromised patient: Suggested algorithm to guide microbial investigation.

SUGGESTED READINGS

American Thoracic Society; Infectious Diseases Society of America: Guidelines for the management of adults with hospital-acquired, ventilator-associated, and healthcare-associated pneumonia, *Am J Respir Crit Care Med* 171:388–416, 2005.

Bartlett JG, Dowell SF, Mandell LA, et al: 2000 Practice guidelines for the management of community-acquired pneumonia in adults. Infectious Diseases Society of America, *Clin Infect Dis* 31:347–382, 2000.

Lim WS, Baudouin SV, George RC, et al: BTS guidelines for the management of community acquired pneumonia in adults: update 2009, *Thorax* 64(Suppl 3):iii1–iii55, 2009.

Mandell LA, Bartlett JG, Dowell SF, et al; Infectious Diseases Society of America: Update of practice guidelines for the management of community-acquired pneumonia in immunocompetent adults, *Clin Infect Dis* 37:1405–1433, 2003.

Niederman MS, Mandell LA, Anzueto A, et al: Guidelines for the management of adults with community-acquired pneumonia. Diagnosis, assessment of severity, antimicrobial therapy, and prevention, *Am J Respir Crit Care Med* 163:1730–1754, 2001.

Ramsdell J, Narsavage GL, Fink JB: American College of Chest Physicians' Home Care Network Working Group: Management of community-acquired pneumonia in the home: an American College of Chest Physicians clinical position statement, *Chest* 127:1752–1763, 2005. (Available at www.chestnet.org.)

Woodhead M, Blasi F, Ewig S, et al: European Respiratory Society; European Society of Clinical Microbiology and Infectious Diseases: Guidelines for the management of adult lower respiratory tract infections, *Clin Microbiol Infect* 17(Suppl 6):E1–E59, 2011. (Available at www.ersnet.org or www.escmid.org.)

Chapter **24**
Community-Acquired Pneumonia

Ilya Berim • Sanjay Sethi

BURDEN OF DISEASE

Pneumonia and influenza remain common causes of death in the United States (ranked 7th) and globally (ranked 6th). More than 60,000 deaths were attributed to pneumonia in 2005 in the United States. In Europe, the incidence of lower respiratory tract infections reached 25.8 million in 2002, yielding only to diarrheal illness as a most common disease. The mean length of hospital stay for pneumonia exceeds 5 days, and readmission rate within 30 days after hospital discharge approaches 20%. The overall economic health care system burden associated with community-acquired pneumonia (CAP) is approximately $40 billion annually in the United States and reaches €10 billion in Europe. According to British Thoracic Society guidelines, age-standardized rate of hospital admissions due to CAP rose by 34% from 1997 to 2004. CAP also is the most common cause of severe sepsis. Admission to the intensive care unit (ICU) is required in up to 20% of cases of CAP. Because the incidence of pneumonia is substantially higher among elderly persons, it is anticipated that in view of the aging population, the incidence and health care burden of pneumonia will only increase. In the United States, approximately 4.2 million outpatient clinic visits for pneumonia were recorded for 2006, and this number has been increasing ever since. At the same time, despite introduction of novel antimicrobials, imaging modalities, and biomarker testing, mortality attributable to CAP has not changed significantly since the introduction of penicillin.

CLINICAL PRESENTATION

The clinical presentation and diagnosis of CAP are complex. Presence of classic symptoms such as fever, generalized fatigue, cough, sputum production, dyspnea, pleuritic chest pain, and hemoptysis is highly variable, and ranges from nearly 90% for cough to less than 15% for hemoptysis. Many factors influence the clinical presentation of CAP, including the patient's age, comorbid conditions, and lifestyle factors, as well as the causative microbe. Presence of certain symptoms, as discussed further on, may help identify the offending organism. However, the significant variability in the clinical presentation of CAP makes it virtually impossible to diagnose the disease, let alone the causative agent, from the clinical presentation alone, and further diagnostic tests are usually needed.

Probability of an atypical presentation, in which the classic symptoms are lacking, increases with patient age and number of comorbid conditions. In general, any compromise of the patient's immune system can lead to silencing of clinical symptoms despite rapidly progressive underlying infection. Absence of fever and cough is common in the elderly population; rather, altered mental status, generalized malaise, tachypnea, and tachycardia are often the only manifestations of pneumonia in this population. Such atypical clinical presentations can delay the correct diagnosis and treatment by several days, which probably leads to increased mortality.

The major causes of pneumonia have been divided into the typical organisms, such as *Streptococcus pneumoniae*, *Haemophilus influenzae*, and *Klebsiella pneumoniae*, and the atypical pathogens, such as *Mycoplasma pneumoniae*, *Chlamydophila* spp., *Coxiella burnetii*, and viruses. Historical descriptions of differences in clinical presentation between these two groups of pathogens have been widely used and still are commonly regarded as important. CAP caused by the typical organisms has been characterized as of more acute onset, with manifestations including fever with intense chills, along with cough, usually productive of purulent or bloody sputum and occasionally associated with pleuritic chest pain. Findings suggestive of pulmonary consolidation (such as dullness to percussion, rales, bronchial breathing) also were thought to be part of the typical presentation, as well as leukocytosis with neutrophil predominance and occasionally presence of circulating immature leukocytes (bands).

By contrast, pneumonia caused by "atypical" pathogens has been described as being of more gradual onset, with lower body temperature, nonproductive cough, and white blood cell counts in the normal to high-normal range. Systemic manifestations such as generalized malaise and muscle aches can dominate the clinical picture.

Unfortunately, studies have failed to demonstrate the accuracy of such purported differences in clinical presentation of CAP in distinguishing between the typical and atypical pathogens. Accordingly, this distinction should not be relied on to make an etiologic diagnosis or decisions about antibiotic treatment.

RISK FACTORS

Certain risk factors are associated with higher frequency of infections with particular pathogens.

Age Increased age favors infection with *S. pneumoniae*, group B streptococci, *Moraxella catarrhalis*, *H. influenzae*, gram-negative bacilli, and *Chlamydophila pneumoniae*. Aspiration pneumonia risk increases with age as well as risk for pneumonia due to multiple organisms. It seems that an apparent decrease in frequency of *Legionella* infection has been noted among persons older than 80 years. Every year over 65 increases the risk for pneumonia. The annual incidence of CAP in noninstitutionalized elderly people is estimated to be 25 to 44 per 1000, compared with 4.7 to 11.6 per 1000 in the general population. The risk of infection severe enough to necessitate hospital admission also increases markedly with age, ranging from 1.6 per 1000 adults 55 to 64 years of age to 11.6 per 1000 after age 75. Age is one of the main predictive factors for mortality associated with CAP. The death rate for pneumonia or influenza has been evaluated at 9 per 100,000 in the elderly population, rising to 217 per 100,000 among patients with one risk factor and to 979 per 100,000 among those with more than one.

Alcoholism Alcohol consumption may potentially lead to impaired level of consciousness, predisposing the drinker to aspiration pneumonia by impairing the cough reflexes, with alterations in the mechanisms of swallowing and mucociliary clearance. Owing to the immunosuppressive effects and impairment of innate lung defenses attributable to high alcohol intake, heavy drinking increases the risk of infection with gram-negative organisms. Alcohol impairs the function of lymphocytes, neutrophils, monocytes, and alveolar macrophages. Each of these factors contributes to the reduced bacterial clearance from the airways in these patients. Whether alcoholism predisposes to increased pneumonia severity in general is controversial; however, *S. pneumoniae* infections tend to be more severe in alcoholic patients. Also, infections caused by gram-negative bacilli and *L. pneumophila* occur more frequently in heavy drinkers.

Airway Colonization Airway colonization is common in patients with chronic obstructive pulmonary disease (COPD), as is impairment of innate lung defense mechanisms. Patients with COPD appear to be at increased risk for CAP, and pathogens such as *H. influenzae* and *M. catarrhalis* become more prevalent. Very pronounced decrease in forced expiratory volume in 1 second (FEV$_1$), along with bronchiectasis, predisposes affected patients to infection with *Pseudomonas aeruginosa*. Invasive aspergillosis has been described as an often fatal complication of high-dose corticosteroid treatment of exacerbations of COPD in patients with severely compromised lung function. Conditions leading to altered level of consciousness (narcotic use, alcohol consumption, cerebrovascular disease, dementia), poor dental hygiene, history of head and neck surgery affecting swallowing mechanisms, and upper gastrointestinal tract disease all are predisposing factors for development of aspiration pneumonia. Usual culprit organisms include anaerobes and members of the oral and enteric flora.

Organisms such as *S. pneumoniae*, *S. aureus*, group B streptococci, and *H. influenzae* frequently cause superinfections after viral illnesses such as influenza and RSV infection.

Altered Immunity Patients with a compromised immune system are at increased risk for development of CAP. The list of possible pathogens is long and only increases with worsening degree of immunodeficiency. Immunosuppression achieved with medications predisposes to infections with otherwise rare pathogens such as *Pneumocystis jiroveci*, *Mycobacterium avium* complex, *Histoplasma* spp., *Coccidioides* spp., *Cryptococcus neoformans*, Mucoraceae spp., and *Toxoplasma*, to name a few. Some examples of comorbid conditions leading to an immunocompromised state are chronic liver disease, heart failure, cancer, diabetes, lymphoproliferative disease, human immunodeficiency virus (HIV) infection/acquired immunodeficiency syndrome (AIDS), and immunoglobulin deficiencies.

Malnutrition, which frequently accompanies such conditions, also leads to alterations in cellular immunity and decreased levels of secretory immunoglobulin A (IgA), increasing the chance of airway colonization and/or infection with gram-negative bacilli.

Environmental Factors Geographic location and professional history also seem to play a role in susceptibility to CAP. Occupations associated with exposure to dusts, fumes, and various chemicals (such as construction work, painting, and mining, to name a few) increase the risk of acquiring CAP in general, with *S. pneumoniae* being the most likely pathogen. Exposure to contaminated water supply and cooling towers of air-conditioning units increases the chance of acquiring Legionnaire's disease. *Legionella* organisms thrive in warm water, and could then be spread in water mist. Contact with animals may lead to pneumonia due to *Yersinia pestis* (plague, for which rodents constitute a natural reservoir), *Francisella tularensis* (tularemia, with rabbits, voles, and muskrats as carriers), *C. burnetii* (Q fever, transmitted by sheep, dogs, and cats), *Rhodococcus* (present in horses) or *Chlamydophila psittaci* (psittacosis, transmitted by birds).

In certain settings, bioterrorism must be considered as well. Potential agents utilized for such purposes include those organisms causing anthrax, tularemia, and plague.

Institutionalization Both the frequency and the severity of pneumonia increase in institutionalized patients. Oropharyngeal colonization by gram-negative bacilli or *S. aureus* plays a major role here. Epidemics of viral infections also are frequent in this patient population. The main microorganisms isolated in cases of pneumonia diagnosed in institutional environments are, in order of decreasing frequency, *S. pneumoniae*, *S. aureus*, gram-negative bacilli, and *H. influenzae*.

Nutrition Susceptibility to infection is increased by a number of malnutrition-related phenomena, such as a decreased level of secretory IgA, a failure of macrophage recruitment, and alterations in cellular immunity. As a result, the frequency of respiratory tract colonization by gram-negative bacilli is increased in patients with malnutrition and the incidence and severity of respiratory infections are increased. Malnutrition acts in association with other comorbid conditions frequently found in patients with pneumonia, such as alcohol consumption, COPD, chronic respiratory failure, and neurologic disease.

Smoking Smoking alters mucociliary transport, humoral and cellular defenses, and epithelial cell function and increases adhesion of *S. pneumoniae* and *H. influenzae* to the oropharyngeal epithelium. Also, smoking predisposes to infection by influenza viruses, *L. pneumophila*, and *S. pneumoniae*. Smoking itself, however, is not a risk factor for pneumonia severity.

PATIENT EVALUATION/DIAGNOSTICS

Clinical presentation of CAP can be rather nonspecific, especially in elderly and debilitated persons. Risk factors for specific causative agents, such as history of recent travel into endemic areas, is an important part of the clinical history in a patient with suspected CAP. Because of the inaccuracy of a purely clinical diagnosis, additional investigations are required to confirm the diagnosis, identify the causative pathogen, and initiate appropriate treatment. These are discussed in Chapter 23. **Table 24-1** summarizes the American Thoracic Society/

Table 24-1 | **Clinical Indications for Diagnostic Testing for Community-Acquired Pneumonia**

Indication	Blood Culture	Sputum Culture	*Legionella* UAT	Pneumococcal UAT	Other
Intensive care unit admission	X	X	X	X	X*
Failure of outpatient antibiotic therapy		X	X	X	
Cavitary infiltrates	X			X	X†
Leukopenia	X		X		
Active alcohol abuse	X	X	X	X	
Chronic severe liver disease	X		X		
Severe obstructive/structural lung disease		X			
Asplenia (anatomic or functional)	X		X		
Recent travel (within past 2 weeks)			X		X
Positive *Legionella* UAT result		X‡	NA		
Positive pneumococcal UAT result	X	X		NA	
Pleural effusion	X	X	X	X	X¶

*Endotracheal aspirate if patient is intubated, possibly bronchoscopy or nonbronchoscopic bronchoalveolar lavage.
†Fungal and tuberculosis cultures.
‡Special media for *Legionella* culture.
¶Thoracentesis and pleural fluid cultures.
NA, not applicable; *UAT*, urinary antigen test.
From Mandell LA, Wunderink RG, Anzueto A, et al: Infectious Diseases Society of America/American Thoracic Society consensus guidelines on the management of community-acquired pneumonia in adults, *Clin Infect Dis* 44(Suppl 2):S27–S72, 2007.

Infectious Diseases Society of America (ATS/IDSA) recommendations of tests proven to be useful in different settings for investigating and treating CAP.

SPECIFIC PATHOGENS

Streptococcus Species

S. pneumoniae is the most common bacterium isolated from patients with CAP. It is a saprophyte of the respiratory tract, which can easily proliferate as soon as natural defenses decline (as with increasing age, alcoholism, diabetes, smoking, or immunosuppression). In the classic presentation, the onset of pneumococcal pneumonia is abrupt, characterized by intense and prolonged chills and considerable pleuritic chest pain. Symptoms and signs are rapidly progressive, with high fever (core body temperature close to 40° C [104° F]), tachycardia, and tachypnea; cough is common, as are oliguria and cyanosis. At this stage, a nasolabial herpes simplex lesion may develop, crackles are heard, and chest radiographs show homogeneous lobar or segmental consolidation. Without antibiotic treatment, cough persists, with eventual production of rust-colored sputum. Leukocytosis is frequent, and blood cultures are positive in 10% to 20% of patients if specimens are obtained before antibiotic therapy. Arterial blood gas analysis reveals decreases in PaO_2 and $PaCO_2$. Recrudescence of symptoms may occur after a few days; then the fever resolves and an abundant diuresis ensues. Radiologic and physical signs characteristically regress rapidly and considerably. The rapid rate of multiplication of *S. pneumoniae*, together with the high risk for secondary complications (e.g., empyema, meningitis, septicemia), makes any case of *S. pneumoniae* pneumonia a medical emergency.

Streptococcal species other than *S. pneumoniae* rarely cause pneumonia, but among these, *S. pyogenes* most often is involved, more in the young than in the elderly. Pneumonia caused by *S. pyogenes* occurs after viral infections such as measles, varicella, or rubella in infants and after influenza, measles, or varicella in

adults. The clinical presentation is that of typical pneumonia. Pleural effusion and empyema frequently develop, and other complications include pneumothorax, pericarditis, mediastinitis, and bronchopleural fistula.

Staphylococcus Species

The severity of *Staphylococcus* infection is due to the prevalence of its resistance to multiple antibiotics and to lung tissue lysis as part of the infection, leading to formation of bullae and their subsequent rupture into the pleura (pneumothorax, pneumopyothorax), with consequent serious ventilatory defects and septicemia. Staphylococcal infection is acquired by inhalation or aspiration through the airways or occurs by hematogenous spread. Airborne contamination may follow a viral infection such as influenza or measles, or it may be linked to comorbidity (COPD, carcinoma, laryngectomy, seizure); hematogenous spread is the result of bacteremia (endocarditis, infective foci with discharge into the bloodstream). Direct bloodstream infection caused by intravenous drug abuse is the most common cause in many inner-city hospital emergency departments. The clinical presentation may be unusual compared with typical pneumonia when the infection develops through vascular dissemination (e.g., dyspnea, cough, and purulent sputum might be masked by symptoms of endocarditis or the primary infective focus) or when the infection is causing a pleural effusion, empyema, or lung abscess. The chest radiograph may show two possible features: central or segmental consolidation secondary to aspiration or multiple infiltrates that are generally nodular early on and can subsequently progress to parenchymal consolidation with or without cavitation after vascular spread of the infection. Abscess, pleural effusion, and empyema are frequent, as well as septicemia. Overall outcome depends on associated diseases, spread of infection, and resistance of *Staphylococcus* to antibiotics.

Community-acquired methicillin-resistant *Staphylococcus aureus* (MRSA) has emerged as a frequent infectious agent associated with skin and soft tissue infections in the community setting. Community-acquired MRSA also can cause severe pulmonary infections, including necrotizing pneumonia and empyema. It is more virulent than health care–associated MRSA isolates. Community-acquired MRSA usually contains the gene encoding Panton-Valentine leukocidin and the SCC*mec* type IV element and belongs to the USA300 pulsed-field gel electrophoretic pattern. Panton-Valentine leukocidin is a toxin that creates lytic pores in the cell membranes of neutrophils and induces the release of neutrophil factors that promote inflammation and tissue destruction. Community-acquired MRSA typically is more susceptible to a wider class of antibiotics than those with activity against health care–associated MRSA. The optimal antibiotic treatment for Panton-Valentine leukocidin-positive community-acquired MRSA infection is unknown; however, antibiotics with activity against MRSA and the ability to inhibit toxin production may be optimal (linezolid or clindamycin for susceptible isolates).

Haemophilus influenzae

Most invasive infections due to *H. influenzae* result from encapsulated, typable strains rather than from nonencapsulated, nontypable strains. An exception is in patients with COPD, in whom the nontypable strains often are the etiologic agents of pneumonia and occasionally even cause an associated bacteremia. A history of upper respiratory tract infection is common. Small pleural effusions can occur, but empyema and cavitation are rare.

Mycoplasma pneumoniae

Mycoplasma pneumoniae pneumonias usually occur in small epidemics, particularly in closed populations. The clinical presentation commonly is that of an atypical pneumonia, as described earlier. *M. pneumoniae* infections mimic, to some extent, the presentation of viral respiratory infections, but the incubation period is longer (10 to 20 days) than for viruses, and the fever generally is of mild to moderate severity, with core body temperature below 39° C (102.2° F). Within a few days, most symptoms subside, although the low-grade fever and cough frequently persist. A history of a preceding upper respiratory tract infection may be found in up to 50% of patients. A variety of extrapulmonary manifestations may be encountered, including arthralgia, cervical lymphadenopathy, bullous myringitis, diarrhea, immune hemolytic anemia, meningitis, meningoencephalitis, myalgia, myocarditis, hepatitis, nausea, pericarditis, skin eruptions, and vomiting. Diffuse crackles occasionally are heard. Infiltrates usually are localized in the lower lobes and regress very slowly over 4 to 6 weeks. Pleural effusions and mediastinal lymphadenopathy are rare.

Chlamydia Species

Psittacosis is a pneumonia caused by an intracellular bacterium, *Chlamydia psittaci*, which is responsible for ornithosis in domestic fowl. *C. psittaci* can be transmitted to humans by inhalation from infected birds, including canaries, parakeets, parrots, pigeons, and turkeys. The clinical presentation is that of an atypical pneumonia. After a 7- to 14-day incubation period, the onset may be abrupt. Fever with temperatures of 38° to 40° C (100.4° to 104.0° F), possibly with chills, is associated with arthralgia, headache, myalgia, dyspnea, and thoracic pain. Cough may be severe, and sputum, if any, usually is mucoid. Splenomegaly and a macular rash are evocative of psittacosis. The radiographic appearance is variable but typically includes lower lobe infiltration. Hepatitis, phlebitis, encephalitis, myocarditis, renal failure, and intravascular

coagulation are unusual complications. Despite the efficiency of antibiotics such as tetracycline and erythromycin, psittacosis is associated with a mortality rate of approximately 1%. Relapse is prevented by continuing treatment for 2 weeks after return to a normal temperature.

Previously known as the TWAR (*Taiwan acute respiratory*) agent, *Chlamydia pneumoniae* has been recognized as a pathogen responsible for pneumonia since 1985. The incidence of pneumonia caused by *C. pneumoniae* is uncertain because of the lack of reliable diagnostic tests. However, it does appear to be an important cause of pneumonia in all age groups. The clinical presentation is that of an atypical pneumonia in young adults; in elderly persons, the course may be severe, particularly if comorbid conditions are present. Sore throat may precede the onset of fever (with temperatures in the range of 37.7° to 39° C [100° to 102.2° F]) and a nonproductive cough. The chest radiograph shows subsegmental infiltrates, which usually clear over 2 to 4 weeks.

Legionella pneumophila

Legionella organisms are aerobic gram-negative intracellular bacilli; approximately 30 species have been identified, the most common being *L. pneumophila*. Water- and air-conditioning systems are their natural reservoirs; spread of the bacilli occurs by air, but no transmission between human beings has been reported. *L. pneumophila* infection may cause an asymptomatic seroconversion, a single episode of pyrexia, and mild to severe pneumonia. The nonpneumonic illness is known as Pontiac fever and is associated with fever, chills, headache, and upper respiratory tract symptoms. Pneumonia occurs either sporadically or in small epidemics and is more likely to occur in immunocompromised persons. After 2 to 8 days of incubation, headache, myalgia, high fever, and chills precede pneumonia by a few days. Initially, there is a nonproductive cough that may become productive of watery or even purulent sputum. Dyspnea, hemoptysis, and chest pain are frequent manifestations. Extrapulmonary symptoms and signs are numerous and include abdominal pain, agitation, watery diarrhea, arthralgia, confusion, skin rash, headache, hematuria, hyponatremia, hypophosphatemia, myalgia, nausea, oliguria, proteinuria, renal failure, seizures, splenomegaly, and vomiting. Leukocytosis, neutropenia, lymphopenia, and hepatic inflammation may be observed. The chest radiograph shows consolidation, often unilateral and dense, initially localized and then spreading gradually. Pleural effusion frequently is present; cavitation is rare. The outcome depends on the early clinical recognition and treatment and on comorbid conditions. Mortality is increased in immunosuppressed patients and in those who have complications of the infection.

Gram-Negative Bacilli

Gram-negative bacilli include various members of the families Enterobacteriaceae and Pseudomonadaceae, in particular *K. pneumoniae*, *Escherichia coli*, *Pseudomonas aeruginosa*, and *Acinetobacter* spp. Gram-negative bacilli are more often responsible for nosocomial pneumonia than for CAP. CAP attributable to these agents may result from their colonization of the oropharynx, followed by inhalation or microaspiration of the organisms; however, most of these patients meet criteria for health care–associated pneumonia, such as residence in long-term care facilities. Comorbidity is usual in patients who acquire these pneumonias. The clinical presentation is that of a typical pneumonia. The prognosis is poor, particularly in cases featuring immunodepression, alcoholism, neutropenia, and old age.

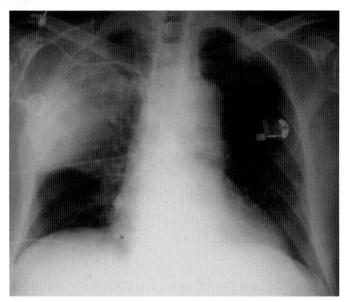

Figure 24-1 *Klebsiella* pneumonia. Chest radiograph shows a bulging fissure. *(From Rabbat A, Huchon G: Bacterial pneumonia. In Albert RK, Spiro SG, Jett JR, editors: Clinical respiratory medicine, ed 3, Philadelphia, 2008, Mosby.)*

Friedländer's pneumonia (caused by *K. pneumoniae*) typically occurs in men older than 40 years; alcoholism, diabetes mellitus, and chronic lung disease are predisposing factors. Historically, patients were thought to produce particularly large volumes of thick and bloody sputum; they were likely to present with prostration and hypotension and to have multiple patches of consolidation, particularly in the upper lobes, with bulging fissures (**Figure 24-1**) and multicavitation on chest radiographs (i.e., an expanding pneumonia).

E. coli pneumonia and *P. aeruginosa* pneumonia typically occur in chronically ill patients; hemoptysis is rare, and the lung infection usually involves the lower lobes. Abscessation and empyema occur frequently. *Acinetobacter* pneumonia progresses very quickly, with development of severe hypoxemia, shock, bilateral consolidation, and empyema and even death within a few days.

Pseudomonas pseudomallei, which causes melioidosis, is an aerobic, gram-negative bacillus found in soil, vegetation, and water in tropical regions. Infection of the lung occurs more commonly as a result of spread through the bloodstream after cutaneous infection than as a result of inhalation. The clinical presentation may be either acute or chronic. Acute melioidosis manifests with high fever, dyspnea, chest pain, cough with purulent sputum, and hemoptysis. Local cellulitis and lymphangitis may be seen at the place of cutaneous inoculation. The chest radiograph shows diffuse miliary nodules, infiltrates, or cavitation. Chronic melioidosis may occur years after contraction of the infection in an endemic area. Signs and symptoms either are absent or may resemble those of pulmonary tuberculosis: asthenia, anorexia, weight loss, low-grade fever, productive cough, and hemoptysis. Chest radiographs show apical infiltrates, possibly with cavitations.

Anaerobic Bacteria

Anaerobic bacterial pneumonia results from aspiration; therefore, it typically occurs in situations involving alcoholism, coma, seizure, and general anesthesia. Chronic dental infection; head, neck, and lung cancer; and bronchiectasis are additional risk factors. Anaerobic pneumonia begins as a typical pneumonia with pleuritic pain; pulmonary infiltrations preferentially involve the lower lobes, particularly the right lower lobe. If patients aspirate while lying supine, the segments involved typically are the posterior segment of the right upper lobe and the apical segment of the right lower lobe. Necrosis and suppuration follow, and fever with temperatures higher than 39° C (102.2° F), dyspnea, and pleuritic pain persist. Sputum is purulent and fetid, which often is obvious on entering the patient's room. Leukocytosis is high, and segmental infiltrations with small transparent areas of necrosis are seen. Abscess and empyema occur frequently. The outcome is closely related to treatment—delay in antibiotic treatment or inappropriate antibiotic choice probably will result in necrotizing pneumonia, abscess formation, and empyema, which increases the fatality rate.

Coxiella burnetii

C. burnetii is the causative agent of Q fever and is the most frequent pathogen responsible for pneumonia among the rickettsial organisms. Ticks are vector agents, and various wild and domestic animals (cattle, sheep, goats) are infected with no evidence of disease; *C. burnetii* multiplies in the placenta of pregnant animals and spreads during parturition. Although *C. burnetii* is present in numerous species of ticks, the main route of transmission is by inhalation of infectious aerosols. *C. burnetii* is particularly resistant to chemical and physical agents. The clinical presentation is that of an atypical pneumonia. The onset occurs after a 2- to 4-week incubation period. Patients present with high fever (i.e., body temperature of 40° C [104° F] or more), chills, myalgia, and headache, all of abrupt onset; cough usually is nonproductive. Abdominal and thoracic pain, pharyngitis, and bradycardia also may be features. There usually is no rash, in contrast with other rickettsial infections. Hepatomegaly and splenomegaly may be found on physical examination. The chest radiograph shows dense nodular infiltrates; pleural effusion and linear atelectasis may be seen. Leukocytosis is not a feature, and mild hepatitis may be found. The course usually is benign.

Nocardia Species

Nocardia asteroides and, to a lesser extent, *Nocardia brasiliensis* are responsible for most cases of *Nocardia* pneumonia. Nocardiae are aerobic, gram-positive bacilli present mainly in soil. Approximately 50% of patients have no underlying disease. The others tend to have predisposing problems such as immunosuppression, malignancy, or long-term corticosteroid therapy. The onset of the infection is usually subacute, but it can be fulminant; in the latter case, there is a high fatality rate. Symptoms include fever, asthenia, anorexia, productive cough, and chest pain. Multiple subcutaneous abscesses may be present, as well as neurologic signs when there is central nervous system involvement. Chest radiograph abnormalities vary, ranging from infiltration to lobar consolidation; cavitation, nodules, abscesses, and pleural effusion also may be seen. The prognosis depends on whether the infection disseminates, but it is usually good in the case of isolated lung disease. Metastatic infection may occur anywhere but is particularly common in the central nervous system and the skin. Infection also may reach the pleura and the chest wall.

Actinomyces israelii

Both *Actinomyces* and *Arachnia* can cause actinomycosis, but *Actinomyces israelii* is the main responsible organism. These are

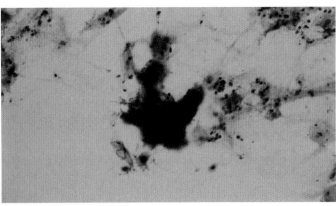

Figure 24-2 Sputum Gram stain showing *Actinomyces* organisms (center). *(From Rabbat A, Huchon G: Bacterial pneumonia. In Albert RK, Spiro SG, Jett JR, editors:* Clinical respiratory medicine, *ed 3, Philadelphia, 2008, Mosby.)*

anaerobic, gram-positive, filamentous, branching bacilli (**Figure 24-2**) that were incorrectly thought to be fungi for many years. They normally reside in the oropharynx and become invasive pathogens when there is a defect in the anatomic barrier or when they are inhaled, at which time the infection may extend directly from one place to an adjacent area. Bad dentition, bronchiectasis, and COPD are risk factors for pulmonary infection. Men are far more frequently affected than women. The clinical presentation suggests tuberculosis, carcinoma, or chronic fungal infection; asthenia, anorexia, weight loss, and low-grade fever may precede cough and chest pain by months. Cervicofacial and thoracic involvement coexists rarely. When infection progresses to the pleural space and chest wall, the opening of a sinus tract may disclose pus. Radiographic features are variable and include small cavitary nodules confined to one segment; cavitary infiltration; extension of infection to the interlobar fissure, chest wall, bone, or pleura; and empyema.

Pasteurella multocida

Pasteurella multocida is a gram-negative coccobacillus present in the oropharynx of mammals. It causes cutaneous infection in humans after animal bites. Pneumonia has been reported in patients with chronic pulmonary diseases. The clinical presentation is nonspecific and includes fever, cough, purulent sputum, and dyspnea. Chest radiographs show lower lobe infiltrates; pleural effusion and empyema may occur.

Francisella tularensis

Francisella tularensis is a gram-negative bacillus found in various mammals and insects of the Northern Hemisphere. Tularemia occurs after the bite of, or contact with, an infected animal. The onset of pneumonia is abrupt; fever, chills, and malaise precede dyspnea, cough, and chest pain. Painful ulceroglandular infection with adenopathy may be found at the site of bacterial inoculation. The chest radiograph shows signs of pneumonia, possibly with hilar adenopathy or pleural effusion.

Yersinia pestis

Yersinia pestis (formerly called *Pasteurella pestis*) is a short gram-negative rod that causes plague. It is a disease of rodents (squirrels, rabbits, rats) that is transmitted to humans by flea bites or by person-to-person contact through aerosol inhalation. Initial signs and symptoms are chills, fever, prostration, delirium, headache, vomiting, and diarrhea. There are three forms of plague: bubonic, septicemic, and pneumonic. Bubonic plague

consists of lymphadenopathy, with palpable masses forming in the cervical, axillary, femoral, and inguinal areas. Signs of septicemia are those of shock and petechial hemorrhages. Plague pneumonia results from either metastatic infection or inhalation of the pathogen. Pneumonia occurs within a week of initial exposure and is characterized by chest pain, productive cough, dyspnea, and hemoptysis. The chest radiograph shows lower lobe infiltrates, possibly nodules, lymphadenopathy, and pleural effusions.

Bacillus anthracis

Bacillus anthracis is a large gram-positive rod that causes anthrax. *B. anthracis* is found in the soil, water, and vegetation and infects cows, sheep, and horses, which in turn infect humans after contact with contaminated materials. Fever and malaise usually appear progressively. Three forms of anthrax are found: cutaneous, intestinal, and pneumonic. Inoculation of *B. anthracis* into superficial wounds or skin abrasions causes cutaneous anthrax, which is characterized by a black-crusted pustule on a large area of edema. Intestinal anthrax results from ingestion of contaminated material, and the resulting illness can be severe. Pneumonic anthrax is due to inhalation of the contaminated material. Nonproductive cough and chest pain precede dyspnea, stridor, tachypnea, cyanosis, and edema of the neck and anterior chest. Peribronchovascular edema, enlargement of the mediastinum, and pleural effusions usually are seen on the chest radiograph.

Brucella Species

Brucella organisms are gram-negative coccobacilli found in the genitourinary tract of cows, pigs, goats, and dogs. Brucellosis results from contact with infected animals or from ingestion of unpasteurized milk products. The pathogen then spreads through the body by way of the bloodstream. General symptoms include fever, malaise, and headache. Hepatic enlargement and splenomegaly are common, as is lower back pain. Respiratory symptoms are less frequent than abnormalities on the chest radiograph, which include nodules, miliary infiltrates, and lymphadenopathy.

Moraxella catarrhalis

Moraxella catarrhalis, formerly named *Branhamella catarrhalis*, is a gram-negative diplococcus that commonly is found in the oropharynx of normal persons. *M. catarrhalis* pneumonia is seen in patients with underlying chronic diseases such as COPD, congestive heart disease, or malignancy. Symptoms and radiographic findings are nonspecific. Leukocytosis is common, and the course usually is favorable.

TREATMENT

SITE OF CARE DECISION

A crucial decision in the treatment of CAP is whether or not the patient's condition warrants hospital admission. Numerous factors contribute to such decision making, including risk of death from the pneumonia, disease severity, presence of comorbid conditions, need for advanced diagnostics, ability to take oral medications, and the degree of social support. In the past, hospital admission was an instinctive "knee jerk" response to the diagnosis of CAP. However, hospitalization is associated with an increased risk of acquiring multidrug-resistant nosocomial bacterial strains, increased risk for thromboembolic events, up to a 75-fold increase in cost, and less patient satisfaction.

Box 24-1 American Thoracic Society Criteria for Admission of Patients with Community-Acquired Pneumonia to an Intensive Care Unit

Major Criteria
Invasive mechanical ventilation
Vasopressor use

Minor Criteria
Hypotension requiring aggressive fluid resuscitation
Hypothermia (core body temperature <36° C)
Thrombocytopenia (platelet count <100,000/dL)
Leukopenia (white blood cell count <4000/dL)
Uremia (BUN >20 mg/dL)
Confusion or disorientation
Multilobar radiographic involvement
PaO_2/FIO_2 ratio <250
Respiratory rate ≥30 breaths/minute

BUN, blood urea nitrogen.
Modified from Mandell LA, Wunderink RG, Anzueto A, et al: Infectious Diseases Society of America/American Thoracic Society consensus guidelines on the management of community-acquired pneumonia in adults, *Clin Infect Dis* 44(Suppl 2):S27-S72, 2007.

Informed practitioners have therefore mounted a vigorous effort to reduce unnecessary admissions for CAP, primarily by better identification of patients who can be safely treated at home.

Several outcome tools have been developed to predict prognosis in CAP, and these are now being used to identify patients at low risk of mortality and appropriate for treatment at home rather than in hospital. Among the well-validated ones are the Pneumonia Severity Index (PSI) and the CURB-65 and CRB-65 indices. These are summarized in Chapter 23, Figures 23-5 and 23-6.

CURB-65 or CRB-65 (which is CURB-65 without the blood urea nitrogen level) indices are significantly more user-friendly scoring systems requiring consideration of four or five readily assessed variables (see Chapter 23, Figure 23-6).

Another sometimes challenging decision is whether and when to admit the patient to an ICU. Generally, patients with high scores on mortality prediction indices (such as class V PSI or group 3 CURB-65) are likely to benefit from early ICU admission. Emerging data suggest that early admission to the ICU in appropriate patients can improve outcomes. The challenge is identifying these patients among the larger group of patients at risk for higher mortality. Latest ATS/IDSA guidelines defined need for ICU admission as the presence of one of the major criteria (need for invasive mechanical ventilation or hemodynamic instability requiring vasopressor use) or three of nine minor criteria listed in **Box 24-1**. Several scoring systems (CURXO, SMART-COP, and CAP-PIRO) tested criteria similar to the ATS minor criteria set and found them to be similar in terms of predicting need for admission to intensive care. All of the aforementioned scoring systems, however, are not without limitations, especially when applied in younger populations. Development and validation of a dedicated scoring system to predict need for ICU treatment will be useful.

These scoring systems have contributed significantly to the objective assessment of the severity and prognosis prediction of CAP. Such systems, however, should not be used as the sole parameter for determining the need for hospital admission. In practice, as many as 40% of patients with CAP who are at low risk for dying as assessed by these scores get admitted for management of the pneumonia. In many of these patients, comorbid conditions requiring inpatient management or social factors that make home treatment unsafe necessitate hospital care. A combination of a prognostic scoring system and assessment for comorbidity and risk factors related to the patient's social situation should guide decisions about site of care for CAP.

ANTIMICROBIAL TREATMENT

Eradication of the offending pathogen from the lower respiratory tract is the goal of antimicrobial CAP therapy. Ideally, the identity and the antimicrobial susceptibility of the pathogen should be known before initiation of treatment, so that an antibiotic that has the narrowest antimicrobial spectrum, least side effects, and the lowest cost can be prescribed. However, diagnostic testing able to identify causative organisms so rapidly that the results would be available before initiation of antimicrobial therapy are still lacking. The lack of sensitivity and specificity of current diagnostic testing is also a concern. Biomarkers and molecular detection may ultimately provide the necessary diagnostic tools to support pathogen directed treatment, but are not adequately validated for clinical use at present. Furthermore, there is evidence that earlier administration of appropriate antimicrobial therapy (with one or more antibiotics effective in vitro against the causative pathogen and given in adequate doses) improves outcomes in CAP. Therefore, delay in initiation of antimicrobial therapy while awaiting the results of microbiologic studies, or even for obtaining such studies (e.g., waiting for the patient to produce an adequate sputum sample) could have deleterious effects on patient outcome.

These considerations have prompted the current emphasis on broad-spectrum empirical therapy, with or without subsequent adjustment of antimicrobial spectrum once diagnostic results become available. Empirical choice of antimicrobials depends on factors such as severity of illness, knowledge of the most common pathogens associated with the patient's condition, local resistance patterns, and the growing understanding that CAP frequently can be a polymicrobial infection, most commonly consisting of a combination of a virus or an atypical pathogen with a typical bacterial pathogen. In view of the lack of sensitivity of current diagnostic testing, hesitation to adjust the antibiotic regimen is common if the patient is responding to therapy, even if diagnostic data support narrowing of the antimicrobial spectrum. Current recommendations also emphasize rapid administration of antibiotics in CAP, with retraction of previous guidelines on specific time intervals at which antibiotics should be administered. Therefore, current guidelines do not include specific timing for administration of antibiotics for CAP, except that antibiotics should be started in the emergency department if that is the facility admitting the patient to the hospital.

A major consideration determining empirical antibiotic choice in the current ATS/IDSA guidelines is the site of care, which serves as a surrogate marker for disease severity (outpatient, inpatient, and ICU settings) (**Box 24-2** and **Table 24-2**). In the outpatient setting, choice of antibiotics is influenced primarily by presence of comorbid conditions and by recent antibiotic use. These two risk factors portend poor outcomes and infection by drug-resistant pathogens. Recent antibiotic use (within 3 months) should prompt choice of an agent from an antibiotic class other than the one to which the patient has already been exposed. Local resistance patterns also should be

Table 24-2 ATS/IDSA Recommendations for Empirical Antibiotic Treatment of Community-Acquired Pneumonia

In-Hospital Setting	Antibiotic Regimen	
	Outpatient	Inpatient
Non-ICU setting		
Absence of risk factors	Macrolide (preferred) OR Doxycycline	Respiratory fluoroquinolone (moxifloxacin, gemifloxacin, or levofloxacin 750 mg) OR Beta-lactam + macrolide
Presence of risk factors: chronic heart, lung, liver, or renal disease; diabetes mellitus; alcoholism; malignancy; asplenia; immunosuppressive condition/medications; use of antimicrobials in past 3 months	Respiratory fluoroquinolone (moxifloxacin, gemifloxacin, or levofloxacin 750 mg) OR Beta-lactam + macrolide	
ICU setting		Beta-lactam + either azithromycin or respiratory fluoroquinolone (aztreonam + respiratory fluoroquinolone in penicillin-allergic patients)

ATS/IDSA, American Thoracic Society/Infectious Diseases Society of America; ICU, intensive care unit.
Data from Mandell LA, Wunderink RG, Anzueto A, et al: Infectious Diseases Society of America/American Thoracic Society consensus guidelines on the management of community-acquired pneumonia in adults, Clin Infect Dis 44(Suppl 2):S27–S72, 2007.

Box 24-2 Most Common Etiologic Agents of Community-Acquired Pneumonia*

Outpatient
Streptococcus pneumoniae
Mycoplasma pneumoniae
Haemophilus influenzae
Chlamydophila pneumoniae
Respiratory viruses; influenza A and B viruses, adenovirus, respiratory syncytial virus, parainfluenza virus

Inpatient Non-ICU
S. pneumoniae
M. pneumoniae
C. pneumoniae
H. influenzae
Legionella
Aspiration flora
Respiratory viruses (see above)

Inpatient ICU
S. pneumoniae
S. aureus
Legionella
Gram-negative organisms
H. influenzae

*As designated by the American Thoracic Society and the Infectious Diseases Society of America.
ICU, intensive care unit.
Modified from Mandell LA, Wunderink RG, Anzueto A, et al: Infectious Diseases Society of America/American Thoracic Society consensus guidelines on the management of community-acquired pneumonia in adults, Clin Infect Dis 44(Suppl 2):S27–S72, 2007.

kept in mind in choosing agents for empirical antimicrobial therapy; for example, high-level macrolide resistance (minimum inhibitory concentration [MIC] of 16 μg/mL or higher) at a prevalence of 25% or more should discourage macrolide use as a single agent. Of the multitude of potential causative agents, five or six pathogens typically account for a majority of cases of CAP; nevertheless, the possibility of unusual pathogens should always be kept in mind. A thorough recent travel or exposure history and an awareness of specific pathogen

association with certain epidemiologic settings are necessary to consider these unusual pathogens in CAP.

With respect to management, inpatients with CAP treated in the non-ICU setting are quite similar to the outpatients with equivalent risk factors. Pathogen spectra for these patient groups also are similar, except that Legionella and aspiration are more common in inpatients. Parenteral therapy is the preferred mode in the hospitalized patients.

With CAP severe enough to warrant admission to an ICU, an expanded list of likely pathogens has been reported. Although S. pneumoniae remains the most common, Legionella, S. aureus, and gram-negative bacilli including P. aeruginosa are identified with increasing frequency and warrant consideration for empirical coverage (**Table 24-3**). Those patients with CAP admitted to the ICU are by definition severely ill, and available data point to improved outcomes with use of antibiotic combinations in these patients; thus, monotherapy with fluoroquinolones or beta-lactams is not indicated. All patients should receive antibiotic combinations active against the most likely offending organisms. Presence of certain comorbid conditions such as bronchiectasis and severe COPD and other factors such as frequent antibiotic and systemic corticosteroid use are associated with increased probability of infection with P. aeruginosa; in such instances, empirical treatment effective against this pathogen is warranted. If S. aureus infection is suspected, coverage for community-acquired MRSA with agents such as vancomycin or linezolid should be provided. If necrotizing pneumonia is evident, clindamycin should be added to the regimen.

ROUTE AND DURATION OF THERAPY; HOSPITAL DISCHARGE

Most patients with CAP severe enough to warrant hospital admission are treated with intravenous antibiotics. Switching to oral therapy should be considered once the patient has achieved clinical stability (**Box 24-3**), is able to tolerate oral medications, and has a functioning gastrointestinal tract. In general, either the same agent or same class of antimicrobials should be used for the oral therapy regimen. Early initiation of oral therapy leads to earlier hospital discharge and overall

Table 24-3 Empirical Coverage for Uncommon Pathogens Causing Community-Acquired Pneumonia

Suspected Pathogen	Special Considerations
Pseudomonas	Piperacillin-tazobactam, cefepime, imipenem, or meropenem PLUS either ciprofloxacin or levofloxacin (750 mg) OR Aminoglycoside and azithromycin OR Aminoglycoside and antipneumococcal fluoroquinolone OR Substitute beta-lactam (piperacillin-tazobactam, cefepime, imipenem, or meropenem) with aztreonam in patients allergic to penicillin
Community-acquired methicillin-resistant *Staphylococcus aureus*	Vancomycin (+ clindamycin in patients with necrotizing pneumonia) OR Linezolid

Data from Mandell LA, Wunderink RG, Anzueto A, et al: Infectious Diseases Society of America/American Thoracic Society consensus guidelines on the management of community-acquired pneumonia in adults, *Clin Infect Dis* 44(Suppl 2):S27–S72, 2007.

Box 24-3 Criteria for Clinical Stability in Management of Community-Acquired Pneumonia

- Temperature ≤37.8° C
- Heart rate ≤100 beats/minute
- Systolic blood pressure ≥90 mm Hg
- Respiratory rate ≤24 breaths/minute
- Oxyhemoglobin saturation ≥90% or PO_2 ≥60 mm Hg on preadmission level of oxygen supplementation

Modified from Mandell LA, Wunderink RG, Anzueto A, et al: Infectious Diseases Society of America/American Thoracic Society consensus guidelines on the management of community-acquired pneumonia in adults, *Clin Infect Dis* 44(Suppl 2):S27–S72, 2007.

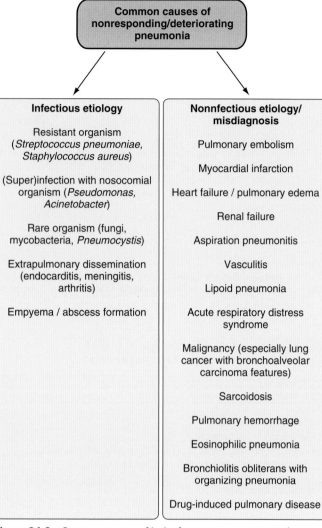

Figure 24-3 Common causes of lack of response to treatment in patients with community-acquired pneumonia (CAP).

COMPLICATIONS/FAILURE TO RESPOND TO THERAPY

A lack of response to empirical therapy is observed in up to 10% of outpatients and 15% of patients hospitalized with CAP. Challenges remain in the definition of nonresponse and treatment failure; however, the general consensus is that treatment adjustments probably should be withheld in the first 72 hours unless the patient's condition is deteriorating. Failure to achieve clinical stability using the aforementioned criteria within the first 3 days is suggestive of nonresponse to therapy, although in up to 25% of patients (especially those of advanced age and with multiple comorbid conditions), 6 days or longer may be needed to meet these criteria.

Several factors may potentially lead to lack of response to empirical therapy, including misdiagnosis of CAP, infection or superinfection with resistant organisms, infection dissemination with or without abscess formation, and others (**Figure 24-3**). However, no apparent cause for lack of response can be identified in up to 30% to 44% of such cases, with suggested reasons including comorbidity and possibly variations in inflammatory response.

Failure of empirical antimicrobial therapy usually results in a combination of further diagnostic testing, broadening of the antibiotic treatment regimen and/or transfer to higher-level care. An aggressive and complete reevaluation is still required

decreased number of adverse events. In-hospital observation before discharge is unnecessary after the switch to oral medications if the patient meets at least four of the five stability criteria (see Box 24-3), is free from comorbid conditions of clinical significance, and has adequate social supports in place.

In an effort to decrease the rate of adverse events of antibiotic therapy along with cost optimization, shorter durations of antimicrobial therapy have been considered, with current ATS/IDSA guideline recommendations denoting 5 days as minimal duration of therapy. Antibiotics can be discontinued once clinical stability has been achieved and maintained for 48 to 72 hours. Biomarker-guided determination of therapy duration has been attempted, suggesting that even 3-day therapy may be a viable option; however, further studies are needed to validate such an approach.

More than 7 to 10 days of total antibiotic administration is rarely required, unless extrapulmonary infections such as endocarditis or meningitis are present, initial therapy was not active against a subsequently identified offending pathogen, or *P. aeruginosa* infection, *S. aureus* bacteremia, or tissue necrosis was present.

in nonresponding and especially deteriorating patients. Exhaustive review of the findings on the history and physical examination, with increased attention to risk factors including personal habits and environmental, occupational, social, and travel history, is indicated. Reevaluation of patient's immune status could be helpful if compromise of any sort is suspected (e.g., HIV infection, common variable immunodeficiency). Valuable information occasionally can be obtained from the patient's social contacts, rather than directly from the patient.

Obtaining repeat microbiologic studies with evaluation for less common pathogens might be of benefit, although one must be aware of decreased sensitivity of bacterial studies obtained during antimicrobial therapy. Abscesses (if present) and pleural effusions should be drained, acquired fluid sent for microbiologic studies. Alternative sources of infection should be excluded. If no explanation emerges from these measures, bronchoalveolar lavage (BAL) could be considered, with differential cell count often providing important clues to the possible cause of nonresponse. For example, neutrophil-predominant BAL fluid is suggestive of bacterial infection and possibly bronchiolitis obliterans; lymphocyte-predominant BAL fluid is common in tuberculosis, sarcoidosis, and hypersensitivity pneumonitis; hemosiderin-laden macrophages are seen in alveolar hemorrhage; and a predominance of eosinophils is suggestive of fungal, *Pneumocystis*, or drug-induced diseases and eosinophilic pneumonia. In intubated patients, tracheal aspirates should be carefully examined. Absence of multidrug-resistant pathogens in the aspirate suggests that such organisms are less likely to be responsible for the lack of clinical improvement; however, the reverse is not true because of high rates of colonization by such pathogens in intubated patients.

Radiologic evaluation with a computed tomography (CT) scan of the chest with contrast simultaneously assess the lung parenchyma, pulmonary vasculature, and the pleural space and could provide valuable clues for the reason for nonresponse. For example, presence of nodules with a halo sign may suggest invasive aspergillosis complicating CAP in a patient with COPD on systemic corticosteroids.

Empirical escalation of antibiotic therapy could be considered, especially in patients with risk factors for potentially untreated pathogens; however, little evidence points to better outcomes with this approach. Severity of illness at presentation and comorbid conditions seem to be responsible for the failure to respond to guidelines-based therapy in a majority of such cases of CAP.

SPECIFIC COMPLICATIONS

ASPIRATION PNEUMONIA

Mendelson originally described the syndrome of aspiration of gastric contents in 1946 in 61 obstetric patients in whom aspiration pneumonia developed after ether anesthesia. Manifestations appear very rapidly after the event and include cough (dry or productive of pink sputum from bronchoalveolar hemorrhage), tachypnea, tachycardia, fever, diffuse crackles, cyanosis, and bronchospasm in some cases. The chest radiograph shows extensive atelectasis and infiltrates, and arterial blood gas analysis reveals hypoxemia and normocapnia or hypocapnia. In the most severe cases, the $PaCO_2$ may be elevated, and a metabolic acidosis may be present.

A number of clinical features help distinguish aspiration pneumonia from other CAPs. Aspiration pneumonia tends to have a more insidious course, such that the patient may have

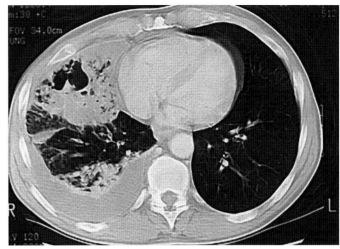

Figure 24-4   Necrotizing aspiration pneumonia. Chest computed tomography scan demonstrates involvement of the entire right middle lobe (which suggests pulmonary gangrene) and an effusion, which was found to represent an empyema.   *(From Rabbat A, Huchon G: Bacterial pneumonia. In Albert RK, Spiro SG, Jett JR, editors:* Clinical respiratory medicine, *ed 3, Philadelphia, 2008, Mosby.)*

an empyema, lung abscess, or necrotizing pneumonia at the time medical care is first sought. The sputum may be putrid because of anaerobic bacteria, and weight loss is common. Chest imaging commonly shows necrotizing infiltrates or multiple abscesses, typically located in dependent regions of the lung (**Figure 24-4**).

LUNG ABSCESS

The incidence of pulmonary abscess has decreased over the past decade. Lung abscess is associated with several conditions, including poor dental status or periodontal disease, chronic alcoholism, intravenous drug use, and head and neck cancer. Lung abscess may complicate bronchiectasis (**Figure 24-5**) and the course of aspiration pneumonia in persons with impaired consciousness, dysphagia and gastroesophageal reflux, or acute or chronic neurologic diseases, but it also may occur with bronchial obstruction by a foreign body or bronchial carcinoma.

Pulmonary abscesses usually are polymicrobial, with a predominant anaerobic flora, such as *Streptococcus intermedius*, *Streptococcus salivarius*, *Streptococcus constellatus*, *Fusobacterium* spp., *Prevotella* spp., or *Bacteroides* spp.

Clinical manifestations usually develop insidiously, particularly before onset of frank necrosis. This period may last several weeks after an initial aspiration. By the time of diagnosis of the lung abscess, patients may have lost weight and have a high fever, chills, putrid expectoration, and chest pain. Pleural involvement with an empyema is a frequent complication of lung abscess. Laboratory findings include a very high white cell count and considerable elevation of inflammatory and catabolic markers.

Radiologic features of lung abscess typically consist of a peripheral cavity more than 2 cm in diameter in the dependent lung regions. CT is useful to distinguish empyema with bronchopleural fistula from lung abscess.

Appearance of the sputum Gram stain often is misleading. Bronchoscopic sampling such as bronchial aspiration, protected specimen brush procedures, or BAL should be performed with inoculation onto anaerobic media. Percutaneous fluoroscopic or ultrasound or CT-guided fine needle aspiration may be a useful diagnostic technique. Aspirates should be grown on

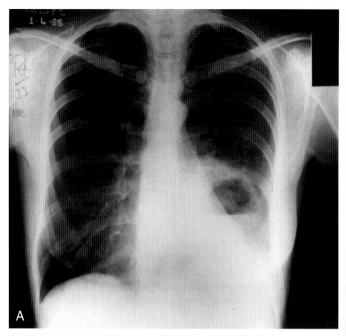

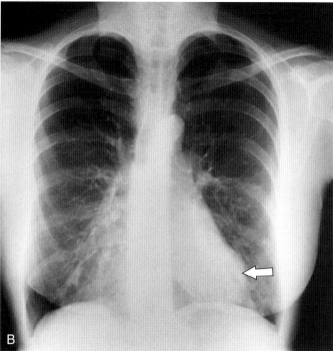

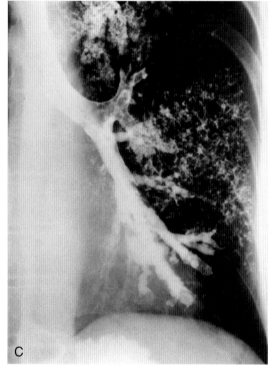

Figure 24-5 Radiographic appearance in left lower lobe pneumonia. **A,** Lung abscess associated with lower lobe pneumonia. **B,** At 3 months after resolution of the lung abscess, widened airways with thickened walls are apparent in the left lower lobe *(arrow).* These bronchiectatic changes were consequent to the pneumonia. **C,** Fiberoptic bronchoscopic bronchogram of the left lower lobe confirms gross dilatation of the airways, typical of postinfective bronchiectasis. *(From Rabbat A, Huchon G: Bacterial pneumonia. In Albert RK, Spiro SG, Jett JR, editors:* Clinical respiratory medicine, *ed 3, Philadelphia, 2008, Mosby.)*

anaerobic media, and samples should be sent promptly to the laboratory for specific anaerobic cultures.

PARAPNEUMONIC EFFUSION AND EMPYEMA

The signs and symptoms suggestive of a parapneumonic collection are increased breathlessness, swinging pyrexia, and raised levels of inflammatory markers. The chest radiograph usually demonstrates the collection of fluid. A lateral radiographic view or an ultrasound scan is useful to confirm the presence of fluid.

All pleural fluid specimens should be submitted for Gram stain and culture, because the identification of significant bacterial cultures confirms the diagnosis of infection and aids in antibiotic choice. Unfortunately, approximately 40% of infected

pleural effusions are culture negative, and in this situation, biochemical pleural fluid markers (pH, lactate dehydrogenase, white blood cell count, and glucose) are central to establishing a diagnosis. Fluid drainage by means of a chest tube and prolonged antibiotic therapy is necessary in all cases of complicated parapneumonic pleural effusion and empyema. (See Chapter 69 for a more detailed description of these two clinical entities.)

BRONCHOPLEURAL FISTULA

A bronchopleural fistula is caused by a connection between the pleural space and the consolidated lung; it can complicate either an empyema or a lung abscess. The bronchopleural fistula causes a pyopneumothorax (i.e., air-fluid level in the pleural space), so that, on drainage of an empyema, not only pus but also air comes out through the chest drain. A bronchopleural fistula will not seal unless infection is controlled. Initial treatment is conservative, with antibiotics and tube drainage, to allow healing of the fistula. If this approach fails, surgery may be necessary to attempt primary closure of the fistula or closure of the potential space with other living tissues, such as muscle flaps. The management of bronchopleural fistulas that do not close with conservative treatment requires the surgical skills of a thoracic specialist.

ORGANIZING PNEUMONIA

Organizing pneumonia, sometimes known as *cryptogenic organizing pneumonia* (now the preferred designation for *bronchiolitis obliterans organizing pneumonia* [BOOP]), is a condition in which an organizing inflammatory exudate with fibroblast proliferation occurs after an episode of pneumonia. The consolidation often is patchy and may be fleeting. Organizing pneumonia subsequent to a bacterial infection is suggested when a residual consolidation (often fleeting) is observed despite adequate antibiotic treatment. Investigation includes examination of sputum or bronchial washings to exclude infection. CT may help to visualize the consolidation and exclude other causes. The definitive investigation is an open lung biopsy showing the typical histologic changes, which along with highly suggestive clinical findings constitute sufficient evidence for a confident diagnosis. A course of steroids usually leads to resolution. When the steroids are stopped, however, relapse may occur; in such cases, treatment for several months may be necessary (see Chapter 50).

Table 24-4   Recommendations for Vaccine Prevention of Community-Acquired Pneumonia

Factor	Pneumococcal Polysaccharide Vaccine	Inactivated Influenza Vaccine	Live Attenuated Influenza Vaccine
Route of administration	Intramuscular injection	Intramuscular injection	Intranasal spray
Type of vaccine	Bacterial component (polysaccharide capsule)	Killed virus	Live virus
Recommended groups	All persons ≥65 years of age	All persons ≥50 years of age	Healthy persons 5-49 years of age,* including health care providers and household contacts of high-risk persons
	High-risk persons 2-64 years of age	High-risk persons 6 months–49 years of age	
	Current smokers†	Household contacts of high-risk persons Health care providers Children 6-23 months of age	
Specific high-risk indications for vaccination	Chronic cardiovascular, pulmonary, renal, or liver disease	Chronic cardiovascular or pulmonary disease (including asthma)	Avoid in high-risk persons
	Diabetes mellitus	Chronic metabolic disease (including diabetes mellitus)	
	Cerebrospinal fluid leaks	Renal dysfunction	
	Alcoholism	Hemoglobinopathies	
	Asplenia	Immunocompromising conditions/medications	
	Immunocompromising conditions/ medications	Compromised respiratory function or increased aspiration risk	
	Native Americans and Alaska natives	Pregnancy	
	Long-term care facility residents	Residence in a long-term care facility	
		Aspirin therapy in persons ≤18 years of age	
Revaccination schedule	One-time revaccination after 5 years for (1) adults ≥65 years of age, if the first dose is received before age 65 years; (2) persons with asplenia; and (3) immunocompromised persons	Annual revaccination	Annual revaccination

*Avoid use in persons with asthma, reactive airway disease, or other chronic disorders of the pulmonary or cardiovascular system; persons with other underlying medical conditions, including diabetes, renal dysfunction, and hemoglobinopathies; persons with immunodeficiencies or who receive immunosuppressive therapy; children or adolescents receiving salicylates; persons with a history of Guillain-Barré syndrome; and pregnant women.
†Vaccinating current smokers is recommended by the Pneumonia Guidelines Committee but is not currently an indication for vaccine according to the Advisory Committee on Immunization Practices statement.
From Mandell LA, Wunderink RG, Anzueto A, et al: Infectious Diseases Society of America/American Thoracic Society consensus guidelines on the management of community-acquired pneumonia in adults, *Clin Infect Dis* 44(Suppl 2):S27–S72, 2007. (Adapted from Harper SA, Fukuda K, Uyeki TM, et al: Prevention and control of influenza: recommendations of the Advisory Committee on Immunization Practices [ACIP], *MMWR Recomm Rep* 54:1-40, 2005.)

BRONCHIECTASIS

Permanent dilatation of the bronchus can be a sequela of severe pneumonia, causing localized bronchiectasis. CT scanning during or after an episode of acute pneumonia may show bronchial dilatation, so the diagnosis cannot be made with confidence until after the pneumonia has completely resolved. The presence of bronchiectasis is suggested by continual cough productive of sputum or recurrent infections in one part of the lung. Investigation consists of sputum examination, when organisms associated with bronchiectasis such as *H. influenzae* or *P. aeruginosa* may be isolated. The diagnostic test of choice is a thin-section, high-resolution CT scan. Management consists of postural drainage of the infected lobe and antibiotic treatment for any acute infection. In patients who have coexisting airflow obstruction, treatment with bronchodilators or inhaled steroids may be helpful. (See Chapter 45 for a full description of this clinical entity.)

PREVENTION

Administration of vaccines targeting *S. pneumoniae* and influenza viruses and risk factor modification such as smoking cessation, aspiration precautions, and cessation of alcohol abuse constitute the main preventive measures for CAP (**Table 24-4**). Vaccination status should be assessed at the beginning of the hospitalization, and vaccination may be performed either at discharge or during outpatient follow-up if needed. Vaccination at discharge is preferred in patients in whom compliance with outpatient follow-up care is likely to be unreliable.

CONTROVERSIES AND PITFALLS

Whether empirical treatment of atypical pathogens, specifically *C. pneumoniae* and *M. pneumoniae*, is essential and clearly beneficial in all patients with CAP is an area of controversy. This is reflected in American guidelines recommending coverage for atypical pathogens in all patients, in contrast with European recommendations making such coverage optional at the discretion of the treating physician.

Health care–associated pneumonia (HCAP) is a more recent designation for a form of pneumonia acquired in the community but warranting treatment more like that for nosocomial pneumonia, because of risk factors that predispose affected patients to infections by pathogens that usually are found in the local hospital setting (see Chapter 27). Current criteria used to distinguish HCAP from CAP are in question as being too broad in scope, potentially leading to excessive use of broad-spectrum antibiotics. It is likely that refinement of these criteria in the near future will redefine the boundaries between HCAP and CAP.

Acknowledgment

In preparation of this chapter, we retained some material from Chapter 27 on bacterial pneumonias, by Antoine Rabbat and Gérard J. Huchon, in the third edition of this book. The contribution of these authors is gratefully acknowledged.

SUGGESTED READINGS

Bochud PY, Moser F, Erard P, et al: Community-acquired pneumonia. A prospective outpatient study, *Medicine (Baltimore)* 80:75–87, 2001.

Christ-Crain M, Opal SM: Clinical review: the role of biomarkers in the diagnosis and management of community-acquired pneumonia, *Crit Care* 14:203, 2010.

Feikin DR, Schuchat A, Kolczak M, et al: Mortality from invasive pneumococcal pneumonia in the era of antibiotic resistance, 1995-1997, *Am J Public Health* 90:223–229, 2000.

File TM Jr, Marrie TJ: Burden of community-acquired pneumonia in North American adults, *Postgrad Med* 122:130–141, 2010.

Kee C, Palladino S, Kay I, et al: Feasibility of real-time polymerase chain reaction in whole blood to identify *Streptococcus pneumoniae* in patients with community-acquired pneumonia, *Diagn Microbiol Infect Dis* 61:72–75, 2008.

Lim WS, Baudouin SV, George RC, et al: BTS guidelines for the management of community acquired pneumonia in adults: update 2009, *Thorax* 64(Suppl 3):iii1–iii55, 2009.

Mandell LA, Marrie TJ, Grossman RF, et al: Canadian guidelines for the initial management of community-acquired pneumonia: an evidence-based update by the Canadian Infectious Diseases Society and the Canadian Thoracic Society. The Canadian Community-Acquired Pneumonia Working Group, *Clin Infect Dis* 31:383–421, 2000.

Mandell LA, Wunderink RG, Anzueto A, et al: Infectious Diseases Society of America/American Thoracic Society consensus guidelines on the management of community-acquired pneumonia in adults, *Clin Infect Dis* 44(Suppl 2):S27–S72, 2007.

Schuetz P, Christ-Crain M, Thomann R, et al: Effect of procalcitonin-based guidelines vs standard guidelines on antibiotic use in lower respiratory tract infections: the ProHOSP randomized controlled trial, *JAMA* 302:1059–1066, 2009.

Waterer GW, Rello J, Wunderink RG: Management of community-acquired pneumonia in adults, *Am J Respir Crit Care Med* 183:157–164, 2011.

Chapter **25**
Viral Pneumonia

Ganapathi Iyer Parameswaran • Sanjay Sethi

Despite increasing recognition of the role of viruses in causing pneumonia in adults, either as sole pathogens or as copathogens with bacteria, diagnosis and treatment of viral pneumonias remain difficult clinical problems. Progress has been made in development of precise laboratory tests to diagnose lower respiratory tract infections of viral origin. Wider availability of such tests is likely to spur recognition and give impetus to development of new therapies.

BURDEN OF DISEASE

VIRAL COMMUNITY-ACQUIRED PNEUMONIA

The proportion of pneumonias in adults that are caused by viruses is difficult to quantify with any precision. This lack of certainty is not surprising, because in approximately 50% of pneumonias, an identifiable pathogen cannot be established by conventional laboratory testing. Molecular techniques such as polymerase chain reaction (PCR) analysis improve this number but are rarely performed in routine clinical care. Difficulties in obtaining adequate specimens for viral cultures or molecular testing add to the problem. However, several recent studies have made efforts to quantify the burden of viral community-acquired pneumonias in adults and are summarized in **Table 25-1**. Although the proportion of viral pneumonias varies in these studies owing to differences in study populations and rigor of testing for viruses, it is clear that viruses cause a significant proportion of pneumonias. Overall, in immunocompetent adults hospitalized with pneumonia, viruses are the responsible pathogens in 15% to 30% of the cases, either by themselves or as copathogens with bacteria. Lower respiratory secretions such as bronchoalveolar lavage (BAL) fluid, tracheal aspirates, or good-quality induced sputum are preferable as specimens for diagnosis of viral pneumonia. Such specimens are more difficult to obtain, however, and most studies have used nasopharyngeal wash samples or swabs for culture and molecular testing. Presence of established pathogens such as influenza virus in such upper respiratory tract samples in a patient with pneumonia most probably implies that the virus is a sole or copathogen in causation of pneumonia; however, this general rule may not be applicable to other viruses. Presence of such viruses as rhinovirus might imply only upper respiratory infection in a patient with pneumonia due to another pathogen. Findings on studies of viral pneumonias must therefore be interpreted with some caution.

VIRAL PNEUMONIA IN IMMUNOCOMPROMISED PATIENTS

Patients who have undergone hematopoietic stem cell transplantation (HSCT) or solid organ transplantation or who are undergoing intensive chemotherapy for leukemias exhibit a higher incidence of viral upper respiratory infections than that in normal control subjects, as well as more frequent involvement of the lower respiratory tract, more severe pneumonias, and higher rates of death from viral pneumonia. All of the pathogens mentioned in Table 25-1 are represented in these patients. Respiratory syncytial virus (RSV), adenovirus, and parainfluenza virus, which usually cause only mild illness in immunocompetent persons, can cause severe pneumonias with high mortality rates in this high-risk patient population. Extrapulmonary manifestations of influenza infection, such as myocarditis, are not unusual in this population. RSV is the most common viral pathogen of the lower respiratory tract in patients who have undergone hematopoietic stem cell or solid organ transplantation, as reported in many series. Fulminant, disseminated adenoviral infections have been reported in patients with advanced human immunodeficiency virus (HIV) disease. Cytomegalovirus (CMV) infection is a major problem in stem cell and solid organ transplant recipients and probably is the most common viral pneumonia among patients who are not on prophylaxis or preemptive treatment regimens.

PATHOGENS

Although some variability has been documented in the frequency with which different viral pathogens are diagnosed as the etiologic agent of pneumonia in specific series, the most frequent pathogens are influenza A virus, influenza B virus, and RSV. In addition, parainfluenza viruses 1, 2, and 3 and adenovirus, coronaviruses, and rhinovirus also may cause pneumonia. Human metapneumovirus (hMPV) and, more recently, bocavirus have been recognized as pathogens. Rarer pathogens are CMV, varicella-zoster virus (VZV), herpes simplex virus (HSV), rubeola virus (the measles virus), and hantavirus.

INFLUENZA VIRUSES

The most frequent viral pathogen implicated in causing pneumonia and increased mortality, influenza virus serotypes A and B, especially A, are responsible for outbreaks of respiratory

Table 25-1 Summary of Selected Clinical Studies of Viral Pneumonia

Study	Population/Viral Studies	Results	Comments
Jennings et al, 2008	304 hospitalized adults Nasopharyngeal swab viral culture, DFA, and real-time PCR analysis	Viral etiology established in 88/304 (29%)	Microbial etiology established in 177/304 (58%) Rhinovirus most frequent, followed by influenza virus and RSV
Johnstone et al, 2008	300 adults hospitalized with pneumonia 193 patients had nasopharyngeal swabs, DFA, and NAAT (NASBA and real-time PCR analysis)	Viral etiology established in 29/193 (15%)	Microbial etiology established in 75/193 (39%) Of viruses, influenza virus, hMPV, and RSV most frequent
de Roux et al, 2004	1356 nonimmunocompromised adults hospitalized with pneumonia 338 had paired serologic sample testing for viruses (influenza virus, parainfluenza virus, RSV, adenovirus)	Positive results on paired serologic samples in 61/338 (18%); in 31 (9%) of these, virus established as sole pathogen	Microbial etiology established in. 518/1356 (38%) Influenza A and B viruses most frequent viruses
Marcos et al, 2006	198 hospitalized adults Viral culture, serologic testing, IFA, and nasopharyngeal swab real-time PCR analysis	Positive results on viral testing in 46/198 (23%)	Microbial etiology established in 112 (57%) Influenza A virus, RSV, and adenovirus most frequent
Johansson et al, 2010	184 hospitalized adults with community-acquired pneumonia Nasopharyngeal culture and PCR assay	Virus established as sole or copathogen in 53/184 (29%)	Influenza virus, rhinovirus, RSV, and parainfluenza viruses most frequent

DFA, direct fluorescent antibody test; hMPV, human metapneumovirus; IFA, indirect fluorescent antibody test; NAAT, nucleic acid amplification test; NASBA, nucleic acid sequence–based amplification; PCR, polymerase chain reaction; RSV, respiratory syncytial virus.

illness each winter. Minor changes in hemagglutinin and neuraminidase proteins of the virus causing "antigenic drift" are responsible for seasonal influenza outbreaks. Although people of all ages are exposed to infection, the consequences of influenza-specific respiratory infection are more severe in certain groups of patients—elderly persons, nursing home residents, infants, those with severe coexisting cardiac and respiratory diseases such as congestive heart failure and chronic obstructive pulmonary disease (COPD), pregnant women, patients with immunosuppression due to hematologic malignancies, and those with HIV disease. Most of the deaths attributable to seasonal influenza occur in these groups. In addition, obesity has been associated with more severe disease and higher mortality in the recent H1N1 pandemic.

Major mutations in hemagglutinin and neuraminidase result in "antigenic shifts" and are responsible for pandemics. The most recently described is the current H1N1 (swine origin) virus pandemic starting in 2009. In contrast with seasonal influenza, the proportion of deaths in younger patients (18 to 65 years) has increased during pandemics. This increased mortality has been attributed to lack of previous exposure to a similar strain of the virus, with corresponding lack of protective antibodies, in patients who were not alive at the time of an earlier outbreak with a similar virus. This pattern has been seen in the current H1N1 pandemic.

Thus, influenza-related pneumonia occurs each year during the fall, winter, and spring seasons as a consequence of infection with circulating seasonal influenza viruses. Distinct from this pattern, pandemic influenza viruses cause pneumonias in explosive outbreaks. Such pandemic viral pneumonias differ from the seasonal disease in several ways: (1) Patients 18 to 65 years of age, especially those in the 20- to 45-year-old age group, are affected more often than in seasonal disease; (2) mortality due to influenza-related pneumonia is increased among adults 20 to 45 years of age; (3) the proportion of primary viral pneumonias is higher than in seasonal disease, in which most influenza-related pneumonias are due to bacteria;

(4) viral influenza–related illness occurs outside of the usual influenza season; and (5) special risk factors for severe disease and mortality have been recognized, such as pregnancy and severe obesity. The recent H1N1 pandemic has infected more than 50 million persons in the United States alone, and caused approximately 18,000 deaths worldwide. Severe infections, consisting of pneumonia and acute respiratory distress syndrome (ARDS), typically have been seen in adults, with a median age of 40 years.

The true incidence of pneumonia in influenza respiratory infection is unknown, because most patients with influenza-related illness are evaluated and managed as outpatients without radiographs. Of a group of elderly adults with a high vaccination rate (greater than 90%), 2% to 6% were hospitalized with influenza-related illness; of these, only 5% had radiographically confirmed pneumonia. A significant proportion of such patients will have other illnesses, such as congestive heart failure, that precipitate hospitalization. Pneumonia developing during influenza infection can be one of two types: primary viral pneumonia or postinfluenza bacterial pneumonia. Louria and co-workers, reporting on the 1957-1958 pandemic, described four syndromes of lower respiratory tract illness due to influenza in New York City: (1) influenza illness with physical signs of lower respiratory involvement, but no infiltrates on the chest film; (2) influenza illness followed by bacterial pneumonia; (3) acute, rapidly progressive pneumonia due to influenza virus; and (4) concomitant viral and bacterial pneumonia. The histopathologic changes of influenza-related viral infection of the lower respiratory tract consist of desquamation of tracheobronchial epithelium, alveolar duct dilatation, hyaline membrane covering alveolar surfaces, and hemorrhage and inflammatory infiltrate in the alveolar spaces and interstitium.

Pathogenesis of Bacterial Pneumonia in Influenza

The association of influenza lower respiratory infection with bacterial pneumonia is striking. Such influenza-associated bacterial pneumonias, caused by *Streptococcus pneumoniae*, *Haemophilus influenzae*, and *Staphylococcus aureus*, including methicillin-resistant strains, are more frequent and severe than primary bacterial pneumonias due to the same pathogens. The seasonal incidence of *S. pneumoniae* infection in a community parallels the incidence of influenza illness. The mechanisms underlying the increased frequency and severity of these influenza-associated bacterial pneumonias are mostly unclear at present, but emerging evidence suggests roles for multiple viral and host factors. Increased apoptosis and desquamation of airway epithelial cells infected with influenza virus exposes multiple surface adhesins for pathogenic bacteria. Influenza viruses expressing PB1-F2, a proapoptotic protein that interferes with mitochondrial function and increases epithelial cell apoptosis, increase susceptibility to *S. pneumoniae* infection. When infected with viral strains lacking PB1-F2, mice were less susceptible to bacterial pneumonia, compared with those infected with wild-type viral strains. Moreover, influenza infection decreases the efficacy of airway mucociliary clearance, and thus clearance of pathogenic bacteria.

Viral neuraminidase increases bacterial growth and dissemination, and adherence of *S. pneumoniae* to airway epithelial cells in mouse models. Influenza strains with high neuraminidase activity are associated with higher mortality after bacterial infection. Influenza virus inhibits neutrophil chemotaxis and phagocytic capacity; inhibits, through induction of IFN-γ, macrophage receptor with collagenous structure (MARCO) production by macrophages. MARCO is a scavenger protein involved in macrophage recognition and killing of bacteria. Influenza virus also causes desensitization of Toll-like receptors (TLRs), and this desensitization persists for several weeks.

Primary Influenza-Related Viral Pneumonia

The true incidence of primary influenza pneumonia is unknown, because many patients do not undergo radiography or detailed clinical evaluation. It originally was considered that most of the deaths in the 1918 influenza pandemic were due to primary viral pneumonia. Later analysis of multiple data sources, however, strongly suggested that a majority of deaths (approximately 80%) from influenza-related pneumonia were due to secondary bacterial (postinfluenza) pneumonias, caused primarily by *S. pneumoniae* and *H. influenzae* and other gram-negative organisms such as *Klebsiella pneumoniae* and *Escherichia coli*. A series of 33 patients with influenza-related pneumonias and deaths from the 1957-1958 pandemic again showed that a majority of deaths were due to bacterial pneumonia. Of 33 patients, 15 had acquired bacterial pneumonia after influenza illness; six had primary viral pneumonia with isolation of influenza virus, but no bacterial pathogen, from lung tissue; and nine had concomitant bacterial and viral pneumonia. In the recent (2009) H1N1 virus pandemic, initial reports suggested that deaths were mostly due to viral pneumonia. Further analysis of autopsy lung specimens showed that in approximately 30% of these deaths, a bacterial pathogen could be identified by molecular studies. However, the proportion of viral pneumonia (approximately 70%) is striking and higher than in previous pandemics. Moreover, *S. aureus*, especially methicillin-resistant *S. aureus* (MRSA), was found in a significant proportion of bacterial pneumonias, with high mortality, especially among teenage patients. Therefore, in summary, primary viral as well as secondary bacterial infections, including those due to MRSA, must be considered in every case of influenza-related pneumonia and treated presumptively until full identification of the pathogens involved is obtained.

The typical clinical course of primary viral pneumonia is described as progression of the initial upper respiratory tract symptoms to shortness of breath, increased cough and sputum, and respiratory failure, as compared with secondary bacterial pneumonia, in which a period of improvement after the initial influenza infection is followed by new and worsening respiratory symptoms due to pneumonia. The sputum often is thin and blood-stained in primary viral pneumonia. Radiographs usually show bilateral interstitial or infiltrative opacities, which may mimic the appearance of congestive heart failure.

RESPIRATORY SYNCYTIAL VIRUS

Long considered to be a pathogen of children only, RSV is now recognized as a significant pathogen in elderly and immuno-compromised adults. It is the second most common pathogen in most series of viral pneumonias. Similar to the influenza viruses, RSV causes winter outbreaks of respiratory illness. It is estimated that in most populations of nursing home residents, approximately 10% develop RSV respiratory infections each year. Most of these are self-limiting upper respiratory infections; the remaining 10% or so develop pneumonia. Centers for Disease Control and Prevention (CDC) surveillance data suggest that RSV infections are responsible for about 10,000 deaths annually in elderly patients living in the community. In one prospective series of elderly adults, RSV was the responsible pathogen in 11% of patients hospitalized with pneumonia during winter months. Chest radiographs often show bilateral fluffy infiltrates.

HUMAN METAPNEUMOVIRUS

Since being described as a cause of respiratory illness in children in 2001, hMPV is now recognized to cause pneumonias in adults, especially elderly patients with cardiopulmonary diseases. A prospective study, using reverse transcriptase PCR testing of nasopharyngeal samples, found evidence of hMPV infection in 4% of 193 adults hospitalized with pneumonia during an influenza season. Evidence of hMPV infection was present, by PCR analysis of nasopharyngeal aspirate and/or paired serologic samples, in 4% of adults visiting an emergency department in Canada with pneumonia or exacerbation of COPD.

PARAINFLUENZA VIRUSES 1, 2, AND 3

Parainfluenza viruses 1, 2, and 3 cause upper respiratory infections as well as pneumonia in elderly adults, especially nursing home residents. A study in Sweden found serologic evidence for recent parainfluenza virus infection in approximately 10% of community-acquired pneumonias in elderly persons.

CORONAVIRUSES

Several coronavirus strains cause the common cold during winter months. Pneumonia has been described in elderly persons and immunocompromised patients; the frequency of such infections is not known. In 2002, a novel strain, SARS-CoV, spread around the globe, causing an acute pneumonia and ARDS.

RHINOVIRUS

The most frequent cause of the common cold was thought to be not a pathogen in the lower respiratory tract. However, the advent of molecular methods such as real-time PCR analysis has demonstrated that in many patients, especially in those with chronic respiratory diseases such as COPD or immuno-suppression, rhinovirus is present in the lower airways during pneumonia. The role of rhinovirus as a sole pathogen in causation of pneumonia is still a matter of debate and research.

VARICELLA-ZOSTER VIRUS

Pneumonia associated with chickenpox in adults is a well-recognized complication and continues to occur each year in the United States. When chickenpox occurs in adults, the incidence of pneumonia as a complication is increased by approximately 25-fold over that in children. Except in rare instances, such pneumonia is associated with the rash typical of the disease. A study of military recruits revealed that radiographic lung abnormalities are much more common than signs and symptoms of pneumonia—that is, most lung involvement is subclinical. Mortality rates for severe pneumonia leading to respiratory failure have decreased over the last few decades owing to improvements in ventilatory support and prompt therapy with acyclovir.

CLINICAL FEATURES

Viral pneumonias in general have the same clinical symptoms (cough, shortness of breath, increased sputum, and chest pain) and signs (radiographic consolidation, fever, tachycardia, tachypnea, reduced arterial oxygen saturation) as those of bacterial pneumonias. Some clinical features occur more often in viral pneumonias than in bacterial pneumonias, although this distinction is not precise enough for a diagnosis to be made on clinical evaluation without further testing, except in rare situations. Patients with viral pneumonias tend to be older and frailer, with other comorbid conditions such as cardiac failure and COPD; have less chest pain, tachycardia, and fever; and show lower levels of leukocytosis than in the characteristic clinical picture in bacterial pneumonias. Features such as rhinitis, conjunctivitis, and pharyngitis or a typical rash for varicella or measles can point to a viral etiology for pneumonia. Gastrointestinal complaints often accompany influenza-related infections. RSV infections are more likely to be associated with wheezing than influenza virus infections. Chest radiographs show lobar infiltrates or basal atelectasis–like patterns, and infiltrates often are bilateral; these features are not specific enough, however, to allow clinical differentiation between viral and bacterial pneumonia. Varicella pneumonia often causes nodular lung lesions on chest films, although interstitial infiltrates also are described. The difficulties in differentiating between viral and bacterial pneumonias on clinical features alone are illustrated by a study that compared findings on the chest radiograph in children with community-acquired pneumonia. In children with alveolar infiltrates, 71% had a bacterial cause; in those with proven bacterial pneumonia, 72% had alveolar infiltrates; and in those who had only interstitial infiltrates, approximately 50% had a bacterial cause. CT scans show a variety of appearances—ground glass opacities, nodules, and lobular and segmental infiltrates.

Serum procalcitonin levels are being increasingly used to guide decisions regarding the need for antibacterial therapy. A very low level may indicate a low likelihood of bacterial infection in lower respiratory infections. This association, however, does not imply that the cause is viral. To establish a viral cause, another diagnostic method (culture or PCR assay) is still necessary.

DIAGNOSIS

The accuracy of clinical features in predicting a viral infection depends on the pretest probability of viral respiratory infection in a given population. In one series of 258 patients seeking emergency or urgent care for acute respiratory symptoms during influenza season, clinical judgment had sensitivity and specificity of 29% and 92%, respectively, in diagnosing influenza; the figures improved to 67% and 96% if patients presented within 48 hours of symptom onset. Patients with viral pneumonia, however, often do not have accompanying upper respiratory symptoms, and the symptoms and signs overlap with those of bacterial pneumonia.

Attempts at precise definition of the roles and frequency of these viruses in causing pneumonia have been hampered by difficulties in viral culture, and by a nihilistic attitude among medical professionals stemming from lack of effective therapy against many of these viruses. Precise diagnosis of viral causes for pneumonia has multiple benefits: (1) Public health measures against spread of highly infective viruses such as influenza viruses and RSV can be better coordinated. (2) Attempts at development of effective therapies can be supported with increasing recognition of the etiologic roles of these viruses. (3) Unnecessary antibiotic therapy can be curtailed. (4) Infection control and prophylaxis measures can be implemented in hospitals and nursing homes.

A variety of clinical specimens are suitable for diagnosis of viral pneumonia. These include, in order of preference, lung tissue and BAL fluid, nasopharyngeal wash sample, nasopharyngeal swabs, and sputum. BAL often is avoided because of its invasive nature but nevertheless is desirable in immuno-compromised and critically ill patients, in whom a specific diagnosis is necessary and co-infections are common. Diagnosis of viral infection in a patient with pneumonia can be attempted by one or more of four methods, as summarized in **Table 25-2**.

Culture of virus from clinical specimens, using tissue culture cells, remains the standard diagnostic modality. However, it is labor-intensive, requires expertise in culture techniques and recognition of the effects of virus on cells, and is not always available except in large laboratories. Sending specimens out to reference laboratories is problematic, because many viruses tolerate such transportation poorly. Moreover, some viruses such as rhinovirus, hMPV, and some coronaviruses grow poorly in tissue cultures, and the results of viral culture take several days to become available. With all of these caveats, if a suitable specimen is available, culture should be attempted on samples obtained in patients suspected to have viral pneumonia. Shell vial cultures, especially when combined with immunofluorescent antibody staining of cells, has higher sensitivity than that of tube culture.

Serologic testing had been a mainstay in retrospective diagnosis of viral infections and remains an important epidemiologic tool. However, owing to the requirement for paired samples separated by 4 weeks to demonstrate a significant increase in IgG titers, serologic studies are now rarely used in clinical diagnosis of viral pneumonia.

Antigen detection can be performed in most respiratory secretions using direct fluorescent antibody (DFA) and enzymatic immunoassay (EIA) tests. DFA testing, performed by treating samples with a virus-specific antibody tagged with a fluorophore and a fluorescence microscope, often is used in conjunction with shell vial culture of viruses from respiratory secretions. EIAs are available for detection of influenza A virus in kit form

Table 25-2 Commonly Used Methods for Diagnosis of Viral Lower Respiratory Infection

Method	Tests	Specimen(s)	Comments
Culture	Inoculation of cultured human or primate cells; shell vial culture	NP wash, NP swab, sputum, BAL fluid, lung tissue	"Gold standard"; labor-intensive; some viruses grow poorly
Serologic testing	IgG and IgM assays; paired (acute and convalescent) IgG titers	Blood	Paired titers not useful in clinical diagnosis of acute infection
Antigen detection	DFA, EIA	NP wash, NP swab, BAL fluid, sputum; DFA with shell vial culture	Poor to moderate sensitivity, except for DFA with shell vial culture
Molecular methods	PCR assay; RT-PCR; real-time PCR analysis: NASBA	NP wash, NP swab, sputum, BAL fluid, lung tissue	Sensitivity better than that of culture; high specificity

BAL, bronchoalveolar lavage; DFA, direct fluorescent antibody test; EIA, enzymatic immunoassay; IgG, IgM, immunoglobulins G and M; NP, nasopharyngeal; PCR, polymerase chain reaction; RT-PCR, reverse transcriptase PCR.

(Rapid Influenza Diagnosis Test [RIDT]). Although highly specific (90% to 95%), these rapid tests have lower sensitivity (approximately 70%) compared with viral culture and molecular methods, especially when the viral load is low. A rapid antigen detection test is available for RSV; its sensitivity is very low compared with that of culture—only about 10%.

Molecular methods depend on detection of virus-specific genetic material. Reverse transcriptase PCR (RT-PCR), nucleic acid sequence–based amplification (NASBA), and real-time RT-PCR methods have been used. These methods have sensitivity (97% to 99%) and specificity (90% to 95%) similar to and often better than viral culture. Real-time PCR results are available the same day and can distinguish between strains such as H1N1 and H3N2. Commercially available tests using multiple primers, allowing testing for a panel of viruses, are becoming more common in large laboratories. The x-TAG RVP assay, approved by the U.S. Food and Drug Administration (FDA), tests for 12 viruses commonly implicated in respiratory illness. Even broader tests, using panviral gene microarrays, are being used as research tools and may soon be available for clinical use.

Patients suspected on clinical grounds to have influenza pneumonia should be tested for influenza using RIDT. If the result of this test is negative, viral culture of respiratory secretions (nasopharyngeal swab or wash sample, BAL fluid, endotracheal aspirate) should be performed. If available, a nucleic acid amplification test such as PCR assay should be performed on these specimens. In patients suspected to have other (or unknown) viral pneumonias, viral culture and, if available, a multiplex viral PCR assay are indicated.

TREATMENT

With pneumonias caused by the aforementioned viruses, effective treatment is available for those due to influenza A and B viruses, VZV, and possibly RSV. Available antiviral drugs are (1) adamantanes (amantadine and rimantadine); (2) neuraminidase inhibitors (oseltamivir, zanamivir, and, provided by the CDC on a case-by-case basis, peramivir); (3) ribavarin; and (4) acyclovir and its derivatives valganciclovir and famciclovir.

The adamantanes—amantadine and rimantadine—are no longer recommended for treatment of influenza owing to widespread resistance of the virus strains and should not be used in treatment of viral pneumonias. Of the neuraminidase inhibitors, oseltamivir is available orally only; zanamivir as an inhaled powder; and peramivir as an intravenous formulation. Ribavirin is available in oral formulation and as a liquid for aerosol administration and has been used intravenously in small series of patients.

The neuraminidase inhibitors are effective in reducing duration of symptoms for outpatients with influenza-related upper respiratory infection, when started within 48 hours of onset of symptoms. Efficacy against influenza pneumonia is unclear. A large Canadian study of adults hospitalized with seasonal influenza–related infections showed reduction in mortality and hospital stay when oseltamivir was started even later than 48 hours. The CDC currently recommends neuraminidase inhibitor treatment for all adults with severe influenza-related illness. It seems reasonable, therefore, to use one of these agents for any patient suspected to have influenza-related pneumonia, whatever the duration of symptoms, while etiologic investigations are under way. This approach also means that any patient with possible viral pneumonia during seasonal influenza season or during an influenza pandemic should receive oseltamivir while appropriate studies are undertaken to identify the specific etiologic agent of pneumonia.

Zanamivir is an alternative to oseltamivir. It is available only as an inhalant. Zanamivir can provoke wheezing and clog nebulizers (the CDC advises against using this agent in a nebulizer) and probably should be avoided in patients with respiratory compromise. Increasing resistance to oseltamivir is being reported in influenza A virus. These strains remain sensitive to zanamivir and peramivir. Oseltamivir is less active against influenza B virus than against influenza A virus; zanamivir is preferred if influenza B virus is known to be the etiologic agent, in the absence of contraindications to its use. The incidence of resistance to oseltamivir in the United States remains low, as reported by the CDC (less than 1% for H1N1 and H3N2) in April 2011 (http://www.cdc.gov/flu/weekly/).

In patients who do not respond to or who deteriorate while on oseltamivir, and if drug resistance is suspected, intravenous peramivir is available from the CDC. A recent uncontrolled case series shows promising results in such patients with use of intravenous peramivir. Drug sensitivity testing for cultured viral strains is available in reference laboratories and at the CDC.

Ribavirin is active against RSV. However, efficacy in RSV-related lower respiratory infections in adults is unproved. Limited evidence for efficacy comes from small case series of patients with immunocompromised states such as hematopoietic stem cell transplantation and patients undergoing chemotherapy for leukemia. Its use in adults critically ill with pneumonia and proven RSV infection should be considered carefully, with involvement of a physician who has some experience in using ribavirin in such situations. Ribavirin aerosol often is combined with intravenous immunoglobulin to treat severe RSV infections in immunocompromised patients. In addition, testing and, during the wait for results, initial treatment for bacterial pneumonias should be added. Ribavirin can cause hemolytic anemia. Aerosol use introduces hospital staffing problems, because this agent is teratogenic in animal experiments, and accidental exposure of women of reproductive age must be avoided. In VZV pneumonia, antiviral treatment with intravenous acyclovir should be given.

In every patient with suspected influenza-related lower respiratory infection, bacterial pneumonia due to *S. pneumoniae*, *H. influenzae*, or *S. aureus* including MRSA is a major consideration. Bacterial cultures should be performed, and antibiotics effective against these pathogens should be prescribed.

CONTROVERSIES AND PITFALLS

Probably the major reason for underdiagnosis of viral pneumonia is an inappropriately low level of clinical suspicion and corresponding lack of laboratory testing. During influenza season or a pandemic outbreak, the clinical management plan for every patient with pneumonia should include consideration of viral pneumonia. Similarly, any pneumonia in an immunosuppressed patient or elderly nursing home resident should raise suspicion for a viral cause. In patients with suspected influenza-related pneumonia, bacterial infection, especially due to *S. pneumoniae*, *H. influenzae*, or *S. aureus* including MRSA, should be a consideration in laboratory testing and initial treatment, because it is not possible to distinguish between viral and bacterial pneumonia with certainty on clinical examination alone.

Diagnosing viral lower respiratory infections using upper respiratory samples such as nasopharyngeal washings inevitably raises the question of whether the identified virus is involved in the lower respiratory infection. This remains an area to be explored. Pending further data, clinical judgment of whether the virus detected from upper respiratory samples might be responsible for pneumonia is necessary. When serious pathogens such as influenza virus are detected in a patient with pneumonia, the prudent approach is to assume that the patient has a viral and possibly a secondary bacterial pneumonia and treat accordingly. The situation is much less clear cut for less well-established lower respiratory tract pathogens such as hMPV, bocavirus, and rhinovirus. Recent evidence shows that high viral load in nasopharyngeal samples, as determined using quantitative PCR assay, correlates with an increased chance that the lower respiratory disease is due to the virus. Such tests are not commonly available.

Although good evidence supports the efficacy of antiviral drugs in treatment of influenza-related pneumonia, treatment of RSV infections in adults with ribavirin is controversial. There are no high-quality, controlled trials of ribavirin in adults to date. Based on small uncontrolled case series, expert opinion favors use of ribavirin and intravenous immunoglobulin in hematopoietic stem cell transplant recipients with RSV-related lower respiratory infections. Although it may be reasonable to extend this approach to patients with other serious immunocompromising conditions such as solid organ transplantation and prolonged steroid therapy, ribavirin use in elderly patients with no identified immunocompromising conditions is based on anecdotal reports and has to be approached on a case-by-case basis with advice from a physician who is experienced in treatment of RSV infections.

CONCLUSIONS

Advances in molecular methods of diagnosis have increased awareness and recognition of the role of viruses in causing pneumonia in immunocompetent as well as immunosuppressed adults. The list of viruses capable of causing such pneumonias is increasing. Although current therapeutic options are mostly limited to influenza infection, increasing recognition of viral pneumonias and underlying pathogenetic mechanisms would spur research and development of more effective and varied therapies.

SUGGESTED READINGS

Centers for Disease Control and Prevention (CDC): Bacterial coinfections in lung tissue specimens from fatal cases of 2009 pandemic influenza A (H1N1)—United States, May-August 2009, *MMWR Morb Mortal Wkly Rep* 58:1071–1074, 2009.

Bautista E, Chotpitayasunondh T, Gao Z, et al: Clinical aspects of pandemic 2009 influenza A (H1N1) virus infection, *N Engl J Med* 362:1708–1719, 2010.

Falsey AR, Walsh EE: Viral pneumonia in older adults, *Clin Infect Dis* 42:518–524, 2006.

Falsey AR, Hennessey PA, Formica MA, et al: Respiratory syncytial virus infection in elderly and high-risk adults, *N Engl J Med* 352:1749–1759, 2005.

Hall CB: Respiratory syncytial virus and parainfluenza virus, *N Engl J Med* 344:1917–1928, 2001.

Johansson N, Kalin M, Tiveljung-Lindell A, et al: Etiology of community-acquired pneumonia: increased microbiological yield with new diagnostic methods, *Clin Infect Dis* 50:202–209, 2010.

Louria DB, Blumenfeld HL, Ellis JT, et al: Studies on influenza in the pandemic of 1957–1958. II. Pulmonary complications of influenza, *J Clin Invest* 38:213–265, 1959.

Mahony JB: Detection of respiratory viruses by molecular methods, *Clin Microbiol Rev* 21:716–747, 2008.

McGeer A, Green KA, Plevneshi A, et al: Antiviral therapy and outcomes of influenza requiring hospitalization in Ontario, Canada, *Clin Infect Dis* 45:1568–1575, 2007.

Perez-Padilla R, de la Rosa-Zamboni D, Ponce de Leon S, et al: Pneumonia and respiratory failure from swine-origin influenza A (H1N1) in Mexico, *N Engl J Med* 361:680–689, 2009.

Rello J, Pop-Vicas A: Clinical review: primary influenza viral pneumonia, *Crit Care* 13:235, 2009.

Shah JN, Chemaly RF: Management of RSV infections in adult recipients of hematopoietic stem cell transplantation, *Blood* 117:2755–2763, 2011.

Chapter **26**

Nonbacterial Infectious Pneumonia

William Graham Carlos III • Chadi A. Hage

Nonbacterial causes of infectious pneumonia are important diagnostic considerations in the evaluation of patients who are immunocompromised, who have recognized structural lung disease, or who do not respond to appropriate antibiotic therapy for presumed bacterial pneumonia. A detailed clinical history can assist the astute clinician in making the diagnosis of a nonbacterial cause of infectious pneumonia in these circumstances. Important information to gather includes travel history, geographic location, occupational history, and recreational activities. This chapter presents an overview of common fungal and parasitic causes of pneumonia, including clinical presentation, diagnostic considerations, and treatment options.

FUNGAL PNEUMONIAS

ASPERGILLOSIS

Aspergillus organisms are ubiquitous saprophytic fungi. They grow well in soil and decaying vegetation. These fungi also have been found in hospitals, ventilation and water systems, and dust associated with construction activity. Disease manifestations depend on the immune status and lung structure of the host. Clinical manifestations include allergic disease, airway colonization, aspergilloma formation, tracheobronchial disease, chronic necrotizing pneumonia, and invasive disseminating disease. Allergic disease generally is seen in immunocompetent patients and may encompass airway hyperreactivity, allergic bronchopulmonary aspergillosis (ABPA), and hypersensitivity pneumonitis. Airway colonization occurs in patients with impaired mucociliary clearance or distorted lung structure such as in bronchiectasis. Aspergillomas, or "fungus balls," thrive in cavitary lung lesions such as those associated with tuberculosis. Tracheobronchial aspergillosis and chronic necrotizing pneumonia (locally invasive aspergillosis) are manifestations found in patients with acquired immunodeficiency syndrome (AIDS), recipients of transplanted organs (especially lungs), and patients with obstructive lung disease who use inhaled or systemic steroids. Finally, invasive or disseminated aspergillosis develops in the context of profound and protracted granulocytopenia (**Figure 26-1**).

Fungal culture and histopathologic examination constitute the "gold standard" for the diagnosis of aspergillosis. The diagnosis has been simplified by the advent of the galactomannan detection assay, which confers a high degree of sensitivity and specificity. The treatment of aspergillosis is tailored to the disease manifestation. Allergic manifestations are managed with routine asthma care that includes avoidance of allergen exposures and maintenance bronchodilators. Steroids are reserved for severe cases. ABPA mandates treatment with corticosteroids initially and may require the addition of itraconazole. Aspergillomas can be followed clinically and generally remain dormant but can manifest with massive hemoptysis necessitating embolization or surgical resection. Voriconazole is the preferred agent for treatment of invasive aspergillosis. Liposomal amphotericin B, posaconazole, and echinocandins are reserved for salvage therapy.

HISTOPLASMOSIS

Histoplasmosis is the most prevalent endemic mycosis in North America. *Histoplasma capsulatum* is a dimorphic fungus existing as a mold in nature. It forms spores that become aerosolized, facilitating inhalation. After inhalation, *H. capsulatum* grows as yeast forms in the host.

The clinical manifestations of histoplasmosis are variable and depend on the intensity of exposure along with the immune status and underlying lung architecture of the host. The Mississippi and Ohio River valleys are highly endemic. Histoplasmosis also is endemic to parts of Central America, South America, Africa, and Asia. Moist soil is an ideal habitat for *Histoplasma*, especially when supplemented with bird or bat guano. Activities that can lead to infection include spelunking (caving), excavation, demolition, and cleaning of chicken coops or old buildings. After inhalation, the spores are converted into yeasts, which are phagocytosed by macrophages. The organism is able to survive and proliferate inside macrophages, allowing it to disseminate. Within 2 weeks, however, a protective cellular immune response usually develops, which contains the fungus by forming granulomas (often seen as calcified granulomas on chest radiographs). Most otherwise healthy persons infected with a low inoculum remain asymptomatic (i.e., the infection is subclinical) or are minimally symptomatic. Patients with impaired immunity that fails to contain the infection can develop progressive disseminated histoplasmosis, with involvement of the bone marrow, liver, spleen, adrenal glands, gastrointestinal tract, and central nervous system (CNS). This manifestation typically is seen in persons with AIDS or patients taking immunosuppressive medications such as prednisone, methotrexate, and anti-TNF-α agents. Common clinical manifestations of disseminated disease include fever, weight loss, hepatosplenomegaly, pancytopenia, meningitis, focal brain lesions, ulcerations of the oral mucosa, gastrointestinal ulcerations, and adrenal insufficiency. Disseminated histoplasmosis carries a high mortality rate unless promptly diagnosed and appropriately treated (**Table 26-1**).

Patients who inhale larger inocula of *Histoplasma* conidia during outbreaks or in an enclosed space may develop severe

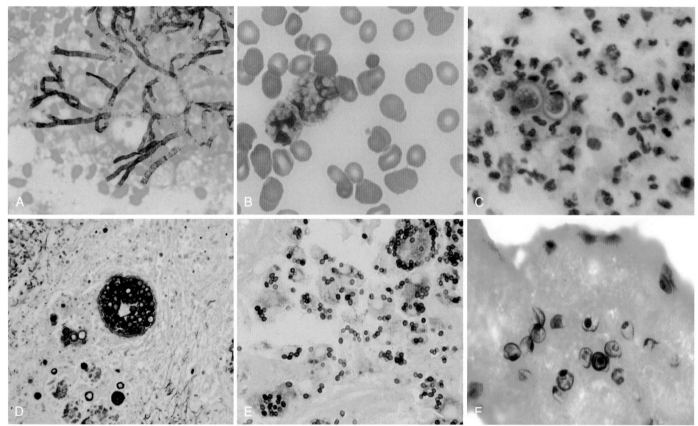

Figure 26-1 Examples of pulmonary fungal pathogens. **A,** *Aspergillus fumigatus* hyphae in BAL fluid from a neutropenic patient with invasive aspergillosis (Gomori methenamine silver nitrate [GMS] stain). **B,** *Histoplasma capsulatum* seen inside phagocytes on a peripheral blood smear from a patient with AIDS complicated by disseminated histoplasmosis (Giemsa stain). **C,** Large, broad-based budding *Blastomyces dermatitidis* yeasts in BAL fluid from a patient with pulmonary blastomycosis (Giemsa stain). **D,** *Coccidioides immitis* spherule containing numerous small spores in a lung biopsy specimen from a patient with acute pulmonary coccidioidomycosis. **E,** Cluster of narrow based-budding, small *Cryptococcus neoformans* yeasts, extracellularly located, in BAL fluid from a patient with AIDS complicated by disseminated cryptococcosis (GMS stain). **F,** Extracellularly located *Pneumocystis jiroveci* cysts (GMS stain) in BAL fluid from a patient with AIDS who presented with respiratory failure. *AIDS,* acquired immunodeficiency syndrome; *BAL,* bronchoalveolar lavage.

pulmonary disease with a flulike illness that can lead to respiratory failure. When the infection occurs in the context of structural lung disease (bullous emphysema), it may not be effectively contained, and patients can develop chronic cavitary histoplasmosis with upper lobe infiltrates, cavitations, and pleural thickening. Other late manifestations of histoplasmosis include fibrosing mediastinitis (a late complication associated with high morbidity), calcification of mediastinal nodes, and broncholithiasis.

Identification of *H. capsulatum* is accomplished using a combination of tests. Fungal culture remains the "gold standard." However, *H. capsulatum* may require up to 4 weeks to be grown in culture, limiting its utility in severe cases. Rapid diagnostic testing using antigen detection in serum or urine samples is useful in patients with moderate to severe disease. Antigen detection in bronchoalveolar lavage (BAL) fluid may help make the diagnosis of pulmonary histoplasmosis. Rapid diagnosis also can be achieved through cytopathologic examination, albeit with lower sensitivity than that attained with culture or antigen detection. *Histoplasma* serologic testing (immunodiffusion and complement fixation) is particularly useful in chronic (cavitary) and subacute disease, because detectable levels of antibody appear after 4 weeks of infection.

Treatment for histoplasmosis is reserved for patients with chronic pulmonary, disseminated, or acute moderate to severe disease. Liposomal amphotericin B followed by itraconazole is the preferred regimen for severe cases. Mild to moderate disease can be treated with itraconazole exclusively. Corticosteroids also may be useful in cases of severe, life-threatening acute pulmonary histoplasmosis. The duration of treatment for acute pulmonary histoplasmosis is 6 to 12 weeks, whereas that for disseminated and chronic pulmonary histoplasmosis is 12 to 18 months.

Fibrosing mediastinitis and broncholithiasis represent chronic reactions to past infection and do not respond to antifungal therapy. Treatment consists of endoscopic or surgical removal of partially or completely eroded broncholiths. Placement of endovascular stents may be required in advanced fibrosing mediastinitis causing obstruction of major mediastinal vessels. Obstruction of central airways or the esophagus also can occur and may necessitate balloon dilatation or stenting.

BLASTOMYCOSIS

Blastomyces dermatitidis is a dimorphic fungus that causes pulmonary and systemic disease. Most cases of blastomycosis have been reported in North America, where it occurs predominantly in the Midwestern states and Canadian provinces surrounding the Great Lakes. In the United States, the endemic region overlaps significantly with that of *H. capsulatum* along the Mississippi and Ohio River valleys. Cases have been reported from Africa and India as well. When outbreaks occur, they usually are associated with outdoor recreational activities or

Table 26-1 Types of Fungal Pneumonia

Fungal Disease	Pulmonary Manifestation(s)	Risk/Host Factor(s)	Diagnostic Test(s)	Treatment
Histoplasmosis	Acute and subacute pulmonary histoplasmosis	Normal host, occupational or recreational exposure	Serologic studies, antigen test, BAL fluid cytopathologic analysis	Itraconazole Amphotericin B
	Chronic cavitary pulmonary histoplasmosis	Emphysema	Serologic studies, sputum or BAL fluid culture	Itraconazole
	Progressive disseminated histoplasmosis	Immunosuppression (AIDS, anti-TNF, organ transplant recipients)	Antigen test, blood and BAL fluid culture, BAL fluid cytopathologic analysis	Amphotericin B Itraconazole
	Mediastinal histoplasmosis (granulomatous and fibrosing mediastinitis and broncholithiasis)	Normal host	Serologic studies	No antifungal therapy, antiinflammatory agent
Blastomycosis	Acute pulmonary blastomycosis	Recreational exposure, normal host	Antigen test, sputum cytopathologic analysis and culture	Itraconazole Amphotericin B
	Chronic pulmonary blastomycosis		Lung biopsy	Itraconazole
Coccidioidomycosis	Acute pulmonary coccidioidomycosis	Normal host, occupational or recreational exposure	Serologic studies, antigen test, sputum and BAL fluid culture, cytopathologic analysis	Fluconazole Amphotericin B Itraconazole
	Chronic cavitary pulmonary coccidioidomycosis		Serologic studies, sputum and BAL fluid culture	Fluconazole
	Disseminated coccidioidomycosis	Immunosuppression (AIDS)	Antigen test, serologic studies, BAL fluid culture, cytopathologic analysis	Amphotericin B Fluconazole
Aspergillosis	Invasive pulmonary aspergillosis	Neutropenic, leukemia, hematopoietic stem cell transplant recipient	*Aspergillus* galactomannan, BAL fluid cytopathologic analysis and culture	Voriconazole Amphotericin B Echinocandins
	Chronic necrotizing pneumonia	AIDS, COPD, chronic steroid use, solid organ transplant recipient	*Aspergillus* galactomannan, BAL fluid cytopathologic analysis and culture	Voriconazole Amphotericin B Echinocandins
	Tracheobronchial aspergillosis	COPD, inhaled steroids	Bronchoscopy, bronchial biopsy	Voriconazole Amphotericin B
	Allergic bronchopulmonary aspergillosis	Normal host	Serologic testing, peripheral eosinophilia	Itraconazole and systemic corticosteroids
	Mycetoma	Upper lobe cavitary lung disease	Radiographic diagnosis	No antifungal therapy
Pneumocystis infection	*Pneumocystis* pneumonia	Immunosuppression (AIDS)	BAL fluid cytopathologic analysis	Trimethoprim/ sulfamethoxazole, clindamycin-primaquine Pentamidine, dapsone, atovaquone

AIDS, acquired immunodeficiency syndrome; *BAL*, bronchoalveolar lavage; *COPD*, chronic obstructive pulmonary disease; *TNF*, tumor necrosis factor.

work around waterways. As with histoplasmosis, the mechanism of infection involves inhalation of the spores, which are then converted to the yeast form in the lung; however, polymorphonuclear cells are abundant in blastomycosis lesions, mimicking pyogenic infections.

Blastomycosis can manifest clinically in a variety of ways. The most common presentation is pulmonary disease, followed by involvement of the skin, bone, joints, and CNS. *Acute* pulmonary blastomycosis resembles community-acquired pneumonia and often is mistakenly treated for bacterial pneumonia before the correct diagnosis is made. Signs and symptoms include fever, chills, productive cough, and chest pain. Radiographic findings include consolidation, cavities, nodules, and miliary patterns. Mediastinal adenopathy and pleural effusions are uncommon. Acute blastomycosis can progress to acute respiratory distress syndrome (ARDS), even in immunocompetent patients. Risk factors for severe infection include diabetes and diffuse pulmonary involvement. *Chronic* pulmonary blastomycosis mimics lung cancer or tuberculosis and can be insidious in onset and progression and minimally symptomatic. Skin lesions often are mistaken for squamous cell carcinoma or pyoderma gangrenosum.

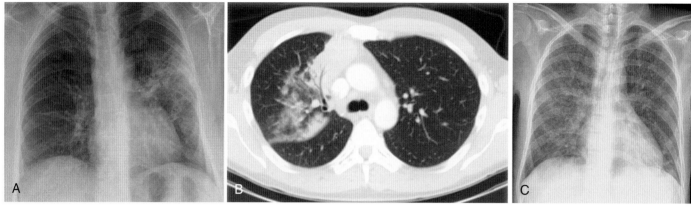

Figure 26-2 **A,** Acute pulmonary blastomycosis in a 51-year-old woman. The chest film shows a left upper lobe infiltrate. **B,** Acute pulmonary coccidioidomycosis in an otherwise healthy man. Chest computed tomography (CT) scan shows area of consolidation in the right upper and middle lobes. **C,** Progressive disseminated histoplasmosis in a 35-year-old patient with AIDS. The chest film shows bilateral reticulonodular interstitial infiltrates. *AIDS,* acquired immunodeficiency syndrome.

Definitive diagnosis requires growth of *Blastomyces* from sputum, BAL fluid, or biopsy material. Rapid identification is made by visualization of the characteristic broad-based budding yeast in clinical specimens. Typically, blastomycosis is diagnosed when a presumed community-acquired bacterial pneumonia fails to respond to antimicrobial therapy or if a mass suspicious for malignancy is detected. When the clinical presentation includes cutaneous manifestations, the diagnosis can be secured by skin biopsy. *Blastomyces* antigen can be found in the urine, serum, or BAL fluid, providing a reliable means for establishing a rapid diagnosis, especially in severe cases. The current antigen assays do not differentiate histoplasmosis from blastomycosis, as a consequence of cross-reactivity. Histopathologic and cytopathologic analysis can be helpful in differentiating histoplasmosis from blastomycosis and should be routinely ordered with invasive testing procedures.

In view of the cross-reactivity of the antigen assay, it is fortunate that the treatment for severe life-threatening blastomycosis is similar to that for histoplasmosis. Intravenous administration of amphotericin is the treatment of choice, and corticosteroids may be added in cases of ARDS. Non–life-threatening cases can be managed with itraconazole. In patients who are intolerant of itraconazole or who have CNS involvement, fluconazole can be used. Almost all patients with blastomycosis should be treated (**Figure 26-2**), although patients with self-limited disease may not require treatment.

COCCIDIOIDOMYCOSIS

Coccidioidomycosis, also known as "valley fever," is caused by the dimorphic soil-dwelling fungus *Coccidioides*. It is endemic in the southwestern United States and northern Mexico. Recent surges in case numbers have been recently reported in Arizona, where 60% of the cases occur. The mechanism of infectivity is similar to that for histoplasmosis and blastomycosis, involving inhalation of spores, leading to neutrophilic inflammatory responses. Case clusters have occurred in patients 2 weeks after they were exposed to dust in endemic areas while excavating or rock hunting, or during a windstorm.

Most patients who become infected with *Coccidioides* are asymptomatic or have a self-limited illness. Patients who become symptomatic usually experience a flulike illness with symptoms including fever, chills, arthralgia, myalgia, and headaches. In addition, cough, pleuritic chest pain, dyspnea, and

rarely hemoptysis may occur. Cutaneous manifestations often are reported with acute pulmonary coccidioidomycosis and may include maculopapular rash, erythema nodosum, and erythema multiforme. Chest radiographs initially show one or more areas of consolidation, with hilar or mediastinal lymphadenopathy. Fibrocavitary lesions can result from progressive disease. Areas of pneumonitis may heal by the formation of a coinlike lesion called a *coccidioidoma* that can persist for life.

Primary progressive coccidioidomycosis with diffuse pneumonia occurs in settings of intense environmental exposure or immunosuppression and often is associated with fungemia and respiratory compromise. Several months after the infection manifests, disseminated coccidioidomycosis may develop, with involvement of skin, bones, joints, genitourinary system, and the meninges. Risk factors for extrapulmonary dissemination include African American or Filipino ancestry, pregnancy during the second or third trimester, and depressed cellular immunity.

The gold standard for the diagnosis of coccidioidomycosis is culture or direct visualization of the fungus in tissue or respiratory secretions. Serologic testing plays an important role in establishing the diagnosis of coccidioidomycosis, in view of its speed and simplicity. Serologic studies are more likely to be positive in patients with disseminated disease and chronic disease. In contrast with *Histoplasma* and *Blastomyces*, *Coccidioides* grows within 3 to 7 days of culture.

The treatment of coccidioidomycosis is similar to that of histoplasmosis and blastomycosis and relies on triazoles (itraconazole or fluconazole) for diffuse pulmonary or nonmeningeal disseminated disease. Amphotericin B generally is reserved for immunocompromised patients with severe or disseminated disease unresponsive to triazoles as well as for pregnant women. For uncomplicated primary pneumonia in a normal host close observation often is all that is needed.

PARACOCCIDIOIDOMYCOSIS

Paracoccidioidomycosis, formerly named "South American blastomycosis," is caused by a fungus endemic to South and Central America, *Paracoccidioides brasiliensis*. Paracoccidioidomycosis is highly endemic in Brazil, Colombia, Venezuela, and Ecuador, with reported infectivity rates as high as 50% to 75% in some areas. Like the other thermal dimorphic fungi, *P. brasiliensis* is inhaled and undergoes transformation in the alveoli. Most cases are subclinical, and only a minor proportion of hosts will develop signs or symptoms weeks after inhalation. Reactivation of disease can occur years after inoculation, and the condition may disseminate hematogenously to the adrenal glands, gastrointestinal tract, and other viscera.

Pulmonary disease frequently is seen in chronic paracoccidioidomycosis. Chest imaging typically reveals pulmonary opacities that can cavitate, in a pattern involving both medial pulmonary fields and resembling a "butterfly wing." The diagnosis of paracoccidioidomycosis can be reliably made by histopathologic examination of clinical specimens revealing characteristic yeast cells with multiple buds. Definitive diagnosis relies on culture of the organism. Serologic testing can suggest the diagnosis and monitor the response to treatment. In severe or disseminated cases of paracoccidioidomycosis, amphotericin B is recommended. Itraconazole is the drug of choice for milder disease.

CRYPTOCOCCOSIS

Cryptococcus neoformans is a yeast with a thick capsule. Two species of *Cryptococcus* are recognized to cause disease in humans: *Cryptococcus gattii* and *Cryptococcus neoformans*. *C. neoformans* has emerged as a leading cause of CNS infection in patients with AIDS. Recent outbreaks of *C. gattii* infection causing pulmonary disease in immunocompetent persons have been reported from the northwestern United States and neighboring Vancouver Island in Canada. The two species of *Cryptococcus* have geographic and clinical differences. Whereas *C. gattii* typically is associated with flowering eucalyptus trees, *C. neoformans* can be found around bird guano throughout the world. Overall, cryptococcosis is a rare infection and usually is asymptomatic and self-limited in immunocompetent patients. In those who have impaired cell-mediated immunity, it may cause lung infection and meningitis. Cryptococcosis is emerging as the third leading fungal infection behind candidiasis and aspergillosis in recipients of organ transplants.

The CNS is the most common site of disease activation. Symptoms of cryptococcal pneumonia include fever, malaise, cough, and chest pain. The chest radiograph may show large, nonspecific nodules or infiltrates, sometimes associated with lymphadenopathy. Pulmonary infections have a tendency toward spontaneous resolution and frequently are asymptomatic. Hematogenous spread to the brain can lead to lesions in gray matter and basal ganglia. CNS disease can manifest as meningoencephalitis with papilledema and high cerebrospinal fluid opening pressure. A patient with AIDS presenting with fever and headache should prompt consideration of a diagnosis of cryptococcal meningitis. Lumbar puncture with an increased opening pressure and India ink smear of centrifuged cerebrospinal fluid is useful in this scenario. In patients who do not have AIDS, levels of cerebrospinal fluid glucose are low, and protein levels are high and can correlate with a lymphocytic pleocytosis. Cryptococcal capsular antigen usually is detected in cerebrospinal fluid or serum by latex agglutination testing, with sensitivity and specificity approaching 90%.

Treatment of cryptococcosis is tailored to the site of involvement and severity. Severe pulmonary disease and CNS involvement require amphotericin B with flucytosine. Mild to moderate disease can be effectively treated with fluconazole.

PNEUMOCYSTIS

Pneumocystis jiroveci is a fungus known to cause pneumonia in patients that are immunocompromised. It is a ubiquitous organism. Commonly found in patients with human immunodeficiency virus (HIV) infection or AIDS, infection is rare in normal hosts. Infection with *Pneumocystis* should be considered in any immunocompromised patient presenting with bilateral infiltrates on chest radiographs. Computed tomography (CT) generally reveals ground glass shadowing in affected areas, and sparing of the pleural surfaces has been noted frequently. The diagnosis of pneumocystosis is readily made through demonstration of the organism using fungal stains. Diagnostic specimens typically are obtained by BAL. Rarely, dissemination can occur, causing renal disease, cutaneous popular skin lesions, choroiditis, and intestinal plaques.

The treatment of pneumocystosis depends on the severity of hypoxemia once the organism has been identified. Patients with a PaO_2 less than 70 mm Hg on room air require treatment with steroids in addition to intravenous trimethoprim-sulfamethoxazole or pentamidine. Mild cases can be treated with trimethoprim-sulfamethoxazole, dapsone, pentamidine, atovaquone, or clindamycin plus primaquine. Various prevention regimens are available for patients who are severely immunosuppressed (e.g., persons with AIDS whose $CD4^+$ counts are less than 200 cells/μL, patients on long-term immunosuppressants). They include trimethoprim-sulfamethoxazole, dapsone, and aerosolized pentamidine.

PARASITIC PNEUMONIAS

AMEBIASIS

Entamoeba histolytica is endemic in tropical developing countries, particularly Mexico, India, and nations of Central and South America, tropical Asia, and Africa. The disease is acquired predominantly after ingestion of contaminated food or water. After intestinal infection, trophozoites can invade intestinal vasculature and reach the liver through the portal venous system. From the liver, the infection may disseminate to the lungs or brain. Liver abscess is the hallmark of invasive disease. Peripheral liver abscesses can erode through the diaphragm, causing pleuropulmonary disease.

Symptomatic amebiasis is predominantly an intestinal infection causing diarrhea and abdominal cramps to dysentery or even intestinal perforation because of mucosal ulcerations. Pleuropulmonary signs and symptoms include cough, dyspnea, and pleuritic pain (usually right-sided) associated with fever and chills, diaphoresis, and weight loss. The chest radiograph may show elevation of the right hemidiaphragm, pleural effusion, atelectasis, lung consolidation (which usually affects the right lower lobe), or lung abscess. Hepatobronchial fistulas have been reported in patients who have pleuropulmonary complications of amebiasis; this finding is associated with the production of copious volumes of chocolate-colored sputum. Pericardial involvement also may be observed in such patients. The diagnosis can be readily established by demonstrating amebic cysts or trophozoites in the stool, pleural fluid, or bronchial secretions. Serologic tests are highly sensitive and specific in invasive disease. Metronidazole is the agent of choice for treatment of invasive amebiasis.

MALARIAL LUNG

Severe falciparum malaria often is complicated by noncardiogenic pulmonary edema, which can develop despite effective antimalarial therapy. This syndrome of malarial lung carries a high mortality rate. Pulmonary involvement is a manifestation of the cytokine storm that follows heavy infection and destruction of red cells. It often leads to ARDS, with capillary congestion, pulmonary edema, and alveolar hemorrhage. Bilateral pulmonary infiltrates and pleural effusions are seen on chest radiographs. It is commonly associated with cerebral disease and high levels of parasitemia. The diagnosis of malaria is established after demonstration of asexual forms of the parasite inside erythrocytes on peripheral blood smears stained with Giemsa or Wright stain. Besides quinine-based antimalarial therapy, exchange transfusion and supportive care with supplemental oxygen and mechanical ventilation are required for severe cases.

PULMONARY ASCARIASIS

Ascaris lumbricoides is the largest intestinal nematode parasite of humans. *Ascaris* is widely distributed in tropical and subtropical areas. Most infected persons are asymptomatic. After egg ingestion, larvae hatch in the jejunum, invade the mucosa, and migrate to the lungs, causing a pneumonitis 1 to 2 weeks after ingestion. The presentation is that of eosinophilic pneumonitis (Löffler-like syndrome), with cough, occasional hemoptysis, wheezing, dyspnea, and high-grade fever. The illness usually is self-limited. Abdominal symptoms and cutaneous reactions also may be present. The chest radiograph can show unilateral or bilateral patchy, migratory, peribronchial infiltrates. The diagnosis is easily established by demonstrating characteristic *Ascaris* eggs in stool. During the transpulmonary migratory phase (eosinophilic pneumonitis), larvae can be found in sputum or gastric aspirates before the eggs appear in the stool. Antihelmintic treatment usually is not required for pulmonary ascariasis, because it usually is self-limited. Symptomatic treatment with bronchodilators and oxygen therapy and potentially corticosteroids is appropriate.

STRONGYLOIDIASIS

Strongyloides typically is found in tropical climates and is especially common in Southeast Asia, sub-Saharan Africa, and Brazil. The southeastern United States has endemic regions as well. *Strongyloides stercoralis* is unique among helminths in that it is capable of replicating in the human host. This feature allows the worm to autoinfect the host, where it may persist for decades. Infection begins when the filariform larvae in contaminated soil penetrate the exposed skin of the host. The larvae migrate through the lymphatic and venous circulation and eventually settle in the capillaries and alveoli of the lungs. Eventually the larvae ascend the tracheobronchial tree to the larynx, are swallowed, and mature into adult egg-laying females. Eggs hatch in the mucosa and pass with feces into the soil. Eggs can transform within the intestine into filariform larvae, which can penetrate the bowel wall and reenter the circulation. These larvae can carry bacteria as they penetrate through the gastrointestinal tract, causing polymicrobial bacteremia, septicemia, or hyperinfection in immunosuppressed patients.

Strongyloidiasis may have a variety of clinical manifestations. Although uncomplicated disease may remain subclinical for years, some patients will develop mild pulmonary disease in the form of cough and bronchospasm, whereas others will progress to ARDS. Recurrent urticaria and larva currens, or "running larva," can cause raised skin lesions. Nonspecific abdominal pain and colitis can develop, as can bowel obstructions. Eosinophilia is common during parasitemia. Radiographic abnormalities can range from a diffuse pneumonitis to chronic migratory pulmonary opacities. Immunosuppressed persons (e.g., patients with AIDS, glucocorticoid users) are susceptible to hyperinfection, with ensuing gram-negative sepsis, pneumonia, or meningitis. In patients with massive infection, pulmonary involvement can be extensive, leading to respiratory failure and pulmonary hemorrhage. Pleural effusions, pulmonary cavitations, and abscesses also have been documented, usually in cases associated with higher burdens of organisms.

The diagnosis of strongyloidiasis can be readily established by demonstrating rhabditiform larvae in stool as well as in sputum, BAL fluid, or biopsy specimens in disseminated disease. Serologic testing may help establish the diagnosis in chronic cases. Even in asymptomatic patients, a diagnosis of strongyloidiasis warrants treatment, in view of the potential for autoinfection and the fatal hyperinfection syndrome. Ivermectin is the preferred therapeutic agent, given daily for 1 or 2 days or up to 7 days in cases of disseminated disease.

VISCERAL LARVA MIGRANS (TOXOCARIASIS)

Visceral larva migrans is caused by *Toxocara* spp. These nematodes are parasitic for nonhuman hosts but do not mature in humans. Consequently, most infections in humans remain subclinical. However, the larvae occasionally may travel through host tissues, where they can elicit profound eosinophilic inflammation, resulting in the syndrome of visceral larva migrans. All feline and canine species can carry *Toxocara*. Nursing mothers can pass larvae to suckling puppies, and pregnant bitches can infect their pups transplacentally. In puppies, the larvae can develop into adult worms, which produce eggs released in their feces. Humans (usually preschool children) acquire toxocariasis by ingesting soil contaminated by pup feces.

Although most infections are subclinical, the infection can progress as the larvae invade the liver, lungs, CNS, and other sites. In such cases, the ensuing intense eosinophilic granulomatous response may be associated with fever, malaise, cough, wheezing, and rashes. Radiographic manifestations consist of migratory infiltrates. Rarely, death results from severe neurologic, pulmonary, or cardiac involvement.

The diagnosis of toxocariasis is made by serologic testing or histologic examination of infected tissues. Stool examination is not helpful, because the larvae do not develop into egg-producing adults in humans. Although most infections with *Toxocara* are self-limited, requiring no treatment, steroids may be warranted for cases associated with severe inflammation. The anthelmintic albendazole given for 5 days appears to be effective in eradicating the organism.

TROPICAL PULMONARY EOSINOPHILIA

Tropical pulmonary eosinophilia develops after infection with lymphatic filarial species (*Wuchereria bancrofti* or *Brugia malayi*) that are found in tropical and subtropical areas. The infection is transmitted by mosquitos. Circulating filariae are cleared from the bloodstream by the lungs, releasing antigens that cause a pulmonary hypersensitivity reaction.

Clinical manifestations include paroxysmal cough and wheezing (usually nocturnal), weight loss, fever, adenopathy, and peripheral eosinophilia and elevated serum immunoglobulin E (IgE) levels. Chest radiographs may show bilateral interstitial infiltrates and vascular congestion. The diagnosis is based on clinical findings. The clinician must rule out similar entities such as asthma, Löffler syndrome, ABPA, Churg-Strauss syndrome, chronic eosinophilic pneumonia, and the idiopathic hypereosinophilic syndrome. Daily administration of diethyl-carbamazine for 2 to 3 weeks is the standard therapy. Signs and symptoms usually resolve within 5 to 7 days after the initiation of therapy. Corticosteroids and antihistamines may also be used to control symptoms.

PARAGONIMIASIS

Paragonimus species such as *Paragonimus westermani* are hermaphroditic flukes that are endemic in Southeast Asia, South America, and South Africa. They are rarely found in North America and Europe. They infect humans who ingest undercooked crabs or crayfish that contain the encysted parasite. In many endemic regions, these crustaceans are consumed raw or pickled. The organisms penetrate the gut wall and travel to the lung by way of the peritoneal cavity, diaphragm, and pleural space. Mature flukes can be found in bronchioles surrounded by cysts. Parasite eggs are expectorated with sputum or swallowed and expelled with feces. The life cycle is then completed in snails or freshwater crustaceans.

Although some infections remain subclinical, the illness occurs during the first weeks of infection when the parasite is migrating from the intestine to the lung. Signs and symptoms include abdominal pain, diarrhea, hypersensitivity reactions (urticaria, eosinophilia, and fever), chest pain, cough, and hemoptysis. In most cases, however, no clinical manifestations emerge until the adult parasite begins to produce eggs in the lung, causing local inflammation with formation of cavities and cysts. Pulmonary signs and symptoms may include cough productive of rusty-brown sputum or frank hemoptysis. Sometimes the disease is mistaken for tuberculosis or lung cancer. Areas of fibrosis or pleural thickening are common. Pleural effusions are uncommon, but when they occur are characterized by high eosinophil counts in the pleural fluid. Of note, although eosinophilia is common in paragonimiasis, its absence does not rule out this disease.

The diagnosis is based on demonstrating eggs in bronchial secretions, pleural fluid, or feces. A number of serologic tests also are available. The preferred treatment is with praziquantel.

SCHISTOSOMIASIS

Pulmonary schistosomiasis develops when *Schistosoma* eggs are trapped in the pulmonary circulation, causing either pulmonary hypertension or formation of lung nodules. Skin is the portal of entry. The immature parasites migrate in the bloodstream and mature in venous plexuses. Eggs are then released and deposited in organs, where they cause a granulomatous reaction. Pulmonary hypertension is the most frequent and significant pulmonary manifestation of infection with *Schistosoma mansoni* or *Schistosoma japonicum*. The diagnosis is established by visualizing the characteristic eggs in organ biopsy specimens. Serologic tests also are available. Praziquantel is the preferred agent for treatment of schistosomiasis.

ECHINOCOCCOSIS

Echinococcosis is caused by the larval stage of *Echinococcus granulosus* or *E. multilocularis*, both of which may produce cystic lesions in any organ, mainly the liver and lungs. The infection is acquired through the ingestion of eggs. The parasite is transported in the bloodstream to the end organs. Pulmonary symptoms most often are related to compression of adjacent structures. Occasionally cysts may rupture into the airways or pleural space, causing an allergic reaction or superinfection. Chest CT typically shows sharply demarcated cysts with calcified borders and numerous smaller daughter cysts. The diagnosis is based on clinical and epidemiologic data. Serologic test findings are supportive, and aspiration of the cyst should be avoided, to limit the possibility of dissemination and associated hypersensitivity reactions. Surgical resection with complete removal of the cysts is the treatment of choice. Surgery should be done by experienced operators. Postoperative albendazole prophylaxis is recommended.

SUGGESTED READINGS

Carmona EM, Limper AH: Update on the diagnosis and treatment of *Pneumocystis* pneumonia, *Ther Adv Respir Dis* 5:41–59, 2011.

Chapman SW, Dismukes WE, Proia LA, et al: Clinical practice guidelines for the management of blastomycosis: 2008 update by the Infectious Diseases Society of America, *Clin Infect Dis* 46:1801–1812, 2008.

Dutkiewicz R, Hage CA: *Aspergillus* infections in the critically ill, *Proc Am Thorac Soc* 7:204–209, 2010.

Galgiani JN, Ampel NM, Blair JE, et al: Infectious Diseases Society of America: Coccidioidomycosis, *Clin Infect Dis* 41:1217–1223, 2005.

Hage CA, Wheat LJ, Loyd J, et al: Pulmonary histoplasmosis, *Semin Respir Crit Care Med* 29:151–165, 2008.

Kuzucu A: Parasitic diseases of the respiratory tract, *Curr Opin Pulm Med* 12:212–221, 2006.

Taylor WR, White NJ: Malaria and the lung, *Clin Chest Med* 23:457–468, 2002.

Wheat LJ, Freifeld AG, Kleiman MB, et al: Infectious Diseases Society of America: Clinical practice guidelines for the management of patients with histoplasmosis: 2007 update by the Infectious Diseases Society of America, *Clin Infect Dis* 45:807–825, 2007.

Chapter **27**
Nosocomial Respiratory Infections

Gianluigi Li Bassi • Miquel Ferrer • Antoni Torres

DEFINITIONS

The designation *nosocomial respiratory infection* refers to tracheobronchitis and pneumonia caused by pathogens highly prevalent in hospital settings and developing at least 48 hours after hospital admission. Nosocomial tracheobronchitis is characterized by signs of respiratory infection, such as an increase in the volume and purulence of respiratory secretions, fever, and leukocytosis, without radiologic infiltrates suggestive of consolidation on the chest film. Nosocomial pneumonia comprises pneumonia developing in nonintubated patients, ventilator-associated pneumonia (VAP), and health care–associated pneumonia (HCAP). VAP commonly develops in patients who receive invasive mechanical ventilation. HCAP is a more recently recognized clinical entity that is defined in the latest guidelines of the American Thoracic Society for the diagnosis and treatment of nosocomial pneumonia. HCAP develops in patients who are not hospitalized but are at risk for colonization by pathogens present in hospital settings, including multiple drug–resistant (MDR) microorganisms.

EPIDEMIOLOGY

INCIDENCE

Nosocomial tracheobronchitis occurs in 3% to 10% of tracheally intubated patients and often precedes the development of VAP. Nosocomial pneumonia is the second most common nosocomial infection and the leading cause of death from hospital-acquired infections in critically ill patients. Most recent studies report a VAP density rate of approximately 9 to 10 cases per 1000 ventilator days; nevertheless, those rates differ greatly according to the characteristics of the studied population. The risk of VAP is approximately 1% per day on mechanical ventilation and changes over time, being 3% the first 5 days on mechanical ventilation, 2% from days 5 to 10, and 1% for the remaining days.

IMPACT ON OUTCOMES

Nosocomial tracheobronchitis in hospitalized patients is associated with longer duration of mechanical ventilation and intensive care unit (ICU) stay. Indeed, tracheobronchitis is associated with increased sputum production, which often leads to weaning difficulties and extubation failure. Nevertheless, tracheobronchitis is not associated with worse survival.

The crude mortality rate for nosocomial pneumonia may be as high as 30% to 70%, although several cofactors influence mortality, making it extremely difficult to determine the true disease-attributable mortality. Indeed, the heterogeneity between patient populations, microbial patterns, antibiotic treatment, and diagnostic methods challenge precise estimate of mortality. Several case-matching studies have estimated that one third to one half of all VAP-related deaths are a direct result of the infection, with a higher mortality rate in cases caused by *Pseudomonas aeruginosa* or *Acinetobacter* spp. and associated with bacteremia. Higher mortality is associated in particular with late-onset VAP, specifically when the initial empirical antimicrobial therapy regimen is inadequate.

PATHOGENESIS

ROLE OF ENDOTRACHEAL TUBE

Pulmonary aspiration of colonized oropharyngeal secretions across the tracheal tube cuff is the main pathogenic mechanism for development of tracheobronchitis and VAP. The endotracheal tube (ETT), commonly used in the ICU for long-term mechanically ventilated patients, includes a high-volume, low-pressure (HVLP) cuff, which is approximately two to three times larger than the trachea; hence, when the cuff is inflated within the trachea, folds invariably form along the cuff surface, which leads to aspiration of oropharyngeal secretions. Several respiratory defense mechanisms are severely impaired after tracheal intubation: (1) The ETT completely bypasses the anatomic barrier provided by laryngeal structures, creating a direct conduit by which bacteria can be aspirated and reach lower airways; (2) presence of the tube hinders cough; and (3) inflation of the ETT cuff within the trachea drastically lowers mucociliary velocity.

Additionally, the ETT is commonly made of polyvinylchloride (PVC). With this material, bacteria easily adhere to the internal surface of the tube to form a complex structure called biofilm. Bacteria present within the biofilm have survival advantages and may be a source of persistent infection.

SOURCES OF COLONIZATION

Exogenous Versus Endogenous Sources

Patients can be colonized exogenously by contaminated respiratory equipment, the hospital environment, and the hands of the attending staff. Thus, health care personnel should be adequately trained in infection control and preventive strategies; strict sterilization protocols and hand washing with alcohol-based solutions should be implemented; and finally, lower patient-nurse ratios can be expected to promote optimal care with consequent lower colonization rates.

Nevertheless, endogenous colonization is believed to be the primary pathogenic mechanism for nosocomial respiratory infection development. In the hospitalized patient, the oral flora may shift to a predominance of aerobic gram-negative pathogens, *P. aeruginosa*, and methicillin-resistant *Staphylococcus aureus* (MRSA). After aspiration of bacteria-laden oropharyngeal secretions and colonization of the airways, the occurrence of respiratory infection depends on the size of the inoculum, the patient's functional status, and the competency of host defenses.

Stomach

According to the gastropulmonary hypothesis of colonization, the stomach of patients being treated in ICUs often is colonized by pathogens as a consequence of alkalinization of gastric contents by enteral nutrition and drugs. Continuous gastroesophageal reflux facilitates translocation of microbes into the oropharynx, which are then aspirated across the ETT cuff. Early studies have shown that in tracheally intubated patients, gastric pH higher than 4 is consistently associated with pathogenic colonization of the stomach. Conclusive evidence is still lacking, however, for an association of gastric colonization with increased risk of pneumonia, and some investigators have not found a relationship with bacteria causing lung infection as first originating in the stomach.

ETIOLOGIC AGENTS

Nosocomial respiratory infections may be caused by a variety of pathogens, and often more than one pathogen may be isolated. Microorganisms responsible for those infections differ according to the studied population, the duration of hospital stay, and the specific diagnostic methods used. Nosocomial respiratory infections are commonly caused by aerobic, gram-negative bacilli, such as *P. aeruginosa*, *Escherichia coli*, *Klebsiella pneumoniae*, or *Acinetobacter* spp., whereas *Streptococcus aureus* is the predominant isolated gram-positive pathogen. In a recent report by Esperatti and colleagues, the etiology of nosocomial pneumonia was investigated for invasively versus noninvasively ventilated patients managed in the ICU. Of interest, no significant differences were found, except for a higher proportion of *S. pneumoniae* in the noninvasively ventilated patients. These results imply that prevalence rates for nosocomial pathogens are similar in intubated and nonintubated patients, and that the use of empirical therapy likely to be active against them is warranted.

Underlying diseases may predispose patients to infection with specific organisms. For instance, patients with chronic obstructive pulmonary disease (COPD) are at increased risk for *Haemophilus influenzae*, *Moraxella catarrhalis*, *P. aeruginosa*, or *S. pneumoniae* infections; patients with acute respiratory distress syndrome (ARDS) are at higher risk for development of VAP caused by *S. aureus*, *P. aeruginosa*, and *Acinetobacter baumannii*. Finally, patients with traumatic injuries and neurologic disorders are at increased risk for *S. aureus*, *Haemophilus*, and *S. pneumoniae* infections.

Identification of pathogens resistant to multiple drugs is extremely important, in order to guide appropriate antibiotic treatment. Potential MDR pathogens are *P. aeruginosa*, MRSA, *Acinetobacter* spp., *Stenotrophomonas maltophilia*, *Burkholderia cepacia*, and extended-spectrum beta-lactamase–producing (ESBL-positive) *K. pneumoniae*. Conversely, *S. pneumoniae*, *H. influenzae*, methicillin-sensitive *S. aureus*, and antibiotic-sensitive Enterobacteriaceae organisms are not considered to be MDR pathogens. The incidence of MDR pathogens is closely linked to local factors and varies widely from one hospital to another. Accordingly, practitioners must be aware of the most prevalent microorganisms in their own clinical facilities and geographic regions to avoid the administration of initial inadequate antimicrobial therapy.

Legionella pneumophila as a cause of nosocomial pneumonia should be considered, particularly in immunocompromised patients. Anaerobes may potentially cause nosocomial infections, but often those pathogens are identified in association with aerobic pathogens, and their role is still considered controversial. Nosocomial infections are rarely caused by a fungus. *Candida* spp. and *Aspergillus fumigatus* are the most common isolated fungi, predominantly in immunocompromised patients. Finally, herpes simplex virus type 1 and cytomegalovirus (CMV) are the most common viruses identified as a cause of respiratory infections in hospitalized patients; of note, CMV pneumonia was found to be consistently associated with worse outcomes in patients managed in the ICU.

PREVENTION

Nosocomial respiratory infections are associated with high morbidity and mortality and constitute an important burden for the health care system; therefore, appropriate preventive strategies, summarized in **Box 27-1**, should be implemented to reduce overall incidence of those diseases. Approaches with proven efficacy in reduction of nosocomial respiratory infections should be grouped and implemented as a bundle, because together they are expected to result in a better outcome than when implemented individually.

Box 27-1 Preventive Strategies for Nosocomial Pneumonia

- Implementation, as a bundle, of nosocomial pneumonia–preventive strategies that have proven efficacy in reducing morbidity and mortality
- Implementation of educational programs for caregivers and frequent performance feedbacks and compliance assessment
- Strict alcohol-based hand hygiene
- Avoidance of tracheal intubation and use of noninvasive ventilation when indicated
- Daily sedation vacation and implementation of weaning protocols
- No ventilatory circuit tube changes unless the circuit is soiled or damaged
- Use of tracheal tube with cuff made of novel materials and shapes
- Use of silver-coated tracheal tube
- Application of low level of PEEP during tracheal intubation
- Aspiration of subglottic secretions
- Internal cuff pressure maintained within the recommended range and carefully controlled during transport of patients outside ICU setting
- Oral care with chlorhexidine
- Avoidance of stress ulcer prophylaxis in patients at very low risk for gastrointestinal bleeding, with use of sucralfate considered when indicated
- Semirecumbent patient positioning
- Continuous lateral rotation therapy
- Postpyloric feeding in patients who have impaired gastric emptying
- SDD for patients requiring mechanical ventilation for longer than 48 hours

ICU, intensive care unit; *PEEP*, positive end-expiratory pressure; *SDD*, selective digestive decontamination.

GENERAL PROPHYLACTIC MEASURES

Maintaining high levels of current knowledge on pathophysiology of nosocomial infections and preventive strategies in clinical health care personnel can be effective in reducing incidence of those diseases. Respiratory care practitioners and nurses should be the primary recipients of ongoing education programs, and frequent performance feedback and compliance assessment should be undertaken.

The World Health Organization (WHO) has endorsed hand hygiene as the single most important element of strategies to prevent health care–associated infections. Overall, most of the studies conducted in ICUs have shown consistent reduction in nosocomial infection rates through implementation of alcohol-based hand hygiene.

Daily interruption or lightening of sedation, as a strategy to avoid consistent impairment of respiratory defenses, as well as the avoidance of paralytic agents, is highly recommended.

Noninvasive Ventilation

Tracheal intubation and mechanical ventilation constitute the main risk for nosocomial respiratory infections and should be avoided whenever possible. Noninvasive ventilation is an attractive alternative for patients with acute exacerbations of COPD or acute hypoxemic respiratory failure, and for some immunocompromised patients with pulmonary infiltrates and respiratory failure.

Tracheal Tube Cuff

Novel ETT cuffs made of polyurethane, silicone, and latex have been developed and tested in laboratory and clinical trials. Particularly, the polyurethane cuff forms smaller folds on its inflation, so that the risk of aspiration of secretions above the cuff is less. The shape of the cuff may also play a role in prevention of aspiration. In comparison with standard cuffs with cylindrical shape, cuffs designed with a smooth tapering shape allow elimination of folds for a full section of the trachea-cuff contact zone, irrespective of the cuff material. Nevertheless, the clinical evidence on the efficacy of these novel tapered cuffs is still lacking.

It is important to maintain the internal pressure of the endotracheal tube cuff pressure between 25 to 30 cm H_2O, particularly when low levels of positive end-expiratory pressure (PEEP) are applied, in order to prevent both "macroleakage" of contaminated secretions into the lower airways and tracheal injury.

Tracheal Tubes Coated With Antimicrobial Agents

Coating the ETT with antimicrobial agents, such as silver, is a promising strategy to prevent biofilm formation within the tube with consequent VAP. The North American Silver-Coated Endotracheal Tube (NASCENT) randomized trial studied 2003 patients, expected to require mechanical ventilation for more than 24 hours, who were randomized to be intubated with either a silver-coated or a conventional tube. Use of the silver-coated ETT was associated with a lower incidence of microbiologically confirmed VAP, for a relative risk reduction of 35.9%.

Aspiration of Subglottic Secretions

Preventive aspiration of colonized subglottic secretions through dedicated ETTs reduces hydrostatic pressure exerted above the cuff, potentially preventing macroleakage across the cuff. Subglottic secretion drainage has been shown to reduce the incidence of VAP by nearly half, primarily by reducing both early- and late-onset pneumonia.

Body Position

Intubated patients are at higher risk for gastropulmonary aspiration when placed in the supine position (0 degrees) than in a semirecumbent position, particularly when they are enterally fed. The American and European guidelines strongly suggest that intubated patients should be preferentially kept in the semirecumbent position (30 to 45 degrees) rather than supine (0 degrees) to prevent aspiration, especially when the patient is receiving enteral feeding.

Stress Ulcer Prophylaxis in Intubated Patients

In the ICU, stress ulcer prophylaxis usually is achieved with either sucralfate, histamine type 2 receptor blockers (H_2 blockers), or proton pump inhibitors (PPIs). Sucralfate is the only agent that potentially prevents stress gastrointestinal ulceration without raising gastric pH. Clinicians must weigh the potential benefit of sucralfate (with potentially less VAP and more gastrointestinal bleeding) against that of H_2 blockers or PPIs (with potentially more VAP and less gastrointestinal bleeding) and probably should limit stress ulcer prophylaxis to high-risk patients.

Modulation of Oropharyngeal and Gastrointestinal Colonization

Extensive efforts have been devoted to modulate oropharyngeal flora of hospitalized patients and reduce the risk for aspiration of pathogens. Oropharyngeal decontamination with chlorhexidine effectively reduces VAP, particularly among patients managed in cardiothoracic ICUs. Results in noncardiac ICU populations are more uncertain, and significant reductions in VAP rates have been achieved only when chlorhexidine was used at concentrations of 2%.

Selective decontamination of the digestive tract (SDD) has been used as a preventive strategy against nosocomial pneumonia for almost 3 decades. The SDD regimen comprises a combination of nonabsorbable antibiotics active against gram-negative pathogens (e.g., tobramycin, polymyxin E), plus either amphotericin B or nystatin, administered into the gastrointestinal tract in order to prevent oropharyngeal and gastric colonization with aerobic gram-negative bacilli and *Candida* spp. while preserving the anaerobic flora. Some regimens include a short course of systemic antibiotics (most commonly cefotaxime) in addition to nonabsorbable gastrointestinal antibiotics. SDD reduces the incidence of VAP, and it is the only VAP-preventive strategy that has shown survival benefits in patients managed in the ICU. The long-term effects of SDD on emergence of bacterial resistance and risk of superinfections are still controversial.

DIAGNOSIS

Nosocomial pneumonia should be suspected in patients with a new or progressive infiltrate on lung imaging associated with at least two of the following clinical features:

- Fever
- Leukocytosis or leukopenia
- Purulent airway secretions

The presence of these clinical signs, without a new infiltrate on the chest film, suggests nosocomial tracheobronchitis. In patients managed in the ICU, clinical signs suggestive of pneumonia often are too nonspecific to be of diagnostic value. Moreover, the chest radiograph often is difficult to interpret in those

Table 27-1 | **Clinical Pulmonary Infection Score (CPIS)***

Criterion	Scoring Factor		
	0	1	2
Tracheal secretions	Absent	No purulent	Abundant and purulent
Infiltrates on chest radiograph	No	Diffuse	Localized
Temperature (°C)	≥36.5 and ≤38.4	≥38.5 or ≤38.9	≥39 or ≤36
Leukocytes (cells/μL)	≥4000 and ≤11000	<4000 or >11000	<4000 or >11000 + bands >50% or >500
Pao_2/Fio_2	>240 or ARDS		≤240, no ARDS
Microbiology*	Negative		Positive

*CPIS of 6 or higher is considered positive for infection.
ARDS, acute respiratory distress syndrome.
Modified from Pugin J, Auckenthaler R, Mili N, et al: Diagnosis of ventilator-associated pneumonia by bacteriologic analysis of bronchoscopic and nonbronchoscopic "blind" bronchoalveolar lavage fluid, *Am Rev Respir Dis* 143:1121–1129, 1991.

patients; indeed, when infiltrates are evident, it is challenging to differentiate among cardiogenic and noncardiogenic pulmonary edema, pulmonary contusion, atelectasis, and pneumonia. Clinical variables often are evaluated as a group, to improve specificity of the clinical diagnosis. The Clinical Pulmonary Infection Score (CPIS) is based on clinical assessments, pulmonary radiographic findings, and semiquantitative culture of tracheal aspirate, each worth between 0 and 2 points (**Table 27-1**). A minimum value of 6 is the threshold to identify patients with pneumonia. Nevertheless, the value of CPIS remains to be validated in a large prospective study, especially in patients with bilateral pulmonary infiltrates.

The presence of bacteria in the lower airways of intubated patients is not sufficient to diagnose true lung infection, because the tracheobronchial tree of mechanically ventilated patients frequently is colonized by enteric gram-negative bacilli. Many sampling procedures are available, such as sputum collection, endotracheal aspiration, bronchoalveolar lavage (BAL), and protected specimen brush (PSB) procedures. In addition, several microbiologic techniques can be used, including Gram staining and intracellular organism count from specimens obtained by tracheal aspiration and BAL. Each diagnostic technique has advantages and limitations and provides different levels of diagnostic specificity and sensitivity.

Qualitative cultures of endotracheal aspirates yield a high percentage of false-positive results owing to frequent bacterial colonization of the proximal airways. Conversely, quantitative culture techniques of endotracheal aspirates may have an acceptable overall diagnostic accuracy. When patients develop pneumonia, pathogens are present in the lower respiratory tract secretions at concentrations of at least 10^5 to 10^6 colony-forming units (CFU)/mL, and contaminants generally are present at less than 10^4 CFU/mL. The current proposed VAP diagnostic threshold is 10^6, 10^4, and 10^3 CFU/mL for tracheal aspirates, BAL fluid, and PSB samples, respectively. Likewise, in a patient without radiographic pulmonary infiltrates, tracheal aspirates colonized at a concentration of at least 10^6 CFU/mL may suggest tracheobronchitis.

DIAGNOSTIC STRATEGIES FOR NOSOCOMIAL RESPIRATORY INFECTION

An ideal diagnostic strategy for patients suspected on clinical grounds to have nosocomial respiratory infection should achieve the following objectives:

- Accurately identify patients with true pulmonary infection and isolate the causative microorganisms, to allow prompt initiation of appropriate antimicrobial treatment and then optimization of therapy based on susceptibility studies of the pathogens
- Identify patients with extrapulmonary sites of infection
- Withhold and/or withdraw antibiotics in patients without infection

The diagnosis of nosocomial pneumonia begins with clinical suspicion triggered by suggestive findings. The presence of a new or progressively worsening radiographic infiltrate plus clinical criteria constitutes a firm basis for further investigation. Either of two diagnostic algorithms can be used: clinical or bacteriologic. The *clinical approach* recommends treating every patient suspected to have a pulmonary infection with new antibiotics even when the likelihood of infection is low (**Figure 27-1**). Nevertheless, samples of respiratory secretions such as endotracheal aspirate or sputum should be obtained before the initiation of antibiotic treatment. In this strategy, the selection of appropriate empirical therapy is based on risk factors and local resistance patterns. The etiology in each case of pneumonia is defined by semiquantitative cultures of endotracheal aspirates or sputum, often with additional microscopic examination of the Gram stain. Antimicrobial therapy is adjusted according to culture results or clinical response. Semiquantitative culture of tracheal aspirates has the advantage that no specialized microbiologic techniques are required, and the sensitivity is high. This clinical strategy provides antimicrobial treatment to a majority of the patients with suspected pneumonia and yields a low rate of false-negative results. Still, if the tracheal aspirate culture does not demonstrate pathogens and the patient has not received new antibiotics within the previous 72 hours, the diagnosis of pneumonia is unlikely. The main drawback of this strategy is that the high sensitivity of semiquantitative cultures of tracheal aspirates leads to overtreatment, with institution of unnecessary antibiotics in patients with false-positive results.

The *bacteriologic strategy* is based on the results of quantitative cultures of lower respiratory secretions (**Figure 27-2**). The procedure used to collect the samples (endotracheal aspirate, BAL fluid, or PSB) may be invasive (bronchoscopic) or noninvasive (blind procedures). The strategy reduces risks for overuse of antibiotics, because quantitative cultures yield fewer microorganisms above the threshold in comparison with

Figure 27-1 Clinical noninvasive strategy for the diagnosis and management of ventilator-associated pneumonia (VAP). *LRT,* lower respiratory tract. *(Modified from American Thoracic Society: Guidelines for the management of adults with hospital-acquired, ventilator-associated, and healthcare-associated pneumonia,* Am J Respir Crit Care Med *171:388-416, 2005.)*

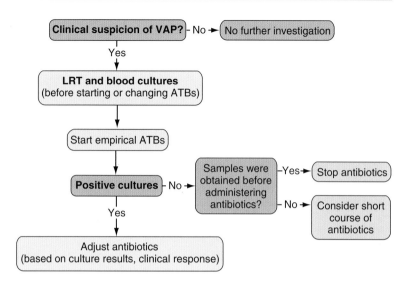

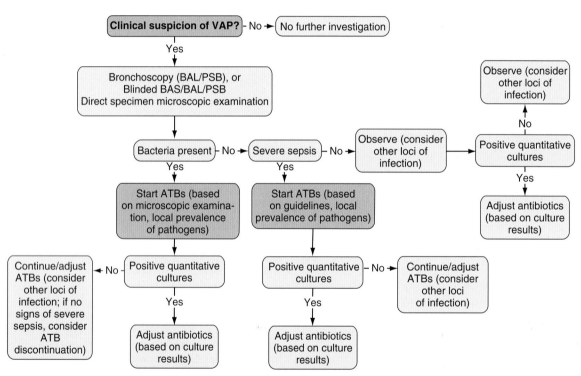

Figure 27-2 Invasive and quantitative culturing strategy for the diagnosis and management of ventilator-associated pneumonia (VAP). *ATB,* antibiotic; *BAL,* bronchoalveolar lavage; *BAS,* bronchial aspiration; *PSB,* protected specimen brushing. *(Modified from American Thoracic Society: Guidelines for the management of adults with hospital-acquired, ventilator-associated, and healthcare-associated pneumonia,* Am J Respir Crit Care Med *171:388-416, 2005.)*

semiquantitative cultures. Among the disadvantages of the bacteriologic strategy is the possibility of obtaining false-negative results, which leads to delayed antibiotic treatment in patients with pneumonia. Moreover, results obtained using the microbiology strategy may lack reproducibility, and often no microbiologic information is available at the time of initiation of empirical antibiotic therapy.

PRACTICAL IMPLEMENTATION OF A DIAGNOSTIC STRATEGY IN SUSPECTED NOSOCOMIAL RESPIRATORY INFECTION

In practice, the development of local clinical guidelines can combine both clinical and bacteriologic strategies. In mechanically ventilated patients, the presence of an infiltrate on the chest radiograph differentiates between the possible presence of pneumonia and tracheobronchitis. The next step is to obtain samples from the lower respiratory tract, before initiation of antibiotic treatment or change in regimen, even though it should not delay the administration of antibiotic therapy, particularly for septic patients. When indicated, additional samples should be collected for microbiologic analyses, such as blood, pleural fluid, and, in case *L. pneumophila* or *S. pneumoniae* infections are suspected, urine should be obtained. With clinical findings suggestive of pneumonia, CPIS should be calculated, to improve objective assessment of the clinical parameters (see Table 27-1).

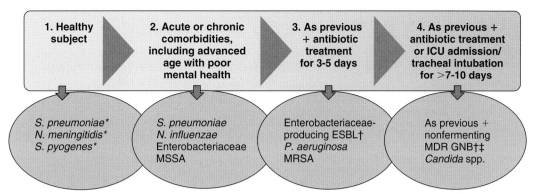

Figure 27-3 Evolution of the potentially pathogenic microorganisms present in the oropharyngeal flora, related to comorbidity, antibiotic treatment, and colonization pressure. Implicated species include *Neisseria influenzae, Neisseria meningitidis, Pseudomonas aeruginosa, Streptococcus pneumoniae,* and *Streptococcus pyogenes,* as well as drug-resistant/susceptible staphylococci. *ESBL,* extended-spectrum beta-lactamase; *GNB,* gram-negative bacilli; *ICU,* intensive care unit; *MDR,* multidrug-resistant; *MRSA,* methicillin-resistant *Staphylococcus aureus; MSSA,* methicillin-sensitive *S. aureus.* *Transiently present in healthy carriers. †Producers of extended-spectrum beta-lactamase or with type ampC chromosomal beta-lactamases. ‡*P. aeruginosa, Stenotrophomonas* spp., *Acinetobacter* spp., *Burkholderia* spp.

TREATMENT

Once the clinical decision to initiate antimicrobial therapy for nosocomial respiratory infection has been made, the following issues should be considered, both to achieve the best antimicrobial efficacy and to reduce overuse of antibiotics:

- The most likely etiologic microorganisms
- Choice of the empirical antimicrobials likely to be active against these microorganisms
- The adjustment of therapy after microbiologic results are in and with duration of treatment

An important point is that the indiscriminate administration of antimicrobial agents may contribute to the emergence of multiresistant pathogens and increase the risk of severe superinfections with increased morbidity and mortality, as well as exposing the patient to antibiotic-related adverse effects and higher costs. On the other hand, correct and prompt treatment of nosocomial respiratory infections results in better patient survival.

THE LIKELY ETIOLOGIC MICROORGANISMS

The selection of initial antimicrobial therapy needs to be tailored to the local prevalence of pathogens and antimicrobial patterns of resistance of the institution. The dynamics of change of oropharyngeal flora during hospital stay is depicted in **Figure 27-3.** Changes in oropharyngeal flora tend to occur progressively, so that the presence of microorganisms during one stage often overlaps with the next stage.

CHOICE OF THE EMPIRICAL ANTIMICROBIALS LIKELY TO BE ACTIVE AGAINST CAUSATIVE MICROORGANISMS

The latest guidelines of the American Thoracic Society and the Infectious Diseases Society of America (ATS/IDSA) for the management of adult patients with nosocomial pneumonia recommend that the selection of empirical antibiotic therapy for each patient should be based on the timing of onset and presence of risk factors for MDR pathogens—antimicrobial therapy in preceding 90 days; current hospitalization of 5 days or more; high frequency of antibiotic resistance in the community or in the specific hospital unit; hospitalization for 2 days or longer within the preceding 90-day period; residence in a

Table 27-2 **Initial Empirical Antibiotic Treatment in Nosocomial and Ventilator-Associated Pneumonia of Early Onset in Patients Without Risk Factors for Infection by Multidrug-Resistant Pathogens**

Probable Pathogen	Recommended Antibiotic
Streptococcus pneumoniae	Ceftriaxone
Haemophilus influenzae	OR
Methicillin-sensitive	Levofloxacin, moxifloxacin
Staphylococcus aureus	OR
Enteric gram-negative bacilli	Ampicillin/sulbactam
Escherichia coli	OR
Klebsiella pneumoniae	Ertapenem
Enterobacter spp.	
Proteus spp.	
Serratia marcescens	

Modified from American Thoracic Society: Guidelines for the management of adults with hospital-acquired, ventilator-associated, and healthcare-associated pneumonia, *Am J Respir Crit Care Med* 171:388–416, 2005.

nursing home or extended care facility; home infusion therapy (including antibiotics); chronic dialysis within 30 days; home wound care; MDR pathogen carrier status or infection in a family member; and immunosuppressive disease and/or therapy. The antibiotics recommended in the current ATS/IDSA guidelines are shown in **Tables 27-2** and **27-3.** Broad-spectrum empirical antibiotic therapy should be rapidly deescalated as soon as microbiologic data become available, to limit the emergence of resistance in the hospital.

Patients with Late-Onset Pneumonia or Early-Onset Pneumonia with Risk Factors for Multidrug-Resistant Bacteria

Patients with late-onset pneumonia or early-onset pneumonia with risk factors for MDR bacteria may be infected with resistant gram-negative bacilli. Priority should be given to treatment with a beta-lactam. Choice of the beta-lactam agent should take into account the following factors: (1) in vitro susceptibility of *P. aeruginosa* in the ICU, (2) the prevalence of Enterobacteriaceae organisms producing ESBL, (3) the results of previous cultures, and (4) antibiotics already received by the patient.

Table 27-3	Initial Empirical Antibiotic Treatment for Nosocomial and Ventilator-Associated Pneumonia of Late Onset or in Patients with Risk Factors for Infection by Multidrug-Resistant Pathogens and Any Degree of Severity

Probable Pathogen	Combined Antibiotic Treatment
Microorganisms from Table 27-2 PLUS: *Pseudomonas aeruginosa* *Klebsiella pneumoniae* (ESBL-positive)* *Acinetobacter* spp.* Other nonfermenting GNB Methicillin-resistant *Staphylococcus aureus* (MRSA) *Legionella pneumophila*†	Antipseudomonal cephalosporin (ceftazidime or cefepime)‡ OR Carbapenem (imipenem, meropenem)‡ OR Beta-lactam/beta-lactamase inhibitor (piperacillin-tazobactam)‡ + Antipseudomonal fluoroquinolone (ciprofloxacin, levofloxacin)§ OR Aminoglycoside§ (amikacin) ± Linezolid or vancomycin¶

ESBL, extended-spectrum beta-lactamase; *GNB*, gram-negative bacilli; *ICU*, intensive care unit.

*If an ESBL-positive strain such as *K. pneumoniae*, or *Acinetobacter*, is suspected, a carbapenem is the agent of first choice.

†If *L. pneumophila* is the suspected pathogen, the combination antibiotic regimen should include a macrolide (e.g., azithromycin), or a fluoroquinolone (e.g., ciprofloxacin or levofloxacin) should be used rather than an aminoglycoside.

‡The choice of beta-lactam is made as follows: Patients who have not received any antipseudomonal beta-lactam within the last 30 days should be administered piperacillin-tazobactam or an antipseudomonal cephalosporin. Patients who have received these drugs should be given empirical therapy with a carbapenem. Patients with infection by ESBL-producing microorganisms should be treated with carbapenem regardless of the results of the antibiogram.

§For combined empirical therapy for multidrug-resistant GNB, an antipseudomonal fluoroquinolone should be given in cases of renal failure or with concomitant use of vancomycin. In other settings, combined empirical therapy with amikacin is initiated and maintained for a 5-day period.

¶Empirical therapy aimed against MRSA is initiated in patients with proven colonization, previous infection by this microorganism, or implementation of mechanical ventilation for more than 6 days. The antibiotic of choice is either vancomycin (except in persons allergic to this medication, those with serum creatinine values of 1.6 mg/dL or greater, or patients presenting with signs of empirical treatment failure after 48 hours of antibiotic therapy) or linezolid.

NOTE: For epidemiologic surveillance, nasal and perineal cultures should be performed on admission and at 1-week intervals thereafter during the ICU stay.

An antipseudomonal beta-lactam regimen would include a third-generation cephalosporin (ceftazidime or cefepime), piperacillin-tazobactam, or a carbapenem (imipenem or meropenem) (see Table 27-3).

ANTIMICROBIAL THERAPY IN SPECIAL SITUATIONS

The addition of antibiotics with activity against MRSA depends on the local prevalence of MRSA, the presence of risk factors for MRSA, and the severity of infection. In geographic areas with documented presence of community-acquired MRSA, severe pneumonia with radiologic images of cavitation and presence of gram-positive cocci in respiratory secretions, empirical treatment with linezolid or vancomycin may be appropriate. Infections by *L. pneumophila* serogroup 1 can be diagnosed by a *Legionella* urinary antigen test. A fluoroquinolone or a macrolide would be an appropriate agent for treatment of *L. pneumophila* infection.

MODIFICATIONS OF THERAPY AND DURATION OF TREATMENT

After 72 hours, treatment should be adjusted in accordance with the microbiologic results. The initial beta-lactam should be continued if the microorganism is susceptible to the empirical beta-lactam originally prescribed. If it is not, another beta-lactam, possibly a carbapenem, may be introduced. The empirical antibiotic active against MRSA should be discontinued if the presence of this pathogen is not confirmed by cultures. Discontinuation of the fluoroquinolone and especially the aminoglycoside should be considered after 3 to 5 days of treatment. The bactericidal activity of aminoglycosides and fluoroquinolones leads to a rapid reduction in the bacterial load during the first days of treatment. Thereafter, monotherapy may be sufficient. This approach would decrease emergence of resistant mutants and minimize nephrotoxicity caused by aminoglycosides.

A majority of infections can be effectively treated with regimens lasting up to 8 days. Four special situations may justify prolonged treatment: (1) infection by microorganisms that may multiply in the cellular cytoplasm, such as *Legionella* spp.; (2) the presence of biofilms or prosthetic devices; (3) the development of tissue necrosis, the formation of abscesses, or infection within a closed cavity, such as empyema; and (4) persistence of the original infection (such as with perforation or endocarditis). If the clinical course from the pneumonia is favorable within the first 3 to 5 days of antimicrobial therapy, treatment may be withdrawn after the completion of 8 days. In cases of pneumonia produced by nonfermenting gram-negative bacilli, the eradication of these microorganisms from the bronchial secretion can be achieved with a longer regimen of up to 14 days.

In patients originally suspected on clinical grounds to have ICU-acquired pneumonia but whose CPIS is lower than 6 on the third day of drug therapy, treatment may be withdrawn. In this setting, the patient probably did not have pneumonia, or the pneumonia was sufficiently mild that prolonged antibiotic treatment is not required (**Figure 27-4**).

IMPORTANT INSIGHTS FOR TREATMENT OF NOSOCOMIAL RESPIRATORY INFECTIONS

Studies have proved beneficial effects of antimicrobial treatment for patients with nosocomial tracheobronchitis being cared for in an ICU. In these patients, antibiotics can have an impact on ICU mortality rate, duration of mechanical ventilation, and ICU stay and ultimately hinder progression of the infection to VAP. Of importance, patients with airway colonization but without local and systemic signs of infection should not be treated. Additionally, aerosolized antibiotics can be a feasible option in such patients.

There is evidence that appropriate and timely antibiotic treatment can improve outcome in patients with VAP. Guidelines can play a significant role in accomplishing this aim. To achieve significant reductions in morbidity and mortality, however, two important principles should be followed: (1) the guidelines should be implemented in specific clinical settings, and (2) antibiotic treatment regimens should be tailored to specific risk factors for acquiring MDR pathogens. Although implementation of such guidelines is difficult, the available

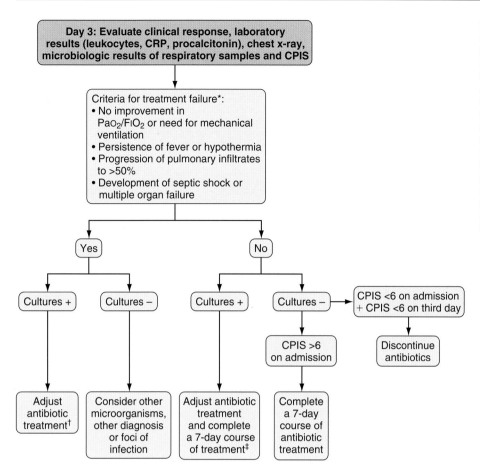

Figure 27-4 Suggested flowchart for follow-up evaluation in patients with nosocomial pneumonia and ventilator-associated pneumonia (VAP). *Criteria of treatment failure. †In cases in which the etiologic agent is *Pseudomonas aeruginosa* or *Acinetobacter* spp., the treatment should be maintained for 14 days. ‡Patients with criteria for treatment failure and in whom methicillin-resistant *S. aureus* (MRSA) is isolated should be administered linezolid. If a gram-negative bacillus is isolated, consultation with an infectious diseases specialist is recommended. *(Modified from American Thoracic Society: Guidelines for the management of adults with hospital-acquired, ventilator-associated, and healthcare-associated pneumonia, Am J Respir Crit Care Med 171:388–416, 2005.)*

evidence demonstrates improvement in both management and outcome.

SUGGESTED READINGS

American Thoracic Society: Guidelines for the management of adults with hospital-acquired, ventilator-associated, and healthcare-associated pneumonia, *Am J Respir Crit Care Med* 171:388–416, 2005.

The Canadian Critical Care Trials Group: A randomized trial of diagnostic techniques for ventilator-associated pneumonia, *N Engl J Med* 355:2619–2630, 2006.

Craven DE, Hjalmarson KI: Ventilator-associated tracheobronchitis and pneumonia: thinking outside the box, *Clin Infect Dis* 51(Suppl 1):S59–S66, 2010.

Esperatti M, Ferrer M, Theessen A, et al: Nosocomial pneumonia in the intensive care unit acquired by mechanically ventilated versus nonventilated patients, *Am J Respir Crit Care Med* 182:1533–1539, 2010.

Kollef MH, Afessa B, Anzueto A, et al: Silver-coated endotracheal tubes and incidence of ventilator-associated pneumonia: the NASCENT randomized trial, *JAMA* 300:805–813, 2008.

Lacherade JC, De Jonghe B, Guezennec P, et al: Intermittent subglottic secretion drainage and ventilator-associated pneumonia: a multicenter trial, *Am J Respir Crit Care Med* 182:910–917, 2010.

Rello J, Sa-Borges M, Correa H, et al: Variations in etiology of ventilator-associated pneumonia across four treatment sites: implications for antimicrobial prescribing practices, *Am J Respir Crit Care Med* 160:608–613, 1999.

Schweickert WD, Gehlbach BK, Pohlman AS, et al: Daily interruption of sedative infusions and complications of critical illness in mechanically ventilated patients, *Crit Care Med* 32:1272–1276, 2004.

Torres A, Ewig S, Lode H, Carlet J, European HAP Working Group: Defining, treating and preventing hospital acquired pneumonia: European perspective, *Intensive Care Med* 35:9–29, 2009.

Vincent JL, Rello J, Marshall J, et al: International study of the prevalence and outcomes of infection in intensive care units, *JAMA* 302:2323–2329, 2009.

Chapter **28**

Pneumonia in the Non–HIV-Infected Immunocompromised Patient

Jennifer Quint • Jeremy S. Brown

OVERVIEW

The respiratory tract is continually exposed to a range of microorganisms that normal immune responses generally prevent from causing infection. Hence, it is not surprising that patients with significantly impaired immunity frequently develop lung infections. Immunodeficient patients also frequently have several other risk factors that contribute to an increased risk for development of pneumonia, including low-level microaspiration of oropharyngeal contents, mucosal damage caused by cytotoxic therapy, underlying lung damage, and poor nutrition. As a consequence, lung infections are a common and frequently serious complication in patients with significant impairment of the immune system. Pulmonary infiltrates occur in 25% of patients with neutropenia developing after chemotherapy, and up to 5% of patients undergoing hematopoietic stem cell transplantation (HSCT) will die as a result of pneumonia. The range of potential pathogens causing lung infections in immunocompromised patients is much broader than for the usual pathogens causing community-acquired pneumonia and includes organisms such as *Aspergillus fumigatus* and human cytomegalovirus (CMV); the diagnosis of infections due to these microbes can be difficult, and the required therapies frequently are toxic. The large number of potential pathogens and the background disease together make management of lung infection in immunocompromised patients considerably more complex, and the use of invasive diagnostic tests such as bronchoscopy frequently is necessary. This chapter focuses on the common causative pathogens and the clinical approach to pulmonary infections in patients who have been severely immunocompromised by chemotherapy, organ transplantation, or hematologic disease (**Box 28-1**) but not human immunodeficiency virus (HIV) infection (discussed in Chapter 29). Pneumonia in patients with milder degrees of immunosuppression due to myeloma, low-dose cytotoxic therapy, or disease-modifying agents administered for rheumatologic conditions generally should be managed as community- or hospital-acquired pneumonia, but with recognition that the disease could be due to various opportunistic pathogens, as discussed in this chapter.

GENERAL PRINCIPLES OF THE CLINICAL APPROACH

Potential pathogens causing lung infection in the immunocompromised patient are listed in **Table 28-1**. Empirical therapy that is active against all these possible pathogens is not feasible,

especially given the potential toxicity of some treatments. Hence, the challenge in managing these patients is to (1) reduce the scope of the differential diagnosis to include the most likely problems and thus allow relatively targeted empirical therapy and (2) identify when and which type of invasive diagnostic test(s) should be used to provide the most useful data. The likely potential causative pathogens can be defined by ascertaining the following:

- The clinical and radiologic presentation
- The speed of onset of the infection
- The type, duration, and severity of the patient's immune defect
- Positive results on microbiologic studies
- Associated factors of importance, including any recent local infective epidemics and the patient's prophylaxis regimen, ethnic background, and travel history

The exact type of immune defect is determined by a combination of the disease and the treatment received and, fortunately, can generally be predicted (**Table 28-2**). The three main categories of immune defect are absolute or functional neutropenia, defects in cell-mediated immunity, and deficiencies in antibody responses (a clinically less severely affected category). Each is associated with a particular range of pathogens (see Table 28-2). Patients with neutropenia are mainly at risk for infection with extracellular pathogens such as pyogenic bacteria and filamentous fungi. Defects in cell-mediated immunity tend to predispose affected patients to development of infections with intracellular pathogens such as viruses and mycobacteria, as well as some unusual extracellular infections such as *Pneumocystis* pneumonia (PCP). Deficiencies in antibody responses result in a high incidence of infections due to encapsulated bacteria such as *Streptococcus pneumoniae* and to herpesviruses. Individual patients may have a combination of these immune defects; for example, lymphoma can cause impairment of cell-mediated immunity that can be combined with neutropenia if the patient receives chemotherapy.

HSCT, especially for allograft recipients, is particularly associated with lung complications, including infections with a daunting range of pathogens. The immune defects associated with HSCT depend on the conditioning regimen and type of graft, and evolve with time. In phase I, the preengraftment phase (15 to 45 days after transplantation), prolonged neutropenia and breaks in the mucocutaneous barrier increase the risk of bacterial and fungal infections. Herpes simplex virus reactivation also can occur during this phase. In phase II, the

Box 28-1 Diseases and Conditions Associated With Severe Immunocompromise*

Lymphoma/leukemia
Hematopoietic stem cell transplantation (HSCT)
Aplastic anemia
Solid organ transplantation
Other causes of neutropenia (fewer than 1500 cells/mL)
Inherited disorders of immune function (e.g., chronic granulomatous disease, recent chemotherapy)
High-dose corticosteroid treatment (greater than 30 mg prednisolone for 21 days or longer)
Treatment with immunosuppressive therapy (e.g., tacrolimus, cyclosporine)
Treatment with cytotoxic therapy (e.g., cyclophosphamide, mycophenolate)

*As defined in this chapter.

Table 28-1 Range of Pathogens Commonly Associated With Pneumonia in the Non–HIV-Infected Immunocompromised Patient

Pathogen	Cases (%)
Gram-Negative Pyogenic Bacteria	
Escherichia coli	6
Proteus, Enterobacter, Serratia, and Citrobacter spp.	2
Haemophilus influenzae	<1
Klebsiella pneumoniae	<1
Pseudomonas aeruginosa	8
Acinetobacter spp.	2
Stenotrophomonas maltophilia	<1
Gram-Positive Pyogenic Bacteria	
Streptococcus pneumoniae	2
Viridans streptococci	<1
Staphylococcus aureus	12
Enterococcus spp.	4
Other Bacteria	
Anaerobes	<1
Legionella pneumophila	2
Chlamydia spp.	2
Mycoplasma pneumoniae	<1
Mycobacterium tuberculosis	4
Nontuberculous mycobacteria	<1
Nocardia spp.	2
Fungi	
Pneumocystis jirovecii	3
Candida spp.	9
Aspergillus spp.	24
Rarer molds (e.g., Mucor, Penicillium, Fusarium)	2
Endemic fungi (e.g., Histoplasma, Coccidioides)	<1
Protozoa	
Toxoplasma gondii	<1
Helminths	
Strongyloides stercoralis	<1
Viruses	
Cytomegalovirus	6
Herpes simplex virus, varicella-zoster virus	2
Respiratory viruses (respiratory syncytial virus, adenovirus, influenza virus, parainfluenza virus, human metapneumovirus)	8

Modified from Rañó A, Agustí C, Jimenez P, et al: Pulmonary infiltrates in non-HIV immunocompromised patients: a diagnostic approach using non-invasive and bronchoscopic procedures, *Thorax* 56:379–387, 2001.

immediate post-engraftment phase at around 30 to 100 days after transplantation, infections relate primarily to impaired cell-mediated immunity and include those due to herpesviruses (particularly CMV) and PCP unless the patient is given prophylaxis. During phase III, the late phase (beyond 100 days), common pathogens again include herpesviruses, but there is also a marked increased incidence of infection with encapsulated bacteria such as *S. pneumoniae*, perhaps relating to impaired humoral immunity. Graft-versus-host disease also is associated with ongoing susceptibility to *Aspergillus* during phases II and III. For recipients of nonmyeloablative hematopoietic stem cell transplants, substantial differences may be observed during phase I, but susceptibility to infections during phases II and III is about the same. The risk of disease from community-acquired respiratory viruses is elevated in all three phases.

By combining the clinical pattern of presentation with knowledge of the patient's immune defect, a differential diagnosis of likely pathogens can be suggested. For example, infections developing rapidly over 1 to 3 days with a marked rise in serum inflammatory markers such as C-reactive protein (CRP), pronounced fever, and focal radiologic changes are very likely to be due to infection with pyogenic bacteria. In a patient with a defect in cell-mediated immunity, however, widespread ground glass infiltrations in both lungs developing over several days could represent CMV pneumonitis or PCP. In general, the more severe and prolonged the immune defect, the greater the range of possible causative pathogens and the less typical the clinical presentation for a particular pathogen, prompting the need for early invasive investigation if the initial therapy is failing to effect improvement. Furthermore the character of the disease can be dictated by the severity of the immune defect. For example, infections due to filamentous fungi such as *Aspergillus* progress faster with increasing severity of neutropenia, but may regress and become more focal when the neutrophil count recovers. **Table 28-3** shows the common conditions that should be considered for different presentations of lung complications in immunocompromised patients. Many patients will be found to have dual pathologic processes, either involving two separate pathogens or with simultaneous noninfective (fluid overload being the most common) and infective problems, which will be responsible for separate elements of the clinical picture.

Previous results of microbiologic tests need to be reviewed, because these may provide a strong indication of the cause of the present lung infection. For instance, infected indwelling vascular and urinary catheters can form foci of infection that can metastasize to the lungs, and previous *Aspergillus* infection may recur during new episodes of immunosuppression. Knowledge of previous and present CMV status identifies patients at risk for development of CMV pneumonitis, and positive

Table 28-2 Type of Immune Defect According to Disease/Treatment and Range of Pathogens Commonly Associated With Infections in Patients with Such Immune Defects

Immune Defect	Cause	Associated Pathogens
Neutropenia/functional neutrophil defects	Chemotherapy Early HSCT* Acute leukemia Chronic myelocytic leukemia Aplastic anemia Marrow infiltrations Azathioprine/mycophenolate[†] High-dose corticosteroids[†] Chronic granulomatous disease[†] Other inherited phagocyte defects[†]	Pyogenic bacteria and anaerobes Filamentous fungi (*Aspergillus*, rarer molds) *Candida* spp.
Cell-mediated immunity	HSCT Chronic lymphocytic leukemia Lymphoma Tacrolimus/sirolimus for organ transplant recipients Cyclosporine for organ transplant recipients Azathioprine/mycophenolate High-dose corticosteroids Graft-versus-host disease Inherited disorders of lymphocyte function	*Pneumocystis jirovecii* Herpesviruses Respiratory viruses *L. pneumophila* Mycobacteria and *Nocardia* Agents of endemic mycoses *T. gondii* *S. stercoralis*
Antibody deficiency	HSCT Chronic lymphocytic leukemia Lymphoma Myeloma	Encapsulated bacteria (e.g., *Streptococcus pneumoniae*, *Haemophilus influenzae*), herpesviruses

*Allografts up to 1 month, autografts usually less than 14 days.
[†]Patients usually have a normal neutrophil count but have defects in their function and/or a poor response to infection.
HSCT, hematopoietic stem cell transplantation.

sputum surveillance cultures for methicillin-resistant *Staphylococcus aureus* (MRSA) or *Pseudomonas aeruginosa* may indicate likely causes of a new pneumonia. In addition, positive samples from other patients also may be helpful, because local epidemics of respiratory virus infections are not uncommon in hospitals, and more rarely, clusters of nosocomial *Aspergillus*, *Nocardia* (both of which may be associated with ongoing construction on the hospital site), or *Legionella* infection can occur.

Other important factors that need to be taken into account include the patient's present antibiotic prophylaxis regimen, travel history, and ethnic background. A patient compliant with co-trimoxazole prophylaxis will rarely develop PCP, and fluconazole prophylaxis predisposes to non-albicans *Candida* infection. Patients with certain ethnic backgrounds or a pertinent travel history are more at risk of TB, endemic mycoses such as histoplasmosis, or parasitic diseases such as disseminated strongyloidiasis. Finally, the patient's background lung structure and function should be considered, because existing

structural abnormalities may make certain pathogens more likely. For example, bronchiectasis could predispose affected persons to pneumonia caused by *P. aeruginosa* (**Figure 28-1**), and preexisting lung cavities to *Aspergillus* infection.

CLINICAL ASSESSMENT AND DIAGNOSTIC PROTOCOLS

The combination of new respiratory symptoms and/or new radiologic findings with pyrexia suggests lung infection, although incidental radiologic or microbiology results may also identify active lung infection in an asymptomatic patient. The patient should undergo careful clinical assessment, including a review of previous laboratory and radiologic findings; the high mortality associated with lung infections in immunocompromised patients requires that this is initiated rapidly. The level of oxygenation will characterize the immediate risk to the patient and can also suggest likely pathogens as severe hypoxia is more likely with a bacterial lobar pneumonia, extensive PCP or viral infections. Chest radiographs are an essential first line investigation and are useful for monitoring progress. However, with the exception of lobar consolidation chest radiographs may not be sufficiently sensitive to make an accurate assessment of the pattern of lung shadowing. Ultimately a computed tomography (CT) scan of the thorax often is required. CT scans are approximately 20% more sensitive than chest radiographs at identifying lung involvement and also define whether new changes on a chest radiograph represent consolidation, nodules, ground glass infiltrates, or "tree-in-bud" changes.

All patients with suspected new lung infection require blood and sputum cultures, as well as routine blood tests, and in many cases nasopharyngeal aspirate studies for identification of viruses, assessment of CMV status, and serum testing for fungal antigens (galactomannan or β-D-glucan). An important question for the respiratory physician is when to utilize more invasive investigations, either bronchoscopy with bronchoalveolar lavage (BAL) and possibly transbronchial biopsy, percutaneous radiologically guided biopsy, or, on occasion, surgical biopsy, usually video-assisted thoracoscopic surgery (VATS). Which test should be used and when will depend to a large extent on the type of radiologic presentation—consolidation, diffuse ground glass infiltrates, tree-in-bud changes, and nodules—in accordance with the algorithms for each provided in Figures 28-2, 28-4, 28-6, and 28-7, respectively. These suggested protocols balance the likelihood and necessity of a positive yield against the clinical probability that a particular disease will be identified with the potential complications of the investigations. These protocols are for general guidance; atypical presentations and dual pathology are not uncommon, and an individual patient often will require a modified approach. Immunocompromised patients are also at high risk for development of a range of noninfective causes of lung disease, including pulmonary edema, idiopathic pneumonia syndrome (IPS), and diffuse alveolar hemorrhage (see Chapter 59). These conditions should always be considered in the differential diagnosis for new lung disease. The protocols are discussed in detail next.

INVESTIGATION OF CONSOLIDATION

Rapidly developing focal consolidation usually is due to bacterial pneumonia and initially can be treated empirically with broad-spectrum antibiotics (**Figure 28-2**). The most likely reason for a lack of improvement in the patient's condition within 48 to 96 hours is infection with bacteria resistant to

Table 28-3   **Differential Diagnosis for Computed Tomography (CT) Pattern and Rate of Development of Clinical Problem**

Predominant CT Pattern	Rate of Progression		
	Acute (days)	Subacute (days to weeks)	Chronic (weeks)
Consolidation/focal ground glass infiltration	Bacterial pneumonia Aspiration Diffuse alveolar hemorrhage Acute respiratory distress syndrome (ARDS)*	Cryptogenic organizing pneumonia Aspiration Mycobacteria[†] *Nocardia*[†] Invasive filamentous fungi[†]	Cryptogenic organizing pneumonia Lymphoma Mycobacteria[†] *Nocardia*[†]
Diffuse ground glass infiltration	CMV pneumonia Viral pneumonia Diffuse alveolar hemorrhage ARDS*	CMV pneumonia PCP Idiopathic pneumonia syndrome (IPS) Drug reactions	Drug reaction
Nodules	Metastatic infection Invasive filamentous fungi	Metastatic infection Invasive filamentous fungi *Nocardia* Mycobacteria	Lymphoma Lymphoproliferative disease *Nocardia* Mycobacteria
Multiple nodules (>10)	Metastatic infection	Metastatic infection Mycobacteria	Lymphoma Lymphoproliferative disease Mycobacteria
Bronchiolitis/"tree-in-bud" changes	Viral bronchiolitis *Chlamydia pneumoniae* *Mycoplasma pneumoniae* Bacterial exacerbation bronchiectasis	Viral bronchiolitis *C. pneumoniae* *M. pneumoniae* Nontuberculous mycobacteria *Aspergillus* tracheobronchitis[†] Bacterial exacerbation bronchiectasis	Bronchiectasis Nontuberculous mycobacteria

*Extensive, patchy, mainly posterior.
[†]Usually focal patches.

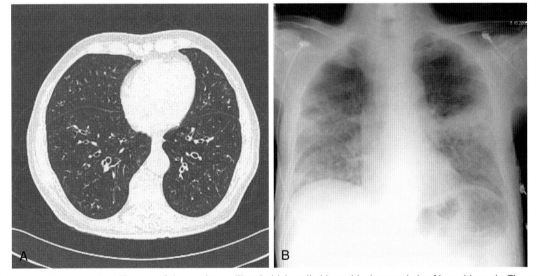

Figure 28-1   A, Computed tomography (CT) scan of thorax shows dilated, thick-walled bronchi, characteristic of bronchiectasis. The patient, who had a long history of chronic lymphatic leukemia and immunoglobulin deficiency, produced purulent sputum daily, culture of which grew *Pseudomonas aeruginosa*. **B,** A chest radiograph obtained in the same patient, whose clinical presentation included high fever, productive cough, and marked hypoxia, shows consolidation (most marked in the left middle zone) due to *P. aeruginosa* pneumonia.

first-line antibiotics. At this point, treatment with second-line antibiotics effective against likely resistant organisms should be started. Consideration also should be given to starting antibiotics that are effective against MRSA and anaerobic pathogens if this has not been done already. In patients at high risk for invasive fungal infection, especially those with CT evidence of associated nodular disease or patchy or infarct-shaped consolidation, failure of first-line therapy warrants testing for fungal antigens (galactomannan or β-D-glucan) and either fiberoptic bronchoscopy (FOB) with BAL or percutaneous CT-guided biopsy (mainly for evaluation of dense consolidation adjacent to the pleura). These investigations also will be necessary in patients whose pneumonia fails to respond to second-line antibiotic therapy or those with subacute or chronic consolidation in whom sputum microbiologic or cytologic testing is nondiagnostic. With progressive disease and lack of a definitive diagnosis after the foregoing tests, surgical biopsy should be seriously considered.

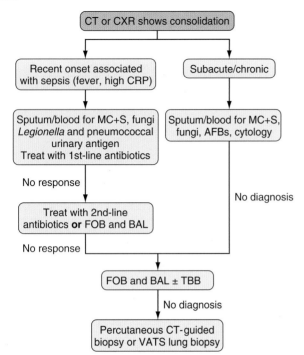

Figure 28-2 diagram: CT or CXR shows consolidation → Recent onset associated with sepsis (fever, high CRP) and Subacute/chronic → Sputum/blood for MC+S, fungi *Legionella* and pneumococcal urinary antigen Treat with 1st-line antibiotics / Sputum/blood for MC+S, fungi, AFBs, cytology → No response → Treat with 2nd-line antibiotics **or** FOB and BAL → No response / No diagnosis → FOB and BAL ± TBB → No diagnosis → Percutaneous CT-guided biopsy or VATS lung biopsy

Figure 28-2 Investigation of consolidation in the immunocompromised patient. *AFBs,* acid-fast bacilli; *BAL,* bronchoalveolar lavage; *CRP,* C-reactive protein; *CT,* computed tomography; *FOB,* fiberoptic bronchoscopy; *MC+S,* microbial culture and sensitivity [testing]; *TBB,* transbronchial biopsy; *VATS,* video-assisted thoracoscopic surgery.

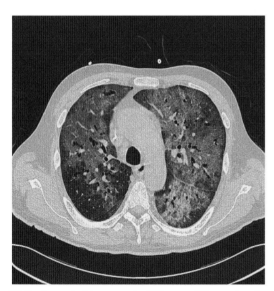

Figure 28-3 Computed tomography (CT) scan of thorax showing widespread bilateral ground glass infiltration in a hematopoietic stem cell transplant recipient. The differential diagnosis for this imaging appearance is broad in scope, including cytomegalovirus pneumonia, *Pneumocystis* pneumonia, drug reactions, and idiopathic pneumonia syndrome, and early invasive investigation typically is required even though with such widespread lung disease the patient is likely to have significant hypoxia.

INVESTIGATION OF DIFFUSE GROUND GLASS INFILTRATION

The differential diagnosis for ground glass infiltrates and centrilobular nodules (**Figures 28-3** and **28-4**) is wide in scope and includes CMV infection, viral pneumonias, PCP, extensive bacterial infection, and noninfective causes such as acute

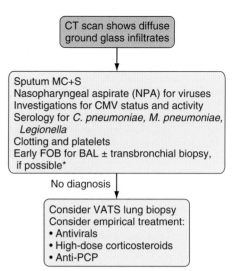

Figure 28-4 diagram: CT scan shows diffuse ground glass infiltrates → Sputum MC+S / Nasopharyngeal aspirate (NPA) for viruses / Investigations for CMV status and activity / Serology for *C. pneumoniae, M. pneumoniae, Legionella* / Clotting and platelets / Early FOB for BAL ± transbronchial biopsy, if possible* → No diagnosis → Consider VATS lung biopsy / Consider empirical treatment: • Antivirals • High-dose corticosteroids • Anti-PCP

*Significant hypoxia often precludes FOB.

Figure 28-4 Investigation of diffuse ground glass infiltrates in the immunocompromised patient. *BAL,* bronchoalveolar lavage; *CMV,* cytomegalovirus; *FOB,* fiberoptic bronchoscopy; *MC+S,* microbial culture and sensitivity [testing]; *PCP, Pneumocystis* pneumonia; *VATS,* video-assisted thoracoscopic surgery.

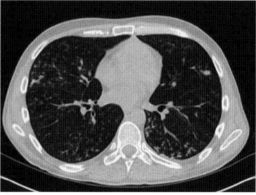

Figure 28-5 Computed tomography (CT) scan showing widespread bilateral "tree-in-bud" changes in a hematopoietic stem cell transplant recipient. This appearance is caused by marked small airway inflammation secondary to respiratory virus infection, bacterial bronchitis (e.g., *Mycoplasma pneumoniae, Chlamydia pneumoniae, Pseudomonas aeruginosa,* or *Haemophilus influenzae* infection), and, when more focal, *Aspergillus* tracheobronchitis or mycobacterial infection.

respiratory distress syndrome (ARDS), drug toxicity, and IPS associated with HSCT (see Chapter 77). As a consequence, unless nasopharyngeal aspirate studies identify a respiratory viral infection, early FOB with BAL and, if possible, transbronchial biopsy should be attempted. Often, however, these patients are markedly hypoxic, increasing the risk associated with the procedure. Negative results on FOB do not exclude infective causes, and a decision then needs to be taken about empirical treatment versus VATS lung biopsy. CT-guided biopsy for investigation of diffuse lung disease carries a high risk of complications coupled with low diagnostic yield and therefore is not appropriate in this setting.

INVESTIGATION OF TREE-IN-BUD CHANGES

Tree-in-bud changes (**Figures 28-5** and **28-6**) suggest small airway pathology, which in immunocompromised patients is

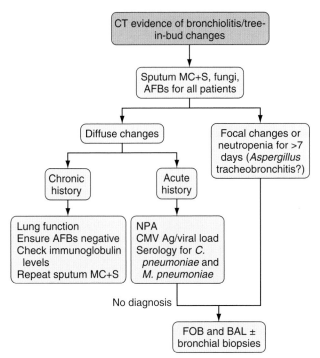

Figure 28-6   Investigation of "tree-in-bud" pattern associated with bronchiolitis in the immunocompromised patient. *AFBs*, acid-fast bacilli; *BAL*, bronchoalveolar lavage; *CMV*, cytomegalovirus; *CT*, computed tomography; *FOB*, fiberoptic bronchoscopy; *MC+S*, microbial culture and sensitivity [testing].

likely to be caused by respiratory virus infection, *Chlamydia pneumoniae*, *Mycoplasma pneumoniae*, or, especially if the changes are focal and associated with nodular changes, *Aspergillus* tracheobronchitis. Subacute or chronic changes also could reflect bacterial infection in bronchiectasis or nontuberculous mycobacteria infection. If results of nasopharyngeal aspirate studies are negative, then early FOB for BAL and bronchial biopsy of macroscopically inflamed bronchial mucosa should be performed. *Aspergillus* tracheobronchitis usually is obvious at FOB and is readily confirmed by culture and cytologic examination of bronchial washings and by bronchial biopsy. Infections due to respiratory viruses, *C. pneumoniae*, and *M. pneumoniae* often are difficult to diagnose but usually are either self-limiting illnesses or readily controlled with macrolide therapy.

INVESTIGATION OF PULMONARY NODULES

Considerations in the differential diagnosis for pulmonary nodules include infection with *Aspergillus* (or other invasive filamentous fungi), *Nocardia*, or mycobacteria (**Figure 28-7**). *Aspergillus* and *Nocardia* tend to cause a small number of nodules, whereas mycobacteria also can cause large numbers of small nodules. In addition, blood-borne spread of bacteria or *Candida* from infected indwelling devices can cause a variable number (often numerous) of pulmonary nodules. Serum testing for fungal antigens (galactomannan or β-D-glucan) should be performed. Nodules caused by pyogenic bacterial and viral pneumonia tend to be associated with other radiographic changes findings such as ground glass infiltrates or consolidation. The

Figure 28-7   Investigation of pulmonary nodules in the immunocompromised patient. *AFBs*, acid-fast bacilli; *BAL*, bronchoalveolar lavage; *CMV*, cytomegalovirus; *CT*, computed tomography; *FOB*, fiberoptic bronchoscopy; *GVHD*, graft-versus-host disease; *MC+S*, microbial culture and sensitivity [testing]; *VATS*, video-assisted thoracoscopic surgery.

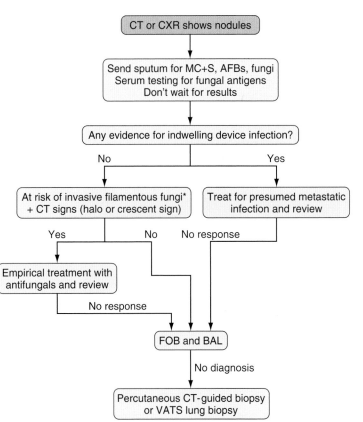

*Neutropenia >7 days, high-dose steroids, GVHD, previous episode invasive aspergillosis. Even with halo or crescent signs present on the CT scan there should be a low threshold for performing BAL to identify the fungal species.

other major causes of nodules are underlying malignant disease and lymphoproliferative disorders secondary to prolonged immunosuppression. In the absence of CT signs suggestive of invasive filamentous fungal infection (the halo and crescent signs), nodules in patients with line infections or a positive blood culture may be treated empirically as for metastatic infection. For a majority of other patients with lung nodules, FOB with BAL is necessary, although for patients at high risk for infection with invasive filamentous fungi, if CT changes suggestive of *Aspergillus* infection are present, then empirical antifungal therapy is a reasonable alternative strategy, especially if the result of fungal antigen testing is positive. If FOB findings are unhelpful, the patient should progress to percutaneous CT-guided or VATS lung biopsy, because infections due to fungi, *Nocardia*, or mycobacteria are accompanied by specific histopathologic changes, and biopsy frequently is diagnostic.

BRONCHOSCOPY

Although many immunocompromised patients with pneumonia are hypoxic and have low platelet counts and/or abnormal clotting, FOB generally is safe and has a diagnostic yield of 30 to 50%. Exclusion of active infection is necessary to make a diagnosis of IPS after HSCT, so even a negative result can be useful. In our own experience, peroral FOB can be performed without significant bleeding in patients with a platelet count of 10,000/mL. BAL should be performed in patients with marked hypoxia or severe tachypnea only after careful consideration of risk versus benefit, because the procedure commonly reduces PaO_2 by 20 mm Hg and may precipitate the need for intubation and mechanical ventilation. Transbronchial biopsy improves the diagnostic yield of FOB by perhaps 5% to 10% but often is not possible, because the patient needs to be able to tolerate the potential complication of a pneumothorax and have a platelet count above 50,000/mL.

SPECIFIC CLINICAL ENTITIES

BACTERIAL PNEUMONIA

General Considerations

Pneumonia due to bacterial pathogens is the most common lung infection in the immunocompromised patient, causing about 40% to 50% of infective episodes. The main risk factor is neutropenia, but cell-mediated immune defects and functional defects in phagocyte responses due to cytotoxic or immunosuppressive therapy also will markedly increase the risk for development of pneumonia. Antibody deficiencies associated with lymphoproliferative disorders, myeloma, and HSCT predispose affected patients to development of pneumonia with encapsulated organisms such as *S. pneumoniae* and *Haemophilus influenzae*. Many cases of bacterial pneumonia are nosocomial infections in patients who have been hospitalized for long periods and who previously have been treated with antibiotics so that the normal oropharyngeal flora has been replaced mainly by gram-negative bacteria. As a consequence, the range of potential organisms causing bacterial pneumonia is very different from that seen in community-acquired pneumonia, with a high frequency of resistant organisms such as *P. aeruginosa* and MRSA (see Table 28-1).

Clinical Features and Diagnosis

Bacterial pneumonia often manifests with a clinical picture similar to that seen in immunocompetent patients, with new-onset fever, cough, chest and radiologic signs of lobar consolidation, and a rapid rise in the level of inflammatory markers such as CRP. However, a more insidious or diffuse presentation that is more difficult to differentiate from viral or fungal infection is not uncommon. CT scans showing dense focal consolidation with a lobar distribution are helpful in differentiating bacterial from fungal or viral pneumonia (**Figure 28-8**), and blood cultures will be positive in about 20% of cases. Antigen testing of the urine may identify *Legionella pneumophila* or *S. pneumoniae* infections. Patients with an atypical clinical presentation or those who do not respond to first- or second-line antibiotics should have FOB and BAL, which has a reasonably high diagnostic yield for bacterial pneumonia. Protected specimen brush procedures probably add little information over and above that obtained with directed BAL. Histologic examination is unlikely to reveal specific features, and lung biopsy is mainly used to exclude other causes of lung infiltrates.

Management

Oxygen therapy to maintain a normal PaO_2 is essential and may require continuous positive airway pressure (CPAP) support. Intubation may be necessary if the patient's underlying disease

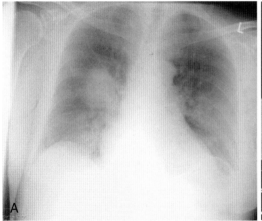
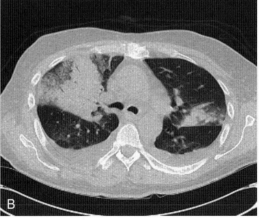

Figure 28-8 **A,** Chest radiograph showing a mass-like consolidation in the right middle lung zone in a patient with acute myeloid leukemia recently treated with chemotherapy and presenting with a high temperature but no respiratory symptoms after 9 days of neutropenia. **B,** Computed tomography (CT) scan of thorax in the same patient, showing that the shadowing is due to dense consolidation in the right upper lobe, with a smaller area of consolidation in the left upper lobe. The blood cultures grew *Escherichia coli*, and the patient improved rapidly on appropriate antibiotics, suggesting that the consolidation was a hospital-acquired pneumonia due to *E. coli*.

does not preclude mechanical ventilation but is associated with a poor prognosis in immunocompromised patients (up to a 95% mortality rate). Initial antibiotic therapy should be effective against the local pattern of hospital-acquired infections and will therefore probably include extended-range beta-lactams, aminoglycosides, or ciprofloxacin. Lack of response within 72 to 96 hours should prompt a switch to another broad-spectrum parenteral antibiotic (e.g., a carbapenem) in case the causative pathogen is resistant to first-line agents. Treatment for infections due to MRSA or other resistant gram-positive organisms also should be considered. Carbapenems and extended-range beta-lactams usually have good efficacy against anaerobic organisms.

Prevention

Antibacterial prophylaxis with a fluoroquinolone (e.g., levofloxacin) often is used during the neutropenic phase after HSCT. Prolonged antibiotic prophylaxis with penicillin V against encapsulated organisms is necessary for patients rendered functionally asplenic by their disease or therapy. Antibiotic prophylaxis also may be indicated in patients with chronic graft-versus-host disease, immunoglobulin deficiencies, and bronchiectasis. Vaccination against *S. pneumoniae* is recommended for all hematopoietic stem cell transplant recipients, and the conjugated vaccine probably should be used because of its stronger immunogenicity. Concern has emerged about the risk of whooping cough in recipients of hematopoietic stem cell transplants, who perhaps should receive vaccination against *Bordetella pertussis* and prophylaxis with azithromycin if exposed to an infected case.

MYCOBACTERIAL INFECTIONS

Mycobacterial infections usually are associated with defects in cell-mediated immunity and tend to develop subacutely. The risk for *Mycobacterium tuberculosis* infection is strongly dependent on the ethnic background and country of origin of the patient. Tuberculosis should be considered in at-risk patients with a cell-mediated immune defect or patchy or nodular lung shadowing, particularly those with a high-risk ethnic background. Nontuberculous mycobacterial infections (e.g., *Mycobacterium kansasii* or *Mycobacterium avium* complex [MAC]) are infrequent complications in immunocompromised patients. Exclusion of the diagnosis by negative culture takes too long to be clinically useful in patients with progressive disease. Therefore, with significant clinical suspicion of mycobacterial infection, invasive investigations are necessary to obtain material for a rapid diagnosis by identification of acid-fast bacilli, specific histopathologic changes, or possibly polymerase chain reaction (PCR) assay for samples obtained from sterile sites. Treatment is with the standard chemotherapy regimens.

NOCARDIAL INFECTIONS

Nocardia are gram-positive aerobic organisms found in soil and stagnant water. They grow relatively slowly as branching filaments. Immunocompromised patients should avoid gardening or occupations that result in exposure to soil and plants. Infection occurs through inhalation, so patients who wish to continue gardening may minimize exposure by wearing protective clothing such as an N-95 mask and gloves. The organisms most commonly causing human infection belong to the *Nocardia asteroides* complex, but other *Nocardia* spp. also can cause disease. Around 2% of lung infections in immunocompromised patients are due to *Nocardia*, and like mycobacterial infections, nocardial infections tend to affect patients with defects in cell-mediated immunity. In hematopoietic stem cell transplant recipients, the median time to onset is approximately 200 days after transplantation. Risk factors for disease also include corticosteroid use, active graft-versus-host disease, and concomitant opportunistic infections, especially with CMV.

Nocardia infection can manifest as a relatively acute pneumonia or as a more indolent disease similar to infection with *Mycobacteria* or *Aspergillus*. Radiologic changes include patches of consolidation, large nodules, often with cavitation, and pleural involvement in up to a third of cases. Hematogenous spread to other organs such as the brain, joints, and soft tissues occurs in up to 50% of patients. Microscopy or histologic examination can make the diagnosis rapidly through identification of characteristic beaded, branching, gram-positive and weakly acid-fast filaments. Respiratory and occasionally blood cultures can be positive but require prolonged aerobic culture. Most *Nocardia* strains are sensitive to co-trimoxazole as well as carbapenems, amikacin, third-generation cephalosporins, tetracyclines, and co-amoxiclav, but treatment needs to be very prolonged, lasting up to 12 months in immunocompromised patients. Mortality is high, reportedly up to 70%.

CYTOMEGALOVIRUS INFECTION

General Considerations

CMV infection is one of the most important complications in patients with defects in cell-mediated immunity such as transplant recipients and patients receiving potent immunosuppressive drugs such as fludarabine or alemtuzumab. CMV is the largest member of the Herpesviridae family of human double-stranded DNA viruses. It has a 230-kb genome that encodes over 200 products, which are expressed during replication in three overlapping phases over 24 hours termed immediate-early, early, and late.

Primary CMV infection is common in the general population, occurring mainly in children or young adults, but usually is asymptomatic or causes only mild disease. Previous infection is identified by serologic studies and leads to asymptomatic latent infection that can be reactivated in immunocompromised persons. Reactivation can be initiated by the cytokine tumor necrosis factor and stress catecholamines, so the virus often will be detected in transplant recipients 3 to 4 weeks after an infective episode involving another pathogen. Around 60% of immunocompromised patients with negative results on serologic testing for CMV who then receive transplants or blood products containing leukocytes from CMV-positive donors will develop CMV infection, which tends to be more severe than disease due to CMV reactivation. CMV-negative immunocompromised patients also can rarely develop primary infection after exposure to someone with active CMV infection.

Clinical Features and Diagnosis

The potential effects of CMV reactivation in immunocompromised patients are varied and include (1) clinically asymptomatic infection, which is common even in immunocompromised patients; (2) a CMV syndrome, defined as fever, a 50% fall in the leukocyte count, and a 2.5-fold increase in transaminases; (3) organ-specific infection, including the liver, central nervous system (CNS), gastrointestinal system, and lungs, often associated with more severe involvement of the transplanted organ; (4) accentuated rejection-related damage to the target organ (e.g., bronchiolitis obliterans in lung transplant recipients);

(5) impaired host immunity with increased incidence of opportunistic infections including pneumonia due to *Aspergillus*, *Pneumocystis jirovecii*, gram-negative bacteria, and *Nocardia*; and (6) increased incidence of EBV-associated lymphoproliferative disease.

CMV pneumonitis commonly manifests with insidious onset of fever, malaise, cough, and dyspnea with hypoxia. The chest radiograph may be normal in appearance or show nonspecific diffuse bilateral infiltrates. CT scan is more sensitive at identifying pulmonary infiltrates and classically shows bibasal symmetric ground glass opacities, septal line thickening, and multiple small centrilobular nodules (**Figure 28-9**). More asymmetric changes, consolidation, and effusions are not uncommon, however. The main considerations in the differential diagnosis are IPS, drug-induced pneumonitis, and, in patients not receiving effective prophylaxis, PCP. Serologic determination of either IgG or IgM has no place in the diagnosis of CMV disease, because these antibodies merely reflect previous exposure. However, CMV reactivation is nowadays readily detected by identifying significant viremia through either measuring the level of pp65 antigenemia or CMV DNA using PCR assay in the blood. CMV viremia usually is detectable 2 to 5 days before any clinical manifestations. Unfortunately, CMV viremia is not always present in patients with CMV pneumonitis; conversely, evidence of reactivation does not necessarily mean that new lung infiltrates are due to CMV pneumonitis. The chance that CMV infection is responsible for new lung infiltrates is proportional in part to the level of CMV in the blood, especially if the viral load increased rapidly. Definitive confirmation that CMV is causing pneumonia requires identification of CMV in the respiratory tract by FOB for BAL and preferably a transbronchial biopsy, or possibly a VATS lung biopsy. The presence of "owl's eye" intranuclear inclusions on cytologic examination is pathognomonic for CMV infection and although this modality is rapid, it is a relatively insensitive test. CMV can be cultured from respiratory samples using fibroblast cell culture to look for the distinctive cytopathogenic effect, but this takes at least a week and therefore is of little clinical benefit. The main diagnostic techniques for CMV pneumonitis are the relatively sensitive rapid tests for CMV antigens using BAL samples directly, or indirectly by probing cell cultures inoculated with the samples after 24 to 48 hours incubation (the shell vial or early antigen detection assays). Quantitative PCR assay on BAL fluid has been used to improve the predictive value for the diagnosis of CMV pneumonitis but requires further investigation. Despite this range of diagnostic techniques, a well-validated standard for identifying CMV pneumonitis is lacking, except for VATS biopsy.

Treatment

The currently available antiviral agents for treatment of CMV infection and disease are acyclovir, valacyclovir, ganciclovir, valganciclovir, foscarnet, and cidofovir (**Table 28-4**). A regimen based on the purine analogue ganciclovir is the preferred treatment; this agent, once phosphorylated within infected cells, competitively inhibits viral DNA polymerase. Ganciclovir has significant marrow-depressant effects and may be too toxic for use in hematopoietic stem cell transplant recipients or in patients with existing pancytopenia. Oral absorption is poor, but oral therapy with the valine ester valganciclovir has excellent bioavailability. The second-line agent foscarnet also inhibits the activity of viral DNA polymerase (by binding to the pyrophosphate-binding site). Foscarnet frequently causes significant renal toxicity. Alternatively, cidofovir has a broad activity against DNA viruses including CMV, acting as a competitive inhibitor of viral DNA polymerases. Cidofovir causes both myelosuppression and renal toxicity, and patients should be prehydrated and given probeniced before initiation of treatment. Patients with CMV disease also are frequently given hyperimmune intravenous immunoglobulin (IVIG) as passive vaccination therapy. Very few studies have compared these drugs for efficacy in CMV pneumonia. Treatment lasts from 14 to 21 days and should be guided by blood tests measuring the level of CMV viremia. Patients at risk for such infection often are given antiviral prophylaxis such as with valganciclovir. The mortality rate for established CMV pneumonia is up to 50% in hematopoietic stem cell transplant recipients but is less in other types of immunocompromised patients. Detection of CMV viremia frequently leads to preemptive therapy before symptomatic CMV infection develops, increasing the numbers of patients requiring treatment but improving overall outcome.

LUNG INFECTIONS DUE TO OTHER HERPESVIRUSES

Herpes simplex virus (HSV) and varicella-zoster virus (VZV) are rare causes of lung infection in immunocompromised patients, with a presentation similar to that for CMV pneumonia, but patients also may have the characteristic skin involvement. Microbiologic diagnosis relies on isolation of the virus from skin lesions or BAL fluid, and treatment is with high-dose acyclovir. Human herpesvirus type 6 (HHV6) may be an important pathogen causing infection after HSCT. Patients with HHV6 viremia have more CMV reactivation and unexplained fever and rash compared with patients without HHV6 viremia, and high-level HHV6 viremia (up to 25,000 copies/mL) has been associated with culture-negative pneumonitis.

INFECTIONS WITH RESPIRATORY VIRUSES

General Considerations

Lower respiratory tract infections with respiratory viruses are relatively common in immunocompromised patients. The common relevant viruses are respiratory syncytial virus (RSV), parainfluenza virus (PIV) (90% serotype III), influenza A virus, adenovirus, human metapneumovirus, coronavirus, and possibly rhinovirus. Infection is acquired by inhalation of infected respiratory droplets from other infected patients or mildly affected immunocompetent contacts. Consequently, immunocompromised patients should avoid contact with social

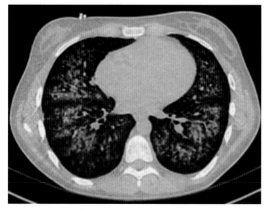

Figure 28-9 Computed tomography (CT) scan of thorax showing changes due to cytomegalovirus pneumonitis in a patient who had undergone hematopoietic stem cell transplantation for lymphoma 3 months previously.

Table 28-4	Treatment Options for Viral Lung Infections			
Treatment	**Dose**	**Mode of Action**	**Viruses**	**Role/General Comments**
Ganciclovir	2.5-5 mg/kg IV 2-3×/day	Inhibitor of viral DNA polymerase	CMV, HSV, HHV6	First-line agent; myelosuppressive; good efficacy
Valganciclovir	900 mg PO 1-2×/day	Prodrug of ganciclovir	CMV, HSV, HHV6	Better oral availability than ganciclovir
Foscarnet	60 mg/kg IV 3×/day	Inhibitor of viral DNA polymerase	CMV	Second-line agent; good efficacy; nephrotoxic
Acyclovir	10-15 mg/kg IV 3×/day	Inhibitor of viral DNA polymerase	HSV, VZV, HHV-6	Toxicity relatively uncommon
Cidofovir	1-5 mg/kg IV once weekly	Inhibitor of viral DNA polymerase	Adenovirus Possibly CMV	Third-line agent for CMV infection; efficacy against adenovirus unclear; nephrotoxic
Ribavarin	0.8 mg/kg inhaled	Nucleoside analogue	RSV, PIV, influenza virus, adenovirus, human metapneumovirus	Questionable benefit; nebulizer requires a scavenger tent because of potential toxicity; given over 12 to 18 hours
IVIG	E.g., 500 mg once daily	Passive vaccination	CMV, RSV	Combination treatment with antiviral agent
Palivizumab	15 mg/kg IV	Humanized anti-RSV monoclonal antibody	RSV	Efficacy unclear; used in combination with ribavarin
Amantidine	100 mg PO 2×/day	M2 inhibitor	Influenza A virus	Efficacy unclear; lowers incidence of progression to pneumonia?
Zanamivir	10 mg inhaled 2×/day	Neuraminidase inhibitor	Influenza virus	Probably reasonable efficacy
Oseltamivir	75 mg PO 2×/day	Neuraminidase inhibitor	Influenza virus	Probably reasonable efficacy

CMV, cytomegalovirus; *HHV-6*, human herpesvirus-6; *HSV*, herpes simplex virus; *PIV*, parainfluenza virus; *RSV*, respiratory syncytial virus; *VZV*, varicella-zoster virus.

contacts or members of the hospital staff clearly suffering from upper respiratory tract infections. Nosocomial epidemics of respiratory viruses readily occur, so infected patients should be effectively isolated. Respiratory viral infections are associated with defects in cell-mediated immunity and generally are a late complication after HSCT.

Clinical Features and Diagnosis

Respiratory virus lung infections often cause a bronchiolitis, manifesting with cough, fever, wheeze, and inspiratory squeaks. They frequently are preceded by a few days of coryzal symptoms. The chest radiograph may be normal in appearance, but a CT scan will show evidence of small airway involvement, with widespread tree-in-bud changes (**Figure 28-10**). The main considerations in the differential diagnosis in this clinical scenario are *Chlamydia* or *Mycoplasma* infection, extensive bacterial bronchitis (usually associated with bronchiectasis), and possibly *Aspergillus* tracheobronchitis. With more severe disease associated with significant pneumonitis, CT evidence will include small, poorly defined centrilobular nodules and usually bilateral patchy areas of peribronchial ground glass opacity and consolidation. The differential diagnosis in such cases is much broader in scope, including bacterial pneumonia, CMV pneumonitis, PCP, and noninfective causes of pneumonitis. In many patients, the diagnosis of respiratory viral infection can be rapidly confirmed by noninvasive testing using nasopharyngeal aspirate samples for either immunofluorescence for viral antigens or PCR assay for viral nucleic acids. A negative result on nasopharyngeal aspirate studies should lead to FOB, because these tests are more sensitive with BAL fluid than with nasopharyngeal aspirate samples. Respiratory viral infections in immunocompromised patients are often very prolonged but

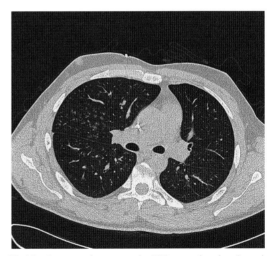

Figure 28-10 Computed tomography (CT) scan showing "tree-in-bud" changes (most obvious in the right upper lobe) due to PIV serotype 3 bronchiolitis in a patient with relapsed acute myeloid leukemia who had completed chemotherapy 25 days previously and presented with coryzal symptoms, cough, and a mild fever. *PIV*, parainfluenza virus.

not too severe, with symptoms and positive results on nasopharyngeal aspirate studies persisting for several weeks.

Treatment and Special Considerations with Specific Viruses

With the exception of influenza, treatment options for respiratory viruses are limited and depend on the underlying virus (see Table 28-4). In the absence of pneumonia, the mortality associated with respiratory virus infection in immunocompromised patients is relatively low, and patients can be given supportive therapy only. By contrast, pneumonia due to respiratory viruses after HSCT is associated with significant mortality (up to 40%). Secondary infections are common, and patients frequently need concurrent treatment with antibiotics.

Influenza Viruses Infection after HSCT with influenza viruses is perhaps surprisingly less common than infection with RSV and PIV. First-line therapy is with neuraminidase inhibitors (zanamivir or oseltamivir), which do seem to be effective at limiting disease severity and duration. An alternative agent for treatment of influenza virus infection is amantidine, but its efficacy is not clear. Transplant recipients (and their family members or household contacts) should receive lifelong seasonal influenza vaccination with the trivalent inactivated vaccine. If an outbreak occurs with a nonvaccine influenza strain, chemoprophylaxis with zanamivir or oseltamivir should be considered.

Parainfluenza Virus Although infection with PIV probably is among the most common causes of respiratory viral infection after HSCT, currently data on effective treatments are scarce. Ribavarin and IVIG may have activity against PIV infection but have not yet been shown to be beneficial in clinical practice. No useful vaccine is generally available as yet.

Respiratory Syncytial Virus Hematopoietic stem cell transplant recipients, particularly those who are pre-engraftment and lymphopenic or those who have preexisting obstructive airway disease, are at highest risk for severe RSV pneumonia. Therapies for RSV infection include systemic or aerosolized ribavirin, passive immunization with high-RSV-titer immunoglobulin, and monoclonal antibody directed at the RSV F antigen (palivizumab). No randomized trial has been completed to test the efficacy of these strategies, and efficacy data are limited. Some centers provide monthly palivizumab prophylaxis for hematopoietic stem cell transplant recipients during the RSV season (November to April in the Northern Hemisphere), particularly for pediatric recipients. Preemptive aerosolized ribavirin may be effective in those transplant recipients with lymphopenia and preexisting impaired lung function who develop RSV upper respiratory tract infection before the emergence of evidence that the infection has spread to the lungs.

Human Metapneumovirus Human metapneumovirus (hMPV) is a relatively recently identified RNA paramyxovirus related to RSV. It has been increasingly associated with lower respiratory tract infection and pneumonia in hematopoietic stem cell transplant recipients, with mortality rates of up to 50%. IVIG and ribavirin have in vitro activity against hMPV, but no recommendations on treatment are currently available owing to lack of data.

Adenovirus Adenovirus infections can occur in patients with impaired cell-mediated immunity due to reactivation or de novo acquisition. Many different adenovirus serotypes exist, so pretransplant serology is not helpful. In HSCT, the risk of adenovirus infection is increased for allograft recipients, after T cell depletion or treatment with antithymocyte globulin (alemtuzumab), and for patients with graft-versus-host disease receiving systemic steroids. Clearance of adenovirus has been shown to be associated with recovery of adenovirus-specific T cell immunity. Few antiviral agents have in vivo activity against adenoviruses, and no randomized, placebo-controlled study of antiviral drug therapy for adenoviral infection has been performed. The available data suggest that cidofovir or ribavirin may have some efficacy.

Respiratory Viruses and Lung Allograft Syndromes

Respiratory viral infection early after hematopoietic cell transplantation can be a predictor for the development of alloimmune lung syndromes such as progressive airways obstruction due to bronchiolitis obliterans, perhaps as they sensitize the respiratory epithelium for lung involvement by graft-versushost disease. Clinically, patients will present with rapidly progressive airway obstruction in the context of active respiratory viral infection and will require aggressive immunosuppression to prevent progression to respiratory failure.

INVASIVE ASPERGILLOSIS

General Considerations

Invasive infections with *Aspergillus* constitute a common and important cause of lung infection in immunodeficient patients. *Aspergillus* organisms are saprophytic filamentous fungi that are found ubiquitously in the environment. They propagate by dispersal of airborne spores, which are 2 to 3 μm in diameter and can therefore reach the distal airway. Exposure to airborne spores is essentially continuous, but this rarely causes a clinical problem unless the host's immune response is impaired. In a patient with impaired macrophage or neutrophil function, however, the spores can germinate and form a colony of branching multicellular hyphae that gradually expands and penetrates through host tissue, causing invasive pulmonary aspergillosis (IPA). The usual site of infection is the respiratory tract, including the sinuses, but blood-borne spread to internal organs (especially the CNS), bone, and skin is common. The most frequently isolated species causing infection are *A. fumigatus* (66% of cases), *Aspergillus flavus* (14%), *Aspergillus niger* (7%), and *Aspergillus terreus* (4%).

Clinical Features

IPA is mainly a disease that affects patients with hematologic malignancies receiving chemotherapy, persons with aplastic anemia, or transplant recipients in the early phase after HSCT. Significant persistent neutropenia is the strongest risk factor, with the incidence proportional to the depth and duration of neutropenia, so that more than 50% of patients with neutropenia lasting for over 4 weeks will develop IPA. Patients at high risk also include those receiving high-dose systemic corticosteroid therapy and/or have graft-versus-host disease (causing IPA in the late phase after HSCT), lung and liver transplant recipients, and patients with inherited disorders of phagocyte function such as chronic granulomatous disease (CGD), in which mutations in genes encoding the NADPH oxidase system impair the phagocyte oxidative burst. Various genetic polymorphisms affecting Toll-like receptors (TLRs) and cytokines seem to modify the risk of invasive aspergillosis for patients in the above risk groups.

The speed of development of IPA is proportional to the level of immunosuppression, but the disease usually evolves relatively slowly over days and weeks. Fever may be the only symptom of IPA, although cough, pleuritic chest pain, and hemoptysis are common. Chest radiographs show expanding patches of irregular consolidation (often infarct shaped) or nodules that can cavitate. CT scans are very helpful, because they will define the nodular nature of infiltrates, may show specific signs associated with IPA, and can identify the lung as

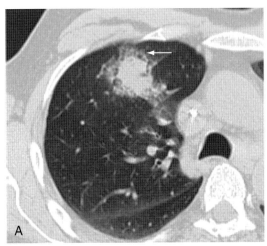

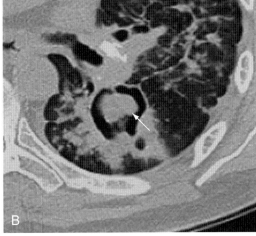

Figure 28-11 **A,** Computed tomography (CT) scan showing a nodule surrounded by an area of lower attenuation ground glass infiltration (the halo sign, indicated by the *white arrow*) suggestive of invasive aspergillosis. **B,** CT scan showing an area of invasive aspergillosis that has cavitated. Within the cavity, a mycetoma (*white arrow*) is evident.

the source of infection in patients with pyrexia and a normal chest radiograph. Specific CT appearances for IPA include the *halo sign,* an area of lower attenuation shadowing around a nodule or patch of consolidation reported in 50% of cases of IPA and usually occurring in the first week of infection (**Figure 28-11**); the *air crescent sign,* a partial cavity formed by infarcted necrotic lung, which is a very specific but later-onset sign occurring around the third week of infection; and an *intrapulmonary cavity containing a fungal ball,* especially associated with recovery of the patient's neutrophil count (see Figure 28-11). The halo sign may be detected in other infections, with neoplasms (adenocarcinoma, bronchoalveolar carcinoma, Kaposi sarcoma, and metastases), and in vasculitis. *Aspergillus* has a predilection for growing into blood vessels, and patients with IPA may suffer fatal massive hemorrhage. Other manifestations of invasive *Aspergillus* infections affecting the lung include *Aspergillus* tracheobronchitis, chronic necrotizing pulmonary aspergillosis (CNPA), and chronic cavitary pulmonary aspergillosis (CCPA).

With *Aspergillus* tracheobronchitis, infection is restricted to the tracheobronchial tree and manifests with a severe unremitting cough and pyrexia. CT scans may show focal areas of bronchial wall thickening and tree-in-bud small airway disease (**Figure 28-12**). FOB usually is diagnostic, with a distinctive macroscopic appearance of patchy, highly inflamed mucosa with necrotic white slough. *Aspergillus* can be found in cultures and/or cytology of bronchial washings, and there may be evidence of fungal invasion of the respiratory mucosa in bronchial biopsy specimens.

The more indolent forms of invasive aspergillosis such as CCPA or CNPA are increasing in incidence and are associated with milder degrees of immunosuppression, including steroid and cytotoxic therapies, chronic lung disease or cystic fibrosis. Affected patients present with a long history of cough and marked systemic symptoms of malaise, fatigue, and weight loss. On chest radiographs, CNPA manifests as an indolent patch of consolidation with or without cavitation that progresses over weeks or months (**Figure 28-13**), whereas CCPA manifests with an expanding upper lobe dry cavity with a thickened and irregular wall. There may be associated pleural thickening. *Aspergillus* infection also can cause a progressive upper lobe fibrosis.

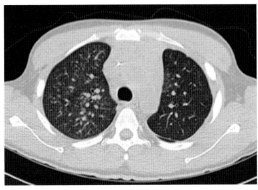

Figure 28-12 Computed tomography (CT) scan of thorax in a patient with acute lymphocytic leukemia treated with chemotherapy who presented with persistent cough and fever. The scan shows asymmetric "tree-in-bud" and nodular changes mainly affecting the right upper lobe, which were caused by *Aspergillus* tracheobronchitis.

Microbiologic Diagnosis

Investigations that can be helpful in making the diagnosis of IPA are described in **Table 28-5**. In high-risk patients with a compatible clinical syndrome and CT findings highly suggestive of IPA (halo and crescent signs), the diagnosis can be made clinically and may not require confirmation by invasive investigations. However, some *Aspergillus* species (e.g., *A. terreus*) are resistant to amphotericin B, and a clinical presentation similar to that in IPA can be caused by rarer filamentous fungi with drug sensitivities that differ from those demonstrated for *Aspergillus.* Hence, microbiologic confirmation is reassuring, because it ensures that appropriate treatment is given. A microbiologic diagnosis of IPA can be made by culture, cytologic, or histologic appearances in BAL or lung biopsy specimens, or by the detection of fungal cell wall antigen (galactomannan or β-D-glucan) or DNA (by PCR assay) in blood or BAL fluid. Isolation of *Aspergillus* from BAL in a high-risk immunodeficient patient is highly predictive of IPA but is relatively insensitive, identifying only 50% of cases of IPA. Culture from sputum is even less sensitive, and blood cultures are only rarely positive. Percutaneous CT-guided or VATS biopsy is highly sensitive, because

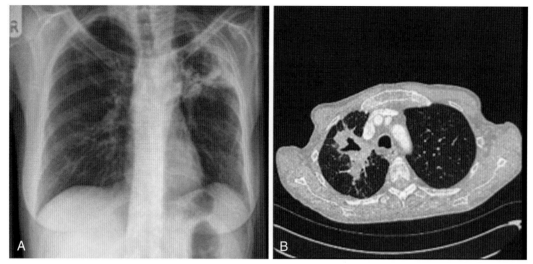

Figure 28-13 Slowly invasive aspergillosis in patients without severe immunosuppression. **A,** Chest radiograph showing a large irregular cavity in the left upper lobe with marked pleural thickening on a background of chronic obstructive pulmonary disease; the diagnosis was chronic cavitary pulmonary aspergillosis (CCPA), confirmed by surgical resection. **B,** Computed tomography (CT) scan showing a thick-walled dry cavity due to chronic necrotizing pulmonary aspergillosis (CNPA) in a patient with long-standing rheumatoid arthritis that was treated with a variety of immunosuppressive therapies. The diagnosis was confirmed by histologic identification of *Aspergillus* hyphae invading lung tissue in a biopsy sample obtained at video-assisted thoracoscopic surgery.

Table 28-5 Types and Roles of Diagnostic Tests for Invasive Aspergillosis

Test	Sample	Time Needed	Method	Role and General Comments
Culture	Sputum, BAL fluid, CSF, biopsy specimen	2-4 days	Culture on fungal media	Low sensitivity (50% for BAL) and does not necessarily improve invasive disease (can be colonizing the respiratory tract)
Cytologic examination	BAL fluid, biopsy specimen	6 hours	Microscopy for fungal elements	May not distinguish between fungal species
Histologic examination	Biopsy specimen	24-48 hours	Visualization of dichotomous branching septate hyphae	Fungal stains necessary; may not distinguish between fungal species
Antigen testing	Serum, BAL fluid	6 hours	Galactomannan detection	Cell wall antigen for *Aspergillus* and *Penicillium* spp.; sensitive; false positives occur
Antigen testing	Serum, BAL fluid	6 hours	β-D-Glucan detection	Cell wall antigen for *Candida, Aspergillus, Penicillium,* and *Pneumocystis* spp.; sensitive; false positives occur
PCR assay	Blood, BAL fluid	24 hours	Amplification of target DNA	Role not yet established, probably highly sensitive
CT appearance	—	Instant	Identification of halo or crescent sign, intracavitary mycetomas	Specific for invasive filamentous fungal infection but does not identify fungal species

BAL, bronchoalveolar lavage; *CSF,* cerebrospinal fluid; *CT,* computed tomography; *PCR,* polymerase chain reaction.

histopathologic examination of the sample can readily identify fungal hyphae infiltrating through lung tissue if fungal stains are used. Hence, strong consideration should be given to biopsy of lung nodules not responding to conventional antibacterial antibiotics, especially if BAL was nondiagnostic. To decrease mortality by allowing rapid identification of cases of IPA before the fungal load is high, several noninvasive tests have been developed. These include detection of galactomannan or β-D-glucan cell wall antigen in the blood (or BAL fluid if FOB has been performed), or PCR assay for *Aspergillus* DNA from the blood or BAL fluid. These tests are highly sensitive and when used as surveillance in high-risk patients could lead to preemptive antifungal therapy before clinically apparent disease has developed, leading to an improved mortality. However, detection of fungal DNA in a single sample of peripheral blood is a poor indicator of early invasive fungal infection, and galactomannan antigen is not specific for *Aspergillus* spp., frequently giving false-positive results (especially in patients treated with piperacillin-tazobactam or in young children). Despite these caveats, a negative galactomannan assay result makes active IPA infection unlikely. Serologic tests for antibodies to *Aspergillus* usually yield negative results in immunocompromised patients with IPA.

Diagnosing chronic forms of IPA in less immunocompromised patients often is difficult owing to lack of sensitivity of culture and the lack of data on the predictive values for antigen testing. CT-guided or VATS biopsy frequently is necessary to exclude malignancy and to confirm fungal invasion of lung tissue. *Aspergillus* IgG levels usually are raised in patients with CCPA, but not necessarily so in those with CNPA.

Treatment

The treatment options for invasive aspergillosis have been considerably improved by the introduction of new azoles, voriconazole and more recently posaconazole, and a new class of antifungal agents, the echinocandins, the first example of which is caspofungin. Doses, modes of action, and common toxicities for the different treatment options are given in **Table 28-6**. Voriconazole may be more effective than amphotericin B for treating IPA, but which drug is used depends on the patient's tolerance for that agent and any preexisting medical conditions (e.g., amphotericin B should be avoided in patients with renal problems, and azoles in patients with liver disease). Itraconazole is less efficacious and should be reserved for oral treatment in patients recovering from IPA after induction treatment with amphotericin B, caspofungin, or voriconazole or for the long-term treatment required for chronic forms of invasive aspergillosis. Drug levels probably should be monitored for patients receiving itraconazole, voriconazole, and posaconazole, at least for patients on prolonged therapy. The role of combination therapy remains unclear, but this strategy is potentially attractive in view of different mechanisms of action for the three effective classes of drugs. Urgent surgical resection should be considered in patients with major hemoptysis, because fatal bleeding is not uncommon. Elective resection can be used as primary therapy for single lesions due to IPA, especially those containing an intracavitary mycetoma that might lead to reactivation of IPA during subsequent immunosuppression. Treatment of IPA for several weeks often is necessary, followed by prophylactic therapy in cases with persisting radiologic changes. Treatment of CNPA and CCPA will need to be continued for months if not years (and even lifelong). Owing to a combination of uncontrolled infection and the underlying disease, the mortality rate for IPA is around 50%, and with chronic forms of aspergillosis, the infection rate remains as high as 33%.

Azoles can be used for prophylaxis in at-risk groups, including hematopoietic stem cell transplant recipients. Fluconazole is not effective at preventing mold infections such as IPA, and despite its efficacy against *Aspergillus*, voriconazole seems to offer no clinical benefit over prophylaxis with fluconazole. However, prophylaxis with the newer extended-spectrum triazole posaconazole reduced the incidence of invasive aspergillosis in patients with prolonged neutropenia, from 7% to 1%. Acquired resistance of *A. fumigatus* to posaconazole has emerged during the course of therapy, which may potentially limit its use for prophylaxis.

OTHER FUNGAL INFECTIONS

Infections Due to Non-*Aspergillus* Filamentous Fungi

Although *Aspergillus* spp. dominate infections due to molds, other filamentous fungi can cause invasive pulmonary infections in immunocompromised patients, including *Fusarium*, *Zygomycetes*, *Scedosporium*, and *Penicillium*. These infections often are clinically similar to invasive aspergillosis but have a different spectrum of susceptibilities to antifungal agents. Hence, non-*Aspergillus* filamentous fungal infection needs to be considered in patients with a clinical diagnosis of IPA who are not responding to antifungal therapy. Diagnosis is made by culture from respiratory samples or lung biopsy, and mortality is very high. Galactomannan and β-D-glucan cell wall antigen test results are negative in patients infected with zygomycetes. Treatment is with surgical débridement combined with amphotericin and, for infections due to *Fusarium* and *Scedosporium* but not zygomycetes, voriconazole or posaconazole.

Infections Due to *Candida* Spp.

Infection with *Candida* rarely manifests as a pneumonia, but candidemia may lead to metastatic lung infection that causes

Table 28-6 Treatment Options for Invasive Aspergillosis

Treatment	Dose	Mode of Action	Role and General Comments	Toxicity
Amphotericin B	1-1.5 mg/kg IV once daily	Binds to ergosterol in the fungal cell membrane	Effective; cheap; withdrawn in a third of patients due to toxicity	Fever and chills; phlebitis; hypokalemia, hypomagnesemia; uremia; bronchospasm; gastrointestinal disturbance; muscle pain
Lipid formulations of amphotericin B	1-5 mg/kg per day IV	As above	Expensive; much improved toxicity profile	As above (much lower incidence)
Itraconazole	200 mg once daily or 2-3×/day IV or PO	Inhibits ergosterol biosynthesis	Poor efficacy in acute IPA; poor absorbance (check levels)	Gastrointestinal disturbance; elevated hepatic transaminases; fluid retention; neuropathy
Voriconazole	6 mg/kg 2× on day 1; then 4 mg/kg IV once daily 200 mg PO 2×/day	Inhibits ergosterol biosynthesis	Effective; expensive; good absorption	Elevated hepatic transaminases; visual and CNS disturbances
Posaconazole	200 mg 3×/day PO (no intravenous formulation)	Inhibits ergosterol biosynthesis	Effective; expensive; good absorption	Elevated hepatic transaminases; paresthesia; tremor; visual disturbances Availability maximized with fatty food
Caspofungin	70 mg loading dose; 50 mg IV once daily	Inhibits fungal cell wall synthesis	Expensive; effective	Generally well tolerated; flushing; gastrointestinal disturbance
Surgery	—	—	For life-threatening hemoptysis or removal of single lesions	Pleural dissemination of *Aspergillus* as well as the usual postoperative complications

CNS, central nervous system; *IPA*, invasive pulmonary aspergillosis.

pyrexia and is associated with radiologic evidence of lung nodules that often are peripheral in location and sometimes very large. Neutropenic patients with mucositis or indwelling lines are at risk for invasive candidemia, which usually is caused by dissemination of endogenous colonizing *Candida* spp. The frequent use of fluconazole for prophylaxis has led to increasing isolation of non-*albicans* species such as *Candida glabrata* and *Candida parapsilosis*. Treatment is with caspofungin, amphotericin, voriconazole, or posaconazole.

Infections Due to *Cryptococcus* and Endemic Fungi

Cryptococcus neoformans infections are acquired by inhalation of the fungal spores. Although respiratory infection often is asymptomatic, cryptococcal disease can cause multifocal consolidation and severe pneumonia in patients with defects in cell-mediated immunity and carries a mortality rate of 30%. The diagnosis is made by microscopic identification or culture of *C. neoformans* from respiratory tract samples. Treatment is with intravenous amphotericin B in combination with flucytosine, followed by oral fluconazole. Reactivation of latent infection with endemic fungi such as *Histoplasma* and *Coccidioides* should be considered in patients with defects in cell-mediated immunity presenting with multifocal lung shadowing who have lived in relevant geographic areas, especially if there is evidence of extrapulmonary involvement. Diagnosis generally requires identification of the fungus in tissues samples.

Pneumocystis jirovecii Infection

In addition to its close association with HIV infection, PCP is an important type of pneumonia in non–HIV-infected immunocompromised patients with defects in cell-mediated immunity or who are receiving systemic corticosteroid therapy equivalent to greater than 20 mg daily of prednisolone. The clinical presentation generally is insidious in onset, with cough and progressive dyspnea developing over weeks, but can be more fulminant. Impaired gas transfer and hypoxia on exertion with progression to respiratory failure are common. The chest radiograph usually shows bilateral infiltrates but may be normal in appearance. Generally the CT scan will show ground glass infiltrates, which classically mainly affect the upper lobes and spare the lung peripheries (**Figure 28-14**). On rare occasions, however, even the CT scan may show only minimal abnormalities. The diagnosis is made by recognition of the clinical picture

in an at-risk patient and should be confirmed by cytologic identification of the characteristic *P. jirovecii* cysts in BAL fluid. Diagnosis can be improved using immunohistochemistry assay for *Pneumocystis* antigens, and perhaps by PCR analysis, although the latter will have a significant false-positive rate as a consequence of colonization in the absence of disease.

First-line treatment is with high-dose co-trimoxazole and adjuvant steroids given according to the protocols used for PCP in HIV-infected patients. Myelosuppression due to co-trimoxazole means that many patients with hematologic disorders have to switch to second-line therapy with clindamycin and primaquine. In non-HIV immunocompromised patients, PCP is associated with intubation and mortality rates of around 30% each. PCP prophylaxis usually is prescribed for several months after allograft HSCT or organ transplantation, and occasionally longer in patients who continue to receive immunosuppressive drugs. Patients recovering from PCP should continue on chemoprophylaxis until their immunosuppression is resolved, although there are no clear parameters for defining this endpoint. Consensus is lacking on the requirement for PCP prophylaxis after autograft HSCT and for severe non–transplantation-related immunosuppression. Cotrimoxazole prophylaxis given either daily or three times per week is very effective (greater than 90% efficacy) and provides some protection against other pathogens, including *Toxoplasma*, *Nocardia*, and bacteria.

CONTROVERSIES AND PITFALLS

- Exactly when bronchoscopy should be used for diagnosing respiratory infections in immunocompromised patients remains controversial, with no clear consensus on early versus late bronchoscopy. The approach described in this chapter based on the type of lung shadowing aims to target bronchoscopy to the patients for whom it may be most helpful.
- CMV pneumonitis is an especially difficult diagnosis to confirm; the specific diagnostic tests often are inconclusive, and the clinician is left with presumptive evidence of involvement of CMV consisting of the combination of a pneumonitis with blood test results indicating reactivation of the virus.
- A major pitfall to avoid is failure to consider noninfective causes of respiratory problems in the non-HIV-infected immunocompromised patient; pulmonary edema, alveolar hemorrhage, ARDS, drug-related or idiopathic pneumonitis, and rapidly progressive airway obstruction due to lung graft-versus-host disease (often precipitated by respiratory viral infections) often need to be included in the differential diagnosis.
- Although most infective causes of lung problems in the non–HIV-infected immunocompromised patient generally have fairly characteristic presentations and affect selected risk groups, considerable overlap between clinical presentations for illnesses due to specific infectious agents is typical. This is especially true for the more severely immunosuppressed patient, in whom the usual clinical presentations become less characteristic.
- Finally, the clinician needs to remember that non–HIV-infected immunocompromised patients often have two simultaneous pathologic conditions (e.g., a bacterial pneumonia complicated by ARDS, or a respiratory viral infection with lung graft-versus-host disease).

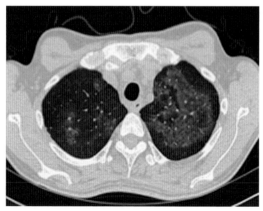

Figure 28-14 Computed tomography (CT) scan showing an upper lobe ground glass infiltrate with peripheral sparing. This pattern is highly suggestive of *Pneumocystis* pneumonia in patients with a defect in cell-mediated immunity.

SUGGESTED READINGS

Boeckh M: The challenge of respiratory virus infections in hematopoietic cell transplant recipients, *Br J Haematol* 143:455–467, 2008.

Denning DW, Riniotis K, Dobrashian R, et al: Chronic cavitary and fibrosing pulmonary and pleural aspergillosis: case series, proposed nomenclature change, and review, *Clin Infect Dis* 1(Suppl 3):S265–S280, 2003.

Freemantle N, Tharmanathan P, Herbrecht R: Systematic review and mixed treatment comparison of randomized evidence for empirical, pre-emptive and directed treatment strategies for invasive mould disease, *J Antimicrob Chemother* 66(Suppl 1):i25–i35, 2011.

Hope WW, Walsh TJ, Denning DW: Laboratory diagnosis of invasive aspergillosis, *Lancet Infect Dis* 5:609–622, 2005.

Kanne JP, Godwin JD, Franquet T, et al: Viral pneumonia after hematopoietic stem cell transplantation: high-resolution CT findings, *J Thorac Imaging* 22:292–299, 2007.

Maertens J, Meersseman W, Van Bleyenbergh P: New therapies for fungal pneumonia, *Curr Opin Infect Dis* 22:183–190, 2009.

Maschmeyer G, Beinert T, Buchheidt D, et al: Diagnosis and antimicrobial therapy of pulmonary infiltrates in febrile neutropenic patients, *Ann Hematol* 82(Suppl 2):S118–S126, 2003.

Rañó A, Agustí C, Jimenez P, et al: Pulmonary infiltrates in non-HIV immunocompromised patients: a diagnostic approach using noninvasive and bronchoscopic procedures, *Thorax* 56:379–387, 2001.

Rubin RH: The pathogenesis and clinical management of cytomegalovirus infection in the organ transplant recipient: the end of the 'silo hypothesis,' *Curr Opin Infect Dis* 20:399–407, 2007.

Tomblyn M, Chiller T, Hermann E, et al: Guidelines for preventing infectious complications among hematopoietic cell transplantation recipients: a global perspective, *Biol Blood Marrow Transplant* 15:1143–1238, 2009.

Chapter **29**

Pulmonary Infections in Patients with Human Immunodeficiency Virus Disease

Robert F. Miller • Marc C.I. Lipman • Alison Morris

EPIDEMIOLOGY, RISK FACTORS, AND PATHOPHYSIOLOGY

HUMAN IMMUNODEFICIENCY VIRUS INFECTION: BACKGROUND

It is now more than 30 years since the first report from Los Angeles, in the United States, of an "outbreak" of *Pneumocystis* pneumonia (PCP) among homosexual men that heralded the onset of the global human immunodeficiency virus (HIV) pandemic. Since the early 1980s, HIV infection has steadily spread throughout the world and caused an estimated 25 million deaths. At the end of 2009, according to the United Nations Program on HIV/AIDS (UNAIDS), 33.3 million people worldwide were HIV-infected, a majority of these living in resource-poor countries. In 2008, the Centers for Disease Control and Prevention (CDC) reported that in the United States, 1,178,350 persons 13 years of age or older were living with HIV infection, and more than 40,000 were newly infected each year. In the United Kingdom, the Health Protection Agency estimated that in 2009, 86,500 persons were living with HIV infection and 6630 were newly diagnosed. Over the previous 10 years, the proportion of U.K. residents older than 50 years of age who were living with HIV infection had increased from 1 in 20 to 1 in 5.

Current antiretroviral therapy (ART) regimens have the potential to suppress HIV replication for decades. In 2011, persons with newly diagnosed HIV infection living in nations such as the United States and the United Kingdom that provide access to treatment and care have an expectation that on ART their life expectancy will approach that for an age-matched HIV-uninfected population. Their clinicians now manage HIV-infected populations whose medical complications reflect age-related comorbidity. Unfortunately, these observations do not apply to a majority of people worldwide with HIV infection, who live in financially impoverished environments with little access to comprehensive health care prevention and treatment programs.

Respiratory disease remains an important contributor to morbidity and mortality, and more than two thirds of HIV-infected persons have at least one respiratory episode during the course of their illness. With relatively preserved immune responses, infectious agents are similar to those seen in the general population, although at a higher frequency. With progressive HIV disease, subjects are at an increased risk for opportunistic disease. For example, the North American Prospective Study of Pulmonary Complications of HIV Infection (PCHIS), a multicenter cohort drawn from all HIV risk groups at various stages of immunocompromise, revealed that over an 18-month study period, of approximately 1000 subjects who were not using ART, 33% reported an upper respiratory tract infection, 16% had an episode of acute bronchitis, 5% acute sinusitis, 5% bacterial pneumonia, and 4% developed PCP.

The immune dysregulation that arises from HIV infection means that bacteria, mycobacteria, fungi, viruses, and protozoa can all cause disease in patients with advanced infection. **Box 29-1** shows the organisms that typically infect the lung in HIV disease. Of these, the agents of bacterial infections, tuberculosis, and PCP are the most important. In the West, 40% of diagnosed AIDS cases are due to PCP. This chapter provides a brief general overview of the epidemiology and pathogenesis of HIV infection, followed by a more detailed discussion of other important aspects of the disease and its infectious pulmonary complications.

It is reported that by the end of 2009, 33.3 million people worldwide had acquired HIV infection (**Figure 29-1**). Of these, over 40% are thought to have developed AIDS (for definition of AIDS, see **Tables 29-1** and **29-2** and **Box 29-2**). Globally, 2.6 million people acquired HIV infection in 2009, and 1.8 million died of AIDS. The developing world has been most affected. Sub-Saharan Africa is the current epicenter of the pandemic (accounting for two thirds of all infections; here, nearly 6% of adults are HIV-infected. South and Southeast Asia are responsible for almost a fifth of the estimated HIV global burden. In Central-Eastern Europe and Central Asia, there are currently 1.4 million HIV-infected persons. In the developed world, North America and Western Europe account for approximately 1.5 million and 820,000 infections, respectively. The vast majority of these are spread through sexual contact, although vertical (mother-to-child) and blood-borne infections are common. In the developing world, heterosexual transmission is the norm. In North America and Europe, men who have sex with men constitute the largest group of HIV-infected persons.

VIROLOGY AND IMMUNOLOGY OF THE HUMAN IMMUNODEFICIENCY VIRUS

HIV was first isolated in 1983 from patients with symptoms and signs of immune compromise. Two subtypes, HIV-1 and HIV-2, have subsequently been identified. HIV-1 (hereafter referred to as HIV) is responsible for a majority of infections, is associated with a more aggressive clinical course, and is the focus of this chapter.

HIV is a human retrovirus belonging to the lentivirus family. Cell-free or cell-associated HIV infects through attachment of its viral envelope protein (gp120) to the CD4 antigen complex on host cells. The CD4 receptor is found on several cell types, although the T helper lymphocyte is the main site of HIV infection in the body. Additionally, HIV gp120 also must bind to the cell surface protein co-receptor chemokine receptor 5 (CCR5), or to other co-receptors, including CXCR4, depending on the host cell type. Polymorphisms in genes coding for CCR5 may affect disease progression by reducing the ability of

HIV to enter and infect cells. At a population level, this effect appears to be small.

Once HIV is inside the cell, it uses the enzyme reverse transcriptase (RNA-dependent DNA polymerase) to transcribe its own RNA into a DNA copy that translocates into the nucleus and integrates with host cell DNA using its viral integrase. The virus (as proviral DNA) remains latent in many cells until the cell itself becomes activated. This may arise from cytokine or antigen stimulation. The viral genetic material is then transcribed into new RNA, which, in the form of newly created virions, bud from the cell surface and infect other host CD4-bearing cells.

HIV infection directly attacks the immune system, and in particular the T helper cells that underpin the coordinated immune response. This leads to progressive immune dysfunction, with an inability to react to opportunistic pathogens as well as persistent, unregulated immune activation. The etiopathogenic process is not well defined, although at the time of primary infection it is thought that HIV spreads to regional lymph nodes, circulating immune cells, and thymus. The result is a massive viral infection of the human host, which, despite a relatively potent immune response, targets specific memory T cells responsible for sustaining long-term protective immunity. Without therapeutic intervention, progressive immune failure is inevitable. This occurs through a combination of direct cell killing caused by HIV replicating within cells and the negative effects of chronic immune activation. Ultimately, in most cases the infection produces immune system destruction and dysfunction, which is reflected in a reduction in circulating absolute blood CD4+ cell count, a decrease in the percentage of T cells expressing CD4 markers, and a fall in the CD4+-to-CD8+ T cell ratio. Patients present with clinical disease indicating profound immunodeficiency.

Box 29-1 Etiologic Agents of Human Immunodeficiency Virus (HIV)-Related Pulmonary Infections

Bacteria
Streptococcus pneumoniae
Haemophilus influenzae
Staphylococcus aureus
Pseudomonas aeruginosa
Nocardia asteroides
Rochalimaea henselae
Mycobacterium tuberculosis
Mycobacterium avium-intracellulare
Mycobacterium kansasii

Fungi
Pneumocystis jirovecii
Cryptococcus neoformans
Histoplasma capsulatum
Aspergillus spp.
Penicillium marneffei

Parasites
Toxoplasma gondii
Leishmania spp.
Strongyloides stercoralis

Viruses
Cytomegalovirus
Influenza A viruses

NATURAL HISTORY OF HUMAN IMMUNODEFICIENCY VIRUS INFECTION

Intervention with ART, as well as specific preventive (prophylactic) therapy for opportunistic infections has changed the

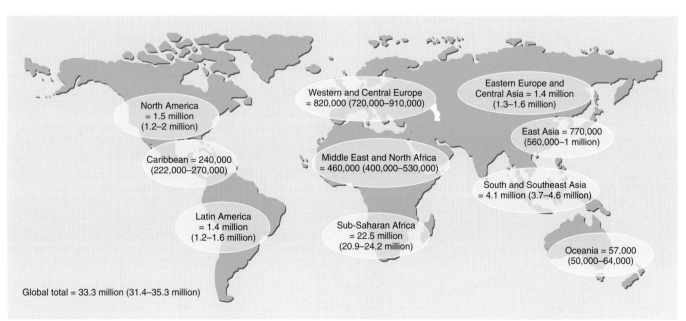

Figure 29-1 Estimated number of adults and children with human immunodeficiency virus (HIV) infection (for December 2009) by regions of the world. *(From UNAIDS: AIDS epidemic update: December 2009, Geneva, World Health Organization, 2009. www.unaids.org/en/dadataanalysis/epidemiology/2009aiddsepidemiologyupdate/, accessed 10/03/2012.)*

clinical presentation of HIV disease in countries in which these interventions are available. Death rates for HIV-infected cohorts have fallen precipitously. In the absence of ART, in the developed world the median interval between HIV seroconversion and progression to AIDS is estimated to be 10 years and is shorter in cash-poor countries. Untreated, almost all cases of HIV infection progress to full-blown AIDS; without ART, 95% of affected patients will die within 5 years. Globally, in 2011 the main causes of death among HIV-infected patients (a majority of whom were not receiving ART) included tuberculosis, enteric bacterial infection, bacterial pneumonia, and PCP.

The clinical course of untreated HIV infection evolves in several reasonably distinct stages. First, acquisition of the virus, next, seroconversion, which (in the minority) may be associated with a clinical illness (primary HIV infection), then follows a clinically silent period lasting several months to years which leads to symptoms and signs indicating progressive HIV-induced immune compromise, ultimately resulting in AIDS (e.g., PCP).

Acute Primary Human Immunodeficiency Virus Infection

The time from acquisition of HIV infection to development of detectable antibodies (the "window" period) usually is about 6 to 8 weeks. For 30% to 70% of people who become infected, a seroconversion illness is typical. Antibodies to HIV antibody normally are detectable within 2 to 3 weeks of onset of these symptoms, though this can take longer. HIV RNA in peripheral blood is detectable before the appearance of antibodies and often is used to confirm infection.

The nonspecific features of primary "seroconversion" HIV infection usually are self-limiting, and the infection typically mimics a flu-like illness or glandular fever. Nearly all persons with primary HIV infection spontaneously recover within 4 weeks, irrespective of their acute symptoms. A small proportion develop persistent (symmetric) generalized lymphadenopathy. The prognosis for this group is no different from that for asymptomatic HIV-positive persons.

Table 29-1 CDC Classification of HIV Infection

Group	Infection
I	Acute primary
II	Asymptomatic
III	Persistent generalized lymphadenopathy
IV	Other disease
Subgroup A	Constitutional disease (e.g., weight loss >10% of body weight or >4.5 kg; fevers with temperatures >38.5° C for >1 month; diarrhea lasting >1 month)
Subgroup B	Neurologic disease (e.g., HIV encephalopathy, myelopathy, peripheral neuropathy)
Subgroup C	Secondary infectious diseases
Subgroup C1	AIDS-defining secondary diseases (e.g., *Pneumocystis jirovecii* pneumonia, cerebral toxoplasmosis, cytomegalovirus retinitis)
Subgroup C2	Other specified secondary infectious diseases (e.g., oral candidiasis, multidermatomal varicella zoster)
Subgroup D	Secondary cancers (e.g., Kaposi sarcoma, non-Hodgkin lymphoma)
Subgroup E	Other conditions (e.g., lymphoid interstitial pneumonitis)

AIDS, acquired immunodeficiency syndrome; *HIV*, human immunodeficiency virus.

Box 29-2 Adult AIDS Indicator Diseases*

Candidiasis of esophagus, trachea, bronchi, or lungs
Cervical carcinoma, invasive
Coccidioidomycosis, disseminated or extrapulmonary
Cryptococcosis, extrapulmonary
Cryptosporidiosis, with diarrhea for longer than 1 month
Cytomegalovirus disease (not in liver, spleen, or lymph nodes)
Cytomegalovirus retinitis
Encephalopathy caused by HIV (AIDS dementia complex)
Herpes simplex: ulcers for >1 month, or bronchitis, pneumonitis, esophagitis
Histoplasmosis, disseminated or extrapulmonary
Isosporiasis, with diarrhea for >1 month
Kaposi sarcoma
Lymphoma: Burkitt, or immunoblastic, or primary in CNS
Mycobacterium avium complex or *Mycobacterium kansasii*, disseminated or extrapulmonary
Mycobacterium tuberculosis, any site (pulmonary or extrapulmonary)
Mycobacterial infections due to other species or unidentified species, disseminated or extrapulmonary
Pneumocystis jirovecii pneumonia
Pneumonia recurrent within a 12-month period
Progressive multifocal leukoencephalopathy
Salmonella (nontyphoidal) septicemia, recurrent
Toxoplasmosis of brain
Wasting syndrome caused by HIV

*1993 data.
AIDS, acquired immunodeficiency syndrome; *CNS*, central nervous system; *HIV*, human immunodeficiency virus.
Centers for Disease Control: 1993 revised classification system for HIV infection and expanded surveillance case definition for AIDS among adolescents and adults, *MMWR* 41 (No.RR-17), 1992.

Table 29-2 CDC Classification System for Human Immunodeficiency Virus (HIV) Infection: Clinical Categories*

CD4+ Count (cells/μL)	A: Acute (Primary) HIV Infection, Asymptomatic or With Persistent Generalized Lymphadenopathy	B: Symptomatic (not A or C)	C: AIDS Indicator Conditions
≥500	A1	B1	C1
200-499	A2	B2	C2
<200	A3	B3	C3

*Patients are stratified clinically (A-C) and immunologically (1-3). Category B consists of symptomatic conditions that are not included within AIDS indicator diseases (category C) but either can be attributed to or are complicated by HIV infection. Examples are persistent candidiasis, thrombocytopenia, and peripheral neuropathy.
AIDS, acquired immunodeficiency syndrome; *CDC*, Centers for Disease Control and Prevention.

Chronic Human Immunodeficiency Virus Infection

Although a proportion of HIV-seropositive persons remain completely well without ART for an extended period (approximately 20%, after 10 years), many infected persons have minor symptoms and signs suggesting immune dysfunction. Oral candidiasis and constitutional symptoms (e.g., malaise, idiopathic fever, night sweats, diarrhea, weight loss) are the strongest clinical predictors of progression to AIDS.

The term AIDS was originally created as an epidemiologic tool to capture specific clinical presentations, which early in the HIV epidemic appeared to suggest significant immune deficiency. Over the past 30 years, the definition has been modified to incorporate the expanding spectrum of diseases affecting HIV-infected patients, including cervical carcinoma and recurrent bacterial pneumonia (see Box 29-2). The 1993 CDC classification included an immunologic criterion for AIDS (CD4$^+$ count below 200 cells/μL or CD4$^+$ percentage less than 14% of total lymphocytes) regardless of clinical symptoms (see Table 29-2). These data are used to define a point at which the risk for severe opportunistic infection rises dramatically.

Apart from cervical carcinoma, AIDS indicator diseases differ little between men and women. Injection drug users in the United States and the United Kingdom have a high incidence of recurrent bacterial pneumonia and tuberculosis. Geographic differences occur that reflect the opportunistic pathogens present in the local environment (e.g., histoplasmosis or visceral leishmaniasis usually are found only in patients from endemic areas). In the developed world, survival differences after an AIDS diagnosis mainly arise from variation in ease of access to and provision of medical care. It is clear that better treatment outcomes are associated with specialist care provided by treatment centers with extensive experience in the management of HIV-infected persons.

In countries in which ART is available, the spectrum of HIV-related disease has changed over the past 30 years. In the HIV Outpatient Study (HOPS), a prospective multicenter observational study in the United States, between 1994 and 2007, opportunistic infections associated with very low CD4$^+$ counts (e.g., cytomegalovirus retinitis, *Mycobacterium avium* complex [MAC] infection) declined rapidly after introduction of ART and stabilized at low levels during the period 2003 to 2007. In the EuroSIDA cohort (a pan-European prospective study of HIV infection), between 1994 and 2004, opportunistic infections were observed less frequently over time, and malignant disease, such as non-Hodgkin lymphoma, increased as an AIDS-defining event.

Although death rates have fallen in ART-treated populations, there has been a rise in the proportion of non-AIDS deaths. In some series, this category accounts for a majority of events. Causes include liver disease (often due to viral hepatitides) and cancer, as well as cardiovascular disease and drug-related toxicity. In such circumstances, AIDS deaths usually occur among patients who have not accessed medical care regularly and who present with advanced HIV disease.

A new manifestation of opportunistic infection has been described in patients commencing ART. The immune reconstitution inflammatory syndrome (IRIS) (the pathogenesis of which is discussed later under treatment for tuberculosis) may cause severe if temporary clinical illness as the patient's immunity recovers. Patients appear to experience a relapse of their original (and often incompletely treated) disease. IRIS often is seen in MAC infection, tuberculosis, hepatitis B, CMV retinitis, and herpesvirus infection. In the developed world, metabolic complications of ART, such as ischemic heart disease, hypertension, diabetes, and cerebrovascular disease, are increasingly encountered by clinicians providing care. A significant number of persons receiving ART also experience drug toxicity. An increasing number of patients also are surviving to manifest symptoms associated with chronic hepatitis B and C virus infection. HIV-associated nephropathy (often with chronic kidney disease) is common among black Africans and is a significant cause of long-term morbidity.

PROGNOSTIC MARKERS

Laboratory markers and clinical symptoms (e.g., oral candidiasis or thrush) can independently reflect the immune changes that lead to serious disease. Staging systems have been developed that can predict the risk of progression to severe opportunistic disease (AIDS). The fall in absolute blood CD4$^+$ T lymphocyte count is the most widely used prognostic marker, although CD4$^+$ counts may be affected by a number of factors apart from HIV, including intercurrent infection, cigarette smoking, exercise, time of day, and laboratory variation. The percentage of CD4$^+$ cells and the ratio of CD4$^+$ to CD8$^+$ cells are more stable measures and may be used if the CD4$^+$ absolute counts appear to vary widely between routine clinical assessments.

Measurement of plasma HIV RNA "viral load" provides important prognostic information that can both guide therapy and suggest long-term outcome. It is of particular value in patients who have high CD4$^+$ counts but are clinically well, because it gives an indication of the expected speed of clinical progression.

PULMONARY IMMUNE RESPONSE DURING HUMAN IMMUNODEFICIENCY VIRUS INFECTION

It is clear from the frequency with which HIV-related respiratory disease occurs that the pulmonary immune response is profoundly compromised. Evidence from simian immunodeficiency virus (SIV)-infected primates indicates that within the lung acute retroviral infection causes a rapid increase, followed by a decline in SIV RNA. Intrapulmonary replication is "compartmentalized," in that plasma SIV levels correlate poorly with those in bronchoalveolar lavage (BAL) fluid. In humans, comparison of HIV replication in blood and in alveolar lining fluid indicates that little intrapulmonary HIV replication occurs when patients are asymptomatic. This process increases significantly with development of pulmonary disease, and in some instances, local HIV replication is greater than in plasma. Other studies, however, show no consistent change in HIV levels in BAL fluid as the patient's clinical status alters. Pulmonary memory CD4$^+$ cells are not as extensively infected by HIV compared with those within the gastrointestinal tract. Alveolar macrophages appear to carry a much lower HIV "viral load" than macrophages obtained from other body sites.

HIV affects both the humoral and cellular components of innate immunity. These alterations are apparent even in patients with (near) normal CD4$^+$ counts and undetectable HIV loads, and include a BAL CD8$^+$ lymphocytosis. HIV-induced impairment of innate immune function, particularly when there is additional CD4$^+$ cell depletion, likely contributes to the pathogenesis of opportunistic pulmonary infections, for example, the increased risk of *mycobacterium tuberculosis* infection and bacterial pneumonia.

Phagocytosis of bacteria by human alveolar macrophages does not appear to be influenced by HIV infection, suggesting that other mechanisms are important. In the general population deficiencies in signaling through Toll-like receptors (TLRs) are associated with an increased risk of, or an adverse outcome from, a number of infections. Activation of HIV-infected human macrophages by TLR4 results in impaired tumor necrosis factor-α release compared to that from uninfected macrophages; as interleukin (IL)-10 release is not impaired, this effect appears specific.

Intra-pulmonary immune responses after ART initiation are not as well described as those occurring during untreated HIV infection. Detection of HIV in BAL fluid is less likely in subjects on ART. Starting such therapy is associated with a delayed but significant decrease in the absolute number and percentage of alveolar CD8+ lymphocytes. Successful virologic control leads to a reduction in activated intrapulmonary CD8+ cells and increases in CD8+-naive and central memory cells—implying that the intrapulmonary CD8+ lymphocyte pool is repopulated from the peripheral circulation.

ART also induces a marked reduction in concentrations of proinflammatory cytokines and chemokines in BAL fluid. Despite this, both IFN-γ and IFN-γ inducible chemokines (inducible protein [IP]-10, monokine induced by IFN-γ [MIG]) remain detectable and appear to contribute to recruitment of memory cells into the lung.

On the basis of these findings, it is hypothesized that ART-naive patients have uncontrolled intrapulmonary HIV replication, which results in nonspecific cellular activation and augmented cytokine and chemokine expression. These changes promote an influx of inflammatory cells into the alveoli. With institution of ART, intrapulmonary HIV load and cellular activation are reduced and nonspecific cytokine secretion resolves, although persistent, low-level IFN-γ production from resident memory cells maintains IFN-γ–inducible chemokine levels. As a result, normal intrapulmonary trafficking of these cells occurs, resulting in more clear-cut evidence of innate and acquired immune control. The former includes ART reducing mononuclear cell chemokine production with a subsequent impact on TLR2-mediated signaling.

RISK FACTORS FOR RESPIRATORY DISEASE

An individual patient's risk for respiratory disease is determined by the medical history (e.g., receipt of effective preventive therapy or ART), place of residence and travel history (e.g., the influence of geography on mycobacterial and fungal disease), and immunity status. Falling blood CD4+ counts or high plasma HIV RNA "viral loads" increase the chance of respiratory infection, with an increased spectrum of potential organisms associated with greater degrees of immunosuppression. For example, HIV-infected patients with a CD4+ count below 200 cells/μL are four times more likely to have one episode of bacterial pneumonia per year than those with higher CD4+ cell counts. More exotic organisms are found in subjects with very low CD4+ counts. These include bacteria such as *Rhodococcus equi* and *Nocardia asteroides* and fungi such as *Aspergillus* spp. and *Penicillium marneffei*. Just as with *P. jirovecii*, this increased susceptibility reflects the importance of T cell depletion and macrophage dysfunction in the loss of host immunity (a process that has been confirmed by animal experiments).

Among HIV-infected patients, injection drug users are at greatest risk for development of bacterial pneumonia and tuberculosis. Persons who have had previous respiratory episodes (PCP or bacterial pneumonia) appear to be at increased risk for subsequent episodes of such disease. Whether this susceptibility

relates to host or environmental factors is not certain, although structural lung damage and abnormal pulmonary physiology are likely to be contributing factors. This argument is supported by the increased rates of pneumonia in HIV-infected smokers compared with nonsmokers. Recent work has shown that chronic obstructive pulmonary disease (COPD) and lung cancer occur more frequently and at a younger age among HIV-infected patients, than in the general population. In view of the large number of HIV-infected persons who smoke heavily, targeting this population for smoking cessation obviously is a pressing need. This goal is reinforced by the association between smoking and an increased risk for bacterial pneumonia and more rapid progression to first AIDS illness and death.

CLINICAL FEATURES

BACTERIAL INFECTION

Bronchitis

The clinical presentation in bronchitis mimics that in bacterial exacerbations of chronic obstructive lung disease; most patients have a productive cough and fever. The pathogens commonly identified are similar to those in the general population (e.g., *Streptococcus pneumoniae* and *Haemophilus influenzae*). However, patients with advanced disease may be infected with *Pseudomonas aeruginosa* or *Staphylococcus aureus*. Response to appropriate antibiotic therapy in conventional doses is good, although relapses are common.

Bronchiectasis

Bronchiectasis is increasingly recognized in HIV-infected patients with advanced HIV disease and low CD4+ lymphocyte counts. It probably arises secondary to recurrent bacterial, mycobacterial or *P. jirovecii* infections. The diagnosis most often is made by high-resolution (thin-section) computed tomography (CT) scanning (**Figure 29-2**). Its prevalence has not been accurately determined, although with improved survival from both opportunistic infections and HIV disease, it can be expected to be increasingly common in clinical practice. The pathogens isolated in patients with bronchiectasis are those seen in bronchitis. In addition, *Burkholderia cepacia* and *Moraxella catarrhalis* have been described.

Pneumonia

Community-acquired bacterial pneumonia occurs more frequently in HIV-infected patients than in the general population. It is especially common in HIV-infected injecting drug

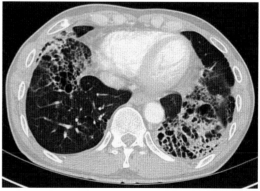

Figure 29-2 Computed tomography scan of thorax showing widespread bronchiectasis in a patient with a previous history of multiple episodes of bacterial pneumonia.

users. The spectrum of bacterial pathogens is similar to that in non–HIV-infected persons (see Box 29-1). *S. pneumoniae* is the most commonly identified pathogen, followed by *H. influenzae*. HIV-infected patients with *S. pneumoniae*–related pneumonia frequently are bacteremic. In one study, the rate of pneumococcal bacteremia in HIV-infected patients was 100 times that for an HIV-negative population. More recent work has confirmed this to be the case for all causes of HIV-related bacterial pneumonia. Typically, blood cultures have a 40-fold increased pick-up rate in HIV-positive patients. The widespread use of ART has led to some decrease in rates of bacterial pneumonia and bacteremia, although they are still considerably higher than in a non–HIV-infected population.

Bacterial pneumonia has a similar presentation in HIV-infected patients and in uninfected persons. Chest radiographs frequently are atypical in appearance, mimicking that in PCP in up to half of the cases (**Figure 29-3**). By contrast, radiographic lobar or segmental consolidation also may be seen in a wide range of bacterial organisms (**Figure 29-4**); these include

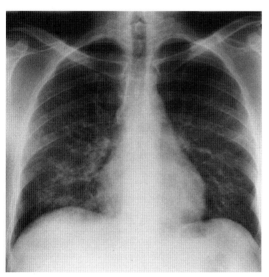

Figure 29-3 Chest radiograph showing bilateral, diffuse, interstitial infiltrates mimicking the changes of *Pneumocystis jirovecii* pneumonia. The etiologic agent was *Streptococcus pneumoniae*.

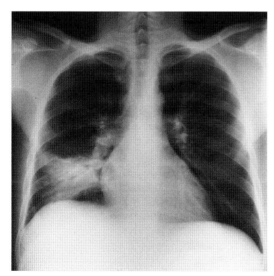

Figure 29-4 Chest radiograph showing lobar consolidation. The etiologic agent was *Salmonella choleraesuis*.

S. pneumoniae, *P. aeruginosa*, *H. influenzae*, and *M. tuberculosis*. PCP also may manifest with lobar or segmental consolidation. In patients with more advanced HIV disease and low CD4+ lymphocyte counts, *P. aeruginosa* and *S. aureus* also can cause pneumonia.

Complications of bacterial pneumonia are frequent, and pleural effusions are twice as likely in HIV infection (often occurring with *S. aureus* infection); empyema and intrapulmonary abscessation are present in up to 10% of patients. Inevitably, the mortality rate is high (approximately 10%).

Other Bacterial Infections

***Nocardia asteroides* Infection** *N. asteroides* has been reported as a cause of infection in patients with advanced HIV disease and low CD4+ lymphocyte counts. The widespread use of trimethoprim-sulfamethoxazole (TMP-SMX) for prophylaxis against PCP may have reduced the incidence of infection due to this organism. The clinical presentation often is indistinguishable from that with other bacterial infections. Chest radiographic appearance may mimic that in tuberculosis (see later). The diagnosis is made by identification of the organism in sputum or BAL fluid or lung tissue.

***Rhodococcus equi* Infection** *R. equi* usually produces pneumonia in patients who have advanced HIV infection and have been in contact with farm animals or with soil from fields or barns where animals are housed. The presentation is subacute, with 2 to 3 weeks of cough, dyspnea, fever, and pleuritic chest pain. The chest radiograph typically shows consolidation with cavitation. Pleural effusions are common. The diagnosis usually is made by culture of sputum or blood; bronchoscopy with BAL or pleural aspiration may be necessary in some cases.

***Bartonella henselae* Infection** *B. henselae* is a gram-negative bacillus that causes bacillary angiomatosis in HIV-infected patients. Clinically, the cutaneous lesions may mimic Kaposi sarcoma, from which they may be distinguished by demonstration of organisms in tissue using Warthin-Starry silver stain. Bacillary angiomatosis also may infect the lungs, where it produces endobronchial red or violet polypoid angiomatous lesions, which may resemble those of Kaposi sarcoma. Biopsy is necessary to confirm the diagnosis.

MYCOBACTERIAL INFECTIONS

Tuberculosis

HIV infection is associated with a 20- to 40-fold increased risk for development of active tuberculosis disease in a person with latent tuberculosis infection (LTBI) over that in noninfected subjects. Taken together with its ability to infect both the immunocompromised and the immunocompetent, tuberculosis is perhaps therefore the single most important disease associated with HIV infection. It is estimated that each year, 1.1 million new cases of active tuberculosis occur in HIV-infected patients. Accordingly, tuberculosis is a major cause of HIV-related morbidity and mortality. It also is a clear driver in both resource-rich and poor countries for the current overall increase in tuberculosis rates. Where HIV infection is endemic, tuberculosis control at a population level is almost impossible if treatment for both infections is not available.

In the United Kingdom, many centers routinely offer HIV antibody testing to all patients with tuberculosis, regardless of risk factors for HIV infection. In the United States, the CDC now recommends HIV testing as a routine part of health care for all patients 13 to 64 years of age seeking medical services. The benefit of treating HIV co-infection is indisputable. Moreover, strategies that reduce high-risk behavior and cut ongoing HIV transmission can be introduced. Unfortunately, offering HIV testing in tuberculosis clinics has not been routine practice in many countries, and integration with HIV infection–related services is poor. This disconnect leads to both diagnostic delay of HIV infection and potentially suboptimal, uncoordinated care, with potentially disastrous outcomes.

Active tuberculosis can occur at any stage of HIV infection and, unlike almost every other HIV-related infection, may do so despite effective ART. In the United States, the United Kingdom, and most European countries, reporting of tuberculosis in both HIV-infected and non–HIV-infected patients is mandatory.

Clinical disease in HIV-infected patients may arise in several different ways: by reactivation of latent tuberculosis, by rapid progression of pulmonary infection, and by reinfection from an exogenous source.

Pulmonary disease is the most common presentation, and clinical manifestations are determined by the patient's level of immunity. For example, persons with reasonably well-preserved CD4+ counts exhibit clinical features similar to those of "normal" adult postprimary disease (**Table 29-3**). Signs and symptoms typically include weight loss, fever with sweats, cough, sputum, dyspnea, hemoptysis, and chest pain. These patients may have no clinical features to suggest associated HIV infection. The chest radiograph frequently shows upper lobe consolidation, and cavitary change is common (**Figure 29-5**). If performed, the tuberculin skin test (TST), using purified protein derivative (PPD), usually gives a positive result, and the likelihood that spontaneously expectorated sputum or BAL fluid will be smear-positive for acid-fast bacilli is high.

In persons with advanced HIV disease (i.e., low CD4+ lymphocyte counts and clinically apparent immunosuppression), it may be difficult to diagnose tuberculosis. The clinical presentation here often is with nonspecific symptoms. Fever, weight loss, fatigue, and malaise may be mistakenly ascribed to HIV infection itself. In this context, pulmonary tuberculosis is often similar to primary infection, with the chest radiograph showing diffuse or miliary-type shadowing (**Figure 29-6**), hilar or mediastinal lymphadenopathy, or pleural effusion; cavitation is

unusual, with no upper zone chest radiographic predominance. In up to 10% of patients, the chest radiograph may appear normal; in others, the pulmonary infiltrate can be bilateral, diffuse, and interstitial in pattern, thus mimicking PCP. Hilar lymphadenopathy and pleural effusion also may be manifestations of pulmonary Kaposi sarcoma or lymphoma, with which *M. tuberculosis* may coexist. The TST result usually is negative, and spontaneously expectorated sputum and BAL fluid samples often are smear-negative (although they are culture-positive).

In addition to pulmonary tuberculosis, extrapulmonary disease occurs in a high proportion of HIV-infected persons with low CD4+ lymphocyte counts (less than 150 cells/μL). Mycobacteremia and generalized lymph node infection (**Figure 29-7**) are common, but involvement of bone marrow, liver, pericardium, meninges, and brain also has been described.

Evidence of extrapulmonary tuberculosis should be sought in any HIV-infected patient with suspected or confirmed pulmonary tuberculosis, by culture of stool, urine, and blood or bone marrow. Traditional solid phase culture and speciation techniques may take 6 to 10 weeks. Liquid culture methods (e.g., BACTEC, Becton Dickinson, Towson, Maryland) that

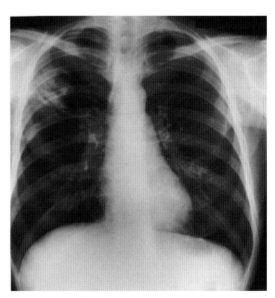

Figure 29-5 Chest radiograph showing pathologic changes of pulmonary tuberculosis in early-stage human immunodeficiency virus infection. Upper lobe infiltrates and cavities are seen.

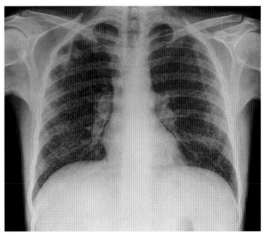

Figure 29-6 Chest radiograph showing pathologic changes of miliary tuberculosis. The patient's CD4+ count was 80 cells/μL.

Table 29-3 Tuberculosis and Human Immunodeficiency Virus (HIV) Infection

Diagnostic Feature	Stage of HIV Disease	
	Reasonable Immunity	Impaired Immunity
Chest radiographic appearance	Upper zone infiltrates and cavities (cf postprimary infection)	Lymphadenopathy, effusions, miliary or diffuse infiltrates (cf primary infection) Normal
Sputum or bronchoalveolar lavage "smear-positive"	Frequently	Less commonly
Disease site	Localized	Widely disseminated
Tuberculin test–positive	Frequently	Less commonly

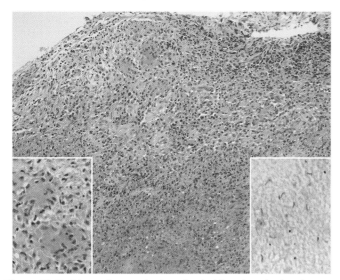

Figure 29-7 Photomicrograph of mediastinal lymph node showing necrotic tissue surrounded by areas of poorly developed granulomatous inflammation (*left inset*). A Ziehl-Neelsen stain showed numerous acid-fast bacilli (*right inset*). *(Reproduced from Miller RF, Shahmanesh M, Talbot MD, et al: Progressive symptoms and signs following institution of highly active antiretroviral therapy and subsequent antituberculosis therapy: immune reconstitution syndrome or infection? Sex Transm Infect 82:111–116, 2006.)*

detect early growth provide a faster diagnosis (usually in 2 to 3 weeks). Molecular diagnostic tests using *M. tuberculosis* genome detection (e.g., by polymerase chain reaction [PCR]) offer the possibility of yet more rapid diagnosis (within hours). The original concerns that "high-tech" systems may not be practical in a field setting are now being challenged. The World Health Organization (WHO) has endorsed the Xpert TBRIF assay, which is portable and simple to use with sputum samples. This kit is expensive, however, although it may be of use in high-prevalence tuberculosis/HIV infection settings, in which prompt treatment initiation is critical to infection control. Current data suggest that such tests are of value, although less sensitive in HIV-infected subjects (in whom sputum samples generally have a lower bacterial load). The availability of simple but highly sensitive and specific methods that utilize the inoculation of large quantities of the sample (e.g., sputum) onto microscopic plates with subsequent rapid detection (in days) of both mycobacterial growth and resistance patterns (i.e., microscopic observation drug susceptibility [MODS] assay) is of great potential significance.

Until the results of culture and speciation are known, acid-fast bacilli identified in respiratory samples, biopsy tissue, an aspirate, or blood in an HIV-infected patient, regardless of the CD4+ lymphocyte count, should be regarded as being *M. tuberculosis*, and conventional antituberculosis therapy should be commenced. If culture fails to demonstrate *M. tuberculosis* and instead another mycobacterium (see later) is identified, then the treatment regimen can be modified.

Drug-Resistant Tuberculosis

Multiple drug–resistant (MDR) tuberculosis—that is, disease caused by *M. tuberculosis* strains resistant to isoniazid and rifampicin (rifampin), with or without other drugs—is now an important clinical problem in HIV-infected patients in the United States, where it is responsible for approximately 3% of all cases of tuberculosis in this population. Outbreaks of MDR tuberculosis have occurred in both HIV-infected and non–HIV-infected persons in the United States in prison facilities, hostels, and hospitals. Similar incidents also have been documented among HIV-infected patients in Europe. Inadequate treatment (including case management and supervision of medication) of tuberculosis and poor patient compliance with antituberculosis therapy are the most important risk factors for development of MDR tuberculosis. Other cases have arisen through exogenous reinfection of profoundly immunosuppressed HIV-infected patients who are already receiving treatment for drug-sensitive disease.

Despite antituberculosis therapy, the median survival in HIV-infected persons with MDR tuberculosis initially was only 2 to 3 months. Recently this has improved, largely because of an increased awareness of the condition with early initiation of suitable therapy as determined by drug sensitivity testing.

The advances in molecular diagnostics are not confined to rapid mycobacterial speciation. Commercial kits are available which can detect the commonest mutations that confer rifampicin and isoniazid resistance with good sensitivity. These are of great potential value in infection control in tuberculosis-endemic areas. They can guide initial therapy, assess for resistance in unexpected poor clinical response and significantly improve treatment outcomes. Next generation tests will also incorporate drug resistance profiles for other important agents such as fluoroquinolones.

Extensively Drug-Resistant Tuberculosis

Extensively drug-resistant (XDR) tuberculosis—that is, *M. tuberculosis* resistant to isoniazid and rifampicin (rifampin), plus any fluoroquinolone and one or more of the three injectable second-line drugs (capreomycin, kanamycin, and amikacin)—is an increasing clinical problem. Originally described in South Africa in association with HIV infection, XDR tuberculosis has now been identified worldwide. The current picture mirrors early reports of MDR tuberculosis in HIV infection in that mortality is very high among HIV-infected patients: In the original South African study from KwaZulu Natal, survival was less than 3 weeks from the time of receipt of the first sputum sample. Earlier suspicion and prompt initiation of therapy have improved survival, although the outcome often is poor and treatment is extremely expensive.

Infections Due to Mycobacteria Other Than Tuberculosis

***Mycobacterium avium* Complex Infection** Before the widespread availability of ART, disseminated MAC infection developed in up to 50% of HIV-infected patients. It remains a problem in patients with advanced HIV disease who are not receiving such therapy and who have CD4+ lymphocyte counts below 50 cells/μL. Clinical presentation is nonspecific and may be confused with the effects of HIV infection itself. Fever, night sweats, weight loss, anorexia, and malaise are common. Anemia, hepatosplenomegaly, abdominal pain, and chronic diarrhea are frequent findings. The diagnosis of disseminated MAC infection is based on culture of the organism from blood, bone marrow, lymph node, or liver biopsy specimens. Also, MAC frequently is identified in BAL fluid, sputum, stool, and urine, but detection of the organism at these sites is not diagnostic of disseminated infection. Evidence of pulmonary MAC infection is not usually obtained from a chest radiograph, which may be negative or show nonspecific infiltrates. Rarely, focal consolidation, nodular infiltrates, and apical cavitation (resembling the changes of *M. tuberculosis* infection) have been reported.

***Mycobacterium kansasii* Infection** *M. kansasii* infection is the second most common nontuberculous opportunistic mycobacterial infection in HIV-infected persons and usually appears late in the course of HIV infection in patients with CD4$^+$ lymphocyte counts below 100 cells/μL. The most frequent presentation is with fever, cough, and dyspnea. In approximately two thirds of persons with *M. kansasii* infection, the disease is localized to the lungs; the remainder have disseminated disease that affects bone marrow, lymph node, skin, and lungs. The diagnosis is made by culture of the organism from respiratory secretions or from bone marrow, lymph node aspirate, or skin biopsy. Focal upper lobe infiltrates with diffuse interstitial infiltrates are the most common radiographic abnormalities; thin-walled cavitary lesions and hilar adenopathy also have been reported.

***Mycobacterium xenopi* Infection** *M. xenopi* may occasionally be isolated from sputum or BAL fluid samples, but its significance is uncertain. Patients have low CD4$^+$ counts, and *M. xenopi* usually is accompanied by a copathogen such as *P. jirovecii*. Treatment of PCP is associated in most cases with resolution of symptoms. Some evidence suggests that starting ART prevents disease recurrence, provided that an adequate immune response is retained.

Pneumocystis jirovecii Pneumonia

The development of PCP is largely related to underlying states of immunosuppression induced by malignancy or treatment thereof, organ transplantation, or HIV infection. In 2011 in the United States, the United Kingdom, Europe, and Australasia, PCP was largely seen only in HIV-infected persons unaware of their serostatus or in those reported to be intolerant of or noncompliant with anti–*P. jirovecii* prophylaxis and ART.

P. jirovecii originally was regarded as a protozoan, as suggested by its morphology and the lack of response to antifungal agents such as amphotericin B. The organism is now thought to be a fungus. The demonstration of antibodies against *P. jirovecii* in most healthy children and adults suggests that infection is acquired in childhood and persists in the lungs in a dormant phase. Subsequent immunosuppression (e.g., as a result of HIV infection) allows the fungus to propagate in the lung, causing clinical disease. This "latency hypothesis," however, is challenged by several observations: *P. jirovecii* cannot be identified in the lungs of immunocompetent persons; "case clusters" of PCP in health care facilities suggest recent transmission; different genotypes of *P. jirovecii* are identified in each episode in HIV-infected patients who have recurrent PCP; genotypes of *P. jirovecii* in patients who have PCP correlate with place of diagnosis and not with their place of birth, suggesting infection has been recently acquired. Taken together, these data suggest that PCP arises by reinfection from an exogenous source.

The clinical presentation of PCP is nonspecific, with onset of progressive exertional dyspnea over days or weeks, together with a dry cough, with or without expectoration of minimal quantities of mucoid sputum. Patients often report an inability to take a deep breath, which is not due to pleurisy (**Table 29-4**). Fever is common, yet patients rarely complain of temperature-related signs and symptoms including sweats. In HIV-infected patients, the presentation usually is more insidious than in those receiving immunosuppressive therapy. The median time to diagnosis from onset of symptoms is more than 3 weeks in those with HIV infection, compared with less than 1 week in non–HIV-infected patients. In a small proportion of HIV-positive patients, the disease course of PCP is fulminant, with an interval of only 5 to 7 days between onset of symptoms and progression to development of respiratory failure. In others, it may be much more indolent, with respiratory symptoms that worsen almost imperceptibly over several months. Rarely, PCP may manifest as a fever of undetermined origin without respiratory symptoms.

Clinical examination usually is remarkable only for the absence of physical signs; occasionally, fine, basal, end-inspiratory crackles are audible. Features that would suggest an alternative diagnosis include a cough productive of purulent sputum or hemoptysis, chest pain (particularly pleural pain), and signs of focal consolidation or pleural effusion (see Table 29-4). Of note, infection with more than one pathogen occurs in almost one fifth of these patients, so symptoms may be related to infection with any of several agents.

The chest radiographic appearance in PCP typically is unremarkable initially. Later, diffuse reticular shadowing, especially in the perihilar regions, is seen and may progress to widespread alveolar consolidation that resembles that in untreated pulmonary edema or with presentation late in disease. At this stage,

Table 29-4 **Clinical Presentation in *Pneumocystis jirovecii* Pneumonia**

Examination	Typical Presentation	Atypical Presentation
Symptoms	Progressive exertional dyspnea over days or weeks	Sudden onset of dyspnea over hours or days
	Dry cough ± mucoid sputum	Cough productive of purulent sputum Hemoptysis
	Difficulty taking in a deep breath not related to pleuritic pain	Chest pain (pleuritic or "crushing")
	Fever ± sweats Tachypnea	
Signs	Normal breath sounds or fine end-inspiratory basal crackles	Wheeze, signs of focal consolidation or pleural effusion
Chest radiographic appearance	*Early:* perihilar "haze," or bilateral interstitial shadowing	Pleural effusion, lobar or segmental consolidation
	Late: alveolar-interstitial changes or "whiteout" (marked alveolar consolidation with sparing of apices and costophrenic angles)	
Arterial blood gases	Pao$_2$: *early:* normal; *late:* low	
	Paco$_2$: *early:* normal or low; *late:* normal or high	

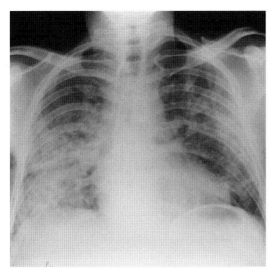

Figure 29-8 Chest radiograph showing diffuse bilateral interstitial infiltrates in a patient with severe *Pneumocystis jirovecii* pneumonia.

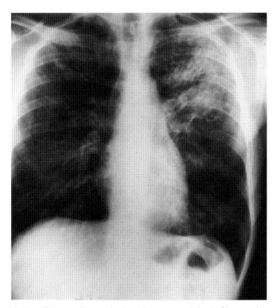

Figure 29-9 Chest radiograph showing upper lobe infiltrates in a patient with *Pneumocystis jirovecii* pneumonia. The patient had received nebulized pentamidine.

the lung may be grossly consolidated and almost airless (**Figure 29-8**). Up to 20% of chest radiographs are atypical in appearance, showing lobar consolidation, honeycomb lung, multiple thin-walled cystic air spaces (pneumatoceles), intrapulmonary nodules, cavitary lesions, pneumothorax, and hilar and mediastinal lymphadenopathy. Predominantly apical changes, resembling those of tuberculosis, may occur in patients with PCP that developed subsequent to anti–*P. jirovecii* prophylaxis with nebulized pentamidine (**Figure 29-9**). All of these radiographic changes are nonspecific; similar changes occur with other pulmonary pathogens, including pyogenic bacterial, mycobacterial, and fungal infection, as well as Kaposi sarcoma and nonspecific interstitial pneumonitis. Respiratory symptoms in an immunosuppressed, HIV-infected patient with a normal-appearing chest radiograph should not be discounted, however, because radiographic abnormalities may not appear until 2 to 3 days later.

The diagnosis of PCP is made by demonstration of the organism in induced sputum, BAL fluid, or lung biopsy material using histochemical or immunofluorescence techniques.

Molecular detection tests for *P. jirovecii* using a variety of primers have been reported using BAL fluid, induced sputum and oropharyngeal wash (OPW) specimens. In general PCR-based tests have increased sensitivity, but a reduced specificity when compared to visualization of the organism using histochemical stains. This reduced specificity results from the finding that *P. jirovecii* DNA may be detected in respiratory samples from HIV-infected patients who do not have PCP (such as with tuberculosis or bacterial pneumonia) but are colonized with the organism. One study compared two PCR-based assays; these had sensitivities of 97% and 98%, but specificities were only 68% and 66%. The sensitivity of molecular detection techniques is lower if OPW rather than BAL fluid is used.

FUNGAL INFECTIONS

Many fungal infections of the lung are confined to specific geographic regions, although with widespread travel they may occur in patients outside these areas. *Candida, Aspergillus*, and *Cryptococcus* spp. are ubiquitous and are found worldwide.

Candidal Infection

In contrast with infections of the oropharynx and esophagus, candidal infection of the trachea, bronchi, and lungs is rare in HIV-infected patients, as are candidemia, disseminated candidiasis, and deep focal candidiasis. The clinical presentation of pulmonary candidal infection has no specific features. Chest radiography is equally nonspecific—the radiographic appearance may be normal or show patchy infiltrates. Isolation of *Candida* from sputum may simply represent colonization and does not mean that the patient has candidal pneumonia. Indirect evidence may be obtained from positive cultures or rising antibody titers. However, in HIV-infected patients a high antibody titer alone is a less reliable indicator, and antibodies may be absent in proven cases of invasive candidal infection. Some correlation occurs between identification of large quantities of *Candida* species in BAL fluid and *Candida* spp. as the cause of pneumonia. Definitive diagnosis is made by lung biopsy.

Aspergillus Infection

Unlike in patients immunosuppressed and rendered neutropenic by systemic chemotherapy, infection with *Aspergillus* species is relatively rare in HIV-positive patients. Risk factors for aspergillosis are neutropenia, which commonly is drug-induced (e.g., in chemotherapy), and use of corticosteroids. Fever, cough, and dyspnea are the most common presenting manifestations, but pleuritic chest pain and hemoptysis are found in approximately one third of patients.

Patterns of pulmonary disease include cavitating upper lobe disease, focal radiographic opacities resembling bacterial pneumonia, bilateral diffuse and patchy opacities (nodular or reticular-nodular in pattern), pseudomembranous aspergillosis (which may obstruct the lumen of airways), and tracheobronchitis. Diagnosis of pulmonary aspergillosis is made by the identification of fungus in sputum, sputum casts, or BAL fluid in association with respiratory tract tissue invasion (**Figure 29-10**). Serum (1,3)-β-D-glucan levels may be elevated (see further on).

Cryptococcal Infection

Infection may manifest in one of two ways: either as primary cryptococcosis or complicating cryptococcal meningitis as part of disseminated infection with cryptococcemia, pneumonia, and cutaneous disease (umbilicated papules mimicking

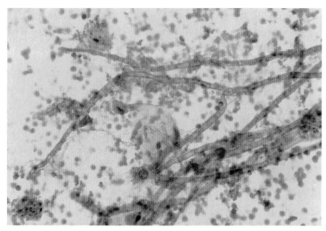

Figure 29-10 Bronchoalveolar lavage fluid containing *Aspergillus fumigatus* organisms.

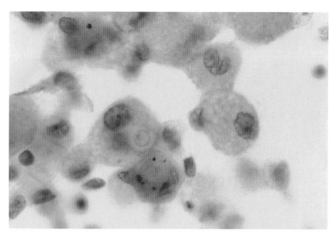

Figure 29-12 Bronchoalveolar lavage fluid containing *Cryptococcus neoformans* organisms.

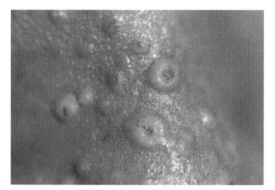

Figure 29-11 Skin changes in disseminated cryptococcosis. The multiple, umbilicated lesions resemble those of molluscum contagiosum.

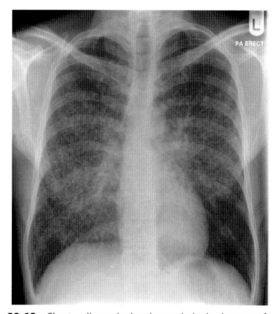

Figure 29-13 Chest radiograph showing pathologic changes of histoplasmosis.

molluscum contagiosum) (**Figure 29-11**). Primary pulmonary cryptococcosis presents in a very nonspecific way and is frequently indistinguishable from other pulmonary infections. In disseminated infection, the presentation frequently is overshadowed by headache, fever, and malaise (caused by meningitis). The time to onset may range from only a few days to several weeks. Examination may reveal skin lesions, lymphadenopathy, and meningism. In the chest, signs may be absent or crackles may be audible. Arterial blood gas analysis may reveal normal findings or show hypoxemia. The most common abnormality on the chest radiograph is focal or diffuse interstitial infiltrates. Less frequently, masses, mediastinal or hilar lymphadenopathy, nodules, and effusion are noted.

The diagnosis of cryptococcal pulmonary infection (**Figure 29-12**) is made by identification of *Cryptococcus neoformans* (by staining with India ink or mucicarmine, and by culture) in sputum, BAL fluid, pleural fluid, or lung biopsy tissue. Cryptococcal antigen may be detected in serum using the cryptococcal latex agglutination (CrAg) test. Titers usually are high but may be negative in primary pulmonary cryptococcosis, in which case BAL fluid (CrAg) is positive. In patients with disseminated infection, *C. neoformans* also may be cultured from blood and cerebrospinal fluid.

Endemic Mycoses

The endemic mycoses caused by *Histoplasma capsulatum*, *Coccidioides immitis*, and *Blastomyces dermatitidis* are found in HIV-infected patients living in North America (especially the Mississippi and Ohio River valleys). Histoplasmosis also is found in Southeast Asia, the Caribbean Islands, and South America. Coccidioidomycosis is endemic in the southwest United States (southern California), northern Mexico, and in parts of Argentina and Brazil. Blastomycosis has a similar distribution, with an extension north into Canada.

Histoplasmosis

Progressive, disseminated histoplasmosis in patients with HIV typically manifests with a subacute onset of fever and weight loss; approximately 50% of patients have mild respiratory symptoms with a nonproductive cough and dyspnea. Hepatosplenomegaly frequently is noted on examination, and a rash (similar to that produced by *Cryptococcus* spp.) may be seen. Rarely, the presentation may be rapidly fulminant, with clinical features of the sepsis syndrome including anemia or disseminated intravascular coagulation. The chest radiograph may be normal in appearance (in up to one third of patients), although characteristic abnormalities consist of bilateral, widespread nodules 2 to 4 mm in size (**Figure 29-13**). Other radiographic features are nonspecific and include interstitial infiltrates, reticular nodular shadowing, and alveolar consolidation. The diagnosis is made reliably by identification of the organism in Wright-stained peripheral blood or by Giemsa staining of bone marrow, lymph node, skin, sputum, BAL fluid, or lung tissue. It is important that identification be confirmed by detection of *H. capsulatum* var. *capsulatum* polysaccharide antigen by radioimmunoassay, which has a high sensitivity. False-positive results are possible in patients infected with *Blastomyces* and *Coccidioides* spp. Testing for *Histoplasma* antibodies by complement fixation or immunodiffusion techniques may give a negative result in immunosuppressed, HIV-positive patients. Serum (1,3)-β-D-glucan levels may be elevated (see further on).

Coccidioidomycosis

The clinical presentation of coccidioidomycosis is highly variable. The chest radiograph may show focal pulmonary disease with alveolar infiltrates, adenopathy, and intrapulmonary cavities or, alternatively, diffuse reticular shadowing. Diagnosis is made by isolation of the organism in sputum or BAL fluid. Disseminated disease is identified by isolating the fungus in blood, urine, or cerebrospinal fluid. Serologic tests also may be used for diagnosis.

Blastomycosis

Blastomycosis presents in patients who have advanced HIV infection, when CD4$^+$ lymphocyte counts are usually less than 200 cells/μL. Clinical signs and symptoms include cough, fever, dyspnea, and weight loss. Patients may present late in respiratory failure. Disseminated disease can occur with both pulmonary and extrapulmonary features. Involvement of multiple body systems including the skin, liver, brain, and meninges is common. Chest radiographic abnormalities include focal pneumonic change, miliary shadowing, or diffuse interstitial infiltrates. Diagnosis is made by culture from BAL fluid, skin, and blood. In this infection, early cytologic or histologic diagnosis is important, because culture of the organism may take 2 to 4 weeks. The mortality rate is high for disseminated infection.

Penicillium marneffei Infection

P. marneffei infection is particularly common in Southeast Asia. Most HIV-infected patients present with disseminated infection and solitary skin or oral mucosal lesions, or with multiple infiltrates in the liver or spleen, or bone marrow (leading to presentation with pancytopenia). Pulmonary infection has no specific clinical features, and chest radiographs may be normal-appearing or show diffuse, small nodular infiltrates. Diagnosis is made by identifying the organism in bone marrow, skin biopsy specimens, blood films, or BAL fluid. The differential diagnosis for *P. marneffei* infection includes both PCP and tuberculosis.

VIRAL INFECTIONS

Community-Based Respiratory Viral Infections

Influenza A

HIV-infected persons do not have a greater incidence of influenza A but may be at increased risk for more severe disease. This susceptibility is due to associated medical comorbid conditions.

HIV-infected patients with seasonal or H1N1 influenza typically present with an acute respiratory illness (e.g., coryzal symptoms) with fever, headache, and myalgia. Vomiting and diarrhea occur more often with H1N1 influenza than with seasonal influenza. Some patients with seasonal or H1N1 influenza may not have fever. Careful clinical assessment, together with awareness of local surveillance data on circulating influenza viruses and other community-prevalent respiratory pathogens, is important in the differential diagnosis for patients presenting with an influenza-like illness. In some HIV-infected patients, especially those with low CD4$^+$ cell counts (less than 100 cells/μL), the illness may progress rapidly (**Figure 29-14**) and can be complicated by secondary bacterial pneumonia. The diagnosis is made by detection of viral antigen or RNA, or by culture of nasopharyngeal aspirate or nasal swab.

CYTOMEGALOVIRUS INFECTION

CMV frequently is isolated from BAL fluid from patients with CD4$^+$ counts below 100 cells/μl; however, the role of CMV in causing disease in this context is unclear (see later).

In patients in whom CMV is the sole identified pathogen, clinical presentation and chest radiographic abnormalities (usually diffuse interstitial infiltrates) are nonspecific. Diagnosis of CMV pneumonitis is made by identifying characteristic intranuclear and intracytoplasmic inclusions, not only in cells in BAL fluid but also in lung biopsy specimens (**Figure 29-15**).

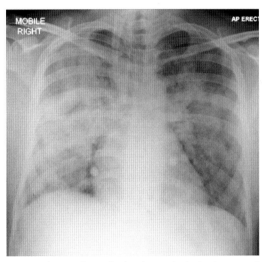

Figure 29-14 Chest radiograph showing pathologic changes of severe H1N1 influenza.

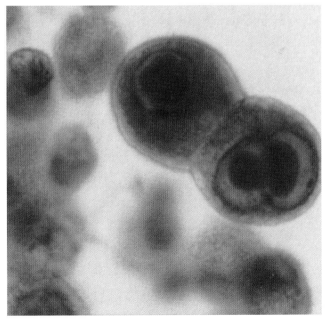

Figure 29-15 Bronchoalveolar lavage fluid containing cytomegalovirus inclusions.

PROTOZOAL INFECTIONS

Leishmaniasis

Pulmonary involvement with *Leishmania* spp. may rarely occur as part of the syndrome of visceral leishmaniasis in HIV-infected patients. Patients usually have advanced HIV disease with CD4+ lymphocyte counts below 300 cells/µL and present with fever, splenomegaly, and leukopenia. Respiratory symptoms often are absent. Diagnosis of visceral leishmaniasis most often is made by staining and culture of splenic or bone marrow aspirate. Occasionally the parasite is found by chance in a skin or rectal biopsy specimen or BAL fluid taken for other purposes. The chest radiograph may be normal in appearance or show reticular-nodular infiltrates.

Toxoplasmosis

Toxoplasma gondii infection in HIV-infected patients usually occurs as a result of reactivation of latent, intracellular protozoa acquired in a primary infection. Toxoplasmic pneumonia frequently manifests with nonproductive cough and dyspnea. Chest radiographic abnormalities include diffuse interstitial infiltrates indistinguishable from those of PCP (**Figure 29-16**), as well as micronodular infiltrates, a coarse nodular infiltrate, cavitary change, and lobar consolidation. The diagnosis is made by hematoxylin-eosin or Giemsa staining of BAL fluid, which reveals cysts and trophozoites of *T. gondii*. Staining of BAL fluid is not always positive; the diagnostic yield is increased either by staining of transbronchial biopsy material or by performing PCR assay to detect *T. gondii* DNA in BAL fluid.

Strongyloidiasis

The nematode *Strongyloides stercoralis* is endemic in warm countries worldwide. In immunosuppressed patients, the organism has an increased ability to reproduce parthenogenetically in the gastrointestinal tract without the need for repeated exposure to new infection—so-called autoinfection. This enhanced reproductivity results in a great increase in worm load, and a hyperinfective state ensues; massive acute dissemination with *S. stercoralis* may occur in the lungs, kidneys, pancreas, and brain. Although infection with *S. stercoralis* is more severe in immunocompromised patients, it is no more common in patients who have HIV infection. Presentation with hyperinfection may be with fever, hypotension secondary to bacterial sepsis, or disseminated intravascular coagulation. The clinical features of respiratory *S. stercoralis* infection are very nonspecific. *S. stercoralis* in sputum or BAL fluid (**Figure 29-17**) may be identified in HIV-positive patients in the absence of symptoms elsewhere; this can predate disseminated infection and as such requires prompt treatment.

DIAGNOSIS

It is apparent from the foregoing discussion that HIV-related pneumonias of any cause may present in a very similar manner. A wide range of investigations are available to aid diagnosis. These are listed in **Box 29-3**. If the subject is producing sputum,

---

Box 29-3 **Tests Available to Aid Diagnosis of Human Immunodeficiency Virus (HIV) Infection-Related Pneumonia**

Physiologic
Transcutaneous pulse oximetry
Arterial blood gas analysis
Lung function testing

Radiologic
Chest radiography
Computed tomography scan of thorax

Histopathologic
Serologic studies (antigen or antibody testing)
Serum lactate dehydrogenase measurement
Microscopy and culture of body fluid/tissue (e.g., sputum, blood, bronchoalveolar lavage fluid, lung tissue) obtained by:
    Sputum induction
    Bronchoscopy and bronchoalveolar lavage
    Bronchoscopy and transbronchial biopsy
    VATS lung biopsy
Nucleic acid detection of specific organisms (e.g., by polymerase chain reaction assay for *Pneumocystis jirovecii* in bronchoalveolar lavage fluid or induced sputum)

VATS, video-assisted thoracoscopic surgery.

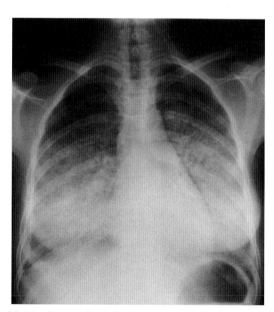

Figure 29-16 Chest radiograph showing pathologic changes of *Toxoplasma gondii* pneumonia. The diffuse bilateral infiltrates resemble those in *P. jirovecii* pneumonia. *(Reproduced from Miller RF, Lucas SB, Bateman NT: Disseminated* Toxoplasma gondii *infection presenting with a fulminant pneumonia,* Genitourin Med *72:139–143, 1996.)*

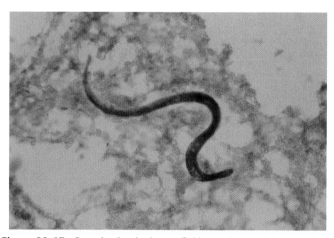

Figure 29-17 Bronchoalveolar lavage fluid sample containing an adult *Strongyloides stercoralis* roundworm.

it is important to obtain samples for bacterial and mycobacterial detection. In up to one third of cases, these will assist in diagnosis. Obtaining three samples on consecutive days (preferably either with overnight or early morning production) is the crucial first step in the diagnosis of pulmonary tuberculosis. This is considerably easier and safer for health care personnel than obtaining hypertonic saline–induced sputum or BAL fluid. Blood cultures also are important, because very high rates of bacteremia have been reported in both bacterial and mycobacterial disease (see earlier).

A patient who presents with symptoms and signs consistent with pneumonia should have chest radiography and arterial oxygen assessments performed at the first consultation. The question at this stage usually is whether this infectious episode is due to bacterial infection, tuberculosis, or PCP. In general, alveolar and interstitial shadowing is taken as evidence for PCP, although important caveats apply.

Until tuberculosis has been ruled out, the patient should be segregated from other people in hospital and community environments and should be made aware of personal infection control measures such as "cough hygiene."

ARTERIAL OXYGEN ASSESSMENTS

Transcutaneous pulse oximetry and arterial blood gas analysis are useful tests for hypoxemia. They can be used to distinguish an alveolar condition (i.e., PCP) from bacterial pneumonia. The alveolitis produces a greater impairment of oxygen transfer (especially during exercise), such that for a given clinical situation there will be more hypoxemia and a wider alveolar-arterial oxygen gradient (i.e., $PO_2[A-a]$) in those with PCP. With use of pulse oximetry, this manifests as low oxygen saturation at rest that decreases further with exercise. In general, more information can be obtained from arterial blood gas analysis, although this advantage is offset by the need for direct arterial puncture.

Of patients with PCP, fewer than 10% have a normal PaO_2 and a normal $PO_2(A-a)$. These measures are sensitive, although not particularly specific for PCP, and similar results may occur with bacterial pneumonia, pulmonary Kaposi sarcoma, and *M. tuberculosis* infection. The diagnostic value of identifying exercise-induced desaturation, measured by transcutaneous oximetry, has been validated only in HIV-infected patients who have PCP and a normal or near-normal appearance on the chest radiograph. The test's value has not been confirmed in patients with radiographic abnormalities due to PCP or other pathogens. Exercise-induced desaturation may persist for many weeks after treatment and recovery from PCP, even in the absence of active pulmonary disease.

LUNG FUNCTION TESTING

Abnormalities of lung function are well documented with HIV infection. The most common of these relate to tests measuring gas exchange, rather than the size of the conducting airways. In general, an overall reduction in diffusing capacity for carbon monoxide (DLCO) occurs at all stages of HIV infection, with the largest changes found in HIV-infected patients with PCP. A normal DLCO in a patient with symptoms but a normal-appearing or unchanged chest radiograph makes the diagnosis of PCP extremely unlikely. Data from the North American Pulmonary Complications of HIV Infection Study (PCHIS) suggest that patients with rapid rates of decline in DLCO are at an increased risk for development of PCP. A recent

cross-sectional study of HIV-infected patients showed 47% had respiratory symptoms. Almost two thirds of patients had diffusion impairment, which was associated with a history of past or present smoking ("ever smoking") and receipt of PCP prophylaxis. Approximately 21% had irreversible airway obstruction. This finding was associated with pack-years smoked and injection drug use and with receipt of ART.

COMPUTED TOMOGRAPHY SCANNING

High-resolution (thin-section) CT scanning of the chest may be helpful when the chest radiographic appearance is normal, unchanged, or equivocal. The characteristic appearance of an alveolitis (i.e., areas of ground glass attenuation through which the pulmonary vessels can be clearly identified) may be present, which indicates active pulmonary disease (**Figure 29-18**). This feature, however, is neither sensitive nor specific for PCP, although its sensitivity can be improved if evidence for reticulation or small cystic lesions is added. Hence, a negative test result implies an alternative diagnosis.

BIOCHEMICAL ASSAYS

Lactate Dehydrogenase

In an HIV-infected patient who presents with an acute or subacute pneumonitis, an elevated serum lactate dehydrogenase (LDH) level is strongly suggestive of PCP. In interpreting such results, it is important to recognize that other pulmonary disease processes (e.g., pulmonary embolism; nonspecific pneumonitis; fungal, bacterial, and mycobacterial pneumonia) and extrapulmonary disease (Castleman disease and lymphoma) also may cause elevations of LDH and may need to be considered in the correct clinical context.

Plasma or Serum S-Adenosylmethionine

The rationale behind use of the plasma or serum S-adenosylmethionine (SAM or AdoMet) assay is that *Pneumocystis* was thought to be unable to metabolize SAM, because it lacks a SAM synthetase and therefore scavenges this from its host. According to this hypothesis, patients with PCP might be expected to have low SAM levels. Some studies have shown that plasma AdoMet levels can be used to distinguish HIV-infected patients with PCP from those with other-cause pneumonia (e.g., bacterial pneumonia or tuberculosis) and found no

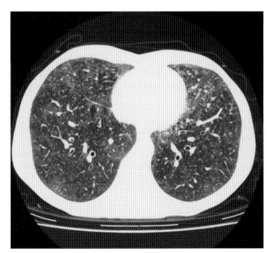

Figure 29-18 Computed tomography scan of thorax showing diffuse bilateral ground glass shadowing typical of *Pneumocystis* pneumonia.

overlap in AdoMet levels between those with and those without PCP. Another study that measured serum AdoMet reported overlapping levels in HIV-infected patients with PCP and other-cause pneumonia. Currently measurement of serum or plasma AdoMet is not used for diagnosis of PCP.

Serum (1,3)-β-D-Glucan

In all fungi, including *Pneumocystis*, (1,3)-β-D-glucan is a cell wall component. Serum (1,3)-β-D-glucan levels are higher in patients with PCP (with or without underlying HIV infection) when compared to patients without PCP. The sensitivity and specificity of this assay are maximal using a cutoff of 100 pg/mL (for diagnosis of PCP). Because serum (1,3)-β-D-glucan levels may be elevated in pneumonia caused by several fungal pathogens, this test does not permit discrimination among potential etiologic disorders (e.g., PCP, *Aspergillus* infection, histoplasmosis). Additionally, case reports of false-positive results in patients with pulmonary infection due to *P. aeruginosa* further limit diagnostic utility. Among patients with confirmed PCP, use of serum (1,3)-β-D-glucan levels to monitor response to therapy requires further evaluation.

From the preceding discussion, it is evident that noninvasive tests cannot reliably distinguish the different infecting agents from each other but may be useful in excluding acute opportunistic disease. Thus, the clinician is left with either proceeding to diagnostic lung fluid or tissue sampling (using either induced sputum collection or bronchoscopy and BAL with or without transbronchial biopsy) (**Table 29-5**) or treating an unknown condition empirically. ART also has altered the investigation of respiratory disease. The numbers of invasive procedures performed are falling, and such procedures tend to be used in patients not taking antiretroviral drugs (usually to exclude PCP), or in whom no response to empirical antibiotic therapy (regardless of the CD4+ count) has been observed.

INDUCED SPUTUM

Spontaneously expectorated sputum is inadequate for diagnosis of PCP. Sputum induction by inhalation of ultrasonically nebulized hypertonic saline may provide a suitable specimen (see Table 29-5). The technique requires close attention to detail and is much less useful when samples are purulent. Sputum induction must be carried out away from other immunosuppressed patients and health care workers, ideally in a room with separate negative-pressure ventilation, to reduce the risk of nosocomial transmission of tuberculosis. Although very specific (at a rate greater than 95%), the sensitivity of induced sputum varies widely (55% to 90%), and therefore a negative result for *P. jirovecii* prompts further diagnostic studies. The use of immunofluorescence staining enhances the yield of induced sputum compared with standard cytochemistry.

BRONCHOSCOPY

Fiberoptic bronchoscopy with BAL commonly is used to diagnose HIV-related pulmonary disease. When a good "wedged" sample is obtained, the test has a sensitivity of greater than 90% for detection of *P. jirovecii* (**Figure 29-19**). Just as with induced sputum, fluorescent staining methods increase the diagnostic yield, which makes bronchoscopy the procedure of choice in most centers. More technically demanding (both of the patient and of the operator) than induced sputum collection, bronchoscopy and BAL have the advantage that direct inspection of the upper airway and bronchial tree can be performed and, if necessary, biopsy specimens taken. Transbronchial biopsy may marginally increase the diagnostic yield of the procedure. This is relevant for the diagnosis of mycobacterial disease, although the relatively high complication rate in HIV-infected persons (pneumothorax and the possibility of significant pulmonary hemorrhage in up to 10%) outweighs the advantages of the technique for routine purposes.

Samples of BAL fluid are examined for bacteria, mycobacteria, viruses, fungi, and protozoa. Inspection of the cellular component also may provide etiologic clues—cooperation of a pathology department with experience in opportunistic infection diagnosis is vital. The drug interactions associated with antiretroviral protease inhibitor therapy mean that special care should be exercised with use of sedation with either benzodiazepine or opiate drugs. Prolonged sedation and life-threatening arrhythmias have been reported.

A diagnostic strategy therefore includes sputum induction and, if results are nondiagnostic or if the test is unavailable, bronchoscopy and BAL. If this approach does not yield a result, consideration is given to either a repeat bronchoscopy and BAL

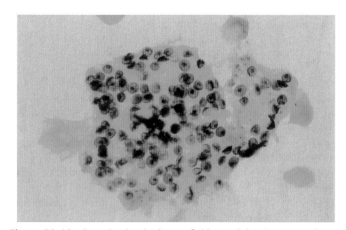

Figure 29-19 Bronchoalveolar lavage fluid containing *Pneumocystis jirovecii* organisms. (Grocott silver stain.)

Table 29-5	Induced Sputum, Bronchoalveolar Lavage, and Surgical Biopsy in Diagnosis of *Pneumocystis jirovecii* Pneumonia			
Technique	**Ease of Procedure**	**Diagnostic Sensitivity (%)**	**Cost**	**Comments**
Induced sputum	Simple—once technique established	50-90	Low	Requires dedicated health care worker(s) and facility Risk to health care workers from expectorated aerosol
Bronchoalveolar lavage	Moderate	90->95	Moderate	Risk of deterioration after procedure Risk to health care workers from coughed secretions Sensitivity may be increased by two-lobe lavage
Surgical biopsy	Complex	>95	High	Requires health care workers with surgical expertise

with transbronchial biopsy or video-assisted thoracoscopic surgery (VATS) for biopsy.

EMPIRICAL DIAGNOSIS AND THERAPY

Although empirical therapy usually is reserved for the management of presumed bacterial pneumonias and initially may appear unwise when the underlying disease may be an opportunistic infection, in reality PCP is almost invariably a diagnosis of exclusion, and certain clinical and laboratory features may guide the assessment of an HIV-infected patient's risk for this condition. The likelihood that *P. jirovecii* is the causative organism increases if the person is not taking effective anti-*Pneumocystis* drug prophylaxis or has a previous medical history with clinical or laboratory features suggestive of systemic immunosuppression (i.e., recurrent oral thrush, long-standing fever of unknown cause, clinical AIDS, or blood CD4+ count less than 200 cells/μL). Hence, some centers advocate use of empirical therapy for HIV-infected patients who present with symptoms and chest radiographic and blood gas abnormalities typical of mild PCP, without the need for bronchoscopy. Invasive measures are reserved for patients with an atypical radiographic presentation, those who fail to respond to empirical therapy by day 5, and those who exhibit clinical deterioration at any stage.

Most clinicians in the United States and the United Kingdom would seek to obtain a confirmed diagnosis in every case of suspected PCP. In practice, both strategies discussed above appear to be equally effective, although a number of caveats should be borne in mind when empirical treatment is given for PCP. Patients who have PCP typically take 4 to 7 days to show clinical signs of improvement, so a bronchoscopically proven diagnosis ensures that the treatment being given is correct, particularly in the first few days of therapy, when the drug regimen may not be well tolerated. In addition, the diagnosis of PCP has implications for the infected person, because it may influence the decision to start either ART or anti-*Pneumocystis* prophylaxis. Finally, empirical therapy requires the patient to be maximally adherent with treatment, because nonresolution of symptoms may be seen as a failure of therapy, rather than of compliance.

TREATMENT

Persons infected with HIV, compared with the non–HIV-infected general population, have an increased likelihood of adverse reactions to therapeutic agents. Such agents include TMP-SMX (see later on) and other antibacterial and antimycobacterial agents. In addition, complex drug interactions with other medications, particularly components of ART, have been reported. Before institution of therapy for any infectious complication in an HIV-infected patient, it is important to consult with a physician experienced in the care of such patients and to seek advice from a specialist pharmacist.

TREATMENT OF BACTERIAL PNEUMONIA

The main organisms causing pneumonia in HIV-infected persons are similar to those found in the general population with community-acquired pneumonia. Thus, bacterial pneumonia in HIV-infected patients should be treated in a manner similar to that in HIV-negative persons, using published American Thoracic Society (ATS) and British Thoracic Society (BTS) guidelines. In addition, expert advice on local antibiotic resistance patterns should be sought from infectious disease or microbiology colleagues, because treatment usually is begun on an empirical basis before the causative organism is identified and antibiotic sensitivities are known. The same clinical and laboratory prognostic indices that are described for the general population apply to HIV-infected patients and should be documented on presentation.

Response to appropriate antibiotic therapy usually is rapid and is similar to that seen in the non–HIV-infected person. Early relapse of infection after successful treatment is well described. Those HIV-infected patients who have presumed PCP and are being treated empirically with high-dose TMP-SMX, and who have infection with either *S. pneumoniae* or *H. influenzae*, rather than *P. jirovecii*, also may improve. In addition, in those patients who are treated with benzylpenicillin for proven *S. pneumoniae* pneumonia but do not respond, and penicillin resistance can be discounted as the cause, it is important to consider the possibility of a second pathologic process, such as PCP. Copathogens are reported in up to 20% of cases of pneumonia.

TREATMENT OF PNEUMOCYSTIS JIROVECII PNEUMONIA

Before institution of treatment, assessment of the severity of PCP should be performed, to include a thorough history, physical examination, arterial blood gas analysis, and chest radiography. On the basis of the findings, patients can then be stratified into those with mild, moderate, or severe disease (**Table 29-6**).

Table 29-6 **Grading Severity of *Pneumocystis jirovecii* Pneumonia**

Clinical Feature	Disease Severity		
	Mild	**Moderate**	**Severe**
Symptoms and signs	Dyspnea on exertion with or without cough and sweats	Dyspnea on minimal exertion and occasionally at rest; cough and fever	Dyspnea and tachypnea at rest; persistent fever and cough
Oxygenation			
Pao_2 on room air, at rest (mm Hg)	>83	61-83	≤8.0; ≤60
Sao_2 on room air	>96	91-96	<91
Sao_2 with exercise	>90	<90	<90
$Po_2(A–a)$ (mm Hg)	<35	35-45	>45
Chest radiographic appearance	Normal or minor perihilar shadowing	Diffuse interstitial shadowing	Extensive interstitial shadowing with or without diffuse alveolar shadowing

This classification is important, because some drugs are of unproven benefit and others are known to be ineffective for the treatment of severe disease. In addition, adjuvant glucocorticoid therapy may be given to patients with moderate or severe pneumonia. Before (or as soon as feasible after) starting therapy with TMP-SMX, dapsone, or primaquine, patients should be tested for glucose-6-phosphate dehydrogenase deficiency, because these drugs increase the risk of hemolysis.

Trimethoprim-Sulfamethoxazole

Several drugs are effective in the treatment of PCP. TMP-SMX is the drug of first choice (**Tables 29-7** and **29-8**). Overall, it is effective in 70% to 80% of patients when used for first-line therapy. Adverse reactions to TMP-SMX are common and usually become apparent between days 6 and 14 of treatment.

Neutropenia and anemia (in up to 40% of patients), rash and fever (up to 30%), and biochemical abnormalities of liver function (up to 15%) are the most frequent adverse reactions. Hematologic toxicity induced by TMP-SMX is neither attenuated nor prevented by coadministration of folic or folinic acid. Furthermore, the use of these agents may be associated with reduced therapeutic success. During treatment with TMP-SMX, monitoring with full blood counts, liver function testing, and measurements of urea and electrolytes at least twice weekly is indicated.

It is not known why HIV-infected patients, especially those with higher CD4$^+$ counts, experience such a high frequency of adverse reactions to TMP-SMX. The optimal strategy for management of an HIV-infected patient who has PCP and who becomes intolerant of high-dose TMP-SMX has not been

Table 29-7 Treatment of *Pneumocystis jirovecii* Pneumonia According to Disease Severity

Regimen Category	Effective Agent or Regimen		
	Mild Disease	**Moderate Disease**	**Severe Disease**
First choice	Trimethoprim-sulfamethoxazole	Trimethoprim-sulfamethoxazole	Trimethoprim-sulfamethoxazole
Second choice	Clindamycin-primaquine OR Trimethoprim-dapsone OR Atovaquone	Clindamycin-primaquine OR Intravenous pentamidine OR Trimethoprim-dapsone	Clindamycin-primaquine OR Intravenous pentamidine
Adjuvant corticosteroids	Benefit not proven	Benefit proven	Benefit proven

Table 29-8 Treatment Schedules for *Pneumocystis jirovecii* Pneumonia*

Drug	Dosage	Comments
Trimethoprim-sulfamethoxazole (TMP-SMX)	Trimethoprim 15-20 mg/kg IV q24h plus sulfamethoxazole 75-100 mg/kg IV daily in divided doses, q6h or q8h	Give IV for moderate to severe disease, can change to oral formulation after clinical improvement
	Same daily dose of TMP-SMX as above, given in divided doses q8h for 21 days OR 1920 mg (two TMP-SMX double-strength tablets) PO q8h for 21 days	Given for mild disease
Clindamycin-primaquine	Clindamycin 600-900 mg IV q6h-q8h plus primaquine 15-30 mg PO q24h for 21 days OR Clindamycin 300-450 mg PO q6h-q8h plus primaquine 15-30 mg PO q24h for 21 days	Methemoglobinemia less likely if primaquine dose of 15 mg PO q24h is used
Pentamidine	4 mg/kg IV q24h for 21 days	Diluted in 250 mL of 5% dextrose in water and infused over 60 minutes 3 mg/kg IV q24h for 21 days used by some clinicians to reduce toxicity
Trimethoprim-dapsone	Trimethoprim 15 mg/kg PO q24h in divided doses q8h plus dapsone 100 mg PO q24h for 21 days	
Atovaquone	750 mg PO q12h for 21 days	Give with food to increase absorption
Glucocorticoids	Prednisolone 40 mg PO q12h on days 1-5, then 40 mg PO q24h on days 6-10, then 20 mg PO q24h on days 11-21 OR Methylprednisolone IV at 75% of dose given above for prednisolone	Regimen recommended by CDC/NIH/IDSA; widely used in United States
	Methylprednisolone 1 g IV q24h on days 1-3, then 0.5 g IV q24h on days 4-6, then prednisolone 40 mg PO q24h, tapered to 0 over days 7-16	Regimen widely used in United Kingdom

*NOTE: None of these regimens for adjuvant glucocorticoids therapy have been compared in prospective clinical trials.
CDC, Centers for Disease Control and Prevention; *NIH*, National Institutes of Health; *IDSA*, Infectious Diseases Society of America.

established. Many physicians advocate "treating through" minor rash, often adding an antihistamine and a short course of oral prednisolone (30 mg every 24 hours, tapering to zero over 5 days).

Other Therapeutic Agents

If treatment with TMP-SMX fails, or is not tolerated by the patient, several alternative therapies are available (see Tables 29-7 and 29-8).

Clindamycin-Primaquine

The combination of clindamycin and primaquine is widely used for treatment of PCP whatever the severity. The combination is as effective as oral TMP-SMX and oral trimethoprim-dapsone for the treatment of mild and moderate-severity disease. As a second-line treatment it is effective in up to 90% of patients. Methemoglobinemia due to primaquine occurs in up to 40% of patients. If a once-daily dose of 15 mg rather than 30 mg of primaquine is used, the likelihood of methemoglobinemia is reduced. Diarrhea develops in up to 33% of patients receiving clindamycin. In such instances, stool samples should be analyzed for the presence of *Clostridium difficile* toxin.

Trimethoprim-Dapsone

This oral combination is as effective as oral TMP-SMX and oral clindamycin plus primaquine (see earlier) for treatment of mild and moderate-severity PCP. The combination has not been shown to be effective in patients who have severe PCP. Most patients experience methemoglobinemia (caused by dapsone), which usually is asymptomatic. Up to one half of patients have mild hyperkalemia caused by trimethoprim.

Atovaquone

Atovaquone is licensed for the treatment of mild and moderate-severity PCP in patients who are intolerant of TMP-SMX. In tablet formulation (no longer available), this drug was less effective but was better tolerated than TMP-SMX or intravenous pentamidine for treatment of mild or moderate-severity PCP (see Tables 29-7 and 29-8). There are no data from prospective studies that compare the liquid formulation (which has better bioavailability) with other treatment regimens. Common adverse reactions include rash, fever, nausea and vomiting, and constipation. Absorption of atovaquone is increased if it is taken with food.

Intravenous Pentamidine

Intravenous pentamidine is now seldom used for the treatment of mild or moderate-severity PCP because of its toxicity. Intravenous pentamidine may be used in patients who have severe PCP, despite its toxicity, if other agents have failed (see Tables 29-7 and 29-8). Nephrotoxicity develops in almost 60% of patients given intravenous pentamidine (indicated by elevation in serum creatinine), leukopenia develops in approximately half, and up to 25% have symptomatic hypotension or nausea and vomiting. Hypoglycemia occurs in approximately 20% of patients. Because of the long half-life of the drug, this effect may emerge up to several days after the discontinuation of treatment. Pancreatitis also is a recognized side effect.

Caspofungin

The echinocandin caspofungin inhibits (1,3)-β-D-glucan synthase and is effective against *Aspergillus* and *Candida*. Case reports and small case series show that a regimen of caspofungin, used alone or in combination with other therapy, may be

effective therapy for PCP in patients not responding to or tolerating first-line therapy. It has not been prospectively evaluated against TMP-SMX or other therapeutic agents for first-line therapy.

Adjuvant Glucocorticoids

For patients who have moderate and severe PCP, adjuvant glucocorticoid therapy reduces the risk of respiratory failure by up to half, and the risk of death by up to one third (see Tables 29-7 and 29-8). Glucocorticoids are given to HIV-infected patients with confirmed or suspected PCP who have a PaO_2 less than below 70 mm Hg or a $PO_2(A-a)$ greater than greater than 33 mm Hg. Oral or intravenous adjunctive therapy is given at the same time as (or within 72 hours of starting) specific anti–*P. jirovecii* therapy. Clearly, in some patients treatment is commenced on a presumptive basis, pending confirmation of the diagnosis. If glucocorticoids are started at a later time, the benefits are less clear, although most clinicians would use these agents in patients with moderate or severe PCP. In prospective studies, adjuvant glucocorticoids have not been shown to be of benefit in patients with mild PCP. However, it would be difficult to demonstrate this, given that survival in such cases approaches 95% with standard treatment.

General Management of *Pneumocystis jirovecii* Pneumonia

Mild PCP may be treated on an outpatient basis with oral TMP-SMX if the patient is able to manage at home, is willing to attend the outpatient clinic for regular review, and exhibits clinical and radiographic evidence of recovery. If the patient is intolerant of oral TMP-SMX despite clinical recovery, either the drug is switched to an intravenous formulation or the regimen may be changed to oral clindamycin plus primaquine. All patients with moderate and severe PCP should be hospitalized and given intravenous TMP-SMX or intravenous clindamycin and oral primaquine (plus adjuvant steroids). Patients with moderate or severe disease who show clinical and radiographic response by days 7 to 10 of therapy may be switched to oral TMP-SMX to complete the remaining 14 days of treatment. If the patient has failed to respond within 7 to 10 days or deteriorates before this time, while receiving TMP-SMX, then treatment should be changed to clindamycin and primaquine, or intravenous pentamidine.

Deterioration in the Patient with *Pneumocystis jirovecii* Pneumonia

Deterioration in a patient who is receiving anti–*P. jirovecii* therapy may occur for several reasons (Table 29-9). Before deterioration is ascribed to treatment failure necessitating a change in therapy, these alternatives should be evaluated carefully. It also is important to consider treating for any copathogens present in BAL fluid and to perform bronchoscopy if the diagnosis was made empirically, and to repeat the procedure or carry out open lung biopsy to confirm that the diagnosis is correct.

Prognosis

The prognosis for patients with severe PCP with respiratory failure requiring admission to the ICU has improved over the last decade. This improvement probably is due to better management of respiratory failure and ARDS, rather than to specific improvements in PCP care or to use of ART (see further on). Factors associated with poor outcome include increasing patient

Table 29-9   **Causes of Clinical Deterioration in a Human Immunodeficiency Virus (HIV)-Infected Patient with *Pneumocystis jirovecii* Pneumonia**

Cause	Comments
Severe progressive pneumonia	
Side effects of therapy	Drug-induced anemia Drug-induced methemoglobinemia
Iatrogenic	Pulmonary edema due to fluid overload
Postbronchoscopy	Sedation Pneumothorax
Pneumothorax	Spontaneous
Copathology in lung	Bacterial infection CMV infection Intercurrent pulmonary embolism
Wrong diagnosis	When diagnosis of PCP is empirical and is in fact bacterial pneumonia
Inadequate therapy	Wrong dose or route of administration Adjuvant glucocorticoids omitted in moderate or severe disease

CMV, cytomegalovirus; *PCP*, *Pneumocystis* pneumonia.

age, need for mechanical ventilation, and development of a pneumothorax. The last factor reflects both the association between this complication and PCP and the subsequent difficulty in successful mechanical ventilation of such patients.

Timing of Initiation of Antiretroviral Therapy in a Patient with *Pneumocystis* Pneumonia

The optimal timing of initiation of ART after PCP remains to be determined; some clinicians start ART immediately, whereas others prefer to see a clinical response to PCP treatment. One randomized trial of patients with opportunistic infection, approximately two thirds of whom had PCP, demonstrated that ART was associated with a significant reduction in mortality but no evidence of increased IRIS when ART was initiated early (within 2 weeks) compared with deferred therapy (i.e., at 4 weeks or later after initiation of treatment for the opportunistic infection. Although this study supports early ART, it does not show whether immediate treatment at time of PCP diagnosis or waiting for a response to PCP treatment (usually within 4 to 7 days) is the best strategy. Furthermore, the study excluded those with severe laboratory abnormalities and required patients to be able to take oral medication, so mechanically ventilated patients were not studied, suggesting possible selection bias in favor of less sick patients.

TREATMENT OF MYCOBACTERIAL DISEASES

Treatment of Tuberculosis

The treatment of HIV-related mycobacterial disease is complex. Not only do patients have to take prolonged courses of relatively toxic agents, but also these antimycobacterial drugs have side effects similar to those of other prescribed medications, especially those used for ART. Drug-drug interactions also are extremely common.

Overlapping Toxicity

In the developed world, isoniazid-related peripheral neuropathy is rare in HIV-negative subjects taking pyridoxine. The

nucleoside reverse transcriptase inhibitors (RTI) didanosine and stavudine, which are now less rarely used in the United States and the United Kingdom, but which frequently are seen in the developing world can also cause a painful peripheral neuropathy. This complication develops in up to 30% of patients if stavudine and isoniazid are coadministered. Rash, fever, and biochemical hepatitis are common adverse events with rifamycins, pyrazinamide, and isoniazid (occurring more frequently in patients with tuberculosis who have HIV infection with hepatitis C coinfection). The non-nucleoside RTI drugs (e.g., nevirapine) have a similar toxicity profile. If treatment for both HIV and tuberculosis is coadministered, then ascribing a cause may be problematic.

Drug-Drug Interactions

Drug-drug interactions between medications used to treat tuberculosis and HIV infection occur because of their common pathway of metabolism, through the hepatic cytochrome P-450 enzyme system. Rifampin is a potent inducer of this enzyme (rifabutin less so), which may result in subtherapeutic levels of non-nucleoside RTI and protease inhibitor antiretroviral drugs, with the potential for inadequate suppression of HIV replication and the development of resistance to HIV. In addition, the protease inhibitor class of antiretroviral drugs inhibits the metabolism of rifamycins, which leads to increases in their plasma concentration and is associated with increased drug toxicity. The non-nucleoside RTI drugs are inducers of this enzyme pathway. Coadministration of rifabutin with efavirenz requires an increase in the dose of rifabutin to compensate for the increase in its metabolism induced by efavirenz (see later). The newer classes of ART such as integrase inhibitors (e.g., raltegravir) or second-generation non-nucleoside RTI (e.g., rilpivirine) also are significantly affected by rifamycins.

Type and Duration of Therapy for Tuberculosis

The optimal duration of treatment of tuberculosis, using a rifamycin-based regimen, in a patient who has HIV infection is unknown. Current recommendations from the BHIVA and the ATS/CDC/Infectious Diseases Society of North America (IDSA) are to treat tuberculosis in HIV-infected patients in the same way as for the general population (i.e., for 6 months for drug-sensitive pulmonary tuberculosis). In addition, ATS/CDC/IDSA guidelines recommend that treatment be extended to 9 months in patients who have cavitation on the original radiograph, continuing clinical signs, or a positive culture after 2 months of therapy.

Risk for development of rifampin monoresistance in HIV-infected patients receiving the drug has been reported. This association is especially strong if intermittent regimens are used and may be related to a lack of efficacy of the other drugs present in the combination (e.g., intermittent isoniazid). Hence, daily medication regimens are recommended and should be closely supervised in all HIV-positive patients. In clinical practice, rifabutin usually is given thrice weekly with ritonavir-boosted protease inhibitors. This regimen appears generally to achieve adequate rifamycin levels, although therapeutic drug failure and rifamycin resistance have recently been reported in patients who demonstrated appropriate adherence to prescribed treatment. Some clinicians now routinely prescribe daily rifabutin at its thrice-weekly dose and monitor drug levels. Little additional toxicity is reported, although the regimen is more expensive and has not been fully evaluated.

Directly observed therapy (DOT) is an important although fairly labor-intensive strategy that has the support of the WHO.

It is of undoubted value in populations at risk for nonadherence, such as substance abusers, the homeless, and people with mental health problems, and can be integrated with addressing other health care needs. This approach can help to offset what might appear punitive to persons in DOT programs.

Timing of Initiation of Antiretroviral Therapy for Tuberculosis

Recent data are available that can guide the optimal time to start ART in patients being treated for tuberculosis. Initial decision analysis showed that early treatment with antiretroviral therapy led to a marked reduction in further opportunistic disease. Against this was balanced the risk of needing to discontinue antituberculosis therapy or ART because of drug toxicity or drug-drug interactions. IRIS was reported to be more likely if these treatments were started at the same time.

These findings have now been confirmed in several studies from around the world, predominantly in developing nations. In essence, deferred ART (i.e., given at least 8 weeks after starting antituberculosis therapy) was associated with significantly increased mortality, when compared to treatment started within 4 weeks. Although IRIS was several times more frequent in the latter population, its morbidity generally was manageable and mortality was low. The survival benefit of early treatment was most pronounced in post hoc analyses in subjects with the lowest CD4+ counts (that is, less than 50 cells/µL).

Delaying the start of antiretroviral therapy can simplify patient management and may reduce or prevent adverse drug reactions and drug-drug interactions; plus also reduce the risk of IRIS. Based on current guidance for general ART initiation, patients with CD4+ counts above 350 cells/µL, who are at low risk of HIV disease progression or death during 6 months of treatment for tuberculosis, could defer ART until treatment for tuberculosis is completed or well under way. In these patients, the CD4+ count should be closely monitored. In patients who have CD4+ counts of 349 to 100 cells/µL, many centers currently delay starting ART until after the first 2 months of treatment for tuberculosis have been completed, and patients are given concomitant PCP prophylaxis. In those with CD4+ counts below 99 cells/µL, ART is started as soon as possible after initiation of treatment for tuberculosis.

Two options exist for starting antiretroviral therapy in a patient already being treated for tuberculosis. First, the rifampin-based regimen is continued and ART is commenced—for example, with a combination of two nucleoside RTIs and a non-nucleoside RTI such as efavirenz (if the patient weighs more than 60 kg, the efavirenz dose often is increased to 800 mg given once daily, to compensate for rifampin-induced metabolism of efavirenz). Alternatively, the rifampin is stopped and rifabutin is started: Antiretroviral therapy is given, with a combination of two nucleoside RTI drugs and either a single ritonavir-boosted protease inhibitor or a non-nucleoside RTI. Here the dose of rifabutin is adjusted to take into account the pharmacokinetic effect of the coadministered drug. With a boosted protease inhibitor, it usually is prescribed at a dose of 150 mg thrice weekly, and with efavirenz, it is increased to 450 mg once a day, although as discussed earlier, some centers will use 150 mg rifabutin once daily.

Immune Reconstitution Inflammatory Syndrome

Before the advent of ART, physicians treating patients with tuberculosis recognized that an apparent response to the antimycobacterial treatment would sometimes be followed by a short period of clinical deterioration. This paradoxical reaction (in the context of overall treatment response) was seen as an interesting and probably immune-based phenomenon directed against residual mycobacterial antigen, of generally little consequence. The widespread introduction of ART has led to an increased awareness by clinicians of similar but generally more severe events in HIV-infected persons. In the context of HIV infection, a reaction of this type is now termed *immune reconstitution inflammatory syndrome* (IRIS), or immune reconstitution disease.

Such reactions can manifest in a number of ways, and in association with a range of opportunistic conditions. Perhaps the most common of these is similar to a paradoxical reaction. In this instance, after initiation of ART in a patient being treated for tuberculosis, for example, the original symptoms and signs or new features develop. These often are of an inflammatory nature and may be associated with marked radiographic changes. Manifestations of IRIS may include fever, dyspnea, lymphadenopathy, effusions, parenchymal pulmonary infiltrates, or expansion of cerebral tuberculomas. This form of IRIS is seen most frequently with disease due to mycobacteria (commonly *M. tuberculosis* or MAC), fungi (notably, *Cryptococcus*), and viruses (hepatitis viruses and Herpesviridae).

IRIS develops in up to one third of HIV-infected patients being treated for tuberculosis when ART is started. The median time to onset of tuberculosis-related IRIS is about 4 weeks from beginning antituberculosis treatment or 2 weeks from commencing ART. It appears to be more likely in patients who have disseminated tuberculosis (and hence presumably more stimulating antigen present as well as more potential for significant inflammatory reactions); and a lower baseline blood CD4+ count. A rapid fall in HIV load as well as a large increase in CD4+ counts in response to ART may also predict IRIS; as might circulating inflammatory cytokines such as interferon-γ or markers such as C-reactive protein. The relationship between early use of ART and low blood CD4+ counts suggests that care must be taken when antiretrovirals are started in patients with tuberculosis at sites where rapid expansion of an inflammatory mass could be life-threatening. Examples of this are cerebral, pericardial, or peritracheal disease (**Figure 29-20**).

An important point is that IRIS currently is a diagnosis of exclusion. No specific laboratory test is available to assist with this, and it should be made only after progressive or (multi) drug-resistant tuberculosis, poor drug adherence (to either antituberculosis or antiretroviral agents) and drug absorption, or an alternative pathologic process has been excluded as an explanation for the presentation. Criteria have been drawn up that seek to provide clinical diagnostic guidelines (**Box 29-4**).

The mechanism leading to IRIS is unclear. It is not due to failure of treatment of tuberculosis or to another coexistent disease process, and if anything it is most likely to represent an exuberant and uncontrolled response to mycobacterial antigens (from both dead and alive organisms).

Current treatments include nonsteroidal antiinflammatory drugs and glucocorticoids. The latter are undoubtedly effective although they can lead to hyperglycemia and hypertension. Recurrent aspiration of lymph nodes or effusion also may be needed. Although IRIS often is self-limiting, it may persist for several months. Rarely, temporary discontinuation of ART is required. In this situation there may be precipitous falls in CD4+ counts, and patients are at risk of other opportunistic infections.

Attention also has focused on an issue of possibly greater concern—the form of IRIS referred to as the "unmasking phenomenon": In some persons with presumably latent

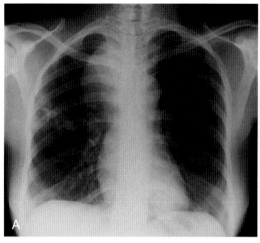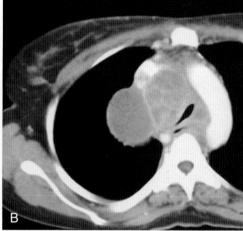

Figure 29-20 Chest radiograph (**A**) and CT scan (**B**) showing massive mediastinal lymphadenopathy in a patient with IRIS due to *Mycobacterium tuberculosis.* *(Reproduced from Buckingham SJ, Haddow LJ, Shaw PJ, Miller RF: Immune reconstitution inflammatory syndrome in HIV-infected patients with mycobacterial infections starting highly active anti-retroviral therapy, Clin Radiol 59:505–513, 2004.)*

Box 29-4	**Diagnostic Criteria for Immune Reconstitution Inflammatory Syndrome in Human Immunodeficiency Virus-Infected Patients with Tuberculosis**

Evidence Supporting Diagnosis
1. Initial diagnosis of tuberculosis confirmed by laboratory methods or by appropriate response to treatment
2. Development of new clinical phenomena temporally associated with start of ART, including but not limited to:
   - New or enlarging lymphadenopathy, cold abscesses, or other focal tissue involvement
   - New or worsening central nervous system disease
   - New or worsening radiologic features of tuberculosis
   - New or worsening serositis (pleural effusion, ascites, pericardial effusion, or arthritis)
   - New or worsening constitutional symptoms such as fever, night sweats, and/or weight loss
   - Retrospective review indicating that clinical or radiologic deterioration occurred in the absence of change in tuberculosis treatment regimen
3. Immune restoration (e.g., a rise in CD4+ lymphocyte count in response to ART)
4. A fall in HIV "viral load" in response to ART

Alternative Diagnoses to Be Excluded
Progressive underlying infection
Treatment failure due to drug resistance (MDR or XDR)
Treatment failure from poor adherence
Adverse drug reaction
Comorbidity—another, coexistent diagnosis (e.g., non-Hodgkin lymphoma)

ART, antiretroviral treatment; *MDR,* multidrug-resistant; *XDR,* extensively drug-resistant.

---

tuberculosis infection who start ART, systemic active (and often infectious) tuberculosis develops within a 3-month period. Although the patient's disease probably would have manifested in time anyway, and some reported cases may in fact represent progression of previously subclinical tuberculosis, reflecting ascertainment bias, the current view is that this phenomenon is real and constitutes an adverse effect of ART. In view of the fact that persons most at risk live in countries with limited facilities for pre-ART screening, this issue has major implications for ART rollout programs in resource-poor areas. It has led to heightened need for intensified screening using simple algorithms that seek to exclude mycobacterial infection and disease before institution of ART. One consequence of this added awareness is the increased use of regimens to treat LTBI, plus the increased detection of subclinical active tuberculosis cases.

Treatment of Disseminated *Mycobacterium avium* Complex Infection

Combination antimycobacterial therapy by itself does not cure MAC infection. A commonly used regimen is oral clarithromycin 500 mg once daily or every 12 hours with oral ethambutol 15 mg/kg once daily with or without oral rifabutin 300 mg once daily. If clarithromycin is not used, oral rifabutin 600 mg once daily is given—the lower dose adjusting for yet more drug-drug interactions. Use of three drugs has no impact on overall outcome, although it reduces the risk of resistance and possibly enhances early mycobacterial killing. In patients whose clinical status is severely compromised by symptoms, intravenous amikacin 7.5 mg/kg once daily for 2 to 4 weeks also is given. Trough blood levels must be measured to ensure that toxic accumulation of amikacin does not occur. Fluoroquinolones such as moxifloxacin or levofloxacin may be extremely useful because they have good antimycobacterial activity with limited side effects. At present, many of these agents are not licensed for this indication. In view of the concerns regarding XDR tuberculosis, it is important to ensure that patients are adherent to such treatment regimens, thereby reducing the risk for development of fluoroquinolone resistance.

Mycobacterium kansasii Infection

A frequently used regimen consists of rifampin, isoniazid, and ethambutol in conventional doses; all drugs are given by mouth.

TREATMENT OF FUNGAL INFECTIONS

The treatment regimens for fungal infections complicating HIV infection are shown in **Table 29-10**.

Cryptococcosis

After initial treatment of cryptococcal infection there is a high likelihood of relapse of infection; hence, lifelong secondary preventive therapy is needed unless ART is commenced and

Table 29-10 Treatment of Fungal Pulmonary Infection in Human Immunodeficiency Virus (HIV)-Infected Patients

Infectious Agent	Drug	Comments
Aspergillus spp.	Voriconazole 6 mg/kg IV q12h on day 1, then 4 mg/kg IV q12h, then 200 mg PO q12h	Change to oral therapy once evidence of clinical recovery
	OR Liposomal amphotericin 5 mg/kg IV q24h	Use for severely ill patients, monitor renal function
Cryptococcus neoformans	Liposomal amphotericin 4-6 mg/kg IV q24h plus	Monitor renal function
	Flucytosine 50 mg/kg IV q6h for 2-4 weeks	Monitor blood count, liver and renal function
	OR Fluconazole 300-400 mg PO q12h for 2-4 weeks	
Histoplasma capsulatum	Liposomal amphotericin 3 mg/kg IV q24h , then itraconazole 200 mg PO q8h for 3 days, then 200 mg PO q12h	Use for severely ill patients Monitor renal function Change to oral therapy after 2 weeks or after clinical improvement obtained Monitor itraconazole levels
	Itraconazole 200 mg PO q8h for 3 days, then 200 mg PO q12h for 6-12 weeks	Use for less severely unwell patients Monitor itraconazole levels
Coccidioides immitis	Amphotericin B 0.5-1 mg/kg q24h for 2-4 weeks OR Liposomal amphotericin 4 mg/kg IV q24h for 2-4 weeks	Monitor renal function
Penicillium marneffei	Liposomal amphotericin 3 mg/kg IV q24h for 2 weeks, THEN Itraconazole 400 mg PO q24h for 10 weeks	Use for severely ill patients Monitor renal function Monitor itraconazole levels
	Itraconazole 400 mg PO q24h for 4-6 weeks	Use for mild disease Monitor itraconazole levels

results in sustained improvements in CD4$^+$ counts (greater than 250 cells/µL) and suppression of HIV load in peripheral blood. Secondary prophylaxis most often is with oral fluconazole, 200 to 400 mg four times daily. Just as with mycobacterial disease, "late" IRIS events can occur after months or even years. These should be investigated to exclude active disease and other conditions.

Histoplasmosis

Oral itraconazole 200 mg twice daily is the current treatment of choice. The dose is adjusted to achieve blood trough drug levels that are above the standard lowest effective concentration. There are no data on the impact of ART on which to base decisions about discontinuation of secondary prophylaxis.

Coccidioidomycosis

Treatment of coccidioidomycosis is difficult. After initial treatment with amphotericin B, either itraconazole or fluconazole may be given for long-term suppression. The overall prognosis is poor, with a 40% mortality rate despite therapy. There are no data on the impact of ART on which to base decisions about discontinuation of secondary prophylaxis.

Penicillium marneffei Infection

Oral itraconazole has now replaced amphotericin B as the treatment of choice for *P. marneffei* infection, apart from the subgroup of patients who are acutely unwell. Fluconazole is less effective than itraconazole. After initial treatment, lifelong suppressive therapy with itraconazole is needed. There are no data on the impact of ART on which to base decisions about discontinuation of secondary prophylaxis.

TREATMENT OF PARASITIC INFECTIONS

The treatment regimens are shown in **Table 29-11**.

Toxoplasmosis

A combination of sulfadiazine and pyrimethamine is the regimen of choice for *T. gondii* infection. The most frequent dose-limiting side effects are rash and fever. Adequate hydration must be maintained to avoid the risk of sulfadiazine crystalluria and obstructive uropathy. Alternative regimens are given in Table 29-11. Once treatment is completed, lifelong maintenance is necessary to prevent relapse, unless ART achieves adequate immune restoration (blood CD4$^+$ count above 250 cells/µL and undetectable HIV load).

Visceral Leishmaniasis

Visceral leishmaniasis usually is treated with liposomal amphotericin B, although this therapy is associated with a high rate of relapse. Second-line therapy (or first-line in cash-poor environments) is to use sodium stibogluconate (see Table 29-11).

Strongyloides stercoralis Infection

The agent of choice for treatment of *S. stercoralis* infection is ivermectin. Risk of treatment failure with thiabendazole in HIV-infected persons is higher than that in non–HIV-infected patients.

TREATMENT OF VIRAL INFECTIONS

Cytomegalovirus Infection

Cytomegalovirus pneumonitis is treated with intravenous ganciclovir 5 mg/kg every 12 hours, for 14 days. Drug-induced

Table 29-11 Treatment of Parasitic Infections in Human Immunodeficiency Virus (HIV)-Infected Patients

Infectious Agent	Drug	Comments
Toxoplasma gondii		
First choice	Sulfadiazine 1-1.5 g PO q6h plus pyrimethamine 200 mg PO q24h on day 1, then 50 mg (in patients weighing <60 kg) or 75 mg (in patients weighing >60 kg) plus folinic acid 15 mg PO q24h for 14-28 days	Rash and fever are common
Second choice	Clindamycin 600 mg PO or IV q6h plus pyrimethamine and folinic acid (doses as above) for 14-28 days	If diarrhea develops, analyze stool for *Clostridium difficile*
Leishmania spp.		
First choice	Liposomal amphotericin B 2-4 mg/kg IV q24h for 10 days	
Second choice	Sodium stibogluconate 20 mg/kg IV or IM q24h for 3-4 weeks	
Strongyloides stercoralis	Ivermectin 200 μg/kg PO q24h for 4 doses over 16 days	

neutropenia is managed with granulocyte colony-stimulating factor. Some centers use valganciclovir, an oral formulation of ganciclovir, at a dose of 900 mg orally every 12 hours, to treat CMV pneumonitis. Side effects and their management are as for ganciclovir. Phosphonoformate (foscarnet) can be used for treatment of CMV end-organ disease (e.g., pneumonitis), although it has an extensive toxicity profile.

Influenza A

HIV-infected patients presenting with documented or suspected influenza A and duration of symptoms for 48 hours or less should receive the neuraminidase inhibitor oseltamivir, in a dose of 75 mg given orally twice a day, or zanamivir, in a dose of 10 mg given by inhalation twice a day, both given for 5 days (assuming that a majority of circulating strains in a given flu season are susceptible). Additionally, in patients with documented influenza A and a CD4+ count below 200 cells/μL, a neuraminidase inhibitor may be given in absence of fever or if duration of symptoms is longer than 48 hours. In patients with H1N1, treatment often is given regardless of duration of symptoms.

CLINICAL COURSE AND PREVENTION

Within the past several years, advances in drug therapy have radically altered the depressingly predictable nature of progressive HIV infection. Combinations of prophylaxis against specific opportunistic infections and ART can reduce both the incidence of common conditions and the associated mortality. The observational North American Multicenter AIDS Cohort Study (MACS) demonstrated that the risk of PCP in patients with blood CD4+ counts less than 100 cells/μL can be reduced almost four-fold (from 47% to 13%) if both specific prophylaxis and ART are taken. However, as common conditions are prevented, other less treatable illnesses may arise.

It has become apparent that specific infection prophylaxis also may confer protection against other agents. This "cross-prophylaxis" is seen particularly with the use of TMP-SMX for PCP which also provides cover against cerebral toxoplasmosis and several common bacterial infections (although not those caused by *S. pneumoniae*), and with use of macrolides for MAC infection, which further reduces the incidence of bacterial disease and also PCP. Use of large amounts of antibiotic raises the possibility of future widespread drug resistance. This concern clearly is of clinical import, and recent reports suggest that indeed in some parts of the world, the incidence

of pneumococcal TMP-SMX resistance is rising. Current preventive therapies pertinent to lung disease focus on *P. jirovecii*, MAC, *M. tuberculosis*, and certain bacteria (**Table 29-12**).

PNEUMOCYSTIS JIROVECII *PNEUMONIA PROPHYLAXIS*

Numerous studies have demonstrated the greatly increased risk of PCP in persons with blood CD4+ counts below 200 cells/μL who do not take adequate drug therapy. Clinical symptoms also constitute an independent risk factor for PCP; accordingly, the current guidelines recommend lifelong prophylaxis against *P. jirovecii* in HIV-infected adults who have had previous PCP, CD4+ counts below 200 cells/μL, constitutional symptoms (documented oral thrush or fever of unknown cause with temperatures above 37.8° C that persists for more than 2 weeks), or clinical AIDS. The importance of secondary prophylaxis (i.e., used after an episode of PCP) becomes clear from historical data, which indicate a 60% risk of relapse in the first 12 months after infection.

The increases in systemic and local immunity that occur with ART have led to several studies evaluating the need for prolonged prophylaxis in persons with sustained elevations in blood CD4+ counts and low HIV RNA load. In summary, it appears that both primary and secondary PCP prophylaxis can be discontinued once CD4+ counts are above 200 cells/μL for more than 3 months. A caveat to this is that the patient should have a low or undetectable HIV RNA load, that the CD4+ percentage is stable or rising and is greater than 14% and that the patient plans to continue ART over the long term with good adherence.

Recent data accrued from a cohort study, a retrospective review and a case series show a low incidence of PCP among patients who discontinued or never started PCP prophylaxis, who were receiving ART and had CD4+ counts between 100 and 200 cells/μL and plasma HIV viral loads of less than 50 to 400 copies/mL. Although these data imply that primary PCP prophylaxis can be safely discontinued in certain patients with CD4+ counts between 100 and 200 cells/μL, with some experts recommending this approach for their patients, this has not been widely adopted.

Trimethoprim-Sulfamethoxazole

As with treatment strategies, TMP-SMX is the drug of choice for prophylaxis of PCP (**Table 29-13**). It has the advantages of being highly effective for both primary and secondary prophylaxis (with the 1-year risk of PCP during therapy with this

Table 29-12 Prevention of Respiratory Infections in Human Immunodeficiency Virus (HIV)-Infected Adults

Organism	Preventive Method	Specific Agent	Indications	Cost	Comments
Pneumocystis jirovecii	Regular drug	Trimethoprim-sulfamethoxazole (daily)	Persistent thrush, fever, AIDS, CD4$^+$ count <200 cells/μL	Cheap	Provides cross-protection May lead to resistance
Mycobacterium tuberculosis	Regular drug	Isoniazid (6-12 months)	Purified protein derivative positive Close contact with active case	Cheap	Compliance a potential problem, therefore resistance possible
Mycobacterium avium complex	Regular drug	Clarithromycin (daily) or azithromycin (weekly)	CD4$^+$ count <50 cells/μL	Expensive	Provides cross-protection May lead to resistance
Streptococcus pneumoniae	Immunization	23-valent capsular polysaccharide (single dose)	All subjects at diagnosis and at 5 years	Cheap	Uncertain protection Transient increase in HIV "load"
Influenza virus	Immunization	Whole or split virus (yearly)	All subjects	Cheap	Uncertain protection Transient increase in HIV "load"

AIDS, acquired immunodeficiency syndrome

Table 29-13 Primary and Secondary Prophylaxis Regimens for *Pneumocystis jirovecii* Pneumonia

Drug	Dose	Comments
Trimethoprim-sulfamethoxazole	1 double-strength* tablet PO q24h	*Other options for primary prophylaxis*: 1 double-strength* tablet PO q24h 3×/week OR 1 single-strength† tablet PO q24h Protects against toxoplasmosis and certain bacteria
Dapsone	100 mg PO q24h	With pyrimethamine (25 mg PO q24h 3×/week) Protects against toxoplasmosis
Pentamidine	300 mg given by Respirgard II (jet) nebulizer every 4 weeks	Less effective in subjects with CD4$^+$ <100 cells/μL Provides no cross-prophylaxis
Atovaquone	750 mg PO q12h	Absorption increased if administered with food Protects against toxoplasmosis

*160 mg trimethoprim plus 800 mg sulfamethoxazole.
†80 mg trimethoprim plus 400 mg sulfamethoxazole.

agent being 1.5% and 3.5%, respectively). It is cheap, can be taken orally, acts systemically, and provides some cross-prophylaxis against other infections, such as toxoplasmosis and infections due to *Salmonella* spp., staphylococci, and *H. influenzae*. Its main disadvantage is that adverse reactions are common (see earlier), occurring in up to 50% of patients taking the prophylactic dose.

The standard dose of TMP-SMX is one double-strength tablet (containing 160 mg of trimethoprim plus 800 mg of sulfamethoxazole) per day. Other regimens have been tried; these include one "double-strength" tablet thrice weekly and one single-strength tablet per day. In general, when used for primary prophylaxis, these regimens are tolerated well (if not better than the standard) and appear to be as efficacious as one double-strength tablet per day. The data are less clear in secondary prophylaxis, in which subjects are at a much higher risk for recurrent PCP. Attempts to desensitize patients who are intolerant of TMP-SMX have met with some success.

Dapsone

In patients who cannot tolerate TMP-SMX, dapsone is a safe and inexpensive alternative. It has been studied in a number of trials as both primary and secondary prophylaxis and is effective at an oral dose of 100 mg/day. When combined with pyrimethamine (25 mg three times per week), it provides a degree of cross-prophylaxis against toxoplasmosis. Before starting dapsone, patients are tested for glucose-6-phosphate dehydrogenase deficiency.

Pentamidine

Nebulized pentamidine has largely fallen from use as a prophylactic agent. Initial advantages included better clinical tolerance and efficacy similar to that of TMP-SMX for primary preventive therapy. The associated breakthrough rate for this agent, however, is higher in patients who have lower CD4$^+$ counts (i.e., below 100 cells/μL) and in those who take it as secondary prophylaxis. Other disadvantages include delivery equipment costs and complexity (alveolar deposition is crucial, so the nebulizer system used is important), the risk of transmission of respiratory disease (e.g., tuberculosis) to other patients and staff during the nebulization procedure, altered clinical presentation of PCP during pentamidine therapy (increased frequency of radiographic upper zone shadowing, increased incidence of pneumothorax), and a lack of systemic protection against *Pneumocystis* and other infectious agents. In addition, an acute bronchoconstriction effect during nebulization has been noted. Long-term follow-up studies have not demonstrated any significant negative effect on lung function.

Atovaquone

Atovaquone oral suspension is used as a second-line prophylactic agent in patients intolerant of TMP-SMX. It appears to be similar in efficacy to dapsone (given together with weekly pyrimethamine), with a reduced incidence of side effects, of which the most frequent are rash, fever, and gastrointestinal disturbance.

Predictors of *Pneumocystis* Prophylaxis Failure

A low blood CD4+ count (less than 50 cells/μL) is the current best laboratory predictor of prophylaxis failure. This correlation is not particularly surprising because the median blood CD4+ count of subjects not on prophylaxis who develop PCP is below 50 cells/μL. Persistent fever of unknown cause is an important clinical risk factor for PCP. Used as preventive therapy, TMP-SMX significantly reduces the chance for development of *Pneumocystis*. It is therefore vital that subjects who are most vulnerable be encouraged to use this drug on a regular basis.

BACTERIAL INFECTION PROPHYLAXIS

The effective and safe (i.e., replication-incompetent) bacterial vaccines that are available would be expected to be widely used to prevent HIV-related disease. In fact, clinical acceptance of both pneumococcal and the *H. influenzae* type b (Hib) vaccines is poor (current estimates for the former are at most only 40% of the infected population for use of the recommended 23-valent vaccine). One reason for this low uptake rate may be that the protection conferred by vaccination (90%) in the general population is not seen in immunosuppressed HIV-infected persons, reflecting their inability to generate adequate memory B cell responses (especially those with CD4+ counts below 200 cells/μL). In North America, however, the CDC/IDSA recommendation is to give the pneumococcal vaccine as a single dose as soon as HIV infection is diagnosed, with a booster at 5 years, or if an individual patient's blood CD4+ count was less than 200 cells/μL and subsequently increased on ART. Several studies show that pneumococcal immunization reduces the risk of invasive pneumococcal infection in this population. This does not appear to be the case in a developing nation setting, where not only is the 23-valent vaccine ineffective against both invasive and noninvasive pneumococcal disease but the overall incidence of pneumonia is increased. Conjugated pneumococcal vaccines confer enhanced protection but are currently much more expensive. Cost-benefit analyses are awaited.

Infection with Hib is less common in HIV-infected adults. Accordingly, immunization with Hib vaccine is not routinely recommended.

There is little evidence to suggest that the high frequency of bacterial infections in the HIV population is related to bacterial colonization. Therefore, continuous antibiotics are rarely indicated, although both TMP-SMX and the macrolides (clarithromycin and azithromycin) given as long-term prophylaxis for opportunistic infection have been shown to reduce the incidence of bacterial pneumonia, sinusitis or otitis media, and infectious diarrhea. The use of TMP-SMX also confers a survival advantage in many studies performed in resource-poor settings. There is little evidence, however, showing that TMP-SMX protects against pneumococcal infection.

PREVENTION OF INFLUENZA A

All HIV-infected persons, regardless of CD4+ count, should be offered annual immunization against influenza A.

MYCOBACTERIUM TUBERCULOSIS *PROPHYLAXIS*

The interaction between HIV and tuberculosis is of fundamental importance because the annual risk for the development of clinical tuberculosis in a given patient is estimated to be 5% to 15% (i.e., similar to a non–HIV-infected subject's *lifetime* risk). The concern that HIV-infected patients may develop disseminated infection after bacillus Calmette-Guerin (BCG) administration means that despite its undoubted potential protective value in many parts of the world where HIV infection is rife, clinicians may be wary of using it routinely. As such, effective case finding (largely for active infectious disease, though increasingly for LTBI) becomes even more relevant to tuberculosis control. The distinction between LTBI (i.e., clinically asymptomatic disease with a normal appearance on the chest radiograph and negative mycobacterial sputum cultures) and active tuberculosis disease is distorted by HIV. *M. tuberculosis* can be isolated from asymptomatic persons, while active disease symptom screens are so all-encompassing that they are poorly specific.

HIV-infected patients with pulmonary tuberculosis are less likely to be AFB smear–positive than their HIV-negative counterparts, although they are still infectious and can transmit tuberculosis. One of the problems with standard methods of tuberculosis contact tracing when applied to HIV infected subjects is that both TST results and chest radiology may be unreliable. However, in the absence of BCG immunization, a positive PPD (e.g., greater than 5 mm induration with 5 tuberculin units) indicates a greatly increased risk of future active disease (6- to 23-fold compared with nonanergic, PPD-negative, HIV-infected subjects).

The introduction of commercial mycobacterial interferon gamma release assays (IGRAs), which are highly sensitive indicators of mycobacterial infection and are reasonably specific for detection of *M. tuberculosis* (although unaffected by BCG), has renewed interest in screening strategies for LTBI. The tests have some clear advantages over TST (including reducing false positives due to BCG, less potential for reporter error when the TST is read, and no need for a return visit by the subject under investigation if the IGRA result is negative). Because IGRAs detect host immunity, however, they are inevitably affected by HIV infection and are less sensitive in subjects with declining immunity (and low blood CD4+ counts). They cannot discriminate between recent and past infection, so they yield a positive result in large numbers of people in tuberculosis-endemic areas. They do not test for active disease, and results generally do not revert to negative after successful treatment of LTBI or active tuberculosis. In low-tuberculosis-prevalence settings, such as the United States and the United Kingdom, IGRAs may offer a cost-effective means of identifying persons who are at high risk for development of active tuberculosis and hence should be offered LTBI treatment.

The WHO recommends at least 6 months of isoniazid (together with pyridoxine to prevent peripheral neuropathy). This drug is safe and well-tolerated, although compliance is a problem (especially if treatment is for longer than 6 months). There is little evidence to suggest that this single-agent regimen leads to isoniazid resistance, which probably reflects the low mycobacterial load present in such patients. In view of the concerns regarding undertreatment of subclinical active disease, however, some workers are now advocating use of molecular diagnostic methods as part of an initial screen before initiation of LTBI therapy.

Recent studies performed in tuberculosis-endemic settings have shown useful and comparable efficacy of rifapentine plus isoniazid weekly for 3 months, or twice-weekly rifampin and isoniazid also for 3 months, and of 6 months or longer of isoniazid alone. A 36-month monotherapy regimen of isoniazid was superior to a 6-month regimen in a study performed in Botswana. Of note, the benefit of treatment (in preventing the development of active disease) was apparent only in subjects who were TST-positive before LTBI treatment, suggesting that the longer course was not merely preventing exogenous, newly acquired infection.

Secondary LTBI prophylaxis after treatment for active disease generally is not recommended, because ART will reduce the risk of tuberculosis by 50% to 80% after 3 months of therapy and should be encouraged. ART also appears to have an additive (and similar-sized) effect to that of specific antituberculosis therapy in reducing the risk of progression to tuberculosis disease during primary prophylaxis.

MYCOBACTERIUM AVIUM *COMPLEX PROPHYLAXIS*

Data from North America indicate that the prevention of disseminated MAC infection has an effect on survival (25% reduction in mortality rate in subjects taking clarithromycin). The U.S. guidelines advise prophylaxis with a macrolide (either clarithromycin 500 mg orally twice per day or azithromycin 1250 mg orally once a week) in all HIV-infected persons with blood CD4+ counts >50 cells/μL. In Europe, where the prevalence of disseminated MAC infection probably is lower (perhaps because of previous BCG vaccination), this may be less relevant. Here, surveillance cultures of blood may be more cost effective in the at-risk HIV population with low CD4+ counts. Routine stool and sputum cultures probably do not add much to this strategy because disseminated MAC is much more common than isolated organ disease.

Single-agent prophylaxis may lead to antibiotic resistance. This does not seem to be reduced by the addition of a second drug (rifabutin) to the prophylactic regimen. The latter is now a second-line prophylactic agent, largely as a result of its rather worse protective effect and its adverse interaction profile with protease inhibitors. As mentioned earlier, if the patient sustains a rise in CD4+ count above 100 cells/μL for longer than 6 months, it is safe to discontinue prophylaxis.

PROGNOSIS

PNEUMOCYSTIS JIROVECII *PNEUMONIA*

Several clinical and laboratory features have prognostic significance in HIV-infected patients with PCP (**Box 29-5**). Severity scores based on the patient's age, use of injection drugs, serum albumin, serum bilirubin, and $PO_2(A–a)$, or the patient's age, hemoglobin, PaO_2, presentation with a second or third episode of PCP, the presence of medical comorbidity and of pulmonary Kaposi sarcoma can predict survival reasonably accurately, with the highest scores indicating the worst outcome. In the era of ART the mortality from an episode of PCP is approximately 10%.

BACTERIAL INFECTION

In general, the outcome with bacterial respiratory infection in HIV-infected patients is similar to that seen in the HIV-negative population. Clinical and laboratory markers of disease severity that have been defined in the adult general population (e.g., those described in the ATS, or the BTS guidelines for the

---

Box 29-5 Prognostic Factors Associated with Poor Outcome in *Pneumocystis jirovecii* Pneumonia

On Hospital Admission
Older age
Reduced body mass index
No previous knowledge of HIV serostatus
Tachypnea (respiratory rate higher than 30 breaths/minute)
Second or subsequent episode of *Pneumocystis jirovecii* pneumonia
Poor oxygenation: PaO_2 <53 mm Hg or $PO_2(A–a)$ >30 mm Hg
Low serum albumin (<35 g/dL)
Low hemoglobin (<12.0 g/dL)
Peripheral blood leukocytosis (>10.8 × 10⁹/L)
Elevated serum lactate dehydrogenase levels (>300 IU/L)
Elevated serum bilirubin
Elevated C-reactive protein level
CD4+ count <50 cells/μL
Marked chest radiographic abnormalities: diffuse bilateral interstitial infiltrates with or without alveolar consolidation
Medical comorbid or other coexistent condition (e.g., pregnancy)

After Hospital Admission
At bronchoscopy:
1. In bronchoalveolar lavage fluid: detection of
   ● copathogens: CMV, bacteria
   ● neutrophilia (>5% neutrophils on differential count)
2. Detection of pulmonary Kaposi sarcoma
Serum lactate dehydrogenase levels that remain elevated
Development of pneumothorax
High APACHE II score on ICU admission
Need for mechanical ventilation

APACHE II, Acute Physiology and Chronic Health Evaluation [study] II; *CMV*, cytomegalovirus; *HIV*, human immunodeficiency virus; *ICU*, intensive care unit.

---

management of community-acquired pneumonia in adults) apply to HIV-infected patients. These are confusion, raised respiratory rate, abnormal renal function, and low blood pressure. Recurrent pneumonia is common (reported in up to 55% of cases) and may lead to chronic pulmonary disease (see earlier).

MYCOBACTERIUM TUBERCULOSIS *INFECTION*

Although tuberculosis normally responds to standard multiple-drug therapy, work from Africa has highlighted the increased mortality rate in HIV-infected compared with non–HIV-infected persons. A relationship also has been described between risk of death and blood CD4+ count: HIV-infected patients with CD4+ counts below 200 cells/μL have a mortality rate of 10%, compared with 4% in those with CD4+ counts of 200 to 499 cells/μL. As discussed previously, early use of ART (i.e., within the first 4 weeks of treatment) is now recommended in subjects with low blood CD4+ counts.

MYCOBACTERIUM AVIUM *COMPLEX INFECTION*

Several case-control studies have indicated that in the absence of effective treatments, MAC-infected patients have a reduced survival compared with CD4+ count–matched control subjects (approximately 4 months versus 9 months, respectively). Currently available treatment regimens may reduce this difference, although severe anemia appears to be an independent predictor of death in patients with this infection.

CONTROVERSIES AND PITFALLS

ANTIRETROVIRAL THERAPY AND OPPORTUNISTIC INFECTIONS

The introduction of ART, together with the wide availability of accurate methods of determining plasma RNA viral load, has led to profound changes in both clinical practice and outcome with HIV disease. Respiratory disease, in particular, bacterial pneumonia and tuberculosis, still occurs more frequently than in HIV-seronegative subjects, despite apparently effective ART. Overall, however, data indicate that clinical progression is rare in subjects who are able to adhere rigorously to at least 95% of their antiretroviral drug regimen. Mortality rates have fallen by 80% for almost all conditions, and it seems that a damaged immune system can, to a clinically significant extent, be reconstituted for a period of at least several years. Thus, clinicians need to consider not only opportunistic infection or malignancy within the diagnostic workup but also the effects of drug therapy itself. The adverse effect profile of ART (e.g., metabolic and mitochondrial toxicities, liver damage, and neuropsychiatric disorders), as well as the large number of drug-drug interactions, makes this a highly complex area of clinical management. The best-characterized example of this issue is HIV-related tuberculosis. Here, not only is there overlap between toxicity and pharmacologic interaction, but IRIS is common. Research is needed to address this area. Studies should inform the decision on when to start ART in patients already on antituberculosis medication: For example, should ART begin at much higher blood CD4+ counts than those currently recommended? What are good and simple predictors of an individual patient's risk for IRIS? Other work needs to focus on elucidation of why full pulmonary immunity is not restored with ART.

PREDICTORS OF DISEASE

Despite the benefits of ART, it is likely that in the long term, HIV infection will progress to severe disease. Currently, little work has been conducted in this area. Research should focus on developing strategies that are cost-effective and practicable in both high and low tuberculosis burden settings. This is important, because in the latter, respiratory disease such as tuberculosis remains a common problem, even in subjects of known HIV serostatus. For example, recent U.K. guidance on screening for LTBI in HIV infection has not been evaluated at a national level.

As discussed previously, immune-based tests have shown promise in immunocompetent patients with LTBI. If these tests can be refined to work consistently in HIV infection at a reasonable cost, the possibility emerges for targeting persons at risk for future tuberculosis, or for predicting tuberculosis "unmasking" after initiation of ART. The recent descriptions of whole genome sequencing and microarrays of host immune signatures to distinguish LTBI from active disease are important in this respect.

Rapid diagnostics that are not exorbitant in cost and complexity are urgently needed. A common clinical scenario is that in which the patient presents with nonspecific signs and symptoms potentially associated with any of numerous entities in an extensive differential diagnosis. Often, the best treatment regimen is multiple and empirical—as, for example, in a patient from an endemic tuberculosis area with low blood CD4+ counts who has both pulmonary and central nervous system disease: Is the clinical problem tuberculosis, toxoplasmosis, cryptococcosis, or viral or bacterial infection? Any such test for tuberculosis would also have to distinguish between the different states of old (treated), old (inactive), old (latent) and active. Although not insurmountable, at present, such distinction is not possible. Some encouraging data have been derived from urine lipoarabinomannan (LAM) assays, which are of less value in HIV-negative subjects than in the HIV-infected. This difference is due to the large amount of renally cleared LAM associated with the overall increased bacterial load present in HIV-related tuberculosis. Utilizing such specific aspects of tuberculosis or HIV pathology may encourage development of novel and specific tests.

Rapid diagnostic assays that assess organism viability also are important. If the clinician can receive early feedback on whether treatment is producing a suitable killing effect, then therapy can be tailored to the individual patient. This feedback enables regimens to be "dose-adjusted" as needed and removes the element of concern that often is present when patients are slow to respond. Such delayed response is well recognized in the treatment of PCP or other fungal or mycobacterial disease, for example.

BACTERIAL INFECTIONS

The frequency of bacterial infection (often recurrent) with its attendant sequelae makes effective strategies for vaccination an important priority. The reason for the observed differential response to vaccination is unclear—even in the United States, African Americans do not seem to derive the same benefit as that observed in whites. This difference merits further research, together with more emphasis on identifying the local immune response present in the lung in such patients.

Bacterial infections may be clinically indistinguishable from other pathogens, and only two thirds of all respiratory infections are formally diagnosed. Improved methods to address this problem are needed. The use of rapid antigen tests may be one way forward. Rapid availability of results is especially important in view of the high incidence of (potentially fatal) bacteremia present in populations of affected patients. For maximum benefit, such screening requires a system that is simple and cheap and hence suitable to both resource-rich and resource-poor countries.

MYCOBACTERIAL DISEASES

M. tuberculosis is globally the most important HIV-related pathogen. Strategies of control and prevention are vital to ensure that millions of people do not become co-infected and that those who are do not go on to develop clinical disease. Rapid diagnostics are critical. The encouraging reports of the simple and cheap MODS assay and also user-friendly molecular techniques, both to diagnose tuberculosis and then to provide resistance data in field settings (see earlier), argue for large-scale rollout and evaluation.

Beyond public health measures such as infection control, rapid case finding, DOTs, use of fixed-dose combination drugs, case management, and education, research needs to improve on current drug therapy. Long-acting preparations such as rifapentine show promise but, as the problem with rifampicin monoresistance demonstrates, much work remains to be done. Several antimycobacterial drugs are now in clinical trials. Initial data are promising, and several agents have novel mechanisms of action. The Global Alliance and the WHO "Stop TB" campaigns have been crucial in this regard. The fluoroquinolones moxifloxacin and gatifloxacin are now widely available. These potent drugs possess considerable ability both to kill mycobacteria and also to "sterilize" infected sites. Trials of treatment-shortening regimens are ongoing worldwide. These drugs also are important as part of treatment protocols and stratagems that will effectively tackle the estimated 500,000 new cases of MDR tuberculosis, in addition to benefiting the 50,000 persons who have currently almost untreatable XDR tuberculosis across the world.

Vaccination against *M. tuberculosis* using BCG has been attempted with caution in immunosuppressed HIV-infected populations. However, a safe vaccine may be the only affordable way of protecting large parts of the world from tuberculosis. So far there appears to be more success with vaccines to either enhance or replace the primary protective effects of BCG.

PNEUMOCYSTIS JIROVECII *DISEASE-RELATED ISSUES*

Newer methods of diagnosis (e.g., PCR tests on oral rinse samples) may prove invaluable for quick and easy disease confirmation, although their applicability to routine samples needs further evaluation.

Despite the efficacy of TMP-SMX for *P. jirovecii* prophylaxis, compliance remains a problem. One concern with widespread use of prophylaxis is that resistance to TMP-SMX will start to emerge. Reports have indicated that certain mutations in the *P. jirovecii* dihydropteroate synthase gene confer resistance. These mutations seem to be increasing over time, although they do not appear to be present in many patients in whom treatment for PCP with TMP-SMX lacks efficacy. The implications of this observation are uncertain but could include a greater likelihood of treatment failure and the possibility of worsening patterns of global bacterial drug resistance.

SUGGESTED READINGS

Crothers K, Thompson BW, Burkhardt K, et al: Lung HIV Study: HIV-associated lung infections and complications in the era of combination antiretroviral therapy, *Proc Am Thorac Soc* 8:275–281, 2011.

Huang L, Cattamanchi A, Davis JL, et al: International HIV-Associated Opportunistic Pneumonias (IHOP) Study; Lung HIV Study: HIV-associated *Pneumocystis* pneumonia, *Proc Am Thorac Soc* 8:294–300, 2011.

Kaplan JE, Benson C, Holmes KH, et al: Centers for Disease Control and Prevention (CDC); National Institutes of Health; HIV Medicine Association of the Infectious Diseases Society of America: Guidelines for prevention and treatment of opportunistic infections in HIV-infected adults and adolescents: recommendations from CDC, the National Institutes of Health, and the HIV Medicine Association of the Infectious Diseases Society of America, *MMWR Recomm Rep* 58(RR-4):1–207, 2009.

Morris A, Crothers K, Beck JM, Huang L: American Thoracic Society Committee on HIV Pulmonary Disease: An official ATS workshop report: emerging issues and current controversies in HIV-associated pulmonary diseases, *Proc Am Thorac Soc* 8:17–26, 2011.

Pozniak AL, Coyne KM, Miller RF, et al: BHIVA Guidelines Subcommittee: British HIV Association guidelines for the treatment of TB/HIV coinfection 2011, *HIV Med* 12:517–524, 2011.

Chapter **30**

Noninfectious Conditions in Patients with Human Immunodeficiency Virus Infection

Thomas Benfield

Although most complications affecting the lungs during the course of HIV infection arise from the viral infection itself, especially as reported early in the epidemic, HIV-infected patients may present with or subsequently develop complications related to alterations in immune regulation. A marked CD8+ T cell infiltrate in the lung may be caused by HIV in both symptomatic and nonsymptomatic patients. The effects of the virus on the pulmonary microenvironment include a progressive decline in local immunocompetence that results in failure to mount a protective immune response against opportunistic infections. The spectrum of noninfectious complications associated with HIV infection encompasses other idiopathic conditions and pulmonary malignancies, which include Kaposi sarcoma, Hodgkin and non-Hodgkin lymphomas, and solid tumors (**Table 30-1** and **30-2**).

RESPIRATORY SYMPTOMS AND PULMONARY FUNCTION

Respiratory symptoms, impaired diffusion, emphysema, airway obstruction, and small airway disease related to HIV infection are common clinical findings. In a recent study of 167 HIV-1–infected persons, nearly two thirds were found to have diffusion impairment and one fifth had irreversible airway obstruction. The most common symptoms and signs were dyspnea and a cough. Severe symptoms such as shortness of breath at rest were less frequent. Patients with respiratory symptoms were more likely to be current or past injection drug users and smokers. Approximately one fourth reported using respiratory inhaler medication. Smoking and the number of pack-years smoked increased the risk of diffusion impairment and airway obstruction. Prophylaxis for *Pneumocystis jirovecii* pneumonia and low CD4+ cell counts increased the risk for impaired diffusion, and treatment with cART increased the risk for airway obstruction. These associations may be a proxy for the duration of HIV-1 infection and severity of the underlying immunodeficiency. The correlation with low CD4+ cell counts supports this possibility. Overall, the HIV-infected population appears to be more susceptible to noninfectious disease for a number of reasons. Smoking cessation counseling certainly offers one possibility of reducing the increased susceptibility.

NEOPLASIA

Cancer incidence is higher in persons with immunodeficiency of all causes. In HIV-1 infection, cancers that are uncommon in the general population predominate and include mainly lymphoma and Kaposi sarcoma. Other, more common cancers are now seen with increasing frequency; however, as HIV-1 infection has become controllable with antiretrovirals.

KAPOSI SARCOMA

Epidemiology, Risk Factors, and Pathogenesis

In the general population, Kaposi sarcoma is a rare benign skin tumor that develops in the skin of the lower extremities in elderly men from the Mediterranean area. The disease, originally described in 1872 by the Hungarian physician Moricz Kaposi, is 100 to 1000 times more frequent in persons with HIV-1 infection than in the general population and is associated with an aggressive course. The incidence of AIDS-associated Kaposi sarcoma has, however, declined substantially over the past 2 decades. Before the advent of cART, incidence rates ranged from 25 to 50 cases per 1000 person-years of follow-up (PYFU) but have steadily declined, so that the incidence in a cART-treated population is less than 5 per 1000 PYFU. Approximately 5% to 10% of all diagnosed cases of AIDS are based on a finding of Kaposi sarcoma. HIV-1–infected men who have sex with men have a 20 times higher risk for development of this tumor than in persons in other transmission groups. Frequency increases with lower CD4+ T cell counts, but the disease can occur at all levels of immunodeficiency. Thus, when Kaposi sarcoma is the AIDS-defining illness, it may occur at a relatively higher CD4+ T cell count than other such illnesses.

Kaposi sarcoma is an angioproliferative inflammatory condition that is associated with infection with human herpesvirus type 8 (HHV-8). Gene expression profiling shows that the lesions consist of aberrant endothelial and inflammatory cells of lymphatic origin. HHV-8, a γ-2 herpesvirus of the *Rhadinovirus* genus, has been demonstrated in all forms of Kaposi sarcoma, and in situ hybridization has demonstrated the presence of HHV-8 RNA and DNA in spindle, endothelial, and mononuclear cells of the tumor. HHV-8 DNA is detectable in peripheral blood before the development of the tumor, and increased viral replication is evident before onset of symptoms.

Table 30-1	Noninfectious Pulmonary Conditions Associated With Human Immunodeficiency Virus Type 1 Infection
Disease Category	**Specific Disease(s)**
Neoplastic disease	Kaposi sarcoma Castleman disease Non-Hodgkin lymphoma Primary effusion lymphoma Lung cancer
Inflammatory disease	Nonspecific interstitial pneumonitis Lymphocytic interstitial pneumonitis Lung fibrosis
Airway disease	Chronic obstructive pulmonary disease Emphysema
Pulmonary vascular disease	Pulmonary hypertension
Miscellaneous	Antiretroviral treatment–induced respiratory disease

Table 30-2	Association of Noninfectious Pulmonary Conditions with Degree of Immunodeficiency
Degree of Immunodeficiency	**Noninfectious Pulmonary Condition**
Severe (CD4$^+$ cell count less than 50 cells/μL)	Kaposi sarcoma Castleman disease Non-Hodgkin lymphoma Primary effusion lymphoma Lung cancer Nonspecific interstitial pneumonitis Lymphocytic interstitial pneumonitis Chronic obstructive pulmonary disease Pulmonary hypertension Antiretroviral treatment–induced respiratory disease
Moderate to severe (CD4$^+$ cell count 50-200 cells/μL)	Kaposi sarcoma Non-Hodgkin lymphoma Lung cancer Nonspecific interstitial pneumonitis Lymphocytic interstitial pneumonitis Chronic obstructive pulmonary disease Pulmonary hypertension Antiretroviral treatment–induced respiratory disease
Moderate (CD4$^+$ cell count 200-350 cells/μL)	Non-Hodgkin lymphoma Lung cancer Chronic obstructive pulmonary disease Pulmonary hypertension Antiretroviral treatment–induced respiratory disease
Normal (CD4$^+$ cell count greater than 350 cells/μL)	Lung cancer Chronic obstructive pulmonary disease Pulmonary hypertension

More than 80% of patients with AIDS-associated Kaposi sarcoma have antibodies to HHV-8. HHV-8 may exert its oncogenic potential in several ways. The HHV-8 genome contains several genes that are homologues to human genes. Among these is a latent nuclear antigen that binds to p53 and associates viral DNA to human DNA during mitosis; a viral cyclin that activates cyclin-dependent kinases to prevent human cells from remaining in a G_1 phase; a constitutively expressed receptor (viral interleukin-8 receptor) that may be involved in angiogenesis; a Bcl-2 like protein that prevents apoptosis; and viral homologues to cytokines (viral macrophage inflammatory protein [MIP] and viral interleukin-6) that may be responsible for some of the constitutive symptoms associated with Kaposi sarcoma. Cytokines are required for HHV-8–infected endothelial cells to acquire their phenotype and for continued growth of the tumor. The HIV-1 Tat protein upregulates cytokines and metalloproteinases that further promotes the oncogenic potential of Kaposi sarcoma cells.

Genetics

Genetic polymorphisms of the Fc-γ receptor IIIA, the interleukin-6 and interleukin-8 promoter regions have been associated with an increased risk for development of Kaposi sarcoma. Some human leukocyte antigen (HLA) types also have been associated with this disease.

Clinical Features

Cutaneous and mucocutaneous manifestations of AIDS-associated Kaposi sarcoma are the more common and usually precede visceral disease by months to years. Skin and visceral lesions appear as red or violet macules, papules, or nodules that may coalesce to form plaque-like lesions. Lesions may affect any area of the skin and involve any organ system. Lymphadenopathy is frequent.

Pulmonary Kaposi sarcoma may cause nonproductive cough, hemoptysis, shortness of breath, chest pain, and fever. In rare instances, involvement of the larynx or trachea may cause airway obstruction. Extrapulmonary involvement is frequent, but 15% of cases of Kaposi sarcoma occur without skin lesions. CD4$^+$ cell counts are low (0 to 100/μL) at the time of diagnosis. Examination of the lungs usually shows no abnormalities. Chest radiograph may be normal in appearance but commonly shows singular or multiple peribronchovascular nodules (**Figure 30-1**, *A* and *B*). Diffuse infiltration and air space consolidation also may be present. Pleural effusion is common. Hilar and mediastinal lymphadenopathy may be visible on chest films but are better visualized with computed tomography (CT) scanning. With pulmonary disease, CT scans typically reveal peribronchovascular nodules that are larger than 1 cm in diameter. The role of magnetic resonance imaging (MRI) or positron emission tomography (PET) in the diagnosis and management of pulmonary Kaposi sarcoma is not clear.

Diagnosis

Pulmonary Kaposi sarcoma is highly likely in a HIV-1–infected person with a CD4$^+$ cell count of less than 100/μL, the characteristic cutaneous or mucocutaneous lesions, and pulmonary symptoms. Bronchoscopy is useful to visualize typical endobronchial lesions (see Figure 30-1, C). These are flat or slightly raised and occur throughout the tracheobronchial tree but are seen most frequently at airway bifurcations. Pleural effusions usually are exudative and may be serous or serosanguineous. Serum lactate dehydrogenase may be elevated. Histologic verification is usually not required for a diagnosis of Kaposi sarcoma. Endobronchial biopsy may confer a substantial risk of severe bleeding, but biopsy may be necessary in cases in which bronchial involvement is lacking. In such cases, transbronchial or percutaneous needle biopsy is useful. In cases of pleural Kaposi sarcoma, video-assisted thoracoscopy can be used to visualize pleural lesions and to perform biopsy. Open lung biopsy in this

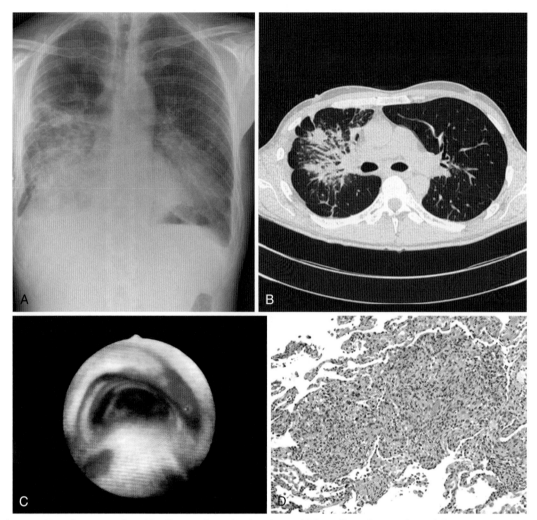

Figure 30-1 Pulmonary Kaposi sarcoma. **A** and **B,** Chest radiographs showing multiple peribronchovascular nodules. **C,** Typical violet-red endobronchial nodule visualized through a fiberbronchoscope. **D,** Transbronchial biopsy specimen of pulmonary Kaposi sarcoma lesion. *(C, Courtesy Dr. L. Huang. D, Courtesy Dr. J. Junge.)*

setting is obsolete because of the associated complications. Lung biopsy specimens show typical features of Kaposi sarcoma, which include a tumor-like infiltrate with a peribronchovascular distribution of spindle cells. Slitlike spaces without endothelium contain extravasated erythrocytes (see Figure 30-1, *D*). In situ hybridization and immunostaining usually are positive for HHV-8. HHV-8 DNA is detectable in bronchoalveolar lavage fluid (BAL) cells.

Treatment

All patients with Kaposi sarcoma should be treated with cART, but immune reconstitution may induce an inflammatory reaction and flare of the disease within 2 to 8 weeks of initiation of this therapy. Cutaneous and mucocutaneous lesions of AIDS-associated Kaposi sarcoma usually regress with cART without chemotherapy but may require additional local radiotherapy. Visceral Kaposi sarcoma, however, will necessitate chemotherapy. Concomitant use of cART increases the response rate to chemotherapy. All patients should be offered *P. jirovecii* prophylaxis regardless of their CD4+ cell count. Pegylated liposomal doxorubicin or liposomal daunorubicin are used for first-line treatment of Kaposi sarcoma, in addition to cART. In randomized multicenter trials, response rates and adverse effect profiles to both agents given as monotherapy proved to be superior to conventional chemotherapy.

Liposomal anthracyclines are well tolerated overall. Myelosuppression is the most important dose-limiting toxicity. The risk of drug-drug interactions with antiretroviral agents is low for anthracyclines. The taxane paclitaxel, in combination with granulocyte colony-stimulating factor (G-CSF), is approved for second-line treatment of Kaposi sarcoma. Experience with paclitaxel and pulmonary Kaposi sarcoma is limited, and the use of paclitaxel is associated with more severe adverse effects than those reported with anthracyclines. Paclitaxel has potential serious drug-drug interactions with antiretroviral drugs.

Due to the high cost of anthracyclines and taxanes their use may be limited in resource-poor settings. Alternatively, the most widely used regimen for the treatment of pulmonary Kaposi sarcoma, a combination regimen of doxorubicin (Adriamycin), bleomycin, and vincristine (ABV) may be used. Vincristine may be replaced with vinblastine in patients with polyneuropathy. The combination is given every 2 weeks. Response is evaluated after four to six series of chemotherapy. Response rates are 30% to 50%. Adverse side effects include anemia, neutropenia, thrombopenia, neuropathy, mucositis and alopecia. There are potential drug-drug interactions between vincristine or vinblastine and antiretroviral agents.

Investigational agents include thalidomide, imatinib, mTOR inhibitors, IL-12, and fumagilin.

Clinical Course and Prevention

Untreated pulmonary Kaposi sarcoma is associated with a median survival of less than 6 months. Combination ART improves survival in HIV-1–infected patients with pulmonary Kaposi sarcoma receiving chemotherapy to 50% and above. Severe immunodeficiency (CD4$^+$ cell count below 100/μL), pleural effusion and/or hypoxia are associated with a particularly rapid course of this disease. Prevention is best accomplished through treatment of the underlying HIV-1–related immunodeficiency with cART.

MULTICENTRIC CASTLEMAN DISEASE

Epidemiology, Risk Factors, and Pathogenesis

Castleman disease is a rare lymphoproliferative disease characterized by angiofollicular proliferation. Three histologic variants—hyaline vascular, plasma cell, and mixed—and two clinical types, localized and multicentric, have been described. The incidence of Castleman disease is increased in patients with HIV-1 infection. Multicentric Castleman disease (MCD) is associated with concomitant AIDS-associated Kaposi sarcoma. One study found HHV-8 DNA in 14 of 14 cases of HIV-1–associated MCD but in only 7 of 17 non–HIV-1–infected cases. HHV-8 DNA was detected in only 1 of 34 lymph node biopsy specimens from HIV-1–uninfected patients with localized disease. MCD frequently transforms to the non-Hodgkin form of lymphoma. Pulmonary involvement in Castleman in HIV-1 infection is exceedingly rare but probably also is underdiagnosed.

Clinical Features

The localized form of Castleman disease usually manifests as mediastinal lymph node hyperplasia without systemic symptoms. Signs and symptoms of multicentric disease include fever, generalized lymphadenopathy, fatigue, hepatosplenomegaly, and pancytopenia. Symptoms are thought to be related in part to cytokine disarray by viral homologues of IL-6 and IL-10 encoded by the HHV-8 genome. Symptoms and signs of pulmonary involvement include shortness of breath, cough, and bilateral crackles. Worsening of symptoms often is preceded by HHV-8 viremia. CD4$^+$ cell counts vary, ranging from normal to extremely low, indicating severe immunodeficiency. Chest radiographs and CT scans may show noduloreticular interstitial infiltration, mediastinal lymphadenopathy, or pleural effusions.

Diagnosis

Bronchoscopy findings usually are normal. Analysis of BAL fluid cells may show hypercellularity and lymphocytosis. A lung biopsy is required to confirm the diagnosis. HHV-8 DNA usually is detected in biopsy specimens by immunostaining or in situ hybridization techniques.

Treatment

Localized disease is cured by surgical resection. Treatment of MCD is difficult and may include corticosteroids, chemotherapy, immune therapy, and/or radiation therapy. Specific antiherpesvirus therapy with ganciclovir or foscarnet to reduce the HHV-8 replication has been shown to be of some use. Treatment with rituximab (anti-CD20 monoclonal antibody) for HIV-associated MCD is now considered the "gold standard." The most significant adverse effect may be progression of concomitant Kaposi sarcoma. Mild to moderate infections may occur.

Clinical Course and Prevention

Survival rates are poor but have improved in the era of cART, with a 5-year overall survival of approximately 50%. Patients with multicentric Castleman disease often develop non-Hodgkin lymphoma, discussed next.

NON-HODGKIN LYMPHOMA

Epidemiology, Risk Factors, and Pathogenesis

In the pre-cART era, non-Hodgkin lymphoma (NHL) represented the second most common HIV-1–associated cancer after Kaposi sarcoma. With the introduction of cART, rates of NHL have declined by 40% to 70% for most histologic subtypes. Despite the decline in incidence, NHL is now one of the most common initial AIDS-defining illnesses: The risk of low-grade lymphoma (although not AIDS-defining) is increased 4-fold, the risk of high-grade lymphoma is increased 600-fold, and the risk of primary brain lymphoma is increased 3600-fold with HIV-1 infection over corresponding risks in the absence of infection. Recognized risk factors for development of NHL include concomitant infection with Epstein-Barr virus (EBV) and/or HHV-8, as well as male gender, increased age, and immunodeficiency. A diagnosis of AIDS usually precedes primary pulmonary lymphoma.

Most AIDS-related NHLs belong to one of three categories of high-grade B cell lymphomas: Burkitt lymphoma, centroblastic lymphoma, and immunoblastic lymphoma. Burkitt and Burkitt-like lymphomas tend to occur in patients with relatively high CD4$^+$ cell counts, as compared with centroblastic large cell and immunoblastic lymphomas, which occur at low CD4$^+$ cell counts. The incidence of Burkitt lymphoma is unchanged in the era of cART. Pulmonary NHL can manifest either as primary or secondary involvement. Dissemination is common for NHL, but primary pulmonary lymphoma is a rare condition, accounting for less than 0.5% of HIV-1–related lymphomas.

The pathogenesis of NHL is complex and involves immune dysfunction together with dysregulation of cytokine responses, chronic antigen stimulation, and co-infection with EBV and HHV-8.

Genetics

Somatic mutations of immunoglobulin, c-Myc, Bcl-6, and p53 genes are associated with transformation into lymphoma. Overexpression of Bcl-2 is associated with resistance to chemotherapy and a poor prognosis. Persons heterozygous for the CCR-5 chemokine Δ32 mutation may be at reduced risk for NHL, whereas the stromal cell–derived factor 1 (SDF1)-3'A chemokine variant may be associated with an increased risk for NHL.

Clinical Features

Patients may present with nodal or extranodal disease and may have systemic symptoms. Clinical signs of advanced NHL with pulmonary involvement include fever, night sweats, and weight loss (B symptoms). Manifestations of primary pulmonary involvement include shortness of breath, cough, and chest pain. Primary pulmonary lymphoma is associated with CD4$^+$ cell counts less than 50/μL. Anemia, thrombocytopenia, and leukopenia are frequent findings. Serum lactate dehydrogenase often is elevated with secondary but not primary pulmonary involvement. Chest radiographs and CT scans commonly show isolated or multiple central or peripheral nodules (**Figure 30-2, A**). Mediastinal lymphadenopathy and pleural effusion are less common.

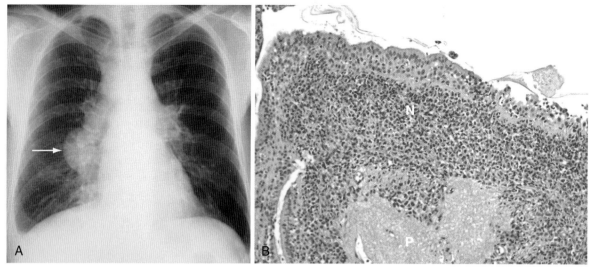

Figure 30-2 Primary pulmonary non-Hodgkin lymphoma. **A,** Chest radiograph showing a single, large central nodule (*arrow*). **B,** Transbronchial biopsy specimen of non-Hodgkin lymphoma (*N*). The patient also had *Pneumocystis jirovecii* pneumonia (*P*). *(Courtesy Dr. J. Junge.)*

Diagnosis

Fiberoptic bronchoscopy usually is normal. Cytologic examination of BAL fluid may reveal lymphoma cells, but biopsy is required to establish a histologic diagnosis. Transbronchial biopsy has reasonable diagnostic yield for secondary but not primary pulmonary lymphoma. Percutaneous thoracic needle biopsy is the most commonly used method to obtain tissue for diagnosis. In rare cases, video-assisted thoracoscopic or open lung biopsy may be necessary. Histologically, the lymphoma invades the alveolar septa and vascular walls (see Figure 30-2, *B*). Necrosis is frequent. Most tumors are high-grade centroblastic or immunoblastic large B cell lymphomas that are EBV-positive and overexpress Bcl-2.

Treatment

There is no evidence to indicate that primary or secondary pulmonary NHL should be treated differently from NHL in general. Chemotherapy regimens that include cyclophosphamide, doxorubicin, vincristine (Oncovin), and prednisone (CHOP), or CHOP-rituximab (CHOP-R), or etoposide, prednisone, vincristine (Oncovin), cyclophosphamide, and doxorubicin (EPOCH) are used in conjunction with cART. CHOP-R may be beneficial in primary pulmonary lymphoma because these often overexpress bcl-2. No significant drug-drug interactions occur between commonly used cART regimens and CHOP. Use of cART is associated with less anemia, thrombocytopenia, and other adverse effects of chemotherapy.

Clinical Course and Prevention

The median survival from primary pulmonary lymphoma is less than 4 months with chemotherapy alone. Survival from lymphoma has improved in the cART era.

PRIMARY EFFUSION LYMPHOMA

Epidemiology, Risk Factors, and Pathogenesis

Primary effusion lymphoma (PEL), or body cavity–associated lymphoma, is a rare type of non-Hodgkin lymphoma that occurs almost exclusively with HIV-1 infection. PELs grow mainly in the body cavities (pleural, pericardial, and peritoneal) as lymphomatous effusions without an identifiable contiguous tumor mass. PEL occurs predominantly in men who have sex with men and are seropositive for HHV-8. In contrast with NHL, PEL lacks c-myc gene rearrangements. PEL is positive for HHV-8 and Epstein-Barr virus, expresses CD45, exhibits clonal immunoglobulin gene rearrangements, and lacks *bcl2*, *bcl6*, *ras*, and *TP53* gene alterations.

Clinical Features

PEL is associated with progressive immunodeficiency and consequently low $CD4^+$ cell counts. Patients usually have a previous diagnosis of Kaposi sarcoma. Clinical manifestations include fever, generalized lymphadenopathy, and fatigue. Symptoms and signs of pleural involvement include shortness of breath and cough. Chest radiographs show unilateral or bilateral effusion. CT scans are useful to rule out localized masses representing NHL, Kaposi sarcoma, or other neoplastic disease. PEL usually remains localized to the body cavity of origin.

Diagnosis

The diagnosis is based on the demonstration of morphologic, immunophenotypic, immunogenotypic, viral and molecular characteristics of pleural fluid. Demonstration of HHV-8 often is necessary.

Treatment

Treatment follows guidelines for treatment of NHL and should include chemotherapy together with cART.

Clinical Course and Prevention

PEL has an aggressive clinical course and is associated with a high mortality rate. The 1-year overall survival rate is 40%.

LUNG CANCER

Epidemiology, Risk Factors, and Pathogenesis

The risk for development of small cell carcinoma, non–small cell carcinoma, and bronchoalveolar carcinoma is two to five times greater among persons with HIV-1 infection than in the general population, and such cancers appear at a younger age. Adenocarcinoma accounts for a majority of cases. Men are affected more often than women. The risk is increased with a $CD4^+$ cell count less than 500/µL. From 60% to 80% of HIV-1–infected persons are smokers, and this factor contributes significantly to the excess risk. Epidemiologic modeling, however, shows that smoking alone cannot account for the excess risk, suggesting that other cofactors are at play. It is possible that smoking may additively or synergistically together with HIV-1 infection affect the lung more severely than in non–HIV-1–infected persons. HIV-1 may enhance lung damage, leading to increased oxidative stress.

Clinical Features

Clinical features do not differ from those of lung cancer in general, but HIV-1–infected patients tend to be younger at presentation. Symptoms and signs of localized disease may be subtle but may include persistent cough, shortness of breath, chest pain, and weight loss as the disease develops. Chest radiographs and CT scans may show nodular or diffuse infiltrates, hilar or mediastinal lymphadenopathy, or pleural effusion.

Diagnosis

Fiberoptic bronchoscopy may reveal bronchial invasion. Biopsy is required to establish a histologic diagnosis, and specimens can be obtained by transbronchial, percutaneous thoracic, open lung, or video-assisted thoracoscopic techniques.

Treatment

Treatment of HIV-1–associated lung cancer follows current guidelines for treatment of non–HIV-1–associated lung cancer, as described in Chapter 67.

Clinical Course and Prevention

Patients with HIV-1 infection tend to present with more advanced disease. Studies indicate that overall survival is shortened for persons with HIV-1 infection and lung cancer compared with the general population.

INFLAMMATORY PULMONARY DISORDERS

NONSPECIFIC INTERSTITIAL PNEUMONITIS

Epidemiology, Risk Factors, and Pathogenesis

Nonspecific interstitial pneumonitis (NIP), also known as chronic interstitial pneumonitis, is a common cause of pulmonary disease in adults with advanced, untreated HIV-1 infection. Half of HIV-1–infected adults without pulmonary symptoms and with CD4$^+$ T lymphocyte counts below 200 cells/μl show histopathologic changes characteristic of NIP. The incidence of NIP at different CD4$^+$ strata is unknown. NIP is rare in children.

The etiology of NIP is unknown. There is evidence of HIV-1 RNA expression in pulmonary CD4$^+$ T lymphocytes and macrophages. Cytotoxic CD8$^+$ T cells are the predominant lymphocyte type, and it is speculated that these cells induce pulmonary inflammation. Other mechanisms of lung damage include increased levels of inflammatory mediators (e.g., cytokines and leukotrienes) and release of superoxide anion from activated alveolar macrophages.

Clinical Features

The signs and symptoms of NIP are unspecific and resemble many clinical manifestations of HIV-1 infection such as cough, shortness of breath, and fever. Extrapulmonary involvement is rare. Examination of the lungs usually yields normal findings. There may be subtle hypoxia that further increases on exercise. Chest radiographs and CT scans may be normal in appearance or show diffuse alveolar, nodular, or interstitial infiltrates that are indistinguishable from those typically seen in other common HIV-1–associated infections (**Figure 30-3**, *A*). Pleural effusion is less common.

Diagnosis

Suspicion of NIP should arise when standard histocytologic studies, microbiologic staining and culture, and molecular techniques do not yield a pathogen. Thus, NIP is a diagnosis of exclusion. Tissue specimens are required to establish the diagnosis and may be obtained by bronchoscopy, fine needle aspiration, or open lung biopsy procedures. Transbronchial biopsy specimens characteristically show various degrees of perivascular, peribronchial, and pleural lymphocyte and plasma cell infiltration. Edema, fibrin deposition, pneumocyte hyperplasia, and thickening of alveolar septa are common; alveolar septal infiltration is uncommon (see Figure 30-3, *B*). Lymphoid aggregates are frequently seen. BAL fluid analysis shows lymphocytosis and a decrease in relative and absolute numbers of alveolar macrophages. Because of the risks involved with biopsy procedures, some clinicians make a presumptive diagnosis after

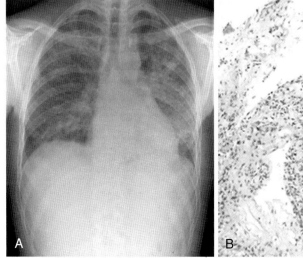
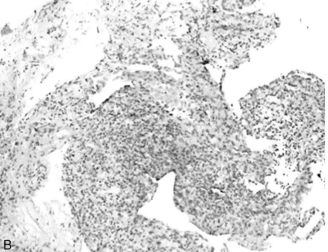

Figure 30-3 Nonspecific interstitial pneumonitis. **A,** Chest radiograph showing noninfectious bilateral diffuse infiltration before start of combination antiretroviral therapy. **B,** Transbronchial biopsy specimen. *(Courtesy Dr. J. Junge.)*

ruling out an infectious cause for the patient's pulmonary symptoms.

Treatment

Symptoms may resolve without therapy. In view of the association of NIP with severe immunodeficiency, however, initiation of cART is almost always indicated. Data from several case series indicate that cART leads to resolution of symptoms and the pathologic changes.

Clinical Course and Prevention

The natural course of NIP without cART is chronic and rarely leads to respiratory failure. Some individuals may be asymptomatic. NIP is best prevented by initiating cART before the development of moderate to severe immunodeficiency.

LYMPHOCYTIC INTERSTITIAL PNEUMONITIS

Epidemiology, Risk Factors, and Pathogenesis

Lymphocytic interstitial pneumonitis (LIP) is a disease of unknown etiology associated with HIV-1 infection and autoimmune disease. LIP occurs predominantly and not infrequently among untreated infants and children, in whom LIP is an AIDS-defining illness. LIP is rare among adults. An association has been observed between LIP and advanced HIV-1 disease. As with NIP, HIV-1 RNA expression in pulmonary CD4$^+$ T lymphocytes and macrophages has been reported.

Clinical Features

As with NIP, the symptoms of LIP are unspecific and include non-productive cough, shortness of breath, and fever. Extrapulmonary involvement of lymph nodes is common and generalized lymphadenopathy is frequent. Peripheral CD8$^+$ T lymphocytosis is characteristic. Clubbing has been reported among children. Chest radiographs may be normal but commonly show diffuse alveolar, nodular, or interstitial infiltration. Pleural effusion is common. CT scans may reveal peribronchial nodules or a diffuse ground glass appearance.

Diagnosis

Similar to NIP, LIP is an exclusion diagnosis that requires tissue samples to establish the diagnosis. Transbronchial biopsy is characterized by peribronchial, perivascular, and pleural infiltration of lymphocytic and plasma cells. These findings are also characteristic of NIP. However, septal infiltration differentiates LIP from NIP. Lymphoid aggregates are common.

Treatment

Treatment of LIP is directed at the underlying immunodeficiency caused by HIV-1. Initiation of cART is associated with resolution of pulmonary symptoms.

Clinical Course and Prevention

The natural course of LIP is variable and ranges from spontaneous remission to respiratory failure. LIP is best prevented by initiating cART before the development of moderate to severe immunodeficiency.

CRYPTOGENIC ORGANIZING PNEUMONIA

The presenting clinical features of cryptogenic organizing pneumonia (COP) in HIV-infected patients may be dramatic, with the development of a flulike illness with acute or subacute symptoms (fever, malaise, anorexia, weight loss, nonproductive cough, and dyspnea). Usually this syndrome develops in immunocompromised patients with infections or malignancy. Physical examination often reveals bibasal crackles, and the chest radiograph shows multiple bilateral alveolar opacities. Linear or nodular opacities also may be present. In patients with typical COP, alveolar lavage may demonstrate an alveolitis characterized by CD8$^+$ T lymphocytes, foamy macrophages, and a small increase in neutrophils, eosinophils, and mast cells. Treatment with glucocorticosteroids causes a remission or stabilization of the disease. However, relapse is common if the steroids are withdrawn.

CHRONIC AIRWAY DISEASE AND EMPHYSEMA

Epidemiology, Risk Factors, and Pathogenesis

HIV-1–infected smokers are 10% to 25% more likely than smokers without infection to have chronic obstructive pulmonary disease (COPD). Several factors that increase the risk for development of COPD are frequent among HIV-1–infected patients, including a high prevalence of tobacco smoking, intravenous drug use, and recurrent bacterial and opportunistic infections. COPD develops at younger age and is more prevalent among African Americans. Currently, it is unknown whether HIV-1 infection per se or the increased life expectancy associated with cART, or a combination of the two factors, accounts for the increased prevalence of COPD. Evidence appears to support all three possibilities. Ongoing viral replication and activation of pulmonary cytotoxic T lymphocytes may lead to parenchymal destruction by mechanisms similar to the effects of tobacco smoking. Advanced HIV-1 disease is associated with impairment of lung function. Some studies suggest a synergistic effect of HIV-1 and smoking, which may explain why HIV-1–infected patients may develop COPD at a younger age. HIV-1–infected intravenous drug users have reduced FEV$_1$, FVC, and diffusing capacity of carbon monoxide (DLCO) compared with persons in other transmission categories. This respiratory impairment may be explained in part by the fact that these patients more frequently are heavy smokers and suffer from recurrent lower respiratory infections. Pulmonary bacterial and opportunistic infections (e.g., *P. jirovecii* pneumonia) are associated with permanent reductions in FEV$_1$, FVC, FEV$_1$/FVC, and DLCO after recovery from the infection.

Chapter 41 deals with COPD in detail.

Genetics

Mutations in the α_1-antitrypsin gene predispose affected persons to the development of emphysema.

Clinical Features

Signs and symptoms of COPD do not differ between persons with and those without HIV-1 infection and include cough, sputum production, shortness of breath, wheezing, and chest tightness. HIV-1–infected patients may be younger.

Diagnosis

Spirometry is central to the diagnosis. Reductions in FEV$_1$, FVC, and FEV$_1$/FVC will confirm the diagnosis and establish the severity of the condition. A radiograph is useful to distinguish between COPD or emphysema and other lung and heart conditions manifesting with similar symptoms. Arterial blood gas analysis is performed to confirm hypercapnia or to establish the need for oxygen treatment.

Treatment

Treatment does not differ from COPD treatment in general. Therapy includes bronchodilators, inhaled glucocorticosteroids, and pulmonary rehabilitation. Influenza and pneumococcal vaccination is recommended and does not confer any increased risk for HIV-1 disease progression. Oxygen treatment follows general guidelines.

No important drug interactions between antiretrovirals and bronchodilators have been noted, except between some protease inhibitors and theophylline. There is the potential of drug interactions between protease inhibitors and inhaled glucocorticosteroids, but not with nucleoside and non-nucleoside analogues. Nicotine can be used to treat tobacco dependency together with antiretrovirals. There is a potential drug interaction with bupropion and protease inhibitors and non-nucleoside analogues. Similar interactions may occur with vareniclin.

Clinical Course and Prevention

The clinical course usually is not any different from that for COPD in the general population. Smoking cessation is central to successful prevention of further disease progression. Care also should be taken to avoid secondary smoke exposure. Avoidance of lung irritants is important. COPD is not believed to affect HIV-1 disease progression. Antiretroviral management of HIV-1 infection should follow national and international guidelines and should not be delayed.

HIV-1–ASSOCIATED PULMONARY HYPERTENSION

Non–HIV-1–associated pulmonary hypertension is described in detail in Chapter 58.

Epidemiology, Risk Factors, and Pathogenesis

Pulmonary hypertension is an infrequent cause of pulmonary disease among HIV-1–infected patients. However, the incidence (approximately 0.5%) is higher than for non–HIV-1–infected persons (about 0.02%), and the risk increases with age. A careful examination is required to distinguish between primary and secondary forms of pulmonary hypertension. HIV-1 infection per se is assumed to induce vascular changes associated with primary pulmonary hypertension, whereas drug use (with associated foreign particle microembolism), COPD, interstitial pulmonary disease, essential hypertension, ischemic heart disease, chronic thromboembolism, and valvular heart disease contribute to secondary pulmonary hypertension. Some reports have implicated concurrent infection with HHV-8 in the pathogenesis of pulmonary hypertension.

The pathogenesis remains unclear. Remodeling of the media and adventitia of the arterial pulmonary tree, the extracellular matrix and plexiform lesion characterize HIV-1–related and non–HIV-1–related sporadic forms. The increase in pulmonary vascular resistance may be caused by vascular growth factors, mechanical obstruction of the pulmonary arteries, hypoxia, or other stimuli. Chronic changes may remain even after the initiating insult or factor is removed. Pulmonary vascular resistance increases right ventricular systolic pressure, with consequent dilatation and dysfunction, ultimately leading to right ventricular failure.

Genetics

Familial primary pulmonary hypertension is characterized by autosomal dominant inheritance and incomplete penetrance. A mutation in the type II bone morphogenetic protein receptor (BMPR II) has been associated with this disorder.

Clinical Features

The predominant symptom is dyspnea, particularly exertional dyspnea. This symptom is nonspecific, so the diagnosis often is made late in the clinical course. Other common symptoms and signs may include other nonspecific complaints and findings such as fatigue, angina, syncope or near syncope, and peripheral edema. Pulmonary hypertension may occur at any CD4$^+$ cell count.

Diagnosis

A full diagnostic evaluation is crucial to rule out non–HIV-1–related causes, because they may necessitate other specific therapy. The chest radiograph shows cardiomegaly and enlarged central pulmonary arteries, or signs of emphysema suggestive of chronic obstructive pulmonary disease, or interstitial infiltration suggestive of parenchymal disease. Echocardiogram usually confirms right axis deviation and right ventricular hypertrophy (P pulmonale). Echocardiography provides imaging of right atrial and ventricle enlargement, tricuspidal regurgitation and reduced left ventricular size. Arterial blood gases commonly demonstrate hypoxia. Pulmonary function test is helpful to distinguish between obstructive or restrictive underlying pulmonary causes. Perfusion lung scans or CT performed with use of intravenous contrast can rule out central and peripherally located thrombi. Additionally, the lung parenchymal CT images may establish alternative diagnoses. Magnetic resonance pulmonary angiography is promising because it also provides assessment of right ventricular function. Eventually, cardiac catheterization will be necessary to measure pulmonary artery pressure, cardiac output, and left ventricular filling pressure.

Treatment

HIV-1–associated pulmonary hypertension has been treated with epoprostenol, inhaled prostacyclin, inhaled iloprost, bosentan (an endothelin receptor antagonist), and sildenafil. The effect of each agent is variable, but these drugs generally improve dyspnea and exercise tolerance. The effect is temporary, however, and concerns have emerged regarding adverse effects. Combination ART is associated with improved hemodynamics and survival. Use of anticoagulation is not supported by available evidence.

Clinical Course and Prevention

Pulmonary hypertension progresses to heart failure over 1 to 2 years despite therapy and is associated with a poor survival rate. Higher CD4$^+$ cell counts have been associated with better survival.

MISCELLANEOUS CONDITIONS

ANTIRETROVIRAL THERAPY AND RESPIRATORY SYMPTOMS

Antiretroviral treatment may cause unexpected respiratory symptoms. Lactic acidosis and hepatic steatosis with hepatic failure are rare but severe complications associated with therapy with nucleoside reverse transcriptase inhibitors (RTIs), particularly stavudine, didanosine, and zidovudine, that may occur after a few to several months of treatment. Lactic acidosis carries a high mortality rate. Patients with elevated serum lactate levels may be asymptomatic or critically ill or may report nonspecific symptoms such as dyspnea, tachypnea, fatigue, nausea, diarrhea, vomiting, and abdominal pain.

Another nucleoside RTI, abacavir, can produce a hypersensitivity reaction with fever, rash, and myalgias. Respiratory signs and symptoms, including cough, dyspnea, and pharyngitis, frequently accompany the hypersensitivity reaction. Hypersensitivity is associated with the HLA-B5701 tissue type.

The non-nucleoside RTI analogues (efavirenz and nevirapine) also may cause a hypersensitivity reaction including pulmonary hypersensitivity.

Immune reconstitution inflammatory syndrome (IRIS) may occur weeks to months after initiation of cART. IRIS is an inflammatory reaction to asymptomatic or residual opportunistic pathogens that may cause serious clinical conditions or aggravation of symptoms. Examples of such pulmonary pathogens are the HIV-1 virus, *Mycobacterium avium* complex, *Mycobacterium tuberculosis*, and *P. jirovecii*. Associated noninfectious conditions include sarcoidosis, vasculitis, and other autoimmune disease. Any inflammatory symptoms should be evaluated and treatment instituted when necessary. Optimal therapy has not been determined. Antiinflammatory therapy may attenuate symptoms, but many cases resolve spontaneously.

AGING AND PULMONARY DISEASE

Aging HIV-infected persons are at an increased risk for several chronic diseases including noninfectious pulmonary diseases. A recent observation was that in addition to COPD, lung cancer, and pulmonary hypertension, HIV-infected patients also are at increased risk for development of lung fibrosis. After controlling for smoking, the risk was found to be highest among persons older than 50 years. At present, it is unknown whether lung fibrosis is caused by HIV, by specific interstitial disease, by scarring from previous infection, or by adverse effects of antiretrovirals.

CONTROVERSIES AND PITFALLS

Noninfectious pulmonary complications of HIV-1 infection very often constitute a diagnosis of exclusion, because pulmonary infectious complications are many times more frequent than noninfectious complications. Therefore, extensive microbiologic and histopathologic workup often is required to rule out HIV-related infections such as *Pneumocystis* pneumonia (PCP).

In view of the extended life expectancy with cART and high prevalence of smoking, non–AIDS-related pulmonary malignancies are expected to increase in frequency. Many clinicians have been reluctant to refer HIV-1–infected patients to oncology services because of the dismal prognosis associated with HIV-1 infection, pulmonary cancer, and the adverse effects of aggressive chemotherapy. Recent studies, however, indicate that chemotherapy is better tolerated and response rates are higher with concomitant cART.

Another matter of some controversy is whether or not to initiate cART for nonspecific pulmonary inflammatory disease, COPD, pulmonary hypertension, and other non-AIDS pulmonary disease. In cases associated with immunodeficiency (CD4$^+$ cell count below 350 to 500/μL) or constitutional symptoms, cART should always be offered according to national and international guidelines. In other cases, initiation of cART is prudent if the underlying condition leading to pulmonary inflammatory disease, COPD, pulmonary hypertension, or another disorder is believed to be the HIV-1 infection. Most adverse effects of cART, drug interactions, and compliance issues are easily managed today with the introduction of less toxic compounds and once-daily dosing regimens.

WEB RESOURCES

AIDS Malignancy Program of the National Cancer Institute: www.cancer.gov/dctd/aids
Antiretroviral treatment guidelines: www.aidsinfo.nih.gov
HIV drug interactions: www.hiv-druginteractions.org

SUGGESTED READINGS

Aboulafia DM: The epidemiologic, pathologic, and clinical features of AIDS-associated pulmonary Kaposi's sarcoma, *Chest* 117:1128–1145, 2000.

Bower M, Collins S, Cottrill C, et al: British HIV Association guidelines for HIV-associated malignancies 2008, *HIV Med* 9:336–388, 2008.

Crothers K, Huang L, Goulet JL, et al: HIV infection and risk for incident pulmonary diseases in the combination antiretroviral therapy era, *Am J Respir Crit Care Med* 183:388–395, 2011.

Gingo MR, George MP, Kessinger CJ, et al: Pulmonary function abnormalities in HIV-infected patients during the current antiretroviral therapy era, *Am J Respir Crit Care Med* 182:790–796, 2010.

Grubb JR, Moorman AC, Baker RK, Masur H: The changing spectrum of pulmonary disease in patients with HIV infection on antiretroviral therapy, *AIDS* 20:1095–1107, 2006.

Guiguet M, Boué F, Cadranel J, et al; Clinical Epidemiology Group of the FHDH-ANRS CO4 cohort: Effect of immunodeficiency, HIV viral load, and antiretroviral therapy on the risk of individual malignancies (FHDH-ANRS CO4): a prospective cohort study, *Lancet Oncol* 10:1152–1159, 2009.

Guihot A, Couderc LJ, Rivaud E, et al: Thoracic radiographic and CT findings of multicentric Castleman disease in HIV-infected patients, *J Thorac Imaging* 22:207–211, 2007.

Rosen MJ, Beck JM: *Human immunodeficiency virus and the lung*, New York, 1998, Marcel Dekker.

Nador RG, Cesarman E, Chadburn A, et al: Primary effusion lymphoma: a distinct clinicopathologic entity associated with the Kaposi's sarcoma-associated herpes virus, *Blood* 88:645–656, 1996.

Ray P, Antoine M, Mary-Krause M, et al: AIDS-related primary pulmonary lymphoma, *Am J Respir Crit Care Med* 158:1221–1229, 1998.

Sitbon O, Lascoux-Combe C, Delfraissy JF, et al: Prevalence of HIV-related pulmonary arterial hypertension in the current antiretroviral therapy era, *Am J Respir Crit Care Med* 177:108–113, 2008.

Chapter **31**
Tuberculosis and Nontuberculous Mycobacterial Infections

Nicholas Walter • Charles L. Daley

The genus *Mycobacterium* consists of slow-growing organisms that are widely disseminated throughout the world and range from species that cause no human disease to those such as *Mycobacterium tuberculosis* and *Mycobacterium leprae* that are responsible for enormous morbidity and mortality. Mycobacteria are aerobic bacilli with high concentrations of lipids in their cell wall, which make them impermeable to most common stains. However, because of their ability to retain carbolfuchsin dye despite decolorization attempts with acid alcohol, they are referred to as acid-fast bacilli (AFB). Although mycobacteria can produce disease in almost any site, two groups of mycobacteria have a propensity for causing pulmonary infections: certain members of the *M. tuberculosis* complex and the nontuberculous mycobacteria (NTM).

Tuberculosis (TB) is the disease caused by bacteria of the *M. tuberculosis* complex, which includes the clinically relevant species *M. tuberculosis*, *Mycobacterium bovis*, and *Mycobacterium africanum*. Although *M. tuberculosis* is the most common cause of TB worldwide, both *M. bovis* and *M. africanum* can produce clinically indistinguishable forms of disease. The tubercle bacilli have been around for thousands of years, with evidence of human infection dating back to Neolithic, pre-Columbian, and early Egyptian times. Not until the Industrial Revolution, however, did TB become a major cause of human disease and death. It is estimated that approximately 25% of all adults died from TB in Europe during the 17th and 18th centuries. Throughout this period, the etiology of TB was hotly debated, with some of these early investigators arguing for a hereditary cause and others for a transmissible etiology. Finally, in 1882, Robert Koch presented his momentous discovery: The tubercle bacillus was the cause of TB. Early attempts at therapy, including the sanatorium movement, surgery, and lung collapse therapy, provided little relief from TB, and it was not until the discovery of paraaminosalicylic acid (PAS) and streptomycin in the 1940s that the age of antituberculosis chemotherapy began. Since that time, additional drugs have been developed, and most of the world treats TB with the same four-drug regimen administered for 6 months. More recently, however, co-infection with human immunodeficiency virus (HIV) and the emergence of drug-resistant strains of *M. tuberculosis* have conspired to complicate clinical management and to create barriers to global TB control.

The NTM group consists of nonlepromatous organisms that are not members of the *M. tuberculosis* complex. The NTM have been referred to as "mycobacteria other than tuberculosis" (MOTT), atypical mycobacteria, and environmental mycobacteria. The last designation refers to their widespread presence in the environment. The NTM have several features that distinguish them from *M. tuberculosis*: They have a wide range of pathogenicity, are not always associated with disease, and, unlike *M. tuberculosis*, are not transmissible from human to human. Of note, however, the incidence of NTM disease is increasing in many areas of the world, and the cause for this increase is unknown. Unfortunately, the pathogenic NTM are relatively drug resistant compared with *M. tuberculosis*, so NTM infections typically are difficult to treat. Because of the current poor understanding of the transmission and pathogenesis of these infections, little insight into their prevention has emerged, so no public health strategy for the control of disease caused by these ubiquitous organisms has been formulated.

TUBERCULOSIS

EPIDEMIOLOGY, RISK FACTORS, AND PATHOGENESIS

EPIDEMIOLOGY

The World Health Organization (WHO) estimates that 30% of adults worldwide are infected with organisms in the *M. tuberculosis* complex. From this large reservoir of infected people, an estimated 9 million new cases of TB occurred in 2009, leading to approximately 1.3 million deaths. In 2008, TB was estimated to be the seventh leading cause of death worldwide, and it is the number one killer of HIV-infected patients.

The burden of TB varies significantly throughout the world, with more than 90% of cases occurring among people residing in developing countries (**Figure 31-1**). The highest incidence rates for TB are in sub-Saharan Africa, particularly in the southern region of the continent. Not surprisingly, the highest prevalence of HIV co-infection also is in this region. Worldwide, approximately 23% of all persons with TB have underlying HIV co-infection; however, in sub-Saharan Africa, an estimated 50% of persons with TB have HIV/AIDS.

Recent reports of outbreaks of multidrug-resistant TB (MDR TB) and extensively resistant TB (XDR TB) have highlighted the importance of providing effective antituberculosis therapy to patients. MDR TB refers to disease caused by isolates of *M. tuberculosis* that are resistant to at least isoniazid (INH) and rifampin, whereas XDR TB refers to that due to MDR TB isolates that also are resistant to fluoroquinolones and at least one second-line injectable agent (amikacin, capreomycin, or

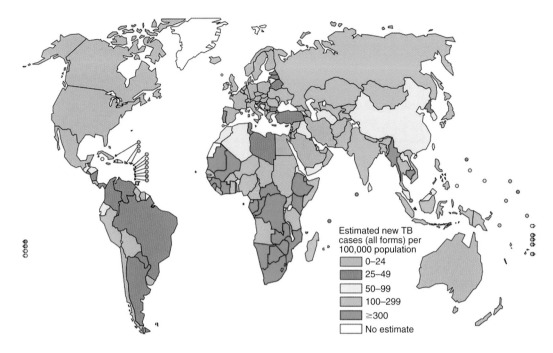

Figure 31-1 Tuberculosis (TB) notification rates, 2009. The legend depicts the number of notified TB cases, which includes both new and relapse cases per 100,000 population. *(From* Global tuberculosis control 2010, *Geneva, World Health Organization, 2010.)*

kanamycin). Surveys have documented that approximately 4.6% of TB cases worldwide are MDR TB, and 5.4% of these cases are XDR TB. More cases of drug-resistant TB exist today than in all of recorded history, and this trend is likely to continue unless more effective TB control measures are implemented globally.

In the United States, the TB case rate declined by 3% to 5% per year from 1953 to 1984. Between 1986 and 1992, the numbers of TB cases increased by approximately 20%. This increase in the number of cases was the result of at least three major factors: (1) inadequate public health measures, (2) immigration from countries where TB is prevalent, and (3) co-infection with HIV. Fortunately, case numbers have declined since 1992 and are now at a historic low. In 2010, a total of 11,181 cases of TB were reported in the United States, for an incidence of 3.6 per 100,000 population. TB case rates declined an average of 4.5% each year during 2000 to 2010. TB rates were 11 times higher among foreign-born persons than among U.S.-born people. Among U.S.-born persons, blacks were 7 times more likely to have TB than whites. Approximately 1% of new cases in the country had MDR TB, approximately 90% of whom were foreign-born. Of these MDR TB cases, approximately 1% to 2% were XDR TB.

RISK FACTORS

Certain people are at higher risk for development of TB simply because they are more likely to be exposed to and thus infected with *M. tuberculosis* (Table 31-1). For example, approximately 60% of reported TB cases in the United States occur among foreign-born people who come from areas where the disease is endemic. Other populations with an increased prevalence of TB infection include certain racial and ethnic groups, low-income populations, the homeless, and injection drug users.

Table 31-1	Criteria for a Positive Reaction on Tuberculin Skin Testing
Induration Size	**Risk Groups**
≥5 mm	HIV-infected persons Close contact with an infectious tuberculosis case Abnormal-appearing chest radiograph* consistent with previous tuberculosis Immunosuppressed patients receiving the equivalent of ≥15 mg/day of prednisone for at least 1 month
≥10 mm	Foreign-born persons recently arrived (<5 years) from high-prevalence countries Medical conditions† that increase the risk of tuberculosis Injection drug users Medically underserved, low-income populations (e.g., homeless persons) Residents and staff of long-term care facilities (e.g., nursing homes, correctional institutions, homeless shelters) Health care workers Children <4 years of age Tuberculin skin test converters (increase of ≥10 mm induration within a 2-year period)
≥15 mm	All others; these persons should not be screened in the absence of indication

*The predominant chest radiographic finding consistent with previous tuberculosis is presence of fibrotic lesions; other changes such as pleural thickening or isolated calcified granulomas are not related.
†Medical conditions and factors associated with increased risk for development of active disease in a patient with latent tuberculosis infection include silicosis, end-stage renal disease, malnutrition, diabetes mellitus, carcinoma of the head or neck and lung, immunosuppressive therapy, lymphoma, leukemia, weight loss of more than 10% ideal body weight, gastrectomy, and jejunoileal bypass.

Anyone infected with *M. tuberculosis* can develop TB disease, but certain groups are at higher-than-normal risk for progression to active disease (see Table 31-1). Patients who have been recently infected with *M. tuberculosis* and those with medical conditions associated with significant immunosuppression are at particularly high risk for development of TB. HIV co-infection is the strongest known risk factor for the development of TB and is estimated to increase the risk of progression to TB by 50- to 100-fold. Inhibitors of tumor necrosis factor-α (TNF-α) may increase the risk for development of TB by up to 10-fold, and patients taking TNF-α blockers frequently present with disseminated disease. This association appears to be stronger for infliximab and adalimumab than for etanercept. Other medical conditions are associated with a more modest increase in risk for development of disease.

PATHOGENESIS

TB is spread from person to person almost exclusively through the air by droplet nuclei, which are particles 1 to 5 μm in diameter that contain viable tubercle bacilli. Droplet nuclei are expelled into the air when patients with infectious TB create an aerosol by talking, coughing, or singing. Three factors determine the likelihood of transmitting TB: the number of bacilli expelled into the air, the concentration of organisms in the air, and the duration of contact with (i.e., breathing of) the infected air. Whether an inhaled tubercle bacillus establishes an infection in the exposed person's lung depends on both bacterial virulence and host immune defenses.

The tubercle bacillus grows slowly, dividing approximately every 18 to 24 hours. Tubercle bacilli spread through the lymphatics to the hilar lymph nodes or through the bloodstream. Small numbers of bacilli are deposited in other organs, which may then become sites of extrapulmonary disease. An adaptive immune response occurs after 2 to 8 weeks.

Once cell-mediated immunity develops, collections of activated T cells and macrophages form granulomas that wall off the mycobacterial organisms (**Figure 31-2**). For most persons with normal immune function, infection with *M. tuberculosis* seems to be arrested once cell-mediated immunity develops, even though small numbers of viable bacilli remain within the granuloma. Although a primary complex can sometimes be seen on chest radiograph, most TB infections are asymptomatic and can be detected only indirectly with a tuberculin skin test (TST) or interferon-γ release assay (IGRA). Persons with "walled-off" TB infection who do not have active disease are not infectious and thus cannot spread the disease to others.

If cell-mediated immunity does not contain the tubercle bacilli, the initial infection progresses to active disease. Without treatment, infected persons have approximately a 5% chance of developing TB in the first 1 to 2 years after infection and an additional 5% chance of developing TB during the remainder of their lifetime (**Figure 31-3**). By contrast, persons who are co-infected with HIV have a 5% to 10% annual risk of active disease developing. When active TB develops soon after infection, the disease is referred to as *primary* TB. By contrast, when TB develops years or even decades after the initial infection, the disease is referred to as *postprimary* or *reactivation* disease. Exogenous reinfection, involving acquisition of a second strain of *M. tuberculosis*, also can lead to disease and seems to be more common in HIV-infected patients.

GENETICS

Both susceptibility and resistance to developing TB have long been thought to have a genetic component. Epidemiologic and genetic studies, including those in animal and human models, support this hypothesis. Recent investigations of specific candidate genes and genome-wide scans have identified people at increased risk for TB. Although polymorphisms in more than 10 genes have been associated with active TB, only polymorphisms in the human leukocyte antigen (HLA)-DR molecules and in the genes for the vitamin D$_3$ receptor, SCL11A-1, IFN-γ promoter, and mannose-binding lectin all have been associated with increased susceptibility to *M. tuberculosis*. Because each association has been relatively modest at the individual level, the genetic susceptibility is likely to be polygenic in nature. Ultimately, whether an individual with TB infection progresses to disease will depend on the interplay among host, infecting organism, and environment.

CLINICAL FEATURES

The clinical manifestations of TB are protean. Patterns of disease vary depending on whether the disease is primary or reactivation in nature, the host's immune status, and possibly the strain of *M. tuberculosis*. Of note, the clinical features of active TB are the result of a balance between host defenses and bacterial virulence; therefore, a continuum of disease is likely, and the clinical presentation of disease may be altered in severely immunocompromised patients. Most patients initially are seen with pulmonary disease, which is classically divided into primary disease and postprimary disease.

PULMONARY TUBERCULOSIS

The initial infection in the lung, referred to as *primary* infection, causes formation of an inflammatory infiltrate, which may be seen on a chest radiograph, often in the middle or lower lung zones. The draining lymph nodes may enlarge and compress adjacent bronchi, particularly in infants and children. Parenchymal disease usually clears as cell-mediated immunity develops, and it tends to clear more rapidly than nodal involvement. If the parenchymal disease persists beyond the development of

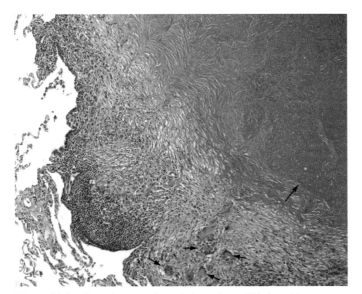

Figure 31-2 Caseating granuloma in lung tissue. This lung biopsy specimen contains a caseating granuloma. The *large arrow* highlights the caseous center. The *smaller arrows* point out giant cells, typical of granulomatous inflammation.

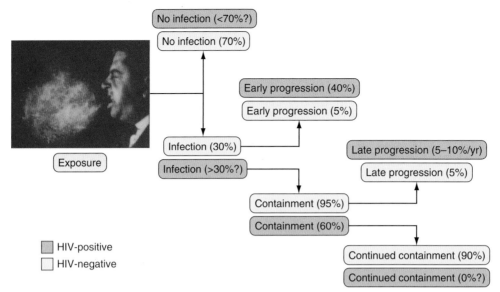

Figure 31-3 Pathogenesis of tuberculosis. After exposure to an infectious case of tuberculosis, approximately 30% of close contacts become infected with *Mycobacterium tuberculosis*. Of the contacts who become infected, approximately 5% will develop active tuberculosis in the first year after infection and an additional 5% will develop active tuberculosis over the course of their lifetime. Therefore, approximately 90% of infected people will not develop tuberculosis. When tuberculosis is introduced into an HIV-infected population, its pathogenesis is altered. Although susceptibility is difficult to establish conclusively, HIV-infected people appear to be more susceptible to initial infection than HIV-negative contacts. In outbreak settings, approximately 40% of HIV-infected contacts develop tuberculosis within the first year of exposure. After tuberculosis infection, HIV-infected people develop active tuberculosis at a rate of 5% to 10% per year. *HIV*, human immunodeficiency virus.

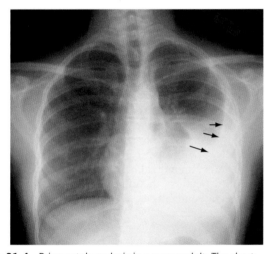

Figure 31-4 Primary tuberculosis in a young adult. The chest radiograph demonstrates a large, left-sided pleural effusion (arrows).

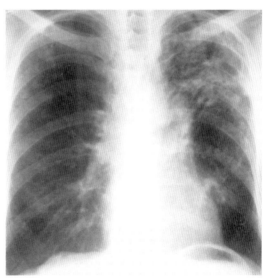

Figure 31-5 Postprimary tuberculosis. The chest radiograph shows upper lobe air space opacities with cavitation. Bronchial spread of the infection is evident in the lower lung zones.

cell-mediated immunity, cavitation may occur, although this finding is uncommon. Pleural effusions are a common manifestation of primary TB and presumably result when a peripheral, caseous focus ruptures into the pleural space (**Figure 31-4**). Pleuritis caused by TB may manifest as an acute illness characterized by cough, fever, and pleuritic chest pain.

During most initial infections with *M. tuberculosis*, small numbers of organisms are disseminated hematogenously, and some become seeded in the apices of the lung. The organisms seem to grow preferentially in this well-oxygenated environment, with progression to active disease occurring months or years after the initial infection. This accounts for the characteristic radiographic location of reactivation disease, which in most cases occurs in the apical or posterior segments of the upper lobes (**Figure 31-5**). In areas of chronic infection or areas of caseation, fibrosis may occur. Fibrocaseous lesions may contain live mycobacteria for many years, and these are the lesions that may reactivate years later.

EXTRAPULMONARY TUBERCULOSIS

As tubercle bacilli spread throughout the body during the initial infection, they can lodge in any organ and produce a focus of disease. Approximately 17% of HIV-uninfected patients with TB have an extrapulmonary form of disease only. An extrapulmonary site of infection is more likely to develop in HIV-infected patients than in HIV-seronegative persons, and the risk of extrapulmonary TB increases as the CD4+ lymphocyte count decreases. The two most commonly involved extrapulmonary sites are peripheral lymph nodes and the pleura, but any site or organ can be involved. Other common sites for extrapulmonary TB are within well-vascularized areas such as the kidney, the meninges, the spine, and the growing ends of long bones.

TUBERCULOUS LYMPHADENITIS (SCROFULA)

Lymphadenitis is the most common form of extrapulmonary TB, accounting for approximately 25% of extrapulmonary disease. Lymphadenitis usually manifests as a painless, erythematous, firm mass most commonly involving the anterior and posterior cervical nodes or supraclavicular fossa. In HIV-uninfected people, the mass usually is unilateral, not associated with other sites, and systemic symptoms are absent. However, in HIV-infected patients, tuberculous lymphadenitis often is associated with multifocal disease and systemic symptoms. Without treatment, the mass will enlarge and a fistulous tract may develop.

Diagnosis of tuberculous lymphadenitis usually involves fine needle aspiration or excisional biopsy with histopathologic examination, examination for acid-fast organisms, and culture for mycobacteria. Histopathologic evidence of mycobacterial infection, including caseating granulomas, is seen in nearly all cases, but the smear is positive in only approximately 25% to 50% of cases and the culture in approximately 70% to 80%.

PLEURAL TUBERCULOSIS

Pleurisy usually is a manifestation of primary TB and results when a subpleural caseous focus ruptures into the pleural space. The resulting delayed-type hypersensitivity reaction produces pleural liquid that has a high protein concentration. Most patients are initially seen with chest pain, fever, and a nonproductive cough. If left untreated, the pleural effusion will resolve spontaneously over 2 to 4 months. The rate of reactivation, however, is approximately 65% within the next 5 years.

Diagnosis of tuberculous pleural disease begins with sampling of the pleural fluid. Early in the course of disease, the fluid may have a polymorphonuclear predominance, but in almost all cases, mononuclear cells become the majority. Cell counts typically are in the 100 to 5000 cells/μL range, and the cells are almost all lymphocytes; the presence of mesothelial cells and/or eosinophils makes the diagnosis of TB unlikely.

Pleural fluid AFB smears are seldom positive, and pleural fluid cultures are positive in only approximately 20% to 40% of cases. M. tuberculosis can be isolated from 30% to 50% of induced sputum specimens from patients with TB pleuritis; such specimens should therefore be obtained in all patients. Pleural biopsy specimens provide the highest diagnostic yield, with positive culture results in up to 80% to 90% of cases when at least three specimens are obtained. Thoracoscopic biopsies are nearly always diagnostic, but the procedure is invasive, costly, and often not available.

Other tests that may be helpful in the diagnosis of pleuritis are adenosine deaminase and interferon-γ (IFN-γ) assays. The enzyme marker adenosine deaminase has been shown to have high sensitivity but variable specificity. A recent metaanalysis suggested that pleural fluid IFN-γ concentration has sensitivity of 89% and specificity of 97% for pleural TB in HIV-uninfected patients. Sensitivity and specificity also are high in HIV-infected patients.

When faced with a lymphocytic exudative pleural effusion in a patient with a positive TST reaction or IGRA result, the clinician should strongly consider TB. Whether to start treatment empirically or proceed with a pleural biopsy will depend on the certainty of the diagnosis and whether or not the patient is at risk for drug-resistant TB. In the latter situation, pleural tissue should be obtained for smear and culture to direct drug susceptibility testing.

GENITOURINARY TUBERCULOSIS

Genitourinary disease is responsible for approximately 15% of extrapulmonary cases of TB and can affect either the kidneys or genitals. Renal disease may manifest with local symptoms that include dysuria, hematuria, urinary frequency, and flank discomfort. In many cases, however, the patient may be asymptomatic. Urine examination may demonstrate sterile pyuria, hematuria, or both. M. tuberculosis can be isolated from urine in 80% to 95% of patients who provide three morning urine specimens for culture. In patients with pulmonary TB, urine cultures have been reported to be positive in approximately 5% of cases. An intravenous pyelogram may show evidence of destructive changes in the kidney or ureteral abnormalities such as strictures and hydronephrosis. Computed tomography (CT) often demonstrates renal enlargement with abscess formation.

Genital involvement is common in patients with renal TB. Men usually present with a slowly enlarging mass in the seminal vesicles, prostate, or epididymis. TB usually is diagnosed using fine needle aspiration or urine culture. In female patients, the fallopian tube is the primary site of involvement. Women tend to present with pelvic pain, abnormal uterine bleeding, irregular menses, amenorrhea, or infertility. Genital TB is diagnosed using urine culture and endometrial biopsy or curettage. Unfortunately, infertility is common even after successful treatment.

BONE AND JOINT TUBERCULOSIS

Skeletal involvement is thought to arise from reactivation from foci that were seeded at the time of initial infection. The infection begins in the subchondral region of the bone and then spreads to cartilage, synovium, and joint space. Although weight-bearing bones are the most likely to be affected, any bone or joint may be involved. In most series, TB of the spine, or Pott's disease, accounts for more than 50% of cases. In children, the upper thoracic spine is the most frequently affected site, whereas in adults, the lower thoracic and upper lumbar vertebrae typically are involved. After the spine, the hips and knees are the most common sites of skeletal TB.

Most patients initially are seen with pain in the involved joint. Systemic symptoms usually are absent, and delays in diagnosis are common. Tuberculous involvement of the joint usually is first suspected after a radiograph shows changes suggestive of the diagnosis. Typical findings include metaphyseal erosion and cysts, loss of cartilage, and narrowing of the joint space. In Pott's disease, two vertebral bodies and the intervening joint space usually are involved. CT and/or magnetic resonance imaging (MRI) should be obtained to better define the pattern and extent of involvement. Confirmation of the diagnosis requires aspiration of joint fluid or of periarticular abscesses or biopsy of affected bone or synovium. Acid-fast smears are positive in 20% to 25% of joint fluid aspirates, with isolation of mycobacteria in 60% to 80%. Histopathologic evidence of granulomatous inflammation is almost always present in bone and synovial biopsy specimens.

CENTRAL NERVOUS SYSTEM TUBERCULOSIS

Meningitis is the most common form of central nervous system (CNS) TB, with tuberculomas occurring less commonly.

Tuberculous meningitis, although less common than in the past, is still associated with the highest rates of morbidity and mortality for any form of TB, with a mortality rate of approximately 20%. Patients usually are initially seen with some combination of headache, abnormal behavior, confusion, fever, cranial nerve abnormalities, and occasionally seizures.

CT and MRI studies may provide evidence for a basilar meningitis or show hydrocephalus or tuberculous abscesses. To confirm the diagnosis, however, cerebrospinal fluid (CSF) must be sampled for examination and culture. CSF protein is usually elevated, and glucose concentration decreased. Very high protein concentrations are associated with a worse prognosis. White blood cell counts are elevated, with values of 100 to 1000 cells/μL, most of which are lymphocytes. As with pleural effusions, however, a polymorphonuclear predominance may be noted early in the disease. AFB smears of cerebrospinal fluid are positive in only 10% to 25% of cases, and cultures are positive in approximately 55% to 80%. An RD-1 antigen–specific ELISPOT assay in combination with other rapid tests (Gram staining and cryptococcal antigen assay) was reported to be a good "rule-in" test for TB meningitis, with a sensitivity of 82% and specificity of 100%.

GASTROINTESTINAL TUBERCULOSIS

Gastrointestinal disease is an uncommon manifestation of extrapulmonary TB, although it is more common in HIV-infected patients. Classically, ileocecal involvement and tuberculous peritonitis are the most common forms. Patients with ileocecal involvement may present with abdominal pain simulating appendicitis or intestinal obstruction. Diagnosis of ileocecal TB can be difficult and often is made at the time of surgery.

Tuberculous peritonitis often manifests with abdominal pain and swelling. Fever, weight loss, and anorexia are also common. Ascitic fluid usually is high in protein. Ascitic fluid white blood cell count typically is more than 150 cells/mm³ with a lymphocytic predominance. AFB smears are seldom positive, and cultures are positive in approximately 50% to 80% of cases; the higher yield has been reported when 1 L of fluid was cultured. Laparoscopic biopsy usually is required to make the diagnosis of peritoneal TB.

PERICARDIAL TUBERCULOSIS

Tuberculous pericarditis is a relatively uncommon manifestation of extrapulmonary TB. The clinical presentation is quite variable and determined by the stage of disease. Early in the clinical course, fever and chest pain may predominate. Some patients present with large-volume pericardial effusions and signs and symptoms of tamponade. Other patients present with constrictive pericarditis. The pericardial fluid usually is serosanguineous and occasionally grossly bloody. It typically is a lymphocytic exudative fluid with white blood cell counts in the range of 5000 to 7000 cells/μL, although counts up to 50,000 have been reported. AFB smears of the fluid are seldom positive, and cultures are positive in less than a third of cases. Often pericardial biopsy samples show histopathologic evidence consistent with a mycobacterial infection, but in some cases nonspecific inflammatory findings are described.

MILIARY TUBERCULOSIS

Miliary or disseminated TB occurs when tubercle bacilli spread throughout the body, through the bloodstream, resulting in

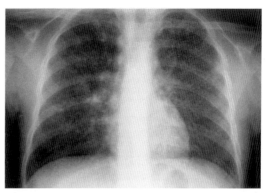

Figure 31-6 Miliary tuberculosis in an older child. The chest radiograph demonstrates diffuse small nodules 2 to 3 mm in diameter. The patient was diagnosed with disseminated tuberculosis with meningitis.

small (approximately 1 to 2 mm) granulomatous lesions. Miliary TB is seen more commonly in infants, children less than 4 years old, and in immunocompromised people. Disease can result from early dissemination after infection or later after reactivation and dissemination. Disseminated TB usually develops insidiously with systemic symptoms such as fever, weakness, weight loss, fatigue, and anorexia. Cough and dyspnea also may be prominent symptoms. The mean duration of symptoms approaches 16 weeks, but some patients may go undiagnosed for more than 2 years. The chest radiograph typically shows the classic "miliary" pattern of diffuse small nodules (**Figure 31-6**). Sputum AFB smears are positive in 20% to 25% of cases, and sputum is culture-positive for *M. tuberculosis* in up to 65% of cases. Bronchoscopy should be considered in patients who are unable to produce sputum or who have produced negative sputum smears. Other potential sources include urine, which is culture-positive in up to 25% of patients, and liver and bone marrow, which are culture-positive in up to 25% to 40%.

DIAGNOSIS

To diagnose TB, the disease must first be suspected. TB should be suspected in certain high-risk groups reviewed previously (see Table 31-1) and when the clinical and/or radiographic presentation is consistent with TB. The medical history should elicit whether or not the person suspected of having TB has been exposed to *M. tuberculosis* or has a previous history of TB infection or disease. Symptoms at presentation will vary depending on the sites(s) of involvement and extent of disease as described previously. Guidelines suggest that all persons with an unexplained cough lasting 2 to 3 weeks or more be evaluated for TB. Of note, up to 20% of patients with pulmonary disease are asymptomatic. Findings at physical examination are rather nonspecific and will vary, depending on the site of involvement. Among HIV-infected patients, TB should be considered when any respiratory infection or fever of unknown origin occurs, because the risk for TB in this group is substantially elevated, and signs and symptoms of TB often are atypical.

TUBERCULIN SKIN TEST AND INTERFERON-γ RELEASE ASSAYS

The TST (discussed in more detail later on), which uses purified protein derivative (PPD), is the most common way to identify persons with latent tuberculosis infection (LTBI) but should not be used in the diagnosis of active TB. In general, the sensitivity of the TST for detection of active TB ranges from 65% to 94%, but in critically ill patients with disseminated disease, the sensitivity decreases to only 50%. Thus, a negative TST reaction can never exclude a diagnosis of TB.

IGRAs measure the release of IFN-γ in whole blood in response to stimulation by *M. tuberculosis* antigens. Whole blood is incubated overnight with early secretory antigen target 6 [ESAT-6], culture filtrate protein 10 [CFP10], TB7.7, and control antigens; lymphocytes sensitized by previous exposure to *M. tuberculosis* release IFN-γ. IGRAs currently available include the QuantiFERON-TB (QFT-TB) Gold and QFT-TB Gold In-Tube (QFT-GIT), which measure IFN-γ in the serum using enzyme-linked immunosorbent assay (ELISA) (Cellestis Limited, Carnegie, Victoria, Australia) and the T-Spot.*TB* test, which uses enzyme-linked immunospot (ELISPOT) methodology (Oxford Immunotec, Oxford, United Kingdom) to identify IFN-γ–producing cells.

The reported sensitivity of QFT-GIT in patients with active TB has varied, ranging from 62% to 94%, with a pooled sensitivity of 80%, whereas the T-Spot.*TB* test has a sensitivity of 35% to 100%, with a pooled sensitivity of 81%. By contrast, the TST has a pooled sensitivity of 65% in patients with TB. Although the IGRAs have improved sensitivity compared with the TST, the values are still too low to rule out active TB with confidence, and neither test can differentiate latent from active TB.

RADIOGRAPHIC EXAMINATIONS

Plain chest radiography is a sensitive but nonspecific test to detect pulmonary TB. Radiographic manifestations of TB vary, depending on whether the patient has primary or postprimary TB and whether co-infection with HIV is present. Patients who have primary pulmonary TB at initial evaluation may demonstrate radiographic opacities in the lower lung zones and an associated pleural effusion (see Figure 31-4). TB caused by reactivation typically involves the apical and posterior segments of the upper lobes or superior segment of the lower lobe (see Figure 31-5). Cavitation and volume loss are common in reactivation disease but unusual in primary disease. Findings on the chest radiograph in patients co-infected with HIV depend on the severity of immunosuppression. Early in the course of HIV disease, the radiograph may show a typical reactivation pattern with cavitation (**Figure 31-7**), but as the CD4+ cell count declines, the radiographic appearance is more like the pattern seen in primary TB (**Figure 31-8**). Patients co-infected with HIV may sometimes have a normal-appearing chest radiograph despite being sputum AFB smear–positive.

BACTERIOLOGIC EXAMINATION

Sputum Microscopy

Diagnosis of pulmonary TB begins with obtaining two or three spontaneously expectorated sputum samples collected at 8- to 24-hour intervals, with at least one collected in early morning. Two methods are commonly used for acid-fast staining: the carbolfuchsin methods (Ziehl-Neelsen and Kinyoun methods) and a fluorochrome procedure that uses auramine O or auramine-rhodamine dyes (**Figure 31-9**).

Approximately 5,000 to 10,000 bacilli/mL are necessary to allow detection of these organisms in stained smears. The sensitivity of sputum AFB smears ranges from 50% to 80%, depending on the extent of disease; patients with cavitary

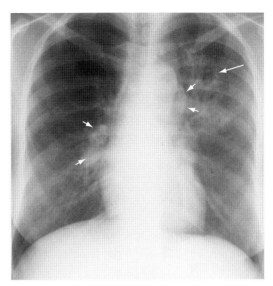

Figure 31-7 Tuberculosis in a human immunodeficiency virus (HIV)-infected patient. The chest radiograph demonstrates a left upper lobe cavitary process (*large arrow*). In addition, bilateral hilar adenopathy and aortopulmonary window adenopathy (*small arrows*) are evident.

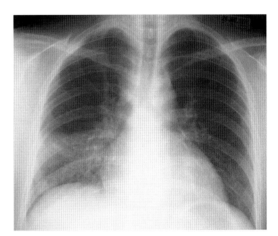

Figure 31-8 Primary-type presentation of tuberculosis in a human immunodeficiency virus (HIV)-infected patient. The chest radiograph demonstrates right lower lobe and right middle lobe air space consolidation with likely right hilar and paratracheal adenopathy.

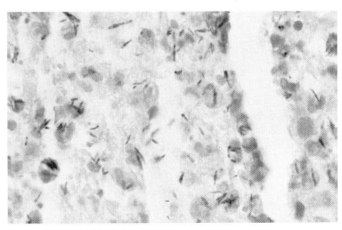

Figure 31-9 Acid-fast stain in tissue showing *Mycobacterium tuberculosis*. (Ziehl-Neelsen stain.)

disease are more likely than those without cavities to expectorate tubercle bacilli. Light-emitting diode (LED)–based fluorescence microscopy allows for more rapid evaluation of specimens and may increase the sensitivity slightly over that for conventional light microscopy. If patients are unable to produce sputum or have negative sputum smears, additional diagnostic tests may be indicated. In such circumstances, either sputum induction or biopsy using fiberoptic bronchoscopy (FOB) may provide adequate specimens. Studies suggest that sputum induction with hypertonic saline and FOB with bronchoalveolar lavage produce similar yields in smear-negative cases. The primary role of FOB is in smear-negative HIV-infected TB suspects, in whom this technique also can help identify alternative causes of the illness.

Mycobacterial Cultures and Identification

Culture of *M. tuberculosis* remains the "gold standard" modality for diagnosis of TB, and isolation of the organism is necessary for drug susceptibility testing and genotyping. Thus, all clinical specimens suspected of containing mycobacteria should be inoculated onto culture media. There are three different types of traditional culture media: egg-based (Lowenstein-Jensen or Ogawa), agar-based (Middlebrook 7H10 or 7H11), and liquid (Middlebrook 7H12) media. Growth in the liquid media is faster than that in solid media, and automated commercial broth systems allow for growth detection within 1 to 3 weeks compared with solid media, for which growth takes 3 to 8 weeks. However, solid media allow for observation of colony morphology and the detection of mixed infections. Because only 10 to 100 organisms are required to detect *M. tuberculosis*, cultures are more sensitive than smears, with reported sensitivity ranging from 80% to 93%. The tubercle bacilli can be identified from cultures and distinguished from NTM species by chemical means or with molecular methods.

Molecular Assays

Nucleic acid amplification assays (NAAs) amplify and detect *M. tuberculosis*–specific nucleic acid sequences in clinical specimens within 24 to 48 hours. Two U.S. Food and Drug Administration (FDA)-approved NAAs are available in the United States: the AMPLICOR *M. tuberculosis* (Roche Diagnostic Systems, Inc., Branchburg, New Jersey) and the Amplified Mycobacterium Tuberculosis Direct (MTD) Test (Gen-Probe, Inc., San Diego, California). The enhanced MTD (E-MTD) assay is approved for use with both smear-negative and smear-positive specimens, but the AMPLICOR assay is approved for use with smear-positive specimens only. The assays show sensitivities of at least 80% to 90% in most studies, with specificities of approximately 98% to 99% in smear-positive specimens. The E-MTD assay has been shown to have a sensitivity and specificity close to 100% in smear-positive specimens, and in smear-negative specimens the sensitivity is 90% and specificity is 99%.

NAAs are particularly valuable for rapidly distinguishing TB from NTM infection. When both the NAA and AFB smear are positive, pulmonary TB is almost certain and TB therapy should be initiated. If the NAA result is negative but the sputum smear is positive, testing the sputum for inhibitors and repeating the NAA is advised. If inhibitors are not detected and a second sputum specimen is NAA-negative but smear-positive, the patient probably has an NTM infection. If smears are negative but the clinical suspicion is intermediate to high, an NAA should be ordered, because a positive NAA result in this setting is likely to indicate TB. However, a negative NAA result in a smear-negative patient does not exclude TB. NAA tests should not be performed on sputum specimens from patients at low risk for development of TB. NAAs have been shown to reduce time to diagnosis, to accelerate contact investigations, and to reduce nonindicated TB treatment and are considered a standard component of the TB-diagnostic armamentarium.

Use of NAA for testing extrapulmonary specimens has been systemically reviewed. The sensitivity of commercial assays for detecting *M. tuberculosis* in CSF and pleural fluid has been approximately 60%, with a specificity of 98%. Therefore, NAAs may be useful in confirming a diagnosis of CNS or pleural TB, but because of the low sensitivity, they cannot be used to rule out disease.

The Xpert MTB/RIF (Cepheid, Sunnyvale, California) is an automated diagnostic system that performs real-time PCR to amplify an MTB-specific sequence of the *rpoB* gene, which is probed with molecular beacons to identify rifampin resistance. The device, which provides results within two hours, indicates both the presence of *M. tuberculosis* and the presence of rifampin resistance. In a large multicountry study, the Xpert MTB/RIF correctly identified 98% of patients with smear-positive and culture-positive TB. The sensitivity for smear-negative, culture-positive disease was 72%.

Drug Susceptibility Testing

Drug susceptibility studies should be performed on all initial isolates and only by laboratories that have experience in culturing mycobacteria. Drug susceptibility testing also should be performed on patients whose treatment is failing or who have a recurrence. The agar proportion method and the liquid radiometric or chemoluminescence methods are the ones most commonly used in the Unites States. Automated radiometric procedures for drug susceptibility testing offer more rapid results but often require confirmation with solid media.

More rapid methods of detection of drug resistance are now available. The WHO recommends that rapid methods of drug susceptibility testing for INH and rifampin or rifampin alone be used over conventional testing. The Xpert MTB/RIF test described previously correctly identified 98% of rifampin resistance. Since rifampin resistance rarely occurs in isolation and is generally accompanied with INH resistance, rifampin resistance frequently indicates MDR TB. Thus, Xpert MTB/RIF can provide a presumptive diagnosis of MDR TB within 2 hours. Unlike the Xpert MTB/RIF, other molecular methods are able to identify mutations in the *M. tuberculosis* genome that confer resistance to multiple agents. Line-probe assays like the Genotype MTBDR*plus* (Hain Lifesciences, Nehren, Germany) can detect mutations that confer resistance to rifampin and INH whereas the MTBDRsi test also can identify resistance to fluoroquinolones, aminoglycosides, and ethambutol. In the United States, the Molecular Detection of Drug Resistance program at the Centers for Disease Control and Prevention (CDC) uses DNA sequencing to identify mutations that confer resistance to rifampin, INH, fluoroquinolones, kanamycin, amikacin, and capreomycin. With previous authorization, this service accepts and tests isolates from patients at particularly high risk for MDR or XDR TB.

TREATMENT

Identifying and treating patients with TB is the most effective way of preventing transmission in the community. TB must be treated with at least two drugs to which the organism is susceptible, to prevent the emergence of drug resistance. Dosages

Table 31-2 First-Line Antituberculosis Drug Regimens for Adults and Children

Drug	Preparation	Doses Daily	1×/wk	2×/wk	3×/wk
		Adults (max.):			
Isoniazid	Tablets (50 mg, 100 mg, 300 mg); elixir (50 mg/5 mL); aqueous solution (100 mg/mL) for intravenous or intramuscular injection	5 mg/kg (300 mg)	15 mg/kg (900 mg)	15 mg/kg (900 mg)	15 mg/kg (900 mg)
		Children (max.):			
		10-15 mg/kg (300 mg)	—	20-30 mg/kg (900 mg)	—
Rifampin	Capsule (150 mg, 300 mg); powder may be suspended for oral administration; aqueous solution for intravenous injection	*Adults* (max.):			
		10 mg/kg (600 mg)	—	10 mg/kg (600 mg)	10 mg/kg (600 mg)
		Children (max.):			
		10-20 mg/kg (600 mg)	—	10-20 mg/kg (600 mg)	—
Rifabutin	Capsule (150 mg)	*Adults* (max.):			
		5 mg/kg (300 mg)	—	5 mg/kg (300 mg)	5 mg/kg (300 mg)
		Children (max.):			
		Appropriate dosing for children unknown	Appropriate dosing for children unknown	Appropriate dosing for children unknown	Appropriate dosing for children unknown
Rifapentine	Tablet (150 mg, film-coated)	*Adults:*			
		—	10 mg/kg (continuation phase) (600-900 mg)	—	—
		Children:			
		Drug not approved for children	Drug not approved for children	Drug not approved for children	Drug not approved for children
Pyrazinamide	Tablet (500 mg, scored)	*Adults:*			
		20-25 mg/kg (2 g)	—	35-50 mg/kg (4 g)	30-40 mg/kg (3 g)
		Children:			
		15-30 mg/kg (2 g)	—	50 mg/kg (4 g)	—
Ethambutol	Tablet (100 mg, 400 mg)	*Adults:*			
		15-20 mg/kg (1.6 g)	—	35-50 mg/kg (4 g)	20-35 mg/kg (2.5)
		Children:			
		15-20 mg/kg (1 g)	—	50 mg/kg (4 g)	—

of commonly used first-line and second-line drugs are shown in **Tables 31-2** and **Table 31-3**, respectively. In the United States, a regimen consisting of INH and rifampin given for 6 months, plus pyrazinamide for the initial 2 months, is considered standard short-course therapy. Ethambutol should be added to the treatment regimen for the first 2 months of therapy, but once a drug-susceptible isolate has been demonstrated, ethambutol can be stopped (**Table 31-4**). After the first 2 months of treatment, one of several regimens can be chosen for the continuation phase of treatment. For HIV-negative patients who have a documented negative AFB smear after 2 months of therapy and have no evidence of cavitation on the initial chest radiograph, a once-weekly regimen consisting of rifapentine and INH is effective. The total duration of therapy should be 6 months, but in patients whose 2-month culture remains positive and whose chest radiograph shows evidence

of cavitation, the continuation phase should be extended by 3 months, to complete a 9-month treatment course (**Figure 31-10**).

Some patients may be intolerant of a first-line drug or have underlying drug-resistant disease. In such cases, addition of a second-line drug may be necessary (see Table 31-3). These medications include the fluoroquinolones, PAS, ethionamide, cycloserine, clofazimine, and injectables such as kanamycin, capreomycin, and amikacin. The duration of treatment for drug-resistant TB will be determined by the drugs used, the site, and the extent of the disease. Expert consultation should be obtained for treating drug-resistant TB.

To prevent acquired drug resistance, clinicians must prescribe an adequate regimen and ensure that patients adhere to therapy. Directly observed therapy (DOT) should be used whenever possible. If DOT is not available, combination

Table 31-3 Second-Line Antituberculosis Drug Regimens for Adults and Children

Drug	Preparation	Daily	1×/wk	2×/wk	3×/wk
Cycloserine	Capsule (250 mg)	*Adults* (max.): 10-15 mg/kg/d (1.0 g in two doses), usually 500-750 mg/d in two doses *Children* (max.): 10-15 mg/kg (1 g)	*	*	*
Ethionamide	Tablet (250 mg)	*Adults* (max.): 15-20 mg/kg/d (10 g/d), usually 500-750 mg/d in a single daily dose or two divided doses *Children* (max.): 10-20 mg/kg (1 g)	*	*	*
Streptomycin	Aqueous solution (1-g vials) for intravenous or intramuscular administration	*Adults* (max.): 15 mg/kg (1 g) *Children* (max.): 20-40 mg/kg (1 g)	— —	15-20 mg/kg (1.5) 20 mg/kg	15-20 mg/kg (1.5) —
Amikacin/ kanamycin	Aqueous solution (500-mg and 1-g vials) for intravenous or intramuscular administration	*Adults* (max.): 15 mg/kg (1 g) *Children* (max.): 15-30 mg/kg (1 g)	— —	15-20 mg/kg (1.5) 15-30 mg/kg	15-20 mg/kg (1.5) —
Capreomycin	Aqueous solution (1-g vials) for intravenous or intramuscular administration	*Adults* (max.): 15 mg/kg (1 g) *Children* (max.): 15-30 mg/kg (1 g)	— —	15-20 mg/kg (1.5) 15-30 mg/kg	15-20 mg/kg (1.5) —
Paraaminosalicylic acid (PAS)	Granules (4-g packets) can be mixed with food; tablets (500 mg) are still available in some countries, but not U.S.; a solution for intravenous administration is available in Europe	*Adults* (max.): 8-12 g/d in two or three doses *Children* (max.): 200-300 mg/kg in two to four divided doses	*	*	*
Levofloxacin	Tablets (250, 500, 750 mg); aqueous solution (500-mg vials) for intravenous injection	*Adults/children* (max.): 500-1000 mg daily Optimal dose not known	*	*	*
Moxifloxacin	Tablets (400 mg); aqueous solution (400 mg/250 mL) for intravenous injection	*Adults/children* (max.): 400 mg daily Optimal dose not known	*	*	*

*There are no data to support intermittent administration.

preparations that include INH and rifampin, or INH, rifampin, and pyrazinamide, should be used.

Persons with active untreated pulmonary TB are infectious, particularly those for whom AFB are identified in a sputum specimen. Treatment of TB rapidly renders these patients non-infectious. According to the CDC, patients are not considered infectious if they are on adequate therapy for 2 or more weeks, have a favorable clinical response to therapy, and have three consecutive negative sputum smear results from sputum collected on different days.

SPECIAL CIRCUMSTANCES

Human Immunodeficiency Virus Co-infection

Despite being immunocompromised, HIV-infected patients with TB respond well to regimens containing INH and rifampin. Thus, the current recommendations are to begin the same antituberculosis regimen as used in HIV-seronegative cases. A recent study from San Francisco, however, noted that the relapse rate among HIV-infected patients was 9.3 per 100 person-years versus 1.0 in HIV-uninfected patients or those with unknown

Table 31-4 Drug Regimens for Culture-Positive Pulmonary Tuberculosis Caused by Drug-Susceptible Organisms

		Initial Phase			Continuation Phase	
Regimen	Drugs	Interval and Dose Number (minimal duration)	Regimen	Drugs	Interval and Doses (minimal duration)	
1	INH RIF PZA EMB	7 d/wk for 56 doses (8 wk) OR 5 d/wk for 40 doses (8 wk)	1a	INH/RIF	7 d/wk for 126 doses (18 wk) OR 5 d/wk for 90 doses (18 wk)	
			1b	INH/RIF*	2×/wk for 36 doses (18 wk)	
			1c	INH/RPT†	1×/wk for 18 doses (18 wk)	
2	INH RIF PZA EMB	7 d/wk for 14 doses (2 wk), then 2×/wk for 12 doses (6 wk) OR 5 d/wk for 10 doses (2 wk), then 2×/wk for 12 doses (6 wk)	2a	INH/RIF*	2×/wk for 36 doses (18 wk)	
			2b	INH/RPT†	1×/wk for 18 doses (18 wk)	
3	INH RIF PZA EMB	3×/wk for 24 doses (8 wk)	3a	INH/RIF	3×/wk for 54 doses (18 wk)	
4	INH RIF EMB	7 d/wk for 56 doses (8 wk) OR 5 d/wk for 40 doses (8 wk)	4a	INH/RIF	7 d/wk for 217 doses (31 wk) OR 5 d/wk for 155 doses (31 wk)	
			4b	INH/RIF	2×/wk for 62 doses (31 wk)	

EMB, ethambutol; *HIV*, human immunodeficiency virus; *INH*, isoniazid; *PZA*, pyrazinamide; *RIF*, rifampin; *RPT*, rifapentine.
*Not recommended for HIV-infected patients with CD4$^+$ cell count below 100 cells/μL.
†Should be used only in HIV-seronegative patients who have negative sputum smears at the time of completion of 2 months of therapy and who do not have cavitation on the initial chest radiograph.

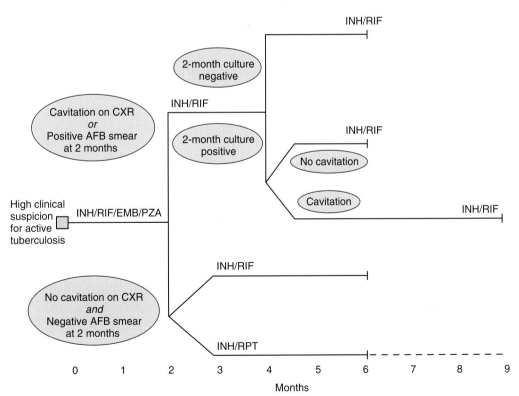

Figure 31-10 Treatment of pulmonary tuberculosis. Patients suspected to have tuberculosis whose chest radiograph (*CXR*) shows no evidence of cavitation and who have negative acid-fast bacilli (*AFB*) sputum smears after 2 months of therapy can be treated in the continuation phase with isoniazid (*INH*) and rifampin (*RIF*) to complete a 6-month duration of therapy. Alternately, they may be treated with INH and rifapentine (*RPT*) administered once weekly. If cultures remain positive after 2 months of therapy, treatment duration should be extended by 3 months. TB suspects who have evidence of cavitation on the chest radiograph or who have a positive AFB smear after 2 months of therapy should be treated with INH and RIF. If the 2-month culture is negative, they can be treated for a total of 6 months. If the 2-month culture is positive and there is no evidence of cavitation on the CXR, they can be treated for 6 months. However, if cavitation is present, the continuation phase should be lengthened by 3 months. *EMB*, ethambutol; *PZA*, pyrazinamide. *(From American Thoracic Society; CDC; Infectious Diseases Society of America: Treatment of tuberculosis, MMWR Recomm Rep 52[RR-11]:1–80, 2003.)*

serostatus. In addition, HIV-infected patients treated with a 6-month regimen were four times as likely to relapse as those treated longer. Studies have demonstrated that intermittent therapy is also associated with a higher rate of relapse and acquired rifampin resistance. Therefore, HIV-infected patients should not be treated with highly intermittent treatment regimens, particularly if they have advanced HIV disease.

The treatment of TB in HIV-infected patients is more complicated because of the potential for drug interactions between the rifamycins and antiretroviral agents, such as the protease inhibitors and non-nucleoside reverse transcriptase inhibitors (NNRTIs), the risk of an immune reconstitution syndrome, and the propensity to develop acquired drug resistance. The rifamycins are inducers of the cytochrome P-450 pathway (rifampin > rifapentine > rifabutin) and thus can increase the metabolism of some antiretroviral drugs. Some combinations of these drugs are contraindicated, and for other combinations, dosages must be adjusted. Therefore, consultation with an expert in the field is necessary to determine the best treatment regimens for HIV-infected patients with TB.

Antiretroviral treatment should be started for all HIV-infected patients with TB, regardless of CD4$^+$ count. For patients who are antiretroviral-naive, the timing of antiretroviral initiation has been controversial because of the concern for interactions with TB medications and immune reconstitution syndrome. A recent trial in South Africa demonstrated that "integrated" therapy (in which antiretrovirals are started during TB therapy) was associated with a 56% reduction in mortality relative to "sequential" therapy (in which antiretrovirals are started at the completion of TB therapy). A trial in Cambodia compared initiation of antiretrovirals 2 weeks or 8 weeks after starting TB therapy in patients with CD4$^+$ count less than 200 cells/μL. Earlier initiation of antiretrovirals was associated with a 34% reduction in mortality.

Extrapulmonary Tuberculosis

In general, treatment of extrapulmonary TB follows the same principles as those for pulmonary disease. However, both surgery and the use of corticosteroids may be needed more often in extrapulmonary TB. Corticosteroids should be considered in patients with confirmed CNS or pericardial TB. Corticosteroids have been demonstrated to improve the outcomes of tuberculous pericarditis in both acute and later phase disease. In neither setting, however, is there a significant decrease in progression to constriction or need for pericardiectomy. In CNS TB, use of corticosteroids has been shown to decrease the frequency of neurologic sequelae in children. Treatment duration should be prolonged in patients with bone and joint disease to 6 to 9 months and for CNS disease to 9 to 12 months.

Children

Children should be treated with the same regimens as those recommended for adults, but doses should be adjusted appropriately. Although some experts do not recommend the use of ethambutol in children, it seems to be safe and should be used whenever underlying drug resistance is suspected. In addition, some experts recommend increasing the duration of therapy to 9 to 12 months in children with disseminated or meningeal disease. HIV-infected children should receive at least 9 months of therapy.

Pregnancy and Breastfeeding

Pregnant and breastfeeding women with active TB must be treated, because the potential for untreated TB in the fetus or infant is always of greater concern than any small risks associated with therapy. Pyrazinamide currently is not recommended in the United States in pregnant women because of a lack of data regarding teratogenicity, but the drug is recommended by the WHO and the International Union Against Tuberculosis and Lung Disease (IUATLD).

Drug-Resistant Tuberculosis

New guidelines for the programmatic management of drug-resistant TB were recently published by the WHO. The recommendations were formulated on the basis of the results of several large systematic reviews commissioned by the WHO. In patients with MDR TB, four second-line drugs that are likely to be effective, as well as pyrazinamide, should be used in the intensive phase of therapy. Regimens should include pyrazinamide, a later-generation fluoroquinolone, an injectable agent, ethionamide (or prothionamide), and either cycloserine or PAS if cycloserine cannot be used. No second-line parenteral agent was found to be superior to another. Because of its low cost, kanamycin was favored, although amikacin could be used in place of kanamycin. Streptomycin is not recommended. An intensive phase (injectable phase) of at least 8 months' duration is recommended, with a total duration of at least 20 months. Cure rates for treatment of MDR TB have averaged around 60% to 70% (range of 30% to 95%) in programmatic settings. XDR TB is associated with a high mortality rate and cure rates ranging from 30% to 60%. In view of the complexity of therapy and possible need for surgical resection, experts in the management of drug-resistant TB should be consulted early in the course of therapy.

CLINICAL COURSE AND PREVENTION

MONITORING FOR ADVERSE REACTIONS AND RESPONSE TO THERAPY

All patients receiving antituberculosis therapy must be educated about possible drug-related adverse reactions. The patients should be warned about insignificant side effects, such as the orange discoloration of urine from rifampin, as well as the symptoms of potentially serious side effects. Baseline measurements of hepatic enzymes, bilirubin, serum creatinine, and blood urea nitrogen, as well as a complete blood cell count including platelets, are obtained before initiation of drug therapy. A serum uric acid level is obtained if pyrazinamide is included in the drug regimen. Visual acuity and red-green color discrimination are monitored in patients receiving ethambutol. Although routine laboratory monitoring for drug toxicity may not be necessary, many centers repeat liver function tests after 1 month of therapy and thereafter if symptoms develop or the liver function tests are elevated significantly.

Sputum examinations at monthly intervals are important to monitor response to therapy. Smears and cultures should be negative after 2 to 3 months of therapy. If the sputum smear remains positive after 3 months, the patient must be reevaluated; special attention is given to monitoring adherence and ruling out acquired drug resistance. Drug susceptibility tests are repeated, and the appropriateness of the drug regimen is reassessed.

PREVENTION

The best method of preventing TB is to identify active cases and treat them to cure, thus preventing transmission to others.

Unfortunately, most transmission has occurred before diagnosis and initiation of therapy, so other methods are needed to prevent the development of TB. Two methods are used to do this. The first is to vaccinate patients with the only available TB vaccine, bacillus Calmette-Guérin (BCG). Although BCG is the most widely used vaccine in the world, serious shortcomings with this approach are recognized (as discussed later on). The second is to diagnose LTBI and treat affected patients with antituberculosis drugs to prevent progression to active disease.

DIAGNOSIS OF LATENT TUBERCULOSIS INFECTION

Most people who are infected with *M. tuberculosis* are able to arrest the development of active disease with adequate cell-mediated immunity. As noted previously, however, approximately 10% of infected people have TB develop during their lifetime. Treatment of LTBI is a pillar of TB prevention in lower incidence countries like the United States because treatment can reduce the risk of progression to TB by up to 92%. Testing for LTBI should be targeted at people with clinical and epidemiologic risks for TB (**Figure 31-11**). Until recently, the only method to detect LTBI was the TST. Recently, blood-based assays have been developed that provide an alternative to the TST.

Tuberculin Skin Test

The traditional test to diagnose LTBI for more than 100 years has been the TST. The reaction to intradermally injected tuberculin is a classic example of a delayed-type hypersensitivity reaction, characterized by a peak reaction at 48 to 72 hours

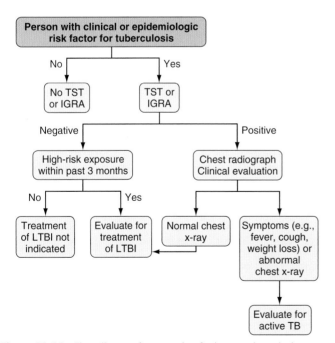

Figure 31-11 Flow diagram for screening for latent tuberculosis infection (LTBI). In persons with clinical or epidemiologic risk factors for tuberculosis (TB), a tuberculin skin test (TST) or interferon-γ release assay (IGRA) should be performed. A positive test result warrants clinical evaluation and chest radiograph. If either yields abnormal findings, the patient should be evaluated for the possibility of active TB. If the chest radiograph is normal in appearance, the patient is a candidate for LTBI treatment. If the initial TST reaction or IGRA result is negative but the patient has had contact with infectious cases of TB, treatment may still be indicated.

marked by induration and, rarely, vesiculation and necrosis. The standard tuberculin test consists of intradermal administration of 0.1 mL (5 tuberculin units) of PPD, usually given in the volar surface of the forearm. Sensitization is induced by infection with *M. tuberculosis* or other cross-reacting mycobacteria antigens. The TST reaction should be read by trained readers 48 to 72 hours after injection. The basis of the reading is the degree of induration present, not erythema.

Over time, delayed-type hypersensitivity resulting from mycobacterial infection may wane in some people, resulting in a nonreactive TST despite the fact that they are truly infected. The stimulus of this initial negative TST reaction in these persons may "boost" or increase the size of the reaction to a second test administered later, resulting in a positive TST reaction and incorrectly suggesting tuberculin conversion. This ability of the TST to recall the waned reactivity is known as the booster phenomenon.

Because of the difficulty in distinguishing boosting (indicating previous infection many years ago) from tuberculin conversion (indicating recent infection), two-step testing is recommended in persons who require annual TSTs and persons older than 55 years of age.

TST is not entirely specific for the diagnosis of infection with *M. tuberculosis* and false-positive tests can occur from either infection with NTM or BCG vaccination. In a patient who has received BCG, the likelihood that a positive TST reaction represents a false-positive result due to BCG rather than LTBI depends on the age at vaccination. In 24 studies that involved almost 250,000 subjects vaccinated in infancy with BCG, only 1% had a positive TST attributable after 10 years. BCG vaccination after infancy had a more significant and lasting impact on the TST reaction. In practice, most clinicians ignore previous BCG vaccination when interpreting the results of TSTs if at least several years have elapsed since the time of vaccination.

Three different thresholds—5, 10, and 15 mm—have been set for defining a positive tuberculin reaction, depending on the individual or population being tested (see Table 31-1). For persons at highest risk for development of TB, a cutoff of 5 mm or more is recommended. This group includes persons known or suspected of being HIV-infected, close contacts of active TB cases, persons with an abnormal-appearing chest radiograph showing fibrosis consistent with previous TB (**Figure 31-12**), and other immunosuppressed patients. A cutoff of 10 mm of induration or greater is classified as positive for people at intermediate risk for TB. The remaining group consists of persons at low risk for TB who have no risk factors. In these persons, TST reactions are classified as positive if the induration is 15 mm or more across; in general, such patients should not be screened.

Recent TST converters also are at high risk for development of TB and have therefore been identified as a high-priority group for treatment of LTBI. In the United States, conversion is defined as an increase in induration of at least 10 mm within a 2-year period.

Interferon-γ Release Assays

As noted previously, there are three new T cell–based tests for the diagnosis of LTBI: QFT-TB Gold, QFT-GIT, and T-Spot.*TB* test. The QFT-TB Gold assays use an ELISA method to measure antigen-specific production of IFN-γ, whereas the T-Spot.*TB* test uses ELISPOT to measure the number of cells that produce IFN-γ. The CDC has recommended that these assays be used in any situation in which the TST is used, whereas the U.K.

National Institute for Clinical Excellence has suggested that the IGRAs be used as confirmatory tests to the TST.

Numerous studies have assessed the test characteristics of these assays by use of different versions of the tests, in different populations, and under different laboratory conditions. Overall, the specificity rates for QFT-GIT, T-Spot.*TB*, and TST are approximately 99.8%, 97.8%, and 88.7%, respectively. Of note, however, a "gold standard" test for LTBI is lacking, so the true test characteristics of these assays are unknown. In studies assessing the correlation with degree of exposure, both IGRAs correlated with exposure better than the TST, and neither was affected by previous BCG vaccination.

The advantages of IGRAs compared with the standard TST are several: These blood-based tests have less cross-reactivity from vaccination with BCG and NTM, are less susceptible to reader variability that occurs with TST interpretation, require only one patient visit to obtain results, and may be more specific for identifying *M. tuberculosis* infection. Additionally, IGRAs may be more predictive of the development of active disease than the TST. The rate of progression to active disease among patients who tested positive for LTBI and who refused preventive therapy has ranged from 2.3% to 3.3% for TST, 2.8% to 14.3% for QFT-GIT, and 3.3% to 10.0% for T-Spot.*TB*.

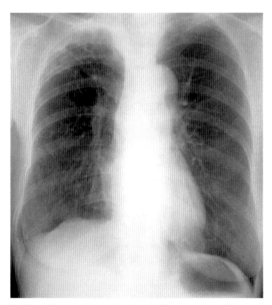

Figure 31-12 Chest radiograph obtained in a patient with previous tuberculosis. Changes include right upper lobe linear and nodular opacities with pleural thickening. In addition, note the elevation of the right hemidiaphragm and superior retraction of the right hilum secondary to volume loss.

TREATMENT OF LATENT TUBERCULOSIS INFECTION

Treatment is not recommended for all persons with LTBI. Instead, therapy should be provided to those persons at higher risk for TB infection and/or TB. For persons who are at increased risk of progressing to disease, treatment of latent infection is indicated, regardless of age. It is critical that patients being considered for LTBI therapy receive a clinical and radiographic evaluation to exclude the possibility of active disease. The two most commonly used drugs for the treatment of LTBI are INH and rifampin (**Table 31-5**).

INH was evaluated in randomized controlled trials conducted by the United States Public Health Service that included more than 70,000 participants encompassing a variety of populations. In these studies, the effectiveness of the drug compared with placebo in reducing the incidence of active TB averaged approximately 60%, with a range of 25% to 92%, the higher values being associated with better adherence to the drug. On the basis of these studies, the American Thoracic Society (ATS) and the CDC recommend that INH be administered as a single daily dose or twice weekly. Completion of treatment is based on the total number of doses administered and not on duration of therapy alone.

Hepatitis is the most important adverse reaction related to INH. Although liver enzyme abnormalities are relatively common in persons taking INH, symptomatic hepatitis is uncommon. The rate of INH-related hepatitis is estimated to be 1 per 1000 persons and increases with age. The most important cofactor for the development of INH hepatitis is alcohol consumption, so patients should be advised not to drink alcohol when they are taking INH. In addition, all persons taking INH should be educated about the signs and symptoms of hepatitis, including nausea, vomiting, extreme fatigue, abdominal pain, dark urine, and jaundice, so that they can be evaluated before the hepatitis becomes severe.

The other potential side effect of INH is peripheral neuropathy that is caused by interference with the metabolism of pyridoxine. In persons predisposed to neuropathy (such as patients with diabetes, uremia, malnutrition, and HIV infection), in pregnant women, and persons with seizure disorders, pyridoxine (at a dose of 25 or 50 mg/day) should be given concurrently with INH.

Rifampin alone for 4 months is an alternative option for treatment of LTBI although only one large randomized trial has evaluated the efficacy of rifampin monotherapy for LTBI. This trial, conducted among patients with silicosis at extremely high risk for LTBI, found that 3 months of daily rifampin was as efficacious as 6 months of daily INH. Nonetheless, approximately 10% of the patients in each treatment group progressed

Table 31-5   Recommended Drug Regimens for Treatment of Latent Tuberculosis Infection in Adults

Drug	Duration (months)	Dosing Interval	Minimum No. of Doses	Comments
Isoniazid	9	Daily	270	*Preferred*: 9 months of isoniazid
		Twice weekly	76	*Acceptable alternative*: 6 months of isoniazid OR 4 months of rifampin
Isoniazid	6	Daily	180	Not indicated for HIV-infected persons, those with fibrotic lesions on chest radiograph, or children
		Twice weekly	52	
Rifampin	4	Daily	120	For persons who are contacts of patients with isoniazid-resistant, rifampin-susceptible tuberculosis
Rifapentine/ isoniazid	3	Once weekly	12	Newly recommended regimen using directly observed therapy

HIV, human immunodeficiency virus.

to active TB. Subsequent nonefficacy trials indicate that 4 months of daily rifampin monotherapy is associated with fewer serious adverse effects and better rates of treatment completion than 9 months of daily INH. Rifampin alone has a very low rate of hepatotoxicity. Rifampin should be used for patients who are intolerant of INH or who are presumed to have infection with INH-resistant strains of *M. tuberculosis*.

Weekly rifapentine plus INH for 3 months is a third option for treatment of LTBI in low-incidence settings. In 2011, the CDC released results of the PREVENT TB trial, a 10-year multinational study in which more than 8000 patients with LTBI at high risk for progression to active disease were randomized to receive once-weekly, directly observed rifapentine plus INH for 3 months or standard daily self-administered INH for 9 months. The once-weekly rifapentine plus INH group had equivalent efficacy (7 TB cases versus 15 in the INH-only group), was safe and tolerable, and was associated with better adherence (82% completion versus 69% completion in the INH group). A critical point to emphasize is that the PREVENT-TB trial evaluated directly observed rifapentine plus INH, and the effectiveness of this regimen in practice if self-administered is unknown.

CLINICAL MONITORING

Baseline laboratory testing of liver enzymes is not routinely indicated but is recommended in the following patient groups: HIV-infected persons, pregnant women and those within 3 months post partum, patients with a history of liver disease, and persons who use alcohol regularly. Follow-up laboratory testing of liver enzymes is indicated only if baseline liver enzyme tests are abnormal or when symptoms of hepatitis occur. Drugs should be withheld if a patient's serum transaminase level is greater than three times normal if associated with symptoms and five times normal if asymptomatic.

SPECIAL CIRCUMSTANCES

CO-INFECTION WITH HUMAN IMMUNODEFICIENCY VIRUS

All HIV-infected persons should be screened for TB and LTBI. HIV-infected persons with LTBI should receive 9 months of INH once active TB has been ruled out. Rifampin should be used with caution in HIV-infected persons taking PIs or NNRTIs because of drug interactions described previously. In HIV-infected persons taking these antiretroviral drugs who have LTBI, rifabutin (often at an adjusted dose) can be substituted for rifampin in some circumstances.

ABNORMAL-APPEARING CHEST RADIOGRAPHS

In patients with evidence of LTBI who have an abnormal-appearing chest radiograph with parenchymal fibrotic lesions (see Figure 31-12) who have not been previously treated, sputum should be collected to exclude active TB. Once active TB has been excluded, treatment options for LTBI include INH for 9 months and rifampin for 4 months.

PREGNANCY AND LACTATING WOMEN

Although INH can be given safely during pregnancy, most clinicians wait until after delivery to begin treatment for LTBI, unless the woman has HIV infection or has been in known contact with an infectious case.

Infants and Children

Once infected, infants and children younger than 5 years of age are at high risk for progression of the initial infection to active TB and should receive INH for 9 months.

Contacts with Drug-Resistant Cases

Contacts of patients with INH-resistant, rifampin-susceptible TB should be treated with rifampin for 4 months. The treatment of persons in recent contact with an MDR TB case is challenging, however, and needs to be individualized on the basis of the susceptibility pattern of the source patient's organism, the probability that infection has occurred, and risk factors for progression to active TB. Treatment of contacts of patients with MDR TB often entails the administration of two drugs (to which the source case's isolate is susceptible) for 9 to 12 months.

VACCINATION WITH BACILLUS CALMETTE-GUÉRIN

BCG is a live attenuated vaccine derived from a strain of *M. bovis*. BCG is used to vaccinate children and, in some cases, adolescents and adults throughout much of the world. Although the vaccine seems to be protective in children, it confers little protection in adults, who are the ones who usually transmit disease. Data suggest that BCG vaccination decreases the risk of disseminated disease in young children—the primary reason for its use today. In countries in which BCG vaccination was suspended, TB rates did not increase significantly.

As noted previously, BCG vaccination can influence the results of tuberculin skin testing because of cross-reaction with PPD. The effects of BCG vaccination on tuberculin reactivity vary, depending on the specific vaccine used, age at vaccination, and interval between vaccination and skin testing. Despite widespread use of BCG vaccination, it has been difficult to demonstrate significant impact on TB control globally. New vaccines are urgently needed.

DISEASES CAUSED BY NONTUBERCULOUS MYCOBACTERIA

NTM comprise more than 135 different species that are widely distributed throughout the environment. The list of mycobacterial species has grown dramatically over recent years because of the availability of DNA sequencing, and because organisms that differ in sequence by 1% or more from all known species are defined as new species.

The NTM were not widely recognized as a cause of human disease until the late 1950s. In 1959, Runyon reported a classification system that organized NTM organisms into four groups on the basis of microbiologic characteristics, including the formation of pigment and the speed of growth. This system has become less useful with the development of rapid molecular methods of diagnosis, but differentiating NTM species on the basis of their rate of growth is still used today. NTM typically are divided into rapidly and slowly growing species (Table 31-6).

EPIDEMIOLOGY, RISK FACTORS, AND PATHOGENESIS

EPIDEMIOLOGY

NTM have been isolated from soil and water, including both natural and treated water sources, from throughout the world.

Table 31-6	Clinically Significant Nontuberculous Examples of Mycobacteria by Rate of Growth	
Slowly Growing (>7 days of incubation for mature growth)	**Rapidly Growing (≤7 days of incubation for mature growth)**	
Mycobacterium avium	Mycobacterium fortuitum	
Mycobacterium intracellulare	Mycobacterium peregrinum	
Mycobacterium kansasii	Mycobacterium abscessus	
Mycobacterium xenopi	Mycobacterium massiliense	
Mycobacterium simiae	Mycobacterium bolletii	
Mycobacterium szulgai	Mycobacterium chelonae	
Mycobacterium scrofulaceum	Mycobacterium mucogenicum	
Mycobacterium malmoense		
Mycobacterium haemophilum		
Mycobacterium genavense*		
Mycobacterium marinum*		

*This organism often grows within 7 to 10 days.

Because these organisms do not seem to be transmitted from human to human, the source of human infection is thought to be through environmental exposures. Skin test surveys of U.S. Navy recruits in the 1960s demonstrated higher rates of reactivity in those from the southeastern United States than from the northern states, suggesting higher rates of infection. Studies evaluating antibody to lipoarabinomannin (LAM) have demonstrated anti-LAM antibodies beginning early in life and rapidly rising through age 12.

Epidemiologic data on NTM infections are largely lacking, because unlike TB, NTM infections are not routinely considered reportable to public health authorities. The median rates of pulmonary NTM isolation have been estimated to be approximately 6.2 per 100,000 population in North America, 8.3 per 100,000 in Europe, 15 per 100,000 in Asia, and 7.2 per 100,000 in Australia. Studies from Oregon have reported that the prevalence of NTM infections was higher in females than males (6.4 per 100,000 versus 4.7 per 100,000) and was highest in persons aged more than 50 years (15.5 per 100,000). Among four integrated health care systems in the United States, the annualized prevalence ranged from 1.4 to 6.6 per 100,000 and among persons aged 60 years or more, the annualized prevalence was 26.7 per 100,000.

Recent data support the view that the incidence of NTM infections is increasing. Studies from Canada, Australia, Taiwan, the Netherlands, and the United States have reported increases in the incidence or prevalence of NTM. In a retrospective cohort review from 1997 to 2003 in Ontario, Canada, 222,247 pulmonary isolates from 10,231 patients were identified. The prevalence was 9.1 per 100,000 in 1997 and increased to 14.1 per 100,000 by 2003 ($P < .0001$), with an average annual increase of 8.4%. Increases were noted among *Mycobacterium avium* complex (MAC), *Mycobacterium xenopi*, rapidly growing mycobacteria, and *Mycobacterium kansasii*. Of note, the rate of TB declined 4.0% over the study period. Of 200 patients who were evaluated in more detail, 33% fulfilled the clinical, radiologic, and bacteriologic ATS criteria. In the United States, pulmonary hospitalizations for NTM infections increased significantly among both males and females between 1998 and 2005.

The most common pathogenic NTM vary geographically. MAC is the most common cause of NTM-related pulmonary disease in almost all studies. The next most common NTM species depends on the origin of reported data. For example, in the United States, *M. kansasii* is the second most common cause of pulmonary disease, followed by *Mycobacterium*

abscessus. In Canada, and some parts of Europe, *M. xenopi* is the second most common, whereas in northern Europe and Scandinavia, *Mycobacterium malmoense* is second.

RISK FACTORS

Skin test reactivity to mycobacterial antigens has ranged in prevalence from 11% to 33% in the United States. Predictors of skin test reactivity have included residence in the southeastern region of the country, male gender, black race, birth outside of the United States, and degree of soil exposure. Of note, however, many of the patients who develop pulmonary disease related to NTM do not have these characteristics. For example, patients with the nodular-bronchiectatic form of pulmonary disease (see "Pulmonary Disease" further on) frequently are white, postmenopausal women who were born in the United States.

Patients who have pulmonary infections caused by NTM often have structural lung disease such as chronic obstructive pulmonary disease, bronchiectasis, cystic fibrosis, pneumoconiosis, previous TB, alveolar proteinosis, and chronic aspiration. A study from France noted that more than 50% of the patients who met ATS disease criteria (except for those with *M. kansasii*) had underlying predisposing factors such as preexisting pulmonary or immune deficiency. HIV-infected patients and those with abnormalities in the IFN-γ or interleukin-12 (IL-12) pathways are predisposed to severe NTM infections.

PATHOGENESIS

Although little is known about the pathogenesis of NTM infections, several observations have provided some insight into this disease. First, in HIV-infected patients, disseminated NTM infections typically occur only after the CD4+ lymphocyte count falls below 50 cells/μL, suggesting that specific T cell products or activities are required for mycobacterial resistance. Second, in HIV-uninfected patients, certain genetic syndromes have been identified that are associated with disseminated NTM infections. These syndromes have been traced to mutations in IFN-γ and IL-12 synthesis and response pathways. Third, a striking association has been noted among bronchiectasis, nodular pulmonary NTM infections, and a particular body habitus, predominantly in postmenopausal women. In the last instance, it remains to be seen whether or not these women have some sort of subtle immune deficiency that predisposes them to NTM pulmonary infections, or whether their predisposition is related to ineffective mucociliary clearance or poor tracheobronchial secretion drainage. Investigators have hypothesized that decreased leptin, increased adiponectin, and/or decreased estrogen may account for the increased susceptibility in these latter patients. In addition, in those with the distinctive morphotype, abnormalities in fibrillin have been hypothesized to further increase the susceptibility to NTM infections through expression of the immunosuppressive cytokine tumor growth factor-β.

NTM do not seem to live in a state of dormancy like that for *M. tuberculosis*. Moreover, unlike with TB, simply isolating an NTM from a respiratory specimen does not mean that the patient has NTM-related disease. For years the term *colonization* has been used to describe the infective status of patients who have a single or small number of positive cultures over time and in whom progressive disease cannot be demonstrated. With longer follow-up, however, many of these patients do, in fact, demonstrate clinical and/or radiographic progression of disease, so it may be more appropriate to think of these patients as having indolent infection.

GENETICS

The genetics of NTM infection are not well understood. Studies from Japan and South Korea have not found an association of such infections with mutations in genes encoding IFN-γ, IL-12, or HLA. However, associations with NTM pulmonary disease and mutations in the major histocompatibility complex class I chain–related A (MICA) gene and natural resistance-associated macrophage protein 1 gene (*Nramp1*) have been reported. The role of Toll-like receptor-2 remains controversial.

CLINICAL FEATURES

The most common clinical manifestation of NTM infection is chronic lung disease. However, lymphatic, skin or soft tissue, and bone or joint involvement, as well as disseminated disease, also is important. The propensity for a specific manifestation varies with the NTM species and certain host factors. For example, HIV-infected patients typically are seen with disseminated disease caused by *Mycobacterium avium*, whereas elderly white women often have pulmonary disease caused by *Mycobacterium intracellulare*.

PULMONARY DISEASE

Chronic pulmonary disease is the most common clinical presentation of NTM disease, and patients usually present with chronic cough, fatigue, malaise, dyspnea, fever, hemoptysis, chest pain, and weight loss. Patients should be evaluated for possible gastroesophageal disorders that lead to aspiration, lipoid pneumonia, cystic fibrosis, and α_1-antitrypsin anomalies. Physical examination may identify certain morphologic characteristics in postmenopausal women, and occasionally men, that include thin body habitus, scoliosis, pectus excavatum, and mitral valve prolapse.

NTM pulmonary infections manifest with two prototypical radiographic patterns: fibrocavitary disease, consisting of upper lobe opacities with cavities and volume loss, and nodular bronchiectatic disease, consisting of nodules and bronchiectasis.

Classically, *fibrocavitary disease* was recognized in older men with underlying lung disease (**Figure 31-13**). This radiographic pattern mimics that of TB, and NTM infection frequently is identified in the course of evaluation for TB. By contrast, *nodular bronchiectatic disease* typically occurs among women without known structural lung disease. Chest radiographs reveal opacities in the middle and lower lung fields. High-resolution CT scans demonstrate bronchiectasis often in the middle lobe and lingula, with evidence of small noncavitating nodules, centrilobular in location (**Figure 31-14**). It is important to recognize that there is a great deal of overlap between the two classic radiographic presentations and between the patterns of disease produced by the various NTM species.

Patients with *M. kansasii* infection usually present with upper lobe cavitary opacities, and the cavities typically are thin-walled (**Figure 31-15**). The chest radiograph in patients with rapidly growing mycobacterial infections usually shows multilobar, patchy, reticulonodular or mixed interstitial alveolar opacities, with an upper lobe predominance (**Figure 31-16**). Cavitation is reported to occur in 15% to 40%. High-resolution CT scans will show bronchiectasis and small nodules, similar to those in MAC infection.

LYMPHADENITIS

In children, the most common form of NTM disease is cervical lymphadenitis. *M. avium* is the most common etiologic agent, accounting for 80% of culture-proven cases. *Mycobacterium scrofulaceum* is the second most common cause of lymphadenitis in the United States and Australia, whereas *M. malmoense* and *Mycobacterium haemophilum* are in Scandinavia, the United Kingdom, and other areas of northern Europe. *M. tuberculosis* is isolated in only 10% of cases of culture-proven mycobacterial cervical lymphadenitis in the United States, but in adults, 90% are due to TB.

Infection usually involves the submandibular, submaxillary, cervical, and preauricular lymph nodes in children between 1 and 5 years of age. The disease is of insidious onset and is rarely associated with systemic symptoms. Involvement of the lymph nodes usually is unilateral, and affected tissue is nontender. The lymph nodes may enlarge and eventually rupture, producing sinus tracts just as in tuberculous lymphadenitis. Diagnosis

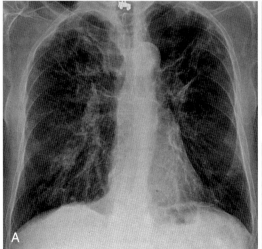
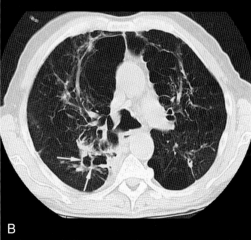

Figure 31-13   A, Chest radiograph obtained in a patient with upper lobe emphysema and severe lung disease caused by *Mycobacterium avium* complex. **B,** Chest computed tomography from the same patient demonstrates severe emphysema with cavitation posteriorly (*arrows*) in the right lower lobe.

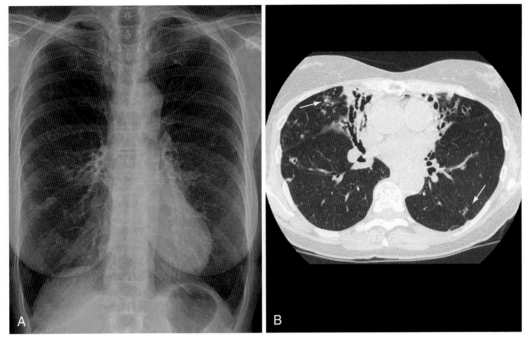

Figure 31-14 **A**, Chest radiograph showing right middle lobe and lingular bronchiectasis in a patient with *Mycobacterium avium* complex and *Mycobacterium simiae* infection. **B**, Chest computed tomography from the same patient demonstrating bronchiectasis in the right middle lobe and lingula. Note also the nodular opacities and tree-in-bud opacities (*arrows*).

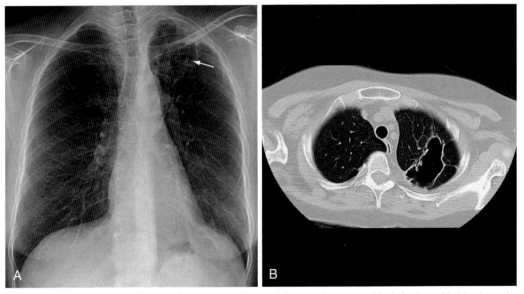

Figure 31-15 **A**, Chest radiograph showing a thin-walled cavity (*arrow*) in the left upper lobe caused by infection with *Mycobacterium kansasii*. **B**, Chest computed tomography from the same patient demonstrating a thin-walled cavity in the left upper lobe.

usually is made by fine needle aspiration or surgical excision of the involved lymph nodes. Only 50% to 82% of excised nodes will be culture positive. Treatment for most cases of NTM-related cervical lymphadenitis is surgical excision.

SOFT TISSUE, SKIN, AND BONE INFECTIONS

Although virtually any NTM can cause skin, soft tissue, and bone infections, the most common species to do so are the rapid growers *Mycobacterium marinum* and *Mycobacterium ulcerans*. Rapid growers often produce infections at the site of punctures or surgery. Joint and bone infections have occurred after surgery and traumatic injuries. Tissue biopsy is the most sensitive way to diagnose these infections.

DISSEMINATED INFECTIONS

Disseminated infections are most commonly associated with HIV infection and other forms of severe immunosuppression. More than 90% of reported cases of disseminated infection in HIV-infected patients are due to MAC, and almost all of these are due to *M. avium*. The next most common cause of disseminated NTM disease in HIV-infected patients is *M. kansasii*, but a number of other species also have been implicated. Most patients have advanced HIV disease at clinical presentation and complain of fever, night sweats, and weight loss. Abdominal pain and diarrhea also may be reported. In non–HIV-infected patients, fever of unknown origin is a common presentation. Diagnosis usually is through detection of the causative

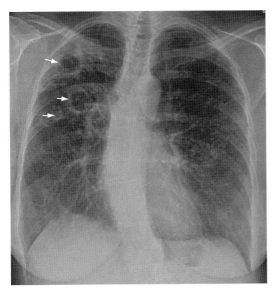

Figure 31-16 Chest radiograph obtained in a patient with infection caused by *Mycobacterium abscessus*. Note the multiple cavities (*arrows*), diffuse nodular opacities, and kyphoscoliosis.

organism in the blood. In HIV-infected patients, *M. avium* can be isolated in more than 90% of cases.

DIAGNOSIS

INTEGRATION OF CLINICAL, MICROBIOLOGIC, AND RADIOGRAPHIC DATA

Patients suspected of having a NTM infection should be evaluated with a chest radiograph or high-resolution CT, or both, particularly in the absence of evidence of cavitation on the radiograph. If radiographic abnormalities are consistent with an NTM infection, at least three sputum specimens should be obtained for AFB examination and mycobacterial culture. TB, as well as other disorders, should be excluded.

To diagnose NTM infection, the clinician must weigh clinical, bacteriologic, and radiographic information (**Box 31-1**). NTM pulmonary infections should be suspected when a patient presents with a compatible clinical picture and nodular or cavitary opacities on the chest radiograph or multifocal bronchiectasis with multiple small nodules on a high-resolution CT scan. In addition to these clinical criteria, the patient should have at least two positive cultures from separate sputum specimens or a positive culture from at least one bronchial wash or lavage procedure. Additional diagnostic criteria include transbronchial or other lung biopsy specimens with mycobacterial histopathologic features and culture-positive for NTM, or a biopsy specimen showing mycobacterial histopathologic features and one or more sputum or bronchial washings that are culture-positive. In patients who do not meet the preceding definition for disease, close follow-up is indicated, because many will demonstrate progression over time.

LABORATORY DIAGNOSIS

The same methods that are used to stain and grow *M. tuberculosis* are used for NTM. Both solid and liquid culture media support growth of the NTM, and both are recommended for use in the clinical laboratory. Although cultures in broth media have a higher yield and provide a more rapid result, they do not allow for observation of colony morphology, growth rates,

---

Box 31-1 Clinical and Microbiologic Criteria for Diagnosis of Lung Disease Due to Nontuberculous Mycobacteria

Clinical*
1. Pulmonary symptoms, nodular or cavitary opacities on the chest radiograph, or multifocal bronchiectasis with multiple small nodules on a high-resolution computed tomography scan
AND
2. Appropriate exclusion of other diagnoses

Microbiologic
1. Positive culture results from at least two separate expectorated sputum samples. If results are nondiagnostic, consider repeat sputum acid-fast bacilli (AFB) smears and cultures.
   OR
2. Positive culture result from at least one bronchial wash or lavage.
   OR
3. Transbronchial or other lung biopsy with mycobacterial histopathologic features (granulomatous inflammation or AFB) and positive culture for nontuberculous mycobacteria (NTM) or biopsy showing mycobacterial histopathologic features (granulomatous inflammation or AFB) and one or more sputum or bronchial washings that are culture-positive for NTM.

*Presence of both clinical criteria is required.
Modified from Griffith DE, Aksamit T, Brown-Elliott BA, et al; ATS Mycobacterial Diseases Subcommittee, American Thoracic Society; Infectious Diseases Society of America: An official ATS/IDSA statement: diagnosis, treatment, and prevention of nontuberculous mycobacterial diseases, *Am J Respir Crit Care Med* 175:367-416, 2007.

---

and recognition of mixed cultures, as do solid media. For most mycobacteria, the optimum temperature for growth is 28° to 37° C, and most clinically significant NTM organisms grow at 35° to 37° C. However, some NTM species—*M. marinum*, *Mycobacterium chelonae*, *M. ulcerans*, and *M. haemophilum*—require lower temperatures for optimum growth. Others, such as *M. xenopi*, grow best at higher temperatures. Some species require special media, such as iron or heme for *M. haemophilum* and mycobactin J for *Mycobacterium genavense*. Most NTM organisms grow within 2 to 3 weeks on subculture, but it may take up to 8 to 12 weeks to grow *M. ulcerans* and *M. genavense*. Rapidly growing mycobacteria usually grow within 7 days on subculture.

Species identification can be performed biochemically or, more commonly, with high-performance liquid chromatography (HPLC), genetic probes, and/or 16S ribosomal DNA sequencing. Genetic probes are commercially available only for *M. tuberculosis*, *M. kansasii*, *M. avium*, *M. intracellulare*, and *Mycobacterium gordonae*. These probes have a sensitivity of between 85% and 100%, with a specificity of 100%. HPLC is a practical and rapid way to detect differences in mycolic acid content between NTM species, although this method cannot differentiate some species of NTM. DNA sequence analysis is able to differentiate strains on the basis of two hypervariable sequences.

An alternative approach to the clinical problems of rapidly distinguishing pulmonary MAC infection from TB and distinguishing MAC disease from MAC colonization has been proposed by Japanese investigators who have developed an enzyme immunoassay (EIA) for a MAC-specific glycopeptidolipid. This assay identified MAC pulmonary disease with 84% sensitivity and 100% sensitivity. Although promising, this assay is not widely available and awaits validation in additional clinical cohorts.

DRUG SUSCEPTIBILITY TESTING

The role of in vitro susceptibility in management of patients with NTM disease is controversial because, with the few specific exceptions mentioned further on, in vitro susceptibility results are not demonstrated to correlate with clinical response to therapy. This is in contrast with *M. tuberculosis*, for which susceptibility results have clear clinical implications.

Macrolide resistance in MAC infection is an important instance in which susceptibility results have prognostic and therapeutic implications. Development of macrolide resistance is associated with azithromycin or clarithromycin monotherapy and portends a poor prognosis. Macrolide resistance is an indication for aggressive therapy including the use of an aminoglycoside and surgical resection if feasible. Current ATS guidelines recommend clarithromycin testing for new, previously untreated MAC isolates, those who fail macrolide-based treatment regimens, or prophylaxis regimens.

Rifampin resistance among previously untreated *M. kansasii* isolates represents a second instance in which in vitro susceptibility informs management, because rifampin resistance has been correlated with poor outcomes. Isolates resistant to rifampin also should be tested against rifabutin, ethambutol, isoniazid, clarithromycin, fluoroquinolones, amikacin, and sulfonamides.

The role of testing for macrolide susceptibility with *M. abscessus* is unclear. *M. abscessus* isolates routinely appear to be macrolide-susceptible on in vitro testing but patients with *M. abscessus* infections are noted to have poor clinical responses to macrolides. This discrepancy may be explained with discovery of the *M. abscessus* erm(41) gene, which confers inducible macrolide resistance. A subset of isolates classified as *M. abscessus* on routine testing are shown with molecular methods to be *Mycobacterium massiliense*. *M. massiliense* has a deletion in the erm(41) gene that makes it nonfunctional, and a better clinical response to macrolide-based therapy was demonstrated in patients infected with *M. massiliense* than in those infected with *M. abscessus*.

In summary, because NTM susceptibility results do not always correlate with clinical response and interpretation differs for different organisms, results should be interpreted with caution and, if possible, in consultation with clinicians expert in the care of NTM infections.

TREATMENT

When the patient's culture specimen grows *M. tuberculosis,* treatment is always indicated, assuming that the isolate was not due to laboratory cross-contamination. With NTM infections, however, isolation should not always lead to treatment. The decision to treat is based on the potential risks and benefits for the individual patient. Thus, management of patients with NTM infections is complicated and requires a great deal of individualization of therapy. In addition, because in vitro susceptibility results for many NTM species do not correlate well with clinical response to antimicrobial therapy, clinicians should use such data with a clear understanding of the limitations.

PULMONARY INFECTIONS

Mycobacterium avium Complex

Before the availability of the newer macrolides, the long-term cure rate for patients treated with antituberculosis regimens was approximately 50%. Small, noncomparative studies of azithromycin- and clarithromycin-containing regimens suggest higher bacteriologic response rates, but long-term follow-up data often are lacking. The ATS currently recommends that the treatment regimen be based on the presence or absence of cavitary disease and whether or not the patient has been treated previously (**Table 31-7**). For patients with noncavitary nodular bronchiectasis disease, a three-times-a-week regimen may be considered. For patients with cavitary or advanced disease and

Table 31-7 Nontuberculous Mycobacteria and Recommended Therapy

Common Etiologic Agents	Recommended Antimicrobial Therapy	Other Etiologic Mycobacterial Species
M. avium complex		*M. simiae*
Nodular bronchiectasis	Clarithromycin 1000 mg 3×/wk OR azithromycin 500-600 mg 3×/wk; rifampin 600 mg 3×/wk; ethambutol 25 mg/kg 3×/wk	*M. szulgai* *M. celatum* *M. asiaticum*
Cavitary disease	Clarithromycin 1000 mg daily OR azithromycin 250 mg daily; rifampin 450-600 mg daily; ethambutol 15 mg/kg daily Also consider amikacin 15 mg/kg (for the first 2-3 mo) 3×/wk	*M. haemophilum* *M. smegmatis* *M. chelonae*
Previously treated	Clarithromycin 1000 mg daily OR azithromycin 250 mg daily; rifampin 450-600 mg daily OR rifabutin 150-300 mg daily; amikacin 15 mg/kg (for the first 2-3 months) 3×/wk	*M. fortuitum* *M. scrofulaceum* *M. shimodei*
M. kansasii	Isoniazid 300 mg/day; rifampin 600 mg/day; ethambutol 15 mg/kg/day Can add aminoglycoside in severe disease	
M. abscessus	Clarithromycin 1000 mg/daily OR azithromycin 250 mg/daily; cefoxitin max. 12 g/d divided in 3-4 doses/day OR imipenem 500-1000 mg q8-12 h PLUS amikacin 15 mg/kg 3×/wk	
M. xenopi	Clarithromycin 1000 mg daily OR azithromycin 250 mg daily; rifampin 450-600 mg daily; ethambutol 15 mg/kg daily Also consider isoniazid and/or amikacin 15 mg/kg (for the first 2-3 mo) 3×/wk	
M. malmoense	Clarithromycin 1000 mg daily OR azithromycin 250 mg daily; rifampin 450-600 mg daily; ethambutol 15 mg/kg daily	

in those who have been treated previously, daily therapy is recommended. An aminoglycoside should be considered in patients, at least for the first 2 to 3 months of therapy, if they have cavitary disease or if previous treatment has failed. Surgery should be considered in patients in whom the infection is due to a macrolide-resistant strain of MAC, in whom treatment has failed, or in whom cavitary disease is localized and potentially resectable.

Mycobacterium kansasii

Patients with lung disease caused by *M. kansasii* should be treated with INH, rifampin, and ethambutol (see Table 31-7). Substitution of clarithromycin for INH has been associated with good short-term outcomes, and in one study, no relapses were seen at follow-up evaluation after 46 months. As with other NTM infections, the treatment duration should encompass 12 months of negative sputum cultures. For patients whose isolate is resistant to the rifamycins, a three-drug regimen is recommended on the basis of data for in vitro susceptibility to clarithromycin or azithromycin, moxifloxacin, ethambutol, sulfamethoxazole, or streptomycin. Surgical resection is almost never necessary in patients infected with *M. kansasii*.

Mycobacterium malmoense

Mycobacterium malmoense is the second most common cause of pulmonary NTM disease in some areas of northern Europe. The clinical relevance of *M. malmoense* seems to vary, because 70% to 80% of the European patients in whom *M. malmoense* is isolated meet ATS criteria for disease, whereas in the United States, this organism rarely causes pulmonary disease.

Current recommendations are to treat *M. malmoense* pulmonary disease with two to four drugs including ethambutol and rifampin. In a randomized clinical trial conducted by the British Thoracic Society, a regimen consisting of clarithromycin, ethambutol, and rifampin had a more favorable outcome than a regimen containing ciprofloxacin instead of the macrolide. However, overall mortality was not different between regimens.

Mycobacterium xenopi

M. xenopi is one of the most common causes of NTM lung disease in Canada, the United Kingdom, and some parts of Europe. Disease usually occurs in persons with underlying lung disease and often is cavitary at the time of clinical presentation. The optimal treatment is not known. In the British Thoracic Society clinical trial just described, the same two treatment regimens were evaluated in patients with *M. xenopi* pulmonary disease. No differences were noted in the treatment success, failure, or relapse rates. All-cause mortality was high and slightly greater in the ciprofloxacin-containing regimen. With use of various treatment regimens, 58% of patients with lung disease due to *M. xenopi* were cured in a report from the Netherlands. Current recommendations are to treat patients with ethambutol, rifampin, and a macrolide, with the possible addition of INH and an aminoglycoside for severe disease.

Rapidly Growing Mycobacteria

M. abscessus is the third most frequently encountered NTM respiratory pathogen in the United States and accounts for 80% of cases of lung disease due to rapidly growing mycobacteria. Treatment outcomes with *M. abscessus* generally are poor, in part because the organism is susceptible to only a few antimicrobials, including the macrolides, imipenem, cefoxitin, amikacin, tigecycline, clofazimine and occasionally linezolid. In vitro

susceptibility testing is recommended for selection of a treatment regimen. As noted previously, although *M. abscessus* may be macrolide-susceptible in vitro, induction of the *erm(41)* gene may result in clinical resistance. The impact of such resistance on the efficacy of the treatment regimen is unknown, so macrolides are still recommended for treatment. Unfortunately, no antibiotic regimen has demonstrated predictable long-term sputum conversion in patients with pulmonary disease. Recent studies from South Korea and the United States reported culture conversion rates of at least 12 months in approximately 50% to 60% of patients. Current recommendations are to provide periodic drug administration of multidrug therapy, including a macrolide, and one or more parenteral agents such as amikacin, cefoxitin, or imipenem for 2 to 6 months to help control symptoms and prevent progression (see Table 31-7). For patients who are good candidates, surgical resection should be considered but only if done by an experienced surgeon and after a period of intensive antimicrobial therapy. In two studies, outcomes were better in patients who underwent surgical resection in addition to antimicrobial therapy.

M. chelonae typically is susceptible to tobramycin, macrolides, linezolid, imipenem, and amikacin and may demonstrate susceptibility to fluoroquinolones and doxycycline. Isolates usually are resistant to cefoxitin. Treatment should consist of at least two drugs to which in vitro drug susceptibility has been demonstrated. The duration should be for at least 12 months of culture negativity.

Mycobacterium fortuitum isolates typically are susceptible to newer macrolides, fluoroquinolones, doxycycline, minocycline, sulfonamides, cefoxitin, and imipenem. As with *M. abscessus*, however, *M. fortuitum* harbors an *erm* gene, so the clinical efficacy of macrolides is uncertain. Therapy should be with at least two agents with in vitro activity for at least 12 months of culture negativity.

LYMPHADENITIS

Cervical lymphadenitis usually is caused by MAC or *M. scrofulaceum* infection. Surgical excision of the involved lymph nodes without chemotherapy usually is curative, with success rates of approximately 95%. In patients who have surgical excision fail, a macrolide-based treatment regimen with or without repeat excision is usually successful.

SKIN, SOFT TISSUE, AND BONE/JOINT INFECTIONS

For most patients with MAC infection, a combination of surgical excision plus multidrug chemotherapy is usually successful. The optimal duration of therapy is not known but probably should be 6 to 12 months. For serious infections caused by rapidly growing mycobacteria, a newer macrolide should be combined with a parenteral medication (amikacin, cefoxitin, or imipenem) or perhaps another oral agent in the case of *M. fortuitum* infection. Therapy should continue for a minimum of 4 months for skin infections and at least 6 months for bone infections. Surgery generally is indicated for extensive disease, and removal of foreign objects such as breast implants, percutaneous catheters, and joint prostheses will be necessary.

DISSEMINATED INFECTIONS

Treatment of disseminated MAC infection in HIV-infected patients should include clarithromycin, 500 mg twice daily, and ethambutol, 15 mg/kg daily with or without rifabutin 300 mg, once daily. Azithromycin, 500 mg daily, could be used as an alternative to clarithromycin. Treatment should be considered to be lifelong, unless immune restoration is achieved by anti-retroviral therapy. Anti-MAC treatment can be stopped for patients who are asymptomatic and have achieved a CD4$^+$ lymphocyte count of more than 100 cells/μL for at least 12 months. Prophylaxis should be reintroduced if the count falls below 100 cells/μL.

The treatment for disseminated disease caused by *M. kansasii* is the same as for pulmonary disease. Unlike with MAC infection, no effective prophylactic regimen is available.

CLINICAL COURSE AND PREVENTION

The clinical course will depend on the specific species of NTM causing disease, the severity and extent of disease, and the treatment regimen used. Untreated *M. kansasii* infection usually is progressive, much like TB. With appropriate treatment, however, almost all patients respond well, and both treatment failure and relapse are uncommon. Untreated MAC pulmonary disease is quite variable in its progression. In some patients, progression can be seen over a matter of months, and in others, it may take years to demonstrate progressive disease. Treatment responses in MAC infections also are variable, with cure rates ranging from 60% to 85%. Genotyping data suggest that reinfection is common in women with nodular bronchiectasis, so a patient in whom cure is achieved may become infected again. The clinical course of untreated *M. abscessus* infection generally is slow and progressive, but more rapidly progressive presentations have been described, particularly in patients with cystic fibrosis or esophageal disorders associated with aspiration. Treatment of *M. abscessus* disease is complicated, and cure is uncommon. The mortality rate with *M. xenopi* infection has been reported to be as high as 57%, but this probably reflects the organism's predilection for patients with severe underlying structural lung disease.

PREVENTION

Strategies for preventing NTM infections are difficult to formulate because of the current poor understanding of the transmission and pathogenesis of these infections. In at least two or three situations, methods to potentially prevent NTM disease have been recognized. The first is among patients with advanced HIV infection. Preventive therapy for disseminated MAC infection is recommended for HIV-infected patients with fewer than 50 CD4$^+$ lymphocytes/μL. Azithromycin given in a dose of 1200 mg once weekly is the preferred agent. An acceptable alternate regimen is clarithromycin, 500 mg, twice daily, or rifabutin, 300 mg daily. Primary prophylaxis should be discontinued when patients have responded to highly active antiretroviral therapy (HAART) with an increase in CD4$^+$ lymphocyte count to more than 100 cells/μL for more than 3 months. Prophylaxis should be reintroduced if the count falls to less than 50 to 100 cells/μL.

A second way to prevent NTM infections is through good clinical practices in health care settings, where contamination of water sources, biologicals, and multidose vials has been implicated in postsurgical infections. In these settings, tap water should not be used to wash wounds or equipment, and multidose vials should be avoided for injections.

Prevention of community-acquired pulmonary infections remains elusive. The organisms have been isolated in tap water and water distribution systems, survive well at water temperatures of 45° C, and are resistant to typical decontamination methods. Therefore, it is not clear how to best decrease environmental exposure.

CONTROVERSIES AND PITFALLS

TB remains one of the most important public health problems in the world. Despite effective treatment and preventive regimens, TB continues to spread, particularly in resource-poor countries, where both HIV co-infection and drug-resistant *M. tuberculosis* disease create additional barriers to control. Delays in the diagnosis and initiation of effective antituberculosis chemotherapy lead to higher morbidity and mortality in affected patients and continued transmission to others. The first step in preventing these scenarios is timely diagnosis and initiation of therapy, which begins with the recognition of TB as a potential cause of the patient's illness. Because of the increased frequency of drug-resistant TB, more rapid diagnostics are urgently needed, particularly in areas where HIV co-infection is common. Current treatment regimens require that multiple drugs be administered over a prolonged treatment course. Poor adherence to therapy, which has resulted in poor outcomes including the development of drug-resistant disease, remains a barrier to completion of therapy. New drugs that would allow for shorter treatment regimens, ideally administered intermittently, could improve our ability to treat patients to cure.

As the United States and other industrialized countries move toward the goal of TB elimination, improved diagnostics for detecting LTBI and ideally for identifying patients at increased risk for progression to active disease will be needed. It remains to be seen whether the new IGRAs will provide us with such tools. With 12 weekly doses of rifapentine plus INH, the PREVENT-TB has offered the long-awaited promise of a shorter course of therapy for LTBI, but the trial was performed with directly observed therapy. Implementation of this strategy in routine practice will require careful consideration of logistics and costs. Finally, BCG vaccination has failed as a significant TB control measure, because it does not prevent infection from occurring and it does not prevent the development of active TB in adults, thereby allowing continuation of the cycle of transmission. New vaccines are urgently needed if TB is to be eliminated on a global scale.

As the incidence of TB declines in many countries, NTM infections are increasing to fill the ecologic void. The reasons for this and just how much NTM exists are not really known because of the lack of epidemiologic and surveillance data. Much research effort should be directed at elucidation of the natural history of NTM infections and how and where people become infected. Because of the difficulty in distinguishing colonization from disease, it is important to develop better diagnostic tests and to develop new drugs and better treatment regimens for these resistant and difficult-to-treat infections. Current knowledge about the treatment of these infections is remarkably deficient. Which macrolide is superior? Which rifamycin is superior? Does addition of an aminoglycoside improve outcomes? What is the role of the fluoroquinolones? Of importance as well, how can these infections be prevented? Only better epidemiologic data and clinical trials can answer these questions.

WEB RESOURCES

American Thoracic Society: www.thoracic.org
Centers for Disease Control and Prevention: www.cdc.org
Francis J. Curry National Tuberculosis Center: www.nationaltbcenter.org

Heartland National Tuberculosis Center: www.heartlandntbc.org

International Union Against Tuberculosis and Lung Disease: www.iuatld.org

Northeastern Regional Training and Medical Consultation Consortium: www.umdnj.edu/globaltb/home.htm

Southeastern National Tuberculosis Center: sntc.medicine.ufl.edu

World Health Organization, Stop TB Partnership: www.stoptb.org

SUGGESTED READINGS

American Thoracic Society: Diagnostic standards and classification of tuberculosis in adults and children, *Am J Respir Crit Care Med* 161:1376–1395, 2000.

American Thoracic Society: Targeted tuberculin testing and treatment of latent tuberculosis infection, *Am J Respir Crit Care Med* 161: S221–S247, 2000.

American Thoracic Society; CDC; Infectious Diseases Society of America: Treatment of tuberculosis, *MMWR Recomm Rep* 52(RR-11):1–80, 2003.

American Thoracic Society; Centers for Disease Control and Prevention; Infectious Diseases Society of America: American Thoracic Society/Centers for Disease Control and Prevention/Infectious Diseases Society of America: controlling tuberculosis in the United States, *Am J Respir Crit Care Med* 172:1169–1227, 2005.

Centers for Disease Control and Prevention (CDC): Updated guidelines for the use of nucleic acid amplification tests in the diagnosis of tuberculosis, *MMWR Morb Mortal Wkly Rep* 58:7–10, 2009.

Griffith DE, Aksamit T, Brown-Elliott BA, et al; ATS Mycobacterial Diseases Subcommittee, American Thoracic Society; Infectious Diseases Society of America: An official ATS/IDSA statement: diagnosis, treatment, and prevention of nontuberculous mycobacterial diseases, *Am J Respir Crit Care Med* 175:367–416, 2007.

Jensen PA, Lambert LA, Iademarco MF, Ridzon R; Centers for Disease Control and Prevention: Guidelines for preventing the transmission of *Mycobacterium tuberculosis* in health-care settings, 2005, *MMWR Recomm Rep* 54(RR-17):1–141, 2005.

Mazurek GH, Jereb J, Vernon A, et al; Centers for Disease Control and Prevention (CDC): Updated guidelines for using interferon gamma release assays to detect *Mycobacterium tuberculosis* infection—United States, 2010, *MMWR Recomm Rep* 59(RR-5):1–25, 2010.

World Health Organization: *Guidelines for the programmatic management of drug-resistant tuberculosis, 2011 update*, ed 3, Geneva, 2011, World Health Organization.

World Health Organization: *Treatment of tuberculosis, guidelines*, ed 4, Geneva, 2010, World Health Organization.

Chapter **32**

Invasive Mechanical Ventilation

Lukas Brander • Arthur S. Slutsky

The ancient Greek physician and philosopher Claudius Galen (129 to 210 CE) was the first to describe artificial ventilation of an animal. With the exception of a few historical anecdotes, mechanical ventilation did not become a widely used therapeutic intervention in clinical medicine until the outbreak of the poliomyelitis epidemic in Europe and the United States in the 1940s and 1950s, during which negative-pressure ventilators were made available to many of the patients with polio-related breathing impairment. Since then, there have been many developments in the technology of ventilators, and mechanical ventilation has become a commonly used, lifesaving procedure for patients with respiratory failure.

Ventilators initially were used in conjunction with neuromuscular blocking agents to provide controlled ventilation. Recognition that abolition of spontaneous breathing rapidly leads to deconditioning of the respiratory muscles stimulated the development of ventilatory strategies designed to deliver assistance in synchrony with the patient's spontaneous breathing efforts. The first mode to allow a patient to initiate and terminate a predefined level of pressure support was introduced in the early 1980s, initiating a process that led to a growing awareness of the complexity and consequences of patient-ventilator interactions and more recently to the development of ventilatory modes that allow individualization of the assist on a breath-by-breath basis.

This chapter outlines the indications for and contraindications to invasive mechanical ventilation, illustrates the operation of various ventilatory modes, describes the essentials of mechanical ventilation in patients with obstructive and with restrictive pulmonary disease processes, and summarizes the potential complications of mechanical ventilation.

INDICATIONS AND CONTRAINDICATIONS

The goals of mechanical ventilation include decreasing the oxygen cost of breathing by unloading the respiratory muscles and maintaining adequate gas exchange, while minimizing potential complications associated with ventilation, including ventilation-induced lung injury (VILI), patient-ventilator asynchrony, hemodynamic compromise, and negative effects on other nonpulmonary organs. Mechanical ventilation is indicated when the patient is unable to maintain the function of their respiratory system as a result of underlying pulmonary disease, failure of the respiratory muscles, instability of the chest wall, increased metabolic demand, or the requirement for deep sedation or for neuromuscular blockade, and when noninvasive ventilation has failed or is contraindicated (e.g., in an unconscious patient, during surgery, with rapid progression of respiratory failure).

A number of methods can be used to monitor mechanical ventilation, including clinical assessment (e.g., respiratory pattern, auscultation, patient-ventilator interaction) and assessment of gas exchange (e.g., arterial blood gases, pulse oximetry, carbon dioxide tension in exhaled air). Monitoring the pressure waveforms and flow applied to the airways allows calculation of the variables of respiratory system mechanics; chest radiography or computed tomography helps assess the underlying disease process or some complications of mechanical ventilation (e.g., displacement of the endotracheal tube, pneumothorax); and monitoring the function of nonpulmonary organs (e.g., cardiac performance, central nervous system function, urinary output) may indicate adequacy of global and regional oxygen delivery. For safety reasons, virtually all ventilators contain adjustable alarm limits for the various functional components, such as upper and lower limits of applied ventilator pressure (i.e., pressure wave forms [P_{VENT}]), ventilatory rate, tidal volume (V_T), minute ventilation, and other variables.

TECHNIQUES

MODES OF INVASIVE MECHANICAL VENTILATION

Most mechanical ventilators are capable of delivering ventilation in a fully controlled manner, to assist spontaneous breathing, and to facilitate nonassisted spontaneous breathing (**Figure 32-1**). Normally, the means by which inhalation is terminated (cycled off) is used to classify the ventilatory modes. Common mechanisms to cycle off the inhalation include volume, pressure, airflow, and time. Initiation of an inhalation (i.e., trigger-on) can be based either on predefined time intervals or on systems in which the patient's inspiratory effort has to exceed a specific threshold. Most frequently, pneumatic systems are used that require a predefined, adjustable change in pressure or airflow within the ventilator circuit to trigger the initiation of an inhalation by the ventilator. Alternative trigger-on and cycling-off methods, such as changes in pleural pressure (P_{PL}) (as can be assessed by esophageal pressure [P_{ES}] measurements) or changes in the amplitude of the diaphragm electrical activity (Edi), are currently entering clinical practice.

With *volume-cycled* ventilation, the ventilator delivers a predefined V_T with a frequency that is either predefined or set by the patient's inspiratory effort. The pressure used to deliver the V_T depends on the mechanical properties of the two major components of the respiratory system (see also further on): (1) the resistance of the inspiratory limb of the ventilator circuit (including the endotracheal tube) and the central airways and (2) the compliance of the respiratory system, consisting of the lung and chest wall.

		Controlled modes		Controlled/assisted combined modes				Assisted modes			Nonassisted spontaneous breathing
		VCV	PCV	SIMV	PRVC	VS	BiPAP, APRV	PSV	PAV	NAVA	CPAP
Termination of the breath is determined by	volume	✓	x	✓	✓	✓	x	x	x	x	x
	pressure	x	✓	✓	x	x	✓/x	x	x	x	x
	flow	x	x	x	x	x	x	✓	x	x	x
	time	x	(✓)/x	x	x	x	✓	x	x	x	x
Initiation of the breath by time/by patient effort		✓/✓	✓/✓	✓/✓	✓/✓	x/✓	✓/(✓)	x/✓	x/✓	x/✓	x/✓
Neurally triggered/cycled		x	x	x	x	x	x	x	x	✓	x
Predefined level of assist		x	x	✓	x	x	x	✓	x	x	x
Assist is proportional to the patient's respiratory effort		x	x	x	x	x	x	x	✓	✓	x

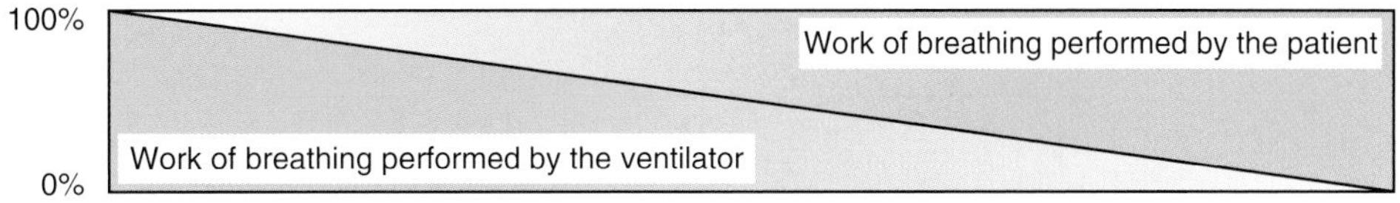

100% — Work of breathing performed by the patient
0% — Work of breathing performed by the ventilator

Figure 32-1 Characteristics of available modes of mechanical ventilation including the method used to terminate (cycle-off) the inhalation and the method to initiate (trigger-on) the inhalation. The available modes include time-cycled, volume-targeted, or pressure-targeted (or -controlled) modes (volume-targeted" or "-controlled" ventilation [*VCV*], pressure-targeted" or "-controlled" ventilation [*PCV*]); modes combining controlled ventilation with assist to spontaneous breathing (synchronized intermittent mandatory ventilation [*SIMV*], pressure-regulated volume control [*PRVC*], volume support [*VS*], airway pressure release ventilation [*APRV*], bilevel positive airway pressure [*BiPAP*]); modes of pure assist to spontaneous breathing (pressure support [*PSV*], proportional assist ventilation [*PAV*], neurally adjusted ventilatory assist [*NAVA*]); and finally, modes that do not deliver assist to the patient but allow unrestricted breathing while delivering a constant pressure (continuous positive airway pressure [*CPAP*]). The work of breathing can completely or largely be taken over by the ventilator during controlled modes of ventilation, whereas during modes that assist spontaneous breathing, the load on the respiratory muscles is shared between the patient and the ventilator.

With *pressure-cycled* ventilation, the ventilator will stop delivering pressure as soon as a predefined pressure level is reached. With this system, the delivered V_T depends on the respiratory system mechanics, and minute ventilation is not guaranteed.

With *flow-cycled* ventilation, the ventilator will cease delivery of pressure as soon as the airflow drops to a predefined level of its maximum. For example, with pressure support ventilation, a preset pressure is applied as soon as the patient's effort exceeds the trigger-on threshold. The ventilator will stop delivering pressure when the inspiratory flow has decreased to a predetermined percentage of its peak value.

With *time-cycled* ventilation, the ventilator will deliver a predefined level of pressure for a predefined time.

MODES THAT TARGET VOLUME OR PRESSURE

Controlled modes of ventilation (i.e., volume- or pressure-targeted or -controlled ventilation) normally are used when deep sedation or muscle paralysis is required (e.g., during surgery), when the patient is making no breathing efforts (e.g., after drug overdose), as a last resort when sufficient synchrony between the ventilator and the patient cannot be achieved, or when maximal reduction of the oxygen cost of breathing and complete unloading of the respiratory muscles from the work of inspiration are desired (e.g., respiratory muscle fatigue, severely altered mechanics of the respiratory system, or severely compromised oxygenation). Adaptation of the patient to controlled mechanical ventilation may require deep sedation and occasionally muscle paralysis.

Volume-Targeted (or -Controlled) Ventilation

With time-cycled, volume-targeted (i.e., volume-controlled) ventilation (VCV), V_T is preset, and the minute ventilation is guaranteed by the ventilator, depending on the ventilatory rate. Triggering delivery of additional breaths with the preset V_T occurs when the patient's breathing efforts exceed a caregiver-defined trigger-on threshold. Volume assist-control (A/C) refers to a variation of VCV in which the patient initiates delivery of a fixed V_T by the ventilator, whereas a VCV backup rate ensures that the patient receives a minimum minute ventilation. Parameters that can be modified with most of the ventilators are the rate of inspiratory flow or ratio of the inspiratory to expiratory times (I/E ratio), the inspiratory rise time, the duration of the end-inspiratory pause time, and with some ventilators, the flow pattern during inhalation (**Figure 32-2**). The effects of changes in these parameters on the pressure and flow waveforms are demonstrated in Figure 32-2, *B* and *C*.

Pressure-Targeted (or -Controlled) Ventilation

With pressure-controlled ventilation (PCV), a maximum inspiratory pressure is targeted by the caregiver. The ventilator increases the pressure to this level during each breath. The flow pattern is decelerating; flow is high initially but decreases as the P$_{VENT}$ limit is approached. Inhalation is terminated when a predefined time limit or flow level is reached. The applied V_T depends on the relative stiffness (elastance) of the respiratory system (e.g., V_T is lower if pulmonary edema develops or if the patient contracts the abdominal or chest wall musculature) and on the resistance to airflow (e.g., V_T will be lower if secretions markedly increase airway

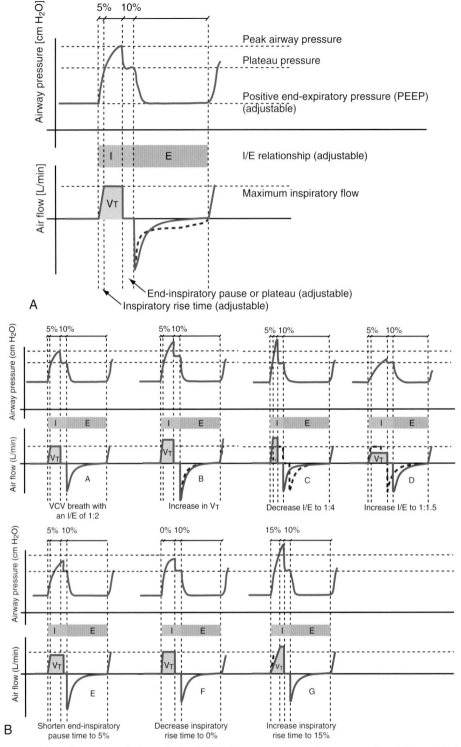

Figure 32-2 **A,** Volume-targeted (or volume-controlled) ventilation (VCV) with a square-wave flow pattern. The delivered tidal volume (VT) is calculated by integrating the area under the flow curve, as indicated by the *blue-shaded area*. During the end-inspiratory pause, the inspiratory and expiratory valves of the ventilator are closed for a predefined time interval (expressed as a percentage of the entire breath period). Ideally, at the end of expiration, the full tidal volume applied during inhalation (minus that lost during gas exchange) has left the lung and the airflow is reduced to zero. This may not be the case in a patient with dynamic collapse of the airways during expiration (e.g., in a patient with chronic obstructive pulmonary disease), where dynamic hyperinflation of the lungs may result from incomplete exhalation of the applied VT and persistence of expiratory airflow is detectable at end expiration (*dashed line*). The inspiratory flow pattern can be varied with many of the modern ventilators to constant (square-wave), decelerating (ramp), or sinusoidal. **B,** Changes in the adjustable parameters with volume-controlled ventilation (*VCV*) result in characteristic changes of the pressure and volume waveforms. The plotted curves demonstrate isolated changes in parameters, under conditions in which all other ventilatory parameters, as well as the mechanical characteristics of the respiratory system, are assumed to remain unchanged. The area under the inspiratory flow curve reflects the tidal volume (VT). A, Baseline conditions. B, An increase in VT results in an increase in the maximum inspiratory flow and hence in an increased peak airway pressure and end-inspiratory plateau pressure. C, Decreasing the I/E ratio results in a prolongation of expiration, while the maximum inspiratory flow and hence the peak airway pressure both increase. D, An increase in the I/E ratio has the exact opposite effect. E, A reduction in the inspiratory pause time reduces the maximum inspiratory flow and hence the peak airway pressure, while the plateau pressure and the inspiratory and expiratory times remain unchanged. F, When the time to reach the maximum inspiratory flow (inspiratory rise time) is shortened, the maximum inspiratory flow and the peak airway pressure will both decrease, whereas prolongation of the inspiratory rise time, G, has the opposite effect. In both situations, the end-inspiratory plateau pressure and the inspiratory and expiratory times do not change.

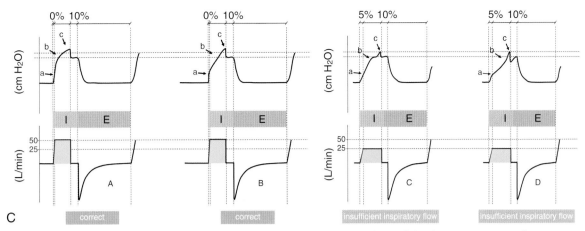

Figure 32-2, cont'd C, Airway pressure tracings during volume-controlled ventilation. The shape of the airway pressure waveform may provide an indication of whether settings of inspiratory flow are adequate. *A* and *B* are normal waveforms: *a*, fast pressure increase; *b*, convex or straight pressure shoulder; *c*, peak pressure. The interrupted (*C*) or even concave (*D*) segments *a* and *b* of the pressure waveform indicate that the maximal inspiratory flow falls short of the patient's actual demand. This may be the case in patients with high respiratory drive, such as in hypermetabolic states, sepsis, and delirium.

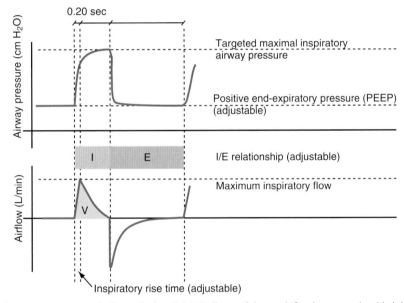

Figure 32-3 Pressure-targeted (or pressure-controlled) ventilation (PCV). Delivery of the predefined pressure level is initiated after a trajectory defined by the preset ventilatory rate. Additional triggering-on also is possible when the patient's effort exceeds a predefined trigger-on threshold. The delivered tidal volume (VT) is calculated as the time integral of the flow curve. The inspiratory rise time defines how quickly the maximal airflow is reached. Inspiration is terminated after a caregiver-specified time interval that results from choosing a ratio of inspiratory-to-expiratory times (I/E ratio) and a ventilatory rate or, alternately, from choosing an absolute inspiratory time.

resistance). The adjustable parameters are the targeted PVENT, the inspiratory rise time, and, in some ventilators, the inspiratory time (**Figure 32-3**).

MODES THAT DELIVER ASSISTANCE TO SPONTANEOUS BREATHING

Patients often are ventilated with volume- or pressure-targeted modes (i.e., controlled ventilation) in the early phase of the disease process, whereas modes delivering assistance to spontaneous breathing usually are applied later. Assistance to spontaneous breathing is used to prevent respiratory muscle atrophy as well as to maintain physiologic feedback and intrinsic defense mechanisms, such as the Hering-Breuer reflex, based on the hypothesis that integration rather than abolition may help to minimize VILI. This approach should be better suited than "caregiver-controlled" mechanical ventilation to accommodate

the typically rapid changes in lung mechanics and metabolic demands in critically ill patients. Ventilatory modes in which patients breathe spontaneously early in the course of the acute lung injury (ALI) process may have certain advantages, such as improved pulmonary ventilation-perfusion (V/Q) matching (**Figure 32-4**), increased oxygenation, preserved cardiac function, reduced need for excessive sedation, prevention of ventilation-associated respiratory muscle dysfunction, and ventilation at lower mean airway pressure, compared with controlled modes of ventilation. Induction of respiratory muscle fatigue or failure secondary to increased work of breathing is a potential disadvantage, but this frequently can be minimized with use of the appropriate level of positive end-expiratory pressure (PEEP) and adjustment of inspiratory flow rates. Of interest, recent data suggest that early neuromuscular blockade for 48 hours in patients with ALI may decrease mortality (see further on).

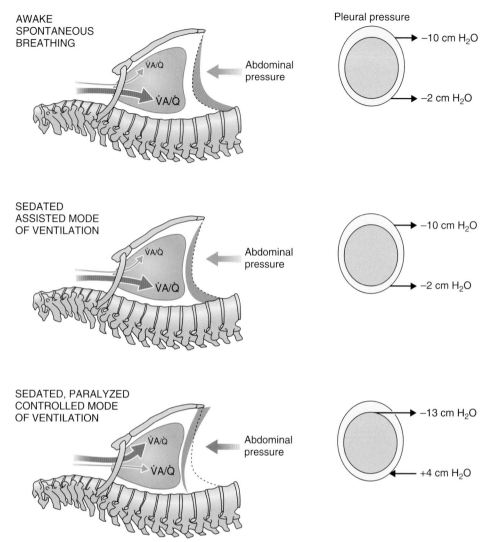

Figure 32-4 Ventilation-perfusion (V̇A/Q̇) distribution during spontaneous breathing and during mechanical ventilation. In a classic article, Froese and Bryan demonstrated that with spontaneous breathing (in either an awake or sedated patient), dorsal excursions of the diaphragm were more pronounced than ventral excursion. The active diaphragm generates a greater negative pressure in the dorsal pleural space, thereby increasing the pressure gradient between the central airways and the pleural space (transpulmonary pressure); this promotes alveolar recruitment and ventilation of the dependent lung regions. Ventilation of dependent, usually well-perfused parts of the lungs, along with an increase in blood flow to previously minimally perfused or nonperfused areas, helps to convert shunt units to units with normal V̇/Q̇ distribution, thereby increasing oxygen content of arterial blood, and to lower pulmonary vascular resistance. During application of positive-pressure ventilation with inactive or only minimally active inspiratory muscles (e.g., with neuromuscular blockade or with hyperventilation), gas is preferentially distributed toward the ventral regions of the lungs, where the impedance to airflow is lower than in the dependent, partially atelectatic regions. Generation of positive pressure in the dorsal pleura promotes collapse of alveoli in the dorsal lung regions and the V̇/Q̇ mismatch becomes worse. *(Data from Froese AB, Bryan AC: Effects of anesthesia and paralysis on diaphragmatic mechanics in man, Anesthesiology 41:242-255, 1974; Warner DO, Warner MA, Ritman EL: Atelectasis and chest wall shape during halothane anesthesia, Anesthesiology 85:49-59, 1996; Hedenstierna G, Lichtwarck-Aschoff M: Interfacing spontaneous breathing and mechanical ventilation. New insights, Minerva Anestesiol 72:183-198, 2006; Oczenski W, editor: Atmen-Atemhifen, Stuttgart, Georg Thieme Verlag, 2006.)*

Pressure Support Ventilation

Pressure support ventilation is patient-triggered and, normally, flow-cycled, allowing the patient to actively control the start of each breath. Once the patient's inspiratory effort exceeds the trigger-on threshold, a caregiver-defined level of PVENT is delivered to the airways (**Figure 32-5**, **A**). After a high initial airflow that is required to rapidly approach the targeted pressure, the airflow progressively decreases. Once a predefined percentage of the maximum inspiratory flow is reached, the ventilator terminates inhalation and opens the expiratory valve. Parameters that can be adjusted with pressure support ventilation are the trigger-on threshold, the inspiratory rise time, and the pressure level (see Figure 32-5, B). To better match termination of the inhalation with the patient's individual demand,

the cycling-off airflow threshold can be varied in some ventilators.

Analogous to all pressure-targeted ventilation modes, pressure support ventilation does not guarantee a specific VT or minute ventilation. Changes in VT and minute ventilation can be achieved by adjusting the level of pressure support and/or the cycling-off criteria.

Difficulties with Conventional Modes of Assistance to Spontaneous Breathing

It is sometimes assumed that assisting spontaneous breathing will decrease respiratory effort; however, unless the ventilator settings are selected to satisfy the patient's demand, such a mode can actually result in the opposite. Ideally, assistance

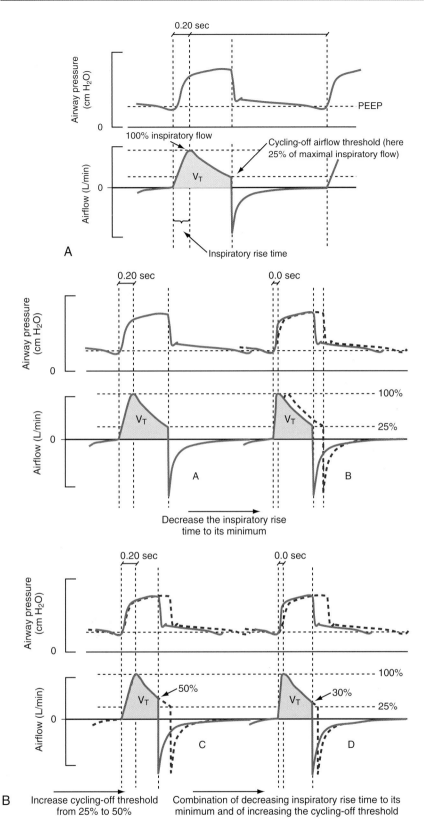

A

Decrease the inspiratory rise time to its minimum

B   Increase cycling-off threshold from 25% to 50%   Combination of decreasing inspiratory rise time to its minimum and of increasing the cycling-off threshold

Figure 32-5   A, Pressure support ventilation (PSV). The delivered tidal volume (VT) is calculated by integrating the area under the flow curve, as indicated by the *blue-shaded area*. The inspiratory rise time defines how fast the maximal airflow (100%) is achieved. Thereafter, the inspiratory airflow continuously decreases because, once the pressure target is reached, maintaining this level requires progressively less air to flow into the lungs. As soon as the cycling-off airflow threshold (i.e., a preset percentage of maximal air flow) is reached, the ventilator ceases to deliver inspiratory flow, and the expiratory valve is opened to allow passive exhalation. **B,** Changes in the parameters of pressure support ventilation result in characteristic changes of the pressure and volume curves. Panels *A* to *D* demonstrate isolated changes of parameters assuming that all other ventilatory parameters and the mechanical characteristics of the respiratory system remain unchanged. *A,* PSV breath with an inspiratory rise time of 0.20 second. *B,* After reducing the inspiratory rise time to its minimum, the peak inspiratory flow and consequently also the cycling-off airflow threshold are both reached earlier. Decreasing the inspiratory rise time results in a shorter inspiratory time, while the VT remains unchanged. Note that although the inspiratory rise time is decreased to 0 seconds, the peak inspiratory flow is reached with a small delay. *C,* Increasing the cycling-off airflow threshold from 30% to 50% similarly shortens the inspiratory time; however, VT decreases in this case. *D,* A combination of a maximal decrease in the inspiratory time and a moderate increase in the cycling-off airflow threshold shortens the inspiratory time, whereas the loss in VT is only minimal. Such an approach can be used to achieve a prolongation of the expiratory time in patients at risk for dynamic hyperinflation because of expiratory flow limitation (e.g., patients with COPD) (see also Figure 32-19). *COPD,* chronic obstructive pulmonary disease.

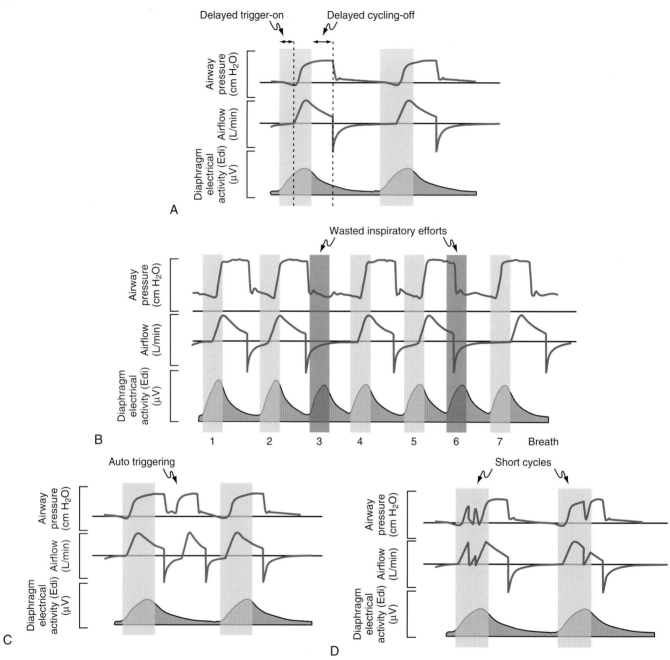

Figure 32-6 Examples of patient-ventilator asynchrony. **A,** Both the initiation and the termination of the assist delivered by the ventilator are delayed relative with the patient's respiratory demand, as reflected by the electrical activity of the diaphragm (Edi). Note that the neural expiration normally starts at approximately 70% to 80% of the maximum Edi. **B,** The ventilator delivers assist in response to the breathing efforts *1* and *2*, whereas effort *3* fails to trigger the ventilator. Wasted inspiratory efforts frequently occur when settings for the trigger threshold are inadequate, when excessive inspiratory efforts are required because of auto-PEEP, when delay in cycling-off is excessive, or when the respiratory muscles are too weak to translate a neural inspiratory effort into an effective breath. **C,** Auto triggering may occur when the generation of airflow or negative pressure in the expiratory limb of the ventilatory circuit is not related to an inspiratory effort (e.g., transmission of pressure oscillations because of cardiac activity, leaks in the ventilator circuit). Auto triggering often occurs when the trigger-on threshold is set at a level that is too sensitive. **D,** Short cycles. Delivery of assist by the ventilator is prematurely terminated and immediately resumed as the patient makes an inspiratory effort. For example, short cycles may occur when the airflow is impeded by a high resistance within the ventilator circuit (e.g., secretion in the endotracheal tube or in the trachea) or when the patient actively blocks inspiratory airflow that might be delivered in excess of the patient's demand.

should be delivered in synchrony with and in proportion to the patient's actual respiratory demand (i.e., both the timing and magnitude of the assist delivered by the ventilator are synchronized to the patient's inspiratory effort).

Although important improvements have been made in the trigger-on characteristics and the cycling-off characteristics of ventilators, ideal synchrony between the ventilator and the

patient has not been achieved with most modes of ventilation, and patient-ventilator asynchrony is common (**Figure 32-6**). Patient-ventilator asynchrony may result in increased inspiratory and expiratory muscle activity and may introduce an unnecessary burden, in terms of work of breathing, in patients whose respiratory muscles are already under stress. Technologies that allow delivery of assistance in proportion to the patient's demand on a breath-by-breath basis have only recently been developed (e.g., proportional assist ventilation [PAV] and neurally adjusted ventilatory assist [NAVA], as described later on).

Variables that can be adjusted to improve synchrony between the patient and the ventilator include the trigger-on threshold, the inspiratory rise time or flow rate, and the cycling-off airflow threshold. The mechanisms used to initiate a breath (trigger-on) detect changes in airflow or pressure in the ventilatory circuit. Hence, negative deflections of short duration (pneumatic trigger mechanisms) may be detectable in the airway pressure and/or flow tracings when a breath is triggered by the patient's effort. Delivery of the assistance is terminated either after a predefined time has elapsed (time-cycled) or after a prespecified cycling-off airflow threshold (flow-cycled) has been reached (see Figure 32-5). Rise time refers to the time required by the ventilator to increase the inspiratory airflow from zero to peak. As demonstrated in **Figure 32-7**, the rise time changes the slope of the increase in pressure during early inspiration. Generally, rise time (or the inspiratory flow pattern) should be set to ensure that air is delivered rapidly (fast increase in airway pressure) after initiation of a breath. By establishing an optimal inspiratory rise time, synchrony to the patient's respiratory demand can be optimized and work of breathing can be reduced.

The fact that conventional modes of ventilation always deliver a uniform, predefined level of assist but do not take into account the physiologic variability of the breathing pattern stimulated the development of the PAV and NAVA modes, which deliver pressure assistance in proportion to the patient's demand.

Proportional Assist Ventilation

PAV, the first patient-triggered mode that adapted the level of assist to the patient's inspiratory effort, was introduced in 1987. With PAV, the ventilator delivers positive pressure throughout inspiration in proportion to the inspiratory airflow and volume generated by the patient (**Figure 32-8**). The magnitude of unloading is based on measuring elastance and resistance of the respiratory system. Whereas with conventional modes of ventilation the VT or the delivered PVENT is relatively constant from breath to breath, with PAV only the relationship between delivered PVENT and the inspiratory effort of the patient is constant, whereas VT and the delivered PVENT become dependent variables. Although PAV requires that the patient always assume a portion of the respiratory work, this mode has been demonstrated to effectively unload the respiratory muscles.

Limitations of PAV include the necessity to determine elastance and resistance of the respiratory system (a task that is not easy to perform in spontaneously breathing patients) and the occurrence of runaway phenomena at high levels of assist.

Neurally Adjusted Ventilatory Assist

A relatively new strategy of mechanical ventilation, NAVA, uses the Edi to control the ventilator (**Figure 32-9**). Because breathing signals originate from the brain and reach the diaphragm by way of the phrenic nerves, Edi represents the neural respiratory effort with respect to both timing and amplitude. During NAVA, positive pressure is applied to the airway opening in direct proportion to the Edi amplitude, so defining a target pressure or volume is not required. The patient's respiratory control mechanisms, including feedback from mechanoreceptors and chemoreceptors, adjust the Edi and thereby

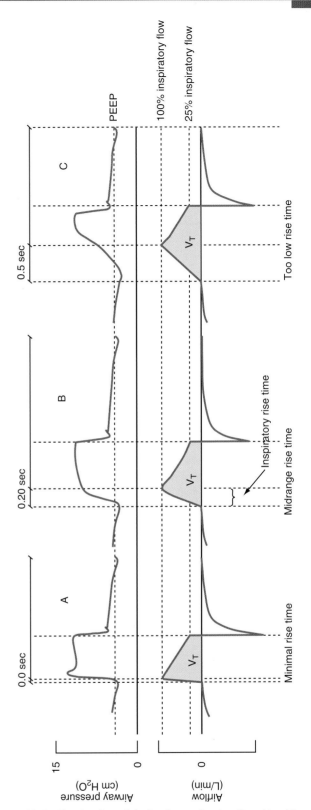

Figure 32-7 The rise time of the inspiratory flow is adjustable with most current ventilators. **A,** A pressure spike in early inspiration may indicate inspiratory flow in excess of the patient's demand or an obstruction in the central airways including the tracheal tube. **B,** No deformation of the inspiratory pressure waveform is visible with a midrange rise time. **C,** A concave deformation of the inspiratory pressure waveform indicates that the patient is making an inspiratory effort, because demand is higher than the flow provided by the ventilator. *(Modified from Branson RD, Campell RS: Pressure support ventilation, patient ventilator synchrony and ventilator algorithms,* Respir Care *43:1045-1047, 1998.)*

Figure 32-8 Proportional assist ventilation (PAV) as volume assist. **A,** With PAV, the assist is delivered in proportion to inspiratory effort. The pressure delivered to the airways increases until the end of inspiration. **B,** An increase in volume assist results in a higher pressure delivered for the same tidal volume. Note that with PAV delivered as flow assist, the waveforms appear different, although the basic principles are very similar to those for delivery of PAV as volume assist. (*Modified from Oczenski W, editor: Atmen-Atemhilfen, Georg Thieme Verlag, 2006.*)

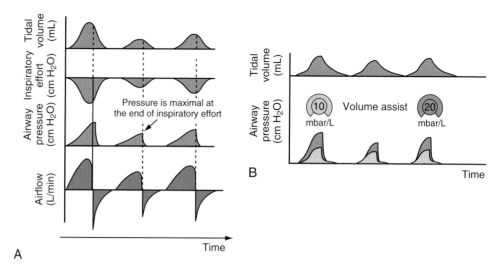

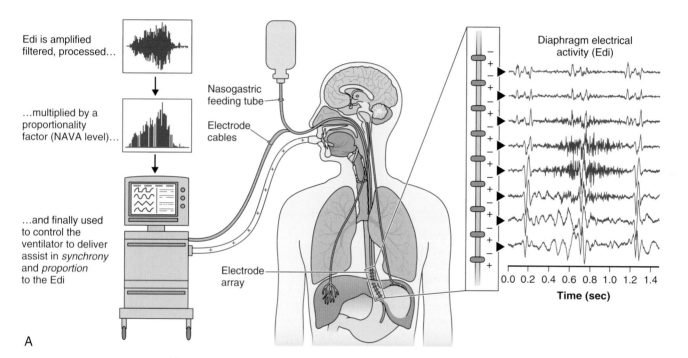

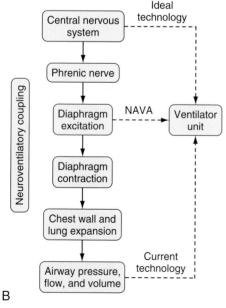

Figure 32-9 **A,** With neurally adjusted ventilatory assist (NAVA), the electrical activity of the diaphragm (Edi) is derived by use of an array of electrodes mounted on a nasogastric tube. The signals from each electrode pair on the array are differentially amplified, filtered, and multiplied by a proportionality factor (NAVA level) before the signal is used to control the pressure generated by the ventilator. Hence, with NAVA, the pressure delivered to the patient is synchronous and (virtually) instantaneously proportional to the patient's Edi. **B,** Neuromechanical coupling and control of the ventilator. Chain of steps necessary to transform central respiratory drive into an inspiration (neuromechanical coupling) that ultimately results in delivery of assist by the ventilator (neuroventilator coupling). The current technology requires transmission of the electrical excitation into a contraction of the respiratory muscles (e.g., the diaphragm) and in generation of a pneumatic signal (pressure or flow at the airway opening) that is sufficient in magnitude to exceed the trigger-on threshold of a sensor within the ventilator. With NAVA, the Edi is used to control the ventilator. Hence, with NAVA, control of the ventilator is independent of the force generated by the respiratory muscles and also is independent of leaks in the ventilator circuit. (*A and B, Modified from Sinderby C, Navalesi P, Beck J, et al: Neural control of mechanical ventilation in respiratory failure, Nat Med 5:1433-1436, 1999.*)

regulate the pressure and delivered volume. Animal data and a number of clinical studies suggest that NAVA is applicable in the ICU environment, efficiently delivers assistance synchronous to the subject's demand, unloads the respiratory muscles, maintains gas exchange, and preserves cardiac performance during invasive ventilation and also during noninvasive ventilation even with use of an excessively leaky interface. Simultaneous measurement of the Edi (which reflects the patient's neurally generated effort) and the delivered assist allows monitoring the patient's ability to translate a neural effort into ventilation, referred to as *neuroventilatory efficiency*. NAVA does not require measurement of respiratory system mechanics, and runaway phenomena are unlikely to occur.

PAV and NAVA both depend on presence of an intact respiratory drive. Although the concept of delivering assistance in proportion to the patient's demand is appealing, and although data from experimental and clinical studies are promising, these modes need to be tested in clinical trials to better define their indications and limitations.

COMBINED MODES

Airway Pressure Release Ventilation

With airway pressure release ventilation (APRV) (**Figure 32-10**), the pressure in the ventilator circuit alternates between a high and a lower level (normally the higher pressure level is of longer duration than the lower pressure level) and spontaneous breathing is allowed in any phase of the cycle. The high- and low-pressure levels, the rate of change between the two levels, the respiratory system compliance, and the airway resistance to flow are the main determinants of the "mechanical ventilation" portion with APRV, whereas the complementary "spontaneous breathing" portion mainly depends on the patient's respiratory drive. In contrast with continuous positive airway pressure (CPAP), APRV interrupts P_{VENT} briefly to augment spontaneous minute ventilation and thereby increases alveolar ventilation and CO_2 removal without increasing the work of breathing. Spontaneous efforts during APRV are not actively assisted except for those breaths that happen to occur during the change from the lower to the upper pressure level. Total minute ventilation with APRV is the sum of the mechanical, pressure-controlled ventilation and the complementary

spontaneous breathing. APRV *without* spontaneous breathing is essentially the same as PCV.

APRV has a number of interesting features. First, APRV overcomes shortcomings inherent in many modes of assisted spontaneous breathing related to triggering-on and cycling-off the ventilator by simply avoiding inspiratory and expiratory valves in the ventilator circuit. However, the time-cycled release and reestablishment of the high P_{VENT} is not synchronized to the patient's breathing efforts, so patient-ventilator asynchrony may result. Second, the application of CPAP recruits some atelectatic areas, increases lung volume, and allows spontaneous breathing to occur on a portion of the pressure-volume curve where impedance to airflow is low and only a small transpulmonary pressure change is required to produce the V_T. Third, APRV maintains P_{VENT} at high levels for a prolonged period. Because alveoli are continually recruited along the inspiratory limb of the pressure-volume curve, recruitment may be more efficient with APRV than with shorter-application positive pressure (e.g., with pressure support ventilation).

Bilevel Positive Airway Pressure Ventilation

With BiPAP ventilation, two levels of continuous positive pressure are used, as with APRV, and unrestricted spontaneous breathing is allowed on both pressure levels (**Figure 32-11**, *A*). As an additional option, assistance to spontaneous breathing efforts can be provided at the lower pressure level (see Figure 32-11, *B*), at the higher pressure level, or at both levels. The transition from the low-pressure to the high-pressure level is coordinated with the patient's breathing effort. The designations Bi-Vent, DuoPAP, and Bi-level used by ventilator manufacturers are synonymous with BiPAP.

Despite the theoretical advantages of APRV and BiPAP, trials showing clinically relevant benefits are currently lacking. Further work is needed before these modes can be recommended for specific patient conditions or phases in the process of mechanical ventilation.

Synchronized Intermittent Mandatory Ventilation

Synchronized intermittent mandatory ventilation (SIMV) combines volume- or pressure-targeted breaths at a caregiver-defined rate (mandatory breaths) with unassisted spontaneous breathing (**Figure 32-12**). Because ideally the mandatory

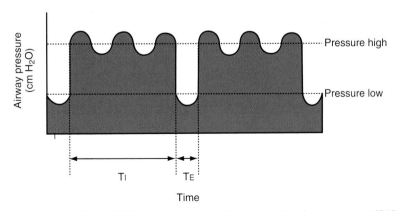

Figure 32-10 With airway pressure release ventilation (APRV), two levels of continuous positive airway pressure (CPAP) are delivered by the ventilator. The higher pressure level is maintained until the inspiratory time (TI) has elapsed; the pressure is then changed to the lower pressure level, usually for a short period of time (TE, typically 0.5 to 1.5 second), before the high-pressure level is resumed. The duration of TI and TE is defined by the caregiver. Spontaneous breathing is allowed in any phase of the cycle. Because the pressure release periods are of short duration, a residual expiratory positive airway pressure (intrinsic PEEP) will be maintained in the lung compartments with a high time constant (slow passive exhalation), preventing end-expiratory collapse of these lung regions. While preventing end-expiratory collapse of the lungs, this helps improve oxygenation as a result of a better match between ventilation and perfusion, and periodic release of the airway pressure assists in removal of carbon dioxide.

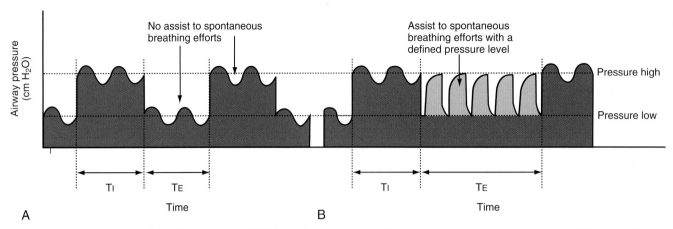

Figure 32-11 **A,** With bilevel positive airway pressure (BiPAP) ventilation, two levels of continuous positive airway pressure are delivered by the ventilator. The pressure levels and the relationship between inspiratory and expiratory times (TI and TE) are both defined by the caregiver. **B,** Delivery of assist to individual spontaneous breathing efforts is optional; this modality can be combined with BiPAP to compensate for the additional inspiratory work imposed by the flow resistance of the endotracheal tube. Of note, changes between the lower and the higher pressure levels are synchronized to the patient's efforts. The major difference between BiPAP and airway pressure release ventilation (APRV) is the longer duration at the low-pressure level with BiPAP, with a higher probability of derecruitment of lung regions. *(Modified from Oczenski W, editor:* Atmen-Atemhifen, *Stuttgart, Georg Thieme Verlag, 2006.)*

Figure 32-12 Synchronized intermittent mandatory ventilation (SIMV) with unassisted spontaneous breathing between two volume-targeted breaths. Within a short period before starting the next mandatory breath, a trigger window allows synchronization of the controlled breath to the patient's breathing effort. When the patient's breathing effort does not exceed the trigger-on threshold during this trigger window, the ventilator will deliver a mandatory breath (either volume- or pressure-targeted as defined by the caregiver) after the maximal time interval for intermittent mandatory ventilation (IMV) has elapsed. This time interval is defined by the preset rate for IMV. *PEEP,* positive end-expiratory pressure. *(Modified from Oczenski W, editor:* Atmen-Atemhifen, *Stuttgart, Georg Thieme Verlag, 2006.)*

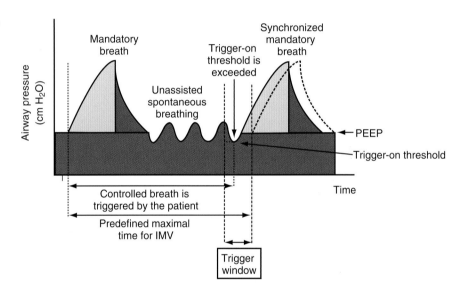

breaths should be synchronized to the patient's own breathing effort, SIMV requires that the ventilator settings for the trigger-on threshold be adequate for this purpose.

The main differences between SIMV and BiPAP are that SIMV does not allow spontaneous breathing during the mandatory breaths, whereas spontaneous breathing is possible during all phases with BiPAP, and that with SIMV, all mandatory breaths are volume- or pressure-targeted, whereas BiPAP provides only pressure-targeted breaths. Despite its name, concerns similar to those with all pneumatically triggered modes of mechanical ventilation, regarding the delivery of ventilator assistance in synchrony and in proportion to the patient's demand, apply for SIMV as well.

Pressure-Regulated Volume Control and Volume Support

Pressure-regulated volume control (PRVC) and volume support (VS) use either pressure-targeted ventilation (for PRVC) or pressure support ventilation (for VS) to achieve a predefined VT. Basically, both modes first deliver a test breath at a low-pressure level, measure the achieved VT, and calculate the necessary adjustments in the inspiratory pressure to achieve the targeted VT in the subsequent breath. The same procedure is repeated for every breath. It has been suggested that these modes may be useful in weaning the patient from the ventilator on the basis of the rationale that the stronger the respiratory muscles (e.g., the higher the share of the VT produced by the inspiratory effort of the patient), the lower the level of assistance needed by the ventilator. The major concern with both PRVC and VS is that if the patient's breathing efforts increase because of an increased respiratory demand (e.g., hypoxemia, fever, increased metabolism), the level of assistance will paradoxically decrease. Also, spontaneous breathing patterns in critically ill patients often are highly variable, and the required VT may vary on a breath-by-breath basis. Again, PRVC and VS are designed such that the level of assist paradoxically decreases during periods of high demand, and vice versa.

MODES THAT FACILITATE SPONTANEOUS BREATHING

Continuous Positive Airway Pressure

With CPAP, a caregiver-defined level of positive pressure is maintained by the ventilator while the patient is breathing spontaneously (**Figure 32-13**). Of note, because the patient's

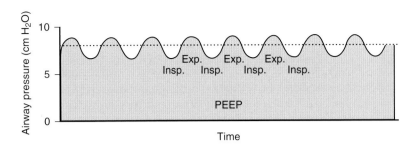

Figure 32-13 With continuous positive airway pressure (CPAP), a caregiver-defined level of pressure within the ventilatory circuit is maintained. Changes in the airway pressure with inspiration and expiration are constantly compensated for by pressure generated by the ventilator. *PEEP*, positive end-expiratory pressure.

breathing efforts are not assisted with CPAP, the patient must have adequate respiratory drive and adequate respiratory muscle function. CPAP helps to increase and maintain the functional residual capacity (FRC) and thereby to increase the lung units available for gas exchange (reduction of intrapulmonary right-to-left shunt), prevent end-expiratory airway collapse, and counter the effects of auto-PEEP or intrinsic PEEP.

Positive End-Expiratory Pressure

PEEP refers to the airway pressure (relative to atmospheric pressure) at the end of a breath. PEEP can be applied with most ventilation modes. Patients with respiratory failure from asthma or chronic obstructive pulmonary disease (COPD) who require mechanical ventilation have increases in FRC and in alveolar pressure at the end of exhalation that exceeds atmospheric pressure (i.e., auto-PEEP or intrinsic PEEP), thereby increasing the inspiratory work of breathing. Applying PEEP counters the effect of auto-PEEP on work of breathing. Patients with the acute respiratory distress syndrome (ARDS), acute lung injury (ALI), or hypoxemic respiratory failure from obesity have a reduced FRC that leads to alveolar and/or airway collapse. In these patients, PEEP is used to restore FRC, to recruit regions with collapsed alveoli or airways, to prevent derecruitment of open alveoli, to redistribute fluid within the lung, and to make dependent lung regions available for ventilation. All of these effects can improve the match between ventilation and perfusion, improve oxygen saturation, and decrease the need for high fractions of inspired oxygen. PEEP also has been used in patients with flail chest to stabilize the chest wall.

All of the aforementioned beneficial effects of PEEP are lost and adverse or even harmful effects may occur when excessive levels of PEEP are used. For example, excessive PEEP may increase dead space by over-distending alveoli and concomitantly decreasing alveolar capillary blood flow or may add to the hyperinflation of the lungs in patients with COPD or asthma. High levels of PEEP may reduce pulmonary blood flow by impeding venous return, thereby increasing pulmonary vascular resistance (i.e., decreasing cardiac output in the face of constant pulmonary arterial and venous pressure translates to an increased pulmonary vascular resistance). If pulmonary vascular pressures are kept constant relative to the level of PEEP, however (as will be the case unless cardiac output decreases), the effect of increasing lung volume on pulmonary vascular resistance is small. Of note, the effects of PEEP on cardiac performance are more pronounced during hypovolemia and can partially be reversed by ensuring adequate intravascular fluid volume.

In the past, PEEP was used mainly to increase oxygenation, thereby improving oxygen transport; however, there has been a change in the rationale underlying the use of PEEP, with a greater focus on its use to minimize cyclic air space opening and closing (i.e., atelectrauma) and hence to decrease ventilator-induced lung injury, rather than simply to improve oxygenation.

Table 32-1 Combinations of Inspiratory Oxygen Fraction (FIO_2) and Positive End-Expiratory Pressure (PEEP) in Patients with Acute Lung Injury or Acute Respiratory Distress Syndrome to Achieve Oxygenation Goals*

FIO_2	PEEP (cm H_2O)
0.3	5
0.4	5
0.4	8
0.5	8
0.5	10
0.6	10
0.7	10
0.7	12
0.7	14
0.8	14
0.9	14
0.9	16
0.9	18
1.0	18
1.0	20
1.0	22
1.0	24

*Partial pressure of arterial oxygen (PaO_2) of 55 to 80 mm Hg or oxyhemoglobin saturation measured by pulse oximetry (SpO_2) of 88% to 95%. Modified from Ventilation with lower tidal volumes as compared with traditional tidal volumes for acute lung injury and the acute respiratory distress syndrome. The Acute Respiratory Distress Syndrome Network, *N Engl J Med* 342:1301-1308, 2000.

Given the current lack of tools to monitor both alveolar overdistention and collapse, and given the heterogeneity of the distribution of most disease processes within the lung, identification of the "best PEEP?" level is not straightforward in clinical practice. In fact, the gravitational gradient in pleural pressure and end-expiratory lung volume that exists in both normal subjects and patients requiring mechanical ventilation implies that there cannot be a single level of PEEP that is "best" for all regions of the lung. Pending further clarification on how to set PEEP, a pragmatic approach for daily clinical practice in patients with ALI is to adhere to the algorithm used in the large Acute Respiratory Distress Syndrome Network (ARDSNet) trial (Table 32-1) and to carefully observe the effect of changes in PEEP on parameters such as blood oxygenation, cardiac performance, and expiratory flow limitation. Of note, in patients with stiff chest walls (e.g., massive ascites), higher levels of PEEP are warranted.

PRINCIPLES OF RESPIRATORY SYSTEM MECHANICS RELEVANT TO MECHANICAL VENTILATION

Adjusting ventilator parameters to the patient's individual condition and interpreting pressure and airflow tracings requires an understanding of the fundamental principles of respiratory system mechanics in ventilated patients. Although these general principles apply to the entire respiratory system, regional inhomogeneities (e.g., lower end-expiratory lung volumes, airway closure, and/or atelectasis in dependent regions) and regional differences in disease processes result in ventilation is never distributed uniformly within the lungs in mechanically ventilated patients. The compliance of a specific alveolar region and the resistance of the associated airways ultimately determine the portion of the VT received by a particular lung region.

AIRWAY RESISTANCE AND LUNG ELASTANCE

To a simplified approximation, the patient-ventilator unit can be considered as an in-series mechanical system that consists of a resistive element (ventilator and endotracheal tubing + central airways) and an elastic element (lung-thorax compartment). During inflation, the pressure applied to the tube inlet (PVENT) is equal to the sum of the pressure required to overcome the resistive elements (PRESIST) and the pressure required to distend the lung and chest wall (PELAST). The flow through the resistive element is a function of the difference in pressure between the tube inlet and the tube outlet (PRESIST) and the resistance of the tubing system (i.e., flow [L/min] = PRESIST [cm H₂O]/resistance [cm H₂O × min/L]). For example, forcing air at a low flow rate through a large-bore tube requires less pressure than if a high flow is applied to a small bore tube. Because PRESIST is used to overcome the resistive element, only PELAST is applied across the respiratory system (i.e., the lungs and the chest wall). **Figure 32-14** demonstrates the relationship between PVENT and the pressure within the central airways (PAW) throughout a respiratory cycle.

PELAST is made up of two components: the pressure required to distend the lung and the pressure required to distend the chest wall (which includes both the ribcage and the diaphragm, along with the abdomen). The elastance (1/Compliance = applied pressure [PELAST] divided by the applied VT) of the chest wall (ECW) and that of the lung (EL) are mechanically in series, and their sum equals the elastance of the entire respiratory system (ERS). In clinical practice, PVENT measured either at the airway opening or in the ventilator circuit is considered to be the "driving pressure," and PVENT typically is used to assess the propensity for induction of VILI. Such an approach has important shortcomings, however, and may yield misleading results. PVENT is referenced to ambient pressure and therefore reflects the pressure gradient across the entire respiratory system (i.e., across both the lung and the chest wall). The key variable defining the degree of lung distention and the propensity for induction of VILI, however, is only the pressure across the lung (i.e., the transpulmonary pressure [PL]).

The relative stiffness (or elastance) of the lung and the chest wall define what proportion of PAW is used to distend the chest wall and what proportion is used to distend the lung (**Figure 32-15**). For example, if the elastance of the chest wall is twice that of the lung, then two thirds of PAW is used to distend the

chest wall and only one third is used to distend the lung. The fractions EL/ERS and ECW/ERS determine how PAW is apportioned between the lung (PL = PAW × EL/ERS) and the chest wall (PCW = PAW × ECW/ERS). Predicting PL on the basis of PAW without information on the elastance of the lung and the chest wall is not possible. Furthermore, lung and chest wall elastance vary among individuals and may also change over time during critical illness (e.g., with accumulation of edema or ascites). Although calculating the elastance of the entire respiratory system (ERS) is relatively easy (ERS = PVENT/VT), calculating the elastance of the lung and the chest wall separately is unfortunately not straightforward and requires knowledge of PL. **Figure 32-16** illustrates the intrabreath changes in PL during unassisted spontaneous breathing and during volume-targeted ventilation.

PL equals the difference between the alveolar pressure (PALV) and the pleural pressure (PPL). Because PVENT closely approximates PALV during an end-inspiratory and end-expiratory airway occlusion, PL can be calculated as PL = PVENT – PPL after performance of an appropriate maneuver to occlude the airways. Because direct measurement of PPL is invasive, and because the pressure in the lower third of the esophagus closely approximates that in the adjacent pleura, measurement of Pes (by means of inflatable latex balloons) can be used to estimate PPL. Hence, PL can be estimated as PL = PVENT – Pes (with a number of caveats, such as the effect of mediastinal weight on Pes in a supine patient, gravitational gradients, and spatial heterogeneity of PPL). Accordingly, approximation of PPL from measured Pes is not widely used currently in routine clinical practice.

Patients with ALI or ARDS may demonstrate an increase in ERS that is mainly attributed to an alteration in the EL. Some studies suggest, however, that the increase in EL results from presence of fluid filling a large portion of the lung such that the tidal volume delivered now expands the ventilated lung to a higher end-inspiratory lung volume (requiring a higher distending pressure, which is reflected in a greater EL). An increase in ERS also could be due to an increase in ECW. Of note, the chest wall in this context comprises not only the thoracic cage but also its caudal boundary, the diaphragmatic-abdominal compartment. ECW is increased in patients with severe obesity, chest wall injury, surgical dressings, and ascites and after major abdominal surgery. For example, in a patient with ALI associated with abdominal surgery, ECW may increase when intraabdominal hypertension (e.g., bowel edema, ascites) develops, even when the lung mechanics are normal. With the assumption that PVENT remains unchanged in the patient described previously, the pressure distending the lung actually decreases, because a greater share of PVENT is used to distend the chest wall (i.e., to displace the diaphragm toward the abdomen). Thus, arbitrarily limiting PVENT to a specific uniform value may not be necessary to prevent VILI in patients with high ECW but may potentially even cause harm by leading to marked reductions in tidal volume, insufficient ventilation, and severe hypoxemia.

PRACTICAL APPROACH TO VENTILATING PATIENTS WITH OBSTRUCTIVE AIRWAY DISEASE

An increase in airway resistance leading to expiratory airflow limitation and gas trapping is the major pathophysiologic abnormality in patients with asthma or COPD. With healthy lungs, the elastic recoil forces are sufficient to promote passive exhalation until FRC is reached. Partial loss of the elastic lung

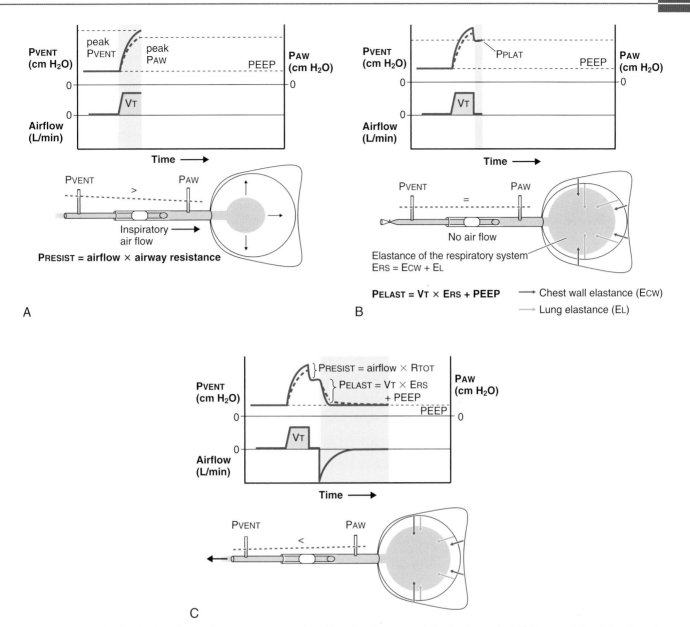

Figure 32-14 **A,** During inspiration, the ventilator generates pressure (PVENT) to force a predefined volume of air (VT) in a predefined time into the lungs of the patient. The pressure loss over the total resistance of the endotracheal tube and of the central airways (PRESIST) defines what proportion of the PVENT reaches the central airways (PAW). **B,** Because the pressure within the respiratory system and the central airways equilibrates when the inspiratory and expiratory valves are closed, assessment of the respiratory system elastance (ERS) is possible during an end-inspiratory hold. For a given VT, the ERS defines the plateau pressure (PPLAT) at the end of inspiration. Note that because of the inhomogeneity of the time constants among different lung regions, the duration of the end-inspiratory plateau (normally approximately 10% of the breath cycle) often is too short for sufficient equilibration of the pressure across all lung regions. Hence, an end-inspiratory hold of longer duration (e.g., longer than 5 seconds) is necessary to adequately assess respiratory system mechanics. **C,** The expiration is passive (not actively supported by the ventilator) and driven only by the elastic recoil of the lungs and the chest wall. *PEEP,* positive end-expiratory pressure.

recoil in patients with COPD further aggravates this problem. Patients with limitation of expiratory airflow often activate expiratory muscles in an attempt to force the inspired volume through the partially collapsed or constricted central airways.

DYNAMIC HYPERINFLATION AND AUTO-PEEP

Dynamic hyperinflation occurs when expiratory flow has not emptied alveoli to their resting FRC values by the end of exhalation. The residual positive pressure within the lungs referenced to atmospheric pressure or to PEEP applied through a ventilator is referred to as *auto-PEEP* (or *intrinsic PEEP*). Although auto-PEEP usually implies dynamic hyperinflation,

the two are not synonymous, because lung volume at end-expiration can be normal when expiratory muscles are highly activated. The presence of auto-PEEP results in the underestimation of mean pressure within the lung as measured by PVENT, and hence in misinterpretation, if assessment of lung mechanics is solely based on PVENT.

Classically, dynamic hyperinflation is present in patients with COPD, in whom the unstable airways collapse during exhalation (**Figure 32-17**), and in patients with asthma, in whom increased bronchomotor tone impedes exhalation. Exacerbation of the disease process such as bronchospasm in asthma or bronchitis with thickening of the mucosa in COPD worsens the condition. Of note, auto-PEEP also may develop in patients with more restrictive disease processes such as ARDS, in which intrapulmonary time constants are widely inhomogeneous, or when low VT settings at high ventilatory rates are used. A narrow-diameter or kinked endotracheal tube, inspissated secretions, an obstructed filter in the expiratory limb of the ventilatory circuit, a highly variable respiratory rate, or tachypnea will further predispose the respiratory system to development of auto-PEEP.

Persistent airflow at the end of exhalation, especially in combination with consistent failure to trigger the ventilator with inspiratory efforts, should heighten clinical suspicion for the presence of dynamic hyperinflation. Measurement of auto-PEEP requires equilibration of the pressure across the entire lung during occlusion of the expiratory valve at end-expiration (**Figure 32-18**), ideally performed during muscle paralysis (but paralysis usually should not be undertaken solely to make this measurement). Measurement of auto-PEEP during spontaneous breathing is difficult and often unreliable, because

the inspiratory and expiratory efforts interfere with the procedure, and studies have shown that expiratory muscle contraction can occur. These contractions may be difficult to detect clinically.

Dynamic hyperinflation can markedly increase the oxygen cost of breathing in a spontaneously breathing patient (**Figure 32-19**). Because the compliance of the respiratory system is lower at high lung volumes, more energy is required to expand the lungs. Furthermore, with dynamic hyperinflation the patient needs to produce large pleural pressure swings to overcome the auto-PEEP before pressure in the ventilator circuit decreases below the applied PEEP level and before pneumatic trigger systems located in the ventilator can be excited. Because generation of force by the inspiratory muscles is impaired during hyperinflation (decreased resting length of the diaphragm requires a higher-than-normal respiratory drive to lower pleural pressure), triggering the ventilator becomes challenging for patients with COPD and especially for those who have weakness or fatigue of the respiratory muscles—both of these conditions are difficult to distinguish from the effects of trying to inhale while breathing at a lung volume near total lung capacity (TLC).

Dynamic hyperinflation increases resistance of the inferior vena cava and increases pleural and juxtacardiac pressures, thereby impeding venous return to the right atrium, leading in turn to a decrease in cardiac output. Recognition that auto-PEEP and not cardiac dysfunction is the main cause of impaired cardiac performance under such circumstances is important, because treatment strategies are markedly different.

Inappropriate settings during mechanical ventilation can worsen dynamic hyperinflation, especially when high ventilatory rates and/or high VT settings resulting in excessive minute ventilation are used, when the assist is delivered asynchronous to the patient's demand (**Figure 32-20**), or when PEEP levels higher than those needed to counterbalance auto-PEEP are used.

The first approach to minimizing dynamic hyperinflation in a patient with obstructive airway disease is to decrease the resistance in the expiratory airways by removing any

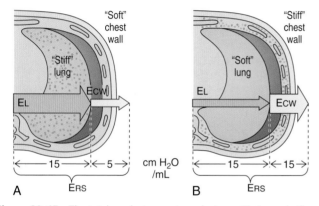

Figure 32-15 The total respiratory system elastance (ERS) equals the sum of its components: ERS = elastance of the lungs (EL) + elastance of the chest wall (ECW). The same ERS may arise from a high EL and a low ECW elastance (**A**) or from identical EL and ECW (**B**). *(Modified from Gattinoni L, Chiumello D, Carlesso E, Valenza F: Bench-to-bedside review: chest wall elastance in acute lung injury/acute respiratory distress syndrome patients,* Crit Care 8:350-355, 2004.)

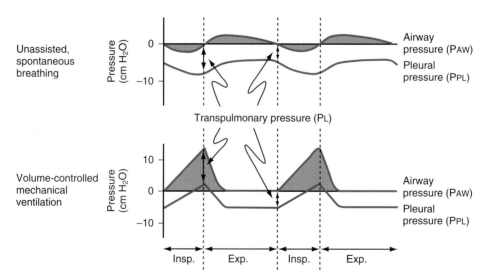

Figure 32-16 Transpulmonary pressure (PL). The pressure applied to the lungs (i.e., PL) equals the intrapulmonary pressure minus the intrapleural pressure: PL = PAW − PPL. The changes of PL from inspiration to expiration, and hence the propensity for development for ventilator-induced lung injury (VILI), are greater with volume-controlled mechanical ventilation than with spontaneous breathing. *(Modified from Oczenski W, editor:* Atmen-Atemhilfen, *Stuttgart, Georg Thieme Verlag, 2006.)*

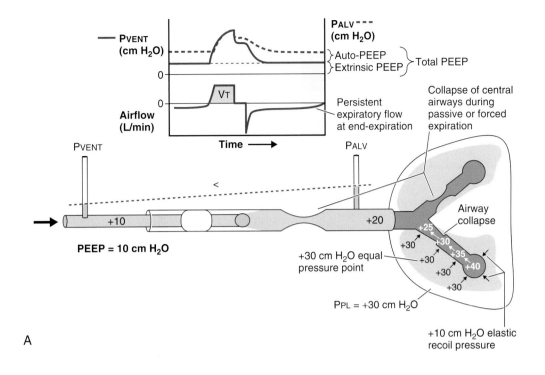

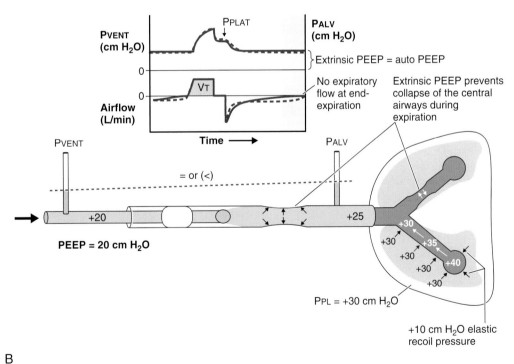

Figure 32-17 **A,** Ideally there is no airflow at the end of the expiration, and hence alveolar pressure (PALV) is in equilibrium with the pressure in the ventilator (PVENT), and the respiratory system has returned to its functional residual capacity (FRC). Unstable airways collapse during passive or during forced expiration when the pressure surrounding the airways exceeds the intraluminal pressure, resulting in expiratory flow limitation. Consequently, air may be trapped within the lung, and a pressure gradient between the alveoli (PALV) and the ventilator circuit (PVENT) may be established (auto-PEEP) if the expiratory phase is too short to allow complete exhalation. **B,** Application of extrinsic PEEP partially counters the collapse of the airways, reduces the resistance to expiratory airflow, and may help with triggering of the ventilator by the patient. Note that peak and plateau pressure did not change, because extrinsic PEEP partially replaced auto-PEEP without adding to it. Note that expiratory flow may be impeded when an extrinsic PEEP level in excess of the auto-PEEP level is used. *PEEP,* positive end-expiratory pressure.

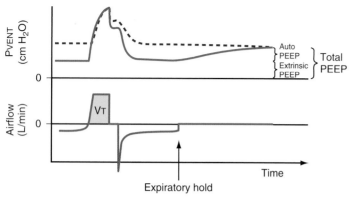

Figure 32-18 Expiratory hold technique to estimate the level of auto-PEEP. The exhalation valve is closed during an expiratory hold. When the expiratory flow equals zero, airway pressure rises to the auto-PEEP level. After reopening of the expiratory valve, flow continues, and the additional exhaled volume equals the volume of trapped gas. Of note, inspiratory and expiratory muscle activity interferes with the measurement of intrinsic PEEP. *PEEP,* positive end-expiratory pressure. *(Modified from MacIntyre NR: Intrinsic PEEP,* Prob Respir Care *4:45, 1991.)*

mechanical obstruction and by treating bronchospasm and airway inflammation. The most effective and abrupt way to decrease auto-PEEP is to reduce minute ventilation, although this may lead to an increase in an already elevated arterial PCO_2 ($PaCO_2$). Alternatively, adding extrinsic PEEP (**Figure 32-21**) will decrease the work of breathing, thereby reducing CO_2 production and lowering the $PaCO_2$ even if alveolar ventilation is unchanged. Because patients with COPD with chronically elevated $PaCO_2$ levels retain sufficient bicarbonate to normalize arterial pH, minute ventilation should not be adjusted to maintain a normal $PaCO_2$. In addition, the inspiratory phase should be shortened (thereby allowing maximum time for exhalation), as demonstrated in Figures 32-19 and 32-20. Of note, the variability in the duration of the expiratory phase and, hence, in the expired volume per breath increases when switching from a controlled mode of ventilation to a mode that delivers assistance to spontaneous breathing. This may result in modification of the degree of dynamic hyperinflation on a breath-by-breath basis and can induce patient-ventilator asynchrony because of wasted inspiratory efforts, especially when high levels of assist are used (see Figure 32-6).

The principles of a ventilatory strategy in acute asthma are very similar to those described for COPD—that is, adjusting the ventilatory rate to low frequencies and using low V_T while accepting hypercapnic acidosis. A pH as low as 7.20 normally is well tolerated in these patients, and such an approach helps minimize hyperinflation.

PRACTICAL APPROACH TO VENTILATING PATIENTS WITH RESTRICTIVE PULMONARY DISEASE

A decrease in lung compliance and in FRC is the major pathophysiologic abnormality in patients with restrictive pulmonary disease processes such as pulmonary fibrosis, interstitial pneumonias, sarcoidosis, bronchiolitis obliterans organizing pneumonia, and those with ALI and ARDS.

The challenge in ventilating patients with restrictive diseases is to provide adequate oxygenation, while at the same time not causing further lung injury. Although mechanical ventilation clearly leads to improved survival in patients with ALI or ARDS, its ability to improve survival in patients with other

restrictive processes (particularly idiopathic pulmonary fibrosis) is limited at best. The required approach is one of maintaining adequate oxygenation while trying not to overinflate the lung at end-inhalation (see later).

COMPLICATIONS OF MECHANICAL VENTILATION

Complications and side effects of intubation or of invasive mechanical ventilation include upper airway trauma (e.g., vocal cord injury), aspiration of gastric contents, barotrauma (e.g., pneumothorax or pneumomediastinum), disruption of normal host defense mechanisms, reduction in the ability to heat and humidify inspired gases, local tracheal ischemia induced by the cuff of the endotracheal tube, impairment of communication and of swallowing, and the perceived need by health care providers for sedatives and occasionally neuromuscular blocking drugs. Although use of a cuffed endotracheal tube helps prevent gross aspiration, pharyngeal secretions that pool at the top of the cuff may still seep into the lungs, increasing the probability of development of nosocomial pneumonia. An endotracheal tube greatly impairs the patient's inherent cough mechanisms by preventing closure of the glottis.

Mechanical ventilation itself can induce or aggravate lung injury that is clinically, functionally, and histologically indistinguishable from ALI or ARDS. Also, applying positive pressure to the airways may adversely affect cardiac performance and result in hemodynamic compromise.

VENTILATOR-INDUCED LUNG INJURY

Diseased lungs are more susceptible than healthy lungs to the development of VILI. VILI also can initiate and propagate cascades (e.g., upregulation of a systemic inflammatory response) that ultimately culminate in multiple system organ failure (MSOF) (**Figure 32-22**). A ventilatory strategy that uses low V_T and limited $PVENT$ is not only protective to the lung but also has the potential to reduce the incidence of MSOF. Exposure to excessive mechanical stresses can result in damage to lung tissue and cell integrity from either of two primary factors: (1) overdistention of the lung (i.e., volutrauma) and (2) repetitive air space recruitment and derecruitment (atelectrauma). The critical feature defining induction of VILI secondary to volutrauma seems to be the degree of regional lung distention, rather than the absolute $PVENT$ reached. High pressures per se in the respiratory system do not necessarily result in VILI. For example, trumpet players repeatedly generate very high airway pressures (more than 150 cm H_2O) without incurring lung damage, because no excessive lung distention occurs.

Alveolar overdistention and shear forces can stimulate lung and immune cells to produce and release inflammatory cytokines and chemokines—that is, biotrauma. Biotrauma encompasses the release of numerous biologic (including inflammatory) mediators into the pulmonary interstitial and alveolar spaces. Concomitant disruption of lung tissue and cell integrity and disruption of lung epithelial and endothelial barriers facilitates the spillover of lung-derived inflammatory mediators, endotoxin, and even bacteria into the bloodstream, resulting in initiation, exacerbation, or propagation of a systemic inflammatory response. In view of the vast aerated surface area of the lung, it is conceivable that release of even small quantities of inflammatory mediators per cell could lead to a large quantity of mediators that could potentially enter the circulation.

The typically heterogeneous distribution of disease in patients with ALI or ARDS puts them at a high risk for VILI,

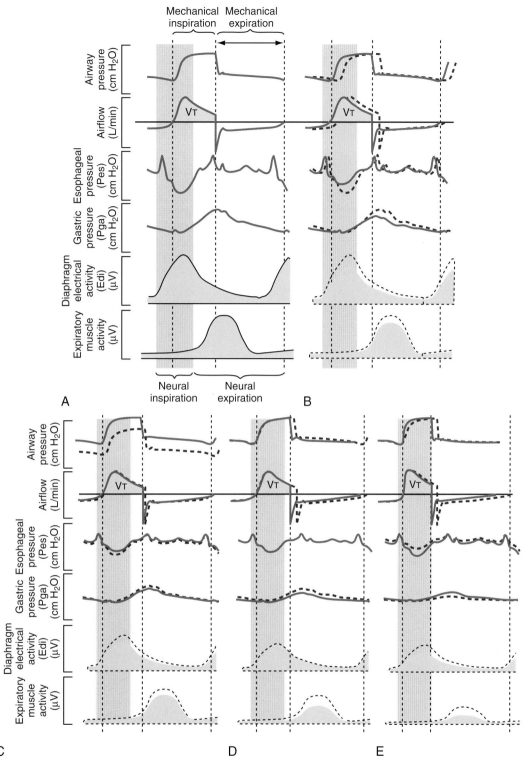

Figure 32-19 **A,** Demonstration of delivery of assist with pressure support ventilation (PSV) in a patient with expiratory flow limitation resulting in dynamic hyperinflation. There is substantial asynchrony (delayed triggering-on and cycling-off) between the assist delivered by the ventilator and the patient's (neural) respiratory demand, as reflected by the electrical activity of the diaphragm (Edi). The high amplitudes for the Edi and for esophageal pressure (Pes) deflections indicate that the inspiratory muscles are highly active during delivery of pressure by the ventilator, whereas the high amplitudes for the expiratory muscle activity and for the gastric pressure (Pga) deflections indicate that the patient uses his expiratory muscles to counter delivery of pressure by the ventilator during neural expiration. **B,** After optimizing the trigger-on threshold, delivery of assist starts earlier (requiring less inspiratory effort) and also ceases earlier (requiring less activation of the expiratory muscles). **C,** Adjusting the level of extrinsic PEEP to compensate for auto-PEEP allows earlier detection of the inspiratory effort by the ventilator (see Figure 32-21) and helps to further reduce the inspiratory workload. **D,** Increasing the cycling-off airflow threshold results in earlier termination of the assist. Hence, expiratory muscle activity can be reduced. Note that the ventilator inspiratory time, as well as the delivered tidal volume (VT), decreases when the cycling-off airflow threshold is increased, whereas the expiratory time increases (provided the respiratory rate remains unchanged). **E,** When the inspiratory rise time is reduced, the peak inspiratory flow and thus the cycling-off airflow threshold both are reached earlier, and the inspiratory time is further shortened. After completion of all steps as demonstrated here (**B** to **E**), ventilator assist is delivered in synchrony with the patient's neural respiratory demand, and unloading of the inspiratory muscles is achieved as reflected by minimization of the amplitudes for Edi and for Pes deflections. Expiration is driven only by the elastic recoil of the lung and the chest wall, as reflected by minimization of the amplitudes for expiratory muscle activity and for Pga deflections. *PEEP,* positive end-expiratory pressure.

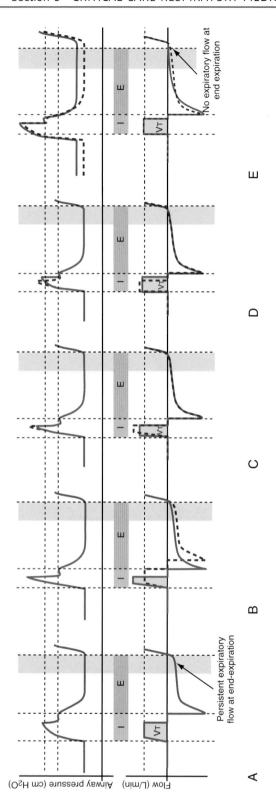

Figure 32-20 Adjustment of ventilatory parameters with volume-targeted ventilation in a patient with expiratory flow limitation and dynamic hyperinflation. **A,** Baseline condition with persistent flow at end-expiration. **B,** Shortening the inspiratory phase by reduction of the inspiratory-expiratory times relationship allows longer expiration provided the ventilatory rate remains unchanged. A higher maximal inspiratory airflow and hence a higher peak pressure during inspiration are required to force the same tidal volume (VT) into the lungs in a shorter period of time. Of note, a high inspiratory flow may result in a moderate increase in the respiratory rate, which will necessitate careful monitoring of the net effect on the duration of the expiration. **C** and **D,** Decreasing the inspiratory rise time (here, from 5% to 0% of the respiratory cycle) while shortening the time of the inspiratory pause at end-inspiration (here from 10% to 5% of the respiratory cycle) allows more time to deliver the tidal volume and hence results in lower maximal flow and lower peak pressure. **E,** Increasing the extrinsic PEEP partially counteracts the dynamic collapse of airways during expiration and diminishes the impedance to expiratory flow. *PEEP,* Positive end-expiratory pressure.

both alveolar overdistention during lung inflation and alveolar collapse at the end of lung deflation.

STRATEGIES TO PREVENT VENTILATOR-INDUCED LUNG INJURY IN CLINICAL PRACTICE

Although mechanical ventilation is only one of multiple factors contributing to the pathogenesis of multiple organ dysfunction syndrome (MODS), clinical trials have clearly shown that lung-protective mechanical ventilation decreases mortality among patients with ARDS.

The large ARDSNet study demonstrated that a VT of 6 mL/kg predicted body weight (PBW) was associated with decreased mortality compared with use of 12 mL/kg PBW in patients with ALI. It is important in applying this approach to base VT on the PBW, not on measured body weight. For a male patient, PBW = 50 + 0.91 × (cm of height − 152.4); for a female patient, PBW = 45.5 + 0.91 × (cm of height − 152.4). The VT should be lowered if necessary to reduce PPLAT to less than 30 cm H2O. Some investigators suggest that a ventilatory strategy that keeps PPLAT below 30 cm H2O is sufficient to ensure lung protection. However, a safe upper limit of PPLAT in patients with ALI or ARDS is not known. A recent post hoc analysis demonstrated that lowering PPLAT even further to values less than 30 cm H2O could potentially decrease mortality.

The beneficial effects of using relatively low VT, and possibly also higher levels of PEEP, probably are related to the two main components—reduction of VILI and prevention of nonpulmonary organ dysfunction—as suggested by many preclinical and smaller clinical studies. In support of this mechanism, a recent large clinical study by Mascia and colleagues demonstrated that a lung-protective ventilatory strategy using VT of 6 to 8 mL/kg PBW combined with higher levels of PEEP prevented the decline of pulmonary function in brain-dead organ donors and roughly doubled the number of lungs available for transplantation. Another recent large clinical study demonstrated that pharmacologic neuromuscular blockade for 48 hours early in the course of ARDS resulted in both better survival and less time spent on the ventilator, compared with the use of placebo. Possible mechanisms by which neuromuscular blockade might lead to improved outcome are summarized in **Figure 32-23**.

In a number of studies, the investigators used *permissive hypercapnia* (i.e., allowing the PaCO2 to increase if necessary to maintain a sufficiently low VT) in the absence of any specific

because the consolidated lung regions are susceptible to atelectrauma and the better or normally aerated regions are prone to volutrauma. Barotrauma and volutrauma are likely to occur when volumes and pressures meant for the entire lung (e.g., a VT of approximately 10 mL/kg) are forced into only a small portion of functional lung (the "baby lung"). In addition, shear forces at the interface between the open and closed lung units result in atelectrauma when PEEP levels insufficient to prevent end-expiratory alveolar collapse are used. Hence, ideally, a ventilatory strategy in patients with ALI or ARDS should prevent

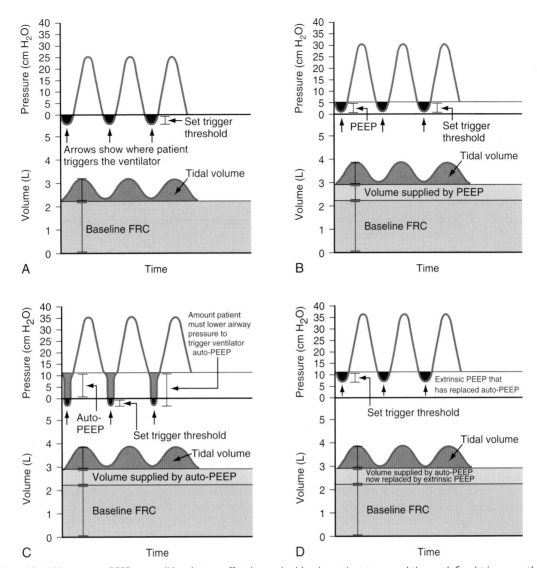

Figure 32-21 **A** and **B**, Without auto-PEEP, a small inspiratory effort is required by the patient to exceed the predefined trigger-on threshold (here, 1 to 2 cm H_2O below extrinsic PEEP). **C**, In the presence of auto-PEEP, the patient first needs to lower alveolar pressure to overcome auto-PEEP before the pressure in the ventilator circuit can be reduced sufficiently to exceed the trigger threshold below extrinsic PEEP. **D**, Applying extrinsic PEEP brings the trigger threshold closer to the alveolar pressure level at end-expiration. Now only a small inspiratory effort is required to exceed the trigger-on threshold. *PEEP*, positive end-expiratory pressure. *(Modified from Howman SF: Mechanical ventilation: a review and update for clinicians, Hosp Physician 35:26–36, 1999.)*

contraindications (e.g., increased intracranial pressure). The concept is that the detrimental effects of the acute hypercapnia are less than the use of higher VT. How to treat the accompanying respiratory acidosis is still a matter of debate, but decreases in pH to approximately 7.20 to 7.25 usually are well tolerated and probably do not have to be addressed unless detrimental physiologic consequences of the acidosis develop.

How to adjust PEEP in patients with ARDS continues to be widely debated. Three recent large studies on higher versus lower PEEP levels in patients with ALI and ARDS, as well as two metaanalyses, found that random application of either higher or lower levels of PEEP in an unselected population does not significantly improve outcome. However, both metaanalyses suggested that in the subgroup of patients with severe, hypoxemic ARDS (as opposed to those without ARDS), higher levels of PEEP might be associated with a reduction in mortality. Some workers have suggested that in the aforementioned clinical studies, a potentially beneficial effect of higher PEEP in some ("lung-recruitable") patients might have been negated

by a detrimental effect occurring in others (i.e., "non–lung-recruitable"). In fact, a cohort study recently demonstrated that the effect of PEEP on lung recruitment is closely associated with the percentage of potentially recruitable lung as determined by computed tomography.

Pending further clarification of how to define optimal PEEP levels in individual patients, a pragmatic approach for daily clinical practice is to adhere to the algorithm used in the large ARDSNet trial (see Table 32-1). Determining optimal ventilator setting in an individual patient with ALI or ARDS is always a continuous, iterative process of evaluation, intervention, and reevaluation that must take into account changes in the disease process over time.

VENTILATOR-INDUCED DIAPHRAGM DYSFUNCTION

Acquired neuromuscular disorders, referred to as critical illness polyneuromyopathy (CIPM), are frequently encountered in critically ill patients. The inability of the patient to resume the

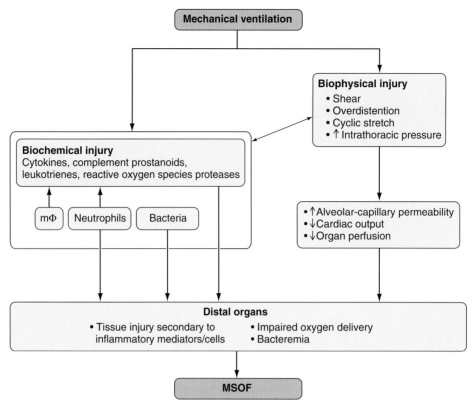

Figure 32-22 Postulated mechanisms whereby mechanical ventilation may contribute to multiple system organ failure (MSOF). *mΦ*, macrophages. *(Modified from Slutsky AS, Tremblay LN: Multiple system organ failure. Is mechanical ventilation a contributing factor?* Am J Respir Crit Care Med *157:1721–1725, 1998.)*

entire work of breathing due to reduced respiratory muscle strength and endurance, with consequent difficulties in weaning from mechanical ventilation, is a hallmark of the syndrome and may be the first symptom to alert the clinician of the disorder. In fact, many patients who experience weaning failure display diaphragmatic weakness as manifested by reduced pressure generation by the diaphragm after supramaximal magnetic stimulation of the phrenic nerves.

It has been suggested that in addition to the well-established risk factors for CIPM (i.e., corticosteroids, neuromuscular blocking agents, severe sepsis, MODS and severe pulmonary diseases), the use of controlled modes of mechanical ventilation may be another factor that contributes to the development of respiratory muscle weakness. For example, two recent studies demonstrated that about 1 to 3 days of complete diaphragm inactivity in brain-dead organ donors (i.e., in absence of any spontaneous muscle activity) associated with mechanical ventilation resulted in a roughly 50% reduction in the cross-sectional areas of diaphragm muscle fibers and in a marked decrease in diaphragm force generation during phrenic nerve stimulation. By contrast, the early and preferential use of ventilation modes that assist spontaneous breathing (i.e. the work of breathing is shared between the ventilator and the patient) has been suggested to help prevent or delay the development of respiratory muscle weakness. However, how much such assistance would adequately meet the patient's demand and would thus prevent both respiratory muscle disuse atrophy and fatigue has not been established.

LUNG RECRUITMENT

Recruitment maneuvers can decrease the heterogeneities present in the lung, improve gas exchange, and potentially mitigate VILI by reducing cyclic air space opening and closing. Recruitment refers to the process of reopening collapsed alveoli by transiently increasing PVENT. This can be accomplished by maintaining a static PVENT of 40 cm H_2O for 40 seconds or by increasing PEEP transiently. Although animal studies seem to indicate that recruitment maneuvers are effective in decreasing VILI, human data indicating improved clinical outcomes are not available. This may be because recruitment maneuvers are likely to be effective in patients who have "recruitable" lungs, and none of the studies to date have stratified patients on the basis of lung recruitability. If recruitment maneuvers are used, it is important to monitor for adverse effects such as hypotension, barotraumas, and arrhythmias.

ALTERNATIVE APPROACHES TO LUNG RECRUITMENT

Prone positioning and high-frequency ventilation (HFV) represent alternative ways of attaining lung recruitment.

Placing patients with ARDS in a prone position improves PaO_2 in approximately 70% of patients and also may decrease VILI by improving the homogeneity of end-expiratory lung volume. Recent large clinical trials have been unable to confirm a specific survival benefit for prone positioning in diverse populations of patients with ALI and ARDS. However, posttrial studies and metaanalyses indicate that the subgroup of patients with severe hypoxemia, defined by baseline PaO_2/FIO_2 below 100 mm Hg, but not in patients with less severe hypoxemia, may indeed benefit from prone positioning. The optimal duration of prone positioning has not been established. In clinical practice, an empirical trial of such positioning may be attempted when severely impaired oxygenation fails to respond to usual measures, including sedation, recruiting maneuvers, and high PEEP; during such trials, every possible effort should be made

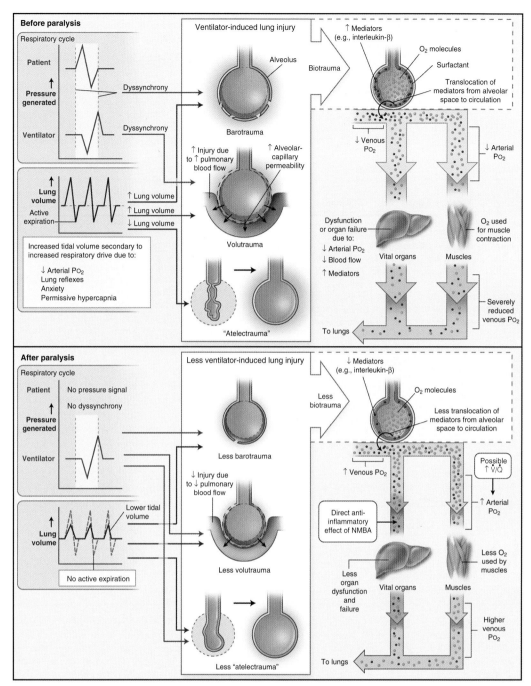

Figure 32-23 Possible mechanisms by which use of neuromuscular blocking agents (NMBAs) may lead to improved survival in patients with the acute respiratory distress syndrome (ARDS). Before induction of paralysis (*top*), increased respiratory drive from multiple causes can lead to increased tidal volumes (VT) and patient-ventilator asynchrony, all of which can potentially worsen various forms of ventilator-induced lung injury (VILI). VILI combined with impaired cardiac performance and consequent decrease in oxygen delivery to vital organs may lead to increased organ dysfunction and ultimately death. After paralysis is obtained (*bottom*), lower VT and improved patient-ventilator synchrony allow for better lung-protective ventilation, less VILI, and less impairment of cardiac performance. VILI also may be lessened by reduced pulmonary blood flow from decreased oxygen consumption. NMBAs also may indirectly improve arterial oxygenation by decreased muscular oxygen consumption and by improving the distribution of ventilation relative to perfusion (V̇/Q̇). Finally, NMBAs may have direct antiinflammatory effects. *(From Slutsky AS: Neuromuscular blocking agents in ARDS,* N Engl J Med *363:1176-1180, 2010.)*

to prevent misadventures associated with postural changes (e.g., displacement of endovascular lines or of the endotracheal tube).

HFV encompasses a number of ventilatory modes, including high-frequency positive-pressure ventilation (HFPPV), high-frequency jet ventilation (HFJV), high-frequency flow interruption (HFFI), and high-frequency oscillatory ventilation (HFOV), all of which use substantially higher ventilatory frequencies (i.e., in the range of 1 to 25 Hz) and much lower VT than with conventional modes (**Figure 32-24**). During HFV, the VT typically is less than the dead space. Gas transport is accomplished by various aspects of convection and diffusion. With HFV, a high mean PVENT is used to recruit alveoli and maintain lung volume above FRC. Thus, in contrast with controlled modes of ventilation, HFV maintains lung volume at a relatively constant level and uses very small VT to accomplish

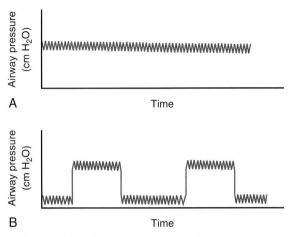

Figure 32-24 With high-frequency ventilation (HFV), extremely small tidal volumes (typically 1 to 3 mL/kg) are applied at very high ventilatory rates (typically 60 to 1500/minute, equivalent to 1 to 25 Hz). HFV allows maintenance of a relatively high mean airway pressure, whereas tidal excursions, and hence alveolar recruitment and derecruitment, are minimized. HFV can be applied either with a constant mean airway pressure (**A**) or alternating between lower and higher mean airway pressures (**B**).

ventilation. Intermittent sighs or sustained inflations are optionally used to recruit collapsed lung regions and to avoid atelectasis.

HFV is a potentially interesting ventilatory approach in patients with ARDS, because the small VT and the small pressure excursions allow the use of a relatively high mean PVENT without overdistending the lungs or allowing cyclic collapse to occur. Recent clinical studies in infants and adults with ARDS suggest that HFV may be as effective as conventional mechanical ventilatory support, but no studies have demonstrated that it reduces mortality.

WEANING FROM MECHANICAL VENTILATION

"Weaning" often is used interchangeably with "liberation" from mechanical ventilation and refers to the transition from full ventilatory support to resumption of unassisted spontaneous breathing by the patient.

All mechanically ventilated patients should be allowed to progress to spontaneous breathing at the earliest possible time, because unnecessary prolongation of ventilation is associated with increased risk for adverse effects such as ventilation-associated pneumonia, VILI, or perhaps respiratory muscle atrophy. On the other hand, premature discontinuation of ventilatory support in a patient not yet ready to assume the entire work of breathing also entails potential harm, including complications related to reintubation. Conventional weaning predictors measure the patient's ability to breathe without assistance but do not assess the ability to clear respiratory tract secretions or to protect the lower airways from aspiration.

Initiation of weaning requires that the patient can and will trigger the ventilator, a prerequisite that often can be achieved only when the level of sedation is reduced or when the $PaCO_2$ is allowed to increase by reducing the minute ventilation. It is not surprising that "protocolized" interruption of sedation on a daily basis reduces the total time spent on mechanical ventilation.

Good clinical judgment in this regard is essential: Only patients with a reasonable likelihood of being able to breathe on their own are suitable candidates for attempts at weaning.

Box 32-1 Criteria for Initiation of a Spontaneous Breathing Trial*

- Evidence of some reversal of the underlying cause of respiratory failure
- Adequate oxygenation: PaO_2/FIO_2 ratio ≥150-200, required PEEP ≤5-8 cm H_2O, FIO_2 ≤0.4-0.5, and pH ≥7.25
- Hemodynamic stability as defined by the absence of active myocardial ischemia and the absence of clinically significant hypotension—that is, a condition requiring no vasopressor therapy or therapy with only low-dose vasopressors (e.g., dopamine or dobutamine given at a dose of less than 5 µg/kg/minute).
- The patient is able to initiate an inspiratory effort.
  The decision to use these criteria for initiation of a spontaneous breathing trial must be individualized.

*Some patients in whom not all of these criteria are satisfied (e.g., patients with chronic hypoxemia values below the thresholds cited) may be ready for attempts to discontinue mechanical ventilation.
PaO_2/FIO_2, ratio of arterial partial pressure of oxygen to fraction of inspired oxygen; *PEEP*, positive end-expiratory pressure.
Modified from MacIntyre NR, Cook DJ, Ely EW Jr, et al: Evidence-based guidelines for weaning and discontinuing ventilatory support: a collective task force facilitated by the American College of Chest Physicians; the American Association for Respiratory Care; and the American College of Critical Care Medicine, *Chest* 120(suppl):375-395, 2001.

Although measuring a variety of physiologic variables may help guide this decision, the process often entails a "trial and error" component. Careful monitoring of the patient's comfort, gas exchange, respiratory mechanics, and hemodynamics during a trial of spontaneous breathing is mandatory. The protocol-based use of spontaneous breathing trials (SBTs) is recommended to identify patients who are likely to be able to breathe spontaneously without assistance (**Figure 32-25**). Criteria to initiate an SBT as recently recommended by a consensus conference are summarized in **Box 32-1** (for details, see the cited source paper authored by MacIntyre and co-workers), but each patient must be evaluated for specific factors that might modify the recommendation or mandate an alternate approach.

A formal SBT often is not required after short-term ventilation (e.g., in patients ventilated for less than 24 hours as, for example, in the postoperative period), whereas an SBT should be performed on a daily basis during a daily interruption of sedation in those patients who meet certain criteria (see Box 32-1). Conventionally, an SBT is performed with use of a minimal level of assist (i.e., 0 to 7 cm H_2O, preferably 0 cm H_2O), an FIO_2 of 0.5, and a PEEP level of 5 to 7.5 cm H_2O. An initial brief period of spontaneous breathing can be used to assess the advisability of continuing on to a formal SBT. The criteria used to assess the patient's readiness to continue tolerance during SBTs are the respiratory pattern, the adequacy of gas exchange, hemodynamic stability, and subjective comfort. Tolerating an SBT for 30 to 120 minutes warrants discontinuation of the ventilator. Removal of the artificial airway is a separate consideration and is based on assessing airway patency and the ability of the patient to protect the airway.

When an SBT fails, the cause should be determined. Once reversible causes for failure are corrected, and if the patient still meets the criteria listed in Box 32-1, subsequent SBTs should be performed at least every 24 hours. Patients who fail an SBT should receive a stable, nonfatiguing, comfortable form of ventilatory support. Anesthesia and sedation strategies and ventilator management aimed at early extubation should be used in postsurgical patients. Weaning protocols designed for non-physician health care professionals should be developed and

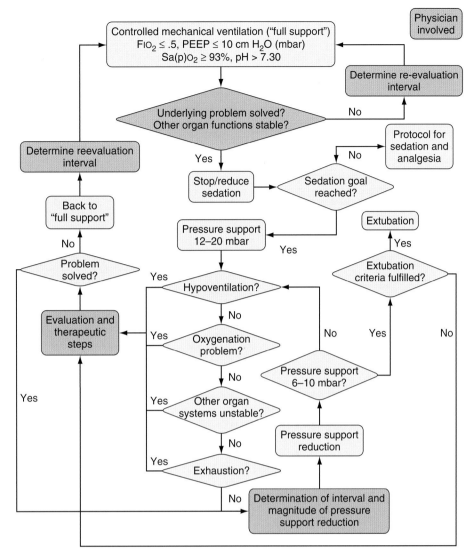

Figure 32-25 Example of a protocol for gradual reduction in the assist level during weaning. *(Modified from Jakob SM, Lubszky S, Friolet R, et al: Sedation and weaning from mechanical ventilation: effects of process optimization outside a clinical trial,* J Crit Care *22:219-228, 2007.)*

implemented by intensive care units (ICUs). Protocols aimed at optimizing sedation also should be developed and implemented.

FAILURE TO WEAN FROM MECHANICAL VENTILATION

A number of factors may be involved in failure to wean a patient from mechanical ventilation, including mismatch between respiratory muscle strength and endurance and the respiratory load (e.g., with CIPM), altered mechanical properties of the respiratory system (e.g., with restrictive or obstructive pulmonary diseases or obesity), inability of the patient to sufficiently clear secretions and to maintain patency of the airways, or presence of a neuropsychological disorder (e.g., delirium, anxiety).

A frequently underrecognized predisposing factor in unsuccessful weaning is cardiac failure after removal of positive-pressure delivery during mechanical ventilation. A combination of several mechanisms may be involved and may result in either preferential right or left ventricular failure, or both. Consequences include myocardial ischemia in predisposed patients, arterial hypotension, cardiogenic pulmonary edema, and a mismatch between increased work of breathing and global oxygen

delivery. Right ventricular failure most frequently results from increased right ventricular load due either to increased return of venous blood to the right ventricle or to increased pulmonary vascular resistance secondary to hypoxemia, hypercapnia, pulmonary edema, elevated intrinsic PEEP, or a combination of these factors. Left ventricular failure may be related to increased afterload (e.g., as a result of removing the positive intrathoracic pressure or arterial hypertension), to impaired filling due to right ventricular distention (interventricular dependence), or to diastolic dysfunction, which may be worsened by arterial hypertension or by catecholamines discharged during a stressful SBT or extubation period. In patients in whom cardiac dysfunction is suspected during weaning from mechanical ventilation, close monitoring (e.g., pulmonary artery pressure, pulmonary capillary wedge pressure, cardiac stroke volume, mixed venous oxygen saturation using a pulmonary artery catheter, or echocardiography) may be helpful to differentiate the mechanisms involved and to closely monitor the effect of therapeutic interventions.

Tracheotomy should be considered after an initial period of stabilization on the ventilator when it becomes apparent that the patient will require prolonged ventilator assistance. Unless there is evidence for clearly irreversible disease (e.g., high spinal cord injury or advanced amyotrophic lateral sclerosis), a patient requiring prolonged mechanical ventilatory support for respiratory failure should not be considered permanently ventilator-dependent until 3 months of weaning attempts have failed. Weaning strategies in patients requiring prolonged mechanical ventilation should be slow-paced and should include gradual lengthening of SBTs.

CONTROVERSIES AND PITFALLS

Better understanding of the potential harm of mechanical ventilation, of the interaction between the patient and the ventilator, and of the importance of optimizing treatment processes associated with mechanical ventilation (e.g., sedation and weaning protocols) has fostered the development of many technical and conceptual improvements in recent years. Nevertheless, further advances are required in numerous areas, including the development of ventilatory strategies that individualize ventilation to the specific patient at a specific point in time and that minimize VILI and its systemic consequences, improvement of alternative approaches to protecting the lung during mechanical ventilation, improving patient-ventilator interactions, and prevention of respiratory muscle deconditioning during mechanical ventilation. Current controversies include the precise role of recruitment maneuvers and ways to individualize PEEP levels, as well as the indications for invasive versus noninvasive ventilation.

Although further research is likely to provide new insights, an important challenge for researchers and clinicians alike is to identify elements of the current knowledge that can be incorporated into daily clinical management to improve outcomes for patients who require ventilatory assistance. In general, a protocolized approach is more likely to result in lasting improvement in care for ventilated patients. Implementing such protocols requires adequate resources, and institutions must make a commitment not only to develop protocols but also to the iterative process of implementation, reassessment, and refinement.

WEB RESOURCES

Guidelines/Protocols

http://ardsnet.org—provides information on completed and on future research projects related to various aspects of ARDS

http://www.ccmtutorials.com/rs/mv/index.htm—provides an illustrative tutorial on mechanical ventilation

SUGGESTED READINGS

Briel M, Meade M, Mercat A, et al: Higher vs lower positive end-expiratory pressure in patients with acute lung injury and acute respiratory distress syndrome: systematic review and meta-analysis, *JAMA* 303:865–873, 2010.

dos Santos CC, Slutsky AS: The contribution of biophysical lung injury to the development of biotrauma, *Annu Rev Physiol* 68:585–618, 2006.

Fan E, Needham DM, Stewart TE: Ventilatory management of acute lung injury and acute respiratory distress syndrome, *JAMA* 294:2889–2896, 2005.

Gattinoni L, Caironi P: Refining ventilatory treatment for acute lung injury and acute respiratory distress syndrome, *JAMA* 299:691–693, 2008.

Gattinoni L, Caironi P, Cressoni M, et al: Lung recruitment in patients with the acute respiratory distress syndrome, *N Engl J Med* 354:1775–1786, 2006.

Jaber S, Petrof BJ, Jung B, et al: Rapidly progressive diaphragmatic weakness and injury during mechanical ventilation in humans, *Am J Respir Crit Care Med* 183:364–371, 2011.

Levine S, Nguyen T, Taylor N, et al: Rapid disuse atrophy of diaphragm fibers in mechanically ventilated humans, *N Engl J Med* 358:1327–1335, 2008.

MacIntyre NR, Cook DJ, Ely EW Jr, et al: Evidence-based guidelines for weaning and discontinuing ventilatory support: a collective task force facilitated by the American College of Chest Physicians; the American Association for Respiratory Care; and the American College of Critical Care Medicine, *Chest* 120(suppl):375–395, 2001.

Mascia L, Pasero D, Slutsky AS, et al: Effect of a lung protective strategy for organ donors on eligibility and availability of lungs for transplantation: a randomized controlled trial, *JAMA* 304:2620–2627, 2010.

Papazian L, Forel JM, Gacouin A, et al: Neuromuscular blockers in early acute respiratory distress syndrome, *N Engl J Med* 363:1107–1116, 2010.

Sud S, Friedrich JO, Taccone P, et al: Prone ventilation reduces mortality in patients with acute respiratory failure and severe hypoxemia: systematic review and meta-analysis, *Intensive Care Med* 36:585–599, 2010.

Tobin MJ, Laghi F, Jubran A: Ventilator-induced respiratory muscle weakness, *Ann Intern Med* 153:240–245, 2010.

Tremblay LN, Slutsky AS: Ventilator induced lung injury: from the bench to the bedside, *Intensive Care Med* 32:24–33, 2006.

Ventilation with lower tidal volumes as compared with traditional tidal volumes for acute lung injury and the acute respiratory distress syndrome. Acute Respiratory Distress Syndrome Network, *N Engl J Med* 342:1301–1308, 2000.

Chapter **33**
Noninvasive Mechanical Ventilation
Paolo Carbonara • Stefano Nava

Noninvasive ventilation (NIV) is mechanical ventilatory support delivered to the airways in the absence of invasive devices such as an endotracheal tube or tracheotomy cannula. The most common devices used to establish the ventilator-patient interface are nasal, oronasal, and full face masks, along with nasal pillows and helmets. The role of NIV has grown steadily in recent years, and in expert hands, it now represents an extremely valuable tool for the management of acute respiratory failure (ARF). The key factors in successful use of NIV are proper patient selection and a high level of competence and experience in both medical and adjunctive personnel on the respiratory care team. It has been shown that in the appropriate setting, NIV is effective in improving gas exchange and alveolar ventilation, as well as in avoiding intubation in patients with ARF. A role for this ventilatory mode also has been proposed in the management of chronic hypercapnic respiratory failure in chronic obstructive pulmonary disease (COPD), although its use is associated with more controversial results.

In general, the main goal of NIV is to provide adequate ventilatory support while avoiding the risks related to tracheal intubation (laryngeal and tracheal damage, lower-airway infections, accidental extubation, higher risk of barotrauma, and volutrauma), as well as sparing the patient the level of pharmacologic sedation commonly required for intubation. In addition, NIV can be performed outside the intensive care unit (ICU)—for example, in step-down units or the emergency department, or on respiratory care wards. On the other hand, it is obvious that NIV cannot guarantee the level of airway control provided by invasive ventilation in terms of leak avoidance, effective delivery of flow and pressure to the airways, and control of minute ventilation. Accurate positioning of the interface device is crucial to minimize air leaks, and patients should be constantly monitored for timely detection of signs of worsening that may necessitate a prompt switch to invasive ventilation.

INDICATIONS FOR IMPLEMENTATION OF NONINVASIVE VENTILATION

In general, NIV is indicated in patients showing clinical and functional signs of acute respiratory distress, in particular:

- Poor alveolar gas exchange level (as indicated by PaO_2/FIO_2 less than 200 mm Hg)
- Ventilatory pump failure with hypercapnia and respiratory acidosis ($PaCO_2$ greater than 45 mm Hg and pH below 7.35)
- Severe dyspnea accompanied by use of accessory respiratory muscles

- Tachypnea (with respiratory rate greater than 24 breaths/minute)

These signs indicate a combination of increased work of breathing and decline in respiratory pump efficiency and point to the need for ventilatory support to relieve the rapidly worsening inspiratory muscle fatigue and to restore acceptable levels of gas exchange and alveolar ventilation. In the presence of these conditions, NIV should be initiated as soon as possible.

It also is important to bear in mind the conditions that preclude use of NIV and dictate prompt intubation with no delay—severely impaired neurologic state as evidence by a Kelly score (a scale specifically devised to assess patient responsiveness) higher than 4, respiratory arrest, shock, severe cardiovascular instability, and presence of excessive airway secretions. Facial lesions that prevent the fitting of nasal or facial masks also will prevent the use of NIV.

MODES

This chapter focuses exclusively on positive-pressure ventilation, which can be broadly defined as the intermittent delivery of pressure to the airways by means of a machine connected to the airway opening. The modes more frequently used for noninvasive ventilation are pressure support ventilation (PSV) and proportional assist ventilation (PAV), often with the addition of extrinsic positive end-expiratory pressure (PEEP); the use of continuous positive airway pressure (CPAP) in the acute setting is confined mainly to the treatment of hypoxemic respiratory failure, especially if the cause is related to cardiogenic pulmonary edema.

EQUIPMENT

VENTILATORS

A simple, informal way of classifying mechanical ventilators on the basis of their performance distinguishes three main types:

1. *Typical ICU ventilators*, powered by compressed gas, usually from wall outlets, and interfaced to the patient exclusively by means of a double circuit, with separate inspiratory and expiratory limbs. These systems are equipped with a screen to allow complete monitoring of ventilatory parameters and graphic display of flow, volume, and pressure curves. They typically are used for invasive ventilation. When set for pressure ventilation, they function on the PSV/PEEP algorithm, in which, as mentioned, the PSV level is superimposed on

the PEEP, with total inspiratory pressure thus resulting from the sum of PSV and PEEP.

2. *Portable home ventilators* (bilevel ventilators), electrically powered and providing only a single circuit for both inspiration and expiration. These machines are used exclusively for noninvasive ventilatory support. They function on the IPAP/EPAP algorithm, in which the inspiratory positive airway pressure (IPAP) is not superimposed on the expiratory pressure (EPAP).

3. *"Hybrid" ventilators,* usually powered by electricity, allowing both single- and double-circuit options. They use the PSV/PEEP algorithm. They can be used for both invasive as well as noninvasive ventilation.

INTERFACES

Patient-circuit interfaces for NIV can be nasal (nasal mask or nasal pillows or plugs), oral (mouthpiece), or facial (oronasal mask, full face mask, helmet). The choice of the appropriate interface is crucial to ensure the success of the treatment and patient compliance. In general, the nasal mask is better tolerated by patients, because it allows expectoration and creates less overall discomfort and is associated with less subjective claustrophobia. In acutely ill patients, face masks usually are preferred over nasal masks by most clinicians, because they provide better control of air leaks, especially in view of the difficulty of breathing exclusively through the nose for patients with acute respiratory failure. In fact, leak control is a key determinant of success for NIV, because it has been shown that air leaks represent the single most important cause of patient-ventilator asynchrony, even when such leaks are relatively modest. On the other hand, placement of nasal or oronasal masks should never be too tight, to prevent development of severe pressure skin lesions, especially frequent across the bridge of the nose, and to improve tolerability. The marked difference in internal volume associated with different interfaces does not usually affect NIV outcome in terms of clinical response and gas exchange variables, when the treatment is delivered by an experienced staff, as shown by a randomized prospective study that compared full face masks, oronasal masks of various sizes, and mouthpieces.

CLINICAL INDICATIONS

In the past decade, the role of NIV has steadily grown, so that it has now become a first-line intervention in a number of clinical conditions. In particular, on the basis of solid evidence gathered over the past 2 decades, NIV has been established as a first-choice intervention in the treatment of acute respiratory failure in the setting of COPD exacerbations and cardiogenic pulmonary edema. The role of NIV also appears to be well established in the management of respiratory failure developing in immunocompromised patients. Finally, NIV has been used as a weaning strategy and to reduce extubation failure.

EXACERBATIONS OF CHRONIC OBSTRUCTIVE PULMONARY DISEASE

Acute respiratory failure frequently complicates COPD exacerbations for a number of reasons deeply rooted in the pathophysiology of the disease. In particular, a combination of airway disease and loss of elastic recoil contributes to the generation of airflow limitation, which in turn can lead to air trapping and lung hyperinflation. As a consequence, the diaphragm is flattened, with loss of optimal length of its muscle fibers and diminished contractile efficiency. Moreover, intrinsic positive end-expiratory pressure (PEEPi) often is present, as a result of the nonreversible airflow limitation. PEEPi places a further burden on inspiratory muscles, because it has to be overcome before a negative alveolar pressure, necessary to the initiation of inspiratory airflow, can be generated.

The contraction of the diaphragm initially is isometric, and only after PEEPi has been counterbalanced can chest expansion begin. The combined effect of increased work of breathing and loss of contractile efficiency places the diaphragm at risk for development of fatigue, a precursor to acute alveolar hypoventilation with hypercapnia and respiratory acidosis. The first studies on the role of noninvasive ventilation in patients with COPD experiencing acute hypercapnic respiratory failure were conducted in the late 1980s. Since then, several controlled randomized studies have shown that NIV added to standard medical treatment is effective in reducing mortality, avoiding intubation, relieving dyspnea, and reducing length of hospital stay in patients with COPD with acute respiratory failure when compared with medical management plus oxygen therapy alone.

A randomized controlled study conducted on 236 patients showed that the rate of success with NIV was especially high in subjects with mild acidosis (pH greater than 7.30), whereas patients with more severe acidosis did not fare equally well and were more likely to require intubation. These findings point to the need for an early and accurate differentiation between patient subgroups on the basis of severity of illness, to allow prompt initiation of the most effective treatment. Patients with mild to moderate acidosis can receive NIV in hospital units outside the ICU, so long as they are staffed with trained personnel. More severely affected patients can still undergo a NIV trial, but only under strict management in an ICU setting, where they can be intubated with no delay in case signs of failure become apparent. Patients treated with NIV, irrespective of their initial severity status, had lower rates of infectious complications (ventilator-associated pneumonia, sepsis). A recent prospective study conducted in the United Kingdom in 9716 inpatients with COPD exacerbation and ARF managed in general clinical practice showed an overall mortality rate of 25% for patients receiving NIV—significantly higher than rates reported in the randomized controlled trials (RCTs). The study pointed to several potential explanations, including inaccurate selection of candidate patients for NIV, including, in some cases, patients with mixed acidosis or prevailing metabolic acidosis; the use of NIV as a "ceiling" of treatment in subjects with very severe disease; and substantial delays in initiating the ventilatory treatment. In addition, patients with mild acidosis (those in which the effectiveness of NIV is higher) appeared to be a minority among the overall group and often do not receive NIV at all. These results highlight the need for better implementation, in general clinical practice, of proper use of NIV in accordance with the evidence gathered from the RCTs.

CARDIOGENIC PULMONARY EDEMA

Cardiogenic pulmonary edema is a consequence of left ventricular failure. It frequently leads to a reduction in lung compliance, with decreased functional residual capacity, regional atelectasis, ventilation-perfusion mismatch and poor gas exchange, resulting in lung failure with hypoxemic respiratory failure. The latter condition is characterized by PaO_2/FIO_2 of less than 300. Treatment with CPAP has long been known to improve survival rate and to lower the need for intubation in patients with cardiogenic pulmonary edema, compared with those receiving conventional medical treatment plus oxygen therapy.

CPAP has the advantage of being practical and relatively easy to use; in most cases treatment with CPAP is administered directly in the emergency department.

In hypoxemic patients, conventional NIV has not produced significant improvements over those achieved with CPAP, although it can be effective in patients with cardiogenic pulmonary edema exhibiting hypercapnia. These data were recently questioned by a multicenter trial comparing oxygen therapy alone, CPAP, and NIV. The investigators concluded that with NIV, the physiologic improvements were faster than with oxygen alone, but without any significant effect on intubation or mortality rates. However, the very low intubation rate in this study (less than 3%) raises questions regarding whether the patient population was comparable to that of other studies.

RESPIRATORY FAILURE IN IMMUNOCOMPROMISED PATIENTS

An immunocompromised status, irrespective of its specific cause (hematologic neoplasms, use of immunosuppressant drugs, AIDS) often leads to lung infections of serious entity which may result in severe hypoxemic respiratory failure. Immunocompromised patients can potentially benefit significantly from NIV, especially because they are particularly at risk for infectious complications related to endotracheal intubation and invasive ventilation. In fact, it has been shown that NIV, especially when applied early, can significantly ameliorate the respiratory symptoms of these patients and reduce need for intubation and overall mortality. According to Principi and colleagues, NIV can even be administered to these patients, by trained personnel, outside the ICU, so as to avoid the risks related to exposure to the ICU environment. These data provide a rationale for a timely use of NIV as an effective means of treatment for respiratory failure in these patients.

ROLE OF NONINVASIVE VENTILATION IN HYPOXIC PATIENTS

One of the major confounders of these studies was the marked variability of the case mix; patients with different underlying disorders and pathophysiologic pathways were included under the same generic definition of having hypoxemia. Confalonieri and associates evaluated NIV in patients with ARF (PaO_2/FiO_2 below 250) consequent to community-acquired pneumonia, including both those with and those without COPD. Compared with standard treatment alone, NIV produced a significant reduction in respiratory rate, need for endotracheal intubation, and ICU stay. A subgroup analysis, however, showed that the benefits of NIV occurred only in those patients with COPD.

Antonelli and co-workers compared NIV with conventional ventilation provided using an endotracheal tube in selected patients with hypoxemic ARF. Sixty-four consecutive patients were enrolled. After 1 hour of mechanical ventilation, the PaO_2/FiO_2 ratio had improved in both groups. Ten patients in the NIV group required intubation. Patients randomized to receive conventional ventilation more frequently developed serious complications and, in particular, infections secondary to endotracheal intubation. Among survivors, the duration of mechanical ventilation and ICU stay were shorter in patients randomized to receive NIV. It should be kept in mind, however, that this single study was conducted in selected patients in one well-experienced center.

A study performed in three European ICUs with considerable expertise with NIV clarifies the issue of "real-life" use of NIV in this setting. This study showed that only 16.5% of patients admitted with ARDS can be successfully treated with this technique. In two years' time, 479 patients were hospitalized for this disorder, a large majority of whom (69%) were already intubated at admission, so that only 147 were eligible for the study. NIV improved gas exchange and avoided intubation in 54% of this subset of patients, for an overall success rate of less than 20%. In these patients NIV was associated with less ventilator-associated pneumonia and a lower ICU mortality rate (6% versus 53%). It should be noted, however, that the study was conducted in three ICUs with solid expertise with NIV. In summary, the use of NIV as an alternative to invasive ventilation in severely hypoxemic patients generally is not advisable and should be limited to hemodynamically stable patients who can be closely monitored in an ICU.

Major surgery is sometimes complicated by the occurrence of atelectasis and pneumonia, which lead to hypoxemia and respiratory distress during the early postoperative period.

One randomized study showed that nasal CPAP delivered through a helmet decreased atelectasis and prevented pneumonia more effectively than did standard therapy alone during an episode of mild respiratory failure after upper abdominal surgery. In another study, NIV significantly ameliorated gas exchange and pulmonary function abnormalities after gastroplasty in obese patients.

NIV may be used in the early treatment of ARF secondary to lung resection, a fatal complication in up to 80% of cases. Auriant and colleagues showed that NIV is safe and effective for reducing the need for intubation and improving survival.

The use of NIV for severe acute respiratory syndrome (SARS) and other airborne diseases has generated debate. Two observational studies from China found no evidence of viral spread to caregivers who took appropriate precautions. In the event of a bird flu pandemic, ventilator resources are likely to be severely strained, and NIV may offer a means of supporting some of the afflicted, mainly those with initial respiratory failure. Some investigators, however, consider NIV to be contraindicated in respiratory failure from communicable respiratory airborne diseases unless it is used in a negative-pressure isolation room and strict precautions are taken against pathogen transmission.

In conclusion, the outcome of NIV in patients with hypoxemic ARF for whom endotracheal intubation is not mandatory yet depends primarily on the type and evolution of the underlying disorder. The high rate of failure of NIV in community-acquired pneumonia and acute respiratory distress syndrome suggests that for patients with these disorders, a cautious approach consisting of early treatment and avoidance of delay of needed intubation is advisable, and patients should be monitored in an ICU setting to assess progression toward the need for invasive ventilation.

ROLE OF NONINVASIVE VENTILATION IN THE PREVENTION OF POSTEXTUBATION FAILURE

Postextubation failure occurs in a percentage of patients varying from 2% to 20%. Necessity for reintubation usually becomes apparent 48 to 72 hours after extubation and is associated with a high mortality rate, as well as a high risk for lower respiratory tract infections. NIV has been applied as a mean of preventing extubation failure with a variable degree of success, depending on the nature and severity of the underlying disease. Recently an RCT conducted on 106 patients with chronic pulmonary disease and hypercapnic respiratory failure who were treated either with NIV for 24 hours after extubation or with oxygen therapy alone, showed a significant effect of NIV in reducing the incidence of postextubation respiratory failure, the need for reintubation, and the overall 90-day mortality. This study seems to confirm a potential role for early NIV treatment in the prevention and treatment of post-extubation failure, at least in patients with chronic respiratory disease.

NONINVASIVE VENTILATION AND WEANING

The first randomized controlled study of an NIV strategy was performed in severely ill patients with COPD ventilated through an endotracheal tube. Patients who failed the T-piece trial were randomized to undergo either extubation, with immediate application of NIV, or continued weaning with the endotracheal tube in place. The study showed that the likelihood of weaning success is increased, while the duration of mechanical ventilation and ICU stay are decreased, when NIV is used as a weaning technique.

A second randomized controlled study was conducted in patients with chronic respiratory disorders, intubated for an episode of ARF. This study also found a shorter duration of invasive mechanical ventilation in the group weaned noninvasively, although no differences were found in ICU or hospital stay or 3-month survival rate.

In a third randomized controlled trial, patients who failed spontaneous breathing trials on three consecutive days were randomized to be extubated and receive NIV or to remain intubated and continue a conventional weaning protocol. Most of the patients were affected by hypercapnic respiratory failure. The duration of conventional mechanical ventilation, time spent in the ICU, and duration of hospitalization were significantly reduced in the NIV group. Patients treated with NIV also had lower rates of nosocomial pneumonia and septic shock and better 90-day survival.

In a recent report, unselected patients who failed trials with a spontaneous-breathing T-piece were randomized either to undergo extubation and NIV or to attempt a traditional weaning trial during invasive ventilation. The percentage of complications in the NIV group was lower, with lower frequency of pneumonia and tracheotomy. Length of stay in the intensive care unit and mortality were not statistically different between the groups. Further studies are clearly needed to assess the real benefits of NIV in weaning with other forms of respiratory failure, such as acute respiratory distress syndrome, postsurgical complications, or cardiac impairment.

In conclusion, in accord with the results of a recent meta-analysis, NIV may be safely and successfully used in the ICU setting to shorten the process of liberation from mechanical ventilation in clinically stable patients recovering from an episode of hypercapnic ARF who had previously failed a weaning trial.

PHYSIOLOGIC EFFECTS OF NONINVASIVE VENTILATION

NIV has been proved to achieve a variety of effects in patients with ARF, largely irrespective of the ventilator mode (PSV or PAV). In particular, in patients with hypercapnia, NIV can restore acceptable levels of alveolar ventilation, significantly reducing $PaCO_2$ and decreasing respiratory acidosis. Alveolar gas exchange also is significantly improved, as evidenced by an increase in PaO_2, which appears to be more rapid and dramatic in patients with cardiogenic pulmonary edema. The improvement in gas exchange seems to involve multiple mechanisms: increased functional residual capacity (FRC) with positioning of the lung volume along the linear part of the pressure-volume curve, facilitating the distensibility of lung parenchyma, and rendering areas of atelectasis or dystelectasis more accessible to ventilation; more uniform overall ventilation with improvement in the ventilation-perfusion ratio; and a higher alveolar pressure opposing fluid extravasation from the capillary bed.

A variable degree of inspiratory muscle rest also usually is obtained, although total diaphragm rest is almost never achieved with NIV because the required inspiratory pressure level would be too high, leading to excessive air leaks and gastric overdistention. Work of breathing is almost constantly reduced, as signaled by a marked reduction in the amplitude of esophageal pressure inspiratory shift (ΔPes). Diaphragmatic rest during noninvasive ventilation is also shown by a reduction in the pressure-time product and of diaphragm electrical activity as measured by electromyography.

Amelioration of diaphragm fatigue and improvement in alveolar ventilation as indicated by reduction in the level of hypercapnia are associated with a more normal breathing pattern, with reduction in breathing frequency. In patients with COPD, NIV increases dynamic compliance (usually decreased in this condition as a consequence of ventilation inhomogeneity and pendelluft), thus allowing a more uniform distribution of ventilation.

Moreover, NIV effectively prevents the increase in $PaCO_2$ often induced by oxygen therapy in ARF due to COPD exacerbations.

In addition to these favorable effects on respiratory mechanics and gas exchange, the potential for unfavorable hemodynamic effects also should be considered. In particular, even in normal persons, positive pressure, especially when applied throughout the entire ventilatory cycle, can reduce venous return to the heart, resulting in reduction in cardiac output. This effect has been demonstrated both in patients with "stable" COPD and during COPD exacerbations.

FUTURE DIRECTIONS

As reviewed in this chapter, the accumulating evidence seems to point to a number of more specific indications for the use of NIV. Several RCTs favor the use of this mode of ventilation. Smaller observational and pilot studies suggest the benefit of NIV in certain disease states; however, further large-scale trials are needed to confirm these findings. In certain geographic areas, old age is considered a barrier to ICU admission. Among patients older than 75 years, the use of NIV rather than standard therapy has been shown to significantly reduce mortality rate.

Some observation studies also have demonstrated that NIV may be successfully used to treat, rather than prevent, an episode of overt respiratory failure during exacerbations of a neuromuscular disease, cystic fibrosis, trauma, obesity-associated hypoventilation, and pancreatitis and eventually as a bridge to lung transplantation.

Indeed, other investigations suggested that NIV may be used in the weaning process in hypoxic patients, and in the treatment of postextubation failure in the subset of hypercapnic patients.

CONTROVERSIES AND PITFALLS

Despite the growing evidence for a role for NIV in the management of ARF, still unresolved are a few questions concerning its optimal utilization in clinical practice. The main controversy concerns the safety of NIV when applied outside the ICU setting, specifically in emergency departments and on regular wards. Although some evidence shows that NIV can be performed with good results in regular respiratory wards, the limiting factor for its success is the availability of specifically trained staff (doctors, nurses, and respiratory therapists). Such availability is far from consistent across hospitals and countries, so the experiences of different groups often are difficult to compare and to generalize. Availability of skilled and experienced staff is obviously crucial for proper patient selection and monitoring, appropriate handling of the equipment, and timely recognition of signs of worsening that might require escalation to invasive ventilation.

The same observations apply in the emergency department, where most patients with ARF who could potentially benefit from NIV initially are evaluated. In fact, many of these patients, for logistical reasons (such as shortage of ICU beds), first receive NIV in this setting, where monitoring is critical for ensuring success, because a delay in switching from noninvasive to invasive ventilation when necessary may result in increased mortality. Accordingly, knowledge and proper evaluation of the predictors of NIV outcome are extremely important.

As indicated by the foregoing considerations, the effectiveness of NIV is strictly dependent on location of implementation, timing, and staff training. Its success or failure will therefore depend on careful, case-by-case judgment that is firmly rooted in the reality of the available resources.

CONCLUSIONS

In summary, the past 2 decades have witnessed a dramatic increase in the use of NIV, which has become a clear-cut first-line treatment in the management of ARF in conditions as diverse as COPD and cardiogenic pulmonary edema and, in many instances, in immunocompromised patients. Moreover, NIV is no longer confined to the ICU, but in expert hands, it has crossed ever more often into the regular ward, thus broadening the spectrum of options available for the treatment of respiratory failure. Current research is focusing on improving the quality and safety of the devices and establishing new ventilatory modes to extend even further the indications for use of NIV, as well as improving its rate of success.

SUGGESTED READINGS

Ambrosino N, Nava S, Torbiki A, et al: Haemodynamic effect of pressure support and PEEP ventilation by nasal route in patients with stable chronic obstructive pulmonary disease, *Thorax* 48:523–528, 1993.

Antonelli A, Conti G, Esquinas A, et al: A multiple-center survey of the use in clinical practice of non invasive ventilation as a first line intervention for acute respiratory distress syndrome, *Crit Care Med* 35:18–25, 2007.

Antonelli M, Conti G, Rocco M, et al: A comparison of non-invasive positive pressure ventilation and conventional mechanical ventilation in patients with acute respiratory failure, *N Engl J Med* 339:429–435, 1998.

Auriant I, Jallot A, Hervé P, et al: Noninvasive ventilation reduces mortality in acute respiratory failure following lung resection, *Am J Respir Crit Care Med* 164:1231–1235, 2002.

Beltrame F, Lucangelo U, Gregori D, Gregoretti C: Noninvasive positive pressure ventilation in trauma patients with acute respiratory failure, *Monaldi Arch Chest Dis* 54:109–114, 1999.

Bott J, Carrol MP, Conway JH, et al: Randomised controlled trial of nasal ventilation in acute ventilatory failure due to chronic obstructive airways disease, *Lancet* 341:1555–1557, 1993.

Brochard L, Isabey D, Piquet J, et al: Reversal of acute exacerbations of chronic obstructive lung disease by inspiratory assistance with a face mask, *N Engl J Med* 323:1523–1530, 1990.

Burns KE, Adhikari NK, Keenan SP, Meade M: Use of non-invasive ventilation to wean critically ill adults off invasive ventilation: meta-analysis and systematic review, *BMJ* 338:b1574, 2009.

Celikel T, Sungur M, Cayhan B, Karakurt S: Comparison of noninvasive positive pressure ventilation with standard medical therapy in hypercapnic acute respiratory failure, *Chest* 114:1636–1642, 1998.

Cheung TM, Yam LY, So LK, et al: Effectiveness of non-invasive positive pressure ventilation in the treatment of acute respiratory failure in severe acute respiratory syndrome, *Chest* 126:670–674, 2004.

Collins SP, Mielniczuk LM, Whittingham HA, et al: The use of non-invasive ventilation in emergency department patients with acute cardiogenic pulmonary edema: a systematic review, *Ann Emerg Med* 48:260–269, 2006.

Confalonieri M, Potena A, Carbone G, et al: Acute respiratory failure in patients with severe community-acquired pneumonia. A prospective randomized evaluation of non invasive ventilation, *Am J Respir Crit Care Med* 160:1585–1591, 1999.

Crimi C, Noto A, Princi P, et al: A European survey of non-invasive ventilation practice, *Eur Respir J* 36:362–369, 2010.

Diaz O, Iglesia R, Ferrer M, et al: Effects of noninvasive ventilation on pulmonary gas exchange and hemodynamics during acute hypercapnic exacerbations of chronic obstructive pulmonary disease, *Am J Respir Crit Care Med* 156:1840–1845, 1997.

Dikensoy O, Ikidag B, Filiiz A, Bayram N: Comparison of non-invasive ventilation and standard medical therapy in acute hypercapnic respiratory failure: a randomised controlled trial at a tertiary health centre in SE Turkey, *Int J Clin Pract* 56:85–88, 2002.

Elliott MW: *European Respiratory Society Interactive course on non-invasive positive pressure ventilation: consensus, controversies and new horizons,* Hanover, Germany, February 12–14, 2009.

Fauroux B, Burgel PR, Boelle PY, et al: Chronic Respiratory Insufficiency Group of the French National Cystic Fibrosis Federation: Practice of noninvasive ventilation for cystic fibrosis: a nationwide survey in France, *Respir Care* 53:1482–1489, 2008.

Fernandez R, Blanch LP, Valles J, et al: Pressure support ventilation via face mask in acute respiratory failure in hypercapnic COPD patients, *Intensive Care Med* 19:456–461, 1993.

Ferrer M, Esquinas A, Arancibia F, et al: Noninvasive ventilation during persistent weaning failure: a randomized controlled trial, *Am J Respir Crit Care Med* 168:70–76, 2003.

Ferrer M, Valencia M, Carrillo A, et al: Non-invasive ventilation after extubation in hypercapnic patients with chronic respiratory disorders: randomized controlled trial, *Lancet* 374:1082–1088, 2009.

Ferrer M, Valencia M, Nicolas JM, et al: Early non-invasive ventilation averts extubation failure in patients at risk. A randomized trial, *Am J Respir Crit Care Med* 173:164–170, 2006.

Fraticelli AT, Lellouche F, L'her E, et al: Physiological effects of different interfaces during noninvasive mechanical ventilation for acute respiratory failure, *Crit Care Med* 37:939–945, 2009.

Girault C, Daudenthun I, Chevron V, et al: Noninvasive ventilation as a systematic extubation and weaning technique in acute-on-chronic respiratory failure: a prospective, randomized controlled study, *Am J Respir Crit Care Med* 160:86–92, 1999.

Gray A, Goodacre S, Newby DE, et al: Noninvasive ventilation in acute cardiogenic pulmonary edema, *N Engl J Med* 359:142–151, 2008.

Han F, Jiang YY, Zheng JH, et al: Noninvasive positive pressure ventilation treatment for acute respiratory failure in SARS, *Sleep Breath* 8:94–106, 2004.

Hess DR, Pang JM, Camargo CA Jr: A survey of the use of noninvasive ventilation in academic emergency departments in the United States, *Respir Care* 54:1306–1312, 2009.

Hilbert G, Gruson D, Vargas F, et al: Noninvasive ventilation in immunosuppressed patients with pulmonary infiltrates, fever and acute respiratory failure, *N Engl J Med* 344:481–487, 2001.

Jaber S, Chanques G, Sebbane M, et al: Noninvasive positive pressure ventilation in patients with respiratory failure due to severe acute pancreatitis, *Respiration* 73:166–172, 2006.

Joris JL, Sottiaux TM, Chiche JD, et al: Effect of bi-level positive airway pressure (BiPAP) nasal ventilation on the postoperative pulmonary restrictive syndrome in obese patients undergoing gastroplasty, *Chest* 111:665–670, 1997.

Kallet RH, Diaz JV: The physiologic effects of noninvasive ventilation, *Respir Care* 54:102–114, 2009.

Kroschinsky F, Weise M, Illmer T, et al: Outcome and prognostic features of intensive care unit treatment in patients with hematological malignancies, *Intensive Care Med* 28:1294–1300, 2002.

Masip J, Rocha M, Sanchez B, et al: Non invasive ventilation in acute pulmonary edema. Systematic review and meta-analysis, *JAMA* 294:3124–3130, 2005.

Meduri GU, Conoscenti CC, Menashe P, Nair S: Noninvasive face mask ventilation in patients with acute respiratory failure, *Chest* 95:865–870, 1989.

Nava S, Ambrosino N, Clini E, et al: Noninvasive mechanical ventilation in the weaning of patients with respiratory failure due to chronic obstructive pulmonary disease. A randomized, controlled trial, *Ann Intern Med* 128:721–728, 1998.

Nava S, Carbone G, Dibattista N, et al: Noninvasive ventilation in cardiogenic pulmonary edema: a multicenter, randomized trial, *Am J Respir Crit Care Med* 168:1432–1437, 2003.

Nava S, Grassi M, Fanfulla F, et al: Non-invasive ventilation in elderly patients with acute hypercapnic respiratory failure: a randomised controlled trial, *Age Ageing* 40:444–450, 2011.

Nava S, Gregoretti C, Fanfulla F, et al: Noninvasive ventilation to prevent respiratory failure after extubation in high risk patients, *Crit Care Med* 33:2465–2470, 2005.

Navalesi P, Fanfulla F, Frigerio P, et al: Physiologic evaluation of non-invasive mechanical ventilation delivered with three types of masks in patients with hypercapnic respiratory failure, *Crit Care Med* 28:1785–1790, 2000.

O'Brien G, Criner GJ: Mechanical ventilation as a bridge to lung transplantation, *J Heart Lung Transplant* 18:255–265, 1999.

Park M, Sangean MC, Volpe MS, et al: Randomized, prospective trial of oxygen, continuous positive airway pressure, and bilevel positive airway pressure by face mask in acute cardiogenic pulmonary edema, *Crit Care Med* 32:2407–2415, 2004.

Pérez de Llano LA, Golpe R, Ortiz Piquer M, et al: Short-term and long-term effects of nasal intermittent positive pressure ventilation in patients with obesity-hypoventilation syndrome, *Chest* 128:587–594, 2005.

Peter JV, Moran JL, Phillips-Hughes J, et al: Effect of non-invasive positive pressure ventilation on mortality in patients with acute cardiogenic pulmonary oedema: a meta-analysis, *Lancet* 367:1155–1163, 2006.

Philip-Joet FF, Paganelli FF, Dutau HL, Saadjan AY: Hemodynamic effect of bilevel nasal positive airway pressure ventilation in patients with heart failure, *Respiration* 66:136–143, 1999.

Plant PK, Owen JL, Elliot MW: A multicentre randomised controlled trial of the early use of non-invasive ventilation in acute exacerbation of chronic obstructive pulmonary disease on general respiratory wards, *Lancet* 335:1931–1935, 2000.

Plant PK, Owen JL, Elliott MW: Early use of non-invasive ventilation for acute exacerbations of chronic obstructive pulmonary disease on general respiratory wards: a multicentre randomised controlled trial, *Lancet* 355:1931–1935, 2000.

Principi T, Pantanetti S, Catani F, et al: Noninvasive continuous positive airway pressure delivered by helmet in hematological malignancy patients with hypoxemic acute respiratory failure, *Intensive Care Med* 30:147–150, 2004.

Roberts CM, Stone RA, Buckingham RJ, et al; National COPD Resources and Outcome Project implementation group: Acidosis, non-invasive ventilation and mortality in hospitalised COPD exacerbations, *Thorax* 66:43–48, 2011.

Rothaar RC, Epstein SK: Extubation failure: magnitude of the problem, impact on outcomes, and prevention, *Curr Opin Crit Care* 9:59–66, 2003.

Squadrone V, Coha M, Cerutti E, et al: Continuous positive airway pressure for treatment of postoperative hypoxemia, *JAMA* 293:589–595, 2005.

Thys F, Roeseler J, Reynaert M, et al: Noninvasive ventilation for acute respiratory failure: a prospective randomised placebo-controlled trial, *Eur Respir J* 20:545–555, 2002.

Trevisan CE, Vieira SR; Research Group in Mechanical Ventilation Weaning: Noninvasive mechanical ventilation may be useful in treating patients who fail weaning from invasive mechanical ventilation: a randomized clinical trial, *Crit Care* 12:R51, 2008.

Valipour A, Schneider F, Kossler W, et al: Heart rate variability and spontaneous baroflex sequences in supine healthy volunteers subjected to nasal positive airway pressure, *J Appl Physiol* 99:2137–2143, 2005.

Vianello A, Bevilacqua M, Arcaro G, et al: Non-invasive ventilatory approach to treatment of acute respiratory failure in neuromuscular disorders. A comparison with endotracheal intubation, *Intensive Care Med* 26:384–390, 2000.

Vignaux L, Vargas F, Roeseler J, et al: Patient-ventilator asynchrony during non-invasive ventilation for acute respiratory failure: a multicenter study, *Intensive Care Med* 35:840–846, 2009.

Winck JC, Azevedo LF, Costa-Pereira A, et al: Efficacy and safety of non-invasive ventilation in the treatment of acute cardiogenic pulmonary edema—a systematic review and meta-analysis, *Crit Care* 10:R69, 2006.

Wood KA, Lewis L, Von Harz B, Kollef MH: The use of non-invasive positive pressure ventilation in the emergency department: results of a randomized clinical trial, *Chest* 113:1339–1346, 1998.

Chapter **34**
Airway Management in the Intensive Care Unit*

Michael Spiro • Alan McGlennan

The decision to instrument the airway of a patient is one of the most crucial taken; this approach to airway management, although often required in an emergency situation, requires considerable skill, experience, and knowledge of the different types of procedures available. The main reasons to instrument the airway are (1) failure of oxygenation, (2) failure of ventilation, and (3) protection of the airways.

Patients with a variety of medical and surgical diseases may require ventilatory assistance or improved airway control. Such patients include those with primary respiratory failure or with respiratory insufficiency secondary to other pathologic conditions. Implementation of respiratory support may be undertaken semielectively or on an emergency basis.

Airway instrumentation should be performed only by a skilled physician who has assessed the patient thoroughly addressing the risks and benefits for that patient. A vital step in this assessment is prediction of the ease with which intubation is likely to be possible, with identification of an appropriate alternative approach to use in case difficulties arise. An important point to remember is that patients die not because of a failure to intubate but as a result of failure to oxygenate; therefore, recurrent failed attempts to gain airway control should be avoided. Problems with ventilation can quickly lead to severe hypoxia, brain damage, or death.

INDICATIONS FOR AIRWAY SUPPORT

The most common indication for ventilatory support in intensive care is acute respiratory failure, resulting in hypoxia, hypercapnia, or increased work of breathing, necessitating the need for positive-pressure ventilation. This can be provided as noninvasive ventilation (NIV) or as invasive ventilation requiring intubation. Intubation also may be indicated with loss of airway reflexes associated with a reduced level of consciousness, meaning that the patient is unable to protect their airway. Airway protection may be needed in cases of airway soiling or excessive secretion with inadequate cough. The neurosurgical patient managed in the ICU may require ventilation to regulate $PaCO_2$ for control of intracranial pressure. Endotracheal intubation also may be needed when swelling or trauma to the upper respiratory tract results in impending airway loss.

NONINVASIVE VENTILATION

Patients with respiratory failure and preserved airway reflexes may benefit from NIV. The rationale for this application, most commonly seen in acute exacerbations of chronic obstructive pulmonary disease (COPD), is that NIV may reduce the work of breathing and help to correct hypercapnic or hypoxic respiratory failure. NIV is contraindicated, however, with cardiovascular or respiratory instability, compromised ability to handle secretions, aspiration risk, or inability to tolerate a tight-fitting face mask (see Chapter 33 on NIV).

AIRWAY ASSESSMENT

Before instrumentation of the patient's airway, a thorough assessment should be performed to ascertain the likelihood of difficulty in achieving airway control. Several specific aspects of this assessment are considered next.

PREDICTORS OF DIFFICULT MASK VENTILATION

Difficult mask ventilation is encountered in 8% of patients. Patients at risk for such difficulty include those with preexisting partial airway obstruction, snorers, those with facial asymmetry, the obese, persons with Mallampati class IV airway anatomy (complete lack of epiglottis visualization), and the edentulous. Management of patients with facial hair, which often hides a receding mandible and in itself makes a seal for mask ventilation difficult, can present significant problems.

PREDICTORS OF DIFFICULT INTUBATION

Difficult intubation is common in the ICU population, with frequency of reported difficulty between 6.6% and 22%. A history of airway problems should be sought—for example, snoring, sleep apnea, congenital diseases (such as Down or Pierre-Robin syndrome), and previous anesthetic problems.

Examination of the patient should determine the following: ability to protrude the mandible, range of neck movement, atlantooccipital flexion and extension, interincisor distance (less than 3 cm indicates a high likelihood of difficulty), and modified Mallampati test (**Figure 34-1**). Other predictors of difficult intubation include thyromental distance of less than 7 cm (Patil's test) and obesity. Further investigations when indicated could include the view of the larynx obtained at nasal

---

*Additional content for this chapter can be found on Expert Consult.

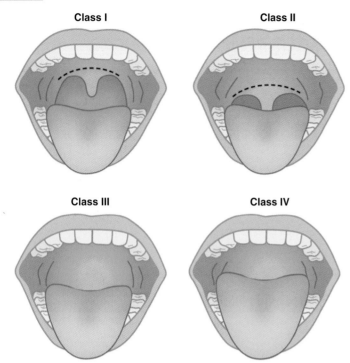

Class I   Class II

Class III   Class IV

Figure 34-1 Mallampati test to classify view of the pharynx. For this test, the patient is asked to protrude the tongue fully while opening the mouth maximally, with the head in the neutral position. *Class I:* The pharyngeal pillars, soft palate, and uvula are visible. *Class II:* Only the soft palate and uvula are visible. *Class III:* Only the soft palate is seen. *Class IV:* Only the hard palate is seen. Mallampati class correlates with Cormack and Lehane grade for the view at laryngoscopy (see Figure 34-5). Increasing class suggests more difficult laryngoscopy.

Box 34-1   **Risk Factors for Aspiration at Time of Intubation**

Instrumentation before postprandial interval of less than 6 hours
Obesity
Pregnancy
Hiatus hernia
Intraabdominal pathology
Vomiting
Symptomatic reflux

---

endoscopy, which may predict the view at laryngoscopy; chest radiographs, which may show tracheal deviation or mediastinal masses; and CT scans, which may be useful when abnormal anatomy is suspected—for example, in association with tracheal stenosis.

ASPIRATION RISK

Aspiration of gastric contents can cause significant morbidity and mortality. Evidence suggests that reducing gastric volume and increasing pH of gastric contents will limit the risk of disorders associated with aspiration. Acid aspiration may lead to a chemical pneumonitis, but aspiration of food particles can result in physical obstruction of the bronchial tree with secondary bacterial pneumonia (**Box 34-1** and **Table 34-1**).

BASIC AIRWAY MANEUVERS AND AIRWAY ADJUNCTS

Patients with complete or partial airway obstruction may benefit from basic airway maneuvers to open the airway.

Table 34-1   **Drugs to Reduce Aspiration Risk**

Drug Class	Specific Agent	Mechanism of Action
Histamine H$_2$ receptor antagonists	Ranitidine 50 mg IV	Increases pH and decreases gastric volume
Proton pump inhibitors	Omeprazole 40 mg IV	Irreversibly binds H$^+$/K$^+$-ATPase; increases pH and decreases gastric volume
Nonparticulate antacids	0.3 M sodium citrate, 10 mL	Neutralizes gastric pH but increases volume. Very effective at increasing gastric pH if given within 30 minutes
Prokinetics	Metoclopramide 10 mg	Reduces gastric volume

Depending on the cause of airway compromise, suctioning may be needed to remove foreign bodies. Neck flexion with extension at the atlantooccipital joint and a chin lift can be used when upper airway tone is reduced; a jaw thrust should be used with in-line stabilization when cervical spine injury is suspected. In patients with a reduced level of consciousness, insertion of an appropriately sized oropharyngeal or nasopharyngeal airway may be helpful.

ENDOTRACHEAL INTUBATION WITH MUSCLE RELAXATION

POSITIONING

Putting the patient in the optimal position is the first and most important step. Appropriate positioning allows good access to the airway and allows efficient preoxygenation. Other advantages include improvement of the laryngoscopic view and, with the head held slightly up, a reduced risk for aspiration of gastric contents. The "head-up" position also increases functional residual capacity by allowing better diaphragmatic excursion, thereby increasing oxygen reserves. The patient should be positioned with the neck flexed on a pillow, but with the head extended, so long as cervical spine injury is not suspected. Positioning is of particular importance in the obese patient (**Figure 34-2**).

BAG MASK VENTILATION

In an elective setting, patients who are adequately fasted may be anesthetized and administered a nondepolarizing muscle relaxant. While awaiting the onset of muscle relaxation, the patient is oxygenated by positive-pressure bag mask ventilation before endotracheal intubation. In other circumstances, a profoundly hypoxic patient may need bag mask ventilation before intubation—for example, in a cardiac arrest scenario. Implementation of this ventilatory mode is therefore a key, lifesaving skill for all physicians to possess. Successful bag mask ventilation requires an open airway, a good seal with the face mask, and the application of positive pressure achieved by compressing the reservoir bag connected to high-flow oxygen.

In patients at risk for aspiration, *rapid sequence induction* can be performed. With the classic technique, the initial step is formal preoxygenation of the patient, followed by the administration of a predetermined dose of rapid-onset general anesthetic agent and then a rapid-onset muscle relaxant. Cricoid pressure is applied, and the patient is intubated as soon as muscle relaxation has occurred.

Table 34-2 Drugs Used in Airway Management in the Intensive Care Unit

Drug	Dose	Action	Comments
Thiopental	3-5 mg/kg	General anesthesia	Barbiturate with rapid onset and offset after bolus administration Potent anticonvulsant
Propofol	1.5-2.5 mg/kg	General anesthesia	Rapid onset, offset slower than with thiopental bolus; causes more hypotension Pain on injection
Suxamethonium	1-2 mg/kg	Relaxation within 30 seconds	Rapid offset, multiple unwanted effects Myalgia, hyperkalemia, arrhythmias, allergy, "suxamethonium apnea"
Rocuronium	1 mg/kg	Muscle relaxation within 60 seconds	Long duration of action, risk of allergic reactions
Suggamadex	2-16 mg/kg	Rapid reversal of rocuronium	Reversal of muscle relaxation in I to 2 minutes Reports of bradycardia

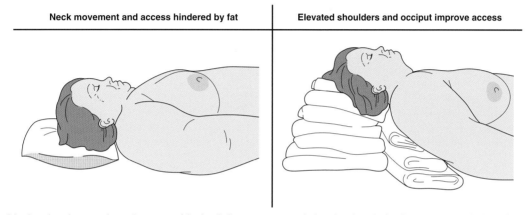

Neck movement and access hindered by fat | Elevated shoulders and occiput improve access

Figure 34-2 Positioning the obese patient. Correct positioning is important to optimize the view during laryngoscopy. Flexion of the lower cervical spine brings the trachea in line with the pharynx, and extension at the atlantooccipital joint aligns the trachea with the oral cavity. With the obese patient in the supine position, neck movement and access with a laryngoscope are hindered by fat. When the patient is repositioned with the shoulders elevated and the occiput further elevated so that the head assumes a "sniffing" position, access to the airway is facilitated. *(From Wiener-Kronish JP, Shimabukuro DW: Airway management. In Albert RK, Spiro SG, Jett JR, editors: Clinical respiratory medicine, ed 3, Philadelphia, 2008, Mosby.)*

PREOXYGENATION

Before induction of anesthesia, the patient should be fully preoxygenated. The patient breathes 100% oxygen through a tight-fitting face mask for 3 minutes. In an emergency, five vital capacity breaths of 100% oxygen can be used in an attempt to fill the functional residual capacity lung compartment with oxygen, thereby significantly raising the alveolar PO_2. This step prolongs the time to desaturation after the onset of apnea, affording the operator significant time to manage the airway safely (**Table 34-2**).

CRICOID PRESSURE

A major concern with an emergency intubation is the risk of aspiration of gastric contents. Cricoid pressure can be applied to prevent passive regurgitation of stomach contents, with subsequent airway soiling. The assistant exerts firm pressure (equivalent to 30 newtons [N] of backward pressure) on the cricoid cartilage to compress the esophagus against the body of the sixth cervical vertebra as the level of consciousness diminishes (**Figure 34-3**). Cricoid pressure should be removed only if the patient actively vomits (associated with risk for esophageal rupture) or in specific instances of inability to oxygenate (see the difficult intubation algorithm presented in Figure 34-7).

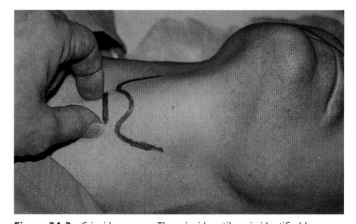

Figure 34-3 Cricoid pressure. The cricoid cartilage is identified by palpation below the thyroid cartilage. Firm pressure is placed on this structure to occlude the esophagus against the body of the sixth cervical vertebra. Pressure is maintained until after intubation is accomplished and airway control is achieved. *(From Wiener-Kronish JP, Shimabukuro DW: Airway management. In Albert RK, Spiro SG, Jett JR, editors: Clinical respiratory medicine, ed 3, Philadelphia, 2008, Mosby.)*

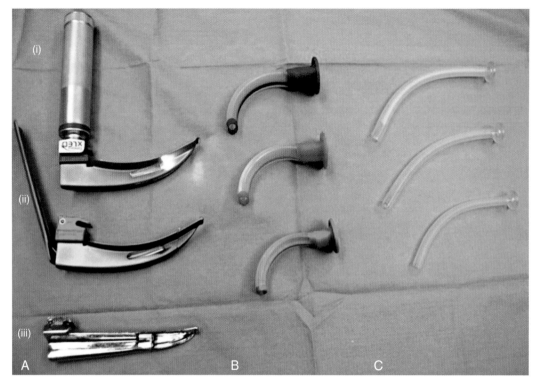

Figure 34-4 Airway management equipment. **A,** Laryngoscope blades: *(i),* The Macintosh blade size 3, the most commonly used blade for intubating an adult. *(ii),* The McCoy blade size 3. Note the hinged tip, which can be activated by depressing the lever; this can be used to elevate the epiglottis when the view of the laryngeal inlet is obscured. *(iii),* The Miller blade size 3, a straight blade that is used to lift the epiglottis directly with the tip, to obtain a view of the larynx. **B,** Oropharyngeal airways in the most common sizes used in adult patients: size 4 *(red),* 3 *(orange),* and 2 *(green).* **C,** Nasopharyngeal airways in different sizes, from *top:* 8.5F, 7.5F, and 6.5F. The size chosen will depend on the size of the patient and appropriate length.

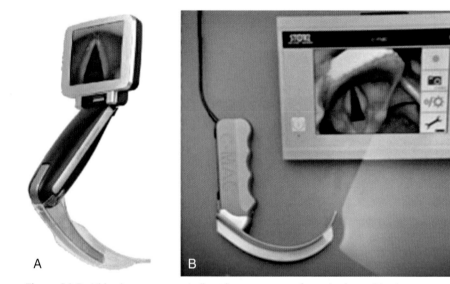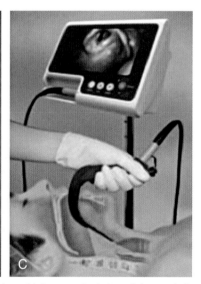

Figure 34-5 Video laryngoscopes. Indirect laryngoscopy performed using a video laryngoscope allows intubation with less manipulation of the cervical spine and often provides an improved view of the laryngeal inlet when problems have been encountered with direct laryngoscopy. **A,** The Venner AP Advance, a handheld laryngoscope with a screen built into the handle. **B,** The Storz C-Mac scope. **C,** The Glidescope. The instruments shown in **B** and **C** both are handheld laryngoscopes with a separate video display screen.

EQUIPMENT

The most common laryngoscope blade used for intubation in adults is the curved Macintosh blade (**Figure 34-4**). This is inserted into the right side of the mouth to displace the tongue laterally. The tip of the blade sits in the vallecula and is lifted forward to elevate the epiglottis and expose the laryngeal inlet. The McCoy blade is a variant of the Macintosh and has a hinged tip to further lift the epiglottis. A straight Miller blade can be useful in adults in whom the epiglottis is difficult to displace. This blade is inserted further to directly lift the epiglottis. Where laryngoscopy may be difficult a video laryngoscope can be used. There are now a variety of different models available on the market (**Figure 34-5**). They require less manipulation of the cervical spine and allow intubation in a seated

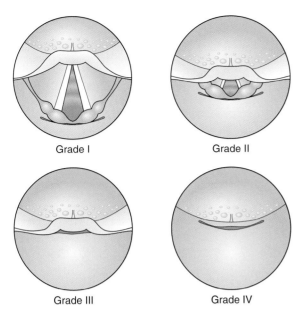

Figure 34-6 Cormack and Lehane grading of laryngoscopic views: *Grade I*: The entire laryngeal inlet is visible. *Grade II*: The arytenoids and posterior vocal cords are seen. *Grade III*: Only the epiglottis is visible, *Grade IV*: The epiglottis is not visualized. Grade III and grade IV views suggest difficulty in passing an endotracheal tube. They often will mandate the use of a bougee or an alternative intubation technique.

position, reducing the aspiration risk (Videos 1-4). Awake fiberoptic intubation may be used were visualization of the larynx may be difficult by other means or if access to the mouth is restricted.

LARYNGEAL ANATOMY

The view of the laryngeal inlet obtained at direct laryngoscopy can be graded in accordance with the Cormack and Lehane classification (**Figure 34-6**). Grade I and grade II views indicate straightforward intubation. A grade III view frequently necessitates the use of a gum elastic bougee to "railroad" the endotracheal tube (ETT) into position, whereas a grade IV view often will mandate a different strategy to achieve successful intubation.

Awake Fiberoptic Intubation

Awake intubation is used in patients with a predicted difficult airway or an unstable cervical spine. This technique allows patients to maintain their own airway until intubation is achieved, thereby greatly reducing the risk for aspiration: risk. No manipulation of the cervical spine is needed. If problems are encountered at any stage, the procedure can be safely abandoned.

The nostrils are prepared with local anesthetic and a vasoconstrictor. An endotracheal tube is mounted on a fiberoptic bronchoscope, which is then maneuvered through the nose, the nasopharynx, and finally the larynx until the scope is situated superior to the carina. Once appropriately positioned, the endotracheal tube is railroaded over the scope. The cuff is inflated and tube position is confirmed before induction of anesthesia.

Gaseous Induction

In patients with stridor or in other situations characterized by partial airway obstruction, a gas induction can be performed. The patient breathes volatile anesthetic, often sevoflurane, through a tight-fitting face mask until anesthesia is induced. This aspect of the technique keeps the patient spontaneously

breathing and maintains a degree of airway tone, preventing airway loss. Tracheal intubation is then performed with the patient under deep inhalational anesthesia. Muscle relaxants are given only after the trachea is intubated and airway control has been established.

Confirming Intubation

Correct ETT placement is confirmed clinically by visualizing the tube's passage through the vocal cords and observation of fogging of the ETT, symmetric chest movement, and bilateral air entry. The "gold standard" modality for such confirmation is measurement of end-tidal CO_2 on ventilation. In critical care, a chest radiograph is performed to confirm ETT position above the carina. Provision must always be made for unexpected difficult intubation.

RESCUE TECHNIQUES

Whenever the decision is taken to intubate, the physician should always have an alternative plan to use if any difficulties are encountered. In the United Kingdom, the difficult intubation algorithm produced by the Difficult Airway Society is used (**Figure 34-7**).

MASK VENTILATION

When intubation is difficult or impossible, oxygenation of the patient remains the main priority. Mask ventilation (with application of cricoid pressure if aspiration is a risk) with 100% oxygen should be attempted. If this proves to be difficult, an airway adjunct, such as a Guedel oropharyngeal airway, should be inserted. A four-handed technique may be used, with two hands holding the mask and maintaining the patient's airway while an assistant operates the bag used to ventilate the patient.

LARYNGEAL MASK AIRWAY

The laryngeal mask is a supraglottic device that has revolutionized anesthesia in the past 25 years. It is inserted orally and when inflated sits in the posterior hypopharynx, pushing the tongue base anteriorly and keeping the glottis open. Its design has been modified and improved over time. Using the laryngeal mask airway (LMA) to ventilate a paralyzed patient in the operating room is now considered acceptable, particularly since the advent of such masks with a gastric port to allow venting of any refluxed gastric secretion. The use of LMAs in resuscitation is promoted in certain practice areas owing to its ease of insertion.

The LMA is extremely useful in clinical situations in which mask ventilation would be difficult or when intubation is impossible. It can be used to maintain oxygenation while a plan for definitive airway control is made, or it can be used as a conduit for access to the larynx. A fiberoptic scope can be inserted through the LMA and an ETT passed over the scope into the trachea. The intubating LMA is specifically designed to facilitate tracheal intubation; special features include an epiglottic elevating bar facilitating access to the trachea. It can be useful in patients in whom neck movement is limited (**Figure 34-8**).

SURGICAL AIRWAYS

CRICOTHYROIDOTOMY

In situations in which it is not possible to either intubate or ventilate the patient, an emergency cricothyroidotomy should be performed (**Figure 34-9**). The cricothyroid membrane is an

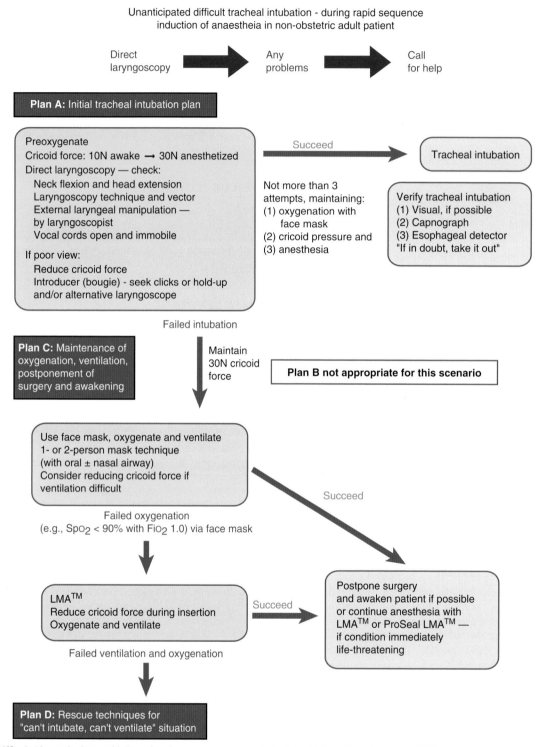

Figure 34-7 Difficult Airway Society guidelines for airway management. If the initial intubation plan (*Plan A*) fails, no more than three attempts at direct laryngoscopy should be performed; an alternative method should be used to facilitate tracheal intubation and maintain oxygenation. Should these techniques fail, then oxygenation is the main priority while the patient is woken up, if appropriate (*Plan C*). Should it be impossible to intubate or ventilate the patient using any of these methods, emergency transtracheal ventilation or cricothyroidotomy should be performed (*Plan D*). (*Courtesy Difficult Airway Society, Association of Anaesthetists of Great Britain and Ireland, London.*)

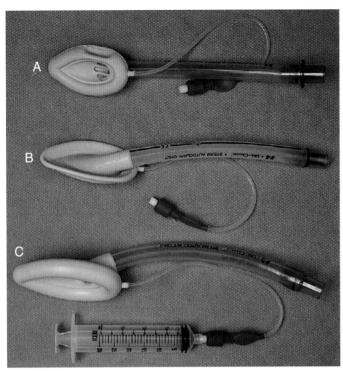

Figure 34-8 Laryngeal mask airway (LMA), available in sizes 1 to 5. Usually, the LMA is inserted fully deflated, with the tongue and mandible gently pulled anteriorly, with continuous pressure posteriorly until a firm end point is reached. Position is confirmed after cuff inflation by the ability to ventilate the patient, as noted by chest rise and auscultation. Most adults will accept a size 4 or 5 airway. The LMA allows ventilation and placement of an endotracheal tube by means of a fiberoptic bronchoscope if direct laryngoscopy has failed. **A,** Size 3, partially inflated. **B,** Size 4, completely deflated. **C,** Size 5, completely inflated. *(From Wiener-Kronish JP, Shimabukuro DW: Airway management. In Albert RK, Spiro SG, Jett JR, editors:* Clinical respiratory medicine, *ed 3, Philadelphia, 2008, Mosby.)*

avascular membrane joining the thyroid cartilage to the cricoid cartilage. A purpose made kink-resistant cannula can be inserted through the cricothyroid membrane into the trachea, and then the patient is jet ventilated through this tube. Larger cricothyroidotomy devices can be used that allow the patient to be ventilated in a conventional fashion. Surgical cricothyroidotomy requires more skill and involves dissection down to the cricothyroid membrane, followed by insertion of an appropriately sized endotracheal tube (6-mm inner diameter) into the trachea. Cricothyroidotomy is associated with multiple complications, including airway loss, esophageal trauma, bleeding, false passage formation, pneumothorax, and surgical emphysema.

TRACHEOSTOMY

Surgical tracheostomy requires a skilled surgeon. It can be performed to sidestep impending upper airway loss in the awake patient with use of local anesthesia. It is not suitable as a rescue technique because it is time-consuming. **Boxes 34-2** and **34-3** lists the indications for and possible complications of surgical tracheostomy.

PERCUTANEOUS TRACHEOSTOMY

Percutaneous tracheostomy is favored by many intensive care physicians because it can be performed at the bedside—useful

---

Box 34-2   Indications for Tracheostomy

Emergency
Impending airway obstruction

Elective
Aid weaning (reduce dead space)
Reduce sedation requirement
Improve oral care
Reduce damage to glottis
Improve patient comfort

Box 34-3   Complications of Tracheostomy

Early
Bleeding
Pneumothorax
Surgical emphysema
Airway loss and hypoxia
Esophageal trauma
Laryngeal trauma

Late
Airway blockage
Dislodged tracheostomy tube
Tracheomalacia
Infection

---

when an unstable patient is too ill for transfer to the operating room—and because the tracheostomy cannula can be inserted by physicians, thus avoiding the logistics of arranging for a surgeon. Other advantages include less tissue damage, lower risk of bleeding, and lower infection rates. Factors making percutaneous tracheostomy an unsuitable choice include difficult anatomy, short neck, and abnormal vascular anatomy.

The intubated patient is positioned with the neck extended while being preoxygenated with 100% oxygen. Two skilled operators are required, one to perform the procedure and another to manage the airway. Local anesthetic is infiltrated and a small incision is made below the cricoid cartilage. Blunt dissection is performed until the trachea is easily palpable to the operator. A fiberoptic bronchoscope is inserted down the ETT, and a needle attached to a syringe is inserted into the trachea between the second and third tracheal rings under direct vision. Air is aspirated through the syringe, and a wire is threaded through the needle into the trachea. A dilator is passed over the wire to enlarge the tract. The tracheostomy tube is then inserted over the wire.

CONTROVERSIES AND PITFALLS IN AIRWAY MANAGEMENT

The rapid sequence induction technique with application of cricoid pressure is a relatively recent introduction to anesthesia. It is widely adhered to in many countries (e.g., the United Kingdom) for cases in which aspiration of stomach contents is a risk during induction. Many countries, however, do not use cricoid pressure to help prevent aspiration (e.g., France). No agreement has emerged regarding which approach is safer. This lack of uniformity worldwide is set to be complicated by the advent of newer drugs. Suggamadex is a gamma cyclodextrin that directly binds aminosteroidal nondepolarizing muscle relaxants in the plasma. Suggamadex allows the rapid reversal

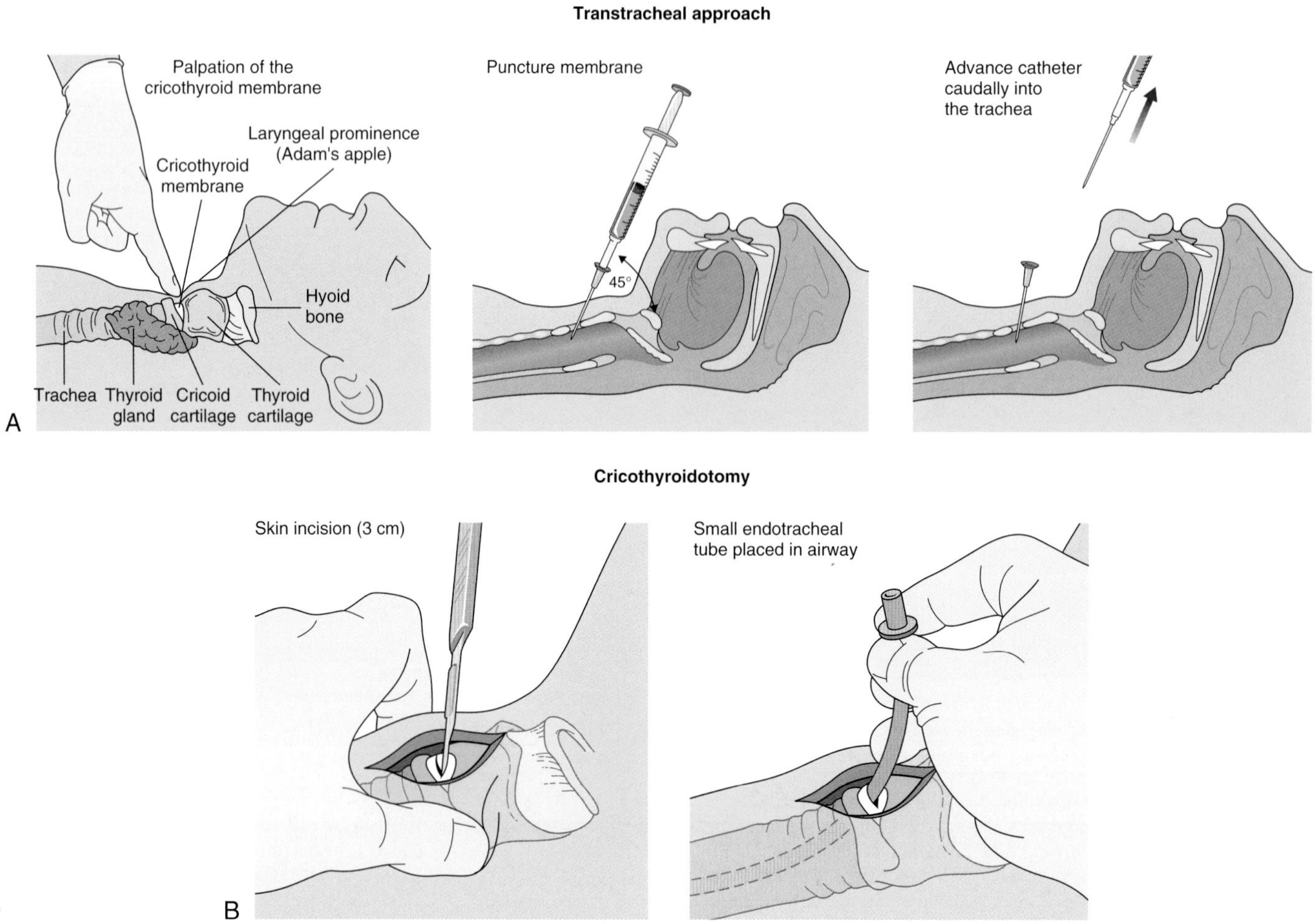

Transtracheal approach

Cricothyroidotomy

Figure 34-9 A, Transtracheal ventilation. The cricothyroid membrane is palpated below the laryngeal prominence of the thyroid cartilage. The membrane is punctured with a catheter while aspirating for air. The catheter is advanced caudally into the trachea after the needle is removed. The catheter is then attached to a high-pressure oxygen delivery system. Exhalation is passive, relying on a patent upper airway. **B,** To perform a cricothyroidotomy, a 3-cm vertical skin incision is made below the thyroid notch; then the cricothyroid membrane is incised with a scalpel blade and the opening dilated with use of the handle, and a small endotracheal tube is placed in the airway.   *(From Wiener-Kronish JP, Shimabukuro DW: Airway management. In Albert RK, Spiro SG, Jett JR, editors:* Clinical respiratory medicine, *ed 3, Philadelphia, 2008, Mosby.)*

of rocuronium-induced muscle relaxation and deep levels of blockade. This may make suxamethonium redundant in anesthesia, since it is used because of its rapid onset, and more important, rapid offset of effects. Suxamethonium also has a considerably worse side effect profile than does rocuronium.

Thiopental has been superseded in most countries by propofol as an induction agent, particularly because of its smoother postoperative profile. Thiopental is retained for rapid-sequence inductions by some operators, however, because of not only its rapid and predictable onset, with a definite end point, but also its rapid offset (generally 5 minutes)—a boon in failed intubation scenarios. In a classic rapid sequence induction, opioids should not be given before the trachea is intubated, mainly because of the increased time to return of spontaneous respiration, which may be dangerous with failure of intubation. Nevertheless, use of these agents is advocated in cases in which a large degree of cardiac stability is needed.

WEB RESOURCE

Difficult Airway Society guidelines for airway management: http://www.das.uk.com/guidelines

SUGGESTED READINGS

Aitkenhead AR, Smith G, Rowbotham DJ: *Textbook of anaesthesia,* ed 5, Edinburgh, 2007, Churchill Livingstone.

Al-Shaikh B, Stacey S, editors: *Essentials of anaesthetic equipment,* ed 3, Philadelphia, 2007, Churchill Livingstone.

Cook T, Woodall N, Frerk C; Fourth National Audit Project: *Major complications of airway management in the UK: results of the Fourth National Audit Project of the Royal College of Anaesthetists and the Difficult Airway Society,* London, 2011, Oxford University Press.

Lim MS, Hunt-Smith JJ: Difficult airway management in the intensive care unit: practical guidelines, *Crit Care Resusc* 5:8–9, 2003.

Savva D: Prediction of difficult tracheal intubation, *Br J Anaesth* 73:149–153, 1994.

Chapter **35**
Hemodynamic Monitoring in Critical Illness

Mark Lambert • Phil Bearfield

The cardiovascular system is subject to rapid and profound changes during critical illness. Tissue hypoperfusion and hypoxia constitute an important cause of organ dysfunction in critically ill patients. Such pathophysiologic changes often are encountered in the setting of shock states attributable to inadequate cardiac output. Therapeutic maneuvers aimed at raising cardiac output have the potential to increase oxygen delivery to the whole body, as can be described by the simplified oxygen flux equation:

$$\dot{D}O_2 = CO \times CaO_2$$

where $\dot{D}O_2$ is whole-body oxygen delivery, CO is cardiac output, and CaO_2 is arterial oxygen content. Increasingly, for the patient as a whole, flow is seen as a more important therapeutic target than pressure, although in certain organs, adequate perfusion pressure is known to be crucial (e.g., brain, heart, kidneys).

Monitoring of cardiovascular parameters allows clinicians to make informed decisions on how to optimize cardiac and circulatory function in order to maintain adequate tissue perfusion. Knowledge of the relevant anatomy and physiology is an essential prerequisite for correct interpretation of the data generated by any monitor.

CIRCULATION MODEL

The circulatory system can be modeled as a hydraulic circuit with a pulsatile pump representing the heart. Cardiac output is the product of heart rate and left ventricular stroke volume. Stroke volume is dependent on preload, left ventricular contractility and afterload. Despite increasingly sophisticated monitoring systems, obtaining accurate quantification of these variables at the bedside remains difficult.

In critical care units, cardiac output monitors are used to measure the hemodynamic impact of a therapeutic intervention. When such equipment is used in this manner, precise measurement rather than accurate measurement may be a more desirable property of any hemodynamic monitor (i.e., precise, reproducible measurement of the *change* in cardiac output is more useful than accurate but imprecise values).

MONITORING DEVICES

Central venous catheters, arterial catheters, and pulse oximeters are used routinely in the critical care setting. In addition, pulmonary arterial catheters, ultrasound-based cardiac output monitors, and devices that measure cardiac output by analysis of the morphology of the arterial pressure waveform also may be used. Despite advances in monitoring technology, significant complications are associated with their use, and to date, evidence for any consequent improvement in survival is lacking. This section addresses the indications, complications, and interpretation of data from the monitoring devices in common use.

ARTERIAL PRESSURE MONITORING

Systolic, mean, and diastolic systemic arterial pressures are routinely measured. Mean arterial pressure (MAP) is a function of cardiac output (CO) and systemic vascular resistance (SVR).

$$MAP = CO \times SVR$$

Because vascular tone and thus SVR are independently controlled, it is not possible to use mean arterial pressure values alone to make assumptions about cardiac output. An adequate systemic blood pressure does not equate to adequate cardiac output or adequate flow in discrete tissue beds.

The systemic arterial pulse wave is generated in the left ventricle and is transmitted through the arterial tree at 6 to 10 meters/second. It comprises an incident pressure wave (from the contraction of the left ventricle) and a reflected pressure wave (from the periphery). As the pulse wave advances through the vascular tree, the systolic pressure is seen to increase as a result of an increase in the magnitude of the reflected wave. Therefore, measured systolic arterial pressure varies depending on the site of measurement. Mean arterial pressure may be a more useful marker than systolic blood pressure, because its value is less dependent on site of measurement, is least altered by damping, and is more relevant in determination of blood flow to vital tissue beds such as the brain and kidneys.

Noninvasive Arterial Blood Pressure Monitoring

Noninvasive arterial blood pressure (NIBP) measurements in critical care most commonly are taken using an automated oscillometric device. This consists of a circumferential pneumatic cuff applied to the arm or leg. The cuff is inflated to a pressure above systolic arterial pressure, followed by controlled slow deflation of the cuff. As the cuff pressure falls below systolic arterial pressure, turbulent flow occurs in the artery beneath the cuff, causing oscillations in cuff pressure, which become maximal at MAP (**Figure 35-1**). Processing software allows determination of systolic, mean, and diastolic pressures in accordance with the amplitude of these oscillations.

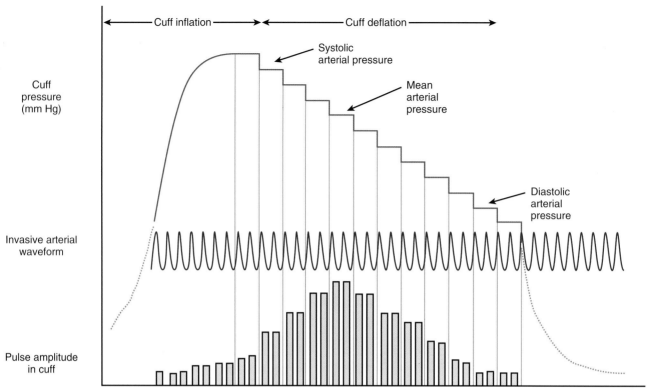

Figure 35-1 Oscillation in blood pressure cuff showing maximum amplitude of cuff oscillation corresponds with mean arterial pressure (MAP).

This technique allows frequent measurement of blood pressure and can be used when continuous monitoring of arterial pressure is not required. It also provides useful confirmation of the reliability of invasive arterial measurement. Measurements in the normotensive range are considered to be accurate but tend to underestimate hypertensive values and overestimate hypotensive values. Measured values are less accurate in the presence of arrhythmia and with incorrect cuff sizing. Cuff width should be 20% greater than arm diameter, with use of a narrow cuff associated with a tendency toward erroneously high values.

Relative contraindications to cuff use include severe peripheral vascular disease, arteriovenous fistulas, local absence of lymph nodes consequent to resection, and local skin or muscle damage.

Complications are rare, but obtaining repeated measurements over short periods may lead to local skin ulceration or bruising. Injury to the ulnar nerve also has been reported.

Invasive Arterial Pressure Monitoring

Under conditions of hemodynamic instability or during therapeutic manipulation of the cardiovascular system, intermittent monitoring of blood pressure provides insufficient clinical information. An indwelling arterial catheter allows direct and continuous measurement of arterial blood pressure, as well as graphical display of the arterial waveform. Arterial blood sampling from the catheter also can be performed, allowing information to be obtained about metabolic status and respiratory function.

The radial, brachial, axillary, femoral, and dorsalis pedis arteries can be used for cannulation, with the radial artery most commonly used. Use of a 20-gauge cannula is recommended to reduce the incidence of vessel occlusion; a cannula of this size also has the most favorable physical properties for accurate pressure measurement. Insertion is performed under conditions

Box 35-1	Complications of Arterial Cannulation

Thrombosis
Embolization (proximal or distal)
Infection (local or systemic)
Hemorrhage (disconnection)
Damage to adjacent structures (nerves, arteriovenous fistula, false aneurysm)
Inadvertent drug administration

of strict asepsis using either direct cannulation or a modified Seldinger technique. Distal perfusion should be periodically assessed after cannulation to ensure that arterial occlusion has not occurred.

The arterial cannula is connected by a continuous column of saline to a pressure transducer which takes atmospheric pressure at the level of the right atrium as its zero reference point. The system is continuously flushed from a pressurized saline source at a rate of 2 to 3 mL/hour to prevent aggregation of thrombus and subsequent occlusion of the cannula. Modifications to the transducer system and maneuvers promoting formation of clots or air bubbles should be avoided, because these can cause loss of energy from the system and "damping" of the measured signal.

Complications of arterial cannulation are listed in **Box 35-1**.

CENTRAL VENOUS CATHETERIZATION

Central venous catheters allow measurement of central venous pressure (CVP) and provide vascular access for blood sampling and administration of vasoactive drugs or parenteral nutrition. Common sites for catheterization include the internal jugular vein, subclavian vein, and femoral vein, although the brachial and cephalic veins also may be used. The chosen site will depend on the patient's anatomy and clinical condition and on the experience of the operator. Two dimensional (2D) ultrasound imaging is readily available in many units and can be used in conjunction with Doppler color flow studies to define the venous anatomy before the procedure. Ultrasound imaging also may be used during the procedure to provide real-time guidance. The U.K. National Institute for Health and Clinical Excellence recommends the use of 2D ultrasound guidance for central venous cannulation. Correct catheter placement is indicated by the characteristic central venous pressure waveform and the radiographic appearance of the line tip positioned at the level of the carina on a plain chest radiograph.

CVP is measured continuously via a pressure transducer, and the CVP waveform may be displayed graphically. The availability and falling cost of disposable transducers have rendered intermittent manometry measurements obsolete. In health, CVP correlates with right ventricular end-diastolic pressure and pulmonary artery occlusion pressure (PAOP). It can therefore be used as an indicator of preload. In critical illness, the normal relationship between right- and left-sided heart pressures may not be maintained. This discrepancy may be the result of many factors, including changes in ventricular compliance, pulmonary hypertension, or pulmonary embolism. Isolated measurements of CVP are poor markers of intravascular volume status; however, dynamic measurements may still be useful. A sustained rise in CVP after a fluid challenge implies that a further increase in preload may not provide an increase in cardiac output.

The complications of central venous cannulation are listed in **Box 35-2**. Despite advances in catheter technology such as antimicrobial coating, risk for microbial contamination is significant. The corresponding risk of catheter-related sepsis may be mitigated by minimizing the time during which the catheter remains in situ. The benefits of changing the catheter must be weighed against the risks associated with catheter reinsertion (**Box 35-3**).

PULMONARY ARTERY CATHETERIZATION

The pulmonary artery flotation catheter (PAFC) is a multilumen central venous catheter that is guided by flow to rest in the pulmonary artery (**Figure 35-2**). It allows measurement and derivation of a wide variety of hemodynamic variables, which are listed in **Box 35-4**. Indications for its use include the following:

- Determination of the cause of hemodynamic insufficiency
- Discrimination between cardiogenic and noncardiogenic pulmonary edema

---

Box 35-2 Complications of Central Venous Catheter Insertion

Arterial puncture
Arrhythmia
Infection
Hemorrhage
Pneumothorax
Hemothorax
Chylothorax
Air embolism
Venous thrombosis
Loss of guidewire
Nerve injury

Box 35-3 Indications for Central Venous Catheter Exchange

Cellulitis
Pus observed at the insertion site
Suspected catheter-related sepsis in the hemodynamically unstable patient
High clinical suspicion for catheter-related infection
Positive fungal blood cultures
Emergency insertion under conditions in which aseptic technique not ensured

---

Box 35-4 Data Obtained with the Pulmonary Artery Flotation Catheter

Measured
Pressures (right atrial, right ventricular, pulmonary artery, pulmonary occlusion pressures)
Cardiac output
Mixed venous oxygen saturation, core temperature

Derived
Systemic vascular resistance
Pulmonary vascular resistance
RV and LV stroke work index
Mean PAP, MRVP
LV and RV coronary perfusion pressure
Cardiac index
Stroke volume index
SVRi, PVRi

LV, left ventricular; *MRVP*, mean right ventricular pressure; *PAP*, pulmonary artery pressure; *PVRi*, peripheral vascular resistance index; *RV*, right ventricular; *SVRi*, systemic vascular resistance index.

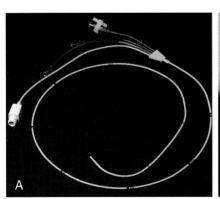
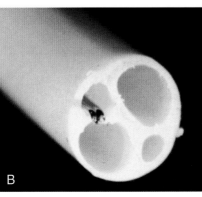

Figure 35-2 Pulmonary artery flotation catheter. **A,** Red channel for balloon inflation; blue channel to proximal port (for right atrial pressure and injectate); yellow channel to distal port (for measurement of pulmonary artery pressure and pulmonary capillary wedge pressure); bright yellow thermistor connection. **B,** Cross section of pulmonary artery catheter. *Clockwise from left:* thermistor wire, distal port channel, balloon channel, proximal port channel.

- Measurement of cardiac output and pulmonary artery pressures (for example, in pulmonary hypertension or hepatopulmonary syndrome)
- Guidance in use of inotrope, vasopressor, or vasodilator therapy in critical illness or after major surgery

Use of the PAFC has declined in recent years owing to concerns over the potential for complications. Recent systematic analysis suggests that the use of the PAFC is associated with neither improved survival nor increased mortality, although some data support a reduction in mortality associated with PAFC use in the most critically ill patients. Further studies are required to precisely define a role for the PAFC in modern critical care; in some centers, its use continues as a monitoring tool in critical illness and during major surgery.

INSERTION

An introducer sheath is placed using a Seldinger technique into a central vein; the internal jugular and subclavian veins are most commonly used. The lumens and balloon of the PAFC should be tested before insertion. The PAFC is passed through the sheath into the right atrium with continuous pressure waveform monitoring from the distal lumen. Once in the right atrium, the balloon is inflated with 1.5 mL of air. This adjustment helps to guide the balloon along the direction of blood flow through the heart and also affords some protection to the myocardium. With careful advancement of the catheter, characteristic pressure waveforms of the right ventricle, pulmonary artery, and pulmonary artery occlusion are sequentially encountered. The waveforms observed during passage of the catheter are shown in **Figure 35-3**.

MEASURING PULMONARY ARTERY OCCLUSION PRESSURE

Accurate measurement of PAOP requires readings to be taken at end expiration and end diastole. Inflation of the balloon at the tip of the PAFC effectively "wedges" the catheter tip in a branch of the pulmonary artery. This creates a continuous column of blood from the catheter tip to the pulmonary venous system. As a consequence of its proximity to the left atrium, the pressures observed can be considered to correlate with left atrial pressure. Left atrial pressure approximates to left ventricular end-diastolic pressure (LVEDP) and therefore may be considered to represent an index of preload. Many factors, including changes in intrathoracic and intraabdominal pressures, catheter position outside West zone 3, mitral valve disease, and changes in left ventricular compliance, may impair the usefulness of PAOP as a predictor of preload (**Table 35-1**).

MEASURING CARDIAC OUTPUT USING THE PULMONARY ARTERY FLOTATION CATHETER

Adding a sensitive thermistor to the PAFC allows calculation of cardiac output by modification of the Stewart-Hamilton equation:

$$M = Q \int Ct \cdot dt$$

Rapid bolus injection of cold fluid into the right atrium causes a change in temperature of the blood in the pulmonary artery, which varies with time (Ct). Because all of the cold fluid (M) must pass through the pulmonary artery, M is equal to the sum of the temperature changes at each interval (t) multiplied by the flow (Q). Rearranging this equation allows calculation of flow (i.e., cardiac output) through the pulmonary artery.

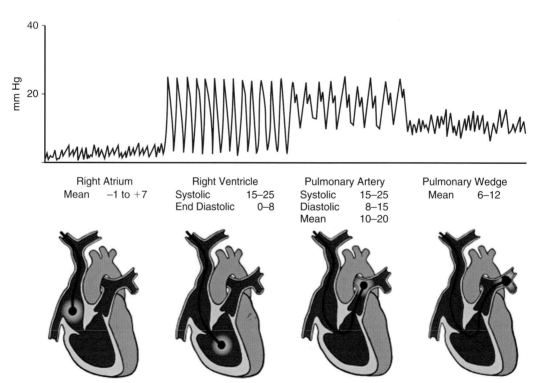

Right Atrium		
Mean	−1 to +7	

Right Ventricle		
Systolic	15–25	
End Diastolic	0–8	

Pulmonary Artery		
Systolic	15–25	
Diastolic	8–15	
Mean	10–20	

Pulmonary Wedge		
Mean	6–12	

Figure 35-3 The changing pressure waveform observed with insertion of pulmonary artery flotation catheter. *(From Gabbe SG, Niebyl JR, Simpson JL, editors: Obstetrics: normal and problem pregnancies, ed 5, Philadelphia, Churchill Livingstone, 2007.)*

Table 35-1 Complications of Pulmonary Artery Flotation Catheter (PAFC) Insertion

Complication	Risk Factor	Prevention
Arrhythmia	Catheter coiling in RV Catheter reentry from PA to RV	Ensure balloon inflation during passage from RA to PA Defibrillator/transcutaneous pacing available Minimize insertion time
Complete heart block	LBBB	Avoid insertion in patients with LBBB Consider pacing electrode placement
Catheter knotting	Dilated RV, excessive catheter length	Monitor pressure waveform during insertion; withdraw catheter if no change after advancing 15 cm Avoid forceful insertion
Valve damage	Knotting of catheter around papillary muscle, balloon inflation during withdrawal	Inflate balloon during forward passage and ensure balloon deflation during catheter withdrawal
Pulmonary infarction	Prolonged balloon occlusion, distal catheter migration, pulmonary hypertension, anticoagulation, prolonged duration of insertion	Minimize wedge procedures, <15-second balloon inflation during PAOP measurements Withdraw catheter if spontaneous wedging or wedging achieved with <1.25 mL of air
Pulmonary artery rupture	As for pulmonary infarction	As for pulmonary infarction
Air embolism	Balloon rupture	Avoid repeat attempts to inflate balloon
Infection	Prolonged insertion	Aseptic insertion Remove PAFC when no longer required

LBBB, left bundle branch block; *PA*, pulmonary artery; *PAOP*, pulmonary artery occlusion pressure; *RA*, right atrium; *RV*, right ventricle.

$$Q = \frac{V \cdot (Tb - Ti) \cdot K1 \cdot K2}{Tb(t)dt}$$

where Q is cardiac output, V is volume injected, Tb is blood temperature, Ti is temperature of the injectate, K_1 and K_2 are constants relating to the specific heat capacity of injectate and equipment dead space volumes, and Tb(t)dt is the change in blood temperature as a function of time.

The decrease in temperature in the pulmonary artery can be plotted against time, as shown in **Figure 35-4**. As the foregoing equation indicates, cardiac output is inversely proportional to the area under this curve

Bolus thermodilution measurements of cardiac output are repeated three times and a mean value is calculated (**Box 35-5** and **Table 35-2**). Using a thermal indicator has several advantages over dye dilution techniques in that the indicator is nontoxic and does not accumulate or recirculate. Cold fluid does, however, cause a transient fall in heart rate, thus reducing cardiac output over the period measured.

In some PAFC designs, a thermal filament wrapped around the PAFC allows semicontinuous measurement of cardiac output. The filament heats the blood in a pulsatile fashion, and the resultant fluctuations in temperature are detected at a downstream thermistor. Comparison of the filament heating time and thermistor output allows calculation of cardiac output. This has been shown to be comparable in accuracy to bolus thermodilution methods and may avoid some of the human error associated with bolus injection of cold fluid.

ARTERIAL WAVEFORM ANALYSIS

PULSE CONTOUR ANALYSIS

If SVR and the mean arterial blood pressure are known, it is possible to calculate the cardiac output:

Table 35-2 Archetypical Hemodynamic Abnormalities in Variables Measured by Pulmonary Artery Flotation Catheter

Circulatory Condition	Hemodynamic Variable		
	CI	PAOP	SVRi
Hypovolemic shock	Low	Low	High
Cardiogenic shock	Low	High	High
Distributive shock (sepsis, anaphylaxis)	High	Normal	Low
Obstructive shock (pulmonary embolism, tension pneumothorax, tamponade)	Low	High	High

CI, cardiac index; *PAOP*, pulmonary artery occlusion pressure; *SVRi*, systemic vascular resistance index.

Box 35-5 Causes of Inaccurate Bolus Thermodilution Cardiac Output Measurement

Malposition
Respiratory pattern
Cardiac shunt
Tricuspid valve regurgitation
Arrhythmia
Injectate temperature misrecorded
Rapid intravenous infusions
Injectate port in introducer sheath
Extremes of cardiac output
Slow injection
Incorrect injectate volume

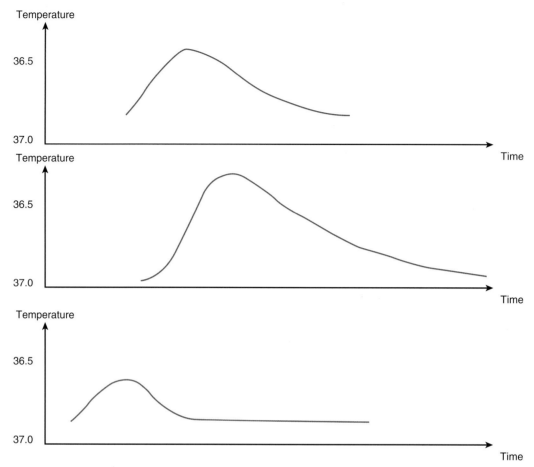

Figure 35-4 Thermodilution curves in normal and low- and high–cardiac output states (*top* to *bottom*, respectively): Changes in the thermodilution waveform with changes in cardiac output. The area under the curve is inversely proportional to cardiac output.

$$CO = \frac{MAP}{SVR} \cdot k$$

Analysis of various components of the arterial waveform, including pulse wave velocity, pulse pressure, and diastolic pressure decay, permits estimation of the SVR. These principles have been understood for more than a century and refined with increasing sophistication over the last few decades. The complexity of the necessary mathematical algorithms, however, has meant that their development into clinically useful bedside instruments has been possible only with the advent of the microprocessor. Modern understanding of the arterial waveform is in terms of two superimposed waves: an incident wave related to left ventricular ejection and another wave reflected back from the peripheral arterial tree. The characteristics of the resultant waveform change with stroke volume, arterial compliance, site of measurement, and the physiologic state of the subject. Furthermore, the impedance of the aorta (its tendency to oppose *pulsatile* arterial flow) changes not only with arterial compliance but also with cardiac output. As a result of all of these factors, devices in current clinical practice use different proprietary algorithms, require periodic calibration for accurate use, and may be used without calibration to estimate the effect of interventions on hemodynamic variables.

PULSE POWER ANALYSIS

The law of conservation of mass and energy can be applied to the problem of estimating stroke volume from analysis of the arterial waveform. This method is based on the assumption that with every left ventricular ejection, the power change is related to the balance between the mass of blood entering (stroke volume) and the mass of blood leaving the aorta (dissipating to the periphery). Assuming also that power is a function of flow, the change in blood pressure over the course of each arterial pulse wave can be used to determine stroke volume. The constant of proportionality describing this relationship changes with blood pressure, and the mathematical technique has been termed *autocorrelation*.

$$\frac{\Delta V}{\Delta BP} = calibration \times 250 \times e^{-k \cdot BP}$$

Potential advantages of this technology over pulse contour analysis include a reduction in the tendency of damping to affect accuracy and the facility to use any anatomic site for waveform analysis.

Devices using pulse contour and pulse power analysis can be used to demonstrate beat-to-beat changes in stroke volume and pulse pressure. Stroke volume variation (SVV) and pulse pressure variation (PPV) are features of the cyclic change in venous return to the heart during the respiratory cycle. The application of positive pressure to the thorax during mechanical ventilation effectively splints the right ventricle, exaggerating this tendency to variation in left ventricular ejection. High SVV and PPV have been shown to be useful predictors of fluid responsiveness in fully ventilated patients.

TRANSPULMONARY INDICATOR DILUTION

Calibration of arterial waveform analysis systems relies on indicator dilution techniques and application of the Stewart-Hamilton equation. The indicators are administered into a vein and detected at a systemic arterial catheter after passing through the four heart chambers and the pulmonary circulation. Further analysis can be performed on the indicator dilution curves to provide information on additional cardiovascular indices, such as intrathoracic blood volumes and extravascular lung water.

Transpulmonary Thermodilution With Arterial Waveform Analysis

The technique of transpulmonary thermodilution with arterial waveform analysis uses a central venous bolus of cold injectate with the change in blood temperature detected at a thermistor in the femoral, axillary, or brachial artery. A temperature change–versus–time curve is constructed from which cardiac output can be calculated using the Stewart-Hamilton equation. The thermodilution curves are longer and flatter than those seen for the PAFC, which reflects their thermal equilibrium with a larger blood volume. Further analysis of the morphology of a semilogarithmic transformation of the thermodilution waveform allows calculation of intrathoracic thermal volume (ITTV) and pulmonary thermal volume (PTV). A marker of cardiac preload, the global end-diastolic volume (GEDV), is calculated from the difference between ITTV and PTV. This technique also allows calculation of the extravascular lung water, which provides information on the degree of pulmonary edema and is a correlate of the severity of illness (**Box 35-6**). Cardiac output calculations from the thermodilution curve are used to calibrate continuous cardiac output monitoring by pulse contour analysis (**Figure 35-5**).

Because a thermistor is necessary for calibration, a special-purpose arterial catheter is required. The cold injectate must also be administered via a central vein, necessitating central venous access.

Transpulmonary Lithium Indicator Dilution and Arterial Waveform Analysis

The technique of transpulmonary lithium indicator dilution and arterial waveform analysis gives continuous cardiac output monitoring through pulse power analysis of the arterial waveform with calibration performed using indicator dilution with lithium. A bolus of lithium is injected intravenously and detected at an external lithium ion–sensitive electrode connected to the arterial cannula. A plasma lithium concentration–versus–time curve is obtained from which cardiac output can be derived using the Stewart-Hamilton method. Because the lithium electrode is external, blood is continuously sampled during the calibration process from a standard arterial line. Of note, plasma sodium also affects the potential across the electrode, so a correction must be made. Lithium distributes only in the plasma compartment; thus, a correction for hematocrit also must be made.

Calibration is performed every 24 hours but may be required more frequently if significant changes in arterial compliance are suspected or the waveform becomes damped. Some models also include a decision-making algorithm to guide fluid administration or therapeutic maneuvers.

These devices can be used in the presence of a "standard" radial arterial catheter, and the lithium bolus can be administered either centrally or peripherally. Ongoing lithium therapy and use of nondepolarizing muscle relaxants can cause errors in calibration. Blood sampled during calibration also must be discarded owing to measurement at an external electrode.

ESOPHAGEAL DOPPLER MONITORING AND ULTRASOUND IMAGING

The Doppler effect refers to the change in observed frequency of a wave function when the source is moving relative to the

---

Box 35-6 | **Hemodynamic Indices Determined With Use of Transpulmonary Thermodilution Techniques**

Cardiac output
Systemic vascular resistance
Pulmonary vascular resistance
Intrathoracic blood volume
Global end-diastolic volume
Extravascular lung water
Stroke volume variation
Global ejection fraction

Sources of Error
■ Intracardiac shunts
■ Large abdominal aortic aneurysm
■ Pulmonary embolism
■ Acute volume change in compartments

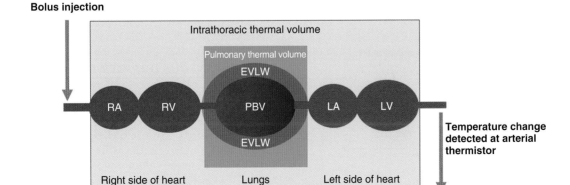

Figure 35-5 Intrathoracic compartments in transpulmonary thermodilution. *EVLW*, extravascular lung water; *LA*, left atrium; *LV*, left ventricle; *PBV*, pulmonary blood volume; *RA*, right atrium; *RV*, right ventricle. The intrathoracic thermal volume is the volume between points of injection and detection. The pulmonary thermal volume is PBV + EVLW. *(Courtesy Pulsion Medical Systems AG, Munich, Germany.)*

observer. The magnitude of this effect is proportional to the velocity of the moving object. Applying this principle to ultrasound waves allows measurement of velocity of red blood cells in the descending thoracic aorta using the following equation:

$$v = \frac{c \cdot f_D}{2 \cdot f_T \cdot \cos\theta}$$

where v is the velocity of red blood cells, c is the speed of ultrasound waves through body tissues, f_D is the observed frequency shift of the reflected ultrasound waves, f_T is the transmitted frequency of the ultrasound wave, and $\cos\theta$ is the cosine of the angle of insonation between the axis of the sound beam and the direction of blood flow.

A flexible probe containing an ultrasound transceiver is passed into the lower esophagus, where the thoracic aorta and the esophagus are closely apposed. Ultrasound waves are emitted from the probe, which is focused on the aorta by the operator, with the probe positioned to obtain the maximum peak velocity. The change in observed frequency of the reflected ultrasound waves from the red blood cells allows calculation of blood velocity in the descending aorta. The spectrum of red cell velocities is plotted against time and displayed as shown in **Figure 35-6**. The esophageal Doppler monitor traces the maximum velocity waveform to permit calculating the area under this curve during systole. This area is the *stroke distance*, or the distance over which a column of blood moves in the aorta during systole. Aortic red blood cell velocity is measured in the descending thoracic aorta distal to the origin of the left subclavian artery. To estimate left ventricular stroke volume from this measurement, two factors must be known or otherwise accounted for: First, the cross-sectional area of the aorta is required for stroke distance to be converted into volume, and probes have been developed with an M-mode echocardiographic transducer to facilitate this step. Second, a proportion of the cardiac output has left the aorta proximal to the transducer; in a resting healthy adult, this is approximately 30% and must be compensated for. One manufacturer (Cardio-Q ODM, Deltex Medical, Chichester, United Kingdom) uses a nomogram based on the patient's age, height, and weight to directly calibrate descending aorta blood flow velocity to total cardiac output. The process is based on in vivo measurements from an esophageal Doppler monitor and a thermodilution pulmonary artery catheter in an ICU patient population and removes the need to separately account for the fraction of cardiac output distributed into the upper body.

The width of the base of the velocity waveform represents the systolic ejection time and is displayed as the corrected flow time (FTc). The flow time is corrected to a heart rate of 60 beats/minute to allow comparison of flow times despite the increasing ratio of systolic time to diastolic time at increased heart rates. Variation in FTc may reflect changes in preload and afterload. A low FTc may reflect hypovolemia as ventricular ejection is short with a low left ventricular end-diastolic volume (LVEDV). Changes in SVR (afterload) also will alter the FTc, because they determine the resistance to flow in the arterial system. FTc is inversely correlated with SVR. The peak velocity and mean acceleration of the velocity waveform may provide information regarding the contractile state of the myocardium.

The esophageal Doppler monitor can be used to assess fluid responsiveness by detecting changes in stroke volume after administration of a fluid bolus. After the fluid challenge, a change in stroke volume of greater than 10% suggests that further fluid boluses may result in additional increases in stroke volume—the implication being that the ventricle lies on the steep part of its Starling curve.

The Doppler probes are small, minimally invasive, easy to insert, and allow rapid acquisition of data. Operation of the device can be learned quickly. Contraindications to probe insertion include esophageal pathology (e.g., varices) and facial trauma. Abnormalities of aortic and esophageal anatomy may inhibit probe focusing, limiting the usefulness of the device. The esophageal Doppler monitor cannot be used in the presence of aortic balloon counterpulsation.

In calculation of cardiac output, the esophageal Doppler monitor relies on several assumptions that may not hold true in critical illness. Only flow in the descending aorta is measured (approximately 70% of cardiac output), and a correction is applied to allow calculation of stroke volume. Changes in the regional distribution of the circulation that occur in critical illness may limit the accuracy of the calculated values. Turbulent flow (as associated with anemia or hyperdynamic circulation) in the aorta may alter velocity measurement, leading to inaccurate results. Some nomograms assume a constant and circular aortic area, whereas changes in descending aortic diameter have been shown in patients with hypotension. The esophagus and the aorta may not run parallel, leading to deviation from the assumed angle of insonation of 45 degrees. Probe position can easily be lost, making consistent trend measurements difficult. Nasal and oral probes are available; however, the probe may be uncomfortable for nonsedated patients, which can limit its use. Nevertheless, when used appropriately to assess the immediate impact of a therapeutic intervention, the esophageal Doppler monitor is a precise and safe device that is relatively easy to use.

TRANSCUTANEOUS DOPPLER MONITORING

Using principles similar to those for the esophageal Doppler monitor, blood velocity in the ascending aorta can be calculated from data obtained with an ultrasound probe positioned in the suprasternal notch. With knowledge of the area of the aortic outflow tract, the flow in the ascending aorta can be calculated, thus allowing stroke volume and cardiac output to be measured. This method is noninvasive and allows measurements to be taken at the aortic root, which are therefore not affected by alterations distribution of cardiac output between the upper and lower body. Its use is limited by difficulties in identifying the aortic root, maintaining alignment of the ultrasound probe

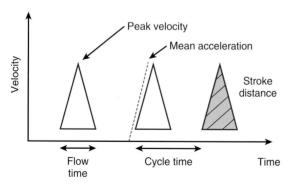

Figure 35-6 Schematic of the esophageal Doppler waveform showing stroke distance, mean acceleration, peak velocity, and flow time. *(From Parrillo JE, Dellinger P, et al, editors: Critical care medicine, ed 3, Philadelphia, Mosby, 2007.)*

with the ascending aorta, and discomfort in nonsedated patients. These limitations predispose the system to a high degree of interobserver variability, so it is infrequently used as a monitoring tool in critical care.

ECHOCARDIOGRAPHY

Both transthoracic and transesophageal echocardiography techniques can be used to measure end-diastolic and end-systolic ventricular volumes for calculating left ventricular stroke volume. The use of these modalities for hemodynamic monitoring is limited by availability of equipment and trained operators. Because measurements can be made only intermittently, these techniques are not used for routine critical care monitoring.

SUGGESTED READINGS

Bland JM, Altman DG: Statistical methods for assessing agreement between two methods of clinical measurement, *Lancet* 1:307–310, 1986.

Connors AF Jr, Speroff T, Dawson NV, et al: The effectiveness of right heart catheterisation in the initial care of critically ill patients. SUPPORT Investigators, *JAMA* 276:889–897, 1996.

Dellinger RP, Levy MM, Carlet JM, et al: Surviving Sepsis Campaign: International guidelines for management of severe sepsis and septic shock 2008, *Crit Care Med* 36:296–327, 2008.

Erlanger J, Hooker DR: An experimental study of blood-pressure and of pulse-pressure in man, *Bull Johns Hopkins Hosp* 12:145–378, 1904.

Gattinoni L, Brazzi L, Pelosi P, et al: A trial of goal-oriented hemodynamic therapy in critically ill patients, *N Engl J Med* 333:1025–1032, 1995.

Harvey S, Harrison DA, Singer M, et al: Assessment of the clinical effectiveness of pulmonary artery catheters in management of patients in intensive care (PAC-Man): a randomised controlled trial, *Lancet* 366:472–477, 2005.

Morris CG, Pearse RM: Pro-con debate: we should not measure cardiac output in critical care, *JICS* 10:10–12, 2009.

Mythen MG, Webb AR: Perioperative plasma volume expansion reduces the incidence of gut mucosal hypoperfusion during cardiac surgery, *Arch Surg* 30:423–429, 1995.

Pearse RM, Ikram K, Barry J: Equipment review: an appraisal of the LiDCO plus method of measuring cardiac output, *Crit Care* 8:190–195, 2004.

Remington JW, Noback CR, Hamilton WF, Gold JJ: Volume elasticity characteristics of the human aorta and prediction of the stroke volume from the pressure pulse, *Am J Physiol* 153:298–308, 1948.

Pearse R, Dawson D, Fawcett J, et al: Early goal-directed therapy after major surgery reduces complications and duration of hospital stay. A randomised, controlled trial, *Crit Care* 9:687–693, 2005.

Singer M, Clarke J, Bennett ED: Continuous hemodynamic monitoring by esophageal Doppler, *Crit Care Med* 17:447–452, 1989.

Swan HJ, Ganz W, Forrester J, et al: Catheterisation of the heart in man with use of a flow-directed balloon-tipped catheter, *N Engl J Med* 283:447–451, 1970.

Chapter **36**
Acute Respiratory Distress Syndrome

Jesús Villar • Demet S. Sulemanji • Robert M. Kacmarek

The acute respiratory distress syndrome (ARDS) is an inflammatory disease process of the lungs that is a response to both direct and indirect insults, characterized clinically by severe hypoxemia, reduced lung compliance, and bilateral radiographic infiltrates. Although much has evolved in the current understanding of its pathogenesis and factors affecting patient outcome, there is still no specific treatment for ARDS.

In 1967, Ashbaugh and colleagues published an article in *The Lancet* in which they described for the first time a clinical syndrome that they termed the "adult respiratory distress syndrome" for its similarity to the well-recognized infant respiratory distress syndrome. From a cohort of 272 patients who were receiving respiratory support, these investigators identified 12 patients with a constellation of specific pulmonary findings: The respiratory distress in these patients was defined as sudden and catastrophic and often associated with a multiorgan system insult that led to tachypnea, hypoxemia, decreased lung compliance, and bilateral pulmonary infiltrates on the chest radiograph, in the absence of cardiogenic pulmonary edema. In this study, respiratory support consisted of oxygen therapy delivered by nasal prongs or face mask and mechanical ventilation. The mortality rate was 58%, and on histopathologic examination, the lungs of the nonsurvivors were heavier than normal and exhibited atelectasis with interstitial and alveolar edema and hyaline membranes. Since that time, the hallmarks of this syndrome, now known as ARDS, have been recognized to consist of (1) a risk factor for the development of acute respiratory distress (e.g., sepsis, trauma, pneumonia, aspiration, pancreatitis), (2) severe hypoxemia despite a relatively high fraction of inspired oxygen (FIO_2), (3) decreased lung compliance, (4) bilateral pulmonary infiltrates, and (5) lack of clinical evidence of cardiogenic pulmonary edema. Acute lung injury (ALI) resulting in ARDS also can occur in the setting of left ventricular failure, but this is very difficult to diagnose without careful serial measurements of pulmonary artery and capillary (wedge) pressure. Although ALI/ARDS had been recognized for more than a century and was referenced in published data from the Second World War, it was not until the landmark paper by Ashbaugh's group that broad clinical interest in ARDS began to emerge. In the subsequent years, very few acronyms have received as much attention in critical care medicine.

ARDS usually occurs in previously healthy people. Characteristically, there is a latent period between the insult and the development of the full-blown clinical syndrome, which usually is 18 to 24 hours in duration. After this interval, tachypnea, labored breathing, and cyanosis are observed, and arterial blood gas analysis confirms hypoxemia. The abnormalities in lung mechanics and oxygenation are assessed once the patient is intubated and receiving mechanical ventilation. The chest radiograph classically shows diffuse, bilateral, interstitial alveolar infiltrates (**Figure 36-1**). Resolution of the infiltrates, if it occurs at all, is much slower than with cardiogenic pulmonary edema.

PATHOPHYSIOLOGY, HISTOPATHOLOGY, AND ETIOLOGY

ARDS is caused by an insult to the alveolar-capillary membrane that results in increased permeability and subsequent interstitial and alveolar edema. The mechanisms whereby a wide variety of insults can lead to this syndrome are not clear. ALI includes injury to both the pulmonary capillary endothelium and the alveolar epithelium. In the ARDS lung, an influx of protein-rich edema fluid into the air spaces occurs as a consequence of increased permeability of the alveolar-capillary barrier. The degree of alveolar epithelial injury is an important determinant and predictor of outcome. The normal alveolar epithelium has two types of cells. The type I cells make up 90% of the alveolar surface area and are easily injured. The type II cells make up the remaining 10% of the alveolar surface area and are more resistant to injury; their functions include surfactant production, ion transport, and proliferation and differentiation to type I cells after injury.

The loss of epithelial integrity in ARDS has several consequences. First, under normal conditions, the epithelial barrier is much less permeable than the endothelial barrier; thus epithelial injury can contribute to alveolar flooding. Second, the loss of epithelial integrity and injury to type II cells serve to disrupt normal epithelial fluid transport, impairing the removal of edema fluid from the alveolar space. Third, injury to type II cells reduces the production and turnover of surfactant. Fourth, loss of epithelial barrier can lead to sepsis in patients with bacterial pneumonia. Finally, in severe alveolar epithelium injury, pulmonary fibrosis can develop. Independent of the clinical disorders associated with ARDS (**Box 36-1**), it is useful to think of the pathogenesis of ARDS as a result of two different pathways: a direct insult to lung cells and an indirect insult occurring as a result of an acute systemic inflammatory response. The host's inflammatory response to the initial direct (pulmonary) or indirect (nonpulmonary) insult is a key factor in determining the development and progression of the acute injury to the lung. Despite ongoing elucidation of the role of cellular and humoral components of the inflammatory responses in the lung, the precise sequence of events leading to lung damage is still unknown. As with any form of inflammation, ALI during ARDS represents a complex process in which multiple cellular signaling pathways can propagate or inhibit damage to the lung.

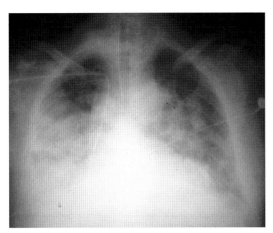

Figure 36-1 Chest radiograph showing diffuse, bilateral, interstitial, and alveolar infiltrates in a patient with acute respiratory distress syndrome (ARDS). The patient, a 54-year-old man, developed ARDS as a result of a severe bacterial pneumonia and required intubation and mechanical ventilation. His initial PaO_2/FIO_2 ratio was 113 mm Hg while he was receiving $FIO_2 = .6$ on PEEP of 10 cm H_2O. *PEEP*, positive end-expiratory pressure.

Box 36-1 | **Most Common Clinical Disorders Associated with Development of Acute Respiratory Distress Syndrome (ARDS)**

Direct Lung Injury
Common Causes
- Pneumonia
- Aspiration of gastric contents

Less Common Causes
- Pulmonary contusion
- Near-drowning
- Inhalational injury
- Fat emboli
- Reperfusion pulmonary edema

Indirect Lung Injury
Common Causes
- Sepsis
- Multiple trauma

Less Common Causes
- Acute pancreatitis
- Drug overdose
- Cardiopulmonary bypass
- Transfusions of blood products

The typical histopathologic features of ARDS are collectively known as *diffuse alveolar damage*. The early phase of ALI—the exudative phase—is characterized by leakage of protein-rich edema fluid into the lung and inflammatory cellular alveolar infiltrates. During this phase, a cytokine storm and an array of inflammatory mediators are released into the interstitium and alveolar space, perpetuating inflammation and promoting the development of atelectasis and structural damage to the lung architecture. In addition, damage to the alveolar-capillary barrier enhances the difficulty in removing the excess of extravascular lung fluid. An important source of these inflammatory mediators is neutrophils, which play a key role in the pathogenesis and progression of ALI. Human and animal studies have demonstrated migration and activation of neutrophils in the lungs, where they cause cell damage through the production of free radicals, inflammatory cytokines, and proteases. It is well accepted, however, that a single mediator does not predominate, and that several parallel and simultaneously interacting mechanisms may be involved. Clinically, this initial phase is manifested as marked hypoxemia and reduced lung compliance. Eventually, these changes evolve to a fibroproliferative phase in which capillary thrombosis, lung fibrosis, and neovascularization take place. Most nonsurvivors of ARDS die during this phase, despite aggressive ventilatory support with high inspiratory concentrations of oxygen and positive end-expiratory pressure (PEEP). However, only a small proportion of patients with ARDS die of hypoxemia. Rather, lung injury appears to predispose patients to the development of a systemic inflammatory response that culminates in multiple system organ dysfunction. A plethora of evidence suggests that the development of multiple extrapulmonary organ dysfunction is due to alveolar epithelial-endothelial barrier disruption and the migration of cytokines produced in the lungs into the systemic circulation.

More than 50 specific conditions associated with the development of this syndrome are recognized. The risk for development of ARDS depends on the predisposing clinical condition (i.e., some events are more likely than others to progress to ARDS) but also increases with the number of predisposing factors. Sepsis, bacterial pneumonia, multiple trauma, and aspiration pneumonia are the most common predisposing factors, accounting all together for more than 70% of cases; infection is the most frequent cause. Many invading organisms can trigger host innate and acquired immune systems to initiate the inflammatory cascade. The risk for development of ARDS also depends on patient characteristics. For example, alcoholism is a predisposing factor, and new data suggest the possibility of a genetic predisposition. Overall mortality from ARDS has not decreased substantially since the publication of the 1967 report, and the current survival rate approximates to 45% in all major epidemiologic series. Sepsis-related ARDS is characterized by a higher overall disease severity, poorer recovery from lung injury, and higher mortality than non–sepsis-related ARDS. Among patients with ARDS associated with combined pulmonary and nonpulmonary sources of infection, mortality is even higher. Approximately 80% of all deaths in patients with ARDS occur within 2 to 3 weeks after the onset of the syndrome. Death traditionally has been attributed to the underlying disease, the presence of sepsis, and the failure of vital organ systems other than the lung.

DEFINITION, INCIDENCE, AND SEVERITY

Because it is difficult to measure changes in capillary and alveolar permeability at the bedside, diagnosis of ARDS is based on a combination of clinical, oxygenation, hemodynamic, and radiographic criteria. These criteria allow the inclusion of a highly heterogeneous group of critically ill patients, because various types of lung injury can lead to a similar pulmonary response. Despite general agreement on the overall criteria on which to base a definition of ARDS (i.e., severe hypoxemia, marked decreased of lung compliance), the specific values of these variables and the preferred conditions of measurement vary greatly among clinicians and scientists. Thus, the original description of ARDS has proved to be incapable of identifying a uniform group of patients. Several of the patients in the original report of Ashbaugh and co-workers would not be classified as having ARDS today, because fluid overload was an important etiologic factor in those cases. Some investigators have questioned whether ARDS is a distinct entity. Others have suggested that ARDS should not be considered a separate syndrome but should be seen as part of the multiple system organ dysfunction syndrome. From a clinical perspective, a strict definition of ARDS may not be required, because current management is supportive. From a therapeutic standpoint, however, a more precise definition probably is necessary, because the effects on outcome of certain ventilatory and adjunctive techniques may presumably vary depending on the degree of lung injury. In terms of prognosis, a number of investigators have examined whether various parameters of oxygenation and lung mechanics would be useful in predicting outcome. In the context of research on ARDS, a very strong argument can be made for a universal definition: It would help standardize experimental and clinical studies evaluating the natural history, incidence, pathophysiology, treatment, and outcome of ARDS. It also would help in the comparison of data among various clinical studies and centers.

A good example of the problems inherent in formulation of a definition for ARDS is the wide disparity in the literature on the incidence. Reported data in the United States suggest an occurrence rate greatly in excess of that expected from current clinical experience in Europe. The most common figure cited for the annual incidence of ARDS is 75 cases per 100,000 population. This is based on an American Lung Program Task Force of the National Heart and Lung Institute in 1972. This internal report suggested that there were about 150,000 cases per year of ARDS in the United States, a value similar to the number of all new cases of cancer. In 1988, Webster and colleagues in England estimated an incidence of 4.5 cases per 100,000 population, and in 1989, Villar and associates in Spain calculated the incidence as 3.5 new cases per 100,000 population per year. Most epidemiologic studies report an ARDS incidence ranging from 4 to 8 cases per 100,000 population per year.

In an attempt to overcome some of these problems, Murray and colleagues proposed an expanded definition of ARDS that takes into account various pathophysiologic features of the syndrome. Their definition uses a "lung injury score" (LIS) to characterize the acute pulmonary damage by considering four components: assessment of the chest radiograph, degree of hypoxemia (determined as the ratio of arterial partial pressure of oxygen to the fraction of inspired oxygen, PaO_2/FIO_2), level of PEEP, and the value of lung compliance, when available (**Table 36-1**). The final injury score is obtained by dividing the total score by the number of components that were used. A score of 0 indicates no lung injury, a score of 1 to 2.5 indicates mild to moderate lung injury, and a score greater than 2.5 indicates severe lung injury or ARDS. The LIS is not specific for ARDS, however, and has not been validated, because it is not clear whether patients with identical LIS have similar degrees of lung injury. Furthermore, patients with a major component of cardiogenic edema may be mislabeled as having ARDS, and a postoperative patient with moderate atelectasis and mild fluid overload may fit the LIS criteria for ARDS.

Because severe hypoxemia is the hallmark of ARDS, it should be crucial to the assessment of the severity of ARDS, for predicting the development and evolution in any given patient, and for assessing the response to treatment. To better characterize the severity of lung damage, in 1994 an American-European Consensus Conference (AECC) defined ALI and ARDS as follows:

Table 36-1 Lung Injury Scoring System

Chest Radiograph Infiltration		PEEP (cm H₂O)	
Nil	0	≤5	0
1 Quadrant	1	6-8	1
2 Quadrants	2	9-11	2
3 Quadrants	3	12-14	3
4 Quadrants	4	≥15	4
Hypoxemia: PaO₂/FIO₂ (mm Hg)		Compliance* (cm H₂O)	
≥300	0	≥80	0
225-299	1	60-79	1
175-224	2	40-49	2
100-174	3	20-39	3
<100	4	≤19	4

Final score: Divide sum by number of components used.

No lung injury	0
Mild-moderate injury	0.1-2.5
Severe lung injury (ARDS)	>2.5

From Murray JE, Matthay MA, Luce JM, Flick MR: An expanded definition of the adult respiratory distress syndrome, *Am Rev Respir Dis* 138:720-723, 1988.
*If measured.
ARDS, acute respiratory distress syndrome; *PEEP*, positive end-expiratory pressure.

Box 36-2 **American-European Consensus Definitions for Acute Lung Injury (ALI) and for Acute Respiratory Distress Syndrome (ARDS)**

- Acute onset
- Severe hypoxemia (PaO_2/FIO_2 <300 mm Hg for ALI OR ≤200 mm Hg for ARDS)
- Diffuse bilateral pulmonary infiltrates on frontal chest radiograph
- Absence of left atrial hypertension OR pulmonary artery wedge pressure <18 mm Hg if measured

---

(i) acute and sudden onset of severe respiratory distress; (ii) bilateral infiltrates on frontal chest radiograph and (iii) the absence of left atrial hypertension (a pulmonary capillary wedge pressure <18 mm Hg or no clinical signs of left ventricular failure; and (iv) severe hypoxemia (assessed by the PaO_2/FIO_2 ratio).

According to these guidelines, ALI exists when the PaO_2/FIO_2 ratio is 300 mm Hg or less regardless of the level of PEEP and FIO_2, and ARDS is present when the PaO_2/FIO_2 ratio is 200 mm Hg or less regardless of the PEEP setting and FIO_2 (**Box 36-2**). Although this definition formalized the criteria for the diagnosis of ARDS and is simple to apply in the clinical setting, it has been challenged over the years in several studies. Such definitions have limitations: The physiologic thresholds do not require standardized ventilatory support, and the use of PEEP can improve oxygenation indices sufficiently to convert the patient's status from meeting the definition of ARDS to not meeting the ARDS definition and also can change the physiology in the lung such that the patient does not meet the criteria for ARDS. Therefore, the ARDS criteria may be met when the PaO_2 is measured with zero PEEP but not when

Table 36-2 Definitions of Acute Respiratory Distress Syndrome in Several Published Reports

Published Study	Criteria
Montgomery et al: *Am Rev Respir Dis* 132:485–489, 1985	PaO_2/FIO_2 <150 mm Hg PCP <18 mm Hg
Villar et al: *Am Rev Respir Dis* 140:814–816, 1989	PaO_2 ≤75 mm Hg on FIO_2 ≥0.5 PCP <18 mm Hg
Bone et al: *Chest* 96:849–851, 1989	PaO_2/FIO_2 ≤150 mm Hg (with ZEEP) OR PaO_2/FIO_2 ≤250 mm Hg with PEEP PCP ≤18 mm Hg
Amato et al: *N Engl J Med* 338:347–354, 1998	Lung injury score ≥2.5 and PCP <16 mm Hg
Stewart et al: *N Engl J Med* 338:355–361, 1998	PaO_2/FIO_2 <250 mm Hg on PEEP of 5 cm H_2O
Brochard et al: *Am J Respir Crit Care Med* 158:1831–1838, 1998	Lung injury score >2.5
Villar et al: *Intensive Care Med* 25:930–935, 1999	PaO_2/FIO_2 ≤150 mm Hg on PEEP ≥5 cm H_2O
ARDSNet: *N Engl J Med* 342:1301–1308, 2000	AECC
Gattinoni et al: *N Engl J Med* 345:568–573, 2001	PaO_2/FIO_2 ≤200 mm Hg on PEEP ≥5 cm H_2O PCP ≤18 mm Hg
Villar et al: *Crit Care Med* 34:1311–1318, 2006	PaO_2/FIO_2 ≤200 mm Hg on PEEP ≥5 cm H_2O and FIO_2 ≥0.5
Meade et al: *JAMA* 299:637–645, 2008	PaO_2/FIO_2 <250 mm Hg
Mercat et al: *JAMA* 299:646–655, 2008	PaO_2/FIO_2 ≤200 mm Hg PCP ≤18 mm Hg

AECC, American-European Consensus Conference; *PCP,* pulmonary capillary pressure; *PEEP,* positive end-expiratory pressure; *ZEEP,* zero PEEP.

measured at a PEEP of 5 or 10 cm H_2O, making patient comparisons difficult. Furthermore, most of the randomized controlled studies did not use the same definition for ARDS, nor did they evaluate the same ventilatory approaches. Diversity among ARDS definitions is apparent in a large number of studies (**Table 36-2**).

GENETICS

Critical care physicians have long recognized that some patients progress despite therapy, whereas others do better than predicted. It is now well accepted that these responses may be related to variations in the genome. Little is known, however, about the genes that are responsible for susceptibility to and outcome of ARDS. The search for genetic variants determining susceptibility and predicting outcome is still a developing field. The identification of important associations between genotype and clinical outcomes will have an impact on the development of more efficient genotype- or phenotype-guided therapies for patients with ALI or ARDS. The current understanding is that the pathogenesis of ARDS has a fundamental inflammatory component eliciting a response similar to that observed against any pathogen. In addition, common genetic risk factors with modest effects may be associated with disease susceptibility. Many studies have searched for genetic variations underlying ARDS susceptibility. Owing to the impracticality of classical genetic approximation in ARDS, association studies comparing unrelated ARDS cases with controls for genetic variants at specified locations of the human genome represent the prevailing study design for detecting such loci. The genetic variants explored usually are single base changes in the DNA, known as single-nucleotide polymorphisms (SNPs), because they are the most common variants across the genome. The genetic studies of ARDS have focused largely on candidate genes involved in the response to external stimulus and cell signal

transduction, because those genes are assumed to be important in the immune response.

Extensive cross-species gene expression pattern comparisons in experimental models of ALI/ARDS have revealed that IL-6, an acute-phase response cytokine with pleiotropic effects, is highly upregulated. This finding is consistent with clinical studies indicating that IL-6 and other cytokines are released from the lungs in patients with ARDS; increased IL-6 concentrations are found in the bronchoalveolar lavage fluid and serum of these patients. IL-6 levels have been correlated with clinical outcome and implicated in the development of multiple system organ failure. A G/C SNP located at position −174 of the promoter region of the IL-6 gene has been shown to functionally affect the activity of the IL-6 gene promoter in vitro. To date, assessing the SNP variation for virtually all common variants of the gene has allowed subsequent studies to reveal a consistent picture for the association of the IL-6 gene with ALI and ARDS.

In case-control studies of patients with severe sepsis and ARDS, several investigators have explored variants of the gene encoding the lipopolysaccharide-binding protein (LBP) and serial measurements of the LBP in serum to relate them with risk gene variants. It has been reported that (1) a four-SNP risk haplotype of the LBP gene is associated with mean serum LBP concentrations within the first week of the disease process; (2) LBP levels at 48 hours are much higher in patients with ARDS than in those with ALI; and (3) a subsequent increase of LBP levels at 48 hours is associated with a four-fold increase in mortality rate. A positive association with ARDS susceptibility and/or outcome has been reported for several other genes, including surfactant pulmonary-associated protein B (*SFTPB*), angiotensin-converting enzyme (*ACE*), tumor necrosis factor (*TNF*), vascular endothelial growth factor (*VEGF*), *IL-10*, pre-B cell–enhancing factor (*PBEF*), chemokine CXC motif ligand 2 (*CXCL2*), mannose-binding lectin-2 (*MBL2*), myosin

Table 36-3	Positive Genetic Association Studies With Susceptibility to and/or Outcome of Acute Respiratory Distress Syndrome (ARDS)*			
Gene	**Variant(s)**	**Sample Size (case/control) or Cohort**	**Population**	**Year of Publication**
SFTPB	T/C −1580	52/46	European	2000
IL-6	G/C −174	96	European	2002
ACE	I/D intron 16	96/2168	European	2002
SFTPB	Intron 4 TR	189 at risk for ARDS	Multiethnic	2004
TNF	G/A −308	212/441	European	2005
VEGF	C/T +936	117/240	European	2005
IL-10	A/G −1082	211/429	European	2006
ACE	I/D intron 16	101/348	Chinese	2006
PBEF	T/G −1001	375/787	European	2007
CXCL2	−665 TR	183	European	2007
MBL2	Gly54Asp	212/442	European	2007
NFKB1	Ins/del ATTG −94	103	European	2007
VEGF	C/T +936	394	European	2007
F5	Arg506Gln	106	European	2008
LBP	Haplotype −1978 to −763	175	European	2009
DIO2	Thr92Ala		European	2011

*See text for complete names of gene abbreviations.

light chain kinase (*MLCK*), nuclear factor κ light polypeptide gene enhancer in B cells (*NFKB1*), coagulation factor V (*F5*), and type 2 deiodinase (*DIO2*) (**Table 36-3**). These genes are involved mainly in the response to external stimulus and cell signal transduction.

Altogether, significant progress has been made in the studies of genetic associations for ARDS. Because all studied candidate genes await repetitive validation in independent studies using larger samples, the search for genetic variants determining susceptibility and outcome in ARDS still needs to grow, to identify associations between genotype and clinical outcomes. The identification of genetic risk factors might allow the development of a new classification of patients and a more accurate determination of patient outcome.

VENTILATOR-INDUCED LUNG INJURY

Unequivocal evidence from both experimental and clinical research shows that mechanical ventilation can damage the lungs and initiate an inflammatory response, possibly contributing to extrapulmonary organ dysfunction. This type of injury, referred to as *ventilator-induced lung injury* (VILI), resembles the syndromes of ALI and ARDS. VILI can trigger a complex array of inflammatory mediators, resulting in a local and systemic inflammatory response. Substances produced in the lungs can be translocated into the systemic circulation as a result of injury to the pulmonary epithelium and to the capillary endothelium. This type of injury forms the basis for the use of low tidal volumes (in the range of 4 to 8 mL/kg of predicted body weight) during mechanical ventilation of patients with ALI or ARDS. The recognition of VILI has prompted a number of investigators to suggest that ALI and ARDS may in part be a product of efforts to mechanically ventilate patients, rather than representing progression of the underlying disease. On the other hand, current scientific evidence supports a link between VILI and the development of extrapulmonary organ dysfunction, in a manner similar to that in which severe cases of sepsis manifest clinically. In addition, functional genomic approaches using gene array methodology to measure lung gene expression have identified patterns of genes differentially expressed in animal models of VILI, similar to those gene pathways activated during experimental and clinical sepsis.

Ventilators are intended to deliver air or oxygen at tidal volumes and frequencies sufficient to provide adequate alveolar ventilation, to reduce the work of breathing, and to enhance oxygenation (see also Chapter 32). However, mechanical ventilation is a nonphysiologic process, and complications are associated with its application, including increased risk for pneumonia, impaired cardiac performance, and lung injury. During mechanical ventilation, pressures, gas volumes, ventilatory rates, and concentrations of inspired oxygen often are applied at levels that exceed those normally experienced by healthy lungs during spontaneous breathing. VILI is not a new concept—it is the designation historically applied to macroscopic injuries associated with alveolar rupture due to overdistention resulting from application of high inspiratory pressures. Clinical manifestations include interstitial emphysema, pneumothorax, pneumomediastinum, and pneumoperitoneum. The concept of VILI has shifted somewhat from pressure-induced (really volume-induced) injury to increased vascular permeability, accumulation of lung fluid, "atelectrauma," and inflammation induced by mechanical ventilation.

In 1998 Tremblay and Slutsky coined the term *biotrauma* to describe the pulmonary and systemic inflammatory response triggered by lung cell distention, alveolar disruption, and/or necrosis after the application of mechanical ventilation. Although a Consensus Conference in 1994 recommended that plateau pressure generally should be limited to 35 cm H_2O, little change in ventilator practice occurred until publication of an ARDS Network study demonstrating that a lung-protective strategy using a tidal volume of 6 mL/kg of predicted body weight and moderate levels of PEEP decreased mortality in patients with ALI. This study confirmed that VILI was not just an interesting experimental entity but also was an important clinical entity. This recognition led to the widespread, albeit not universal, use of lung-protective strategies in patients with ALI. Unequivocal evidence from both experimental and clinical data has proved that mechanical ventilation can cause or aggravate ALI. Many of the pathophysiologic consequences of VILI mimic those of ARDS. A number of specific forms of injury caused by the trauma of mechanical ventilation have been identified: barotrauma, volutrauma, atelectrauma, and biotrauma. Current experimental and clinical evidence supports a link between VILI and the development of extrapulmonary organ dysfunction, by mechanisms similar to those whereby most severe cases of sepsis are clinically manifested (**Figure 36-2**).

PATHOPHYSIOLOGY OF VENTILATOR-INDUCED LUNG INJURY

Lung volumes for all mammals scale with a common function based on body mass. In spontaneously breathing mammals, tidal volumes are approximately 6 to 7 mL/kg of body weight (**Figure 36-3**), yet historically, tidal volumes of 12 to 15 mL/kg were used in mechanically ventilated patients with acute respiratory failure, and peak alveolar pressures were allowed to increase above 40 cm H_2O. This "one tidal volume fits all"

approach was formulated in the 1960s, because anesthesiologists and critical care pioneers had demonstrated that ventilation with small tidal volume resulted in a gradual loss of lung volume (i.e., atelectasis) and hypoxemia. Large-tidal-volume ventilation was useful to prevent this negative physiologic consequence. Since the mid-1970s, experimental studies have

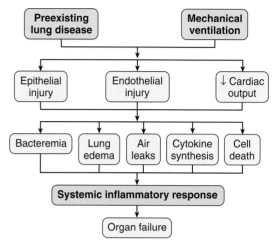

Figure 36-2 Mechanical ventilation and multiple system organ failure: Postulated mechanism by which mechanical ventilation with or without sepsis may contribute to multiple system organ failure.

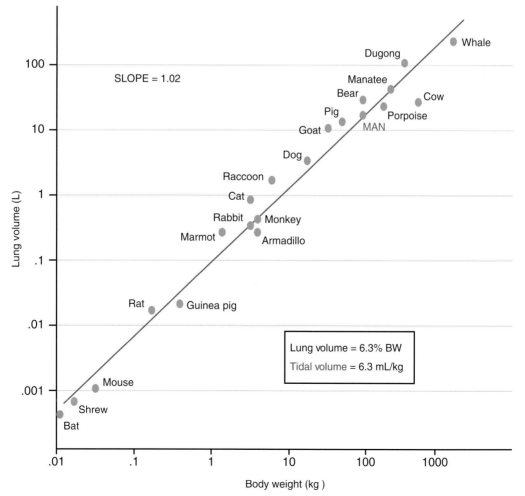

Figure 36-3 Scaling of the lung in mammals. *BW*, body weight. *(From Villar J, Kacmarek RM, Hedenstierna G: From ventilator-induced lung injury to physician-induced lung injury: why the reluctance to use small tidal volumes?* Acta Anaesth Scand *48:267–271, 2004.)*

described the onset of pulmonary edema in rats and larger mammals ventilated with high peak alveolar pressures.

Experimental evidence and advances in lung imaging techniques and bedside ventilator waveform analysis are providing support for the concept that any tidal volume, regardless of how small, has the potential to damage the preinjured lung. Limitation of tidal volume to 6 to 7 mL/kg and plateau pressure to a maximum of 30 cm H_2O represents the standard for mechanical ventilation in patients with ALI or ARDS. However, tidal hyperinflation may occur in some patients despite limiting tidal volume to 6 mL/kg and plateau pressure to 30 cm H_2O. Current evidence suggests that lung-protective ventilation strategies (in the absence of a priming pulmonary insult) cause significant gene expression in the lung. These changes can be detected even after 90 minutes of mechanical ventilation. In patients with ARDS, a further reduction of tidal volume to levels lower than 6 mL/kg in some instances minimizes tidal hyperinflation and attenuated pulmonary inflammation, as evaluated by pulmonary cytokines and computed tomography.

VILI is a dynamic process that is hard to capture at a single point in time. The damage observed in VILI reflects the primary injurious stimuli and the secondary complex interactions of inflammatory mediators on alveolar epithelial and capillary endothelial cells. Alveolar overinflation elicits a well-coordinated response that contributes to cellular proliferation and inflammation. As the epithelium is progressively stretched, a nonreversible opening of water-filled channels between alveolar cells occurs, resulting in free diffusion of small solutes and albumin across the epithelial barrier. The pulmonary endothelium is a metabolically active surface that provides a regulatory interface for the continual processing of blood-borne vasoactive molecules; it plays an active role in homeostasis and immunologic and inflammatory events, regulates vascular tone, and interacts with inflammatory cells and neighboring vascular cells. Mechanical forces originating within the alveolus can cause endothelial disruption and hemorrhagic injury, even in the absence of preexisting inflammation. Cell deformation by mechanical forces directly causes conformational changes in molecules within the cell membrane, leading to activation of downstream messenger systems. Mechanical ventilation can trigger a complex array of pro- and antiinflammatory mediators that may lead to either greater injury or enhanced lung healing and quicker restoration of pulmonary function. Some ventilatory strategies, however, can cause an acute imbalance in this normal stress response, altering lung cellular function and producing a local and a systemic response. Two mechanisms are believed to be responsible for this mechanical ventilation–induced cytokine release (biotrauma). The first is *direct trauma* to the cell with disruption of the membranes, resulting in translocation of cytokines into both the alveolar space and the systemic circulation. The second mechanism has been termed *mechanotransduction*. In vitro studies have shown that most pulmonary cells can produce cytokines in response to cyclic stretch. A large number of genes differentially expressed in the lung by mechanical ventilation have been identified in in vivo animal models of VILI, including genes involved in immunity and inflammation, stress response, metabolism, and transcription processes. However, the sensing mechanism of these physical forces and the translation into intracellular signals is largely unknown.

Mechanical ventilation with large tidal volumes results in extracellular matrix remodeling in patients. This effect suggests a potential contributory role of mechanical ventilation in causing lung fibrosis (**Figure 36-4**). In elective surgical patients,

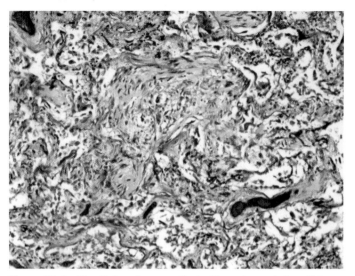

Figure 36-4 Fibrotic lung from a patient with acute respiratory distress syndrome after 10 days of mechanical ventilation. (Gomori trichrome staining technique: *blue* represents fibrosis, *purple* represents the nuclei of the cells (mostly fibroblasts), and red blood cells are stained in *red*.) 100× magnification.

mechanical ventilation with a tidal volume of 12 mL/kg and no PEEP promote procoagulant changes, leading to fibrin deposition within airways; such changes can be prevented by use of low Vt and high-level PEEP.

MECHANICAL VENTILATION–INDUCED SEPSIS

Sepsis originating from pulmonary and nonpulmonary infections is the most frequent cause and complication of ARDS. First described by Hippocrates in 400 BCE, sepsis is a controversial topic eliciting various hypotheses for its immunopathophysiology. The controversy surrounding sepsis is a result of the way it is defined, because its etiology and pathogenesis remain unclear, and because it is defined by inflammation, regardless of the source.

Sepsis describes a complex clinical syndrome occurring as a result of a systemic inflammatory response to live bacteria or bacterial products. Sepsis develops when the initial, appropriate host response to an infection becomes amplified and is then deregulated. According to the current definition, sepsis represents a disease continuum that proceeds from infection to a systemic inflammatory response syndrome and finally to severe sepsis. The clinical management of sepsis remains very complicated because of the nonhomogeneous nature of patient populations and because of the difficulties in precise clinical classification of patients with the disorder. Whether the sepsis is treated or not, potential outcomes include multiple system organ dysfunction, shock, and death.

Because an all-encompassing single mechanism for sepsis remains elusive, mechanical ventilation–induced inflammation may be a root cause, by amplifying the sepsis cascade of microbial or nonmicrobial origin. Most pulmonary cells express a large repertoire of genes under transcriptional control that are modulated by biomechanical forces and bacterial infections. The highly integrated pulmonary defense system is capable of initiating rapid and intense immune responses to invading microbes or cell debris, resulting in profound local and systemic inflammation. Healthy experimental animal and human lungs ventilated with small, moderate, and large tidal volumes evoke early inflammatory responses similar to those evoked by endotoxin or those seen during infections (activation of nuclear factor κB [NFκB] and cytokine release). Gene expression profiles obtained from microarrays across different experimental models of VILI also suggest that the response triggered by alveolar overdistention might mimic an innate immune inflammatory response against pathogens. Mechanical ventilation enhances lipopolysaccharide (LPS)-induced expression of TNF-α. When used with moderate tidal volumes, it augments the innate immune response to bacterial products in the lung and may play a role in the perpetuation of a septic state. Ventilator-associated pneumonia is a frequent complication of mechanical ventilation and an important contributor to morbidity and mortality in critically ill patients. Endotracheal intubation may be the most important factor leading to pneumonia, because the endotracheal tube directly interferes with the barrier between the oropharynx and the lower respiratory tract, by preventing glottic closure, leading to an ineffective cough mechanism. It is not surprising that pulmonary bacterial colonization and infection are associated with a higher risk for development of ARDS, because the lung, with the largest epithelial surface area of the body, is repeatedly exposed to airborne particles and microorganisms.

As with the association of bacteria and their products translocating from the gut and leading to sepsis, injurious mechanical ventilation may be responsible for translocation of bacteria and their products from the alveoli into the bloodstream and be a major factor in the development of systemic infection and multiple organ dysfunction. In the absence of a pulmonary infection, however, mechanical ventilation–induced epithelial and endothelial damage could be responsible for the translocation of soluble mediators derived from pathogens or tissue other than bacteria or endotoxin. In some cases, those pathogen-associated molecules could come from pathogens that are colonizing rather than infecting the airway.

VILI and sepsis involve more mediators than was previously thought. Essential components of the innate immune system are the Toll-like receptors, which recognize not only microbial products but also degradation products released from damaged tissue, providing signals that initiate inflammatory responses. Toll-like receptor agonists circulate in the bloodstream both attached to microorganisms and also separately. Because the pulmonary epithelial and endothelial barriers are damaged during ALI, lung cytokines and bacterial products can be trafficked from the alveoli and the interstitium into the systemic circulation, leading to inter- or intracellular signaling impairments in the functional metabolic properties of those populations of cells. It has been found that mechanical ventilation, in the absence of infection, can induce upregulation of the Toll-like receptor-4 signaling pathway (a receptor related to endotoxin signal transduction), resulting in an increase in proinflammatory cytokine levels in the lungs and in the systemic circulation.

MULTIPLE SYSTEM ORGAN DYSFUNCTION: A COMMON END FOR VENTILATOR-INDUCED LUNG INJURY AND SEPSIS

Approximately 80% of all deaths in patients suffering from ARDS occur within 2 to 3 weeks after its onset. The exact cause of death remains elusive; no autopsy studies have revealed why patients with ARDS die. Death has traditionally been attributed to the underlying disease, the presence of sepsis, and/or the failure of vital organ systems other than the lung. The association of ARDS with multiple system organ dysfunction is not inevitable, but it certainly is common.

The relationship of ARDS with multiple system organ dysfunction is complex, with at least three possible pathophysiologic models: (1) Although sepsis may cause similar local injury (e.g., increased capillary leak), the functional implications of this injury in the lung are greater because of the exquisite susceptibility of the gas exchange apparatus of the lung to edema; (2) local injury to the lungs (trauma, aspiration, gas inhalation) may set up a secondary diffuse inflammatory response resulting in damage to other organs; or (3) infection and sepsis set off the chain of events leading to ARDS and multiple system organ dysfunction. Among those three models, the classic accepted scenario is that ARDS is complicated by sepsis, which results in multiple system organ dysfunction. A fourth possibility has emerged in light of current evidence on VILI: Ventilator-induced inflammatory response may alter cellular pathways that are important for the normal function of tissues and organs.

Multiple system organ dysfunction is a cumulative sequence of organ dysfunctions in patients suffering from the same diseases often found in patients with ARDS. Still to be resolved is why in most studies on sepsis, at least a third of the patients do not have a truly identified source of the septic process. Among several possible reasons, one of the most frequently offered is that antibiotics, administered early, have suppressed the growth of bacteria, as borne out by results of blood culture. It is plausible that mechanical ventilation could be partially responsible for the development of sepsis or a sepsis-like syndrome in critically ill patients, even if blood cultures are negative. Several investigators have suggested that the mechanical ventilation–induced inflammatory response may be a contributing factor in multiple system organ dysfunction by initiating or propagating a malignant, systemic inflammatory response (see Figure 36-2). ARDS and acute kidney injury are frequent complications in critically ill patients with multiple system organ dysfunction. Although the functional changes seen in septic patients are known to affect primarily the lungs, the cardiovascular system, and the kidneys, the gut has long been established as an important component of the immune barrier. An emerging consensus implicates the gut flora in the pathogenesis of sepsis. The gut is a reservoir of pathogens and pathogen-associated molecular patterns from microbes, and translocation of these molecular patterns and toxins other than endotoxin also induces a systemic inflammatory response (probably through Toll-like receptors and NFκB signaling pathways), contributing to the development of a systemic infection and multiple organ dysfunction in critically ill patients.

IMPLICATIONS OF THE SEPSIS–VENTILATOR-INDUCED LUNG INJURY CONNECTION

What conclusions can be drawn from the VILI story? First, the available evidence strongly indicates that patients with ARDS must be ventilated with a tidal volume of 4 to 8 mL/kg of predicted body weight. Second, although data are too limited to support the conclusion that all critically ill patients must be ventilated with a tidal volume of 4 to 8 mL/kg, using small tidal volumes in patients without ARDS may be a reasonable strategy, with little risk for harm, if clinical issues related to maintenance of sufficient PEEP, and possibly the respiratory acidosis that may arise, are addressed appropriately. Third, in view of the relationship between mechanical ventilation and lung injury, an increasingly pertinent consideration is that ARDS may be a consequence of clinical efforts to ventilate the patient, rather than of progression of the underlying disease.

Injurious ventilatory strategies have been shown to increase alveolar-capillary leak, to worsen oxygenation, to cause pulmonary infiltrates, to decrease lung compliance, and to cause an increase in lavage fluid and systemic cytokines—all hallmarks of ALI and ARDS. In the context of increased alveolar-capillary leak, use of excessive intravenous fluids—often administered to treat shock in patients at risk for ALI—can cause increased lung water and likewise impair pulmonary mechanics and gas exchange, leading to worse clinical outcomes. It may not be a coincidence that ARDS was first described in the late 1960s, at the time of the Vietnam conflict, when it was called "Da Nang lung" or "shock lung," in the setting of aggressive resuscitation in the battlefield. Finally, endotracheal intubation affects host defense and can lead to development of colonization or pneumonia, a predisposing factor for ALI and ARDS. Thus, ALI-ARDS may be largely a "man-made" syndrome, arising as a consequence of the aggressive regimens adopted to treat acutely treat patients. If this is so, an inflection point is needed in which ALI-ARDS is no longer a syndrome that must be treated but an iatrogenic illness that should be prevented.

VENTILATORY MANAGEMENT FOR ACUTE RESPIRATORY DISTRESS SYNDROME

Ventilation is an essential function of life and also one of the first to be replicated by artificial means. Mechanical ventilation is the second most frequently performed therapeutic intervention after treatment of cardiac arrhythmias in the intensive care unit (ICU), and it is the most important aspect of the supportive care of patients with respiratory failure. As part of the therapy for the underlying disease, patients with ARDS invariably require endotracheal intubation and mechanical ventilation to decrease the work of breathing and to improve oxygen transport. An improvement in oxygenation can be obtained in many patients with ARDS by an increase in PEEP. To date, the only proven, widely accepted method of mechanical ventilation for ARDS is protective lung ventilation using a low-tidal-volume strategy (4 to 8 mL/kg of predicted body weight) and medium to high PEEP to keep alveoli open throughout the ventilator (respiratory) cycle.

Early interest in low-tidal-volume ventilation was prompted by animal studies in the 1970s showing that mechanical ventilation with large tidal volumes and high peak alveolar pressures resulted in the development of ALI characterized by formation of hyaline membranes and inflammatory infiltrates. Although tidal volumes of 10 to 15 mL/kg had traditionally been used in a majority of patients with respiratory failure, it was recognized in the mid-1980s that ARDS resulted in a significant reduction in the amount of normally aerated lung tissue. The ARDS "baby lung" concept—in which only a small portion of the lung is actually available for ventilation—describes marked overdistention by high tidal volumes.

The effect of different lung-protective ventilatory strategies in patients with ALI or ARDS has been investigated in randomized controlled trials. In the late 1990s, four such trials were conducted to evaluate the benefit of low tidal ventilation in ARDS patients compared with traditional tidal volume ventilation (**Table 36-4**). Only one of these trials, performed in Brazil by Amato and colleagues, showed a significant reduction in mortality in the experimental treatment group. Patients randomized to receive tidal volumes of 6 mL/kg of actual body weight or lower and driving pressures of less than 20 cm H$_2$O were significantly less likely to die during the 28-day study period than were patients randomized to receive the traditional

12 mL/kg of actual body weight tidal volumes and unlimited driving pressures. Because all four studies had limited statistical power owing to small sample sizes, a large trial was needed to definitively determine the effect of low-tidal-volume ventilation in patients with ARDS.

In response to this need, the National Heart, Lung, and Blood Institute ARDS Network enrolled 861 patients at 10 institutions between 1996 and 1999 in a randomized controlled trial known as the Respiratory Management in Acute Lung Injury/ARDS (ARMA) trial. This study compared a ventilatory protocol using tidal volumes of 4 to 8 mL/kg of predicted body weight and maintaining plateau pressures of 30 cm H$_2$O or less with conventional mechanical ventilation using 12 mL/kg of predicted body weight tidal volumes. The lower tidal volume protocol in the ARMA study achieved more pronounced differences between the intervention and control groups in tidal volume (6.2 versus 11.8 mL/kg of predicted body weight) and plateau pressure (25 versus 33 cm H$_2$O) than those achieved in previous studies. The hospital mortality rate was significantly reduced in the low-tidal-volume group, with a nearly 9% reduction in the absolute risk of death from that the control group (31% versus 39.8%; $P = .007$). Although it has been postulated that the mortality benefit demonstrated in the ARMA study was attributable to a high mortality rate in the control group resulting from tidal volumes that were higher than the standard of care, several observational studies performed later indicated that no uniform standard of care existed at the time of the ARMA trial.

Therefore, it is recommended that critical care physicians utilize the ventilation protocol outlined by the Acute Respiratory Distress Syndrome Clinical Network (ARDSNet) investigators. This protocol involves the following principles:

1. High tidal volumes and high plateau pressures are to be avoided.
2. Tidal volume size should be based on *predicted* body weight, calculated from gender and height—50 + 0.91 × (height in cm − 152.4) for men and 45.5 + 0.91 × (height in cm − 152.4) for women—rather than on actual body weight.
3. Tidal volumes should be systematically adjusted (from 4 to 8 mL/kg of predicted body weight) to maintain a plateau pressure of 30 cm H$_2$O or less.
4. The respiratory rate should be titrated as needed (over a range of 10 to 35 breaths/minute) to maintain a pH of 7.3 to 7.45.
5. An appropriate combination of FIO$_2$ and PEEP should be used to achieve adequate oxygenation (PaO$_2$ of 55 to 85 mm Hg, or SpO$_2$ of 90% or greater).

Since the publication of ARMA, however, despite the statistically significant decrease in mortality rates, widespread use of this therapy remains elusive. Significant barriers to the implementation of low-tidal-volume mechanical ventilation include unwillingness to accept or lack of knowledge of the published data, failure to recognize patients as having ARDS, perceived contraindications to low-tidal-volume ventilation, concerns regarding patient discomfort, and presence of hypercapnia or acidosis.

THE USE OF POSITIVE END-EXPIRATORY PRESSURE IN ACUTE RESPIRATORY DISTRESS SYNDROME

PEEP has become an essential component of the care of many critically ill patients who require ventilatory support. The

Table 36-4 **Randomized Controlled Trials Evaluating Pressure- and Volume-Limited (PVL) Ventilation for Patients With Acute Respiratory Distress Syndrome (ARDS)**

Study*	Inclusion Criteria[†]	Strategy (No. of Patients) PVL Ventilation	Control Strategy	Mortality Rate (%): PLV vs. Control	P Value
Amato et al, 1998	LIS ≥2.5	<6 mL/kg actual BW PEEP above LIP (N = 29)	12 mL/kg actual BW (N = 24)	37.9 vs. 70.8	.026
Brochard et al, 1998	LIS >2.5 for <72 hours Single organ failure	6-10 mL/kg actual BW Plateau pressure ≤30 cm H₂O (N = 58)	10-15 mL/kg actual BW (N = 58)	46.5 vs. 37.9	.452
Stewart et al, 1998	PaO₂/FIO₂ <250 mm Hg at PEEP 5 cm H₂O	≤8 mL/kg ideal BW PIP ≤30 mm H₂O (N = 60)	10-15 mL/kg ideal BW PIP ≤50 mm H₂O (N = 60)	50 vs. 46.7	.855
Brower et al: *Crit Care Med* 27:1492-1498, 1999	PaO₂/FIO₂ ≤200 mm Hg	5-8 mL/kg ideal BW Plateau pressure <30 cm H₂O (N = 26)	10-12 mL/kg ideal BW Plateau pressure <55 mm H₂O (N = 26)	50 vs. 46.1	1
Ranieri et al: *JAMA* 282:54-61, 1999	PaO₂/FIO₂ ≤200 mm Hg	6-9 mL/kg actual BW PEEP above LIP (N = 18)	10-12 mL/kg actual BW PEEP ≤10 mm H₂O (N = 19)	38.9 vs. 57.9	.330
ARDSNet, 2000 (ARMA study)	PaO₂/FIO₂ ≤300 mm Hg	4-8 mL/kg ideal BW Plateau pressure ≤30 cm H₂O (N = 432)	12 mL/kg ideal BW Plateau pressure ≤50 mm H₂O (N = 429)	31 vs. 39.8	.007
Brower et al: *N Engl J Med* 351:327-336, 2004 (ALVEOLI trial)	PaO₂/FIO₂ ≤300 mm Hg	4-8 mL/kg ideal BW PEEP according to scale (N = 273)	4-8 mL/kg ideal BW PEEP according to scale (N = 276)	27.5 vs. 25	.560
Villar et al, 2006 (ARIES study)	PaO₂/FIO₂ ≤200 mm Hg at PEEP ≥5 cm H₂O, FIO₂ ≥0.5	5-8 mL/kg ideal BW PEEP above LIP (N = 50)	9-11 mL/kg ideal BW PEEP ≥5 cm H₂O (N = 45)	32 vs. 53.3	.040
Meade et al, 2008 (LOV study)	PaO₂/FIO₂ <250 mm Hg	6 mL/kg ideal BW PEEP according to scale (N = 508)	6 mL/kg ideal BW PEEP according to scale (N = 475)	40.3 vs. 36.4	.213
Mercat et al, 2008 (ExPress trial)	PaO₂/FIO₂ ≤200 mm Hg	6 mL/kg ideal BW PEEP for plateau = 28 cm H₂O (N = 382)	6 mL/kg ideal BW PEEP based on PaO₂ (N = 385)	39 vs. 35.3	.296
Talmor et al: *N Engl J Med* 359:2095-2104, 2008	PaO₂/FIO₂ ≤300 mm Hg	6 mL/kg ideal BW PEEP for a transpulmonary pressure 0-10 cm H₂O (N = 30)	6 mL/kg ideal BW PEEP according to scale (N = 31)	17 vs. 39	.05

*See Table 36-2 for publication information on studies not "formally" cited in this column.
[†]In addition to having a risk factor for ARDS and bilateral pulmonary infiltrates.
ALVEOLI, Assessment of Low Tidal Volume and Elevated End-Expiratory Pressure to Obviate Lung Injury; *ARIES*, Acute Respiratory Insufficiency: España Study; *ARMA*, Respiratory Management in Acute Lung Injury/ARDS; *BW*, body weight; *ExPress*, Expiratory Pressure; *LIP*, lower inflection point; *LOV*, Lung Open Ventilation; *PEEP*, positive end-expiratory pressure; *PIP*, peak inspiratory pressure.

rationale for the use of PEEP in ALI coincides with the theoretical basis for loss of lung volume and compliance in patients with ARDS. With the application of PEEP, the baseline end-expiratory pressure in mechanically ventilated patients is elevated above atmospheric pressure. The application of PEEP is expected to improve lung mechanics and gas exchange, because it maintains recruited lung volume open. PEEP should be utilized in patients with ARDS to decrease the proportion of nonaerated lung, resulting in improved oxygenation. PEEP prevents complete alveolar collapse and improves oxygenation by increasing functional residual capacity, probably by preventing airway closure and keeping open the previously recruited unventilated alveoli. Conversely, the increase in functional residual capacity also may increase lung compliance. In general,

PEEP is applied to improve oxygenation, which usually is not observed except with a concomitant increase in functional residual capacity. The application of PEEP is expected to increase PaO₂ and to decrease intrapulmonary shunt, alveolar-arterial O₂ pressure difference, and arteriovenous O₂ content difference because greater lung volumes are recruited. Four mechanisms have been proposed to explain the improved pulmonary function and gas exchange with PEEP: (1) increased functional residual capacity; (2) alveolar recruitment; (3) redistribution of extravascular lung water; and (4) improved ventilation-perfusion matching. The increase in lung volume is the result of three separate effects. First, PEEP increases lung volume as a result of distention of already patent airways and alveoli by an amount dependent on system compliance.

Table 36-5	Oxygenation Scale for Application of Positive End-Expiratory Pressure (PEEP)*												
Low PEEP													
FIO₂	0.3	0.4	0.4	0.5	0.5	0.6	0.7	0.7	0.7	0.8	0.9	0.9	0.9	1.0
PEEP (cm H₂O)	5	5	8	8	10	10	10	12	14	14	14	16	18	18-24
High PEEP													
FIO₂	0.3	0.3	0.3	0.3	0.3	0.4	0.4	0.5	0.5	0.5-0.8	0.8	0.9	1.0
PEEP (cm H₂O)	5	8	10	12	14	14	16	16	18	20	22	22	22-24

*NOTE: These tables were used for the first time in the ALVEOLI study but lack a physiologic basis because the data are based on surveys of clinicians' practice. *ALVEOLI*, Assessment of Low Tidal Volume and Elevated End-Expiratory Pressure to Obviate Lung Injury; *FIO₂*, fraction of inspired oxygen.
Data compiled for Brower RG, Lanken PN, MacIntyre N, et al; National Heart, Lung, and Blood Institute ARDS Clinical Trials Network: Higher versus lower positive end-expiratory pressures in patients with the acute respiratory distress syndrome, *N Engl J Med* 351:327, 2004.

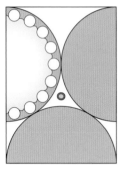 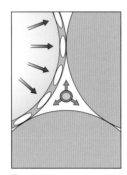

A Low lung volume   B High lung volume

Figure 36-5 As a result of increasing lung volume with PEEP **(B)**, alveolar capillaries are stretched and compressed (*arrows*). Extraalveolar and corner vessels between alveoli are expanded, which increases the flux of fluid into the interstitial space. Without PEEP **(A)**, these changes are reversed. *PEEP*, positive end-expiratory pressure. (*From Kacmarek RM: Positive end-expiratory pressure. In Pierson DJ, Kacmarek RM, editors: Fundamentals of respiratory care, New York, 1992, Churchill Livingstone, pp 891–920.*)

Therefore, the stiffer the system, the smaller the volume change. Second, application of PEEP prevents alveolar collapse during expiration. Dependent, small airways tend to collapse at low lung volumes. Third, PEEP levels above 10 cm H₂O recruit collapsed alveoli in the acutely injured lung. Alveolar recruitment describes reinflation of previously collapsed alveoli. The application of PEEP allows recruitment of flooded alveoli and improves oxygenation without diminishing lung water content, supporting the conclusion that PEEP redistributes lung water from alveoli to the perivascular space. In general, by increasing intraalveolar pressure, PEEP moves fluid from the interstitial space of alveolar vessels to the interstitial space around extraalveolar vessels. In addition, PEEP increases the transmural pressure across corner (in the peribronchial area) and extraalveolar vessels, thereby increasing flux into the interstitial space (**Figure 36-5**).

Although PEEP is well recognized to improve oxygenation in selected patients, its beneficial effects on morbidity and mortality have not been conclusively demonstrated. Early observations that PEEP greatly improves oxygenation in patients with ARDS led to its widespread use in such patients, but the level of PEEP needed to achieve maximum benefit with minimal complications has never been established. Traditionally, PEEP values of 5 to 12 cm H₂O have been used in the ventilation of patients with ARDS. In the ARMA trial, PEEP levels in both the experimental and control groups were adjusted according to the required FIO₂ and ranged between 5 cm H₂O (when FIO₂ was 0.3) and 18 to 24 cm H₂O (when

FIO₂ was 1.0) (**Table 36-5**). On average, patients in the low-tidal-volume ventilation group were treated with levels of PEEP that were no different than those utilized in the high-tidal-volume group. However, it remains unclear whether these values are ideal because randomized controlled trials have not clearly shown that higher levels of PEEP lead to a reduction in mortality rate.

Several randomized controlled trials have evaluated the efficacy of high levels of PEEP in the treatment of ARDS. Thus far, a total of seven published randomized controlled trials have examined the effects of higher levels of PEEP in patients with ALI or ARDS, or both. Those trials have tested higher versus lower PEEP strategies during low-tidal-volume ventilation and lower tidal volume and PEEP titrated to above the lower inflection point of the individual pressure volume curve versus higher-tidal-volume ventilation and lower PEEP (see Table 36-4). At first look, the pooled results of a metaanalysis of these trials suggest that the application of either low or high PEEP levels in patients with ALI or ARDS does not influence outcome. However, this is not what the data show. First, because the ALI-ARDS population was not homogeneous in all the trials, the benefit of higher levels of PEEP could not be appropriately evaluated. Second, in some trials, a PEEP level of 5 cm H₂O was a permissible setting in the higher PEEP group. Therefore, a patient with a PaO₂ of 60 mm Hg on a FIO₂ of 0.3 and 5 cm H₂O of PEEP satisfied the AECC inclusion criteria. It is difficult to accept that in these patients there is a need to test the effects of high levels of PEEP. Finally, some trials (e.g., the Assessment of Low Tidal Volume and Elevated End-Expiratory Pressure to Obviate Lung Injury [ALVEOLI] and Expiratory Pressure [ExPress] trials) (see Table 36-4) included patients with ALI (without ARDS), who did not benefit and more often experienced adverse effects from higher levels of PEEP, suggesting that both trials failed to focus on the patients at highest risk. If the subjects in a trial have a very low risk for the condition that the intervention is hypothesized to prevent, the trial—regardless of sample size—will not verify the value of the experimental intervention under study. In the study of a protective ventilation strategy by Amato and Villar and their respective colleagues, PEEP was significantly higher in the intervention group than in the control group (13 to 14 cm H₂O versus 9 cm H₂O, respectively). Although both trials reported a significantly lower mortality in the intervention group, these findings cannot be solely attributed to higher levels of PEEP, because the intervention strategies in these trials also included both low tidal volumes and high levels of PEEP.

To determine the isolated benefit of high levels of PEEP in patients with ARDS, the ARDSNet conducted a large randomized controlled trial known as the ALVEOLI trial. Patients ventilated with low tidal volumes (4 to 8 mL/kg of predicted body weight) were randomized to a ventilator protocol utilizing high levels (12 to 24 cm H_2O) or low levels of PEEP (5 to 24 cm H_2O). In the first 7 days of ventilator support after initiation of treatment, patients in the high PEEP group received 13 to 15 cm H_2O of PEEP and patients in the low PEEP group, 8 to 9 cm H_2O of PEEP. Although patients in the high PEEP group experienced better improvement in oxygenation, the duration of mechanical ventilation and hospital mortality were similar in the two groups.

The speculation of many investigators regarding the lack of expected benefit from higher PEEP in the ALVEOLI, Lung Open Ventilation (LOV), and ExPress trials (see Table 36-4) is that in a substantial proportion of patients in those trials, the severity of lung injury was modest. In two other trials, Amato and colleagues and Villar and associates enrolled only patients with severe, established ARDS, and both groups found that the application of higher levels of PEEP was associated with a better outcome. By contrast, in the rest of the trials, the investigators studied an unselected, mixed population of ALI and ARDS and, as a result, missed the opportunity to test whether the use of higher levels of PEEP is beneficial in patients with persistent ARDS. Patients in the ALVEOLI, LOV, and ExPress trials had similar PaO_2/FiO_2 ratios at study entry (about 140 ± 50 mm Hg). It is conceivable, however, that a disproportionate number of patients meeting ALI criteria on standard ventilatory settings ended up in the control group, negating the beneficial effect of the treatment because of a lower mortality rate (20% or less in most series). A critical review of the two most recently published trials on the effects of PEEP in ARDS leads to an alternative interpretation. In both trials (the LOV study and the ExPress trial), patients who received higher PEEP were

less likely to require rescue therapy. In addition, a lower PEEP was associated with significantly fewer ventilator-free and organ failure-free days, which may be the reason for a 4% mortality difference in favor of the high PEEP groups ($P = .10$).

Of note, current published metaanalyses including some or all of the available trials reported conflicting results and are biased because they do not deal with all comparisons between tidal volume and PEEP (Table 36-6). The first metaanalysis from Oba and colleagues, which considered five trials (reported by Amato, Brower, Meade, Mercat, and Villar and their co-workers), showed a decrease in in-hospital mortality ($P = .03$) and a trend toward significance for the 28-day mortality ($P = .06$) with higher PEEP and without an increase in barotrauma. A second meta-analysis, by Phoenix and colleagues, included an additional study (by Ranieri and co-workers) and showed a reduction in mortality (pooling together the in-hospital and the 28-day mortality rates, $P = .007$) with higher PEEP. In a subsequent metaanalysis, Putensen and colleagues analyzed the five trials included in the Oba metaanalysis. Data from three of these trials—those reported by Brower, Meade, and Mercat and their co-workers—were pooled together for comparison of lower versus higher PEEP at low tidal volume ventilation. The remaining two studies (by Amato and Villar and their co-workers) were used for the comparison of higher tidal volume and lower PEEP versus lower tidal volume and higher PEEP. Despite opposite results from the two previous metaanalyses, the comparison between lower and higher levels of PEEP at low tidal volume ventilation showed similar hospital mortality rates ($P = .08$). However, the risk of in-hospital mortality was reduced only with the combination of a lower tidal volume and higher PEEP, compared with higher tidal volume and lower PEEP ($P = .005$). Thus, the beneficial effect of PEEP

Table 36-6 Metaanalysis of Data From Randomized Controlled Trials Comparing Lower and Higher Levels of Positive End-Expiratory Pressure (PEEP) in Patients With Acute Lung Injury (ALI) or Acute Respiratory Distress Syndrome (ARDS)

Study Feature	Oba et al: *Respir Med* 103:1171, 2009	Phoenix et al: *Anesthesiology* 110:1098, 2009	Putensen et al: *Ann Intern Med* 151:566, 2009	Briel et al: *JAMA* 303:865, 2010
Trials included in the metaanalysis*	Amato et al, 1998 Brower et al, 2004 Villar et al, 2006 Meade et al, 2008 Mercat et al, 2008	Amato et al, 1998 Ranieri et al, 1999 Brower et al, 2004 Villar et al, 2006 Meade et al, 2008 Mercat et al, 2008	Amato et al, 1998 Brower et al, 2004 Villar et al, 2006 Meade et al, 2008 Mercat et al, 2008	Brower et al, 2004 Meade et al, 2008 Mercat et al, 2008
High PEEP, no. deaths/no. patients (%)	408/1215 (33.6)	415/1233 (33.6)	429/1163 (36.9) at low V_T (Brower et al + Meade et al + Mercat et al) 30/79 (38) (Amato et al + Villar et al)	374/1136 (32.9) 324/951 (34) for ARDS 50/184 (27.2) for ALI
Low PEEP, no. deaths/no. patients (%)	464/1232 (37.6)	482/1251 (38.5)	378/1136 (33.3) at low V_T (Brower et al + Meade et al + Mercat et al) 42/69 (60.9) (Amato et al + Villar et al)	409/1163 (35.2) 368/941 (39) for ARDS 44/220 (19.4) for ALI
Overall effect	$P = .038$	$P = .007$	$P = .08$ high vs. low PEEP at low V_T $P = .005$ high PEEP + low V_T vs. low PEEP + high V_T	$P = .25$ (hospital mortality) $P = .01$ (ICU mortality) $P = .049$ (beneficial for ARDS only) $P = .07$ (harmful for non-ARDS)

*See Tables 36-2 and 36-4 for publication information on cited studies.
ICU, intensive care unit; *V_T*, tidal volume.

may have been due to a simultaneous reduction in the tidal volume and an increase in the level of PEEP. Finally, a fourth metaanalysis from Briel and colleagues (see Table 36-6) was performed on the individual data for 1136 patients (with higher PEEP) and 1163 patients (with lower PEEP) from trials that compared lower and higher PEEP values at a low-tidal-volume ventilation. The individual data analysis showed that a nonsignificant difference was found in hospital mortality rates between the higher and lower PEEP groups (32.9% versus 35.2%; $P = .25$). In conclusion, these metaanalyses of individual patient data suggest that higher levels of PEEP may be associated with lower mortality in patients who meet ARDS criteria, whereas such a benefit is unlikely in patients who have less severe lung injury.

RESCUE STRATEGIES FOR REFRACTORY HYPOXEMIA

A number of alternative techniques (currently available worldwide or under evaluation) can be used to improve oxygenation and ventilation in patients with ALI or ARDS who have refractory hypoxemia. Today, refractory hypoxemia is rare and an infrequent cause of death (accounting for less than 15% of ARDS-related deaths). There is no standard definition for refractory hypoxemia in terms of a predetermined PaO_2 value under a specific oxygen concentration (FIO_2) and applied PEEP level for a specific period of time. In most reports, it has been defined as having a PaO_2 below 60 mm Hg on an FIO_2 0.8 to 1.0 and PEEP 10 to 20 cm H_2O for more than 12 to 24 hours.

RECRUITMENT MANEUVERS

As described previously, ARDS is characterized by collapsed and consolidated alveoli. Recruitment maneuvers are intended to reopen these alveoli and to attenuate the injurious effects of the repetitive opening and closing of the alveolar unit. In general, a recruitment maneuver is defined as applying a pressure higher than that applied during a normal breath either intermittently (for 2 to 3 minutes) or sustained for a short period of time (up to about 40 seconds). A recruitment maneuver usually improves oxygenation and may influence ventilation by reducing $PaCO_2$. Recruitment occurs during the whole period of inspiration, and the amount of recruited lung area correlates with the inspiratory pressure applied. The amount of potentially recruitable lung tissue seems to correlate well with the severity of ARDS. With respect to hemodynamics, the acute and substantial increase in intrathoracic pressure during the recruitment maneuver often induces a decline in cardiac output and tissue oxygenation. Therefore, it is essential to stabilize the patient hemodynamically before a recruitment maneuver procedure. Although the potential for barotrauma is a concern during a recruitment maneuver, when recruiting pressures are maintained at or below 50 cm H_2O peak alveolar pressure, barotrauma has been rarely reported.

The ALVEOLI trial also evaluated the safety and efficacy of recruitment maneuvers in the first 80 patients randomized to receive high-level PEEP. Continuous positive airway pressure (CPAP) of 35 to 40 cm H_2O was applied for 30 seconds, and the results were compared with those of a sham recruitment maneuver. Because the interventions resulted in only small and transient increases in oxygenation, they were discontinued. Such maneuvers have been associated with transient hypotension and hypoxemia, and their long-term benefit remains unproved. In a metaanalysis of seven clinical trials involving 1170 patients with ALI/ARDS, there was no significant difference in survival between groups receiving an "open lung" ventilatory strategy that included recruitment maneuvers and groups given standard ventilatory care. The main limitation of that systematic review, however, was the design of the trials, in that they either did not isolate recruitment maneuvers from other variables or assessed only short-term outcomes, and few of these trials determined the patient-specific PEEP level (by decremental trial) after the recruitment maneuvers—a key to the successful use of such maneuvers. Most recent data suggest that a recruitment maneuver performed in the early phase of ARDS might be more effective than in late-stage ARDS.

EXTRACORPOREAL MEMBRANE OXYGENATION

Extracorporeal membrane oxygenation (ECMO) is a technique that originally was applied in patients with acute respiratory failure of such severity that it was impossible to provide adequate oxygenation by conventional mechanical ventilation. To supplement gas exchange, a portion of the cardiac output must go through the ECMO circuit. During ECMO, CO_2 is removed by the extracorporeal circuit, but this technique usually is supplemented with conventional mechanical ventilation at low ventilatory rates, high PEEP levels, and tidal volumes adequate to maintain a plateau pressure below 30 cm H_2O. Most long-term adult ECMO procedures are performed using the venovenous approach. Access for both blood removal and return is by way of the femoral, saphenous, or jugular vein. Despite the excitement generated by earlier reports of success, the results of ECMO trials led to a loss of enthusiasm for its use in acute respiratory failure. Some investigators, however, believe that there exists a role for ECMO in young adult patients with single organ system failure who are deemed to have potentially reversible pulmonary dysfunction when all other conventional modalities have failed.

Recently a large multicenter adult ECMO trial was completed. Referred to as the CESAR trial (Conventional Ventilatory Support versus Extracorporeal Membrane Oxygenation for Severe Adult Respiratory Failure), this randomized controlled trial assessed the effectiveness of extracorporeal lung assist in 180 patients with severe ARDS. The findings of this study represent the first positive results for adult ECMO application in severe respiratory failure. Survival at 6 months or absence of severe disability was achieved in 63% of the patients on ECMO, compared with 47% of the control group ($P = .03$). However, a number of major concerns and limitations with this study have been identified: First, patients allocated to conventional management (control group) were treated with conventional mechanical ventilation or with high-frequency ventilation. Second, patients in the control group were ventilated with a nonstandardized protocol; to ensure the collaboration of participating centers, physicians were allowed to choose any ventilatory strategy. Third, 30% of patients in the control group were not ventilated with a lung-protective strategy. Fourth, no data regarding ventilatory parameters at study entry and during the mechanical ventilation period are presented. Fifth, all patients receiving ECMO were treated in the same center. Sixth, the ECMO center did not treat patients randomized to the conventional management group. Seventh, many patients randomized to receive ECMO did not receive ECMO. In fact, 103 patients who were screened for eligibility were excluded because a bed was unavailable for ECMO, and 22 patients (25%) assigned to be transferred to the ECMO center never received ECMO (16 of these improved with conventional management). Finally, a more critical analysis of outcomes data for patients who actually received ECMO (68 of 90) compared with those who were treated with mechanical ventilation for whom information about mortality was available (87 plus 22) showed that the mortality rates were similar in both groups (48.5% for ECMO versus 43.1% for mechanical ventilation) ($P = .64$, by our own calculations). In addition, the length of ICU stay and hospital stay was more than twice as high in the ECMO group.

The highly specialized equipment and knowledge required to provide ECMO make this technique available only in specific medical centers.

HIGH-FREQUENCY OSCILLATORY VENTILATION

Some clinicians have proposed that high-frequency oscillatory ventilation (HFOV) is an ideal mode of ventilation for patients with ARDS, because it is the natural culmination of low-tidal-volume ventilation. Current understanding of the mechanisms and importance of ventilator-induced lung injury has advanced considerably over the past 3 decades. HFOV should theoretically be an ideal mode to ventilate patients with severe lung damage, because it achieves gas exchange by delivering very small tidal volumes that typically are 1 to 3 mL/kg (often less than the anatomic dead space) at frequencies ranging from 3 to 10 Hz around a relatively constant mean airway pressure. HFOV is not a difficult technique. In fact, it is easier than conventional mechanical ventilation: It incorporates fewer and simpler controls that are not interrelated as they are in conventional mechanical ventilators. Recent prospective, observational studies have reported that HFOV is a feasible and efficient method of ventilation that results in rapid and sustained improvement in oxygenation in patients with severe ARDS. However, a critical examination of randomized controlled trials comparing HFOV with conventional ventilation demonstrates that there is equivalence between conventional ventilation and HFOV. Specifically, there is no evidence that conventional mechanical ventilation with low tidal volumes, high-level PEEP, and limited plateau pressures is more harmful that HFOV. All of the randomized controlled trials to date have compared HFOV with a less-than-optimal approach to conventional ventilation. Several ongoing trials, however, are comparing HFOV with low-tidal-volume ventilation.

PRONE POSITIONING

Changes in posture can have profound effects on the pulmonary function of patients with severe respiratory failure. Most changes in pulmonary physiology with posture occur as a consequence of the influence of gravity and chest wall shape on the mechanical properties of the lung. By tradition, patients with respiratory failure are cared for supine. In critically ill patients, the supine posture is associated with a fall in functional residual capacity to below closing capacity, resulting in ventilation-perfusion mismatching and a drop in PaO_2. During acute respiratory failure, a reduction of functional residual capacity results in supine hypoxemia regardless of age. Because most lung infiltrates in patients with ARDS are seen in dependent lung regions, it was postulated that prone positioning of patients redistributes blood flow and ventilation to the least affected areas of the lung, promotes secretion clearance, and shifts the weight of the mediastinal contents anteriorly, to assist in the recruitment of atelectatic regions. Thus, the proposed mechanisms by which prone positioning improves oxygenation include an increase in functional residual capacity, a change in regional diaphragm motion, redistribution of perfusion to better-ventilated lung units, redistribution of ventilation to better-perfused lung units, and improved secretion clearance.

Since 1974, prone positioning has been proposed as a technique to improve oxygenation. The practice of turning prone seems to be inexpensive and safe, with the possible exception of an increased risk of regurgitation or inadvertent extubation. However, the act of turning is labor-intensive; at least four experienced staff members are required for this maneuver to avoid the loss of vascular accesses or the airway during turning. Meticulous care must be used in positioning the patient. Placing a neck roll or a pillow under the patient's shoulders and turning the head to one side constitutes the recommended way to support the patient when prone. In addition, prone positioning may be associated with an increased need for sedation. Automated prone positioning uses special devices operated by one nurse, and therapy can be individualized in accordance with the patient's needs and responses. Most complications, such as skin injury, facial edema, catheter removal or compression, hypotension, arrhythmias, and inadvertent extubation, are associated with manual positioning. The risk of developing pressure ulcers is ever-present, as the patient is immobile and pressure on bony prominences may be prolonged. If the patient's tongue becomes edematous to the point of the teeth cutting into it, a dental mouth prop should be used to prevent injury. Facial edema, although only temporary, can be very disturbing for the patient's family to view and can be minimized with application of ice packs.

Although sufficient data have accumulated to permit the conclusion that oxygenation frequently improves when patients with ARDS are turned prone (in about 70% of patients), prone positioning is still not widely implemented. Three recent systematic reviews and metaanalysis in patients with ALI or ARDS have shown that in general, prone positioning does not reduce mortality or duration of mechanical ventilation despite improved oxygenation and a decreased risk of pneumonia. By stratifying patients according to their PaO_2/FIO_2 ratio, however, the most recent metaanalysis has found that in patients with severe ARDS, as defined by a PaO_2/FIO_2 ratio less than 100 mm Hg, prone positioning was able to cause a significant reduction (16% decrease in the relative risk) of all-cause mortality. Thus, prone positioning should be considered to represent a rescue maneuver, and it should be reserved only for patients with severe acute hypoxemic failure in the early phase of the disease process. In such circumstances, the potential for life-threatening complications of prone positioning, including accidental dislodgment of the endotracheal tube or central venous catheters and endotracheal tube obstruction, should be weighed against the short-term benefit of improved oxygenation. Unfortunately, no recommendations can be offered on the optimal timing or duration of prone positioning until large randomized controlled trials in patients with severe hypoxemia provide more information. Extended prone positioning seems to be most beneficial when maintained 18 to 20 hours daily.

INHALED VASODILATORS

Antiinflammatory agents and vasodilators have been tried experimentally in animals and humans for prophylaxis or treatment of ARDS. Prostaglandins, ibuprofen, pentoxifylline, inhaled nitric oxide (iNO), inhaled prostacyclin, almitrine, and corticosteroids all have been tried. None of them have shown any major benefit on outcome in large randomized human trials, even though significant improvements of oxygenation have been observed with some of these agents.

Nitric oxide (NO) is important for the regulation of pulmonary vascular smooth muscle tone. NO appears to be pivotal in acute and chronic hypoxic pulmonary vasoconstriction. Pulmonary hypertension is a typical feature of ARDS and is a bad prognostic factor in respiratory failure. Inhaled NO selectively dilates pulmonary vasculature without systemic effects. Over the past two decades, an increasing number of clinical studies have been published assessing different aspects of inhaled NO in patients with ARDS and addressing the ability of NO to attenuate ALI. Despite the fact that many clinicians consider inhaled NO to be a useful rescue treatment for patients with ARDS, no randomized controlled trial has demonstrated an outcome benefit. A systematic review and metaanalysis of 12 randomized controlled trials including a total of 1237 patients with severe ALI or ARDS found that overall, NO is associated with limited improvement in oxygenation at 24 hours of therapy, has no effect on duration of ventilation, does not confer mortality benefits, and may cause harm.

IMPLICATIONS OF RESCUE THERAPIES FOR CLINICAL PRACTICE

Use of rescue therapies carries a number of implications for clinical practice. First, not enough evidence from well-performed randomized controlled trials has been accumulated to support routine use of ECMO for rescue therapy in adults with severe ARDS. Second, no specific ventilatory mode (including high-frequency oscillatory ventilation) has been proved to be superior to limiting end-inspiratory plateau pressures and tidal volumes and appropriately setting PEEP. Third, although altering body position is part of routine clinical care in most patients with respiratory failure, evidence to support the routine use of prone positioning is lacking. However, prone ventilation seems to reduce mortality in patients with severe acute hypoxemic respiratory failure. Fourth, none of the pharmacologic therapies evaluated in patients with ALI or ARDS, including inhaled vasodilators, have been shown to reduce morbidity or mortality when compared with placebo or conventional treatment. The good news is that none of these therapies that improve oxygenation significantly increase morbidity or mortality. Accordingly, when conventional therapy fails, all such interventions may be tried. Nevertheless, clinicians should consider that the only thing these therapies may accomplish is increasing cost.

SUPPORTIVE TREATMENT

SEDATION

Patients with ARDS who are being ventilated with low tidal volumes should be managed with the same sedation strategies recommended for all critically ill mechanically ventilated patients. Specifically, sedation protocols using standardized sedation scales and sedation goals have been proved to reduce the duration of mechanical ventilation. Preference should be given to the daily interruption of sedation and the use of intermittent boluses, rather than continuous infusions, when tolerated.

MUSCLE PARALYSIS

Neuromuscular blocking agents have commonly been used in clinical practice for patients with marked ventilator asynchrony

and in a large but highly variable proportion of patients with ARDS. Current guidelines indicate that neuromuscular blocking agents are appropriate for facilitating mechanical ventilation when sedation alone is inadequate, most notably in patients with severe gas exchange impairment. The mechanisms by which these agents may benefit patients with ARDS are not completely understood but presumably involve improvement in patient-ventilator synchrony and limiting of excessive airway pressures. Prevention of barotrauma is another mechanism by which neuromuscular blockade may improve outcome.

Previous publications suggesting that the use of neuromuscular blockade agents may lead to increased incidence of ICU-acquired weakness or other complications raised concerns about long-term side effects with routine use of paralytic agents for ARDS. However, the latest information on the use of neuromuscular blockade in the treatment of patients with severe ARDS showed promising results. In a multicenter, double-blind trial conducted in France, 340 patients with severe ARDS within the previous 48 hours were randomly assigned to receive, for 48 hours, either the neuromuscular blocking agent cisatracurium besylate (178 patients) or placebo (162 patients). Severe ARDS was defined as a PaO_2/FIO_2 ratio less than 150 mm Hg, with a PEEP of 5 cm H_2O or less and a tidal volume of 6 to 8 mL/kg of predicted body weight. The primary outcome was death either before hospital discharge or within 90 days after study enrollment, as reflected in the 90-day in-hospital mortality rate. The hazard ratio for death at 90 days in the cisatracurium group, as compared with the placebo group, was 0.68 ($P = .04$) after adjustment for both the baseline PaO_2/FIO_2 and plateau pressure. The crude 90-day mortality rate was 31.6% in the cisatracurium group and 40.7% in the placebo group ($P = .08$); the mortality rate at 28 days was 23.7% with cisatracurium and 33.3% with placebo ($P = .05$). In addition, treatment with the neuromuscular blocking agent cisatracurium for 48 hours early in the course of severe ARDS increased the numbers of ventilator-free days and days outside the ICU, and decreased the incidence of barotrauma during the first 90 days. The rates of ICU-acquired neuromuscular weakness did not differ significantly between the two groups. Additional work is needed to determine whether the use of neuromuscular blocking agents for only 48 hours is beneficial in selected patients. The beneficial effect of the neuromuscular blocking agent on survival was confined to the two thirds of patients with a PaO_2/FIO_2 ratio below 120 mm Hg.

FLUID MANAGEMENT IN ACUTE RESPIRATORY DISTRESS SYNDROME

Until recently, the optimal strategy for fluid management in patients with ARDS was unclear. Animal and human data suggest that when lung capillary permeability increases, lung water accumulates to a greater degree than usual at lower pulmonary artery occlusion pressures. Human trials show improved physiologic end points with various diuretic approaches to reduce lung water, including diuresis without vascular pressure measurements, intravascular pressure–targeted diuresis, and diuresis guided by direct measurements of lung water. Abundant data suggest that prompt resuscitation of hemodynamically unstable patients improves outcome, whereas the same resuscitative efforts given later may not be helpful and may potentially be harmful.

The ARDSNet published in 2006 the results of a large randomized trial comparing two fluid management strategies in 1000 patients with ALI or ARDS. Subjects were randomized to management with either a conservative (−136 ± 491 mL) or a liberal (6992 ± 502 mL) approach. In other words, the conservative fluid management group had a net fluid balance of about zero over the first 7 days of the protocol, whereas the liberal fluid management group had an average daily fluid gain of approximately 1 L. Fluid and diuretic management was dictated by a highly protocolized regimen, and all patients received respiratory support using a low-tidal-volume, plateau pressure–limited ventilation strategy. Although no significant difference was noted in the primary outcome of 60-day mortality, the conservative approach improved lung function and shortened the duration of mechanical ventilation and ICU stay without increasing the rate of nonpulmonary organ failure. These data provide reassurance and support for the use of a conservative fluid management strategy in patients with ARDS.

CORTICOSTEROIDS

Corticosteroids would seem to be an ideal therapy for ALI, in view of their potent antiinflammatory and antifibrotic properties. Several clinical trials have evaluated the utility of corticosteroids in preventing ARDS and in treating either early-stage (inflammatory) or late-stage (fibrotic) ARDS. None of them have demonstrated a mortality benefit. Despite failed studies of prevention or early treatment, great interest remains in the use of corticosteroids for so-called salvage therapy in patients with persistent ALI. The ARDSNet performed the largest randomized, blinded trial of methylprednisolone versus placebo in patients with ARDS of at least 7 days' duration. No survival benefit was noted in the steroid group (29.2% versus 28.6%); however, methylprednisolone increased the number of ventilator-free days, shock-free days, and ICU-free days during the first month. Also, it was associated with a significant increase in 60-day and 180-day mortality rates among patients enrolled after 13 days from onset of ARDS. This study argues against the use of corticosteroids to treat patients with ARDS. However, a metaanalysis of selected trials showed that prolonged administration of systemic steroids is associated with favorable outcomes and a survival benefit when given before day 14 after onset of ARDS. The latter finding prevailed when data for subgroups from the ARDSNet were reanalyzed according to time of treatment initiation. Nevertheless, the questionable benefit of steroids in patients with ARDS should not preclude the use of a low-dose regimen in acutely ill patients with sepsis, including those with ARDS.

PROGNOSIS AND LONG-TERM SURVIVAL

Prognosis with ARDS depends primarily on the underlying cause of lung injury. In an analysis of the ARDSNet database, survival to home discharge was lowest in patients with sepsis, intermediate in patients with pneumonia, and highest in patients with trauma and ARDS.

Very few studies have evaluated the long-term outcome of patients with ARDS. Patients who are treated for this condition often face long-term physical and psychological complications that result from their prolonged hospitalization. Studies have considered long-term outcomes in patients with ARDS in terms of respiratory function, exercise tolerance, loss of muscle mass, and cognitive effects. In 2001, a 1-year follow-up study of patients with ARDS in the United States found that a significant percentage of deaths occurred between day 28 and 4 months, which raised the potential for longer monitoring in the evaluation of new interventions or therapies. One-year

predictors of death were advanced age and the premorbid functional status. Anxiety, depression, and posttraumatic stress disorder were frequent in that study.

Patients with ARDS lose a significant amount of body weight during their hospital stay. Most patients gradually recover this weight but still remain below admission weight after 12 months. In addition, most patients complain of proximal muscle weakness, with a decrease in distance covered on the 6-minute walk test. A long-term prospective study from Canada found that patients exhibited impairment on pulmonary function testing, seen as a mild restrictive pattern, with subsequent clinical improvement over the course of a year to near-normal levels. No patients required oxygen at rest after 12 months, and only 6% of patients required oxygen with ambulation. Similarly, marked impairment in exercise tolerance is typical; with the reestablishment of muscle mass, however, this impairment levels off by the end of 1 year, but no significant gains were made in the second year. Radiographic abnormalities were present in 80% of cases at 12 months. Of note, half of all patients who contracted ARDS had returned to work by 1 year, with most returning to their original employment position.

On the basis of this cumulative evidence, a patient surviving hospitalization for ARDS can be expected to return to a similar lifestyle over the course of a year, with some lingering physical and psychological challenges. Therefore, in the absence of significant comorbid conditions, the long-term outcome data are sufficient to warrant aggressive treatment for ARDS.

CONTROVERSIES AND PITFALLS

In patients with acute coronary syndromes, the working diagnosis is based on the presence of acute chest pain that is accompanied by abnormalities on the electrocardiogram (ECG) and the biomarker troponin. Troponin is the biomarker for detection of heart injury, and troponin levels serve as the basis for risk stratification and therapeutic interventions in patients with coronary artery disease. By contrast, pathognomonic laboratory or clinical features are lacking in patients with ARDS. There are no data that link a particular PaO_2/FIO_2 ratio to predictable structural changes in the alveolar-capillary membrane, probably because ARDS represents a common pathway of diverse events and disease entities. Also, current guidelines for ARDS management do not follow a strict stratification, as used in patients with coronary artery diseases. Stratification of respiratory and ventilatory variables at the onset of ARDS could be a useful strategy for identifying and selecting patients for clinical trials with various levels of mortality risk. Using demographic, pulmonary, and ventilatory data collected at ARDS onset, a simple prediction model based on a stratification of variables into low, intermediate, and high categories of risk assists in predicting patient outcome. Tertile distribution for age, plateau airway pressure, and PaO_2/FIO_2 ratio at ARDS onset is able to identify subgroups with markedly different mortality rates.

Lack of specific knowledge of the molecular mechanisms responsible for ARDS represents the most important obstacle to the successful diagnosis and treatment of affected patients. In comparing the management of acute chest pain with ARDS, the former is based on an emergency medical model of awareness of a life-threatening condition and the importance of adherence to predefined decision algorithms. No comparable awareness and emergency decision algorithms are available for the care of patients with ARDS. It is plausible that a new definition based on specific biochemical criteria of lung

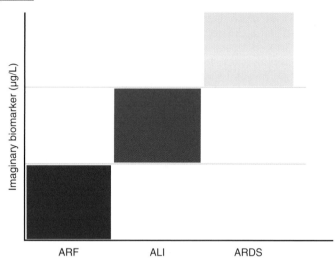

Figure 36-6 Use of a hypothetical biomarker for the diagnosis of ARDS. *ALI*, acute lung injury; *ARDS*, acute respiratory distress syndrome; *ARF*, acute respiratory failure.

inflammation, rather than on clinical parameters, is likely to provide clinicians with a better stratification and identification of a more homogeneous population of patients with ALI and ARDS. Thus, stratification of patients with ARDS should be linked to two measures of severity: one that specifically quantifies the severity of ALI and ARDS and another that quantifies the overall physiologic response along with comorbidity and premorbid health. Adding objective measures, such as levels of biologic markers, could facilitate recognition of ALI and ARDS.

The use of simple thresholds for the diagnosis of disease processes of increasing prevalence in the general population is common. This is the case with the use of blood sugar for diabetes and hemoglobin for anemia. It appears improbable that in the case of ARDS, a biomarker alone will resolve this issue. Instead, a clinical prediction model or a combination of such a predictor model with a biomarker would provide a better definition of ALI and ARDS (**Figure 36-6**). Ideally, such a biomarker should be (1) 100% sensitive, (2) 100% specific, (3) easy to measure in blood, exhaled air, or any other biologic sample, (4) affected by treatment, and (5) cost-effective. There have been recent efforts to identify biologic markers in pulmonary edema fluid and in blood collected from patients with and without ARDS. It has been postulated that owing to increased permeability of the alveolar-capillary barrier, proteins leak into the circulation. Patients at risk for ARDS who have higher levels of interleukin-8 in bronchoalveolar lavage fluid subsequently progress to ARDS. Serial LBP measurements may offer a clinically useful biomarker for identification of patients likely to experience the worst outcomes and with the highest probability for development of sepsis-induced ARDS. A combination of biologic markers that reflect endothelial and epithelial pulmonary injury, inflammation, and coagulation will be superior to clinical predictors or biomarkers alone for predicting

mortality or stratifying patients with ALI or ARDS. Finally, serial elevation of plasma levels of functionally relevant cell proteins (above a critical threshold) could be used for the differential diagnosis for ALI and ARDS. The measure of those biomarkers may inform clinicians of the development of ALI or ARDS.

An interesting direction for research would be identification of reliable biomarkers that are specific for the noninfectious, septic-like syndrome of VILI. It is hoped that the rapidly evolving sciences of genomics, proteomics, and computational biology can be used to model VILI and to tailor mechanical ventilation strategies to create an ideal inflammatory environment for minimal injury, tissue repair, cell regeneration, and organ function. Such a strategy would not only mitigate VILI but also decrease the incidence of other ventilator-induced complications.

SUGGESTED READINGS

Ashbaugh DG, Bigelow DB, Petty TL, Levine BE: Acute respiratory distress in adults, *Lancet* 2:319–323, 1967.

Bernard GR, Artigas A, Brigham KL, et al: Consensus Committee: The American-European Consensus Conference on ARDS, *Am J Respir Crit Care Med* 149:818–824, 1994.

Briel M, Meade M, Mercat A, et al: Higher vs lower positive end-expiratory pressure in patients with acute lung injury and acute respiratory distress syndrome: systematic review and meta-analysis, *JAMA* 303:865–873, 2010.

Murray JE, Matthay MA, Luce JM, Flick MR: An expanded definition of the adult respiratory distress syndrome, *Am Rev Respir Dis* 138:720–723, 1988.

Sud S, Friedrich JO, Taccone P, et al: Prone ventilation reduces mortality in patients with acute respiratory failure and severe hypoxemia: systematic review and meta-analysis, *Intensive Care Med* 36:585–599, 2010.

Tomashefski JF Jr: Pulmonary pathology of acute respiratory distress syndrome, *Clin Chest Med* 21:435–466, 2000.

Ventilation with lower tidal volumes as compared with traditional tidal volumes for acute lung injury and the acute respiratory distress syndrome. The Acute Respiratory Distress Syndrome Network, *N Engl J Med* 342:1301–1308, 2000.

Villar J, Kacmarek RM, Pérez-Méndez L, Aguirre-Jaime A: A high positive end-expiratory pressure, low tidal volume ventilatory strategy improves outcome in persistent acute respiratory distress syndrome: a randomized, controlled trial, *Crit Care Med* 34:1311–1318, 2006.

Villar J, Pérez-Méndez L, Basaldúa S, et al: HELP network: Age, plateau pressure and PaO$_2$/FIO$_2$ at ARDS onset predict outcome, *Respir Care* 56, 2011.

Villar J, Pérez-Méndez L, Kacmarek RM: Current definitions of acute lung injury and the acute respiratory distress syndrome do not reflect their true severity and outcome, *Intensive Care Med* 25:930–935, 1999.

Villar J, Pérez-Méndez L, López J, et al: HELP Network: An early PEEP/FIO$_2$ trial identifies different degrees of lung injury in patients with acute respiratory distress syndrome, *Am J Respir Crit Care Med* 176:795–804, 2007.

Ware LB, Matthay MA: The acute respiratory distress syndrome, *N Engl J Med* 342:1334–1349, 2000.

Chapter **37**

Upper Airway Disease: Rhinitis and Rhinosinusitis

Glenis K. Scadding • Harsha H. Kariyawasam

UPPER AIRWAY

The upper airway is a continuous structure that extends from the nasal vestibule to the alveolar units of the lung. Although the airway traditionally has been divided into upper and lower segments by an arbitrary line drawn at the level of the vocal cords, airway disease does not restrict itself to such specific anatomic regions. In fact, upper and lower airway disease frequently coexist, and upper airway manifestations of disease often can precede lower airway involvement. Such recognition has led to the sobriquet "the United Airway," with an emphasis on approaching patients with disease from a combined perspective on both the upper and lower airways.

RHINITIS

Rhinitis is defined as the presence of two or more symptoms of nasal discharge (anterior or posterior), blockage with sneeze, or itch for more than 1 hour on most days. It is an umbrella term that encompasses multiple diseases with distinct immunopathogenic mechanisms and correspondingly specific diagnostic and treatment strategies (**Figure 37-1**). Although rhinitis is subdivided into two broad categories of allergen-induced rhinitis and nonallergic rhinitis, disease overlap is common. Thus, a careful history and directed investigations are required to establish the exact diagnosis. In practice, inflammatory changes usually are continuous from nasal to sinus mucosa (see Figure 37-1); therefore, the designation *rhinosinusitis* is more accurate, although its use may lead to clinical confusion with the separate group of diseases that are historically classified under *sinusitis*. Apart from viral colds, allergic rhinitis (AR) is the most common cause of nasal symptoms.

EPIDEMIOLOGY, RISK FACTORS, AND PATHOPHYSIOLOGY

Allergic Rhinitis

Up to 30% of adults and 40% of children are affected, and worldwide the prevalence of AR continues to increase (**Figure 37-2**). The condition has marked effects on quality of life and is responsible for reduced school and workplace attendance (by 3% to 4%) and performance (by 30% to 40%). The resulting economic burden is high, and rhinitis and related AR are common. It is estimated that nearly 500 million people worldwide have AR, and it is one of the most common reasons for attendance with a primary care practitioner.

The predisposition to develop AR is both genetic and environmental. Identical monozygotic twins demonstrate a 40% to 50% concordance rate, whereas dizygotic twins have a 25% concordance rate. Thus, persons with an affected parent or sibling are at increased risk but as-yet undefined environmental factors must interact with genetic predisposition for disease occurrence. Western lifestyle seems to be associated with an increased prevalence of allergic disorders in general, including asthma and eczema. Studies to identify the exact genes involved are still limited in AR, and the findings have been difficult to interpret because of lack of replication in separate population cohorts. As in asthma, multiple genes are involved, many of which code for epithelial molecules concerned with innate immunity, suggesting that an impaired mucosal barrier is relevant to development of AR, as is now confirmed in eczema.

The key immunologic event that initiates AR is binding of allergen to specific IgE on mast cells found in the nasal mucosa. Cross-linking of two or more high-affinity IgE molecules in response to allergen binding leads to mast cell activation and degranulation with release of mediators, initiating an immune cascade (**Figure 37-3**). This is termed the immediate response. With the release of histamine, leukotrienes, prostaglandins, bradykinin, and other mediators (platelet-activating factor, substance P, tachykinins) comes the immediate onset of symptoms of sneezing, itching, and "running," typically seen in instances of intermittent allergen contact—for example, with hay fever. An additional immunologic event in up to 70% of affected persons is a further influx of inflammatory cells consisting predominantly of eosinophils, basophils, and T cells expressing T_H2 cytokines such as interleukin (IL)-4 (B cell IgE class switching) and IL-13 (mucus hypersecretion). Clinically this process is characterized by further obstruction, decreased olfaction, and mucosal irritability with immunopathologic changes similar to those seen in chronic asthma (see Figure 37-3). Local mucosal allergen–specific IgE production by nasal B cells is now confirmed and leads to local (skin prick test–negative) rhinitis. Emerging evidence also indicates that activated nasal epithelium–derived cytokines such as thymic stromal lymphopoietin (TSLP), IL-25 (i.e., IL-17E), and IL-33 can further promote disease through initiation, enhancement, and maintenance of T_H2 inflammation at the mucosal surface where allergen deposition and sampling occur. In addition, the potential for innate mucosal immune mechanisms such as Toll-like receptor (TLR) signaling system to drive or skew T_H2 responses is increasingly recognized.

Common aeroallergens that can initiate AR include plant pollen, house dust mite, fungal spores, cockroach aeroallergens, and dander from domestic pets. AR was formerly categorized as seasonal, perennial, and occupational; however, the World Health Organization (WHO) Allergic Rhinitis and Impact in Asthma (ARIA) guidelines suggest that intermittent and persistent rhinitis are better subdivisions, because they are globally applicable, even in geographic regions that lack specific seasons.

In the United Kingdom and other North European countries, symptoms in the spring are frequently caused by allergy to tree pollens. The peak period for tree pollens ranges from mid-February for alder to early April. Silver birch, oak, ash, elm, willow, and poplar release pollen from late March or early April to the middle of May. Pine trees pollinate from late April to early July. In late spring and early summer—the classic hay fever season—AR results from allergy to grasses such as rye, timothy, and cocksfoot. In late summer, weed pollens, such as nettle and mugwort, are responsible, whereas in autumn, the fungi *Cladosporium* spp., *Alternaria* spp., and *Aspergillus* spp.

provoke symptoms. In the United States, ragweed pollen allergy is a common cause of rhinitic symptoms, usually from mid-August to mid-September. Grass pollen is the most common seasonal allergen in the United Kingdom, and symptoms correlate with the presence of high airborne pollen counts.

Perennial rhinitis—in which symptoms occur throughout the year—in the United Kingdom most commonly is caused by allergy to the fecal pellets of the house dust mite (*Dermatophagoides pteronyssinus*), which flourishes in warm, humid environments and lives in bedding and soft furnishings. The major house dust mite allergen *Der p 2* is now recognized as demonstrating molecular mimicry to the mammalian lipid-binding protein (LBP) MD-2. This feature allows *Der p 2* to bind bacterial lipopolysaccharide (LPS) airway TLR-4 signaling complex, which is highly expressed on epithelium, and facilitates TLR signaling. Such signaling is important for the development of allergen-driven T_H2 signaling pathways. Allergy to dander from domestic pets (such as cats, dogs, rabbits, and hamsters) can account for perennial rhinitis, whereas allergens encountered in the workplace are responsible for occupational rhinitis. Examples are sensitization to latex, flour, and grain (bakers); allergies to small mammals among laboratory workers; and allergy to wood dust, biologic products (such as antibiotic powder and enzyme-enhanced detergents), and rosin (colophony) from solder flux.

Constant or very-high-level allergen contact produces chronic obstructive symptoms, with reduced olfaction and nasal hyperreactivity, the allergic nature of which may not be recognized, because hyperreactivity to nonspecific irritants, such as inhaled fumes, dusts, and cold air, may lead to an erroneous diagnosis of "vasomotor" rhinitis. True food allergy is rarely the cause of isolated rhinitis but may be relevant in small children with multisystem allergy.

Infectious Rhinitis

The nasal and sinus mucosa can be infected by all types of organisms: viruses, bacteria, fungi, and protozoa. Of such infections, viral infections are the most frequent.

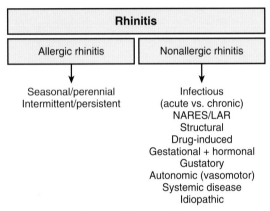

Figure 37-1 Classification of rhinitis. *NARES/LAR*, nonallergic rhinitis with eosinophilia syndrome/local allergic rhinitis.

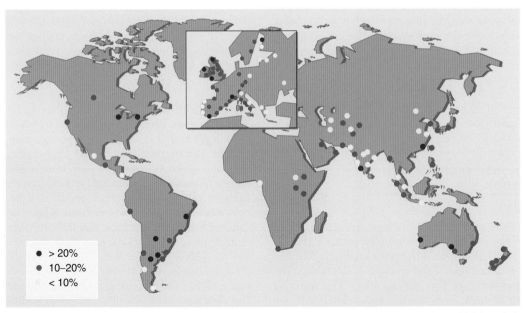

Figure 37-2 Global prevalence of hay fever in 13- to 14-year-olds. *(From Strachan D, Sibbald B, Weiland S, et al: Worldwide variations in prevalence of symptoms of allergic rhinoconjunctivitis in children: the International Study of Asthma and Allergies in Childhood [ISAAC],* Pediatr Allergy Immunol *8:161–176, 1997.)*

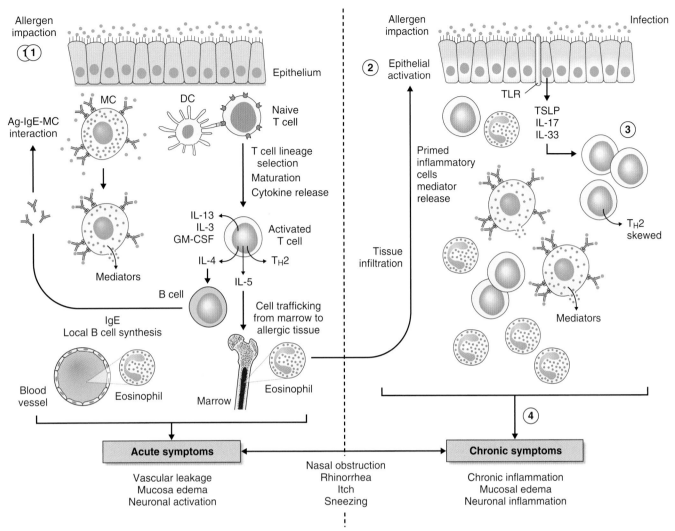

Figure 37-3 Immunopathogenesis of allergic rhinitis. 1, Allergen impaction on the mucosal surface leads to its solubilization and diffusion to sites of mast cell (MC) residence, where cross-linking of two or more high-affinity (FcεRI) IgE receptors lead to MC activation and subsequent degranulation and release of mediators, such as histamine and leukotrienes, that initiate the immediate rhinitis symptoms (acute inflammation). Dendritic cells (DC) also take up allergen and present processed allergen peptide in the context of MHC class II to naive T cells, which then undergo activation, leading (2) to the release of T$_H$2 cytokines. IL-5 in particular is essential for the maturation, release, and trafficking of eosinophils from the bone marrow. 3, Intense cellular infiltration characterizes the late nasal response, which leads to (4) chronic inflammation of the epithelium and submucosa with structural cell activation, edema, and neural hyperreactivity. TLR signaling and epithelial activation, along with TSLP, IL-17, and IL-33 signaling, will further promote T$_H$2 signaling. Chronic symptoms of rhinitis develop. *Ag,* antigen; *GM-CSF,* granulocyte-macrophage colony-stimulating factor; *IgE,* immunoglobulin E; *IL,* interleukin; *MHC,* major histocompatibility complex; *TLR,* Toll-like receptor; *TSLP,* thymic stromal lymphopoietin.

The Common Cold (Acute Coryza)

Most people have approximately three colds per year, but small children have from six to eight. Humans spend 2 years of their lives with colds, of which 50% result from rhinoviruses, a further 20% from coronaviruses, and a further 20% from influenza virus, parainfluenza virus, adenoviruses, and respiratory syncytial virus; the remainder are caused by other viruses, including enteroviruses. Viral invasion occurs at the point of infection, usually in the posterior nasopharynx, and results in transient vasoconstriction of the mucous membrane, followed by vasodilatation and edema with mucus production. A leukocytic inflammatory infiltrate develops, followed by desquamation of mucous epithelial cells. Initially, a clear watery secretion is produced, but this is followed by epithelial desquamation with opacification of secretions—not necessarily an indication of bacterial infection, which complicates only approximately 2% of colds. Resolution occurs in a few days in uncomplicated viral infections; however, compared with nonatopic persons,

allergic patients have more colds of greater severity. With rhinovirus infections in asthmatic children exposed to allergens to which they are sensitized, the odds ratio for hospitalization with asthma approaches 20.

Nonallergic Rhinitis

Nonallergic, Noninfectious Rhinitis

By definition, patients with nonallergic rhinitis (NAR) are skin prick–negative for common aeroallergens. NAR occurs in around 25% of persons with rhinitis symptoms. However, mixed rhinitis (a combination of allergic and nonallergic forms) can occur in up to 44% to 87% of patients. NAR incidence is higher in women. The nonallergic form of rhinitis incorporates a very heterogeneous group of conditions, and it is possible to further subclassify NAR into etiologic subtypes: a group for which the etiology is known and one for which it cannot be established, termed idiopathic rhinitis. The latter type is a diagnosis of exclusion, and approximately 60% of NAR cases will

Box 37-1 Differential Diagnosis for Rhinitis

Polyps
Mechanical factors
    Deviated septum
    Adenoidal hypertrophy
    Foreign bodies
    Choanal atresia
Tumors
    Benign
    Malignant
Granulomas
    Wegener granulomatosis
    Sarcoid
    Infectious
    Malignant-midline destructive granulomas
Ciliary defects
Cerebrospinal rhinorrhea

Box 37-2 Drugs Commonly Associated With Rhinitis*

Known Mechanism
Inflammatory
Aspirin and nonsteroidal antiinflammatory drugs (NSAIDs)

Neuronal
Peripherally acting sympatholytics:
Doxazosin
Prazosin
Indoramin
Phentolamine
Guanethidine
Centrally acting sympatholytics:
Methyldopa
Clonidine
Reserpine
Ganglion-blocking sympatholytics:
Trimethaphan

Vasodilator (phosphodiesterase inhibition)
Sildenafil

Unknown Mechanism/Idiopathic
Psychotropics
Chlordiazepoxide
Risperidone
Amitriptyline

Antihypertensives/Other
Beta blockers (including ocular formulation)
Angiotensin-converting enzyme inhibitors
Calcium channel blockers
Amiloride
Hydralazine

Hormones
Estrogen/oral contraceptives

*Although it is possible to explain the mechanism of drug-induced rhinitis for certain groups of medications, several other types of drugs have an as-yet unexplained mechanism.

fall into this category. A summary of considerations in the differential diagnosis for NAR is presented in **Box 37-1**. An essential division is between NAR with eosinophilic inflammation in the upper airway and that without.

Nonallergic Rhinitis with Eosinophilia Syndrome

Nonallergic rhinitis with eosinophilia syndrome (NARES) was described in 1981. The presence of eosinophils in nasal smears (more than 5% to 25%, according to different authorities) characterizes NARES, which probably is the counterpart of intrinsic asthma and may precede nasal polyposis and aspirin sensitivity. It typically is rapidly responsive to topical nasal corticosteroids. Recent progress in identifying local airway mucosal production of allergen-specific IgE has implications for future disease classification, and an entity termed *local allergic rhinitis* (LAR) has been described recently. What overlap NARES will have with LAR is not yet defined, but it is likely that with further investigation of these two NAR subtypes, common disease mechanisms will be found and the classification terminology will change further.

Aspirin hypersensitivity, or aspirin-exacerbated respiratory disease (AERD), develops usually in adult life in patients with rhinitis (often NARES), with subsequent development of nasal polyps and asthma. Mast cell and eosinophil degranulation are seen in biopsy specimens, and polyclonal local IgE production stimulated by superantigens from staphylococci has been described. Cyclooxygenase-1 (COX-1) inhibition by aspirin or other nonsteroidal antiinflammatory drugs (NSAIDs) promotes leukotriene production, while inhibiting that of prostaglandins, including PGE_2, a bronchodilator. Leukotrienes cause bronchoconstriction, mucosal swelling, and excess mucus production, and sensitivity to their effects is high in aspirin sensitivity, probably because of increased numbers of specific receptors. The clinical picture often is one of aggressive eosinophilic polyposis, severe asthma with life-threatening reactions to aspirin and other NSAIDs, and frequent need for oral corticosteroids. A subgroup reacts also to "E number" foods (i.e., additives and preservatives, such as sulfites in wine), as well as high-salicylate foods such as some herbs, spices, dried fruit, and jams.

Nonallergic Rhinitis Without Eosinophilia
Autonomic Rhinitis The nasal mucosa receives a rich efferent innervation from both the parasympathetic and sympathetic nervous system. Nasal glandular secretion is largely mediated by the parasympathetic fibers, the main postganglionic neurotransmitter being acetylcholine (ACh) acting through muscarinic receptors (predominantly the M_3 subtype). The sympathetic fibers mediate vascular tone and can regulate nasal airflow by potent effects on venous erectile tissue. The primary neurotransmitter is norepinephrine (noradrenaline). In autonomic rhinitis, there is no evidence of nasal inflammation, but of autonomic dysfunction or imbalance. Nasal and, in some patients, cardiovascular reflexes are abnormal, and there may be association with the chronic fatigue syndrome. Topical ipratropium is useful in decreasing watery rhinorrhea; capsaicin applications also may relieve symptoms for several months after a few weeks of treatment. Epinephrine (adrenaline) and other sympathomimetics lead to vasoconstriction of the nasal mucosa, with increased nasal patency. Both α- and β-adrenergic blockers increase nasal resistance and can produce symptoms of nasal stuffiness (**Box 37-2**). Stimulation of the parasympathetic system leads to an increase in nasal secretions. However, patients who have this condition also have increased responsiveness to both histamine and methacholine, which results in nasal blockage and rhinorrhea. It also is associated with hypertrophy of the inferior turbinates, and nasal polyps are sometimes present. Certain stimuli such as cold air, exercise, mechanical or thermal factors, and humidity changes result in rhinorrhea and other symptoms of rhinitis, and a period of nasal

hyperresponsiveness often follows viral infection. This observation is consistent with general neuronal dysregulation leading to excessive and troublesome neural hyperreactivity and imbalance with certain environmental exposures.

Drug-Induced Rhinitis

The main drugs implicated in pharmacologic rhinitis are listed in Box 37-2. This entity is mostly noninflammatory—for example, antihypertensives, particularly beta blockers, can cause nasal obstruction by abrogation of the normal sympathetic tone, which maintains nasal patency. Exogenous estrogens in oral contraceptives or hormone replacement therapy also evoke rhinitis in some patients. Overuse of α-agonists results in rhinitis medicamentosa: a tachyphylaxis of α-receptors to extrinsic and intrinsic stimuli. The mucosa becomes swollen and reddened. Aspirin hypersensitivity is an inflammatory form of drug-induced rhinitis (see earlier).

Hormonal Rhinitis

Hormonal rhinitis is seen in pregnancy, occasionally in relation to menstruation, and at puberty. Rhinitis is more common in the later stages of pregnancy and may be more frequent in women who smoke. The exact pathogenesis is unknown, but the effects of estrogens on nasal mucosal homeostasis in relation to vascular tone and glandular secretion are relevant, with the potential for effects on nasal tissue remodeling as well. The symptoms disappear soon after the affected woman gives birth. Chronic nasal obstruction is associated with hypothyroidism and acromegaly.

Food-Induced Rhinitis

Gustatory Rhinitis

Rapid induction of nasal hypersecretion in relation to consumption of food, particularly spicy food, is termed gustatory rhinitis. Although the exact mechanism is uncertain, the stimulation of afferent neural fibers—for example, by capsaicin—leads to excessive efferent activation of parasympathetic nasal neural pathways. Thus, intranasal blockade of acetylcholine with an ipratropium spray before eating often is effective.

Food Allergen-Induced Rhinitis

Much rarer than is popularly supposed, food allergy rarely causes isolated rhinitis. In early infancy, milk or egg allergy can cause rhinitis as part of a spectrum that can include atopic dermatitis, gut symptoms, asthma, and failure to thrive. AR is sometimes accompanied by the oral allergy syndrome, in which sensitization to pollen results in oral reactivity to the same components in fresh fruit and vegetables. In Northern Europe, the reactions usually are mild, typically consisting of itching of the lips, mouth, and throat on consumption of the offending food; cooked food is tolerated without reaction, because the major allergen involved is heat-labile profilin. Southern Europeans, however, in whom the immune system recognizes lipid transfer proteins, can experience more severe reactions, including anaphylaxis. Allergy to food may be confused with food intolerance (in which IgE-mediated mechanisms are not involved). Some foods are rich in histamines (e.g., cheese, some fish, some wines) that may result in flushing, headache, and rhinitis and the same may occur with tyramine-rich foods (e.g., bananas). Food additives and coloring agents (such as sulfites, benzoates, and tartrazine) also may provoke reactions, especially in aspirin-sensitive subjects. Finally, alcohol or spicy, hot food containing capsaicin may irritate C fibers, thereby nonspecifically provoking rhinitic symptoms.

Atrophic Rhinitis

Atrophic rhinitis is characterized by atrophy of mucosa plus the bone beneath. The nose is widely patent, but crusting and an unpleasant odor are characteristic. *Klebsiella ozaenae* has been found in many patients, and cure with long courses of ciprofloxacin has been reported. Uncertain, however, is whether this condition is primarily infective. It may follow extensive surgery, radiation therapy, chronic granulomatous disease, or trauma. Possibly the primary problem is failure of normal mucociliary clearance mechanisms.

Granulomas/Vasculitis

A number of granulomatous diseases may involve the nose and sinuses as part of the generalized disease, and nasal symptoms may be the first manifestation. These include Wegener granulomatosis, Churg-Strauss syndrome, and sarcoidosis, particularly in persons of Afro-Caribbean ancestry. Mucous membrane infiltration and thickening with granulomas may be present and may involve the septum, inferior turbinates, and occasionally the sinuses. Nasal congestion is a prominent symptom, sometimes with epistaxis and marked crusting. Sufferers feel unwell, with fatigue and malaise. Infective granulomatous disease may involve the nose and sinuses; examples are tuberculosis, leprosy, syphilis, blastomycosis, histoplasmosis, and aspergillosis.

Occupational Rhinitis

Occupational rhinitis can be allergic or nonallergic, with the former nearly always preceding or developing concurrently with occupational asthma.

Idiopathic or Intrinsic Rhinitis

Idiopathic or intrinsic rhinitis is a diagnosis of exclusion, with no evidence for any of the aforementioned causes. Symptoms tend to be perennial, and local allergy has been suggested as a cause, on the basis of histologic findings of mast cells and eosinophils in resected turbinates and on positive responses to local nasal allergen challenge in a subgroup of patients. Direct release of mediators from mast cells or neurogenic mechanisms may be involved here. Finally, emotional factors may play a part, ranging from stress to sexual arousal that compounds nasal blockage and discharge to emphatic or consistent complaints of gross nasal symptoms, despite the absence of abnormal findings on examination. Such effects may be mediated through autonomic dysfunction. Gastroesophageal reflux extending above the vocal cords is thought to be a cause of rhinitis, especially in small children. Chronic exposure to dry air or occupational irritants—for example, those found in the shipbuilding industry—can lead to nasal mucosal changes, often with squamous cell abnormalities.

DIFFERENTIAL DIAGNOSIS FOR RHINITIS

A summary of considerations in the differential diagnosis for rhinitis is provided in Box 37-1. Neoplasms, foreign bodies, and trauma all can produce obstruction, pain, purulent discharge, and epistaxis. In adults, the possibility of neoplasm should always be considered in patients who have persistent symptoms, particularly if these are unilateral. In children, the presence of a foreign body should be considered if the nasal discharge is unilateral and foul-smelling. Local disease in the pharynx and larynx also may involve the nose and paranasal sinuses (e.g., enlarged adenoids), as may dental disease (e.g., maxillary dental root infection), which may spread to the maxillary sinus.

RHINOSINUSITIS

Evolutionary developments in humans have meant that the head is now held upright, so that sinuses, which reach down to the level of the top jaw, drain at the level of the nasal bridge, against gravity. This process is dependent on efficient mucociliary clearance and a patent ostiomeatal (sinus drainage point) complex and is easily compromised by mucosal swelling or mucociliary failure from any cause. The sinus drainage pathways are illustrated in **Figure 37-4**.

Rhinosinusitis, which means inflammation of the lining of the nose and sinuses, is another umbrella term that incorporates a large and heterogeneous group of upper airway disorders. It is a common condition, affecting up to 15% of the population in Western countries, and is associated with significant morbidity as well as substantial socioeconomic and health care costs.

The 2007 European position paper (EP₃OS-2007) defines rhinosinusitis as inflammation of the nose and paranasal sinuses characterized by two or more symptoms, one of which should be nasal obstruction (blockage, congestion) or nasal discharge (anterior or posterior), together with either facial pressure or pain or reduction in or loss of smell. Sinus and nasal examination accomplished by endonasal inspection or CT scanning is important to confirm the diagnosis. Sinusitis is subclassified as acute or chronic disease. *Chronicity* is arbitrarily defined by the persistence of symptoms beyond 12 weeks. Chronic rhinosinusitis (CRS) is further broadly subdivided into CRS without nasal polyps (CRSsNP) and with nasal polyps (CRSwNP).

Acute Rhinosinusitis

Acute rhinosinusitis (ARS) is common. It can be mild, moderate, or severe. Whereas a simple upper airway viral infection often will resolve after 5 days, with ARS the symptoms worsen by then or persist beyond 10 days. In the absence of confounding factors such as allergic inflammation or anatomic abnormalities, for example, full resolution is expected within a month.

Although the nose harbors bacteria, the sinuses normally are largely sterile, possibly because of the nitric oxide (NO) concentrations therein and continuous mucociliary clearance. ARS rarely occurs directly after trauma, dental infections, and diving into polluted water but usually arises from a bacterial infection secondary to the common cold. The mucous membranes of the nose and sinuses become swollen, which leads to blockage of the ostiomeatal complex and bacterial infection of the sinuses, particularly with *Haemophilus influenzae* and *Streptococcus pneumoniae*, with other causative bacteria identified as *Staphylococcus aureus*, *Moraxella catarrhalis*, *Streptococcus pyogenes*,

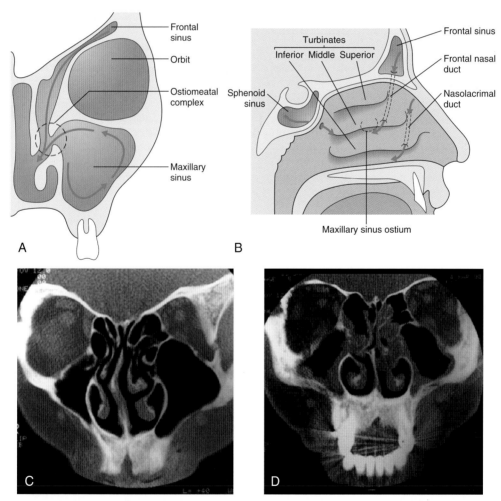

Figure 37-4 Sinus drainage pathways. **A** and **B**, In these diagrams, the ostiomeatal complex is seen to drain the frontal, anterior ethmoid, and maxillary sinuses. **A**, Coronal section. **B**, Lateral view. **C** and **D**, Computed tomography (CT) scans. **C**, On a coronal image, the paranasal sinuses are clear in a patient with a deviated nasal septum. **D**, On a lateral view, significant thickening of the mucosal lining is evident. CT changes do not correlate well with nasal symptoms but do relate to eosinophil counts in blood and sputum and to pulmonary function in accompanying asthma. (**C** and **D**, Courtesy Ian Mackay.)

and gram-negative bacteria such as *Klebsiella* and *Pseudomonas*. Anaerobic organisms also may be involved.

Chronic Rhinosinusitis

Failure to correctly subclassify the different subtypes of CRS has prevented confirmation of their exact incidence and prevalence, but CRS without nasal polyps (CRSsNP) accounts for a majority of cases seen.

Although CRS probably occurs after failure of resolution of ARS with the same bacterial pathogens involved, other factors often are present, such as eosinophilic inflammation (in both allergic and nonallergic forms of rhinosinusitis), immune deficiency (innate or adaptive), or structural abnormalities; the role of pathogens is disputed. One possibility is persistence of organisms as a biofilm that continually stimulates a damaging mucosal immune response.

Immune Defects

Panhypogammaglobulinemia is a severe condition with variable absence of all classes of immunoglobulin; it manifests with bacterial and other infections at many sites. Initial presentation may be to the otorhinolaryngologist with symptoms of recurrent acute or chronic rhinosinusitis. It is important to make the diagnosis early before irreversible damage occurs at other sites (the lungs) and so that appropriate immunoglobulin therapy can be instituted.

Total or relative *absence of IgA* may be present in the absence of any obvious clinical disease. However, IgA deficiency is now known to be associated in some patients with IgG2 subclass deficiency, and such persons may be more prone to episodes of sinusitis caused by encapsulated bacteria such as *H. influenzae* and *S. pneumoniae*.

Acute, chronic, and recurrent forms of sinusitis are common in persons with human immunodeficiency virus infection, the most common causative organisms being *S. pneumoniae* and *H. influenzae*. A tendency to chronicity and to relapse has been described, and in addition, fungal (*Cryptococcus* spp., *Alternaria* spp., and *Aspergillus* spp.) and viral (cytomegalovirus) sinusitis may occur.

Mucus Clearance Defects

The nose and paranasal sinuses are lined with ciliated epithelium, which in a coordinated fashion moves a mucus blanket toward the nasopharynx. This mucus is important for the entrapment and removal of particulate material and toxic substances, which include bacteria and allergens. The integrity of the mucociliary clearance pathway is vital to the appropriate drainage and ventilation of the paranasal sinuses and the nose (see Figure 37-4). Primary ciliary dyskinesia is inherited as an autosomal recessive trait and is characterized by the presence of sinusitis, bronchiectasis, situs inversus (Kartagener syndrome, present in 50% of these patients), and male infertility that results from dyskinetic sperm. Various ciliary structural defects have been described (e.g., absence of inner or outer dynein arms or both), but some cilia appear normal (Young syndrome). Recent work suggests that deficiency of inducible nitric oxide synthase (iNOS) may be the common underlying abnormality. Presentation is with chronic sinusitis, bronchiectasis or bronchitis, and obstructive azoospermia.

Secondary ciliary defects may arise after viral or bacterial infections. A number of mechanisms are involved:

- Mucous membranes become swollen and inflamed, which may result in blockage of the sinus ostia, thus preventing

clearance (this is particularly critical at the ostiomeatal complex).
- If viruses or bacteria damage the epithelial cell layer, the integrity of cilial clearance is destroyed.
- Some bacteria produce toxins that inhibit cilial clearance mechanisms.
- Mucus during infection becomes thick and difficult to clear.

Chronic Rhinosinusitis With Nasal Polyps

Chronic rhinosinusitis with nasal polyps (CRSwNP) represents a more distinct immune phenotype with better characterization. Nasal polyps (**Figure 37-5**) result from prolapse of the mucous membranes lining the nose and on examination are seen as pale, grapelike swellings arising predominantly from the middle meatus. These lesions are insensitive to pain but cause blockage and hyposmia and often are associated with asthma and aspirin hypersensitivity. They also may be infection-related, being common in persons with cystic fibrosis. Classification of polyps is similar to that of rhinitis (**Box 37-3**).

Nasal polyposis demonstrates a strong heritable component, with a relative risk of 18 times the normal rate of 4% in the population and 6 times the normal rate with an affected father and mother, respectively. A strong association of AERD with CRSwNP is recognized. A number of genes have been found to be associated with AERD (e.g., leukotriene C4 synthase promoter region); these vary among different populations. HLA-DQB1 is associated with allergic fungal sinusitis. The genetics of cystic fibrosis are discussed in Chapter 46; heterozygotes for cystic fibrosis are overrepresented in the chronic rhinosinusitis population. Primary ciliary dyskinesia is also genetic, with an incidence of approximately 1 in 20,000. Various structural ciliary defects have been described, but one

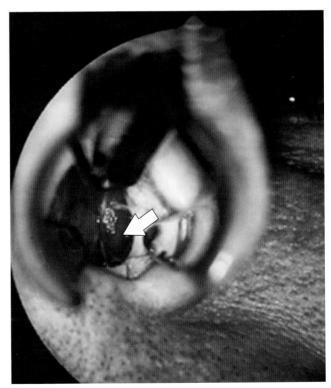

Figure 37-5 Speculum examination of nostril shows a pale watery-looking polyp (*arrow*). Polyps are insensate and grayish, unlike turbinates, which are sensitive and bluish pink. (*Courtesy St. Mary's Hospital Audio-Visual Department.*)

Box 37-3 Classification of Nasal Polyps

Allergic
(Eosinophil-rich; results of skin prick tests may be negative)
Allergic fungal
Sinusitis
Aspirin-sensitive
Churg-Strauss syndrome

Infective
(Neutrophil-rich)
Cystic fibrosis
Immune deficiency

Structural
Antrochoanal

Other
Malignancy

common defect—a lack of iNOS in nasal mucosa—has recently been found.

CLINICAL FEATURES

Allergic Rhinitis

AR manifests in two major patterns: (1) watery discharge, sneezing, or itching and (2) nasal blockage. Affected persons have been called "runners" (or "sneezers" or "itchers") and "blockers," respectively.

Running/Sneezing/Itching

With the "running/sneezing/itching" pattern of AR, symptoms tend to be intermittent and changeable and often are closely related to allergen exposure during the day. Severity varies, with symptoms ranging from trivial to extremely disabling. In addition, itching and injection of the conjunctivae may occur, with watery discharge and conjunctival swelling, and itching in the mouth, oropharynx, and ears. This form of AR tends to be a disorder of children and young adults, and up to one third of patients have associated asthma.

Blockage

The nasal passages are chronically obstructed, with little in the way of immediate allergic symptoms. Other symptoms may include facial ache, headache, nasal hyperreactivity, and loss of sense of smell. Examination of the nose reveals pale or bluish mucosa, which is boggy and swollen, and a watery discharge may be present. Careful clinical inspection of the nose is important to exclude the concomitant presence of polyps, septal deviation, prominent turbinates, and evidence of other systemic disease and tumors.

Secondary symptoms may include disturbed sleep, pharyngitis, poor concentration, cough, and exacerbation of lower respiratory tract problems.

Considerable overlap between causes of rhinitis is not uncommon, adding to the usual rhinitic symptoms; for example, AR characterized by sneezing, itching, and watery discharge results in considerable mucosal swelling, which may result in reduced sinus drainage and contribute to development of secondary infection. Both allergic and infective forms of inflammatory rhinosinusitis may be exacerbated by the presence of anatomic and mechanical defects, such as a deviated nasal septum or enlarged turbinates. It also is important to consider

the possibility of serious underlying conditions, early recognition of which may be necessary to prevent later damage (e.g., defects of immunity, impaired cilial motility, vasculitic and granulomatous disease).

Rhinosinusitis frequently is associated with lower respiratory disease; for example, approximately one third of patients who have bronchiectasis also have chronic sinusitis, and patients who have cystic fibrosis invariably have sinusitis and frequently have nasal polyps develop. Rhinitis is practically ubiquitous in asthmatic persons, with 10% of adults with late-onset asthma exhibiting aspirin hypersensitivity, often with nasal polyps (Samter's triad). Most asthma exacerbations begin with rhinitis, either infective or allergic, or both.

Nonallergic Rhinitis

Infection

Acute Coryza (The Common Cold) The prodrome of the common cold typically consists of a feeling of dryness, itching, and heat in the nose, which may last for a few hours and often is followed by a dry, sore throat; sneezing; watery nasal discharge; and constitutional symptoms of fever and malaise. This phase is followed in a day or so by symptoms of nasal obstruction and mucopurulent discharge, which along with the fever and malaise, may continue until resolution after 5 to 10 days. The initial symptoms of AR and coryza may be difficult to distinguish from each other.

NONINFECTIVE RHINITIS

Symptoms of noninfective rhinitis are similar to those of the blockage pattern of AR, as mentioned previously. Differentiation from AR depends on skin prick or other allergy testing.

Clinical Presentations That Warrant Physician Referral

Patients with unilateral symptoms, bloody discharge, polyps manifesting for the first time, or systemic illness should be seen by an otorhinolaryngologic surgeon. Orbital cellulitis and sinusitis with severe headache or vomiting warrant urgent referral.

Acute Rhinosinusitis

Acute maxillary rhinosinusitis is characterized by facial pain, localized to the cheek, but also present in the frontal area or around the teeth, that is made worse by stooping down or straining. The pain can be unilateral or bilateral, and tenderness may be elicited over the sinus. Acute frontoethmoidal sinusitis may cause pain around the eye and in the frontal region, with overlying tenderness and erythema of the skin. There is usually fever, and toxemia may occur. The differential diagnosis for facial pain is wide in scope and includes dental disease and the numerous causes of headache. Recently, all of the clinical signs and symptoms described here have been shown to be unreliable as diagnostic aids to identify acute sinusitis; instead, the combination of erythrocyte sedimentation rate (ESR) and C-reactive protein (CRP) is the best guide.

Chronic Rhinosinusitis

CRS frequently is pain-free and manifests with a sensation of congestion, poor concentration, tiredness, and malaise. Other signs and symptoms of CRS include purulent nasal discharge (often postnasal), sore throat, and a productive cough, especially in children, in whom misdiagnosis of asthma is not uncommon. Loss of the sense of smell and halitosis are additional features.

DIAGNOSIS, EVALUATION, AND TESTS

EXAMINATION

It frequently is possible to arrive at a diagnosis of rhinitis and rhinosinusitis on the basis of a good detailed history. Physical examination should never be omitted, and it is vitally important that chronic symptoms be appropriately investigated. Observation of the patient's face may reveal an allergic crease or salute, deviation of the nose from midline, or more sinister collapse of the nasal bridge.

Anterior rhinoscopy performed with use of a bright light or head mirror along with a Thudicum speculum allows simple examination of the anterior nasal cavity. In addition, the mucous membrane can be viewed, and the presence of nasal polyps and disorders of the anterior part of the nasal septum can be ascertained.

Nasal endoscopy performed using either a rigid or a fiberoptic flexible endoscope allows more detailed examination and assessment. Congenital defects such as cleft palate and atresia, septal deviation and perforation, abnormalities of the turbinates, compromised state of the mucous membranes, presence of purulent secretions, polyps, neoplasms, and foreign bodies can be identified with this examination.

Coryza

Coryza normally is diagnosed on the basis of the patient's history, and further investigations are rarely required. Viral culture or immunofluorescent techniques can identify specific viruses.

Acute Rhinosinusitis

On examination, red, swollen nasal mucous membranes are present, and pus may be seen in the middle meatus. Endoscopy, together with imaging techniques, allows assessment of the severity and extent of involvement (diagnostic antral puncture and lavage are now rarely required). Middle meatal swabs provide material for bacteriologic culture. Immunoglobulin classes and subclasses are checked in cases of recurrent or chronic sinusitis.

IMAGING TECHNIQUES

Radiography is rarely needed for diagnosis, unless a tumor is suspected. A high incidence of imaging abnormalities in the general population has been recognized: One third of unselected adults and 45% of children will have such abnormalities. After a cold, computed tomography (CT) scans show changes for at least 6 weeks. The role of imaging is largely to provide a road map for the surgeon after failure of medical treatment.

Since the advent of CT, plain sinus radiographs now have only a very limited role in the diagnosis of acute rather than chronic sinusitis, because opacification or a fluid level may be seen in a sinus or gross soft tissue swelling may be evident. The imaging investigation of choice is CT, which is the best technique to demonstrate mucosal disease and underlying anatomic abnormalities (see Figure 37-4). The detailed anatomy of both bone and soft tissue is well delineated, and axial and coronal sections can be obtained. The coronal cuts provide views of the ostiomeatal complex, important for planning surgery for acute and chronic sinusitis (**Figure 37-6**). Preoperatively, coronal sections at 3 to 4 mm give maximal anatomic detail, whereas axial views provide vital information regarding the relation of the optic nerve to the posterior ethmoidal and sphenoid sinuses. Magnetic resonance imaging (MRI) is of very limited value,

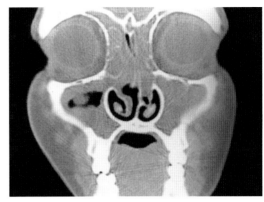

Figure 37-6 Computed tomography scan of paranasal sinuses. This coronal image shows almost complete opacification of maxillary and ethmoid sinuses with polyps that obstruct the ostiomeatal complex. *(Courtesy Ian Mackay.)*

because bone is not well imaged. MRI is useful, however, in distinguishing one type of soft tissue from another and has the advantage of avoiding irradiation.

MUCOCILIARY FUNCTION TESTING

For the simplest test, known as the saccharin clearance test, one quarter of a grain of saccharin is placed on the lateral nasal wall, 1 cm behind the anterior end of the inferior turbinate. A sweet taste is detected within 20 minutes if cilial function is normal—that is, the mucociliary mechanism is able to transport the particle to the nasopharynx and the pharynx, where taste is detected. If cilial function is abnormal, more sophisticated tests of cilial activity in cells detached by brushings taken from the turbinate can be undertaken with use of phase contrast microscopy. Significant abnormalities on this test constitute an indication for electron microscopic examination of cilia. Confirmation of reports of very low nasal NO in primary ciliary dyskinesia means that a nasal NO concentration of greater than 250 parts per billion (ppb) excludes this diagnosis with 95% sensitivity.

NASAL AIRWAY TESTS

Dynamic tests include nasal inspiratory peak flow measurement (for which the patient, wearing a mask attached to a peak flow meter, sniffs hard with a closed mouth) and rhinomanometry. The latter technique is used to assess nasal airway resistance by measuring airflow across a pressure gradient with use of a pneumotachograph and face mask. Acoustic rhinometry uses a sound pulse to measure the nasal cross-sectional area.

Nasal airway resistance can change very dramatically within a few minutes. Congestion is produced by engorgement of venous erectile tissue within the nose; the mucous membrane receives dense, autonomic innervation. Nasal resistance falls with administration of epinephrine and other sympathomimetic drugs but also with exercise, rebreathing, and adoption of the erect posture. Nasal resistance increases in rhinitis and, in some persons, with ingestion of alcohol, aspirin, and other drugs, as well as when the supine posture is adopted.

EVALUATION FOR SUSPECTED ALLERGIC RHINITIS

The diagnosis usually is obvious from a careful history and examination but can easily be missed in chronic blockers; thus, skin prick tests should be performed in all patients presenting to the rhinitis clinic. Skin tests that use allergen extracts to elicit IgE-mediated immediate hypersensitivity responses can be used to confirm or exclude atopy. If all of the skin test results are negative, the history may still suggest local nasal allergen-specific IgE driven disease. However, positive results on skin testing do not confirm the diagnosis, because many asymptomatic persons exhibit a positive response to common allergens. Correlation between skin prick tests and history should be sought, because occasionally it is possible to identify an allergen that can be avoided. Measurement of total IgE is not helpful; however, measurement of specific IgE levels to common aeroallergens by means of immunologic testing may be useful, and the results show a good correlation with skin test results. Occasionally, particularly where occupational rhinitis may be a possibility, nasal challenge and provocation tests (with the offending allergen, histamine, aspirin, or methacholine) may be required.

NASAL CYTOLOGY

It may be of value to determine the presence or absence of eosinophils in patients who have perennial rhinitis and negative results on skin testing and who are not atopic. Subsets of these patients have nasal eosinophilia and are more likely to demonstrate allergic features such as sneezing and congestion; they are more likely to respond to topical corticosteroids.

TREATMENT

ALLERGIC RHINITIS

Treatment for AR has five major components:

- Allergen avoidance
- Pharmacotherapy
- Immunotherapy
- Surgery (rarely)
- Patient education (vital)

Identify and Avoid Allergens

In practice, the identification and avoidance of allergens may be extremely difficult. House dust mites are responsible for much perennial AR. Mites flourish at temperatures of approximately 15°C and 60% to 70% relative humidity, conditions present in many homes that contain central heating. They flourish particularly in soft furnishings, mattresses, pillows, and bed covers, as well as in carpets. Allergen avoidance and measures to reduce the load (i.e., wooden floors rather than carpets, regular vacuum cleaning, and barrier covers for mattresses and pillows) effectively reduce rhinitic symptoms. Acaricides that kill the mites do not eliminate the antigen, which is present in the fecal pellets. Removal of a pet may not abolish symptoms, because allergens may persist in rooms for many months, if not years. Avoidance of pollen is difficult, but vacationing away from pollen areas or, failing that, staying indoors when the pollen count is high, closing windows, shutting car windows, and avoiding open grassy spaces may help.

Medical Suppressive Therapy

The classification system and treatment plan for AR according to ARIA are shown in **Figures 37-7** and **37-8**, respectively. Intermittent rhinitis is defined as that accompanied by symptoms for fewer than 4 days per week or fewer than 4 weeks in total. Persistent symptoms are defined as those present for more

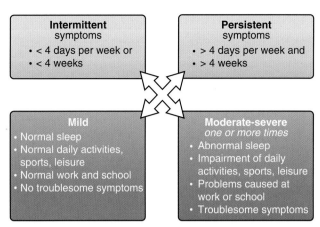

Figure 37-7 Classification of rhinitis by frequency and severity. *(From Bousquet J, Van Cauwenberge P, Khaltaev N, et al: Allergic rhinitis and its impact on asthma,* J Allergy Clin Immunol *108[suppl]:S147–S334, 2001.)*

than 4 days per week and lasting more than 4 weeks in total duration. Classification of disease severity as mild, moderate, or severe is based on effects on day-to-day well-being and ability to sleep or work. Thus, the diagnosis takes into account severity of disease in terms of effects on quality of life, as well as disease duration, which in turn guides pharmacotherapy and immunotherapy intervention. However, in view of the spectrum of respiratory diseases (i.e., NAR) that can manifest with rhinitis symptoms and the possible need for use of allergen-specific immunotherapy, the key concept of *seasonality* is very useful in the diagnostic algorithm and has been retained by several guidelines and standards of care documents such as that from the British Society for Allergy Clinical Immunology (BSACI).

Topical Corticosteroids

Metaanalysis has shown that topical corticosteroids constitute the most effective treatment for AR. Regular use is needed, and preseasonal dosing reduces development of seasonal rhinitis symptoms. For polyps or marked nasal blockage, betamethasone drops or oral corticosteroids for the first 2 weeks of therapy may be needed, followed by a nonabsorbable drop formulation of fluticasone propionate (Flixonase Nasule), particularly in the long term for polyp management (**Figure 37-9**). Side effects of topical corticosteroids include local irritation and minor epistaxis. Systemic steroid absorption is low except with betamethasone and dexamethasone, which should be reserved for only short-term use.

Sodium cromoglycate is less effective when given nasally but may be suitable for small children, whereas severe conjunctival symptoms are best treated with sodium cromoglycate or nedocromil sodium. Corticosteroid eye drops are to be avoided.

Antihistamines

Antihistamines provide excellent relief of sneezing, itching, and rhinorrhea, but not congestion; oral ones have the advantage of being effective for mouth and eye symptoms. Chlorpheniramine is best avoided because it is sedating and reduces driving ability and academic performance. Newer histamine H_1 antagonists are largely nonsedating. Certain molecules—terfenadine, astemizole, and diphenhydramine in particular—can produce QT prolongation and fatal cardiac arrhythmias, especially with high blood levels from overdosing or combination of an antihistamine with another hepatically metabolized drug. Fexofenadine, cetirizine, levocetirizine, and desloratadine seem safe

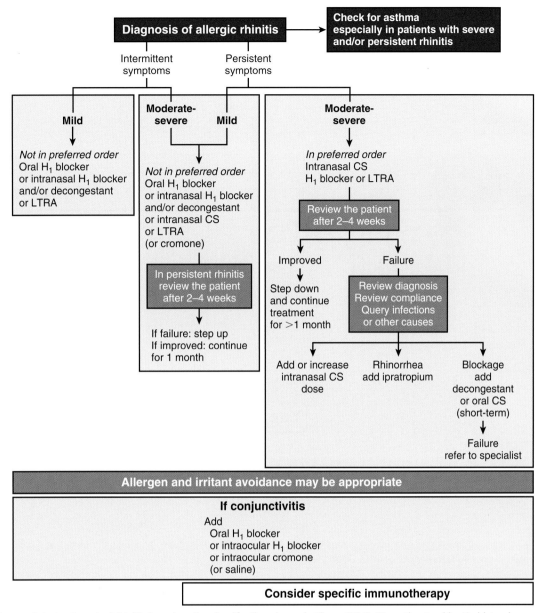

Figure 37-8 Approach to treatment of rhinitis based on the classification shown in Figure 37-7. *CS*, corticosteroids; *H₁*, histamine receptor type H₁; *LTRA*, leukotriene receptor antagonist. *(From Bousquet J, Khaltaev N, Cruz AA, et al: Allergic Rhinitis and Its Impact on Asthma [ARIA] 2008 update [in collaboration with the World Health Organization, GA[2]LEN and AllerGen], Allergy 63[Suppl 86]:8–160, 2008.)*

in this respect and possess some measurable nasal unblocking activity. Azelastine and levocabastine are useful topical antihistamines. Rupatadine can block both histamine and platelet-activating factor.

Other Agents

Vasoconstrictors are useful in the short term for relief of marked congestion, but long-term use must be avoided because of the risk of rhinitis medicamentosa. Anticholinergics such as ipratropium bromide may be useful if extensive, watery secretion is a major problem. Antileukotrienes are similar in efficacy to antihistamines for treatment of AR, with no major benefits from a combination of the two. In some patients with polyps, however, these agents can reduce symptoms and polyp size when used with a topical steroid. Douching the nose with isotonic saline can reduce AR symptoms and improve endoscopic appearance and quality of life in chronic rhinosinusitis.

Immunotherapy

Immunotherapy is the only treatment that has been shown to influence the course of disease. Three years of treatment reduces symptoms for several years thereafter. In children with rhinitis, subcutaneous immunotherapy reduces progression to asthma as determined by follow-up evaluation at 3, 5, and 10 years. Reduction in the rate of new allergic sensitization also has been noted.

Desensitization involves the administration of increasing doses of relevant allergen extract by subcutaneous injection over a period of months and has been shown to effectively diminish symptoms of allergic seasonal rhinitis in response to grass pollen, ragweed pollen, and birch pollen. Some studies also suggest efficacy with house dust mite and some animal danders. Desensitization has largely been superseded by the success of effective medical therapy in the suppression of allergic inflammation and is therefore reserved for nonresponders

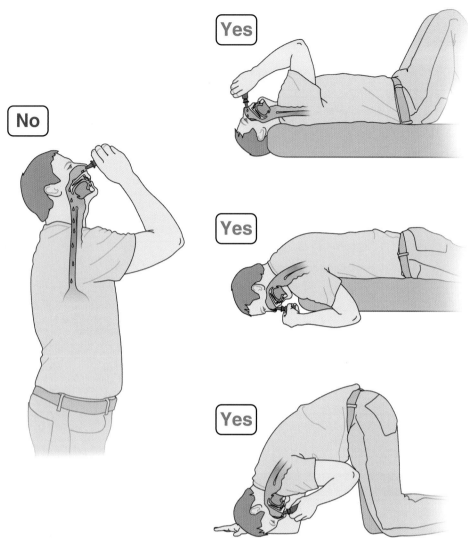

Figure 37-9 Correct instillation of nasal drops. *(Modified from Scadding GK, Durham SR, Mirakian R, et al: BSACI guidelines for the management of allergic and non-allergic rhinitis,* Clin Exp Allergy *38:19–42, 2008.)*

with severe disease. It is not always effective, and concerns have been raised regarding occasional anaphylactic reactions and deaths after the procedure, so it must be undertaken by well-trained personnel in a hospital setting with cardiorespiratory resuscitation facilities at hand.

Safer sublingual approaches have now been demonstrated to be effective, and grass pollen tablets are now available; trials with house dust mite sublingual preparations are ongoing. The first sublingual dose needs to be given under medical supervision; thereafter, each dose is taken every day at home. Eight weeks of preseasonal therapy followed by continuation throughout the pollen season is suggested, with subsequent continuation of this treatment for 3 years. However, pre- and co-seasonal therapy repeated over 3 years may suffice. The benefits of grass pollen sublingual immunotherapy last for at least 2 years after cessation of treatment.

Surgical Intervention

When medical treatment is only partly successful, a full otorhinolaryngologic assessment is performed, because correction of a deviated nasal septum or reduction of hypertrophied mucosa may help relieve the symptoms. With coexistent chronic sinus infection, functional endoscopic sinus surgery (FESS) techniques may be necessary to facilitate sinus drainage, aeration, and access for medications, although a recent study showed that medical therapy with corticosteroids and long-term macrolides was equally effective. Both resulted in improved control of concomitant asthma.

INFECTIONS

Acute Coryza (The Common Cold)

Treatment is essentially symptomatic, with analgesics, antipyretics, rest, and broad-spectrum antibiotics if secondary infection is present. Oral or topical nasal zinc may decrease symptoms and their duration.

NONINFECTIOUS CAUSES

Intrinsic Rhinitis

Anticholinergics (e.g., ipratropium bromide) are useful for troublesome rhinorrhea (i.e., intrinsic rhinitis) (**Figure 37-10**), particularly when eosinophils are absent from nasal secretions. When eosinophilia is present, a response to topical corticosteroid therapy is usual. α-Agonist decongestants, such as pseudoephedrine and xylometazoline, should be used sparingly. Surgical procedures may help if nasal obstruction is predominant.

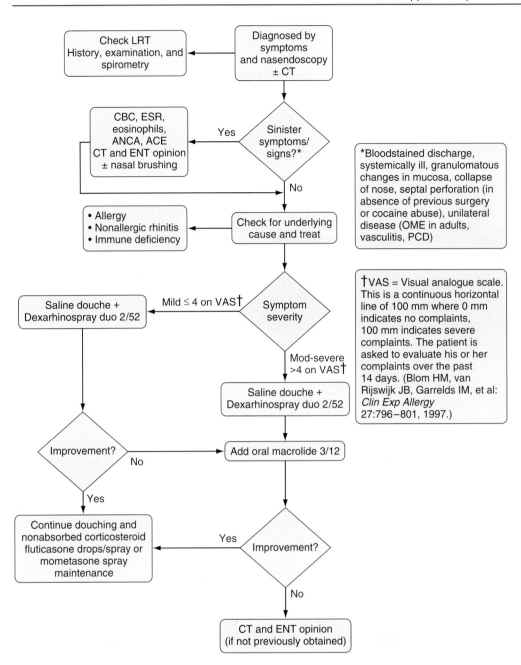

Figure 37-10 Management of chronic rhinosinusitis without nasal polyps (CRSsNP). *ACE*, angiotensin-converting enzyme; *ANCA*, antineutrophil cytoplasmic antibodies; *CBC*, complete blood count; *CT*, computed tomography; *ENT*, ear-nose-throat; *ESR*, erythrocyte sedimentation rate; *LRT*, lower respiratory tract; *OME*, otitis media with effusion; *PCD*, primary ciliary dyskinesia. *(Modified from Scadding GK, Durham SR, Mirakian R, et al: BSACI guidelines for the management of allergic and non-allergic rhinitis, Clin Exp Allergy 38:19–42, 2008.)*

Structural Defects

Occasionally, topical corticosteroid therapy may ameliorate rhinitis secondary to structural defects, but normally surgical correction is required.

Immune Defects

Therapy of immune-related rhinitis is directed toward correction of the underlying defect.

Mucus Clearance Defect

It is not possible to correct the underlying mucus clearance defect, so therapy relies on regular douching, improved drainage and aeration, and prevention of secondary infection.

Granulomas

Appropriate, specific antimicrobial therapy is required for infectious causes of granulomatous disease. Sarcoidosis that involves the nose responds to either local or systemic glucocorticoid therapy. Each case will require a specific targeted approach.

Drug-Induced Disease

A careful drug history must be taken and the incriminated drug excluded.

ACUTE RHINOSINUSITIS

Most cases of ARS resolve spontaneously. Analgesics and antipyretics provide symptomatic relief, but aspirin must be avoided in persons who may be hypersensitive. Acetaminophen (paracetamol) and codeine are satisfactory alternatives. Decongestants such as oxymetazoline and xylometazoline reduce edema but compromise mucociliary activity and are not recommended. Broad-spectrum antibiotics are appropriate for severe disease with a number needed to treat of 8. These antimicrobials must have activity against the most common pathogens, namely *S. pneumoniae*, *H. influenzae*, and *M. catarrhalis*. Agents such as amoxicillin, trimethoprim-sulfamethoxazole (co-trimoxazole), or a macrolide such as clarithromycin are appropriate. Amoxicillin-clavulanate has the added advantage of activity against *S. aureus* and penicillin-resistant *H. influenzae*. If anaerobic infection is suspected, a combination of amoxicillin-clavulanate and metronidazole or clindamycin may be used.

Recent evidence suggests that topical nasal corticosteroids help, either in conjunction with antibiotics or alone, to reduce symptom severity and hasten recovery. There is no suggestion that they lead to more recurrences or to more adverse events. In a number of rhinosinusitis scenarios, acute intervention will be required, as shown in the EPOS guidelines (**Figure 37-11, A** and *B*).

CHRONIC RHINOSINUSITIS

With CRS, the aims of treatment are to remedy any underlying cause (e.g., immunologic defect, anatomic abnormality that prevents drainage) and to restore the integrity of the mucous

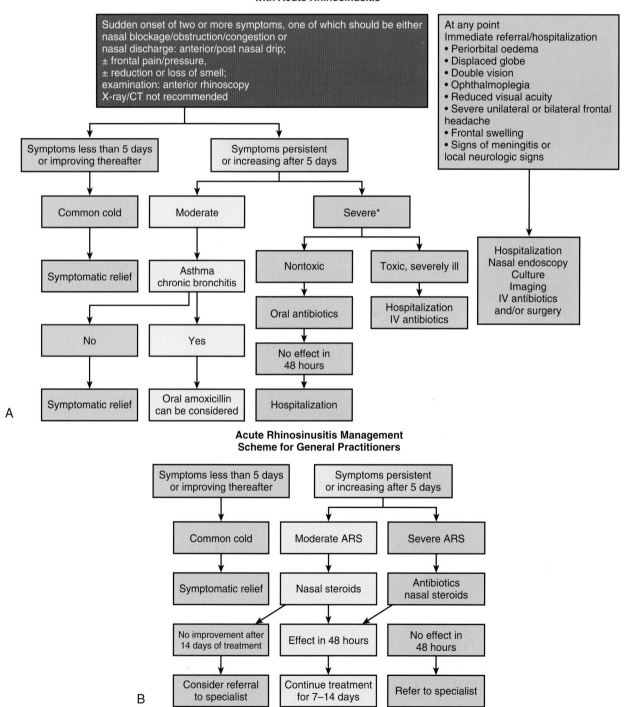

Figure 37-11 Treatment schemes for acute rhinosinusitis (ARS): **A**, in children; **B**, general approach. *CT,* computed tomography; *IV,* intravenous. (*From Fokkens W, Lund V, Mullol J, et al: European position paper on nasal polyps 2007,* Rhinology 45[Suppl 20]:1-136, 2007.)

membranes to allow normal ventilation of the sinuses and drainage. Nasal douching with saline relieves symptoms and improves the endoscopic appearance. Topical corticosteroids may help to reduce mucous membrane swelling and improve drainage. Initially, betamethasone drops taken in the head-down position (see Figure 37-9) are briefly used, but nonabsorbed fluticasone propionate (Flixonase Nasule) is safer for long-term use. Prolonged courses of macrolide antibiotics produced improvements equivalent to those achieved with FESS, possibly because of their antiinflammatory activity. Amphotericin douching is ineffective.

SURGICAL INTERVENTIONS FOR ACUTE AND CHRONIC RHINOSINUSITIS

Major changes have occurred in recent years as a result of the advent of high-resolution CT scans and FESS. Better demonstration of the nasal and sinus anatomy is achieved with CT scans, as well as of the important ostiomeatal complex, the vital region in which sinus drainage by mucociliary clearance occurs.

Obstruction in this zone is very important in the generation of chronic sinus disease. The main aim of FESS is to restore adequate drainage for the frontal, maxillary, and ethmoidal sinuses (see Figure 37-4). When this fails, more radical sinus surgery may be needed, but complete investigation for underlying medical factors (e.g., immune deficiency) should be undertaken first.

Nasal Polyps

Unilateral nasal polyps (**Figure 37-12**) warrant appropriate investigation to exclude transitional cell papilloma, squamous cell carcinoma, encephalocele, or other pathologic conditions. In the absence of contraindications and clinical suspicion regarding the nature of the polyp, a medical polypectomy accomplished with use of prednisolone (0.5 mg/kg, enteric-coated) plus betamethasone drops (two in each nostril three times a day with the head upside down) for 5 days, up to 14 days as indicated by clinical need, can be as effective as surgery and is superior with respect to control of concomitant asthma. This should be followed by long-term corticosteroid drops—

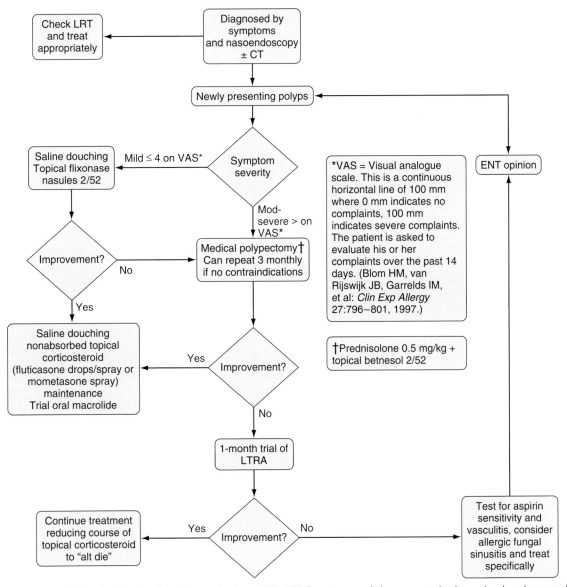

Figure 37-12 Treatment of chronic rhinosinusitis with nasal polyps (CRSwNP). Symptoms and signs are rated using a visual analogue scale. See Figure 37-10. *CT,* computed tomography; *ENT,* ear-nose-throat; *LRT,* lower respiratory tract; *LTRA,* leukotriene receptor antagonist. *(Modified from Scadding GK, Durham SR, Mirakian R, et al: BSACI guidelines for the management of rhinosinusitis and nasal polyposis,* Clin Exp Allergy *38:260–275, 2008.)*

initially betamethasone for 2 weeks, then almost nonabsorbed fluticasone propionate. Subsequently, a trial of a leukotriene receptor antagonist should be undertaken for 2 to 4 weeks, with continuation if beneficial. Other measures being evaluated include regular saline douching and topical lysine aspirin in patients sensitive to this on nasal challenge. Failure of medical treatment is an indication for surgery.

Patients with aspirin-exacerbated respiratory disease should be warned to avoid all COX-1 inhibitors and to watch for exacerbation by similar substances: "E number" foods, preservatives, high-salicylate foods. Most patients can tolerate paracetamol 500 mg or a COX-2 inhibitor.

CLINICAL COURSE AND PREVENTION

RHINITIS

Allergic Rhinitis

The clinical course in AR is variable. With good compliance, allergen avoidance, and regular pharmacotherapy, symptoms usually are minimal. Understandably, patients want a cure. Immunotherapy remains of limited value, but with development in understanding of the mechanism of generation of IgE responses and of ways in which this can be modulated, it may become more useful.

Infections

Coryza: The Common Cold

Unfortunately, avoidance of the common cold is virtually impossible, and prevention by immunization has thus far been a failure. Colds are self-limiting, however, and normally last approximately 5 days. Clinical trial data support the value of zinc in reducing the duration and severity of symptoms of the common cold when administered within 24 hours of the onset of common cold symptoms.

Most asthma exacerbations (80% in children and 60% in adults) start with a viral upper respiratory tract infection. Synergy among allergen sensitization, exposure, and rhinoviral infection leads to an almost 20-fold likelihood that an asthmatic child will require hospitalization. Other complications include acute sinusitis, pharyngitis, otitis media, mastoiditis, and tonsillitis. The common cold frequently leads to lower respiratory infection, including laryngotracheitis, bronchitis, and occasionally pneumonia. Patients who have other cardiorespiratory diseases may also experience exacerbations.

Intrinsic Rhinitis

Intrinsic rhinitis often has an onset in middle age or later and frequently is refractory to treatment. Combinations of therapy may prove helpful.

RHINOSINUSITIS

Acute Bacterial Rhinosinusitis

Before the antibiotic era, acute bacterial rhinosinusitis carried significant morbidity and mortality associated with spread of bacterial sepsis beyond the sinuses. Osteolysis of the sinus wall was common, with abscess formation and direct spread to neighboring structures, in addition to local spread and thrombophlebitis. Local complications include orbital cellulitis with or without abscess formation, cavernous sinus thrombosis, sagittal sinus thrombosis, intracranial abscess formation, meningitis and encephalitis, osteomyelitis, and septicemia. Complications are now rarely seen, because severely affected patients are prescribed broad-spectrum antibiotics.

Chronic Rhinosinusitis

With CRS, the clinical course is again variable, depending on the subtype of disease present. Often addressing any underlying contributing or exacerbating factor will decrease the frequency and severity of exacerbations, but complete resolution of disease is not common.

CONTROVERSIES AND PITFALLS

- Not all patients who have nasal symptoms have AR—neoplasm or foreign body may be the cause.
- Unilateral discharge in children probably indicates the presence of a foreign body, but in adults it may be a sign of carcinoma.
- Unilateral lesions must be biopsied to exclude malignancy.
- Nasal decongestants should be used sparingly, if at all.
- Most medical treatment failures result from poor compliance; once-daily treatment is best, if possible.
- The common cold, a cause of widespread morbidity, remains a major research challenge.
- Intrinsic rhinitis can be troublesome to treat, and further research is required.
- Turbinates and polyps can be difficult to distinguish from one another; in general, however, turbinates are rigid and pain-sensitive, whereas polyps are mobile and insensitive to irritating or painful stimuli.
- Facial pain in the absence of nasal symptoms is rarely caused by sinus disease, so other causes such as migraine, dental problems, and temporomandibular joint syndrome should be considered.
- Chronic refractory sinusitis should stimulate investigation for underlying immune or other defects.
- CT scan is the investigation of choice—plain radiography or magnetic resonance imaging has a limited role.
- Treatment of rhinosinusitis benefits asthma.

SUGGESTED READINGS

Bousquet J, Khaltaev N, Cruz AA, et al: Allergic Rhinitis and Its Impact on Asthma (ARIA) 2008 update (in collaboration with the World Health Organization, GA(2)LEN and AllerGen), *Allergy* 63(Suppl 86):8–160, 2008.

Bousquet J, van Cauwenberge P, Aït Khaled N, et al: Pharmacologic and anti-IgE treatment of allergic rhinitis ARIA update (in collaboration with GA2LEN), *Allergy* 61:1086–1096, 2006.

Ragab S, Scadding GK, Lund VJ, Saleh H: Treatment of chronic rhinosinusitis and its effects on asthma, *Eur Respir J* 28:68–74, 2006.

Scadding GK, Durham SR, Mirakian R, et al: BSACI guidelines for the management of allergic and non-allergic rhinitis, *Clin Exp Allergy* 38:19–42, 2008.

Scadding GK, Durham SR, Mirakian R, et al: BSACI guidelines for the management of rhinosinusitis and nasal polyposis, *Clin Exp Allergy* 38:260–275, 2008.

Thomas M, Yawn BP, Price D, et al; European Position Paper on Rhinosinusitis and Nasal Polyps Group EPOS Primary Care Guidelines: European position paper on the primary care, diagnosis, and management of rhinosinusitis and nasal polyps 2007—a summary, *Prim Care Respir J* 17:79–89, 2008.

Chapter **38**

Asthma: Epidemiology, Pathophysiology, and Risk Factors

Borja G. Cosio • Jaime Rodríguez Rosado • Federico Fiorentino Rossi

Asthma has been described throughout time, beginning with ancient Egyptians. The Georg Ebers Papyrus, found in Egypt in the 1870s, contains prescriptions written in hieroglyphics for more than 700 treatments for the disorder. The inhalation of fumes extracted from the heating of herbs in bricks was one of the remedies available. The term *asthma* comes from the Greek word *aazein*, meaning "to pant, or breathe with the mouth open." Between the 1930s and 1950s, asthma was considered to be a psychosomatic illness. During the 1960s, the emergence of the inflammation theory refuted a psychological origin and proved that asthma is a physical disease. Nonetheless, an association between psychological conditions (e.g., anxiety, depression) and difficult-to-treat asthma has been recognized since that time.

Nowadays, asthma is defined as a chronic inflammatory process characterized by reversible and variable airflow obstruction due to bronchial responsiveness secondary to multiple external stimuli in which genetic factors interact with environmental factors. The Global Initiative for Asthma (GINA) gives an operational description of asthma, as follows:

. . . a chronic inflammatory disorder of the airways in which many cells and cellular elements play a role. The chronic inflammation is associated with airway hyperresponsiveness that leads to recurrent episodes of wheezing, breathlessness, chest tightness and coughing, particularly at night or in the early morning. These episodes are usually associated with widespread, but variable, airflow obstruction within the lung that is often reversible either spontaneously or with treatment.

At present, much research is directed at elucidation of the underlying causes of asthma, which remain unknown. The risk for development of asthma is supported by evidence for a mixture of genetic, environmental, and lifestyle factors. Asthma does not respect age or gender, affecting both children and adults from kindergarten and school through work to retirement. For the moment, there is no cure for this condition, so preventive strategies are being effectively applied at the community level to prevent onset of the condition and to control worsening of asthma symptoms in the future. Nevertheless, some of these approaches have failed to reach the entire spectrum of the community population, for various reasons, such as limited access to information, personal beliefs, religious practices, and ethnicity within emigrational cohorts. Moreover, clinical practice guidelines and their distribution are basic for acute asthma diagnosis, treatment, and control.

EPIDEMIOLOGY

The World Health Organization (WHO) estimates that 300 million people have asthma worldwide, producing significant morbidity and interfering with daily activities and quality of life. During the year 2009, 250,000 people died from this condition in low- to middle-income countries. Furthermore, asthma is the most frequent chronic respiratory condition among children worldwide, and its prevalence is increasing. The Centers for Disease Control and Prevention (CDC) has estimated a significant rise in asthmatic patients of 12.3% since 2001 in the United States. Statistical figures for 2009 show that 24.6 million people had asthma, compared with 20.3 million at the beginning of the decade. This increase has come with a cost to society of $56 billion dollars in medical expenses and lost productivity. No clear explanation for this increased prevalence, however, has emerged, especially in view of the overall reduction in smoking and in second-hand smoke exposure with the implementation of laws banning smoking. The same situation is described outside the United States. From a metaanalysis of data obtained through routine statistics and population surveys, Anderson and co-workers concluded that asthma prevalence increased in the United Kingdom from 1955 to 2004.

Despite a large number of research studies, the reasons for why some people develop asthma and others do not and why asthma has emerged as a public health problem in some populations earlier than in others are not well understand. The main problem in focusing on the epidemiology of asthma is to address a proper operational definition in an attempt to unify the large conclusions of many epidemiologic studies from different areas of the world. The need to derive a practical and tangible definition of asthma for use in large-scale questionnaire-based epidemiologic research has led to a focus on asthma symptoms and their highly subjective expressions as part of the results. In questionnaire surveys, the presence of asthma often is defined on the basis of responses to questions about symptoms of wheeze in the past weeks or months, "wheeze ever," and doctor-diagnosed asthma. This approach has been shown to have good short-term repeatability but may lack specificity, particularly in children, because other causes of wheezing illness, such as viral infection, may be misdiagnosed as asthma. With a focus on symptoms, the most common clinical presentation is one of breathlessness, wheezing, chest tightness, and cough, especially at night, coexisting with asymptomatic periods. Because of the nonspecificity and variability inherent in personal perception of respiratory difficulty, implementation of vital patient educational programs and pharmacologic treatment of asthma symptoms may be delayed. Clinical symptoms vary from one person to another, so a severe asthma exacerbation that necessitates urgent medical attention may not be recognized at first, and consequent delay in getting required treatment may lead to a poorer outcome.

Reported prevalence rates for asthma are widely variable. Despite the difficulty in obtaining a consensus on epidemiologic data, several studies have shown that asthma prevalence is increasing worldwide, with at least 7% to 10% of the population affected. Inclusion of data obtained using nonstandardized methods (questionnaires versus definition agreement) in a majority of the epidemiologic studies to determine asthma prevalence underlies the notable differences in global rates published in contemporary literature. This particular finding has no significance for geographic distribution of asthma, rates for which remain very low in many rural villages, in contrast with data reported for Western populations. Pollution in industrialized civilizations acts like a silent predator on the susceptible airway, leading to asthma in persons with certain respiratory diseases. A "hygiene hypothesis" has been proposed to explain an increased risk in children for the development of asthma that may reflect reduced microbe exposure in early life.

In a morbidity and mortality report from the CDC for the period 2006 to 2008, asthma prevalence was estimated as 7.8% for the U.S. population (**Table 38-1**). Current asthma prevalence was higher among the multiracial (14.8%), Puerto Rican Hispanics (14.2%), and non-Hispanic blacks (9.5%) than among non-Hispanic whites (7.8%). Current asthma prevalence also was higher among children (9.3%) than among adults (7.3%), among females (8.6%) than among males (6.9%), and among the poor (11.2%) than among the near-poor (8.4%) and nonpoor (7.0%).

With respect to the worldwide variability in reported prevalence rates for asthma, different studies have examined the impact on asthma care in two of the most ethnically diverse nations, such as the United Kingdom and the United States. Emigrational cohorts of Mexican Hispanics have demonstrated a lower rate of asthma than that in U.S.-born Hispanics. Moreover, in a comparison of U.K.-born persons of the same ethnic group with those already settled after emigration, the second group demonstrated a lower rate of physician visits for asthmatic symptoms. Nevertheless, Westernization does not explain this variance, and the inequalities also may be influenced by differences in genetics, environmental risk factors, and social activities.

One of the main objectives of the European Community Respiratory Health Survey (ECRHS) was to estimate the variation in prevalence of asthma, asthma-like symptoms, atopic sensitization, and bronchial hyperreactivity, predominantly in Western Europe and many other countries (**Figure 38-1**). The highest rates in Europe were in the United Kingdom (15.2%), and the lowest were in Georgia (0.28%). Another important ongoing multicenter study, the International Study of Asthma and Allergies in Children (ISAAC), had as its main aim to determine the asthma prevalence in children. A comparative survey conducted in Canadian children between 2 and 7 years of age showed an asthma prevalence of 9.8% overall, with a 4.6% higher rate in boys than in girls (**Figure 38-2**). GINA embraced the results of both of these valuable studies in the Global Burden of Asthma report and estimated that by 2025, 400 million people around the world will have a diagnosis of asthma. In the same way, this increase in prevalence is directly related to the augmented rates of rhinitis, eczema, and other atopic disorders.

In relation to mortality, asthma accounts for an estimated 250,000 annual deaths worldwide. Statistical data show large differences between countries, and asthma death rates do not parallel prevalence rates (**Figure 38-3**). Mortality seems to be high in countries where access to essential drugs is low. According to the WHO, many asthma-related deaths are preventable, being a result of suboptimal long-term medical care and delay in obtaining help during the final, fatal attack. In many areas of the world, people with asthma do not have access to basic asthma medications and health care. Nations with the highest death rates are those in which controller medications are not available. In many countries, deaths due to asthma have declined recently as a result of better asthma management. Considerable evidence points to an overall trend of decreasing mortality. For instance, mortality rates in Australia registered by the Australian Institute of Health and Welfare decreased by approximately 70% between 1989 and 2006. Persons older than 65 years of age and people of lower socioeconomic status were at higher risk for dying from asthma, mainly secondary to respiratory infections during winter. Overall, asthma-related mortality in Australia remains uncommon, accounting for 402 (0.30%) in the year 2006 of all deaths (Australian Centre for Asthma Monitoring: *Asthma in Australia 2008*, AIHW Asthma Series no. 3, Cat. no. ACM 14, Canberra, Australian Institute of Health and Welfare, 2008) (**Figure 38-4**).

It is worth emphasizing that many of the deaths secondary to asthma are preventable, and that the high economic costs attributable to this disease can be diminished. The elevated prevalence and mortality rates are associated with not inconsiderable consumption of health-related resources, placing an additional economic load on health care services.

PATHOGENESIS

Asthma is an inflammatory disorder of the airways in which multiple mediators and several types of inflammatory cells are involved. This pattern of inflammation is strongly associated with airway hyperresponsiveness and classic asthma symptoms of wheezing, breathlessness, chest tightness, and coughing.

A genetic predisposition to develop specific immunoglobulin E (IgE) antibodies directed against common environmental allergens, or *atopy*, is the strongest identifiable risk factor for the development of asthma. Intrinsic abnormalities in airway smooth muscle and airway remodeling in response to injury and inflammation add to the effects of airway inflammation in creating the clinical presentation of asthma (**Figure 38-5**).

AIRWAY INFLAMMATION IN ASTHMA

Despite the highly heterogeneous clinical expression of asthma, the presence of airway inflammation remains a consistent feature. Although airway inflammation in asthma is persistent even though symptoms are episodic, no clear relationship between the severity of asthma and the intensity of inflammation has been discovered. The inflammation affects all airways, including in most patients the upper respiratory tract and nose, but its pathophysiologic effects are most pronounced in medium-sized bronchi. The pattern of inflammation in the airways appears to be essentially the same in all clinical forms of asthma, whether allergic, nonallergic, or aspirin-induced, and at all ages.

Table 38-1 Prevalence of Current Asthma Among Children and Adults by Sex, Race/Ethnicity, and Economic Status-Poverty Level*

Characteristic	Prevalence Rate (%)[†]		
	Children	Adults	Total
Race/Ethnicity			
White, non-Hispanic	8.2 (7.6-8.9)	7.7 (7.3-8.0)	7.8 (7.5-8.1)
Black, non-Hispanic	14.6 (13.4-15.9)	7.8 (7.2-8.4)	9.5 (9.0-10.1)
Multiracial	13.6 (11.1-16.6)	15.1 (12.7-18.0)	14.8 (12.7-17.0)
Hispanic, Puerto Rican ethnicity	18.4 (14.9-22.5)	12.8 (10.9-14.9)	14.2 (12.5-16.2)
Sex			
Male	10.7 (10.1-11.4)	5.5 (5.2-5.9)	6.9 (6.6-7.2)
White, non-Hispanic	9.5 (8.6-10.5)	5.9 (5.5-6.4)	6.8 (6.4-7.3)
Black, non-Hispanic	16.5 (14.9-18.2)	5.7 (4.9-6.6)	8.5 (7.7-9.3)
Multiracial	14.6 (10.9-19.5)	11.2 (8.0-15.3)	12.1 (9.4-15.3)
Hispanic, Puerto Rican ethnicity	23.6 (18.0-30.2)	7.0 (4.8-10.1)	11.3 (9.0-14.0)
Female	7.8 (7.2-8.4)	8.9 (8.6-9.3)	8.6 (8.3-9.0)
White, non-Hispanic	6.9 (6.1-7.8)	9.3 (8.8-9.8)	8.7 (8.3-9.1)
Black, non-Hispanic	12.7 (11.0-14.5)	9.5 (8.7-10.3)	10.3 (9.5-11.1)
Multiracial	12.6 (9.2-16.9)	19.1 (15.4-23.4)	17.4 (14.5-20.8)
Hispanic, Puerto Rican ethnicity	13.0 (9.7-17.3)	18.2 (15.5-21.2)	16.9 (14.6-19.4)
Economic Status			
Poor	11.7 (10.6-12.9)	11.0 (10.2-11.9)	11.2 (10.5-12.0)
White, non-Hispanic	10.1 (8.1-12.5)	13.3 (11.9-14.7)	12.5 (11.3-13.8)
Black, non-Hispanic	15.8 (13.7-18.3)	10.9 (9.6-12.4)	12.2 (11.0-13.4)
Multiracial	21.1 (15.4-28.2)	20.2 (14.3-27.8)	20.5 (15.6-26.4)
Hispanic, Puerto Rican ethnicity	23.3 (16.8-31.4)	22.1 (17.6-27.4)	22.4 (18.7-26.7)
Near-Poor	9.9 (8.8-11.0)	7.9 (7.2-8.5)	8.4 (7.8-8.9)
White, non-Hispanic	9.5 (7.8-11.5)	9.1 (8.2-10.0)	9.2 (8.4-10.0)
Black, non-Hispanic	14.3 (12.1-16.9)	8.1 (6.8-9.6)	9.7 (8.5-11.0)
Multiracial	16.1 (10.5-24.0)	12.8 (8.3-19.0)	13.6 (9.7-18.8)
Hispanic, Puerto Rican ethnicity	17.9 (12.0-26.0)	13.9 (9.4-20.1)	14.9 (11.1-19.8)
Nonpoor	8.2 (7.7-8.8)	6.6 (6.3-6.9)	7.0 (6.7-7.3)
White, non-Hispanic	7.6 (7.0-8.3)	6.8 (6.4-7.2)	7.0 (6.7-7.4)
Black, non-Hispanic	13.6 (11.8-15.7)	6.5 (5.8-7.4)	8.4 (7.6-9.2)
Multiracial	9.2 (6.4-13.2)	14.9 (11.5-19.1)	13.4 (10.8-16.6)
Hispanic, Puerto Rican ethnicity	14.0 (10.0-19.3)	9.1 (6.8-12.2)	10.4 (8.3-13.0)
TOTAL	9.3 (8.9-9.7)	7.3 (7.0-7.5)	7.8 (7.6-8.0)

*United States, National Health Interview Survey, 2006 to 2008.
[†]95% confidence interval.
From Moorman JE, Zahran H, Truman BI, Molla MT; Centers for Disease Control and Prevention (CDC): Current asthma prevalence—United States, 2006-2008, *MMWR Surveill Summ* 60(suppl):84-86, 2011.

Inflammatory Cells

Studies using bronchoalveolar lavage and bronchial biopsies have demonstrated that a variety of cells and mediators are involved, with IgE and mast cells implicated in the acute response and eosinophils and eosinophil granule proteins in the late response, with T cells, particularly T_H2 cells, orchestrating these responses through their production of cytokines such as the interleukins IL-4, IL-5, IL-9, and IL-13. Stromal and epithelial cells also are involved in the inflammatory response, as shown by the ability of these cells to respond to T_H2 cytokines with the production of chemokines that initiate and perpetuate tissue inflammatory reactions. As a result, a pathogenetic construct for atopic asthma (and possibly other forms of asthma) has been proposed in which (1) T_H2 cells play a central role in the recognition of antigens and the initiation and perpetuation of inflammation; (2) eosinophils are important

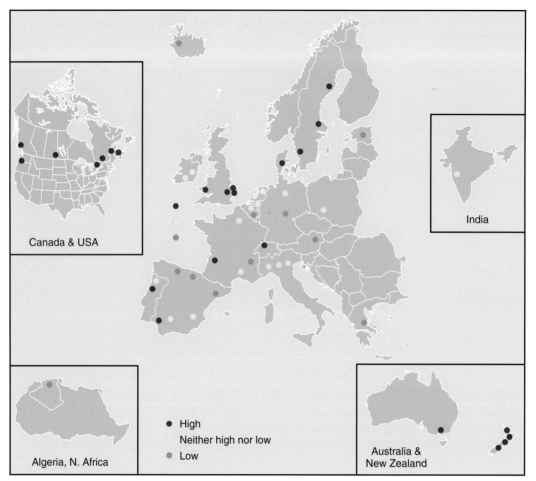

Figure 38-1 Prevalence of asthma in Europe. *(Courtesy European Community Respiratory Health Survey I Centers. Available at: http://www.ecrhs.org/ECRHS%20I.htm.)*

proinflammatory and epithelium-damaging cells; and (3) a variety of cells, including mast cells, epithelial cells, basophils, fibroblasts, smooth muscle cells, and macrophages, contribute through the secretion of cytokines that generate tissue inflammation or influence T_H2 lymphocyte or eosinophil function.

Implicit in the "inflammation theory" of asthma is the belief that inflammation is both necessary and sufficient to account for the complex features of asthma. Although inflammation is undoubtedly a cornerstone of asthma, it is now clear that the asthmatic response is more complex. Also clear from pathologic investigations is that structural alterations exist in the asthmatic airway. Mathematical modeling studies have provided evidence that these alterations contribute to the symptoms and physiologic dysregulation seen in asthma. As a result, it has been proposed that the chronic inflammation that is characteristic of the asthmatic airway leads to a remodeling response, and that the structural alterations induced by this response play an important role in generating the manifestations of the disorder. This conceptual evolution predicts that an enhanced understanding of asthma pathogenesis can be expected when asthma is studied in the context of paradigms of injury and wound healing, as well as the traditional paradigms relevant to the interface of inflammation and airway physiology. It also suggests that studies utilizing this new perspective will identify novel targets against which therapies can be directed and will help to elucidate the biologic basis for the patient-to-patient variability encountered in clinical practice.

Inflammatory Mediators

More than 100 different mediators are now recognized to be involved in asthma and to mediate the complex inflammatory response in the airways. Chemokines are expressed mainly in airway epithelial cells and are important in the recruitment of inflammatory cells into the airways. Eotaxin is relatively selective for eosinophils, whereas macrophage-derived chemokines (MDCs) recruit T_H2 cells.

Cytokines such as IL-1β and TNF-α, which amplify the inflammatory response, and granulocyte-macrophage colony-stimulating factor (GM-CSF), which prolongs eosinophil survival in the airways, orchestrate the inflammatory response in asthma and determine its severity. T_H2-derived cytokines include IL-5, which is required for eosinophil differentiation and survival; IL-4, which is important for T_H2 cell differentiation; and IL-13, needed for IgE formation.

Cysteinyl leukotrienes are potent bronchoconstrictors that act as proinflammatory mediators mainly derived from mast cells and eosinophils. Their inhibition has been associated with an improvement in lung function and asthma symptoms.

The prostaglandin PGD_2 is a bronchoconstrictor derived predominantly from mast cells and is involved in T_H2 cell recruitment to the airways.

Histamine is released from mast cells and contributes to bronchoconstriction and to the inflammatory response.

Nitric oxide (NO) has been associated with the presence of eosinophilic inflammation in asthma. It is produced

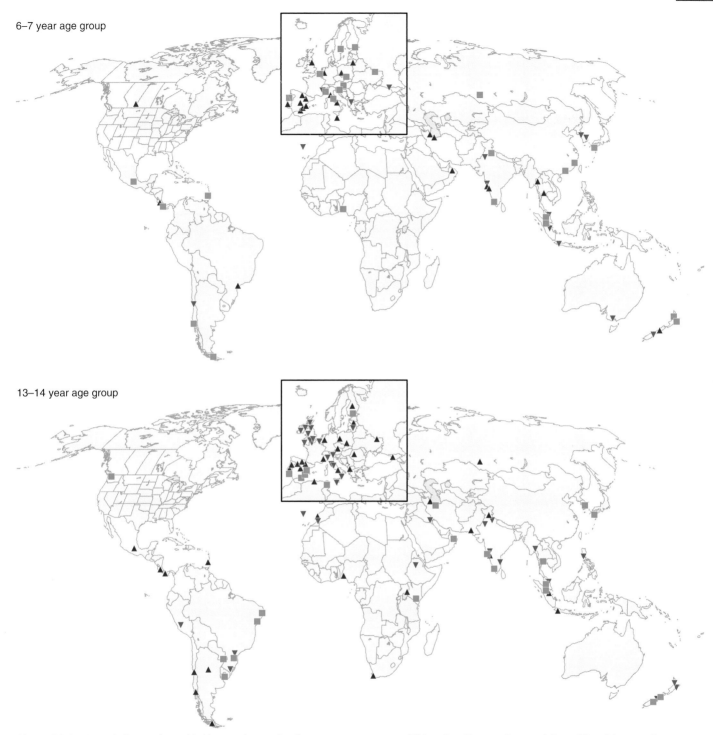

Figure 38-2   Annual changes in worldwide prevalence of asthma symptoms among children 6 to 7 years of age and those 13 to 14 years of age, over a mean of 7 years after phase I of the International Study of Asthma and Allergies in Childhood (which in most participating countries was conducted between 1991 and 1993). *Blue triangles*, locations where prevalence was reduced by at least 1 standard error (SE) per year; *green squares*, locations where there was little change in prevalence (i.e., change of less than 1 SE per year); *red triangles*, locations where prevalence increased by at least 1 SE per year.   *(From Subbarao P, Mandhane PJ, Sears MR: Asthma: epidemiology, etiology and risk factors, CMAJ 181:E181-E190, 2009.)*

predominantly from the action of inducible nitric oxide synthase (iNOS) in airway epithelial cells. Exhaled NO concentration is increasingly being used to diagnose asthma in the context of a compatible clinical history and to monitor the effectiveness of asthma treatment.

PATHOPHYSIOLOGY

Airway narrowing is the final common pathway leading to symptoms and physiologic changes in asthma. As discussed

next, several factors contribute to the development of airway narrowing in asthma (**Figure 38-6**).

Bronchoconstriction   Bronchoconstriction is an abnormal contraction of airway smooth muscle that was presumed to be due to an intrinsic abnormality in the airway myocytes. Nervous system dysfunction with cholinergic and/or tachykinin excess also was proposed as an important pathogenic process. Autonomic dysfunction decreases in response to β-agonist and increases in response to α-agonist activity.

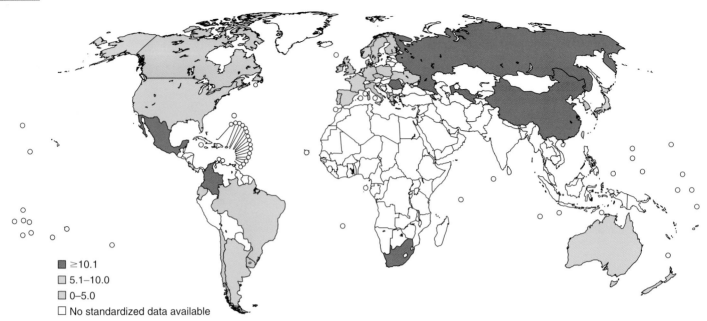

Figure 38-3 World map of asthma case-fatality rates: asthma deaths per 100,000 people with asthma in the 5- to 34-year-old age group. *(From Masoli M, Fabian D, Holt S, Beasley R; Global Initiative for Asthma [GINA] Program: The global burden of asthma: executive summary of the GINA Dissemination Committee Report, Allergy 59:469-478, 2004.)*

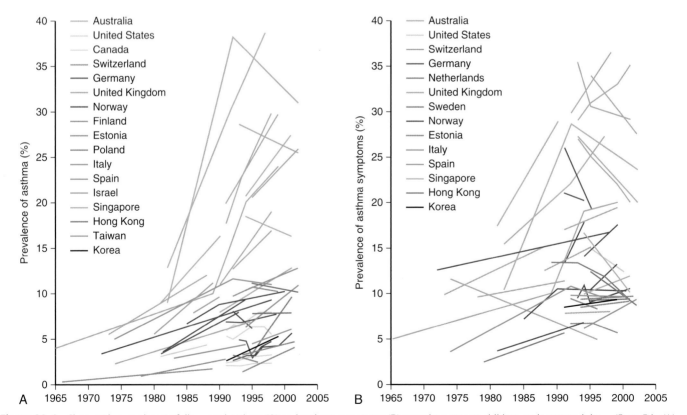

Figure 38-4 Changes in prevalence of diagnosed asthma (**A**) and asthma symptoms (**B**) over time among children and young adults. *(From Eder W, Ege MJ, von Mutius E: The asthma epidemic, N Engl J Med 355:2226-2235, 2006.)*

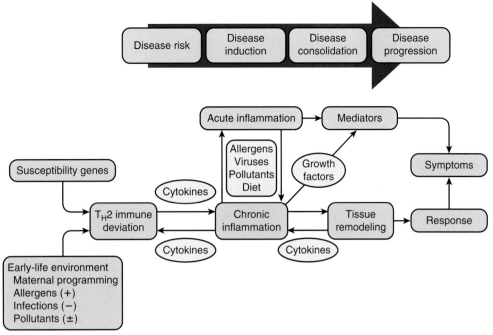

Figure 38-5   Natural history of asthma.   *(From Szefler SJ: The natural history of asthma and early intervention, J Allergy Clin Immunol 109:S550, 2002. Adapted from Holgate ST: The cellular and mediator basis of asthma in relation to natural history, Lancet 350[Suppl 2]:5-9, 1997.)*

Airway Edema   Airway edema is due to increased microvascular leakage occurring in response to inflammatory mediators. This pathomechanism may be particularly important during acute exacerbations.

Airway Remodeling   In addition to the inflammatory response, characteristic structural changes, often described as airway remodeling, are observed in the airways of asthma patients. Some of these changes are related to the severity of the disease and may result in relatively irreversible narrowing of the airways. These changes may represent repair in response to chronic inflammation.

Airway remodeling can be defined as an airflow obstruction despite aggressive antiinflammatory therapies, including regimens of inhaled corticosteroids and systemic corticosteroids. It was first appreciated over 75 years ago by Huber and Koessler in their classic description of fatal asthma. The natural history of airway remodeling is poorly understood, and it does not appear to be a universal finding or a modifiable factor with early treatment.

The effect of bronchoconstriction on airway remodeling has been studied by exposing subjects to a dust mite allergen or repeated methacholine inhalation challenge. Both agents cause bronchoconstriction, although dust mite allergen induces an eosinophilic inflammation. The repetition of the exposure leading to bronchoconstriction after 4 days, observed in bronchial biopsy specimens, established that both the allergen and methacholine groups developed airway remodeling that was independent of inflammation for the second group.

On histopathologic examination, the airway remodeling is associated with a variety of features including airway wall thickening, mucous gland hyperplasia, persistence of inflammatory cellular infiltrates, release of fibrogenic growth factors along with collagen deposition, and elastolysis. Increase in the number and size of vessels in the airway wall is one of the most consistent features of asthma remodeling occurring in the lungs of patients with mild, moderate, and severe asthma. Airway wall thickening is the result of a dense fibrotic response that occurs in the lamina reticularis. The pathologic significance of subepithelial fibrosis is not clear, but this process has been associated with disease severity and correlated with a decline in forced expiratory volume in 1 second (FEV_1).

All components of the airway wall have been reported to be thickened in asthma (**Figure 38-7**). Elements involved in this response are increase in airway smooth muscle, increased myocyte muscle mass, edema, inflammatory cell infiltration, glandular hypertrophy and hyperplasia, and connective tissue deposition. The recently popularized "perturbed equilibrium hypothesis" also suggests that wall thickening can destabilize the dynamic forces that control airway caliber, leading to airway collapse.

Mucus Metaplasia   Mucus hypersecretion, epithelial hypertrophy, mucus metaplasia, and airway obstruction due to bronchial mucus plugging are well-documented features of chronic asthma and status asthmaticus. Epithelial hypertrophy and increased airway mucus can contribute to the airway obstruction seen in asthma.

Airway Hyperresponsiveness   Airway hyperresponsiveness is the characteristic functional abnormality of asthma, resulting in airway narrowing in response to a known or unknown stimulus. In turn, this airway narrowing leads to variable airflow limitation and intermittent symptoms. Airway hyperresponsiveness is linked to both inflammation and repair of the airways and is partially reversible with therapy. Its mechanisms are incompletely understood, although it has been related to increased volume or contractility of airway smooth muscle cells, excessive airway contraction due to inflammatory changes, and exaggerated bronchoconstriction occurring in response to sensory stimuli in sensory nerves sensitized by excessive inflammation.

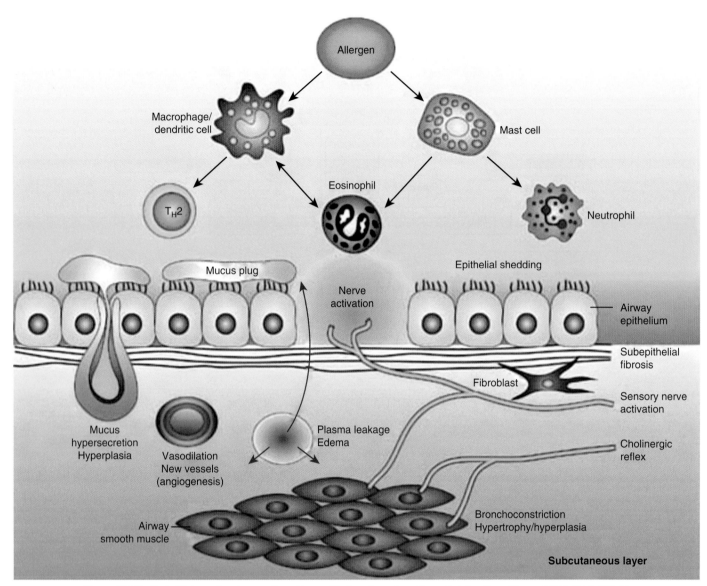

Figure 38-6 Pathobiology of asthma. *(From Barnes PJ: New drugs for asthma,* Nat Rev Drug Discov *3:831–844, 2004.)*

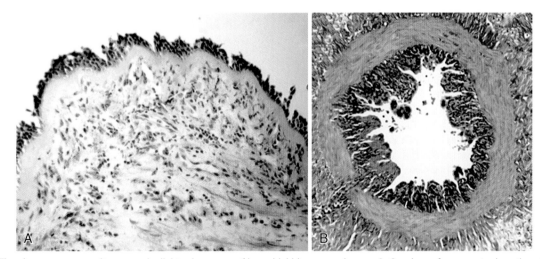

Figure 38-7 The airway mucosa as it appears by light microscopy of bronchial biopsy specimens. **A,** Specimen from an atopic asthmatic patient shows loss of surface epithelium and early thickening and hyaline appearance of the reticular basement membrane (RBM). **B,** Specimen from a patient with severe asthma shows airway remodeling with thickening of the RBM and muscular layer. *(**A,** From Jeffery PK: Remodeling in asthma and chronic obstructive lung disease,* Am J Respir Crit Care Med *164:S28–S38, 2001.)*

Special Circumstances

Acute Exacerbations

Transient worsening of asthma symptoms and underlying inflammation may result from exposure to risk factors for asthma, such as exercise, emotional stress, air pollutants, or occupational exposure. More prolonged worsening usually is due to viral infections of the upper respiratory tract (particularly from rhinovirus and respiratory syncytial virus [RSV]) or allergen exposure leading to increased inflammation in the lower airways (acute or chronic inflammation), which may persist for several days or weeks.

Asthma exacerbations constitute a primary reason for attendance at hospital emergency departments worldwide. Asthma exacerbations have been shown to significantly reduce health-related quality of life in patients classified as having moderate to severe asthma. A multivariable analysis of data from a prospective and multicenter study conducted in Canada that included 695 patients presenting to emergency departments demonstrated that older asthmatic patients with a history of previous hospital admission for asthma in the past 2 years and patients receiving either oral or inhaled corticoids, with an increased need for β_2-agonist puffs among others, are more likely to require hospital admission.

Nocturnal Asthma

Asthma usually worsens at night. The mechanisms accounting for this nocturnal worsening of symptoms are not completely understood but may be driven by circadian rhythms of circulating hormones such as epinephrine, cortisol, and melatonin and neural mechanisms such as cholinergic tone. An increase in airway inflammation at night has been reported. This finding may reflect a reduction in endogenous antiinflammatory mechanisms.

Difficult-to-Treat Asthma

In a minority of patients, asthma may prove difficult to manage and relatively insensitive to the effects of glucocorticosteroids. The reasons are not well understood. Common associations are poor compliance with treatment and psychological and psychiatric disorders. However, genetic factors may contribute in some instances. Many of these patients have difficult-to-treat asthma from disease onset, rather than progressing from milder asthma. In such patients, airway closure leads to air trapping and hyperinflation. Although the histopathologic pattern appears broadly similar to that in other forms of asthma, additional features include an increase in neutrophils, more small airway involvement, and further structural changes. Research over the past 2 decades has identified allergic pathways as being fundamental to asthma pathogenesis with a prominent role played by a subset of T cells (designated T_H2-like) that produce cytokines and chemokines implicated in the regulation of IgE and the maturation, recruitment, priming, and activation of mast cells, basophils, and eosinophils. Allergic pathways that contribute to airway dysfunction in mild-moderate asthma are largely sensitive to corticosteroids. In more severe asthma, however, the inflammatory profile commonly changes, with greater involvement of neutrophils and evidence of tissue destruction and airway remodeling.

Smoking and Asthma

The prevalence of smoking among persons with asthma reflects that in the general population; thus, smokers with asthma comprise a large group of patients with poorly controlled disease. Smoking cessation is an effective intervention for smokers with asthma, but because sustained quitting rates are low, additional or alternative therapies are needed for patients with asthma who smoke.

As seen in patients with chronic obstructive pulmonary disease (COPD), asthmatic patients who smoke may have a neutrophil-predominant inflammation in their airways and exhibit a poor response to glucocorticosteroids. Tobacco smoking makes asthma more difficult to control, results in more frequent exacerbations and hospital admissions, and produces a more rapid decline in lung function with an increased risk of death.

The antiinflammatory actions of corticosteroids are mediated in part by the recruitment of histone deacetylase (HDAC), a nuclear enzyme involved in the switching off of activated inflammatory genes. Cigarette smoke reduces HDAC activity in vitro, which may potentially explain corticosteroid insensitivity in smokers with asthma, as has been observed in COPD.

RISK FACTORS

Asthma is a condition characterized by lung airway inflammation initiated and perpetuated by an inappropriate immune response, increased airway responsiveness, and variable airflow obstruction. These results come from complex interactions between multiple genetics and environmental influences. Although a clear cause-and-effect association is not always possible to demonstrate, numerous risk factors have been identified (Box 38-1).

The asthma risk factors can be divided into genetic and environment factors, including in the latter allergens, nutritional factors, perinatal factors, and tobacco smoke (active and secondhand smoking). In addition, a series of trigger factors, either direct or indirect, also can worsen asthma symptoms.

Box 38-1 Asthma Risk and Trigger Factors

Risk Factors
Genetics
Atopy
Airway hyperresponsiveness
Obesity
Sex

Environmental Factors
Allergens
Diet
Perinatal factors
Tobacco smoke
Infections
Occupational exposure

Trigger Factors
Direct
Respiratory infections
Nonspecific irritants
Weather changes

Indirect
Exercise
Emotional extremes
Food allergens
Medications
Gastroesophageal reflux disease
Menstruation
Pregnancy

Among the direct factors are infections, nonspecific irritants such as tobacco smoke, outdoor air pollution, industrial spills, bonfire smoke, and meteorologic changes (low temperatures, high humidity). Indirect factors are exercise, extremes of emotion, food allergens, medications, menstruation, gastroesophageal reflux disease (GERD), and pregnancy.

GENETICS

Certain components of the asthma phenotype appear to be strongly heritable, such as atopy, airway hyperresponsiveness, obesity, and gender. In fact, a family history of asthma is a clear risk factor for developing asthma. Current data show that multiple genes may be involved in the pathogenesis of asthma, although the specific genes responsible for these inherited components have not yet been identified.

The relative risk for asthma in a first-degree relative of the patient is between 2.5% and 6%; in monozygotic twins, the risk is 60% and in dizygotic twins, 25%. In contrast with other pathologic conditions caused by a unique genetic abnormality (e.g., cystic fibrosis) in which a hereditary pattern can be explained with a simple mendelian pattern, asthma is a heterogeneous disease in which multiple genes interact. The final phenotype depends on the smaller additive actions of these particular genes, combined with and modulated by environmental factors.

One of the most commonly studied genetic factors is atopy. *Atopy* can be defined as the genetic predisposition to develop IgE antibodies against specific allergens. Atopy is considered the main factor contributing to development of asthma. The atopic pattern is characterized by atopic dermatitis, allergic rhinitis, and asthma. Not all atopic patients, however, develop all three conditions. The incidence of atopy in the general population is approximately 30%, whereas that of asthma is much lower—the implication being that not all atopic persons develop asthma, but that almost all asthmatic patients have atopy.

Other areas of the asthmatic phenotype in which a search for genetic factors has been focused are airway hyperresponsiveness, inflammatory responses, and T_H1-T_H2 immune responses. In some cases, a number of chromosomal regions associated with asthma susceptibility have been identified, such as the major locus near the long arm of chromosome 5 (5q), although with inconsistent results.

Obesity is another factor that has been associated with asthma. Asthma is more frequently observed in obese people (body mass index greater than 30) and is more difficult to control in obese asthmatics. The influence of obesity on lung mechanics and the generation of a proinflammatory state in addition to hormonal or neurogenic influences are likely to play a role. This risk may be greater with nonallergic asthma than with allergic asthma.

A clear-cut genetic factor also has been established—asthma is twice as frequent in male children as in females. This predilection reverses by adulthood, when the prevalence of asthma is greater in women than in men, and it reaches its maximal differences when related to severe asthma.

Approximately 20 genome-wide linkage screening studies have been reported in different populations for investigating chromosomal regions that are linked to asthma and atopy, or related phenotypical features such as elevated IgE levels, wheezing, and bronchial hyperresponsiveness. A number of chromosomal regions have been repeatedly identified, across multiple studies, that contain genes of biologic relevance to asthma and allergic disease, including the cytokine cluster on 5q (containing interleukin-3 [IL-3], IL-5, and GM-CSF), *FCER1B* on 11q, *IFNG* (interferon-γ) and *STAT6* on 12q, and *IL4R* (the IL-4Rα chain, also part of the IL-13 receptor) on 16p. Linkage studies followed by positional cloning approaches have resulted in the identification of a handful of novel asthma susceptibility genes, including *CYFIP2*, *DPP10*, *HLAG*, *PHF11*, *GPRA*, and *ADAM33*. *GPRA* (G protein—coupled receptor for asthma) and *ADAM33* (a disintegrin and metalloproteinase domain–containing protein 33) have generated considerable interest, because their expression in bronchial smooth muscle cells suggests roles in the pathobiology of asthma and pulmonary allergic disease.

ENVIRONMENTAL FACTORS

The environment plays a pivotal role in the development of asthma because it interacts with the genetic susceptibility of the subject to develop an asthmatic phenotype. Environmental factors, however, frequently overlap with trigger factors that can precipitate asthma symptoms, and their influence can be additive.

Risk Factors in Childhood
Phenotypes of Asthma
Although some 50% of preschool children have wheezing, only 10% to 15% have a diagnosis of "true" asthma by the time they reach school age. Commonly described phenotypes in early infancy and childhood are transient wheezing, nonatopic wheezing, late-onset wheezing, and persistent wheezing. Only transient wheezing in early infancy has been well characterized, with decreased airflow rates on pulmonary function testing at birth, onset of wheezing within the first year, and resolution by mid-childhood, with no lasting effects on pulmonary function. The other three phenotypes have been described primarily by age at onset in cohort studies, and their genesis in early infancy is largely unknown. A majority of children with persistent wheezing (in whom asthma will subsequently be diagnosed) experience their first symptoms before the age of 3. By 3 years, they have abnormal lung function that persists to adulthood, and by adolescence, most have atopy. Of children with nonatopic and late-onset wheezing, some experience remission, whereas others experience persistent symptoms and exhibit atopy. Distinguishing among these different phenotypes in early childhood is critical to an understanding of the role of risk factors and their timing in early infancy.

Breast-feeding
The influence of breast-feeding on the risk of childhood atopy and asthma remains controversial. Presented next is a review of observational data accumulated to date: Some studies have shown protection, whereas others have reported higher rates of allergy and asthma among breast-fed children. A metaanalysis and several individual studies showed that exclusive breast-feeding for at least 3 months was associated with lower rates of asthma between 2 and 5 years of age, with the greatest effect occurring among those with a parental history of atopy. One of the difficulties in interpreting these data lies in differentiating viral infection–associated wheeze in childhood from the wheeze of atopic asthma. In a longitudinal birth cohort study, breast-feeding was associated with a higher risk of atopic asthma in later childhood, with the greatest influence among children with a maternal history of atopy. The benefit

of avoiding nutritional allergens during breast-feeding also is controversial. In some studies, exclusion of milk, eggs, and fish from the maternal diet was associated with decreased atopic dermatitis in infancy, but other studies found no association. Studies in children from birth to the age of 4 years have demonstrated no effect of maternal dietary restriction during lactation on the subsequent development of atopic diseases, including asthma.

Nutritional Factors
The increase in incidence of asthma and atopy in developed countries has been associated with changes in the nutritional habits (processed foods, low antioxidant intake, high n-6 polyunsaturated fatty acids). Breast-fed infants are less likely to develop wheezing illness during early childhood than are intact cow's milk– or soy protein–fed infants.

Lung Function
Decreased airway caliber in infancy has been reported as a risk factor for transient wheezing, perhaps related to prenatal and postnatal exposure to environmental tobacco smoke. Furthermore, the presence of airways with decreased caliber has been associated with increased bronchial responsiveness and increased symptoms of wheeze. Several studies have suggested an association between reduced airway function in the first few weeks of life and asthma in later life. The magnitude of the effect of this risk factor in isolation (i.e., without concomitant allergy) is unclear; perhaps persons with smaller airways require less stimulus (i.e., airway inflammation) before symptoms become apparent. Children with wheezing (and diagnosed asthma) persisting to adulthood have a fixed decrement in lung function as early as the age of 7 or 9 years. Recent studies of preschool children have documented abnormal lung function in those with persistent wheezing as early as the age of 3 years. However, some infants in whom persistent wheezing develops have normal lung function shortly after birth, which suggests a critical period of exposures within the first few years of life, before the development of these persistent abnormalities in expiratory flow. By contrast, infants who exhibit early transient wheezing exhibit decreased airflow shortly after birth. Maternal smoking with in utero nicotine exposure has been correlated with this type of lung dysfunction, but the effects of other exposures have been less well studied.

Family Structure
Family size and the number and order of siblings may affect the risk of development of asthma. The hygiene hypothesis posits that exposure of an infant to a substantial number of infections and many types of bacteria stimulates the developing immune system toward nonasthmatic phenotypes. This hypothetical scenario may be exemplified in the real world by large family size, whereby later-born children in large families would be expected to be at lower risk for asthma than first-born children because of exposure to their older siblings' infections. Although this theory has been supported by some studies of allergy prevalence, it has been partially refuted by recent studies of this topic suggesting that although large family size (more than 4 children) is associated with a decreased risk of asthma, birth order is not involved. Furthermore, doubt has been cast on simplistic renditions of this hypothesis, in that infections per se cannot explain some epidemiologic patterns (e.g., prevalence rates for allergy and asthma are high in some South American countries, where exposures to infection are higher than in some countries with lower rates of asthma). In addition, not only

allergic but also autoimmune and other chronic inflammatory diseases are increasing, a trend that is difficult to explain using the hygiene hypothesis alone, because allergic and autoimmune diseases are associated with competing immunologic phenotypes.

Socioeconomic Status
Children of parents with lower socioeconomic status have greater morbidity from asthma, but findings with respect to the prevalence of asthma are mixed. Such results may depend both on how socioeconomic status is measured and on the specific outcome examined. Some studies have reported associations of lower socioeconomic status with higher rates of airway obstruction and symptoms but not with a diagnosis of asthma. Whether socioeconomic status is as relevant to the incidence of allergy and asthma as it is to the expression, severity, and management of these diseases remains unclear. Parental stress also has been prospectively associated with wheezing in infancy, and family difficulties have been linked to asthma. Children whose caregivers report high levels of stress and who have difficulties parenting are at greatest risk for development of asthma.

Antibiotics and Infections
The use of antibiotics has been associated with early wheezing and asthma in several studies. One suggested mechanism for this association is immunologic stimulation through changes in the bowel flora, but other studies found no coincident increase in eczema or atopy, despite increased wheezing rates—an observation that argues against this mechanism. Greater antibiotic use also may potentially represent a surrogate marker for a higher numbers of infections (perhaps viral) in early life.

Viral infections of the lower respiratory tract contribute to early childhood wheezing. Whether lower respiratory tract infection promotes sensitization to aeroallergens causing persistent asthma is controversial: Childhood viral infections may be pathogenic in some children but protective in others. Infants of mothers with allergy or asthma have a relatively persistent maturational defect in T_H1 cytokine synthesis in the first year of life, which may play a role in the development of persistent or severe viral infections. Severe viral infection of the lower respiratory tract in genetically susceptible infants who are already sensitized to inhalant allergens may lead to deviation toward T_H2 responses promoting asthma. It is unclear whether these effects of lower respiratory tract infection are virus-specific (e.g., RSV, rhinovirus) or whether synergistic exposures to allergens can induce asthma even in children (or adults) who are not genetically susceptible. Interactions of genes with environmental exposures (including allergens, air pollution, environmental tobacco smoke, and diet) modulate the host response to infections. It remains controversial whether the occurrence or timing of childhood infection is pathogenic or protective for the development and long-term outcome of asthma and allergy and of nonallergic wheeze phenotypes. This controversy relates in part to small sample size, cross-sectional analysis, lack of precise case definition, and incomplete microbial assessment in studies of this phenomenon. Respiratory infections in early childhood are associated with early wheezing, but it is unclear whether infection alone has a role in the development of persistent asthma. Repeated lower respiratory tract infection may affect infants who are already at risk for asthma because of family history or atopy. Severe infection with certain viruses such as RSV and rhinovirus may play a role in persistent wheezing, although other studies have suggested no effect. Considered as a proxy for viral infections, day care attendance is associated with higher incidence of early wheeze but lower incidence of persistent wheeze.

Allergens

Allergens are well known to trigger asthma symptoms and also are considered to be the main environmental risk factors. The exposure to allergens can be outdoor (pollens, fungi, molds, yeasts) or indoor (house dust mite, animal proteins [particularly dog and cat dander], cockroaches, and fungi). Most of the allergens associated with asthma are in the air and to induce a condition of hypersensitivity must be present in abundance over considerable periods of time. As soon as the sensitization occurs, the patient can show extreme reactivity, to the point that minimum quantities of the antigen produce significant exacerbations of the disease.

Total serum IgE level, a surrogate for allergen sensitivity, has been associated with the incidence of asthma. High levels of IgE at birth were associated with greater incidence of both atopy and aeroallergen sensitivity but not necessarily asthma. However, sensitization to aeroallergens, particularly house dust mite, cat, and cockroach allergens, is well documented as being associated with asthma. Immune responses in the developing infant and young child may affect the development of asthma. For example, impairment in interferon-γ production at 3 months was associated with a greater risk for development of wheeze. Immaturity in neonatal immune responses may promote the persistence of the T_H2 immune phenotype and development of atopy, but an association with persistent asthma is as yet unproved. More recent work has focused on the role of the innate immune system in handling and presentation of antigens and suggests that polymorphisms in Toll-like receptors (TLRs) may play a greater role than has been previously recognized in the development of the skewed immune responses associated with persistent asthma.

Exposure to Animals

Although several studies have demonstrated a lower risk of development of atopy and asthma with exposure to farm animals in early life, the findings of studies on the influence of exposure to domestic cats and dogs have been inconsistent. In some studies, exposure to cats was associated with a greater risk of allergic sensitization, whereas other studies showed a lower risk. Exposure to dogs may be protective not only against the development of specific sensitization to dog allergen but also against other sensitization (e.g., to house dust mites) and asthma. Other studies of exposure to dogs have suggested that protection against wheezing may be mediated by high levels of endotoxin.

Perinatal Factors

Several prenatal and perinatal factors are proposed to be associated with the development of asthma. Risk factors in the prenatal period are multifactorial. Assessment is complicated by the variety of wheezing conditions that may occur in infancy and childhood, only some of which evolve to classic asthma. The principal prenatal factor is exposure to maternal smoking. The exposure to smoking during pregnancy increases the risk of acquiring asthma up to 37% at the age of 6 and up to 13% after that age. The exposure is clearly associated with fetus growth retardation with disproportionately small airways relative to the size of the lung parenchyma, which in turn is associated with increased airway hyperreactivity, low pulmonary function, asthma, and increased frequency of emergency department visits for treatment of acute exacerbations.

The perinatal factors studied have been maternal age, diet during pregnancy, prematurity, mode of delivery, and in utero exposure to antibiotics. The incidence of wheezing illnesses during childhood is inversely related to maternal age. In one study evaluating young maternal age as a risk factor for childhood asthma, children born to mothers younger than 20 years of age had the highest risk for development of asthma.

Diet and Nutrition   Observational studies examining prenatal nutrient levels or dietary interventions and the subsequent development of atopic disease have focused on foods with antiinflammatory properties (e.g., omega-3 fatty acids) and antioxidants such as vitamin E and zinc. Several studies have demonstrated that higher intake of fish or fish oil during pregnancy is associated with lower risk of atopic disease (specifically eczema and atopic wheeze) up to the age of 6 years. Similarly, higher prenatal vitamin E and zinc levels have been associated with lower risk of development of wheeze up to the age of 5 years. However, no protective effect against the development of atopic disease in infants has been shown for maternal diets that excluded certain foods (e.g., cow's milk, eggs) during pregnancy. Two recent studies reported an inverse relation of maternal vitamin D levels with onset of wheeze in early life, but no relation with atopy or symptoms in later life. The Mediterranean diet during pregnancy is associated with reduced risk of atopy and asthma.

Prematurity and mode of delivery also have been proposed to be associated with asthma. Delivery by cesarean section has been reported to increase the risk of childhood asthma over that associated with vaginal delivery. The possible explanation—an extension of the hygiene hypothesis—is that microbial exposure and infections during early childhood protect against allergic disease; however, data in support of this extended hypothesis are conflicting. Development of atopy was two to three times more likely among infants delivered by emergency cesarean section, although no such association occurred with elective cesarean section. Potential reasons for these findings include maternal stress and differences in the infant's gut microflora associated with specific modes of delivery.

Prenatal Stress   A number of animal models have suggested that prenatal maternal stress acts through regulation of the offspring's hypothalamic-pituitary-adrenal axis to decrease cortisol levels, which may affect the development of an allergic phenotype. Although a correlation has been found between caregiver stress early in the infant's life and higher levels of IgE in the infant and early wheezing, no studies to date have shown an association with asthma.

Antibiotic Use   The association between prenatal antibiotic treatment and subsequent development of atopic disease has been examined in two ways: (1) with treatment as a dichotomous predictor (i.e., any antibiotic use) and (2) by number of courses of antibiotics during pregnancy. Longitudinal cohort studies examining any antibiotic use showed a greater risk for persistent wheeze and asthma in early childhood and a dose-response relation between number of antibiotic courses and risk of wheeze or asthma.

Adult-Onset Asthma

Asthma in adults may have persisted from childhood, may have occurred as a relapse of earlier childhood asthma (whether or not recalled by the affected patient) or may be true adult-onset asthma, with history of no symptoms earlier in life. New-onset asthma in adulthood may have environmental (especially occupational) causes with or without allergen sensitization. Although adult asthma may develop in relation to treatment with specific drugs (e.g., beta blockers, nonsteroidal antiinflammatory drugs) or, in women, the use of hormone replacement therapy, occupational exposure to sensitizing agents or irritants is more common.

Tobacco Smoke and Environmental Tobacco Smoke Exposure
Active smoking and environmental tobacco exposure are associated with increased bronchial responsiveness, frequent bronchial irritation symptoms, increased sensitization to occupational agents, exaggerated decline in lung function, aggravation of acute symptoms, and decreased response to the treatment.

Secondhand smoke is a combination of the smoke given off by the burning end of a cigarette, pipe, or cigar and the smoke exhaled by the smoker. Maternal smoking is the most important cause of secondhand exposure and is associated with the development of asthma in early life. In adults, secondhand smoke exposure increases the risk of asthma, wheezing, bronchitis, and dyspnea; this risk is significantly higher with a daily exposure of longer than 8 hours.

Occupational Exposure
Occupational asthma is found predominantly in adults, and workplace sensitization is responsible for 1 in 10 cases of asthma among adults of working age (see Chapter 40). High-risk occupations for the development of asthma include farming and agricultural work, painting, plastic manufacturing, and cleaning. IgE- and cell-mediated allergic reactions are involved in its pathobiology.

Infections
Early infections with RSV or parainfluenza virus have clinical features similar to symptoms of asthma. Prospective studies in infants infected with RSV early in life have shown that 40% continue with wheezing or develop asthma in later childhood.

Hygiene Hypothesis
The hygiene hypothesis, proposed by Strachan in 1989, suggested that infection and unhygienic contact with older siblings or through other exposures may confer protection against the development of atopy. The lower exposure to these infections among the youngest family members secondary to the improvement in standard of living, programs of immunization, and the indiscriminate use of antibiotics is suggested to be the origin of the problem.

TRIGGER FACTORS

As mentioned earlier, a number of factors are associated with worsening of symptoms and the development of asthma exacerbations.

DIRECT TRIGGERS
Respiratory Infections
Viral respiratory infections are the main trigger factors associated with exacerbations. In small children, RSV and parainfluenza virus are the most common agents; in older children and adults, rhinovirus and influenza virus are predominant.

Nonspecific Irritants
Smoke and bonfire exposure, industrial spills, and pollution (e.g., nitrogen dioxide, sulfur dioxide, carbon monoxide) are sources of nonspecific irritants. Outbreaks of asthma exacerbations have been shown to occur in relationship to increased levels of air pollution, although the role of pollutants in the development of asthma is less well defined.

Meteorologic Changes
Low temperatures, high humidity, cold, and dry air are common asthma triggers and can cause severe symptoms. Hot, humid air also can trigger asthma symptoms. In certain areas, heat and sunlight combine with pollutants to create ground-level ozone, which can be a strong asthma trigger. Wet weather (which encourages the growth of mold) and windy weather (which blows pollen and mold in the air) also are associated with worsening of symptoms.

INDIRECT TRIGGERS
Exercise
Exercise can induce an asthma attack in people who have no other triggers and do not experience asthma under any other circumstances. People with exercise-induced asthma are believed to be more sensitive to changes in the temperature and humidity of the air. The contrast between the warm air in the lungs and the cold inhaled air or the dry inhaled air and moist air in the lungs, evidently can trigger an attack.

Emotional Extremes
Laughing, weeping, anger, and fear all can provoke hyperventilation and unleash airway hyperreactivity, with consequent development of a bronchoconstrictive crisis.

Food Allergens
Food allergy is frequently associated with asthma. Eggs, peanuts, milk, soybean, shellfish, fish, wheat, chocolate, nuts, or orange, among others, might induce asthma in sensitized patients with an incidence between 3% and 10% of children with asthma.

Medications
Aspirin and other nonsteroidal antiinflammatory agents can exacerbate asthma and can cause severe exacerbations. Beta blocker drugs can induce bronchospasm in patients with asthma, either administered orally or intraocularly. Newer cardioselective beta blockers could be safer in asthmatics with ischemic heart disease although further studies are needed. Also, a number of studies have found an association between regular acetaminophen ingestion in early childhood and asthma. This association comes from the depletion induced by acetaminophen in the antioxidant glutathione in lung tissue. As a result, oxidative damage may occur, prostaglandin E_2 (PGE_2) production increases, and T_H2 processing may be promoted.

Gastroesophageal Reflux Disease
Gastroesophageal reflux disease (GERD) can be silent in about 75% of cases and is a frequent cause of chronic cough and asthma exacerbations. In two series, between 50% and 80% of asthmatic patients reported classic GERD symptoms such as heartburn. The mechanism by which GERD can worsen asthma is mainly the tracheobronchial aspiration of gastric acid contents, resulting in airway inflammation. Different studies have determined that treating GERD in asthmatic patients reduces asthma treatment needs and decreases asthma symptoms,

although no improvement in lung function test variables has been demonstrated. In fact, a systematic review that analyzed different treatment options for GERD symptoms in asthmatic patients concluded that none of the therapeutic interventions resulted in clinical improvement as reflected in reduced bronchial hyperreactivity or asthma-like symptoms.

Pregnancy

Asthma in pregnant women can remain unchanged, improve, or worsen, and it is estimated to be present in 4% to 8% of gestational women, as the predominant chronic respiratory disease during the gestational period. Asthma control and management should be established to ensure adequate fetal growth. The main complications are observed more frequently in patients with poorly controlled asthma, in women with severe asthma, and as a consequence of exacerbations predominantly secondary to viral infections. Although the principal physiopathologic mechanisms leading to changes in asthmatic pregnant women remain unclear, the elevation of different types of hormones (progesterone, cortisol) and the lack of treatment compliance during pregnancy seems to play an important role.

SUGGESTED READINGS

Akinbami LJ, Moorman JE, Liu X: Asthma prevalence, health care use, and mortality: United States, 2005-2009, *Natl Health Stat Rep* 32:1–14, 2011.

Asher MI, Montefort S, Bjorksten B, et al: Worldwide time trends in the prevalence of symptoms of asthma, allergic rhinoconjunctivitis, and eczema in childhood: ISAAC phases one and three repeat multicountry cross-sectional surveys, *Lancet* 368:733–743, 2006.

Bara I, Ozier A, Tunon de Lara JM, et al: Pathophysiology of bronchial smooth muscle remodelling in asthma, *Eur Respir J* 36:1174–1184, 2010.

Bisgaard H, Bønnelykke K: Long-term studies of the natural history of asthma in childhood, *J Allergy Clin Immunol* 126:187–197, 2010.

Breysse PN, Diette GB, Matsui EC, et al: Indoor air pollution and asthma in children, *Proc Am Thorac Soc* 7:102–106, 2010.

Busse WW, Lemanske RF Jr, Gern JE: Role of viral respiratory infections in asthma and asthma exacerbations, *Lancet* 376:826–834, 2010.

D'Amato G, Cecchi L, D'Amato M, Liccardi G: Urban air pollution and climate change as environmental risk factors of respiratory allergy: an update, *J Investig Allergol Clin Immunol* 20:95–102, 2010.

Eder W, Ege MJ, von Mutius E: The asthma epidemic, *N Engl J Med* 355:2226–2235, 2006.

Global Initiative for Asthma: *Global strategy for asthma management and prevention. HHLBI/WHO Workshop report, updated 2011* (article online): http://www.ginasthma.org/; accessed February 2, 2012.

Grainge CL, Lau LC, Ward JA, et al: Effect of bronchoconstriction on airway remodeling in asthma, *N Engl J Med* 364:2006–2015, 2011.

Anderson HR, Gupta R, Strachan DP, Limb ES: 50 years of asthma: UK trends from 1955 to 2004, *Thorax* 62:85–90, 2007.

Lemanske RF Jr, Busse WW: Asthma: clinical expression and molecular mechanisms, *J Allergy Clin Immunol* 125(2 Suppl 2):S95–S102, 2010.

Lloyd A, Price D, Brown R: The impact of asthma exacerbations on health-related quality of life in moderate to severe asthma patients in the UK, *Prim Care Respir J* 16:22–27, 2007.

Murphy DM, O'Byrne PM: Recent advances in the pathophysiology of asthma, *Chest* 137:1417–1426, 2010.

Subbarao P, Mandhane PJ, Sears MR: Asthma: epidemiology, etiology and risk factors, *CMAJ* 181:E181–E190, 2009.

Xepapadaki P, Papadopoulos NG: Childhood asthma and infection: virus-induced exacerbations as determinants and modifiers, *Eur Respir J* 36:438–445, 2010.

Chapter **39**

Diagnosis and Management of Asthma in Adults

Ian D. Pavord • Ruth H. Green • Pranabashis Haldar

Asthma is a disorder of the airways that is characterized by typical symptoms arising from a complex interplay between chronic inflammation and disordered airway function. Worldwide disease prevalence has, until recently, risen steadily, and the condition contributes to a significant amount of morbidity and is responsible for many preventable deaths, particularly in developed countries, where 1 in 10 children and 1 in 20 adults have a diagnosis of asthma. The goals of management of asthma are to make an accurate diagnosis; to quantify current morbidity and assess risk of future morbidity; and to use pharmaceutical and nonpharmaceutical interventions to eliminate or minimize current symptoms and future risk of asthma attacks and accelerated decline in lung function. Because asthma usually is a lifelong disease, good patient education and a collaborative approach to management can be expected to increase the chances of success. Pharmacologic management involves the stepwise use of β-agonist bronchodilators, inhaled corticosteroids, and other agents in dosages usually titrated according to symptom management. Important nonpharmacologic measures include patient education, avoidance of triggers, and smoking cessation. Satisfactory control of asthma is achieved in a majority of patients. However, between 5% and 10% of cases of so-called refractory asthma remain poorly controlled and contribute disproportionately to asthma-related morbidity, health care costs, and mortality. The reasons for this are complex and multifactorial, and many patients with refractory asthma require referral to specialist centers.

DEFINITION AND KEY FEATURES OF ASTHMA

Asthma is derived from the Greek word *aazein*, meaning "to labor in breathing" and was first used by Hippocrates, in 450 BCE, to describe a condition characterized by spasms of breathlessness. The present Global Initiative for Asthma (GINA) definition of the disease (**Box 39-1**) is a lengthy description of histopathologic, pathophysiologic, and clinical features that encompass the major disease characteristics. Fundamental features are airway hyperresponsiveness, chronic airway inflammation, disordered airway mucosal immunity, and structural changes to the airways (airway remodeling).

AIRWAY HYPERRESPONSIVENESS

Airway hyperresponsiveness is considered to be the cardinal pathophysiologic abnormality in asthma. It represents an exaggerated bronchoconstrictor response to a variety of largely exogenous inhaled stimuli causing bronchoconstriction, either by a direct effect on airway smooth muscle or indirectly by interacting with neural pathways or mast cells. Airway hyperresponsiveness is likely to be the basis for the variable airflow obstruction that is responsible for many of the day-to-day symptoms of asthma, including those associated with exercise-induced asthma, nocturnal asthma, and asthma induced by fumes or cold air.

Airway hyperresponsiveness can be objectively demonstrated as a 20% fall in the forced expiratory volume in 1 second (FEV_1) after inhalation of histamine or methacholine) at a concentration below 8 mg/mL. This represents an abnormal effector response of airway smooth muscle, characterized by heightened pharmacologic sensitivity and reactivity to the bronchoconstrictor stimulus (**Figure 39-1**). Naturally occurring airway hyperresponsiveness reflects an abnormally amplified response of airway nerves and mast cells to exogenous stimuli, as well as an intrinsic abnormality of the airway smooth muscle response. The basis for this generalized hyperresponsiveness is not entirely clear, but sensitization of airway nerves, mast cells, and smooth muscle by inflammatory mediators, along with loss of epithelial barrier function, reduced production of bronchoprotective factors, an intrinsic abnormality of airway smooth muscle, and structural changes to the airway, all are likely to play a part (**Figure 39-2**). One key pathologic feature associated with airway hyperresponsiveness in asthma not seen in nonasthmatic eosinophilic bronchitis is infiltration of the bronchial smooth muscle layer by mast cells, implying that the interaction between these cells is fundamentally important in the pathogenesis of airway hyperresponsiveness.

CHRONIC AIRWAY INFLAMMATION

Histopathologic examination of postmortem specimens from patients with fatal asthma show an inflammatory response characterized in many cases by the presence of airway eosinophilia. Typically, eosinophilic infiltration can be found throughout the airway wall, within thick viscid plugs that occlude the airway lumen and often extend into the lung parenchyma and alveolar spaces and even into adjacent blood vessels (see Figure 39-2). In addition, extensive eosinophilic degranulation with deposition of major basic proteins occurs. Associated findings include widespread shedding of the airway surface epithelium, thickening of the reticular basement membrane, and enlargement of airway smooth muscle and submucosal glands. A minority of patients dying from asthma, particularly those with sudden-onset fatal

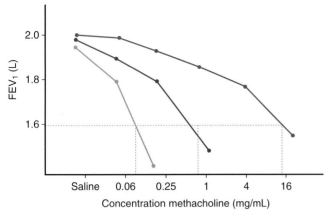

Figure 39-1 Airway responsiveness measured as the fall in forced expiratory volume in 1 second (FEV_1) after increasing inhaled concentrations of methacholine. Severe (*yellow*), moderate (*green*), and mild (*blue*) airway hyperresponsiveness are shown. Note increased airway responsiveness is associated with a lower provocative concentration required to cause a 20% fall in FEV_1 (PC_{20}) (see *green line*), a steeper gradient, and a higher maximum % fall in FEV_1.

Box 39-1   Global Initiative for Asthma (GINA) Description of Asthma

Asthma is a chronic inflammatory disorder of the airways in which many cells and cellular elements play a role, in particular, mast cells, eosinophils, T lymphocytes, neutrophils, and epithelial cells. In susceptible individuals, this inflammation causes recurrent episodes of wheezing, breathlessness, chest tightness, and cough, particularly at night and in the early morning. These episodes are usually associated with widespread airflow obstruction that is typically reversible either spontaneously or with treatment.

From Global Strategy for Asthma Management and Prevention (Update 2009). Available at www.ginaaasthma.org.

asthma, exhibit evidence of eosinophilic inflammation. In these cases it is believed that widespread mast cell degranulation is the primary event with evidence for a relative excess of neutrophils in the distal airways and parenchyma.

Bronchoscopy and bronchial biopsy studies in patients with mild asthma show similar although less dramatic changes. Eosinophil numbers are increased in bronchial biopsy specimens and bronchoalveolar lavage (BAL) fluid, and the eosinophils are activated, with increased concentrations of major basic proteins and leukotrienes found in BAL fluid. Endobronchial biopsy specimens also show increased numbers of $CD4^+$ T cells of T_H2 type, producing the interleukins IL-4, IL-5, and IL-13. These cytokines increase production of IgE and play an important role in the maintenance of eosinophilic airway inflammation.

The limited number of patients studied by bronchoscopy makes it difficult to investigate heterogeneity of the lower airway inflammatory response, but less invasive assessment of airway inflammation using induced sputum analysis has shown that a significant proportion of patients with asthma studied when stable and during an attack have normal eosinophil numbers in induced sputum samples. This sputum cell profile has been reported in patients with severe asthma and in patients who are not treated with inhaled corticosteroids, and the absence of eosinophilic airway inflammation has been confirmed by bronchoscopy studies. Thus, the presence of a distinct noneosinophilic corticosteroid-resistant asthma phenotype across the range of asthma severity seems secure. Noneosinophilic asthma is discussed in more detail later in the chapter.

DISORDERED AIRWAY MUCOSAL IMMUNITY

The airway mucosa in persons with asthma mounts an abnormally amplified immunologic response to a variety of exogenous stimuli, including inhaled allergens, cigarette smoke, infectious agents, and air pollutants. Some or all of these abnormal responses may be the consequence of failure of maturation of the immune response in early life as a result of reduced exposure to pathogens at a critical point in development.

Particular interest has focused in the response to allergen, because atopy is twice as common in patients with asthma as in control subjects without asthma, and inhalation of allergen in a patient with atopic asthma who is sensitized to the allergen results in a marked eosinophilic airway inflammatory response, developing 4 to 6 hours after inhalation associated with airflow obstruction (the late response) and increased airway responsiveness lasting for days and weeks. Common aeroallergens in many Westernized countries include house dust mite, cat fur, grass pollen, ragweed, and *Aspergillus fumigatus* spores. Most patients with childhood-onset asthma are sensitized to one of more of these allergens, and many have extrapulmonary manifestations of allergy, including eczema and allergic rhinitis. Opinions regarding the significance of the response to allergen vary, ranging from a fundamentally important role in the pathogenesis of airway inflammation and dysfunction in asthma to a position in which it is seen as a more peripheral mechanism. The occurrence of histopathologically similar forms of asthma in nonatopic patients and the disappointing therapeutic effect of allergen avoidance and anti-IgE treatment suggest that the latter position is correct, although uncertainty remains.

Growing evidence points to an abnormal airway response to infecting respiratory viruses, resulting in an amplified airway inflammatory response and more pronounced clinical consequences. The molecular mechanisms of this remain uncertain but constitute an active area of current study. There is little doubt that viral infection is an important trigger for acute severe asthma. Smoking and perhaps exposure to other environmental pollutants have been linked to worsening of symptoms, an increased risk of asthma attacks, and the development of fixed airflow obstruction. This association may reflect an abnormality of the innate immune response; patients with asthma who smoke or are exposed to environmental pollutants tend to have noneosinophilic, neutrophilic airway inflammation.

STRUCTURAL CHANGES TO THE AIRWAY

Structural changes in airway morphology (airway remodeling) probably occur as a result of chronic airway inflammation and dysfunction. These changes are likely to be the basis for the accelerated lung function decline and fixed airflow obstruction seen in some patients with asthma. Key features of airway remodeling include thickening of the subepithelial basement membrane caused by abnormal deposition of collagen, increased airway smooth muscle bulk, increased mucus-secreting cells, and increased airway vascularity (see Figure 39-2). In severe asthma, bronchiectasis, small airway fibrosis, and emphysema may be features. The bronchiectasis is associated with sensitization to *Aspergillus*.

PATHOPHYSIOLOGIC BASIS OF ASTHMA

Asthma is a complex condition in which it is not always obvious which of the various pathophysiologic abnormalities is

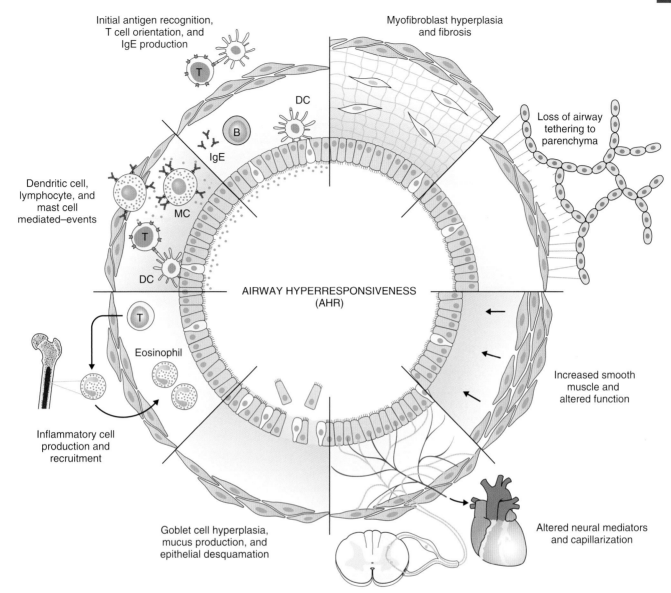

Figure 39-2   Schematic diagram of the inflammatory and remodeling processes in the airway that may potentially contribute to airway hyperresponsiveness and airflow obstruction.   *(Courtesy Professor Mark Inman.)*

responsible for morbidity at any one time. In order to make some sense of this complexity, it can be helpful to consider five potentially important pathophysiologic factors, presented in alphabetical array for convenience:

- Airway hyperresponsiveness
- Bronchitis
- Cough reflex hypersensitivity
- Damage to the airways and surrounding lung
- Extrapulmonary factors.

These abnormalities are likely to be linked, but the mechanism is complex, and cross-sectional and longitudinal correspondence among them is not close. Accordingly, each is best considered as a relatively independent factor.

It is likely that these factors contribute to airflow obstruction and morbidity in different ways (**Figure 39-3**). Airway hyperresponsiveness is responsible for short-term, bronchodilator-responsive variable airflow obstruction which is the basis for many of the day-to-day symptoms experienced by patients and is suppressed by bronchodilator therapy, and to a lesser extent corticosteroids. Bronchitis, which may be eosinophilic and corticosteroid-responsive or neutrophilic and corticosteroid-unresponsive, manifests with cough and sputum and a relatively bronchodilator-resistant but potentially corticosteroid-responsive airflow obstruction of more gradual onset. Inflammation-mediated airflow obstruction is particularly important in the pathogenesis of asthma attacks. Cough and a small amount of sputum production is common in asthma. It probably reflects airway inflammation but also may be due to cough reflex hypersensitivity, a common but poorly understood and difficult-to-treat aspect of asthma and other airway diseases. Airway damage may manifest with disability caused by bronchodilator and corticosteroid-resistant airflow obstruction or mucus retention and infection as a result of airway and lung parenchymal damage. Extrapulmonary conditions linked to the inflammatory airway disease or independent of it also may contribute to symptoms (**Box 39-2**).

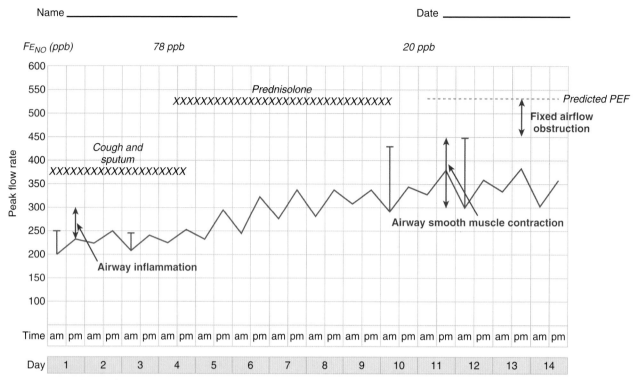

Figure 39-3 Peak expiratory flow (PEF) chart illustrating airflow obstruction due to at least three discrete mechanisms: airway smooth muscle contraction (note good acute response to inhaled salbutamol); airway inflammation (note loss of acute bronchodilator response but gradual increase in PEF with oral prednisolone); and airway damage (bronchodilator and steroid-unresponsive airflow obstruction).

Box 39-2	**Differential Diagnosis of Asthma in Adults With and Without Airflow Obstruction***

Without Airflow Obstruction
Chronic cough syndromes
Hyperventilation syndrome
Vocal cord dysfunction
Rhinitis
Gastroesophageal reflux
Cardiac failure
Pulmonary fibrosis

With Airflow Obstruction
COPD
Bronchiectasis[†]
Inhaled foreign body[†]
Obliterative bronchiolitis
Large airway stenosis
Lung cancer[†]
Sarcoidosis[†]

*FEV_1 <70% predicted, FEV_1/FVC <0.7.
[†]May also be associated with nonobstructive spirometry values.
COPD, chronic obstructive pulmonary disease; FEV_1, forced expiratory volume in 1 second; *FVC*, forced vital capacity.

ASTHMA HETEROGENEITY AND CLINICAL SUBGROUPS OF PATIENTS WITH ASTHMA

Asthma has long been recognized as a heterogeneous disease. As early as 1918, Francis Rackemann identified clear clinical subgroups on the basis of history, skin tests, and response to "a clinical experiment such as a change in residence, a restriction in diet or an elimination of some supposedly offending substance." He made a distinction between "extrinsic asthma" due to "hypersensitivity to some foreign substance outside of the body and

"intrinsic asthma . . . implying the essential cause of the trouble is inside of the body." The subdivision of extrinsic (atopic) and intrinsic (nonatopic) asthma remains popular. The most obvious difference is that the peak age at onset of atopic asthma is in childhood, whereas nonatopic asthma often manifests first in adults. It has not been possible to identify consistent histopathologic differences. In general, patients with atopic asthma exhibit more airway hyperresponsiveness and better responses to inhaled corticosteroids than those with nonatopic asthma. Nonatopic asthma is associated with greater heterogeneity of the lower airway inflammatory response, because a majority of patients with noneosinophilic asthma are nonatopic.

Asthma also has been classified according to the dominant clinical characteristic. Exercise-induced asthma, premenstrual asthma, and seasonal asthma are examples. These subdivisions help to remind the clinician of the dominant trigger but do not identify patients with a distinct pathologic process or treatment response. Important exceptions are aspirin-induced asthma, asthma in endurance athletes, and occupational asthma. These conditions are considered later.

Current interest is in categorization of asthma by the pattern of lower airway inflammation. The development of induced sputum as a means to non-invasively assess airway inflammation has made it possible to do this. Cross-sectional studies show that 20% to 40% of patients with symptomatic asthma do not have sputum evidence of eosinophilic airway inflammation. Many have a sputum neutrophilia and evidence of airway release of cytokines linked to the innate immune response. This sputum profile is evident in corticosteroid-naive as well as corticosteroid-treated persons and is consistently seen in patients with asthma, suggesting it is not always an artifact related to infection or treatment. Noneosinophilic asthma is clinically important, because response to corticosteroids is less pronounced in patients with this inflammatory profile than in persons with more typical sputum features. Noneosinophilic asthma has been associated with smoking, obesity, high-level endurance training in athletes, menopause, occupational endotoxin exposure, and recurrent bacterial bronchitis. Treatment and management approaches have not been investigated extensively, but aggressive corticosteroid therapy is unlikely to be helpful. Preliminary evidence indicates that long-term macrolide antibiotics may be of benefit.

Cross-sectional sputum studies also have shown that some patients with cough have eosinophilic airway inflammation but normal airway function (eosinophilic bronchitis). Eosinophilic bronchitis is closely related to "atopic cough," a condition described in Japan and characterized by cough, atopy, and evidence of large airway eosinophilic inflammation. Cough variant asthma initially was described as asthma manifesting with a bronchodilator-responsive chronic cough. More recently, this entity has been extended to encompass patients presenting with cough and objective evidence of asthma (i.e., variable airflow obstruction and/or airway hyperresponsiveness). All of these conditions are characterized clinically by a corticosteroid-responsive chronic cough.

GENETICS OF ASTHMA

Asthma has long been known to run in families. Studies of monozygotic and dizygotic twins, which control for environmental exposure, have estimated heritability of 30% to 70%. Considerable effort and resources have been put into identifying the genetic basis of asthma. This work is inevitably compromised by the rather general and imprecise definition of the disease, and results have been mixed and often are inconsistent. A better understanding of different phenotypes of asthma and a stronger focus on aspects of the disease (i.e., fixed airflow obstruction, airway hyperresponsiveness, atopy, eosinophilic airway inflammation), rather than on the syndrome, may be the way forward. Despite these limitations, some consistent genetic associations have been identified.

Functionally important polymorphisms of the prostaglandin D_2 (PGD_2) receptor gene have been associated with asthma in case control studies in racially diverse populations. PGD_2 is an important product of mast cells, and the receptor is involved in T cell recruitment. Mice deficient in this gene do not develop airway inflammation in response to allergen. Interest in this receptor has increased recently, because preliminary evidence indicates that PGD_2 receptor antagonists have useful therapeutic effects in asthma. Positional cloning studies have identified a consistent association between asthma and multiple single nucleotide polymorphisms of the ADAM33 gene, particularly when asthma is associated with airway hyperresponsiveness or fixed airflow obstruction. This gene may be involved in control of airway structure and myogenesis. The minor allele (G) of the functional variant of the promoter region of the matrix metalloproteinase 12 gene (MMP12) has been associated with better lung function in patients with asthma and in smokers, suggesting a role for MMP12 in maintaining lung function and raising the possibility of a common mechanism for the development of fixed airflow obstruction in smokers and in patients with asthma. Polymorphisms of the genes for IL-13 and FcεR1B, which modifies the activity of the high-affinity IgE receptor, may have a closer link with atopy, IgE, eosinophilic airway inflammation, and mucus production. Other genetic associations with asthma such as polymorphisms of the gene for the microbial pattern recognition receptors CD14, Toll-like receptor-1 (TLR-1), and this should be T cell immunoglobulin

mucin-like domain-1 (TIM-1) may operate primarily by modifying innate immunity and the maturation of the immune system.

Genetic polymorphisms also may potentially influence the response to treatment. Variation in the gene for the β_2-adrenergic receptor (ADRB2) has been the subject of much interest, because persons who are Gly16 homozygotes or heterozygotes have a diminished acute bronchodilator response compared with Arg16 homozygotes. On the other hand, Arg16 homozygotes are more susceptible to β_2-receptor downregulation and may potentially be at risk for an adverse response to regular use of β_2-agonists. Evidence for such an effect, however, has not been seen consistently, particularly with long-acting β_2-agonists. Important genetic diversity in the response to corticosteroids has been more difficult to establish, in part because the response to this treatment is more difficult to quantify. The response to leukotriene antagonists has been associated with the C allele of the LTC4 synthase gene promoter (A-444C) polymorphism. This polymorphism is also associated with aspirin-induced asthma, an asthma variant associated with increased airway production of cysteinyl leukotrienes.

DIAGNOSIS

One of the problems facing clinicians and epidemiologists is the absence of a "gold standard" modality for defining or diagnosing asthma. Characteristic clinical features (**Box 39-3**) coupled with objective demonstration of variable airflow obstruction and/or airway hyperresponsiveness usually will provide sufficient evidence to make the diagnosis.

HISTORY

Asthma symptoms typically are variable reflecting variability in airflow obstruction and other aspects of the disease.

Box 39-3	**Factors Affecting Likelihood of Asthma as Cause of Respiratory Symptoms***

Factors Associated With Increased Probability of Asthma
More than one of the following symptoms: cough, breathlessness, wheeze, chest tightness
Symptoms worse at night and in the early morning
Symptoms occurring in response to exercise, allergen exposure, and cold air
Symptoms developing after taking aspirin or beta blockers
History of atopic disorder
Family history of asthma and/or atopic disorder
Variable wheeze heard on auscultation of the chest
Variable PEF (see Clinical Examination Section)
Otherwise unexplained low PEF

Factors Associated With Lower Probability of Asthma
Prominent dizziness, light-headedness, peripheral tingling
Isolated cough
Repeatedly normal physical examination of chest when symptomatic
Normal PEF when symptomatic
Voice disturbance
Symptoms with colds only
Chronic productive cough
Significant smoking history (i.e., more than 20 pack-years)
Cardiac disease

---

*Presence of any one factor is sufficient evidence for or against a diagnosis of asthma.
PEF, peak expiratory flow [rate].

Exaggerated diurnal variation in physiologic bronchomotor tone causes airflow obstruction and symptoms at night, maximally at 4 AM. Other symptoms reflect airway hyperresponsiveness to a multitude of possible trigger factors. Symptoms occurring after exercise, after exposure to allergens, and in response to inhaled noxious fumes such as cigarette smoke are most commonly reported. Box 39-3 lists some of the symptoms that increase and decrease the probability of asthma. An assessment of disease severity can be made from the frequency of daily symptoms, exercise limitation, nocturnal wakening, and exacerbation frequency (Table 39-1).

The pattern of daytime symptoms and seasonal variations can help identify common triggers. In patients with adult-onset symptoms, the possibility of occupational asthma or an alternative diagnosis should be carefully explored. Symptoms that worsen at work but remit outside of the workplace should alert the clinician to the possibility of occupational asthma.

CLINICAL EXAMINATION

Findings on the clinical examination frequently are normal in persons with well-controlled symptoms. Patients with persistent symptoms may display features of obstructive airway disease, notably a hyperinflated and hyperresonant chest and diffuse polyphonic expiratory wheeze. These signs are indistinguishable from those found in chronic obstructive pulmonary disease (COPD). Physical examination is helpful for identifying features of an alternative diagnosis.

Measuring Airflow Obstruction

The demonstration of obstructive spirometry in patients with a history suggestive of asthma strongly supports the diagnosis and is a strong basis to commence therapy. Spirometry is the preferred method for demonstrating airflow obstruction, because it is less effort-dependent than peak expiratory flow. Airflow obstruction is defined as an FEV_1/FVC ratio of less than 0.7.

Measuring Variability in Airflow Obstruction

The spirogram frequently is normal in patients with asthma who are asymptomatic at the time of testing. In this clinical scenario, measurement of *variability* in airflow obstruction will provide useful additional information. A number of different methods exist to measure variability:

Diurnal variation in peak expiratory flow (PEF): Calculated from serial PEF measurements (see Figure 39-3); typically expressed as the difference between the highest and lowest daily readings as a percentage of the mean (see Table 39-1)

Assessment of the bronchodilator response: Measured as the change (improvement) in FEV_1 or PEF from baseline with either a short-acting bronchodilator (bronchodilator responsiveness) or after a therapeutic trial of corticosteroid (steroid responsiveness)

Assessment of airway responsiveness: Measuring the fall in FEV_1 in response to bronchoconstrictor stimuli, including pharmacologic agents (methacholine or histamine challenge tests), exercise, and allergen challenge (see Figure 39-1)

The measurement characteristics of the various tests to assess variable airflow obstruction and asthma in general are outlined in Table 39-1. An algorithm for the assessment of patients with suspected asthma is presented in **Figure 39-4.**

DIAGNOSTIC PATHWAY

The diagnostic pathway followed will depend on the pretest probability for the diagnosis, response to therapy, and level of clinical suspicion for an alternative diagnosis. The scope of the differential diagnosis is quite different in patients with and without airflow obstruction (see Box 39-2), and the main diagnostic question also is different. In the former, the clinician often is seeking support for a clinical diagnosis of asthma and the initiation of antiasthma therapy; in the latter, the evidence for an airway problem is more clear-cut, and the question is not whether inhalers should be used but how intensive the corticosteroid component of that therapy should be.

The key point in the history is to establish that symptoms are variable and linked to airflow obstruction and/or variable eosinophilic airway inflammation. Problems arise when symptoms are clearly associated with infections. A prolonged post-viral cough is common in otherwise healthy persons but also can be the presenting manifestation of asthma. Recurrent bouts of bronchitis in a patient with a long-standing chronic productive cough and focal coarse crackles should raise the possibility of bronchiectasis. Prominent dizziness, panic, peripheral tingling, light-headedness, and chest tightness are very suggestive of dysfunctional breathing.

Vocal cord or glottic dysfunction is an important condition that can cause serious diagnostic difficulty in both adolescents and adults and, if not recognized, unnecessary overtreatment. Wheezing that arises from the glottis is heard throughout the lung fields but also is easy to hear without the stethoscope, with prominent noises arising from the neck. Direct visualization of the glottis by laryngoscopy may reveal the characteristic inspiratory apposition of the cords. Sometimes persons who have asthma make this noise, because they subconsciously feel the need to impress on the examiner the severity of their condition. In other patients, the noise occurs for purely psychological reasons, and no evidence of asthma is found. Patients may be of either gender but are often women in the age range of 16 to 50 years, who may have a paramedical background. Their "asthma" seems "resistant" to standard treatments, and often they have been hospitalized on many occasions and been treated unsuccessfully with large doses of corticosteroids and other treatments. Home peak flow readings and attempts at spirometry may be variable but show little correlation with attacks or treatment. Flow-volume curves may show a characteristic "fluttering" of the inspiratory curve. Measurement of total airway resistance in a body plethysmograph may be diagnostic, because the panting maneuver necessary for such measurement abolishes the vocal cord adduction, and airway resistance can be shown to be normal. Occasionally patients end up being mechanically ventilated because of "severe" asthma, but once pharmacologic paralysis is achieved, it can be seen that airway resistance is normal and that there is no necessity for high inflation pressures.

Vocal cord dysfunction probably is much more common than has been appreciated and if the condition is underdiagnosed or the relevant symptoms are mistaken for asthma, overtreatment is likely. Correct diagnosis is essential, and if vocal cord dysfunction is the sole or major part of the wheezing disorder, speech therapy can be helpful.

Diagnostic Strategy in Patients With Normal Spirometry Findings

In patients with normal spirometry findings, the primary considerations in the differential diagnosis are non–bronchodilator-,

Table 39-1   **Summary of Tests Used to Assess Asthma**

Measurement	Methodology	Measurement Characteristics	Comments
Spirometry	Enables clear demonstration of airflow obstruction FEV_1 largely independent of effort and highly repeatable Less applicable in acute severe asthma Assesses only one aspect of the disease state	Normal ranges widely available and robust Short-term (20-minute) 95% range for repeat measure of FEV_1 <160 mL; FVC <330 mL, independent of baseline value	Good for short- and longer-term reversibility testing in subjects with preexisting airflow obstruction >400-mL increase in FEV_1 highly suggestive of asthma Less helpful in subjects with normal pretreatment values because of ceiling effect
Peak expiratory flow (PEF)	Widely available and simple Applicable in a wide variety of circumstances including acute severe asthma PEF variability can be determined from home readings in most subjects PEF effort dependent and not as repeatable as FEV_1 Assesses only one aspect of the disease state	Normal ranges of PEF are wide, and currently available normative tables are outdated and do not encompass ethnic diversity Change in PEF more meaningful than absolute value >60 L/min increase in PEF suggested as best criteria for defining reversibility Normal range of PEF variability defined as amplitude % highest <8% or <20% depending on number of readings and degree of patient coaching	Useful for short- and longer-term reversibility testing in subjects with preexisting airflow obstruction Less helpful in subjects with normal pretreatment values because of ceiling effect Little information on the use of PEF variability as an index of treatment response PEF monitoring may improve asthma control in patients with more severe disease and in those with poor perception of bronchoconstriction
Asthma Control Questionnaire	Response to 7 questions, 5 relating to symptoms, 1 rescue treatment use and 1 FEV_1 Response usually assessed over the preceding week Shortened, five-question symptom only questionnaire is just as valid	Well-controlled: ≤0.75; inadequately controlled: ≥1.5 95% range for repeat measure ± 0.36 Minimal important difference 0.5	
Mini Asthma Quality of Life Questionnaire (AQLQ)	Response to 15 questions in 4 domains (symptoms, activity limitations, emotional function, environmental stimuli) Response usually assessed over the preceding week Closely related to larger 32-item Asthma Quality of Life Questionnaire	95% range for repeat measure ± 0.36 Minimal important difference 0.5	Well-validated quality of life questionnaire Could be used to assess response to longer term treatment trials
Airway responsiveness	Responsive to change (particularly indirect challenges such as inhaled mannitol) Less of a ceiling effect Not applicable in patients with impaired lung function (i.e., FEV_1/FVC <0.7 and <70% predicted)	Normal methacholine PC_{20} >8 mg/mL 95% range for repeat measure ± 1.5-2 doubling doses	Has not been widely used to monitor disease and assess treatment responses
Exhaled nitric oxide (FeNO)	Measurements can be obtained in almost all adults Results immediately available Reasonably close relationship between FeNO and eosinophilic airway inflammation, which is independent of gender, age, atopy, and inhaled corticosteroid use Not closely related to other measures of asthma morbidity	Normal range <25 ppb at exhaled flow of 50 mL/sec. 95% range for repeat measure 4 ppb >50 ppb highly predictive of a positive response to corticosteroid therapy <25 ppb highly predictive of a poor response to corticosteroids or successful step down in corticosteroid therapy	Evidence that FeNO can be used to guide corticosteroid treatment is mixed. Protocols for diagnosis and monitoring have not been well defined, and more work is needed Low FeNO (<25 ppb) may be of particular value in identifying patients who can step down corticosteroid treatment safely
Sputum eosinophil differential count	Information available in 80-90% of patients, although immediate results not available Sputum eosinophil count not closely related to other measures of asthma morbidity	Normal range <2%; 95% range for repeat measure ± 2-3 fold	Close relationship between raised sputum eosinophil count and corticosteroid responsiveness Use of sputum eosinophil count to guide corticosteroid therapy associated with reduced exacerbations in patients with more severe disease

FEV_1, forced expiratory volume in 1 second; *FVC*, forced vital capacity; PC_{20}, provocative concentration of inhaled substance required to cause a 20% fall in FEV_1; *ppb*, parts per billion.

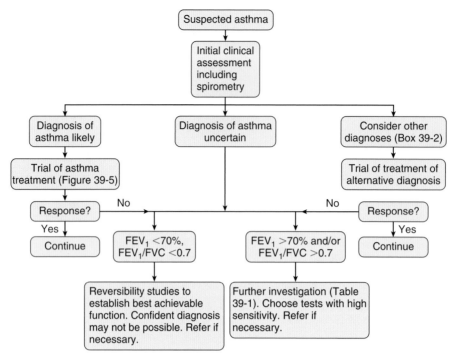

Figure 39-4 Algorithm for the initial investigation of suspected asthma. *FEV₁*, forced expiratory volume in 1 second; *FVC*, forced vital capacity.

non–corticosteroid-responsive conditions. All tests of variable airflow obstruction lack sensitivity in this setting, meaning that negative findings are not particularly helpful. Positive findings are obtained more frequently with repeated testing or if care is taken to perform the assessment when the patient is symptomatic. Assessment of airway hyperresponsiveness is a more sensitive test, so the absence of airway hyperresponsiveness should prompt careful consideration of an alternative diagnosis.

Diagnostic Strategy in Patients With Obstructive Spirometry

In patients with obstructive spirometry, tests of airway responsiveness and reactivity are less specific for a diagnosis of asthma. The measurement of airway hyperresponsiveness is therefore not helpful. Bronchodilator challenge tests and therapeutic trials of corticosteroid treatment may aid diagnosis, because larger changes in FEV₁ (i.e., more than 400 mL) are very suggestive of asthma. In many cases it may not be possible to assign a precise diagnostic label, although bronchodilator and steroid reversibility studies do help guide the intensity of therapy with these agents.

Other Investigations

Further investigations are helpful if an alternative diagnosis or presence of an additional disorder that may aggravate asthma symptoms is suspected. Further imaging of the upper airway, esophageal pH monitoring, a computed tomography (CT) chest scan, and sputum culture may help in selected cases. Objective assessment of atopy with skin prick testing or measurement of IgE and allergen-specific IgE may help support a diagnosis of atopic asthma and will provide an important guide to allergen avoidance strategies, anti-IgE treatment, and antifungal therapy (see further on). A raised blood eosinophil count commonly is seen in asthma; in the absence of an obvious systemic explanation (e.g., eczema), it is a specific but not sensitive marker of eosinophilic airway inflammation.

One of the most important recent advances in the field of assessment of airway disease has been the development of techniques to assess airway inflammation that are safe and feasible in most patients (i.e., inflammometry, as described later on). Two techniques are in widespread use: induced sputum analysis, in which differential and total cell counts are used to determine the characteristics and intensity of the lower airway inflammatory response, and measurement of exhaled nitric oxide (FENO), whereby the concentration of nitric oxide in exhaled air is used to provide information about the presence of potentially corticosteroid responsive airway inflammation. Measurement of FENO is particularly relevant to primary care practice, because the instruments needed for this assessment have become affordable, the technique is simple, and it provides an immediate result, making it ideal for monitoring purposes. A raised sputum eosinophil count or FENO concentration is sufficiently common in untreated asthma to be of diagnostic value, but abnormal results are nonspecific, occurring in up to a third of patients classified as having cough and COPD. The real value of these techniques is that raised values are strongly associated with a positive response to corticosteroid treatment irrespective of the context in which the abnormal test result occurs.

MANAGEMENT OF STABLE ASTHMA

AIMS

Three major consequences of clinical importance in asthma are recognized, as reflected in the following management goals:

1. Control of asthma symptoms
2. Prevention of asthma attacks
3. Preservation of normal lung function

Both pharmacologic and nonpharmacologic measures play an important role in achieving these aims (**Box 39-4**; **Figures 39-5 and 39-6**).

Control of Symptoms

Asthma symptoms are a cause of both physical and psychological morbidity that exert considerable impact on quality of life. Any of several well-validated questionnaires can be used to assess the control of asthma symptoms (see Table 39-1).

Prevention of Asthma Attacks

Asthma attacks are defined as periods of poor asthma control manifested by an increase in symptoms and deterioration in lung function that are not adequately managed by the individual patient's usual therapeutic regime. They frequently are precipitated by allergen exposure or viral infections. Severe attacks lead to hospitalization and constitute the primary cause of asthma-related death. The management of asthma attacks is considered later in this chapter.

Box 39-4 Goals of Asthma Management

- Minimal (ideally no) chronic symptoms, including nocturnal symptoms
- Minimal (infrequent) exacerbations
- No emergency visits
- Minimal (ideally no) use of β₂-agonist on an as-needed basis
- No limitations on activities, including exercise
- PEF circadian variation of less than 20%
- (Near-) normal PEF
- Minimal (or no) adverse effects

PEF, peak expiratory flow.

Addressing Lung Function Decline

Chronic asthma is associated with accelerated decline in lung function that is considered to be a function of persistent airway inflammation. Clinically important decrease in lung function may occur early in the disease, presenting a challenge to efforts at prevention. The rate of decline in adults is more marked in those with severe adult-onset disease, in smokers, and in patients with frequent exacerbations. Although interventions preventing decline are poorly understood, smoking cessation, early removal from occupational sensitizers, and possibly optimal corticosteroid therapy are likely to be effective.

PHARMACOTHERAPY IN ASTHMA

Inhaled pharmacologic therapies are central to asthma management. The range of available drugs may be categorized mechanistically into bronchodilators and antiinflammatory agents.

Bronchodilators

β₂-*Agonists*

β₂-Agonists act by a common final pathway of increased intracellular cyclic adenosine monophosphate (cAMP) in smooth muscle cells that inhibits contractility, leading to improvements in lung function and decrease in airway hyperresponsiveness. The primary role of bronchodilators is in the relief and prevention of symptoms, by means of short- and long-acting agents, respectively. Additionally, the regular use of long acting bronchodilators can lead to sustained improvements in lung

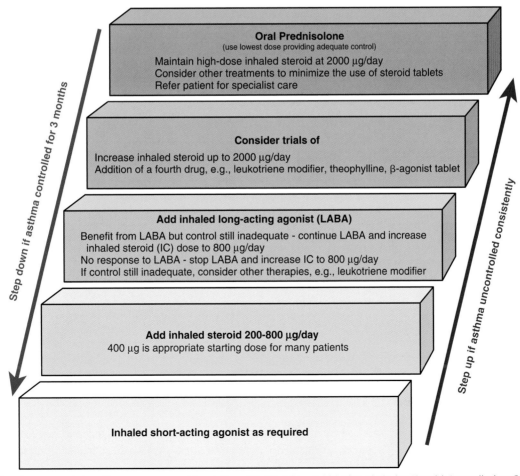

Figure 39-5 Stepwise approach to asthma management in adults. *(Modified from British Thoracic Society/Scottish Intercollegiate Guidelines Network.)*

		Control of asthma symptoms	Prevention of exacerbations	Preservation of lung function
Pharmacologic	Inhaled and oral corticosteroids	+++	+++	?
	Long-acting β agonists	++	+(*)	
	Antileukotrienes	+	+	
	All bronchodilators	++		
Nonpharmacologic	Patient education	++	+	
	Trigger avoidance	++	+	
	Smoking cessation	+++	?	+
	Breathing retraining techniques	++		

Figure 39-6 The effect on management options on the goals of asthma therapy. *The prevention of exacerbations with long-acting β-agonists is only in conjunction with inhaled corticosteroids.

function and may reduce exacerbations, particularly less severe events.

Short-acting β_2-agonists are widely used for rescue symptomatic therapy. At present, long-acting β_2-agonists, such as salmeterol and formoterol, generally are recommended as agents of first choice for patients who have symptoms that persist despite regular inhaled corticosteroids. Salmeterol is a partial agonist of the β_2 receptor, whereas formoterol is a full agonist. These agents appear to have similar clinical effects, but formoterol has a more rapid onset of action. Side effects of tachycardia, tremor, and muscle cramps are rarely a problem unless these drugs are given in high doses. Tolerance to the effects of long-acting β_2-agonists with loss of bronchodilator activity after the subsequent administration of both short- and long-acting β_2-agonists has been reported but is of uncertain clinical relevance.

As with short-acting β_2-agonists, these agents work primarily through the relaxation of airway smooth muscle, with additional inhibitory effects on mast cells and vascular permeability. Long-acting β_2-agonists have no measurable effects on eosinophilic airway inflammation, and their use as first-line agents in patients with asthma is not recommended. When added to inhaled steroids, long-acting β_2-agonists control daytime and nighttime symptoms and reduce the need for rescue β_2-agonists more than other treatment options. The generalizability of the clinical trials showing this has been questioned, however, because most recruited only patients who demonstrated large acute improvements in FEV_1 after use of inhaled bronchodilators.

Theophylline

Theophylline has been used for many years in relatively high doses as a bronchodilator, but owing to its narrow therapeutic window and recognized adverse effects, it often has been reserved for use in patients with more severe asthma. Gastrointestinal upset is particularly common, but tachycardia and arrhythmia also can occur, and measurements of serum concentration generally are advised with high-dose treatment. Recent interest has focused on the use of lower-dose theophylline, because side effects are less of an issue, and the combination of low-dose inhaled corticosteroids and theophylline has been shown to result in asthma control comparable with that achieved with higher doses of inhaled corticosteroids and may provide slightly greater improvements in lung function. A metaanalysis has suggested that long-acting β_2-agonists are more effective than theophylline in patients taking low doses of inhaled corticosteroids and result in fewer side effects. Unlike long-acting β_2-agonists, however, theophylline has been shown to have possible antiinflammatory activity and may therefore have a role in the management of some patients with corticosteroid-resistant disease.

Antiinflammatory Therapies

Inhaled Corticosteroids

Inhaled corticosteroids are the mainstay of asthma pharmacotherapy. They act topically in the large- and medium-sized airways, binding to glucocorticoid receptors that are expressed ubiquitously by cells. The antiinflammatory effects of corticosteroids are mediated by the direct repression of transcription factors such as nuclear factor κB. The poor systemic bioavailability of inhaled corticosteroids minimizes systemic side effects, although chronic treatment with higher doses of potent steroid may be associated with mild adrenal suppression and stunted growth in children. Corticosteroids effectively suppress eosinophilic inflammation, which is associated with a decrease in symptoms, lower rate of exacerbations, and reduced asthma mortality.

Inhaled corticosteroids are less effective for managing severe asthma and may not be useful to treat severe asthma exacerbations, perhaps because of the intensity and site of airway inflammation. Oral therapy is believed to be more effective in these circumstances.

Patients often are concerned about the possibility of adverse effects of inhaled corticosteroids, and in some parts of the world, notably North America, this concern has led to their relative underuse. At low doses, up to 800 μg daily of beclomethasone dipropionate (BDP) or budesonide or 500 μg daily of fluticasone, side effects are not usually significant, but they do become an issue at doses above this. Furthermore, there is little additional therapeutic benefit beyond the point at which local and systemic side effects become common, and it is becoming clear that use of an alternative drug is a better strategy than increasing the dose of inhaled steroid in most patients.

Dysphonia commonly occurs as a consequence of deposition of inhaled corticosteroid particles locally in the oropharynx and local side effects such as oral candidiasis and hoarseness of voice may also develop. Use of a large-volume spacer device and careful rinsing of the mouth after the use of inhaled corticosteroids will reduce the risk of these local effects. Systemic side effects include bruising and atrophy of the skin, cataract formation, glaucoma, and reduced bone mineral density. Suppression of the adrenocortical axis can occur with high-dose inhaled corticosteroids, and specific advice on use of corticosteroid replacement therapy during intercurrent illness should be considered in patients who genuinely require long-term high-dose therapy. Systemic effects occur partly as a result of gastrointestinal absorption of swallowed particles and partly due to systemic absorption via the airways. The use of spacer devices, dry powder mechanisms, and mouth rinsing after inhaler use will minimize adverse effects. Another approach to minimize local side effects is to use ciclesonide, a prodrug that is activated by contact with the lower airway epithelium. Drugs with high first pass metabolism in the liver such as budesonide and fluticasone have less systemic side effects than beclomethasone, but at high doses (more than 800 to 1000 μg daily of BDP/budesonide or more than 500 μg daily of fluticasone), systemic absorption through the buccal and airway mucosa becomes increasingly important.

Antileukotrienes

Antileukotrienes act by inhibiting different levels of the lipoxygenase pathway, which is involved in the formation of leukotrienes from arachidonic acid. Leukotrienes are important proinflammatory mediators in asthma that also promote bronchoconstriction. Leukotriene receptor antagonists (e.g., montelukast) reduce exercise-induced asthma and have a modest suppressive effect on asthma symptoms. They appear to work best in patients not taking inhaled corticosteroids and, because of their excellent safety profile, often are considered for use in children. Inhibitors of leukotriene biosynthesis may offer an advantage over receptor antagonists in that they inhibit production of the noncysteinyl leukotriene LTB_4. Whether this results in important clinical advantages has not been clearly defined, and concerns have been raised about liver toxicity with the only available inhibitor, zileuton.

Oral Corticosteroids and Corticosteroid-Sparing Agents

A further group of patients have severe persistent asthma that remains difficult to control despite the aforementioned measures as outlined. In these circumstances, treatment with oral corticosteroids, usually in the form of daily prednisolone, may be required to minimize symptoms and prevent severe asthma exacerbations. Although courses of oral corticosteroids are unquestionably a vital part of the management of acute exacerbations, careful consideration should be made before they are administered on a long-term basis because of the high associated risk of significant adverse effects. When they are required, the lowest dose that maintains asthma control should be given. Preventive therapy for osteoporosis should be considered, and patients should be monitored for the development of

hypertension, diabetes, cataracts, glaucoma, and adrenal suppression. Obesity, thinning and bruising of the skin, and myopathy also are important concerns. Inhaled corticosteroids should always be continued, because these agents are likely to allow a reduction in the oral corticosteroid dose; this may be one situation in which higher-dose inhaled steroids are justified.

Corticosteroid-sparing agents include methotrexate, gold, and cyclosporine. Some evidence suggests that these agents have steroid-sparing effects in asthma, but each comes with its own safety concerns, and use of these agents should be confined to specialist units. The risk of adverse effects from the use of long-term oral corticosteroids and the lack of safe alternatives necessitate careful monitoring of the response to treatment. A small minority of patients with severe asthma demonstrate resistance to corticosteroid treatment despite apparently good compliance. The mechanisms for this resistance are not fully understood but may relate to transcriptional regulation of genes associated with steroid-responsive inflammation.

Anti-IgE Monoclonal Antibody

IgE has an important role in the development of allergic diseases in atopic persons, and suppression of IgE is therefore a potential target in the management of atopic asthma. The monoclonal antibody omalizumab blocks the interaction of IgE with mast cells and basophils. It is given as a subcutaneous injection at doses titrated to serum IgE levels and patient weight. Clinical trials have shown improved symptom control, fewer exacerbations, and greater reductions in inhaled corticosteroid dose with no apparent adverse effects. The therapy is expensive, however, and the efficacy and cost-effectiveness of treatment in unselected patients remain uncertain. Omalizumab therefore appears to be a potentially useful antiinflammatory agent in patients with atopic asthma.

STEPWISE ALGORITHM FOR ASTHMA TREATMENT

Guidelines recommend the titration of therapy for asthma in a stepwise manner, with the primary aim of satisfactorily controlling symptoms at the lowest dose of corticosteroid (see Figure 39-5). Changes in therapy should be reviewed every 3 months until stability is achieved. This algorithm assumes clinical control is concomitantly associated with control of underlying airway inflammation and therefore fulfillment of all three targets of care.

Of note, step 3 of the British Thoracic Society (BTS) treatment pathway recommends the addition of a long-acting β-agonist to low-dose corticosteroid therapy over an increase in corticosteroid dose. There is molecular evidence for a synergistic effect between the two drug classes. In clinical practice, the strategy achieves clinical improvement, as indicated by reduction of symptoms, optimization of lung function, and a fall in exacerbation frequency, comparable with that provided by a dose escalation in corticosteroid alone. Combination inhalers of long-acting β-agonists and inhaled corticosteroids have been developed and are now commonly prescribed. They have the advantage of patient convenience but do not allow independent dose alterations of the component drugs.

Monitoring Asthma Control and Guided Self-Management Plans

A number of potential tools are available to assess asthma (see Table 39-1). All such tools assess different aspects of the disease, and it is likely that they provide complementary information. Objective symptom scores are particularly useful, because

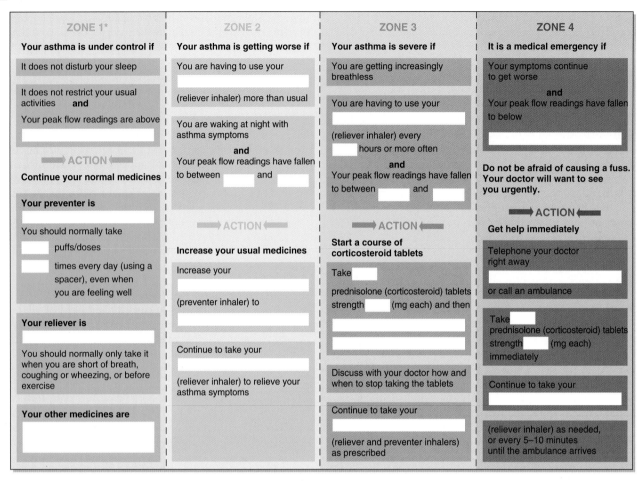

*If you are persistently in this zone, your doctor may reduce your usual medication.

Figure 39-7 Page from a typical preprinted self-treatment plan. *(From Partridge MR: Asthma: clinical features, diagnosis, and treatment. In Albert RK, Spiro SG, Jett JR, editors: Clinical respiratory medicine, ed 3, Philadelphia, Mosby, 2008.)*

patients may adjust to their impairment and not question symptoms that are potentially reversible. The extent to which these assessments allow risk stratification is unclear; this is an important area for further study. Table 39-1 outlines the characteristics of some of the most common methods used to assess asthma.

Regular review appointments also provide an opportunity to review patient education, inhaler technique, and self management skills. Self-management plans are individualized written protocols instructing patients in recommended courses of action on the basis of their asthma control that is graded and risk-stratified according to symptoms or peak flow (**Figure 39-7**). They are attractive for being patient-centered. Both symptom- and peak flow–guided plans lessen asthma morbidity and reduce the frequency of hospitalizations and unscheduled doctor visits. Although little evidence has been found for the superiority of one strategy over another, a peak flow–based plan may be more appropriate in patients with impaired perception of airflow obstruction.

Referral to a Specialist

Asthma often is managed very successfully in primary care. Patients for whom referral for specialist care typically will be required fall into three broad groups:

- Patients with suspected occupational asthma
- Patients with treatment-refractory asthma, defined as those failing to achieve control despite appropriate high-dose therapy (BTS step 4 or 5). Although constituting 5% to 10%

of the asthma population, this group accounts for over 60% of health care resource utilization for asthma in the United Kingdom. The reasons for a poor therapeutic response are multifactorial (**Box 39-5**).
- Patients at higher risk for asthma-related death (**Box 39-6**). Relative risk is additive; accordingly, patients with several minor risk factors, as well as those with a single major risk factor, require referral.

NONPHARMACOLOGIC ASPECTS OF ASTHMA CARE

Patient Education

Appropriate patient education is essential for the provision of care based on self-management. Several aspects of this component of the management program have been identified:

- Identifying and avoiding asthma triggers, the most important of which is smoking.
- Understanding the role of different prescribed therapies—that is, distinguishing between therapy for immediate relief from symptoms ("relievers") and therapy to prevent or reduce the frequency of symptoms ("preventers"), to support compliance with therapy, which is a considerable problem in asthma care
- Encouraging compliance with medication
- Ensuring correct inhaler technique
- Recording and monitoring peak flow
- Following a self-management plan

Patient Factors

Poor inhaler technique and incorrect use of inhalers
Poor compliance with therapy
- Particularly in younger patients and those with psychological disorders
Persistent exposure to sensitized allergen
- Occupation
- Pets
Smoking
- Associated with increased symptoms, accelerated decline in lung function, and impaired steroid responsiveness
Obesity
- Associated with increased symptoms and impaired steroid responsiveness
Concomitant psychological morbidity
- Both anxiety and depression can heighten perception of breathlessness, leading to increased symptoms

Disease Factors

Coexistent aggravating disorders
- Dysfunctional breathing disorders
- Rhinosinusitis
- GERD
- Cardiac failure
Aspergillus-associated asthma
- Associated with more intense eosinophilic airway inflammation and bronchiectasis
Churg-Strauss syndrome
True steroid-resistant asthma
- This subgroup constitutes a minority of patients with refractory asthma
- High doses of oral or parenteral steroid usually overcome the impaired response to conventional therapy
Absence of demonstrable eosinophilic airway inflammation (noneosinophilic asthma)
- Patients with this condition have corticosteroid resistance, so escalation of steroids unlikely to be helpful
- Best management uncertain

GERD, gastroesophageal reflux disease.

Box 39-6 Risk Factors for Severe Asthma

Major Risk Factors

Previous mechanical ventilation for asthma
Previous admission to intensive care unit
Recent hospital admission for asthma

Minor Risk Factors

Asthma requiring oral steroids or theophylline for control
High β-agonist consumption
Factors associated with poor compliance
- Lower socioeconomic class
- Coexistent psychopathology
- History of drug abuse or alcohol dependence
- Adolescence

Specialist asthma nurses are central providers of information and education for patients. Regular follow-up with an asthma nurse reinforces key messages and leads to superior asthma control.

Smoking Cessation and Allergen Avoidance

Approximately 25% of patients with asthma smoke. Smoking in this population is associated with increased symptoms and accelerated lung function decline. Smoking cessation studies have shown a significant improvement in the control of symptoms and lung function within weeks of stopping.

Allergen sensitization and exposure are common and often contribute to increased asthma symptoms. Simple measures such as limiting contact with household pets, notably cats, should be advised. Evidence is lacking for a proven benefit of more intensive and often expensive measures to lower the burden of ubiquitous allergens (e.g., house dust mite). Regular use of antihistamines may be helpful when there is a clear association between allergen exposure and deteriorating asthma control (e.g., loss of control with concomitant hay fever).

Breathing Retraining Techniques

Disordered breathing patterns such as hyperventilation frequently coexist with asthma and may contribute significantly to the clinical expression of asthma-like symptoms. The diagnosis should be suspected in patients with prominent symptoms that do not follow a predictable or episodic pattern and are out of proportion to objective evidence of airway dysfunction. Physiotherapy-based breathing retraining programs can be effective and may avoid the inappropriate escalation of pharmacotherapy.

RECENT DEVELOPMENTS IN ASTHMA MANAGEMENT

The failure to optimize asthma control in some patients highlights deficiencies in current therapeutic modalities and strategies. Four key areas of ongoing research are likely to influence future asthma care, particularly in subgroups of patients with refractory disease:

- Inflammation-guided management (inflammometry)
- The use of a single inhaled combination treatment for relief and maintenance therapy
- The development of monoclonal antibody therapies as targeted antiinflammatory agents
- Novel techniques for treating airway dysfunction

Inflammometry

Several important observations have increased interest in the use of inflammometry in the clinical assessment of asthma and other airway diseases. First, the presence of eosinophilic, corticosteroid-responsive airway inflammation is not closely related to either the pattern or the severity of the airway dysfunction or symptoms. A raised sputum eosinophil count is seen in 70% to 80% of corticosteroid-naive patients with asthma, 50% of corticosteroid-treated patients with symptomatic asthma, 30% to 40% of patients with cough, and up to 40% of patients with COPD. Within diagnostic groups, a weak correlation has been noted between the presence of eosinophilic airway inflammation and the severity of symptoms or disordered airway function. Thus, little can be deduced about the presence and severity of eosinophilic airway inflammation from a standard clinical assessment, and if this information is required, then measurement of the sputum eosinophil count is informative.

Second, the presence of eosinophilic airway inflammation is more closely associated with a positive response to corticosteroids than any other clinical measure. Moreover, a positive response to corticosteroids is seen irrespective of the pattern of airway disease in which eosinophilic airway inflammation occurs. Thus, if the clinical question were whether a patient with chronic respiratory symptoms should receive corticosteroid treatment, then the identification of a raised sputum eosinophil count or FeNO would be a better basis for making this decision than the findings of other tests.

Third, the sputum eosinophil count is a better marker for titrating corticosteroid therapy than are standard clinical measures. Studies in asthma and COPD have shown that use of management strategies in which decisions about corticosteroid use and dose are guided by the sputum eosinophil count results in a lower frequency of exacerbations and more economical use of corticosteroids in comparison with management guided by traditional clinical measures. FENO measurements also have been used to guide corticosteroid treatment, but with more mixed results. Studies thus far have suggested that FENO-based management may allow more economical use of corticosteroids by more accurately identifying patients in whom reduced doses will suffice.

The link between eosinophilic airway inflammation and corticosteroid responsiveness, together with the development of inexpensive nitric oxide monitors, has opened the way for a new approach to the management of airway disease in clinical practice, with the emphasis more on assessing airway inflammation than on diagnostic labeling. **Figure 39-8** outlines an approach to assessment of patients presenting with new-onset airway disease whereby decisions about the use of corticosteroids are based on assessment of eosinophilic airway inflammation or FENO, rather than on recognition of patterns of symptoms and airway dysfunction.

Single-Inhaler Therapy

The combination of budesonide and formoterol is licensed for use in a single combination inhaler for relief of symptoms and maintenance of asthma control. This dual role is made possible because formoterol is a long-acting β-agonist with a rapid onset of action, comparable with that of salbutamol. Thus, the frequency of inhaler use will be governed by the severity and frequency of symptoms, ensuring higher doses of corticosteroid during periods of poor control. This is appropriate if deteriorating symptoms are associated with worsening underlying airway inflammation. Studies have shown improvements in lung function, reduction in exacerbation frequency, and better symptom control with this approach. It may be particularly applicable in patients with variable treatment adherence.

Monoclonal Antibody Therapies

A growing number of monoclonal antibodies are being developed to target key proinflammatory mediators of the T_H2 pathway that are considered important for perpetuating inflammation in asthma. Of these, mepolizumab, a monoclonal antibody blocking IL-5 (a key cytokine responsible for eosinophil maturation and recruitment) has been shown to reduce the frequency of severe exacerbations in patients with severe asthma and eosinophilic airway inflammation. Trials exploring blocking antibodies to IL-4 and IL-13 and oral antagonists of the PGD_2 receptor $CRTH_2$ also are under way. It is likely that all of these agents will work best in the subgroup of patients with an eosinophilic T_H2-type pattern of airway inflammation and that the main benefits of treatment will be a reduction in frequency of asthma attacks. Identification of these patients by means of inflammometry will become increasingly important.

Bronchial Thermoplasty

Bronchial thermoplasty offers a nonpharmacologic approach to asthma treatment. The technique is targeted at the airway smooth muscle, which is considered central to airway dysfunction in asthma. Thermal energy is applied bronchoscopically to the bronchial wall using a wire basket. (A video of the procedure is available on Expert Consult.) Bronchial thermoplasty is thought to prevent bronchoconstriction by disrupting airway smooth muscle bundles. A sham-controlled study has shown improvement in asthma-related quality of life and reduced exacerbation numbers for at least a year after the procedure.

MANAGEMENT OF IMPORTANT PATIENT SUBGROUPS

SEVERE ASTHMA

A proportion of patients will have persistent symptoms despite appropriate treatment for moderate persistent asthma as just outlined. Although representing a relatively small minority, these patients experience much morbidity, consume significant health care resources, and probably are best managed in specialist settings. Severe asthma can be defined simply as asthma that continues to cause significant morbidity despite high-level anti-asthma therapy (i.e., step 4 of the BTS asthma management guidelines) (see Figure 39-5).

Figure 39-8 Suggested algorithm for assessment of airways disease. Eosinophilic airway inflammation can be assessed using induced sputum eosinophils or FENO. *Potentially treatable aggravating factors include rhinitis, anxiety-hyperventilation syndrome, vocal cord dysfunction, bronchiectasis, and gastroesophageal reflux disease. †Symptomatic therapy includes short- and long-acting bronchodilator therapy, oral theophylline, and mucolytics, as well as specific treatments for the aggravating factors. ‡As supported by limited evidence, some patients with symptoms suggesting airways disease have raised FENO that is not reflective of eosinophilic airway inflammation and is not corticosteroid-responsive. Therefore, a persistently raised FENO after corticosteroid treatment should prompt a more thorough assessment of airway inflammation using induced sputum specimens when available. The suggested cutoff points for "high" and "low" FENO in adults are 25 ppb and 50 ppb, respectively, but this is a very loose guideline. The interpretation of FENO in the range of 25 to 50 ppb varies between individual patients, and in some instances, different cutoff points may apply.

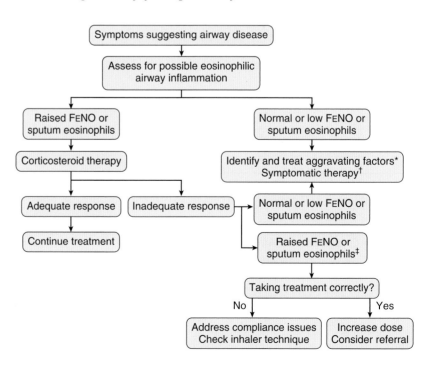

Before additional therapeutic measures are considered, it is important to accurately confirm the diagnosis, to ensure that persistent symptoms are due to asthma, rather than to other aggravating or coexisting factors such as dysfunctional breathing, vocal cord dysfunction, obesity, bronchiectasis, COPD, rhinitis, or gastroesophageal reflux (see Box 39-5). Box 39-3 lists some features that increase the probability that non–asthma-related factors are responsible for persistent morbidity. Next, it is important to assess compliance with existing therapy, ideally using relatively objective measures such as prescription refill rates and blood theophylline and/or prednisolone levels. Poor adherence is very common in patients with severe asthma and has been linked with poor outcomes, notably an increased risk of fatal and near-fatal attacks. The best means to detect poor treatment adherence and to tackle it have yet to be established. This is an important area for further study.

Once these issues have been addressed, current guidelines advocate a step up in treatment, usually to regular oral steroids. The response to oral steroids, however, is known to be mixed, and side effects are an important issue; moreover, the efficacy of alternative drugs in patients with severe asthma often has not been well established. Much of the current research effort in severe asthma focuses on patients with severe asthma, and there is increasing realization that new treatments are unlikely to be helpful in all patients. The future is likely to be individualization of treatment based on a more complete understanding of the mechanism of persistent morbidity and the ways in which this can be modulated.

Recently there have been attempts to identify clinically important groups of patients using mathematical techniques such as factor analysis and cluster analysis. **Figure 39-9** shows the results of one of the first attempts to phenotype patients with asthma recruited from primary care practices and from a severe asthma cohort being seen in a specialist hospital clinic. The main finding was that patients with severe asthma had more marked discordance in expression of symptoms and airway inflammation. The presence of these discordant phenotypes in patients with refractory asthma in particular suggests that a management approach which relies on symptoms to guide antiinflammatory treatment would result in suboptimal outcomes in a significant number of patients and that management guided by an objective measure of corticosteroid-responsive inflammation (i.e., eosinophilic airway inflammation) may be better. This is exactly what has been found in trials that have compared inflammation-guided use of steroids with symptom-guided use. The main outcome of these trials has been a reduction in the frequency of asthma attacks, suggesting that the main clinical benefit of controlling eosinophilic airway inflammation is to reduce the risk of attacks.

The recognition of these various groups of patients not only helps to guide corticosteroid treatment but also may identify patients for whom alternative noncorticosteroid treatments may be helpful. Long-term low-dose macrolide antibiotics may be particularly effective in patients with refractory noneosinophilic asthma. Bronchial thermoplasty, a treatment that specifically targets airway smooth muscle but has no known effect on

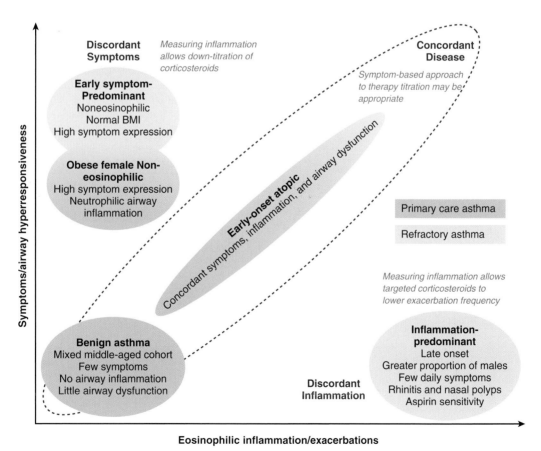

Figure 39-9   Clinical phenotypes of asthma: A summary of phenotypes identified using cluster analysis in primary and secondary care asthma populations. The clusters are plotted according to their relative expression of symptoms and inflammation, because these are the two clinically pertinent and modifiable dimensions of the disease. The plot highlights greater discordance to be a feature of secondary care asthma. Although reasons for this dissociation are unclear, the use of measures of airway inflammation in these subgroups is clinically informative. *BMI,* body mass index.   *(Reproduced with permission from Haldar P, Pavord ID, Shaw DE, et al: Cluster analysis and clinical asthma phenotypes,* Am J Respir Crit Care Med *178:218-224, 2008.)*

airway inflammation, may also be a helpful treatment in patients with predominant airway dysfunction. Patients with inflammation-predominant disease, without much in the way of day-to-day symptoms or disordered airway function, may benefit from specific antiinflammatory treatments such as anti-IL-5, omalizumab, and, if they are sensitized to *Aspergillus*, antifungal treatment. Mepolizumab, the monoclonal antibody against IL-5, is a particularly attractive treatment option, because it is a very specific and effective inhibitor of the eosinophilic airway inflammation.

ASPIRIN-INDUCED ASTHMA

Around 5% of adults with asthma develop significant bronchoconstriction, often with rhinorrhea and urticaria, after ingesting aspirin and other cyclooxygenase inhibitors. Bronchoconstriction occurs as a consequence of inhibition of production of bronchoprotective prostaglandin E_2 and unchecked production of cysteinyl leukotrienes. Aspirin-induced asthma usually is seen in patients with nonatopic, adult-onset disease, many of whom have, in addition, rhinitis and nasal polyps (i.e., Samter's triad). Patients tend to have severe eosinophilic airway inflammation that often is difficult to control with inhaled corticosteroids alone, and a high proportion of patients require, and do well with, oral corticosteroids taken either intermittently or continuously. Drugs blocking the production and action of leukotrienes may be particularly helpful in patients with aspirin-induced asthma.

CHURG-STRAUSS SYNDROME

Churg-Strauss syndrome is characterized by vasculitis and histologic evidence of extravascular granulomas in a patient with asthma and allergic rhinitis. The criteria for diagnosis of Churg-Strauss syndrome are summarized as follows:

- Presence of asthma
- Peripheral blood eosinophilia (presence of more than 1.5 × 10^9 cells/L)
- Systemic vasculitis involving two or more extrapulmonary organs

Biopsy of easily accessible affected tissue can be helpful to confirm the presence of vasculitis and extravascular granuloma (**Figure 39-10**) but should not delay institution of treatment. Antineutrophilic cytoplasmic antibodies (ANCA) are present in two thirds of cases, but this finding is not specific. The key to prompt diagnosis is maintaining clinical awareness of the condition, especially in an adult patient who presents with allergic rhinitis, sinusitis, asthma, or an eosinophilia (which can be marked), together with systemic features such as fever, rash (especially lower limb purpura), weight loss, or arthralgia. Other features include pulmonary infiltrates, peripheral neuropathy, cranial and other isolated nerve palsies, cerebrovascular accidents, abdominal pain, bloody diarrhea, and, occasionally, intestinal perforation. Renal disease is uncommon, but cardiac involvement can occur and is a serious complication potentially leading to heart failure and sudden death. These manifestations of disease may develop over a short period, emphasizing the importance of a prompt diagnosis. The differential diagnosis clearly depends on the specific manifestation of Churg-Strauss syndrome occurring in the individual patient, but pulmonary manifestations may need differentiating from allergic bronchopulmonary aspergillosis, other pulmonary eosinophilias, pulmonary sarcoidosis, Wegener

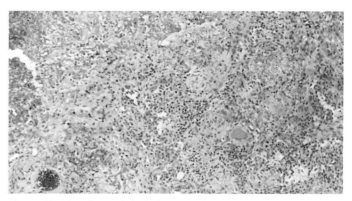

Figure 39-10 Histopathologic features of Churg-Strauss syndrome (CSS). This photomicrograph shows a combination of parenchymal necrosis and focally marked tissue eosinophilia in CSS. The inflammatory infiltrate includes a combination of eosinophils and variable numbers of epithelioid histocytes in a vaguely granulomatous appearance. *(From Partridge MR: Asthma: clinical features, diagnosis, and treatment. In Albert RK, Spiro SG, Jett JR, editors: Clinical respiratory medicine, ed 3, Philadelphia, Mosby, 2008.)*

granulomatosis, microscopic polyangiitis, and polyarteritis nodosa.

In many cases, the response to steroids alone may be very good, and it is possible to achieve long-term control with low-dose prednisolone. With more aggressive disease, additional treatment with cyclophosphamide is necessary. Prognosis reflects the degree of severity of the disease and its manifestations, with the worst outcomes in patients with cardiac decompensation or cerebrovascular manifestations. The association of Churg-Strauss syndrome with the use of leukotriene antagonists has recently attracted attention. Although theoretically any drug may potentially induce a hypersensitivity vasculitis, the most likely reason for development of relevant problems after initiation of leukotriene antagonist is that improved control of the patient's asthma has led to a reduction in oral steroid dose with subsequent unmasking of a previously silent systemic condition.

ASPERGILLUS-ASSOCIATED ASTHMA

The fungus *Aspergillus* is globally distributed and found in soil and decaying leaf mold and vegetable matter. Fungal spores are dispersed by the wind, and peak levels are found during the autumn and winter. Some patients with asthma develop an IgE- and IgG-mediated response to *Aspergillus* and other molds on repeated exposure. Patients who are highly atopic, have long-standing disease, and exhibit evidence of airway damage are at particular risk. Some develop the arbitrarily defined condition *allergic bronchopulmonary aspergillosis* (ABPA), which features, in addition to asthma and *Aspergillus* sensitivity, pulmonary eosinophilia and infiltration with an intense allergic reaction in the proximal airways. This reactivity can result in bronchial occlusion, which may give rise to segmental or lobar collapse and, especially if untreated, significant bronchial wall damage and development of bronchiectasis of the proximal airways (**Figure 39-11**). It is becoming clear that less well-developed forms of this condition are common, and the term *Aspergillus*-associated asthma is preferred. Up to 40% of patients with severe asthma have *Aspergillus* sensitization, and many grow *Aspergillus* in their sputum when this organism is looked for specifically.

The following features should alert the clinician to the possibility of *Aspergillus*-associated asthma:

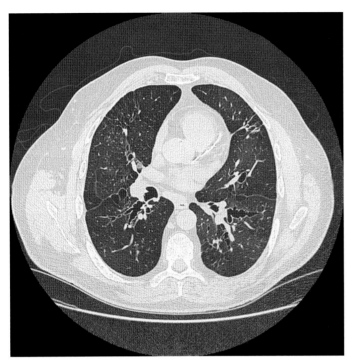

Figure 39-11 Computed tomography scan of the thorax of a patient with bronchopulmonary aspergillosis. Significant proximal airway bronchiectasis is evident. *(From Partridge MR: Asthma: clinical features, diagnosis, and treatment. In Albert RK, Spiro SG, Jett JR, editors:* Clinical respiratory medicine, *ed 3, Philadelphia, Mosby, 2008.)*

- A marked peripheral blood and sputum eosinophilia
- Demonstration of a positive result on immediate skin prick testing or RAST for *A. fumigatus*
- Positive precipitins (i.e., IgG antibodies) to *A. fumigatus*
- *A. fumigatus* grown on sputum culture
- A raised total immunoglobulin E level
- Lung imaging showing lobar collapse, infiltrates, and bronchiectasis, which is classically worst in the proximal airways in this condition (see Figure 39-11)

The combination of *Aspergillus* sensitization and colonization may be an important and potentially modifiable factor responsible for airway damage and the development of fixed airflow obstruction, and there is increasing interest in screening for this condition in patients with more severe disease. The acute syndrome associated with pulmonary infiltration is undoubtedly helped by oral corticosteroid therapy, and a maintenance regimen of inhaled steroids between attacks probably prevents recurrent attacks and preserves lung function. Long-term maintenance oral corticosteroid therapy may be necessary. Increasing evidence suggests that antifungal drugs (e.g., itraconazole 200 mg twice daily for 4 months) are effective in patients with aspergillus-associated asthma.

OCCUPATIONAL ASTHMA

Approximately 15% of patients with adult-onset asthma are thought to have occupational asthma. The causes, diagnosis, investigation, and management of occupational asthma are discussed in more detail in Chapter 40. The key point in the history is that symptoms are worse at work and better away from work, particularly with prolonged work absence during holidays. It should be possible to document this work effect objectively with PEF measurements done at work and away

from work. A computerized analysis system is available online (see under "Web Resources"); this has been shown to be a valid means of diagnosing occupational asthma provided accurate and frequent (i.e., every 2 hours during waking hours) PEF readings are available. Occupational asthma results in considerable expense to the patient as a result of lost productivity, estimated to be in the order of £13 million in the United Kingdom over the course of his or her lifetime. Society contributes a similar amount, so reducing the incidence of occupational asthma is an important priority.

Work can aggravate preexisting asthma because of exposure to irritant stimuli (e.g., cold air) or can cause new-onset disease because the worker becomes sensitized to an occupational high- or low-molecular-weight sensitizer. Occupational asthma due to exposure to a sensitizer often occurs after the worker has been exposed for some time and is classically preceded by work-related rhinitis. This latent period is not seen with work-aggravated asthma. If the condition is recognized early, then removal of the worker from the occupational sensitizer can lead to complete remission; cessation of exposure is an important priority even if complete remission is not achieved. Environmental control with appropriate management of underlying asthma often is all that is needed in work-aggravated asthma. Asthma also can develop after sudden accidental exposure to a high concentration of toxic fumes, resulting in the so-called reactive airway dysfunction syndrome (RADS).

ASTHMA IN ATHLETES

A high proportion of endurance athletes report symptoms suggesting asthma and have abnormalities of airway function consistent with this condition. Up to 50% of Olympics-standard swimmers and winter sport athletes report use of asthma treatment. The prevalence may be highest in athletes participating in these sports, because endurance exercise occurs in challenging environments. The pathophysiologic basis of airway dysfunction is incompletely understood but the injurious effect of pollution and cold air on the airway mucosa is likely to be important. Athletes with asthma tend to have noneosinophilic airway inflammation and respond poorly to inhaled corticosteroid treatment.

ASTHMA IN PREGNANCY

Asthma may worsen, stay the same, or improve during pregnancy. The pattern may be repetitive in subsequent pregnancies. For women who experience a worsening of asthma, this is likeliest in the second and third trimesters; problems during labor are extremely unusual. Treatment for asthma should be the same during pregnancy as in the nonpregnant state, except that leukotriene antagonists should not be initiated during pregnancy. In the absence of appropriate advice, those with asthma may stop their medication on discovering they are pregnant, and it is important that pregnant women are reassured as to the safety of usual asthma treatment. After delivery, breast-feeding should be encouraged; none of the commonly used asthma medications are secreted in breast milk to the degree that any alteration in treatment is necessary.

ASTHMA ATTACKS

Asthma attacks are the third leading cause of preventable admissions to the hospital, and are responsible for more than 5000 deaths per year in the United States and 1500 deaths per year in the United Kingdom. Attacks are often not acute. In around half of patients the asthma attack has often been developing for days or weeks and there have been many opportunities to alter their treatment to prevent deterioration to crisis levels. Thus, undertreatment or inappropriate therapy is an important contributor to asthma morbidity and mortality.

People who have asthma die because they, their loved ones, or their doctors underestimate the severity, because of delays in seeking medical treatment, and because of underuse of oxygen and corticosteroid tablets. The severity of an exacerbation must therefore be carefully assessed, and the outcome determines the therapy given and the optimal treatment setting. **Box 39-7** and **Table 39-2** show features associated with exacerbations of asthma of mild, moderate, severe, or critical nature. All but the mildest attacks require treatment with bronchodilators, corticosteroids, and oxygen, with careful follow-up and assessment of responses to each intervention (**Figure 39-12**). Non–life-threatening asthma can be treated initially with four to six puffs of salbutamol from a pressurized metered dose inhaler (pMDI) with a large-volume spacer plus ipratropium, four puffs from a pMDI with large-volume spacer, both repeated as necessary every 10 to 15 minutes. A good response with symptom relief and an improvement in PEF to greater than 80% of the patient's best is followed by continuing regular β-agonists every 4 hours for 24 to 48 hours, a four-fold increased dose of inhaled corticosteroids for at least 7 days, and careful review of the patient's disease control status within days.

In life-threatening asthma, bronchodilators (albuterol [salbutamol] 5 to 10 mg and ipratropium bromide 0.5 mg) are administered by a nebulizer. All patients with life-threatening asthma and patients with non–life-threatening asthma who have an incomplete response (PEF 50% to 80% of predicted or

---

Box 39-7 Recognition and Assessment of Acute Severe Asthma in the Hospital Setting

Features of Acute Severe Asthma
Peak expiratory flow rate (PEFR) 50% of predicted (or patient's best) or less
Cannot complete sentences in one breath
Respiratory rate 25 breaths/minute or greater
Pulse greater than 110

Life-Threatening Features
PEFR less than 33% of predicted or best
Silent chest, cyanosis, or feeble respiratory effort
Bradycardia or hypotension
Exhaustion, confusion, or coma
If arterial saturation of oxygen is less than 92% or a patient has any life-threatening features, measure arterial blood gases

Blood Gas Markers of a Very Severe, Life-Threatening Attack
Normal (36-45 mm Hg) or high arterial partial pressure of carbon dioxide ($PaCO_2$)
Severe hypoxia, with PaO_2 less than 60 mm Hg irrespective of treatment with oxygen
A low pH (or high H^+)

No other investigations are needed for immediate management.

Caution: Patients experiencing severe or life-threatening attacks may not appear distressed and may not demonstrate all or even most of these abnormalities. The presence of any listed factor, however, should strongly signal this possibility to the clinician.

From Partridge MR: Asthma: clinical features, diagnosis, and treatment. In Albert RK, Spiro SG, Jett JR, editors: *Clinical respiratory medicine*, ed 3, Philadelphia, Mosby, 2008.

Table 39-2 Guide to Severity of Asthma Exacerbations

Symptoms Imminent	Mild	Moderate	Severe	Respiratory Arrest
Breathless	Walking Can lie down	Talking Prefers sitting	*At rest*: hunched forward	
Talks in	Sentences	Phrases	Words	
Alertness	May be agitated	Usually agitated	Usually agitated	Drowsy or confused
Respiratory rate	Increased	Increased	Often >30 breaths/min	
Use of accessory muscles and suprasternal retractions	Usually not	Usually	Usually	Paradoxical thoracoabdominal movement
Wheeze	Moderate, often only end expiratory	Loud	Usually loud	Absence of wheeze
Pulse	<100	100-120	>120	Bradycardia
Peak expiratory flow rate after initial bronchodilator (% predicted or % personal best)	>80	~60-80	<60 (<100 L/min in adults) or response lasts < 2 hour	
Arterial partial pressure of oxygen (PaO_2)—on air	Normal Test not usually necessary	>60 mm Hg	<60 mm Hg Possible cyanosis	
Arterial partial pressure of carbon dioxide ($PaCO_2$)*	<45 mm Hg	<45 mm Hg	>45 mm Hg Possible respiratory failure (see text)	
Arterial oxygen saturation (%)—on air	>95	91-95	<90	

*Hypercapnia (hypoventilation) develops more readily in young children than in adults and adolescents.
From Partridge MR: Asthma: clinical features, diagnosis, and treatment. In Albert RK, Spiro SG, Jett JR, editors: *Clinical respiratory medicine*, ed 3, Philadelphia, Mosby, 2008. Adapted from National Heart, Lung, and Blood Institute/World Health Organization Works.

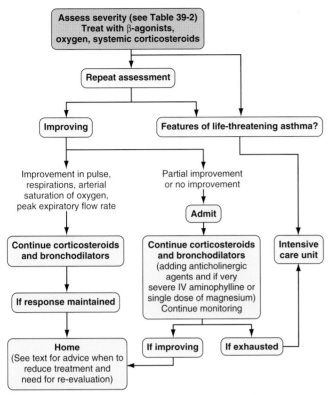

Figure 39-12 Algorithm for management of patient with acute severe asthma presenting for emergency care. *IV*, intravenous. *(From Partridge MR: Asthma: clinical features, diagnosis, and treatment. In Albert RK, Spiro SG, Jett JR, editors:* Clinical respiratory medicine, *ed 3, Philadelphia, Mosby, 2008.)*

best) with persistent symptoms require continuation of β-agonists every 2 to 4 hours and prompt addition of oral corticosteroids (prednisolone 30 to 40 mg once daily for 7 to 14 days). Either hospitalization is arranged or the patient is seen again urgently (the same day or the next morning).

A chest radiograph is indicated and should be performed if there is suspicion of additional intrathoracic pathology such as a pneumothorax or infective consolidation that will require additional therapeutic measures, if the patient fails to respond or deteriorates after initial therapy, or if the asthma attack is life-threatening or mechanical ventilation is being considered. If the blood oxygen saturation (SaO_2) does not reach 92% with the patient breathing room air or if the PEF is less than 100 L/min, arterial blood gas analysis is indicated. Patients with features of severe disease (see Table 39-2) should be referred urgently for intensive care monitoring. The first warning of this level of acuteness may be a normal or raised arterial partial pressure of carbon dioxide ($PaCO_2$) on blood gas sampling. Repeat blood gas sampling should be done in patients who are not clearly improving or appear to be deteriorating.

A single dose of magnesium sulfate (1.2 to 2 g intravenous infusion over 20 minutes) has also been shown to be safe and effective in severe asthma attacks and there is preliminary evidence that inhaled magnesium can be helpful when added to nebulized salbutamol. Intravenous aminophylline, 250 mg given slowly over 20 minutes followed by an infusion of 0.5 mg/kg/hour, is widely used if the patient is not taking regular oral theophyllines, although this practice is not strongly evidence-based.

Once clinical recovery has been achieved, the following criteria for successful management should be ascertained at discharge of the patient from the hospital:

- The patient has been on discharge medication for 24 hours.
- Inhaler technique has been checked.
- PEF should be greater than 75% of predicted or better and PEF rate diurnal variability should be less than 25%, unless the patient's respiratory physician confirms otherwise.
- Treatment with oral and inhaled corticosteroids in addition to bronchodilators has been prescribed.
- The patient has a PEF meter for home use, along with a written asthma action plan.
- Local follow-up evaluation has been arranged for within a week.
- A follow-up appointment in the chest clinic within 4 weeks has been scheduled.

The reason(s) for the exacerbation and admission must be determined and details sent to the primary care physician, together with a discharge plan and potential best PEF. Patients need to be given clear advice on how long to continue corticosteroid tablets, which should be continued in full dose until clinical stability is achieved and then either stopped suddenly (if the patient was not previously on corticosteroids and has taken them for less than 2 weeks) or tapered off.

Every attack of severe asthma and every hospital admission or emergency department visit must be regarded as a sign of failure of that patient's previous asthma management. Patients presenting with acute severe asthma are at high risk for recurrent attacks and have a poor prognosis, often reflecting poor self-management skills. After successful medical management of the attack, a full review of the lessons that can be learned from the attack is warranted, and a self-management plan for the future should be formulated and communicated to the primary care physician. The most important elements of the management plan are illustrated in Figure 39-7.

CONTROVERSIES AND PITFALLS

A growing view is that the current "one size fits all" guidelines approach to diagnosis and management is not appropriate with such a poorly defined entity as asthma. Much of the evidence on which guideline management suggestions are based is derived from clinical trials conducted in relatively homogeneous populations bearing little resemblance to the population receiving treatment for asthma in the community. The future is likely to see increasing individualization of therapy, with management decisions based on a rigorous analysis of the mechanism of the patient's morbidity and an accurate assessment of the risk of attacks, rather than a desperate and largely futile attempt to shoehorn different cases into a diagnostic category and then follow the relevant guideline. This individualized therapy approach requires more thorough evaluation of patients with suspected asthma, which includes an assessment of airway inflammation.

The development of new drugs has been a slow and frustrating process, with few therapeutic advances in the past 15 to 20 years. In part, this limitation reflects the problems with asthma as a diagnostic entity, as outlined previously. There needs to be a wider appreciation that new and existing treatments may be efficacious only in certain subgroups of patients and are likely to modulate only particular aspects of the syndrome. These subgroups and the aspects of the syndrome that are modified often are entirely predictable from the mode of action of the treatment. The archetypal example of drug development being adversely affected by unhelpful disease labels is the story of the clinical development of blocking antibodies against IL-5, in particular mepolizumab, which very specifically ablates eosinophils. Eosinophilic airway inflammation is associated with exacerbations of asthma, but not with airway hyperresponsiveness, which causes most asthma symptoms. Yet for 10 years, mepolizumab was tested exclusively against outcomes related to airway hyperresponsiveness in patients identified by the presence of variable airflow obstruction and/or airway hyperresponsiveness. It is therefore not surprising that the results were negative. When the drug was tested in patients with eosinophilic airway inflammation against outcomes associated with an airway eosinophilia (asthma attacks), it worked. Clinical researchers and regulatory authorities need to embrace this new understanding and ensure that future trials assess sensible outcomes in the right populations of patients. Clinicians using these agents need to develop the expertise to identify these potentially treatment-responsive subgroups of patients.

Some patients continue to do badly as a result of poor treatment adherence. Many patients struggle to appreciate that current treatments suppress the disease but do not cure. There is also a failure to understand that asthma is an episodic condition that very rarely remits completely. New and imaginative ways to educate hard-to-reach and nonadherent patients are needed. Clinicians often adopt a safety-first approach to treatment, and a growing view is that a significant number of patients with mild, low-risk disease are overtreated. Confidential enquiries into asthma deaths also continue to highlight undertreatment of high-risk patients. Better risk stratification is needed, and more precise definition and quantification of modifiable risk factors for poor asthma outcomes are urgently needed. Better risk stratification will allow clinicians to target treatment more effectively and also will facilitate discussion with patients. One aspect of asthma that is very poorly understood is the development of irreversible airflow obstruction. Decline is difficult to measure, and how much of a problem it represents has not been established; only a very basic understanding of risk factors has been achieved thus far. More research in this area is urgently required.

Perhaps the most important pitfall is the failure to recognize "pseudoasthma" in a patient whose symptoms are not responding to escalating antiasthma therapy. Clinicians should repeatedly question the validity of the diagnosis in patients who are doing well and should actively seek objective confirmation of the presence of abnormal airway function or airway inflammation. This assessment should be capable of identifying corticosteroid-unresponsive phenotypes of asthma such as noneosinophilic asthma. Box 39-2 lists some features that should alert the clinician to an alternative explanation for asthma-like symptoms.

SUMMARY

- Asthma is a clinical diagnosis that is made on the basis of the history and a demonstration of variable airflow obstruction.
- It is a syndrome, rather than a discrete entity; a growing interest in defining clinically important subgroups of asthma is influencing today's research.
- Bronchial provocation testing with methacholine or histamine should be performed if diagnostic uncertainty remains in patients with normal spirometry findings.
- In patients with fixed airflow obstruction, it may not be possible to make a clear distinction between asthma and

other related conditions, notably COPD. Assessment should focus more on defining mechanisms of airflow limitation, best achievable lung function, and optimal symptom control.
- Treatment goals for asthma are targeted at controlling symptoms, preventing asthma attacks, and preserving normal lung function.
- Asthma pharmacotherapy is broadly categorized into bronchodilator and antiinflammatory agents. These are currently prescribed in a stepwise manner with the primary aim of controlling symptoms.
- From 5% to 10% of patients have treatment-refractory asthma. Alternative or additional diagnoses should be sought in such cases. Newer therapies and different management strategies are being developed, but these agents have a limited spectrum of effects and are likely to work well only in certain subgroups. Assessment of airway inflammation is helpful in patients with severe asthma and may help identify patients who respond to these treatments.

SUGGESTED READINGS

Anderson GP: Endotyping asthma: new insights into key pathogenic mechanisms in a complex, heterogeneous disease, *Lancet* 372:1107–1119, 2008.

Brightling CE, Bradding P, Symon FA, et al: Mast-cell infiltration of airway smooth muscle in asthma, *N Engl J Med* 346:1699–1705, 2002.

British Guideline on the Management of Asthma: A national clinical guideline. British Thoracic Society and Scottish Intercollegiate Guidelines Network, *Thorax* 63:iv1–iv121, 2008

Busse WW, Lemanske RF Jr, Gern JE: Role of viral respiratory infections in asthma and asthma exacerbations, *Lancet* 376:826–834, 2010.

Douwes J, Gibson P, Pekkanen J, Pearce N: Non-eosinophilic asthma: importance and possible mechanisms, *Thorax* 57:643–648, 2002.

Haldar P, Brightling CE, Hargadon B, et al: Mepolizumab and exacerbations of refractory eosinophilic asthma, *N Engl J Med* 360:973–984, 2009.

Haldar P, Pavord ID, Shaw DE, et al: Cluster analysis and clinical asthma phenotypes, *Am J Respir Crit Care Med* 178:218–224, 2008.

Reddel HK, Taylor DR, Bateman ED, et al: An official American Thoracic Society/European Respiratory Society statement: asthma control and exacerbations: standardizing endpoints for clinical asthma trials and clinical practice, *Am J Respir Crit Care Med* 180:59–99, 2009.

Taylor DR, Pijnenburg MW, Smith AD, de Jongste JC: Exhaled nitric oxide measurements: clinical application and interpretation, *Thorax* 61:817–827, 2006.

Wenzel SE: Asthma: defining of the persistent adult phenotypes, *Lancet* 368:804–813, 2006.

WEB RESOURCES

British Thoracic Society/SIGN asthma guidelines: http://www.britthoracic.org.uk/c2/uploads/asthma_fullguideline2007.pdf

Global Strategy for Asthma Management and Prevention, Global Initiative for Asthma (GINA) 2006: http://www.ginasthma.org.

Occupational OASYS computerized occupational PEF software: http://www.occupationalasthma.com/occupational_asthma_pageview.aspx?id=4556

Video of bronchial thermoplasty: http://www.nejm.org/search?q=bronchial+thermoplasty

Asthma action plan resources: http://www.asthma.org.uk/all_about_asthma/publications/be_in_control_perso.html

Chapter **40**

Occupational Asthma

Olivier Vandenplas • Jean-Luc Malo

The workplace environment can lead to the development of different types of work-related asthma (**Figure 40-1**), including occupational asthma (OA) (i.e., asthma *caused* by work) and work-exacerbated asthma (i.e., preexisting or coincident asthma *exacerbated* by nonspecific stimuli at work). OA is defined as a disease characterized by variable airflow limitation and/or bronchial hyperresponsiveness and/or airway inflammation secondary to factors and conditions attributable to a particular working environment and not to stimuli encountered outside the workplace. OA may result either from immunologically mediated sensitization to occupational agents (i.e., "allergic" OA, or "OA with a latency period") or from exposure(s) to high concentrations of irritant compounds (i.e., irritant-induced asthma [IrIA], best typified by the *reactive airways dysfunction syndrome* [RADS]).

In recent years, a growing interest in occupational asthma (OA) has emerged, for several reasons:

- The frequency of asthma has increased progressively during the past 2 decades, with a recent plateau, and occupational exposure may be a contributing factor.
- Epidemiologic data indicate that approximately 18% of cases of asthma in adults are attributable to workplace exposures.
- The number of agents that can cause OA is steadily increasing (www.asthme.csst.qc.ca).
- OA, together with diseases related to exposure to asbestos dust, has become the most prevalent occupational lung disease in many developed countries, resulting in an increased burden to society.
- OA is an excellent model to study the epidemiology, pathophysiology, genetics, and other aspects of asthma in humans.

EPIDEMIOLOGY

CAUSAL AGENTS

The workplace agents causing immunologically mediated OA usually are categorized as either high-molecular-weight (HMW) or low-molecular-weight (LMW) substances (i.e., with molecular weights above or below 5000, respectively). HMW agents are (glyco)proteins of vegetable and animal origin, whereas LMW agents include chemicals, metals, and wood dusts. The intrinsic characteristics of occupational agents that determine their sensitizing potential remain largely uncertain. Of note, however, LMW agents causing OA typically are highly reactive electrophilic compounds that are capable of combining with hydroxyl, amino, and thiol functionalities on airway proteins. Quantitative structure-activity relationship models have identified a number of reactive groups that are associated with a high risk of respiratory sensitization, such as isocyanate ($N{=}C{=}O$), carbonyl ($C{=}O$), and amine (NH_2), particularly when two or more groups are present within the same molecule.

A very large number of substances (more than 400) used at work can cause the development of immunologically mediated OA. The most common causal agents and occupations are listed in **Table 40-1**. A few agents—specifically, flour, diisocyanates, latex, persulfate salts, aldehydes, animals, wood dusts, metals, and enzymes—account for 50% to 90% of OA cases. Nevertheless, the distribution of causal agents may vary widely across geographic areas, depending on the pattern of industrial activities. The highest rates of OA occur in bakers and pastry makers, other food processors, spray painters, hairdressers, wood workers, health care workers, cleaners, farmers, laboratory technicians, and welders.

All agents in exceedingly high concentrations can theoretically cause OA through nonimmunologic mechanisms, especially with agents occurring in vapor or gaseous form, by apposition to dry particles, such as chlorine and ammonia, but fire smoke and alkaline dusts, such as those released during the World Trade Center disaster, also have been incriminated in the development of persistent asthma.

PREVALENCE AND INCIDENCE

Cross-sectional surveys of workforces exposed to sensitizing agents found highly variable prevalence rates of OA. In general, the prevalence of OA caused by HMW agents is less than 5%, and that for LMW agents ranges from 5% to 10%. Cohort studies reported incidence rates of 2.7 to 3.5 cases of OA per 100 person-years among workers exposed to laboratory animals, 4.1 per 100 person-years among those exposed to wheat flour, and 1.8 per 100 person-years among dental health apprentices exposed to natural rubber latex. Estimates of the incidence of OA in the general population provided by voluntary notification schemes, medicolegal statistics, and population-based surveys are summarized in **Table 40-2**. Acute IrIA accounts for about 10% of all reported cases of OA.

RISK FACTORS

OA results from complex interactions between environmental factors and individual susceptibility. The environmental and individual risk factors are summarized in **Table 40-3**, together with the level of evidence supporting their role. The intensity of exposure to sensitizing agents currently is the best-identified and the most important environmental risk factor for the

Figure 40-1 Various types of work-related asthma. *RADS*, reactive airways dysfunction syndrome.

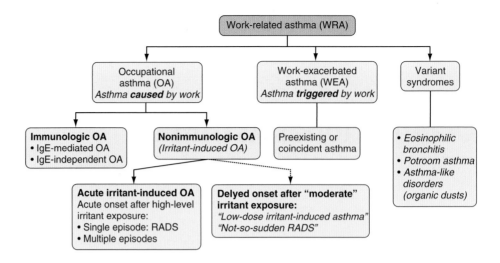

Table 40-1 Principal Agents Causing Immunologic Occupational Asthma

	Agent	Occupation/Industry
High-Molecular-Weight Agents		
Cereals, flour	Wheat, rye, barley, buckwheat	Flour milling, bakers, pastry makers
Latex		Health care workers, laboratory technicians
Animals (food animals, other)	Mice, rats, cows, seafood	Laboratory workers, farmers, seafood processors
Enzymes	α-Amylase, maxatase, alcalase, papain, bromelain, pancreatin	Baking products manufacture, bakers, detergent production, pharmaceutical industry, food industry
Low-Molecular-Weight Agents		
Diisocyanates	Toluene diisocyanate (TDI), methylene diphenyl-diisocyanate (MDI), hexamethylene diisocyanate (HDI)	Polyurethane production, plastic industry, molding, spray painters
Metals	Chromium, nickel, cobalt, platinum	Metal refinery, metal alloy production, electroplating, welding
Biocides	Aldehydes, quaternary ammonium compounds	Health care workers, cleaners
Persulfate salts		Hairdressers
Acid anhydrides	Phthalic, trimellitic, maleic, tetrachlorophthalic acids	Epoxy resin workers
Reactive dyes	Reactive black 5, pyrazolone derivatives, vinyl sulfones, carmine	Textile workers, printers, food industry workers
Woods	Red cedar, iroko, obeche, oak, others	Sawmill workers, carpenters, cabinet and furniture makers

development of OA. Characterization of the relationship between the level of exposure to occupational agents and the development of IgE sensitization and OA has been greatly enhanced by the use of personal sampling techniques, direct analytic methods for chemicals, and immunoassay techniques for the quantification of airborne protein allergens. Exposure-response relationships may be affected by the nature of the sensitizing agent, individual susceptibility, and timing of exposure. Some agents seem to be more potent than others in inducing sensitization; the dose-response relationship for IgE sensitization is steeper for the bakery enzyme alpha-amylase than for wheat allergens. Some evidence indicates that the exposure-response relationships are not linear for certain occupational agents (e.g., laboratory animals, wheat flour), thereby suggesting an unexplained protective effect of high-level exposures. The role of genetic susceptibility markers, such as certain human leukocyte antigen (HLA) class II alleles, may become more apparent at low levels of exposure to occupational agents.

The timing of exposure also may play a role, because the frequency of onset of work-related asthma symptoms is consistently higher within the first 1 to 4 years of exposure to HMW agents, and exposure-response gradients are more clearly documented in this early period of exposure.

A number of studies indicate that exposure to cigarette smoke can increase the risk for IgE-mediated sensitization to some HMW and LMW agents, but the evidence supporting an association between smoking and the development of clinical OA is still very weak. The role of other environmental cofactors, such as non-respiratory routes of exposure and concomitant exposure to endotoxin and pollutants at work, remains largely uncertain.

Atopy has been consistently demonstrated as an important host risk factor for the development of IgE sensitization and OA, but only for HMW agents. Prospective cohort studies of workers entering exposure to occupational sensitizing agents have shown that the presence of rhinitis and nonspecific

Table 40-2 Estimates of Incidence of Occupational Asthma (OA)

Country	Period	Incidence of OA (Cases per 10^6 Workers)
Physician-Based Notification Schemes		
United Kingdom (SWORD)	1989-1992	22
	1992-1993	37
	1992-1097	38 (34-41)*
	1992-2001	87
West Midlands (SHIELD)	1991-2005	42 (37-45)*
United States (SENSOR)		
Michigan	1988-1994	29
	1995	27 (58-204)
California	1993-1996	25 (23-27)*
Canada		
British Columbia	1991	92
Quebec (PROPULSE)	1992-1993	42-79
France (ONAP)	1996-1999	24 (22-25)*
Italy (PRIOR)	1996-1997	24 (18-30)*
South Africa (SORDSA)	1997-1999	18
Australia (SABRE)	1997-2001	31 (27-36)*
Spain		
Catalonia	2002	77 (66-90)*
Belgium (WAB)	2000-2002	24 (19-29)*
Medicolegal Statistics		
Finland	1976	36
	1989-1995	174
Canada		
Quebec	1986-1988	25
	1989-1999	13-24
Sweden	1990-1992	80 (70-90)*
Germany	1995	51
Belgium	1993-2002	29 (28-31)*
Population-Based Surveys		
Finland	1986-1998	Men: 478[†] Women: 419[†]
ECRHS	1990-1995 1998-2003	250-300

*95% confidence interval.
[†]Estimated from the work-attributable fraction of asthma derived through linkage of two national registries—the Medication Reimbursement of the Social Insurance Institution for Asthma and the Finnish Register of Occupational Diseases for Occupational Asthma.
ECRHS, European Community Respiratory Health Survey; ONAP, Observatoire National des Asthmes Professionnels; PROPULSE, Projet Pulmonaire Sentinelle; SABRE, Surveillance of Australian Workplace-Based Respiratory Events; SENSOR, Sentinel Event Notification System for Occupational Risks; SHIELD, Midland Thoracic Society Rare Respiratory Disease Registry Surveillance Scheme of Occupational Asthma; SORDSA, Surveillance of Work-Related and Occupational Respiratory Diseases in South Africa; SWORD, Surveillance of Work-Related and Occupational Respiratory Diseases; WAB, Work-Related Asthma in Belgium.

bronchial hyperresponsiveness at baseline is associated with an increased risk for subsequent IgE sensitization and development of OA.

With the advances in human genetics, research has been directed toward investigating the genetic basis of individual susceptibility to develop OA. Certain HLA class II molecules (i.e., HLA-DR, HLA-DQ, and HLA-DP alleles), which are involved in the presentation of processed antigens to T lymphocytes, were found to confer either susceptibility to or protection against OA due to various LMW and HMW occupational allergens (i.e., isocyanates, red cedar, acid anhydrides, platinum salts, natural rubber latex, and laboratory animals). Other evidence suggests that genes associated with T_H2 cell differentiation (i.e., polymorphism of the IL-4 receptor α chain, IL-13, and CD14 (C159T) genes) may play a role in the development of OA. Genes involved in the protection against oxidative stress, such as glutathione S-transferase (GST) and N-acetyltransferase (NAT), have been associated with an increased risk of isocyanate-induced OA (e.g., GSTM1-null genotype and slow N-acetylator phenotypes) or a protective effect (e.g., GSTP1*Val/Val allele). Overall, the currently available information indicates that the utility of genetic testing is limited for both diagnostic and preventive purposes. In addition, there is convincing evidence that a wide variety of environmental factors can interact with genetic determinants to affect disease susceptibility. For instance, a gene-environment interaction has been demonstrated in platinum refinery workers, in whom the relative risk of sensitization associated with the HLA-DR3 phenotype was more apparent at lower levels of exposure.

PATHOPHYSIOLOGY

OA can be classified according to pathogenic mechanisms as either immunologically or nonimmunologically mediated. Immunologically mediated OA is characterized by a latency period that is necessary for acquiring sensitization, whereas nonimmunologically mediated OA has no latency period.

IMMUNOLOGIC, IMMUNOGLOBULIN E-MEDIATED OCCUPATIONAL ASTHMA

HMW occupational agents act as complete antigens and induce specific IgE antibody production. The best examples are laboratory animals and flour. Some LMW occupational agents, including platinum salts, trimellitic anhydride, and other acid anhydrides, also induce specific IgE antibodies, and some others, specific IgG antibodies. They probably act as haptens and bind with proteins to form complete antigens, which are then recognized by antigen-presenting cells, and mount a CD4+ response, with production of specific IgE antibodies by B cells stimulated by several interleukins.

Reactions between specific IgE and antigens lead to a cascade of events that result in the release of inflammatory mediators and influx of cells in the airway, with consequent airway inflammation and development of airway hyperresponsiveness, as in asthma involving common allergens. Although other classes of antibodies have been postulated to have a role in asthma, evidence for their participation is not available. In the case of diisocyanates, mechanisms of allergic sensitization that are independent of IgE antibody have been postulated. There are no apparent differences in the pathogenetic mechanisms between OA induced by HMW occupational agents and those of allergic nonoccupational asthma.

Table 40-3   Summary of Potential Risk Factors for Development of Occupational Asthma (OA)

Risk Factor	Strength of Evidence	Agents/Settings
Environmental Risk Factors		
High level of exposure	+++	*HMW agents*: Wheat flour, α-amylase, laboratory animals, detergent enzymes, snow crab allergens *LMW agents*: Platinum salts, acid anhydrides
	++	Diisocyanates
Skin exposure	+	Diisocyanates
Cigarette smoking	++	*IgE sensitization*: Laboratory animals, snow crab, shrimp, salmon, psyllium, green coffee, enzymes, acid anhydrides, platinum, reactive dyes
	+	*Clinical OA*: Laboratory animals, enzymes
Individual Risk Factors		
Atopy	+++	*HMW agents*: Flour, laboratory animals, snow crab, psyllium, detergent enzymes, α-amylase
	+	*LMW agents*: Platinum, acid anhydrides
Genetic Markers		
HLA class II alleles	++	*LMW agents*: Diisocyanates, red cedar, acid anhydrides, platinum salts *HMW agents*: Laboratory animals, latex
Antioxidant enzyme* variants	++	Diisocyanates
TLR-4/8551 G variant	+	Laboratory animals
IL-4RA (I50V) II variant	+	Diisocyanates
Preexisting nonspecific bronchial hyperresponsiveness	+	Apprentices exposed to HMW agents (laboratory animals, flour, latex)
Preexisting rhinitis	+	IgE sensitization to HMW agents (laboratory animals, flour, latex)
Work-related rhinitis	+++	Nonoccupational asthma in the general population and OA in cohorts of workers exposed to laboratory animals
Gender—female	+	Snow crab processors

HLA, human leukocyte antigen; *HMW*, high-molecular-weight; *IgE*, immunoglobulin E; *IL-4RA*, interleukin-4 receptor alpha chain; *LMW*, low-molecular-weight; *TLR-4*, Toll-like receptor-4.
*Glutathione *S*-transferase (GSTM) and *N*-acetyltransferase (NAT).

IMMUNOLOGIC, NON-IMMUNOGLOBULIN E-MEDIATED OCCUPATIONAL ASTHMA

Many LMW agents, including diisocyanates and plicatic acid (responsible for red cedar asthma), have been shown to cause OA, yet specific IgE antibodies cannot be detected or are found in only a small percentage of affected persons. Specific IgG antibodies also are found and have been discovered to be significantly associated with the development of OA.

The significance of IgE and IgG antibodies in the pathogenesis of asthma is not clear. Bronchial biopsy specimens from patients with OA obtained at the time of diagnosis have shown activation of T lymphocytes, suggesting that T lymphocytes may play a direct role in mediating airway inflammation. This hypothesis has been substantiated by the finding of proliferation of peripheral blood lymphocytes when stimulated with the appropriate antigen in a proportion of affected persons with nickel-induced asthma and Western red cedar asthma. In isocyanate-induced asthma, an increase in CD8+ cells and in percentage of eosinophils was found in the peripheral blood of patients during a late asthmatic reaction induced by exposure testing. Cloning of T cells from bronchial biopsy specimens of these subjects showed that most of the clones exhibited CD8+ phenotype that produced IL-5, with very few clones producing

IL-4. This finding provides supportive evidence that CD8+ cells may play a direct role in OA without the necessity of producing IgE antibodies.

Early asthmatic reactions induced by occupational allergens probably are associated with smooth muscle contraction and edema induced by inflammatory mediators such as histamine and leukotrienes but not cellular infiltration. Late asthmatic reactions are associated with influx of inflammatory cells. Although both asthma and OA have been identified as diseases in which eosinophilic inflammation plays a key role, the role of neutrophils has recently been examined. Induced sputum examination is a noninvasive means to assess cell profiles and currently is more often used as an interesting investigative tool. Eosinophilic and neutrophilic variants of OA have been found in the case of OA due to LMW agents, especially diisocyanates. Some LMW agents have pharmacologic properties that cause bronchoconstriction. For example, diisocyanates may block the β₂-adrenergic receptor. Diisocyanates and other occupational agents also may stimulate sensory nerves to release substance P and other peptides that have been shown to inhibit neutral endopeptidases necessary for the inactivation of neuropeptides. Neuropeptides affect many cells in the airways and may participate in airway inflammation by causing smooth muscle

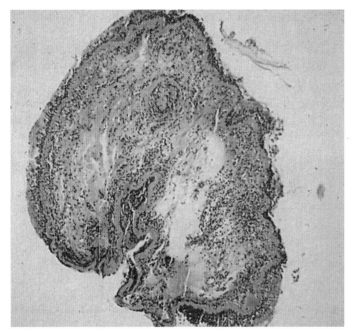

Figure 40-2 Bronchial biopsy specimen from a patient who had occupational asthma caused by exposure to toluene diisocyanates. Even after removal from exposure, partial desquamation of the epithelium, thickened basement membrane, and some cellular infiltration are evident.

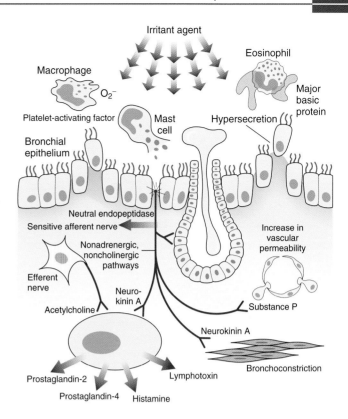

Figure 40-3 Proposed pathophysiology of reactive airways dysfunction syndrome (RADS).

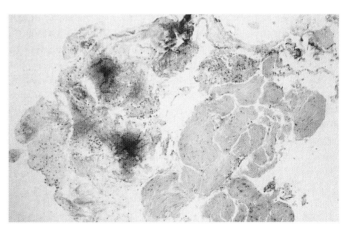

Figure 40-4 Bronchial biopsy specimen taken 3 days after an acute accidental inhalation of a high concentration of chlorine. This preparation shows almost complete desquamation of bronchial mucosa with fibrinohemorrhagic deposit. (Weigert-Masson stain.)

contraction, mucus production, and recruitment and activation of inflammatory cells. Thus, LMW occupational agents such as diisocyanates may have a variety of proinflammatory effects and induce asthma through more than one mechanism. An autopsy study of the lung of a person with isocyanate-induced asthma who died after reexposure showed denudation of airway epithelium, subepithelial fibrosis, infiltration of the lamina propria by leukocytes (mainly eosinophils), and diffuse mucous plugging of the bronchioles, similar to findings in persons who died from non-OA. Bronchial biopsy specimens of 18 patients with proven OA also have shown extensive epithelial desquamation, ciliary abnormalities of the epithelial cells, smooth muscle hyperplasia, and subepithelial fibrosis (**Figure 40-2**). The total cell count, eosinophils, and lymphocytes were increased compared with those in healthy control subjects.

NONIMMUNOLOGIC OCCUPATIONAL ASTHMA

OA resulting from nonimmunologic mechanisms is characterized by the absence of latency. The underlying mechanism of IrIA is not known. It has been postulated that the extensive denudation of the epithelium in these conditions leads to airway inflammation and airway hyperresponsiveness by several mechanisms, including loss of the epithelial cell–derived relaxing factors, exposure of the nerve endings leading to neurogenic inflammation, and nonspecific activation of mast cells with release of inflammatory mediators and cytokines (**Figure 40-3**). Secretion of growth factors for epithelial cells, smooth muscle, and fibroblasts may lead to airway remodeling. Sequential changes in the airways of a patient with IrIA have been described. In the acute phase of IrIA, rapid denudation of the mucosa with fibrinohemorrhagic exudate in the submucosa is followed by regeneration of the epithelium with proliferation of basal and parabasal cells and subepithelial edema (**Figure**

40-4). In the chronic phase of IrIA, marked thickening of the airway wall is seen (**Figure 40-5**). In a study of IrIA caused by multiple exposures to an irritant, inflammatory infiltrate with eosinophils and lymphocytes and diffuse deposition with collagen fibers were found. Similar sequential changes have been reproduced in animal models of IrIA.

CLINICAL FEATURES

OA induced by immunologic mechanisms is a form of asthma that is characterized by the clinical features of hypersensitivity: (1) work-related asthma symptoms develop only after an initial symptom-free period of exposure (i.e., the latency period),

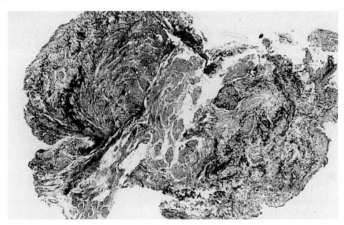

Figure 40-5 Bronchial biopsy specimen taken 2 years after an acute accidental inhalation of chlorine, showing severe desquamation of epithelial cells. Smooth muscle cells are surrounded by reticulocollagenic fibrous tissue. (Weigert-Masson stain.)

which is required to acquire the immunologic sensitization; (2) once OA is initiated, the asthmatic reactions tend to recur on reexposure to the causal agent at concentrations not affecting others who are similarly exposed; and (3) asthma affects only a proportion (usually a minority) of those exposed to the agent.

A typical history of OA includes the appearance or worsening of asthma symptoms at work and their disappearance or improvement away from work. This pattern frequently is obscured, however, because late asthmatic reactions can develop after the workshift, and asthma symptoms can be triggered by nonspecific stimuli outside the workplace. In addition, when affected workers continue to be exposed to the sensitizing agent, remission of symptoms in the evenings or during weekends tends to disappear, and much longer periods off work are necessary for improvement to take place. Thus, OA often remains unrecognized by affected workers and their physicians for long periods, the diagnosis usually being made 2 to 4 years after the onset of symptoms. The latency period typically is within 2 years of starting exposure to sensitizing agents, but OA may develop after much longer periods of exposure.

Some differences in the clinical presentation of subjects with OA caused by HMW and that implicating LMW agents have been noted, with isolated late or atypical asthmatic reactions more frequently observed after specific inhalation challenges with LMW agents. A majority of workers with OA also suffer from occupational rhinitis. Work-related rhinitis symptoms are more frequent and severe when HMW agents are involved. In those patients with associated rhinitis, work-related nasal symptoms frequently precede the onset of OA, especially with exposures to HMW agents.

The acute IrIA originally described by Brooks and colleagues in 1985 under the term *reactive airways dysfunction syndrome* is due to acute airway injury from accidental exposure to a high dose of irritants. In the typical clinical presentation, symptoms of asthma and airway obstruction or nonspecific bronchial hyperresponsiveness develop within a few hours after the acute exposure in a person without a history of respiratory disease, although sometimes the interval to symptom onset is longer. Certain features distinguish IrIA from allergic OA: At the time of the acute event, coughing generally is a predominant symptom. Thereafter, bronchial obstruction, if present, does not respond as well to bronchodilators, which may potentially be explained by the marked airway remodeling that has been documented in bronchial biopsy specimens from patients with IrIA.

DIAGNOSIS

Confirmation of the diagnosis of OA by objective means is necessary for several reasons. The diagnosis of OA has considerable socioeconomic implications for the worker and his or her family; it typically means a change of job in most instances, with its financial and other consequences. Asthma is a common disease, and it has been estimated that up to 50% of workers are exposed at one time or another to agents with sensitizing or irritating properties. The combination of having asthma and working in an environment with an agent known to give rise to OA does not make the diagnosis of OA. An occupational cause should be suspected for all new cases of adult-onset asthma, especially in persons who report worsening of their asthma symptoms at work. A detailed occupational history including past and current exposure to possible causal agents in the workplace, possible episodes of accidental exposures to irritant material, work processes, and specific job duties should be obtained. In addition, the intensity, frequency, and peak concentrations of exposure in the workplace should be assessed qualitatively. Worksite-specific information, including material safety data sheets, also can be requested, although in some instances, the information is incomplete on all constituents of the product, especially those constituents with concentrations less than 1%. Computerized databases and published lists of agents and workplaces are useful. Walk-through visits of the workplace may be necessary. Industrial hygiene data and employee health records can be obtained as well. Open medical questionnaires should be regarded as fairly sensitive but not specific tools for diagnostic purposes. Temporal associations are not sufficient to diagnose work-related asthma.

A person with suspected OA is best evaluated by a specialist in this area of practice. The role of this specialist is to confirm the diagnosis of OA by objective means if possible and to assess for impairment or disability. A delay in referral may jeopardize the chance of confirming the diagnosis with objective measurements, because the subject may have left the workplace and have recovered, or the working conditions may have changed. In cases of OA, however, inhalation challenges with a specific agent generally remain positive even 2 years or more after cessation of exposure.

An algorithm for the clinical investigation of OA is shown in **Figure 40-6**. The advantages and pitfalls of the various tools in confirming the diagnosis of OA are listed in **Table 40-4**. The presence of sensitization to occupational agents can be detected either by skin testing or by radioallergosorbent test (RAST) or enzyme immunosorbent assay (ELISA) techniques. In patients with a compatible clinical history of OA and bronchial hyperresponsiveness, a positive result on a skin test or RAST probably has a diagnostic accuracy close to 80% in the case of HMW agents. Unfortunately, very few standardized testing materials are commercially available for skin tests or for RASTs in OA, and for most LMW agents, an IgE-mediated mechanism has not been confirmed

For HMW agents, skin tests to detect immediate reactivity and measurements of specific IgE antibodies are important tools. The absence of nonspecific bronchial hyperresponsiveness in a subject at the end of 2 weeks of working under the usual conditions virtually excludes the diagnosis of asthma and OA. If nonspecific bronchial hyperresponsiveness is present, further testing is required. Spirometric measurements obtained

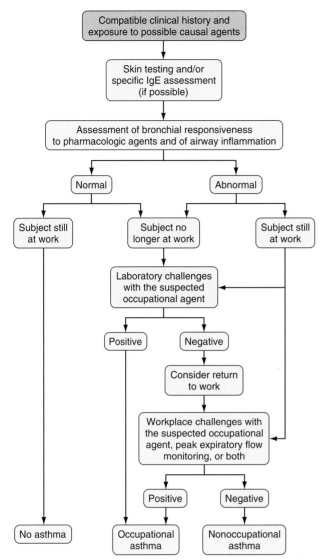

Figure 40-6 Clinical investigation of occupational asthma. *IgE, immunoglobulin E. (From Chan-Yeung M, Malo JL: Occupational asthma, N Engl J Med 333:107-112, 1995.)*

Table 40-4 **Advantages and Disadvantages of Diagnostic Methods in Occupational Asthma**

Method	Advantages	Disadvantages
Questionnaire	Simple, sensitive	Low specificity
Immunologic testing	Simple, sensitive	Only for agents of high molecular weight and for some of low molecular weight; identifies sensitization, not disease; no "standardized" or commercially available agents
Bronchial responsiveness to methacholine/histamine	Simple, sensitive	Not specific for asthma or occupational asthma; occupational asthma not ruled out by a negative test result if subject is no longer exposed
Measurement of forced expiratory volume in 1 second (FEV_1) before and after a work shift	Simple, inexpensive	Low sensitivity and specificity
Assessment of airway inflammation (induced sputum, exhaled nitric oxide [NO])	Addresses physiopathology of asthma; identifies eosinophilic bronchitis	Not specific for occupational asthma; limited to specialized centers
Peak expiratory flow monitoring	Relatively simple, inexpensive	Requires patient's cooperation and honesty; not as sensitive as FEV_1 or a computerized method to assess airway caliber to interpret changes
Specific inhalation challenges in a hospital laboratory	Positive result is confirmatory	Diagnosis not ruled out by a negative result on confirmatory testing (e.g., with use of wrong agent or with cessation of work exposure); expensive; few referral centers
Serial FEV_1 measurement at work under supervision	Negative result rules out diagnosis when patient tested under usual work conditions	A positive result may be obtained in conditions of irritation; requires collaboration of employer

From Chan-Yeung M, Malo JL: Occupational asthma, *N Engl J Med* 333:107-112, 1995.

before and after a work shift have not been found to be sensitive or specific. Two options (controlled exposure and PEF) can be considered for objective confirmation, depending on availability (see Figure 40-6). Exposure to the suspected agent under control conditions in a hospital laboratory can be done as originally described by Pepys and Hutchcroft in 1975. Attempts have been made to improve specific challenge tests by exposing subjects in the laboratory to low and stable levels of dry or wet aerosols and vapors to avoid nonspecific reactions. However, these tests can give false-negative results if an incorrect agent is used for testing or if the subject has been away from work for too long, although such occurrences are rare. In the latter instance, the subject should be instructed to return to the workplace, if feasible, and specific laboratory or worksite challenges should be repeated at a later time.

Burge and co-workers were the first to propose the use of serial measurement of peak expiratory flow (PEF) by use of portable devices in the diagnosis of OA. An example of serial PEF recording is shown in **Figure 40-7**. Although relatively good correlation has been found between the results of serial PEF monitoring and OA as confirmed by specific inhalation challenges in the laboratory, several limitations and pitfalls in

PEF monitoring are recognized (see Table 40-4). When PEF monitoring is suggestive of OA and specific inhalation challenges in the laboratory are not possible or yield negative results, it is advisable to confirm OA by sending a technician to the workplace to record serial spirometric variables throughout a work shift. The use of computerized peak flowmeters is very helpful in overcoming some of the problems of PEF monitoring. Computerized programs to assess changes in PEF are currently available (e.g., OASYS [Occupational Asthma Expert System]). Combining PEF monitoring with serial assessments

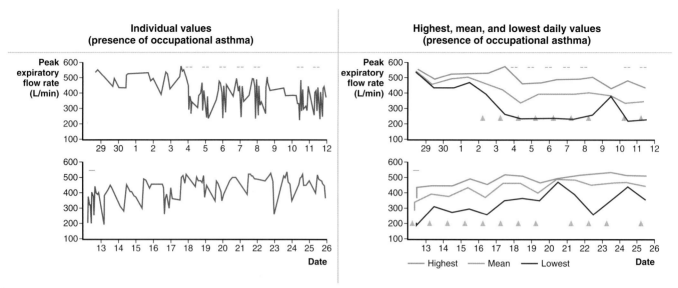

Figure 40-7   Pattern of changes in peak expiratory flows that suggest occupational asthma. The *horizontal lines* show the periods at work; the *triangles* illustrate the need for an inhaled bronchodilator.   *(From Malo JL, Cote J, Cartier A, et al: How many times per day should peak expiratory flow rates be assessed when investigating occupational asthma?* Thorax *48:1211–1217, 1993.)*

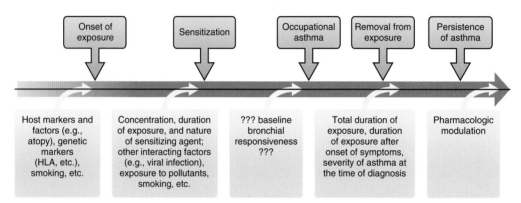

Figure 40-8   Natural history of asthma and occupational asthma. The *boxes* illustrate the steps; the modifying factors before each step are listed under the *horizontal line.* HLA, human leukocyte antigen.   *(From Malo JL, Ghezzo H, D'Aguino C, et al: Natural history of occupational asthma: relevance of type of agent and other factors in the rate of development of symptoms in affected subjects,* J Allergy Clin Immunol *90:937–943, 1992.)*

of nonallergic bronchial responsiveness can provide further objective evidence, although this approach does not add to the sensitivity and specificity of PEF monitoring alone. Finally, assessment of airway inflammation (percent eosinophils) in induced sputum has recently been found to be sensitive and specific in the diagnosis of OA. Such measurements improve the sensitivity and specificity of PEF monitoring. Assessing airway inflammation at work and away from work also can be done by assessing exhaled NO, but the reliability of this technique has not been demonstrated in the investigation of OA.

The main diagnostic criteria for IrIA are (1) the report of at least one inhalational accident (dates, times); (2) the onset of symptoms generally within 24 hours; and (3) the presence of airway obstruction or hyperresponsiveness.

CLINICAL COURSE

Subjects with OA will deteriorate if they continue in the same job without protection. Fatalities in workers who continue to be exposed have been reported. A scheme of the progressive natural history of OA is shown in **Figure 40-8**. Most patients with OA improve but do not recover completely even several years after removal from exposure. Even those subjects apparently cured as indicated by clinical and functional assessments

continue to show airway inflammation and remodeling on subsequently obtained bronchial biopsy specimens. Follow-up studies of various types of OA have shown that persons who became asymptomatic after leaving exposure had better lung function and a lower degree of nonallergic bronchial hyperresponsiveness at the time of diagnosis and a shorter duration of exposure after the onset of symptoms. These findings suggest that they were diagnosed at an earlier stage of the disease. Early diagnosis and removal from exposure are essential in ensuring recovery. Although symptoms subside and lung function improves within 1 year of leaving the job involving exposure, decrease in nonallergic bronchial hyperresponsiveness depends on the length of the interval from cessation of exposure. Specific IgE antibodies decrease even more slowly, with no plateau after 5 years as shown in persons with snow crab–induced asthma. It has been recommended that assessment of permanent respiratory impairment or disability take place after at least 2 years of cessation of exposure. The rate of decline in lung function of patients with OA with continuous exposure is higher than in patients without asthma. Moreover, specific bronchial reactivity to the offending occupational agents often persists after the person has left exposure for 2 or more years. Thus, it is not advisable for these patients to return to the same job after they became asymptomatic. Finally, although fewer follow-up studies are available, the outcome with IrIA seems similar to that with immunologic OA.

A histologic basis for the persistence of symptoms and non-allergic bronchial hyperresponsiveness in patients with OA has been confirmed. Higher total cell count and eosinophils in bronchoalveolar lavage fluid were found in persons with Western red cedar asthma who did not recover than in those who recovered completely after removal from exposure. Saetta and co-workers in 1992 documented some reversal of airway wall remodeling (thickness of subepithelial fibrosis and number of subepithelial fibroblasts) in patients with toluene diisocyanate (TDI)-induced asthma 6 months after cessation of exposure, but no decrease in bronchial inflammation and in the degree of nonallergic bronchial hyperresponsiveness was seen. Signs of airway inflammation and remodeling may persist for intervals of 10 years or more after the cessation of exposure, even in apparently cured workers. The reasons for the persistence of symptoms and nonallergic bronchial hyperresponsiveness, as well as of airway inflammation and remodeling, after removal from exposure are not known.

Some researchers have explored the possibility of further improving clinical outcomes by combining the use of inhaled steroids to reduce the degree of airway inflammation with removal from exposure. Although more improvement in various clinical and functional parameters was shown by comparison with removal from exposure only, no case of cure from asthma was documented. Because most cases of IrIA occur in isolation, it is difficult to study the natural history in a series of such patients. However, the time course of improvement seems to follow the same pattern as for OA caused by sensitization. Cure in the first 2 to 3 years after the inhalational accident has been described in approximately 25% of persons who incurred the exposure, with the remainder still showing airway inflammation and remodeling many years after the inhalational accident.

PREVENTION

Primary prevention aims at reducing the risk of the development of immunologic sensitization to workplace agents and subsequent OA. In view of the strong evidence for an exposure-response relationship, primary preventive efforts should focus on the control of workplace exposures. Various interventions can be implemented to reduce exposure at the workplace, including the elimination of hazardous agents whenever feasible; the modification of sensitizing materials (e.g., encapsulation of detergent enzymes); the substitution of highly sensitizing agents by materials with lower asthmagenic potential (e.g., nonvolatile oligomers of diisocyanates, latex gloves with a lower content of powder and protein allergens); engineering changes to the workplace (e.g., improved ventilation, enclosure of industrial process); implementation of safer work practices; and the use of personal protective equipment. Such primary preventive strategies have been shown to be effective in reducing the incidence of OA resulting from enzymes in the detergent industry and from latex gloves in health care facilities.

Another approach is to identify susceptible persons at the time of preemployment examination and exclude them from employment or from high-risk jobs. Unfortunately, the currently identified markers of individual susceptibility (see Table 40-3) have a low positive predictive value for the development of OA. The high prevalence of these markers among the general population, compared with the relatively low risk of occupational sensitization, precludes such screening from being an effective strategy and would unduly exclude many workers in whom OA would never develop. Accordingly, primary prevention should be directed toward reducing exposure to low-enough levels to prevent the onset of asthma in all workers, irrespective of their individual susceptibility. Nevertheless, physicians caring for adolescents with asthma and allergic diseases may offer useful advice regarding careers in which their underlying atopic status increases the risks for work-related sensitization to HMW agents.

Secondary prevention involves the detection of the disease process at an early (preferably preclinical) stage to prevent the development of overt OA and to minimize long-term respiratory impairment by appropriate interventions, which usually involve removal of the worker from exposure. The rationale underlying secondary prevention is the consistent finding that the outcome of OA is better with early diagnosis and milder asthma at the time of removal from exposure. Reduction in the delay between the onset of respiratory and appropriate assessment and intervention could be achieved by increasing awareness of the disease among workers and health professionals. All workers with new-onset asthma or worsening of existing asthma should be interviewed to discover any temporal relationship between work exposure and their symptoms. In the field of occupational medicine, early identification of OA requires the implementation of periodic health surveillance programs in high-risk industries that may be based on questionnaires, spirometry, and identification of allergen-specific IgE when such tests are available and reliable. Surveillance programs should focus on the very first years of exposure, when the incidence of sensitization is highest. Growing evidence indicates that appropriately designed surveillance programs are effective in identifying OA in subjects with less severe asthma and a more favorable outcome.

TREATMENT

Workers with immunologic OA who remain exposed to the causal agent are likely to experience a worsening of asthma symptoms and nonspecific bronchial hyperresponsiveness, with an accelerated decline in FEV_1 over time. This adverse long-term outcome is not prevented by treatment with inhaled corticosteroids and long-acting β_2-agonists. Thus, the ideal treatment for patients with OA is complete removal from the causal exposure. Nevertheless, OA is associated with substantial long-term morbidity. Complete avoidance of exposure results in an overall improvement in asthma, but asthma symptoms and nonspecific bronchial hyperresponsiveness persist in approximately 70% of the patients with OA several years after removal from the offending environment.

Avoidance of exposure is associated with a substantial adverse socioeconomic impact, because maintaining the affected worker at the same job after elimination of the causal agent from the workplace or accommodation of the worker to an unexposed job often is not feasible.

Reduction in rather than complete avoidance of exposure to causal agents may lead to clinical improvement in terms of asthma symptoms and exacerbations and could be considered as an alternative to complete avoidance, in order to minimize the socioeconomic impact of OA when elimination of exposure is not feasible or when jobs that do not entail exposure are not available. Reducing a worker's exposure can be implemented by various engineering measures (see earlier section, "Prevention") or by relocation of the affected worker to a less exposed area or job in the same company. Nevertheless, the limited available evidence indicates that the option of exposure reduction is less beneficial than cessation of exposure, and that this approach requires careful medical monitoring of the subject to ensure early identification of asthma worsening.

Besides environmental interventions, the pharmacologic treatment of OA should follow the general recommendations for asthma as defined in the Global Initiative for Asthma (GINA) guidelines. Patients with OA should be thoroughly informed about the possibilities for compensation, and established cases should be reported to the appropriate public health authorities, according to national regulations. Patients should be considered as permanently and completely impaired for jobs involving exposure to the sensitizing agent that caused their OA. Evaluation for impairment and disability should take into account all of the special features of asthma and should be based on the level of airway obstruction, the degree of nonspecific bronchial hyperresponsiveness or airway reversibility, the minimum amount of medication required for maintaining control of asthma, and the effects of asthma on quality of life.

Data on the optimal management of IrIA are limited, because most cases occur in isolation. Some evidence from case series indicates that subjects with IrIA should benefit rapidly from treatment with oral and/or inhaled corticosteroids, although the dose and duration of treatment remain unknown. Unlike persons with immunologic OA, workers with acute IrIA may be able to continue in their usual jobs if the risk of accidental high-level exposures is prevented through engineering controls. Persons who develop IrIA may subsequently experience worsening of their asthma symptoms on exposure to irritants in the workplace, which may substantially reduce their capacity to work in polluted or dusty environments.

CONTROVERSIES AND PITFALLS

It is important to have objective evidence that the patient's asthma is due to occupational exposure. Many pitfalls may be encountered in confirming the diagnosis of OA. Although lists of agents causing OA found in published articles and databases are useful to alert the physician, the absence of an agent on such lists does not exclude the possibility of OA, because new proteinaceous materials and chemicals are constantly being introduced into the marketplace. Patients often are asked to leave the job when the diagnosis is suspected. However, one of the objective tests for OA is serial monitoring of PEF by the patient for a period at work and a period away from work. Unless the patient has severe symptoms, it is best to obtain objective evidence first before recommending permanent removal from a specific workplace (i.e., job resignation). PEF monitoring also has limitations, as discussed previously. It should be done properly according to a protocol and with use of a logging device, or together with serial measurements of nonallergic bronchial hyperresponsiveness and airway inflammation. Specific challenge tests have been said to be the "gold standard" modality for diagnosis of OA. When a new agent is

suspected, investigators often use several methods to confirm the diagnosis. Some evidence suggests that work-related asthma remains largely unrecognized and inappropriately investigated. A crucial step for enhancing the diagnosis of OA is to promote the prompt referral of workers suspected of having work-related asthma to specialists who have the expertise and facilities for conducting appropriate investigations. In addition, the relative cost and effectiveness of various diagnostic approaches should be further assessed.

Considerable controversy continues regarding whether exposure to a low level of irritant gases or fumes in the workplace or in the environment can actually induce asthma de novo. Despite a great deal that has been learned about OA over the past several years, many gaps remain in current knowledge. Future research priorities should include further improvement in diagnostic, surveillance methods, and control of exposures to prevent the development of the disease and curtail the psycho-socioeconomic impact.

SUGGESTED READINGS

Becklake MR, Chan-Yeung M, Malo JL: Epidemiological approaches in occupational asthma. In Bernstein IL, Chan-Yeung M, Malo JL, Bernstein DI, editors: *Asthma in the workplace*, ed 3, New York, 2006, Taylor & Francis, pp 37–85.

Dykewicz MS: Occupational asthma: current concepts in pathogenesis, diagnosis, and management, *J Allergy Clin Immunol* 123:519–528, 2009.

Gautrin D, Bernstein IL, Brooks SM, Henneberger PK: Reactive airways dysfunction syndrome and irritant-induced asthma. In Bernstein IL, Chan-Yeung M, Malo JL, Bernstein DI, editors: *Asthma in the workplace*, ed 3, New York, 2006, Taylor & Francis, pp 579–627.

Malo JL, Chan-Yeung M: Agents causing occupational asthma, *J Allergy Clin Immunol* 123:545–550, 2009.

Malo JL, Chan-Yeung M: Occupational asthma, *J Allergy Clin Immunol* 108:317–328, 2001.

Mapp CE, Boschetto P, Maestrelli P, Fabbri LM: Occupational asthma, *Am J Respir Crit Care Med* 172:280–305, 2005.

Newman-Taylor AJ, Yucesov B: Genetics and occupational asthma. In Bernstein IL, Chan-Yeung M, Malo JL, Bernstein DI, editors: *Asthma in the workplace*, ed 3, New York, 2006, Taylor & Francis, pp 87–108.

Nicholson PJ, Cullinan P, Taylor AJ, et al: Evidence based guidelines for the prevention, identification, and management of occupational asthma, *Occup Environ Med* 62:290–299, 2005.

Tarlo SM, Balmes J, Balkissoon R, et al: Diagnosis and management of work-related asthma: American College Of Chest Physicians Consensus Statement, *Chest* 134:1S–41S, 2008.

Vandenplas O, Cartier A, Malo JL: Occupational challenge tests. In Bernstein IL, Chan-Yeung M, Malo JL, Bernstein D, editors: *Asthma in the workplace*, ed 3, New York, 2006, Taylor & Francis, pp 227–252.

Vandenplas O, Malo JL: Definitions and types of work-related asthma: a nosological approach, *Eur Respir J* 21:706–712, 2003.

Vandenplas O, Toren K, Blanc PD: Health and socioeconomic impact of work-related asthma, *Eur Respir J* 22:689–697, 2003.

Chapter **41**

Chronic Obstructive Pulmonary Disease: Epidemiology, Pathophysiology, and Clinical Evaluation

William MacNee

Chronic obstructive pulmonary disease (COPD) is a preventable and treatable chronic lung condition characterized by airflow limitation that is not fully reversible. COPD is increasingly recognized as a major global problem that places a burden on both patients who suffer from this disabling condition and health care resources. Despite significant advances in our understanding of the pathogenesis, physiology, clinical features, and management of COPD in recent years, much remains to be discovered about this condition.

Although hidden by the generic term "chronic obstructive pulmonary disease," COPD is a heterogeneous collection of syndromes with overlapping manifestations, which has led to major difficulties in obtaining an acceptable definition of the condition. In addition, as with many chronic inflammatory conditions, COPD is associated with extrapulmonary effects and comorbidities that affect both morbidity and mortality.

The acceptance that symptoms of breathlessness, cough, and sputum production are part of aging or an inevitable consequence of cigarette smoking, and not related to a disease, results in underdiagnosis despite the diagnosis of COPD being easily made. This underdiagnosis is exacerbated by the belief, reinforced by many definitions, that COPD is an "irreversible" condition and that there is nothing "to reverse" with treatment. This leads not only to underdiagnosis but also to undermanagement.

It is now well recognized that significant responses to treatment do occur, which has led to a much more positive approach to the diagnosis and treatment of COPD. Whereas previous treatments largely focused on patients at the severe end of the disease spectrum, recent guidelines recognize that diagnosis and treatment at an earlier stage can offer significant benefits for patients. Although unable to cure COPD, current treatments can reduce symptoms, improve function, and reduce exacerbations in patients as well as decrease the enormous health care costs associated with COPD.

DEFINITIONS AND DIAGNOSTIC CONSIDERATIONS

In defining COPD, several problems must be considered. First, COPD is not just one disease but a group of diseases. Second, it is difficult to differentiate COPD from asthma; the persistent airways obstruction in older patients with chronic asthma is often difficult or even impossible to distinguish from that of COPD patients, who may demonstrate partial reversibility of their airflow limitation. Indeed, some patients with asthma may develop COPD, or these two common conditions may coexist in the same individual. Therefore the problem often is not whether the patient has asthma *or* COPD, but rather whether *either* asthma or COPD is present.

Chronic bronchitis is defined clinically by the American Thoracic Society (ATS) and the United Kingdom (UK) Medical Research Council as "the production of sputum on most days for at least three months in at least two consecutive years when a patient with another cause of chronic cough has been excluded." This definition does not require the presence of airflow limitation. Chronic bronchitis results from inflammation in the larger airways, with bronchial gland hypertrophy and mucus cell hyperplasia.

Emphysema is defined pathologically as "abnormal, permanent enlargement of the distal air spaces, distal to the terminal bronchioles, accompanied by destruction of their walls and without obvious fibrosis." As with chronic bronchitis the definition of emphysema does not require the presence of airflow limitation. As emphysema progresses, the consequent loss of lung elastic recoil contributes to the airflow limitation in COPD.

Bronchiolitis or *small airways disease* also occurs in COPD, where chronic inflammation in the smaller bronchi and bronchioles less than 2 mm in diameter leads to airway remodeling, resulting in airflow limitation. Although relatively little is known of the natural history, bronchiolitis may contribute increasingly, as it progresses, to the airflow limitation in COPD.

The relative contributions made by large or small airways abnormalities or emphysema to the airflow limitation, in individual patients with COPD, is difficult to determine. Thus the term "chronic obstructive pulmonary disease" was introduced in the 1960s to describe patients with incompletely reversible airflow limitation caused by a combination of airways disease and emphysema, without defining the contribution of these conditions to the airflow limitation.

In the statement on the standards for diagnosis and care of patients with COPD by ATS and European Respiratory Society (ERS), COPD is defined as "a preventable and treatable disease state characterized by airflow limitation that is not fully reversible. The airflow limitation is usually progressive and is associated with an abnormal inflammatory response in the lungs to noxious particles or gases, primarily caused by cigarette smoking. Although COPD affects the lungs, it also produces significant systemic consequences." This is similar to the definition produced by the World Health Organization (WHO) Global Initiative on Obstructive Lung Disease (GOLD), which first introduced the concept of COPD as an inflammatory disease into its definition.

The diagnosis of COPD should be considered in any person with the following:

- A history of chronic progressive symptoms: cough, wheeze, and/or breathlessness, with little variation in these symptoms
- A history of exposure to risk factors: cigarette smoke, occupational and environmental dust, and gaseous exposure

The diagnosis requires objective evidence of airflow limitation assessed by spirometry. A postbronchodilator forced expiratory volume in the first second (FEV_1)/forced vital capacity (FVC) ratio of less than 0.7 confirms the presence of airflow limitation that is not fully reversible.

A number of specific causes of airflow limitation, such as cystic fibrosis, bronchiectasis, and bronchiolitis obliterans, are not included in the definition of COPD, but these should be considered in its differential diagnosis. COPD is considered primarily as a lung disease. However, the extrapulmonary effects and comorbidities should also be considered in patients with COPD.

PATHOLOGY

The pathologic changes in COPD are complex and occur in the central conducting airways, the peripheral airways, the lung parenchyma, and the pulmonary vasculature.

Inflammation initiated by exposure to particles or gases underlies most of the pathologic lesions associated with COPD and represents the innate and adaptive immune responses to a lifetime exposure to noxious particles, fumes, and gases, particularly cigarette smoke. Enhanced inflammation also contributes to disease exacerbations, in which acute inflammation is superimposed on the chronic disease. There is good evidence that all smokers have inflammation in their lungs. However, there is individual susceptibility in the inflammatory response to tobacco smoking, and those who develop COPD show an enhanced or abnormal inflammatory response to inhaled toxic agents.

Although the clinical and physiologic presentation of chronic asthma may be indistinguishable from COPD, the pathologic changes are distinct from those in most cases of COPD, largely because of cigarette smoking. The histologic features of COPD in the 15% to 20% of COPD patients who are nonsmokers have not yet been studied in detail. Although complex, the pathology of COPD can be simplified by considering separate disease sites in which pathologic changes occur in smokers to produce a clinical pattern of largely fixed airflow limitation (**Box 41-1**). The clinicopathologic picture is complicated because chronic bronchitis, bronchiolitis, and emphysema may exist in an individual patient, resulting in the clinical and pathophysiologic heterogeneity seen in patients with COPD.

CHRONIC BRONCHITIS

Mucus is produced by mucous glands present in the larger airways and by goblet cells in the airway epithelium. Chronic bronchitis is characterized by hypertrophy of the mucous glands (**Figure 41-1**). Goblet cells that occur predominantly in the surface epithelium of the larger airways increase in number

---

Box 41-1 Chronic Obstructive Pulmonary Disease (COPD): Pathologic Changes

Proximal Airways (cartilaginous airways >2 mm in diameter)
Macrophages and CD8 T lymphocytes
Few neutrophils and eosinophils (neutrophils increase with progressive disease)
Submucosal bronchial gland enlargement and goblet cell metaplasia (results in excessive mucus production or chronic bronchitis)
Cellular infiltrates (neutrophils and lymphocytes) of bronchial glands
Airway epithelial squamous metaplasia, ciliary dysfunction, increased smooth muscle and connective tissue

Peripheral Airways (noncartilaginous airways <2 mm in diameter)
Bronchiolitis at early stage
Macrophages and T lymphocytes (CD8$^+$ > CD4$^+$)
Few neutrophils or eosinophils
Pathologic extension of goblet cells and squamous metaplasia into peripheral airways
Luminal and inflammatory exudates
B lymphocytes, lymphoid follicles, and fibroblasts
Peribronchial fibrosis and airway narrowing with progressive disease

Lung Parenchyma (respiratory bronchioles and alveoli)
Macrophages and CD8$^+$ T lymphocytes
Alveolar wall destruction caused by loss of epithelial and endothelial cells
Development of emphysema (abnormal enlargement of air spaces distal to terminal bronchioles)
Microscopic emphysematous changes
  Centrilobular (dilation and destruction of respiratory bronchioles, often found in smokers and predominantly in upper zones)
  Panacinar (destruction of whole acinus, typically found in α_1-antitrypsin deficiency and more common in lower zones)
Macroscopic emphysematous changes
  Microscopic changes progress to bullae formation, defined as an emphysematous air space >1 cm in diameter.

Pulmonary Vasculature
Macrophages and T lymphocytes

Early Changes
Intimal thickening
Endothelial dysfunction

Late Changes
Vascular smooth muscle
Collagen deposition
Destruction of capillary bed
Development of pulmonary hypertension and cor pulmonale

---

and change in distribution, extending more peripherally. Bronchial biopsy studies confirm findings in resected lungs and show bronchial wall inflammation in chronic bronchitis. Activated T lymphocytes are prominent in the proximal airway walls, with a predominance of the CD8 suppressor T lymphocyte subset, rather than the CD4 subset, as seen in asthma. Macrophages are also prominent. Sputum volume correlates with the degree of inflammation in the airway wall. Neutrophils are present, particularly in the bronchial mucus-secreting glands (Figure 41-1), and become more prominent as the disease progresses. In stable chronic bronchitis, the high percentage of intraluminal

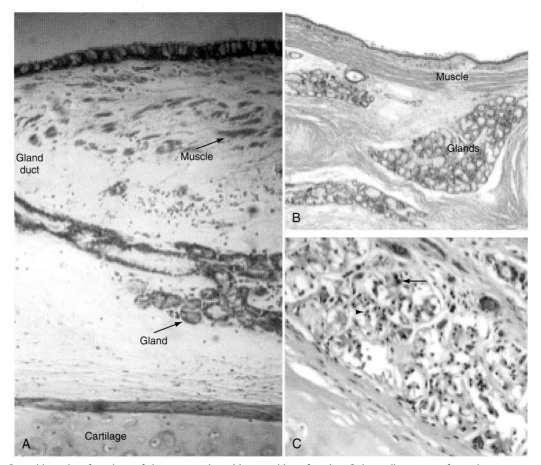

Figure 41-1   A, Central bronchus from lung of cigarette smoker with normal lung function. Only small amounts of muscle are present, and epithelial glands are small. This contrasts sharply with **B,** bronchus from patient with chronic bronchitis, where the muscle appears as a thick bundle and the glands are enlarged. **C,** Enlarged glands at higher magnification, showing evidence of chronic inflammation in glands involving polymorphonuclear leukocytes *(arrowhead)* and mononuclear cells, including plasma cells *(arrow).   (Courtesy Dr. J. C. Hogg.)*

neutrophils is associated with the presence of neutrophil chemotactic factors, including interleukin-8 (IL-8) and leukotriene B_4 (LTB_4). Elastase released from these cells is a potent stimulant for the secretion of mucus. Macrophages and CD8+ T cells also accumulate in the mucous glands.

Evidence indicates that the airway inflammation in patients with chronic bronchitis persists after smoking cessation, particularly if the production of sputum persists, although cough and sputum improve in most smokers who quit. Airway wall changes include squamous metaplasia of the airway epithelium, loss of cilia and ciliary function, and increased smooth muscle and connective tissue.

SMALL AIRWAYS DISEASE AND BRONCHIOLITIS

The smaller bronchioles (<2 mm in internal diameter) normally contribute relatively little to the total airway resistance, because there are so many airways of this size in parallel. Considerable narrowing of these airways can occur before pulmonary function becomes impaired and symptoms develop. Small airways inflammation is one of the earliest changes in asymptomatic cigarette smokers. The inflammatory cell profiles in the small airways are similar to those in larger airways, including the predominance of CD8+ lymphocytes, increase in CD8/CD4 ratio, and increased macrophages. Mucosal ulceration, goblet cell hyperplasia, and squamous cell metaplasia may be present, as well as mesenchymal cell accumulation and fibrosis. With progression of the condition, structural remodeling may occur,

characterized by increased collagen content and scar tissue formation that narrows the airways and produces fixed airway obstruction (**Figure 41-2**).

EMPHYSEMA

Pulmonary emphysema is defined as abnormal permanent enlargement of air spaces distal to the terminal bronchioles, accompanied by destruction of bronchiolar walls. The major types of emphysema are recognized according to the distribution of enlarged air spaces within the *acinar unit,* the part of lung parenchyma supplied by a single terminal bronchiole, as follows:

- Centrilobular (or centriacinar) emphysema, in which large air spaces are initially clustered around the terminal bronchiole (Figure 41-3, *A*).
- Panlobular (or panacinar) emphysema, where the large air spaces are distributed throughout the acinar unit (Figure 41-3, *B*).

Air space enlargement can be identified macroscopically when the enlarged space reaches 1 mm. A *bulla* is a localized area of emphysema, conventionally defined as greater than 1 cm in size.

Centrilobular and panlobular emphysema can occur alone or in combination. The association with cigarette smoking is clearer for centrilobular than panlobular emphysema, although smokers can develop both types. Those with centrilobular emphysema appear to have more abnormalities in the small

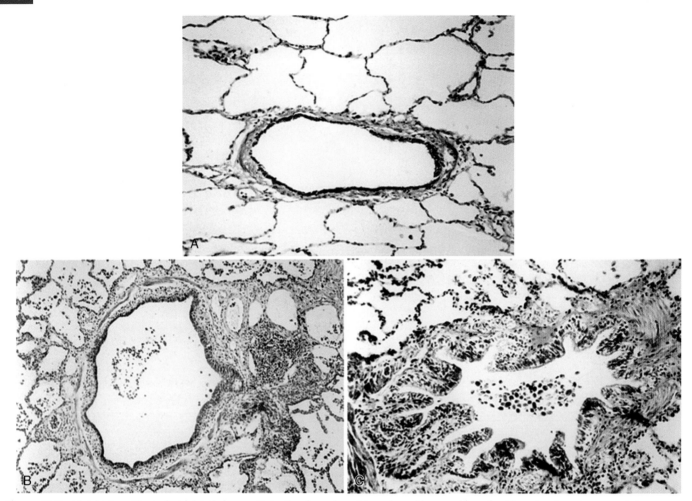

Figure 41-2 Histologic sections of peripheral airways. **A,** Section from cigarette smoker with normal lung function, showing near-normal airway. **B,** Section from patient with small airways disease, showing inflammation in wall and inflammatory exudate in airway lumen. **C,** More advanced case of small airways disease, with reduced lumen, structural reorganization of airway wall, increased smooth muscle, and deposition of peribronchiolar connective tissue. *(Courtesy Dr. J. C. Hogg.)*

airways than those with panlobular emphysema. Panacinar emphysema appears more severe in the lower lobes, in contrast to centriacinar emphysema, which usually concentrates in the upper lobes. Panlobular emphysema is associated with α_1-antitrypsin deficiency, but can also be found in patients with no identified genetic abnormality.

Other types include *paraseptal* (periacinar or distal acinar) emphysema, in which enlarged air spaces occur along the edge of the acinar unit, but only where it abuts against a fixed structure such as the pleura or a vessel. Mixed types of emphysema occur in COPD patients.

The bronchioles and small bronchi are supported by attachment to the outer aspect of adjacent alveolar walls. This arrangement maintains the tubular integrity of the airways. Loss of these attachments and consequent loss of lung elastic recoil may lead to distortion or irregularities of the airways, which contributes to the airflow limitation. The inflammatory cell profile in the alveolar walls is similar to that described in the airways and persists throughout the disease.

PULMONARY VASCULATURE

Changes in the pulmonary vasculature occur early in the course of COPD; thickening of the intima is followed by increase in smooth muscle and infiltration of the vessel wall with inflammatory cells, including macrophages and CD8+ T lymphocytes. As the disease progresses, greater amounts of smooth muscle, proteoglycans, and collagen accumulate, thickening the arterial wall. The development of chronic alveolar hypoxia in patients with COPD results in hypoxic vasoconstriction and subsequently leads to structural changes in the pulmonary vasculature, pulmonary hypertension, and right ventricular hypertrophy and dilation (cor pulmonale).

ETIOLOGY

RISK FACTORS

Cigarette Smoking

Cigarette smoking is the single most important identifiable etiologic factor in COPD. The cause-and-effect relationship between cigarette smoking and COPD derives from several well-controlled population studies over the last four decades.

Maternal smoking is associated with low birth weight and decreased lung function at birth, which may lead to decreased level of function in early adulthood, increasing the risk of developing COPD depending on lifestyle, particularly smoking history. Further, smoking by either parent is associated with an increase in respiratory illness in the first 3 years of life, which may contribute to airflow limitation in later life.

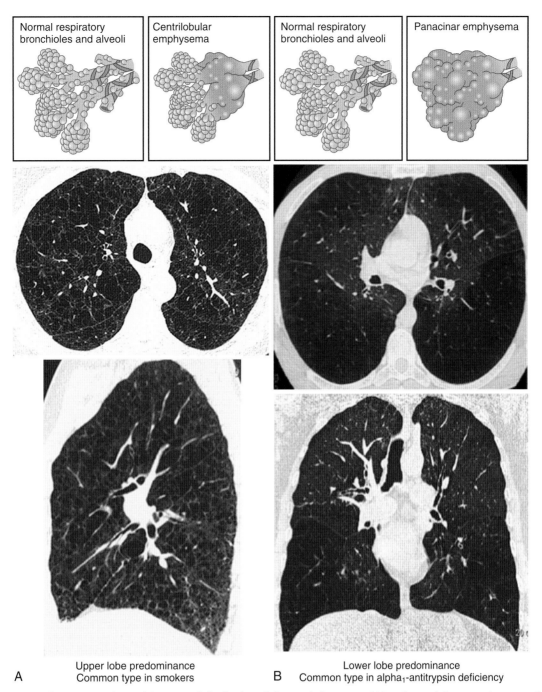

Figure 41-3   Diagrammatic representation and CT scans of distribution of abnormal air spaces within acinar unit in two major types of emphysema. **A,** Acinar unit in normal lung *(left top)* and in centrilobular emphysema, showing focal enlargement of air spaces around respiratory bronchiole. CT scans show patchy centrilobular emphysema. **B,** Panlobular (panacinar) emphysema, showing confluent, even involvement of acinar unit. CT scans show diffuse, low-attenuation areas of panlobular emphysema.

Mild airflow limitation and a reduced increase in lung function occur in smoking adolescents. In addition, the plateau FEV_1 in the third decade of life is also shortened considerably by cigarette smoking, which results in the initiation of FEV_1 decline years earlier than in those who do not smoke.

In adulthood the effect of smoking on FEV_1 decline is well known. In general there is a significant dose-response effect, with smokers having lower lung function the more and the longer they smoke. There is, however, considerable variation. Most longitudinal studies indicate that the decline in FEV_1 in smokers ranges from 45 to 90 mL per year, in contrast to the normal 30 mL/yr (**Figure 41-4**). However, values vary

considerably among individuals, and some experience significantly greater decline, at least temporarily, which may explain why COPD may seem to surface over a short period in the fifth and sixth decades of life. Some nonsmokers have impaired lung function, and 15% to 20% of COPD patients are lifelong nonsmokers. Conversely, some heavy smokers are able to maintain normal lung function, although the frequently quoted "15% to 20%" of smokers who are thought to develop clinically significant COPD is probably an underestimate. About 35% of smokers with normal lung function initially developed COPD during a 25-year follow-up in the Copenhagen City Heart Study.

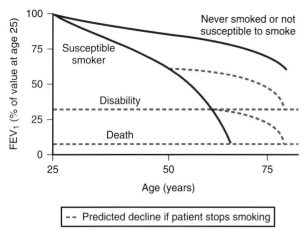

Figure 41-4 Decline in forced expiratory volume in 1 second (FEV$_1$) in smokers and nonsmokers. Horizontal dashed lines represent level of FEV$_1$ consistent with disability or death; curved dashed lines represent change in FEV$_1$ decline with smoking cessation.

Pipe and cigar smokers have significantly greater morbidity and mortality from COPD than nonsmokers, although the risk is less than that from cigarettes. There is a trend to an increased relative risk of chronic airflow limitation from passive smoking, but the effect is not powerful enough to demonstrate clinical significance. Epidemiologic studies have associated cessation of smoking with a decrease in the prevalence of respiratory symptoms and improvement in the subsequent decline in FEV$_1$ (Figure 41-4). The first effect on lung function after smoking cessation is a small increase of 50 to 100 mL in FEV$_1$. There is some debate on whether decline in FEV$_1$ after smoking cessation completely normalizes, although in general those who quit smoking continue to have an FEV$_1$ decline slightly larger than in those who never smoked.

Air Pollution

Air pollution has been recognized as a risk factor in chronic respiratory disease in association with various air pollution episodes in the past. The introduction of air quality standards in the 1950s and 1960s led to a decrease in smoke and sulfur dioxide levels, which produced less discernible peaks of pollution related to morbidity and mortality. However, more recent studies show an association between respiratory symptoms, general practitioner consultations and hospital admissions in patients with airways disease, including COPD, at levels of particulate air pollution below 100 µg/m³, levels currently experienced in many urban areas in Western countries.

The role of long-term exposure to *outdoor* air pollution as a risk factor for the development of COPD is still debated. Air pollution does appear to be a risk factor for mucus hypersecretion, although the association with airflow limitation and accelerated decline in FEV$_1$ is less clear. Air pollution may affect the development of lung function in childhood, which may influence the risk of COPD in adulthood. It is also recognized that *indoor* air pollution, derived from the combustion of biomass fuel in fires and stoves, is an important etiologic factor in COPD and is a particular problem among women in developing countries. Exposure to biomass smoke is thought to increase the risk of COPD two-fold to three-fold.

Occupational Exposure to Dusts

There is a causal link between occupational dust exposure and the development of mucus hypersecretion. In addition, longitudinal studies in workforces exposed to dust show an association between dust exposure and a more rapid decline in FEV$_1$. Selection bias must be considered in these associations, resulting from the "healthy worker effect," with those having respiratory symptoms or lower lung function excluded before entering the occupation. An estimated 15% to 20% of COPD cases are caused by occupational dusts, which increases to 30% in never-smokers. A study of male workers in the Paris area exposed to occupational dusts showed a 5 to 15 mL/yr successive decline in FEV$_1$ from dust exposure. Exposure to welding fumes is also associated with a small but significant risk of developing COPD, from a study in shipyard workers. Workers exposed to *cadmium* have an increased risk of emphysema.

Chronic Mucus Hypersecretion

Population studies of respiratory symptoms indicate a higher prevalence of cough and sputum among smokers than non-smokers. Cessation of smoking is associated with cessation of sputum production in most cases. Earlier studies of working men in London showed that smoking accelerated the decline in FEV$_1$, but failed to show a correlation between the degree of mucus hypersecretion and an accelerated decline in FEV$_1$ or mortality. By contrast, mortality was strongly related to the development of a low FEV$_1$. Data from a more general population study in Copenhagen between 1976 and 1994 suggested that mucus hypersecretion was associated with increased risk of hospital admission and excessive decline in FEV$_1$ of 10 to 15 mL. Moreover, as FEV$_1$ decreases, the association between mucus hypersecretion and mortality becomes stronger.

Chronic Bronchopulmonary Infection

The "British hypothesis" suggested that chronic sputum production (chronic bronchitis) predisposed patients to recurrent bronchopulmonary infections, which subsequently resulted in biologic changes in the airways and alveoli, causing the progression of chronic airflow limitation. In the 1960s and 1970s, Fletcher and Peto refuted this hypothesis, showing no relationship between recurrent infective exacerbations of bronchitis and the decline in lung function in men with chronic bronchitis. This has been challenged more recently in the Lung Health Study, which showed an association in continued smokers between lower respiratory tract infection and a faster rate of decline in lung function. This is supported by more recent studies of patients with COPD.

Cough and sputum production in adulthood is more often reported in those with a history of chest illness in childhood. The association between childhood respiratory illness and ventilatory impairment in adulthood is probably multifactorial. Low economic status, greater exposure to passive smoking, poor diet and housing, and residence in areas of high pollution may all contribute to this finding.

HOST FACTORS

Lung Growth

Several studies indicate that mortality from chronic respiratory diseases and adult ventilatory function correlate inversely with birth weight and weight at 1 year of age. Thus, impaired growth in utero may be a risk factor for the development of chronic respiratory diseases, including COPD. Any factor that affects lung growth during gestation or in childhood, and thus subsequent attainment of maximum lung function, has the potential to increase the risk of developing COPD.

Diet

Diet may influence the development of COPD. Because oxidative stress is thought to have a role in the pathogenesis of COPD, dietary antioxidants such as vitamins A, C, and E should have a protective effect in smokers. The Seven Countries Study found an inverse relationship between baseline intake of fruit and fish and subsequent COPD mortality. In the U.S. Third National Health and Nutrition Examination Survey (NHANES-III), dietary factors, particularly a low intake of vitamin C and low plasma levels of ascorbic acid, were related to a diagnosis of bronchitis. Two British studies also showed that dietary intake of vitamins C and E influences lung function in adults. Studies further suggest a decreased risk of COPD in subjects with a high intake of omega-3 fatty acids.

Atopy and Airway Hyperresponsiveness

The "Dutch hypothesis" proposed that smokers with chronic, largely irreversible airflow limitation and subjects with asthma shared a common constitutional predisposition to allergy, airway hyperresponsiveness, and eosinophilia. Smokers tend to have higher levels of immunoglobulin E (IgE) and higher eosinophil counts than nonsmokers, but not as high a level as in asthmatic patients. Studies in middle-aged smokers with a degree of airflow limitation found a positive correlation between accelerated decline in FEV_1 and increased airway responsiveness to either methacholine or histamine. Over a range of studies, the presence of airway hyperresponsiveness adds approximately 10 mL/yr to decline in FEV_1.

Bronchodilator reversibility has been suggested as a proxy for airway hyperresponsiveness, and some studies suggest reversibility as a predictor of FEV_1 decline. However, these studies have not been adjusted for the actual value of the post-bronchodilator FEV_1; when this is done, minimal association appears to exist between reversibility and FEV_1 decline.

Whether airway hyperresponsiveness is a cause or consequence of COPD remains a subject of debate. Although asthma has been considered confusingly as a risk factor for COPD, good evidence supports that asthmatic patients have a more rapid decline in FEV_1 than nonasthmatic patients, as well as an increased mortality, primarily from COPD. Poorly controlled asthma will likely lead to airway remodeling and fixed airflow obstruction, fulfilling the definition of COPD.

Genetic Factors

Chronic obstructive pulmonary disease is a prime example of a condition of gene-environment interaction. The observation of a familial association for an increased risk of airflow limitation in smoking siblings of subjects with severe COPD suggests a genetic component to this disease. Genetic linkage analysis has identified several sites in the genome that may contain susceptibility genes, such as chromosome 2q. Genetic association studies show that a number of candidate genes are associated with the development of COPD or with rapid decline in FEV_1. However, the associations are not consistent in different populations (**Box 41-2**).

Because COPD is a complex and heterogeneous condition, COPD-related phenotypes may differ between different genetic subtypes of COPD. Several studies suggest polymorphisms in various genes related to emphysema severity or distribution of emphysema. A genetic predisposition to the development of COPD exacerbations has also been suggested.

Many genes with unknown functions likely contribute to the pathogenesis of COPD, and until recently, it has not been

---

Box 41-2   Candidate Genes in Chronic Obstructive Pulmonary Disease

Epoxide hydrolase
Glutathione-*s*-transferase
Heme oxygenase-1
Catalase
Tumor necrosis factor (TNF)
Transforming growth factor beta-1
Serpine-2
Matrix metalloproteinase (MMP-1)
Interleukins (IL-4RA); IL-6; IL-8A-251T; IL-IRN
Nicotine acetylcholine receptor (CHRNA5)

Table 41-1   Alpha₁-Antitrypsin Phenotypes: Frequency in UK Population, Concentration, and Emphysema Risk

Phenotype	Frequency (%)	Average Concentration* (g/L)	Risk Factor for Emphysema
MM	86	2	No
MS	9	1.6	No
MZ	3	1.2	No
SS	0.25	1.2	No
SZ	0.2	0.8	Yes
ZZ	0.03	0.4	Yes

*Serum α_1-protease inhibitor.

---

practical to interrogate the entire genome. Genome-wide association studies may provide a better alternative to candidate gene approaches. Recent genome-wide association studies have identified a single nucleotide polymorphism (SNP) on chromosome 15 that has a significant association with COPD. Multiple genes of interest are present near the most likely associated SNP, including subunits of the nicotinic acetylcholine receptor (CHRNA3 and CHRNA5) and an iron-binding protein (IREB2). A further genome-wide association study identified four SNPs on chromosome 4q, which is strongly associated with FEV_1/FVC. Thus, although genome-wide association studies are at an early stage, chromosome 4 and 15 genetic associations appear to be most significant in COPD.

The most consistent association with COPD is *alpha₁-antitrypsin* (α_1-proteinase inhibitor) *deficiency*. Alpha₁-antitrypsin is a glycoprotein that is the major inhibitor of serine proteases, including neutrophil elastase. More than 75 biochemical variants of α_1-antitrypsin have been described relating to their electrophoretic properties, giving rise to the *phase inhibitor* (Pi) nomenclature (**Table 41-1**). The most common allele in all populations is PiM, and the most common genotype is PiMM, which occurs in 93% of the alleles in subjects of Northern European descent. PiMZ and PiMS are the next two most common genotypes and are associated with α_1-proteinase inhibitor levels of 15% to 75% of the mean levels of PiMM subjects. Similar levels occur in the much less common PiSS type. The most important other type is PiSZ, in which basal levels are 35% to 50% of normal values. The threshold point for increased risk of emphysema is a level of about 80 mg/dL, which is about 30% of normal.

The homozygous PiZZ type, in which serum levels are 10% to 20% of the average normal value, is the strongest genetic risk factor for the development of emphysema. This recessive trait is most frequently seen in individuals of Northern European descent. Such individuals, particularly if they smoke, are likely to develop COPD, usually panlobular emphysema, at an early age. The onset of disease occurs at a median age of 50 in non-smokers and 40 years in smokers.

The defect resulting in α_1-antitrypsin deficiency is related to a single point mutation at position 342, where the nucleotide sequence for this codon is changed from GAG to AAG, resulting in an amino acid change from glutamic acid to lysine. In the PiZZ subject, α_1-antitrypsin protein accumulates in the endoplasmic reticulum of the liver. The structure of the protein reveals that the defect results in the development of abnormal protein polymers, which prevents the α_1-antitrypsin passing through the endoplasmic reticulum and thus prevents the secretion of the protein. These polymers may also be chemotactic for inflammatory cells and may thus contribute to the increased elastase burden. It is postulated that a deficiency in α_1-proteinase inhibitor results in excess activity of neutrophil elastase and therefore tissue destruction and emphysema.

Studies of U.S. blood donors identify a 1:2700 prevalence of PiZZ subjects, the majority of whom had normal spirometry. An estimated 1:5000 UK children are born with the homozygous deficiency (PiZZ). However, the number of subjects identified with disease is much lower than predicted from the known prevalence of the deficiency. It is therefore by no means inevitable that all individuals with homozygous deficiency will develop respiratory disease.

OTHER FACTORS

An association between COPD patients' economic status, education, and lung function and COPD hospitalization has been shown in a Danish study, despite relatively small differences among social classes. However, social risk factors are likely multifactorial and may relate to intrauterine exposure, childhood infections, childhood environment, diet, housing conditions, and occupational factors.

The role of gender as a risk factor for COPD remains unclear. Previous studies typically showed greater COPD mortality in men than women, but more recent studies show that COPD now has almost equal prevalence in men and women, probably reflecting the change in tobacco smoking. Women may be more susceptible to the effects of tobacco smoke than men, but this is still debated.

EPIDEMIOLOGY

Although COPD is a leading cause of morbidity and mortality worldwide, its prevalence varies across countries. The imprecise, variable definitions of COPD and the lack of spirometry to confirm the diagnosis make it difficult to quantify morbidity and mortality. In addition, prevalence data underestimate the total disease burden because COPD typically is not diagnosed until it is clinically recognized, usually at a moderately advanced stage. Mortality from COPD is also likely to be underestimated because it is often cited as a "contributory factor" rather than a cause of death.

PREVALENCE

In the past, imprecise definitions of COPD and underdiagnosis have resulted in underreporting of the condition. Prevalence studies of COPD vary depending on the survey method employed, including self-report of physician diagnosis of COPD, prebronchodilator or postbronchodilator spirometry, and respiratory symptom questionnaires. The lowest prevalence figures come from physician self-reporting; most national surveys indicate that about 6% of the general population has been diagnosed with COPD. This figure probably reflects the underrecognition of COPD, particularly in the early stages, when symptoms are not recognized as representing a disease.

Studies based on standardized spirometry suggest that 25% of subjects over age 40 have airflow limitation (FEV_1/FVC <0.7). However, prevalence data vary depending on the spirometric criteria used to define COPD. The use of a postbronchodilator, fixed FEV_1/FVC (<0.7) leads to potential underdiagnosis in younger adults and overdiagnosis in older adults (>50). Other prevalence studies are based on percent predicted FEV_1. In a UK population survey, 10% of men and 11% of women age 18 to 64 years had an FEV_1 greater than 2 standard deviations (SD) below their predicted values; the numbers increased with age, particularly in smokers. In current smokers 40 to 65 years old, 18% of men and 14% of women had an FEV_1 greater than 2 SD below normal, compared with 7% and 6% of male and female nonsmokers, respectively.

Approximately 14 million people in the United States have COPD, increasing by 42% since 1982. The best data available come from the 1988-1994 NHANES-III study. Prevalence of mild COPD (defined as FEV_1/FVC <0.7 and FEV_1 >80% predicted) was 6.9% and prevalence of moderate COPD (defined as FEV_1/FVC <0.7 and FEV_1 ≤80% predicted) was 6% for those age 25 to 75. The prevalence of both mild and moderate COPD was higher in males than females, in whites than in blacks, and increased steeply with age. Airflow limitation affected an estimated 14.2% of current white male smokers, 6.9% of ex-smokers, and 3.3% of never-smokers. Airflow limitation occurred in 13.6% of white female smokers, 6.8% of ex-smokers, and 3.1% of never-smokers. Less than 50% of COPD patients, based on the presence of airflow limitation, had a physician diagnosis of COPD.

Data from five Latin American cities in five different countries showed the presence of COPD (FEV_1/FEC ratio <0.7) increased sharply with age. The highest prevalence was in the over-60 age-group and ranged from 18.4% in Mexico City to 31.1% in Montevideo, Uruguay. In 12 Asian-Pacific countries, prevalence of moderate to severe COPD in those over age 30 was 6.3%. However, prevalence rates ranged from 3.5% to 6.7% across the Asia-Pacific region.

The UK national study reported abnormally low FEV_1 in 10% of males and 11% of females age 60 to 65 years. In England and Wales, an estimated 900,000 people have a diagnosis of COPD, although because of underdiagnosis, the true number is likely closer to 1.5 million. The mean age at diagnosis in the UK was 67 years, and prevalence increased with age. COPD was more common in men than in women and was associated with socioeconomic deprivation. The prevalence of diagnosed COPD has increased in the UK in women from 0.8% in 1990 to 1.4% in 1997, but did not change over the same period in men. Similar trends are found in the United States, again probably reflecting differences in smoking habits. National surveys of consultations in British general practices found a modest decline in the number of middle-aged men with symptoms of COPD and a slight increase in middle-aged women. These trends are confounded by changes over the years in the application of the diagnostic labels for this condition, particularly the overlap between COPD and asthma.

MORBIDITY AND SOCIOECONOMIC IMPACT

Morbidity data in patients with COPD are less available and less reliable than mortality data, but the number of physician visits, emergency department (ED) visits, and hospitalizations in COPD patients increases with age, is greater in men than women, and is likely to increase with the aging population.

The ERS White Book provides data on the mean number of consultations for major respiratory diseases across 19 European countries. In most, consultations for COPD equal the number for asthma, pneumonia, lung cancer, and tuberculosis combined. In the United States in 2000, there were 8 million physician office/hospital outpatient visits for COPD, 1.5 million ED visits, and 673,000 hospitalizations.

The disability-adjusted life years (DALYs) for a condition is the sum of years lost because of premature mortality and years of life lived with disability, adjusted for the severity of the disability. In 1990, COPD was the 12th leading cause of DALYs in the world, about 2.1% of the total. COPD is projected to be the fifth leading cause of DALYs worldwide in 2020.

In the UK, emergency admissions for exacerbations of COPD increased from 0.5% of all hospital admissions in 1991 to 1% in 2000. Morbidity from COPD increases with age and is greater in men than women. COPD morbidity also may be affected by comorbidities (e.g., ischemic heart disease, diabetes mellitus) and may impact health status. Airway diseases (chronic bronchitis and emphysema, COPD, and asthma) account for a calculated 24.4 million lost working days per year in the UK, which represents 9% of all certified sickness absence among men, and 3.5% of the total in women. Respiratory diseases in the UK rank as the third most common cause of days of certified incapacity, with COPD accounting for 56% of these days lost in men and 24% in women. Most admissions are in the over-65 age-group and patients with advanced disease, although admissions recur at all stages. About 25% of patients diagnosed with COPD are admitted to the hospital, and 15% of all outpatients are admitted each year. In 2002-2003, there were 110,000 hospital admissions for COPD exacerbations in England, representing 8% of all emergency admissions. The burden in primary care is even greater, providing 86% of COPD care. Patients with COPD average six or seven visits annually to their general practitioner.

MORTALITY

Chronic obstructive pulmonary disease is the fourth leading cause of death in the United States and Europe and is projected to be the third leading cause of death (now fifth) worldwide by 2020, a result of the increase in smoking in the developing world and the changing demographics in those countries with increasing longevity of their populations. Large international variations in mortality for COPD cannot be entirely explained by differences in diagnostic patterns, diagnostic labels, or smoking habits. Death certification figures underestimate mortality because as previously stated, COPD is often cited as a contributory factor to the cause of death. COPD death rates are low under age 45 and increase steeply with age. Although mortality from COPD in men has been falling slightly, mortality in women has increased. U.S. data (2000-2005) indicate that COPD accounts for 5% of all deaths, with age-standardized mortality rate stable at approximately 64 deaths per 100,000 population; however, mortality in males fell from 83.8 in 2000 to 77.3 per 100,000 in 2005 and increased in females from 54.4 to 56.0 per 100,000.

In the UK in 2003, an estimated 26,000 persons (14,000 men, 12,000 women) died from COPD, 4.9% of all deaths, 5.4% of all male deaths, and 4.2% of all female deaths. Mortality from COPD in the UK has fallen in men but risen in women over the last 25 years, except in the over-75 age-group. In American women the decline in mortality which was recorded until 1975 has reversed and has increased substantially between 1980 and 2000, from 20.1 to 56.7 per 100,000, whereas the increase in men has been more modest, from 73.0 to 82.6 per 100,000. These trends presumably relate to the later peak prevalence of cigarette smoking in women compared with men. In the UK, age-adjusted death rates from chronic respiratory diseases vary by a factor of 5 to 10 in different geographic locations. Mortality rates tend to be higher in urban areas than in rural areas.

In the UK, COPD reduces life expectancy by an average of 1.8 years (76.5 vs. 78.3). The reduction in life expectancy increases with age, from 1.1 year in mild disease to 1.7 years in moderate disease and 4.1 years in patients with severe disease.

NATURAL HISTORY AND PROGNOSIS

Chronic obstructive pulmonary disease is generally progressive, particularly if the patient's exposure to noxious agents continues. However, the natural history of COPD is variable; not all individuals follow the same course. Stopping exposure to noxious agents, such as cigarette smoke, may result in some improvement in lung function and may slow or halt progression of the disease.

The airway obstruction in susceptible smokers develops slowly because of an accelerated rate of decline in FEV_1 that continues for years. As noted previously, impaired lung function development during childhood and adolescence as a result of recurrent infections or exposure to tobacco smoke may lead to lower maximally attained lung function in adulthood. This failure in lung growth, often combined with a shortened plateau phase in teenage smokers, increases the risk of COPD (**Figure 41-5**). In never-smokers the FEV_1 declines at a rate of 20 to 30 mL/yr (see Figure 41-4). Smokers as a population have a faster rate of decline, and reported changes in FEV_1 in patients with COPD exceed 50 mL/yr. However, decline in COPD patients varies considerably. The initial level of FEV_1 is related to the annual rate of decline in FEV_1, and individuals in the highest or lowest FEV_1 percentiles remain in the same percentiles over subsequent years. This suggests that susceptible cigarette smokers can be identified in early middle age by a reduction in FEV_1.

Longitudinal data from the Lung Health Study in the United States show that stopping smoking, even after significant airflow limitation is present, can result in some improvement in function, and that it will slow or even stop the progression of airflow limitation. Men who quit smoking at the beginning of the study had an FEV_1 decline of 30.2 mL/yr, whereas for those who continued to smoke throughout the study, the decline was 66.1 mL/yr. Similar findings were seen in women.

The FEV_1 is a strong predictor of survival. Less than 50% of patients whose FEV_1 has fallen to 30% of the predicted values are alive 5 years later. The best association between FEV_1 and survival is the postbronchodilator FEV_1, rather than prebronchodilator. Other clinical parameters shown to be important prognostic indicators independent of FEV_1 include weight loss, a poor prognostic sign. Other unfavorable prognostic factors include severe hypoxemia, raised pulmonary arterial pressure,

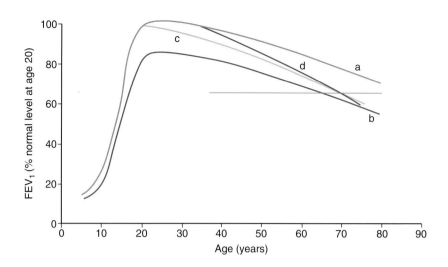

Figure 41-5 Different patterns of obtaining abnormally low forced expiratory volume in 1 second (FEV₁) in middle age. FEV₁ plotted as a percentage of maximal at age 20 against years of age. Line *a*, normal age-related decline in FEV₁ in healthy subjects; *b*, abnormal growth rate but normal age-related decline in FEV₁; *c*, premature or early decline; *d*, accelerated decline in lung function. *(From Weiss ST, Ware JH: Am J Respir Crit Care Med 154:s208–s211, 1996.)*

and low carbon monoxide transfer, which become apparent in patients with severe disease.

PATHOGENESIS

Central to the pathogenesis of COPD is an enhanced inflammatory response to inhaled particles or gases. The following pathogenic processes are involved in this inflammatory response (**Figure 41-6**):

- Increased air space inflammation
- Increased protease burden and decreased antiprotease function
- Oxidant/antioxidant imbalance and oxidative stress
- Defective lung repair

AIR SPACE INFLAMMATION

Inflammation is present in the lungs, particularly in the small airways, of all smokers. This inflammatory response is thought to be a normal, protective, innate immune response to inhaled toxins. This response is amplified in patients who develop COPD, through mechanisms not fully understood. COPD does develop in some patients who do not smoke, but the inflammatory response in these patients is not well characterized. The abnormal inflammatory response in COPD leads to tissue destruction, impairment of defense mechanisms that limit such destruction, and defective repair mechanisms. In general, the inflammatory and structural changes in the airways increase with disease severity and persist even after smoking cessation.

The *innate* inflammatory immune system provides primary protection against the continuing insult from inhalation of toxic gases and particles. The first line of defense consists of the mucociliary clearance apparatus and macrophages that clear foreign material from the lower respiratory tract; both are impaired in COPD. The second line of defense of the innate immune system is the exudation of plasma and circulating cells into both large and small conducting airways and the alveoli. This process is controlled by an array of proinflammatory chemokines and cytokines (**Box 41-3**). COPD is characterized by increased neutrophils, macrophages, T lymphocytes (CD8 > CD4), and dendritic cells in various parts of the lungs (see Box 41-2). Generally, the extent of inflammation is related to degree of airflow limitation. These inflammatory cells are capable of

---

Box 41-3 Inflammatory Mediators in COPD

Leukotriene B₄ (LTB₄)
   Neutrophil and T cell chemoattractant
   Produced by macrophages, neutrophils, and epithelial cells
Chemotactic factors
   CXC chemokines, interleukin-8 (IL-8), growth-related oncogene-α
   Produced by macrophages and epithelial cells
   Attract cells from circulation; amplify proinflammatory responses
Proinflammatory cytokines
   Tumor necrosis factor alpha (TNF-α)
   Interleukin-1beta (IL-1β) and IL-6
Growth factors
   Transforming growth factor beta (TGF-β)
   May cause fibrosis in airways directly or through release of another cytokine, connective tissue growth factor

COPD, chronic obstructive pulmonary disease.

---

releasing a variety of cytokines and mediators that participate in the disease process. This inflammatory cell pattern is greatly different from that found in asthma.

An *adaptive* immune response is also present in the lungs of patients with COPD, as shown by the presence of mature lymphoid follicles, which increase in number in the airways according to disease severity. Their presence has been attributed to the large antigen load associated with bacterial colonization or frequent low respiratory tract infections, or possibly an autoimmune response. Dendritic cells are major antigen-presenting cells, are increased in the small airways, and provide a link between the innate and adaptive immune responses.

Both central airways and peripheral airways are inflamed in smokers with COPD. Smokers with chronic bronchitis have greater inflammation in bronchial glands. Recent studies characterizing the inflammation show increased infiltration of mast cells, macrophages, and neutrophils in smokers with chronic bronchitis (see Box 41-1). An increase in T lymphocytes, mainly in the CD8+ subset, occurs, in contrast to the predominance of the CD4 T cell subset in asthma. CD8 lymphocytes may have a role in apoptosis and destruction of alveolar wall epithelial cells, through the release of perforins and tumor necrosis factor alpha (TNF-α). Excessive recruitment of CD8 T lymphocytes may occur in response to repeated viral infections, damaging the lungs in susceptible smokers.

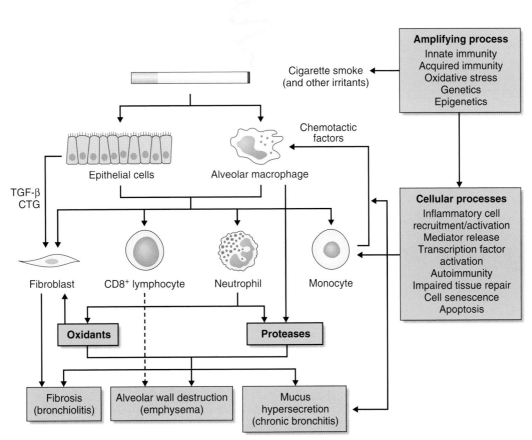

Figure 41-6   Overview of pathogenesis of chronic obstructive pulmonary disease. Cigarette smoke activates macrophages in epithelial cells to produce chemotactic factors that recruit neutrophils and CD8+ cells from the circulation. These cells release factors that activate fibroblasts, resulting in abnormal repair processes and bronchiolar fibrosis. Imbalance between proteases released from neutrophils and macrophages and antiproteases leads to alveolar wall destruction (emphysema). Proteases also cause the release of mucus. Increased oxidant burden resulting from smoke inhalation or release of oxidants from inflammatory leukocytes causes epithelial and other cells to release chemotactic factors, inactivates antiproteases, directly injures alveolar walls, and causes mucus secretion. Several processes are involved in amplifying the inflammatory responses in COPD. *TGF-β,* Transforming growth factor beta; *CTG,* connective tissue growth factor.   *(From MacNee W: Pathology and pathogenesis. In* ABC of COPD, *ed 2, London, 2011, Blackwell.)*

PROTEINASE/ANTIPROTEINASE IMBALANCE

Important for understanding the pathogenesis of COPD, an association was seen between α_1-antitrypsin deficiency and development of early-onset emphysema. Alpha$_1$-antitrypsin is a potent inhibitor of serine proteases and has greatest affinity for the enzyme neutrophil elastase. It is synthesized in the liver and increases from its usual plasma concentration as part of the acute-phase response. The activity of this protein is critically dependent on the methionine-serine sequence at its active site. Table 41-1 provides the average α_1-antitrypsin plasma levels for the more common phenotypes.

A deficiency in alpha$_1$-antitrypsin levels, particularly the inability to increase levels in the acute response, results in unrestrained proteolytic damage to lung tissue, leading to emphysema, which develops at an earlier age than in the patient with the more common emphysema in COPD. Cigarette smoking is a cofactor in the development of emphysema in alpha$_1$-antitrypsin–deficient patients, probably as a result of oxidation and thus inactivation of the remaining functional α_1-antitrypsin by oxidants in cigarette smoke. Hypothetically, under normal circumstances, the release of proteolytic enzymes

from inflammatory cells, which migrate to the lungs to fight infection or after cigarette smoke inhalation, does not cause damage because of inactivation of these proteolytic enzymes by an excess of inhibitors. In conditions of excessive enzyme load or with absolute or functional deficiency of antiproteinases, however, an imbalance develops between proteinases and antiproteinases that favors proteinases, leading to uncontrolled enzyme activity and degradation of lung connective tissue in alveolar walls, resulting in emphysema. Cigarette smoke and inflammation produce oxidative stress, which primes several inflammatory cells to release a combination of proteases and to inactivate several antiproteases by oxidation.

This simplified protease/antiprotease theory is complicated by the presence of other antiproteases (e.g., antileukoprotease) and other proteases (e.g., metalloproteases) released from macrophages (**Table 41-2**).

ELASTASE SYNTHESIS AND REPAIR

An abnormality of elastin synthesis and repair may be involved in the pathogenesis of emphysema. Severe starvation has been reported to cause COPD in both humans and animals;

Table 41-2 Proteinases and Antiproteinases in COPD

Proteinases	Antiproteinases
Serine proteinases	α_1-Antitrypsin
Neutrophil elastase	α_1-Antitrypsin
Cathepsin G	Secretory leukoprotease inhibitor
Proteinase 3	Elafin
Cysteine proteinases	Cystatins
Cathepsins: B, K, L, S	
Matrix metalloproteinases (MMP-8, MMP-9, MMP-12)	Tissue inhibitor of MMPs (TIMP-1 to TIMP-4)

COPD, chronic obstructive pulmonary disease.

in addition, starvation can exacerbate proteinase-induced emphysema in animal models. Whether the milder malnutrition that occurs in emphysematous patients has a role in the pathogenesis is unknown.

Certain disorders of connective tissues, including Ehlers-Danlos syndrome and cutis laxa (generalized elastolysis), have been associated with the development of emphysema. Emphysema also develops in some animal models with genetic defects in tissue metabolism.

OXIDANT/ANTIOXIDANT IMBALANCE

Considerable evidence supports the presence of an imbalance between oxidants and antioxidants that favors the oxidants (oxidative stress) in patients with COPD. Cigarette smoke itself produces a huge oxidant burden in the air spaces, and oxidants are released in increased amounts from the activated inflammatory cells that migrate into the air spaces in response to smoking, as noted earlier. Important antioxidants such as glutathione may also be affected by inhalation of cigarette smoke. Smoking initially depletes glutathione, but a subsequent rebound of levels occurs, presumably as a protective mechanism against the effects of cigarette smoking.

Studies have measured increased markers of oxidative stress, such as products of lipid peroxidation reactions, in biologic fluids of patients with COPD as indirect measurements of reactive oxygen species activity. Evidence shows increased markers of oxidative stress in bronchoalveolar lavage (BAL) fluid, sputum, exhaled breath, and breath condensate as well as systemically in the blood and skeletal muscle in patients with COPD, supporting a role for oxidative stress in its pathogenesis. Oxidative stress can directly damage cells, increase air space epithelial permeability, inactivate antiproteases, and importantly, trigger an enhanced inflammatory response by activating redox-sensitive transcription factors (e.g., NF-κB, AP-1). Also, oxidative modification of target molecules occurs more in the lungs in patients with COPD than in smokers without COPD.

Histone deacetylase-2 (HDAC2) is modified by oxidative stress in COPD, resulting in decreased level and activity. Decrease in HDAC2 results in acetylation of the lysine residues and DNA, resulting in uncoiling of DNA and increasing the accessibility of transcription factors and RNA polymerase to the transcriptional machinery, thus increasing gene transcription. Studies of resected lungs indicate that HDAC2 protein and activity is reduced in lung tissue in COPD as a result of oxidative modification of the molecule and is associated with

an increase in histone-4 acetylation at the IL-8 promoter and increased IL-8 mRNA expression. This mechanism may be responsible for perpetuating inflammation in COPD.

The transcription factor *nuclear erythroid-related factor 2* (Nrf2) controls the expression of several of the most important antioxidant enzymes. COPD lungs have decreased expression of Nrf2 transcriptional activity, which may result in reduced protection against oxidative stress.

OTHER MECHANISMS

Autoimmunity, apoptosis, and cell senescence also may be involved in the pathogenesis of emphysema (Figure 41-6). Studies show that *apoptosis* occurs in emphysematous lungs, predominantly involving endothelial cells in the alveolar walls and resulting from a decrease in vascular endothelial growth factor (VEGF) or VEGF signaling, also shown to occur in association with emphysema in human lungs. These data led to the concept of an "alveolar maintenance program" required for the structural preservation of the lungs. Cigarette smoke is thought to cause disruption of this maintenance program, resulting in emphysema. The lung destruction or tissue destruction of emphysema is therefore caused by the mutual interaction of alveolar cell apoptosis, oxidative stress, and protease/antiprotease imbalance.

Similar features between pulmonary emphysema and lung aging led to the hypothesis that both conditions share underlying mechanisms, including oxidative stress, inflammation, and apoptosis. The cellular equivalent of aging is *senescence*, which is characterized by a nonproliferative stage in which cells are metabolically active and apoptosis resistant. Mechanisms associated with cell senescence include accumulation of DNA damage, impairment of DNA repair, epigenetic modifications in nuclear DNA, protein damage, oxidative stress, and telomere attrition. Telomere length is decreased in cells from emphysematous lungs, as are antiaging molecules such as sirtuins, suggesting a role for accelerated aging and cell senescence in the pathogenesis of emphysema.

Considerable evidence supports the role of the adaptive immune response in the progression of COPD. The presence of autoantibodies to lung structural cells and elastase suggests involvement of autoimmune mechanisms in pathogenesis of COPD.

Both oxidants and proteases such as elastase are important secretagogues for mucus and thus may be involved in the hypersecretion of mucus that occurs in chronic bronchitis. Airway mucus synthesis is regulated by the epidermal growth factor receptor (EGFR) system. Cigarette smoke upregulates EGFR expression and activates EGFR tyrosine phosphorylation, causing mucus synthesis in epithelial cells by a mechanism that probably involves oxidative stress.

PATHOPHYSIOLOGY

AIRFLOW LIMITATION AND HYPERINFLATION

The characteristic physiologic abnormality in COPD is a decrease in maximum expiratory flow, which results from (1) loss of lung elasticity and (2) increase in airway resistance in small airways.

The main site of airflow limitation in COPD occurs in the small conducting airways (<2 mm in diameter) and results from inflammation, narrowing (airway remodeling), and inflammatory exudates in the small airways, features that correlate

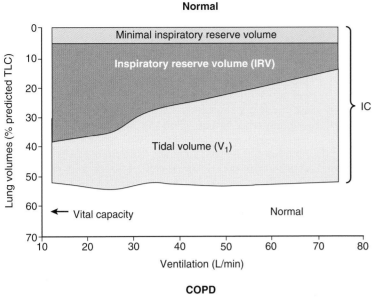

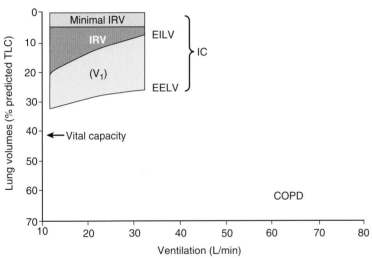

Figure 41-7 In health, the body meets the increased oxygen demand produced by exercise by using some of the inspiratory reserve volume of the lungs to increase tidal volume. *COPD*, chronic obstructive pulmonary disease. *EELV*, end-expiratory lung volume; *EILV*, end-inspiratory lung volume; *IC*, inspiratory capacity; *IRV*, inspiratory reserve volume; *TLC*, total lung capacity. *(Data from O'Donnell DE et al:* Am J Respir Crit Care Med *164:770, 1999.)*

with the reduction in FEV_1. Other factors contributing to the airflow limitation include loss of the lung elastic recoil (caused by destruction of alveolar walls) and destruction of alveolar support (from alveolar attachments). The resultant airway obstruction causes progressive trapping of the air during expiration, resulting in hyperinflation at rest and dynamic hyperinflation during exercise. Lung hyperinflation reduces the inspiratory capacity, and thus functional residual capacity (FRC) increases, particularly during exercise (**Figure 41-7**). These features are thought to occur early in the course of the disease and result in the breathlessness and limited exercise capacity typical of COPD. Bronchodilators reduce air trapping and thus decrease lung volumes, improving symptoms and exercise capacity. Tests of overall lung mechanics (e.g., FEV_1, airway resistance) are usually abnormal in patients with COPD when breathlessness develops.

Residual volume, FRC, and (in some cases) total lung capacity (TLC) increase. Maximum expiratory flow-volume curves show a characteristic convexity toward the volume axis, with preservation of peak expiratory flow initially. The uneven distribution of ventilation in advanced COPD causes a reduction in "ventilated" lung volume, and thus the carbon monoxide transfer factor (TLCO) is almost always reduced, although

the lung diffusing capacity for carbon monoxide (DLCO), normalized to ventilated alveolar volume (DLCO/VA/KCO), may remain relatively well preserved in patients without emphysema.

The ability to draw air through the conducting airways during inspiration depends on the strength of the respiratory muscles, which in turn depends on their resting length; the compliance of the respiratory system (lung and chest wall); and the resistance of the airways. Exhalation is normally passive and results from the elastic recoil of the lungs. The characteristic changes in the static pressure-volume curve of the lungs in COPD are an increase in static compliance and a reduction in static transpulmonary pressure at any given lung volume. These changes are generally thought to indicate emphysema.

The resistance to airflow depends on the length and diameter of the airways and the physical properties of the respirable gas. At a constant airway diameter, airflow on inhalation is proportional to the difference between atmospheric gas pressure and alveolar pressure. During exhalation, airflow depends on the difference between alveolar and atmospheric pressures. Throughout inhalation and during the initial portion of exhalation, this relationship is constant. However, at a certain point during exhalation, flow cannot increase despite further

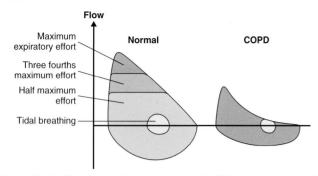

Figure 41-8 Flow-volume loop over normal individual and patient with chronic obstructive pulmonary disease (COPD). Patients who have COPD may reach airflow limitation even during tidal breathing. *(From Celli B. In Albert R, Spiro SG, Jett JR, editors:* Comprehensive respiratory medicine, *St Louis, 1999, Mosby.)*

increases in alveolar pressure. This is a result of dynamic compression of the airways, which limits flow, as illustrated by the flow-volume loop (**Figure 41-8**). During exhalation from TLC, flow increases to a point beyond which additional expiratory effort has no effect. During tidal breathing, expiratory flow is well below that attainable during maximum expiration. In COPD, however, the flow-volume loop is different. The major site of the fixed airway narrowing in COPD is in peripheral airways of diameter less than 2 mm. Loss of lung elastic recoil pressure is also an important mechanism of airway obstruction, resulting from a reduction in the distending force applied to the intrathoracic airways. Dynamic expiratory compression of the airways is enhanced by loss of lung recoil and by atrophic changes in the airways and loss of support from the surrounding alveolar walls, allowing flow limitation at lower driving pressure and flow.

In addition to a decrease in peak expiratory flow, the later expiratory portion of the flow-volume curve is concave relative to the volume axis in patients with COPD. In severe disease the flow generated during tidal breathing may actually reach the maximum possible flow (Figure 41-8). Such patients, in response to the increased metabolic demands of exercise, for example, are unable to increase ventilation. Increased respiratory rate results in gas trapping from incomplete alveolar emptying, so-called dynamic overinflation. This increased lung volume increases the elastic recoil and is associated with an increase in the end-expiratory alveolar pressure. The result is an increase in the work of breathing because pleural pressure must drop below alveolar pressure before inspiration of air can occur.

PULMONARY GAS EXCHANGE

Ventilation-perfusion (V/Q) mismatching (as a result of decreased alveolar ventilation without a corresponding reduction in perfusion) is the most important cause of impaired pulmonary gas exchange in COPD. Other causes, such as impaired alveolar-capillary diffusion of oxygen and increased shunt, are much less important. In general, gas exchange worsens as the disease progresses. The distribution of ventilation is uneven in patients with COPD. Mechanisms that reduce blood flow include local destruction of vessels in alveolar walls as a result of emphysema, hypoxic vasoconstriction in areas of severe alveolar hypoxemia, and passive vascular obstruction from increased alveolar pressure and distention.

RESPIRATORY MUSCLES

In patients with severe COPD, a combination of lung overinflation and malnutrition results in muscle weakness, reducing the capacity of the respiratory muscles to generate pressure over the range of tidal breathing. In addition, the load against which the respiratory muscles need to act is increased because of the increase in airway resistance. Overinflation of the lungs leads to shortening and flattening of the diaphragm, impairing its ability to generate force to lower pleural pressure. During quiet tidal breathing in normal subjects, expiration is largely passive and depends on the elastic recoil of lungs and chest wall. Patients with COPD increasingly need to use their rib cage muscles and inspiratory accessory (e.g., sternocleidomastoid) muscles, even during quiet breathing. During exercise, this pattern may be even more distorted and may result in paradoxical motion of the rib cage.

Patients with COPD have impaired values of global function of the respiratory muscles, such as maximum inspiratory mouth pressure (PE_{max}), although these measurements are effort-dependent. Diaphragmatic function can be assessed during inspiration by measurement of transdiaphragmatic pressure (Pdi), using balloon-tipped catheters with small transducers in the esophagus and stomach. Pdi values are reduced in patients with COPD.

PULMONARY HYPERTENSION

Pulmonary hypertension complicating COPD is generally defined by a mean *pulmonary artery pressure* (Ppa) greater than 20 mm Hg. This is different from the definition of idiopathic hypertension (Ppa >25 mm Hg). In the natural history of COPD, pulmonary hypertension is often preceded by an abnormally large increase in Ppa (>30 mm Hg) during exercise.

The term *cor pulmonale* is often used synonymously with pulmonary hypertension in COPD. However, cor pulmonale is defined as right ventricular (RV) hypertrophy (enlargement) resulting from disease that affects the structure or function of the lungs. This is a pathologic definition and thus of limited value in clinical practice, because the diagnosis of RV hypertrophy is difficult to make. Pulmonary hypertension is the cause of cor pulmonale, so it is best to use the term *pulmonary hypertension* in COPD rather than cor pulmonale.

There are few data on the prevalence of pulmonary hypertension resulting from COPD, because large studies of right-sided heart catheterization or Doppler echocardiography have not been undertaken. An estimate of the prevalence of pulmonary hypertension in COPD can be obtained from calculating the number of subjects with significant hypoxemia who require long-term oxygen therapy. Significant hypoxemia (PaO_2 <55 mm Hg, FEV_1 <50% of predicted) occurs in 0.3% of the UK population 45 or older. Extrapolation from this figure suggests that in England and Wales, 60,000 patients may be at risk of pulmonary hypertension and eligible for long-term oxygen therapy. Extrapolating these figures to the United States, 300,000 COPD patients are at risk of pulmonary hypertension. **Box 41-4** lists the factors leading to pulmonary hypertension in patients with COPD.

Pulmonary artery hypertension occurs late in the course of COPD, concurrent with the development of hypoxemia. Alveolar hypoxia is the most important functional factor in the development of pulmonary hypertension in COPD. Acute hypoxia causes pulmonary vasoconstriction, and chronic

Box 41-4 **Factors Leading to Increased Pulmonary Vascular Resistance in COPD**

Functional Factors
Alveolar hypoxia
    Acute hypoxia (vasoconstriction)
    Chronic hypoxia (remodeling of pulmonary vascular bed)
Hypercapnia, acidosis
Hyperviscosity (polycythemia)

Structural Factors
Destruction of pulmonary vascular bed
Thromboembolic lesions
Fibrosis
Emphysema
Compression of alveolar vessels

COPD, chronic obstructive pulmonary disease.

hypoxia induces structural changes or remodeling of the pulmonary vasculature, leading to sustained pulmonary hypertension.

The pulmonary hypertension in COPD is precapillary, because of an increased pressure difference between Ppa and pulmonary capillary wedge pressure, reflecting the increased pulmonary vascular resistance. Pulmonary hypertension in COPD is mild to moderate, with a resting Ppa in the stable stage of the disease ranging between 20 and 35 mm Hg. Ppa of 40 mm Hg or greater is unusual in COPD patients, except when measured during an acute exacerbation or during exercise; approximately 1% of patients exhibit severe pulmonary hypertension (Ppa >40 mm Hg). These patients are characterized by less severe airflow limitation but profound hypoxemia and hypocapnia. These patients may have an increased reactivity of the pulmonary arteries to hypoxia or coexisting idiopathic pulmonary hypertension. COPD patients with severe pulmonary hypertension in COPD have a poorer prognosis.

The progression of pulmonary hypertension is slow in COPD patients, and Ppa may remain stable for several years. The mean change in Ppa in a cohort of COPD patients is small (0.5 mm Hg/yr). Also, symptoms and physical signs are of little help in the diagnosis of pulmonary hypertension in COPD patients. The sensitivity of electrocardiography in diagnosing pulmonary hypertension is poor as well. Doppler echocardiography is the best method for the noninvasive diagnosis of pulmonary hypertension. However, right-sided heart catheterization remains the "gold standard" for diagnosing pulmonary hypertension.

The Ppa value is a good indicator of prognosis in patients with COPD. Five-year survival in a group of patients with initial Ppa less than 25 mm Hg was 66%, whereas in those with initial Ppa greater than 25 mm Hg, survival was only 36%.

The development of structural changes in the pulmonary arteries results in persistent pulmonary hypertension and RV hypertrophy/enlargement and dysfunction. Cor pulmonale is the major cardiovascular complication of COPD and is associated with a poor prognosis. Peripheral edema results from a combination of increased venous pressure and renal hormonal changes, leading to increased salt and water retention.

SYSTEMIC EFFECTS AND COMORBIDITIES

Although primarily a disease of the lungs, it is increasingly recognized that, as in many chronic diseases, COPD results in

important systemic features that may affect morbidity and mortality. Comorbid conditions are frequently observed in patients with COPD at all stages, and many patients have multiple comorbidities.

The prevalence of COPD morbidity varies among studies. In a cohort of 1522 patients with COPD, 50% had one or two comorbidities, 15.8% had three or four comorbidities, and 6% had five or more. Comorbidities not only are highly prevalent but also have important prognostic implications. In the Lung Health Study of patients with mild to moderate COPD, deaths from respiratory disease were relatively uncommon (7%); lung cancer was the most common cause of death (33%). Coronary artery disease (CAD) accounted for 10.5%, and cardiovascular disease (including CAD) accounted for 22% of deaths. In a large, pharmacologic intervention study, with cause of death assessed by independent review panel, 27% of deaths were related to COPD, 26% to cardiovascular disease, and 21% to lung cancer.

In a large cohort of COPD patients, the presence of diabetes, hypertension, or cardiovascular disease significantly increased the risk of hospitalization or mortality. Furthermore, combinations of multiple comorbid diseases in an individual resulted in an even higher risk of death. Systemic inflammation in patients with COPD is thought to contribute to these systemic effects and comorbidities.

SKELETAL MUSCLE DYSFUNCTION/WASTING AND WEIGHT LOSS

Peripheral muscle dysfunction is a prominent contributor to exercise limitation, increases health care utilization, and is an independent indicator of morbidity and mortality in COPD.

Weight loss is common in patients with COPD. A decreased body weight is reported in 49% of patients referred to a UK center for pulmonary rehabilitation. The prevalence of muscle wasting in COPD is probably underestimated, as extrapolated from body weight measurements, because fat-free mass (FFM) may be reduced despite preservation of body weight. Independent of body mass index (BMI) and disease severity, FFM index can predict mortality in COPD patients. The prevalence of FFM depletion was about 30% in patients with an FEV_1 of 30% to 70% of predicted and is associated with impaired peripheral muscle strength. Weight loss and loss of muscle mass result from the effects of systemic inflammation, an imbalance between muscle protein synthesis and breakdown, muscle apoptosis, and muscle disuse. Increased systemic inflammatory mediators (e.g., TNF-α, IL-6, O_2 free radicals) may mediate some systemic effects.

Osteoporosis is recognized as one of the systemic effects of COPD. In the TORCH study (Towards a Revolution in COPD Health), 18% of men and 30% of women had osteoporosis, and 42% of men and 41% of women had osteopenia, based on bone mineral density (BMD) assessments. The etiology of osteoporosis in COPD is complex. Several risk factors for osteoporosis are common features in COPD patients, including aging, limited physical activity, vitamin D deficiency, cigarette smoking, hypogonadism, and systemic corticosteroid use. A consequence of osteoporosis is that prevalence of vertebral fractures in COPD patients is 20% to 30%. This can result in increased kyphosis, compromising pulmonary function.

Osteoporosis is related to emphysema and to arterial wall stiffness. Moreover, the osteoprotegerin (OPG)/receptor activator of nuclear factor κB (RANK)/RANK ligand (RANKL) system has been identified as a possible mediator of arterial calcification, suggesting common links between osteoporosis and vascular diseases.

CARDIOVASCULAR DISEASE

Cardiovascular disease is one of the most important comorbidities related to COPD. A study that included 11,943 COPD patients reported a two-fold to four-fold increase in mortality risk from cardiovascular disease over a 3-year follow-up compared with an age-matched and gender-matched control group without COPD. In a cohort of patients with mild COPD in the Lung Health Study, cardiovascular complications accounted for 22% of all deaths during follow-up and for 42% of first hospitalizations. In this study, for every 10% increase in FEV_1, cardiovascular mortality increased by 28%, and nonfatal cardiovascular events increased by almost 20%, after adjustments for relevant confounders such as age, gender, smoking status, and treatment. There is strong epidemiologic evidence that reduced FEV_1 is a marker of cardiovascular mortality. A systematic review and meta-analysis included more than 80,000 patients identified and almost a twofold risk of cardiovascular mortality in patients with the lowest versus the highest lung function quintiles. COPD is an important risk factor for atherosclerosis, ischemic heart disease, cerebrovascular accident (stroke), and sudden cardiac death. Underlying mechanisms that contribute to the increased risk of atherosclerosis in COPD patients are not well understood and probably multifactorial, including low-grade systemic inflammation, endothelial dysfunction, and arterial stiffness.

ANEMIA

Although hypoxemia in COPD can be associated with secondary polycythemia, as a compensatory mechanism to improve oxygen transport to the tissues, polycythemia is present in only 6% of COPD patients, whereas anemia is present in 13% to 33%. The anemia in COPD is normochromic, normocytic, and is likely mediated by shortened red blood cell survival, decreased erythropoietin, and dysregulation of iron homeostasis. Anemia contributes to impaired oxygen transport to the tissues and exercise intolerance and has been associated with increased mortality in COPD patients.

DEPRESSION

Depression has been reported in 10% to 80% of patients with COPD, 2% to 5% higher than in the normal age-matched population. Depression is part of a vicious cycle involving poor health status, isolation, sedentary lifestyle, and worsening health status, resulting in the development of a *reactive* depression. Depression may also precede the development of COPD. Systemic inflammation may also contribute to development of depression.

LUNG CANCER

Lung cancer is three to four times more common in COPD patients than in the general population and constitutes an important mortality risk in COPD patients. Patients with COPD have a higher incidence of lung cancer independent of the history of cigarette smoking. COPD is associated with the risk of developing small cell and squamous cell carcinoma, although no relationship seems to exist between COPD and the risk of developing adenocarcinoma.

DIABETES

The prevalence of diabetes in COPD patients has ranged from 1% to 16% of patients in different studies. Smoking is also a risk factor, and quitting smoking reduces the risk of diabetes. A reduction in lung function has also been associated with diabetes. Inflammatory markers such as TNF-α, IL-6, and C-reactive protein (CRP) have been associated with diabetes, and these inflammatory markers are elevated in COPD and may mediate insulin resistance by blocking signaling through the insulin receptor. The metabolic syndrome also appears to be more common in COPD patients, reflecting concomitant diabetes and cardiovascular disease with airway obstruction.

GASTROESOPHAGEAL REFLUX

An increase in gastroesophageal reflux disease (GERD) has been identified in COPD patients, being more common in those patients with an FEV_1 less than 50% predicted. GERD also appears to be a precipitant of exacerbations of COPD.

CLINICAL FEATURES

SYMPTOMS

Patients with COPD characteristically complain of the symptoms of breathlessness on exertion, chest tightness, wheeze, chronic cough, and lower respiratory tract infections. The cough is often, but not invariably, productive. *Breathlessness* is the symptom that usually causes the patient to seek medical attention and is the most disabling symptom.

Patients often date the onset of their illness to an acute exacerbation of *cough* with sputum production, which leaves them with a degree of chronic breathlessness. Close questioning, however, usually reveals a cough with small amounts of mucoid sputum (usually <60 mL/day), often in the morning for many years. A productive cough occurs in up to 50% of cigarette smokers and may precede the onset of breathlessness. Many patients may dismiss this as simply "smoker's cough." The frequency of nocturnal cough does not appear to be increased in stable COPD. Paroxysms of coughing in the presence of severe airflow limitation generate high intrathoracic pressures, which can produce syncope and "cough fractures" of the ribs.

Breathlessness is usually first noticed on climbing hills or stairs, or hurrying on level ground, which later becomes progressive and persistent. It usually heralds at least moderate impairment of expiratory flow. Patients may adapt their breathing pattern and their behavior to minimize the sensation of breathlessness. The perception of breathlessness varies greatly among patients with the same impairment of ventilatory capacity. However, when the FEV_1 has fallen to 35% or less of the predicted value, breathlessness is usually present on minimal exertion. Severe breathlessness is often affected by changes in environmental temperature or occupational exposure to dust and fumes. Some patients have severe orthopnea, relieved by leaning forward, whereas others find greatest ease when lying flat. The impact of breathlessness can be assessed on the UK Medical Research Council (MRC) Dyspnea Scale (**Table 41-3**).

Wheeze (wheezing) is common but not specific to COPD because it results from turbulent airflow in large airways from any cause.

Chest tightness is also common in patients with COPD, resulting from the disease itself, underlying ischemic heart disease, or GERD. Chest tightness is a frequent complaint

Table 41-3 Modified MRC Dyspnea Scale for Assessing Breathlessness

Grade	Degree of Breathlessness Related to Activities
1	Not troubled by breathlessness, except on strenuous exercise.
2	Short of breath when hurrying or walking up a slight hill.
3	Walks slower than contemporaries on level ground because of breathlessness, or has to stop for "breather" when walking at own pace.
4	Stops for breath after walking about 100 m or after a few minutes on level ground.
5	Too breathless to leave the house, or breathless when dressing or undressing.

Data from UK Medical Research Council.

Table 41-4 Modified Borg Scale for Assessing Breathlessness

Scale	Severity Experienced by Patient
0	Nothing at all
0.5	Very, very slight (just noticeable)
1	Very slight
2	Slight (light)
3	Moderate
4	Somewhat severe
5	Severe (heavy)
6	Very severe Very, very severe (almost maximal) Maximal

during periods of worsening breathlessness, particularly during exercise and exacerbations, and this is sometimes difficult to distinguish from ischemic cardiac pain. Pleuritic chest pain may suggest concurrent pneumothorax, pneumonia, or pulmonary infarction. Hemoptysis can be associated with purulent sputum and may be caused by inflammation or infection. However, blood-tinged sputum should also suggest bronchial carcinoma.

OTHER ASPECTS OF THE HISTORY

As part of the assessment of patients with COPD, the following factors need to be determined from the history:

- Current medications
- History of other medical conditions
- Symptoms of anxiety and depression
- Sleep quality
- Frequency of exacerbations; number of courses of corticosteroids and antibiotics in preceding year
- Hospital admissions
- Occupational and environmental exposure to dust, chemicals, gases, and fumes
- Exposure to biomass fuel
- Previous respiratory problems (chronic asthma or tuberculosis)
- Number of days missed from work
- Social and family support
- Anorexia and weight loss
- Current smoking status and number of pack-years (1 pack-year is defined as 20 cigarettes [1 pack] smoked per day for 1 year)

Several conditions should be considered in the differential diagnosis in patients with COPD. Asthma can be particularly difficult; scales (e.g., the modified Borg scale) can be used to assess the degree of breathlessness (**Table 41-4**).

CLINICAL SIGNS

Patients with COPD typically present in the fifth decade of life. The physical examination may be completely negative early in the disease course. The physical signs are not specific and depend on the degree of airflow limitation and pulmonary overinflation. Because of the heterogeneity of COPD, patients may show a range of phenotypic clinical presentations. The

sensitivity of physical examination to detect or exclude moderately severe COPD is rather poor.

PATIENT ASSESSMENT

GENERAL EXAMINATION

The respiratory rate may be increased. A breathing pattern with a prolonged expiratory phase, with or without pursing of the lips, is characteristic of patients with COPD. A forced expiratory time greater than 5 seconds strongly suggests the presence of airflow limitation. Use of accessory muscles of respiration, particularly the sternocleidomastoids, is often seen in advanced disease, and these patients often adopt a posture in which they lean forward, supporting themselves with their arms to fix the shoulder girdle. This allows use of the pectoral muscles and the latissimus dorsi muscle to increase chest wall movement.

Tar-stained fingers indicate the smoking habit in many patients. In advanced disease, cyanosis may be present, indicating hypoxemia, but it may be masked by anemia or accentuated by polycythemia, and is a fairly subjective sign. The "flapping tremor" associated with hypercapnia is neither sensitive nor specific, and papilledema associated with severe hypercapnia is rare.

As described earlier, weight loss may also be apparent in advanced disease, as well as a reduction in muscle mass. The body mass index (BMI; weight/height^2) should be calculated. Finger clubbing is not a feature of COPD and should suggest the possibility of complicating bronchial neoplasm, pulmonary fibrosis, or bronchiectasis.

CHEST EXAMINATION

In the later stages of COPD, the chest is often barrel-shaped with a kyphosis, resulting in an increased anterior/posterior chest diameter, horizontal ribs, prominence of the sternal angle, and a wide subcostal angle. The distance between the suprasternal notch and the cricoid cartilage (normally 3 finger-breadths) may be reduced because of the elevation of the sternum. These are all signs of overinflation. An inspiratory tracheal tug may be detected, attributed to contraction of the low, flat diaphragm. The horizontal position of the diaphragm also acts to pull the lower ribs in during inspiration (Hoover sign). The xiphisternal angle widens, and abdominal protuberance results from forward displacement of the abdominal contents, giving the appearance of weight gain. Increased intra-thoracic pressure swings may result in indrawing of the supra-sternal and supraclavicular fossae and intercostal muscles.

Decreased hepatic and cardiac dullness on percussion indicates overinflation. A useful sign of gross overinflation is the absence of a dull percussion note, normally caused by the underlying heart, over the lower end of the sternum. Breath sounds may have a prolonged expiratory phase or may be uniformly diminished, particularly in the advanced stages of COPD. Wheezing may be present both on inspiration and expiration but is not an invariable sign. Crackles may be heard, particularly at the lung bases, but are usually scant and vary with coughing.

CARDIOVASCULAR EXAMINATION

Air trapping decreases venous return and compresses the heart. Accordingly, tachycardia is common in COPD patients. The presence of positive alveolar pressure at the end of exhalation (i.e., intrinsic positive end-expiratory pressure, or auto-PEEP) results in the need to create a more negative pleural pressure than usual, manifested by paradoxical pulse. Overinflation makes it difficult to localize the apex beat and reduces the cardiac dullness. The characteristic signs that indicate the presence or consequences of pulmonary hypertension may be detected in advanced cases. The heave of RV hypertrophy may be palpable at the lower left sternal edge or in the subxiphoid regions. Heart sounds are usually soft, although the pulmonary component of the second heart sound may be exaggerated in the second left intercostal space, indicating pulmonary hypertension. An RV gallop rhythm may be detected in the fourth intercostal space to the left of the sternum. The jugular venous pressure can be difficult to estimate in patients with COPD because it swings widely with respiration and is difficult to discern if there is prominent accessory muscle activity. There may be evidence of functional tricuspid incompetence, producing a pansystolic murmur at the left sternal edge. The liver may be tender and pulsatile, and a prominent v wave may be visible in the jugular venous pulse. The liver may also be palpable below the right costal margin as a result of overinflation of the lungs.

Peripheral vasodilation accompanies hypercapnia, producing warm peripheries with a high-volume pulse. Pitting peripheral edema may also be present as a result of fluid retention.

PHYSIOLOGIC ASSESSMENT

The degree of airflow limitation cannot be predicted from the symptoms and signs noted on clinical evaluation. Accordingly, the degree of airflow limitation should be assessed in every patient. At an early stage of the disease, conventional spirometry may reveal no abnormality. Results of tests of small airways function, such as the frequency dependency of compliance and closing volume, may be abnormal. However, these tests are difficult to perform, have high coefficient of variation (CV), and are valid only when lung elastic recoil is normal and there is no increase in airway resistance. These tests therefore are *not* recommended in normal clinical practice.

Spirometry

Spirometry is the best test of airflow limitation in patients with COPD. Spirometric measurements have a well-defined range of normal values. A postbronchodilator FEV_1/VC ratio less than 0.7 is a diagnostic criterion for COPD. The rate of decline of

the FEV_1 can be used to assess susceptibility in cigarette smokers and progression of disease.

It is important that a volume plateau is reached when performing the FEV_1 maneuver, which can take 15 seconds or more in patients with severe airway obstruction. If this maneuver is not carried out, the vital capacity (VC) can be underestimated. FEV_1 within ±20% of predicted value is considered in the normal range. Thus, an FEV_1 of 80% or more of the predicted value is normal. Under usual circumstances, 70% to 80% of the total volume of the air in the lungs (FVC) should be exhaled in the first second. When the FEV_1/FVC ratio falls below 0.7, airflow limitation is present. The reproducibility of the FEV_1 varies by less than 200 mL between maneuvers.

Spirometric measurements are evaluated by comparison of the results with appropriate reference values based on age, gender, height, and race. The presence of a postbronchodilator FEV_1/FVC ratio <0.7 confirms the presence of airflow limitation that is not fully reversible. However, in older adults, values of FEV_1/FVC between 0.65 and 0.7 may be normal. Thus, use of a fixed ratio of FEV_1/FVC <0.7 postbronchodilator leads to overdiagnosis of COPD in elderly patients. FEV_6 measures the volume of air that can be forcibly exhaled in 6 seconds. It approximates the FVC, although in healthy individuals the FEV_6 and FVC are identical. Use of FEV_6 instead of FVC may be helpful in patients with more severe airflow limitation. To avoid the effect of airway collapse in patients with COPD during forced expiration, the clinician should use a slow or relaxed VC measurement, which allows patients to exhale at their own pace. The slow VC is often 0.5 L greater than the FVC.

The FEV_1 as a percentage of the predicted value can be used to assess the severity of disease (**Table 41-5**). FEV_1 does not fully capture the impact of COPD on the patient's functional capabilities, however, and thus other measurements in addition to spirometry are required to assess the effect of COPD on functional ability. Breathlessness can be gauged by the MRC scale (see Table 41-3). Exercise capacity can be objectively measured by a reduction in self-paced walking distance (e.g., 6-minute walking distance [6MWD]), which is a strong predictor of health status impairment and prognosis. A combination of these variables to give a more detailed indication of disease severity has been proposed as the *BODE index*, a composite score of *b*ody mass index, airways *o*bstruction, *d*yspnea, and *e*xercise that appears to be a better predictor of subsequent survival than any of the individual components (**Table 41-6**).

Expiratory Flow

Expiratory flows measured at 75% or 50% of VC have also been used to identify patients with COPD. These measurements

Table 41-5	Spirometric Classification of COPD Severity
Stage	**Characteristics**
I: Mild	FEV_1/FVC <0.7 FEV_1 ≥80% predicted
II: Moderate	FEV_1/FVC <0.7 50% ≤ FEV_1 <80% predicted
III: Severe	FEV_1/FVC <0.7 30% ≤ FEV_1 <50% predicted
IV: Very severe	FEV_1/FVC <0.7 FEV_1 <30% predicted or FEV_1 <50% predicted plus chronic respiratory failure

Table 41-6 Variables and Point Values in Computation of BODE* Index

Variable	Points on BODE Index			
	0	1	2	3
FEV$_1$ (% of predicted)	≥65	50-64	36-49	≤35
Distance walked in 6 minutes (m)	≥350	250-349	150-249	≤149
MMRC dyspnea scale†	0-1	2	3	4
Body mass index	>21	≤21	—	—

*Body mass index, degree of airflow obstruction and dyspnea, and exercise capacity.
†See Table 41-3.

are less reproducible than the FEV$_1$, such that an abnormal value must fall below 50% of predicted value. Flows at lung volume less than 50% of VC were previously considered to be an indicator of small airways function, but probably provide no more clinically useful information than measurements of the FEV$_1$.

Peak expiratory flow can either be read directly from the flow-volume loop or measured with a handheld peak flowmeter. Flowmeters are relatively easy to use and are particularly useful in subjects with asthma, who have variations in serial measurements. In patients with COPD, however, many of the variations are often within the error of the measurement. The peak expiratory flow may underestimate the degree of airflow limitation in COPD and is thus not used as a routine assessment.

Reversibility Testing

Assessment of reversibility to bronchodilators was performed in COPD patients (1) to help distinguish patients with marked reversibility who have underlying asthma and (2) to establish the postbronchodilator FEV$_1$, which is the best predictor of long-term prognosis.

There is no agreement on a standardized method of assessing reversibility, but this is usually quantified on the basis of a change in the FEV$_1$ or peak expiratory flow. However, there may be changes in other lung volumes after bronchodilators (e.g., inspiratory capacity, residual volume) which may explain why some symptoms improve in some patients after a bronchodilator without a change in spirometry. An improvement in FEV$_1$ in response to a bronchodilator is not a good predictor of a symptomatic response.

Bronchodilator reversibility can vary from day to day, depending on the degree of bronchomotor tone. A change in FEV$_1$ that exceeds 200 mL is considered greater than random variation. Therefore, changes should be reported as significant only if they exceed 200 mL. In addition to this absolute change of 200 mL in FEV$_1$, a percentage change of 12% over baseline has been suggested as significant by the ERS/ATS and GOLD guidelines.

Approximately 30% of patients with COPD show significant reversibility of their airflow limitation in response to a bronchodilator. It is usually recommended that reversibility be assessed using a large bronchodilator dose, either with repeated doses from a metered dose inhaler or by nebulization, because this results in more patients with a significant response. In some cases, addition of a second drug, such as an anticholinergic agent to a β$_2$-agonist, further increases FEV$_1$. Reversibility

testing with a bronchodilator is usually indicated only at diagnosis. Although not a requirement for the diagnosis of COPD, postbronchodilator spirometry is recommended to assess for chronic airflow limitation (see earlier discussion). A formal assessment of steroid reversibility is not included in the most recent guidelines for assessment and management of COPD. The most common method is to measure FEV$_1$ before and after treatment with 30 mg of prednisolone for 2 weeks. Although patients with previous response to nebulized bronchodilators are more likely to respond to steroids, individual patient responses cannot be predicted.

Lung Volumes

Static lung volumes such as TLC, residual volume (RV) and FRC, and the ratio RV/TLC are measured in patients with COPD, to assess the degree of overinflation and gas trapping, and are usually increased. These measurements are not necessary in every patient. The standard method of measuring static lung volumes, using the helium dilution technique during rebreathing, may underestimate lung volumes in COPD, particularly in patients with bullous disease, because the inspired helium may not have sufficient time to equilibrate properly in the enlarged air spaces. Body plethysmography uses Boyle's law to calculate lung volumes from changes in mouth and plethysmographic pressures. This technique measures trapped air in the thorax, including poorly ventilated areas, and therefore gives higher readings than the helium dilution technique.

Gas Transfer for Carbon Monoxide

A low DLCO is present in many patients with COPD. Although there is a relationship between the DLCO and the extent of microscopic emphysema, the severity of the emphysema in an individual patient cannot be predicted from the DLCO, and a low DLCO is not specific for emphysema. The usual method is the *single-breath technique*, which uses alveolar volume calculated from the helium dilution during a single-breath test. This method underestimates alveolar volume in patients with severe COPD, however, producing a lower value for the DLCO. This test can be useful to distinguish patients with COPD from those with asthma because a low DLCO excludes asthma.

Arterial Blood Gases

Arterial blood gases (ABGs) are needed to confirm the degree of hypoxemia and hypercapnia that develops in patients with COPD. Hypoxemia and hypercapnia are not usually observed until the FEV$_1$ falls below 50% of predicted. It is essential to record the fraction of inspired oxygen concentration (FIO$_2$) when reporting ABGs. It may take at least 30 minutes for a change in FIO$_2$ to have its full effect on the arterial oxygen partial pressure (PaO$_2$), because of long time constants for alveolar gas equilibration in COPD, particularly during exacerbations. Pulse oximetry is increasingly used to measure the level of oxygenation, but it should not replace ABG assessment in patients with FEV$_1$ below 50% predicted, because measurements of PaCO$_2$ are often required. ABG abnormalities may worsen during exercise and sleep and during exacerbations.

Exercise Tests

Although exercise testing is rarely needed to diagnose COPD, useful functional information may be obtained from doing any of three types of tests.

Progressive symptom-limited exercise tests require the patient to maintain exercise on a treadmill or a cycle until symptoms prevent the person from continuing, while the workload is continuously increased. A maximum test is usually defined as a heart rate greater than 85% of predicted or ventilation greater than 90% predicted. The results are particularly useful when simultaneous electrocardiography and blood pressure monitoring are performed, to assess whether coexisting cardiac or psychological factors contribute to exercise limitation.

Self-paced exercise tests are simple to perform and give information on sustained exercise that may be more relevant to activities of daily living. The 6MWD has approximately 8% CV. A learning effect, however, may influence the result of repeated tests. The 6MWD test is useful only in patients with moderately severe COPD (FEV_1, <1.5 L) who would be expected to have an exercise tolerance of less than 600 m in 6 minutes. There is a weak relationship between 6MWD and FEV_1, although walking distance is a predictor of survival in COPD patients. An alternative test is the *shuttle walking test*, in which the patient performs a paced walk between two points 10 m apart (the shuttle). The pace of the walk is increased at regular intervals, as dictated by bleeps on a tape recording, until the patient is forced to stop because of breathlessness. The number of completed shuttles is recorded.

Steady-state exercise tests involve exercise at a sustainable percentage of maximum capacity for 3 to 6 minutes, during which ABGs are measured, enabling calculation of dead space/tidal volume ratio (V_D/V_T) and shunt. This assessment is seldom required in patients with COPD.

OTHER TESTS

Lung pressure-volume curves are difficult to measure, requiring assessment of esophageal pressure with an esophageal balloon, and are not part of the routine assessment of patients with COPD. These tests may be necessary in special circumstances.

Measurements of small airways function with nitrogen washout test, helium flow-volume loops, or frequency dependence of compliance have poor reproducibility in patients with COPD. Although these tests can differentiate smokers from nonsmokers, they are not useful for predicting in which smokers COPD will develop, and thus are not used in routine practice.

Respiratory Muscle Function Test

The usual tests of respiratory muscle function in COPD are maximum inspiratory and expiratory mouth pressures. These tests can be useful in cases where breathlessness or hypercapnia is not fully explained by other lung function testing or when peripheral muscle weakness is suspected (see Chapter 42).

Sleep Studies

Selected patients should be assessed for the presence of nocturnal hypoxemia. Finding nocturnal hypoxemia, however, provides no further prognostic or clinically useful information in the assessment of patients with COPD, unless coexisting sleep apnea syndrome is suspected.

HEALTH STATUS

Health-related or health status quality of life is a measure of the impact of the disease on daily life and well-being. Breathlessness in patients with COPD limits exercise, reduces expectation, diminishes daily activity, restricts social activities, disturbs mood, and impairs well-being. Several questionnaires are available to assess health status and are used in hospital rehabilitation programs and research. The Chronic Respiratory Disease Index Questionnaire is sensitive to change but is time-consuming and requires training to administer properly. The Breathing Problems Questionnaire is a self-completed test that is easy to complete but relatively insensitive to change.

The *St. George's Respiratory Questionnaire* is a self-completed test with three components—*symptoms* (distress caused by respiratory symptoms), *activity* (disturbance in daily activities), and *impact* (psychosocial function)—summed to give a total score of overall health status. This is the most validated health status tool in COPD. However, a rather poor relationship exists between the St. George's Respiratory Questionnaire and the FEV_1. It is clear from various studies that there can be improvement in health status without any improvement in FEV_1 in response to treatment. An example of this is the response to pulmonary rehabilitation. The threshold of clinical improvement is a change of four units in the St. George's Respiratory Questionnaire. Exacerbations of COPD have a clear detrimental effect on health status.

More recently, the *COPD Assessment Test* (CAT) has been shown to correlate well with the more detailed St. George's Respiratory Questionnaire. The CAT may be useful clinically in assessing functional status, health status, and response to treatment.

OTHER MEASUREMENTS

Erythrocythemia or polycythemia is important to identify in patients with COPD because it predisposes to peripheral vascular, cardiovascular, and cerebrovascular events. *Erythrocythemia* does not develop until there is clinically important hypoxemia (PaO_2 <55 mm Hg) and is not inevitable even at this level. *Polycythemia* should be suspected when the hematocrit is greater than 47% in women and 52% in men, and/or the hemoglobin is greater than 16 g/dL in women or 18 g/dL in men, provided other causes of spurious polycythemia from decreased plasma volume (dehydration, diuretics) can be excluded. A complete blood count may reveal the anemia of chronic disease that occurs in COPD.

Alpha$_1$-antitrypsin deficiency screening with measurements of the level and determination of allelic phenotype are indicated for patients (<45 years old) with early onset of emphysema and in those with a family history of premature emphysema. Because of the potential importance for other family members, some experts recommend that all patients with COPD be screened.

Electrocardiography is not routinely required in the assessment of patients with COPD, except when coexisting cardiac morbidity is suspected. It is an insensitive technique for the diagnosis of cor pulmonale.

Overinflation of the chest increases the retrosternal air space, which transmits sound waves poorly, making echocardiography difficult in patients with COPD. Thus, an adequate examination can be achieved in only 65% to 85% of patients with COPD. Two-dimensional echocardiography has been used in the investigation of right ventricular dimensions. Pulsed-wave Doppler echocardiography is used to assess ejection flow dynamics of the right ventricle in patients with pulmonary hypertension. The tricuspid gradient can be used to calculate the right ventricular systolic pressure. The technique estimates the pressure gradient across the tricuspid regurgitant jet recorded by Doppler ultrasound. The maximum velocity of the regurgitant jet is measured from the continuous-wave Doppler recordings, and the simplified Bernoulli equation is used to calculate the maximum pressure gradient between the right ventricle and the right atrium, $P_{RV} - P_{RA} = 4v^2$, where P_{RV} and P_{RA} are the right ventricular and right atrial pressures and v is the maximum velocity. The right atrial pressure is estimated from clinical examination of the jugular venous pressure.

IMAGING

Plain Chest Radiography

All patients with suspected COPD should have a posteroanterior (PA) chest radiograph performed at diagnosis. COPD does not produce any specific features on plain chest radiography unless features of emphysema are present. There may be no abnormalities, however, even in patients with severe disability. A chest x-ray film is used to discount other causes of respiratory symptoms and to identify complications with COPD, such as bulla formation. The most reliable radiographic signs of emphysema can be divided into those caused by overinflation, by vascular changes, and by bullae (see Computed Tomography). The following radiologic features are indicative of *overinflation:*

- Low, flattened diaphragm; the border of the diaphragm in the midclavicular line on the PA film is at or below the anterior end of the seventh rib, and it is flattened if the perpendicular height from a line drawn between the costal and cardiophrenic angles to the border of the diaphragm is less than 1.5 cm.
- Increased retrosternal air space, visible on the lateral film at a point 3 cm below the manubrium; it is present when the horizontal distance from the posterior surface of the aorta to the sternum exceeds 4.5 cm.
- Obtuse costophrenic angle on the PA or lateral chest radiograph.
- Inferior margin of the retrosternal air space 3 cm or less from the anterior aspect of the diaphragm.

The *vascular changes* associated with emphysema result from loss of alveolar walls and are shown on the plain chest radiograph by the following:

- Reduction in the number and size of pulmonary vessels, particularly at the lung periphery
- Vessel distortion, producing increased branching angles and excess straightening or bowing of vessels
- Areas of increased lucency

Critical to the assessment of vascular loss in emphysema is the quality of the chest radiograph, because increased transradiancy (translucency) may be only an overexposure. The accuracy of diagnosing emphysema on plain chest radiography increases with severity of the disease, reported at 50% to 80% in patients with moderate to severe disease. However, the sensitivity is as low as 24% in patients with mild to moderate COPD.

Computed Tomography

Computed tomography (CT) has been used to detect and quantify emphysema. Techniques can be divided into (1) those that provide a visual assessment of low-density areas on the CT scan, which can be semiquantitative or quantitative, and (2) those that use CT lung density to quantify areas of low x-ray attenuation. These techniques are used to measure macroscopic and microscopic emphysema, respectively. A visual assessment of emphysema on CT scanning shows the following:

- Areas of low attenuation without obvious margins or walls
- Attenuation and pruning of the vascular tree
- Abnormal vascular configurations

Areas of low attenuation correlate best with areas of macroscopic emphysema. Visual inspection of the CT scan can be used to locate macroscopic emphysema, although assessing the extent is insensitive and subject to high intraobserver and interobserver variability. The CT scan can be used to assess different types of emphysema; centrilobular emphysema produces patchy areas of low attenuation prominent in the upper zones, whereas those of panlobular emphysema are diffuse throughout the lung zones (see Figure 41-3).

A more quantitative approach to assessing macroscopic emphysema is by highlighting picture elements (pixels) in the lung fields in a predetermined low-density range, between -910 and -1000 Hounsfield units, the "density mask" technique. Although the choice of the density range is arbitrary, there is good correlation between pathologic emphysema score and the CT density score. This technique may still miss areas of mild emphysema.

Microscopic emphysema can be quantified by measuring CT lung density. CT density is measured on a linear scale in Hounsfield units (water $= 0$ H; air $= -1000$ H). CT lung density is a direct measure of physical density, and thus, as emphysema develops, a decrease in alveolar surface area occurs as alveolar walls are lost, associated with an increase in distal air space size, which would decrease lung CT density. A standardized protocol on either an inspiratory or an expiratory CT scan of the chest is required to measure lung density accurately.

A *bulla* is defined arbitrarily as an emphysematous space greater than 1 cm in diameter. On the plain chest radiograph, a bulla appears as a localized avascular area of increased lucency, usually separated from the rest of the lung by a thin, curvilinear wall. Marked compression of the surrounding lung may be seen, and bullae may also depress the diaphragm. CT is much more sensitive than plain radiography in detecting bullae and can be used to determine the number, size, and position. CT can quantify the extent and distribution of emphysema as part of surgical assessment in bullous disease and for lung volume reduction.

SUGGESTED READINGS

Agusti A: Systemic effects of chronic obstructive pulmonary disease: what we know and what we don't know (but should), *Proc Am Thorac Soc* 4:522–525, 2007.

Calverley PMA, MacNee W, Pride NB, Rennard SI, editors: *Chronic obstructive pulmonary disease*, ed 2, London, 2003, Chapman & Hall.

Celli BR, MacNee W: Standards for the diagnosis and treatment of patients with COPD, *Eur Respir J* 23:841–845, 2004.

Cosio MG, Saetta M, Agusti A: Immunologic aspects of chronic obstructive pulmonary disease, *N Engl J Med* 360:2445–2454, 2009.

Global Initiative for Chronic Obstructive Pulmonary Disease Workshop Report: Medical Communications Resources. www.goldcopd.com, 2008.

Hogg JC, Senior RM: Chronic obstructive pulmonary disease. II. Pathology and biochemistry of emphysema, *Thorax* 57:830–834, 2002.

Hogg JC, Timens W: The pathology of chronic obstructive pulmonary disease, *Ann Rev Pathol* 4:435–459, 2009.

Hogg JC, Chu F, Utokaparch S, et al: The nature of small-airway obstruction in chronic obstructive pulmonary disease, *N Engl J Med* 350:2645–2653, 2004.

MacNee W: Pathogenesis of chronic obstructive pulmonary disease, *Proc Am Thorac Soc* 2:258–266, 2005.

MacNee W, Tuder R: New paradigms in the pathogenesis of chronic obstructive pulmonary disease. 1, *Proc Am Thorac Soc* 6:527–531, 2009.

MacNee W, Maclay J, McAllister D: Cardiovascular injury and repair in chronic obstructive pulmonary disease, *Proc Am Thorac Soc* 5:824–833, 2008.

Management of chronic obstructive pulmonary disease, *Eur Respir Monogr* www.ersnet.org, 38:2006.

Mannino DM, Watt G, Hole D, et al: The natural history of chronic obstructive pulmonary disease, *Eur Resp J* 27:627–643, 2006.

Peinado VI, Pizarro S, Barbera JA: Pulmonary vascular involvement in COPD, *Chest* 134:808–814, 2008.

Rabinovich RA, MacNee W: Chronic obstructive pulmonary disease and its comorbidities, *Br J Hosp Med* 72:137–145, 2011.

Vestbo J, Hogg JC: Convergence of the epidemiology and pathology of COPD, *Thorax* 61:86–88, 2006.

Voelkel NF, MacNee W, editors: *Chronic obstructive lung disease*, ed 2, Hamilton, Ontario, 2008, BC Decker.

Wouters EF: Local and systemic inflammation in chronic obstructive pulmonary disease, *Proc Am Thorac Soc* 2:26–33, 2005.

Chapter **42**

Treatment of the Stable Patient with Chronic Obstructive Pulmonary Disease

Bartolome R. Celli

The airflow obstruction of chronic obstructive pulmonary disease (COPD), as defined by the forced expiratory volume in 1 second (FEV_1), is thought to be only partially irreversible. This physiologic fact has been perpetuated over the years and has generated an unjustified negativist therapeutic attitude in many health care providers. The evidence suggests that the airflow obstruction of COPD *does* reverse with therapy, and that therapies aimed at the extrapulmonary manifestations of the disease *do* improve patient outcomes. An optimistic attitude toward these patients helps relieve fears and misconceptions. In contrast to many other diseases, some forms of intervention in COPD improve survival, such as smoking cessation, long-term oxygen therapy in hypoxemic patients, lung volume reduction surgery in certain patients with inhomogeneous upper lobe emphysema, and even pharmacologic therapy. Other interventions, such as pulmonary rehabilitation, lung transplantation, and bronchodilator therapy, improve symptoms and the quality of a patient's life once the diagnosis of COPD has been established.

Box 42-1 summarizes the available therapeutic options for patients with COPD. This chapter reviews medical management of COPD that centers on three goals: (1) prevent deterioration in lung function, (2) alleviate symptoms, and (3) treat complications as they arise. Once diagnosed, patients with COPD should be encouraged to participate actively in their management; collaborative management improves their self-reliance and self-esteem. All patients should be encouraged to lead a healthy life and exercise regularly. Preventive care is extremely important, and all patients should receive immunizations, including pneumococcal vaccine every 5 years and yearly influenza vaccine. **Figure 42-1** provides an algorithm detailing this comprehensive approach.

MULTICOMPONENT DISEASE

Increasing evidence shows that independent of the degree of airflow limitation, the lung volumes are important in the development of symptoms in patients with more advanced COPD. Studies have demonstrated that dyspnea perceived during exercise, including walking, more closely relates to development of dynamic hyperinflation than to changes in FEV_1. Further, the improvement in exercise brought about by several therapies, including bronchodilators, oxygen, lung reduction surgery, and even rehabilitation, is more closely related to delaying dynamic hyperinflations than by changing the degree of airflow obstruction. *Hyperinflation*, expressed as the ratio of inspiratory capacity to total lung capacity, was shown to predict survival better

than the FEV_1. This not only provides new insights into pathogenesis, but also opens the door for novel ways to alter lung volumes and perhaps impact COPD progression.

The association between COPD and important systemic manifestations in patients with more advanced disease is now accepted. Because of a persistent systemic inflammatory state or other, yet-unproven mechanisms (e.g., imbalanced oxidative stress, abnormal immunologic or reparative response), many patients with COPD may have decreased fat-free mass (FFM), impaired systemic muscle function, anemia, osteoporosis, depression, pulmonary hypertension, and cor pulmonale, all of which are important determinants of outcome. Indeed, dyspnea measured with a simple tool such as the UK Modified Medical Research Council (MMRC) scale, the body mass index (BMI; kg/m^2), and the 6-minute walking distance (6MWD) are all better predictors of mortality than the FEV_1. The incorporation of these variables into the multidimensional *BODE index* (BMI, airflow obstruction, dyspnea, exercise capacity) predicts survival even better. The BODE index is also responsive to exacerbations and, more importantly, acts as a surrogate marker of future outcome after interventions, thus providing clinicians with a useful tool to help determine the comprehensive severity of the disease. Other multidimensional indices (e.g., age, dyspnea, and obstruction [ADO]; dyspnea, obstruction, smoking, and exacerbation [DOSE]), have also shown important outcome predictive capacity and could be used to test novel forms of therapy.

Based on the multidimensional nature of COPD and the availability of multiple effective therapies, the approach shown in Figure 42-1 may more accurately help clinicians evaluate patients and choose therapies than the current approach, using primarily the FEV_1 percentage from reference values.

TREATABLE DISEASE

Current evidence suggests that besides smoking cessation, long-term oxygen therapy in hypoxemic patients, mechanical ventilation in acute respiratory failure, and lung volume reduction surgery for patients with upper lobe emphysema and poor exercise capacity improve survival. The TORCH study (Towards a Revolution in COPD Health) in more than 6000 patients showed not only that the combination of salmeterol and fluticasone improved lung function and health status, but also that the relative mortality risk over the 3 years of the study decreased by 17.5%. This is not exclusive of this drug combination; the Understanding Potential Long-Term Impacts on Function with Tiotropium (UPLIFT) study also observed a decrease in mortality risk over 4 years in patients taking tiotropium, a long-acting

Figure 42-1 Algorithm describing the comprehensive management of patients with chronic obstructive pulmonary disease. *FEV₁*, forced expiratory volume in 1 second; *FVC*, forced vital capacity; *BODE*, body mass index, degree of airflow obstruction and dyspnea, and exercise capacity; *BMI*, body mass index; *MMRC*, Modified Medical Research Council Scale; *6MWD*, 6-minute walking distance.

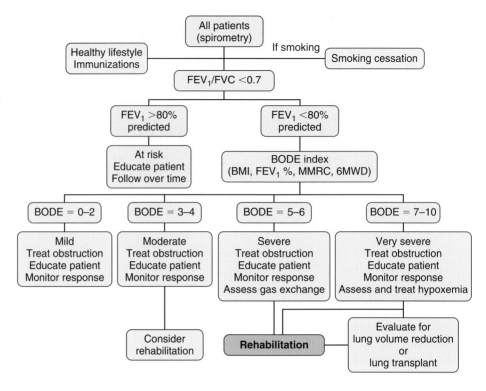

Box 42-1 Therapy of Patients with Symptomatic Stable Chronic Obstructive Pulmonary Disease

Improve Survival
Smoking cessation
Lung volume reduction (select patients)
Noninvasive ventilation (acute or chronic hypercapnic ventilatory failure)

May Improve Survival
Pharmacotherapy
    Salmeterol and fluticasone
    Tiotropium
Pulmonary rehabilitation

Improve Patient-Centered Outcomes
Pharmacotherapy
    Short-acting bronchodilators
    Long-acting antimuscarinics
    Long-acting beta-agonists
    Inhaled corticosteroids
    Theophylline
    Alpha₁-antitrypsin (select patients)
    Antibiotics (select patients)
Oxygen therapy
Surgery
Lung volume reduction
Lung transplantation
Pulmonary rehabilitation

anticholinergic. Other therapies, such as pulmonary rehabilitation and lung transplantation, improve symptoms and quality of life (QOL) once the diagnosis has been established.

RESPIRATORY MANIFESTATIONS

Once diagnosed, the patient with COPD should be encouraged to participate in disease management, confident that if not cured, COPD can certainly be treated.

SMOKING CESSATION AND SMOKE POLLUTANTS

Smoking is the major cause of COPD, and thus smoking cessation is the most important component of therapy for patients who still smoke. Because secondhand smoke is known to damage lung function, limitation of exposure to involuntary smoke, particularly in children, should be encouraged.

Many factors cause patients to smoke, including the addictive nature of nicotine, conditional responses to stimuli surrounding smoking, psychosocial problems such as depression, poor education and low income, and forceful advertising campaigns. Therefore, smoking cessation programs should also involve multiple interventions. The clinician should always participate in the treatment of smoking addiction, because a physician's advice and the appropriate medications (nicotine patch, gum, or inhalers; bupropion; varenicline) help obtain successful results.

Decreased Exposure to Biomass Fuel

The significant burden of COPD in patients exposed to biomass fuel in certain areas of the world should improve by changing to more efficient and less polluting sources of energy.

PHARMACOLOGIC THERAPY OF AIRFLOW OBSTRUCTION

Most patients with COPD require pharmacologic therapy. This should be organized according to the severity of symptoms, the degree of lung dysfunction, and the tolerance of the patient to specific drugs. A stepwise approach similar to that developed for systemic hypertension may be helpful, because medications alleviate symptoms, improve exercise tolerance and QOL, and may decrease mortality. **Tables 42-1** and **42-2** summarize the evidence supporting the effect of individual and combined therapies on outcomes of importance in patients with COPD. Because most patients with COPD are elderly, care must be taken when prescribing drugs for this population. Comorbidities are frequently present in patients with COPD,

Table 42-1 Effect of Single Pharmacologic Agents on Important Outcomes in Chronic Obstructive Pulmonary Disease Patients

Drug	FEV₁	Lung Volume	Dyspnea	QOL	AE	Exercise Endurance	Disease Modifier by FEV₁	Mortality	Side Effects
Albuterol	Yes (A)*	Yes (B)	Yes (B)	NA	NA	Yes (B)	NA	NA	Some
Ipratropium bromide	Yes (A)	Yes (B)	Yes (B)	No (B)	Yes (B)	Yes (B)	No	NA	Minimal
Long-acting β₂-agonists	Yes (A)	Yes (A)	Yes (A)	Yes (A)	Yes (A)	Yes (B)	Maybe	NA	Minimal
Tiotropium	Yes (A)	Yes (A)	Yes (A)	Yes (A)	Yes (A)	Yes (A)	Maybe	NA	Minimal
Inhaled corticosteroids	Yes (A)	NA	Yes (B)	Yes (A)	Yes (A)	NA	Maybe	No	Some
Theophylline	Some (A)	Yes (B)	Yes (A)	Yes (B)	NA	Yes (B)	NA	NA	Important
PDE4 inhibitors	Yes (A)	NA	NA	Yes (B)	Yes (A)	NA	Maybe	NA	Some

AE, adverse events; *FEV₁*, forced expiratory volume in 1 second; *NA*, not applicable; *PDE4*, phosphodiesterase E4; *QOL*, quality of life.
*(A) indicates solid evidence backing the conclusion; (B) indicates moderate evidence supporting the conclusion.

Table 42-2 Effect of Combined Pharmacologic Agents on Important Outcomes in Chronic Obstructive Pulmonary Disease Patients

Drugs	FEV₁	Lung Volume	Dyspnea	QOL	AE	Exercise Endurance	Disease Modifier by FEV₁	Mortality	Side Effects
Salmeterol + theophylline	Yes (B)*	NA	Yes (B)	Yes (B)	NA	NA	NA	NA	Some
Formoterol + tiotropium	Yes (A)	Yes (B)	Yes (B)	Yes (B)	Yes (B)	NA	NA	NA	Minimal
Salmeterol + fluticasone	Yes (A)	Yes (B)	Yes (A)	Yes (A)	Yes (A)	Yes (B)	Yes	Some	Some
Formoterol + budesonide	Yes (A)	Yes (B)	Yes (A)	Yes (A)	Yes (A)	NA	Maybe	NA	Minimal
Tiotropium + salmeterol + fluticasone	Yes (A)	NA	Yes (B)	Yes (B)	Yes (A)	NA	NA	NA	Some

AE, adverse events; *FEV₁*, forced expiratory volume in 1 second; *NA*, not applicable; *QOL*, quality of life.
*(A) indicates solid evidence backing the conclusion; (B) indicates moderate evidence supporting the conclusion.

mandating caution to ensure that therapy takes these into account.

Bronchodilators

Several important concepts guide the use of bronchodilators. In some patients, changes in FEV_1 may be small, and the symptomatic benefit may result from other mechanisms, such as a decrease in hyperinflation of the lung. Some older COPD patients cannot effectively activate metered dose inhalers (MDIs), and clinicians should work with the patient to achieve mastery of the MDI. If this is not possible, use of a spacer or nebulizer to facilitate inhalation of the medication will help achieve the desired results. Mucosal deposition in the mouth will result in local side effects (e.g., thrush with inhaled steroids) or general absorption and its consequences (e.g., tremor after β₂-agonists). The inhaled route is preferred over oral administration, and long-acting bronchodilators are more effective than short-acting agents. The currently available bronchodilators are described next.

Beta₂-Agonists

The β₂-adrenoceptor agonists increase cyclic adenosine monophosphate (cAMP) within many cells and promote airway smooth muscle relaxation. Other nonbronchodilator effects have been observed, but their significance is uncertain. In the minority of COPD patients with mild intermittent symptoms, it is reasonable to initiate drug therapy with an MDI of a short-acting β₂-agonist as needed for relief of symptoms. Patients with persistent symptoms should receive long-acting

β₂-agonists twice daily or once daily if the new ultra-long-acting agents are available. These prevent nocturnal bronchospasm, increase exercise endurance, and improve QOL. The safety profile of salmeterol in the TORCH trial and *formoterol fumarate* in the SUN and SHINE studies, as well as that of the longer-acting *indacaterol*, is reassuring to clinicians, who frequently prescribe selective long-acting β₂-agonists for their patients with COPD.

Anticholinergics

Anticholinergic drugs act by blocking muscarinic receptors known to be functional in COPD. The appropriate dosage of the short-acting *ipratropium bromide* is 2 to 4 puffs three or four times daily, but some patients require and tolerate larger doses. The therapeutic effect is a decrease in exercise-induced increased lung inflation or dynamic hyperinflation. The long-acting *tiotropium* (Spiriva) is effective in inducing prolonged bronchodilation and decreasing lung volume in patients with COPD. In addition, tiotropium improves dyspnea, decreases exacerbations, and improves health-related QOL compared with placebo and even ipratroprium. The results of the large UPLIFT trial confirmed the effectiveness of tiotropium as a disease-modifying agent in that it improved QOL, decreased exacerbation rate, and provided more bronchial dilation when used with regular treatment. These results place tiotropium as a good first-line agent for COPD patients with persistent symptoms. Other new long-acting anticholinergic agents, such as aclidinium bromide and glycopyrrolate, are being developed and will become available to clinicians worldwide.

Phosphodiesterase Inhibitors

Theophylline is a nonspecific phosphodiesterase inhibitor that increases intracellular cAMP within airway smooth muscle. The bronchodilator effects of these drugs are best seen at high doses, which also carry a higher risk of toxicity. Theophylline's potential for toxicity has led to a decline in its popularity. Theophylline is of particular value for less compliant or less capable patients who cannot use aerosol therapy optimally. The previously recommended therapeutic serum levels of 15 to 20 mg/dL are too close to the toxic range and are frequently associated with side effects. Therefore, a lower target range of 8 to 13 mg/dL is safer and still therapeutic in nature. Some research suggests that theophylline could help reestablish the corticosteroid sensitivity that appears to be absent in patients with COPD.

The specific phosphodiesterase E4 (PDE4) inhibitor *roflumilast* has antiinflammatory and bronchodilator effects, with minimal gastrointestinal irritation. Roflumilast has proved useful in decreasing exacerbations in COPD patients with cough and sputum production.

Other Antiinflammatory Therapy

In contrast to their value in asthma management, antiinflammatory drugs have not been documented to have a significant role in the routine treatment of patients with stable COPD. Cromolyn and nedocromil have not been established as useful agents, although they could possibly be helpful if the patient has associated respiratory tract allergy. One study using monoclonal antibodies against interleukin-8 (IL-8) and tumor necrosis factor alpha (TNF-α) failed to detect a response. However, patients were selected according to the degree of airflow obstruction, not the presence or level of the specific targeted molecule. The groups of leukotriene inhibitors useful in asthma have not been adequately tested in COPD, so a conclusion about their potential use cannot be drawn.

Corticosteroids

Glucocorticoids act at multiple points within the inflammatory cascade, although their effects in COPD appear to be more modest compared with bronchial asthma. In outpatients, COPD exacerbations necessitate a course of oral steroids, as discussed later, but it is important to wean patients quickly; older COPD patients are susceptible to complications such as skin damage, cataracts, diabetes, osteoporosis, and secondary infections. These risks do not accompany standard doses of inhaled corticosteroid aerosols, which may cause thrush but pose a negligible risk for other outcomes, such as cataract and osteoporosis.

Several large multicenter trials evaluated the role of inhaled corticosteroids (ICS) in preventing or slowing the progressive course of symptomatic COPD. The results of these earlier studies showed minimal, if any, benefits in the rate of decline of lung function. On the other hand, in the one study that evaluated it, inhaled fluticasone decreased exacerbations and the rate of loss of health-related QOL. Recent retrospective analysis of large databases suggesting a possible effect of ICS on improving survival was not confirmed in the TORCH trial, in which the ICS-only arm did not show improved survival compared with placebo, whereas the combination arm was significantly more effective than ICS alone. In TORCH the combination was superior in terms of all outcomes evaluated. Along with the more frequent development of pneumonia in the patients receiving ICS, this suggests that ICS should not be prescribed alone but rather with a long-acting β2-agonist (LABA).

Combination Therapy

All the studies on combinations of agents show significant improvements over single agents alone, and clinicians should now consider combination therapy as first-line therapy. Initially, the combination of inhaled ipatroprium and albuterol proved effective in the management of COPD. More recently, the combination of tiotropium and formoterol, even when administered once daily, was almost as effective as tiotropium once daily added to the recommended twice-daily dose of formoterol. Similarly, the combination of theophylline and salmeterol was significantly more effective than either agent alone.

The TORCH study showed better effects of the salmeterol-fluticasone combination on survival, FEV$_1$, exacerbation rate, and QOL than placebo and the individual components alone, confirming earlier studies evaluating the combination of beta agonists and corticosteroids. Recent trials compared tiotropium plus placebo with tiotropium plus salmeterol and with tiotropium plus the combination of salmeterol and fluticasone in a large patient group. The number of hospitalizations related to exacerbations, health-related QOL, and lung function were significantly better in the group receiving triple therapy (LABA, long-acting muscarinic antagonist [LAMA], ICS). Thus, the institution of triple therapy for COPD is consistent with good medicine, if the patient has failed less intense therapy.

Mucokinetic Agents

The mucokinetic drugs decrease sputum viscosity and adhesiveness to facilitate expectoration. The only controlled study in the United States suggesting a value for mucokinetics in the chronic management of bronchitis was a multicenter evaluation of organic iodide, which demonstrated symptomatic benefits. Oral acetylcysteine is favored in Europe for its antioxidant effects; however, a recent large trial failed to document any substantial benefit. Genetically engineered ribonuclease seems to be useful in cystic fibrosis but is of no value in COPD patients.

Antibiotics

In patients with evidence of respiratory tract infection, such as fever, leukocytosis, and a change in the chest radiograph, antibiotics have proved effective. If recurrent infections occur, particularly in winter, continuous or intermittent, prolonged courses of antibiotics may be useful. The major bacterial strains to be considered are *Streptococcus pneumoniae*, *Haemophilus influenzae*, and *Moraxella (Branhamella) catarrhalis*. The antibiotic choice will depend on local experience, supported by sputum culture and sensitivities if the patient is moderately ill or requires hospital admission. Two recent randomized multicenter trials of the macrolide antibiotic *clarithromycin* show a beneficial impact on exacerbations, likely from the drug's antiinflammatory action.

Alpha₁-Antitrypsin

Although supplemental weekly or monthly administration of the enzyme α$_1$-antitrypsin may be indicated in nonsmoking, younger patients with genetically determined emphysema, such therapy is difficult to initiate in practice. Evidence shows that the administration of α$_1$-antitrypsin is relatively safe. Although not entirely clear, the most likely candidates for replacement therapy would be patients with mild to moderate COPD.

VACCINATION

Ideally, infectious complications of the respiratory tract should be prevented in patients with COPD by using effective vaccines. Thus, routine prophylaxis with pneumococcal and influenza vaccines is recommended.

SYSTEMIC MANIFESTATIONS

The systemic manifestations of COPD include peripheral muscle dysfunction, malnutrition, cardiovascular compromise, osteoporosis, depression, anemia, and lung cancer. Some may be responsive to pulmonary and exercise therapy and may benefit patients with minimal response to conventional pharmacologic therapy.

PULMONARY REHABILITATION

Pulmonary rehabilitation has gradually become the "gold standard" treatment for patients with symptomatic COPD. By definition, rehabilitation services are provided to patients with symptoms, most of them with advanced lung disease. Because new therapeutic strategies such as surgical and nonsurgical lung volume reduction and lung transplantation require well-conditioned patients, pulmonary rehabilitation is becoming a crucial component of the overall treatment strategy of many patients previously deemed untreatable.

The most important concept in pulmonary rehabilitation is that any program must attempt to treat each patient enrolled as an individual. The variation that arises from the need to individualize therapy from one patient to another is one factor that makes the objective evaluation of each group of patients enrolled in a rehabilitation program difficult.

Because pulmonary rehabilitation is multidisciplinary and uses different therapeutic components, it is difficult to attribute improved global outcomes to the effect of individual elements of a program. Independent of the study design used, conventional pulmonary function tests do not usually change after pulmonary rehabilitation. Nevertheless, well-controlled studies show significant improvement in different outcomes, including increased exercise capacity, improved health-related QOL, and decreased dyspnea and hospital admissions.

Objectives and Goals

The definition of pulmonary rehabilitation provides three major objectives:

1. Control, alleviate, and as much as possible, reverse the symptoms and pathophysiologic processes leading to respiratory impairment.
2. Improve the quality of life, and attempt to prolong the patient's life.
3. Reduce health care use and costs.

Patient Selection

Any patient symptomatic from a respiratory disease with some functional limitation is a candidate for rehabilitation. It is preferable to choose patients with moderate to moderately severe disease, to prevent the disabling effects of end-stage respiratory failure. This is an important issue because it seems intuitive that patients with minimal functional limitation benefit minimally from programs designed to improve function. On the other hand, patients who are "too" advanced along the course of their illness could be considered "unlikely to benefit" from rehabilitation. This is not true; patients with the most severe degree of lung disease, such as those awaiting lung transplantation and lung volume reduction surgery, have shown significant

functional improvement and increased exercise endurance after pulmonary rehabilitation.

The mild COPD state may not justify the intense effort employed to rehabilitate disabled patients. Other barriers to successful rehabilitation are disabling diseases (e.g., severe heart failure, arthritis), low educational level, hazardous occupation, lack of support, and most importantly, motivation. Although it is customary not to consider patients with cancer as candidates for pulmonary rehabilitation, its inclusion in the preoperative conditioning of patients undergoing lung transplantation or lung volume reduction surgery has expanded the list of indications for rehabilitation.

THERAPEUTIC MODALITIES THAT IMPROVE PATIENT PERFORMANCE

Exercise Conditioning

Exercise conditioning is based on three physiologic principles: *specificity* of training, which attributes improvement only for the type of exercise practiced; *intensity* of training, which establishes that only a load higher than baseline will induce a training effect; and *reversal* of the training effect, which states that once discontinued, the training effect will disappear. The first two have been extensively applied in the rehabilitation of patients with severe COPD.

Lower Extremity Exercise

Several controlled trials prove that pulmonary rehabilitation is more effective than conventional treatment in symptomatic COPD patients. Exercise training is the most important component of a pulmonary rehabilitation program. A rehabilitation program that includes lower extremity exercise is better than other forms of therapy, such as optimization of medication, education, breathing retraining, and group therapy.

All studies report an increase in exercise endurance, a modest but significant improvement in work rate or oxygen uptake, and a decrease in the perception of dyspnea. One study randomized 119 patients to education (62) and education with exercise training (57). After 6 months, the trained patients significantly increased their exercise endurance time and peak O_2 uptake and reported an improvement in the perception of dyspnea and self-assessed efficacy for walking compared with controls. A follow-up showed that the gains were lost after 1 year, and that a once-a-month follow-up training visit was not sufficient to maintain the gained effects.

With exercise, patients with COPD may become desensitized to the dyspnea induced by the ventilatory load. However, randomized studies have documented evidence for a true training effect. Muscle biopsies of trained patients, but not those of the controls, manifested significant increases in all enzymes responsible for oxidative muscle function, with important physiologic outcomes, as supported by a reduction in exercise lactic acidosis and minute ventilation after training.

All willing symptomatic patients capable of some exercise are candidates for rehabilitation. In 50 patients with severe COPD evaluated before and after exercise training, an inverse relationship was seen between the baseline 12-minute walking distance and O_2 uptake and the improvement.

Upper Extremity Exercise

Most knowledge about exercise conditioning is derived from programs emphasizing leg training. This is unfortunate, because the performance of many everyday tasks requires not only the hands but also the concerted action of other muscle groups that are also used in upper torso and arm positioning. Some of these serve a dual function (respiratory and postural), and arm exercise will decrease the capacity to participate in ventilation. These observations suggest that if the arms are trained to perform more work, or if the ventilatory requirement for the same work is decreased, as previously shown, this could improve the capacity to perform activities of daily living.

Arm training results in improved performance, which is primarily task-specific. One study compared two forms of arm exercise—gravity resistance and modified proprioceptive neuromuscular facilitation—with no arm exercise in 45 patients with COPD. The 20 patients who completed the program improved performance on the tests specific for the training. The patients also reported a decrease in fatigue for all tests performed.

Unsupported arm training (against gravity) decreases O_2 uptake at the same workload compared with arm-cranking training. Unsupported arm exercise may be more effective to train patients in activities similar to those of daily living. Cystic fibrosis patients who underwent upper extremity training (swimming and canoeing for $1\frac{1}{2}$ hours daily) exhibited increased upper extremity endurance after 6 weeks; most importantly, their increase in maximal sustainable ventilatory capacity was similar to that obtained with ventilatory muscle training. This suggests that arm exercise training programs can train ventilatory muscles.

Because simple arm elevation results in significant increases in minute ventilation ($\dot{V}E$), oxygen uptake ($\dot{V}O_2$), and carbon dioxide production ($\dot{V}CO_2$), my group studied 14 patients with COPD before and after 8 weeks of three-times-weekly 20-minute sessions of unsupported arm and leg exercise. Our study was part of a comprehensive rehabilitation program to test whether arm training decreases the ventilatory requirement for arm activity. There was a 35% decrease in the rise of $\dot{V}O_2$ and $\dot{V}CO_2$ brought about by arm elevation, associated with a significant decrease in $\dot{V}O_2$. Because the patients also trained their legs, we could not conclude that the improvement resulted from the arm exercise. To answer this question, we had 25 patients with COPD undergo either unsupported arm training (11) or resistance breathing training (14). After 24 sessions, arm endurance increased only for the unsupported arm training group. Interestingly, maximal inspiratory pressure increased significantly for both groups, indicating that training the arms may induce ventilatory muscle exercise for rib cage muscles that hinge on the shoulder girdle.

PHYSICAL MODALITIES OF VENTILATORY THERAPY

Physical modalities include controlled breathing techniques (diaphragmatic breathing exercise, pursed-lip breathing, bending forward), chest physical therapy (postural drainage, chest percussion, vibration position), and respiratory muscle endurance or strength training. The benefits of these modalities include less dyspnea, fewer anxiety and panic attacks, and improved well-being. Although strength and endurance training of the respiratory muscle is associated with an increase in exercise endurance, the clinical significance of these effects remains debatable. These modalities require careful instruction by specialists and should be initiated under close supervision until the patient shows thorough understanding of the techniques. It is often necessary to involve the family because many of these modalities require the assistance of another person (e.g., chest percussion).

Breathing Training

Breathing training is aimed at controlling the respiratory rate and breathing pattern, thus decreasing air trapping. It also attempts to decrease the work of breathing and improve the position and function of the respiratory muscles. The simplest maneuver is *pursed-lip breathing*. Patients inhale through the nose and exhale between 4 and 6 seconds through lips pursed in a whistling-kissing position. The exact mechanism by which this maneuver decreases dyspnea is unknown. *Diaphragmatic breathing* is a technique to change the breathing pattern from having the rib cage muscles as the predominant pressure generators to a more normal pattern in which the pressures are generated with the diaphragm. Diaphragmatic breathing is usually practiced for at least 20 minutes two to three times daily. Although most patients report improvement in dyspnea and perception of dyspnea, this technique results in minimal if any changes in oxygen uptake and resting lung volume. Similar to pursed-lip breathing, there is usually a fall in respiratory rate, minute ventilation, and increased tidal volume with diaphragmatic breathing.

Chest Physical Therapy

The goal of chest physiotherapy is that of removing airway secretions, thereby decreasing airflow resistance and bronchopulmonary infection. These techniques include postural drainage, chest percussion, vibration, and directed cough. *Postural drainage* uses gravity to help drain the individual lung segments. *Chest percussion* should be performed with care in patients with osteoporosis or bone problems. The single most important criterion for chest physical therapy is the presence of sputum production.

Ventilatory Muscle Strength and Endurance Training

It has been shown that in normal individuals the respiratory muscles, as with their skeletal counterparts, can be specifically trained to improve their strength or endurance. Subsequently, several studies showed that a training response will occur if there is sufficient stimulus. An increase in inspiratory muscle strength (and perhaps endurance) should result in improved respiratory muscle function by decreasing the ratio of the pressure required to breathe (PI) and the maximal pressure that the respiratory system can generate (PI_{max}). The PI/PI_{max} ratio, which represents the effort required to complete each breath as a function of the force reserve, is the most important determinant of fatigue in loaded respiratory muscles. Because patients with COPD have reduced inspiratory muscle strength, considerable efforts have been made to define the role of respiratory muscle training in these patients.

Studies show an increase in PI_{max} when the respiratory muscles have been specifically trained for strength. Decreasing PI/PI_{max} through respiratory muscle strength training does not appear to be clinically important. However, respiratory muscle strength often increases as a byproduct of endurance training achieved using resistive loads. Some benefits observed after endurance training may relate to the increased strength. Endurance is achieved through low-intensity, high-frequency training programs; the three types are flow resistive loading, threshold loading, and voluntary isocapneic hyperpnea.

Because many studies have not been controlled, it is difficult to attribute their results to the training. Many show an increase in the endurance time during which the ventilatory muscles could tolerate a known load; some show a significant increase in strength and a decrease in dyspnea during the performance of inspiratory load and exercise. Studies of systemic exercise performance found a minimal increase in walking distance or constant-load exercise endurance. Ventilatory muscle training with resistive breathing clearly results in improved ventilatory muscle strength and endurance. In COPD, however, it is not clear whether this effort results in decreased morbidity or mortality or offers any clinical advantage. In many studies, compliance has been low, with up to 50% of all pulmonary patients failing to complete the programs. Larger multicenter studies with clinical outcomes are needed to select the appropriate patients who may benefit from this labor-intensive form of therapy. Currently, ventilatory muscle training is recommended for patients with symptoms and evidence of ventilatory muscle weakness.

Respiratory muscle training results in increased strength and capacity of the muscles to endure a respiratory load. Whether it also results in improved exercise or performance of activities of daily living is debatable. Knowing the respiratory muscle factors that may contribute to ventilatory limitation in COPD might help predict that increases in strength and endurance should help respiratory muscle function. However, this may be important only in the capacity of the COPD patient to handle inspiratory loads, such as during acute exacerbations. It is less likely that ventilatory muscle training will substantially affect systemic exercise performance.

Respiratory Muscle Resting

Respiratory muscles that must work against a large enough load may become fatigued. Experimentally, this has occurred in both normal volunteers and patients with COPD. Clinically, respiratory muscle fatigue seems to play an important role in the acute respiratory failure of patients with COPD. *Noninvasive ventilation* (NIV) should be helpful in patients with acute or chronic respiratory failure and impending respiratory muscle fatigue, as confirmed by several randomized trials evaluating different outcomes, including the rate of intubation, length of intensive care unit (ICU) and hospital stay, dyspnea, and mortality. Although not all showed the same results in mortality, there was uniform agreement that positive-pressure NIV was effective in reversing acute respiratory failure. The most successfully treated patients were able to cooperate and had elevated partial pressure of carbon dioxide in arterial blood ($PaCO_2$) but no other important comorbid problems (no sepsis or severe pneumonia). Because positive-pressure NIV is potentially dangerous, patients considered for this therapy should be closely monitored and treated by clinicians familiar with these ventilatory techniques.

The possibility that the respiratory muscles of patients with stable severe COPD were functioning close to the fatigue threshold led numerous investigators to explore the role of muscle resting using negative-pressure and positive-pressure NIV. With one exception, the controlled trials using both forms of ventilation showed no benefit in most of the outcomes studied. Therefore, routine use of NIV in stable COPD patients remains controversial.

NUTRITION EVALUATION

Many patients with emphysema appear thin and emaciated and may have anemia, leading to a poor prognosis. Although no evidence suggests a plan that would result in unequivocal benefits for the respiratory system, most authorities agree that any deficiencies should be corrected. Correction of factors such as anemia (to improve oxygen-carrying capacity) and electrolyte imbalances (sodium, potassium, phosphorus, magnesium)

could result in improved cardiopulmonary performance. Similarly, simple measures such as encouraging the patient to take small amounts of food at more frequent intervals result in less abdominal distention and decrease dyspnea after meals. My group also recommends evaluating oxygen saturation (SaO_2) during meals. If hypoexmia is present, this can be alleviated by supplementing O_2 at feeding time.

PSYCHOLOGICAL SUPPORT

Most patients with advanced lung disease have minor psychological problems, mainly *reactive depression* and *anxiety*. Fortunately, these problems are likely to improve as the patients become involved in a rehabilitation program that improves activity and performance. Simple measures, such as being able to exercise under the supervision of supportive specialists, frequently result in desensitization to symptoms, including dyspnea and fear. From 15 to 20 rehabilitation sessions that include education, exercise, physical therapy, breathing techniques, and relaxation are more effective in reducing anxiety than a similar number of psychotherapy sessions. Occasionally, patients have major psychological problems and require primary psychiatric evaluation and treatment.

HOME OXYGEN THERAPY

Therapeutic oxygen has been used systemically since the association between hypoxemia and right-sided heart failure was first recognized and the benefit of continuous O_2 delivery to patients with severe COPD was documented. Since then, much has been learned about the effects of oxygen and hypoxemia, and progress has been made in the area of mechanical O_2 delivery devices. The results of the Nocturnal Oxygen Therapy Trial and UK Medical Research Council studies established that continuous home oxygen improves survival in hypoxemic COPD patients, and that survival is related to the number of hours of supplemental O_2 per day. Other beneficial effects of long-term O_2 include reduction in polycythemia (perhaps resulting more from lowered carboxyhemoglobin levels than improved arterial saturation), reduction in pulmonary artery pressure (Ppa), dyspnea, and rapid eye movement–related hypoxemia during sleep. Oxygen also improves sleep and may reduce nocturnal arrhythmias. Importantly, O_2 can also improve neuropsychiatric testing and exercise tolerance, attributed to central mechanisms causing reduced minute ventilation at the same workload, thereby delaying ventilatory limitation. The improved arterial oxygenation enables greater O_2 delivery, reversal of hypoxemia-induced bronchoconstriction, and the effect of O_2 on respiratory muscle recruitment.

Prescribing Home Oxygen

Patients are evaluated for long-term O_2 therapy by measuring the partial pressure of oxygen in arterial blood (PaO_2). Therefore the recommendation is that PaO_2 measurement, not pulse oximetry for SaO_2, should be the clinical standard for initiating long-term O_2 therapy, particularly during rest. Oximetry may be used to adjust O_2 flow settings over time. If hypercapnia or acidosis is suspected, arterial blood gases (ABGs) must be measured. Some COPD patients who were not hypoxemic before their exacerbation will eventually recover to the point they no longer need oxygen. It is therefore recommended that the need for long-term O_2 be reassessed in 30 to 90 days, when the patient is clinically stable and receiving adequate medical management. O_2 therapy can be discontinued if the patient does not meet ABG criteria.

As with any drug, oxygen may have deleterious effects, particularly in older patients. The hazardous effects of O_2 therapy can be considered under three broad headings. First, *physical risks* include fire hazard or tank explosion, trauma from catheters or masks, and drying of mucous membranes caused by high flow rates and inadequate humidification. Second, *functional effects* are related to increased CO_2 retention and absorptive atelectasis. Elevated $PaCO_2$ in response to supplemental O_2 is a well-recognized complication in a minority of patients, traditionally attributed to reductions in hypoxic ventilatory drive. In many patients, however, the decrease in minute ventilation is minimal. The most consistent finding is a worsening of the pulmonary ventilation/perfusion distribution, with an increase in the dead space/tidal volume ratio. This presumably results from oxygen's blockage of local hypoxic vasoconstriction, thereby increasing perfusion of poorly ventilated areas. Third, although possible, *cytotoxic effects* and atelectasis have not been clearly demonstrated with the low flow rates (1-5 L/min; fraction of inspired oxygen [FIO_2] of 24%-36%) typically used for chronic home O_2 therapy in COPD patients.

Oxygen Delivery Systems

Long-term home O_2 therapy is available from three different delivery systems: oxygen concentrators, liquid systems, and compressed gas. Each system has advantages and disadvantages, and the correct system for each patient depends on patient limitations and the clinical application. Oxygen systems were recently compared on the basis of weight, cost, portability, ease of refilling, and availability; the first three factors may be of particular importance in elderly, often debilitated patients.

Administration Devices

Oxygen is typically administered with continuous flow by a nasal cannula. However, because alveolar delivery occurs during a small portion of a spontaneous respiratory cycle (approximately the first sixth), with the rest of the cycle used to fill dead space and for exhalation, the majority of continuously flowing O_2 is not used by the patient and is wasted into the atmosphere. To improve efficiency and increase patient mobility, several devices are available that focus on O_2 conservation and delivery during early inspiration, including reservoir cannulas, demand-type systems, and transtracheal catheters.

Reservoir nasal cannulas and pendants store oxygen during expiration and deliver a 20-mL bolus during early inspiration. Because more alveolar O_2 is delivered, flows may be reduced proportionally, resulting in a 2:1 to 4:1 O_2 savings at rest and with exercise. Cosmetic considerations have traditionally limited patient acceptance of these devices.

Demand valve systems have an electronic sensor that delivers O_2 only during early inspiration or provides an additional pulse early in inspiration as an adjuvant to the continuous flow. By restricting or accentuating O_2 during inspiration, wasted delivery into dead space or during exhalation is minimized. This results in a 2:1 to 7:1 O_2 savings. The effect of mouth breathing on efficacy is not yet clear.

Transtracheal oxygen therapy introduces a thin flexible catheter into the lower trachea for delivery of continuous (or pulsed) O_2. Because O_2 is delivered directly into the trachea, dead space is reduced, and the upper trachea serves as a reservoir of undiluted O_2. This provides a 2:1 to 3:1 O_2 savings over a nasal cannula. However, the widespread use of transtracheal O_2 has been limited by the rate of complications, requiring administration in specialized centers.

EXACERBATIONS, HOSPITALIZATION, AND DISCHARGE CRITERIA

Although acute exacerbations are difficult to define and their pathogenesis is poorly understood, impaired lung function can lead to respiratory failure, requiring intubation and mechanical ventilation. In addition, repeated exacerbations are associated with poor outcome. The purpose of acute treatment is to manage the patient's decompensation and comorbid conditions to prevent further deterioration and readmission (see Chapter 43).

The therapy of an exacerbation is based on the administration of the same medications that are given in the stable patient, with preference for nebulized medications. In addition, the administration of systemic corticosteroids has resulted in improved outcomes. If a bacterial infection is suspected, antibiotics are administered based on the local prevalence of bacteria.

Traditionally, the decision for hospital admission derives from subjective interpretation of clinical features, such as the severity of dyspnea, determination of respiratory failure, short-term response to emergency department (ED) therapy, presence of right-sided heart failure, and presence of complications (e.g., severe bronchitis, pneumonia, comorbidities). This approach to decision making is less than ideal in that up to 28% of patients with an acute exacerbation of COPD discharged from an ED have recurrent symptoms within 14 days. Additionally, 17% of patients discharged after ED management of COPD will relapse and require hospitalization. Few clinical studies have investigated patient-specific objective clinical and laboratory features that identify patients with COPD who require hospitalization. A general consensus supports the need for hospitalization in patients with severe acute hypoxemia or acute hypercarbia; less extreme ABG abnormalities, however, do not assist with decision making.

Other factors that identify high-risk patients include a previous ED visit within 7 days, number of doses of nebulized bronchodilators, use of home oxygen, previous relapse rate, administration of aminophylline, and use of corticosteroids and antibiotics at ED discharge.

Once improved, clinical assessment plans for modifying drug regimens, use of home oxygen, or potential benefits from pulmonary rehabilitation programs should be prepared. The duration of hospitalization for the COPD patient depends at least partly on a multidisciplinary team present to direct respiratory management.

Because of the complex management issues in caring for COPD patients with impending or frank respiratory failure, physician specialists with extensive COPD experience should participate in the care of hospitalized patients who present with underlying severe disease. This includes patients who require invasive or noninvasive mechanical ventilation or who develop hypoxemia unresponsive to FIO_2 of 0.50 or have new-onset hypercarbia, as well as those who require steroids more than 48 hours to maintain adequate respiratory function, undergo thoracoabdominal surgery, or require specialized techniques to manage copious airway secretions.

The indications for hospital admission vary according to local practices and regulations. The expert consensus considers the severity of the underlying respiratory dysfunction, progression of symptoms, response to outpatient therapy, existence of comorbid conditions, necessity of surgical interventions that may affect pulmonary function, and the availability of adequate home care. The severity of respiratory dysfunction dictates the need for ICU admission. Depending on available resources, patients with severe exacerbations of COPD may be admitted to intermediate or special respiratory care units to identify and manage acute respiratory failure successfully. Limited data support the discharge criteria, but the patient's capacity to function independently and lack of comorbidities help in the decision.

CONTROVERSIES AND PITFALLS

The paradigm that COPD is a disease associated with poor therapy response has shifted to the general sense that patients do respond to therapy. However, the following controversies still remain:

1. Should asymptomatic patients who are diagnosed with airflow obstruction by spirometry be treated?
2. Should symptomatic patients with mild obstruction be treated, and if so, what is the best initial choice for therapy?
3. Should most patients with persistent symptoms be treated with double- or triple-drug therapy?
4. If double-agent therapy is selected, is it better to treat with a β_2-agonist plus inhaled corticosteroids or a long-acting β_2-agonist (LABA) and long-acting muscarinic antagonist (LAMA)?
5. For which patients is pulmonary rehabilitation more effective?
6. Do maintenance programs of pulmonary rehabilitation need to be developed? Are they useful?
7. Is there a definitive role for chronic antibiotic therapy for patients with COPD, and if so, which agents in which schedule?

Although such questions remain unanswered, studies are unraveling the mechanistic processes that result in COPD to develop therapies capable of reversing disease progression. Recent evidence proving the presence of stem cells in the lungs indicates that regenerative therapy may help repair damaged lungs.

CONCLUSION

Knowledge of COPD has increased significantly in recent years. Smoking cessation campaigns have resulted in a significant decrease in smoking prevalence in the United States. Similar efforts worldwide should have the same impact. The consequence should be a future decrease in the incidence of COPD. The widespread application of long-term oxygen therapy for hypoxemic patients has resulted in increased survival. An expanded drug therapy armamentarium has effectively improved dyspnea and quality of life, and pulmonary rehabilitation has documented benefits. Noninvasive ventilation has offered new alternatives for the patient with acute or chronic respiratory failure. Surgical and more innovative nonsurgical volume reduction may serve as an alternative to lung transplantation for patients with severe COPD who are still symptomatic after maximal medical therapy. All these options offer new hope for the patient with chronic obstructive pulmonary disease.

SUGGESTED READINGS

Agustí AG, Noguera A, Sauleda J, et al: Systemic effects of chronic obstructive pulmonary disease, *Eur Respir J* 21:347–360, 2003.

Albert RK, Connett J, Bailey WC, et al: Azithromycin for prevention of exacerbations of COPD. COPD Clinical Research Network, *N Engl J Med* 365:689–698, 2011.

Anthonisen NR, Skeans MA, Wise RA, et al: The effects of a smoking cessation intervention on 14.5-year mortality: a randomized clinical trial. Lung Health Study Research Group, *Ann Intern Med* 142:233–239, 2005.

Calverley PM, Anderson JA, Celli B, et al: Salmeterol and fluticasone propionate and survival in chronic obstructive pulmonary disease. TORCH Investigators, *N Engl J Med* 356:775–789, 2007.

Calverley PM, Rabe KF, Goehring UM, et al: Roflumilast in symptomatic chronic obstructive pulmonary disease: two randomised clinical trials. M2-124 and M2-125 study groups, *Lancet* 374:685–694, 2009.

Casanova C, Cote C, de Torres JP, et al: Inspiratory-to-total lung capacity ratio predicts mortality in patients with chronic obstructive pulmonary disease, *Am J Respir Crit Care Med* 171:591–597, 2005.

Celli BR, MacNee W: Standards for the diagnosis and treatment of COPD, *Eur Respir J* 23:932–946, 2004.

Celli BR, Cote CG, Marin JM, et al: The body mass index, airflow obstruction, dyspnea and exercise capacity index in chronic obstructive pulmonary disease, *N Engl J Med* 350:1005–1012, 2004.

Global Initiative for Chronic Obstructive Lung Disease. www.GOLD.org (updated 2010).

National Emphysema Treatment Trial Research Group: A randomized trial comparing lung-volume-reduction surgery with medical therapy for severe emphysema, *N Engl J Med* 348:2059–2073, 2003.

Nici L, Donner C, Wouters E, et al: American Thoracic Society/European Respiratory Society statement on pulmonary rehabilitation. ATS/ERS Pulmonary Rehabilitation Writing Committee, *Am J Respir Crit Care Med* 173:1390–1413, 2006.

Niewoehner DE, Erbland ML, Deupree RH, et al: Effect of systemic glucocorticoids on exacerbations of chronic obstructive pulmonary disease, *N Engl J Med* 340:1941–1947, 1999.

O'Donnell D, Lam M, Webb K: Spirometric correlates of improvement in exercise performance after anticholinergic therapy in chronic obstructive pulmonary disease, *Am J Respir Crit Care Med* 160:542–549, 1999.

Ries et al. [arm exercise].

Tashkin DP, Celli B, Senn S, et al: A 4-year trial of tiotropium in chronic obstructive pulmonary disease. UPLIFT Study Investigators, *N Engl J Med* 359:1543–1554, 2008.

Welte T, Miravitlles M, Hernandez P, et al: Efficacy and tolerability of budesonide/formoterol added to tiotropium in patients with chronic obstructive pulmonary disease, *Am J Respir Crit Care Med* 180:741–750, 2009.

Chapter **43**

Management of Exacerbations in Chronic Obstructive Pulmonary Disease

John R. Hurst • Jadwiga A. Wedzicha

EPIDEMIOLOGY

It would be difficult to exaggerate the importance of exacerbations in patients with chronic obstructive pulmonary disease (COPD). COPD is the fifth leading cause of death worldwide, and the mortality and morbidity are often associated with episodes of symptom deterioration termed *exacerbations*. Furthermore, whereas death rates in other prevalent conditions are falling, mortality from COPD continues to rise. Exacerbations of COPD account for about 1 in 10 emergency medical admissions to the hospital, and the in-hospital mortality is 10%. Exacerbations are consequently responsible for 70% of the direct costs attributable to COPD.

Exacerbations generally become both more frequent and more severe as the severity of the underlying COPD progresses. On average, patients with moderate to severe COPD, typical of those attending secondary care, will have one or two exacerbations requiring additional treatment annually. However, annual exacerbation incidence rates differ greatly among individual patients, and those prone to more frequent exacerbations experience a particular burden of disease (**Figure 43-1**). The best determinant of future exacerbation history is *past* exacerbation frequency, such that some patients appear more intrinsically susceptible and some more resistant to these important events.

PATHOPHYSIOLOGY

The World Health Organization defines COPD as a disease state having a pulmonary component characterized by airflow limitation that is progressive, not fully reversible, and associated with an abnormal inflammatory response to noxious particles or gases. Airway inflammation is even greater at exacerbation, and the assumption has been that this additional inflammation provokes symptoms such as worsening dyspnea and sputum production, through mechanisms relating to airway tone, airway wall edema, and mucus production. The resultant air trapping increases the work of breathing and causes additional impairment to respiratory muscle function. Triggers of increased airway inflammation are therefore the causes of exacerbation, predominantly tracheobronchial infection, with a lesser role for pollutants. However, the effects of increased inflammation at exacerbation require further clarification, because a direct relationship between the clinical severity of the exacerbation and the degree of airway inflammation has never been conclusively demonstrated.

Defining the role of airway infection in causing COPD exacerbation is problematic. Recent advances in molecular biology have isolated respiratory viruses and potentially pathogenic bacteria from the airways of most patients during exacerbations (**Box 43-1**). However, certainly for patients with more severe underlying disease, bacteria also are often present in the stable state (bacterial colonization). Therefore the presence of an organism at exacerbation does not assume a role in causing that exacerbation. More recent studies suggest that a change in the colonizing bacterial strain may be the precipitating cause. However, not all strain changes are associated with exacerbation, and vice versa. Reflecting this, as discussed later, antibiotics are not of universal benefit during exacerbations. Rhinovirus is the most often identified viral pathogen, and thus exacerbations are more common during the winter months, when viral circulation in the community is higher. The role of atypical organisms such as *Chlamydia* and *Mycoplasma* species appears minimal.

Regarding pollutants in causing COPD exacerbation, large epidemiologic studies link rises in pollutant levels with increases in hospital admission for respiratory disease. Particulate matter less than 10 μm in size (PM_{10}) appears particularly important. Pollutants and microorganisms may interact to amplify the risk of exacerbation.

Because some COPD patients seem more susceptible to exacerbations, there may be genetic determinants of exacerbation frequency. In support of this, susceptibility to exacerbation has a familial component, but no single polymorphism has yet been reported to explain the variance in exacerbation frequency observed in COPD patients.

It is now recognized that COPD is associated with upregulated systemic inflammation, and there is now ample evidence to demonstrate heightened systemic inflammation during exacerbations. This may be important given the association between cardiovascular death and elevated systemic inflammatory markers, and because many patients with COPD die from cardiovascular disease. This systemic inflammation is thought to represent "spillover" from the lung.

Understanding the pathophysiology of exacerbations in COPD explains the rationale for the various therapies employed. Bronchodilators may be helpful for increased bronchoconstriction and hyperinflation, corticosteroids may reduce airway inflammation, and antibiotics may be appropriate in exacerbations caused by bacteria (**Figure 43-2**).

CLINICAL FEATURES

The cardinal feature of COPD exacerbation is an increase in respiratory symptoms beyond what is usual for the patient.

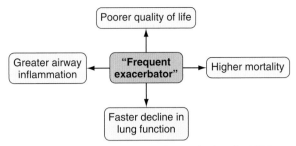

Figure 43-1   Consequences of exacerbations in COPD.

Box 43-1   Common Organisms Isolated at Exacerbation of COPD

Bacteria
Haemophilus influenzae
Moraxella (Branhamella) catarrhalis
Streptococcus pneumoniae
*Pseudomonas aeruginosa**

Respiratory Viruses
Rhinovirus
Influenza
Parainfluenza
Coronavirus
Respiratory syncytial virus
Adenovirus

*In patients with more severe underlying COPD.

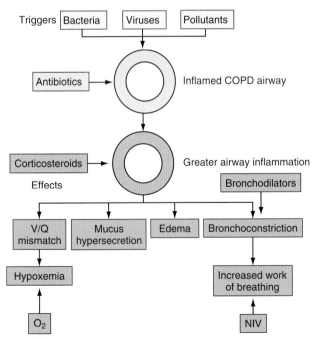

Figure 43-2   Pathophysiology of COPD exacerbation provides rationale for understanding therapies for exacerbations. *NIV*, noninvasive ventilation; *V/Q*, ventilation/perfusion ratio.

Typically, such symptoms include dyspnea, sputum volume, sputum purulence, cough, and wheezing, perhaps accompanied by upper respiratory tract symptoms such as rhinorrhea. Clinical signs are nonspecific but may include tachycardia, tachypnea, cyanosis, use of accessory respiratory muscles, polyphonic expiratory wheeze or crackles on auscultation, and features of carbon dioxide retention or cor pulmonale.

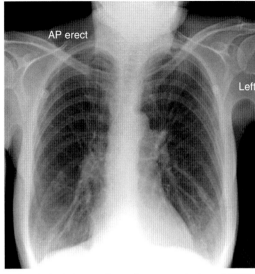

Figure 43-3   Typical chest radiograph at exacerbation of COPD. Note the features of underlying COPD, including hyperexpansion and prominent pulmonary vasculature suggestive of pulmonary hypertension, but no evidence of conditions that may mimic or complicate exacerbation (e.g., pneumothorax, pneumonia, cardiac failure).

Exacerbations are heterogeneous events, and the clinical features vary widely. It may be best to consider the *severity* of the presentation, which represents the combined severity of the underlying COPD and the exacerbation. Patients with mild underlying disease may experience no more than a troublesome worsening of symptoms, whereas those with more severe COPD are at significant risk of respiratory failure. Furthermore, other conditions occurring in patients with underlying COPD may mimic or complicate exacerbations. Proper assessment, as described next, is therefore important.

DIAGNOSIS

Exacerbation of COPD is a clinical syndrome, and there is no confirmatory diagnostic test. Although controversy surrounds how exactly to define an exacerbation, and such differences are important when interpreting study results, it is now widely accepted that an exacerbation is a sustained worsening of a patient's symptoms that is acute in onset, is beyond day-to-day variation, and may necessitate a change in therapy.

Although investigations are not helpful in the diagnosis of exacerbation, diagnostic tests help assess the severity of the presentation and exclude other conditions in patients with underlying COPD that may mimic or complicate exacerbation. Such diagnoses include pneumonia, pneumothorax, pulmonary embolus, and cardiac failure, and appropriate investigations include chest radiography, electrocardiography, oxygen saturation (SaO_2) values, and arterial blood gas (ABG) analysis. Simple venous blood tests include complete blood count, urea and electrolytes, and C-reactive protein. A typical chest radiograph at exacerbation (**Figure 43-3**) should appear much the same as the patient's radiograph in the stable state. Spirometry is not generally helpful because absolute values may be misleading, changes at exacerbation are small, and patients acutely dyspneic have difficulty performing the maneuvers. Sputum microscopy and culture may help to refine empirical antibiotic therapy in those not initially improving. For the patient with mild exacerbation responding to an increase in inhaled bronchodilators, it may be appropriate to omit further investigation.

There is no accepted method of assessing exacerbation severity because it represents the combined severity of the underlying disease and the exacerbation insult. Quantifying changes in symptoms or lung function requires knowledge of the patient at baseline and is difficult to achieve and not generally helpful. Consequently, the degree of health care utilization has been used as a surrogate assessment of severity: *mild* exacerbations require no more than an increase in inhaled bronchodilators, *moderate* exacerbations require antibiotics and corticosteroids in the community, and patients with *severe* exacerbations require hospital admission. The pH is the best indicator of an acute change in alveolar ventilation, and most exacerbations associated with respiratory failure will require hospital assessment. However, the decision to admit a patient depends on more than the severity of the exacerbation and would include, for example, the social circumstances and support available to the patient at home.

TREATMENT

PHARMACOTHERAPY

The principles of therapy at the time of COPD exacerbation are twofold: to modify the course of the event and to support the patient's respiratory function so that disease-modifying therapies can work. Treatment is given in proportion to the clinical severity of the event, and the sequential approach is illustrated in **Figure 43-4**. Many guidelines exist to guide appropriate therapy, including recently updated evidence-based statements from the UK National Institute for Clinical Excellence (NICE). Attention to comorbidities is also important, and in the recovery phase the clinician should consider interventions that may reduce the risk of subsequent exacerbations.

Inhaled Bronchodilators

An increase in the dose or frequency of inhaled short-acting bronchodilators is the mainstay of COPD exacerbation therapy. The bronchodilator effect is similar between the β_2-agonist *albuterol* (salbutamol) and the anticholinergic drug *ipratropium bromide*. Although often used in combination, there is little evidence to suggest an additive benefit. Also, no evidence indicates that nebulization is more effective than administering these drugs by inhaler and large-volume spacer. However, nebulizers are often preferred in dyspneic patients and may be less demanding on nursing time. Nebulizers for COPD should be driven on compressed air.

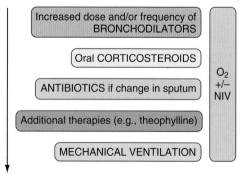

Figure 43-4   Summary of stepwise therapeutic approach to COPD exacerbation, with increasing severity of the exacerbation presentation. *NIV*, noninvasive ventilation.

Patients prescribed long-acting bronchodilators normally continue these therapies, but evidence is minimal to support the introduction of long-acting agents as exacerbation therapy, and short-acting drugs are preferred. The recommended approach is therefore to increase the dose and frequency of either a short-acting β_2-agonist or an anticholinergic, with both drugs used together in the event of inadequate clinical response.

Corticosteroids

Systemic corticosteroids are indicated in all COPD exacerbations except milder events that respond to an increase in inhaled bronchodilators alone. A number of randomized trials, now summarized in systematic reviews, demonstrate a more rapid improvement in FEV_1 after administration of steroids, although effects on outcomes such as oxygenation, hospitalization, and length of stay are more variable, with no definite evidence of a mortality benefit. Guidelines vary in their specific recommendations, generally suggesting oral *prednisone*, 30 to 40 mg for 10 to 14 days. Prolonged courses provide no additional benefit (and increase the risk of side effects), and no evidence suggests that tapering the dose is advantageous. Some physicians choose to give the first dose of prednisone intravenously. Nebulized *budesonide* results in similar improvements in lung function to oral dosing but is more expensive than prednisone.

Intriguingly, the use of systemic steroids may delay the time to subsequent exacerbation. Although initiation of inhaled steroids has no role at exacerbation, inhaled corticosteroids have an important role in exacerbation prevention, as discussed later.

Antibiotics

Anthonisen's seminal work on antibiotics at COPD exacerbation demonstrated benefit only when patients had an increase in at least two of three symptoms: breathlessness, sputum volume, and sputum purulence. Sputum purulence reliably indicates the presence of bacteria at exacerbation. More recently, a meta-analysis has confirmed a small but statistically significant benefit in favor of antibiotics. Local resistance patterns and antibiotic policies will dictate the choice of drug, but coverage should include the common pathogens *Haemophilus influenzae*, *Moraxella (Branhamella) catarrhalis*, and *Streptococcus pneumoniae*. An oral aminopenicillin, macrolide, or tetracycline is therefore an appropriate empirical choice. Comparative data across drug classes are sparse. Intravenous antibiotics are rarely required. Data on the optimal duration of therapy are minimal. Antibiotic use at exacerbation may also prolong the time to subsequent exacerbations, perhaps by modulating airway bacterial load.

OXYGEN THERAPY

Oxygen is indicated to correct the hypoxemic respiratory failure that may result at COPD exacerbation (and is not a treatment for breathlessness). *Hypoxemia* is caused by a combination of increased ventilation-perfusion (V/Q) mismatch and alveolar hypoventilation. Oxygen should be administered in a controlled manner with monitoring of ABG tensions to avoid carbon dioxide (CO_2) retention and development of hypercapnic respiratory failure that may occur in a proportion of patients (those classically said to rely on hypoxic respiratory drive). Studies have shown little risk of hypercapnia if oxygen is titrated to a maximum saturation of 90% to 92%. Failure to correct hypoxemia to over 90% (with fraction of inspired oxygen [FIO_2] >40%) suggests the presence of additional

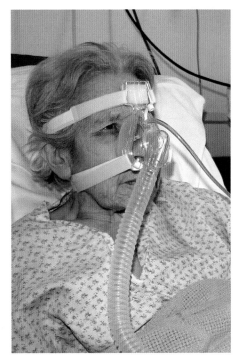

Figure 43-5 Application of noninvasive ventilation by nasal mask in patient with exacerbation of COPD. Note the addition of entrained oxygen.

pathology, such as pulmonary embolus. Achieving adequate oxygenation only at the expense of rising partial pressure of CO_2 in arterial blood ($PaCO_2$) or falling pH is an indication for ventilatory support. Venturi masks provide a more reliable FIO_2 than nasal cannulas, but cannulas may be better tolerated.

NONINVASIVE VENTILATION

Noninvasive ventilation (NIV) refers to the provision of ventilatory support using a nasal or full-face mask and the patient's own upper airway, in the absence of an endotracheal tube. Evidence now supports the use of NIV for patients with hypercapnic respiratory failure caused by exacerbation of COPD. The benefit in mortality with additional reduction in hospital stay and complications may largely be attributed to the reduced need for sedation, intubation, and invasive ventilation. In addition, and in contrast to invasive ventilation, NIV may be used earlier and intermittently, which facilitates communication, nutrition, and physiotherapy. NIV is usually administered as pressure-cycled bilevel positive airway pressure in which the inspiratory and expiratory pressures may be independently varied.

However, NIV is not a substitute for invasive ventilation when required. Therefore, the management plan should consider suitability for invasive ventilation should NIV fail, and some patients may have relative contraindications to NIV or can have respiratory failure of such severity that they should be immediately assessed for invasive ventilation (**Box 43-2**). Most patients suitable for NIV are able to tolerate the treatment (**Figure 43-5**).

INVASIVE VENTILATION

The primary indications for invasive ventilation at exacerbation of COPD are severe hypoxia and acidemia (pH <7.26) in a patient unsuitable or failing NIV. However, although data suggest that patients with COPD have similar outcomes after invasive ventilation as patients with respiratory failure from other causes, the decision to institute invasive ventilation should consider the patient's prior functional status, severity of the current and underlying illness, degree of reversibility of the present deterioration, and presence and severity of comorbidities.

Mortality following invasive ventilation is about 20%, and weaning from the ventilator can be challenging. This is another

setting in which NIV may be valuable. The aim of ventilation is to support gas exchange and respiratory muscle function until other therapies have had sufficient time to be effective. In such circumstances, parenteral corticosteroids and antibiotics are usually given, and bronchodilators may be added to the ventilator circuit from an inhaler and spacer.

OTHER THERAPIES

Methylxanthine drugs such as theophylline have a variety of potentially beneficial effects on respiratory and cardiac function, but a meta-analysis failed to show any benefit in lung function or symptoms with methylxanthines during COPD exacerbations. Despite this and well-recognized problems with drug interactions, side effects, and a narrow therapeutic range necessitating the monitoring of drug levels, theophyllines are still sometimes used in patients who are not demonstrating sufficient progress on otherwise maximal therapy. One action of theophyllines is as phosphodiesterase (PDE) inhibitors, and newer, selective PDE_4 inhibitors are currently undergoing trials (see Chapter 42).

No data support the use of intravenous albuterol (salbutamol) at exacerbation of COPD. Side effects are more common than with the inhaled route, and routine use is not recommended.

Although exacerbations are often associated with an increased volume or tenacity of sputum, no firm evidence currently supports the use of mucolytic drugs at exacerbation of COPD. Also, no evidence supports strategies to facilitate expectoration, such as physiotherapy or saline nebulization, although this largely reflects an absence of *evidence* rather than evidence supporting the absence of benefit. Cough suppressants are contraindicated.

Central respiratory stimulants such as intravenous *doxapram* have now been largely superseded by NIV, a therapy clearly superior in the management of hypercapnic respiratory failure. There remains a limited role for doxapram if NIV is not appropriate, as a bridge to NIV, or (with specialist advice) in conjunction with NIV. The use of doxapram is often limited by side-effects, especially agitation, and any potential benefits do not appear to persist beyond 48 hours.

Although intravenous magnesium may be an effective bronchodilator in exacerbations of asthma, no convincing data are available in COPD, and routine use is not recommended. *Heliox* (helium and oxygen) has a lower viscosity than air and may therefore reduce the work of breathing. However, there remains no evidence of benefit at exacerbation of COPD.

Other supportive measures that should be instituted include appropriate attention to fluid balance and consideration of prophylaxis against venous thromboembolism. For COPD patients not responding to maximal therapy, or for those in whom escalation of therapy is inappropriate, a range of palliative approaches to achieve symptom control should be considered.

CLINICAL COURSE AND PREVENTION

Using analysis of symptoms and lung function changes, the median length of an exacerbation in the COPD patient is 7 to 10 days, although there is wide variability and a proportion of exacerbations take considerably longer. Some patients never seem to recover their preexacerbation lung function. Patients admitted have an in-hospital mortality of about 10%, and for patients with hypercapnic respiratory failure, mortality approaches 50% at 2 years. Some patients may be suitable for early supported discharge, associated with similar outcomes but apparently no more cost-effective than standard care.

Given the importance of exacerbations and having managed the acute event, it is important to consider instituting a range of preventative measures to reduce the risk of further exacerbations in the COPD patient. Mounting evidence suggests that a number of drug classes are able to reduce exacerbation rates, including the long-acting β_2-agonists (LABAs), long acting anticholinergics, and inhaled corticosteroids (ICS), at least for those with moderately severe underlying disease. Combination therapy with LABAs and ICS appears superior to the use of either alone. Oral corticosteroids are ineffective at preventing exacerbations and have no effect on other outcomes measures, so these also are not indicated in stable COPD. Mucolytics may reduce exacerbation frequency in those with milder disease not taking ICS.

Ongoing trials are reexamining the role of antibiotics in reducing exacerbation frequency. Some evidence indicates antibiotic may be effective, but many trials included patients with simple chronic bronchitis; also, the drugs used were older, and any benefit must be balanced against the possibility of promoting drug resistance. Macrolides hold particular promise given their recognized antiinflammatory action.

Vaccination against influenza and pneumococcus *(S. pneumoniae)* is recommended.

Underprescription of long-term oxygen therapy in those requiring such treatment is associated with hospital readmission. Home NIV therapy may reduce admissions in those with chronic hypercapnic respiratory failure, although a specific effect on reducing exacerbations has not been demonstrated. Pulmonary rehabilitation has also been shown to reduce hospitalization in patients with COPD. Furthermore, early treatment that might be included in a patient education program can reduce exacerbation length.

The finding that exacerbation susceptibility varies among COPD patients means it is particularly important to target exacerbation reduction interventions at those most likely to develop these events. The simplest way is to ask patients how many courses of systemic (antibiotic and corticosteroid) therapy they received for exacerbations over the past 12 months. Patients receiving two or more such courses ("frequent exacerbators") are likely to remain frequent exacerbators in the future and should be offered all appropriate exacerbation reduction interventions (see Figure 43-1).

Therefore, a variety of measures may be instituted to reduce the number and consequences of exacerbations, and COPD patients most in need can be identified by asking about prior exacerbation history. For this reason, and for further assessment of patients who present in respiratory failure, it is usually appropriate to review patients in an ambulatory care setting after admission with an acute exacerbation.

CONCLUSION

Research into exacerbations of COPD is moving rapidly. Not many years ago, these events were considered nothing more than "troublesome" deteriorations in symptoms without long-term consequence. We now know this is not true, but many unanswered questions remain. We still understand little about how bacterial and viral pathogens interact. More effective anti-inflammatory agents are required, and the optimal role of antibiotics in preventing exacerbations remains to be defined. We currently have no effective interventions targeting viral pathogens, especially rhinovirus. Understanding why some patients appear more susceptible to exacerbations could lead to the development of new therapeutic approaches. Also, it is now recognized that COPD is associated with systemic inflammation that may cause considerable cardiovascular comorbidity, and ways to assess and manage this may reduce the number and impact of exacerbations in patients with chronic obstructive pulmonary disease.

WEB RESOURCES AND GUIDELINES/PROTOCOLS

World Health Organization (WHO) Global Initiative for Obstructive Lung Disease (GOLD). www.goldcopd.com.

American Thoracic Society (ATS)/European Respiratory Society (ERS) standards for the diagnosis and treatment of COPD. www.ersnet.org.

United Kingdom National Institute for Clinical Excellence (NICE) COPD guidelines. www.nice.org.uk.

Cochrane Airways Group (up-to-date, accurate systematic reviews and meta-analyses). www.cochrane-airways.ac.uk.

SUGGESTED READINGS

Anthonisen NR, Manfreda J, Warren CP, et al: Antibiotic therapy in exacerbations of chronic obstructive pulmonary disease, *Ann Intern Med* 106:196–204, 1987.

Hurst JR, Vestbo J, Anzueto A, et al: Susceptibility to exacerbation in chronic obstructive pulmonary disease, *N Engl J Med* 363:1128–1138, 2010.

Lightowler JV, Wedzicha JA, Elliott MW, et al: Non-invasive positive pressure ventilation to treat respiratory failure resulting from exacerbations of chronic obstructive pulmonary disease: Cochrane systematic review and meta-analysis, *BMJ* 326:185–187, 2003.

Niewoehner DE, Erbland ML, Deupree RH, et al: Effect of systemic glucocorticoids on exacerbations of chronic obstructive pulmonary disease, *N Engl J Med* 340:1941–1947, 1999.

Saint S, Bent S, Vittinghoff E, Grady D: Antibiotics in chronic obstructive pulmonary disease exacerbations. A meta-analysis. *JAMA* 273:957–960, 1995.

Seemungal TAR, Donaldson GC, Bhowmik A, et al: Time course and recovery of exacerbations in chronic obstructive pulmonary disease, *Am J Respir Crit Care Med* 161:1608–1613, 2000.

Sethi S, Evans N, Grant BJB, et al: New strains of bacteria and exacerbations of chronic obstructive pulmonary disease, *N Engl J Med* 347:465–471, 2002.

Wedzicha JA, Martinez FJ, editors: *Lung biology in health and disease*, Vol 228. *Chronic obstructive pulmonary disease exacerbations*, New York, 2009, Informa Healthcare.

Chapter **44**

Cystic Fibrosis

Felix Ratjen • Elizabeth Tullis

Cystic fibrosis (CF) is a common, fatal, autosomal recessive disorder. Its frequency varies among populations, with approximately 1 in 3300 live births in Caucasians, 1 in 15,000 in African Americans, and 1 in 32,000 in Asians. Although reports of CF exist from medieval times, it was first described and recognized as a genetic disease by Anderson in 1938. Although the increase in sweat chloride and sodium concentrations was observed by Saint Agnese in the 1950s, it was not until 1983 that Paul Quinton described the defective chloride transport in sweat glands and respiratory epithelium as the underlying abnormality. The discovery of the causative, mutated gene encoding a defective chloride channel in epithelial cells in 1989 elucidated the pathophysiology of CF and opened up new avenues of treatment. Despite these major advances, however, it is still unclear how mutations in the cystic fibrosis transmembrane regulator *(CFTR)* gene precisely cause the multifaceted manifestations of CF disease.

GENETICS

Cystic fibrosis is caused by mutations in a gene on chromosome 7 encoding the protein subsequently termed the *CFTR* gene. More than 1800 mutations have been reported to the Cystic Fibrosis Genetic Analysis Consortium. Most of these mutations are rare, and only four mutations occur in a frequency of more than 1%. *CFTR* mutations can be grouped into five classes: *CFTR* is not synthesized (I), is inadequately processed (II), is not regulated (III), shows abnormal conductance (IV), or has partially defective production or processing (V). Class I, II, and III mutations are more common and associated with pancreatic insufficiency, whereas patients with the less common class IV and V mutations often are "pancreatic sufficient" (**Figure 44-1**).

The most common mutation worldwide, found in approximately 66% of patients with CF, is a class II mutation caused by a deletion of *phenylalanine* in position 508 (F508del) of *CFTR*. F508del *CFTR* is misfolded and trapped in the endoplasmic reticulum (ER) and subsequently proteolytically degraded. However, small amounts of F508del *CFTR* reach the plasma membrane of epithelial cells and have some functional activity. These findings suggest that F508del *CFTR* rescue from ER degradation may be a potential therapeutic intervention.

The *CFTR* gene belongs to a family of transmembrane proteins called adenosine triphosphate (ATP)–binding cassette (ABC) transporters and functions as a chloride (Cl⁻) channel in apical membranes. However, *CFTR* possesses other functions in addition to being a chloride channel. *CFTR* has been described as a regulator of other membrane channels, including the *epithelial sodium channel* (eNaC) and the *outwardly rectifying chloride channel* (ORCC). *CFTR* also transports or regulates

bicarbonate (HCO_3^-) transport through epithelial cell membranes and may act as a transporter for other proteins, such as glutathione.

A relationship exists between *CFTR* genotype and clinical phenotype in CF. Patients who carry two "severe" mutations (classes I, II, and III) that cause loss of function in *CFTR* have *classic* CF, characterized by pancreatic insufficiency, early age of diagnosis, and elevated sweat chloride. In contrast, patients who have at least one "mild" mutation with partial function in *CFTR* are typically diagnosed at an older age, have sweat chloride values closer to normal, and are pancreatic sufficient.

Whereas classes IV and V *CFTR* mutations are linked with pancreatic sufficiency, attempts to link specific mutations to the severity of lung disease have shown large phenotypic variability. This is best documented for patients homozygous for the F508del mutation who exhibit a wide spectrum in lung disease severity. This wide phenotypic variation suggests that environmental factors and genes other than *CFTR* influence the development, progression, and disease severity of CF (**Figure 44-2**).

PATHOPHYSIOLOGY

Although there is ongoing debate on how *CFTR* mutations cause disease, some of the fundamental questions have been clarified in recent years. *CFTR* is expressed in higher quantities in tissues clinically affected by CF, such as sinuses, lungs, pancreas, liver, gastrointestinal (GI) tract, and reproductive tract, although low levels also occur elsewhere. Because lung disease is the most pertinent clinical feature of CF, the focus here is on its pathophysiology in the respiratory tract.

Airway epithelial cells secrete chloride and absorb sodium chloride (NaCl), the balance of which is regulated through apical channels, including *CFTR* (**Figure 44-3**). Ion secretion and absorption affect water transport, and a balance between secretion and absorption is thought to be important to maintain an adequate layer of *airway surface liquid* (ASL). The ASL supports the thin mucous layer on top of epithelial cells, which is constantly transported out of the lungs through ciliary movement. Lack or dysfunction of *CFTR* leads to reduced chloride secretion and NaCl hyperabsorption with depletion of ASL. In the absence of adequate ASL, respiratory cilia collapse, leading to breakdown of mucociliary transport. Mucus accumulates in the lower airways, and inhaled bacteria are trapped in this viscous mucous layer on top of respiratory epithelial cells.

The spectrum of bacteria that are relevant for CF lung disease is relatively limited. Overall, *Pseudomonas aeruginosa* is the most common isolate, followed by *Staphylococcus aureus* and *Haemophilus influenzae*. Later in the course of disease, multiresistant organisms such as *Stenotrophomonas maltophilia*,

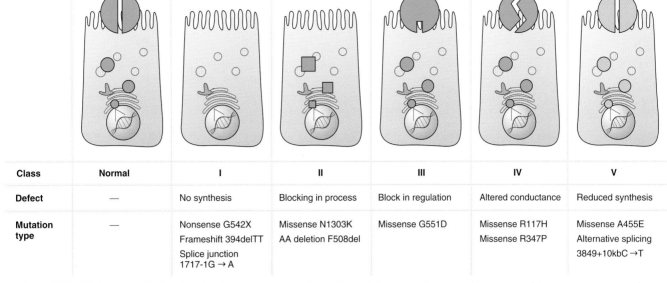

Class	Normal	I	II	III	IV	V
Defect	—	No synthesis	Blocking in process	Block in regulation	Altered conductance	Reduced synthesis
Mutation type	—	Nonsense G542X Frameshift 394delTT Splice junction 1717-1G → A	Missense N1303K AA deletion F508del	Missense G551D	Missense R117H Missense R347P	Missense A455E Alternative splicing 3849+10kbC →T

Figure 44-1 Major classes (I-V) and molecular consequences of cystic fibrosis transmembrane conductance regulator *(CFTR)* gene mutations.

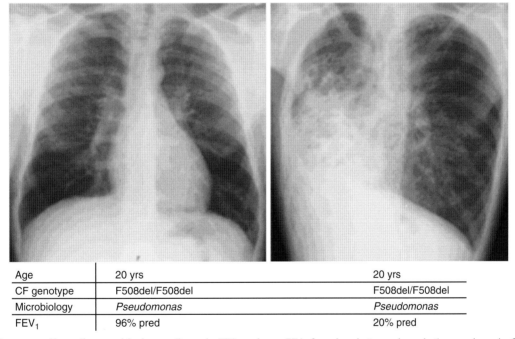

Age	20 yrs	20 yrs
CF genotype	F508del/F508del	F508del/F508del
Microbiology	*Pseudomonas*	*Pseudomonas*
FEV₁	96% pred	20% pred

Figure 44-2 Spectrum of lung disease with chest radiograph, FEV₁, and age. *FEV₁,* forced expiratory volume in 1 second. *pred,* of predicted value.

Achromobacter (Alcaligenes) xylosoxidans, and *Burkholderia cepacia* complex may be isolated. As in other chronic pulmonary diseases, nontuberculous mycobacteria (usually *Mycobacterium avium-intracellulare* or *M. abscessus*) may be isolated. It is challenging to prove whether these organisms are causing ongoing disease requiring treatment, or if they are colonizing only the damaged lung. For a more detailed discussion of nontuberculous mycobacteria (NTM) infections, see Chapter 31.

Stenotrophomonas maltophilia, Alcaligenes xylosoxidans, and *Burkholderia cepacia* complex are isolated in less than 10% of patients with CF. *B. cepacia* complex is an unusual organism that is found in the environment (soil and water) and causes chronic infection in only CF and chronic granulomatous disease. It is inherently multiresistant and difficult to treat and in CF is associated with a significantly worse prognosis. There is evidence for person-to-person spread in patients with CF.

Approximately 15% to 20% of patients with CF who are infected with *B. cepacia* complex will have rapidly progressive deterioration, so-called cepacia syndrome, with necrotizing pneumonia, greatly elevated white blood cell (WBC) counts, bacteremia, and almost 100% mortality.

The mucus in CF lacks oxygen, leading to anaerobic growth conditions for bacteria. Anaerobic bacteria exist in high numbers in CF airways, but their clinical significance is uncertain. The anaerobic growth conditions trigger a switch of *S. aureus* and *P. aeruginosa* from nonmucoid to mucoid cell types, the predominant phenotype in CF lungs. These mucoid strains form biofilms in CF airways that are resistant to killing by the host defense system, resulting in chronic infection. Inflammatory products (e.g., elastase) released by neutrophils stimulate mucus secretion, perpetuating the cycle of mucus retention, infection, and inflammation.

Figure 44-3 Restoring airway surface liquid in cystic fibrosis. *(From Ratjen F: Restoring airway surface liquid in cystic fibrosis, N Engl J Med 354:291–293, 2006.)*

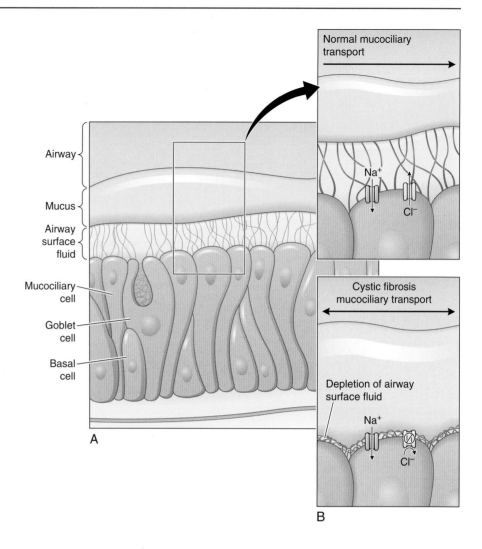

Evidence indicates that inflammation is dysregulated in CF airways. Neutrophilic airway inflammation has been detected in infants with CF in the first months of life, as well as in CF fetal lung tissue. Whether or not inflammation is directly related to the *CFTR* defect is still disputed. However, an exaggerated, sustained, and prolonged inflammatory response to bacterial and viral pathogens is an accepted feature of CF lung disease. The persistent endobronchial inflammation is deleterious for the course of lung disease (**Figure 44-4**).

Exocrine pancreatic insufficiency is present in approximately 85% to 90% of patients with CF, generally in those patients who carry two copies of the class I, II, or III *CFTR* mutations. The exocrine pancreas has great functional reserve, and 98% to 99% of its function must be lost before malabsorption will occur. Patients who are pancreatic sufficient do not have normal pancreatic exocrine function but have sufficient function to prevent fat malabsorption. Pancreatic disease begins in utero and is thought to result from decreased volume of pancreatic secretions with decreased concentrations of HCO_3^-. Without sufficient fluid and HCO_3^-, digestive proenzymes are retained within small pancreatic ducts and are prematurely activated, ultimately leading to tissue destruction, fibrosis, and fatty replacement. The resulting malabsorption contributes to the failure to meet the increased energy demands because of the hypermetabolic state associated with endobronchial

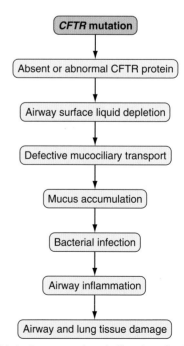

Figure 44-4 Sequence of cystic fibrosis pathophysiology.

infection. Lung infections may lead to anorexia and vomiting, promoting malnutrition. These factors may exacerbate lung infection, leading to a vicious cycle of malnutrition and infection.

CLINICAL FEATURES

Typical signs and symptoms for CF are listed in **Box 44-1**. Symptoms of CF may vary, with monosymptomatic cases often diagnosed late. It is therefore important to be aware of the spectrum of symptoms that may arise and to initiate adequate diagnostic steps.

Although the classic presentation of CF is the combination of chronic productive cough, steatorrhea, and failure to thrive, 10% to 15% of patients do not have pancreatic insufficiency clinically. Because the lungs of patients with CF are normal at birth, pulmonary symptoms may not be obvious. Between 10% and 15% of newborn infants with CF may fail to pass meconium, leading to *meconium ileus*, which is linked to pancreatic insufficiency but not directly associated with more severe clinical disease.

Less common presentations of CF, such as prolonged jaundice in the newborn and rectal prolapse in infants and young children, should trigger diagnostic tests. Occasionally, an infant may have severe malnutrition with anemia, hypoalbuminemia, and edema in the first 4 months of life.

Infertility can be a presenting symptom in adult patients with CF with limited pulmonary symptoms; 98% of males with CF are infertile, with *azoospermia* secondary to atretic or absent vas deferens. Spermatogenesis and sexual potency are normal. Female reproductive function is normal, although a lower rate of fertility has been postulated because of dehydrated cervical mucus.

Initially, pulmonary symptoms of cough will occur only at times of exacerbations, but eventually there is progression to a chronic daily cough productive of sputum. The sputum is initially white, but as infection continues, the mucus becomes thicker and purulent. Minor hemoptysis often occurs at exacerbation. Some patients have an "asthmatic" component to their disease, with wheezing, chest tightness, paroxysmal dry cough, and a degree of reversibility in airflow obstruction with bronchodilators. Over time, as pulmonary function declines, there is increasing dyspnea. Hypoxemia is not usually seen until forced expiratory volume in 1 second (FEV_1) is less than 35% of predicted value, and hypercarbia usually occurs when the FEV_1 is less than 25% or 30% predicted. Cor pulmonale occurs late in the illness.

Pansinusitis is found on sinus radiographs in most patients, although not all will have symptoms of recurrent sinusitis, headache, and postnasal drip. Nasal polyps are seen in approximately 20% of patients and tend to recur even after surgical removal.

DIAGNOSTIC APPROACH

The diagnosis of cystic fibrosis is established by clinical manifestations (see Box 44-1), a history of CF in a sibling, or a positive newborn screening result, in conjunction with laboratory evidence of *CFTR* dysfunction. *CFTR* dysfunction is documented by elevated sweat chloride or characteristic abnormalities in nasal potential difference or by CF-causing mutations in the *CFTR* gene.

A diagnostic algorithm is presented in **Figure 44-5**. Abnormal ion transport is reflected in high sweat NaCl levels, and measurement of chloride concentration in sweat after iontophoresis of pilocarpine is used for diagnosis. Sweat testing must be done using standardized methods, by qualified staff in an experienced laboratory. A sweat chloride concentration greater than 60 mmol/L on repeated analysis is diagnostic for CF; 30 to 60 mmol/L is considered a "borderline" result but may be seen in patients with CF.

Diagnosis can be confirmed by genotyping of the most common *CFTR* mutations, which vary by ethnic origin of the population tested. More than 1800 mutations in *CFTR* have been reported to the *CFTR* database. Most commercial screening panels test for less than 50 mutations and will identify 85% to 90% of CF alleles. Although *CFTR* mutation testing has had no clinical implications in the past, this may change with the introduction of mutation-specific therapy (see later discussion).

The diagnosis of CF requires the presence of two CF-causing mutations. To be considered CF-causing, the mutation must (1) cause a change in the amino acid sequence that severely affects *CFTR* synthesis or function, (2) introduce a premature termination signal (insertion, deletion, or nonsense mutations), (3) alter the "invariant" nucleotides of intron splice sites (first or last two nucleotides), *or* (4) cause a novel amino acid sequence that does not occur in the normal *CFTR* genes from at least 100 carriers of CF mutations from the patient's ethnic group. Of the more than 1800 *CFTR* mutations reported, only approximately 25 are considered disease-causing to date.

If *CFTR* genotyping or sweat test is not diagnostic, a second test of *CFTR* function such as *nasal potential difference* (NPD) measurement can be performed. The transport of Na^+ and Cl^- ions across the nasal mucosa creates a transepithelial electrical potential difference. Changes in NPD in response to stimulation or inhibition of ion channels by nasal perfusion can be measured, and a typical normal or CF response exists. The NPD test is technically difficult, requiring a skilled operator, and therefore is not available in all CF centers. Standard operating procedures and reference values have recently been determined. Other techniques to examine *CFTR* function include analysis of rectal mucosal biopsies in an Ussing chamber.

Box 44-1 **Symptoms and Signs of Cystic Fibrosis (CF)**

Chronic Airway Disease
Chronic productive cough
Airway colonization with CF pathogens (*Staphylococcus aureus*, mucoid *Pseudomonas aeruginosa*)
Persistent chest radiograph abnormalities
Airway obstruction
Digital clubbing
Pansinusitis
Nasal polyps

Gastrointestinal Disease
Meconium ileus
Distal intestinal obstruction syndrome
Rectal prolapse
Pancreatic insufficiency, pancreatitis
Biliary cirrhosis
Failure to thrive
Edema with hypoproteinemia
Deficiency of fat-soluble vitamins

Other
Salt wasting with metabolic alkalosis
Infertility caused by obstructive azoospermia

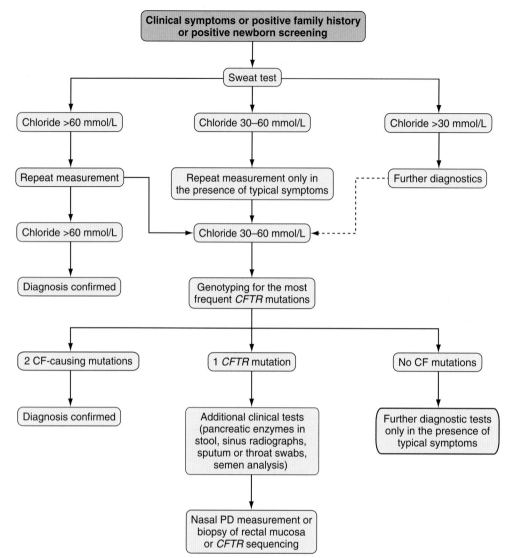

Figure 44-5 Diagnostic algorithm for cystic fibrosis *(CF)*. *PD*, potential difference.

Clinical tests not directly assessing the *CFTR* defect can also aid in the diagnostic process. Most patients with CF are pancreatic insufficient, and a decreased concentration of chymotrypsin or pancreas-specific elastase in feces or 72-hour stool collection with fecal fat analysis can confirm this. Most patients with CF have total opacification of paranasal sinuses, and sinus radiography may be helpful. Bacterial pathogens typical for CF (e.g., mucoid *Pseudomonas*, *S. aureus*) can be detected in sputum or throat swabs and suggest a CF diagnosis. Obstructive azoospermia is found in 98% of men with CF and is a result of *congenital bilateral absence of the vas deferens* (CBAVD). The finding of azoospermia, or lack of vas deferens on careful urologic examination or transrectal ultrasound, suggests CF.

In the past, about 50% of patients with CF in North America were diagnosed by age 6 months and 90% by 8 years. Neonatal screening has been proposed as early diagnosis, and therefore earlier initiation of treatment may improve outcome. A randomized screening program in Wisconsin state found that weight gain and early growth were better in patients diagnosed by neonatal screening. Because good nutrition is linked to a better prognosis, these data would favor the introduction of population-wide neonatal screening. Neonatal screening programs have now been introduced in many countries, most often

based on a two-step approach, with immunoreactive trypsinogen (IRT) in dried blood spots and confirmation by DNA analysis in positive cases. Blood trypsinogen is elevated in pancreatic-insufficient patients in the first weeks of life, but the rate of false-positive results of a single IRT test is high, which can be reduced substantially by inclusions of a second step, including genetic testing for the most common *CFTR* mutations.

DIAGNOSTIC CHALLENGES

In 5% to 10% of patients, the diagnosis of CF is not made until adulthood. Increased awareness continues to result in more adults being diagnosed with CF. Most will not have typical features of CF but rather single-organ disease (CBAVD, recurrent acute pancreatitis, or bronchiectasis) or symptoms that develop later in life. Most patients diagnosed as adults are pancreatic sufficient, have "borderline" sweat chloride tests, and have mutations in the *CFTR* gene that are not considered CF-causing. Commercial genetic screening panels may have diagnostic limitations for patients seen in adulthood by including the more common CF-causing mutations usually seen in childhood diagnosis. Adults are more likely to have less common *CFTR* mutations that are not part of the panel. Complete sequencing of the *CFTR* gene has now become feasible and may offer additional information to assist in the diagnosis of CF, especially for patients with equivocal sweat test results. NPD measurement may be especially helpful in establishing a diagnosis of CF in these patients. Interpretation of these results should be done by an experienced CF physician, who is aware of the limitations of these tests.

Obstructive azoospermia is highly related to mutations in *CFTR*, and the finding of CBAVD should trigger genetic testing for CF, especially because assisted reproductive techniques allow these men to father children. Up to 80% of men with CBAVD may have one or two *CFTR* mutations but no other phenotypic features of CF. A diagnosis of CF should not be made in these cases unless diagnostic criteria are met (sweat test >60 mmol/L or 2 CF-causing mutations). The long-term prognosis for these men is still not certain, including whether typical CF lung disease may develop over time, and thus they should receive appropriate clinical follow-up. The relationship between *CFTR* mutations and recurrent acute pancreatitis, bronchiectasis, or other sinopulmonary disease is not as strong as that seen with CBAVD. However, a higher-than-expected prevalence of *CFTR* mutations is found in these populations.

Despite all these tests, a small number of patients remain in whom a definite diagnosis cannot be made. Typical CF bronchiectasis may be seen in patients who have *CFTR* mutations that are not considered disease-causing and who have a normal or borderline sweat chloride test. Thus, it seems that CF lung disease may occur even with lesser degrees of dysfunction of *CFTR*. The important message is that presence of *CFTR* mutations may put patients at risk for significant CF disease developing later in life, and close follow-up is advised.

This dilemma is further complicated by lack of a common and standardized terminology for patients who have evidence of *CFTR* dysfunction without a definite diagnosis of CF. These patients are being referred to as *atypical* CF, *mild* CF, *nonclassic* CF, or CFTR*opathy*, or if *CFTR* mutations exist in the absence of lung or GI disease, *pre*-CF. The current preferred term for patients with a CF clinical phenotype and evidence of *CFTR* dysfunction but do not meet diagnostic criteria for CF is *CFTR-related disorder.*

CLINICAL COURSE OF LUNG DISEASE AND PRINCIPLES OF THERAPY

The lungs of newborns with CF are normal at birth. Pathologic studies show that the first abnormalities are usually detected in the small airways reflected by mucous plugs and dilation distal to the obstructed airways. These early abnormalities are often focal and do not necessarily produce clinically apparent symptoms. The disconnect between pathologic abnormalities and pulmonary symptoms is now recognized and has important implications for treatment. Studies that use bronchoalveolar lavage fluid show that ongoing airway inflammation is present in patients with mild disease and can be observed early in infancy. The lack of impressive symptoms does not mean that these patients do not have ongoing progressive disease requiring continuous treatment.

Although the traditional approach was to wait for symptoms, a more aggressive strategy is used today. This aggressive approach translates into continuous lifelong treatment, which is time-consuming and labor-intensive for patients and their families. Although the burden for individuals is considerable, it has changed the natural history of disease progression in patients with CF. The classic course of CF was characterized by chronic productive cough and a gradual, but steady, decline in pulmonary function Now most patients with CF maintain their pulmonary function over years, reflected in an annual rate of decline in FEV_1 of less than 2% predicted per year, and many do not regularly expectorate sputum until adulthood. However, it is important to be vigilant about periods of deterioration that present as episodes of pulmonary exacerbations and, unless treated rapidly and aggressively, may lead to an irreversible loss in pulmonary function.

Pulmonary exacerbations in patients with CF are often triggered by viral infections but require prompt treatment with antibiotics directed against pathogens present in respiratory cultures. It is important to recognize the signs of a pulmonary exacerbation early to avoid permanent damage to the lung (**Box 44-2**). In general, any increase in symptoms lasting more than a few days, associated with a decline in FEV_1, requires antibiotic therapy. Because most CF patients are chronically infected with bacteria, suppression rather than eradication of organisms is the primary goal of therapy. Duration of therapy is not guided by changes in sputum bacteriology but rather by improvement in symptoms and pulmonary function.

Because many patients have normal lung function and the annual rate of decline in pulmonary function is minimal, it has become difficult to assess lung disease by lung function alone. Despite this, FEV_1 remains the best predictor of outcome in patients with CF and is therefore used to follow the course of lung disease and to guide treatment. Chest radiographs are performed annually in most centers but have limited sensitivity to detect early abnormalities. High-resolution computed tomography can detect abnormalities not detected by conventional radiography, but CT is associated with a higher cumulative radiation dose and thus not considered part of routine care at present. There is considerable interest in developing more sensitive outcome parameters assessing function, structure,

---

Box 44-2 **Symptoms and Signs of Pulmonary Exacerbation in Cystic Fibrosis Patients**

Symptoms

Increased frequency, duration, and intensity of cough
Increased or new-onset sputum production
Change in sputum appearance
New-onset or increased hemoptysis
Increased shortness of breath; decreased exercise tolerance
Decrease in overall well-being: increased fatigue, weakness, fever, poor appetite

Physical Signs

Increased work of breathing: intercostal retractions and use of accessory muscles
Increased respiratory rate
New-onset or increased crackles on chest examination
Increased air trapping
Fever
Weight loss

Laboratory Findings

Decrease in FEV_1 of 10% or greater compared with best value in previous 6 months
Increased air trapping and/or new infiltrate on chest radiograph
Leukocytosis
Decreased oxygen saturation (SaO_2)

Data from Gibson RL, Burns JL, Ramsey BW: *Am J Respir Crit Care Med* 168:918-951, 2003.
FEV_1, forced expiratory volume in 1 second.

infection, and inflammation to help guide treatment, but currently these tests have a limited role outside of research studies.

Treating bacterial infections and avoiding lung function decline are key to management of CF patients, with regular assessment of clinical status, lung function, and sputum microbiology. Quarterly clinic visits are considered standard in CF care, but some patients require more frequent follow-up.

TREATMENT

GENE REPLACEMENT THERAPY AND PHARMACOTHERAPY

Cystic fibrosis is caused by deficient or absent *CFTR*, and thus gene replacement therapy is a form of curative treatment. Trials so far have targeted the respiratory tract directly. A number of vector systems have been tested in human trials, but adenoviruses and cationic lipids are the two most common vectors. Even though some transient effect on *CFTR* expression and function has been achieved, no study could demonstrate a long-lasting effect. Viral vectors seem to be more efficient than cationic lipids but have the disadvantage of being immunogenic. Although attempts are ongoing to overcome these shortcomings, gene therapy is currently not a therapeutic option for patients with CF.

Another approach to treat the underlying defect is *CFTR* pharmacotherapy aiming to improve trafficking, expression, or function of *CFTR*. For patients carrying class I *stop* mutations, which lead to premature termination codons in the messenger RNA and therefore truncated protein production, treatment with aminoglycosides or its derivative ataluren has been shown to increase *CFTR* expression. Uncontrolled studies also show improved chloride channel function in the nasal epithelium as well as positive trends in lung function. A larger placebo-controlled trial now underway will further clarify clinical benefits of this therapy.

Because most patients do not carry stop mutations, this approach addresses only a small fraction of the CF population. A potentiator of *CFTR* function, VX770, has been tested in patients with the G551D mutation, in which *CFTR* is present on the cell surface but channel function is reduced. Recent studies demonstrate that treatment not only improved lung function, but also reduced sweat chloride concentrations below the threshold clearly diagnostic for CF. A subsequent longer study confirmed these results, and VX770 has become the first *CFTR* modulator to be licensed for clinical use.

For the most common mutation, F508del, misfolded *CFTR* is degraded in the ER before reaching the cell membrane. Because this misfolded *CFTR* does have Cl⁻-conducting function, compounds that affect intracellular trafficking, called *chaperones*, may provide clinical benefit. Some studies have provided proof of concept, and one compound derived from high-throughput screening programs, VX809, is currently tested in clinical trials. Safety has been confirmed in early trials. Because the *CFTR* potentiator VX770 greatly enhanced the effect of *CFTR* corrector therapy in vitro, combination therapy with VX809 is also being tested to enhance therapeutic efficacy.

An alternative to *CFTR* pharmacotherapy is to activate other Cl⁻ channels present in the apical surface of epithelial cells or to inhibit Na⁺ hyperabsorption. This concept seems useful because CF mice lacking *CFTR* do not develop lung disease, which may be caused by better function of alternative Cl⁻ channels. Whether activation of alternative Cl⁻ channels or inhibition of Na⁺ hyperabsorption is a valid treatment option is currently unclear. Denufosol, an activator of alternative chloride secretion, has undergone a full development program and showed promise in improving lung function in both Phase II studies and a 6-month placebo-controlled Phase III trial. However, the second Phase III trial failed to confirm these findings.

SYMPTOMATIC THERAPY

In the absence of a proven curative regimen, symptomatic treatment is still the mainstay of CF therapy. Most of the treatment approaches are directed at interrupting the cycle of mucus retention, infection, and inflammation. Early initiation of therapy is important to avoid permanent damage to the lung.

Airway Clearance

Chest physiotherapy remains the mainstay of airway clearance and is recommended for all patients. Short-term benefits have been demonstrated for many techniques, but long-term efficacy data are limited. The most common techniques are manual percussion, positive expiratory pressure (PEP) mask therapy, and autogenic drainage. In addition, techniques that provide vibration to the airways actively or passively are being used. Debate is ongoing as to which technique provides the best efficacy for patients with CF. Physical activity and exercise are considered important adjuncts to physiotherapy, because impairments in exercise tolerance have been linked to poorer prognosis in CF patients.

Airway secretions in CF patients are highly viscous, indicating the use of drugs that reduce the viscoelasticity of sputum. Classic *mucolytics* such as *N*-acetylcysteine have little effect on lung disease in CF, although they are being revisited because of their potential benefit as antioxidants. Their ineffectiveness as a mucolytic may be because CF mucus contains little mucin and is mainly composed of pus. *Recombinant human deoxyribonuclease* (rhDNase) administered by inhalation reduced sputum viscosity, improved pulmonary function, and reduced the number of pulmonary exacerbations in patients with moderate and with mild lung disease. Data also suggest that rhDNase reduces inflammation in the airways. *Hypertonic saline* has been assessed as another potential drug to improve airway clearance, and recent studies suggest that it may also increase airway surface liquid. The effect on lung function seems to be smaller than that of rhDNase, but these therapies have different mechanisms of action and thus cannot be viewed as virtually exclusive. Hypertonic saline also reduces the frequency of pulmonary exacerbations, an important outcome because these are associated with decreased lung function.

Treatment of Airway Infection

Aggressive treatment of airway infection is a main reason for the increased life expectancy of patients with CF achieved over recent decades. As mentioned, bacterial pathogens in patients with CF are usually limited to a relatively small spectrum, with *S. aureus* or *H. influenzae* the most prominent in younger patients and *P. aeruginosa* in older patients. Most patients go through phases of clinical stability with intermittent pulmonary exacerbations. A set of criteria is used to diagnose pulmonary exacerbations (see Box 44-2), but the threshold for initiating targeted antibiotic therapy should be rather low. Genotyping has shown that the organisms present at exacerbation are the same as when the patient is clinically stable, but with higher bacterial density. Thus, choice of antimicrobial therapy on the basis of the most recent sputum cultures is indicated.

Pulmonary exacerbations are usually treated with intravenous (IV) antibiotic therapy, although oral therapy is used for exacerbations associated with minimal or no drop in lung function. Antistaphylococcal antibiotics are usually administered for 2 to 4 weeks. Patients with CF have differences in drug clearance and require dosages approximately 50% higher than individuals without CF. For patients with *Pseudomonas* infection, combination therapy with a semisynthetic penicillin (e.g., piperacillin), a third-generation cephalosporin (e.g., ceftazidime), or a carbapenem (imipenem or meropenem) with an aminoglycoside (most frequently tobramycin) is administered for 2 to 3 weeks. Oral ciprofloxacin is used for less severe exacerbations.

Treatment of the less common gram-negative organisms such as *B. cepacia* complex, *A. xylosoxidans*, and *S. maltophilia*, can be challenging. These organisms are inherently multiresistant. Although infection with *B. cepacia* complex is clearly associated with a worse prognosis, the relevance of the other gram-negative bacteria is less clear, and currently it is not established whether they are responsible for causing disease. For patients chronically infected with *B. cepacia* complex, trimethoprim-sulfamethoxazole (TMP-SMX) or doxycycline is effective for minor exacerbations. For more severe infections, the best in vitro antibiotics consist of meropenem, and high-dose inhaled tobramycin in combination with either ceftazidime, chloramphenicol, or TMP-SMX. Treatment of exacerbations with *B. cepacia* complex may require prolonged antibiotic therapy (weeks to months) before a clinical response is seen. Use of pulmonary function, WBC count, and markers of inflammation (CRP or ESR) may be helpful to guide therapy. *S. maltophilia* can be treated with TMP-SMX or doxycycline. Because *S. maltophilia* isolates can develop resistance during treatment, TMP-SMX is often combined with a second antibiotic, such as ticarcillin-clavulanate or levofloxacin. *A. xylosoxidans* can be challenging to treat, but options include imipenem and piperacillin. Inhaled colistin may also be effective, because in vitro studies found that high concentrations of colistin inhibit most strains of *A. xylosoxidans*.

Many CF physicians try to eradicate bacteria from CF airways with courses of oral antibiotics even in the absence of symptoms. Prophylactic antistaphylococcal therapy with flucloxacillin initiated at diagnosis is also used in some centers. Although one small study has reported a lower rate of cough and hospital admissions during the first 2 years of life, continuous antistaphylococcal therapy was associated with a higher rate of *P. aeruginosa* acquisition in two other studies, in which mainly cephalosporins were used. *P. aeruginosa* infection increases pulmonary inflammation and has a negative effect on lung function when this pathogen persists. At present, there is insufficient evidence to support the use of prophylactic antistaphylococcal therapy in patients with CF.

Overall, *Pseudomonas aeruginosa* is the major pathogen in CF lung disease. Its prevalence increases with age, and most adult patients are chronically infected with this organism. After an initial transient colonization period with nonmucoid strains, untreated patients generally become chronically infected with mucoid strains of *P. aeruginosa*. Antibiotic therapy usually fails to eradicate mucoid *P. aeruginosa* from the airways. High bacterial counts, low metabolic rate of pathogens in biofilms, poor penetration of antibiotics into airway secretions, and anaerobic conditions in sputum are considered responsible for this finding.

Chronic infection with mucoid strains has a negative impact on the subsequent course of lung disease. Although eradication is virtually impossible in chronic infection, treatment can be effective in the early phase of *P. aeruginosa* infection; a major improvement in patients with CF is early antibiotic therapy. Both inhaled antibiotic therapy with tobramycin alone and combined inhaled antibiotics and oral ciprofloxacin have been used, but more recent evidence suggests that adding ciprofloxacin does not increase therapeutic success. Although the optimal treatment regimen for early *P. aeruginosa* infection has yet to be determined, inhaled tobramycin successfully reduces the incidence of chronic airway infection with *P. aeruginosa* in patients with CF (**Table 44-1**).

To avoid adverse effects and to obtain high drug concentrations in airways, inhaled antibiotic therapy is the treatment of choice for maintenance therapy in patients with *P. aeruginosa* infection. The best evidence currently available is for inhaled *tobramycin*, which has been shown to improve lung function and reduce pulmonary exacerbations in chronically infected patients. In addition, *colistin* is being used "off label" for inhalation. Although colistin has the advantage of low prevalence of resistant strains, its short-term efficacy is inferior to inhaled tobramycin. Inhaled *aztreonam* has been recently licensed as an alternative option to tobramycin based on two controlled clinical trials demonstrating its efficacy. A comparison to inhaled tobramycin also found similar efficacy with aztreonam and suggested superior lung function benefits during therapy; however, most of the patients were previously treated with inhaled tobramycin, which may favor the response to

Table 44-1	**Options for Oral and Inhaled Antibiotic Therapy**	
Antibiotic: **Choose One**	**Pediatric Dose**	**Adult Dose**
Staphylococcus aureus		
Dicloxacillin	6.25-12.5 mg/kg four times daily	250-500 mg four times daily
Cephalexin	12.5-25 mg/kg four times daily	500 mg four times daily
Amoxicillin/ clavulanate	12.5-22.5 mg/kg amoxicillin*	400-875 mg amoxicillin*
Haemophilus influenzae		
Amoxicillin	25-50 mg/kg twice daily	500-875 mg twice daily
Amoxicillin/ clavulanate	12.5-22.5 mg/kg amoxicillin*	400-875 mg of amoxicillin*
Cefuroxime axetil	15-20 mg/kg twice daily	250-500 mg twice daily
Pseudomonas aeruginosa		
Ciprofloxacin	10-15 mg/kg twice daily	750 mg twice daily
Tobramycin[†]	300 mg by nebulizer, twice daily	300 mg by nebulizer, twice daily
Colistin[†]	150 mg by nebulizer, twice daily	150 mg by nebulizer, twice daily

Modified from Gibson RL, Burns JL, Ramsey BW: *Am J Respir Crit Care Med* 168:918-951, 2003.
*Component twice daily.
[†]By inhalation.

aztreonam. Both tobramycin and aztreonam have been studied in cycles of 28 days on and 28 days off, so many clinicians have also started to use both treatments in alternate months to avoid deterioration during the off periods.

Some centers treat chronically infected CF patients with routine IV antibiotic therapy every 3 months, regardless of respiratory symptoms, but this approach has not yet been supported by sufficient evidence.

In addition to inhaled antibiotics, *azithromycin* can improve pulmonary function and reduce pulmonary exacerbations in patients with *P. aeruginosa*–positive disease and more recently has been shown to reduce exacerbations in *P. aeruginosa*–negative patients as well. Although macrolides have no efficacy against *P. aeruginosa* when tested in routine cultures, some evidence suggests macrolides may affect *P. aeruginosa* growing in biofilms. Whether this explains their efficacy or whether this is caused by antiinflammatory properties of macrolides is still unclear (Table 44-1).

Patient-to-patient transmission of bacterial pathogens does occur. Thus, separation regimens have been implemented to prevent cross-infection in patients with CF. This is particularly important with *B. cepacia* complex because person-to-person transmission has been proved, and chronic infection is associated with a worse clinical outcome. Vaccines are being developed against *P. aeruginosa*, but their efficacy is currently unproven.

Inflammation

Cystic fibrosis is characterized by an intense, neutrophil-dominated airway inflammation. Early trials of antiinflammatory treatment have been performed with corticosteroids. Oral prednisone (1-2 mg/kg every other day) was found to reduce lung function decline in *P. aeruginosa*–positive patients, but serious side effects such as glucose intolerance, growth retardation, and cataracts were found in prednisone-treated patients. Inhaled steroids, although widely used in patients with CF, have not been shown to improve lung function and airway inflammation. Therefore, treatment is not indicated unless patients have demonstrated airway hyperreactivity, present in 25% to 40% of patients with CF. High-dose ibuprofen slowed lung function decline in patients with CF in a single-center trial, but its use is still controversial. Even though other drugs targeting specific elements of CF airway inflammation have been studied, none has proved both efficacious and safe.

LUNG TRANSPLANTATION

Double-lung or heart-lung transplantation is a therapeutic option for patients with CF with end-stage lung disease. Determining the timing for transplant remains challenging; many attempts have been made to develop prediction models to facilitate assessment. A patient must be ill enough that there would be a survival benefit from transplant, but not so sick that the patient would die on the waiting list. FEV_1 less than 30% predicted in a patient receiving maximal medical treatment has been found to be the best indicator, because generally it predicts a median survival of 2 years. However, the length of the waiting list for the transplant center must also be considered. Generally, survival is better for adults than children, although a survival benefit through lung transplantation has also been reported in children. Survival is significantly worse for patients infected with *B. cepacia* complex, particularly *B. cenocepacia*, and most centers consider *B. cenocepacia* infection a contraindication for transplantation. However, the Toronto group has

shown that, even in these high-risk patients, transplantation improves survival. Currently, worldwide transplant experience (ISHLT data) has shown a 1-year survival after transplantation of 80%, 5-year survival of 55%, and 10-year survival of 35%.

PANCREATIC INSUFFICIENCY AND MALNUTRITION

Patients with CF with poor nutrition status are more prone to chest infections, and poor nutrition status is linked to worse prognosis. An aggressive approach to maintain normal weight in patients with CF is therefore warranted, by ensuring a high-fat, high-calorie diet with adequate replacement of pancreatic enzymes. If this cannot be achieved through oral intake, enteral feeding by nasogastric or gastrostomy tube is used to maintain adequate nutritional status and normal growth. Malabsorption often is incompletely corrected with pancreatic enzyme replacement and is caused by multiple factors, including incomplete dissolution of the pH-sensitive enteric coating in the proximal small bowel because of lack of neutralization of gastric acid by pancreatic bicarbonate. Use of medications to reduce gastric acidity may improve the effectiveness of enzymes in some patients.

INFERTILITY AND PREGNANCY

Although 98% of men with CF are infertile, with azoospermia secondary to absent vas deferens, spermatogenesis and sexual potency are normal. Men with CF can become fathers with assisted reproductive techniques such as microscopic epididymal sperm aspiration in conjunction with in vitro fertilization.

Female reproductive function is normal, although a lower rate of fertility has been postulated because of dehydrated cervical mucus. In general, women with CF tolerate pregnancy well, and many studies show pregnancy has no negative impact on survival. If women have reasonable lung function (FEV_1 >50% predicted), a stable clinical condition, and adequate nutrition status (BMI >19), the fetal and maternal outcomes are good. It is important to monitor maternal weight gain during pregnancy and check for gestational diabetes each trimester. Genetic testing for CF mutations in the partner is recommended for both men and women with CF who plan to have children.

COMPLICATIONS

PULMONARY COMPLICATIONS

Pneumothorax

Pneumothorax occurs in CF patients with more severe lung disease and lower lung function, usually older children and adults. Treatment is challenging because it may be difficult to expand the fibrotic and infected lung. Pneumothoraces are often recurrent. Chest tube drainage is usually required, and a small-gauge tube is preferred to minimize pain. Good analgesia is necessary to allow chest physiotherapy to continue and prevent worsening pulmonary infection. Chemical pleurodesis with doxycycline, talc, or thoracoscopic surgery may be required to treat recurrent pneumothoraces, although this may not be effective in all cases. If there is an ongoing air leak despite these interventions, surgical pleurodesis may be necessary. Pleurodesis was considered a contraindication to lung transplantation because of problems with removal of the lung at transplant and bleeding complications, but now most centers will perform lung transplant in patients who have had medical or surgical manipulation of the pleural space.

Hemoptysis

Chronic pulmonary infection leads to enlargement of the bronchial artery circulation supplying the lung. Hemoptysis can occur even in patients with mild lung disease and usually indicates infection. Vitamin K deficiency caused by pancreatic insufficiency can contribute to the problem. *Massive* hemoptysis (>250 mL of blood in 24 hours) is less common but occasionally can be life-threatening (see Chapter 20). Hemoptysis is usually treated with antibiotic therapy. Vitamin K and tranexamic acid may also be used. Ongoing massive hemoptysis requires bronchial artery embolization. Angiography is used to locate the abnormal bronchial artery vessels. These vessels are aberrant, and arteries arising from one side may supply contralateral segments of the lung. Because location of the bleeding does not always correlate with origin of abnormal bronchial arteries, bronchoscopy to locate source of bleeding is not helpful. However, bronchoscopy may be necessary to manage the airway in life-threatening hemoptysis. Embolization should be performed by experienced interventional radiologists because of potential complications of bronchial artery embolization, including infarction of the esophagus, lung parenchyma, or chest wall (causing dysphagia or severe chest pain), and transverse myelitis caused by accidental embolization of the spinal arteries.

Allergic Bronchopulmonary Aspergillosis

Although *Aspergillus* is frequently detected in sputum cultures, most of these patients do not have symptoms that can be attributed to the presence of the fungus. About 5% of patients with CF have symptoms caused by hypersensitivity. This entity is called allergic bronchopulmonary aspergillosis (ABPA) and should be suspected in patients who have respiratory deterioration but do not respond well to antibiotic therapy. In addition to symptoms of chronic productive cough, ABPA is usually accompanied by asthmatic features (wheezing), and patients may expectorate gritty brown sputum ("sandy" sputum). Some features of ABPA are difficult to assess in CF, because bronchiectasis, wheezing, productive cough, and presence of *Aspergillus* in the sputum are common features of CF lung disease. Diagnosis is supported by elevated IgE (usually >1000 IU/mL), a positive skin test, and serum precipitins against *Aspergillus* (see aspergilloma, Chapter 53). Treatment of symptoms and decline in lung function requires corticosteroids; high doses (1-2 mg/kg) may be required initially before the dose can be tapered. Adjunctive antifungal therapy with itraconazole may be efficacious in patients without CF who have ABPA, but its efficacy in patients with CF remains unproven. Duration of ABPA therapy is tailored to clinical response, improvement of FEV_1, and normalization of serum IgE levels.

GASTROINTESTINAL COMPLICATIONS

Pancreas

Pancreatic insufficiency is present in most patients from birth, or shortly thereafter, and occurs when more than 98% of the pancreas has been destroyed. Malabsorption of fat leads to malnutrition and deficiency of fat-soluble vitamins (A, D, E, and K). From 10% to 15% of patients have adequate pancreatic function, or pancreatic sufficiency (PS), and thus require no enzyme replacement. Acute pancreatitis develops in 20% of patients with PS and may be recurrent, and some patients have

ongoing destruction of the pancreas and become pancreatic insufficient (PI).

Distal Intestinal Obstruction Syndrome

Undigested fat, mucus from the GI tract, swallowed sputum, and reduced water in the small bowel result in thick, sticky bowel contents. Partial bowel obstruction, usually at the ileocecal junction, can cause recurrent right lower quadrant (RLQ) pain and occasionally altered bowel habit. This condition occurs in 15% to 20% of patients and is called distal intestinal obstruction syndrome (DIOS). The diagnosis is made clinically from the history and palpation of a tender mass in the RLQ along with evidence of fecal collection in the RLQ on abdominal imaging. DIOS rarely causes complete bowel obstruction, elevated WBC count, or fever; if these features are present, other causes of abdominal pain should be considered, such as intussusception, appendicitis or appendiceal abscess, and *Clostridium difficile* colitis. Treatment requires large volumes of intestinal lavage solution (GoLytely, Peglyte) to clear the bowel. Occasionally, enemas with water-soluble osmotic agents such as Gastrografin or Hypaque (diatrizoate sodium) are needed. Prevention of recurrent DIOS should focus on adequate pancreatic enzyme replacement and use of mineral oil or polyethylene glycol.

Intussusception can occur in 1% to 2% of children and young adults with CF and may mimic DIOS. The location of the intussusception is usually ileo-ileo but may be ileo-colic. Intussusception may be recurrent and asymptomatic but can cause small bowel obstruction. It also may be associated with intermittent severe colicky abdominal pain, a palpable mass, and vomiting.

CYSTIC FIBROSIS LIVER DISEASE

Infants may have cholestasis from abnormally concentrated and sticky bile. Fatty infiltration of the liver may be seen, but its significance is uncertain. *CFTR* is expressed in cells of the biliary tract, and plugging of the small intralobular ducts, periductal inflammation, and fibrosis can occur. *Focal biliary cirrhosis* is the most common feature of CF liver disease but is difficult to detect. Autopsy studies suggest that cirrhosis is present in up to 70% of adults with CF. Approximately one third of patients have abnormal liver function tests, but the presence of abnormality does not correlate well with the presence or extent of liver disease. Hepatocellular function is generally preserved. Focal biliary cirrhosis progresses to multinodular cirrhosis and portal hypertension in 5% of patients.

Liver disease is a life-limiting factor in only a few patients, and liver transplantation is rarely indicated, because hepatocellular failure is rare. A small, poorly functioning "microgallbladder" is typically found, and cholesterol gallstones develop in up to 10% of patients with CF. Choledocholithiasis is less common. Ursodeoxycholic acid can normalize elevated liver enzyme levels, but its long-term effect on the evolution of liver disease remains largely unproved.

CYSTIC FIBROSIS-RELATED DIABETES

Langerhans cell function is initially retained, and diabetes mellitus is rare in the first decade of life in patients with CF. The prevalence of glucose intolerance and diabetes mellitus rises continuously with increasing age, and 25% to 30% of adults with CF and PI will have diabetes requiring insulin therapy. CF-related diabetes (CFRD) shares features of both type 1 and

2 diabetes, with a combination of decreased and delayed insulin secretion, as well as insulin resistance. Glucose intolerance can persist for many years before frank diabetes occurs. Control of diabetes is important to prevent protein catabolism and weight loss. Poorly controlled diabetes may increase pulmonary infections. Most patients will require treatment with insulin. During pulmonary exacerbations, increased insulin resistance can temporarily raise insulin needs three-fold to four-fold. Patients with CFRD with poor blood glucose control develop *micro*vascular complications but rarely show *macro*vascular complications.

MALIGNANCY

A review of CF clinics in North America and Europe found an increased prevalence of GI malignancies in patients with CF. The proposed etiology is the chronic injury and inflammation of the GI tract. The increased risk starts in the third decade of life, and the malignancies are found in all parts of the GI tract (colon, esophagus, small bowel, pancreas, liver, biliary tree). The odds ratio for the risk of digestive tract malignancies in patients with CF is 6.5. Screening is difficult because of the widespread nature of the cancers and overall low prevalence but may be indicated in patients referred for lung transplantation, those with a family history of GI cancers, and those with gastroesophageal reflux disease. (GERD) New GI symptoms should trigger appropriate diagnostic tests.

CYSTIC FIBROSIS-RELATED BONE DISEASE

Adults with CF have evidence of decreased bone density, including osteopenia and osteoporosis, as measured by bone dual-energy x-ray absorptiometry (DEXA). Prevalence of low bone density in adults with CF ranges from 40% to 70%, and up to 50% of adults with severe lung disease who are awaiting transplantation will have osteoporosis. The etiology of the decreased bone density is multifactorial, and both failure of normal bone formation and excessive bone loss occur. Malnutrition, vitamin D and K deficiency, hypogonadism, increased bone loss because of elevated inflammatory cytokines from chronic pulmonary infection, and use of corticosteroids all may play a role in the development of low bone density. It is not completely clear whether DEXA scans predict fracture risk in patients with CF. A consensus report suggests treatment with calcium and vitamin D supplementation, treatment of hypogonadism if present, promotion of exercise, treatment of pulmonary infection, and use of bisphosphonates in patients with osteoporosis, in those receiving corticosteroids, and in those on the transplant list.

Hypertrophic pulmonary osteoarthropathy (HPOA) is a chronic proliferative periostitis associated with digital clubbing. It can cause severe bony pain and swelling, especially in knees, ankles, and wrists. It frequently flares at times of pulmonary exacerbations, improving with treatment of the lung infection. Radiography confirms the typical periosteal new bone formation at the distal ends of long bones.

Episodic arthropathy occurs in 5% to 10% of CF patients and presents as transient episodes of acute swelling and joint pain involving single or multiple, large or small joints. These episodes do not necessarily correlate with pulmonary exacerbations. This is a nonerosive arthropathy and responds to nonsteroidal anti-inflammatory drugs or corticosteroids.

About 1% to 2% of patients with CF develop a cutaneous vasculitis, which on biopsy is a *leukocytoclastic vasculitis*. Systemic involvement is rare. It is usually seen on the lower extremities, and the rash consists of usually painless purpura. This typically resolves spontaneously, and specific treatment is not required.

PROGNOSIS

When CF was first described, the median survival was less than 2 years of age. With improvements in therapy, institution of a high-calorie, high-fat diet to optimize growth and nutrition, and establishment of multidisciplinary CF care centers, survival has steadily improved, with national median survival rates of about 36 to 46 years. CF should no longer be thought of as a pediatric disease; in Canada, for example, greater than 50% of patients with CF are now adults.

A number of factors have been shown to influence prognosis in patients with CF. For many decades a gender gap was noted, with males having better survival. Although this gender-related difference in survival is decreasing, it still exists. The etiology is unclear and does not seem to be related to pulmonary function or nutrition status. Other factors influencing survival in CF include socioeconomic status and presence of chronic infection with *P. aeruginosa* or *B. cepacia* complex.

CONTROVERSIES AND PITFALLS

The advances in treatment options for patients with cystic fibrosis over the past 20 years has been welcome and associated with marked improvements in life expectancy, but also leading to new challenges. Better patient outcomes with slower decline in lung function and better survival have made the outcome measures of previous studies difficult to use. The treatment burden for patients has increased, and lifelong therapy with multiple drugs is now the norm. Testing efficacy of new therapies will be difficult because placebo-controlled trials of one therapy alone are no longer possible. Creative study methodologies will be needed to determine which drugs to use in the day-to-day care of patients with CF at different stages of the disease. It will not be acceptable just to keep adding new therapies, because of both the time burden and the financial cost.

With drugs now becoming available to treat the basic defect, investigators need to determine how much correction of *CFTR* function is needed to prevent the progressive lung disease. Long-term follow-up of patients and use of national registries will help address these questions and will require collaboration between countries to obtain the sample sizes needed.

CONCLUSION

Overall, CF treatment has been one of medicine's success stories, because the increase in life expectancy achieved over the recent decades has been impressive. Although the understanding of the disease process has greatly advanced with the definition of the underlying abnormality, treatment is still largely targeted at the "downstream" consequences of the *CFTR* defect: mucus retention, infection, and inflammation. There is considerable promise that in the near future, therapies will become available that will lead to partial or complete correction of *CFTR* function, as well as more efficient symptomatic therapies. Even if these therapies fail in completely correcting the underlying defect, they may be sufficiently efficacious to prevent clinical deterioration. Thus, cystic fibrosis may continue to be a chronic disease requiring long-term treatment but may cease to be life-shortening.

SUGGESTED READINGS

Borowitz D, Baker RD, Stallings V: Consensus Report on Nutrition for Pediatric Patients with Cystic Fibrosis, *J Pediatr Gastroenterol Nutr* 35:246–259, 2002.

Boucher RC: An overview of the pathogenesis of cystic fibrosis lung disease, *Adv Drug Del Rev* 54:1359–1371, 2002.

Davis PB: CF since 1938, *Am J Respir Crit Care Med* 173:475–482, 2006.

Gibson RL, Burns JL, Ramsey BW: Pathophysiology and management of pulmonary infections in cystic fibrosis, *Am J Respir Crit Care Med* 168:918–951, 2003.

Knowles MR, Durie PR: What is cystic fibrosis? *N Engl J Med* 347:439–442, 2002.

Ratjen F, Döring G: Cystic fibrosis, *Lancet* 361:681–689, 2003.

Farrell PM, Rosenstein BJ, White TB: Guidelines for diagnosis of cystic fibrosis in newborns through older adults. Cystic Fibrosis Foundation consensus report, *J Pediatr* 153:S4–S14, 2008.

Rowe SM, Miller S, Sorscher EJ: Mechanisms of disease: cystic fibrosis, *N Engl J Med* 352:1992–2001, 2005.

Chapter **45**
Bronchiectasis
Deborah Whitters • Robert Stockley

Bronchiectasis was first described by Laënnec in 1819 as irreversible dilation and destruction of airways associated with chronic bacterial infection. It is characterized by inflamed and dilated thick-walled bronchi. The clinical features of bronchiectasis include chronic production of often mucopurulent or purulent sputum, persistent bacterial colonization, and recurrent lower respiratory tract infection.

EPIDEMIOLOGY

It is generally believed that the incidence of bronchiectasis has declined since the 1950s, when prevalence in the United Kingdom (UK) was estimated at 100 per 100,000 population, based on mass chest x-ray findings. There are no recent studies in the UK to confirm this belief, and the overall incidence remains unknown. Evidence from other European countries, however, shows a reduction in hospital admissions and new diagnoses of bronchiectasis since the 1970s, attributed to reduced incidence of tuberculosis and more effective treatment of pulmonary infections.

Bronchiectasis remains a significant cause of childhood morbidity in developing countries. Prevalence of non–cystic fibrosis (CF) bronchiectasis in indigenous communities in New Zealand and Australia is reported to be among the highest worldwide, along with Inuit populations of the Northern Hemisphere. Poverty, barriers to medical care (e.g., antibiotic therapy, vaccination), and poor education are contributing factors. Mortality from respiratory disease, including bronchiectasis, is also higher in rural versus urban areas in China; epidemiologic studies are lacking, however, and these populations likely face similar barriers to medical care and therefore antibiotic availability. There are no studies to illustrate the effect of antibiotic therapy or immunization programs on the incidence in countries where it has only recently become available.

PATHOLOGY

The most comprehensive description of bronchiectasis pathology remains that of Whitwell, who examined 200 consecutive resected surgical specimens in 1952. The findings revealed dilated, thickened bronchi, often containing pus with distortion of the bronchial lumen. The inflammatory reaction, visible macroscopically, was shown often to cause complete occlusion of the smaller bronchioles. These findings may be widespread or localized depending on the cause. Microscopically, examination of the bronchial epithelium showed ulceration with granulation tissue in areas where healing had begun. Other specimens had evidence of infiltration of inflammatory cells in the subepithelial tissues and hyperplasia of mucous glands. Supporting connective "elastic" tissues may also be damaged to varying degrees. These features may all be present in varying degrees, in keeping with the varying clinical symptomatology and severity of the disease.

Whitwell classified bronchiectasis into three groups based on pathologic findings—saccular, atelectatic, and follicular—and although these terms may have changed, the descriptions remain the same. *Cylindrical* bronchiectasis is characterized by bronchi showing a regular outline, with dilated airways only and usually ending abruptly. *Varicose* bronchiectasis has similarities to the appearance of varicose veins, with dilation that is deformed by areas of relative constriction. These bronchi also have a distorted and bulbous end. *Cystic* (saccular) bronchiectasis is considered the most severe form of bronchiectasis; its most prominent feature is progressively increasing dilation as the bronchi progress toward the lung periphery and airways, ending in cystlike clusters. These three basic forms of bronchiectasis are demonstrated in **Figure 45-1** by high-resolution computed tomography (HRCT) scanning.

PATHOGENESIS

The cause of non-CF bronchiectasis may only be identifiable in up to 50% of patients. However, a number of recognized conditions and factors are associated with bronchiectasis, and an underlying cause should be assessed in all patients (**Box 45-1**).

The genetic influence on the development of non-CF bronchiectasis is the subject of ongoing research, often on the role of the cystic fibrosis transmembrane conductance regulator *(CFTR)* gene. The most common mutation of this gene, ΔF508 (F508del), is associated with severe CF (see Chapter 44). Numerous other mutations have been identified and associated with a milder clinical phenotype. As a consequence, late first presentation of CF has been described in patients who would otherwise have been considered to have *idiopathic* non-CF bronchiectasis. It is now recognized that mutations of the *CFTR* gene are more frequently observed in patients with bronchiectasis and a normal sweat chloride test than in the general population. Studies show that the spectrum of *CFTR* genotypes is associated with a continuum of *CFTR* dysfunction in the airways. Phenotypes range from patients with bronchiectasis, normal sweat test, and no other features suggestive of CF to those with classic CF. Also, some evidence suggests the *CFTR* mutations are associated with non-CF bronchiectasis and rheumatoid arthritis. Therefore, *CFTR* dysfunction can be identified as a cause of bronchiectasis in patients previously diagnosed with idiopathic non-CF bronchiectasis, but without fulfilling the diagnostic criteria for CF. How this affects patient management is currently unknown.

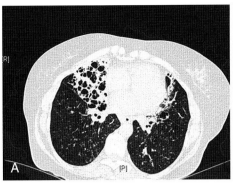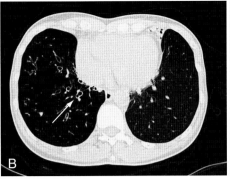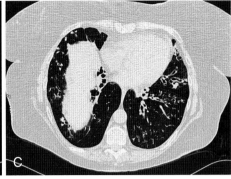

Figure 45-1 **A,** Bilateral *cystic* bronchiectasis. **B,** Moderate *cylindrical* bronchiectasis in right middle lobe, as demonstrated by classic signet ring sign *(arrow)*. **C,** Bilateral severe *varicose* bronchiectasis, more marked on the left side, with associated bronchial wall thickening.

Box 45-1 **Underlying Causes of Bronchiectasis**

Postinfective Causes
Viral infection (adenovirus, measles, human immunodeficiency virus)
Bacterial infection *(Pneumococcus)*
Mycobacterium tuberculosis
Pertussis (whooping cough)
Allergic bronchopulmonary aspergillosis

Host Immune Defects
Humoral immune deficiency (IgA, IgG, IgM)
Selective IgG subclass deficiency
Specific antibody deficiency
Complement deficiency
Chronic granulomatous disease

Mucociliary Clearance Defects
Primary ciliary dyskinesia
Kartagener's syndrome
Young's syndrome

Other Inflammatory Disease
Rheumatoid arthritis
Inflammatory bowel disease
Chronic obstructive pulmonary disease (COPD)

Miscellaneous
Foreign body inhalation
Middle lobe syndrome
Alpha$_1$-antitrypsin deficiency
Toxic inhalation
Gastroesophageal reflux disease (GERD)
Yellow nail syndrome

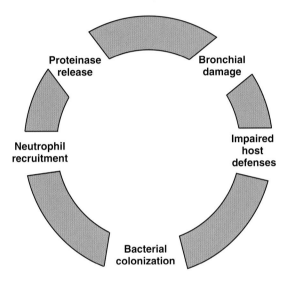

Figure 45-2 Infectious inflammatory cycle of bronchiectasis. Damage to airway results in impaired mucociliary clearance, leading to bacterial colonization, which stimulates neutrophilic inflammation. This not only damages the tissues further, but also disturbs the local immune status, resulting in establishment and maintenance of colonization. Neutrophilic proteinases damage immunoglobulins, reduce antibacterial properties, reduce ciliary beat frequency, and damage airway epithelium, all leading to increased bacterial adherence and retention.

Establishing a cause for bronchiectasis depends on an accurate recollection of events by patients, making it difficult to establish a direct cause and effect in most patients. Nonetheless, an infective insult undoubtedly plays a role in establishing and maintaining the pathologic changes seen in bronchiectasis. This is demonstrated by the falling incidence since the widespread use of antibiotic therapy and immunizations in childhood. The role of infection is further emphasized by the association between the immune defects, and therefore increased susceptibility to infection, and the development of bronchiectasis.

The "vicious cycle" hypothesis of bronchiectasis suggests an initial failure or overwhelmed host defenses, leading to a host-mediated chronic inflammatory response, which in turn causes new or further impairment of mucociliary clearance and defenses, amplifying the problem. This interaction between chronic infection and excessive inflammation, which is predominantly neutrophilic, ensures ongoing damage to the airways and the development and maintenance of the features seen in bronchiectasis. Inflammatory mediators such as the neutrophil chemoattractant interleukin-8 (IL-8) and tumor necrosis factor alpha (TNF-α) are found in bronchial mucosal biopsies and secretions from bronchiectatic airways, in addition to tissue neutrophilia. This initiation of the inflammatory reaction results in the recruitment of phagocytes, dendritic cells, and lymphocytes, which contribute to the adaptive response (**Figure 45-2**).

CLINICAL FEATURES

The severity of clinicopathologic events varies widely in patients with bronchiectasis. At the milder end of the spectrum, patients may have occasional exacerbations, with little or no intervening sputum production. Others have frequent exacerbations with chronic production of purulent sputum, even in the stable state. Symptoms can include *hemoptysis*, especially during exacerbations, and *breathlessness*, characterized by mild to moderate airflow obstruction, lethargy, and reduced health status. Hemoptysis may be only a minor problem, although erosion of mucosal neovascular arterioles during an acute exacerbation can result in massive hemoptysis. Quantitative analysis of HRCT scanning in bronchiectasis shows that the airflow obstruction is primarily linked to disease of small and medium-sized airways and not to bronchiectatic abnormalities in large airways, emphysema, or retained endobronchial secretions. Nonspecific chest pain varying in severity is also reported with increased frequency in bronchiectatic patients.

CLINICAL SIGNS

Finger (digital) clubbing has long been recognized as a sign of chronic suppurative lung disease. Despite previous reports of being frequently encountered in bronchiectasis, clubbing is much less common in more recent studies, perhaps because of a lower threshold for diagnosis of bronchiectasis. Studies report that the prevalence of clubbing is 1% to 2%, both in patients who develop symptoms as adults or in childhood and in adult patients. Overall, this suggests that finger clubbing is now seen only in a minority of patients with non-CF bronchiectasis.

The characteristic clinical finding in bronchiectasis is *coarse crackles* heard on auscultation, consistently reported in up to 73% of patients in more recent studies. Interestingly, an in-depth study of the phenotypes of bronchiectasis found the frequency of crackles to be much less in patients with adult onset of the symptom of chronic productive cough than in those with childhood onset of symptoms (20% vs. 64%). This difference was also associated with a greater amount of sputum production in the childhood-onset group. The crackles typically heard in bronchiectasis occur in the early and middle phases of inspiration, fading by the end of inspiration. Crackles also are usually present at expiration, which differentiates these from the finer crackles in alveolitis or chronic obstructive pulmonary disease (COPD). Although crackles are profuse, this may be reduced with coughing and expectoration. The location and extent of the crackles on physical examination, however, does not necessarily relate to the extent or area of distribution of bronchiectasis on the CT scan.

DIAGNOSIS AND PATIENT ASSESSMENT

RADIOLOGY

Chest radiography is often the first imaging modality used to investigate patients with suspected bronchiectasis. However, radiographs are insensitive as a diagnostic tool for bronchiectasis and suggest the diagnosis in less than 50% of cases in some studies. There is also little evidence for the use of chest radiographs in monitoring patients with bronchiectasis with no change in symptoms.

HRCT is the radiologic modality of choice for establishing the diagnosis of bronchiectasis, although its reported sensitivity and specificity vary. It is difficult to assess fully the accuracy of HRCT in diagnosing all patients with bronchiectasis, but it is believed to be highly specific for the diagnosis of moderate or severe disease. However, the features of early bronchiectasis with bronchial wall thickening are also seen in other conditions (e.g., COPD, asthma), suggesting its specificity is less for frank bronchiectasis. Furthermore, a comparison of thin-section CT with bronchography demonstrated that although bronchial wall thickening is often seen, bronchography shows this is not always bronchiectatic in origin. The increasing use of multi-detector CT scanners, which allow for greater variance in

---

Box 45-2 Diagnostic Testing in Patients with Bronchiectasis

Investigation
Nonspecific inflammatory markers (WBC count, ESR, neutrophils, CRP)
Serum immunoglobulins
Serum electrophoresis
Functional antibodies
Total IgE, specific IgG to *Aspergillus*

In Some Patients
IgG subclasses
Rheumatoid factor
Alpha$_1$-antitrypsin levels
Cystic fibrosis screening

CRP, C-reactive protein; *ESR*, erythrocyte sedimentation rate; *IgE*, immunoglobulin E; *IgG*, immunoglobulin G; *WBC*, white blood cell.

---

section thickness compared to standard HRCT (sections obtained only at 10-mm intervals), may lead to improved detection of bronchiectasis, although this has yet to be assessed for early disease. However, this must be weighed against an increased radiation burden, and at present, standard HRCT remains the recommended investigation for the diagnosis of bronchiectasis.

BLOOD TESTS

Inflammatory markers include white blood cell (WBC) count, neutrophil count, erythrocyte sedimentation rate (ESR), and C-reactive protein (CRP) and can be used as nonspecific tests of disease activity and exacerbation severity. These tests can also be used to guide the need for and response to antibiotics in the absence of changes in clinical state or symptomatology of bronchiectatic patients (**Box 45-2**).

IMMUNOGLOBULINS

Immunoglobulins (IgA, IgG, and IgM) are often elevated in a significant proportion of patients with bronchiectasis, which reflects chronic bronchial infection. *Hypogammaglobulinemia* as a recognized cause of bronchiectasis and antibody deficiency or an inadequate antibody response has been reported in 8% of patients in a large study into causative factors in bronchiectasis. This supports the need for antibody levels (IgA, IgG, IgM) to be checked in patients because they may influence treatment. The role of IgG subclasses is less clear because normal ranges for each subclass have been difficult to establish, and absence or deficiency of a subclass can be found in otherwise healthy individuals, as can IgA deficiency. The inability to produce a response to immunization with a polysaccharide antigen despite normal levels of serum immunoglobulin also suggests a causative but specific immunodeficiency.

Current guidelines recommend that evaluation of antibody deficiency in bronchiectasis should include a universal or targeted assessment of a specific baseline antibody response to peptide and polysaccharide antigens. Routinely, tetanus toxoid, *Streptococcus pneumoniae* and *Haemophilus influenzae* type B are used. If these are low, immunization should occur with the appropriate antigen and levels should be remeasured approximately 21 days later. Whether a response affects the subsequent clinical course remains unknown, and in some cases seems illogical, especially as the *H. influenzae* lung infections are non-typeable *H. influenzae*, not type B.

Allergic bronchopulmonary aspergillosis (ABPA) has been recognized as a cause of bronchiectasis, usually affecting atopic patients and caused by an allergy to *Aspergillus* species. The proximal bronchiectasis, usually affecting the upper lobes, associated with *Aspergillus* is IgG and type 3 immune reaction–related. When ABPA is clinically suspected, elevated total blood eosinophils and IgE suggest an allergic response. Specific IgE in addition to precipitating IgG to *Aspergillus* should be checked.

Rheumatoid factor (RF) is also found to be elevated in some patients in isolation and is a nonspecific finding. However, high RF values can be important in some patients, related to a true arthritic etiology and small airways disease. Nonspecific arthralgia can also be a feature of the exuberant inflammatory reaction related to airway colonization. Treatment of the arthritis or bacterial load can lead to improvement in the related feature.

Alpha$_1$-antitrypsin levels should be guided by clinical suspicion of bronchiectasis, as should genetic testing for CF or its variants (Box 45-2).

MUCOCILIARY FUNCTION

Mucociliary function is assessed in adult patients with suspected *primary ciliary dyskinesia* (PCD). This needs consideration in patients with a history of chronic rhinitis, sinusitis, otitis media, neonatal respiratory symptoms, or situs inversus viscerum (a feature of only 50% of patients with PCD). Male infertility and subfertility in females are also features. PCD is best assessed using the saccharin method or nasal nitric oxide measurements as first-line investigations. Cilia can be obtained for direct examination in patients who require further investigation when these initial investigations are abnormal, although secondary abnormalities can be found in the nasal and bronchial tissues, especially in the patient with chronic infection in the region tested.

NEUTROPHIL FUNCTION

Neutrophil-dominant inflammation is a central feature in bronchiectasis. Neutrophils aggregate quickly at the site of infection. Phagocytosis occurs when the neutrophil moves in response to chemotactic stimuli to the site of bacterial colonization or infection. In particular, leukotriene B$_4$ (LTB$_4$) and IL-8 are major chemoattractants identified, with IL-8 playing a crucial role during acute exacerbations.

The granule proteins of the neutrophil release antibacterial proteins and cytolytic enzymes on activation. Excessive degranulation and activity of cytolytic enzymes such as myeloperoxidase and elastase have been implicated most in host tissue damage and thus may be central to the establishment or amplification of the vicious cycle. The neutrophils also produce reactive oxygen species (ROS) directed at bacterial killing. The release of uncontrolled ROS by neutrophils, however, may also lead to damage to the surrounding tissues, again exacerbating the lung-destructive process. With the genetic defect of chronic granulomatous disease, patients develop a variety of inflammatory complications, including bronchiectasis, as a result of an exaggerated inflammatory response; are unable to produce ROS; and manifest recurrent life-threatening bacterial infections and granuloma formation.

Tests of neutrophil function are not routinely performed in patients with bronchiectasis. However, some studies of immune function have shown oxidative burst to be lower in patients with bronchiectasis. The significance of this abnormality remains to be identified.

Table 45-1 Organisms Isolated in Bronchiectasis

Organism	Frequency
Haemophilus influenzae	14%-35%
Pseudomonas aeruginosa	9%-31%
Staphylococcus aureus	0%-14%
Streptococcus pneumoniae	2%-13%
Moraxella (Branhamella) catarrhalis	0%-20%
Possibly "nonpathogenic organisms" *Corynebacterium* spp., *Neisseria* spp., coagulase-negative *Staphylococcus*, β-hemolytic *Streptococcus*	5%-60%

SPUTUM MICROBIOLOGY

An assessment of lower respiratory tract microbiology is imperative in the investigation and management of bronchiectasis. **Table 45-1** summarizes the most common organisms isolated from the respiratory tract and their frequency in adults with bronchiectasis.

Bronchiectasis is associated with frequent bacterial colonization of the airway. As such, patients, even in the stable state, often produce sputum daily as part of the host defense response. Sputum may be mucopurulent to purulent in appearance, dependent on the neutrophil content. Development or increasing purulence of sputum is often indicative of a bacterial exacerbation. Purulent sputum color can be graded visually and is associated with activity of the underlying markers of bronchial inflammation, such as myeloperoxidase, IL-8, and leukocyte elastase. These factors are central in the ongoing neutrophil-derived inflammation, which, when overexuberant or ineffective, can impair even the competence of lung defenses. Patients with purulent sputum are more frequently found to be colonized than those with persistently mucoid sputum.

The role of quantitative bacterial culture has been important in establishing increased airway inflammation and exacerbation in patients with chronic sputum production. An increase in the bacterial load of more than 10^6 colony forming units (CFUs) is associated with increasing airway neutrophils and inflammation, with a reduction in bacterial load as the exacerbation resolves. Similarly, even in the presence of a background of 10^6 organisms, a further increase in the load may be confirmatory of a change in the bronchiectatic patient's clinical status, requiring intervention even in the absence of other clinical or biochemical markers.

Therefore, identification of colonizing organism is important in patients with bronchiectasis, but quantitative microbiology remains a vital tool for identifying exacerbation status and is a surrogate marker of inflammation that correlates with degree of sputum purulence. Although clinically useful, this is not routinely employed and requires further study and validation.

EXACERBATIONS

ACUTE EXACERBATION

As discussed earlier with microbiologic identification of bronchiectasis exacerbation, presence of bacteria alone does not necessarily indicate an exacerbation requiring antibiotic therapy, in view of the prevalence of colonization in the stable clinical state. A worsening of symptoms from baseline and acute deterioration with a change in bacterial load, however, indicate the

Box 45-3   Features Suggestive of Exacerbation in Bronchiectasis

Change in sputum production (volume, viscosity, or color)
Increasing cough
Increasing dyspnea
Increasing wheeze
Malaise, fatigue
Decreased exercise tolerance
Fever
Decreased pulmonary function (10%)
Radiographic changes indicative of acute process
Change in chest sounds from baseline

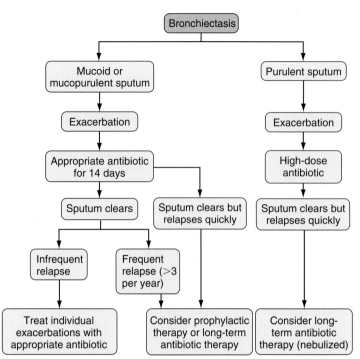

Figure 45-3 The degree of purulence of stable-state sputum must be considered when treating bronchiectasis exacerbation. Patients who relapse quickly or frequently (>3 times in 1 year) with mucoid or mucopurulent sputum are usually managed with short courses (10-14 days) of appropriate antibiotics but may need longer-term preventive therapy. Patients with chronic purulent sputum usually require higher-than-conventional doses of antibiotics and would have a lower threshold for consideration of long-term nebulized antibiotic therapy.

need to introduce or add further antibiotics. **Box 45-3** lists other symptoms suggestive of an acute bacterial exacerbation.

A review of previous microbiology, and thus any change from the stable state, is essential before initiating antibiotic therapy, and ideally, sputum should be obtained for culture, preferably before antibiotic therapy, to guide antibiotic choice.

RECURRENT EXACERBATION

Patients with frequent exacerbations may require longer-term antibiotic therapy. The principle of treatment is to reduce the microbial load and thereby modulate the persistent inflammation characteristic of bronchiectasis, that is, an attempt to break the vicious cycle of bronchiectasis previously described. The aim is to improve the symptoms and subsequent poor health status and quality of life for these patients and reduce the number of exacerbations. The generally accepted cutoff for considering long-term antibiotic therapy is more than three exacerbations in 1 year. This particularly applies to patients colonized with *Pseudomonas aeruginosa*, which is associated with more hospital admissions, poorer quality of life, and more rapidly declining lung function.

Pseudomonas aeruginosa frequently persists in the airways of patients with bronchiectasis after its initial isolation. One feature of *P. aeruginosa* that enhances its ability to colonize the lungs is its ability to form biofilms. A *biofilm* is a community of bacterial cells irreversibly attached to a surface or each other and embedded in a matrix of extracellular polymeric substance (EPS). Existing in biofilms enhances the ability of bacteria to colonize and to evade antimicrobial therapies, thus making it difficult to eradicate these organisms from the lungs of chronically infected patients. The formation of biofilms is multifactorial, but one influential bacterial behavior is *quorum sensing*, a complex cell-to-cell signaling mechanism well characterized in *P. aeruginosa* that modulates bacterial functions, including metabolism, expression of virulence factors, and biofilm formation. This ability to regulate bacterial behavior also enhances the ability of *P. aeruginosa* to invade and colonize the host. Because this pathogen frequently colonizes the lungs of patients with bronchiectasis, its significance in this condition merits further investigation.

Furthermore, the clinical problems associated with *P. aeruginosa* may be further exacerbated by the development of antibodies that reduce bacterial killing. Studies in the 1970s and 1980s of CF patients colonized with *P. aeruginosa* identified a blocking factor in serum that inhibited killing of *Pseudomonas*, subsequently shown to be an IgG$_2$ subclass. Recent work supports the role of inhibitory antibodies in the ability of other bacteria to establish infection within the host. This may partly

contribute to the failure of the host to control infection, and although the role of this mechanism has yet to be established in bronchiectasis, it is worthy of study. However, this ability of organisms to survive will establish ongoing inflammation as a frustrated attempt by the host to eradicate them, leading to proteolytic damage and perpetuation of the vicious cycle illustrated in Figure 45-2. For these reasons, patients should receive longer-term antibiotic therapy as appropriate, if the cycle can be broken (i.e., sputum purulence disappears).

ANTIBIOTIC THERAPY

Figure 45-3 provides a decision-making algorithm for antibiotic therapy of the patient with bronchiectasis.

PATIENT WITH ACUTE EXACERBATION

Prompt antimicrobial therapy is required once an acute exacerbation is identified, guided by the most up-to-date microbiology results and local guidelines. There are not randomized, placebo controlled trials evaluating the effectiveness of antibiotics in exacerbations in bronchiectasis, but in general high-dose, targeted antibiotics are required for effective treatment. The British Thoracic Society guidelines recommend that many patients with bronchiectasis should receive 14 days of antibiotics rather than the conventional dose. The antibiotics most often used for exacerbations have a broad spectrum of activity. Amoxicillin remains the initial choice for many organisms, especially in the UK, but patterns of resistance need to be recognized and management adapted appropriately. *H. influenzae* is usually sensitive to amoxicillin, but the production of

Table 45-2 Antibiotic Guidelines for Bronchiectasis Exacerbation

Organism	Antiobiotic/Dose
Streptococcus pneumoniae β-lactamase –ve *Haemophilus influenzae*	Amoxicillin 500 mg three times daily orally (higher doses may be required in some patients)
β-lactamase +ve organisms *Moraxella catarrhalis* *H. influenzae*	Co-amoxiclav (amoxicillin-clavulanate), 625 mg three times daily orally
Staphylococcus aureus Methicillin sensitive Methicillin resistant	Flucloxacillin, 500 mg three times daily orally Trimethoprim, 200 mg twice daily orally + Rifampicin (based on weight) orally
Pseudomonas aeruginosa	Ciprofloxacin, 500 mg twice daily orally (750 mg twice daily in severe cases) Patient may require intravenous (IV) therapy. Ceftazidime Piperacillin + tazobactam Aztreonam Meropenem *May be combined with:* Gentamicin Tobramycin Colistin

β-lactamase or changes in penicillin-binding proteins increase resistance, and the presence of resistant strains varies from country to country. *Moraxella (Branhamella) catarrhalis* also produces β-lactamase. Antibiotic choices based on current UK guidelines are shown in **Table 45-2**, but local guidelines should be considered.

The decision to give high-dose antibiotics instead of conventional doses is based on clinical judgment and the patient's usual stable state. Those who usually produce purulent sputum in the stable state will often require a higher dose to elicit a clinical response. Furthermore, patients who fail to respond to a conventional dose of antibiotic with an apparently fully sensitive organism may respond only to a higher dose. The failure of sputum to clear (become mucoid) or the occurrence of rapid relapses (within days) indicates a need to consider longer-term therapy. However, the antibiotic regimen should be reviewed early (within 7 days) in patients receiving antibiotics who appear to be failing to respond and in whom sputum remains purulent.

LONG-TERM THERAPY

Long-term antibiotic therapy, either oral or nebulized (inhalational), are considered in patients who exacerbate frequently or have considerable morbidity as a result of their condition. A systematic review of long-term oral antibiotics failed to demonstrate an effect on lung function or exacerbation frequency, although symptoms were improved. Oral antibiotic therapy after detailed assessment of microbiology results most often uses amoxicillin, amoxicillin-clavulanate (co-amoxiclav), and

flucloxacillin. These are used at lower than the standard dose for an acute exacerbation and only with caution. Long-term quinolones alone are not used because of the high risk of resistance in patients colonized with *P. aeruginosa*.

Long-term inhalational (nebulized) antibiotics are used more often because of the low risk of systemic side effects, most frequently in patients chronically colonized with *P. aeruginosa*. Bacterial sensitivities should be assessed before initiation of long-term therapy. Nebulized colistin is often used in patients with *P. aeruginosa* colonization and has been associated with increased quality of life and slower decline in forced expiratory volume in 1 second (FEV_1). However, there remains a paucity of specifically designed studies of colistin in patients with bronchiectasis. Gentamicin and tobramycin are associated with reduced microbial load, and in some cases, tobramycin has been shown to eradicate *P. aeruginosa*. In other patients, however, tobramycin has been associated with significant side effects, precluding its continued use.

PROPHYLACTIC THERAPY

Some antibiotics are used for their potential immunomodulatory properties and ability to mediate the host inflammatory response. *Macrolides* are the most common of these antimicrobials used in clinical practice, although their benefits require further study. Azithromycin, twice weekly for 6 months, has shown positive results, with reduced 24-hour sputum volume and reduced number of exacerbations. Earlier results with erythromycin showed similar effects. However, significant side effects are associated with macrolides, and therefore their long-term use also requires further assessment. Their beneficial effect is thought to result from both their immunomodulatory effect and their inhibitory actions on biofilm formation.

VACCINATION

In keeping with most accepted guidelines, patients with bronchiectasis are routinely vaccinated against influenza. However, no trials provide evidence for or against this intervention or for its role in decreasing the severity or frequency of respiratory exacerbations or decline in lung function. Similarly, evidence is minimal regarding the pneumococcal vaccine, although limited data do support the use of 23-valent pneumococcal vaccine as routine management in adults with bronchiectasis.

ALTERNATIVE THERAPY

As discussed, the role of the neutrophil in bronchiectasis is central to maintaining the inflammation and continued destructive processes of bronchiectasis. Therefore, therapies targeting the actions of the neutrophil provide a potential alternative to conventional therapies. Chemoattractants are required to enable migration of the neutrophil in the airways, and IL-8 is particularly important during exacerbations. The increased activity of IL-8 is associated with increasingly purulent sputum, suggesting cause and effect. With antibiotic therapy, the chemotactic activity decreases as the purulence resolves. However, although targeting this process may be a potential therapeutic option in reducing neutrophilic lung damage, neutrophil recruitment clearly is also necessary as a component of the normal response to infection.

Therefore, modulating this process requires further careful investigation, as would abrogation of the other chemoattractants (e.g., LTB_4). Neutrophil-derived proteinase activity, particularly that of neutrophil elastase, is also crucial in maintenance of inflammation in chronic lung disease and the ongoing destructive process. This is normally counteracted by the actions of antiproteinases (SLPI, α_1-antitrypsin), but overwhelming this central mechanism leads to the ongoing lung destruction. Sputum elastase activity appears to correlate with disease activity, severity, and other inflammatory markers, even in stable-state bronchiectasis. Antielastase therapy may therefore also provide a theoretic disease-modifying therapy for this condition. Indeed, studies of such an approach in CF patients show potential beneficial effects (see Chapter 44).

PHYSIOTHERAPY

It is generally accepted that patients with bronchiectasis should be referred for chest physiotherapy and instruction in chest clearance techniques. Despite minimal evidence to define which patients will benefit or the efficacy of many current interventions, an airway clearance regimen is important in the clinical management of patients with sputum production in the stable state, although no data are available on exacerbations. Further research is required into establishing any true benefits of airway clearance techniques.

MANAGEMENT

SURGERY

With the advent of the antibiotic era, surgery with the aim of symptomatic relief or cure of bronchiectasis is rare. Current indicators for surgery include severe symptoms unrelieved by usual medical management, lung abscess, or major hemoptysis (see Complications). Removal of a segment or lobe would be considered, especially if a proximal obstruction is leading to distal disease. In principle, however, the bronchiectasis should be localized rather than diffuse, and because many patients tend to have multiple segments of the lung affected, "cure" is not possible by limited resection. Perioperative mortality is reported to be low.

TRANSPLANTATION

Lung transplantation has become an option for end-stage lung disease, but data are sparse regarding non-CF bronchiectasis. In general, the guidelines that apply to CF patients are used in patients with non-CF bronchiectasis. General guidelines suggest considering transplantation in patients with FEV_1 of less than 30% predicted, or respiratory deterioration despite maximal medical intervention. Factors such as massive hemoptysis, severe pulmonary hypertension, recurrent admissions, and respiratory failure are all indicators to consider a transplant option.

COMPLICATIONS

HEMOPTYSIS

Hemoptysis occurs in bronchiectasis as a result of erosion of neovascular arterioles and is reported frequently, especially during exacerbations. The definition of massive hemoptysis remains unclear and is thus a subjective term. Many studies use a definition of greater than 200 mL of blood-tinged sputum in 24 hours, which is associated with hemodynamic instability of the patient, or a significant fall in hematocrit during the episode.

However, hemoptysis is associated with mortality greater than 50% and requires prompt and appropriate management. Following stabilization of the patient, percutaneous bronchial artery embolization has been shown to be a safe and effective treatment at controlling hemoptysis in non-CF bronchiectasis. In the event that this is not possible, consideration of surgical intervention is recommended.

Patients with bronchiectasis experience frequent exacerbations and thus are more often subject to the complications associated with respiratory infection, such as pneumonia, empyema, and lung abscess.

RESPIRATORY FAILURE

Respiratory failure and cor pulmonale still occur in severe bronchiectasis. These patients should be treated conventionally, including long-term oxygen therapy (LTOT) and diuretics, in accordance with guidelines.

There is little information on the use of noninvasive ventilation (NIV) either in the acute setting or in the longer term for bronchiectatic patients in respiratory failure. A study of survival in 48 patients admitted to the intensive care unit included those receiving NIV (13) and those who required intubation (26). There was a 19% mortality associated with the first episode of respiratory failure in patients with bilateral bronchiectasis, with mortality of 40% at 1 year, similar to that with COPD. The population studied was at an advanced stage of bronchiectasis, with severe impairment of lung function, frequent use of LTOT, and a high rate of colonization with *P. aeruginosa*, although this alone was not associated with reduced survival. There is a possible overlap with COPD in this group, and although intubation may have been associated with a reduced survival, this likely represented a more severely affected group, making interpretation of the success of NIV in the acute setting less clear. Age and LTOT were also associated with decreased survival.

Comparison of LTOT alone versus that with home nasal mask ventilation in patients with diffuse bronchiectasis and chronic respiratory failure failed to demonstrate an additional benefit on arterial blood gases and survival, although it did reduce hospitalization and improve functional status. Other studies, however, have failed to demonstrate this decrease in hospitalization.

PROGNOSIS

The overall prognosis for patients with bronchiectasis is good, even with a significant risk of mortality at the severe end of the disease spectrum. However, most of the information regarding the prognosis of bronchiectasis is based on a 1990s study in Finland. The prognosis for bronchiectatic patients treated in the hospital was better than that for age-matched and gender-matched COPD patients, but poorer than matched asthmatic patients. Bronchiectasis was the primary cause of death in 13% of bronchiectatic patients.

For patients admitted to the hospital with an acute exacerbation of bronchiectasis, factors associated with an increased mortality risk include male gender, increased creatinine, decreased FEV_1, need for mechanical ventilation, history of smoking, and need for systemic steroids during hospitalization. A U.S. review of mortality in patients admitted with acute exacerbation of bronchiectasis found 9% mortality during admission and 30% at 1 year, with median survival of 46.6 months.

CONTROVERSIES AND PITFALLS

The increasing frequency of HRCT scanning has made it apparent that radiologic changes associated with bronchiectasis are present in a large proportion of patients with COPD. Whether this represents the same pathophysiologic process as in patients with classic non–cystic fibrosis bronchiectasis remains to be determined and will subsequently guide the appropriate treatment for these patients. Furthermore, the experience of successful CF therapies failing (or being detrimental) in patients with non-CF bronchiectasis means that evidence for their use cannot simply be extrapolated. The role of quantitative microbiology, long-term antibiotics, immunization strategies, and mechanical therapies remains based largely on expert opinion rather than evidence. Further studies and clinical trials in patients with non-CF bronchiectasis need to be undertaken.

CONCLUSION

Bronchiectasis is a chronic disease characterized by chronic sputum production and bacterial colonization, regardless of the underlying cause, which should be identified. Conventional management as well as alternative therapies are used to break the vicious cycle that underlies bronchiectatic pathophysiology. Increased understanding of the mechanisms that enhance the ability of bacteria to colonize the lungs of patients with bronchiectasis will also help elucidate the many factors that initiate and perpetuate the damage to the lungs and subsequently to the host defenses.

SUGGESTED READINGS

Asad S, Opal S: Bench-to-bedside review: quorum sensing and the role of cell-to-cell communication during invasive bacterial infection, *Crit Care* 12:236, 2008.

British Thoracic Society Bronchiectasis (non-CF) Guideline Group: Guideline for non-CF bronchiectasis, *Thorax* 65(Suppl 1), 2010. www.brit-thoracic.org.uk.

Cymbala AA, Edmonds LC, Bauer MA, et al: The disease modifying effects of twice weekly azithromycin in patients with bronchiectasis, *Treat Respir Med* 4:117–122, 2005.

Dupont M, Gacouin A, Lena H, et al: Survival of patients with bronchiectasis after the first ICU stay for respiratory failure, *Chest* 125:1815–1820, 2004.

Finklea JD, Khan G, Thomas S: Predictors of mortality in hospitalized patients with acute exacerbation of bronchiectasis, *Respir Med* 104:816–821, 2010.

Hill AT, Campbell EJ, Hill SL, et al: Association between airway bacterial load and markers of airway inflammation in patients with stable chronic bronchitis, *Am J Med* 109:288–295, 2000.

Hornick DB, Fick RB: The immunoglobulin G subclass composition of immune complexes in cystic fibrosis: implications for the pathogenesis of the *Pseudomonas* lung lesion, *J Clin Invest* 86:185–192, 1990.

Jean-Baptiste E: Clinical assessment and management of massive hemoptysis (review), *Crit Care Med* 28:1642–1647, 2000.

Keistenan T, Saynajakangas O, Tuuponen T, et al: Bronchiectasis: an orphan disease with a poorly understood prognosis, *Eur Respir J* 10:2784–2787, 1997.

King PT, Holdsworth SR, Farmer M, et al: Phenotypes of adult bronchiectasis: onset of productive cough in childhood and adulthood, *J COPD* 6:130–136, 2009.

Martinez-Garcia MA, Perpina-Tordera M, Roman-Sanchez P, et al: Quality of life determinants in patients with clinically stable bronchiectasis, *Chest* 128:739–745, 2005.

Martinez Garcia MA, Soler-Cataluna JJ, Perpino-Tordera M: Factors associated with lung function decline in adult patients with non–cystic fibrosis bronchiectasis, *Chest* 132:1565–1572, 2007.

Mikami M, Llewellyn-Jones CG, Bayley D, et al: The chemotactic activity of sputum from patients with bronchiectasis, *Am J Respir Crit Care Med* 157:723, 1998.

Pasteur M, Helliwell SM, Houghton SJ, et al: An investigation into causative factors in patients with bronchiectasis, *Am J Respir Crit Care Med* 162:1277–1284, 2001.

Tsang KW, Chan K, Ho P, et al: Sputum elastase in steady-state bronchiectasis, *Chest* 117:420–426, 2000.

Chapter **46**
Approach to Diagnosis of Diffuse Lung Disease

Athol Wells

The term *diffuse lung disease* (DLD) includes infiltrative lung processes that involve the alveolar spaces or lung interstitium. This definition is fundamentally unsatisfactory because it groups together a variety of diverse disorders, some of which, such as cryptogenic organizing pneumonia, are not actually "diffuse," but rather patchy and sometimes limited in extent. Furthermore, many secondary infiltrative abnormalities, including bacterial infection and malignancy, are excluded, whereas others, such as pulmonary involvement in *connective tissue disease* (CTD), are retained in most DLD classifications. The DLDs are grouped for historical reasons; in early series, DLDs presented most frequently with widespread clinical and chest radiographic abnormalities. However, with increasing clinician awareness of possible DLD, the diagnosis is often made when chest radiographic findings are limited, or disease is apparent only on high-resolution computed tomography (HRCT).

The diagnostic difficulties resulting from the multiple disorders within the DLDs are exacerbated by semantic confusion. Synonymous terms abound for some of the more frequently encountered DLDs, such as the following:

- Cryptogenic organizing pneumonia (bronchiolitis obliterans organizing pneumonia, proliferative bronchiolitis)
- Idiopathic pulmonary fibrosis (cryptogenic fibrosing alveolitis)
- Hypersensitivity pneumonitis (extrinsic allergic alveolitis)

This problem has been partially addressed by the reclassification of the *idiopathic interstitial pneumonias* by a joint American Thoracic Society/European Respiratory Society (ATS/ERS) international consensus committee, discussed in detail in Chapter 47. However, the term *cryptogenic fibrosing alveolitis* (CFA) continues to cause difficulties. As defined in the ATS/ERS reclassification, CFA is strictly synonymous with *idiopathic pulmonary fibrosis* (IPF). The diagnosis of IPF/CFA now requires the presence of usual interstitial pneumonia (UIP) at surgical biopsy or typical appearances on HRCT, in association with a compatible clinical picture. This represents a radical change; in historical series, various disorders presenting with a clinical picture of IPF were grouped together as IPF/CFA. The entity of "clinical CFA syndrome" is still necessary for epidemiologic studies but should not be viewed as a final diagnosis in clinical practice.

In routine practice, a simplified pragmatic approach to diagnosis of DLD is essential; consideration of a checklist of the more common diseases is often useful. The classification of

DLD by their disease burden was addressed most definitively in a study from Bernalillo County, New Mexico, in which the incidence and prevalence of individual DLDs was quantified using a variety of methods (**Table 46-1**). New cases were estimated to occur in 32:100,000 years in males and 26:100,000 years in females; thus, although less common than lung infection, malignant disease or obstructive airways disease, the DLDs are responsible for a considerable disease burden. More recent evidence shows an increase in the prevalence of DLD, especially IPF, which inevitably means that the burden of disease has increased further in the previous one to two decades. Moreover, the workload for the respiratory medicine physician is disproportionate because the diagnosis of individual DLDs is often uncertain, despite more intensive investigation than is generally required in obstructive airways disease, malignancy, or chronic lung suppuration.

A consideration of the differential diagnosis of DLD, based on prevalence alone, is merely a starting point, for two reasons. First, clinical information at initial evaluation profoundly alters diagnostic probabilities; therefore a longer checklist of the DLDs, based on the possible underlying cause, is indispensable. Second, the length to which a specific diagnosis is pursued, with particular reference to surgical biopsy, is critically dependent on the importance of discriminating between *likely* differential diagnoses in individual cases. This crucial point is discussed in detail in the concluding section of this chapter.

INITIAL CLINICAL EVALUATION

Even before chest radiography and HRCT findings are considered, a wealth of diagnostic information can be obtained from initial evaluation. A possible underlying cause is often apparent, although environmental and drug exposures occurring many years earlier and apparently limited exposures are often difficult to interpret in isolation. Much information can often be obtained on the longitudinal behavior of disease from the evolution of symptoms, serial chest radiographic data, and less frequently, serial spirometric volumes. Associated systemic disease and prominent airway-centered symptoms both provide useful diagnostic clues. Less frequently, physical examination may serve to broaden the differential diagnosis. In addition to chest radiography and HRCT, certain noninvasive ancillary tests should be performed in select patients, including autoimmune serology, measurement of precipitins, and echocardiography.

Table 46-1   **Prevalence and Incidence of Interstitial Lung Diseases in Bernalillo County, New Mexico**

Cause	Interstitial Lung Disease (ILD)	Prevalent Cases, N (%)	Incident Cases, N (%)
Occupational and environmental	Pneumoconiosis	8 (3.1)	—
	Anthracosis	3 (1.1)	—
	Asbestosis	17 (6.6)	15 (7.4)
	Silicosis	8 (3.1)	6 (3.0)
	Hypersensitivity pneumonitis	3 (1.5)	—
Drug/radiation	Drug-induced ILD	5 (1.9)	7 (3.5)
	Radiation fibrosis	1 (0.4)	3 (1.5)
Pulmonary hemorrhage syndromes	Goodpasture syndrome	1 (0.5)	—
	Vasculitis	—	1 (0.5)
	Hemosiderosis	2 (0.8)	—
	Wegener granulomatosis	2 (1.2)	6 (3.0)
Connective tissue disease	Mixed connective tissue disease	2 (0.8)	2 (1.0)
	Systemic lupus erythematosus	6 (2.3)	1 (0.5)
	Rheumatoid arthritis	14 (5.4)	10 (5.0)
	Scleroderma	9 (3.5)	3 (1.5)
	Sjögren syndrome	2 (0.8)	1 (0.5)
	Dermatomyositis, polymyositis	—	1 (0.5)
	Ankylosing spondylitis	—	—
Pulmonary fibrosis	Pulmonary (chronic) fibrosis/postinflammatory	43 (16.7)	28 (13.9)
	Idiopathic/interstitial fibrosis	58 (22.5)	63 (31.2)
	Interstitial pneumonitis	8 (3.1)	12 (5.9)
Sarcoidosis		30 (11.6)	16 (7.8)
Other	Alveolar proteinosis	1 (0.4)	—
	Amyloidosis	—	—
	Bronchiolitis obliterans	—	1 (0.5)
	Chronic eosinophilic pneumonia	3 (1.2)	1 (0.5)
	Eosinophilic (granuloma) infiltration	2 (0.8)	—
	Infectious/postinfectious ILD	3 (1.2)	1 (0.5)
	Lymphocytic infiltrative lung disease	1 (0.4)	—
	ILD, not otherwise specified	29 (11.1)	20 (9.8)
TOTAL		258	202

CLINICAL HISTORY

The identification of an *underlying cause* is the single most important contribution made by clinical evaluation. **Table 46-2** provides a checklist of the more important causes of DLD. A careful occupational history is essential and should include details of all previous occupations, including short-term employment. *Asbestos exposure* is often extensive in railway rolling-stock construction, shipyard workers, power station construction and maintenance workers, naval boilermen, garage workers (involved in brake lining), and other occupations in which asbestos exposure is overt; generally, workers in these occupations are well aware of their asbestos exposure. However, other workers, including joiners, electricians, carpenters, and construction workers, who handle asbestos in the form of

roofing and insulation material, are often unaware of significant exposure. Other occupations associated with DLD include coal mining (coal worker's pneumoconiosis), metal polishing (hard metal disease), and sandblasting (silicosis).

A careful history will also disclose exposure to organic antigens known to cause *hypersensitivity pneumonitis*. The two most prevalent forms of hypersensitivity pneumonitis are farmer's (harvester's, thresher's) lung disease, in which the offending antigen, thermophilic actinomycetes *(Thermoactinomyces vulgaris)* is contained within moldy hay, and pigeon (bird) breeder's lung disease (bird fancier's lung), in which avian proteins are inhaled by those breeding birds, or more often, those who keep birds as domestic pets. However, a wide range of other exposures also cause hypersensitivity pneumonitis, and particular attention should be paid to molds (often arising in sites of

Table 46-2   Frequently Encountered Diffuse Lung Diseases with Identifiable Underlying Cause

Cause	Differential Diagnosis	Cause	Differential Diagnosis
Occupational-related or other inhalant-related			Chlorambucil
Inorganic	Aluminum oxide fibrosis		Cyclophosphamide
	Asbestosis		Cytarabine
	Baritosis (barium)		Gold
	Berylliosis		Lomustine
	Coal worker's pneumoconiosis		Melphalan
	Metal polisher's lung/hard metal fibrosis		Methotrexate
	Siderosis (iron oxide)		Mitomycin
	Silicosis		Nitrofurantoin
	Stannosis		Penicillamine
	Talc pneumoconiosis		Phenytoin
Organic	Bird breeder's (fancier's) lung		Propranolol
	Bagassosis (sugar cane)		Sulfasalazine
	Coffee worker's lung		Tocainide
	Farmer's (harvester's) lung	Physical agents/toxins	Cocaine inhalation
	Fishmeal worker's lung		High-concentration oxygen
	Malt worker's lung		Intravenous drug use
	Maple bark stripper's lung		Paraquat toxicity
	Pituitary snuff-taker's lung		Radiation/radiotherapy
	Mushroom worker's lung	Neoplastic disease	Bronchoalveolar cell carcinoma
	Tea grower's lung		Lymphangitis carcinomatosis
	Tobacco grower's lung	Vasculitis-related	Churg-Strauss syndrome
Collagen vascular disease-related	Ankylosing spondylitis		Giant cell arteritis
	Behçet syndrome		Wegener granulomatosis
	Dermatomyositis	Disorders of circulation	Pulmonary edema
	Goodpasture syndrome		Pulmonary venoocclusive disease
	Mixed connective tissue disease	Chronic infection	Aspergillosis
	Polymyositis		Histoplasmosis
	Primary Sjögren syndrome		Tuberculosis
	Rheumatoid arthritis		Parasites, viruses
	Scleroderma	Smoking-induced	Alveolar cell carcinoma
	Systemic lupus erythematosus		Desquamative interstitial pneumonia
Drug-related	Amiodarone		Emphysema
	Azathioprine		Langerhans cell histiocytosis
	Bleomycin		Nonspecific interstitial pneumonia
	Bromocryptine		Respiratory bronchiolitis (alone and with interstitial lung disease)
	Busulfan		
	Carmustine		
	Cephalosporins		

water damage); bathroom molds (as in "basement shower syndrome" and "hot-tub lung" are easily overlooked. Hobbies should also be considered (e.g., cheese-maker's lung, wine-maker's lung). There are now more than 100 known causes of hypersensitivity pneumonitis, and an up-to-date list (e.g., see Bertorelli et al.) of the 50 more frequent causes of hypersensitivity pneumonitis is highly useful.

A detailed drug history is also essential. The drugs most frequently causing DLD are probably amiodarone, methotrexate (at doses used in CTD), and antineoplastic agents, especially bleomycin. However, a wide variety of other agents (>200 at present) cause DLD, although often in only a small number of patients, and the list increases yearly. Fortunately, an international website is now devoted to drug-induced lung disease (www.pneumotox.com), through which all medications should be routinely checked in patients with DLD.

Other therapeutic modalities causing DLD include radiotherapy and exposure to high concentrations of oxygen (especially in those previously receiving bleomycin). Paraquat

ingestion (causing acute or delayed proliferative bronchiolitis), inhalation of crack cocaine or heroin (causing eosinophilic pneumonia, diffuse alveolar hemorrhage, organizing pneumonia or pulmonary edema), and intravenous drug use (causing venoocclusive disease) are also relevant.

Smoking-related DLD is increasingly diagnosed; diseases other than chronic obstructive pulmonary disease caused by smoking include Langerhans cell histiocytosis, *respiratory bronchiolitis associated with interstitial lung disease* (RBILD), desquamative interstitial pneumonia, and nonspecific interstitial pneumonia. Recently, HRCT evaluation has shown that all these processes may coexist in the same patient. Further, both sarcoidosis and hypersensitivity pneumonitis are rare in current smokers. Because RBILD and hypersensitivity pneumonitis often have overlapping clinical and HRCT features, the smoking history is an important discriminator between these two disorders.

Information on likely longitudinal behavior often helps distinguish between acute and chronic disease, because acute infection, heart failure, and disseminated malignancy may all simulate DLD clinically and radiologically. The duration of dyspnea and cough, pattern of symptomatic progression, and previous responsiveness (or nonresponsiveness) to corticosteroid therapy may provide valuable diagnostic clues. Variable dyspnea and cough over several years, responding to steroid therapy, is compatible with hypersensitivity pneumonitis or sarcoidosis, whereas inexorably progressive dyspnea for 2 to 3 years, not responding to steroid therapy, is typical of IPF. Previous chest radiographs may be useful, with unchanging appearances over many years a frequent finding in sarcoidosis, but not in IPF. Previous full pulmonary function tests are seldom available, but serial spirometry may be performed in general practice, because asthma is often suspected when the first symptoms of DLD occur. Thus, useful conclusions may be drawn from the rapidity of decline, or conversely the duration of stability, of spirometric volumes.

Relevant systemic diseases associated with DLD include malignancy (lymphangitis carcinomatosis or multiple metastases) and CTDs complicated by DLD, especially rheumatoid arthritis, systemic sclerosis, systemic lupus erythematosus (SLE), polymyositis or dermatomyositis, and Sjögren syndrome. Lung disease may precede systemic manifestations in all the CTDs (most frequently in polymyositis/dermatomyositis) or may develop concurrently with systemic manifestations. Thus, a full history should include details of arthritis/arthralgia, myositis, skin disorders, Raynaud's phenomenon, and dryness of the eyes or mouth. A subgroup of patients with autoimmune disease who fail to meet formal criteria for an individual disorder are considered to have "undifferentiated connective tissue disease" but may nonetheless develop DLD.

Airway-centered symptoms may help to refine the differential diagnosis. Cough occurs frequently in IPF, but prominent wheeze is more suggestive of hypersensitivity pneumonitis or, less frequently, sarcoidosis. Wheezing is also an important feature of some of the pulmonary vasculitides, especially Churg-Strauss syndrome and occasionally Wegener granulomatosis. Hemoptysis is the most frequent pulmonary symptom at presentation in Goodpasture syndrome; however, the volume is not a good guide to disease severity, because hemoptysis may be trivial or even absent, despite considerable alveolar hemorrhage.

CLINICAL EXAMINATION

Physical examination tends to be less fruitful than the history and HRCT findings in refining the differential diagnosis of DLD. Bilateral predominantly basal crackles on auscultation are a defining feature of IPF and are also common in other forms of idiopathic interstitial pneumonia and asbestosis, but seldom present in sarcoidosis. Digital clubbing is a useful sign strongly indicating IPF or asbestosis; clubbing is rare in sarcoidosis, hypersensitivity pneumonitis, or pulmonary fibrosis associated with connective tissue (except possibly rheumatoid arthritis). However, no diagnostic conclusions can be drawn from the absence of clubbing. Mid- to late-inspiratory "squawks," an underrecognized sign, are strongly indicative of an underlying bronchiolitic disorder, including hypersensitivity pneumonitis, in which the bronchiolitic component may be prominent. Central cyanosis, tachypnea, and pulmonary hypertension are nonspecific findings in end-stage DLD. When pulmonary hypertension is associated with limited DLD, underlying CTD, especially systemic sclerosis and SLE, should be suspected.

DIAGNOSTIC PROCEDURES

BLOOD TESTS

In most cases, specific diagnostic tests for DLD are confined to autoimmune serology and precipitins against organic antigens. Serologic evidence of rheumatoid arthritis and the other major CTDs should be sought in any patient with apparently idiopathic DLD in whom the diagnosis is uncertain. This is particularly important when the diagnosis appears to be cryptogenic organizing pneumonia, because underlying connective disease is common; when present, prognosis is not always good, and prolonged treatment may be required. In the antisynthetase syndrome, characterized by Jo1 antibody positivity, polymyositis or dermatomyositis, and progressive pulmonary fibrosis, lung disease often precedes systemic manifestations. However, although antibodies to extractable nuclear antigens tend to be disease specific, levels of antinuclear antibodies and rheumatoid factor are often moderately increased in idiopathic pulmonary fibrosis and are less useful diagnostically unless titers are greatly elevated.

The presence of *precipitins to organic antigens* increases the likelihood of hypersensitivity pneumonitis but should never be considered diagnostic in isolation. Positive precipitins denote exposure to an antigen, with immune recognition, but alone are not indicative of clinically significant DLD; pigeon and other bird breeders often have avian precipitin positivity without overt lung disease. Moreover, in many patients with convincing exposure histories and a histologic diagnosis of hypersensitivity pneumonitis, the appropriate precipitins are not present; avian antigens, for example, vary between bird species and even between individual birds.

PULMONARY FUNCTION TESTS

Most DLDs are characterized by a restrictive ventilatory defect, a reduction in gas transfer, and variable hypoxia at rest or on exercise. A purely obstructive defect is often present in Langerhans cell histiocytosis and lymphangioleiomyomatosis and is sometimes a feature of fibrotic pulmonary sarcoidosis. A mixed ventilatory defect, which usually denotes an airway-centered component, is often present in hypersensitivity pneumonitis, sarcoidosis, and CTD (in which bronchiolitis or bronchiectasis may coexist with pulmonary fibrosis). Paradoxically, normal lung volumes in association with severe reduction in gas transfer levels are the hallmark of the combination of emphysema and pulmonary fibrosis. The often-cited phenomenon of a marked increase in gas transfer (measured using single-breath techniques) caused by diffuse alveolar hemorrhage is rarely clinically useful because this abnormality persists for only 36 hours after hemorrhage.

The most diagnostically useful pulmonary function pattern is *preservation of gas transfer* in association with *irreversible airflow obstruction*, a combination that points strongly toward intrinsic airways disease (i.e. bronchiolitis) rather than emphysema. However, the pattern of pulmonary function impairment seldom makes a major diagnostic contribution.

CHEST RADIOGRAPHY

With recent attention focused on the diagnostic value of HRCT, it is often forgotten that the plain chest x-ray film provides invaluable information in diffuse lung disease. The chest radiograph points strongly toward a specific diagnosis in some patients. *Sarcoidosis*, the most prevalent DLD encountered in clinical practice, can be diagnosed with confidence from the clinical and chest radiographic features at presentation in many patients. HRCT seldom adds useful diagnostic information in this context.

Several radiographic features have useful positive predictive values (PPVs). The presence of *hilar lymphadenopathy* on chest radiography is particularly strongly predictive of sarcoidosis in the correct clinical context, although the radiographic differential diagnosis includes tuberculosis and malignancy, especially when hilar lymphadenopathy is asymmetric. *Pleural effusions* are an occasional feature of CTD, lymphangioleiomyomatosis, and asbestos-related disease, as well as disease processes that sometimes mimic DLD, including heart failure, infection, and malignancy. The distribution of disease on chest radiography is also diagnostically useful; granulomatous diseases (tuberculosis, sarcoidosis, hypersensitivity pneumonitis) tend to be more prominent in the middle to upper zones, whereas fibrotic diseases (IPF, fibrotic nonspecific interstitial pneumonia, asbestosis) have a predominantly lower-zone distribution.

However, apart from a large subgroup of patients with sarcoidosis, diagnoses based on chest radiography are seldom confident. Chest radiography is sometimes insensitive; in one often-quoted series (Epler et al.), 10% of patients with biopsy-proven DLD had normal chest radiographic appearances. The superior diagnostic accuracy of HRCT over chest radiography has been documented in numerous series, and the increased confidence associated with an HRCT diagnosis is a considerable aid to management. The classification of chest radiographic abnormalities as "nodular, reticulonodular, or reticular" provides relatively little diagnostic information. Predominantly basal *honeycombing* on chest radiography (invariably associated with honeycombing on HRCT) may be diagnostically useful in increasing the likelihood of IPF but is radiographically overt in surprisingly few IPF patients. It is now generally accepted that, except in patients with obvious sarcoidosis, routine HRCT is almost always warranted in DLD, although occasional exceptions exist, including elderly patients with obvious lower-zone honeycombing on chest radiography, indicative of IPF, and patients with long-standing pulmonary fibrosis on serial chest radiography and an obvious underlying cause, such as coal mining.

Two chest radiographic appearances pose particular diagnostic difficulties. *Persistent unexplained multifocal consolidation* has usually been treated unsuccessfully as for community-acquired pneumonia and has a wide differential diagnosis. Serial chest radiography tends to be more useful than HRCT in refining investigation, because the crucial diagnostic distinction lies between *fixed* infiltrates (nonbacterial infection, including tuberculosis, alveolar cell carcinoma, and other malignant processes) and *changing* infiltrates, in which these diagnoses are effectively excluded. However, immunologically mediated diseases, including eosinophilic pneumonia, cryptogenic organizing pneumonia, and vasculitic disorders, may give rise to either fixed or evanescent radiographic abnormalities, and a histologic diagnosis is often warranted. *Diffuse alveolar filling processes* giving rise to widespread air-space consolidation are generally indicative of life-threatening disease. Although this picture may represent DLD (e.g., acute interstitial pneumonitis, acute eosinophilic syndromes, drug-induced pulmonary infiltration), it is essential to broaden the differential diagnosis beyond DLD to include diffuse pulmonary infection, toxic inhalation, severe aspiration, opportunistic infection (especially *Pneumocystis* pneumonia), diffuse alveolar hemorrhage syndromes, mitral

stenosis, and most importantly, heart failure. In both these radiographic presentations, successful management often depends on consideration of a wide differential diagnosis from the outset.

HIGH-RESOLUTION COMPUTED TOMOGRAPHY

High-resolution CT has been the most important diagnostic advance in DLD in the last two decades. Numerous studies have confirmed the overall diagnostic accuracy of HRCT against findings at surgical biopsy, with a striking increase in sensitivity and specificity for individual diseases, compared with chest radiography. However, academic series understate the impact of HRCT, because the most important benefit has been to increase clinician confidence in noninvasive diagnosis, with a corresponding reduction in the numbers of patients needing to undergo surgical biopsy. Before HRCT, diagnoses based on clinical data and chest radiographic findings were seldom confident, and management was necessarily tentative in many cases. The combination of clinical and HRCT information now provides a confident first-choice diagnosis in the majority of patients, and in many other cases, the realistic differential diagnosis is shortened to two or three disorders. This allows surgical biopsy to be reserved for patients in whom the distinction between a small group of possible disorders has important management implications and for occasional patients in whom HRCT appearances are not suggestive of any single disorder. Thus, routine surgical biopsy, as a diagnostic "gold standard," can no longer be justified in the HRCT era.

Histospecific diagnosis aside, HRCT sometimes plays an important role in detecting DLD. The superior sensitivity of HRCT over chest radiography has been an invariable finding in studies of a wide range of disorders. This feature of HRCT is particularly useful when symptoms or lung function impairment are associated with normal chest radiographic appearances. In CTD, pulmonary involvement is now the leading cause of death, and early treatment of progressive lung disease is desirable. By identifying limited pulmonary fibrosis, HRCT allows clinicians to select patients requiring more intensive monitoring, even when immediate treatment is not warranted. In workers previously exposed to asbestos, HRCT often discloses pulmonary fibrosis, which is obscured on chest radiography by concurrent pleural disease. However, it should be stressed that the sensitivity of HRCT occasionally creates its own difficulties. When interstitial abnormalities are limited, their clinical significance is sometimes difficult to rationalize; disease evident only on HRCT should not be extrapolated, in terms of natural history and management, to the more extensive disease described in historical clinical series. It is essential that HRCT findings are integrated with other clinical and investigative features and not interpreted in isolation.

The distinction between predominantly inflammatory and predominantly fibrotic disease can generally be made with reasonable confidence from HRCT. Anatomic distortion and reticular abnormalities are strongly indicative of irreversible fibrotic disease, and this is invariably true of honeycomb change (**Figure 46-1**). Consolidation is usually reversible, although it may occasionally represent dense fibrosis, especially in sarcoidosis. *Ground-glass attenuation* is often more difficult to interpret. In early work, this HRCT sign was shown to identify a substantial increase in the likelihood of significant inflammation, especially in the absence of concurrent reticular abnormalities. However, it is now clear that ground-glass attenuation denotes fine fibrosis in many cases, especially in sarcoidosis and nonspecific

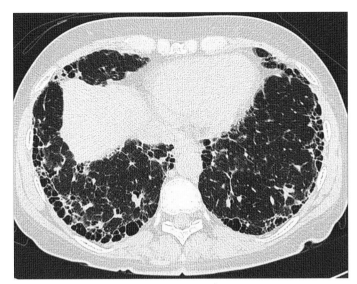

Figure 46-1   High-resolution computed tomography (HRCT) scan in patient with idiopathic pulmonary fibrosis (IPF). There is prominent subpleural honeycombing with no ground-glass attenuation. In the correct clinical context, this image is virtually pathognomonic of IPF.

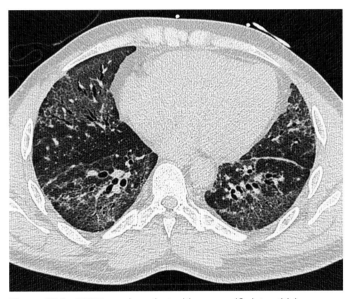

Figure 46-2   HRCT scan in patient with nonspecific interstitial pneumonia. Predominant abnormalities are ground-glass attenuation, with variable admixed fine reticular abnormalities, and traction bronchiectasis. Notably, there is no honeycomb change.

Box 46-1	**High-Resolution Computed Tomography (HRCT) Features of Select Diffuse Lung Diseases (DLDs)**

Idiopathic pulmonary fibrosis: Lower zone, subpleural predominance, maximal posterobasally, predominantly reticular pattern with associated honeycombing.

Nonspecific interstitial pneumonia: Two typical appearances:

1. Variant that overlaps with idiopathic pulmonary fibrosis in disease distribution: ground-glass attenuation predominates, with a variable fine reticular component and traction bronchiectasis, but no honeycombing.
2. Variant that overlaps with cryptogenic organizing pneumonia: consolidation with surrounding ground-glass attenuation and a variable, fine reticular pattern.

Desquamative interstitial pneumonia: Ground-glass attenuation, sometimes diffuse, sometimes basal and peripheral–centered, frequent associated fibrotic cysts with anatomic distortion and traction bronchiectasis.

Acute interstitial pneumonia: Widespread ground-glass attenuation admixed with features of fibrosis, usually with air space consolidation and occasionally with emphysema.

Respiratory bronchiolitis interstitial lung disease: Patchy ground-glass attenuation, poorly defined centrilobular nodules, occasional mosaic attenuation, prominent bronchial wall thickening.

Sarcoidosis: Highly variable; nodules distributed along bronchovascular bundles, interlobular septae, and subpleurally, including the fissure; ground-glass attenuation that may represent either inflammation or fine fibrosis; reticular abnormalities representing fibrosis; distortion most often in upper zones with posterior displacement of upper lobe bronchus; air trapping; associated hilar and mediastinal lymphadenopathy.

Subacute hypersensitivity pneumonitis: Widespread ground-glass attenuation, often containing poorly defined centrilobular nodules, admixed with areas of "black lung" (mosaic attenuation), representing air trapping and enhanced on expiratory HRCT.

Cryptogenic organizing pneumonia: Bilateral patchy consolidation, subpleural and predominantly basal in most cases; occasional peribronchial distribution; associated, often-sparse nodules up to 1 cm in diameter.

Constrictive bronchiolitis: Patchy areas of hyperlucency enhanced on expiration, which may not change in cross-sectional diameter on full expiration; associated bronchiectasis and bronchial wall thickening.

Langerhans cell histiocytosis: Bizarre cyst shapes and associated nodules throughout the lung fields but sparing costophrenic angles and tips of lingula and middle lobes; associated emphysema often seen.

Pulmonary lymphangioleiomyomatosis: Homogeneously distributed, thin-walled parenchymal cysts, varying from a few millimeters to several centimeters in diameter; associated with retrocrural adenopathy, pleural effusion, thoracic duct dilation, pericardial effusion, and pneumothorax.

interstitial pneumonia, in which ground-glass attenuation is the cardinal HRCT feature (**Figure 46-2**). *Traction bronchiectasis* is a key HRCT discriminator because it invariably indicates underlying fibrosis. Thus, reversible inflammatory disease is likely only when ground-glass attenuation is not associated with traction bronchiectasis or admixed with reticular abnormalities.

A wide range of HRCT profiles encompassing the distribution and pattern of DLD strongly suggests individual diseases. **Box 46-1** summarizes the cardinal findings in common DLDs. As with its other applications, it is essential that HRCT findings be integrated with the pretest diagnostic probability, distilled from the history, clinical signs, previous natural history, or treatment course and the investigative findings, especially chest radiography, pulmonary function tests, and serology for

autoimmune disease and environmental antigens. The role of HRCT in diagnosis is critically dependent on the presence or absence of a likely cause. In patients with appropriate environmental antigen or drug exposures (hypersensitivity pneumonitis, pneumoconioses, drug-induced lung disease), malignant disease (lymphangitis carcinomatosis), clinical or serologic evidence of CTD, or a heavy smoking history (Langerhans cell histiocytosis, RBILD), the diagnostic weighting required from HRCT can be reduced. In these contexts, HRCT appearances that are merely compatible (and not classic) often allow a sufficiently confident diagnosis to obviate diagnostic surgical biopsy.

By contrast, as discussed, the diagnostic role of HRCT is much greater in idiopathic disease, but unless the pretest diagnostic probability is high, confident diagnosis requires the presence of typical HRCT appearances. The optimal diagnostic use of HRCT in apparently idiopathic DLD can be distilled in a simple pragmatic algorithm, as follows:

1. The first step is to determine whether HRCT abnormalities are predominantly *fibrotic*, based on the presence of honeycombing, reticular abnormalities, anatomic distortion, or in patients with prominent ground-glass attenuation, the presence of traction bronchiectasis.
2. If disease is fibrotic, as in a large majority of cases, the next important question is whether HRCT findings are typical of *idiopathic pulmonary fibrosis.* As stated in the 2011 American Thoracic Society/European Respiratory Society (ATS/ERS) recommendations, IPF can be diagnosed confidently on HRCT when there is honeycombing with minimal ground-glass attenuation in a predominantly basal and subpleural distribution. It is logical to focus on IPF because it is the most prevalent idiopathic fibrotic disease among patients in whom the diagnosis is not obvious from clinical and chest radiographic findings (most cases of sarcoidosis are diagnosed without recourse to HRCT) (**Figure 46-3**). Further, IPF has a much worse prognosis than other fibrosing processes and therefore is the most important diagnosis to confirm or exclude from the outset. It is now known that HRCT appearances considered typical of IPF by experienced thoracic radiologists have a PPV greater than 95%.
3. If appearances are not typical of IPF, the five most important differential diagnoses (based on prevalence in routine practice) are (a) IPF with atypical HRCT appearances, (b) sarcoidosis, (c) nonspecific interstitial pneumonia, (d) hypersensitivity pneumonitis (with the antigen unknown),

and (e) the fibrotic sequelae of cryptogenic organizing pneumonia. Among these, IPF with atypical HRCT appearances is the most prevalent disorder in most populations; up to 30% of IPF patients have atypical HRCT features. Atypical IPF is especially likely when HRCT appearances are not typical of any of the other four disorders (b-e).

The weighting given to HRCT in the diagnosis of DLD varies from case to case but can usefully be considered in three categories. In some patients, HRCT appearances are virtually *pathognomonic*; this includes many cases of IPF, Langerhans cell histiocytosis, sarcoidosis, and lymphangitis carcinomatosis. Often, HRCT findings are *diagnostic* when combined with clinical information. A good example is the combination of widespread ground-glass attenuation (often with poorly defined centrilobular nodules) in combination with mosaic attenuation, which may be strongly indicative of hypersensitivity pneumonitis in nonsmokers with a compatible exposure history but may also represent RBILD in smokers (**Figure 46-4**). Third, even when not conclusive alone, HRCT may be invaluable when considered with *diagnostic surgical biopsy*. The histologic entity of *nonspecific interstitial pneumonia* (NSIP) is found in a variety of clinicoradiologic contexts, including entities overlapping clinically with IPF, fibrosing organizing pneumonia, and hypersensitivity pneumonitis; HRCT evaluation is key to distinguishing among these variants.

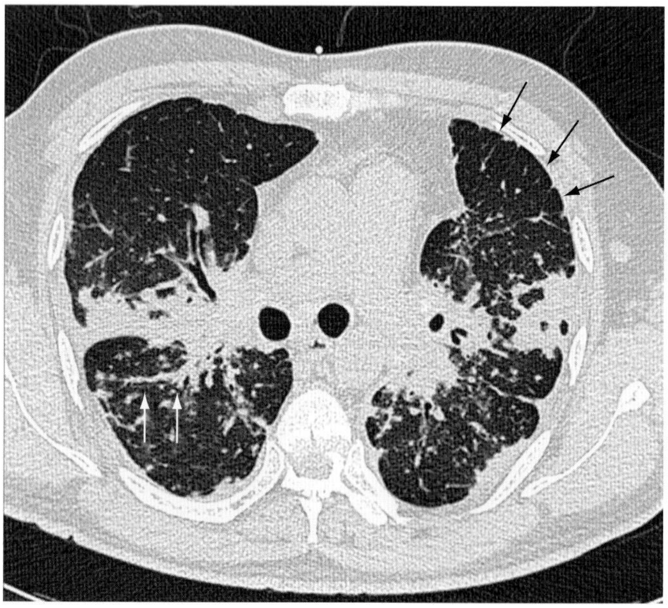

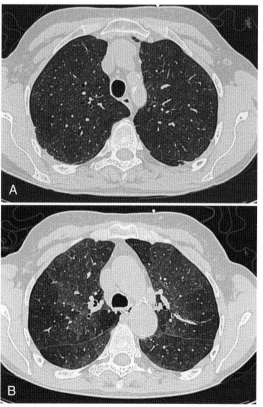

Figure 46-3 HRCT scan in patient with sarcoidosis. Abnormalities suggesting the diagnosis include multiple, well-defined nodules, surrounding bronchovascular beading *(white arrows)*, micronodules (especially in left anterior lung, *black arrows*), septal thickening (by granulomatous infiltration), and areas of dense consolidation, which may be reversible (coalescence of granulomas) or irreversible (fibrosis). This combination of abnormalities is virtually pathognomonic of sarcoidosis.

Figure 46-4 HRCT scans in patient with hypersensitivity pneumonitis. **A,** Abnormalities on inspiratory scan show widespread ground-glass attenuation, often with poorly formed centrilobular nodules, and are often extremely subtle; appearances may be virtually normal. **B,** On expiratory scan, striking regional variation in lung attenuation is often apparent, with areas of darker lung representing gas trapping (from bronchiolitic component of disease).

BRONCHOSCOPIC PROCEDURES

Although endobronchial and transbronchial biopsies are straightforward and relatively noninvasive procedures, the volume of tissue taken is small, with only bronchial and peribronchial tissue sampled. Thus, both procedures have a high yield in diseases with peribronchial distribution, especially sarcoidosis and lymphangitis carcinomatosis. Occasionally, transbronchial biopsy findings can help confirm a diagnosis of hypersensitivity pneumonitis, although bronchoalveolar lavage fluid tends to be more rewarding in this regard. Bronchoscopic biopsy procedures have little or no diagnostic value in the idiopathic interstitial pneumonias.

Hemorrhage and pneumothorax (with transbronchial biopsy) are the important risks associated with bronchoscopic procedures. Major hemorrhage is rare, but pneumothoraces complicate transbronchial biopsies in 1% to 2% of procedures, although intercostal tube drainage is not always required.

In the 1980s, many regarded bronchoalveolar lavage (BAL) as an important part of the diagnostic algorithm in DLD. The distinction between a BAL neutrophilia (suggestive of IPF) and a BAL lymphocytosis (as in sarcoidosis or hypersensitivity pneumonitis) was held to be particularly useful. With experience, however, it became apparent that diagnostic distinctions based on BAL fluid in large groups of patients were insufficiently reliable in individual patients. The advent of HRCT also limited the role of BAL, which had been more influential in the pre-HRCT era, when most noninvasive diagnoses were tentative. There are currently no published evaluations of the diagnostic value added by BAL, once HRCT findings are taken into account.

In recent years, however, use of BAL has increased in some centers. In the 2002 ATS/ERS recommendations, compatible BAL findings (i.e., no lymphocytosis) are a requirement for the noninvasive diagnosis of IPF. Although not formally retained in the 2011 recommendations, this criterion reflects the diagnostic value of BAL findings when HRCT appearances are suggestive of IPF but not definitive. However, a BAL lymphocytosis has an even greater diagnostic impact in some patients with sarcoidosis or hypersensitivity pneumonitis. When significant fibrosis supervenes in these disorders, HRCT appearances often become atypical, and IPF is frequently the preferred diagnosis, before performance of BAL. A BAL lymphocytosis in the setting of fibrotic DLD may be an important justification for diagnostic surgical biopsy. Thus, BAL continues to play a useful diagnostic role in a significant subset of patients, when clinical and HRCT features are inconclusive, although adding little to diagnosis in the majority of DLD patients.

SURGICAL BIOPSY

Surgical biopsy, formerly performed as an open procedure but now widely obtained using video-assisted thoracoscopic surgery (VATS), was once regarded as the diagnostic reference standard and, until recently, was advocated as a routine diagnostic procedure by some authorities. However, routine surgical biopsy is impractical outside referral centers, and in the 1980s, even before HRCT had a significant diagnostic impact, it was performed in less than 15% of patients with IPF in the United Kingdom. Even in referral centers, number of diagnostic surgical biopsies has been radically reduced with the application of HRCT. In one UK referral center, the Royal Brompton Hospital, biopsy was performed in more than 50% of IPF patients in the 1980s but in less than 25% in the mid-1990s. Moreover, it

is increasingly clear that open or VATS biopsy is not a true diagnostic gold standard. Variation between 10 thoracic pathologists in assigning a histologic diagnosis in DLD was recently found to be considerable, with agreement only moderate (kappa coefficient of agreement of 0.38). In more than 20% of biopsies, the first-choice diagnosis was assigned with low confidence.

Thus, although biopsy procedures add invaluable information in select patients, and a pattern of usual interstitial pneumonia is usually diagnostically definitive, a histologic diagnosis alone should no longer be viewed as a diagnostic gold standard.

Sometimes, the histologic diagnosis is at odds with clinical and HRCT information and must be integrated with other information. In some patients with fibrotic hypersensitivity pneumonitis, a histologic pattern of *usual interstitial pneumonia* (which is normally indicative of IPF) is disclosed at biopsy, despite clinical, HRCT, and BAL features of hypersensitivity pneumonitis and an indolent course during follow-up. Similarly, in a cohort of more than 100 patients with IPF or fibrotic NSIP (Flaherty et al., 2003), a combination of histologic and HRCT findings provided more accurate prognostic information than either modality alone. Thus, surgical biopsy is now best viewed, as with HRCT, as a diagnostic "silver standard" that can often be avoided when HRCT and clinical features are typical of an individual DLD.

The morbidity and mortality associated with surgical biopsy in DLD are low in patients with an adequate pulmonary reserve but increase significantly in those with severe disease. In one series (Utz et al.), patients with advanced IPF (mean gas transfer <35% predicted) had a mortality ascribable to biopsy of 15%. Although this figure is generally regarded as an overstatement of the risk of the procedure, based on other series and widespread anecdotal experience, a surgical biopsy should not be performed unless central to management if the gas transfer is less than 30% of predicted. Moreover, in advanced idiopathic fibrotic disease, the prognostic value of a histospecific diagnosis diminishes. In another series (Latsi et al.), mortality was identical in IPF and fibrotic NSIP when the gas transfer was less than 35%, despite major differences in survival in less severe disease.

Thus, in younger patients (<60) presenting with a typical clinical picture of severe IPF and HRCT features suggestive of fibrotic NSIP, immediate referral for consideration of lung transplantation is warranted, without a histologic diagnosis. The exception is the patient presenting with overwhelmingly severe acute DLD, in which the diagnosis is unclear, and realistic differential diagnoses include acute interstitial pneumonia, severe infection (e.g., opportunistic infection), and malignancy. BAL fluid may be required to exclude infection, and occasionally a histologic diagnosis is required to plan management. Both procedures can be performed in ventilated patients, and if disease is slightly less severe, elective mechanical ventilation may be warranted to investigate appropriately.

INTEGRATED DIAGNOSIS IN DIFFUSE LUNG DISEASE

The central diagnostic challenge for the clinician is to integrate the clinical and diagnostic information into a final diagnosis, without overemphasizing any single clinical or investigative feature. Indeed, only the clinician is able to play this latter role, because both histologic and HRCT diagnoses made without reference to other information are seriously flawed in a significant proportion of patients. The most difficult dilemma, when noninvasive evaluation discloses two or more realistic diagnoses, is whether to accept diagnostic uncertainty, without investigating further, or to resort to invasive (surgical biopsy) or semi-invasive (BAL fluid, transbronchial biopsy) procedures.

This decision should be made pragmatically and not by protocol. The value of a specific diagnosis in diffuse idiopathic lung disease is that the clinician is informed of the probable natural history and the likelihood that treatment will play a useful role. From these considerations, the optimal approach to monitoring disease during follow-up usually becomes apparent. Thus, the essential purpose of pursuing a diagnosis is to identify *probable* disease behavior with and without treatment. Broadly, with occasional exceptions, *longitudinal* disease behavior in DLD can be subdivided into five patterns (**Table 46-3**). When a patient can be subclassified confidently into one of these groups, invasive investigation will often add little to short-term and long-term management. Three strands of information are of particular value in making these distinctions: the underlying cause (if any), a morphologic assessment using HRCT (and histologic evaluation in select patients), and observed longitudinal disease behavior.

The identification of an underlying cause is vital because considered with HRCT appearances, it may allow disease to be classified confidently as *self-limited inflammation* (e.g., acute drug-induced lung disease, hypersensitivity pneumonitis, RBILD in smokers), with a good outcome, provided the offending agent is removed. In long-standing disease, knowledge of a cause often allows the clinician to classify fibrotic abnormalities on HRCT as *stable fibrotic disease* (e.g., fibrotic sequelae of nitrofurantoin lung, silicosis, other pneumoconioses); the

confidence of this conclusion is increased by the documentation of stable longitudinal disease behavior, based on previous chest radiographs, symptoms, and occasionally pulmonary function tests. In both self-limited inflammation and stable fibrotic disease, invasive diagnostic investigations are seldom warranted, and potentially toxic treatments can usually be minimized.

A histologic diagnosis is required more frequently in apparently idiopathic disease, to draw two essential distinctions: between inherently stable and potentially progressive fibrotic disease, and between major inflammation (with high risk of evolution to fibrosis with undertreatment) and inexorably progressive fibrotic disease. In both scenarios, therapeutic intervention may be the key to a substantially better outcome. Knowledge of likely intrinsic disease behavior is invaluable because it allows decisive management and increases patient confidence considerably. A confident diagnosis of hypersensitivity pneumonitis, NSIP, or cryptogenic organizing pneumonia associated with significant fibrosis justifies aggressive intervention with a higher risk of drug toxicity, because the treated outcome is often good. By contrast, in IPF, in which the benefits of treatment may be marginal, a more cautious therapeutic approach is often warranted, and in younger patients, the timing in considering transplantation can be planned. As a general principle, BAL and surgical biopsy should always be pursued in patients fit for these procedures, as determined by age, disease severity, and comorbidity, if a confident management strategy based on disease behavior cannot be devised from noninvasive evaluation.

These principles apply especially to the most common presentation of nongranulomatous idiopathic DLD: the cryptogenic fibrosing alveolitis (CFA) clinical syndrome. In previous decades, underlying histologic appearances have tended to be lumped together, but the recent ATS/ERS reclassification of the idiopathic interstitial pneumonias has provided a framework for the separation of a number of disease entities with strikingly diverse natural histories and treated outcomes (**Table 46-4**). In evaluation of biopsy diagnoses in the 1980s of "cryptogenic fibrosing alveolitis" in patients presenting with the CFA clinical syndrome, an alternative histologic diagnosis associated with a much better observed outcome was evident on review in more

Table 46-3 **Most Common Patterns of Longitudinal Disease Behavior in Diffuse Lung Disease (DLD) with Select Underlying Diagnoses***

Pattern	Select Diagnoses
Self-limited inflammation	Drug-induced lung disease (acute onset) Hypersensitivity pneumonitis (usually short-term exposure) Sarcoidosis (distinct subset with, usually, acute onset)
Stable fibrotic disease	Drug-induced lung disease (residual fibrosis after cessation) Hypersensitivity pneumonitis (after prolonged exposure) Nonprogressive pneumoconioses after exposure (e.g., silicosis) Sarcoidosis (residuum of burnt-out disease)
Major inflammation, risk of fibrotic progression	Drug-induced lung disease (unusually florid reactions) Hypersensitivity pneumonitis (usually continuing exposure) Sarcoidosis (prolonged severe inflammation)
Inexorably progressive fibrosis	Drug-induced lung disease (continuing exposure) Hypersensitivity pneumonitis (antigen usually unknown) Progressive pneumoconioses after exposure (e.g., asbestosis) Sarcoidosis (small subset of patients)
Explosive acute DLD	Drug-induced lung disease

*May appear in several categories; excluding idiopathic interstitial pneumonias (see Table 46-4).

Table 46-4 **Idiopathic Interstitial Pneumonias***

Clinicopathologic Diagnosis	Likely Longitudinal Behavior
Idiopathic pulmonary fibrosis/ cryptogenic fibrosing alveolitis	Inexorably progressive fibrosis
Nonspecific interstitial pneumonia (NSIP)	Cellular NSIP: self-limited or major inflammation Fibrotic NSIP: stable or progressive fibrosis
Cryptogenic organizing pneumonia	Self-limited or major inflammation
Desquamative interstitial pneumonia	Self-limited or major inflammation
Respiratory bronchiolitis-associated	Self-limited inflammation interstitial lung disease
Lymphocytic interstitial pneumonia	Self-limited or major inflammation

*American Thoracic Society/European Respiratory Society (ATS/ERS) consensus classification, with most common patterns of longitudinal behavior associated with individual diagnoses.

than 50% of cases. The ATS/ERS classification system is logical and pragmatic because each entity tends to fall into a particular category of longitudinal disease behavior, although a degree of overlap is inevitable. Thus, when a confident noninvasive diagnosis is unattainable in patients with idiopathic interstitial pneumonia, surgical biopsy should always be considered.

In the influential 2004 study of Flaherty et al., in which the final diagnosis was multidisciplinary, two conclusions highly relevant to routine diagnosis were apparent. When a confident prebiopsy diagnosis of IPF was made by clinicians or radiologists, the diagnosis virtually never changed with the addition of *histologic* data. By contrast, in the remaining cases, diagnoses made by clinicians and radiologists changed in approximately 50% of cases when *biopsy* data were considered. However, it should also be stressed that the final diagnosis differed from the histologic diagnosis in 25% of cases. It is now widely accepted that a multidisciplinary diagnosis, negotiated among clinicians, radiologists, and in biopsied cases, pathologists, is the diagnostic reference standard in DLD.

TREATMENT

Key diagnostic distinctions include those that influence the management algorithm. Treatment regimens can be subdivided into those used in predominantly inflammatory disease, in which a treatment response can be expected, and those in which a response is not expected but the primary goal is to prevent or delay the progression of interstitial fibrosis. The broad pragmatic approaches to therapy can best be considered in relation to the broad patterns of disease behavior, as follows:

1. A policy of careful observation without immediate intervention is appropriate if the pattern of behavior is one of self-limited inflammation or stable fibrotic disease.
2. When inflammatory disease is viewed as intrinsically dangerous because of disease severity or is admixed with progressive fibrotic disease, high-dose initial therapy is necessary, with careful definition of the optimal treatment status, as determined by clinical features, imaging, and pulmonary function tests. In the longer term, after initial treatment, best management consists of establishing the minimum level of treatment that serves to preserve the initial gains. However, the specifics of any follow-up treatment protocol depend on the amplitude of the response and the severity of residual irreversible disease.
3. In purely fibrotic diseases, in which stabilization is a realistic long-term goal, initial high-dose corticosteroid or immunosuppressive therapy would not be expected to achieve regression of disease. The key to management lies in finding "civilized" long-term regimens, with toxicity levels acceptable to patients, which prevent further disease progression.
4. In inexorably progressive fibrotic disease, effectively equating with IPF or an IPF-like treatment course in other fibrosing disorders, a "civilized" nontoxic approach is paramount. Delaying disease progression is a realistic goal in some patients, but not at the cost of major toxicity. The importance of distinguishing between IPF and other fibrosing disorders is that in non-IPF diseases, it may be justifiable to take risks with treatment toxicity to attempt to stabilize disease.
5. A final diagnosis is not possible in many patients. The most likely scenario, based on disease prevalence, is probable IPF, but possible fibrotic NSIP or hypersensitivity pneumonitis. Guideline statements written for "definite IPF" do not address this frequent conundrum, and in many elderly patients with major comorbidity or severe lung disease, a surgical biopsy is not practical. In the absence of guideline statements, arguably the most frequent error is to miss an opportunity, and management should be determined by the most optimistic outcome scenario. If NSIP or hypersensitivity pneumonitis is a realistic possibility, a more aggressive approach, as indicated by those diagnoses, is appropriate, even when IPF is clearly the most probable diagnosis.

The optimal diagnostic approach to DLD, as discussed in this chapter, informs all these treatment considerations. In the end, best management consists of reconciling treatments to the predicted and observed patterns of disease behavior. Careful assessment of the many aspects of the DLDs at presentation and during follow-up is indispensable.

CONTROVERSIES AND PITFALLS

CLASSIFICATION OF DISEASE

Given the pivotal importance to management of identifying the likely or observed pattern of disease behavior, with a view to effective management, clinicians need a formalized disease behavior classification of DLDs, as discussed earlier. This approach (1) provides a better understanding of treatment principles by patients and non-DLD clinicians because this classification sidesteps the opaque terminology of DLD, (2) deals with the problem of diagnostic overlap (e.g., probable IPF, possible NSIP, possible hypersensitivity pneumonitis), and (3) provides a simple framework for rational treatment for the large subset of patients who cannot be classified using the current classification approach. An ATS/ERS committee is constructing a preliminary disease behavior classification along these lines.

To achieve a useful system, clinicians need to confront three uncertainties highly relevant to routine practice. First, this type of approach is not a replacement for the current *diagnostic* classification. Best diagnosis and management practice requires that the two classifications be viewed as complementary. A confident histospecific diagnosis establishes which patterns of disease behavior are possible. A diagnosis of IPF, for example, is essentially a statement that management should be as for inexorably progressive fibrosis. A diagnosis of hypersensitivity pneumonitis clarifies that all patterns of disease behavior are possible, and therefore best management should be strongly influenced by many other considerations, as discussed earlier.

A second problem is that in DLD, the current ethos is "definite classification at a single point in time." An approach in which *disease behavior* is the basis for management is limited because such a system is tentative at presentation and becomes increasingly certain as short-term disease behavior, including change with initial therapy, is taken into account. This is actually an advantage because the use of a disease behavior classification perfectly mirrors the way in which experienced clinicians evaluate DLD, with reappraisal of initial impressions and therapies at follow-up. However, formalization of this approach undoubtedly requires a change in mindset.

Third, it is important to consider that although the inflammation/fibrosis dichotomy is the most therapeutically relevant treatment distinction, new antifibrotic agents may ultimately result in partial reversibility of some fibrotic disorders. It may now be timely to design a disease behavior classification around "reversible" versus "irreversible" disease, rather than inflammation and fibrosis. Such an approach would make a classification of disease behavior relevant to rare disorders, such as pulmonary alveolar proteinosis and Langerhans cell histiocytosis, and to clinicians who manage chronic lung and systemic diseases in general, who will appreciate the straightforward rationale of therapies applied to a framework of reversible/irreversible disease.

OPTIMAL DIAGNOSIS AND REGIONAL EXPERTISE

The major shift within DLD to multidisciplinary diagnosis and away from a histologic gold standard does create important practical difficulties outside referral centers. Robust multidisciplinary diagnosis is a process of debate, disagreement, and the reconciliation of divergent views, and this approach cannot work well if one of the three disciplines, whether clinical, radiologic, or histologic, is hegemonic. However, away from referral centers, it is highly unlikely that there will be equivalent expertise in all three disciplines; even within some referral centers, this ideal is not entirely achieved. The act of questioning in a public forum nonetheless undoubtedly leads to improved diagnostic practice, but the importance of maximizing expertise should not be overlooked.

DECISION TO PERFORM BIOPSY

No authoritative guidance on the indications for performing a diagnostic lung biopsy changes that the decision is often nuanced and difficult to make clinically, even before patient concerns are considered. Clinicians know what constitutes a high-risk biopsy and generally know what constitutes a low-risk biopsy. However, many biopsies fall somewhere in-between. Moreover, patients are involved in decisions, especially those associated with increased risk, although expecting a patient to decide whether to undergo a biopsy is unreasonable. One helpful approach is to outline for patients the following five conversations about biopsy and to inform them where they lie in this spectrum:

1. A biopsy is an absolute requirement if a logical management plan can be constructed only with this information, if disease is overtly dangerous, and if there is a real risk of worsening the situation with the wrong treatment approach. Clearly, it is the duty of the physician in this scenario to persuade the patient to undergo the lung biopsy.
2. A biopsy would make management somewhat more precise and might provide benefits in terms of diagnosis and management in the longer term. However, it would be possible to construct a rational, reasonably definitive treatment approach without this information, but without less confidence. The patient can then be informed that a biopsy is strongly recommended, but that the physician could, with some misgivings, construct a logical treatment plan without this information if the patient does not accept the recommendation.
3. The arguments for and against a biopsy are finely balanced ("50/50 call"). In this case, if the patient has strong views as to whether or not to undergo the procedure, the decision is no longer finely balanced.
4. On balance, a biopsy is not needed, and the physician can construct management without this information. However, a biopsy might provide earlier information on the likely

outcome, and the patient needs to be informed that a biopsy might therefore reduce uncertainty, while not changing management. Severe anxiety caused by uncertainty is a valid indication for an invasive diagnostic procedure, and it is appropriate for the patient to choose to undergo the procedure for that reason alone.
5. A biopsy should *not* be performed because the diagnosis is already secure, based on noninvasive data, or because the risks of the procedure are unacceptably high.

The five conversations just summarized do allow a clear statement of the balance of benefit and risk and provide most patients with the information they need to participate in decision making. By contrast, an isolated discussion of the risks of a diagnostic surgical biopsy, although satisfying the demands of clinical governance, fails to make the discussion relevant to the key medical considerations or to engage the patient fully.

SUGGESTED READINGS

American Thoracic Society: Idiopathic pulmonary fibrosis: diagnosis and treatment. International consensus statement, *Am J Respir Crit Care Med* 161:646–664, 2000.

American Thoracic Society, European Respiratory Society: ATS/ERS international multidisciplinary consensus classification of the idiopathic interstitial pneumonias, *Am J Respir Crit Care Med* 165:277–304, 2002.

American Thoracic Society/European Respiratory Society/Japanese Respiratory Society/Latin American Thoracic Society Committee on Idiopathic Pulmonary Fibrosis: An official ATS/ERS/JRS/ALAT statement: idiopathic pulmonary fibrosis: evidence-based guidelines for diagnosis and management. *Am J Respir Crit Care Med* 183:788–824, 2011.

Bertorelli G, Bocchino V, Olivieri D: Hypersensitivity pneumonitis, *Eur Respir Monogr* 14:120–136, 2000.

Coultas DB, Zumwalt RE, Black WC, Sobonya RE: The epidemiology of interstitial lung diseases, *Am J Respir Crit Care Med* 150:967–972, 1994.

Epler GR, McLoud TC, Gaensler EA, et al: Normal chest radiographs in chronic diffuse infiltrative lung disease, *N Engl J Med* 298:934–939, 1978.

Flaherty KR, Thwaite EL, Kazerooni EA, et al: Radiological versus histological diagnosis in UIP and NSIP: survival implications, *Thorax* 58:143–148, 2003.

Flaherty KR, King TE Jr, Raghu G, et al: Idiopathic interstitial pneumonia: what is the effect of a multidisciplinary approach to diagnosis? *Am J Respir Crit Care Med* 170:904–910, 2004.

Hunninghake GW, Zimmerman MB, Schwartz DA, et al: Utility of a lung biopsy for the diagnosis of idiopathic pulmonary fibrosis, *Am J Respir Crit Care Med* 164:193–196, 2001.

Latsi PI, Du Bois RM, Nicholson AG, et al: Fibrotic idiopathic interstitial pneumonia: The prognostic value of longitudinal functional trends, *Am J Respir Crit Care Med* 168:531–537, 2003.

Nicholson AG, Colby TV, du Bois RM, et al: The prognostic significance of the histologic pattern of interstitial pneumonia in patients presenting with the clinical entity of cryptogenic fibrosing alveolitis, *Am J Respir Crit Care Med* 162:2213–2217, 2000.

Utz JP, Ryu JH, Douglas WW, et al: High short-term mortality following lung biopsy for usual interstitial pneumonia, *Eur Respir J* 17:175–179, 2001.

Wells AU: High resolution computed tomography in the diagnosis of diffuse lung disease: A clinical perspective, *Semin Respir Crit Care Med* 24:347–356, 2003.

Chapter **47**

Idiopathic Pulmonary Fibrosis and Other Interstitial Lung Diseases

Amen Sergew • Kevin K. Brown

Interstitial lung diseases (ILDs) are a large and diverse group of pulmonary disorders that affect the interstitium and air space of the lung and are histopathologically characterized by inflammation and/or fibrosis. Many ILDs are of known cause or association, although the most common remain idiopathic. In 2002 the American Thoracic Society/European Respiratory Society (ATS/ERS) International Multidisciplinary Consensus standardized the classification of the *idiopathic interstitial pneumonias* (IIPs) and categorized them into seven distinct disorders: (1) idiopathic pulmonary fibrosis (47%-64% of idiopathic ILDs), (2) nonspecific interstitial pneumonia (14%-36%), (3) cryptogenic organizing pneumonia (4%-12%; formerly bronchiolitis obliterans organizing pneumonia), (4) respiratory bronchiolitis interstitial lung disease, (5) desquamative interstitial pneumonia (10%-17%), (6) acute interstitial pneumonia (<2%), and (7) lymphoid interstitial pneumonia (<2%).

These ILDs differ based on epidemiology, onset of disease, chest imaging findings, histopathology, and most importantly, prognosis and response to treatment. Cryptogenic organizing pneumonia presents and is treated similarly to noncryptogenic presentations of organizing pneumonia, as discussed in Chapter 50. The remaining idiopathic ILDs are discussed in this chapter. **Table 47-1** compares various characteristics and **Figure 47-1** shows some distinct radiologic and histologic patterns of these idiopathic ILDs.

IDIOPATHIC PULMONARY FIBROSIS

Idiopathic pulmonary fibrosis (IPF) is the prototypic chronic, progressive fibrosing interstitial lung disease. In 2011, new ATS/ERS guidelines on the diagnosis, prognosis, and therapy of IPF were published (Raghu et al.). Its prevalence in the United States approaches 100,000 cases with an incidence of 15,000 to 30,000 cases per year. The disease generally affects patients in their sixth decade of life or later, and in patients older than 75 the prevalence increases to 175 per 100,000. There is a slight male predominance.

The cause of IPF is unknown, although risk factors include tobacco use, environmental and occupational exposures, infectious agents such as Epstein-Barr virus (EBV) and hepatitis C virus (HCV), and gastroesophageal reflux disease (GERD). Symptoms are frequently insidious and include cough and shortness of breath, especially with exertion. Symptomatic progression typically occurs over years, although abrupt and otherwise unexplained declines in respiratory symptoms, physiology, and imaging studies (acute exacerbation of IPF) can

occur. On examination, digital clubbing may be present. Chest auscultation reveals mid- to end-inspiratory crackles, most pronounced at the bases. During late stages, patients may show evidence of right-sided heart failure caused by the development of pulmonary artery hypertension.

The diagnostic utility of laboratory testing is limited because no biologic fluid-based biomarkers are currently useful in making a definitive diagnosis. Serum Krebs von den Lugen-6 (KL-6), serum surfactant A and D, serum CCL18, serum brain natriuretic peptide (BNP), plasma and bronchoalveolar lavage (BAL) fluid, and matrix metalloproteinases (MMPs) 1 and 7 are all potential biomarkers. Ongoing studies are evaluating the role of these and other potential biomarkers in diagnosis and disease progression. Laboratory testing is useful in defining the clinical context and excluding alternatives to explain the ILD. In particular, serologic testing for *connective tissue diseases* (CTDs) is recommended in all patients because the distinction between CTD and idiopathic ILD may have prognostic significance. Pulmonary functions tests (PFTs) reveal a restrictive ventilatory defect with a decreased diffusion capacity. BAL findings are nonspecific, and the procedure is not normally required in the diagnostic evaluation. If performed, a mild neutrophilia and mild (<20%) eosinophilia are frequently found. Lymphocytosis, especially greater than 40%, favors an alternate diagnosis.

When a surgical lung biopsy is performed, the histopathologic pattern seen is termed *usual interstitial pneumonia* (UIP). A definite UIP histopathologic pattern diagnosis requires all four of the following features:

1. Extensive fibrosis and architectural distortion, characterized by significant myofibroblasts and fibroblasts and dense collagen in the interstitium. This may be with or without honeycombing.
2. Heterogeneous involvement of the lung with areas of diseased lung, mostly in the subpleural/basilar regions, intermixed with areas of normal lung.
3. Fibroblast foci present.
4. Lack of features inconsistent with UIP:
   - Hyaline membranes
   - Organizing pneumonia
   - Granuloma
   - Extensive interstitial inflammation away from honeycombing
   - Primarily airway-centered
   - Other, atypical features suggestive of an alternate diagnosis

Table 47-1 Comparison of the Idiopathic Interstitial Pneumonias

Onset	Epidemiology	HRCT	Histopathology	Primary Differential	Prognosis
Idiopathic Pulmonary Fibrosis (IPF)					
Insidious over years	Sixth decade of life; male predominance	UIP pattern: peripheral/subpleural and lower lobe–predominant reticular abnormalities; volume loss and architectural distortion; honeycombing and traction bronchiectasis	UIP pattern: dense fibrosis, architectural distortion, fibroblastic foci, subpleural and basilar predominance, minimal inflammation, heterogeneous with areas of normal lung	Familial IPF, chronic HP, CTD-ILD, idiopathic fibrotic NSIP, asbestosis and other toxin exposures, chronic aspiration, Hermansky-Pudlak syndrome	Mortality: 85% in 10 years; mean survival: 4-5 years
Nonspecific Idiopathic Pneumonia (NSIP)					
Subacute to chronic onset over months to years	Fifth to sixth decade of life; slight female predominance	NSIP pattern: reticular abnormalities, ground-glass opacities, subpleural, bibasilar, symmetric	NSIP pattern: Cellular: homogeneous chronic inflammation and few areas of lymphoid granule; type II cell hyperplasia Fibrotic: uniform interstitial fibrosis; chronic interstitial inflammation	CTD-ILD, UIP, chronic HP, sarcoidosis, OP, eosinophilic pneumonia, LIP, DIP, AIP, drugs and toxin, resolving DAD, infection (mycobacteria, PCP, HIV, fungi)	35% (fibrotic predominant) to 100% (cellular predominant) 10-year survival
Respiratory Bronchiolitis Interstitial Lung Disease (RBILD)					
Subacute over weeks to months	Young patients, active smokers (>90%); slight male predominance	RBILD pattern: patchy ground-glass opacities, reticular marking, thickened airways, diffuse centrilobular nodules	RBILD pattern: bronchioles filled with pigmented macrophages; minimal fibrosis, limited to peribronchial areas	Follicular bronchiolitis, HP, infection, talc pneumonitis, chronic aspiration, DIP, NSIP	7-year survival: 75%-100%
Desquamative Interstitial Pneumonia (DIP)					
Subacute over weeks to months	Young patients, generally active smokers (>90%); male predominance	DIP pattern: ground-glass opacities without significant fibrosis; reticular markings; lower lobe and peripheral predominance; rare cysts	Homogeneous, uniform, and diffuse interstitial thickening; diffuse alveolar filling with macrophages	CTD-ILD, infection (e.g., hepatitis, PCP, HIV), PAP, pneumoconiosis, DAH, chronic eosinophilic pneumonia	Mortality: 20%-30%; mean survival: 12 years
Acute Interstitial Pneumonia (AIP)					
Acute onset over days to weeks	Wide age range, with mean of 50 years	DAD pattern: diffuse ground-glass opacification and consolidation; bilateral lobular sparing; late stages: possible traction bronchiectasis	DAD pattern: uniform distribution, hyaline membranes, septal thickening secondary to organizing fibrosis	Environmental, toxic, and drug exposures; infection; ARDS, DAH, hydrostatic edema, AEP, acute exacerbation of underlying ILD, COP, CID-ILD	6-month mortality: 87%-100%
Lymphoid Interstitial Pneumonia (LIP)					
Subacute to chronic over months to rarely years	Wide age range in adults	LIP pattern: basilar reticular opacities or centrilobular nodularity; fibrosis and ground-glass opacities; suggestive perivascular cysts	LIP pattern: interstitial inflammation in alveolar septae, predominantly with histiocytes, plasma cells, and lymphocytes; germinal centers with non-necrotizing granulomas; later stages honeycombing and cysts	HP, CTD-ILD CVID; infection, especially HIV, EBV, and HTLV-1; dysproteinemia; lymphoma	Median survival: 12 years

UIP, Usual interstitial pneumonia; *HP*, hypersensitivity pneumonitis; *CTD-ILD*, connective tissue disease-interstitial lung disease; *DAD*, diffuse alveolar damage; *OP*, organizing pneumonia; *PCP*, *Pneumocystis jirovecii (carinii)* pneumonia; *HIV*, human immunodeficiency virus; *PAP*, pulmonary alveolar proteinosis; *ARDS*, acute respiratory distress syndrome; *DAH*, diffuse alveolar hemorrhage; *AEP*, acute eosinophilic pneumonia; *COP*, cryptogenic pneumonia; *CVID*, common variable immunodeficiency; *EBV*, Epstein-Barr virus; *HTLV-1*, human T-lymphotropic virus type 1.

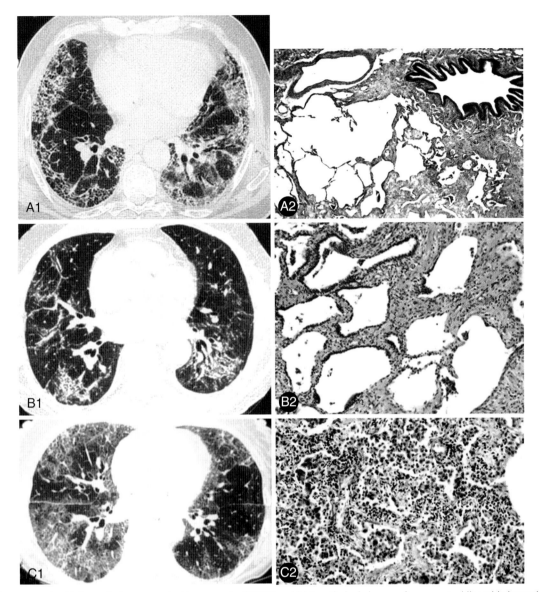

Figure 47-1 Representative high-resolution computed tomography (HRCT) and histopathologic images for common idiopathic interstitial lung diseases (ILDs). *A1*, Usual interstitial pneumonia (UIP) HRCT shows honeycombing, traction bronchiectasis, and fibrosis in subpleural and basilar distribution; *A2*, UIP histology shows heterogeneous findings with some areas of normal alveolar septae as well as areas of severe fibrosis with architectural distortion. *B1*, Nonspecific idiopathic pneumonia (NSIP) HRCT shows reticular abnormalities and ground-glass opacity; *B2*, NSIP histology shows diffuse and homogeneous interstitial inflammation and fibrosis. *C1*, Desquamative interstitial pneumonia (DIP) HRCT shows ground-glass opacities without significant fibrosis or honeycombing; *C2*, DIP histology shows uniform and diffuse interstitial thickening and diffuse alveolar filling with macrophages. *(Histology images courtesy Dr. Dirk Theegasten, Department of Pathology, Ruhr University, Bochum, Germany.)*

The chest imaging or radiologic pattern seen on high-resolution computed tomography (HRCT) scanning in about 50% of patients is also termed UIP. In the other 50% of patients, less well-characterized patterns are seen. When present, a UIP radiographic pattern has a positive predictive value of 90% to 100% for the presence of a UIP histopathologic pattern. Therefore, when this pattern is present, a surgical lung biopsy is rarely if ever needed. A definite HRCT radiologic pattern diagnosis of UIP can be made if all the following characteristics are present:

1. Subpleural/basal predominance
2. Honeycombing with or without traction bronchiectasis
3. Reticular abnormalities
4. Lack of features inconsistent with UIP:

- Distribution that is not localized to subpleural or basilar region (peribronchial, upper lung or midlung predominance)
- Extensive ground-glass opacities
- Diffuse micronodules
- Discrete cysts
- Consolidation
- Air trapping
- Other, atypical features suggestive of an alternate diagnosis

In the clinical context of an idiopathic ILD, the identification of a UIP chest imaging pattern confirms the diagnosis of IPF. In patients with discordant findings in their clinicoradiologic appearances, or if they have atypical features on HRCT,

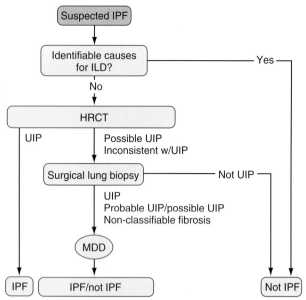

Figure 47-2 Algorithm for diagnosis of idiopathic pulmonary fibrosis *(IPF)*. The initial evaluation of a patient with suspected IPF (typically a patient with cough and chronic progressing dyspnea who has radiographic changes consistent with ILD) rules out other causes of interstitial lung disease *(ILD)*. If no other causes are identified, high-resolution computed tomography *(HRCT)* should be done. If HRCT shows usual interstitial pneumonia *(UIP)*, this is diagnostic. If HRCT is nondiagnostic, surgical biopsy is obtained, followed by multidisciplinary discussion *(MDD)* to make the diagnosis. *(Modified from Raghu G et al: Am J Respir Crit Care Med 183:788-824, 2011.)*

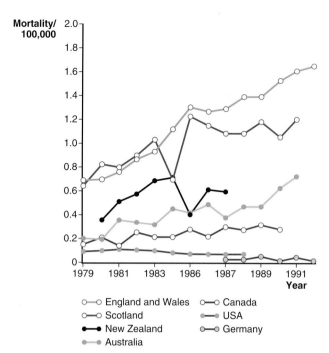

Figure 47-3 Mortality estimates for patients with idiopathic pulmonary fibrosis (IPF) in seven countries (1979-1991). *(Modified from Coultas DB et al: Am J Respir Crit Care Med 150:967-972, 1994.)*

a surgical biopsy is recommended in those who need a definitive diagnosis and are suitable for surgery. Transbronchial biopsies are too small to be diagnostic; therefore when a definitive diagnosis is necessary, a surgical biopsy should be obtained, preferably using video-assisted thoracoscopy, with biopsies from more than one lobe. A UIP histopathologic pattern confirms the diagnosis.

In summary, the new guidelines allow the clinician to establish the diagnosis of IPF based on the following criteria:

1. The clinical context is that of an idiopathic ILD; other potential causes or associations, including infection, drug or environmental exposures, and systemic disorders (e.g., CTDs), have been excluded.
2. The chest imaging and histology show a UIP pattern.

Because the diagnosis of IPF requires combining clinical, radiologic, and often pathologic information, multidisciplinary discussions with chest imagers and pathologists are strongly recommended, especially since a definitive diagnosis cannot be made based on radiologic and histologic findings alone. **Figure 47-2** outlines an algorithm for the diagnosis of IPF.

Patients have complications directly and indirectly related to their IPF. Although the natural history of IPF is generally slow symptomatic and physiologic progression, otherwise unexplained rapid deterioration can occur. *Acute exacerbations* of IPF are defined as the presence of an acute respiratory decompensation of unknown cause and occur in 5% to 10% of patients yearly. Patients tend to present with a viral prodrome and worsening baseline hypoxemia. Invasive mechanical ventilation is often required to maintain oxygenation, but its use is not generally recommended given the poor prognosis associated with acute exacerbations, although it may be appropriate in a minority of patients. Workup should include exclusion of pulmonary embolism, infection, congestive heart failure,

volume overload, pneumothorax, and other causes of lung injury. Imaging studies may show new onset of bilateral diffuse ground-glass opacity or dense consolidation. Lung biopsies show a diffuse alveolar damage (DAD) pattern. Although strong evidence is lacking, treatment with high-dose steroids is provided to most patients, in addition to broad-spectrum antibiotics. The prognosis is poor, with mortality rates of up to 70% or more during the following year.

Pulmonary hypertension is a recognized complication affecting about 10% of IPF patients at diagnosis. Its presence correlates with increased early mortality. With progression of disease, a majority of patients may ultimately develop some clinical evidence of pulmonary hypertension. In patients with worsening symptoms without significant changes in lung imaging studies or in lung volumes or spirometry, pulmonary hypertension should be considered.

Other comorbidities associated with IPF include an increased risk of venous thromboembolic disease, lung cancer, emphysema, GERD, obesity, obstructive sleep apnea, and cardiovascular disease.

A study quantified the mortality rate associated with IPF in 2003 in the United States as 61.2 deaths per 1 million in men and 54.5 per 1 million in women, with 60% of deaths attributed to progressive lung disease. Increased rates are seen in older patients and in the winter months. **Figure 47-3** compares mortality rates (per 100,000 population) from various countries. Although the median survival of symptomatic patients is generally accepted as 3 to 5 years, the survival of individual patients varies widely.

Figure 47-4 shows the natural history of IPF. Relatively stable lung function and slow (most common) or rapid disease progression can all occur. A patient's course is unpredictable, and risk factors for decompensation are poorly understood. No clear consensus exists on a valid staging system for IPF. However, the specific characteristics used at diagnosis to identity patients with risk factors for early mortality include severity of dyspnea, lower forced vital capacity (FVC) or diffusion capacity (DLCO),

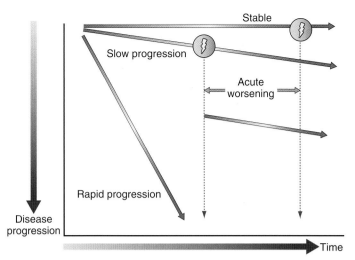

Figure 47-4 Most patients with idiopathic pulmonary fibrosis display a slowly progressive natural history. In a minority of patients, IPF can be stable or rapidly progressive. Some slowly progressive or stable patients may also have acute decompensation *(lightning bolt)*, from a known infection, other lung insult, or an unknown cause, generally with high mortality or resulting in worsened lung function.   *(Modified from Raghu G et al: Am J Respir Crit Care Med 183:788–824, 2011.)*

significant desaturation on 6-minute walking distance (6MWD) testing, and the extent of fibrosis on HRCT. Other suggested risk factors include a shorter 6MWD, presence of significant emphysema, and pulmonary hypertension. Important longitudinal factors associated with an increased risk of early mortality in IPF patients are worsening dyspnea, decline in FVC, decline in DLCO, and increasing extent of disease on HRCT.

Treatment   The 2011 IPF guidelines also review evidence on treatment. To summarize, no medical therapy has proved to provide a survival, quality of life, or functional benefit in patients with IPF, and therefore no specific treatment approach was thought to be useful in the majority of patients. Given this, appropriate patients should be considered for early referral for lung transplantation, as well as referral to research centers to consider prospective therapeutic studies. Beyond this, oxygen therapy for hypoxia at rest, with activity, exercise, and sleep, is frequently used for symptom control. Pulmonary rehabilitation and routine vaccinations are also important to incorporate into disease management. For patients with asymptomatic GERD, therapy is recommended.

Despite inadequate information, many patients will desire medical therapy for IPF. Although convincing evidence of efficacy is lacking, conventional therapy has been considered to be a combination of azathioprine, prednisolone, and *N*-acetylcysteine (NAC). This regimen is has been tested in the prospective, multicenter, placebo-controlled Prednisolone, Azathioprine, and *N*-Acetylcysteine in People with Idiopathic Pulmonary Fibrosis (PANTHER-IPF) trial in the United States. The prednisone + azathioprine + NAC arm of the study was terminated early due to increased mortality and adverse effects when compared to the placebo arm. Thus this regimen is no longer recommended for patients with well-characterized IPF. While the remaining active NAC and placebo arms of the PANTHER-IPF study will hopefully provide a definitive answer, NAC alone is often considered in a minority of patients dosed at 1800 mg daily (split into twice or three times daily doses). *Pirfenidone* is a small-molecule drug thought to be an antifibrotic agent that is approved for use in IPF patients in Japan and Europe. The drug has been tested in multiple trials with

conflicting results, and as a result, the statement does not suggest its use in the majority of patients. A large Phase III trial is now underway in the United States to provide clarity on pirfenidone's usefulness. The Sildenafil Trial of Exercise Performance in Idiopathic Pulmonary Fibrosis (STEP-IPF) studied the effects of *sildenafil* on IPF patients with physiologically severe disease and showed no significant improvement in 6MWD. However, there were some improvements in secondary outcomes such as arterial oxygenation, DLCO, and symptoms of dyspnea and quality of life in the sildenafil group. Further studies would be helpful to assess the risks and benefits of long-term use of sildenafil in IPF patients.

Despite the elevated risk of venous thromboembolic disease, no strong evidence favors prophylactic anticoagulation. Although a small study suggested a potential survival benefit to chronic anticoagulation, a more recent large-scale study of warfarin (Coumadin) in patients with IPF was stopped early for lack of efficacy.

NONSPECIFIC INTERSTITIAL PNEUMONIA

Historically, nonspecific interstitial pneumonia (NSIP) has been the catchall phrase for ILD that does not fit into other categories. In the mid-1990s, NSIP was defined as a specific histopathologic pattern that did not match histopathologic criteria for other idiopathic ILDs. Since then, NSIP has expanded from simply describing a histopathologic pattern to a specific form of an otherwise idiopathic ILD. Because the histopathologic NSIP pattern is not unique, a concerted effort should identify a potentially causative exposure or associated medical condition. When no alternative explanation is identified, the diagnosis of "idiopathic NSIP" can be made.

The epidemiology of NSIP is unknown. Significantly less common than IPF, estimates of the prevalence of idiopathic NSIP range from 1 to 9 per 100,000 population. NSIP presents in a younger population than IPF, with patients in their 40s to 50s and with a female predominance. Symptoms are nonspecific and include cough and dyspnea with a presentation that ranges from subacute (6-12 months) to chronic (up to 3 years); median duration is 18 to 31 months. History and physical examination should be used to evaluate for features suggestive of an alternative explanation for the presence of ILD. For example, the presence of Raynaud's phenomenon, arthritis, and myositis suggests an underlying CTD. Pulmonary examination typically reveals basilar crackles.

Laboratory testing offers limited information and cannot make a definitive diagnosis. However, testing helps define the clinical context and exclude alternative explanations for ILD. Similar to IPF, serologic testing for a CTD is recommended in all patients because the distinction between idiopathic NSIP and the histopathologic pattern of NSIP associated with a CTD may have prognostic significance. PFTs reveal a restrictive ventilatory defect with a decreased DLCO. A minority of patients may present with a mild airflow obstruction. In contrast to IPF, BAL fluid will show lymphocyte predominance in 50% of suspected NSIP patients, generally with a minor proportion of neutrophils and/or eosinophils.

The histopathologic pattern of NSIP is a homogeneously abnormal parenchyma with diffuse interstitial involvement. It can be subdivided based on the amounts of lung fibrosis and inflammation, with *cellular* NSIP consisting almost exclusively of cellular inflammation and *fibrotic* NSIP showing some component of acellular fibrosis. Cellular NSIP has mild to moderate chronic interstitial inflammation with associated type II

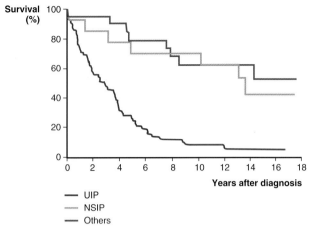

Figure 47-5 Survival curves based on histopathologic subgroups comparing usual interstitial pneumonia *(UIP)*, idiopathic pneumonia *(NSIP)*, and other idiopathic interstitial lung diseases. Patients with UIP pattern have worse prognosis than those with NSIP or other ILDs. *(Modified from Bjoraker JA et al: Am J Respir Crit Care Med 157:199–203, 1998.)*

pneumocyte hyperplasia and few areas of lymphoid aggregates. Fibrotic NSIP results in uniform involvement with dense or loose interstitial fibrosis and a lack of honeycombing or fibroblast foci.

On imaging studies, cellular NSIP has diffuse areas of ground-glass infiltrate, whereas fibrotic NSIP is associated with reticular changes, volume loss, and traction bronchiectasis. The findings are typically symmetric, lower lung predominant, and often the subpleural zone is relatively free of fibrosis. Honeycombing and consolidation are rare findings. The sensitivity and specificity of imaging studies in NSIP are not to the level of being diagnostic. Therefore, when the diagnosis of NSIP is suspected, a surgical lung biopsy should be considered.

Treatment and Prognosis Prospective, controlled therapeutic trials are lacking in the treatment of patients with NSIP, and expert opinion provides the basis for most recommended regimens. Corticosteroids are typically initiated in these patients, with an anticipated transition to steroid-sparing agents such as azathioprine, mycophenolate mofetil, or cyclophosphamide. The prognosis of NSIP is variable, with a minority of patients with progressively fatal disease and others with nearly complete recovery. Patients with a predominantly fibrotic NSIP have a worse prognosis than those with predominantly cellular NSIP. The majority of patients will have relatively stable disease or some mild improvement with therapy. Overall, mortality is better than with UIP. **Figure 47-5** compares the survival curves of patients with NSIP, UIP, and other idiopathic ILD.

RESPIRATORY BRONCHIOLITIS INTERSTITIAL LUNG DISEASE

The histopathologic pattern respiratory bronchiolitis (RB) is a common finding in current or former heavy smokers. However, the overwhelming majority of patients appear to have no related clinical sequelae and it exists as an incidental finding when a patient has lung pathology obtained for other reasons. In contrast, respiratory bronchiolitis interstitial lung disease (RBILD) occurs when a patient with clinical and physiologic evidence of interstitial lung disease has RB as the sole histopathologic finding to account for their ILD. Given the overlapping clinical context, imaging, and pathologic findings, RBILD

appears to be on a spectrum of disease that includes desquamative interstitial pneumonia (DIP).

Patients with RBILD present in their 30s and 40s, with a male predominance of almost 2:1. Patients are almost invariably heavy smokers of at least 30 pack-years. They generally present with dyspnea and cough. Pulmonary findings are similar to DIP, with a mild to moderate reduction in DLCO and a mixed restriction and obstruction. Up to 10% of patients may present with normal physiology, and another 10% show significant bronchodilator response. On chest imaging, as many as 20% of patients may have normal plain chest radiographs. HRCT shows significant airway wall thickening, reticular and centrilobular abnormalities, and small patches of ground-glass opacity. The findings are bilateral and can be found in all five lung lobes and tend to be less extensive and involve less of the lung parenchyma than in DIP. BAL fluid typically shows an excess number of pigmented macrophages with black, golden, or brown inclusions, similar to that seen in otherwise healthy smokers. There may also be a modest neutrophilia.

The diagnosis of RBILD is typically made from the clinical context of a young, heavy smoker and the chest imaging pattern seen on HRCT. If definitive diagnosis is needed, surgical lung biopsy is indicated because transbronchial biopsy and BAL findings cannot provide this level of confidence. The histopathologic pattern is bronchiolocentric, involving first-order and second-order respiratory bronchioles with the peribronchiolar alveoli filled with tightly packed pigmented macrophages. These cells stain positive for periodic acid–Schiff (PAS). The lumen may also be filled with mucus (mucostasis). There is minimal fibrosis, limited to the peribronchial areas.

Prognosis and Therapy The prognosis is generally thought to be good. One study of 32 patients showed 75% of patients had a greater than 7 year survival, with only one patient dying of progressive ILD. Clinical improvement was seen in 28% and physiologic improvement was seen in 10%. In regards to therapy, symptoms may improve with smoking cessation alone and this should always be the initial intervention. If symptoms persist, a trial of corticosteroid therapy is often used, though this is based on expert opinion rather than interventional therapeutic trials.

DESQUAMATIVE INTERSTITIAL PNEUMONIA

Desquamative interstitial pneumonia is thought to be on a continuum of disease with RBILD, and is seen in a similar clinical context, heavy smokers in 60%-87% of cases. In contrast to RBILD, 20% of cases occur in the setting of CTD, viral infections or drug/toxin exposure. The DIP patient population is younger than those with IPF, typically in their 30s to 50s, with a 2:1 male predominance.

The most common pulmonary physiologic finding is a reduced DLCO. The patient may also have mild restriction or mild mixed restrictive-obstructive patterns. HRCT typically shows ground-glass opacities in the lung periphery and bases without significant fibrosis or honeycombing. Other findings include traction bronchiectasis, centrilobular nodules, and cysts, which are typically less than 2 cm in diameter.

Surgical biopsy is required for a definitive diagnosis because BAL fluid and transbronchial biopsy show nonspecific findings. The histopathologic pattern reveals homogeneous and diffuse interstitial thickening. Alveoli are filled with iron-laden macrophages, resulting in the ground-glass pattern. Type II cell hyperplasia and diffuse alveolar septal thickening also are seen. In contrast to RBILD, the patient with DIP has more interstitial fibrosis, lymphoid follicles, giant cells, and eosinophils, although the patterns can show considerable overlap. Unlike UIP, fibroblast foci and honeycombing are not present in DIP. Given the smoking history, some emphysematous changes may also be seen.

Prognosis and Therapy Patients with DIP often show prolonged stability but can progress to end-stage fibrosis. Overall mortality is 6% to 30%, with mean survival of 12 years. Unlike patients with RBILD, patients with DIP can develop acute exacerbations. The main therapeutic intervention is smoking cessation. Corticosteroids and in those that respond, corticosteroid-sparing agents, have been used as an adjunct, but this is based on expert opinion. Patients with ground-glass opacities typically have some improvement of their symptoms and imaging findings, although disease progression occurs in up to 20% of patients. With continued progression, lung transplantation is an option. Interestingly, there have been rare cases of recurrence in the transplanted lung.

ACUTE INTERSTITIAL PNEUMONIA

Acute interstitial pneumonia (AIP) has been known by a variety of names over the years. Hamman and Rich described the first cases in 1935. More recently it was considered an idiopathic form of acute respiratory distress syndrome (ARDS) because their presentation and clinical characteristics are indistinguishable, but they are differentiated by the absence of a known cause or association in AIP. Symptoms include a rapid onset of dyspnea over days to less than 3 weeks, typically following a viral prodrome. Patients routinely develop significant hypoxia and respiratory failure, requiring assisted ventilation. The epidemiology includes a wide age range, with a mean age of 50 years, and affects both genders equally. There is no known association with smoking.

Chest imaging in AIP patients typically shows bilateral ground-glass infiltrates sparing the costophrenic angles and otherwise patchy distribution with associated air bronchograms. Pleural effusions are rare. HRCT in the early phase of disease shows diffuse bilateral ground-glass opacities. In the later stages, bilateral consolidative opacities, especially at the lung bases and in dependent regions are found, as well as bronchial dilation and architectural distortion with honeycombing and cysts.

The diagnosis of AIP is a diagnosis of exclusion. BAL fluid is primarily used to exclude overwhelming infection and reveals increased total cell numbers with red blood cells, neutrophils, and lymphocytes. The histopathologic pattern is diffuse alveolar damage, with hyaline membranes, diffuse septal fibrosis, and type II pneumocyte hyperplasia.

Prognosis and Therapy Mortality in patients with AIP is typically higher than 50%, with most deaths occurring in-hospital within 1 to 2 months from onset of symptoms. Those who survive are at increased risk of recurrence and chronic, progressive fibrotic lung disease, with 6-month mortality of 87% to 100%. There is currently no known specific therapy for AIP. Most experts treat it as ARDS, although corticosteroids are used more often in patients with AIP.

LYMPHOID INTERSTITIAL PNEUMONIA

Lymphoid interstitial pneumonia (LIP) rarely presents as an idiopathic lung disease and is most often seen in the setting of autoimmune disease, genetic abnormalities, infection (especially HIV, EBV, and HTLV-1), or dysproteinemia (e.g., polyclonal and monoclonal gammopathy). When seen as an idiopathic ILD, patients with LIP typically present with cough and progressive shortness of breath over months and rarely up to years. Symptoms can include fever, weight loss, and pleurisy.

Physical examination is consistent with crackles and less frequently digital clubbing (~10% of patients). Pulmonary physiology reveals a restrictive pattern with reduced DLCO. Chest imaging findings can vary and involve basilar reticular opacities, ground-glass opacities, or centrilobular nodularity. Suggestive perivascular cysts are seen in many patients. BAL fluid typically shows a lymphocytosis, but this is not diagnostic. For definitive diagnosis, surgical biopsy is recommended and shows confluent cellular infiltration of the alveolar septae (and less frequently peribronchial and perivascular septae) with lymphocytes, plasma cells, and histiocytes. Germinal centers, occasional non-necrotizing granulomas, and associated multinucleated giant cells are also seen. In later stages of LIP, fibrosis and even honeycombing can be seen. Genetic studies are important to rule out malignancy and monoclonality.

Treatment No randomized trials have identified the treatment for patients with LIP. Anecdotal evidence supports the use of corticosteroids for symptomatic patients and those with a decline in lung function. For those who do not respond or who have side effects, adding a steroid-sparing agent should be considered.

CONTROVERSIES AND PITFALLS

Establishing the correct diagnosis remains the crucial step in the assessment and management of patients with interstitial lung disease, because the diagnosis is the most important determinant of prognosis and appropriate treatment plan. The multidisciplinary approach involving the clinician, chest radiologist, and pulmonary pathologist is critical in piecing together the puzzle. However, this requirement for active multidisciplinary communication is often the rate-limiting step, and the clinician must expend considerable effort to make it work. Beyond the diagnosis, projecting the future disease activity remains an uncertain science, and multiple ongoing studies are underway in an attempt to identify biomarkers predictive of future disease behavior. A number of genetic risk factors for the development of pulmonary fibrosis have been identified, although the utility of these findings in clinical practice is uncertain at present.

Because no therapy used in the treatment of idiopathic pulmonary fibrosis has provided a survival, quality of life, or functional status benefit, the limitations of current treatment options leave plenty of room for controversy. As most interventional treatment trials use purported surrogate end points, the results of these trials will be difficult to interpret and will require the clinician to engage each patient fully to make informed decisions regarding treatment.

SUGGESTED READINGS

American Thoracic Society/European Respiratory Society International Multidisciplinary Consensus Classification of the Idiopathic Interstitial Pneumonias, *Am J Respir Crit Care Med* 165:277–304, 2002; erratum, 166:426, 2002.

Bjoraker JA, Ryu JH, Edwin MK, et al: Prognostic significance of histopathologic subsets in idiopathic pulmonary fibrosis, *Am J Respir Crit Care Med* 157:199–203, 1998.

Coultas DB, Zumwalt RE, Black WC, Sobonya RE: The epidemiology of interstitial lung diseases, *Am J Respir Crit Care Med* 150:967–972, 1994.

Demedts M, Wells AU, Antó JM, et al: Interstitial lung diseases: an epidemiological overview, *Eur Respir J Suppl* 32:2–16, 2001.

Frankel SK, Schwarz MI: Update in idiopathic pulmonary fibrosis, *Curr Opin Pulm Med* 15:463–469, 2009.

Gal AA, Staton GW Jr: Current concepts in the classification of interstitial lung disease, *Am J Clin Pathol* 123:S67–S81, 2005.

Kim DS, Collard HR, King TE Jr: Classification and natural history of the idiopathic interstitial pneumonias, *Proc Am Thorac Soc* 3:285–292, 2006.

Leslie KO: Historical perspective: a pathologic approach to the classification of idiopathic interstitial pneumonias, *Chest* 128(5 Suppl 1):513–519, 2005.

Ley B, Collard HR, King TE Jr: Clinical course and prediction of survival in idiopathic pulmonary fibrosis, *Am J Respir Crit Care Med* 183:431–440, 2011.

Lynch DA, Travis WD, Müller NL, et al: Idiopathic interstitial pneumonias: CT features, *Radiology* 236:10–21, 2005.

Raghu G, Collard HR, Egan JJ, et al: Idiopathic pulmonary fibrosis: evidence-based guidelines for diagnosis and management. ATS/ERS/JRS/ALAT Committee on Idiopathic Pulmonary Fibrosis, *Am J Respir Crit Care Med* 183:788–824, 2011.

Travis WD, Hunninghake G, King TE Jr, et al: Idiopathic nonspecific interstitial pneumonia: report of an American Thoracic Society project, *Am J Respir Crit Care Med* 177:1338–1347, 2008.

Vassallo R, Ryu JH: Tobacco smoke–related diffuse lung diseases, *Semin Respir Crit Care Med* 29:643–650, 2008.

Chapter **48**
Sarcoidosis
Manju Paul • Michael C. Iannuzzi

In the 130 years since Jonathan Hutchinson first described sarcoidosis as a skin disorder, involvement of every organ has been reported. The central abnormality in sarcoidosis is granuloma accumulation, leading to altered organ architecture and function. Although the inciting events in sarcoidosis remain unknown, in general, granulomas form to confine pathogens, restrict inflammation, and protect surrounding tissue. Clinical, epidemiologic, and family-based studies support the hypothesis that sarcoidosis is triggered by airborne exposure in a genetically susceptible person. The diagnosis is established when compatible clinical and radiologic findings are supported by evidence of noncaseating epithelioid cell granulomas in one or more organs in the absence of organisms or particles. Corticosteroids remain the therapeutic cornerstone for patients with organ-threatening or chronic progressive disease.

EPIDEMIOLOGY

Sarcoidosis occurs worldwide and may affect any person at any age, although more than 80% of patients are diagnosed between ages 20 and 50 years. In the United States, African Americans are three and a half times more commonly affected, with an age-adjusted incidence of 35.5 per 100,000 persons, compared with 10.9 per 100,000 in whites. African American women are most commonly affected, with a lifetime risk of approximately 2.7%. African Americans tend to have a more severe form of the disease with greater extrapulmonary involvement. The incidence in most European nations has been reported at less than 1 case per 100,000. In Scandinavian countries such as Sweden and Finland, incidence ranges from 11 to 64 per 100,000. Sarcoidosis is uncommon in Chinese and Southeast Asians; the Japanese, however, have a particular susceptibility to cardiac involvement.

ETIOLOGY AND RISK FACTORS

No single environmental sarcoidosis trigger has been identified. Recently, the multicenter ACCESS (A Case Controlled Etiologic Sarcoidosis Study) report found modestly increased risk with exposure to pesticides or moldy environments or working with building materials, hardware, or industrial organic dusts. Sarcoidosis was not associated with rural living conditions or exposure to wood dusts or heavy metals.

Several microorganisms and viruses have been suggested as potential sarcoid antigens. Mycobacterial catalase protein MkatG is the most promising agent thus far and has been found in tissue obtained from more than 50% of patients with sarcoidosis. A possible explanation for the difficulty in identifying an infectious cause for sarcoidosis is that an insoluble bacterial protein serves as antigen long after the infecting organism has been cleared.

Occupational clustering of sarcoidosis cases has been reported in ship workers, fire fighters, and rescue workers who were involved in the response to the World Trade Center attacks in the United States.

GENETIC FACTORS

Racial differences in incidence rates and disease clustering in families support the hypothesis that heredity contributes to sarcoidosis etiology. Having a first-degree relative with sarcoidosis increases the risk for the disease approximately five-fold. Screening for sarcoidosis among relatives is not recommended, because less than 1% will be found to have the disease. Several human leukocyte antigen (HLA) associations with sarcoidosis have been reported (**Table 48-1**), but HLA seems more likely to influence phenotype than susceptibility. The major histocompatibility complex (MHC) class I allele HLA-B8 is associated with acute sarcoidosis. HLA-DQB1*0201 and HLA-DRB1*0301 are strongly associated with acute disease and good prognosis.

Investigators have studied non-HLA candidate genes that influence antigen processing, antigen presentation, macrophage and T cell activation, and cell recruitment. **Table 48-2** lists non-HLA candidate genes studied to date. Although these candidates are logical on the basis of function, their associations with sarcoidosis have not been consistently reproduced.

To date, two genome scans for sarcoidosis have been reported: one in German whites, with the strongest linkage signals localized to chromosomal short arms 3p and 6p, and the other in African Americans with signals at 5p and 5q. Thus far, two candidate genes from linked regions have been identified: *BTNL2*, located on 6p, encoding butyrophilin-like protein 2, a B7 family member that functions as a negative costimulatory molecule, and *ANXA11*, at chromosomal locus 10q22.2, encoding annexin A11, which may affect apoptosis.

PATHOPHYSIOLOGY

Sarcoidosis is a multisystem inflammatory disease characterized by T lymphocyte infiltration, granuloma formation, and microarchitecture distortion. The events leading to granuloma formation probably begin with antigen presented to T lymphocytes by way of MHC class II peptide in a genetically predisposed host (**Figure 48-1**). Serum amyloid A may have a role in the immune response in sarcoidosis and is capable of eliciting immune responses and triggering cytokine release through interaction with Toll-like receptors (TLRs). The oligoclonal T

Table 48-1 Summary of Human Leukocyte Antigen (HLA) Association Studies of Sarcoidosis

HLA	Risk Alleles	Finding
HLA-A	A*1	Susceptibility
HLA-B	B*8	Susceptibility in several populations
HLA-DPB1	*0201	Not associated with sarcoidosis
HLA-DQB1	*0201	Protection, Löfgren syndrome, mild disease in several populations
	*0602	Susceptibility/disease progression in several groups
HLA-DRB1	*0301	Acute onset/good prognosis in several groups
	*04	Protection in several populations
	*1101	Susceptibility in whites and African Americans
HLA-DRB3	*1501	Associated with Löfgren syndrome
	*0101	Susceptibility/disease progression in whites

cell repertoire in sarcoidosis (α/β and δ/γ receptors) suggests that triggering antigens favor progressive accumulation and activation of selective T cell clones. Initially, macrophages process the antigens, which are then presented to CD4+ T cells by class II MHC molecules. T cell activation occurs by means of T cell receptor (TCR), TLR, or cytokine or chemokine receptors. This leads to signal transduction and activation of transcription factors that promote gene expression controlling T cell proliferation, differentiation, and apoptosis and produce proinflammatory cytokines and chemokines. T cell signal transduction pathways are potential therapeutic targets in sarcoidosis. Macrophages, in the face of chronic cytokine stimulation, differentiate into epithelioid cells, gain secretory and bactericidal capability, lose some phagocytic capacity, and fuse to form multinucleate giant cells. In more mature granulomas, fibroblasts and collagen encase the ball-like cell cluster. As granulomas accumulate, alterations in organ architecture and function occur.

Granulomas can resolve with little clinical consequence or may progress to fibrosis. Acute granulomatous and chronic fibrotic sarcoidosis probably represent different immunopathogenic processes, which remain to be defined (**Figure 48-2**). A

Table 48-2 Non-HLA Candidate Genes Evaluated in Sarcoidosis

Candidate Gene	Findings
Angiotensin-converting enzyme gene (ACE)	Increased risk for ID and DD genotypes Moderate association between II genotype and radiographic progression
CC chemokine receptor 2 gene	Associated with protection/Löfgren syndrome
Chemokine receptor 5 gene	CCR5Δ32 allele more common in patients treated with corticosteroid; refuted with haplotype analysis and larger sample
CD80, CD86 genes	No association detected
Clara cell 10-kDa protein gene	An allele associated with sarcoidosis and with progressive disease at 3-year follow-up
Complement receptor-1 gene	Association with the GG genotype for the Pro1827Arg (C[5507]G) polymorphism
Cystic fibrosis transmembrane regulator gene (CFTR)	R75Q increases risk
Cytotoxic T lymphocyte antigen 4 (CTLA4)	No association with sarcoidosis
Heat shock protein 70-like gene	HSP(+2437)CC associated with susceptibility/Löfgren syndrome
Inhibitor kappa B-alpha gene	Associated with −297T allele Allele −827T in stage II
IL1α gene	The IL-1α -889 1.1 genotype increased risk
IL-4 receptor gene	No association detected
IL-18 gene	Genotype −607CA increased risk over AA
Interferon-γ gene	IFNA17 polymorphism (551T→G) and IFNA10 [60A]– IFNA17 [551G] haplotype increase risk
Macrophage migration inhibitory factor gene	No association with 5-CATT in Irish population
Natural resistance–associated macrophage protein gene (NRAMP)	Protective effect of (CA)(n) repeat in the immediate 5′ region of the NRAMP1 gene
Toll-like receptor-4 gene (TLR4)	Asp299Gly and Thre399Ile mutations associated with chronic disease
Transforming growth factor gene (TGF)	TGF-β2 59941 allele, TGFβ3 4875 A and 17369 C alleles were associated with fibrosis on chest radiograph
Tumor necrosis factor-α gene	Genotype −307A allele associated with erythema nodosum/Löfgren syndrome and −857T allele with sarcoidosis −307A not associated in African Americans
Vascular endothelial growth factor gene	+813 CT and TT genotypes associated with protection
Vitamin D receptor gene (VDR)	BsmI allele associated with sarcoidosis

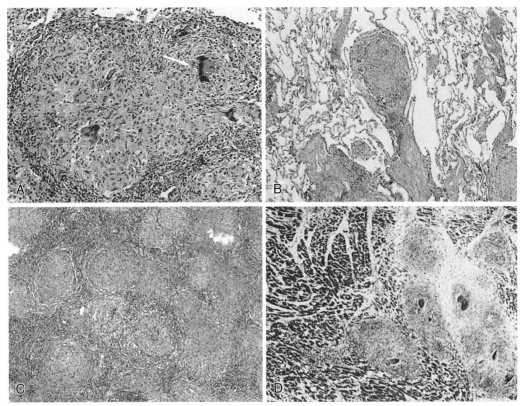

Figure 48-1 Noncaseating granulomatous inflammation in sarcoidosis. **A,** Closeup of epithelioid granuloma with giant cells and mononuclear cell infiltration. **B,** Open lung biopsy specimen showing granulomas, giant cells, and lymphocytic infiltrates in lung parenchyma and within interlobular septal and subpleural regions. **C,** Lymph node biopsy specimen showing extensive replacement with typical sarcoid-type epithelioid granulomas. Fibrinoid necrosis, but not overt caseation, may be seen in the center of granulomas. **D,** Myocardial biopsy specimen showing patchy granulomatous inflammation with giant cells.

switch from T_H1 to T_H2 cytokine profile, along with other mediators such as interleukin-6 (IL-6), transforming growth factor-β (TGF-β), osteopontin, and insulin growth factors (IGFs), is suggested to result in fibrosis. Sarcoidosis may develop or worsen in patients with immune reconstitution during treatment of HIV infection or in those undergoing treatment with interferon.

CLINICAL FEATURES

The clinical presentation of sarcoidosis varies. In up to two thirds of the cases, the patient is asymptomatic, and sarcoidosis is diagnosed incidentally on the basis of radiographic findings of hilar lymphadenopathy. Thoracic involvement is most common (over 90% of patients), followed by skin, eyes, liver, spleen, peripheral lymph nodes, central nervous system (CNS), and heart. Two well-recognized acute, febrile presentations of sarcoidosis are Löfgren syndrome (arthritis, erythema nodosum, and bilateral hilar adenopathy) and Heerfordt syndrome (uveitis, parotid gland enlargement, and facial nerve palsy). These acute presentations portend a good prognosis, with disease resolution within 1 to 2 years. Both syndromes are uncommon in African Americans.

PULMONARY MANIFESTATIONS

More than 90% of patients with sarcoidosis have pulmonary involvement. Common complaints include dry cough, vague chest discomfort, and dyspnea, particularly with exertion. Pleuritic chest pain is uncommon. Wheezing may occur with endobronchial involvement or hyperreactive airways. Sputum production and hemoptysis occur in advanced fibrocystic disease. Pleural involvement is seen in only 2% to 4% of patients and can manifest with pleural effusions, pleural thickening, pneumothorax, and chylothorax. The diagnosis of sarcoidosis often is delayed, especially in patients presenting with predominantly pulmonary symptoms.

Chest auscultation may reveal fine, late, or mid-expiratory crackles, but comparatively less than that heard in pulmonary fibrosis. In view of the marked chest radiographic abnormalities, physical examination of the lungs is surprisingly unrevealing. Clubbing is rare but when present usually is associated with advanced bronchiectasis or liver disease.

Pulmonary Hypertension

The prevalence of pulmonary arterial hypertension and right ventricular dysfunction ranges from 4% to 28%. Pulmonary hypertension is more common in patients with advanced lung disease and has been reported in up to 74% of patients with sarcoidosis who are awaiting a lung transplant. Several potential causes of pulmonary hypertension in sarcoidosis include interstitial lung disease, fibrous destruction of the pulmonary vascular bed, compression of pulmonary arteries by lymphadenopathy, pulmonary venoocclusion, portopulmonary hypertension, myocardial dysfunction, and an intrinsic sarcoid vasculopathy. Patients with pulmonary hypertension are more likely to be listed for a lung transplant and exhibit a 10-fold increase in mortality over that for patients with isolated pulmonary sarcoidosis. Prognosis is poor, with a 5-year survival rate of only 59%. The management of pulmonary hypertension involves

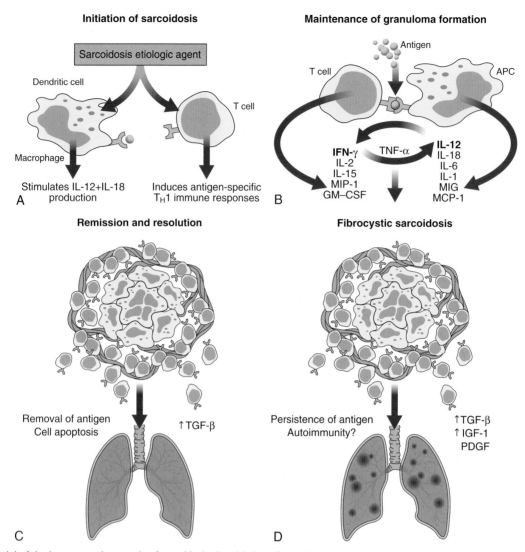

Figure 48-2 Model of the immunopathogenesis of sarcoidosis. **A,** Initiation of sarcoidosis involves stimulation of production of interleukins IL-12 and IL-18 from mononuclear phagocytes and dendritic cells and adaptive T cell immunity to an inciting agent. **B,** Maintenance of granuloma formation by a T_H1 immune response driven by IFN-γ and IL-12 and IL-18. **C,** Resolution of sarcoidosis after removal of stimulating antigen, suppression of T cell responses by TGF-β and other mediators, and granuloma resorption by cell apoptosis. **D,** Fibrotic outcome from persistent, possibly autoimmune antigenic stimulation in the presence of TGF-β and other profibrotic mediators. *APC,* antigen-presenting cell; *GM-CSF,* granulocyte-macrophage colony-stimulating factor; *IFN-γ,* interferon-γ; *IGF-1,* insulin-like growth factor-1; *MCP-1,* monocyte chemotactic protein-1; *MIG,* monokine induced by IFN-γ; *MIP-1,* macrophage inflammatory protein-1; *PDGF,* platelet-derived growth factor; *TGF-β,* transforming growth factor-β; *TNF-α,* tumor necrosis factor-α.

reversal of resting hypoxia. Use of corticosteroids for pulmonary hypertension in sarcoidosis is controversial. The data supporting the benefit of endothelin receptor antagonist and phosphodiesterase-5 inhibitors are very limited.

Chest Radiology

Chest radiographs obtained in patients with sarcoidosis are classified by appearance into four patterns (**Figure 48-3**). Unfortunately, these radiographic patterns have been termed "stages," leading to the erroneous assumption that they represent disease stages rather than chest x-ray patterns.

Stage 0: Absence of radiographic abnormalities
Stage I: Bilateral hilar and/or mediastinal adenopathy without pulmonary parenchymal abnormalities
Stage II: Hilar and/or mediastinal lymphadenopathy with pulmonary parenchymal abnormalities (generally a diffuse interstitial pattern)

Stage III: Diffuse parenchymal disease without nodal enlargement
Stage IV: Pulmonary fibrosis with evidence of volume loss or cystic or honeycomb changes

The initial radiographic pattern at initial presentation generally predicts likelihood of radiographic resolution. Resolution of radiographic abnormalities occurs in approximately 60% to 80% of patients who present with a stage I pattern on the chest radiograph and in 50% to 60% with a stage II pattern, but in less than 30% with a stage III pattern.

Intrathoracic lymphadenopathy and parenchymal infiltrates (stage II chest radiograph) are the most commonly encountered radiographic finding, occurring in 85% of patients. Symmetric hilar adenopathy is most commonly seen. Unilateral hilar adenopathy is unusual and is seen in only 3% to 5%. Mediastinal lymphadenopathy without hilar adenopathy is rare; an alternate diagnosis must be considered in this setting. The

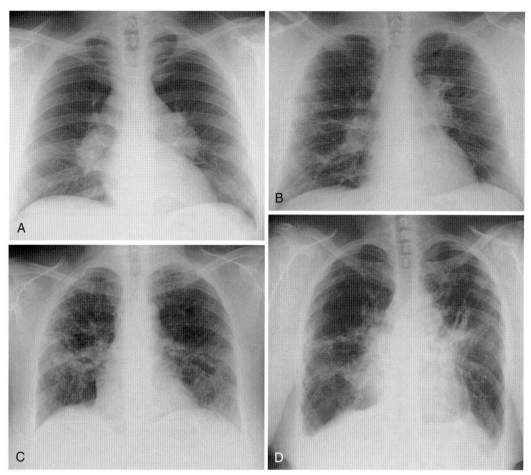

Figure 48-3   Chest radiography stages (patterns) of sarcoidosis. **A,** Stage I pattern on the chest radiograph, with bilateral hilar lymphadenopathy. **B,** Stage II pattern, with bilateral lymphadenopathy and reticulonodular infiltrates. **C,** Stage III pattern, with bilateral infiltrates without adenopathy. **D,** Stage IV pattern, with upward hilar retraction, large cystic and bullous changes, and fibrocystic disease.

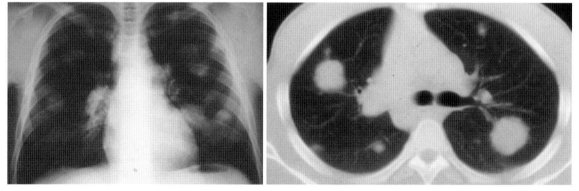

Figure 48-4   Nodular sarcoidosis with multiple bilateral pulmonary nodules. *Left,* Chest radiograph; *right,* computed tomography scan of thorax.

pulmonary parenchymal changes have a strong predilection for the upper lung fields, unlike those noted in other diffuse parenchymal diseases such as pulmonary fibrosis, which are basilar-predominant. High-resolution computed tomography (HRCT) typically demonstrates symmetric mediastinal or hilar lymphadenopathy, parenchymal changes with upper lobe predominance, or multiple small nodules in a perivascular distribution along bronchovascular bundles, interlobular septa, and subpleural regions. Larger, more well-defined nodular infiltrates may mimic malignancy (**Figure 48-4**). Chest computed tomography (CT) also may reveal bronchiectasis (**Figure 48-5**). In patients with fibrocystic lung disease (**Figure 48-6**), mycetomas may

occur. Remarkable discrepancy among radiographic findings, pulmonary function testing abnormalities, and severity of symptoms often exist.

HRCT does not often aid in diagnosis or in guiding therapy when compared with standard chest radiography. HRCT is indicated in the following scenarios: (1) hemoptysis, (2) a radiographic pattern or new finding that does not suggest sarcoidosis, (3) evaluation for transplant candidacy, and (4) search for a mycetoma.

[18]F-fluorodeoxyglucose–labeled positron emission tomography (FDG-PET) can be useful for evaluating activity in sarcoidosis and is more sensitive than gallium scanning. The

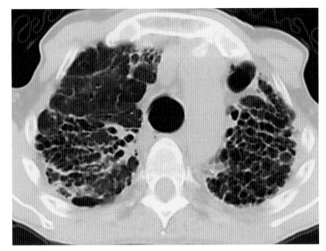

Figure 48-5 Fibrotic bronchiectasis in sarcoidosis. The appearance of the upper lobes with multiple small cystic areas is called honeycombing, readily seen on this computed tomography image.

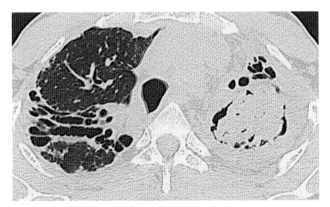

Figure 48-6 Sarcoidosis-related fibrotic honeycombing of upper lobes, with left upper lobe aspergilloma filling a large bulla, is evident on this computed tomography image.

combination of L-[3-^{18}F]-α-methyltyrosine with conventional FDG-PET is useful in discriminating sarcoidosis from malignancy.

Pulmonary Function Testing

Pulmonary function testing assesses the impact of pulmonary sarcoidosis. The two most common abnormalities are reductions in lung volume and vital capacity, representing a restrictive ventilatory defect, with a reduction in diffusing capacity (D$_{LCO}$). A decreased D$_{LCO}$ generally is the first laboratory abnormality detected and the last value to return to normal with disease resolution. A reduction in D$_{LCO}$ is related not only to the restrictive disease but also to sarcoidosis-associated pulmonary hypertension. Obstructive ventilatory defects also may be seen in up to 30% of nonsmokers with sarcoidosis and may represent endobronchial involvement and stenosis, reactivity, or distortion of the airway from parenchymal involvement. Obstructive defects are increasingly seen with fibrosis and bullous transformation. Tests for bronchial hyperreactivity give a positive result in up to 30% of patients.

The prognosis in patients with isolated pulmonary sarcoidosis generally is good. Most patients undergo spontaneous remission or disease stabilization within 2 to 5 years after diagnosis. In a small number of patients, the condition may progress to end-stage lung disease. For those patients with progressive decline in pulmonary function, assessment for oxygen desaturation with exertion should be performed, with consideration of the need for oxygen therapy.

EXTRAPULMONARY SARCOID

Sarcoidosis may affect any organ system. The most commonly involved extrapulmonary organs include the skin (30%), eyes (25%), and lymph nodes, liver, and spleen (20%). Abnormalities in calcium metabolism (hypercalciuria followed by hypercalcemia) are detected in approximately 15% of patients. Clinically apparent cardiac and nervous system involvement have each been reported to occur in about 5% of patients, but magnetic resonance imaging (MRI) and PET scans demonstrate that these organs are more commonly involved. In general, patients who present initially with extrapulmonary disease have a worse prognosis.

Skin

Cutaneous involvement varies and may include erythema nodosum, plaques, nodules, papules, macules, vitiligo, ulcerations, psoriasis-like lesions, and acneiform eruptions. Lesions may be single or occur in crops, may arise in scars and tattoos, and commonly involve the trunk, scalp, nape of the neck, and extremities (**Figure 48-7**). Skin lesions in African American patients frequently leave scars, pits, and pale depigmented areas. Cutaneous involvement usually occurs along with systemic disease, although skin manifestations may precede other organ involvement. Careful examination of the skin is essential at initial presentation, because biopsy of a sarcoidal lesion has a high yield.

Erythema nodosum is a nonspecific hypersensitivity reaction. It occurs in approximately 10% of patients and usually manifests as tender, subcutaneous nodules, often on the anterior tibial surface (**Figure 48-8**). It is more common in women and among persons from Europe, Puerto Rico, and Mexico and is less common in African Americans and Japanese. The onset of erythema nodosum usually is sudden and accompanied by constitutional symptoms such as fever, malaise, and polyarthralgias. The constellation of erythema nodosum, bilateral hilar adenopathy, fever, and polyarthralgias constitutes Löfgren syndrome, an acute form of sarcoidosis that usually is self-limited and carries a good prognosis. Erythema nodosum usually lasts 3 weeks and can recur. Biopsy of the characteristic nodules will show nonspecific septal panniculitis and does not provide histologic support of the diagnosis of sarcoidosis. Biopsy of skin lesions other than those of erythema nodosum usually yields granulomas.

Lupus pernio (**Figure 48-9**), a violaceous, indurated lesion, affects the midface, particularly the nose, nasal alae, malar and periorbital areas, and areas around the eyes. With subsequent erosion into underlying cartilage and bone, as seen in some cases, lupus pernio can be extremely disfiguring. It is more common in women and is associated with chronic disease.

Eyes

Ocular involvement occurs in 25% of patients with sarcoidosis. Any part of the eye can be affected. Black patients and women younger than 40 years are more likely to have ocular involvement. Lacrimal gland involvement is common and usually is asymptomatic (**Figure 48-10**). Conjunctival involvement can manifest as dry or red eyes. The entire uveal tract may be involved. Anterior uveitis (iritis, iridocyclitis) is more common than posterior uveitis (choroiditis). Acute anterior uveitis

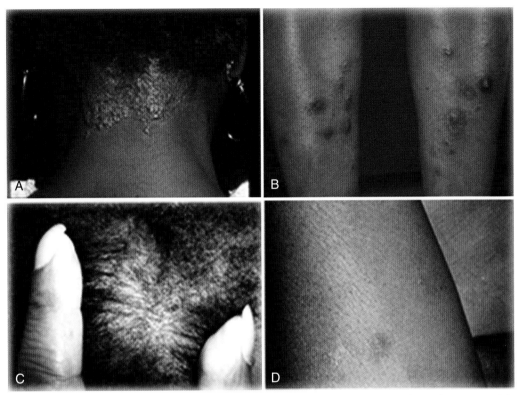

Figure 48-7 Skin lesions in sarcoidosis. **A,** Cluster of waxy papules on nape of the neck. **B,** Raised darkened granulomatous nodules. **C,** Dark, crusting scalp nodules. **D,** Red, nontender nodules.

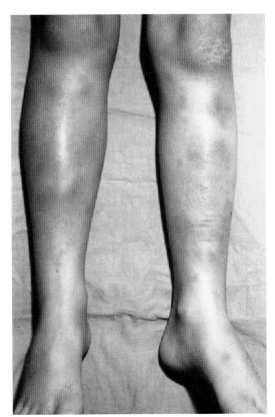

Figure 48-8 Erythema nodosum of the anterior tibia in a patient with sarcoidosis. Raised nodules that were tender to touch are visible on the anterior tibial surface.

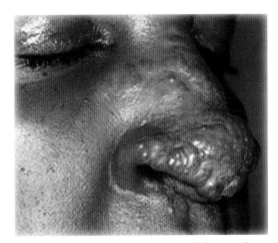

Figure 48-9 Lupus pernio: Raised, bulbous, nodular, crusting, disfiguring nasal granulomas in a patient with sarcoidosis.

manifests with photophobia, eye pain, and blurry vision. Chronic anterior uveitis is more common than acute and may silently result in vision loss and glaucoma. Posterior uveitis can lead to proliferative retinopathy, resulting in loss of vision, and is associated with CNS disease. Approximately 15% of patients with ocular involvement have both anterior and posterior uveitis. Routine dilated funduscopic examination and slit lamp examination by an ophthalmologist are recommended. Biopsy of the conjunctiva and lacrimal glands has a high diagnostic yield.

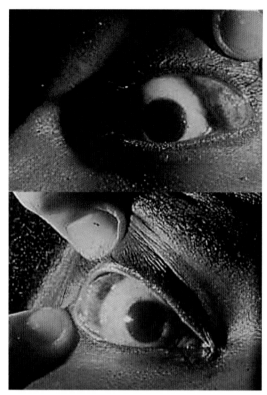

Figure 48-10 Bilateral enlarged nodular lacrimal glands in a patient with sarcoidosis.

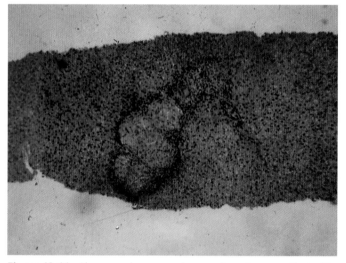

Figure 48-11 Liver granuloma, seen in a specimen from a patient with sarcoidosis.

Liver and Spleen

In up to 80% of patients with sarcoidosis, granulomas will be present on liver biopsy (**Figure 48-11**). Liver involvement in African Americans is at least twice as common as in whites. The liver is palpable in 15% of patients. Sarcoid liver disease manifestations may include asymptomatic liver enzyme elevation, chronic cholestasis, portal hypertension with variceal bleeding, hepatopulmonary syndrome with refractory hypoxemia, and cirrhosis with liver failure. Granulomatous hepatitis in sarcoidosis often results in marked constitutional signs and symptoms such as fever, night sweats, anorexia, right upper quadrant pain, and weight loss. If results of liver function testing are abnormal, tests for viral hepatitis and serum antimitochondrial antibodies to rule out primary biliary cirrhosis should be performed. Alkaline phosphatase and γ-glutamyl transferase are predominantly elevated. Splenomegaly occurs in 6% of patients. Abdominal ultrasound imaging and CT scan may reveal a characteristic hypodense nodular pattern.

Gastrointestinal Tract

Sarcoidosis has been shown to involve the stomach, esophagus, appendix, colon, rectum, and pancreas. Gastric sarcoidosis manifests with epigastric pain, early satiety, and hematemesis secondary to either peptic ulcerations, narrowing of the gastric lumen from granulomatous inflammation, or fibrosis of the gastric wall resulting in pyloric obstruction. Chronic atrophic gastritis with antiparietal cell antibodies resulting in a pernicious anemia–type picture has been reported.

Lymphatics

Although intrathoracic lymph node enlargement is the most common lymphatic manifestation, all lymph node–bearing sites may be involved. Peripheral lymph nodes may be small or grow to several centimeters in diameter and usually are mobile and nontender.

Heart

Cardiac sarcoidosis is most common in Japan, with one autopsy series demonstrating cardiac sarcoidosis in almost half of the cases. In the United States, clinically apparent cardiac involvement occurs in approximately 5% to 10% of patients with sarcoidosis; as suggested by findings with newer imaging techniques such as MRI and PET scanning, however, cardiac inflammation may be more common in North Americans than has been previously appreciated.

The left ventricular free wall is most commonly involved, followed by the basal aspect of the ventricular septum, the right ventricular free walls, and the atrial walls. Conduction abnormalities ranging from first-degree atrioventricular (AV) block to complete heart block are common cardiac manifestations of sarcoidosis. Complete heart block occurs in 30% of affected patients, often heralded by syncope. The most feared extrapulmonary complication is sudden death due to ventricular fibrillation or tachycardia. Because this complication may occur in any patient with sarcoidosis, complaints of dizziness, palpitations, or abnormalities on ECG such as first-degree AV block should trigger cardiac evaluation. Other, less common cardiac manifestations include mitral regurgitation, ventricular aneurysms, pericarditis, pericardial effusions, and tamponade.

Every patient should have a routine electrocardiogram on initial assessment. Further cardiac evaluation may include an echocardiogram, right and/or left cardiac catheterization, electrophysiologic study, and cardiac MRI or PET scan to identify myocardial irritability, left ventricular dysfunction, or pulmonary arterial hypertension. Cardiac biopsy is not useful because sarcoidal granulomas are patchy in distribution and they tend to accumulate in the free left ventricular wall and high interventricular septum, where endomyocardial biopsy generally is avoided. Oral corticosteroid therapy and the need for pacemaker or automatic implantable cardiac defibrillator placement should strongly be considered in patients with arrhythmias or markedly diminished left ventricular function. Because cardiac sarcoidosis mostly occurs in the absence of obvious disease elsewhere, it should be considered as a cause in patients presenting with nonischemic cardiomyopathy, particularly with rhythm disturbances.

Central Nervous System

Neurosarcoidosis occurs in 5% to 15% of patients. The most common manifestation is cranial neuropathy, with unilateral or bilateral seventh nerve palsy seen in 50% to 70% of cases. Cranial neuropathies may resolve spontaneously or with corticosteroid therapy and rarely recur. Optic neuritis, the second most common neuropathy, can result in blurred vision, field defects, and blindness. CNS involvement also includes mass lesions, leptomeningeal disease manifesting as aseptic or chronic meningitis, obstructive hydrocephalus, and hypothalamic and/or pituitary dysfunction. Seizures, headache, change in mental status, confusion, and diabetes insipidus may be presenting manifestations. Spinal cord involvement can produce myelopathies and radiculopathies. Patients with dural lesions, cranial nerve lesions, and nonenhancing brain lesions have a better prognosis than patients with leptomeningeal, enhancing brain parenchymal, and spinal lesions.

Calcium Metabolism

Sarcoid granulomas cause increased conversion of 1-hydroxyvitamin D_3 to the active, 1,25-dihydroxyvitamin D_3 secondary to an increase in 1α-hydroxylase activity. Hypercalcemia is present in 5% of patients, often manifesting as kidney stones. Hypercalciuria is more common than hypercalcemia, and a 24-hour urine collection for total calcium should be included in the initial evaluation. Occasionally, patients present with signs and symptoms of severe hypercalcemia. Typically, calcium abnormalities respond to relatively low doses of corticosteroids.

Other Organ Systems

Patients may complain of nasal and sinus congestion, hoarseness, and noisy breathing, which are secondary to granulomatous infiltration of nasopharyngeal mucosa, sinus, and vocal cord. Sarcoidosis of the upper respiratory tract is associated with chronic disease. Endoscopic sinus surgery may provide symptomatic relief in patients with nasal obstruction or chronic sinusitis secondary to obstruction from sinonasal sarcoidosis. Parotid and salivary gland enlargement occurs in approximately 10% of patients. Bone and muscle involvement often is asymptomatic, but MRI with gadolinium often locates abnormalities in patients with persistent muscle, joint, or bone pain. Direct bone marrow involvement with cytopenia is not uncommon.

QUALITY OF LIFE

Sarcoidosis has a considerable impact on quality of life and is associated with stress, fatigue, pain, and sleep disturbances. One study revealed that 60% of patients reported symptoms of clinical depression. Other studies indicate that quality of life worsens when patients are placed on corticosteroid therapy. Improved communication between physicians and patients is essential, and a multidisciplinary management approach should be considered.

DIAGNOSIS

Because sarcoidosis manifests with nonspecific signs and symptoms, it may be difficult to diagnose. Considerations in the differential diagnosis include infectious causes such as tuberculosis, fungal infections, and other specific infections (e.g., brucellosis, chlamydial infection, tularemia), and autoimmune disorders such as Wegener granulomatosis, Churg-Strauss syndrome, and malignancies. Occupational and environment-induced diseases such as chronic beryllium disease (CBD), hypersensitivity pneumonitis, and drug-induced lung disease also should be considered in the differential diagnosis.

CBD, an occupational hypersensitivity disorder, is elicited by beryllium exposure. Historically, workplace exposure has occurred in the defense, nuclear, aerospace, computer, and electronic industries. CBD is characterized by noncaseating granulomas within affected organs, predominantly lung and skin. Differentiating berylliosis from sarcoidosis can be extremely difficult and relies on a thorough occupational history and demonstrating beryllium sensitization with the beryllium lymphocyte proliferation test. Unsuspected CBD may be misdiagnosed as sarcoidosis, especially in patients with ongoing exposure and presumed corticosteroid resistance. The prognosis with CBD is worse than with sarcoidosis, with an estimated 25% mortality rate. Thus, both establishing the diagnosis of CBD and termination of exposure to beryllium are important, because these measures may lead to resolution of the disease.

In suspected sarcoidosis, a diagnosis should be established with biopsy whenever possible, except in patients presenting with Löfgren syndrome. The key pathologic finding is the noncaseating granuloma. Histologic confirmation can be made noninvasively by the Kveim-Siltzbach test, performed by intradermal injection of a suspension made from the spleen or lymph node of a patient with sarcoidosis. The test result is considered positive if a papule forms at the site of injection within 4 weeks and papule biopsy demonstrates granulomas. This test has a sensitivity of 50% and specificity of 98%. The drawbacks of the test are that it requires 4 to 6 weeks to demonstrate positivity and that it is not widely available. This test is most useful in patients whose lesions are not easily accessible for biopsy and who do not require immediate immunosuppressive therapy.

Fiberoptic bronchoscopy (FOB) is an important tool for diagnosis. FOB can identify endobronchial lesions through direct airway visualization (**Figure 48-12**). The sensitivity of transbronchial lung biopsy, with 4 to 6 pieces collected, ranges from 40% to 90%, and is operator dependent. Additional endobronchial biopsies, transbronchial needle aspiration (TBNA), or endoscopic ultrasonography (EUS)–guided biopsy of lymph nodes can improve yield to up to 90%. Endobronchial ultrasound–guided transbronchial needle aspiration (EBUS-TBNA) has a diagnostic yield of 85% to 92% and has been found to be superior to conventional TBNA sampling in patients with subcentimeter lymph nodes. Because of the high diagnostic yield with EBUS-TBNA, other procedures such as mediastinoscopy are seldom required. The $CD4^+/CD8^+$ ratio in bronchoalveolar lavage (BAL) fluid obtained from patients with sarcoid is greater than 3.5, but BAL cell counts are neither diagnostic nor prognostic.

No specific diagnostic blood test for sarcoidosis exists. Mild anemia, lymphopenia, hypercalcemia, elevated total protein, and abnormalities on liver function testing may be seen. Elevated serum angiotensin-converting enzyme (SACE) levels are present in 50% to 75% of cases, but this finding has low specificity. Observed decline of elevated SACE levels may be used as a marker of corticosteroid therapy compliance. Polymorphisms of the *ACE* gene cause changes in the SACE levels. The polymorphism with insertion (I) or deletion (D) of a portion of gene affects enzyme activity, with DD having higher SACE levels than II polymorphisms. Accordingly, genotype-corrected reference values may be more useful for interpretation.

Figure 48-12 Endobronchial sarcoidosis. **A,** Bronchoscopic view shows extensive nodularity of bronchial mucosa—that is, "cobblestoning" of the airway. Rarely, Wegener granulomatosis, tuberculosis, or fungal disease may be associated with similar airway abnormalities. **B,** Endobronchial biopsy specimen demonstrating several granulomas and giant cells beneath bronchiolar epithelium.

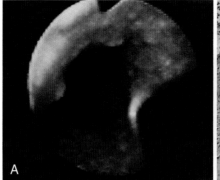
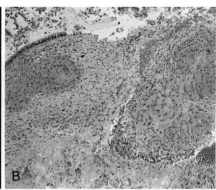

BIOMARKERS OF DISEASE ACTIVITY

Interleukin-2 (IL-2), a T_H1 cytokine that induces T cell proliferation, is elevated in serum and BAL fluid of patients with sarcoidosis and may have prognostic value. Chitotriosidase, which is an enzyme involved in the degradation of chitin, is expressed by activated macrophages. Higher levels of chitotriosidase were found in the serum of patients with active sarcoidosis than in those with inactive disease.

TREATMENT

Sarcoidosis often is a mild, self-limited disease and frequently does not require treatment. Clinical assessment, radiography, and sequential lung function testing with particular attention to any significant decline will establish a basis on which to gauge treatment decisions. **Table 48-3** summarizes the recommended approach to treatment of sarcoidosis.

CORTICOSTEROIDS

Corticosteroid treatment is indicated when patients with sarcoidosis are dyspneic, with commensurately poor values on lung function tests, and in those showing deterioration of health as judged clinically and radiologically, and particularly by progressive impairment of lung function on such testing. Corticosteroids suppress disease activity and produce symptomatic, radiographic, and functional improvement. Uncertainty remains regarding their effect on the overall natural history of the condition. When treatment is required, corticosteroids constitute the first line of therapy.

Long-standing fibrotic lung changes typically show little objective response to these agents, although hypercalcemia and hypercalciuria usually can be controlled with moderate doses of prednisolone. Cessation of short-term corticosteroid treatment is almost always followed by resurgence of the active manifestations. Thus, the effect of corticosteroids usually is one of suppression of the manifestations of sarcoidosis. In a number of controlled situations, the disease progression in patients with pulmonary sarcoidosis receiving specific regimens of corticosteroid treatment has been compared with that of similar groups not receiving corticosteroids. These studies in patients treated for periods of up to 18 months confirmed that corticosteroids could suppress active granulomas and relieve symptoms but did not improve long-term prognosis.

Oral corticosteroid therapy should be strongly considered in the following clinical situations:

- Hypercalcemia or hypercalciuria
- CNS involvement
- Anterior or posterior uveitis that is unresponsive to local therapy
- Active cardiac involvement
- Progressive involvement in any organ system (e.g., progressive respiratory symptoms, abnormal pulmonary function parameters such as reduced diffusion or vital capacity, or worsening radiographic abnormalities)

The optimal dose and duration of corticosteroid treatment have not been determined in randomized, prospective trials. The treatment regimen is individualized on the basis of symptoms and response rate. For pulmonary sarcoidosis, the initial dose generally is 30 to 40 mg/day of prednisone, with 5-mg taper every 2 weeks down to a dose of about 10 to 20 mg/day. Patients should be observed for either symptomatic or pulmonary function improvement at 1 to 3 months. Patients who fail to respond to an initial 3-month course are unlikely to respond to more prolonged therapy. Among responders, treatment should be continued for 9 to 12 months and tapered thereafter if appropriate. Inhaled corticosteroids may be beneficial in patients with endobronchial sarcoidosis with airway hyperreactivity and persistent cough.

Long-term use of corticosteroids is associated with early cataract formation, glaucoma, reduced bone density resulting in osteoporosis, osteonecrosis, and immunosuppression. Judicious use of calcium or vitamin D therapy is important to prevent hypercalcemia and hypercalciuria. Bisphosphonate therapy often is used, especially when bone scans show reduced bone density.

RELAPSE RATES

Relapse rates are higher in patients who achieve medically induced remission than in patients in whom spontaneous remission occurs. Relapse rates were found to be similar in white and in African American patients, but whites maintained a sustained remission with twice the frequency of that in African Americans.

IMMUNOSUPPRESSIVE AND OTHER ALTERNATIVE THERAPIES

Various immunomodulatory and immunosuppressive therapies may be tried if either corticosteroid therapy is poorly tolerated,

Table 48-3 Treatment of Sarcoidosis

Drug Group and Indications	Specific Drug	Dosage and Duration	Side Effects
Corticosteroids for pulmonary or systemic sarcoidosis	Prednisone	*Initial regimen*: 40 mg q24h for 2 weeks 30 mg q24h for 2 weeks 25 mg q24h for 2 weeks 20 mg q24h for 2 weeks 10-15 mg q24h for 6-8 months Taper to 2.5 mg every 2-4 weeks; if relapse occurs, reinstitute lowest previous effective dose	Increased appetite, weight gain Cushingoid habitus Hyperglycemia Adrenal axis suppression Emotional lability, depression Psychosis, pseudotumor cerebri Hypertension Sodium, fluid retention Glaucoma, cataracts Osteoporosis, osteonecrosis Compression fractures Myopathy Pancreatitis Striae, easy bruisability, acne
Antimalarials for mucocutaneous sarcoidosis	Chloroquine phosphate	500 mg q24h for 2 weeks, then 500 mg q48h for 6 months, followed by 6-month drug-free period	Retinopathy Gastrointestinal upset Headache Discoloration of nailbeds
	Hydroxychloroquine sulfate	200 mg q12h or q24h, may be given indefinitely	Reversible dermatitis Retinopathy (rare) Gastrointestinal symptoms Dermatitis
Alternative therapies for:			
Mild disease or as corticosteroid-sparing agent	Pentoxifylline	400 mg q6h or q8h, may be given indefinitely	Gastrointestinal upset Headache
Severe, refractory sarcoidosis and as corticosteroid-sparing agent	Azathioprine	50 mg q24h for 2 weeks Increase by 50 mg every 2-4 weeks Maximum suggested: 150-200 mg q24h	Bone marrow suppression Hepatic toxicity Gastrointestinal toxicity Carcinogenicity Opportunistic infections
	Methotrexate	10-20 mg once a week PLUS folic acid 1 mg/day	Hepatic toxicity Gastrointestinal toxicity Pulmonary toxicity (hypersensitivity pneumonitis) Bone marrow suppression Opportunistic infections (hypersensitivity pneumonitis) Bone marrow suppression Opportunistic infections
Experimental	Doxycycline	200 mg/day	Photosensitivity Gastrointestinal upset
	Minocycline	200 mg/day	
	Thalidomide	100-150 mg qhs	Teratogenicity Peripheral neuropathy Sedation Skin reactions
	Infliximab	Infusion	Infusion reactions Opportunistic infections Tuberculosis, fungal infections, serious infections, sepsis Hypersensitivity reactions
	Etanercept	Injection	Injection site reactions, serious infections, sepsis, death Central nervous system demyelination disorders

or the immunomodulators or other drugs can be used as steroid-sparing agents.

Hydroxychloroquine

The antimalarial drug hydroxychloroquine may be an effective steroid-sparing agent and is particularly useful in patients with neurosarcoidosis, skin involvement, and abnormalities in calcium metabolism. It is contraindicated for use in patients with posterior uveitis, because retinitis is a potential toxic effect. For patients placed on hydroxychloroquine treatment, ophthalmologic examinations should be conducted every 6 months during therapy to monitor for this potential rare ocular toxicity. Women of childbearing age should be counseled to use birth control while taking hydroxychloroquine.

Azathioprine, Methotrexate, Cyclophosphamide, and Mycophenolate Mofetil

Azathioprine, methotrexate, and cyclophosphamide all have been used in the treatment of sarcoidosis. Although these agents benefit selected patients, no studies exist that clearly delineate when these drugs should be used for therapy. Systematic reviews could identify only four randomized trials comparing these agents, and the results were largely inconclusive. The exact mechanism of action of methotrexate (an antimetabolite that reversibly inhibits dihydrofolate reductase) in sarcoidosis is unknown but may involve both cytotoxic and antiinflammatory effects. It has been shown to be useful in uveitis and appears to be a steroid-sparing agent. Mycophenolate mofetil (MMF), a prodrug of mycophenolic acid, which inhibits lymphocyte proliferation, has been reported to be beneficial in patients with cutaneous, neurologic, and renal sarcoidosis. Because MMF does not intercalate into DNA, it has less oncologic potential than azathioprine and cyclophosphamide. MMF also has a rapid onset of action in comparison with other immunosuppressive agents. New agents that are currently being investigated include leflunomide, a methotrexate analogue.

Tetracyclines

Doxycycline and minocycline may be of benefit in some cases of cutaneous sarcoidosis but have not been shown to be effective for management of other organ involvement.

Antitumor Necrosis Factor Therapy

Pentoxifylline

Although pentoxifylline inhibits tumor necrosis factor (TNF), clinical experience indicates that the drug has limited efficacy but may be helpful to lessen systemic symptoms such as fatigue. Gastrointestinal side effects may limit dosing.

Thalidomide

Small clinical series have found that thalidomide may be beneficial in cutaneous sarcoidosis, particularly lupus pernio. Sedation, peripheral neurotoxicity, and teratogenicity limit its usefulness.

Tumor Necrosis Factor-α Blockers

Infliximab, a chimeric monoclonal antibody directed against soluble and membrane-bound TNF-α, recently has been shown to be effective in refractory sarcoidosis, specifically ocular disease. Of interest, etanercept, another TNF-α blocker, was found to be ineffective. Another TNF-α inhibitor, adalimumab, is being investigated for the treatment of cutaneous sarcoidosis. Clinical trials involving cyclosporine, a calcineurin inhibitor, in pulmonary sarcoidosis have not shown any benefit.

The immunomodulatory properties of statins, particularly the suppression of $CD4^+$ T_H1 cell differentiation, which can limit the production of chemokine in alveolar macrophages, appear promising in the treatment of sarcoidosis. A randomized, double-blind, placebo-controlled study is under way at the National Institutes of Health Clinical Center to determine if atorvastatin has steroid-sparing effects in patients being treated for pulmonary sarcoidosis.

LUNG TRANSPLANTATION

Lung transplantation is an appropriate option for patients with sarcoidosis with severe physiologic impairment refractory to medical therapy. Timing of transplantation relative to the disease course is challenging, because mortality rates are high (27% to 53%) among patients with sarcoidosis awaiting a lung transplant. Furthermore, models predicting mortality have not been validated. The most recently published guidelines for lung transplant candidate selection do not delineate disease-specific guidelines for referral. Extrapolating from idiopathic pulmonary fibrosis, the following recommendations for lung transplantation have been suggested: (1) a forced vital capacity (FVC) less than 60% of predicted, (2) diffusing capacity less than 50% of predicted, (3) at-rest or exercise-induced hypoxemia, or (4) failure to maintain lung function despite treatment with steroids or other immunosuppressive agents. These recommendations seem reasonable, because the mortality rate for patients with sarcoidosis on the lung transplant waiting list is similar to that for patients with pulmonary fibrosis.

Specific risk factors for mortality in sarcoidosis patients awaiting lung transplantation have been identified. One study showed an elevated right atrial pressure as the only variable independently associated with mortality in multivariate analysis. A right atrial pressure higher than 15 mm Hg resulted in a 5.2-fold increase in risk of death. Of interest, the mean pulmonary artery pressure (mPAP) at the time of lung transplantation was significantly higher than at the time of listing. Almost all of the patients studied experienced marked progression of pulmonary hypertension while awaiting transplantation, suggesting that more careful right ventricular hemodynamic monitoring can identify those persons who are at increased risk for death. Although repeated right heart catheterizations may not be feasible, repeat echocardiograms and/or monitoring B-type natriuretic peptide (BNP) levels may be helpful to identify worsening pulmonary hypertension.

In a recent review of 405 patients with sarcoidosis listed for lung transplantation in the United Network for Organ Sharing (UNOS) database, no significant difference was found between pulmonary function testing parameters in survivors and those in nonsurvivors. However, underlying pulmonary hypertension, the amount of supplemental oxygen required, and African American race were significant predictors of mortality. Although mPAP was elevated in both survivors and nonsurvivors, mPAP in patients who died while on the waiting list was 33% higher. The marked pulmonary hypertension noted in nonsurvivors was not thought to reflect either cardiac sarcoidosis or chronic left ventricular dysfunction, because of the nearly normal cardiac indices and pulmonary capillary wedge pressures. These data suggest that referral guidelines should be modified to include these particular risk factors, at least until further prospective studies are performed.

Early referral allows for timely evaluation for possible listing. If the risks specific to transplantation in sarcoidosis are considered and carefully evaluated, outcomes match those for other disorders. Recurrence of sarcoidosis in the lung allografts has been reported but does not affect survival or risk for complications.

CLINICAL COURSE

Between 30% and 60% of patients with sarcoidosis are symptomatic. African Americans tend to have more severe disease at presentation. Up to two thirds of patients have spontaneous resolution or improvement in disease activity. Of those with remission, one third have symptom resolution within 1 year and 85% within 2 years. Only 1% to 5% of patients die of sarcoid-related disease, which usually is a result of severe

Box 48-1 Sarcoidosis Risk Factors

Risk Factors Associated With Worsened Outcomes in Sarcoidosis

African-American ethnicity
Lupus pernio
Chronic uveitis
Onset after the age of 40 years
Chronic hypercalcemia
Nephrocalcinosis
Progressive or prolonged symptoms for longer than 6 months
Absence of erythema nodosum
Splenomegaly
Nasal mucosal involvement
Cystic bone lesions
Neurosarcoidosis
Myocardial involvement
Involvement of more than 3 organ systems
Stage III/IV pulmonary disease

Risk Factors Associated With Death of Patient on Lung Transplant Waiting List

Elevated right atrial pressure
Underlying pulmonary hypertension
Higher required levels of supplemental oxygen
African American race

pulmonary, cardiac, or neurologic dysfunction. Sarcoidosis does not affect pregnancy, nor does pregnancy affect sarcoidosis. Corticosteroids, as in asthma, are viewed as safe. Use of other immunosuppressive therapy and hydroxychloroquine is contraindicated in pregnancy. Earlier studies have outlined multiple risk factors associated with worsened prognosis in sarcoidosis (**Box 48-1**). Taken together, the prospect of multisystem involvement and the effect of this illness on the patient's psychosocial well-being highlight the need for a multidisciplinary approach.

CONTROVERSIES AND PITFALLS

The diagnosis of sarcoidosis should be considered early during the evaluation of systemic and respiratory complaints, particularly with additional clues of uveitis, peripheral lymphadenopathy, skin rash, or cranial nerve involvement. To obtain histologic confirmation of the diagnosis, the least invasive approach should be considered. Biopsy of skin, lacrimal gland, peripheral lymph node, and lung or thoracic lymph nodes through bronchoscopy has a high diagnostic yield. Bronchoscopy with endobronchial and transbronchial biopsy, even in patients with a stage I pattern on the chest radiograph, has more than a 60%

yield and should be considered before mediastinoscopy. Lymph node aspiration guided by endobronchial ultrasound imaging will add to the diagnostic yield. Cardiac sarcoidosis should be considered in those patients without risk for coronary artery disease who have unexplained arrhythmias and cardiac dysfunction.

The lack of randomized, controlled treatment trials limits treatment options. Corticosteroids remain the most commonly used therapeutic agents. The role of corticosteroid-sparing medications continues to evolve. When corticosteroids are not tolerated in serious disease, hydroxychloroquine, methotrexate, azathioprine, and anti-TNF agents are used.

WEB RESOURCE

www.sarcoidosis.org

SUGGESTED READINGS

Baughman RP: Lower, steroid-sparing alternative treatments for sarcoidosis, *Clin Chest Med* 18:853–864, 1997.

Hunninghake GW, Costabel U, Ando M, et al: ATS/ERS/WASOG statement on sarcoidosis. American Thoracic Society/European Respiratory Society/World Association of Sarcoidosis and Other Granulomatous Disorders, *Sarcoidosis Vasc Diffuse Lung Dis* 16:149–173, 1999.

Iannuzzi MC, Fontana JR: Sarcoidosis: clinical presentation, immunopathogenesis, and therapeutics, *JAMA* 305:391–399, 2011.

Iannuzzi MC, Rybicki BA, Teirstein AS: Sarcoidosis, *N Engl J Med* 357:2153–2165, 2007.

Judson MA: An approach to the treatment of pulmonary sarcoidosis with corticosteroids: the six phases of treatment, *Chest* 115:1158–1165, 1999.

Judson MA, Baughman RP, Thompson BW, et al: Two year prognosis of sarcoidosis: the ACCESS experience, *Sarcoidosis Vasc Diffuse Lung Dis* 20:204–211, 2003.

Judson MA, Iannuzzi MC, guest editors: *Sarcoidosis: evolving concepts and controversies, Vol 28 of Seminars in Respiratory Critical Care Medicine*, New York, 2007, Thieme Medical Publishers, pp 36–52.

Judson MA, Thompson BW, Rabin DL, et al: The diagnostic pathway to sarcoidosis, *Chest* 123:406–412, 2003.

Koyama T, Ueda H, Togashi K, et al: Radiologic manifestations of sarcoidosis in various organs, *Radiographics* 24: 87–104, 2004.

Morgenthau AS, Iannuzzi MC: Recent advances in sarcoidosis, *Chest* 139:174–182, 2011.

Padilla ML, Schilero GJ, Teirstein AS: Sarcoidosis and transplantation, *Sarcoidosis Vasc Diffuse Lung Dis* 14:16–22, 1997.

Rybicki BA, Iannuzzi MC, Frederick MM, et al: Familial aggregation of sarcoidosis. A case-control etiologic study of sarcoidosis (ACCESS), *Am J Respir Crit Care Med* 164:2085–2091, 2001.

Yeager H, Rossman RD, Baughman RP, et al: Pulmonary and psychosocial findings at enrollment in the ACCESS study, *Sarcoidosis Vasc Diffuse Lung Dis* 22:147–153, 2005.

Chapter **49**
Eosinophilic Lung Disease
Vincent Cottin • Jean-François Cordier

THE EOSINOPHIL LEUKOCYTE AND EOSINOPHILIC PNEUMONIA

The eosinophilic lung diseases are characterized by prominent infiltration of the lung structures by eosinophils, leading to several distinct clinical disorders, especially eosinophilic pneumonia. The most important eosinophilic lung diseases other than eosinophilic pneumonia are allergic bronchopulmonary aspergillosis (ABPA) and hypereosinophilic asthma, which primarily affect the airways.

THE EOSINOPHIL LEUKOCYTE

Eosinophils play a major role in immunity against bacteria, viruses, parasites, and tumors and participate in the pathogenesis of allergic diseases. They also take part in the pathogenesis of numerous inflammatory processes and may be the major cause of tissue injury in eosinophilic disorders. Advances have been made recently in elucidation of the complex role of eosinophils in health and disease through the study of several models of genetically engineered murine cell lines deficient in the eosinophil lineage. Approaches that selectively target the eosinophil lineage in vivo are being developed with a therapeutic perspective, such as use of the humanized antiinterleukin (IL)-5 antibody mepolizumab.

The role of the eosinophil leukocyte as a multifunctional cell is now well appreciated in both innate and adaptive immunity. Eosinophils express Toll-like receptors (TLRs) and participate in the nonspecific inflammatory reaction in tissues in response to various ligands; however, they also play a major role by interacting with T cells. Once perceived as a terminal effector cell in parasitic infections and allergy, the eosinophil is now recognized to be able to modulate T cell responses, by presenting the antigen to naive as well as to antigen-primed T cells, thereby inducing T helper cell type 2 (T_H2) development, cytokine production, and T cell migration to sites of inflammation. T cells can then secrete T_H2-type cytokines (the interleukins IL-4, IL-5, and IL-13), which further enhance the recruitment of eosinophils. Secretion of IL-4 and IL-13 by the eosinophil in turn amplifies the T_H2 response in the lung in a positive loop. In addition, eosinophils may present antigens from the airways or the lung tissue to T_H0 cells in the draining lymph node in the context of major histocompatibility complex (MHC) class II. Eosinophil precursors differentiate in the bone marrow under the action of several cytokines, including interleukin (IL)-5, IL-3, and granulocyte-macrophage colony-stimulating factor (GM-CSF). Eosinophils are recruited in response to diverse stimuli from the circulation into inflammatory foci, including sites in the lung, where they have the potential to modulate immune responses. Recruitment of eosinophils involves cell adhesion and attraction, diapedesis, and chemotaxis by cytokines (mainly IL-5 and eotaxin) and the chemokine receptor CCR3. In tissues, the eosinophils may be triggered through engagement of receptors for cytokines, immunoglobulins, and complement, with ensuing release of active mediators, including proinflammatory cytokines, arachidonic acid–derived mediators, enzymes, reactive oxygen species, complement proteins, chemokines, chemoattractants, metalloproteases, and other toxic granule proteins, especially cationic proteins. Indeed, activation and degranulation of the eosinophil releases specific cationic proteins, including major basic protein (MBP), eosinophil cationic protein (ECP), eosinophil-derived neurotoxin (EDN), protein eosinophil peroxidase (EPO), and MBP homologue. These proteins released mostly by degranulation have proinflammatory properties, through the upregulation of chemoattraction, expression of adhesion molecules, regulation of vascular permeability, contraction of smooth muscle cells, and direct cytotoxicity. The eosinophils also express receptors for cytokines, complement, immunoglobulins, chemokines, and apoptotic signals; regulate mast cell functions; and interact with basophils, endothelial cells, macrophages, platelets, and fibroblasts. However, histopathologic lesions in eosinophilic pneumonias are largely reversible with treatment, with the possible exception of bronchial wall damage in ABPA.

HISTOPATHOLOGIC FEATURES OF EOSINOPHILIC PNEUMONIA

The diagnosis of eosinophilic pneumonia only exceptionally requires lung biopsy, and histopathologic features were described several decades ago. Eosinophilic pneumonia as exemplified by idiopathic chronic eosinophilic pneumonia (ICEP) is characterized by the prominent infiltration of the lung structures by eosinophils. The lung interstitium is infiltrated by eosinophils, and essentially the alveolar spaces are filled with eosinophils and a fibrinous exudate, with conservation of the global architecture of the lung. Immunohistochemical and electron microscopic studies have demonstrated eosinophil degranulation within involved lung tissue.

Some overlap is common between eosinophilic and organizing pneumonia, with organization of the alveolar inflammatory exudate (less prominent than in cryptogenic organizing pneumonia). In addition, eosinophilic microabscesses and a nonnecrotizing vasculitis are common in ICEP and idiopathic acute eosinophilic pneumonia (IAEP). Macrophages and occasional multinucleate giant cells may be present within the infiltrate. The histopathologic pattern in IAEP usually comprises intraalveolar and interstitial eosinophilic infiltrates, diffuse alveolar

Box 49-1 Diagnosis of Eosinophilic Pneumonias

Characteristic Clinical-Imaging Features

■ Chronic eosinophilic pneumonia (onset >1 month earlier)
   OR
■ Acute eosinophilic pneumonia (onset <1 month earlier)
   OR
■ Löffler syndrome (transient mild dyspnea, cough, fever, and pulmonary infiltrates)

Demonstration of Eosinophilia (Preferably Alveolar)

■ Bronchoalveolar lavage (BAL) analysis with >25% eosinophils and preferably >40%
   OR
■ Markedly elevated peripheral blood eosinophilia (eosinophil cell count >1000/µL and preferably 1500/µL)
   OR
■ Lung biopsy demonstrating eosinophilic pneumonia (if performed)

Box 49-2 Clinical Classification of the Eosinophilic Lung Diseases

Eosinophilic Lung Disease of Determined Origin
Eosinophilic Pneumonias of Parasitic Origin
Tropical eosinophilia
Ascaris pneumonia
Larva migrans syndrome
Strongyloides stercoralis infection
Eosinophilic pneumonias in other parasitic infections

Eosinophilic Pneumonias of Other Infectious Causes
Allergic Bronchopulmonary Aspergillosis and Related Syndromes
Allergic bronchopulmonary aspergillosis
Other allergic bronchopulmonary syndromes associated with fungi or yeasts
Bronchocentric granulomatosis

Iatrogenic and Toxic Agent–Induced Eosinophilic Pneumonias
Drugs
Radiation therapy to the breast
Toxic agents

Eosinophilic Lung Disease of Undetermined Origin
Limited to the Lung
Idiopathic chronic eosinophilic pneumonia
Idiopathic acute eosinophilic pneumonia

Associated with Systemic Disease
Churg-Strauss syndrome
Hypereosinophilic syndromes (lymphocytic and myeloproliferative variants)

Lung Diseases with Possible (Usually Minor) Associated Eosinophilia
Organizing pneumonia
Asthma, eosinophilic bronchitis
Idiopathic interstitial pneumonias
Langerhans cell granulomatosis
Sarcoidosis
Lung transplantation

damage, intraalveolar fibrinous exudates, organizing pneumonia, and non-necrotizing vasculitis.

DIAGNOSIS OF EOSINOPHILIC PNEUMONIA

The diagnosis of eosinophilic pneumonia relies on both characteristic clinical-imaging features and the demonstration of alveolar eosinophilia and/or peripheral blood eosinophilia (**Box 49-1**). Bronchoalveolar lavage (BAL) is a noninvasive alternative to lung biopsy in this setting. The percentage of eosinophils in BAL fluid is less than 2% in normal control subjects, and a differential cell count for eosinophils of 2% to 25% may be found in nonspecific conditions. Therefore, a cutoff value of 25% eosinophils or more in BAL fluid, and preferably 40% or more, is recommended for the diagnosis of eosinophilic pneumonia. The presence of marked eosinophilia in BAL fluid obviates the need for lung biopsy in this disorder, especially when the eosinophils are the predominant cell population in BAL fluid (macrophages excepted). Markedly elevated peripheral blood eosinophilia (greater than 1000/µL and preferably 1500/µL) together with typical clinical radiologic features are highly suggestive of the diagnosis of eosinophilic pneumonia, and BAL may not be always mandatory in such patients, although other disorders may be associated with pulmonary infiltrates and peripheral eosinophilia (e.g., bacterial pneumonia, parasitic pneumonia, infiltrates related to lymphoma). Peripheral blood eosinophilia may be absent at presentation, especially in IAEP and in patients receiving corticosteroid treatment.

Eosinophilic pneumonia may be separated into that of undetermined origin, which usually may be included within well-individualized syndromes, and that with a definite cause (mainly infection and drug reaction) (**Box 49-2**). Potential causes must be thoroughly investigated, because identification of a cause may lead to effective therapeutic measures.

EOSINOPHILIC LUNG DISEASES OF KNOWN ORIGIN

EOSINOPHILIC PNEUMONIA IN PARASITIC DISEASES

Parasite infestation is the main cause of eosinophilic pneumonia worldwide. Clinical manifestations are nonspecific. Tropical pulmonary eosinophilia is a disease of decreasing prevalence caused by the filarial parasites *Wuchereria bancrofti* and *Brugia malayi*, deposited in the skin by mosquitoes. The clinical features of tropical eosinophilic pneumonia largely result from an immune response of the host to the antigenic constituents of circulating microfilariae trapped in the lung vasculature (leading to cough that may be associated with fever, weight loss, and anorexia). Patients with tropical pulmonary eosinophilia do not usually have clinical features of lymphatic filariasis. The chest radiograph shows bilateral infiltrative opacities. Blood eosinophilia with counts of more than 2000/µL eosinophils is characteristic of the early stage, occasionally with counts of up to 60,000/µL during the chronic phase of disease. Microfilariae are not detectable in the blood. The diagnosis of filariasis may be established by a strongly positive result on serologic testing in patients residing in an endemic area, with persisting and prominent blood eosinophilia at counts of more than 3000/µL and IgE levels exceeding 10,000 ng/mL. It is further supported by clinical improvement in the weeks after treatment with diethylcarbamazine; the addition of corticosteroids may be beneficial in severe cases.

The nematode *Ascaris lumbricoides* is the most common helminth infecting humans. The disease is transmitted through consumption of food contaminated by human feces containing parasitic eggs. Löffler syndrome (transient mild eosinophilic pneumonia) may develop during the migration of the larvae through the lung. Signs and symptoms often are limited to cough, wheezing, and transient fever, which resolve within a few days, but blood eosinophilia with counts as high as 20,000/μL may be present and last for several weeks. The diagnosis usually is obtained by the delayed finding of the worm or ova in the stools within 3 months of onset of the pulmonary manifestations; larvae may occasionally be found at an earlier stage in sputum or gastric aspirates.

Visceral larva migrans syndrome caused by *Toxocara canis* occurs throughout the world. Humans and especially children become infected after ingestion of eggs released in feces of infected dogs (especially in the soil of urban public playgrounds). Fever, seizures, fatigue, and pulmonary manifestations may occur (cough, dyspnea, wheezes, or crackles heard on pulmonary auscultation and pulmonary infiltrates evident on the chest radiograph). Blood eosinophilia may be present initially or may develop only in the following days. The diagnosis of toxocariasis is obtained by serologic methods, especially enzyme-linked immunosorbent assay (ELISA). Symptomatic treatment is recommended; the use of antihelmintics is controversial.

Strongyloides stercoralis is an intestinal nematode, the larvae of which infect humans through the skin by contact with damp soil. Eosinophilia is present in recently infected persons. Strongyloidiasis may cause severe disease, affecting all organs (hyperinfection syndrome), especially in immunocompromised patients, sometimes years after the initial infection, with or without peripheral eosinophilia and bilateral patchy infiltrates on chest radiograph. The diagnosis of strongyloidiasis depends on the demonstration of larvae in the feces or in any secretion or tissue specimen (including sputum and BAL fluid). Immunodiagnostic assays by ELISA methods may be useful for diagnosis and screening. Treatment with thiabendazole is recommended.

ALLERGIC BRONCHOPULMONARY ASPERGILLOSIS

ABPA occurs mainly in adults with preexisting asthma (with an estimated prevalence of 1% to 2%) and in patients with cystic fibrosis (with an estimated prevalence of up to 7% to 10%). It results from a complex allergic and immune reaction in the bronchi and the adjacent lung parenchyma in response to antigens from *Aspergillus* colonizing the airways of patients with asthma. A pattern of allergic bronchopulmonary mycosis similar to that in ABPA has rarely been reported with infections caused by other fungi or yeasts, including *Penicillium, Drechslera, Torulopsis, Mucor, Candida, Pseudallescheria, Bipolaris, Curvularia, Fusarium, Cladosporium,* and *Saccharomyces.* The immunologic response to the fungus combines both type I and type III hypersensitivity in an allergic host and is mediated by the immunoglobulins IgG, IgE, and IgA, as well as the helper T cell subset 2 (T_H2) CD4$^+$ cells, and by activation and degranulation of mast cells and eosinophils, resulting in progressive damage to the bronchial and surrounding pulmonary tissue. Mucous plugs containing *Aspergillus* obstruct the airways, with subsequent atelectasis, bronchial wall damage, and proximal bronchiectasis predominating in the upper lobes. Of note, IgE sensitization to *Aspergillus* in nonasthmatic patients who do not fulfill criteria for ABPA is associated with reduced lung function. ABPA may be associated with allergic *Aspergillus* sinusitis in a syndrome called sinobronchial allergic aspergillosis. Genetic susceptibility to develop ABPA has been demonstrated, with an increased prevalence of heterozygotic cystic fibrosis transmembrane conductance regulator (CFTR) gene mutations in

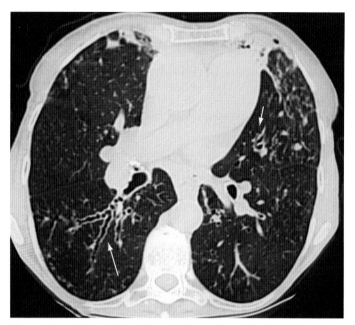

Figure 49-1 Bilateral bronchiectasis in a patient with allergic bronchopulmonary aspergillosis. Affected structures (*arrows*) are well visualized on this computed tomography scan, which also shows some infiltrative opacities.

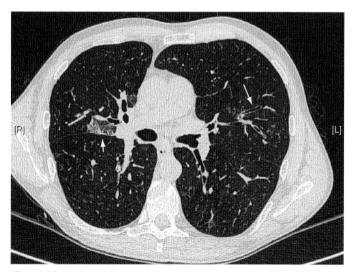

Figure 49-2 Bronchiectasis (*arrows*) in another patient with allergic bronchopulmonary aspergillosis. The computed tomography scan also shows ground glass opacities (*arrowhead*) and centrilobular micronodules.

non–cystic fibrosis patients with ABPA, the association of ABPA with a polymorphism within the IL-4 receptor α-chain gene, and association with certain human leukocyte antigen (HLA) DR subtypes.

Early ABPA is characterized by fever, expectoration of mucous plugs, peripheral blood eosinophilia with counts higher than 1000/μL, and pulmonary infiltrates caused by eosinophilic pneumonia, or segmental or lobar atelectasis caused by mucous plugging. Chronic ABPA is characterized by asthma, eosinophilia, and bronchopulmonary manifestations including bronchiectasis (**Figures 49-1 and 49-2** and **Box 49-3**). The presence of bronchiectasis on computed tomography (CT) images in a patient with asthma is therefore highly suggestive of ABPA; however, typical proximal bronchiectasis may be absent, and such cases are designated ABPA-seropositive. Centrilobular

Box 49-3 Minimal Essential Diagnostic Criteria for Allergic Bronchopulmonary Aspergillosis (ABPA) in Patients With Asthma

Patients With Asthma and Central Bronchiectasis
1. Asthma
2. Central bronchiectasis (involving inner two thirds of chest CT field)
3. Immediate cutaneous reactivity to *Aspergillus*
4. Total serum IgE concentration <417 kU/L (1000 ng/mL)
5. Elevated serum IgE–*A. fumigatus* and/or IgG–*A. fumigatus*
(Infiltrates on chest radiograph and serum precipitating antibodies to *A. fumigatus* may be present but are not minimal essential diagnostic criteria.)

Patients With Asthma and ABPA-Seropositive Status
Patients with the foregoing criteria 1, 3, 4, 5
(Infiltrates may be present on chest radiograph, but this finding does not constitute a minimal essential diagnostic criterion.)

Patients With Cystic Fibrosis
1. Clinical deterioration (increased cough, wheezing, exercise intolerance, increased sputum, decrease in pulmonary function)
2. Immediate cutaneous reactivity to *Aspergillus* or presence of IgE–*A. fumigatus*
3. Total serum IgE concentration <417 kU/L (1000 ng/mL)
4. Precipitating antibodies to *A. fumigatus* or serum IgG–*A. fumigatus*
5. Abnormalities on chest radiograph (infiltrates, mucous plugging, or a change from earlier films)

Box 49-4 Drugs That Can Cause Eosinophilic Pneumonia*

Acetylsalicylic acid
Captopril
Carbamazepine
Diclofenac
Ethambutol
Fenbufen
Granulocyte-macrophage colony-stimulating factor (GM-CSF)
Ibuprofen
L-Tryptophan
Minocycline
Naproxen
Paraaminosalicylic acid (4-aminosalicylic acid)
Penicillins
Phenylbutazone
Piroxicam
Pyrimethamine
Sulindac
Sulfamides, sulfonamides
Tolfenamic acid
Trimethoprim-sulfamethoxazole

*A more detailed list of drugs reported to cause eosinophilic pneumonia may be found at www.pneumotox.com.

nodules and mucoid impaction on CT scan (typically characterized by a V-shaped lesion, with the vertex pointing toward the hilum) also are highly suggestive of ABPA. The expectoration of mucous plugs, the presence of *Aspergillus* in sputum, and late skin reactivity to *Aspergillus* antigen also are common at this stage; however, *Aspergillus* is not reliably identified in sputum or BAL fluid samples of patients with ABPA, and positive cultures are not required for diagnosis. The finding of *Aspergillus* organisms may reflect colonization and thus is not specific for ABPA. Total serum IgE levels of at least 1000 IU/mL constitute a hallmark of ABPA. Peripheral blood eosinophilia is common but is not a required diagnostic criterion.

Identification of immunologic hypersensitivity to *Aspergillus fumigatus* in patients with asthma contributes to the diagnosis of ABPA; it may consist in immediate reaction to prick test for *Aspergillus* antigen, precipitating serum antibodies against *A. fumigatus*, and/or elevated specific serum IgE against *A. fumigatus*. Among approximately 40 antigenic components of *Aspergillus* that can bind with IgE antibodies, specific antibodies to Asp f4 and Asp f6 may be particularly helpful for diagnostic purposes.

Suspicion of ABPA should prompt the measurement of serum total IgE level and skin testing for *Aspergillus*. Early recognition of ABPA allows treatment of exacerbations of ABPA with corticosteroids (with initiation of prednisone at approximately 0.5 mg/kg per day for 2 to 4 weeks then tapered) to prevent the progression of the disease to the irreversible endstage. Inhaled corticosteroids may reduce the need for long-term oral corticosteroids. Oral itraconazole used at a dose of 200 mg twice daily for 4 to 6 months is a useful adjunct to corticosteroids, reducing the burden of fungal antigenic stimulation, allowing reduction of the corticosteroid oral dose, reducing the rate of exacerbations, and possibly improving the long-term outcome. The newer antifungal agent voriconazole has been used as a corticosteroid-sparing agent in ABPA only in isolated case reports and currently is not indicated in ABPA. Omalizumab, an anti-IgE recombinant antibody, has been used successfully in some cases; however, clinical experience is limited.

IATROGENIC EOSINOPHILIC PNEUMONIAS SECONDARY TO DRUGS, TOXIC AGENTS, AND RADIATION THERAPY

Drugs taken in the weeks preceding clinical onset of eosinophilic pneumonia must be thoroughly investigated, including illicit drugs (cocaine or heroin). Eosinophilic pneumonia has been reported in association with many drugs, but causality has been confidently established for fewer than 20 specific agents (**Box 49-4**).

Drug-induced eosinophilic pneumonia may develop progressively and manifest as chronic eosinophilic pneumonia, as a syndrome of transient pulmonary infiltrates with eosinophilia (Löffler syndrome), and occasionally as an acute pneumonia sometimes requiring mechanical ventilation. Acute eosinophilic pneumonia may occur in the context of drug rash with eosinophilia and systemic symptoms (DRESS), with frequent reactivation of human herpesvirus type 6, especially that due to anticonvulsant therapy, antibiotics (minocycline), allopurinol, and nonsteroidal antiinflammatory agents.

Corticosteroids often are given concomitantly with drug withdrawal to accelerate clinical improvement. When present, associated cutaneous rash or pleural effusion increases the likelihood of the diagnosis.

As with ICEP, chronic eosinophilic pneumonia has been described after radiation therapy for breast cancer in women. The clinical syndrome is similar to that for radiation-induced organizing pneumonia.

OTHER LUNG DISEASES WITH ASSOCIATED EOSINOPHILIA

Eosinophilia may be found in other bronchopulmonary disorders in which eosinophilic pneumonia is not prominent.

Eosinophilic inflammation of the airways is a pathologic feature defining a phenotype of asthma. Some mild increase in eosinophils in peripheral blood and BAL fluid differential cell count (usually less than 5%) may be found in patients with asthma. Monitoring of the sputum eosinophil count may help in adapting the treatment and reducing asthma exacerbations and hospital admissions. Patients with the eosinophilic phenotype of asthma are considered to have greater airway remodeling and more frequent exacerbations than those without tissue eosinophilia. Mepolizumab, a humanized monoclonal antibody against IL-5, has been demonstrated to reduce the number of severe exacerbations in patients with refractory eosinophilic asthma (as defined by sputum eosinophil percentage of more than 3% on at least one occasion in the previous 2 years despite high-dose inhaled corticosteroid treatment); mepolizumab also improved the quality of life related to asthma and lowered eosinophil counts in blood and sputum. Some sparing of prednisone therapy and reduction in blood and sputum eosinophil counts also were obtained using mepolizumab therapy in patients with sputum eosinophilia (more than 3% eosinophils) and prednisone-dependent asthma. The therapeutic effect of mepolizumab confirms the role of eosinophils as an effector cell in the minority of asthma patients with the eosinophilic phenotype. More important, blood eosinophilia (i.e., counts of more than 1500/µL) may occasionally occur in the absence of any determined cause or context of systemic disease—a condition referred to as *hypereosinophilic asthma*, which frequently is severe and requires systemic corticosteroid therapy. Hypereosinophilic asthma may evolve to ICEP or overt Churg-Strauss syndrome (CSS), or it may remain solitary, with frequent dependency on oral corticosteroids.

Eosinophilic bronchitis (without asthma) with a high percentage of eosinophils (up to 40%) in sputum is a well-characterized cause of chronic cough responsive to corticosteroid treatment. Bronchial asthma and bronchial hyperreactivity are absent. Patients usually have normal lung function. Eosinophilic bronchitis may exceptionally reveal the myeloid variant of the hypereosinophilic syndrome.

Bronchocentric granulomatosis is a rare condition with nonspecific clinical and radiologic manifestations (fever, cough, and blood eosinophilia with counts generally greater than 1000/µL), diagnosed by lung biopsy. Corticosteroids constitute the mainstay of treatment.

Mildly increased levels of eosinophils may be found on the BAL fluid differential cell count in idiopathic interstitial pneumonias; this finding is associated with a poor prognosis. Focal eosinophilic pneumonia has been reported in cases of usual interstitial pneumonia, nonspecific interstitial pneumonia, and desquamative interstitial pneumonia. The typical clinical and imaging features of cryptogenic organizing pneumonia may closely mimic those of ICEP; some clinical or pathologic overlap between these two diseases is likely, although BAL fluid eosinophilia usually is mild, with differential cell counts less than 20%, in cryptogenic organizing pneumonia. Eosinophilia (usually mild) may be present in pulmonary Langerhans cell histiocytosis and in sarcoidosis.

EOSINOPHILIC LUNG DISEASE OF UNKNOWN ORIGIN

IDIOPATHIC CHRONIC EOSINOPHILIC PNEUMONIA

ICEP is characterized by the progressive development of respiratory and systemic symptoms over several weeks. Cough,

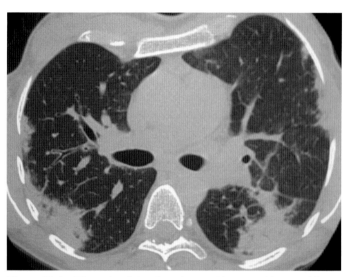

Figure 49-3 Bilateral peripheral patchy opacities are evident on this computed tomography scan of the thorax of a patient with idiopathic chronic eosinophilic pneumonia.

dyspnea, and chest pain are often accompanied by prominent fatigue, malaise, fever, and weight loss. Wheezes or crackles are found in one third of patients. Chronic rhinitis or sinusitis is present in approximately 20% of patients.

Most patients are nonsmokers. ICEP predominates in women (2 : 1 female-to-male ratio), with a mean age of 45 years at diagnosis, and a previous history of atopy in approximately half of the patients. Previous asthma is present in up to two thirds of the patients (it may get worse after the occurrence of ICEP), but it also may occur concomitantly with the diagnosis of ICEP or develop after it. Nonrespiratory minor manifestations are possible in ICEP, suggesting some overlap with CSS; however, any nonrespiratory manifestation (and particularly cardiac manifestations) should systematically prompt further evaluation for possible systemic disease, especially CSS.

Imaging features of ICEP (**Figure 49-3**) characteristically consist of alveolar opacities, with ill-defined margins and variable density, ranging from ground glass to consolidation. Migration of the infiltrates highly suggestive of the diagnosis occurs in approximately a quarter of the cases; however, it also may occur in cryptogenic organizing pneumonia. A peripheral predominance of the lesions (described as the classic pattern of "photographic negative of pulmonary edema") is seen in approximately one fourth of patients. On high-resolution computed tomography (HRCT), the opacities are almost always bilateral and predominate in the upper lobes, with coexisting peripheral ground glass and consolidation opacities. In addition, septal line thickening, bandlike opacities parallel to the chest, or mediastinal lymph node enlargement may be seen. Small pleural effusions are present in only 10% of cases at HRCT.

High-level peripheral blood eosinophilia is the key to the diagnosis (mean blood eosinophil count of approximately 5500/µL) (**Box 49-5**). Alveolar eosinophilia, with BAL fluid differential cell count usually more than 40%, is a hallmark of ICEP. Because the BAL eosinophil cell count drops within days after institution of corticosteroid treatment, assessment for alveolar eosinophilia should be undertaken before any corticosteroid intake. Sputum eosinophilia also may be present; however, its diagnostic value has not been evaluated. C-reactive protein levels are elevated. Total blood IgE level is increased in approximately half the cases.

Lung function tests in ICEP show an obstructive ventilatory defect in approximately half and a restrictive ventilatory defect in half the cases. Usually mild hypoxemia is present in most of the patients.

ICEP responds dramatically to corticosteroid treatment. We use an initial dose of 0.5 mg/kg of oral prednisone per day for 2 weeks, followed by 0.25 mg/kg per day for 2 weeks, then corticosteroids are progressively reduced over a total duration of about 6 months and stopped. Improvement of the symptoms occurs within 2 days, and chest radiograph opacities clear within 1 week and eventually disappear without sequelae in almost all patients. Death resulting from ICEP is extremely rare. Relapses occur in more than half the patients while decreasing or after stopping the corticosteroid treatment and respond very well to resumed corticosteroid treatment; a dose of 20 mg per day of prednisone usually is sufficient to treat the relapses. Most patients need corticosteroids for more than 6 months, and often for several years. Relapses of ICEP may be less frequent in asthmatic patients who receive inhaled corticosteroids after stopping maintenance oral corticosteroids.

IDIOPATHIC ACUTE EOSINOPHILIC PNEUMONIA

IAEP differs from ICEP not only in its acute onset (less than 1 month) and severity but also in the absence of relapse after recovery. This acute pneumonia develops in previously healthy people, with possible respiratory failure, and may be misdiagnosed as infectious pneumonia or acute respiratory distress syndrome (ARDS). Patients with IAEP often are admitted to the intensive care unit. Blood eosinophilia, often lacking at presentation, contrasts with frank alveolar eosinophilia in BAL fluid. Current diagnostic criteria are listed in **Box 49-6.**

IAEP occurs mainly in young adults, with a male predominance and no previous asthma history. In several cases, IAEP developed soon after the initiation of tobacco smoking or change in smoking habits. Potential respiratory exposures within the days before onset of disease have been reported (e.g., cave exploration, heavy dust inhalation, inhalation of smoke), suggesting that exposure to inhaled contaminants or any nonspecific injurious agent may trigger the disease.

IAEP manifests with the acute onset of cough, dyspnea, fever, and chest pain, sometimes with abdominal complaints or myalgias. Tachypnea, tachycardia, and crackles are present on examination. The chest radiograph shows bilateral infiltrates (see **Figure 49-4**), with mixed alveolar interstitial and opacities, especially Kerley lines. Chest CT mainly shows ground glass opacities and air space consolidation, together with poorly defined nodules, interlobular septal thickening, and bilateral pleural effusions (in two thirds of patients)—an imaging pattern

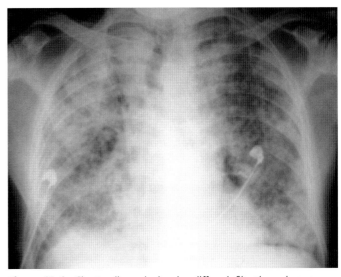

Figure 49-4 Chest radiograph showing diffuse infiltrative pulmonary opacities in a patient with idiopathic acute eosinophilic pneumonia with respiratory failure.

very distinct from that of ICEP that may evoke the diagnosis of IAEP.

Blood eosinophilia usually is lacking at presentation, and the diagnosis of eosinophilic lung disease may not be considered on admission. The finding of BAL fluid eosinophilia usually is sufficient, with differential counts greater than 25%, to obviate the need for lung biopsy; bacterial cultures of BAL fluid are sterile. The peripheral blood eosinophil count often rises over a few days during the initial course of disease—an evolution suggestive of the diagnosis. Eosinophilia also may be found in pleural effusion or sputum samples. High levels of IgE may be present as well.

Lung function tests are performed only in the less severe cases and will show a mild restrictive ventilatory defect, reduced carbon monoxide transfer capacity, and increased alveolar-arterial oxygen gradient, measured as PO₂(A–a). Severe hypoxemia may be present, with most patients fulfilling diagnostic criteria for acute lung injury (including a PaO₂/FIO₂ ratio of 300 mm Hg or less) or for ARDS (PaO₂/FIO₂ ratio of 200 mm Hg or less), with mechanical ventilation necessary in most of them. In marked contrast with ARDS, extrapulmonary organ failure or shock is exceptional; however, a few cases of fatal IAEP have been reported.

Lung biopsy generally is not necessary, and the diagnosis is established on clinical, radiologic, and BAL findings. The histopathologic features of IAEP include acute and organizing diffuse alveolar damage together with interstitial alveolar and bronchiolar infiltration by eosinophils, intraalveolar eosinophils, and interstitial edema. Although recovery may occur without corticosteroid treatment, corticosteroid treatment usually is given for 2 to 4 weeks, with a starting dose of oral prednisone or intravenous methylprednisolone of 1 to 2 mg/kg per day. Complete clinical and radiologic recovery occurs rapidly after initiation of corticosteroids, with no relapse (in contrast with ICEP). A careful search for a potential cause of IAEP is mandatory, especially infectious agents, parasites, and drugs, including illicit and over-the-counter drugs.

CHURG-STRAUSS SYNDROME

CSS (see also Chapter 59) is included in the group of small-vessel vasculitides and is defined as an eosinophil-rich and granulomatous inflammation involving the respiratory tract and necrotizing vasculitis affecting small to medium-sized vessels; it is associated with asthma and eosinophilia. All of the pathologic lesions—initially described from autopsied cases—are seldom found in a single biopsy specimen, and abnormalities often are limited to an eosinophilic perivascular infiltration of the tissues characteristic of the early (prevasculitic) phase of the disease. CSS is one of the pulmonary vasculitides associated with antineutrophil cytoplasmic antibodies (ANCA), together with granulomatosis with polyangiitis (Wegener) and microscopic polyangiitis, with ANCA found only in about 40% of cases of CSS.

CSS is a very rare disorder, occurring especially in the fourth and fifth decades of life, with no gender predominance. About one third of the patients have evidence of allergy, mostly perennial allergies to dust mites. The natural history of CSS usually incorporates three phases: rhinosinusitis and asthma, blood and tissue eosinophilia, and eventual emergence of systemic vasculitis. Eosinophilic rhinitis, present in three fourths of the cases, often is accompanied by relapsing paranasal sinusitis and nasal polyps; however, septal nasal perforation or saddle nose deformity is rare. Asthma becomes progressively cortico-dependent, usually preceding the onset of vasculitis by 3 to 9 years (however, these conditions may be contemporary). The severity of asthma may worsen before onset of the vasculitis, with attenuation thereafter, and further improvement on remission of the vasculitis.

The chest radiograph may remain normal in appearance throughout the course of the disease. Lung opacities, present in more than half of patients, correspond to eosinophilic pneumonia and consist mainly of ill-defined pulmonary infiltrates, sometimes migratory and transient. Pleural eosinophilic exudate, present in approximately one fourth of patients, must be distinguished from the transudate associated with cardiac failure resulting from cardiac eosinophilic involvement with severe cardiomyopathy. HRCT mainly shows areas of ground glass attenuation or air space consolidation, with peripheral predominance or random distribution (**Figure 49-5**). Centrilobular nodules, bronchial wall thickening or dilatation, interlobular septal thickening, and hilar or mediastinal lymphadenopathy are less common. These abnormalities are nonspecific and resemble those seen in ICEP, although the subpleural distribution of consolidation is less pronounced, centrilobular nodules within ground glass opacities are more frequent, and traction bronchiectases are less frequent in CSS than in ICEP. Pulmonary cavitary lesions are exceptional.

Blood eosinophilia, with cell counts greater than 1500 and often 5000/µL, usually parallels disease activity. It disappears

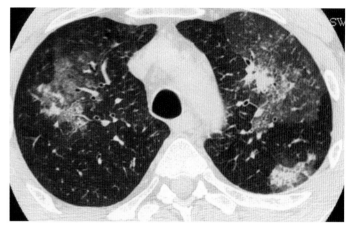

Figure 49-5 Computed tomography scan of the thorax showing ground glass opacity and consolidation with central predominance in a patient with Churg-Strauss syndrome.

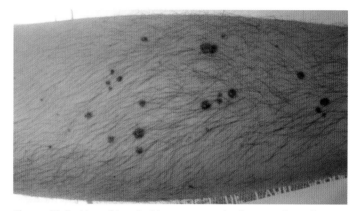

Figure 49-6 Vasculitic palpable purpura on the forearm of a patient with Churg-Strauss syndrome.

with dramatic rapidity after the initiation of corticosteroid treatment. Eosinophilia also is evident on the BAL fluid differential cell count, which may be more than 60%, and sometimes in the pleural fluid. IgE levels usually are markedly increased. High levels of urinary EDN may represent an indicator of disease activity.

Extrapulmonary manifestations of CSS usually include asthenia, weight loss, fever, arthralgias, and/or myalgias. Neurologic involvement typically consists of mononeuritis multiplex or asymmetric polyneuropathy. Cardiac involvement manifesting as eosinophilic myocarditis (or, more rarely, coronary arteritis) often is of insidious onset and asymptomatic and may lead to dilated cardiomyopathy, although marked clinical improvement may follow corticosteroid treatment. Pericardial effusion is common, but tamponade is rare. Endomyocardial fibrosis is rare, in contrast with the idiopathic hypereosinophilic syndrome. Myocardial involvement is a common finding in systematic studies by echocardiography or magnetic resonance imaging (MRI), and its frequency may have been heretofore underestimated. Digestive tract involvement usually manifests as isolated abdominal pain or diarrhea, but intestinal vasculitis (with ulcerations, perforations, or hemorrhage) and cholecystitis may occur. Cutaneous lesions, seen in approximately half of the patients, consist mainly of palpable purpura (**Figure 49-6**) on the extremities, subcutaneous nodules, erythematous rashes, and urticaria. Renal involvement, present in a fourth of the cases, usually is mild.

Table 49-1 **Clinical Phenotypes of Churg-Strauss Syndrome**

Feature	Vasculitic Phenotype	Tissue Disease Phenotype
Respective frequency	~40%	~60%
ANCA	Present (mostly p-ANCA with antimyeloperoxidase specificity)	Absent
Predominant clinical and histopathologic features	Glomerular renal disease Peripheral neuropathy Purpura Biopsy-proven vasculitis	Cardiac involvement (eosinophilic myocarditis) Eosinophilic pneumonia Fever

ANCA, antineutrophil cytoplasmic antibodies; *p-ANCA*, perinuclear ANCA.

Currently used diagnostic criteria for CSS are shown in **Box 49-7**. ANCA also may be considered a major diagnostic criterion when present. Conversely, absence of ANCA does not exclude the diagnosis of CSS. A histopathologic diagnosis of CSS may be obtained by examination of skin, nerve, or muscle biopsy specimens. Lung biopsy and transbronchial biopsy are not helpful. The diagnosis of CSS may be difficult, especially at an early stage, with mild or limited manifestations corresponding to "formes frustes" of CSS. These may consist of cases in which the disease has been partly controlled by corticosteroids given for asthma.

ANCA are found in only approximately 40% of patients and consist mainly of perinuclear ANCA (p-ANCA), with a specificity for myeloperoxidase on ELISA, whereas other ANCA (especially cytoplasmic ANCA [c-ANCA] with proteinase-3 specificity) are very rare in CSS. Of interest, two phenotypes of CSS can be distinguished on the basis of these antibodies (Table 49-1): Patients with ANCA have a vasculitic phenotype (with more frequent vasculitis on biopsy, renal involvement, peripheral neuropathy, and purpura), whereas patients without ANCA have more frequent cardiac and pulmonary involvement. Therefore, patients with CSS seen in respiratory medicine departments or chest clinics are at high risk for cardiac involvement, which can be subclinical (with especially no chest pain) and should be systematically evaluated with measurement of serum troponin, electrocardiogram, echocardiography, and possibly MRI of the heart, which can identify impaired cardiac function and myocardial involvement. Serum measurement of eotaxin-3 and of CCL17/thymus and activation–related chemokine may reflect disease activity and merits further study as a potential biomarker of disease monitoring.

A role for triggering or adjuvant factors such as vaccines or desensitization in the development of CSS has been postulated. Drug-induced eosinophilic vasculitis with pulmonary involvement has been occasionally reported. The possible responsibility of leukotriene-receptor antagonists in the development of CSS is still debated, and these agents must be avoided in patients with asthma and eosinophilia or with extrapulmonary manifestations compatible with smoldering CSS.

Corticosteroids are the mainstay of treatment of CSS, starting with 1 mg/kg per day of prednisone, with progressive tapering over several months. Initial intravenous pulses of methylprednisolone (15 mg/kg/day for 1 to 3 days) are useful in the most severe cases. Approximately half of the patients without poor prognostic factors at onset achieve complete remission with corticosteroid treatment alone and do not experience relapse. Relapses of CSS must be distinguished from relapse or persistence of difficult asthma (generally accompanied by less than 500/µL blood eosinophils). Long-term monitoring of lung function is warranted, because a proportion of patients develop fixed airflow obstruction.

Intravenous pulses of cyclophosphamide (usually up to six pulses) in addition to corticosteroids are indicated in patients with poor prognostic factors at onset (proteinuria with greater than 1 g/day protein excretion; renal insufficiency with serum creatinine greater than 15.8 mg/L; gastrointestinal tract involvement; cardiomyopathy; central nervous system involvement). Immunosuppressive treatment using oral azathioprine also is considered in patients who relapse despite more than 20 mg of prednisone daily. Rituximab, intravenous high-dose immunoglobulins, cyclosporine, and subcutaneous interferon-α have been of recognized benefit in patients with treatment-refractory CSS. The anti-IgE agent omalizumab has been used successfully to treat persistent asthma in patients with CSS; it does not control the systemic disease, however, so careful clinical monitoring is warranted. The prognosis for CSS has improved considerably over the years, with more than 90% of patients alive at 5 years according to current data.

IDIOPATHIC HYPEREOSINOPHILIC SYNDROMES

The historical definition of the idiopathic hypereosinophilic syndromes (HESs) included a persistent eosinophilia with counts greater than 1500/µL for longer than 6 months, a lack of evidence for a known cause of eosinophilia, and presumptive signs and symptoms of organ involvement. Recent studies have demonstrated that HESs fitting this definition may result especially from clonal proliferation of lymphocytes or of the eosinophil cell lineage itself.

HES, as described in older series, was much more common in men than in women (9:1), with an age at onset between 20 and 50 years. The typical clinical presentation includes insidious onset of weakness, fatigue, cough, and dyspnea, with a mean eosinophil count at presentation of up to 20,000/µL. Nonrespiratory manifestations of the HESs mainly target the skin, heart, and nervous system.

Cardiac involvement, present in 60% of patients, manifests mainly as characteristic endomyocardial fibrosis, often associated with development of intracavitary thrombi along the endocardium, and clinically associated with restrictive cardiomyopathy. Echocardiography shows mural thrombus, ventricular apical obliteration, and involvement of the posterior mitral leaflet.

Lung involvement, present in up to 40% of patients, is nonspecific. Cough may be the predominant feature. Asthma, pleural effusion, and pulmonary opacities on the chest CT scan (mostly patchy ground glass attenuation, consolidation, and small nodules) have been reported, and this aspect of HES must be distinguished from pleural effusion secondary to cardiac failure.

The *lymphocytic* variant of HES, which may account for approximately 30% of the cases, is a T cell disorder resulting from the production of chemokines (especially IL-5) by clonal T_H2 lymphocytes bearing an aberrant antigenic surface phenotype (such as $CD3^-CD4^+$). IgE level typically is elevated as a consequence of IL-4 and IL-13 production by T_H2 lymphocytes. Most patients initially have cutaneous papules or urticarial plaques infiltrated by lymphocytes and eosinophils. Diagnosis is obtained by lymphocyte phenotyping and analysis of the rearrangement of the T cell receptor genes in specialized laboratories.

The *myeloproliferative* variant of HES, accounting for approximately 20% of cases, is distinguished on the basis of clinical and biologic features in common with those of chronic myeloproliferative syndromes, including hepatomegaly, splenomegaly, anemia, thrombocythemia, increased serum vitamin B_{12} and leukocyte alkaline phosphatase, and circulating leukocyte precursors. Mucosal ulcerations may be prominent. Severe cardiac manifestations are frequent and may be resistant to corticosteroid treatment. Myeloproliferative HES is attributed to a constitutively activated tyrosine kinase fusion protein (Fip1L1-PDGFRα) due to an interstitial chromosomal deletion in 4q12. Imatinib, a tyrosine kinase inhibitor used to treat chronic myelogenous leukemia, proved to be efficacious in patients with the myeloproliferative variant of HES.

Only approximately half of the patients with HES respond to corticosteroid treatment. Other treatments include chemotherapeutic agents (hydroxyurea, vincristine, etoposide), cyclosporine, interferon-α (particularly for the myeloproliferative variant), and the anti–IL-5 antibody mepolizumab. Imatinib has become the major drug used in patients with the myeloproliferative variant of HES, especially when the FipL1-PDGFRα fusion protein is present. The prognosis with HES has improved markedly, with approximately 70% survival at 1 year.

A large proportion of affected patients have idiopathic HES—no cause can be found despite exhaustive analysis, with neither clonal proliferation of lymphocytes nor fusion protein activity detected. Improvement may be obtained with oral corticosteroids or imatinib. Respiratory manifestations in these patients have not been properly studied but seem to be of generally mild severity.

CONTROVERSIES AND PITFALLS

- The diagnosis of parasitic diseases in patients with eosinophilic pneumonia may be difficult and requires appropriate serologic tests and repeated search for parasites in the feces. Such diseases must be considered in any patient who lived in or visited an endemic area.
- Eosinophilic pneumonia has been reported in association with a variety of drugs, but causality has been confidently established for fewer than 20 specific agents.
- The dose and duration of treatment of ICEP with corticosteroids have not been established. Disease control must be balanced with treatment side effects.
- "Idiopathic" acute eosinophilic pneumonia may be misdiagnosed as severe infectious pneumonia.
- Established diagnostic criteria for CSS currently are lacking. ANCA are found in about 40% of patients, and true vasculitis is a feature in only a minority of cases.
- Asthma is a common denominator in most patients with ICEP and CSS.
- The respiratory manifestations of the lymphocytic and myeloid variants of the HESs have not been described in detail.

SUGGESTED READINGS

Agarwal R: Allergic bronchopulmonary aspergillosis, *Chest* 135:805–826, 2009.

Cottin V, Khouatra C, Dubost R, et al: Persistent airflow obstruction in asthma of patients with Churg-Strauss syndrome and long-term follow-up, *Allergy* 64:589–595, 2009.

Dennert RM, van Paassen P, Schalla S, et al: Cardiac involvement in Churg-Strauss syndrome, *Arthritis Rheum* 62:627–634, 2010.

Kunst H, Mack D, Kon OM, et al: Parasitic infections of the lung: a guide for the respiratory physician, *Thorax* 66:528–536, 2011.

Marchand E, Cordier JF: Idiopathic chronic eosinophilic pneumonia, *Orphanet J Rare Dis* 1:11, 2006.

Marchand E, Etienne-Mastroïanni B, Chanez P, et al: Groupe d'Etudes et de Recherche sur les Maladies Orphelines Pulmonaires: Idiopathic chronic eosinophilic pneumonia and asthma: how do they influence each other? *Eur Respir J* 22:8–13, 2003.

Nair P, Pizzichini MM, Kjarsgaard M, et al: Mepolizumab for prednisone-dependent asthma with sputum eosinophilia, *N Engl J Med* 360:985–993, 2009.

Pagnoux C, Guilpain P, Guillevin L: Churg-Strauss syndrome, *Curr Opin Rheumatol* 19:25–32, 2009.

Patterson K, Strek ME: Allergic bronchopulmonary aspergillosis, *Proc Am Thorac Soc* 7:237–244, 2010.

Sablé-Fourtassou R, Cohen P, Mahr A, et al: Antineutrophil cytoplasmic antibodies and the Churg-Strauss syndrome, *Ann Intern Med* 143:632–638, 2005.

Walsh ER, August A: Eosinophils and allergic airway disease: there is more to the story, *Trends Immunol* 31:39–44, 2010.

Chapter **50**

Organizing Pneumonia

Vincent Cottin • Jean-François Cordier

DEFINITION

Organizing pneumonia (OP) is a histopathologic diagnosis defined by a well-recognized pattern of changes underlying a characteristic clinical-pathologic entity. OP may occur in the absence of etiologic context, in which case it is known as *cryptogenic organizing pneumonia* (COP), or in association with a known causative agent or inflammatory disorder such as connective tissue disease, where it is called *secondary organizing pneumonia*.

Initially described as the specific histopathologic pattern resulting from organization of an inflammatory exudate in the lumen of alveoli of unresolved pneumonia, OP is characterized by intraalveolar buds of granulation tissue with fibroblasts and myofibroblasts intermixed with loose connective matrix (**Figure 50-1**). Similar lesions may be present within the lumen of the bronchioles—hence the formerly synonymous term *bronchiolitis obliterans with organizing pneumonia* ("BOOP"). The latter designation has been abandoned, however, because OP (rather than bronchiolitis) is clearly the major lesion, and furthermore, use of the older term was a potential source of confusion between this entity and bronchiolitis with airflow obstruction occurring, for example, after lung or hematopoietic stem cell transplantation. Although the condition is not strictly interstitial, COP is included in the American Thoracic Society/European Respiratory Society international consensus classification of the idiopathic interstitial pneumonias, because of its idiopathic nature and occasional similarities with interstitial pneumonias.

PATHOGENESIS

OP is a unique condition characterized by intraalveolar accumulation of intermixed fibroblasts and connective matrix, especially collagen, that is reversible with corticosteroids, in contrast with other presentations of pulmonary fibrosis and especially that of usual interstitial pneumonia or idiopathic pulmonary fibrosis.

The first event of the sequence leading to the formation of intraalveolar buds is alveolar epithelial injury with necrosis of pneumocytes (especially type I) (**Figure 50-2**). The epithelial basal laminae are denuded and injured, resulting in formation of gaps. Capillary endothelial injury often is associated. The consequence of alveolar injury is flooding of the alveolar lumen by plasma proteins (permeability edema), including coagulation factors. The balance between coagulation and fibrinolysis is clearly tipped in favor of coagulation (especially because of decreased fibrinolysis), leading to accumulation of fibrin deposits that are soon populated by migratory inflammatory cells and fibroblasts.

Fibroblasts differentiate into myofibroblasts that organize and represent the predominant cell of fibroinflammatory buds. Inflammatory cells and fibrin are progressively replaced by aggregated fibroblasts/myofibroblasts intermixed with a loose connective matrix tissue rich in collagen (especially collagen III) and fibronectin. This process, resembling that of cutaneous wound healing, is similarly reversible, without significant sequelae. It is likely that the relative preservation of the alveolar basal laminae is crucial in determining the reversibility of the lesions. Although COP and secondary OP appear very similar, the microvascular density and the density of collagen fibers within intraalveolar air spaces may be higher in secondary OP than in COP.

Mouse models of intraluminal inflammation have been developed using reovirus infection to induce the histopathologic changes. Lesions similar to OP have been obtained by intranasal inoculation of moderate doses of virus only in a susceptible strain of mice (CBA/J), suggesting that genetic background may contribute to pathogenesis of the condition in mice. Alveolar macrophages and T lymphocytes were implicated in the disease process. Of interest, diffuse alveolar damage with hyaline membrane formation was obtained with the same animal model when higher doses of virus were used. These experimental studies suggest that the intensity of the initial epithelial injury and yet undetermined factors inherent to the host may influence the evolution to either OP or diffuse alveolar damage. Other animal models of OP have been developed in rats inoculated with bacteria and in pigs infected with a circovirus.

The cellular origin of fibroblasts that populate the distal air spaces is unclear. The respective contribution of proliferating lung fibroblasts, fibrocytes or bone marrow–derived fibroblasts, and epithelial-mesenchymal transition has not been evaluated in OP. The mechanism by which corticosteroids facilitate the rapid resolution of OP also is unclear. Several studies have highlighted some characteristics that distinguish the reversible fibrotic budding characteristic of OP from the uncontrolled process of accumulation of fibroblastic foci and collagen deposition seen in usual interstitial pneumonia, including a distinct pattern of expression of metalloproteases, the increased vascularity of fibrotic buds, and a lower apoptotic activity in granulation tissue. In addition, the expression of tumor necrosis factor-α receptor-1 and Fas by alveolar macrophages is higher in patients with OP than in control subjects or patients with idiopathic pulmonary fibrosis. Overall, OP may be considered as a model of normal wound repair, contrasted with the uncontrolled aberrant repair and fibrosing process observed in usual interstitial pneumonia of idiopathic pulmonary fibrosis.

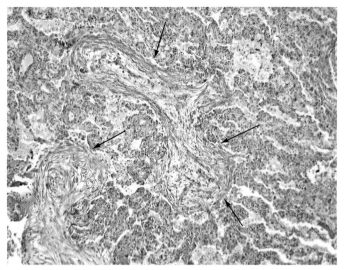

Figure 50-1 Buds of granulation tissue (*arrows*) in the lumen of alveoli. (*Courtesy F. Thivolet-Béjui, Lyon.*)

CLINICAL AND IMAGING FEATURES

CRYPTOGENIC ORGANIZING PNEUMONIA

Clinical Features

The mean age at onset of COP is approximately 50 to 60 years, with no gender predilection. It is more common in nonsmokers or former smokers. The initial manifestations are fever, cough, malaise, anorexia, and progressive weight loss, with a subacute onset over a few weeks. The median duration of the clinical syndrome is less than 3 months. Dyspnea usually is mild. Hemoptysis, chest pain, and severe dyspnea are rare. Crackles may be heard at pulmonary auscultation over involved areas, with clinical features of consolidation in rare instances. Finger clubbing is absent. In many patients, the diagnosis is considered after they have received antibiotics for presumed infectious pneumonia without improvement.

Lung function tests in COP show a mild to moderate restrictive ventilatory pattern and may occasionally yield normal results. The carbon monoxide transfer factor is reduced in most

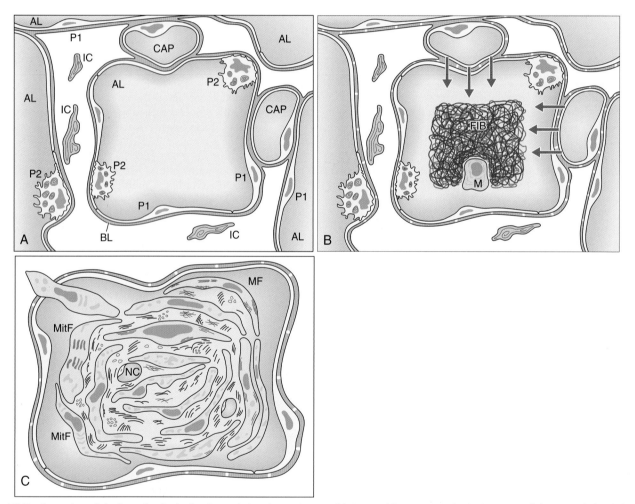

Figure 50-2 Formation of the intraalveolar buds of granulation tissue characterizing organizing pneumonia. **A,** Structure of the normal alveolar space. *AL,* alveolar lumen; *BL,* basal laminae; *CAP,* capillaries; *IC,* interstitial cells; *P1,* type 1 pneumocytes; *P2,* type 2 pneumocytes. **B,** Alveolar injury with alteration and necrosis of alveolar epithelial cells (especially type 1 pneumocytes), denudation of basal laminae with formation of gaps, and leaking of plasma proteins, especially coagulation factors (*arrows*) with formation of fibrin (*FIB*) within the alveolar lumen. Some inflammatory cells and macrophages (*M*) are present. **C,** The intraluminal alveolar fibrin network has been colonized by mitotic fibroblasts (*MitF*), with some acquiring a myofibroblast (*MF*) phenotype characterized by presence of myofilaments beneath the cytoplasmic membrane. Fibroblasts and myofibroblasts have a developed rough endoplasmic reticulum and produce a loose connective matrix (composed of collagen types I and III, fibronectin, and proteoglycans) interspersed between the cells. Neoformed capillaries (*NC*) are present within this intraalveolar bud of granulation tissue, resembling those characteristic of the wound healing process.

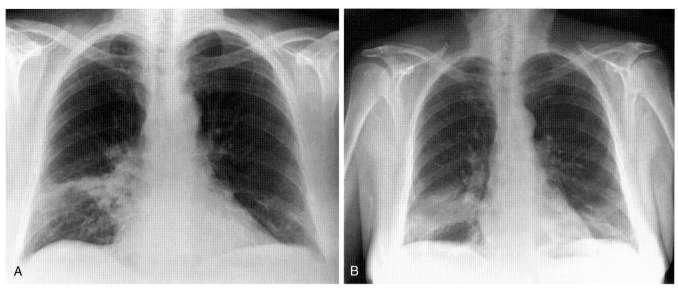

Figure 50-3 Chest radiographs showing the typical imaging pattern in cryptogenic organizing pneumonia. **A,** Patchy alveolar opacity. **B,** Six days later, the distribution of the right lower lobe opacity has changed, with appearance of a new contralateral basal opacity.

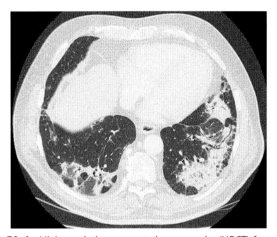

Figure 50-4 High-resolution computed tomography (HRCT) features of typical cryptogenic organizing pneumonia (COP). Patchy bilateral consolidation with peripheral predominance and air bronchogram, associated with ground glass opacities in the right lower lobe, are evident.

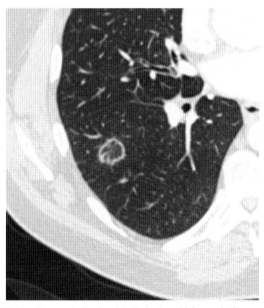

Figure 50-5 Reverse halo sign (atoll sign) on high-resolution computed tomography (HRCT) scan.

patients, whereas the carbon monoxide transfer coefficient (KCO) is within normal limits. Hypoxemia usually is mild. When present, severe hypoxemia may be associated with diffuse infiltrative opacities or right-to-left shunting in perfused areas of lung consolidation.

Blood tests often show moderate leukocytosis and increased C-reactive protein but no significant peripheral blood eosinophilia.

Imaging Features

The imaging features of COP may consist of a variety of high-resolution computed tomography (HRCT) findings, some of which are highly suggestive of the diagnosis. The most typical imaging pattern in COP consists of multiple patchy alveolar opacities (**Figures 50-3 and 50-4**). These usually are bilateral, with a subpleural distribution, and sometimes migratory (with attenuation or clearing in some areas and appearance of new opacities in others), ranging in density from ground glass to consolidation with air bronchogram, with no predominance in cranial versus caudal distribution. The size of the opacities may

vary, ranging from 1 to 2 cm to involvement of an entire lobe. Consolidation at imaging corresponds pathologically with intraalveolar buds of granulation tissue within the distal air spaces, whereas areas of ground glass opacity reflect the cell infiltration of alveolar wall by inflammatory cells, with some OP changes in the distal air spaces. This imaging pattern with multiple patchy alveolar opacities, especially those of a migratory nature, is so characteristic of typical COP that it should immediately suggest the diagnosis. The main other consideration in the differential diagnosis at this stage is idiopathic chronic eosinophilic pneumonia (in the latter, blood eosinophilia with cell counts usually greater than 1500/μL is present; conversely, nodules may be found more frequently in COP than in chronic eosinophilic pneumonia).

Patchy ground glass opacities frequently are observed, usually associated with consolidation. The reverse halo sign or atoll sign (**Figure 50-5**), consisting of a circular consolidation

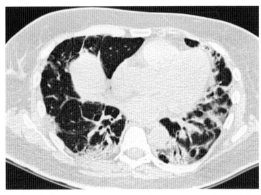

Figure 50-6 High-resolution computed tomography (HRCT) features of progressive organizing pneumonia (OP). The patient had idiopathic inflammatory myopathy. Reticular, hazy, perilobular opacities are evident in the lower lobes.

Box 50-1	**High-Resolution Computed Tomography Patterns in Organizing Pneumonia**

- Multiple patchy alveolar opacities (classic COP pattern)
- Focal pattern
- Nodular pattern
- Bronchocentric pattern
- Linear and bandlike pattern
- Perilobular pattern
- Reverse halo pattern
- Progressive fibrosis pattern

COP, cryptogenic organizing pneumonia.
Modified from King TE: Organizing pneumonia. In Schwarz MI, King TE, editors: *Interstitial lung disease*, ed 5, Shelton, Conn, People's Medical Publishing House, 2011, pp 981–984.

Box 50-2	**Mimics of Cryptogenic Organizing Pneumonia (COP) on Chest Imaging**

Multiple patchy alveolar opacities (classic COP pattern)
  Eosinophilic pneumonia (especially chronic idiopathic)
  Pneumonic-type invasive mucinous adenocarcinoma of the lung
  Primary pulmonary lymphoma (low-grade B cell lymphoma of mucosa-associated lymphoid tissue [MALT])
  Others: infectious pneumonia, tuberculosis or nontuberculous mycobacterial infection, granulomatosis with polyangiitis (Wegener granulomatosis), diffuse alveolar hemorrhage, multiple-infarct lesions, aspiration pneumonia
Solitary focal nodule or mass (focal pattern)
  Lung carcinoma
  Round pneumonia or abscess
  Inflammatory pseudotumors
  Others: all causes of coin lesions or masses
Diffuse infiltrative opacities (progressive or fibrosis pattern)
  Idiopathic interstitial pneumonias, especially nonspecific interstitial pneumonia and idiopathic pulmonary fibrosis (especially acute exacerbation)
  Interstitial pneumonias overlapping with organizing pneumonia
  Others: all causes of infiltrative opacities, especially of infectious or neoplastic origin

pattern (corresponding histopathologically to organizing pneumonia in the distal air spaces) surrounding an area of ground glass opacities (corresponding to alveolar wall inflammation), also is highly suggestive of the diagnosis, although not specific.

Another imaging pattern in COP is a solitary focal nodule or mass-like area of consolidation that may mimic lung carcinoma especially when associated with hypermetabolism on positron emission tomography. It commonly is located in the upper lobes and usually is asymptomatic. An air bronchogram may be present. Diagnosis often is obtained by surgical resection of the lesion in the suspicion of cancer. Solitary focal COP likely represents nonresolving infectious pneumonia in a number of cases.

The infiltrative (or progressive fibrotic) pattern of OP associates interstitial opacities, with small superimposed alveolar opacities on HRCT (with possible perilobular pattern consisting of bowed or polygonal opacities with poorly defined margins bordering the interlobular septa). Honeycombing is not present. Infiltrative or progressive COP may overlap on both histopathologic and imaging studies with idiopathic nonspecific interstitial pneumonia (NSIP), with uniform alveolar and interstitial cellular inflammation (with more or less fibrosis), with the possible presence of foci of organizing pneumonia. Such imaging presentation of OP seems to be particularly frequent in patients with idiopathic inflammatory myopathy (**Figure 50-6**).

Several less common imaging presentations of COP have been occasionally reported, including multiple nodules, cavitary opacities, perilobular opacities, centrilobular or peribronchovascular ill-defined nodules, bronchocentric areas of consolidation, and linear subpleural bands (**Box 50-1**). A few mediastinal lymphadenopathies are not rare in COP. Pleural effusion is uncommon.

Whereas mimics of COP with typical imaging features are few, mimics of COP presenting as nodules, masses, or infiltrative lung diseases are many (**Box 50-2**).

SECONDARY ORGANIZING PNEUMONIA

Most cases of OP occur as a reaction pattern and are considered to represent secondary OP, resulting from a determined cause, often infectious or drug-associated, or occurring in the context of systemic disorders (e.g., connective tissue disease) or other specific conditions. The clinical, laboratory, and imaging features and outcome of secondary OP generally parallel those of COP, with minor differences reported that probably reflect the nature of the underlying disease (e.g., higher lymphocyte percentage on a differential bronchoalveolar lavage [BAL] fluid cell count). A careful etiologic investigation is thus necessary in any patient presenting with OP without evident cause, and especially with relapsing OP. In most cases of secondary OP, corticosteroid treatment is effective.

Secondary Organizing Pneumonia of Known Cause

A histopathologic diagnosis of OP prompts a search for a number of potential underlying causes, including a variety of infectious agents (bacteria, viruses, fungi, parasites) (**Box 50-3**). Diagnosis of the infection (which is no longer active at the time of OP) may be difficult and is based on the clinical history, a rise in antibody titers against the infectious agent, or occasionally direct identification of the infectious agent by use of specific stains and histopathologic analysis of the lung specimens.

Several drugs have been reported to cause OP (**Box 50-4**). All drugs taken in the weeks or months preceding onset of symptoms must be systematically recorded. Any drug suspected to be a cause of OP should be withdrawn if possible

Box 50-3 Infectious Agents Associated With Organizing Pneumonia

Bacteria
Chlamydia pneumoniae
Coxiella burnetii
Legionella pneumophila
Mycoplasma pneumoniae
Nocardia asteroides
Staphylococcus aureus
Streptococcus pneumoniae
Serratia marcescens
Pseudomonas aeruginosa

Viruses
Human immunodeficiency virus
Influenza virus
Parainfluenza virus
Herpesvirus
Hepatitis C virus

Parasites
Plasmodium vivax

Fungi
Cryptococcus neoformans
Penicillium janthinellum
Pneumocystis jiroveci (in AIDS)

Box 50-4 Drugs Commonly Reported as Etiologic Agents of Organizing Pneumonia

5-Aminosalicylic acid	Minocycline
Amiodarone	Nilutamide
Amphotericin B	Nitrofurantoin
Beta blockers	Penicillamine
Bleomycin	Phenytoin
Busulfan	Statins
Carbamazepine	Rituximab
Dihydroergocryptine	Sirolimus
Everolimus	Sulfasalazine
Interferon-α	Tacrolimus
Interferon-β	Thalidomide
Mesalazine	Trastuzumab
Methotrexate	

Box 50-5 Miscellaneous Causes and Clinical Settings Associated With Organizing Pneumonia

Identified Causes
Infections (see Box 50-3)
Drugs (see Box 50-4)
Distal to airway obstruction
Fumes and toxic exposures (e.g., aerosolized textile dye Acramin FWN, mustard gas)

Clinical Settings
Occult aspiration pneumonia
Connective tissue disease
Primary biliary cirrhosis
Inflammatory bowel diseases (ulcerative colitis, Crohn disease)
Transplantation (lung, liver), bone marrow graft
Hematologic malignancies (leukemias: myeloblastic, lymphoblastic, myelomonocytic, T cell; Hodgkin disease)
Cancers and thoracic radiotherapy, especially for breast cancer
Others: common variable immune deficiency, Sweet syndrome, polymyalgia rheumatica, Behçet disease, thyroid diseases, vasculitis, sarcoidosis

Radiation therapy to the breast after resection for cancer may precipitate the development of OP, with an incidence of approximately 2.5% in treated women and a mean delay of approximately 3 to 6 months after the completion of irradiation. In contrast with radiation pneumonitis, the alveolar opacities of OP (often migratory) also may appear in nonirradiated areas of the lungs. The opacities respond well to corticosteroid treatment, but relapses are common when corticosteroids are reduced or stopped. Of interest, radiation therapy to the breast is followed by bilateral lymphocytic alveolitis seen on examination of BAL fluid, with development of OP in only a minority of patients. This observation suggests that a "second trigger" and/or genetic susceptibility may be necessary for OP to occur, in addition to radiation-primed lymphocytic alveolitis.

Secondary Organizing Pneumonia Occurring Within a Specific Context

OP occurs mainly in dermatomyositis or polymyositis and rheumatoid arthritis (it is less common in systemic lupus and Sjögren syndrome and is unusual in systemic sclerosis). Overlapping features of OP and nonspecific interstitial pneumonia seem particularly frequent in patients with dermatomyositis or polymyositis. OP may precede the development of the connective tissue disease or occur concomitantly, although it is seen more frequently during the course of the disease.

Multiple causes of and clinical settings for secondary OP have been reported, a nonexhaustive listing of which is provided in **Box 50-5**.

DIAGNOSIS

A thorascopic lung biopsy is recommended for a definitive histopathologic diagnosis of OP, also ruling out other conditions that may mimic OP.

When nonspecific clinical manifestations associated with typical imaging features suggest the diagnosis of COP, fiberoptic bronchoscopy (which excludes any bronchial obstruction) with BAL is first necessary, and transbronchial biopsy

(and rechallenge should be avoided). The diagnosis of drug-induced OP may be difficult, however, because it has no specific clinical-radiologic presentation.

A recent study surprisingly identified aspiration of food and of other particulate matter as a frequent feature in patients with OP, suggesting that aspiration pneumonia may be a more frequent cause of OP than was previously suspected. Aspiration was suspected on clinical grounds in less than 10% of cases; however, predisposing factors for aspiration frequently were identified (e.g., esophageal or gastric causes, drug use, neurologic conditions). The presence of multinucleate giant cells, acute bronchopneumonia or bronchiolitis, and/or suppurative granulomas on a background of OP changes should therefore direct the pathologist to look for foreign material and particulate matter on the lung biopsy specimen, and should prompt the clinician to evaluate for possible aspiration.

may be contributive. The BAL fluid differential cell count in COP often shows a mixed pattern with increased levels of lymphocytes (20% to 40%), neutrophils (approximately 10%), and eosinophils (5%); some mast cells and plasma cells may be present. The transbronchial lung biopsy specimens may show typical buds of granulation tissue within alveoli. Infectious agents must be systematically searched for on BAL fluid preparations (and on transbronchial biopsy specimens by specific staining, if performed). The combination of a typical clinical-radiologic pattern and a mixed pattern on BAL fluid differential cell count is considered highly suggestive of OP (and of COP in the appropriate clinical context). A decreased ratio of CD4+ to CD8+ lymphocytes in BAL has been reported in COP.

OP is a nonspecific consequence of interstitial inflammation that may be present as an accessory finding in many disorders, including nonspecific interstitial pneumonia, organizing diffuse alveolar damage, aspiration pneumonia, vasculitides, distal obstruction of the airways, and occult aspiration pneumonia. Some histopathologic overlap may exist with chronic eosinophilic pneumonia or the OP-like variant of granulomatous polyangiitis (Wegener granulomatosis). Additional findings suggestive of another diagnosis in secondary OP include necrosis or microabscesses (seen in infectious processes and necrotizing vasculitis) and organic debris (as in occult aspiration pneumonia).

With transbronchial biopsy, the small size of specimens obtained by this method does not allow exclusion of other histopathologic patterns, so the findings should therefore be considered diagnostic of OP only in patients with a typical clinical-imaging profile. The sensitivity and specificity of transbronchial biopsy for the diagnosis of OP have not been rigorously evaluated. Core needle biopsy generally is safe and may be appropriate in a minority of patients with suspected OP, especially with focal consolidation at imaging. Videothoracoscopic lung biopsy remains the most appropriate procedure to obtain specimens of sufficient size both to make a definitive diagnosis of OP and to exclude other processes. When performed, the biopsy should be done before corticosteroids are initiated and should be planned in a preoperative discussion between the surgeon and the physician or a radiologist. Microbiologic analysis also may be performed on the lung specimen.

A reasonable alternative to lung biopsy is to proceed with appropriate management, to include presumptive treatment as indicated, in the absence of confirmation of the histopathologic pattern of OP. Although this approach commonly is used in clinical practice, it carries the risk of misdiagnosing alternative conditions that may mimic OP, including eosinophilic pneumonia, low-grade primary pulmonary lymphoma, and bronchioloalveolar carcinoma (see Box 50-2). Only patients in whom typical findings on imaging studies (e.g., multiple patchy consolidation) are associated with compatible clinical and BAL features should be treated without biopsy; particular attention must be paid to any clue to an alternative diagnosis (e.g., peripheral blood and/or BAL fluid eosinophilia, suggestive microbiologic findings in BAL fluid). When pathologic investigation is not available or consists of only transbronchial biopsy, the diagnosis should be reconsidered whenever the observed clinical response is unusual (especially in case of incomplete response to corticosteroids or relapse despite more than 20 mg/day of oral prednisone).

As in other conditions among the group of idiopathic interstitial pneumonias, the "gold standard" for diagnosis of OP is now the clinical-radiologic-pathologic approach, which effectively ensures that imaging and clinical data, as well as pathology data when available, are consistent with and specific for this entity. Although interobserver agreement for a clinically based diagnosis usually is fair to good, the multidisciplinary approach is particularly useful in cases with histopathologic features overlapping with those of eosinophilic pneumonia, nonspecific interstitial pneumonia, or diffuse alveolar damage. The clinical assessment must include a careful history and evaluation for the presence of comorbid diseases such as connective tissue disease (including formes frustes of connective tissue disease or undifferentiated connective tissue disease), cancer, thoracic radiotherapy for breast cancer, exposure to drugs, inflammatory bowel disease, aspiration, or less common conditions such as common variable immune deficiency (see Box 50-5). A final diagnosis of COP can be made only after all available data including findings on etiologic investigations have been reviewed in a dynamic process requiring close communication among the clinician, the radiologist, and the pathologist.

TREATMENT OF CRYPTOGENIC ORGANIZING PNEUMONIA

Corticosteroid treatment is standard therapy for COP and results in rapid clinical and imaging improvement in typical cases. With institution of therapy, consolidation evolves to ground glass opacities and reticulation and eventually regresses completely within a month; the less frequent linear or reticular opacities may not resolve. The optimal doses and duration of treatment have not been established, and treatment should aim at the best balance between disease control and side effects. We start with prednisone, 0.75 mg/kg per day for 4 weeks, and then continue with progressively decreasing doses for a total duration of treatment of 24 weeks (**Table 50-1**). This regimen limits intense and prolonged corticosteroid treatment with ensuing risk of iatrogenic complications. Other treatment protocols with slower tapering of dosage have been proposed. Parenteral corticosteroid therapy at higher doses often is used as the initial treatment in patients with the progressive or fibrotic variant of COP. Cyclophosphamide or azathioprine may be used in patients whose clinical condition deteriorates despite corticosteroid therapy. Of note, spontaneous improvement has been reported in some cases of COP. Macrolides have been suggested

Table 50-1 Proposed Therapeutic Regimen for Typical Cryptogenic Organizing Pneumonia

Step	Duration	Prednisone Dosage
Treatment of Initial Episode		
1	4 weeks	0.75 mg/kg/d
2	4 weeks	0.5 mg/kg/d
3	4 weeks	20 mg/d
4	6 weeks	10 mg/d
5	6 weeks	5 mg/d
Treatment of Relapse		
1	12 weeks	20 mg/d
2	6 weeks	10 mg/d
3	6 weeks	5 mg/d

for their antiinflammatory properties as an alternative option in patients who are intolerant to corticosteroids or who experience frequent relapses; however, the benefit initially observed in case reports is not confirmed with empirical routine use of these drugs. Secondary OP requires treatment of the underlying condition (connective tissue disease, infection) or withdrawal of the causative drug or exposure. Focal COP does not require corticosteroid therapy after surgical resection (performed for suspected lung cancer).

Most cases of typical COP with alveolar consolidation have a rapid and sometimes dramatic improvement with initiation of corticosteroid therapy, but a minority of patients will have persistent disease, especially those with reticulation on HRCT. Relapses are common (occurring in up to 60% of cases) on decreasing or after stopping treatment and may be treated with prednisone in doses of 20 mg per day given for 2 weeks and then progressively decreased. Relapses of the disease should prompt a search for a persisting cause of OP, especially drug intake. Relapses occurring with daily doses of more than 15 to 30 mg of prednisone (depending on body weight) should prompt extensive reappraisal of the diagnosis and further clinical-radiologic-pathologic consultation, especially when a large sample is not available for histopathologic analysis. The overall prognosis with typical COP is excellent.

SEVERE ORGANIZING PNEUMONIA

Cases of severe COP have been reported, with potentially severe respiratory failure necessitating mechanical ventilation. Such cases only occasionally are found to be associated with "pure OP" histopathologic lesions. They usually represent overlap of COP with one of the following disorders: acute respiratory distress syndrome (ARDS) with pathologic features of diffuse alveolar damage undergoing organization, acute fibrinous and organizing pneumonia (AFOP), or usual interstitial pneumonia exacerbation. In patients with acute exacerbation of idiopathic pulmonary fibrosis, features of diffuse alveolar damage and/or of OP are found in association with preexisting usual interstitial pneumonia. In such cases, the response to corticosteroids is not as favorable as in classic COP. Immunosuppressive agents (especially cyclophosphamide) usually are added to corticosteroids (often used at a higher dose, starting with 1 to 2 mg/kg per day of intravenous methylprednisolone), with variable outcome.

ACUTE FIBRINOUS AND ORGANIZING PNEUMONIA

AFOP is a histopathologic pattern first reported in patients with acute respiratory failure, with predominantly basal and bilateral areas of consolidation at imaging. It is characterized by abundant fibrin deposition within the alveolar air spaces, with hyperplasia of type II pneumocytes, associated organizing-type pneumonia, and absence of hyaline membranes (which constitute the hallmark of diffuse alveolar damage). AFOP currently is considered to be a histopathologic variant of OP that may be associated with more rapid progression of disease. As with OP, AFOP may be encountered in the context of various underlying conditions, including infection.

CONTROVERSIES AND PITFALLS

- OP is defined as a nonspecific histopathologic pattern found in many disorders, especially nonresolving infectious pneumonia. Assessing its clinical significance may be difficult. OP may be difficult to distinguish histopathologically from focal areas of organizing-type pneumonia seen as an accessory finding in another disorder (e.g., nonspecific interstitial pneumonia, organizing diffuse alveolar damage).
- In complex cases, overlap with other recognized histologic patterns may occur, especially with nonspecific interstitial pneumonia (especially secondary OP).
- What differentiates the pathogenic fibrosing process of OP (which resolves with corticosteroids) from that of uncontrolled idiopathic pulmonary fibrosis (resistant to steroids) is poorly understood.
- In cases with typical clinical, radiologic, and BAL findings, initiation of therapy without histopathologic confirmation may be considered; however, the diagnosis must be reconsidered whenever the outcome is unusual. The optimal dose and duration of corticosteroid therapy have not been established. Disease control must be balanced with treatment side effects.
- Whether AFOP represents a variant of OP or a distinct entity is unknown.

SUGGESTED READINGS

American Thoracic Society; European Respiratory Society: American Thoracic Society/European Respiratory Society International Multidisciplinary Consensus Classification of the Idiopathic Interstitial Pneumonias, *Am J Respir Crit Care Med* 165:277–304, 2002.

Beasley MB, Franks TJ, Galvin JR, et al: Acute fibrinous and organizing pneumonia: a histological pattern of lung injury and possible variant of diffuse alveolar damage, *Arch Pathol Lab Med* 126:1064–1070, 2002.

Colby TV: Pathologic aspects of bronchiolitis obliterans organizing pneumonia, *Chest* 102:38S–43S, 1992.

Cordier JF: Cryptogenic organising pneumonia, *Eur Respir J* 28:422–446, 2006.

Cordier JF, Loire R, Brune J: Idiopathic bronchiolitis obliterans organizing pneumonia. Definition of characteristic clinical profiles in a series of 16 patients, *Chest* 96:999–1004, 1989.

Costabel U, Teschler H, Guzman J: Bronchiolitis obliterans organizing pneumonia (BOOP): the cytological and immunocytological profile of bronchoalveolar lavage, *Eur Respir J* 5:791–797, 1992.

Crestani B, Valeyre D, Roden S, et al: Bronchiolitis obliterans organizing pneumonia syndrome primed by radiation therapy to the breast. The Groupe d'Etudes et de Recherche sur les Maladies "Orphelines" Pulmonaires (GERM"O"P), *Am J Respir Crit Care Med* 158:1929–1935, 1998.

Davison AG, Heard BE, McAllister WAC, Turner-Warwick ME: Cryptogenic organizing pneumonitis, *Q J Med* 52:382–394, 1983.

Drakopanagiotakis F, Paschalaki K, Abu-Hijleh M, et al: Cryptogenic and secondary organizing pneumonia, *Chest* 139:893–900, 2011.

Epler GR, Colby TV, McLoud TC, et al: Bronchiolitis obliterans organizing pneumonia, *N Engl J Med* 312:152–158, 1985.

King TE: Organizing pneumonia. In Schwarz MI, King TE, editors: *Interstitial lung disease*, ed 5, Conn, 2011, People's Medical Publishing House, pp 981–984.

Lazor R, Vandevenne A, Pelletier A, et al: Cryptogenic organizing pneumonia. Characteristics of relapses in a series of 48 patients. The Groupe d'Etudes et de Recherche sur les Maladies "Orphelines" Pulmonaires (GERM"O"P), *Am J Respir Crit Care Med* 162:571–577, 2000.

Lee JW, Lee KS, Lee HY, et al: Cryptogenic organizing pneumonia: serial high-resolution CT findings in 22 patients, *AJR Am J Roentgenol* 195:916–922, 2010.

Lohr RH, Boland BJ, Douglas WW, et al: Organizing pneumonia. Features and prognosis of cryptogenic, secondary, and focal variants, *Arch Intern Med* 157:1323–1329, 1997.

Maldonado F, Daniels C, Hoffman EA, et al: Focal organizing pneumonia on surgical lung biopsy. Causes, clinicoradiologic features, and outcome, *Chest* 132:1579–1583, 2007.

Mukhopadhyay S, Katzenstein AL: Pulmonary disease due to aspiration of food and other particulate matter: a clinicopathologic study of 59 cases diagnosed on biopsy or resection specimen, *Am J Surg Pathol* 31:752–759, 2007.

Peyrol S, Cordier JF, Grimaud JA: Intra-alveolar fibrosis of idiopathic bronchiolitis obliterans-organizing pneumonia. Cell-matrix patterns, *Am J Pathol* 137:155–170, 1990.

Vasu TS, Cavallazzi R, Ilirani A, et al: Clinical and radiologic distinction between secondary bronchiolitis obliterans organizing pneumonia and cryptogenic organizing pneumonia, *Respir Care* 54:1028–1032, 2009.

Chapter **51**

Silicosis and Coal Worker's Pneumoconiosis

Cyrielle Jardin • Benoit Wallaert

Pneumoconiosis has been defined as the non-neoplastic reaction of the lung to inhaled mineral or organic dust. Prolonged inhalation of coal mine dust may result in the development of pneumoconiosis, silicosis, and industrial chronic bronchitis and emphysema, either singly or in various combinations. *Coal worker's pneumoconiosis* (CWP) is the term generally applied to interstitial disease of the lung resulting from chronic exposure to coal dust, its inhalation and deposition, and the tissue reaction of the host to its presence, whereas *silicosis* refers to lung disease due to inhalation of dust containing silica. Pneumoconioses differ in a number of ways from acute allergic and toxic interstitial diseases associated with exposure to organic dusts, principally because of their long latency periods (usually 10 to 20 years or more) between exposure onset and disease recognition.

SOURCES OF EXPOSURE

Coal is not a mineral of fixed composition. It is graded by rank, reflecting its carbon content and thus combustibility: Anthracite is the highest-ranked coal, with a carbon content of approximately 98%. Lower-ranked coals, bituminous and subbituminous, have carbon contents of approximately 90% to 95% carbon. The rank of coal has an influence on the risk of disease: Higher-rank coals entail higher risk than lower-rank coals. However, exposure to coal dust with a quartz concentration greater than 15% is associated with a high risk for development of a rapidly progressive form of pneumoconiosis that has the characteristics of silicosis. In open mines, dust levels rarely approach those of underground mines.

The most common form of crystalline silica is quartz. Quartz is almost pure silicone dioxide but often contains traces of other elements. Other crystalline forms of silica are cristobalite and tridymite. The importance of silica as a health hazard is due to its ubiquity (**Table 51-1**). Diatomite is a siliceous sedimentary rock used for filtration; for heat and sound insulation; as an adsorbent and filtering agent; as a filler material in plastics, paper, and insecticides; and in the manufacture of floor coverings.

It seems that development and progression of silicosis depend on the total amount of quartz to which workers are exposed, the time over which that exposure occurs, and the presence of other minerals that may interfere with the toxicity of the quartz.

EPIDEMIOLOGY

CWP was first recognized in Scottish miners in 1830. In recent decades, the incidence of CWP has been declining in industrial countries thanks to improved dust controls, although increased mechanization in the mid-1960s led to a temporary increase in dust levels. In parallel, in a report from the United Kingdom, for the period 1950 to 1980, the annual rate of CWP recognition for state compensation in current and retired miners decreased from approximately 7% to 1% to 2%. The overall prevalence of CWP, which reflects more distant exposure and earlier incidence, declined from approximately 13% to 5%, but regional differences in reported rates were substantial. Similar regional differences and similar declines have been noted in the United States and other countries.

Since the 2000s, however, new sources of silicosis have emerged, especially in developing countries—for example, in Turkey, where the denim industry has been responsible for more than 75 cases thus far. Denim sandblasting is used to give jeans a more "worn-out" appearance and requires highly pressurized sand projection, often performed by young persons without any respiratory protection. In a recent epidemiologic study, among 145 workers recruited from the outpatient clinic at Atatürk University, 77 (53%) presented with radiologic evidence of silicosis.

Other, more anecdotal sources of silica exposure have been described, such as heat-dried mud inhalation in workers engaged in the manufacture of tatami mats in China, and handling quartz-containing fillers by dental supply factory workers in the United States. All of these "new forms" of silicosis underscore the fact that it will always remain a concern for respiratory clinicians worldwide, despite the decline of the mining industry in Western countries.

PATHOPHYSIOLOGY

Three groups of factors are known to influence the character and severity of lung tissue reaction to mineral dusts. The first category is the *intensity and duration of exposure*, followed by *individual susceptibility*, which explains why, among a group of workers exposed to the same dust, only a fraction will develop pneumoconiosis. Finally, the *nature and properties of the dust* are to be considered. For each mineral, geometric and aerodynamic properties, chemistry, and surface properties vary. Particles that can cause pneumoconiosis are aerodynamically and

Table 51-1 Major Industries Associated With Silica Exposure

Occupation	Exposure
Sand blaster	Ship building, oil rig maintenance, preparing steel for painting
Miner	Surface coal mining, roof bolting, shot firing, drilling, tunneling
Miller	Silica flour
Glass maker	Polishing with sand and enamel work
Potter cleaner	Crushing flint and fettling, foundry work, mold making and vitreous enameling, manufacture of cultured quartz crystal
Quarry and stone worker	Cutting of slate, sandstone, and granite
Abrasive worker	Inhalation of fine particles during grinding

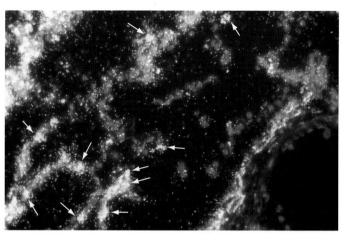

Figure 51-1 Tumor necrosis factor-α messenger RNA (as demonstrated by in situ hybridization) is expressed in alveolar macrophages (*arrows*) in this lung section from a patient with coal worker's pneumoconiosis.

geometrically small enough to reach the respiratory bronchioles and be deposited there—this generally means spherical particles of 0.5 to 5 μm in diameter.

The pathogenesis of pneumoconiosis is similar to that of all interstitial lung diseases. The condition begins as a chronic inflammatory state (alveolitis) in which inflammatory cells are activated, with consequent damage to the pulmonary architecture. Inorganic particles are phagocytosed by alveolar macrophages, causing their activation and the release of inflammatory mediators such as cytokines and arachidonic acid metabolites. These mediators, in turn, induce the recruitment of other inflammatory cells within the alveolar wall and on the alveolar epithelial surface. Toxic oxygen derivatives and proteolytic enzymes are released by the inflammatory cells, which cause cellular damage and disruption of the extracellular matrix.

The inflammatory phase is followed by a reparative phase, in which growth factors stimulate the recruitment and proliferation of mesenchymal cells and regulate neovascularization and reepithelialization of injured tissues. During this phase, abnormal or possibly uncontrolled reparative mechanisms may result in the development of fibrosis. Fibrogenic particles activate proinflammatory cytokine production within the respiratory tract. Tumor necrosis factor (TNF)-α seems to play a key role in the recruitment of inflammatory cells induced by toxic dusts (**Figure 51-1**). In addition, neutrophils recruited in the area of inflammation may contribute to the alveolitis, and respiratory and endothelial cells may play a further role by releasing various chemokines such as interleukin (IL)-8. Finally, growth factors such as platelet-derived growth factor, insulin-like growth factor, fibroblast growth factor, and transforming growth factor-β are involved in the pathogenesis of lung fibrosis and in the proliferative response of type II epithelial cells, which occurs in progressive massive fibrosis (PMF).

GENETICS

More recently, associations of polymorphisms in genes coding for inflammatory cytokines such as TNF-α, IL-6, IL-18, and their receptors with CWP incidence, prevalence, and progression have been reported. In silicosis, a significant association was found between disease severity and the TNF-α −238 variant. Irrespective of disease severity, the TNF-α −308 and IL-1 receptor type A (RA) +2018 variants conferred an increased risk for development of silicotic disease. The TNF-α

polymorphisms in positions 238, 376, and 308 of the promoter region also were found to be associated with severe silicosis in South African miners. In French coal miners differentially exposed to coal dust and cigarette smoke, the TNF-α −308 single-nucleotide polymorphism (SNP) showed an interaction with erythrocyte glutathione peroxidase (GSH-Px) activity in workers with high occupational exposure, whereas the lymphotoxin-α (LTA) *NcoI* polymorphism was associated with CWP prevalence in miners with low blood catalase activity. Certain NFKB1 and FAS-1377 gene polymorphisms also have been described as potential risk factors in a population of Chinese silicotic patients, as compared with a similar group of disease-free silica-exposed miners.

An understanding of genetic variability and environmental factors is crucial to the identification of persons at high risk for development of CWP and to the prevention and treatment of this disease.

HISTOPATHOLOGIC CHANGES

CWP lesions are focal. Simple CWP is associated with macular and nodular lesions, whereas complicated CWP is associated with PMF and lesions of rheumatoid pneumoconiosis (Caplan syndrome, discussed later on).

The pleural surfaces of a coal worker's lung show an irregular pattern of bluish-black pigmentation that corresponds to the junction sites of septal-lymphatic vessels and the pleura. Peribronchial, hilar, and paratracheal lymph nodes are enlarged, black, and firm. The initial lesions in the lung are the coal dust macules, which correspond macroscopically to focal areas of black pigmentation. On microscopic examination, the macule is seen to be composed of coal dust–laden macrophages within the walls of the respiratory bronchioles and adjacent alveoli (**Figure 51-2**). Focal emphysema around the coal dust macule is common and is considered an integral part of the lesion of simple CWP.

The histopathologic hallmark of simple CWP is the nodule. The nodules are rounded lesions with collagenous centers. On microscopic examination, the nodule can be divided into three zones: a central zone composed of whorls of dense, hyalinized fibrous tissue; a middle zone made up of concentrically arranged collagen fibers (onion-skinning); and a peripheral zone of more randomly oriented collagen fibers mixed with dust-laden macrophages and lymphoid cells (**Figure 51-3**). "Old" inactive

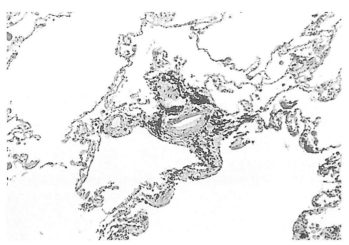

Figure 51-2 Macular lesion of coal worker's pneumoconiosis. This coal macule consists of collections of macrophages, laden with coal dust, seen extending into the connective tissue surrounding the respiratory bronchioles.

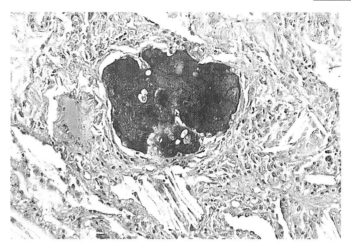

Figure 51-4 Acute silicosis. Infiltration of the alveolar walls by plasma cells and lymphocytes is evident. Note the alveoli filled with an eosinophilic coagulum.

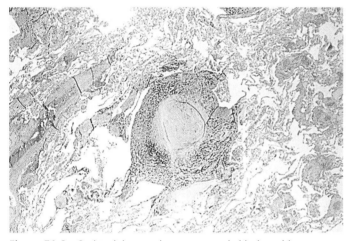

Figure 51-3 Coal nodule, seen here as a rounded lesion with a collagenous center and a peripheral anthracotic pigmented area. The nodule shows a smooth, sharp border, with dust-laden macrophages and laminated collagen deposition within the interstitium of the lung. The small central area is pale and rich in collagen, and the periphery contains a variable amount of fibrogenic dust.

nodules often are relatively acellular. Particles of silica may be demonstrated in the nodules as birefringent particles under polarized light. Nodules represent a form of mixed-dust fibrosis (i.e., coal dust plus silica exposure), usually are found in association with macules, and in some instances may develop from preexisting macules. They are not confined to the respiratory bronchioles but also are seen in the subpleural and peribronchial connective tissues. Nodules tend to cluster and eventually coalesce to produce PMF. Degenerative changes commonly are observed in the nodular lesions, including calcification, cholesterol clefts, and cavitation. In severe silicosis, structural alterations of the pulmonary vasculature may result from the accumulation of dust in the adventitia of large vessels, and involvement of the smaller blood vessels by silicotic nodules also may be seen.

Progressive massive fibrosis is defined as an opacity or fibrotic pneumoconiotic lesion of 1 cm in diameter or greater. These lesions appear as black fibrotic masses that may be round, oval, or irregular in shape. The lung and bronchovascular rays become markedly distorted. Microscopically, the lesions are composed

of bundles of haphazardly arranged hyalinized collagen fibers and/or reticulin fibers and coal dust. Dust particles near the periphery of the lesion are found mainly within macrophages, whereas in the center, the dust tends to lie free in clefts and cavities. The nodules are confluent, emphysematous bullae often surrounding the areas of massive fibrosis. Focal interstitial fibrosis can be observed in the lungs of workers exposed to dust containing a combination of silica and silicates, with sometimes sufficiently advanced lesions to result in honeycombing-type changes. Areas of liquefactive necrosis containing fragments of degenerating collagen as well as cholesterol crystals are frequently observed.

The histopathologic pattern in acute silicosis is quite different from that in the chronic form. Infiltration of the alveolar walls with plasma cells, lymphocytes, and fibroblasts, with some collagenation, is typical. The alveoli are filled with an eosinophilic coagulum (**Figure 51-4**). Electron microscopy shows widening of alveolar walls, with some collagen and clusters of type II cells; the alveolar spaces contain degenerating cells that probably are type II alveolar cells and macrophages. Silica particles may be demonstrated in the lungs and lymph nodes; silicotic nodules are few or absent.

CLINICAL FEATURES AND DIAGNOSIS

CWP and silicosis generally are first recognized from characteristic changes on the plain chest radiograph, which also is critical in evaluating disease progression. Requirements for the diagnosis include a history of significant exposure, radiographic features consistent with these illnesses, and the absence of any other disease that may mimic pneumoconioses (primarily infections with a predominantly miliary radiographic pattern, such as tuberculosis, fungal infections, or sarcoidosis). The radiographic appearances are most usefully described using the coding system devised for classification of findings on standard chest films in pneumoconiosis under the auspices of the International Labour Office (ILO) (**Table 51-2**). In clinical practice, simple CWP is characterized by small rounded opacities (nodules) rather than small irregular opacities, although the latter may be seen in much lesser profusion (as described in Table 51-2, profusion categories 0 to 3 refer to the relative abundance of small opacities apparent on the chest radiograph). For designation of disease characterized by large opacities, either *PMF* or *complicated CWP* is in common use.

Table 51-2	International Labour Organization (ILO) Radiographic Classification of Pneumoconioses		
Small Opacities*		**Regular**	**Irregular**
<1.5 mm in diameter		p	s
>1.5 mm but <3 mm in diameter		q	t
>3 mm but <10 mm in diameter		r	u

Categories

Small Opacities
The four profusion categories, 0 to 3, refer to the concentration (density) of small opacities apparent on the radiograph: category 0, small opacities are absent or less profuse than in category 1; 1, opacities are few in number; 2, opacities are numerous; 3, opacities are very numerous and obscure the normal radiographic markings.

Large Opacities
Complicated pneumoconiosis or progressive massive fibrosis (PMF) is divided into categories A to C based on the size of the large opacities. To be classified as PMF, at least one nodule should be 1 cm or greater in diameter.
A—Sum of diameters of lesions is not more than 50 mm.
B—Total area occupied by lesions is not greater than the area of the right upper zone.
C—Total area occupied by lesions is greater than the area of the right upper zone.

*Small opacities are defined by their average size and profusion.

CLINICAL FEATURES

Simple CWP and category A–complicated CWP are not associated with respiratory symptoms. As in most populations engaged in manual work, breathlessness and cough in coal miners usually are a consequence of cigarette smoking. However, coal mine dust may itself cause chronic bronchitis and chronic obstructive pulmonary disease, which together are known as *industrial bronchitis*. The evidence that coal dust exposure is associated with the development of significant respiratory impairment has led to its designation as a compensable disease despite the absence of CWP.

By contrast, patients with complicated pneumoconiosis (i.e., PMF) of categories B and C may present with undue breathlessness and productive cough. Melanoptysis is the result of necrosis within the conglomerate, coal-containing lesions that characterize PMF. Progressive, undue exertional dyspnea usually is the dominant symptom, but rarely, breathlessness may be present at rest.

No specific abnormal physical signs are found in CWP. Finger clubbing and fine inspiratory crackles are not features of the disease, so if these are present, another explanation should be sought. Only in a small proportion of severe cases of complicated disease does CWP evolve to produce chronic respiratory failure and cor pulmonale.

Other than PMF, CWP may be associated with a number of other disorders—most notably the autoimmune disorders of rheumatoid disease and progressive systemic sclerosis. The combination of rheumatoid disease and CWP is known as *Caplan syndrome* (**Figure 51-5**). This diagnosis is suggested by the association of coal dust exposure, rheumatoid arthritis, and multiple well-defined large, rounded opacities (nodules greater than 10 mm in diameter) on the chest radiograph. Spontaneous disappearance is common, with or without initial cavitation, and new nodules frequently emerge in different locations. The Caplan nodule also is more likely to cavitate, thereby producing

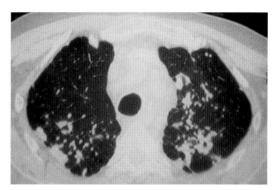

Figure 51-5 Caplan syndrome. High-resolution computed tomography scan obtained at the level of the upper lobes shows bilateral parenchymal micronodules and coalescence in the right upper lobe. Note the cavitation of the nodule in the left upper lobe.

a concentric ring pattern, so this lesion also is known as a necrobiotic nodule. Central necrosis is rare in nodules of CWP, although it may occur in conglomerate lesions.

CWP has been linked with a number of specific infections, the most prominent of which has been tuberculosis. Silicosis is recognized to increase the risk for pulmonary tuberculosis, which can be difficult to diagnose in patients with preexisting abnormalities on plain chest radiographs. Diagnostic skin tests also may show lesser sensitivity in silicotic patients, owing in part to their age and general condition. Silicotic patients can suffer from malnutrition in later stages of the disease because of chronic respiratory failure and elevated metabolism. Protein deficiency may impair immunoglobulin production and thus lessen the skin tests' sensitivity (as they rely on adaptive immune response). In these particular patients, interferon-gamma assays could be used to improve diagnostic performance. In contrast with silicosis, however, CWP does not increase significantly the risk for infection with *Mycobacterium tuberculosis*. The association observed with coal mining (and hence CWP) in some countries appears to have been a consequence only of close contact during long hours of work in the confined mine environment. Nontuberculous mycobacteria, on the other hand, may infect lungs damaged by CWP and other types of pneumoconiosis with greater-than-usual frequency, so CWP does seem to increase the risk for infection with opportunistic organisms. *Mycobacterium avium* probably is the most important of these and is poorly sensitive to antibiotic agents. *Mycobacterium kansasii* and *Mycobacterium malmoense* also may be pathogenic in this setting. It may similarly be difficult to attribute change in the radiographic appearances to advancing infection or worsening PMF. Experimental studies also suggest that mycobacterial infection is a factor that helps explain the progression from simple to complicated pneumoconiosis.

Other opportunistic infections reported in association with CWP have included nocardiosis, sporotrichosis, and cryptococcosis. *Aspergillus* spp. have been noted to colonize cavities in conglomerate lesions of complicated CWP.

A further association with complicated CWP, if manifested by bullous emphysema, is spontaneous pneumothorax. The advanced stages of complicated CWP also are associated with recurrent episodes of acute and subacute bronchitis. Persistent productive cough is common in coal miners in the absence of CWP. No evidence of a causal relationship between silicosis and carcinoma of the lung has been found, although association is consistent for silicotics and limited nonsilicotic workers. The available data leave open the issue of whether silica per se materially increases lung cancer risk in absence of silicosis. In

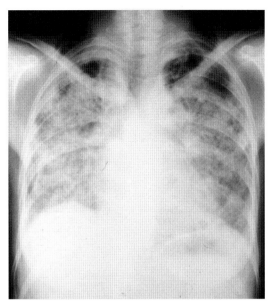

Figure 51-6 Chest radiograph showing alveolar filling in acute silicosis. The patient was a 28-year-old woman who had inhaled fine particles of silica from abrasive powder. The clinical disease that developed was rapidly progressive silicosis, which typically is fatal over the next several years.

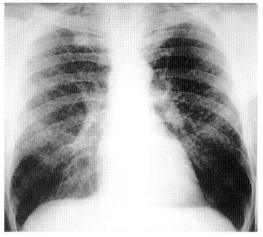

Figure 51-7 Chest radiograph appearance in simple coal worker's pneumoconiosis. The patient was a 55-year-old man who had worked for 18 years in an underground coal mine. He was a nonsmoker with a chronic cough and normal lung function. The radiograph shows a diffuse distribution of small rounded opacities, more prominent in the upper zones than in the lower zones.

1997, the International Agency for Research on Cancer (IARC) classified crystalline silica dust exposure as a known human carcinogen, group 1. Currently, CWP and silicosis should be considered conditions that predispose workers to an increased risk of lung cancer.

Accelerated silicosis is rare and is clinically identical to the classic forms of silicosis, except that the time from initial exposure to the onset of disease is shorter and the rate of progression of disease is dramatically faster.

Acute silicosis is rare. Presenting signs and symptoms include cough, weight loss, and fatigue, with rapid progression to fulminant respiratory failure over several months in some cases. Chest auscultation reveals diffuse crackles, and in patients with this clinical picture, the rapid development of cor pulmonale eventuating in respiratory death is characteristic. Survival after the onset of symptoms often is less than 2 years. Diffuse alveolar filling, most apparent at the bases, is the most prominent finding on the chest radiograph (**Figure 51-6**). Although serial chest radiographs from workers with this illness have been infrequently reported, it seems that the bibasilar filling pattern progresses into large opacities located in the middle zones rather than the upper zones.

CHEST RADIOLOGY

The radiographic pattern in simple CWP typically is one of small rounded opacities that appear first in the upper zones (**Figure 51-7**). The middle and lower zones become involved as the number of opacities increases. The nodules increase in profusion with increasing dust exposure; a change in profusion after dust exposure has ceased is very unusual. Calcification of the nodules may occur (in 10% to 20% of cases).

Complicated pneumoconiosis is defined as presence of a lesion of 1 cm or greater in longest diameter. The large opacities usually are predominant in the upper lobes, may be unilateral or bilateral, and are symmetrically or asymmetrically distributed (**Figure 51-8**). The pattern of change in size is variable and unpredictable. In most but not all cases, PMF occurs on a

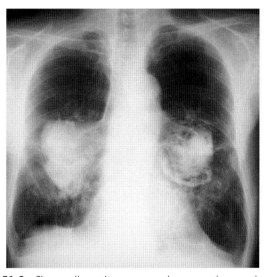

Figure 51-8 Chest radiograph appearance in progressive massive fibrosis. The patient was a 66-year-old man who had worked for 30 years in an underground coal mine. The radiograph shows bilateral masses corresponding to the lesions of progressive massive fibrosis.

background of simple pneumoconiosis, and it may appear after dust exposure has ceased. Cavitation can develop within a PMF lesion (**Figure 51-9**), and occasionally a dense peripheral arc or rim may be seen at its lower pole that represents calcification. Dense calcification with the lesion also is sometimes seen. PMF often is associated with bullous emphysema and fibrotic scarring, leading to distortion of the lung and shift of the trachea and mediastinum to the affected side. Irregular, mainly basal opacities also may be seen on standard radiographs. Eggshell calcification is uncommon in CWP but may occur in intrapulmonary, hilar, or mediastinal lymph nodes, possibly because of concomitant exposure to silica. Pleural effusion is uncommon in CWP. Its presence may be related to an associated infection or an interaction with a systemic collagen vascular disease.

In simple CWP, computed tomography (CT) shows parenchymal lesions that can be detected in miners with normal-appearing chest radiographs. CT thus shows greater sensitivity

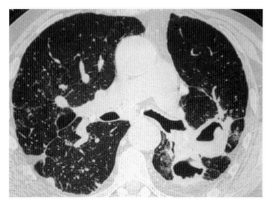

Figure 51-9 Cavitation within progressive massive fibrosis lesion. High-resolution computed tomography scan shows cavitation of the left lung masses. Note the diffuse micronodulation and associated emphysema.

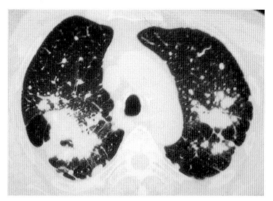

Figure 51-11 Aseptic necrosis. Computed tomography scan shows bilateral masses with necrosis of the right upper lobe mass and bilateral emphysema.

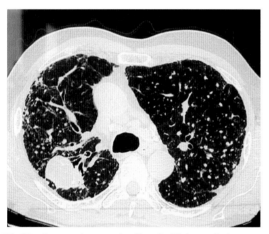

Figure 51-10 Progressive massive fibrosis. High-resolution computed tomography scan shows bilateral masses consistent with progressive massive fibrosis. There is a background of nodules associated with bullous changes around progressive massive fibrosis lesions; this imaging pattern defines paracicatricial emphysema. Note the calcifications within the masses and the lymph nodes.

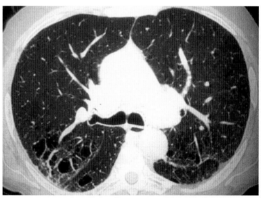

Figure 51-12 Nonbullous emphysema. High-resolution computed tomography scan shows small bullae and low attenuation, without progressive massive fibrosis lesions—an imaging pattern that defines centrilobular or nonparacicatricial emphysema.

than plain radiographs for detection of simple CWP but less obvious benefit with complicated pneumoconiosis. A posterior and right-sided predominance of lesions in the upper zones is evident on these imaging studies.

Nodules usually are observed against a background of parenchymal micronodules and generally are associated with subpleural micronodules. Two categories of lesions can be observed in PMF: lesions with irregular borders that are associated with disruption of the pulmonary parenchyma and lead to typical scar emphysema (**Figure 51-10**) and lesions with regular borders that are unassociated with scar emphysema. When the lesions are greater than 4 cm in diameter, irregular areas of aseptic necrosis can be observed with or without cavitation (**Figure 51-11**).

Two major forms of emphysema occurring in coal workers can be detected on the CT scan: bullous changes around PMF lesions, representing *paracicatricial* or *scar emphysema*, and nonbullous lesions, defined as *irregular emphysema* (**Figure 51-12**). Lesions of diffuse pulmonary fibrosis can be detected on high-resolution CT as honeycombing or areas of ground glass attenuation. Two specific etiopathogenic mechanisms for fibrosis in

coal miners should be considered: (1) a direct effect of deposited coal or silica particles and (2) an indirect effect resulting from an association with scleroderma. In addition, determination of the extent of air trapping on expiratory thin-section CT scans may assess obstructive abnormalities.

LUNG FUNCTION

In all studies of lung function in patients with pneumoconiosis, account should be taken of a number of different and confounding influences; in particular, the effects of smoking need to be considered. It can be stated that simple CWP has no important effect on spirometric measures when previous dust exposure is taken into account and when smoking habits also are considered. Similarly, simple silicosis has no appreciable effect on lung function. In more advanced disease, slight reduction in volumes, compliance, and gas transfer can be present; a predominantly restrictive pattern is seen. Slight reduction in arterial oxygen tension on effort may be observed in advanced disease. Oxygen desaturation is not present when measurements are obtained with the patient at rest or on moderate effort in simple CWP. As in the case of radiographic progression, the changes in pulmonary function are more likely to occur in workers who have had intense exposure to dust. In addition, it must be pointed out that miners who did not have CWP on chest radiography exhibited lower values for forced expiratory volume in 1 second than those measured in control subjects, suggesting the frequent presence of coal dust–induced chronic obstructive pulmonary disease. In PMF, lung function depends on the extent of the lesions and extent of emphysematous changes. Studies of lung function in the more advanced stages of PMF have shown an obstructive and restrictive pattern; therefore, diffusing capacity usually is reduced. Compliance also usually is somewhat decreased. Ultimately, hypoxemic respiratory failure may occur.

SEROLOGIC AND IMMUNOLOGIC FEATURES

No specific biologic features of pneumoconiosis have been identified. However, immunologic abnormalities are now well described: positive circulating antinuclear antibodies or rheumatoid factor. Serum immunoglobulins A and G are present at significantly raised levels in miners with pneumoconiosis. Finally, an increased serum angiotensin-converting enzyme level was observed in 45% of pneumoconiotic coal miners, whatever the radiologic classification of pneumoconiosis. More recently, IL-17–producing lymphocytes have been suspected to induce lung inflammation but not fibrosis in a murine model of experimental silicosis.

BRONCHOALVEOLAR LAVAGE

On bronchoalveolar lavage, no change in differential cell count has been noted, in contrast with a number of other interstitial disorders of the lung. Alveolar inflammatory cells from patients with CWP, especially those with PMF, exhibited spontaneous release of superoxide anions, proinflammatory cytokines, and profibrotic mediators in greater amounts than those measured for cells from control subjects.

CLINICAL COURSE, TREATMENT, AND PREVENTION

PROGNOSIS

Simple CWP is not associated with premature death, but approximately 4% of deaths in coal miners are directly due to complicated pneumoconiosis. In workers with categories 1, 2, and 3 of simple CWP and category A of complicated CWP, life expectancy is the same as that for persons without pneumoconiosis in the general population.

The rate of progression to PMF seems to be influenced chiefly by the age at which the miner begins to show radiographic changes of CWP: The earlier the diagnosis, the more likely there is to be progression reflecting individual susceptibility and the level of cumulative exposure.

MANAGEMENT

No specific treatment affects the course of CWP, although treatment options are available for complications such as tuberculosis, pneumothorax, and chronic hypoxemia.

When a miner is found to have CWP, further dust exposure should be excluded. Simple pneumoconiosis does not necessarily imply complete exclusion from mining, whereas when PMF is detected, all further dusty work should be prevented. Additional information can be obtained from pulmonary function tests, because the development of an obstructive ventilatory defect (resulting from dust exposure) may occur in the absence of CWP. For all smoking patients, appropriate advice and support for smoking cessation should be provided.

After a determination of disability from CWP, the physician should be able to direct the patient toward whatever mechanism exists for compensation. As noted earlier, CWP generally is first recognized from the plain chest radiograph, which also is critical in evaluating disease progression. Requirements for the diagnosis include a history of significant exposure, radiographic features consistent with these illnesses, and the absence of conditions that may mimic these diseases (primarily infections with a predominantly miliary radiographic pattern, such as tuberculosis, fungal infections, or sarcoidosis).

PREVENTION

The prevention of pneumoconiosis depends on controlling exposure concentrations of ambient dust to levels known to be associated with minimal and acceptable risk. Dust control is affected primarily by ventilation, although spraying of water at points of dust generation is a useful measure for dust suppression. The effectiveness of such measures should be monitored by regular measurement of dust concentrations and by regular clinical and radiologic surveillance of the persons in the workforce. Surveillance allows early recognition of workers with simple pneumoconiosis, who are likely to be those with greatest susceptibility, so that ongoing exposure can be restricted (perhaps by transfer to jobs with lower exposure) and the risk of future disablement from PMF reduced.

Variability of individual susceptibility is likely to be an important determinant for CWP, as it is for most occupational disorders, and a number of predictive factors may be useful in identifying miners at higher-than-average risk: initial presence of expiratory wheezes, obstructive pattern of lung function, and more micronodules on CT scan. An alternative approach for the future might involve genetic screening evaluating for polymorphisms in the promoter of various mediators. In any event, control of exposure levels alone is likely to prevent most cases of disabling PMF, and it has been predicted that an exposure concentration over 35 working years that does not exceed an average of 4.3 mg/m^3 is associated with a probability for the development of category 2 or more CWP of no more than 3.4%. This represents a dramatic reduction in risk over the last 50 years.

WEB RESOURCE

International Agency for Research on Cancer website: http://www.iarc.fr/

SUGGESTED READINGS

Akgun M, Araz O: An epidemic of silicosis among former denim sandblasters, *Eur Respir J* 32:1295–1303, 2008.

Attfield MD, Seixas NS: Prevalence of pneumoconiosis and its relationship to dust exposure in a cohort of U.S. bituminous coal miners and examiners, *Am J Ind Med* 27:137–151, 1995.

Begin R, Cantin A, Massé S: Recent advances in the pathogenesis and clinical assessment of mineral dust pneumoconioses: asbestosis, silicosis and coal pneumoconiosis, *Eur Respir J* 2:988–1001, 1989.

Goldsmith DF: Research and policy implications of IARC's classification of silica as a group 1 carcinogen, *Indoor Built Environ* 8:136–142, 1999.

Piguet PF, Collart MA, Grau GE, et al: Requirement of tumour necrosis factor for development of silica-induced pulmonary fibrosis, *Nature* 344:245–247, 1990.

Remy-Jardin M, Remy J, Farre I, Marquette CH: Computed tomography evaluation of silicosis and coal worker's pneumoconiosis, *Radiol Clin North Am* 30:1155–1176, 1992.

Rom WN, Bitterman PB, Rennard SI, et al: Characterization of the lower respiratory tract inflammation of nonsmoking individuals with interstitial lung disease associated with chronic inhalation of inorganic dust, *Am Rev Respir Dis* 136:1429–1434, 1987.

Vanhee D, Gosset P, Boitelle A, et al: Cytokines and cytokine network in silicosis and coal workers' pneumoconiosis, *Eur Respir J* 8:1–9, 1995.

Wouters EF, Jorna TH, Westenend M: Respiratory effects of coal dust exposure: clinical effects and diagnosis, *Exp Lung Res* 20:385–394, 1994.

Yu IT, Tse LA: Exploring the joint effects of silicosis and smoking on lung cancer risks, *Int J Cancer* 120:133–139, 2007.

Yucesoy B, Luster MI: Genetic susceptibility in pneumoconiosis, *Toxicol Lett* 168:249–254, 2007.

Zhai R, Jetten M, Schins RP, et al: Polymorphisms in the promoter of the tumor necrosis factor alpha in coal miners, *Am J Ind Med* 34:318–324, 1998.

Chapter **52**
Asbestosis

Lee S. Newman • Kaylan E. Stinson

Inhalational exposure to asbestos produces both malignant and nonmalignant diseases of the chest. The focus of this chapter is on the two major categories of nonmalignant disease—asbestosis and asbestos-related pleural disorders, listed in **Table 52-1**. These conditions have received a great deal of attention from the scientific and medical communities because of the ubiquitous use of asbestos in modern society and its diverse and pernicious toxicities. Despite major progress in awareness of the issues and in control of exposure, a large burden of asbestos-related disease will continue to accrue as a consequence of ongoing exposure and the characteristic disease latency.

EPIDEMIOLOGY, RISK FACTORS, AND PATHOPHYSIOLOGY

EPIDEMIOLOGY

The first well-documented cases of asbestosis were reported in the early 1900s among asbestos textile workers. Through the 1920s and 1930s, reports emerged of asbestosis, pleural thickening, pleural calcification, and right ventricular failure in asbestos-exposed workers. Radiographic studies that began in the 1930s documented an asbestosis prevalence of 25% to 55% in these workers, especially among those with greater cumulative exposure. Early evidence from these studies suggested that exposure to higher concentrations of asbestos over longer periods of time resulted in increased risk for development of pulmonary fibrosis.

Asbestos use increased extensively in the early 1940s, and this mineral substance was used widely in the United States for the next 30 years. Asbestos use began to diminish when the Occupational Safety and Health Administration (OSHA) regulated workplace asbestos exposure in 1972. It is estimated that between 1940 and 1979, more than 27 million people had potential exposure in the United States alone. Data from a study of sheet metal workers examined between 1986 and 2004, reported by Welch and colleagues, found that asbestosis is continuing to occur even 50 years after first exposure. The study also found that the strongest predictor of nonmalignant asbestos-related disease in the workers was the cutoff year in which employment commenced: Prevalence was lowest among those who began working in the sheet metal industry after 1970 and highest among those who began work before 1949. With thousands of commercial applications and the mineral's resistance to degradation, asbestos remains ubiquitous. Efforts have been made to limit ongoing exposure through abatement programs of asbestos removal from buildings and/or on-site encapsulation. Nevertheless, asbestos-related disability and mortality will continue well into the next decade.

Although the use of asbestos has been curtailed in many developed nations, in less-developed countries this inexpensive but hazardous material continues to be used widely. Many developed countries are now fast replacing the developed ones in the production and use of asbestos. Currently, Russia is the leading producer of asbestos worldwide, followed by China, Brazil, Kazakhstan, and Canada. More than 85% of the world production of asbestos is used to manufacture products in Asia and Eastern Europe. Although asbestos usage in developing countries is increasing, information about asbestos-related disease remains largely obscure. Epidemiologic questions have not been systematically researched.

In keeping with the long latency required before asbestosis becomes clinically apparent, all past and current asbestos workers must be considered to be at risk for development of this fibrosing lung disorder.

ETIOLOGY AND RISK FACTORS

The minerals referred to herein as "asbestos" are a family of naturally occurring, flexible, fibrous hydrous silicates found in soil worldwide. Mined asbestos fibers are categorized as either long and curly (serpentine) or straight and rodlike (amphibole). The serpentine fiber, chrysotile, accounts for most of the commercially used asbestos, favored for its properties of heat resistance, flexibility, and ease of spinning for textiles. Five categories of amphiboles are recognized: crocidolite, amosite, anthophyllite, tremolite, and actinolite. These more rigid fibers are less commonly used but are still pathogenic. All major commercial forms have been associated with development of nonmalignant respiratory disorders and of lung cancer and mesothelioma, as discussed in Chapters 47, 65, and 70.

Asbestosis is the result of either direct or "bystander" exposure to asbestos-containing materials. Major sources of exposure are summarized in **Table 52-2**. During the first half of the 20th century, high-level exposures to asbestos dust occurred in the manufacturing of asbestos textiles and construction materials and in the construction and ship-building trades. Potential exposures still occur in the construction trades and in the process of asbestos abatement. Although the use of asbestos has been curtailed in many developed nations since the 1970s, in less developed countries this inexpensive but hazardous material continues to be used widely. High cumulative, occupational exposures in these settings are still commonplace.

Environmental exposure to asbestiform fibers also is well described as the cause of nonmalignant and malignant asbestos-related lung disease in countries including Turkey, Greece, Japan, and China and the territory of New Caledonia. Exposure in these settings usually occurs when villagers in rural areas

Table 52-1 **Nonmalignant Asbestos-Related Diseases**

Condition	Locus of Pathologic Change	Description
Asbestosis	Parenchyma	Interstitial pulmonary fibrosis
Benign nodules	Parenchyma	Lymphoid or fibrotic nodular scars
Benign pleural effusion	Pleura	Exudative, transient effusion
Pleural plaques	Pleura	Collagenous, hyalinized masses; circumscribed, avascular; usually involving the parietal pleura
Diffuse pleural thickening	Pleura	Collagenous, hyalinized masses; diffuse, avascular; involving the parietal and visceral pleura and interlobular space
Rounded atelectasis	Combined pleura and parenchyma	Scarring of pleura and adjacent lung tissue, resulting in retraction, entrapment, and local partial collapse of lung

disturb natural soil deposits while working in fields or when applying whitewash prepared from these outcrops to their dwellings. In the United States, asbestos-related lung disease caused by nonoccupational exposures is a recently recognized problem, mostly in current and former residents of Libby, Montana. Amphibole asbestos–contaminated vermiculite was mined, milled, and processed near this small town for many years. Personal and commercial use of the contaminated mineral was widespread among residents. During a health screening in 2000 to 2001, nearly 18% of 6668 participants were noted to have pleural thickening on chest radiographs. Less than 1% had findings compatible with asbestosis.

A clear dose-response relationship between asbestos exposure and asbestosis has been recognized, although controversy remains concerning risks at low-level exposure. Risk for asbestosis varies widely among industries, with more disease seen in textile and construction workers than with those in mining. Development of the disease is associated with factors such as respirability of the fiber type, the cumulative dose of exposure, the capacity of the lung to clear the fibers, and the biopersistence of the asbestos. In general, the relative risk for development of asbestosis for asbestos workers increases in proportion to the asbestos exposure levels in the workplace. More severe disease has been associated with higher retention of asbestos fiber in the lungs. Typical asbestos fibers found in the lungs are 20 to 50 μm long and initially are deposited at the bifurcations of conducting airways. Thin fibers, of diameters less than 3 μm,

Table 52-2 **Major Asbestos Uses and Sources of Exposure**

Environment	Type of Exposure	Source of Exposure
Occupational	Asbestos-cement products	Construction industry (sheeting used in roofing and cladding of structural materials, molded into roof tiles, pipes, gutters; filler for wall cracks, cement, joint compound, adhesive, caulking putty)
	Floor tiling	Filler and reinforcing agent in asphalt flooring, vinyl tile, adhesive
	Insulation, fireproofing	Insulators, pipefitters Construction industry (pipes, boiler covers, ship bulkheads, sprayed on walls and ceilings as fireproofing, soundproofing)
	Textiles	Fireproof textiles used in clothing, blankets
	Paper products	Roofing felt, wall coverings, mill board, insulating paper
	Friction materials	Brake linings
	Rubber, plastic manufacture	Filler in rubber and plastics
	Building trades, secondhand exposure	Building maintenance activities, pipefitting, electrical repair, boiler tending and secondhand exposure repair, boiler tending and repair, power station maintenance Carpenters, plumbers, welders
Domestic	"Fouling the nest"	Carrying home asbestos in hair and clothes of exposed workers results in exposure to family members
	Secondhand exposure	Residential remodeling, removal, handling of frayed, friable asbestos in homes can cause environmental exposure
General	Contaminated buildings	Found in low levels in buildings under normal use Elevated exposures from remodeling, renovation, asbestos removal, disturbance of contaminated materials such as acoustic ceiling tiles, vinyl floor tiles, paints, plaster, pipes, boilers, steel beams
	Geologic exposure	Living near asbestos mines or cement factories, or in geographic areas in which naturally occurring asbestos is found in ambient air
	Urban environment	Ambient air levels slightly higher in cities, perhaps because of asbestos shed from automotive brakes in denser traffic, and high concentration of industry and construction

translocate readily into the alveolar space, interstitium, and pleural space. Thicker fibers tend to be incompletely phagocytosed by alveolar macrophages and are retained in the lung, where they can trigger the inflammatory events that lead to fibrosis, as discussed next.

HISTOPATHOLOGY AND GRADING

Asbestosis is defined histopathologically as bilateral, diffuse interstitial fibrosis of the lungs caused by the inhalation of asbestos fibers (**Figure 52-1**). Gray streaks of fibrosis can be seen in the parenchyma along interlobar and interlobular septa. Later, the pleural surface becomes more nodular in appearance, and the parenchyma loses volume and elasticity and forms more fibrotic scars and honeycombing. The gross pathologic changes are most obvious in the lower lung zones bilaterally, with the worst disease nearest to the pleura.

The College of American Pathologists and Pulmonary Pathology Society has modified a 12-point grading scheme that has been shown to be consistently reproducible. The modified grading scheme, based on histologic criteria presented in the 2010 update on the original diagnostic criteria, consists of the following categories of disease severity:

Grade 0—no appreciable peribronchiolar fibrosis, or fibrosis confined to the bronchiolar walls
Grade 1—fibrosis confined to the walls of respiratory bronchioles and the first tier of adjacent alveoli
Grade 2—extension of fibrosis to involve alveolar ducts and/or two or more tiers of alveoli adjacent to the respiratory bronchiole, with sparing of at least some alveoli between adjacent bronchioles
Grade 3—fibrotic thickening of the walls of all alveoli between two or more adjacent respiratory bronchioles
Grade 4—honeycombing changes

Although histologic evidence of pulmonary fibrosis may occasionally be obtained in the course of clinical evaluation, routine lung biopsy and lavage are not recommended, and microscopic evidence is rarely required to diagnose asbestosis.

Occasionally, the determination of asbestos fibers in lung tissue, bronchoalveolar lavage, or sputum may be used to document past exposure, although these measurements are neither usually relied on nor required for the clinical diagnosis of asbestosis. Under light microscopy or by use of transmission electron microscopy, uncoated fibers or fibers coated with proteinaceous material may be detected. These coated fibers—so-called asbestos bodies or ferruginous bodies—are nonspecific, because they can be found in occupationally unexposed people, in occupationally exposed people who have no asbestos-related lung disease, and in workers who have asbestosis. Generally, the most exposed and most severely affected people have higher asbestos fiber counts, but a significant interlaboratory variability is found in these measures.

PATHOGENESIS

Some of the major events thought to be involved in the pathogenesis of asbestosis are summarized in **Figure 52-2**. Within minutes after asbestos fibers have been inhaled, a local tissue response is initiated at the bifurcations of terminal bronchioles and alveolar ducts. The first changes occur in epithelial cells and then in alveolar macrophages as they attempt to engulf and are pierced by the fibers. In addition to cell death, which leads to the release of macrophage contents, asbestos-activated macrophages release reactive oxygen species that directly damage the tissue through peroxidation and direct cytotoxicity. Asbestos also can induce toxicity by mechanisms independent of its ability to promote formation of reactive oxygen species.

Increasing numbers of alveolar macrophages accumulate within 48 hours of first exposure. With chronic inhalation, a localized fibrosing alveolitis in the peribronchiolar region develops, followed by diffuse fibrotic scarring. Increasing the dose of asbestos increases the cellular response. A cascade of events ensues in which the macrophages and neutrophils release various cytokines (such as interleukin-8 and interferon-γ), chemokines, oxidants, and growth factors (such as fibronectin, platelet-derived growth factor, insulin-like growth factor, transforming growth factor-β, tumor necrosis factor-α, and fibroblast growth factor). These attract and alter the function of other inflammatory cells and resident cells, thereby promoting inflammation and fibrosis. The response of fibroblasts to these signals is to proliferate and produce the constituents of extracellular matrix (e.g., collagen, proteoglycans) in the pulmonary interstitium. Resident cells themselves are both targets and perpetrators of the fibrotic response. The pathogenesis of the chronic fibrotic response is complex and remains to be fully elucidated. It is clear, however, that this chronic response is progressive and that, apart from macrophage, neutrophil, and

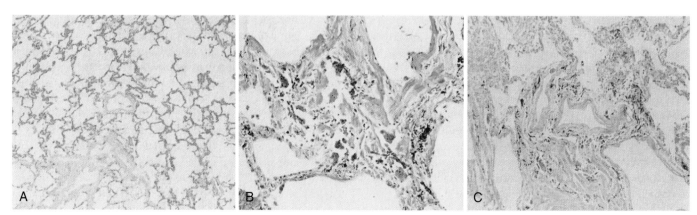

Figure 52-1 Histopathologic features of asbestosis. Disease severity is classified according to a modified grading scheme from the College of American Pathologists, as described in the text. **A,** In this grade 1 lesion, fibrosis is limited to the peribronchiolar tissue and the walls of the respiratory bronchioles. **B,** Enlargement of a grade 1 lesion illustrates presence of asbestos bodies. **C,** In this grade 3 lesion, fibrosis extends into the interstitial space between the respiratory units and into the alveolar ducts. (**A** to **C,** Hematoxylin and eosin stain.) *(Courtesy Dr. Val Vallythan, National Institute for Occupational Safety and Health, Morgantown, West Virginia.)*

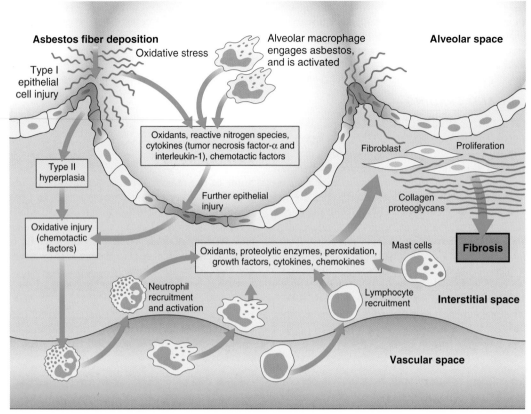

Figure 52-2 Proposed pathogenesis of asbestosis. Asbestos fibers deposit at branch points in the distal airways and alveolar ducts, which prompts an inflammatory cascade characterized by cellular activation, recruitment, and injury. The result is fibroblast proliferation and extracellular matrix deposition in the interstitial space.

epithelial cells, a number of other cell types, such as lymphocytes and mast cells, contribute to the cycle of lung remodeling and fibrosis. Multiple, functionally overlapping, redundant inflammatory events occur in the lung simultaneously during the period of fibrogenesis. The consequence is an irreversible alteration in the structure and function of the lung.

GENETICS

Asbestos exposure is the principal risk factor for the development of nonmalignant asbestos-related disorders. The genetic contribution to this risk is uncertain. A small number of cross-sectional, candidate gene studies have examined the possible contribution of genetic determinants of susceptibility to asbestosis. The glutathione *S*-transferases (GSTs) and *N*-acetyltransferases (NATs) are enzymes that aid in the detoxification of hazardous agents. Several small studies examined GST-null (deletion) polymorphisms and NAT2 slow acetylator genotype in workers with and without asbestosis. Results from these studies, although somewhat inconsistent suggest that people who have a constitutional, homozygous deletion in the *GSTM1* gene that codes for GST class mu, as well as those who are NAT2 slow acetylators, may be at higher risk for asbestosis if exposed to sufficiently high levels of asbestos. On the basis of the premise that asbestos causes DNA damage and alters DNA repair, Zhao and colleagues demonstrated an association between polymorphisms of the DNA repair gene *XRCC1* and the in vitro extent of asbestos-induced DNA damage in Chinese asbestosis cases versus that in nonasbestosis cases. In Spain, patients with asbestosis were more likely than exposed control

subjects to be heterozygous for the α_1-antitrypsin polymorphism Pi*Z.

CLINICAL FEATURES

Asbestosis is the pulmonary fibrotic disease that results from asbestos exposure. It affects the lungs symmetrically and typically is diagnosed on the basis of a consistent occupational or environmental history of asbestos exposure plus evidence of pulmonary fibrosis, usually obtained by chest radiography. The latency period from first exposure to clinical disease is 10 to 20 years but can be up to 40 years or more, with shorter latency and more severe disease seen in those workers with the highest inhalational exposures. In some situations, the exposure history may be difficult to document. If needed, further evidence of occupational exposure can be verified by identifying high numbers of asbestos bodies in bronchoalveolar lavage fluid, sputum, or lung tissue, as discussed previously. Evidence of bilateral pleural plaques is pathognomonic for previous asbestos exposure. The radiographic finding of bilateral interstitial markings in the lower lung zone is sufficient radiographic evidence of asbestosis, although (as discussed in the following section) other tools such as computed tomography (CT) and measures of lung physiology also aid diagnosis.

The most common signs and symptoms of asbestosis are the insidious onset of dyspnea on exertion (and eventually at rest), dry cough that can be paroxysmal, and fatigue. Hemoptysis, chest pain, and weight loss are not common and should raise suspicion for asbestos-related malignancy. Although physical abnormalities are uncommon at the early stages of asbestosis,

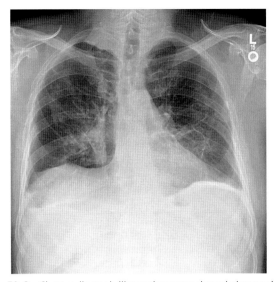

Figure 52-3 Chest radiograph illustrating parenchymal abnormalities in asbestosis. Descriptive designations are from the International Labour Organization (ILO) classification for the radiographic appearance of pneumoconioses (see Chapter 51, Table 51-2). In this case, fine linear opacities of profusion category 1/0 can be seen in the middle and lower lung zones. Calcified pleural plaques are seen along the diaphragm bilaterally.

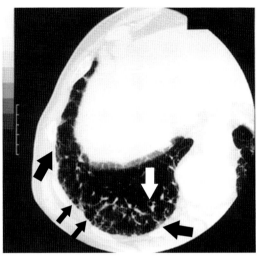

Figure 52-4 Asbestosis. This high-resolution computed tomography (CT) scan of the thorax was obtained in an asbestos-exposed worker with asbestosis and mild pleural thickening. Patchy subpleural accentuation of interstitial markings (*thick arrows*) with honeycombing (*thin arrows*) and traction bronchiectasis (*white arrow*) are classic for the CT appearance in advanced asbestosis.

patients may exhibit such signs later in the clinical course, such as dry, bilateral basilar rales evident on end inspiration, digital clubbing, cyanosis, and signs of cor pulmonale.

RADIOLOGIC FINDINGS

Radiographically, asbestosis typically manifests in the lower lobes with irregular "reticular" markings toward the lung periphery and costophrenic angles (**Figure 52-3**). Linear opacities that resemble extensions of vascular markings may assume a netlike appearance. In early or less severe disease, the middle and upper lung zones may appear relatively spared. With progression, the linear and irregular opacities thicken and spread to the midlung zones, but rarely to the apex. The International Labour Organization (ILO) International Classification of Radiographs of Pneumoconioses characterizes each type of irregular opacity on the basis of increasing size and thickness as either *s, t,* or *u,* and on a scale of profusion (number) of opacities from normal profusion (0/–, 0/0, 0/1) to severe (3/2, 3/3, 3/+) (see Chapter 51, Table 51-2, for classification details). When irregular opacities are seen on the chest radiograph in conjunction with pleural thickening, the radiograph can be considered virtually pathognomonic for asbestosis. However, the chest radiograph lacks sensitivity, because 15% to 18% of symptomatic, biopsy-proven asbestosis cases are associated with a normal appearance on chest radiographs. Focal masses are uncommon except for those caused by rounded atelectasis.

COMPUTED TOMOGRAPHY

Conventional CT and high-resolution CT (HRCT) are more sensitive and specific than radiography for the diagnosis of pleural disease related to asbestos. HRCT, with use of 1- to 3-mm slices, is superior in sensitivity to plain chest radiography for detection of the fine reticular opacities in this disease. Of asbestos-exposed workers who have normal-appearing chest radiographs, 10% to 30% have HRCT scans suggestive of underlying interstitial disease. Thus, the HRCT scan can prove useful when the clinical index of suspicion for asbestosis is high but the chest radiograph appears normal. The most common HRCT findings in asbestosis are short, peripheral septal lines; subpleural curvilinear lines; ground glass attenuation; peripheral cystic lesions (honeycombing); parenchymal bands adjacent to areas of pleural thickening; and bronchiolar thickening (**Figure 52-4**). The density of interstitial abnormalities found on HRCT has been shown to correlate with the symptoms and with physiologic and inflammatory indicators of asbestosis, although in general, findings on both the chest radiograph and the HRCT scan demonstrate only a limited correlation with disease severity measured by assessment of lung physiology.

PULMONARY PHYSIOLOGY ASSESSMENT

The earliest pathophysiologic changes include small airway dysfunction (e.g., decreased forced expiratory flow). As the disease progresses, restriction, evidenced by diminished total lung capacity and forced vital capacity, is observed, as is worsening gas exchange as measured by diffusing capacity and by arterial blood gas partial pressures determined under conditions of exercise and rest. These different parameters do not necessarily show the same degree of abnormality. Measures of gas exchange generally are more sensitive than measures of lung volumes in this disorder. Isolated, severe, obstructive airway disease usually is not attributable to asbestosis alone, although airflow obstruction may be present with or without restriction and occurs even in asbestos-exposed workers who were nonsmokers.

DIAGNOSIS

The long latency between asbestos exposure and development of asbestosis and the gradually progressive nature of the symptoms mean that this disease has a tendency to remain undetected until fairly late in its course. Efforts to conduct workplace surveillance by use of the chest radiograph and ILO readings of these films have improved disease detection. The diagnosis is based on a consistent history of exposure to asbestos, with sufficient duration of latency, and evidence of interstitial fibrosis. A careful work and environmental history holds the key to determining that past exposure has occurred. As discussed previously, the presence of bilateral pleural plaques or demonstration of asbestos bodies in lavage or on biopsy also can aid in the assessment of exposure. Although most algorithms for diagnosis of asbestosis suggest that the combination of histologic analysis plus mineralogic assessment is the most sensitive and specific method of diagnosis, frequently the required biopsy material is unavailable, and such studies are unnecessary in making a probable determination of disease. Even the lung pathophysiologic findings should be considered in context with clinical data. The main considerations in the histologic differential diagnosis include the other pneumoconioses and other causes and agents of pulmonary fibrosis such as pharmaceutical drugs, metal dusts, infectious agents, autoimmune disorders, and idiopathic pulmonary fibrosis.

In the absence of lung histologic and mineralogic analysis, the clinical diagnosis of asbestosis can be made with reasonable confidence on the basis of the following criteria:

- History of significant asbestos exposure
- Appropriate time interval between exposure and disease detection (latency)
- Radiographic evidence of bilateral lung fibrosis by chest radiograph or HRCT (especially with coexisting pleural plaques)

Helpful, but less essential criteria include evidence of restrictive impairment of lung function, abnormalities of gas exchange, bilateral inspiratory crackles (rales), and digital clubbing.

TREATMENT

At present, no cure exists for asbestosis, and no benefit from the use of corticosteroids or other immunosuppressive therapy has been documented. After exposure and early disease have occurred, no prophylactic measures are available.

Medical management in cases of asbestosis focuses on the following interventions:

- Supplemental oxygen therapy in the face of hypoxemia or pulmonary hypertension
- Treatment of intercurrent infections
- Treatment of right ventricular failure in advanced disease
- Immunization for influenza virus and pneumococcal infections
- Appropriate medical documentation of the degree of physical impairment and support and referral of the patient to relevant agencies to apply for workers' compensation benefits if exposure was occupational
- Education on the signs and symptoms of lung cancer and mesothelioma
- Assistance in smoking cessation for current smokers who have asbestosis, to help reduce the risk of lung cancer
- Cessation of ongoing asbestos exposure—always advisable, because it may slow disease progression, as indicated by experimental evidence

In the United States, patients with a diagnosis of asbestosis and occupational exposure to asbestos may apply for workers' compensation benefits. Compensation may be granted on appropriate medical documentation of the degree of physical impairment in combination with employment and exposure requirements. Workers who have evidence of pleural plaques, also referred to as pleural asbestosis, also may be eligible for compensation in some programs, with or without evidence of coexisting pulmonary asbestosis.

CLINICAL COURSE

The prognosis for patients with asbestosis varies widely. It is dependent in part on the magnitude of exposure. In 1906, the disease was almost uniformly fatal by the third decade of life. Today, however, with fewer exposures and shorter exposure times, and with superior detection and supportive care, few patients demonstrate such severe progression of their disease. After removal from exposure, progression usually is slow and occurs in 5% to 40% of patients over approximately a decade of follow-up. Thus, if clinical deterioration occurs over a period of days or weeks, the clinician must look first for other explanations, such as infection or malignancy. Many patients may remain mildly symptomatic for many years and show little or no objective signs of disease progression, whereas others show steady, inexorable decline in lung function, gas exchange, worsening symptoms, development of end-stage respiratory insufficiency, and cor pulmonale with right ventricular failure.

Patients with asbestosis are at increased risk for intercurrent lung infections and lung cancer. The best prognosis is found in those workers who have the lowest ILO profusion scores (i.e., chest radiographs that show the fewest irregular opacities) at the time of termination of exposure. Multiple studies demonstrate that those with the greatest average and cumulative dust exposures tend to have higher initial profusions of small opacities on chest radiographs and more rapid disease progression.

Tobacco smoking also contributes to radiographic evidence of disease severity. Tobacco smoking has been shown to increase risk for development of asbestos-related fibrosis and asbestos-induced lung cancer. Several studies have proposed that smoking enhances the development of interstitial fibrosis in workers exposed to asbestos.

On the basis of National Center for Health Statistics data through 2005, for U.S. residents the age-adjusted mortality rate attributable to asbestosis began to plateau after 2000, but only after having risen from an age-adjusted mortality rate of 0.54 per 1 million population in 1968 to 6.03 per 1 million in 2005. Mortality rates are much higher among men than among women, and the age at which people die of asbestosis has risen from a median of 60 years in 1968 to approximately 79 years in 2005. In 2005, asbestosis resulted in more than 14,000 years of potential lives lost due to reduced life expectancy. Lung cancer is a significant contributing cause of increased mortality rates among patients with asbestosis.

ASBESTOS-RELATED, NONMALIGNANT PLEURAL DISORDERS

The most common pleural changes caused by asbestos are pleural plaques, with or without pleural calcification and diffuse pleural thickening. Presence of pleural thickening is a marker of exposure. Pleural changes are now known to contribute to the lung function abnormalities seen in asbestos-exposed workers. Both types of pleural alteration contribute independently to restrictive lung physiology (reduced vital capacity), reduced lung compliance, and diminished diffusing capacity. Of asbestos-exposed construction workers, 20% to 60% demonstrate chest radiographic evidence of pleural disease, which is remarkable in light of the insensitivity of the radiograph.

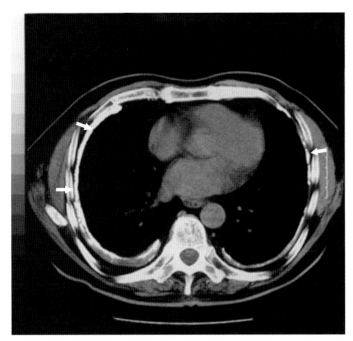

Figure 52-5 Pleural plaque. This conventional computed tomography scan of the thorax, obtained in an asbestos worker, shows extensive bilateral pleural calcifications (*arrows*).

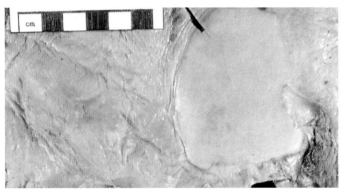

Figure 52-6 The gross pathologic appearance of a pleural plaque adjacent to the diaphragm in a specimen from a construction worker. The benign pleural plaques that form as a consequence of asbestos inhalation have a smooth, shiny appearance and usually are well circumscribed.

Circumscribed pleural plaques that involve the parietal pleura usually are symmetric and bilateral, most commonly between the fifth and eighth ribs toward the posterolateral aspects of the thorax (**Figure 52-5**); they also frequently involve the diaphragmatic pleura (**Figure 52-6**). These lesions remain discrete. Thus, if radiographic evidence of more diffuse thickening is found, either mesothelioma or diffuse pleural thickening must be considered. On histologic examination, pleural plaques are seen to be hyalinized, acellular, avascular masses, and they rarely contain asbestos bodies. They have a tendency to calcify, which can be mistaken for nodular infiltrates on the chest radiograph. Although the ILO classification system has an elaborate section devoted to characterization of pleural abnormalities on the chest radiograph, interreader agreement is relatively low. Because HRCT is more sensitive than chest radiography in the detection of pleural plaques, it helps to determine past asbestos inhalation, because these plaques are pathognomonic for that exposure. Also, HRCT helps to differentiate plaques from extrapleural fat pads. Asbestosis can occur in the absence

of pleural disease, and inversely, pleural disease can occur without underlying pulmonary fibrosis, although autopsy studies suggest that when pleural changes are seen, histopathologic features of asbestosis often are evident even if the radiograph is normal in appearance. Pleural plaques rarely, if ever, undergo malignant transformation.

Diffuse pleural thickening involves both parietal and visceral pleura and is strongly associated with previous, benign asbestos-related pleural effusions. It also may develop when subpleural parenchymal fibrosis extends to the visceral pleura. Diffuse pleural thickening most commonly is located in the lower thorax, can blunt the costophrenic angles, and may be either unilateral or bilateral. Because it is so diffuse, this form of pleural thickening can produce dyspnea on exertion and dry cough, as well as loss of lung function. Other conditions that can induce similar diffuse thickening include past tuberculosis, thoracic surgery, chest trauma with hemorrhage, adverse drug reactions, and infection.

After direct contact of asbestos fibers pleura, an inflammatory, exudative, and often hemorrhagic effusion can develop. It is asymptomatic in two thirds of cases but can be associated with acute chest pain, with or without fever. It can occur in the presence or absence of asbestosis. Its incidence in asbestos-exposed workers has been estimated to be less than 5%. Although it can be the first manifestation of asbestos-related disease, the mean latency period for benign, asbestos-related pleural effusions is 30 years. These effusions often resolve spontaneously but recur in approximately one third of cases. The regression may be associated with pain. The consequences include not only diffuse pleural thickening but also the formation of adhesive fibrothorax. Benign pleural effusion is considered a diagnosis of exclusion.

Rounded atelectasis, although uncommon, is important to recognize because of its tendency to mimic lung tumors. It is thought to occur when visceral pleural thickening invaginates and folds on the lung parenchyma, resulting in atelectasis; CT is the preferred method of detecting its typical cicatricial pattern. Malignancy has only rarely been described in areas of rounded atelectasis. A positron emission tomography scan usually shows no abnormality in rounded atelectasis and may help differentiate the lesion from a lung cancer.

CONTROVERSIES AND PITFALLS

The threshold of asbestos exposure below which asbestosis will not occur is unclear, so any asbestos exposure carries some potential risk of asbestos-related disease. Prevention is superior to treatment of disease, because there is no cure. The best preventive measure is to eliminate inhalational exposure by the following measures or precautions:

- Not working with asbestos
- Not disturbing asbestos in buildings or other locations in which it has been used in the past
- Encapsulating exposed areas of friable asbestos
- Having asbestos removed by personnel experienced in asbestos abatement technologies

Substituting materials that have less toxicity must be considered in industrial applications. When asbestos substitutes are not available, appropriately designed and maintained engineering controls, such as local exhaust ventilation systems, must be in place. Personal respiratory protection is appropriate for short periods of exposure or when other controls are not feasible. Such respirators must be appropriately fitted to the person and tested for the degree of protection they afford the worker by quantitative fit testing. Showering and changing of work clothes at the end of work shifts will help to eliminate take-home exposures. Workers must be educated about the combined risks of asbestos exposure and smoking for lung cancer and must be counseled to avoid future asbestos exposure. Companies that use asbestos must maintain strict compliance with government regulations on permissible exposure limits and appropriate medical surveillance of workers.

SUGGESTED READINGS

American Thoracic Society: Diagnosis and initial management of non-malignant diseases related to asbestos, *Am J Respir Crit Care Med* 170:691–715, 2004.

Burgess WA: Asbestos products, In Burgess WA, editor: *Recognition of health hazards in industry*, New York, 1995, John Wiley & Sons, pp 443–451.

Craighead JE, Abraham JL, Churg A, et al: The pathology of asbestos-associated disease of the lung and pleural cavities: diagnostic criteria and proposed grading scheme, *Arch Pathol Lab Invest* 106:544–595, 1982.

Division of Respiratory Disease Studies: National Institute for Occupational Safety and Health (NIOSH) *Work-related lung disease surveillance report (DHHS [NIOSH] publication no. 2003–2111)*, Washington, DC, 2002, U.S. Government Printing Office.

Hillerdal G: Rounded atelectasis: clinical experience with 74 patients, *Chest* 9:836–841, 1989.

International Labor Office: *International classification of radiographs of pneumoconiosis*, Geneva, Switzerland, 2003, International Labor Organization.

Kamp DW, Weitzman SA: The molecular basis of asbestos induced lung injury, *Thorax* 54:638–652, 1999.

Peipins LA, Lewin M, Campolucci S, et al: Radiographic abnormalities and exposure to asbestos-contaminated vermiculite in the community of Libby, Montana, USA, *Environ Health Perspectives* 111:1753–1759, 2003.

Roggli VL, Gibbs AR, Attanoos R, et al: Pathology of asbestosis—an update of the diagnostic criteria: report of the Asbestosis Committee of the College of American Pathologists and Pulmonary Pathology Society, *Arch Pathol Lab Med* 134:462–480, 2010.

Tossavainen A: International expert meeting on new advances in the radiology and screening of asbestos-related diseases, *Scand J Work Environ Health* 26:449–454, 2000.

Welch LS, Haile E, Dement J, Michaels D: Change in prevalence of asbestos-related disease among sheet metal workers 1986 to 2004, *Chest* 131:863–869, 2007.

Yamamoto S: Histopathological features of pulmonary asbestosis with particular emphasis on the comparison with those of usual interstitial pneumonia, *Osaka City Med J* 43:225–242, 1997.

Zhao XH, Jia G, Liu YQ, et al: Association between polymorphisms of DNA repair gene *XRCC1* and DNA damage in asbestos-exposed workers, *Biomed Environ Sci* 19:232–238, 2006.

Chapter **53**

Connective Tissue Diseases

J.C. Grutters • J.-W.J. Lammers

Connective tissue diseases (CTDs) are generally referred to as a group of systemic disorders with abnormalities in the tissues containing collagen and elastin. Usually, CTDs are characterized by overactivity of the immune system from unknown causes resulting in production of autoantibodies. Pathologic changes are often seen in the lungs of these patients and may be the site of initial manifestation of the systemic disease. All compartments of the respiratory system can be involved, from pleura, airways, and alveolar parenchyma through the pulmonary vasculature. These anatomic regions can be affected either in isolation or in combination, producing a variety of clinical presentations. Furthermore, the pulmonary manifestations of CTDs need to be separated from the effects of therapy (drug reactions, opportunistic infections).

EPIDEMIOLOGY

Specific CTDs include the following:

- *Rheumatoid arthritis* (RA) is the most common CTD and occurs worldwide in approximately 1% of the adult population.
- *Systemic sclerosis* (SSc) has a prevalence of approximately 10 in 100,000 population, with a female/male ratio of 4:1 to 9:1.
- *Polymyositis/dermatomyositis* (PM/DM) is relatively rare, affecting 2 to 10 per 1 million people; has a bimodal age distribution, with an early peak at 5 to 15 years and a later peak at 50 to 60; and occurs three to four times more often in women.
- *Mixed connective tissue disease* (MCTD) has a prevalence that has not been precisely defined but probably approximates 1 in 10,000 people. Mixed disease is more common in women, and most patients present in the second or third decade of life.
- *Systemic lupus erythematosus* (SLE) occurs in up to 1 in 2000 individuals, with a female/male ratio of 10:1.
- *Sjögren syndrome* (SS) has a prevalence of 0.5% to 1% in the general population for primary SS and of 10% to 30% in patients with other autoimmune disorders (secondary SS). SS predominantly affects middle-aged women.

Other CTDs include relapsing polychondritis and ankylosing spondylitis.

PULMONARY INVOLVEMENT

Estimates of the prevalence of pulmonary involvement in CTDs vary widely, depending on the investigated cohort and the methods used to detect lung abnormality. For parenchymal disease, the highest prevalence is seen in histologic or autopsy studies and high-resolution computed tomography (HRCT), which often demonstrates abnormalities not seen on chest radiography.

Systemic sclerosis shows the highest prevalence of *interstitial pneumonia* (IP) (±80% nonspecific) and vascular disease among the CTDs. Autopsy studies indicate that at least some degree of pulmonary fibrosis is present in up to 75% of SSc patients, and vascular disease occurs in approximately 30%. RA and PM/DM also show relatively high prevalence of certain degrees of lung fibrosis, but clinically overt disease occurs less often and is similar to SSc (~5%). Compared with SSc patients, those with RA or PM/DM complicated by lung fibrosis show higher frequency of *usual interstitial pneumonia* (UIP) and *organizing pneumonia* (OP). Of all pulmonary manifestations in CTDs, pleural disease is probably the most common, especially in RA and SLE. **Table 53-1** summarizes the relative frequencies of the major respiratory complications, including IP subtypes, across the various CTDs.

GENETICS

There is increasing evidence of a genetic predisposition for CTDs. For example, RA is strongly associated with the major histocompatibility complex (MHC) Class II gene product HLA-DR4; up to 70% of patients with definite RA express HLA-DR4 versus 28% of control subjects. Evidence for genetic factors in SSc is supported by familial clustering, increased prevalence in twin studies, the high frequency of autoimmune disorders and autoantibodies in family members of SSc patients, and differences in prevalence and clinical manifestations among different ethnic groups. Strong genetic associations have been found between HLA-DRB1*11 and HLA-DPB1*1301 and diffuse SSc, and some evidence suggests an amino acid motif shared by the different MHC Class II susceptibility alleles that may be pivotal in predisposing to autoantibody formation.

GENETIC RISK FACTORS FOR PULMONARY COMPLICATIONS

In SSc and RA in particular, several genetic factors are specifically associated with pulmonary complications. In SSc, carriage of HLA-DRB1*11(04) and DPB1*1301 alleles is associated with lung fibrosis and DRB1*04 and DRB1*08 with pulmonary hypertension, related to the presence of anticentromere autoantibodies (ACAs). ACA positivity has also been shown to associate with carriage of a functional tumor necrosis factor promoter variant (TNF-863A). This and other genetic findings

| Table 53-1 | Relative Frequencies of Pulmonary Manifestations in Connective Tissue Diseases |

Pulmonary Manifestation	RA	SSc	PM/DM	MCTD	SLE	SS
Interstitial pneumonias	++	+++	++	++	+	+
Usual interstitial pneumonia	++	+	+	+	+	+
Nonspecific interstitial pneumonia	+	+++	++	+	+	+
Organizing pneumonia (COP)	+	±	++	+	+	+
Diffuse alveolar damage (AIP)	±		±	±	+	
Lymphocytic interstitial pneumonia	+				±	++
Follicular bronchiolitis	±					+
Constrictive bronchiolitis	+		±	±	±	
Bronchiectasis	++				±	±
Pleural involvement	+++			++	+++	±
Pulmonary hypertension		+++	+	++	++	±
Alveolar hemorrhage	±				+	
Respiratory muscle weakness		±	++		++	

AIP, Acute interstitial pneumonia; *COP,* cryptogenic organizing pneumonia; *MCTD,* mixed connective tissue disease; *PM/DM,* polymyositis/dermatomyositis; *RA,* rheumatoid arthritis; *SSc,* systemic sclerosis; *SLE,* systemic lupus erythematosus; *SS,* Sjögren syndrome.
+++, Common; ++, fairly frequent; +, occasional; ±, rare or very rare.

as yet have no clinical implication, although in the case of TNF-α, they suggest a different pathogenetic role of this cytokine across different SSc subsets. In RA, there is an association between obliterative bronchiolitis (OB) and the expression of histocompatibility antigens HLA-B40 and DR1, which implicates a genetic risk factor.

PATHOGENESIS

INTERSTITIAL FIBROSIS

In CTDs the current concept is that interstitial fibrosis occurs in response to a persistent inflammatory stimulus, causing extended or repetitive tissue damage, and that fibrosis can be considered as an inappropriate response to injury or excessive wound healing. Activation and interaction of both the innate and the adaptive immune system and interaction with extravascular tissue promote the production and secretion of inflammatory mediators, including free radicals, cytokines, and chemokines. Along with growth factors and proteolytic enzymes, together these mediators modulate mesenchymal cell phenotypes and induce synthesis, deposition, and accumulation of extracellular matrix components within the affected tissues. As part of the regulatory process, there is often an upregulation of connective tissue matrix protein breakdown enzymes (e.g., collagenase) and other metalloproteinases and serine proteases (e.g., elastase), which can cause damage to the original architecture. Over time, these processes cause extensive tissue remodeling, with scar tissue substituting for normal tissue architecture and structures.

Numerous lines of evidence suggest that autoimmune antibodies play a key role in the inflammatory process that precedes the development of fibrosis. Reactivity to the nuclear autoantigen topoisomerase I (Scl70) is rarely seen other than with SSc and is strongly associated with lung fibrosis. Recently, the serum of SSc patients was found to contain stimulatory antibodies to the platelet-derived growth factor receptor, which can selectively induce intracellular transcription factors and

reactive oxygen species and stimulate type I collagen-gene expression and myofibroblast phenotype conversion in normal human fibroblasts.

VASCULAR DISEASE

Pulmonary vessels may be involved by inflammation *(vasculitis)* or by concentric fibrosis formation. Vasculitis can affect all levels of the pulmonary circulation. Pulmonary capillaritis usually manifests as diffuse alveolar hemorrhage. The exact pathogenesis of vasculitis is not known, but in some syndromes such as SLE, it is thought to result from immune complex deposition.

Concentric fibrosis of small arterioles will give rise to pulmonary artery hypertension. The pathogenesis of pulmonary hypertension in CTDs is complex, with no single unifying hypothesis at present. Potential etiologies are autoimmune antibodies (e.g., antifibrillarin, antiendothelial, or anticentromere antibodies) and enhanced vasoreactivity. Several reports suggest that dysregulation of the pulmonary vascular tone may contribute to CTD-related pulmonary hypertension ("pulmonary Raynaud's hypothesis"). The observation of decreased nitric oxide (NO) production in the lungs of patients with SSc and pulmonary hypertension supports that endothelial dysfunction contributes to altered regulation of pulmonary vascular tone and development of pulmonary hypertension. Other etiologies might be involved as well, including increased endothelin-1 (ET-1), platelet activation, and oxidant stress.

LUNG PATHOLOGY

AIRWAY PATHOLOGY

The CTDs may affect all parts of the airways. Usually, the pathology is characterized by diffuse inflammatory infiltrates in and around the walls of the larger and smaller airways and sometimes in their lumina. It is usually chronic in nature but may be a mixture of acute and chronic. Persistent inflammatory activity can cause damage to normal airway structures, which may induce wound-healing responses that lead to the accumulation of scar tissue in and around airways. In some conditions, such as relapsing polychondritis, specific anatomic structures may be involved.

Chronic Bronchitis/Bronchiolitis

Chronic bronchitis or bronchiolitis refers to a variable, intense, nonspecific chronic inflammatory cell infiltrate within the bronchial or bronchiolar walls. In SS the infiltrate tends to involve the seromucinous glands, leading to glandular atrophy and a "dry" trachea.

Follicular Bronchitis/Bronchiolitis

Follicular bronchitis or bronchiolitis (FB) is characterized by prominent peribronchial or peribronchiolar lymphoid follicles, with a minor interstitial inflammatory component. Compression of the airway lumina can lead to obstruction and intraluminal acute inflammatory cell infiltrate, plus pneumonia in some cases. FB is part of the spectrum of pulmonary lymphoid hyperplasia, with FB peribronchiolar in localization at one end and *lymphocytic interstitial pneumonia* (LIP) showing interstitial predominance at the other end. Both FB and LIP are rarely found in an idiopathic setting, and their recognition should always prompt investigation for an underlying CTD.

Obliterative Bronchiolitis

Obliterative bronchiolitis (OB) is thought to begin with damage of the respiratory epithelium of terminal bronchioles, leading to the formation of chronic inflammatory granulation tissue, often laid down in a circumferential pattern causing narrowing of the airways. Disease progression leads to obliteration of terminal bronchioles by dense fibrous tissue, with sparing of the respiratory bronchioles and alveoli (**Figure 53-1**).

Organizing pneumonia (OP) is one of the seven entities that constitute IP and has been confused with OB because of the previous term "bronchiolitis obliterans organizing pneumonia" (BOOP). In cryptogenic OP, patchy filling of alveoli with buds of granulation tissue may extend into respiratory bronchioles, but not terminal bronchioles.

Bronchiectasis

Bronchiectasis is defined as permanent abnormal dilation of the airways, usually associated with an inflammatory cell infiltrate. It has many causes, including most CTDs.

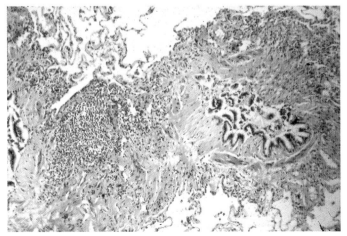

Figure 53-1 Lung biopsy of patient with rheumatoid arthritis (RA), showing constrictive bronchiolitis.

PARENCHYMAL PATHOLOGY

Alveolar parenchymal disease in CTDs usually involves the IPs and sometimes other rare conditions such as alveolar hemorrhage and amyloidosis.

Interstitial Pneumonias

Interstitial pneumonia is now used as a term to indicate the presence of diffuse inflammatory and/or fibrosing lung disease, either idiopathic or in the context of CTDs. In the past the term "fibrosing alveolitis" was often used for this condition. The past decade has seen considerable refinement in the recognition of pathologic IP patterns. For idiopathic IPs, there are presently seven histologic patterns: usual interstitial pneumonia (UIP), nonspecific interstitial pneumonia (NSIP; with a cellular and fibrotic subgroup), cryptogenic organizing pneumonia (COP), acute interstitial pneumonia (AIP; with diffuse alveolar damage [DAD]), lymphocytic interstitial pneumonia (LIP), desquamative interstitial pneumonia (DIP), and respiratory bronchiolitis interstitial lung disease (RBILD). Use of this classification seems consistent and reliable and provides prognostic information for idiopathic disease.

In patients with UIP on lung biopsy and HRCT characteristics compatible with UIP, and with no known cause or association, the diagnosis of idiopathic UIP, *idiopathic pulmonary fibrosis*, is justified and carries a poor prognosis, especially compared with idiopathic NSIP. However, this prognostic difference between idiopathic UIP and NSIP is not necessarily the case in patients with CTD. Those with a UIP pattern on biopsy have a better chance of response to treatment and better prognosis than their counterparts with idiopathic disease.

Both DIP and RBILD are strongly associated with smoking and might not belong in the "idiopathic" IP classification system. Moreover, only small numbers of patients with histologic patterns of DIP and RBILD have been reported in series relating to CTDs, and many of these were smokers. Therefore, these two IP entities are unlikely to be causally related to CTD. **Table 53-2** summarizes the histopathologic characteristics of the IPs typically seen in CTDs.

Other Parenchymal Disorders

Other parenchymal disorders that can sometimes be found in CTDs include diffuse alveolar hemorrhage, amyloidosis, eosinophilic pneumonia, and alveolar proteinosis. In *alveolar hemorrhage*, biopsy shows a combination of intraalveolar hemorrhage and hemosiderosis. The hemosiderin, which provides evidence of previous bleeding, is largely contained within alveolar macrophages but may also impregnate elastin in a blood vessel. Alveolar hemorrhage is usually caused by small-vessel vasculitis of the lung, which is a rare pulmonary manifestation of CTDs, especially in SLE.

Amyloidosis is characterized by extracellular deposition of a proteinaceous substance that can be visualized under polarized light after Congo red staining. Amyloidosis is seen most often in relation to SS, with lymphoid hyperplasia and causing cystic changes.

Eosinophilic pneumonia is characterized by the expansion of alveoli by eosinophils, macrophages, and fibrinous debris, often with eosinophils involving the interstitium, as well as focal intraalveolar organization. This condition is often related to drug exposure in patients with CTD, but has also been attributed to RA itself.

Alveolar proteinosis is marked by accumulation of acellular, finely granular lipoproteinaceous material in alveolar spaces. It has been described in dermatomyositis.

Table 53-2 Interstitial Pneumonias in Connective Tissue Disease: Major Histopathologic Characteristics

Type	Histopathologic Characteristics
Usual interstitial pneumonia (UIP)	Fibrosis with honeycombing, fibroblast foci; anatomic destruction; little inflammatory cell infiltrate; normal/near-normal intervening lung parenchyma (temporal heterogeneity)
Nonspecific interstitial pneumonia (NSIP)	Variable interstitial inflammation and fibrosis; fibroblastic foci absent or scarce; uniformity of changes within biopsy specimen
Organizing pneumonia (OP; or cryptogenic OP)	Patchy filling of alveoli by buds of granulation tissue that may extend into bronchioles (Masson bodies); preservation of lung architecture
Lymphocytic interstitial pneumonia (LIP)	Extensive lymphocytic infiltration in the interstitium often associated with peribronchiolar lymphoid follicles (follicular bronchiolitis)
Diffuse alveolar damage (DAD)*	Diffuse alveolar septal thickening by inflammatory cell infiltrate, hyperplastic pneumocytes, hyaline membranes, air space organization

*In acute interstitial pneumonia (AIP).

PULMONARY HYPERTENSION

The histologic features in CTD-associated pulmonary hypertension vary in relation to the degree of raised pulmonary artery pressure. In mild pulmonary hypertension, the histologic features are typically those of medial hypertrophy. With progression of the disease, marked intimal fibrous thickening and eventually plexiform lesions can be found. These histologic changes are essentially the same as those in idiopathic pulmonary hypertension. Early changes need to be distinguished from secondary changes related to an associated IP.

PULMONARY MALIGNANCY

There is an increased risk for lung cancer in CTDs, especially in patients with lung fibrosis who also smoke. The most common neoplasm in SSc is *adenocarcinoma*, in some cases with a bronchoalveolar pattern. Patients with Sjögren syndrome have an increased risk of pulmonary lymphoma. This is usually a marginal zone, non-Hodgkin lymphoma of mucosa-associated lymphoid tissue (MALT). Preexisting follicular bronchiolitis or LIP is a risk factor (±5% may develop lymphoma).

CLINICAL FEATURES

RHEUMATOID ARTHRITIS

The clinical hallmark of RA is an inflammatory erosive arthritis of small and large joints. Although rheumatoid factor (RF) has a reasonable sensitivity (60%), its specificity is often low (90%). Recently, anticyclic citrullinated peptide (CCP) antibodies have been identified that combine a high sensitivity (75%) with an excellent specificity (97%) for the diagnosis of RA. Extraarticular manifestations of RA are associated with RF, but interestingly not with anti-CCP antibodies. RA can involve any part of the respiratory tract, including the cricoarytenoid joint,

airways, parenchyma, and pleura. Usually, only one of these disorders is predominant in a single individual, although parenchymal changes are often associated with airway disease (on HRCT).

Pleural Disease

Rheumatoid arthritis–associated pleural disease can be asymptomatic, although presenting symptoms and signs can include fever, pleuritic chest pain, and shortness of breath. Pleural effusions are generally small and unilateral, but rarely may occur in large volume or bilaterally. The fluid is exudative, with high protein and lactate dehydrogenase levels and low glucose concentration. Rheumatoid effusions usually have a low pH (<7.2) and are often paucicellular (<10,000/mL), with lymphocytic or polymorphonuclear predominance. Cytologic examination may reveal lipid droplets in the cytoplasm of neutrophils, similar to the phagocytes seen in the joint fluid of arthritic patients and known as RA cells, but these may occur in other conditions. Immunocytochemistry may reveal IgM (RF) and phagocytosed immune complexes in granulocytes and histiocytes. Thoracoscopy may reveal a fine granular appearance to the pleural wall. Histopathologic examination of these micronodules may show a linear granulomatous reaction with the mesothelium replaced by palisading histiocytes. Histologic examination can also show fibrosis with often prominent chronic inflammation, including hyperplastic lymphoid follicles. In general, however, pleural biopsy is especially helpful for exclusion of other causes of pleural disease.

Airways Disease

Bronchiectasis is a frequent finding on HRCT in patients with RA (up to 70%), but in most patients, it is asymptomatic.

Obliterative bronchiolitis is a serious complication of RA, and seems to be more common in women. OB usually occurs in patients who are RF positive and have well-established joint disease. In the past, penicillamine, which is rarely used now, was associated with development of OB in patients with RA. Also, a relationship with gold therapy has been suggested. Patients most often are initially seen with dyspnea and a nonproductive cough, which can worsen rapidly. The chest radiograph is usually normal but may show signs of hyperinflation (**Figure 53-2**) and in later stages fibrobullous degeneration (**Figure 53-3**). The diagnosis of OB should be considered in any patient with RA with progressive dyspnea and cough who has rapidly progressive airflow obstruction. Characteristic HRCT findings of OB consist of areas of decreased attenuation and vascularity with blood flow redistribution, resulting in areas of increased lung attenuation and vascularity ("mosaic perfusion" pattern), which is accentuated on expiratory scans (**Figure 53-4**). The prognosis is poor in RA patients with OB.

Interstitial Pneumonias

The prevalence of clinically significant IP in patients with RA is estimated at 5%. IP is seen more often in men than in women, especially in the context of a high RF titer and severe articular disease. The pathologic patterns are diverse, but in contrast to other CTDs, a UIP pattern is relatively common (**Figure 53-5**). Symptoms are nonspecific and include progressive dyspnea and nonproductive cough. Dyspnea may appear late because of physical inactivity secondary to polyarthritis. Most patients have fine bibasilar crackles, but digital clubbing is less common than in patients with idiopathic pulmonary fibrosis (IPF). Lung function tests usually reveal a restrictive defect with normal airflow and reduced diffusion capacity (DLCO). HRCT is the

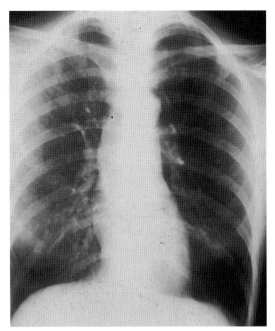

Figure 53-2   Chest radiograph of patient with rheumatoid arthritis showing hyperinflation caused by constrictive bronchiolitis.

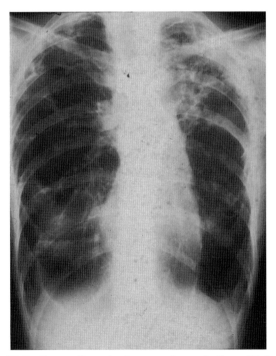

Figure 53-3   Chest radiograph of same patient as in Figure 53-2 a few years later, showing evolution toward fibrosis and bullous degeneration.

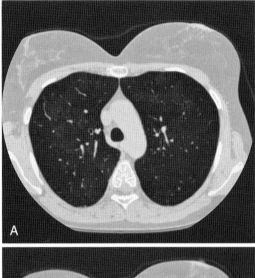

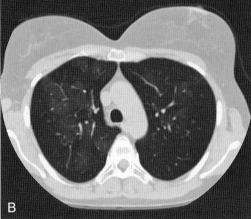

Figure 53-4   Characteristic findings on high-resolution computed tomography (HRCT) in 36-year-old woman with rheumatoid arthritis and severe constrictive bronchiolitis (FEV$_1$ of 35% predicted). **A,** Inspiratory HRCT scan shows geographic pattern, with areas of increased (normal) and decreased (air trapping) attenuation. **B,** This pattern is accentuated on the expiratory scan.

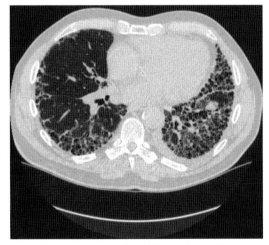

Figure 53-5   Chest CT scan (April 2005) in patient with seropositive rheumatoid arthritis, showing usual interstitial pneumonia (UIP) pattern.

most appropriate investigation to detect IP and is also useful in follow-up. UIP patterns on HRCT appear similar in RA and IPF, but coexisting pleural effusion or (necrobiotic) nodules may help in the differential diagnosis. In general, UIP associated with RA tends to follow a more benign course than the idiopathic form, but patients may develop end-stage respiratory failure (**Figure 53-6**).

Pulmonary Nodules

Pulmonary nodules are an uncommon manifestation in RA. Their occurrence is strongly associated with positive RF and

presence of extrapulmonary (i.e., subcutaneous) rheumatoid nodules. In some cases the nodules may antedate clinical arthritis. Their radiologic appearance is not specific and may mimic malignancy, especially if the lesion is solitary. Nodules may vary in size from millimeters to 7 cm. The nodules are most often

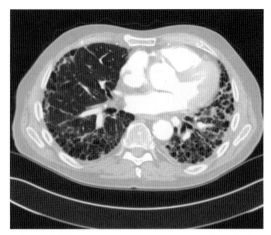

Figure 53-6 Stable lung fibrosis on follow-up chest CT scan (September 2009) of same patient as in Figure 53-5, illustrating a more benign course of usual interstitial pneumonia in rheumatoid arthritis than usually seen in the idiopathic form.

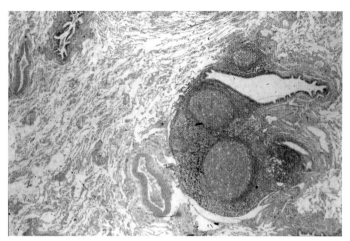

Figure 53-7 Lung biopsy showing hyperplasia of bronchus-associated lymphoid tissue (BALT) in patient with rheumatoid arthritis.

found in the subpleural regions of the upper lung zones but may also be found in other parts of the lung. Histologically, pulmonary nodules show a central zone of fibrinoid necrosis surrounded by a palisading rim of epithelioid histiocytes, together with lymphocytes and plasma cells (*necrobiotic* nodule). Cavitation may occur and can lead to complications such as hemoptysis, secondary infections, and pneumothorax in the case of perforation to the pleura. During follow-up, uncomplicated pulmonary nodules may spontaneously resolve and recur, often in association with the size of extrapulmonary nodules and depending on disease activity status.

Caplan syndrome (rheumatoid pneumoconiosis) is the coexistence of RA with pneumoconiosis, typically coal worker's pneumoconiosis or silicosis. The associated nodules differ from rheumatoid nodules by their large size and the presence of circumferential bands or "arcs of dust" within the necrotic centers of the lesions.

Lymphoid Hyperplasia

Hyperplasia of lymphatic tissue is frequently seen in RA. In particular, lymph nodes, spleen, and bronchus-associated lymphatic tissue (BALT) may be hyperplastic (**Figure 53-7**).

SYSTEMIC SCLEROSIS

Systemic sclerosis can be classified according to American Rheumatism Association criteria. One major criterion and two or more minor criteria (e.g., bibasilar pulmonary fibrosis) are necessary to establish a diagnosis of SSc. A subclassification can be made in *limited* (cutaneous) SSc (lSSc) and *diffuse* (cutaneous) SSc (dSSc). Limited SSc is characterized by skin involvement limited to hands, feet, face, and forearms; presence of anticentromere autoantibodies (ACAs; 60%-70%); Raynaud's phenomenon for years; and a significant incidence of pulmonary hypertension. The acronym CREST (calcinosis, Raynaud's phenomenon, esophageal dysmotility, sclerodactyly, and telangiectasia) fits into this subclassification. Diffuse SSc is characterized by skin involvement on the upper arms and trunk, presence of antitopoisomerase antibodies (Scl70; 40%), and a high incidence of interstitial lung disease (ILD). Furthermore, dSSc is associated with hypertensive crises and renal failure, diffuse gastrointestinal disease, and myocardial involvement.

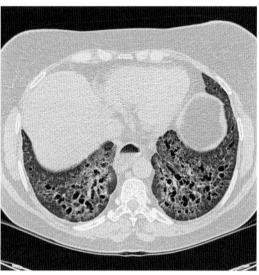

Figure 53-8 Chest high-resolution CT image in patient with systemic sclerosis, showing extensive interstitial fibrosis with traction bronchiectasis (fibrotic nonspecific interstitial pneumonia, fibrotic nonspecific interstitial pneumonia pattern) and ectatic (dilated) esophagus.

Interstitial Pneumonias

Most patients with SSc develop pulmonary manifestations. Patients with diffuse scleroderma and antitopoisomerase-I autoantibodies especially are at high risk for interstitial lung fibrosis. However, the clinical course of it may vary considerably. Although some patients have stable lung function parameters for years, others may have incapacitating or even fatal pulmonary fibrosis.

Lung fibrosis associated with SSc used to be expressed as fibrosing alveolitis (FA) SSc. It was believed that FASSc was indistinguishable from cryptogenic fibrosing alveolitis (CFA) or idiopathic pulmonary fibrosis. The histopathologic substrate of IPF is UIP. Various studies over the past decade, however, clearly demonstrate that histologic and HRCT features of lung fibrosis in SSc are more similar to those found in idiopathic NSIP (**Figure 53-8**).

The most common type of lung fibrosis in SSc is NSIP, with incidence ranging from 55% to 77% of cases. In NSIP, fibrosis and inflammation are more diffuse in involved areas and of the same age throughout the affected lung. On HRCT, fibrotic changes are less coarse, and the proportion of ground-glass opacification is greater than in UIP. A UIP pattern, characterized by honeycomb changes and negligible ground-glass opacity, can also be found in SSc. In contrast to their idiopathic equivalents, SSc patients with UIP or NSIP do not seem to differ in response to immunosuppressive therapy or prognosis, but further studies are needed.

The course of pulmonary fibrosis in SSc is variable and can range from indolent to rapidly progressive. Careful monitoring of longitudinal change of lung function is still regarded as the best means of evaluating disease behavior. Bronchoalveolar lavage (BAL) eosinophilia has also been linked to the progressiveness of lung fibrosis in SSc. The prognosis further depends on the severity of disease at presentation; patients with greater impairment in lung function and more extensive disease on HRCT have higher mortality.

Pulmonary Hypertension

Pulmonary hypertension is typically seen in patients with CREST syndrome. It is usually caused by a precapillary disease process leading to pulmonary artery hypertension. In some patients, pulmonary hypertension is caused by venoocclusive disease or related to severe interstitial fibrosis with hypoxemia. In addition, diastolic dysfunction of the left ventricle, possibly because of cardiac fibrosis, may lead to pulmonary hypertension, defined as mean pulmonary artery pressure higher than 25 mm Hg at rest or higher than 30 mm Hg during exercise in the absence of left-sided heart disease (pulmonary wedge pressure >15 mm Hg). Pulmonary hypertension, both isolated and in association with ILD, occurs in approximately 30% of patients with dSSc and in up to 60% of patients with lSSc (CREST syndrome). In both cases, the presence of pulmonary hypertension significantly worsens the prognosis. Reported survival in patients with SSc and pulmonary hypertension is similar to patients with primary pulmonary hypertension: 2-year survival of approximately 50%.

Other Thoracic Diseases in Sclerosis

In addition to lung fibrosis and pulmonary vascular disease, SSc can be complicated by aspiration pneumonia because of regurgitation of pooled contents from a fibrotic, ectatic esophagus (see Figure 53-8). Aspiration-related infection can be worsened by immunosuppressive therapy, architectural distortion, and traction bronchiectasis caused by fibrotic lung disease, which impairs normal protective clearance mechanisms and increases bacterial colonization of the airways.

Rarely, basal pleural thickening is found, but pleural effusions are unusual.

DERMATOMYOSITIS/POLYMYOSITIS

Polymyositis and dermatomyositis (PM/DM) are rare inflammatory myopathies. Major criteria include symmetric muscle weakness; a muscle biopsy showing inflammatory cell infiltrates and necrosis; elevated muscle enzymes; and a characteristic electromyogram (EMG). The most common pulmonary complications derive indirectly from neuromuscular weakness and directly from diffuse inflammatory manifestations of PM/DM in the lung parenchyma. Furthermore, it may be complicated by pulmonary or extrapulmonary malignancies (PM relative risk, 1.7; DM relative risk, 3.8). Of note, PM/DM may also present as a paraneoplastic syndrome (up to 20% of cases), so it may be difficult to determine which condition arose first.

As in other CTDs, autoantibodies are frequently found in patients with PM/DM. Autoantibodies to a group of cellular enzymes, transfer ribonucleic acid (tRNA) synthetases (anti-Jo1, anti-PL7, anti-PL12) are present in about 30% of patients with PM/DM and are rarely present in other CTDs. Presence of anti-tRNA synthetase antibodies is strongly associated with the occurrence of IPs.

Pulmonary Complications of Muscular Weakness

Muscular weakness can give rise to aspiration pneumonia (as a result of discoordinated swallowing) or respiratory insufficiency (reflecting respiratory muscle dysfunction). Airway protection is critical in patients with PM/DM and severe dysphagia; in severe cases, tracheotomy may be necessary while awaiting the impact of treatment for the underlying myopathy. Clinically significant respiratory muscle weakness has been cited in 7% to 22% of patients with PM/DM, sometimes leading to respiratory insufficiency requiring mechanical ventilatory support or to death. Rarely, bilateral diaphragmatic paralysis has been reported. Respiratory muscle weakness may be the initial presentation of PM/DM, but this is rare. Serial measurements of forced vital capacity (FVC), and maximal static inspiratory and expiratory pressures (PI_{max} and PE_{max}) are useful to diagnose respiratory muscle weakness and monitor the course of the disease.

Interstitial Pneumonias

The most common forms of interstitial lung disease in PM/DM are NSIP and OP. Rarely, other types of IP are found. IP can occur at any point in the disease course. IP onset precedes PM/DM in approximately 20% of cases, but this may be higher, because treatment with immunosuppressive drugs may mask the myopathy, delaying the diagnosis for weeks or even years. Rarely, patients present more acutely, with fevers, dyspnea, and cough evolving over a few days or weeks. In this context, progression to acute respiratory failure may occur. This syndrome resembles idiopathic acute interstitial pneumonia (AIP) and is associated with a histopathologic pattern of DAD (**Figure 53-9**).

In PM/DM, the occurrence of IP is strongly associated with the presence of circulating antisynthetase antibodies (50%-100% of cases). In contrast, antisynthetase antibodies are

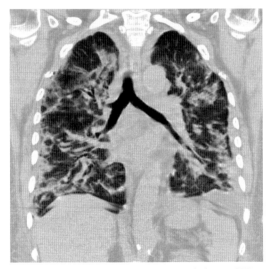

Figure 53-9 High-resolution CT section (coronal plane) of 73-year-old woman presenting with diffuse alveolar damage and organizing pneumonia (proven by video-assisted thoracic surgery lung biopsy) as first manifestation of antisynthetase syndrome (Jo1).

found in less than 5% of patients without diffuse lung disease. This clinical combination, which also includes arthritis, is known as the *antisynthetase syndrome.*

MIXED CONNECTIVE TISSUE DISEASE

Mixed CTD is characterized by the presence of overlapping features of more than one CTD (e.g., Raynaud's phenomenon, synovitis, and/or myositis) and the presence of high titers (>1:1600) of circulating autoantibodies to a nuclear ribonucleoprotein antigen (anti-U1-RNP). Currently, different classification systems are in use for the diagnosis of MCTD, causing difficulty in comparing populations and standardizing clinical evaluation. This is further complicated by the term "overlap syndrome," which is often used for the presence of features of more than one CTD not in the context of high anti-U1-RNP titers, and because some patients have only a few features that defy categorization into one of the major CTDs, but progress to exhibit typical findings of SSc, DM/PM, or SS over time.

Pulmonary complications and their pathologic features resemble those seen in other CTDs. The three most frequent are pleural effusion, interstitial pneumonia, and pulmonary hypertension. Pleural disease in MCTD occurs most frequently in patients with SLE-like clinical features; the pleura are seldom involved in SSc or PM/DM. Interstitial fibrosis most closely resembles interstitial lung involvement in SSc (i.e., showing a histologic pattern of NSIP). OP seems to be relatively infrequent in MCTD, despite a high prevalence in PM/DM. The most serious complication is progressive pulmonary hypertension and cor pulmonale; rapid deterioration and death can occur despite intensive medical intervention. Other causes of pulmonary hypertension include pulmonary vasculitis and pulmonary thromboembolism, especially in MCTD with SLE-like features and circulating antiphospholipid antibodies.

SYSTEMIC LUPUS ERYTHEMATOSUS

Systemic lupus erythematosus is characterized by polyclonal B cell activation and the production of autoantibodies directed against nuclear targets (i.e., double-stranded DNA and anti-Sm antibodies). In contrast, T-cell functions are impaired, resulting in a greater susceptibility to infectious complications.

Pleural disease with or without effusion is the most common pulmonary manifestation of SLE. Diaphragmatic dysfunction or "shrinking lung syndrome" is a rare disorder characterized by reduced lung volumes and normal parenchyma, probably caused by progressive pleural fibrosis or respiratory muscle weakness. Infection is the most common cause of parenchymal disease. Clinically significant IP is a relatively rare complication in patients with SLE (±5%), and usually the course is slowly progressive with stabilization over time. Although difficult to demonstrate, immunohistochemistry may reveal characteristic granular patterns of IgG and complement at the alveolocapillary membrane (**Figure 53-10**). SLE-associated pulmonary hypertension should not be overlooked, especially in the presence of antiphospholipid antibodies, and has been reported in 4% to 14% of patients with SLE, with an overall mortality rate of 25% to 50% at 2 years from the time of diagnosis of pulmonary hypertension. In SLE patients the pulmonary vasculature may be directly involved, or pulmonary hypertension may be related to ILD, diffuse alveolar hemorrhage, airways disease, or thromboembolic disease. Acute lupus pneumonitis/alveolar hemorrhage is a rare pulmonary manifestation in SLE.

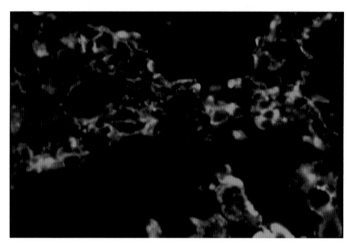

Figure 53-10   Immunohistochemical analysis of lung tissue of patient with systemic lupus erythematosus complicated by interstitial pneumonia, showing characteristic granular patterns of IgG and complement at alveolocapillary membrane.

Antiphospholipid Syndrome

The antiphospholipid syndrome (APS) is a systemic autoimmune disorder characterized by arterial and/or venous thrombosis, recurrent fetal loss (often accompanied by mild to moderate thrombocytopenia), and elevated levels of antiphospholipid antibodies, namely the lupus anticoagulant and/or anticardiolipin antibodies, and/or antibodies to β_2-glycoprotein 1. The APS may be divided into two categories. *Primary* APS occurs in patients without and *secondary* APS occurs in patients with clinical evidence of a major autoimmune disorder (i.e., mainly SLE). Pulmonary manifestations associated with APS include pulmonary embolism and infarction, primary thrombosis of large and small lung vessels, pulmonary capillaritis, pulmonary hypertension, and adult respiratory distress syndrome (ARDS). Also, fibrosing alveolitis has been associated with APS. When multiple organs, systems, and tissues are involved and manifestations develop simultaneously or in less than 1 week, this is known as *catastrophic* APS, which has a mortality greater than 50% despite treatment with full anticoagulation, high-dose corticosteroids and immunosuppressives, and intravenous immune globulin (IVIG). Some evidence suggests therapeutic plasma exchange might improve survival for patients with catastrophic APS.

SJÖGREN SYNDROME

Sjögren syndrome is a slowly progressive autoimmune inflammatory disease affecting the exocrine glands and epithelia in multiple sites, leading to diminished or absent glandular secretions and to a more or less generalized mucosal dryness. SS presents with a wide spectrum, from lacrimal and salivary exocrinopathy to systemic disease, including lung manifestations, and sometimes an associated B cell lymphoma (±5%). The disease can occur alone (primary SS) or in association with almost all of the other CTDs (secondary SS). Pulmonary manifestations have been reported in both the primary and the secondary form. In secondary SS the coexisting CTD influences the pattern of pulmonary expression. **Box 53-1** summarizes the pulmonary manifestations of SS. **Figure 53-11** shows chest HRCT scan consistent with follicular bronchiolitis in a patient with primary SS.

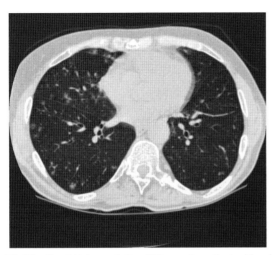

Figure 53-11 Chest high-resolution CT image in patient with primary Sjögren syndrome (SS) and chronic cough, showing pattern consistent with follicular bronchiolitis. Bronchoalveolar lavage (BAL) fluid demonstrated a 57% increase in lymphocytes, and other causes of BAL lymphocytosis were excluded.

Box 53-1 Pulmonary Manifestations in Sjögren Syndrome (SS)

Upper airways disease
    Nasal mucosa infiltration and dryness ("rhina sicca")
    Oral cavity salivary gland involvement (xerostomia)
Lymphocytic infiltration of tracheobronchial submucosal glands
    (xerotrachea)
Subepithelial bronchial and bronchiolar lymphocytic infiltration
    (lymphocytic bronchitis/bronchiolitis)
Lymphoproliferative disorders
    Diffuse lymphoid hyperplasia of lungs (follicular bronchiolitis
      [FB]/lymphoid interstitial pneumonia [LIP])
    Pseudolymphoma
    Lymphomatoid granulomatosis
    Malignant B cell non-Hodgkin lymphoma
Other diffuse interstitial pneumonias
    Usual interstitial pneumonia (UIP)
    Nonspecific interstitial pneumonia (NSIP)
    Organizing pneumonia (OP; or cryptogenic OP)
Multiple lung cysts (often in association with LIP)
Vasculitis and pulmonary hypertension
Pulmonary amyloidosis
Pleural disease (mainly in secondary SS)

RELAPSING POLYCHONDRITIS

Relapsing polychondritis is a rare (<5:1 million) multisystem disease in which recurrent progressive inflammation of cartilaginous structures results in widespread degenerative change. It is considered an autoimmune process, and autoantibodies directed against cartilage and type II collagen have been found. The condition may affect all parts of the body containing cartilage (e.g., nose, ears, joints, ribs). Involvement of the tracheobronchial tree may be found in up to 50% of cases. The diagnosis is generally clinical; **Box 53-2** summarizes the most widely applied diagnostic criteria for relapsing polychondritis. CT may disclose smooth thickening of airway walls, as well as increased airway wall attenuation, with or without calcification. Airway collapse and lobar air trapping can be found in half of patients examined with expiratory CT. Biopsy of affected cartilage is not generally required for a diagnosis but may be pivotal in

---

Box 53-2 Clinical Criteria for Diagnosis of Relapsing Polychondritis*

Bilateral auricular chondritis
Nonerosive, seronegative inflammatory polyarthritis
Nasal chondritis
Ocular inflammation
Respiratory tract involvement (upper/lower)
Cochlear with/without vestibular abnormality

*The presence of three or more criteria is required.

---

atypical cases; auricular biopsy is the most frequent procedure, but rarely biopsy of the tracheal rings may be indicated. Measurement of anti–type II collagen antibody may also be helpful, because it is fairly specific, although only positive in one third of patients with relapsing polychondritis.

Inflammation and destruction of the respiratory cartilage may lead to destruction and obstruction of the glottis, trachea, and bronchi, causing inspiratory and expiratory flow rate limitations, atelectasis, and secondary infections. Pulmonary parenchymal disease is rare, with the exception of vasculitis, which may be present but is often subclinical.

Treatment depends on disease severity. Mild cases may be controlled with nonsteroidal antiinflammatory drugs, whereas relapses may require short-term, high-dose corticosteroids. In life-threatening disease, steroid-resistant disease, and the case of repeated relapses, corticosteroid therapy in combination with an immunosuppressive such as cyclophosphamide should be considered. Tracheostomy may be required for severe glottic or subglottic obstruction, and stenting is occasionally indicated for airway collapse or refractory airway stenosis in the patient with relapsing polychondritis.

ANKYLOSING SPONDYLITIS

Ankylosing spondylitis (AS) is a chronic seronegative spondyloarthritis strongly associated with the MHC antigen HLA-B27, present in 7% of whites and 95% of AS patients. AS is a disease of white males with a prevalence of 0.15%. AS is primarily a chronic inflammatory disease of the vertebral column, but involvement of other parts of the body is common. Nongranulomatous anterior uveitis occurs in up to 25% of patients, and asymptomatic inflammation of the thoracic aorta is present in 20% to 30%. In 10% of patients with AS, clinically important aortic incompetence or dilation of the ascending aorta develops. Pulmonary complications take the form of extrapulmonary restriction or parenchymal disease. Apical fibrobullous disease, with or without cavitation and hilar distortion, is found in some patients, almost exclusively in males. However, AS should always be considered in patients seen with upper lobe fibrosis, present in more than 20% of cases. Of note, a variety of other nonapical parenchymal diseases (e.g., NSIP) may be found in AS patients.

There is no effective treatment against development of apical fibrosis; resistance to corticosteroids is usually seen. In most patients, careful observation without treatment is appropriate, with specific antimicrobial therapy when infectious complications occur. One of the greatest therapeutic dilemmas is the patient with major hemoptysis caused by aspergilloma development in a cavity. First-line treatments include administration of antifungal agents and bronchial artery embolization. When uncontrollable, there may be no option but to proceed to surgical resection of the cavity, usually by lobectomy. However, this surgery carries a high risk of postoperative bronchopleural fistula or empyema and may lead to a fatal outcome.

MARFAN SYNDROME

Marfan syndrome is an inheritable disorder of connective tissue. The condition affects all races and both genders equally, with estimated prevalence of 1 in 5000 (0.02% of population). The mode of inheritance is autosomal dominant with variable penetrance, and 15% to 30% of all cases are caused by de novo mutations. The disorder has been linked to a defect in the *FBN1* gene on chromosome 15, which encodes the glycoprotein fibrillin-1. Fibrillin is essential for the formation of the elastic fibers found in connective tissue, because it provides the scaffolding for tropoelastin.

Patients with Marfan syndrome often have long limbs (arm span/height ratio >1.05) and involvement of the ocular system (e.g., ectopia lentis), cardiovascular (e.g., dilation or dissection of ascending aorta), and skeletal system involvement (e.g., pectus carinatum/excavatum, scoliosis, spondylolisthesis). Pulmonary involvement occurs in approximately 10% of patients and involves apical emphysematous and cystic changes; bullous degeneration may lead to spontaneous pneumothorax. In some cases, upper lobe fibrosis has been described.

BEHÇET SYNDROME

Behçet syndrome is an inflammatory disorder of unknown etiology affecting blood vessels of almost all sizes and types, ranging from small arteries to large vessels and involving veins and arteries. Disease prevalence varies from 1 in 10,000 to 1 in 300,000 worldwide, and it is most common in eastern Mediterranean countries and the Far East. It occurs mainly in young adults with the mean age of onset between 25 and 30 years and is associated with HLA-B51.

Because of the diversity of blood vessels that can be affected, manifestations of Behçet syndrome may occur at many sites throughout the body. Mucocutaneous ulceration is the clinical hallmark, with aphthous oral and genital ulceration seen in almost all patients. Besides ocular lesions (anterior or posterior uveitis or retinal vasculitis) and skin lesions (e.g., erythema nodosum) pseudofolliculitis and papulopustular lesions often occur. Other features include marked arthralgias with synovitis, a predilection to thrombosis, and central nervous system involvement (headaches, meningoencephalitis, cranial nerve palsies, seizures).

Pulmonary involvement is seen in less than 10% of patients with Behçet syndrome. Symptoms include dyspnea, chest pain, and recurrent hemoptysis that can be life threatening. Pathology typically involves aneurysms of the pulmonary artery because of outpouchings of the blood vessel wall caused by inflammation (**Figure 53-12**). Also, arterial and venous thrombosis with pulmonary thromboembolism, pulmonary infarcts, and pleural effusions (in some patients) may occur. In patients with hemoptysis, it is very important to distinguish between aneurysms of the pulmonary artery (with pulmonary-bronchial fistula formation) and pulmonary thromboembolism, because catastrophic pulmonary hemorrhage can occur if the wrong patients are anticoagulated.

Glucocorticoids and other immunosuppressive agents such as cyclophosphamide and azathioprine are the mainstay of therapy to control the vasculitis. In life-threatening situations, lobectomy or pneumonectomy might be considered.

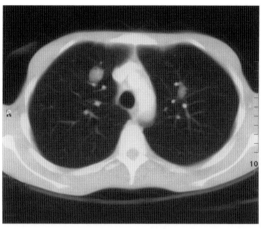

Figure 53-12 CT scan of 27-year-old Moroccan man with Behçet's syndrome initially seen with hemoptysis. The multiple coin-sized consolidations close to central vessels of lung hili proved to be aneurysms on angiography of pulmonary artery.

A forme fruste of Behçet syndrome is known as *Hughes-Stovin syndrome*, defined as the presence of pulmonary artery aneurysm in the setting of systemic thrombosis without extrapulmonary features consistent with Behçet syndrome.

DIAGNOSTIC TESTING

Pulmonary Function Tests

Pulmonary function tests (PFTs) are extremely useful in the identification of clinically relevant parenchymal manifestations of CTDs. Pulmonary fibrosis leads to restrictive lung disease and interferes with gas exchange, resulting in decreased total lung capacity (TLC), vital capacity (VC), and DLCO, but often no decreased flow rates. Follow-up of lung function during the first 6 years of scleroderma symptoms seems helpful for the evaluation of disease progressiveness. The mean percent loss of VC over three 2-year periods in patients with initial PFTs performed during the first 5 years of SSc were 32%, 12%, and 3%, respectively. Thus, careful monitoring of lung function early in the disease, when the greatest loss of lung function occurs, may help identify patients likely to respond to new therapy.

The PFT data also provide important prognostic information. SSc patients with FVC less than 50% predicted have the worst prognosis, with a cumulative 10-year survival close to 50%. Furthermore, DLCO less than 70% predicted in combination with proteinuria and elevated erythrocyte sedimentation rate (ESR) has accurately predicted mortality over 5 years in patients newly presenting with scleroderma.

A reduction in DLCO does not necessarily indicate underlying ILD and can also be a manifestation of pulmonary vascular disease or a combination of both. The VC/DLCO% predicted ratio might be helpful: in pure fibrotic disease, approximately 1; in isolated pulmonary arterial hypertension, usually greater than 1.8; and with a mixture of fibrosis and vasculopathy, VC is moderately decreased but DLCO is even lower, also resulting in an elevated ratio.

Chest Radiography

Chest radiography should be performed in every patient with CTD, regardless of whether they have pulmonary complaints or findings. The pattern of abnormalities might help in the

Table 53-3 Interstitial Pneumonias in Connective Tissue Disease: Major High-Resolution Computed Tomography (HRCT) Imaging Characteristics

Type	HRCT Characteristics
Usual interstitial pneumonia (UIP)	Peripheral, subpleural, and basal distribution; irregular reticular changes with honeycombing; traction bronchiectasis and architectural distortion; minimal ground-glass changes (focal)
Nonspecific interstitial pneumonia (NSIP)	Symmetric, peripheral distribution; basal predominance; more ground-glass attenuation; reticular changes and traction bronchiectasis; honeycombing is not dominant.
Organizing pneumonia (OP; or cryptogenic OP)	Patchy consolidations and/or nodules and/or perilobular opacities; may have a ground-glass component
Lymphocytic interstitial pneumonia (LIP)	Diffuse ground-glass attenuation; centrilobular nodules; septal and bronchovascular thickening; thin-walled cysts
Diffuse alveolar damage (DAD)	Gravity-dependent consolidation; ground-glass opacification, often with lobular sparing; traction bronchiectasis occurs later.

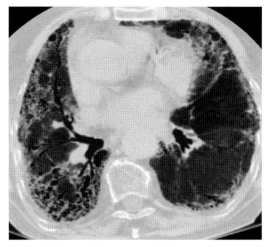

Figure 53-13 High-resolution computed tomography image of usual interstitial pneumonia (UIP) in minimal intensity projection. *(Courtesy Dr. H. W. van Es, St. Antonius Hospital, Nieuwegein, The Netherlands.)*

differential diagnosis of some of the CTDs. If any parenchymal abnormality is seen, HRCT should be performed.

High-Resolution Computed Tomography

Currently, HRCT is the imaging method of choice in evaluating patients with CTD with ILD. It identifies more disease than the chest radiograph, is more specific, and has a greater ability to demonstrate coexisting pleural disease, small airways disease, bronchiectasis, and pulmonary nodules, while also providing diagnostic clues such as esophageal dilation. In addition, HRCT can also be helpful in choosing the best site for open or thoracoscopic lung biopsy. HRCT has revolutionized the subcategorization of IPs in terms of histopathologic-radiologic patterns, especially in idiopathic disease. Similar patterns can be found in CTDs. Recently, 16-slice CT technologies have enabled postprocessing strategies (minimal intensity projection, minIP) that may further improve the evaluation of parenchymal disease patterns. **Table 53-3** summarizes the major characteristics of the different types of IPs, and **Figures 53-13 to 53-16** illustrate HRCT patterns of UIP, NSIP, OP, and LIP.

High-resolution CT also offers particular benefit in the assessment of the severity of diffuse lung and airway diseases. In addition, the pattern of abnormality may frequently be informative in terms of likelihood of response to treatment. A ground-glass pattern denotes predominantly inflammatory disease and is generally associated with improvement. A reticular pattern, particularly honeycombing, correlates well with the presence of established fibrosis.

Bronchoalveolar Lavage

Bronchoalveolar lavage is a valuable diagnostic tool to rule out infection and confirm the presence of (fibrosing) alveolitis, and it can provide a specific diagnosis, as in cases of diffuse alveolar hemorrhage (**Figure 53-17**). Also, BAL fluid can be particularly helpful in the differentiation of follicular bronchiolitis (see Figure 53-11).

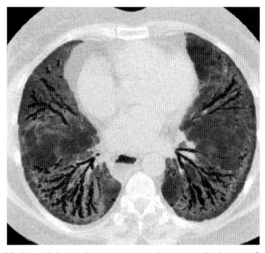

Figure 53-14 High-resolution computed tomography image of nonspecific interstitial pneumonia (NSIP) in minimal intensity projection. *(Courtesy Dr. H. W. van Es, St. Antonius Hospital, Nieuwegein, The Netherlands.)*

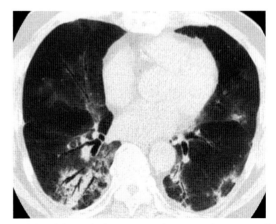

Figure 53-15 High-resolution computed tomography pattern of organizing pneumonia (OP) in minimal intensity projection. *(Courtesy Dr. H. W. van Es, St. Antonius Hospital, Nieuwegein, The Netherlands.)*

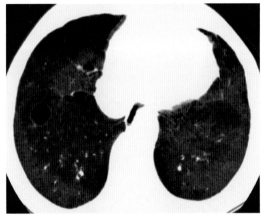

Figure 53-16 High-resolution computed tomography pattern of lymphocytic interstitial pneumonia (LIP). *(Courtesy Dr. H. W. van Es, St. Antonius Hospital, Nieuwegein, The Netherlands.)*

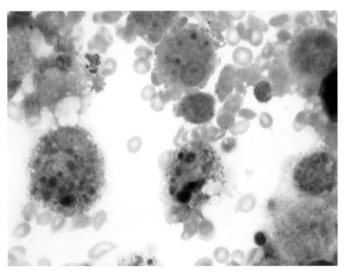

Figure 53-17 May-Grünwald-Giemsa staining of bronchoalveolar lavage fluid in patient with alveolar hemorrhage caused by autoimmune capillaritis. The large cells are hemosiderin-laden alveolar macrophages; the small cells are erythrocytes.

In SSc, differential cell count of BAL is also a valuable prognostic test. In one study of 49 SSc patients with fibrosing alveolitis followed for 2 years, only those with BAL granulocytosis (>3% neutrophils and/or >0.5% eosinophils) at baseline showed a significant disease progression with a marked reduction of DLCO, whereas almost all patients with normal BAL findings or BAL lymphocytosis had stable lung function parameters during the study period.

Lung Biopsy

An important clinical question is when to biopsy for IPs in CTD. If patients are known to have a CTD and have respiratory symptoms, HRCT and lung function testing are most appropriate to detect or exclude with reasonable confidence diffuse ILD. BAL might provide further clues for specific diagnosis and is especially helpful for exclusion of other diagnoses such as infections. In many cases, HRCT findings will also allow, with reasonable confidence, the diagnosis of one of the IP subsets. If this is not the case or HRCT findings are atypical beforehand, a surgical lung biopsy should be considered. However, prognostic data in biopsy specimens from patients with CTD-associated IP are relatively lacking. Therefore, the decision to biopsy

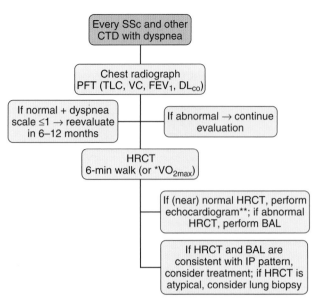

Figure 53-18 Diagnostic flowchart for evaluation of pulmonary manifestations in connective tissue disease *(CTD)*. All patients with systemic sclerosis *(SSc)* and patients with other CTDs and respiratory symptoms can be evaluated for pulmonary complications according to this flowchart. Dyspnea scale is proposed by American Thoracic Society/ European Respiratory Society: *0*, no breathlessness except with strenuous exercise; *I*, shortness of breath when hurrying or walking up a gradually sloping hill; *II*, walking slower than people of the same age because of breathlessness, or stopping for breath when walking at a normal pace on a level surface; *III*, stopping for breath after walking approximately 100 meters, or after a few minutes on a level surface; *IV*, being too breathless to leave the house, or breathless when dressing or undressing. *PFT*, Pulmonary function testing; *HRCT*, high-resolution computed tomography; *BAL*, bronchoalveolar lavage; *IP*, interstitial pneumonia. *VO2max is recommended, because it provides more objective determination of functional capacity and impairment. It identifies factors limiting exercise capacity.
**Routine echocardiography is recommended in SSc because of high risk of cardiac involvement and pulmonary hypertension.

should be primarily reserved for cases with an atypical presentation and when a diagnosis other than IP is being considered (e.g., amyloidosis). Patients may also be taking immunosuppressive drugs, and histopathologic examination may be necessary to distinguish parenchymal manifestations of CTD from drug-induced lung disease or opportunistic infections. Lastly, biopsies may be undertaken to investigate for associated malignancies, especially in LIP.

DIAGNOSTIC FLOWCHART

On the basis of the relatively high prevalence of parenchymal and vascular complications in patients with SSc, routine screening is advisable for these complications at presentation of disease. In other CTDs, evaluation of pulmonary manifestations will usually take place in patients who are symptomatic **(Figure 53-18)**.

TREATMENT

Treatment of pulmonary complications in CTDs is primarily based on the type of lung disease and not on the specific type of CTD. In most cases, no controlled data are available for evidence-based decision making. Because CTDs are autoimmune-based inflammatory diseases and these drugs exert a broad range of immunosuppressive actions, corticosteroids

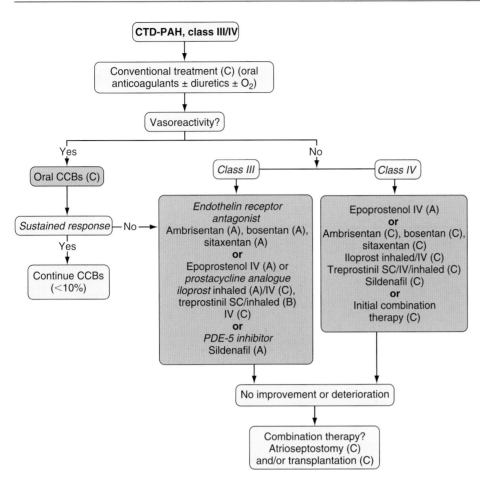

Figure 53-19 Algorithm for the treatment of pulmonary arterial hypertension *(PAH)* in connective tissue disease *(CTD)*, focusing on patients in World Health Organization functional class III or IV. *Class III* patients with PAH have marked limitation of physical activity; they are comfortable at rest; less than ordinary activity causes undue dyspnea or fatigue, chest pain, or near syncope. *Class IV* patients with PAH are unable to carry out any physical activity without symptoms; these patients manifest signs of right-sided heart failure; dyspnea and/or fatigue may even be present at rest; discomfort is increased by any physical activity. *CCBs*, Calcium channel blockers; *IV*, intravenously; *SC*, subcutaneously; levels of evidence (in parentheses): *A*, at least two randomized controlled trials (2 RCTs) that do not contradict; *B*, at least 1 RCT; *C*, efficacy evidence from observational studies, no RCTs available.

remain the mainstay of therapy despite many potential side effects. Other well-known drugs are cyclophosphamide, azathioprine, and methotrexate (MTX). These drugs have immunocytotoxic properties but are also associated with more serious side effects. In particular, MTX has a small (±3%) risk of pulmonary toxicity. Furthermore, cyclosporine A and tacrolimus are of therapeutic value because they can provide strong and specific T cell suppression, but careful monitoring of blood levels is needed to minimize side effects.

DIFFUSE LUNG DISEASE

Corticosteroids are widely used in the treatment of IPs associated with CTDs, although randomized controlled trials (RCTs) offer scant data showing they prevent progression of IPs or reverse fibrosis. Despite this lack of evidence, corticosteroids again remain the mainstay of therapy, with usual doses of prednisone between 0.5 and 1.0 mg/kg in nonacute situations. However, medium-dose corticosteroid therapy (15 mg/day prednisone or equivalent) is associated with the development of *scleroderma renal crisis*, which may lead to irreversible renal failure.

Of the other immunosuppressive drugs, RCTs data are now available in scleroderma diffuse lung disease only for cyclophosphamide. The North American Scleroderma Lung Study investigated the effects of 12 months of 2 mg/kg oral cyclophosphamide versus placebo in patients with signs of interstitial lung fibrosis. Lung function was significantly preserved in the active treatment arm, although absolute changes were small. Interestingly, the skin score improved as well. The cyclophosphamide group had a greater frequency of leukopenia and

neutropenia, but the difference between the two groups in the number of serious adverse events was not significant. Open studies have recently reported mycophenolate mofetil as an alternative to cyclophosphamide.

VASCULAR DISEASE

Treatment options for patients with CTD-associated pulmonary hypertension are similar to those for idiopathic pulmonary hypertension (**Figure 53-19**). Although patients with CTD may not respond as well to therapy as patients with primary pulmonary hypertension, aggressive therapy may improve functional status and quality of life.

Immunomodulatory therapy (corticosteroids with or without cyclophosphamide), long-term plasma exchange, and autologous stem cell transplantation have also been reported to improve or stabilize pulmonary hypertension in patients with CTDs. However, these represent case reports or retrospective case studies, and no prospective study of immunosuppressive therapy has yet been completed.

LUNG TRANSPLANTATION

Lung transplantation is now considered an accepted treatment in patients with end-stage pulmonary or cardiopulmonary disease, although chronic rejection still remains a key problem that precludes long-term survival. According to the recent International Society of Heart Lung Transplantation registry, pulmonary fibrosis caused by systemic diseases, such as scleroderma, sarcoidosis, histiocytosis X, and lymphangioleiomyomatosis (LAM; see Chapter 54), make up approximately 5% of all cases of lung transplantation. Provided that patients with systemic disease have no active disease in other organs, and other organ functions are preserved, the results after transplantation are similar to other diseases (e.g., IPF, emphysema).

CLINICAL COURSE AND PREVENTION

Can early treatment of systemic disease prevent irreversible lung scarring or development of pulmonary hypertension? The widespread use of HRCT has led to increased detection of early lung disease in patients with CTDs. It is unclear what management strategy can be best applied in these patients, who are often asymptomatic and have normal or near-normal pulmonary function. In theory, they might benefit from early introduction of treatment to prevent further irreversible damage. However, most of these cases of subtle disease might never show progression. At present, these patients can only be considered "at risk" for intrinsically progressive disease and should be monitored carefully, especially in the first years after presentation.

Does the clinical course of IPs in the context of CTDs differ from their idiopathic counterparts? Currently, it is not clear that histologic distinctions between IP patterns are as important in CTD as in idiopathic IPs. In limited systemic sclerosis, however, there might be a difference in outcome between UIP and NSIP, justifying lung biopsy in carefully selected cases where HRCT cannot make this distinction, and the patient might benefit from timely referral for lung transplantation.

CONTROVERSIES AND PITFALLS

ACTIVITY VERSUS SEVERITY

In the context of CTDs and lung complications, *disease activity* means "the underlying pathophysiologic process in the pulmonary tissue is still going on and has not (yet) come to a rest (i.e., complete remission)." Complete remission, however, is not synonymous with resolution of disease, because it may have caused severe damage to the tissue leaving scars (i.e., irreversible fibrosis).

Disease severity can best be defined in terms of symptoms and functional limitations of the patient. Pulmonary complications in CTDs may be severe because of direct danger to life, such as diffuse alveolar hemorrhage.

In IPs, treatment decisions are primarily guided by severity of disease. In most of these processes, lung function impairment is the result of the ongoing interstitial inflammatory process and irreversible fibrosis. In some patients, however, the inflammatory phase of disease might have burnt out, leaving only extensive scar tissue. The proportion of active disease will likely determine success of immunosuppressive therapy. At present,

however, no validated biomarkers or imaging technologies can be used to dissect reversible inflammatory disease from irreversible fibrosis. Watchful follow-up of disease evolution is still considered the most important strategy to overcome these limitations.

WEB RESOURCES FOR GUIDELINES/PROTOCOLS

http://www.eustar.org/. This website is an initiative of the European League Against Rheumatism (EULAR) Scleroderma Trials and Research (EUSTAR). The aim is to foster the study and the care of scleroderma and to achieve a consensus on evidence-based standards for the management of patients with scleroderma throughout Europe.

http://www.eular.org/. The European League Against Rheumatism (EULAR) is the organization that represents the patient, health professional, and scientific societies of rheumatology of all the European nations. EULAR endeavors to stimulate, promote, and support the research, prevention, treatment, and rehabilitation of rheumatic diseases.

http://www.rheumatology.org/. American College of Rheumatology.

SUGGESTED READINGS

American Thoracic Society/European Respiratory Society: International multidisciplinary consensus classification of the idiopathic interstitial pneumonias, *Am J Respir Crit Care Med* 165:277–304, 2002.

Badesch DB, Abman SH, Ahearn GS, et al: Medical therapy for pulmonary arterial hypertension, ACCP evidence-based clinical practical guidelines, *Chest* 126:35S-62S, 2004.

Baroni SS, Santillo M, Bevilacqua F, et al: Stimulatory autoantibodies to the PDGF receptor in systemic sclerosis, *N Engl J Med* 354:2667–2676, 2006.

Fagan KA, Badesch DB: Pulmonary hypertension associated with connective tissue disease. In *Pulmonary circulation: diseases and their treatment*, ed 2, London, 2004, Arnold.

Fischer A, Swingris JJ, Groshoug SD, et al: Clinically significant interstitial lung disease in limited scleroderma: histopathology, clinical features, and survival, *Chest* 134:601–605, 2008.

Jimenez SA, Derk CT: Following the molecular pathways toward an understanding of the pathogenesis of systemic sclerosis, *Ann Intern Med* 140:37–50, 2004.

Letko E, Zafirakis P, Baltatzis S, et al: Relapsing polychondritis: a clinical review, *Semin Arthritis Rheum* 31:384–395, 2002.

Saketkoo LA, Asherman DP, Cottin V, et al: Interstitial lung disease in idiopathic inflammatory myopathy, *Curr Rheumatol Rev* 6:108–119, 2010.

Tashkin DP, Elashoff R, Clements PJ, et al: Cyclophosphamide versus placebo in scleroderma lung disease, *N Engl J Med* 354:2655–2666, 2006.

Verleden GM, Demedts MG, Westhovens R, Thomeer M: Pulmonary manifestations of systemic diseases, *Eur Respir Monogr* 34, 2005.

Wells AU, Denton CP: *Pulmonary involvement in systemic autoimmune diseases*, Oxford, England, 2004, Elsevier.

Chapter **54**
Rare Diffuse Interstitial Lung Diseases
Simon R. Johnson • William Y.C. Chang

More than 7000 rare conditions exist, and although individually uncommon, together these diseases affect about 11% of all populations. Most rare diseases are chronic, often progressive, and can therefore form a significant portion of the workload for physicians. The term *orphan disease* is frequently applied to rare conditions and was originally used to suggest a lack of knowledge, research, or specific therapy. In many cases, however, significant progress in understanding the molecular basis of these diseases has resulted in biologically targeted treatments, making a definitive diagnosis especially important for these patients. This chapter describes select rare diffuse lung diseases, either primary or occurring in the context of systemic disease (secondary), likely to be encountered by most physicians, and particularly those for which a firm diagnosis can benefit patient management.

RARE CYSTIC LUNG DISEASES

LYMPHANGIOLEIOMYOMATOSIS

Lymphangioleiomyomatosis (LAM) is a cystic lung disease that affects almost exclusively women and has a prevalence of approximately 5 women per 1 million of most populations. LAM may occur sporadically or as part of the autosomal dominant genetic disorder, *tuberous sclerosis complex* (TSC). In both forms the lungs and lymphatics are infiltrated by LAM cells, an abnormal cell clone harboring biallelic inactivating mutations in the genes associated with TSC, either TSC-1 or more often TSC-2. LAM cells accumulate and cause progressive cystic destruction of the lungs, probably by the elaboration of proteolytic enzymes (**Figure 54-1**). LAM cells form small nodular clumps associated with lymphatic endothelial cells, which in turn form lymphatic channels that allow LAM cells to disseminate throughout the body. LAM cells also infiltrate the axial lymphatics and form the smooth muscle elements of *angiomyolipoma*, a rare tumor of the perivascular epithelioid cell family, present in up to 40% of women with sporadic LAM and almost all patients with TSC-LAM.

Other, extrapulmonary manifestations are related to lymphatic obstruction and include *lymphadenopathy* in up to 30% of patients and *lymphangioleiomyomas*, cystic lymphatic swellings usually in the abdomen, pelvis, or retroperitoneum occurring in up to 20% of patients (**Figure 54-2**). Thoracic and abdominal chylous collections are present in up to 10% of patients. LAM is also associated with a higher prevalence of *meningioma* than the general population. Cystic lung destruction results in recurrent pneumothorax and progressive airflow obstruction, with an average decline in forced expiratory volume in 1 second (FEV_1) of 120 mL per year (normal,

~27 mL/yr). However, the clinical course of patients with LAM varies, with some remaining stable for many years. At present, no features definitively predict which patients will develop progressive disease; however, onset at a younger age, presentation with breathlessness, and poor lung function at presentation suggest more aggressive disease.

Patients with LAM most frequently present with breathlessness or pneumothorax, although chylous pleural effusions, complications of angiomyolipoma, or weight loss can also be the presenting feature. Recurrent pneumothorax or airflow obstruction in younger women, particularly nonsmokers, should raise the possibility of LAM. In most cases the computed tomography (CT) findings of multiple round thin-walled cysts with no zonal predominance suggest the diagnosis. Increasingly, patients are being identified with LAM after investigations for other problems where cystic lung disease is observed on high-resolution CT (HRCT) scanning. In addition, screening for LAM at 18 years of age by CT is recommended for women with TSC; many of these patients have evidence of LAM on CT, but only a minority have respiratory symptoms.

With diagnostic criteria recently formulated by the European Respiratory Society (ERS), a definite diagnosis of LAM can be made based on a characteristic HRCT scan with a renal angiomyolipoma, histologic evidence of LAM cells at other sites (e.g., lymphangioleiomyomas, chylous collections in abdomen or thorax), or the presence of TSC. If TSC or extrapulmonary manifestations are not present, lung biopsy is required for a definitive diagnosis. Transbronchial biopsy can occasionally be helpful, although in most patients, video-assisted thoracoscopic surgery (VATS) is preferred. LAM cells characteristically stain with the monoclonal antibody HMB-45 and also express α–smooth muscle actin, estrogen, and progesterone receptors. The use of these immunohistochemical markers improves identification of LAM cells in lung tissue, including smaller transbronchial biopsies. The recent observation that vascular endothelial growth factor type D (VEGF-D) serum level is increased in about two thirds of patients with LAM has led to its use as a diagnostic marker for LAM. Importantly, a serum VEGF-D level greater than 800 ng/mL can differentiate LAM from other cystic lung diseases, including Langerhans cell histiocytosis, Birt-Hogg-Dube disease, and emphysema.

Patients with sporadic LAM should undergo clinical examination and where necessary, formal screening to exclude tuberous sclerosis complex. Only one third of patients with TSC have the classical triad of epilepsy, learning difficulties, and facial angiofibromas. Many patients with TSC-LAM have normal intelligence and mild skin changes that may be overlooked. Almost all patients with TSC-LAM have renal

667

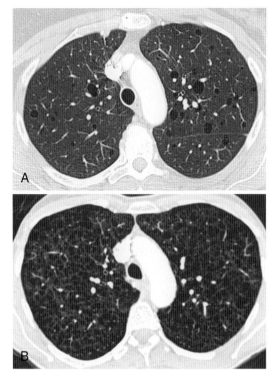

Figure 54-1 High-resolution computed tomography (HRCT) scans showing characteristic radiologic features of patients with lymphangioleiomyomatosis. **A,** HRCT in patient with asymptomatic disease and normal lung function. **B,** Image shows extensive cystic change in patient being considered for lung transplantation.

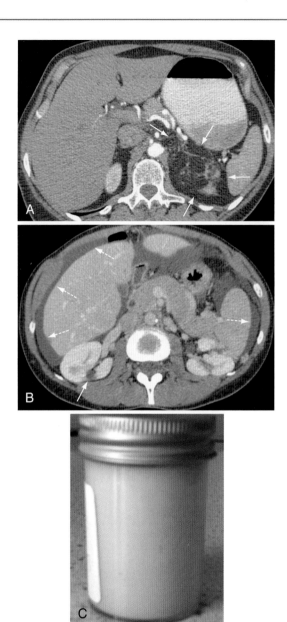

Figure 54-2 **A,** CT image shows a large, left renal angiomyolipoma with areas of fat density (*white arrows*). **B,** CT scan shows chylous ascites and a small, right renal angiomyolipoma (*white arrows*). **C,** Chylous fluid aspirated from pleural collection of patient with lymphangioleiomyomatosis.

angiomyolipomas, which tend to be larger and more frequently multiple and bilateral than in those with sporadic LAM. Making the diagnosis of TSC is important for the management of other aspects of TSC and for the patient's offspring.

To confirm LAM in the presence of cystic lung disease or to evaluate patients for renal angiomyolipoma, a CT scan of the abdomen and pelvis should be performed. Angiomyolipomas greater than 4 cm are prone to growth, rupture, and hemorrhage and should be treated prophylactically when large or in the presence of symptoms.

General management of LAM includes avoidance of estrogen supplementation, including oral contraceptives and hormone replacement therapy. Prophylactic vaccination, pulmonary rehabilitation, and oxygen should be given when appropriate. Bronchodilators are helpful for those with airflow obstruction. Patients with LAM are prone to *pneumothorax,* which occurs in more than 70% of patients and is recurrent in the majority, and early surgical intervention is recommended. Patients considering pregnancy should be warned that the disease may be more active in pregnancy, particularly an increase in pneumothorax. Those with TSC should receive genetic counseling. For patients with severe disease, including those with TSC, lung transplantation can be performed.

Previously, hormone treatment with progesterone or other antiestrogen therapies have been used for these patients, but no evidence indicates there is a benefit for most patients. Studies show that *rapamycin,* an inhibitor of mTOR pathway, is effective in reducing the rate of decline of FEV_1 in patients with impaired lung function. In those with renal angiomyolipoma, including those with TSC, a reduction in tumor volume is seen in those treated with rapamycin. On cessation of therapy, decline in lung function resumes and angiomyolipoma volume increases, and these patients may need long-term

therapy. ERS recommends that mTOR inhibitors for LAM not be used routinely but likely have a role in patients with progressive disease.

LANGERHANS CELL HISTIOCYTOSIS

Langerhans cell histiocytosis (LCH) is a bronchocentric disease categorized by a clonal proliferation of Langerhans cells in the lungs with focal granuloma and small airways destruction resulting in nodules and cystic change. LCH is part of a spectrum of diseases characterized by activated Langerhans cells, including Letterer-Siwe disease (acute disseminated LCH) and Hand-Schüller-Christian disease (chronic idiopathic xanthomatosis). The latter two entities are systemic cancerlike diseases of childhood and are not discussed further here. Adult LCH is generally restricted to the lung, although up to 30% of patients have extrapulmonary features; most often diabetes insipidus

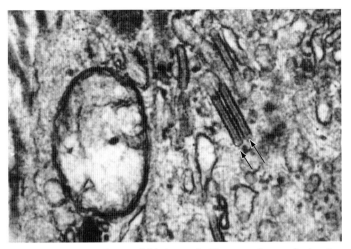

Figure 54-3 Langerhans cell histiocytosis. Electron micrograph showing Birbeck granules *(arrows)*.

caused by pituitary involvement, skin lesions, or bone lesions causing pain and rarely, central nervous system lesions.

Langerhans cell histiocytosis typically affects individuals between 20 and 40 years of age, almost all of whom are current or recent smokers. The infiltrating Langerhans cell clone expresses the surface protein CD1a and has a characteristic appearance on electron microscopy with Birbeck inclusion granules (**Figure 54-3**). LCH may coexist with areas of *desquamative interstitial pneumonitis*, another smoking-related entity characterized by activation of macrophages. Similar to LAM, LCH is of variable severity, with approximately one quarter of LCH patients detected by imaging being asymptomatic. Pneumothorax is the presenting feature in about 20% of patients; the rest present with cough, dyspnea, or weight loss. The chest x-ray film is abnormal in most patients, showing reticular shadowing with midzone and upper-zone predominance (**Figure 54-4**). The CT scan shows a mixture of nodules, cavitating nodules, and cysts, often with thick, irregular walls forming bizarre shapes (**Figure 54-5**); characteristically, the bases of the lungs are relatively spared. As the disease progresses, the cysts tend to amalgamate, and nodules become less common. The diagnosis is usually suspected by the combination of these imaging appearances in younger smokers. Absolute confirmation often requires a surgical biopsy (**Figure 54-6**). However, bronchoalveolar lavage (BAL) fluid with greater than 5% Langerhans cells identified by CD1a positivity, often with increased macrophages and eosinophils, is supportive and can be diagnostic in the correct clinical context.

Lung function is normal in about 15% of LCH patients, although most have airflow obstruction with impaired gas transfer or a mixture of obstructive and restrictive changes. The course of LCH is variable, with spontaneous remission and even resolution in some patients; up to half of patients improve by CT criteria. However, some develop progressive respiratory failure, and a poor outcome is predicted by older age at onset, persistent constitutional symptoms, extrapulmonary involvement, and the presence of pulmonary hypertension. The overall survival for LCH patients is approximately 70% after 10 years, although some will require evaluation for pulmonary transplantation.

Management of LCH is generally supportive. Stopping smoking is the most important intervention and may significantly increase the chance of spontaneous resolution. As a particular feature of LCH, pulmonary hypertension should be

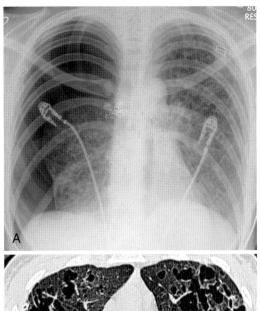

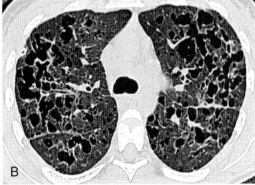

Figure 54-4 A, Chest radiograph of patient with Langerhans cell histiocytosis presenting with a pneumothorax. **B,** CT image from same patient shows multiple irregular cyst and nodules. A chest drain is present in the right hemithorax.

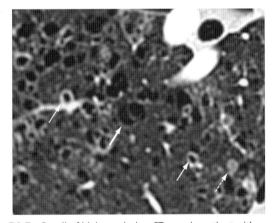

Figure 54-5 Detail of high-resolution CT scan in patient with Langerhans cell histiocytosis showing thin-walled cysts *(thin arrows)*, thick walled cysts *(thick arrow)*, and cavitating nodules *(dashed arrow)*.

screened for in those with active disease and may require specific treatment. In addition, many reports suggest an increased prevalence of lymphoma and lung cancer in patients with LCH. Persisting constitutional symptoms, hemoptysis, or other unexplained features should be thoroughly evaluated before being attributed to LCH alone. For those with active disease, steroids are frequently used, although no evidence supports this. More recently, in individual series, patients with active disease have been treated with 2-chlorodeoxyadenosine (Cladribine), a purine nucleoside analogue with activity

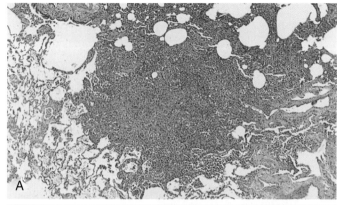

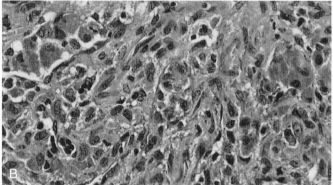

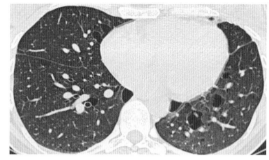

Figure 54-7 High-resolution CT image of patient with Birt-Hogg-Dube syndrome. Cysts are characteristically in a pericardiac distribution.

Figure 54-6 Histopathology of pulmonary Langerhans cell histiocytosis (PLCH). **A,** Low-magnification photomicrograph showing stellate, bronchocentric nodule in PLCH. **B,** High-magnification photomicrograph showing polymorphic, interstitial infiltrate in PLCH. The cellular infiltrate includes a mixture of mononuclear cells and eosinophils. Langerhans cells predominate and are differentiated by highly convoluted nuclei with nuclear grooves, which result in nuclear configurations that resemble crumpled paper or coffee beans.

against lymphocytes and monocytes, with evidence of response in many patients.

BIRT-HOGG-DUBE SYNDROME

Birt-Hogg-Dube (BHD) syndrome was first described as the association of fibrofolliculomas, acrocordons, and trichodiscomas; benign skin-colored papules and skin tags of adult onset; presence of lung cysts; and a predisposition to renal cancer. It is now realized that BHD syndrome may be entirely restricted to the lungs, without cutaneous manifestations, and is caused by either germline or somatic mutations in the folliculin (FLCN) gene, a tumor suppressor of unknown function. Patients with pulmonary disease develop lung cysts predominantly in the central and lower zones of the lungs, characteristically around the heart (**Figure 54-7**). The cysts are 0.2 to 7 cm in size, have thin walls, are often ovoid in shape, and occasionally are multiseptated. The cyst walls have disrupted elastic fibers and are infiltrated by macrophages.

Diagnostic markers of BHD syndrome include a family history of pneumothorax, skin lesions, and early renal cancer. However, less than half of patients will have the triad of skin, renal, and lung features. The main respiratory manifestation is recurrent pneumothorax, generally occurring in adult life. Symptomatic disease is possibly more common in women and those harboring germline rather than somatic mutations. Diagnosis of BHD syndrome is usually made on clinical criteria and the presence of more than five fibrofolliculomas or

trichodiscomas of adult onset or an *FLCN* mutation. Minor criteria are renal cancer before age 50, multiple lung cysts, or a first-degree relative with a germline *FLCN* mutation. In practical terms, particularly with isolated lung disease, diagnosis is best made by screening the patient's blood for *FLCN* mutations in the correct clinical context.

Patients with BHD syndrome tend *not* to develop progressive respiratory failure. The important management is prevention of recurrent pneumothorax; screening for renal cancer, probably best done by yearly magnetic resonance imaging (MRI); and when necessary, cosmetic treatment of dermatologic manifestations.

PULMONARY LIGHT CHAIN DEPOSITION DISEASE

The classic form of light chain deposition disease (LCDD) is caused by a light chain–producing B cell clone, resulting in monoclonal gammopathy, renal deposits, and occasionally, heart and liver nonamyloid light chain deposits; it may be associated with pulmonary nodules. A cystic lung disease caused by a variant LCDD was recently reported. Patients with pulmonary cystic LCDD have no evidence of systemic light chain deposition but develop an aggressive cystic lung disease, resulting in respiratory failure over 3 to 10 years. CT scan initially shows diffuse round cysts that may be associated with micronodules and linear densities, which may enlarge and coalesce over time. The lungs are infiltrated by small CD20-positive B lymphocytes suggestive of an antigen-driven process. Diagnosis is generally made by lung biopsy showing amorphous eosinophilic material in the alveolar walls, small airways, and blood vessels, sometimes associated with reactive giant cells. Congo red staining shows no birefringence, and immunofluorescence is positive for kappa light chains, which are also detectable in serum. Although a rare disorder, most reported patients develop progressive disease that may require pulmonary transplantation. Interestingly, LCDD does not recur in the transplanted lungs, and lung transplantation is associated with a normalization of the serum κ/λ light chain ratio suggesting the disease is located exclusively in the lungs.

EVALUATION OF PATIENTS WITH CYSTIC LUNG DISEASES

In addition to the entities previously described, lung cysts are also seen in *multiple cystic mesenchymal hamartoma,* an entity categorized by a small number of larger, thick-walled cystic lesions prone to hemorrhage. Metastatic endometrial stromal sarcoma can present as lung cysts and can run a deceptively indolent course, in one case diagnosed only after lung transplantation for suspected LAM. Lung cysts are also seen in

Table 54-1   Cystic Lung Diseases: CT Appearance and Clinical Characteristics

| Disease | CT Appearance of Cysts | | | Associated Features |
	Features	Distribution		
Lymphangio-leiomyomatosis	Round, thin walls	All zones		Exclusively women Angiomyolipoma Lymphatic abnormalities and chylous collections Tuberous sclerosis
Langerhans cell histiocytosis	Irregular shapes, thicker walled	Predominantly in middle and upper zones		Positive smoking history Nodules and/or cavitating nodules
LIP/Sjögren syndrome	Round, thin walls, sparse	All zones		Systemic features Interstitial shadowing Serum autoantibodies
Birt-Hogg-Dube syndrome	Ovoid, thin walls	Middle and lower zones; pericardiac		Renal cancer, skin hamartomas *FLCN* mutation
Light chain deposition disease	Mostly round			Nodules and lines serum κ light chains
Cavitating tumors	Round, thicker walls	All zones		History or evidence of primary tumor
Emphysema	Absent walls	Variable pattern		Smoking; inhalational exposure

CT, computed tomography; *LIP*, lymphoid interstitial pneumonia.

lymphocytic interstitial pneumonia (LIP) and patients with acquired immunodeficiency syndrome (AIDS). In these entities, cysts are generally less profuse and associated with interstitial changes.

Diagnosis in patients with cystic lung disease can be difficult. Although imaging and associated features usually suggest the most likely diagnosis, imaging alone is not generally diagnostic (**Table 54-1**). Suspicion of LAM should be followed by abdominal CT, which will show extrapulmonary manifestations in two thirds of patients; LCH by BAL and CD1a staining, and BHD by *FLCN* mutation analysis and renal/skin evaluation. Nonspecific or mixed appearances can be evaluated by autoantibody screening, serum κ/λ light chain ratio and human immunodeficiency virus (HIV) serology. Surgical biopsy may be required but can be avoided in many cases. Because many of these diseases have genetic implications for the patient and family, and specific treatments and clinical trials are available, a definitive diagnosis is often necessary.

OTHER RARE DIFFUSE LUNG DISEASES

PULMONARY ALVEOLAR PROTEINOSIS

Also known as alveolar lipoproteinosis, alveolar phospholipidosis, and pulmonary alveolar phospholipoproteinosis, pulmonary alveolar proteinosis (PAP) is a disease caused by a failure of granulocyte-macrophage colony-stimulating factor (GM-CSF) signaling, which results in a failure of surfactant protein clearance by alveolar macrophages and the accumulation of lipoproteinaceous material in the alveolar spaces. Three categories of PAP have been described: idiopathic, secondary, and congenital.

Idiopathic PAP results from GM-CSF neutralizing autoantibodies and accounts for approximately 90% of cases, with overall prevalence or 4 to 40 per 1 million, dependent on the population studied. It is two to three times more common in men and smokers and has been putatively linked to exposure to flour, cement, wood, chlorine gas, gasoline, and plastics, but a causal link has not been established. Heavy silica dust

exposure was known to cause *silicoproteinosis*, a similar condition, but this is now rarely seen as a result of reduced workplace exposure. Idiopathic PAP usually presents in adulthood, with a mean age at diagnosis of 39 years. Presentation is nonspecific, the most common symptoms being dyspnea, cough, chest pain, hemoptysis, and constitutional upset. Superimposed infection may also be the presenting feature. Examination can be normal, but lung crackles and finger clubbing may be present.

Secondary PAP is not related to GM-CSF autoantibodies but occurs in a small fraction of patients with hematologic disorders (e.g., chronic myelogenous leukemia, myelodysplastic syndromes), immunodeficiency (e.g., HIV, hypogammaglobulinemia, thymic aplasia, IgA deficiency) and *lysinuric protein intolerance*, a genetic disorder caused by an amino acid transporter mutation. *Congenital* PAP is a group of autosomal recessive disorders caused by a variety of GM-CSF receptor and surfactant protein mutations and is invariably fatal in childhood without transplantation.

Chest radiography demonstrates consolidation with thickened intralobular septae (**Figure 54-8**). In a third of cases the changes are asymmetric or unilateral. The pattern is variable and in 50% of PAP patients may be perihilar, resembling the "bat wing" appearance seen in pulmonary edema. The CT appearance of air space shadowing in a geographic pattern with interlobular septal thickening is described as a "crazy paving" pattern (**Figure 54-9**). This appearance is not specific for PAP and may also be seen in cardiogenic pulmonary edema, bronchoalveolar cell carcinoma, *Pneumocystis jirovecii* pneumonia, alveolar hemorrhage, sarcoidosis, cryptogenic organizing pneumonia, nonspecific organizing pneumonia, exogenous lipoid pneumonia, and drug-induced lung diseases. Diagnosis is usually made on the basis of a compatible clinical history and typical radiology and a milky appearance on BAL fluid containing periodic acid–Schiff–positive granular material (**Figure 54-10**). Open-lung biopsy, although rarely essential, shows accumulation of lipoprotein in the alveolar spaces (**Figure 54-11**). Nonspecific increase in serum lactate dehydrogenase (LDH) may also be seen. Lung function is generally restrictive with decreased gas transfer. Anti-GM-CSF antibody

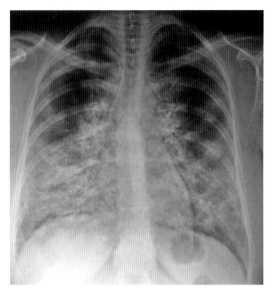

Figure 54-8 Chest radiograph in patient with diffuse bilateral air space shadowing caused by pulmonary alveolar proteinosis (PAP).

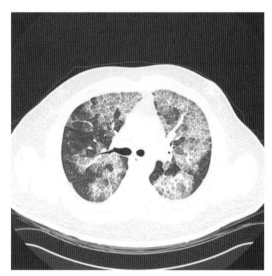

Figure 54-9 High-resolution CT image showing typical "crazy paving" appearance of pulmonary alveolar proteinosis, representing alveolar filling and thickening of secondary pulmonary lobules.

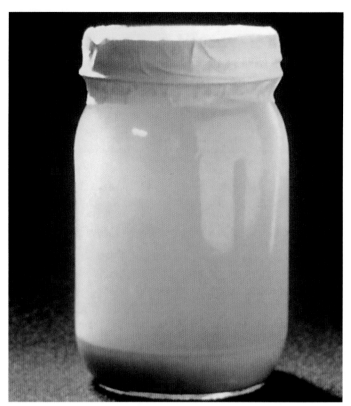

Figure 54-10 Bronchoalveolar lavage (BAL) fluid with classic milky appearance from patient with pulmonary alveolar proteinosis.

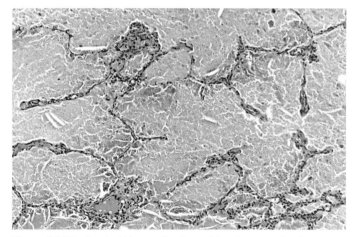

Figure 54-11 Surgical biopsy of patient with pulmonary alveolar proteinosis showing accumulation of lipoprotein in alveoli.

titers also show promise as a diagnostic test in both serum and BAL fluid.

Opportunistic infections can complicate PAP because of impaired macrophage function and host defense. Common organisms include *Nocardia* species, fungi, and mycobacteria. Pulmonary fibrosis has been documented to occur in PAP, but this is rare, and it is unclear as to whether this process is progressive. The treatment of choice for idiopathic PAP is *whole-lung lavage* (WLL) with warmed 0.9% saline performed at specialist centers under general anesthesia using double-lumen endotracheal tube. Lavage is continued until fluid runs clear, typically taking 10 to 12 L of saline per lung. Chest percussion is also sometimes employed to aid clearance of lipoprotein-aceous material. Both multisession WLL and single-session, sequential bilateral WLL are performed. In PAP patients with severe hypoxia, WLL has been performed with extracorporeal membrane oxygenation and in hyperbaric chambers. Complications of WLL include barotrauma and saline thorax. Although there are no randomized controlled trials (RCTs) of WLL, case

series report 85% of patients treated have some improvement in symptoms, lung function, radiology, and survival. The median duration of clinical benefit is 15 months and 60% to 70% will require a repeat lavage. WLL may still be required for secondary PAP, but the mainstay of therapy is to treat the underlying condition. Congenital PAP does not appear to respond well to WLL.

Several small, nonrandomized studies of subcutaneous GM-CSF for idiopathic PAP show an improvement in up to 50% of patients. Inhaled GM-CSF has also undergone trials, but further studies are needed.

In the adult forms of PAP, estimated 5-year and 10-year survival are 75% and 68%, respectively. Approximately one third of cases resolve spontaneously over months to years, one third of patients have stable disease, and another third have progressive disease, with lung transplantation as an option. The overall risk of respiratory death is 10% to 15%. The prognosis is much worse in those under age 5 years with congenital PAP, with 5-year survival of about 14%.

AMYLOIDOSIS

The term *amyloidosis* encompasses a complex group of multisystem conditions that result in the extracellular deposition of *insoluble amyloid*, abnormally folded low-molecular-weight protein molecules, resulting in progressive organ damage. It may be acquired or inherited and present with multisystem or focal disease. Amyloidosis may present to respiratory physicians in a variety of ways. Chronic pulmonary conditions such as bronchiectasis may give rise to systemic AA amyloidosis; systemic amyloidosis itself may result in respiratory symptoms and referral; and localized respiratory tract amyloid deposits may either present with respiratory symptoms or may be found incidentally on chest radiography.

The two most common forms of amyloid to affect the respiratory system are *AL light chain* (AL) amyloidosis, which occurs as a result of deposition of excess immunoglobulin light chain fragments, usually secondary to a plasma cell dyscrasia, or reactive *systemic AA* amyloidosis caused by accumulation of the acute-phase reactant, serum amyloid A, secondary to a variety of other chronic inflammatory conditions. Almost all clinically significant respiratory tract disease is related to AL amyloid. The diagnosis of amyloidosis should be considered with unusual upper airways symptoms in patients with parenchymal changes, unexplained congestive cardiac failure, or nephrotic syndrome suggesting a multisystem disease.

Laryngeal amyloid represents 0.5% to 1% of benign laryngeal disease and may present as discrete nodules or diffuse infiltration; it is often localized and usually relatively benign. Laryngeal amyloid usually affects the supraglottic larynx, and patients present with hoarse voice or stridor, although choking or exertional dyspnea also occur. *Tracheobronchial amyloid* is uncommon, and presenting symptoms include dyspnea, persistent cough, and hemoptysis. Airway narrowing can also cause wheeze, distal atelectasis, recurrent pneumonia, or lobar collapse, and solitary nodules have been mistaken for neoplasia. Amyloidosis can also present with mediastinal and hilar lymphadenopathy although *parenchymal amyloidosis*

presenting as either solitary or multiple nodules or a diffuse alveolar-septal pattern is the most frequently detected respiratory manifestation.

The "gold standard" for diagnosis remains biopsy demonstrating apple-green birefringence with polarized microscopy after staining with Congo red. In some centers, radiolabeled serum amyloid P (SAP) has been used to identify distribution and burden of disease, particularly for solid-organ involvement. With pulmonary involvement, lung function tests may show a restrictive pattern with reduced transfer factor, and in the case of tracheobronchial disease, large airways obstruction may be detected by flow-volume loop. Routine workup excludes an underlying blood cell dyscrasia (e.g., myeloma) and looks for other organ involvement.

Studies on management of respiratory tract amyloid are limited, and management decisions are often made empirically based on symptom management. No treatment may be needed, but local measures such as laser therapy, stenting, and surgical resection have been used for endobronchial and tracheobronchial disease. No evidence shows that steroids have any effect on laryngeal amyloid, and it is thought that repeated endoscopic procedures are safer than repeated open surgery. Many modalities used for myeloma, including chemotherapeutic agents (e.g., melphalan, thalidomide) and autologous bone marrow transplantation, are being tried in systemic AL amyloid, but there have been limited clinical trials.

PULMONARY ALVEOLAR MICROLITHIASIS

Pulmonary alveolar microlithiasis (PAM), first described in 1957, is characterized by the extensive accumulation of intraalveolar calcium phosphate deposits, or "microliths." PAM is an autosomal recessive disease and, although reported worldwide, is most common in Japan, Turkey, and Italy. Presentation is most common in the mid-30s with dyspnea, cough, and chest pain. However, half of patients are asymptomatic, and PAM is detected as an incidental finding on chest radiography or by family screening.

Diagnosis is usually made on the basis of a distinctive calcified micronodular "sandstorm" appearance seen on chest radiography with mid/lower-zone predominance, often obliterating the mediastinal and diaphragmatic contour (**Figure 54-12**). CT scanning, particularly in advanced disease, demonstrates calcified interlobular septa, pleura, and bronchovascular bundles;

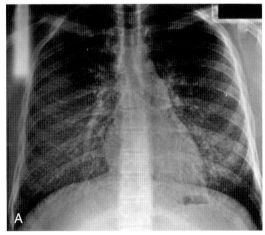
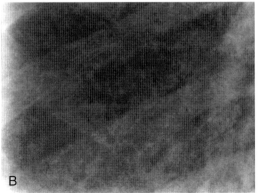

Figure 54-12   Chest x-ray films of patient with pulmonary alveolar microlithiasis. **A,** Numerous tiny opacities are present throughout both lungs. **B,** Magnified view of lower right lung showing numerous opacities (<1 mm in size).

perilobular microliths; and often ground-glass attenuation, areas of consolidation, and subpleural cysts. Lung biopsy reveals characteristic lamellar intraalveolar microliths. Mutations in *SLC34A2*, a gene encoding a sodium-dependent phosphate transporter, highly expressed by alveolar type II cells have been identified in most patients, possibly leading to the aberrant accumulation of calcium phosphate in alveolar spaces.

Longer-term prognosis in patients with PAM is poor, with a mean age of death from respiratory failure of 46 years. Treatment is supportive, including oxygen when required and lung transplantation. Bisphosphonates have been used in children with PAM with some evidence of short-term radiologic and clinical improvement.

PULMONARY MANIFESTATIONS OF RARE SYSTEMIC DISEASES

A number of rare systemic diseases associated with pulmonary manifestations may be encountered by respiratory physicians, including Hermansky-Pudlak syndrome, Erdheim-Chester disease, lysosomal storage disorders (e.g., Gaucher, Niemann-Pick, Fabry), and mucopolysaccharidoses.

HERMANSKY-PUDLAK SYNDROME

Hermansky-Pudlak syndrome (HPS) is an autosomal recessive disorder that results in impaired trafficking of the membrane-bound organelles, melanosomes, platelet-dense bodies, and lysosomes. HPS is most prevalent in Puerto Ricans, in whom it is one of the most common single-gene disorders. The disease segregates to at least seven genes, each with a slightly different phenotype. Clinically, HPS is characterized by the triad of oculocutaneous albinism, platelet aggregation defects causing a bleeding diathesis, and visceral deposition of the fatlike substance ceroid, resulting in pulmonary fibrosis, also involving the gastrointestinal tract, heart, and kidneys. HPS-1 is the most common subtype, with 80% of these patients developing pulmonary fibrosis. Pulmonary fibrosis is more frequent in women, typically presents in the third decade of life, and results in premature death in about half of patients.

No treatment is of proven efficacy, although pirfenidone reduced rate of lung function decline in one small study of patients with HPS-1. Experience with lung transplantation in HPS is limited but can be considered for patients with end-stage disease.

ERDHEIM-CHESTER DISEASE

Erdheim-Chester disease (ECD) is a rare, systemic, non–Langerhans cell histiocytosis of unknown etiology. It occurs predominantly in middle-aged and older adults, most often presenting with bone pain. ECD is characterized clinically and radiologically by bilateral, symmetric osteosclerotic lesions involving the metaphyses and diaphyses of long bones. Approximately half of patients have extraosseous disease, with the lungs affected in 20% to 35% of these. Pulmonary symptoms include cough and progressive dyspnea. The chest x-ray film generally shows diffuse interstitial infiltrates with pleural and interlobular septal thickening; pleural effusions may be present. CT findings include interlobular septal and visceral pleural thickening, patchy reticular and centrilobular opacities, ground-glass changes, and pleural effusions. Diagnosis is generally by biopsy demonstrating CD1a-negative histiocytes around lymphatics and absence of Birbeck granules, although a typical CT scan in combination with the radiologic skeletal findings are highly suggestive of ECD.

Various combinations of treatment have been tried, with the most successful anecdotal cases using a combination of chemotherapeutic agents and steroids. The overall prognosis is poor; one third of ECD patients with pulmonary involvement die within 6 months and about 60% within 3 years.

LYSOSOMAL STORAGE DISORDERS

Lysosomal storage disorders (LSDs) are a group of approximately 50 inherited conditions characterized by a defect in the functional expression of any of the lysosomal enzymes, resulting in the accumulation of their substrates both intracellularly and extracellularly and loss of function in a variety of organ systems, including the lungs. The clinical features depend greatly on the rate and magnitude of accumulation, with a wide spectrum of phenotypes observed, the vast majority presenting in childhood.

Gaucher disease (GD), the most prevalent LSD, is inherited in an autosomal dominant manner and results from a deficiency of glucocerebrosidase activity causing glucocerebroside to accumulate in phagocytic reticuloendothelial cells, called Gaucher cells. Pulmonary involvement is most common in the infantile form (type 2) although adult onset (type 1) is sometimes associated with an interstitial lung disease resulting from accumulation of Gaucher cells in the alveolar spaces and septa. Pulmonary hypertension and hepatopulmonary syndrome are also occasionally seen. Pulmonary involvement is more common in those with severe disease, particularly with neuropathic involvement. Enzyme replacement therapy is currently the mainstay of treatment, but respiratory involvement may not respond well to this.

Niemann-Pick disease is an autosomal recessive disorder characterized by the accumulation of lipid-laden macrophages (Niemann-Pick cells). Lung involvement is relatively frequent in infantile forms but less common in adult forms. The radiologic appearance is typically of reticular or reticulonodular infiltrates. Treatment by WLL may be of some benefit, and bone marrow transplantation has been attempted in some patients.

Fabry disease is an X-linked metabolic disease caused by the absence of α-galactosidase A, resulting in the accumulation of glycosphingolipids. Patients can present with a variety of pulmonary symptoms, including dyspnea, airway obstruction, wheeze, pneumothorax, and hemoptysis. The chest radiograph may be normal, but chest CT may show ground-glass change. Diagnosis is made by bronchial biopsy, bushings, or lavage. Enzyme replacement therapy has been shown to alleviate pulmonary dysfunction in some patients.

MUCOPOLYSACCHARIDOSES

The mucopolysaccharidoses, including *Hurler disease* and *Hunter syndrome*, are a group of inherited multisystem conditions caused by an accumulation of mucopolysaccharides (glycosaminoglycans). Deposition in the upper airway can result in symptoms of sleep apnea as a result of upper airways obstruction, and a number of patients will require nocturnal continuous positive airway pressure (CPAP) support. Deposition in the lungs may result in chronic interstitial changes. Respiratory function may be further compromised by other disease features, such as abnormalities in the shape and structure of the ribs, short neck and immobile jaw, and abdominal organomegaly.

SUGGESTED READINGS

Allen TC, Chevez-Barrios P, Shetlar DJ, Cagle PT: Pulmonary and ophthalmic involvement with Erdheim-Chester disease: a case report and review of the literature, *Arch Pathol Lab Med* 128:1428–1431, 2004.

Colombat M, Stern M, Groussard O, et al: Pulmonary cystic disorder related to light chain deposition disease, *Am J Respir Crit Care Med* 173:777–780, 2006.

Duchateau F, Dechambre S, Coche E: Imaging of pulmonary manifestations in subtype B of Niemann-Pick disease, *Br J Radiol* 74:1059–1061, 2001.

Eng CM, Germain DP, Banikazemi M, et al: Fabry disease: guidelines for the evaluation and management of multi-organ system involvement, *Gent Med* 8:539–548, 2006.

Goitein O, Elstein D, Abrahamov A, et al: Lung involvement and enzyme replacement therapy in Gaucher's disease, *QJM* 94:407–415, 2001.

Huqun, Izumi S, Miyazawa H, et al: Mutations in the *SLC34A2* gene are associated with pulmonary alveolar microlithiasis, *Am J Respir Crit Care Med* 175:263–268, 2007.

Johnson SR: Lymphangioleiomyomatosis, *Eur Respir J* 27:1056–1065, 2006.

Johnson SR, Cordier JF, Lazor R, et al: European Respiratory Society guidelines for the diagnosis and management of lymphangioleiomyomatosis, *Eur Respir J* 35:14–26, 2010.

Kamin W: Diagnosis and management of respiratory involvement in Hunter syndrome, *Acta Paediatr Suppl* 97:57–60, 2008.

Lachmann HJ, Hawkins PN: Amyloidosis and the lung, *Chronic Respir Dis* 3:203–214, 2006.

Pierson DM, Ionescu D, Qing G, et al: Pulmonary fibrosis in Hermansky-Pudlak syndrome: a case report and review, *Respiration* 73:382–395, 2006.

Toro JR, Pautler SE, Stewart L, et al: Lung cysts, spontaneous pneumothorax, and genetic associations in 89 families with Birt-Hogg-Dube syndrome, *Am J Respir Crit Care Med* 175:1044–1053, 2007.

Trapnell BC, Whitsett JA, Nakata K: Pulmonary alveolar proteinosis, *N Engl J Med* 349:2527–2539, 2003.

Vassallo R, Ryu JH, Schroeder DR, et al: Clinical outcomes of pulmonary Langerhans cell histiocytosis in adults, *N Engl J Med* 346:484–490, 2002.

Chapter **55**
Extrinsic Allergic Alveolitis
Kelsey Gray • Cecile Rose

One of the first written descriptions of hypersensitivity pneumonitis (HP), or extrinsic allergic alveolitis (EAA), was in 1713 by Ramazzini, who observed that "minute worms" contained in grain cause a syndrome of dyspnea and cachexia associated with a shortened life span. In 1932, Campbell reported five farmers who developed acute systemic and respiratory symptoms after exposure to moldy hay. In 1944, Pickels named this syndrome "farmer's lung." Farmer's lung and pigeon breeder's disease are the most well studied forms of EAA. Each year, however, new exposure settings and types are added to the list of antigens implicated in the development of EAA.

A heterogeneous disease, EAA has varying clinical presentations associated with the inhalation of antigens, leading primarily to a diffuse mononuclear cell inflammation of the small airways and lung parenchyma. Classifying etiologic antigens into three broad categories is clinically helpful: microbial agents, animal proteins, and low-molecular-weight chemicals (**Table 55-1**). Most particulate antigens are of respirable size, less than 3 to 5 μm in diameter, and deposit in the alveoli. However, some antigens are deposited in airways and then become soluble, as occurs with *Alternaria* spores.

Estimating the true incidence of disease can be challenging, because EAA may be misdiagnosed as an interstitial pneumonia or other pulmonary disorder or may not come to medical attention in individuals with mild disease. Moreover, genetics, coexisting exposures such as smoking, work environments, climates, altitude, and endemic disease (i.e., other granulomatous disorders such as sarcoidosis) vary from country to country, making comparisons of prevalence and incidence challenging. A longitudinal primary care database estimate of the incidence of EAA in the general population was 1 per 100,000 person-years in the United Kingdom. Incidence rates in specific populations with antigen exposure have also been reported. A study in Finnish farmers found 5 cases of EAA per 10,000 farmers who required hospital admission over a 1-year period. A study in Swedish farmers estimated an annual rate of 2 to 3 per 10,000 farmers. Prevalence of EAA among pigeon breeders is estimated at 0.1% to more than 10%, depending on antigen exposure.

RISK FACTORS

It is unclear why some individuals exposed to an antigen develop EAA and others residing or working in the same environment do not. Because only 1% to 15% of persons exposed to etiologic antigens develop EAA, a combination of antigen dose, host-specific factors, and underlying genetics likely contributes to the development of EAA.

Intensity, frequency, and duration of exposure; particle size; antigen solubility; climate; work practices; and use of respiratory protection combine to alter the risk of disease. *Farmer's lung* is associated with exposure to moldy hay, which is more common in harsh winter environments with heavy rainfall, where damp hay is fed to livestock in indoor barns with poor ventilation. *Summer-type EAA*, the most prevalent form of EAA in Japan, occurs in the wet summer months when indoor microbial contamination is at its height. Moreover, EAA associated with bird exposure occurs more frequently during the sporting (bird-hunting) season.

As with other granulomatous disorders, EAA occurs more often in individuals who do not smoke. However, when the disease occurs in smokers, they typically have a more severe course with increased mortality compared to nonsmokers. Concurrent high exposures to carbamate and organochlorine pesticides are associated with a higher risk of developing EAA in at-risk farmers. Pesticide exposure has been shown to activate the immune system, with increased inflammatory cytokine production and differential functional effects on macrophages, which may serve to enhance the inflammatory response to antigen.

There is also evidence that viral infections may be associated with disease development. Dakhama et al. found viral nucleic acids in more than half of the bronchoalveolar lavage (BAL) specimens and alveolar macrophages in subjects with acute EAA; influenza A was isolated in the majority of subjects. Infection with respiratory syncytial virus (RSV) and Sendai virus in mouse models of EAA are associated with a more robust inflammatory response to the inhaled antigens that cause farmer's lung. Fetal microchimerism (fetal cells in maternal tissues) may also be an important mechanism to help explain the observation that EAA is more common in antigen-exposed women who have had children.

Several genetic studies suggest that individuals with certain major histocompatibility complex (MHC) class II haplotypes and alleles as well as tumor necrosis factor alpha (TNF-α) promoter polymorphisms are at increased risk of developing EAA. Specific single nucleotide polymorphisms (SNPs) in the transporter associated with antigen processing (TAP-1) and proteasome subunit beta type 8 (PSMB8) genes, involved in antigen processing and presentation by MHC classes I and II, may have affected disease susceptibility in a population of Mexican patients with EAA. Interestingly, two studies in different populations showed that allelic variants in the promoter region of tissue inhibitor of metalloproteinase 3 (TIMP-3), which inhibits the proteolytic activity of matrix metalloproteinases and thus extracellular matrix turnover, are protective against the development of EAA.

Table 55-1   Three Major Categories of Antigens Causing Extrinsic Allergic Alveolitis (EAA)

Antigen	Exposure	Syndrome
Microbial Agents		
Bacteria		
Thermophilic	Organic dust	Farmer's lung, bagassosis, mushroom worker's lung
Nonthermophilic	Water, hot tubs	Humidifier lung, hot tub lung
Fungi		
Aspergillus spp.	Moldy hay and moldy water Animal bedding Esparto grass	Farmer's lung, ventilation pneumonitis Doghouse disease Espartosis
Trichosporon cutaneum (T. biegelii)	Damp wood and mats	Japanese summer-type EAA
Alternaria spp.	Wood pulp	Wood pulp worker's lung
Cryptostroma corticale	Wood bark	Maple bark stripper's lung
Animal and Plant Proteins		
Animal proteins		
Avian proteins	Bird droppings, feathers (bloom)	Bird fancier's lung, pigeon breeder's lung
Urine, serum, pelts	Rats, gerbils	Animal handler's lung
Plants		
Coffee	Coffee bean dust	Coffee worker's lung
Low Molecular Weight Chemicals		
Toluene diisocyanate (TDI)	Paints, resins, polyurethane foams	Isocyanate (TDI) EAA
Drugs	Amiodarone, gold, procarbazine	Drug-induced EAA
Methylmethacrylate	Dental laboratories	

CLINICAL FEATURES

The clinical presentation of patients with EAA can vary depending on the duration and intensity of exposure. Presentation does not seem to change with the type of antigen (organic vs. inorganic). Traditionally, the clinical presentation of EAA has been classified according to Richerson's scheme, which describes acute, subacute, and chronic forms. Symptoms of *acute* EAA generally occur within 4 to 12 hours of antigen exposure. Flulike symptoms predominate, including fever, cough, dyspnea, chills, malaise, chest tightness, and myalgias. Physical examination frequently reveals fever, tachypnea, tachycardia, and rales. With *subacute* and *chronic* forms, the temporal relationship between antigen exposure and symptom onset is more difficult to assess. Typically, these patients report more insidious onset of progressive dyspnea on exertion, dry or minimally productive cough, fatigue, malaise, anorexia, and weight loss. The physical examination may reveal bibasilar rales; right-sided heart failure and digital clubbing may be present in patients with advanced fibrosis.

Notably, Richerson's classification system was described before the use of computed tomography (CT) and does not correlate well with lung pathology. Lacasse et al., using data from the hypersensitivity pneumonitis (HP) study, used a cluster analysis (e.g., symptomatology, physiology, imaging, BAL data) and found that subacute EAA is likely an attenuated form of acute EAA. Thus, they proposed a binary scheme in which patients are classified according to disease activity, whether active or sequelae. This classification scheme, however, needs further validation before it is integrated into clinical practice.

Table 55-2   Clinical Prediction Rule for Diagnosis of Extrinsic Allergic Alveolitis

Variable	Odds Ratio (95% CI)
Exposure to known antigen	38.8 (11.6-129.6)
Positive precipitating antibodies	5.3 (2.7-10.4)
Recurrent episodes of symptoms	3.3 (1.5-7.5)
Inspiratory crackles	4.5 (1.8-11.7)
Symptoms 4-8 hours after exposure	7.2 (1.8-28.6)
Weight loss	2.0 (1.0-3.9)

From Lacasse Y et al: *Am J Respir Crit Care Med* 168:952-958, 2003.

Several diagnostic criteria have been proposed to differentiate EAA from other interstitial lung diseases (ILDs). A prospective multicenter cohort study of patients who had a pulmonary syndrome with EAA in the differential diagnosis adopted a "clinical prediction rule" for the diagnosis of active EAA (**Table 55-2**). Significant predictors in the final model included exposure to a known offending antigen, positive precipitating antibodies, recurrent episodes of symptoms, inspiratory crackles, symptoms 4 to 8 hours after exposure, and weight loss. These criteria are helpful when combined with BAL and high-resolution CT in determining the likelihood of EAA.

IMAGING

The chest radiograph is often normal in patients with EAA, with an estimated sensitivity of only 10%. In acute

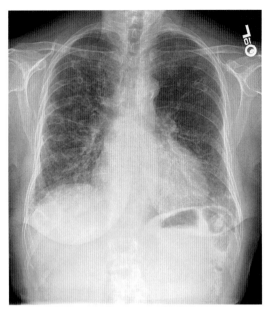

Figure 55-1 Chest radiograph of patient with hot tub lung, showing extensive reticular changes and fibrosis indicative of chronic hypersensitivity pneumonitis, or extrinsic allergic alveolitis (EAA).

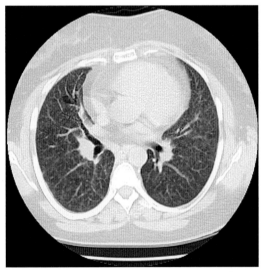

Figure 55-2 Classic high-resolution computed tomography (HRCT) appearance of extrinsic allergic alveolitis, revealing centrilobular nodularity and ground-glass opacities.

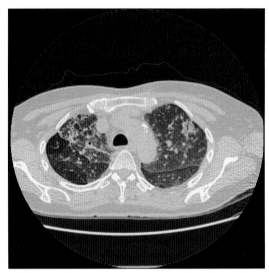

Figure 55-3 High-resolution CT scan of patient with chronic fibrotic extrinsic allergic alveolitis, showing upper-zone fibrosis with mosaic attenuation.

Table 55-3	Radiologic Abnormalities in EAA with Physiologic/Histologic Association	
HRCT Abnormality	**Physiologic Correlate**	**Histologic Correlate**
Centrilobular nodules	None	Cellular bronchiolitis, alveolitis
Ground-glass opacities	Restriction, decreased diffusion capacity	Alveolitis, fine fibrosis, granulomas in alveolar septa
Mosaic attenuation	Obstruction	Bronchiolitis
Emphysema	Obstruction, decreased diffusion capacity	Emphysema, bronchiolar inflammation
Reticulation, honeycomb	Restriction, decreased diffusion capacity	Fibrotic change Traction bronchiectasis

EAA, extrinsic allergic alveolitis; *HRCT*, high-resolution computed tomography.

EAA, radiographs may show diffuse ground-glass or air space consolidation. Patients with subacute EAA may have a combination of nodular or reticulonodular opacities with ground-glass attenuation. Chronic fibrotic EAA usually has the appearance of reticular opacities with honeycombing on chest radiographs (**Figure 55-1**).

High-resolution computed tomography (HRCT) of the chest is the most sensitive imaging study for the detection of subtle changes associated with EAA (**Figures 55-2 and 55-3**). Multiple HRCT abnormalities are seen in patients with EAA that are loosely correlated with histologic and pulmonary function abnormalities (**Table 55-3**). Up to 50% of patients will have mediastinal lymphadenopathy; the nodes are usually smaller than 20 mm and are not detectable on the chest radiograph.

Centrilobular nodules are the most frequent HRCT finding in EAA. The nodules are poorly defined, round, and less than 5 mm in diameter. Nodules predominate in the middle and lower lung zones, although this is not the rule, and are generally of ground-glass attenuation. Histologically, nodules correlate with polypoid intraluminal granulation tissue within the bronchioles (obliterative bronchiolitis [OB], or bronchiolitis obliterans) and reflect an active alveolitis. Centrilobular nodules do not correlate well with pulmonary function abnormalities.

Hazy opacity without obscuration of the underlying bronchovascular margins is most common in acute EAA but may also be seen in the subacute and chronic forms, especially with ongoing antigen exposure. *Ground-glass opacities* typically accompany other CT abnormalities such as centrilobular nodules and air trapping. Histologically, ground-glass opacities correlate with the presence of small granulomas within the alveolar septa, alveolitis, or fine fibrosis. Pulmonary function tests (PFTs) often reveals restrictive physiology with decreased diffusing capacity.

Mosaicism represents a patchwork of regions of differing attenuation caused by ground-glass opacities or air trapping, and often a combination of both in EAA. *Air trapping* reflects a failure of an area to increase in attenuation on expiratory imaging and suggests histologic bronchiolitis. It may also represent the presence of pulmonary hypertension in advanced cases. Obstructive physiology is often present on PFTs when mosaicism is apparent on imaging.

Multiple studies have shown that *emphysema* is more common than fibrosis in chronic farmer's lung, even after adjusting for smoking status. The pattern of emphysema is similar to that caused by tobacco smoke and may be secondary to bronchiolar inflammation and obstruction.

In chronic EAA, the HRCT scan may show patterns typical for nonspecific interstitial pneumonitis (NSIP) or usual interstitial pneumonitis (UIP). Fibrotic EAA is associated with a reticular pattern, honeycombing, and traction bronchiectasis. Honeycomb change is seen in up to 50% of patients with chronic bird fancier's lung and is less common in other forms of EAA. Fibrosis may predominate in the midlung, although a more diffuse distribution has been observed. Imaging features that favor a diagnosis of EAA over idiopathic pulmonary fibrosis (IPF) are upper-zone or midzone predominance, presence of ground-glass opacities, and less honeycomb change. Not surprisingly, the presence of fibrosis on HRCT is correlated with a poor prognosis.

Air space consolidation is rarely seen in EAA patients. Thin-walled cysts, resembling those in lymphocytic interstitial pneumonia, are found in up to 13% of patients with subacute EAA and have an uncertain pathogenesis.

OTHER DIAGNOSTIC TESTING

Laboratory Studies

There are no specific laboratory tests for EAA. Occasionally, nonspecific serum markers of inflammation are elevated, including C-reactive protein, erythrocyte sedimentation rate, rheumatoid factor, and lactate dehydrogenase (LDH). LDH levels are higher in patients with cryptogenic fibrosing alveolitis and EAA than in those with sarcoidosis and correlated with treatment response, as reflected in improving pulmonary physiology. Elevated angiotensin-converting enzyme (ACE) levels have also been correlated with acute symptoms. A neutrophilic leukocytosis with relative lymphopenia may be present in those with acute EAA, whereas leukocyte counts are usually normal in chronic disease. Elevated serum immunoglobulins (IgG and IgM) have also been described.

Serum Precipitins

Serum precipitins are neither specific nor sensitive for EAA. In fact, 10% of asymptomatic farmers and 40% of asymptomatic pigeon breeders have positive precipitating antibodies to causative antigens, but no clinical evidence of disease. In the HP study group's evaluation of diagnostic criteria, 78% of patients with EAA had positive precipitating antibodies. In a patient with a clinical presentation, imaging, physiology, and histology consistent with EAA, the presence of precipitating antibodies can help confirm the diagnosis. Most centers have the ability to test for antigens implicated in pigeon breeder's disease, bird fancier's lung, farmer's lung, and humidifier lung, which include pigeon and parakeet sera, dove feather antigen, *Aspergillus* spp., *Penicillium*, *Saccharopolyspora rectivirgula*, and *Trichiotinus viridans*. Precipitin tests exist for a wider range of antigens but depend on institutional availability and experience.

Pulmonary Physiology

Classically, patients with EAA have a restrictive pattern with decreased forced vital capacity (FVC), total lung capacity (TLC), and diffusion capacity (DL_{CO}). However, patients with farmer's lung more often exhibit obstructive physiology than those with EAA caused by other antigens. About 40% of patients with farmer's lung exhibited obstructive physiology in 6-year follow-up. Patients with subacute and chronic EAA may have a mixed pattern of obstruction and restriction. Methacholine challenge testing is often positive. Gas exchange abnormalities, if present, are characterized by hypoxemia that worsens with exercise. Exercise-induced hypoxemia is usually present early in disease.

In the setting of diagnostic uncertainty, an inhalational challenge using aerosolized material of the suspected causative antigen may be helpful. However, this is not recommended for most patients with suspected EAA. There are no purified, standardized, commercially available antigens to be used for this application, and most centers do not have experience with this technique. Patients may have an immediate reaction, but more frequently a delayed reaction occurs after several hours. In a study of patients with pigeon breeder's disease, which also included normal subjects and those with ILD, all patients with EAA versus approximately 18% of those with ILD and 0% of healthy controls had an increase in body temperature and significant decreases in FVC, arterial oxygen tension (PaO_2), and oxygen saturation (SaO_2) after inhalational challenge with pigeon serum.

Bronchoalveolar Lavage

A *lymphocytic alveolitis* characterizes the BAL fluid of patients with EAA. In fact, a BAL lymphocyte count of less than 30% makes the diagnosis of EAA unlikely, except in smokers and more chronic forms of EAA in which lymphocytosis is less prominent. However, a BAL lymphocytosis is not specific because it may be present in many other conditions, including sarcoidosis, chronic beryllium disease, and several autoimmune lung diseases. Analysis of lymphocyte subsets is variable depending on smoking status, disease stage, and antigen exposure. A predominance of CD8$^+$ T cells is a common feature in non-smokers with acute or subacute EAA, whereas CD4$^+$ predominance is more common in smokers and in those with chronic or fibrotic EAA. Regardless of the subset (CD4, CD8), T lymphocytes are usually activated in patients with EAA, with a polarized type I cytokine profile, as reflected by a predominance of interferon-γ (IFN-γ)–producing T cells.

Histopathology

Findings on transbronchial biopsy are nonspecific and nondiagnostic in 50% of patients with EAA. Proceeding to surgical lung biopsy may be necessary when faced with diagnostic uncertainty, because features of EAA overlap with many other inflammatory lung diseases. The histologic findings vary depending on the stage of disease, although lung biopsies are rarely required in patients with acute EAA. Findings in acute EAA include neutrophilic and eosinophilic alveolar infiltration, small-vessel vasculitis, diffuse alveolar damage, and vascular immunoglobulin and complement deposition. A classic triad of histopathologic features is found in subacute EAA: lymphocytic alveolitis; small, loose non-necrotizing epithelioid cell granulomas; and cellular bronchiolitis (**Figures 55-4 and 55-5**). Foamy macrophages are present in air spaces, while lymphocytes are more prominent in the interstitium. Additionally, foci of obliterative bronchiolitis, intraalveolar fibrosis, and cellular NSIP may be found in subacute EAA.

In chronic EAA, variable stages of interstitial fibrosis may be found. Several patterns may be present, including NSIP,

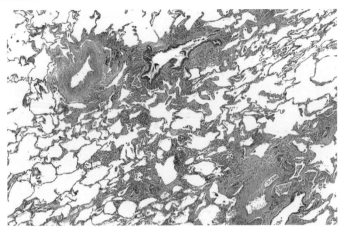

Figure 55-4 Histologic appearance of bronchiolocentric chronic lymphocytic inflammation within the interstitium, along with scattered, poorly formed non-necrotizing granulomas and multinucleated giant cells (hematoxylin-eosin stain [H&E]; magnification 4×).

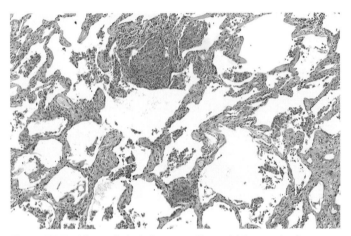

Figure 55-5 Histopathologic features of interstitial expansion by lymphocytes and histiocytes, with poorly formed non-necrotizing granulomas; air spaces contain rare fibrinous exudates and scattered macrophages (hematoxylin-eosin stain [H&E]; 10×).

centrilobular and peribronchiolar fibrosis, bridging fibrosis (between centrilobular and perilobular areas), and a UIP-like pattern. The presence of mild to moderate lymphocytic infiltration, giant cells, poorly formed granulomas, and bridging fibrosis is more specific for EAA and can help differentiate EAA from other fibrotic lung diseases.

Immunopathogenesis

Typically, EAA has been regarded as a T helper cell type 1 (Th1) polarizing inflammatory disease characterized by the production of IFN-γ, TNF-α, interleukin-12 (IL-12), and IL-18. However, there is increasing evidence that IL-17 and TLR6 are also important to the development of EAA and progression of fibrosis in murine models. Moreover, the adoptive transfer of T regulatory cells (CD4+, CD25+) that downregulate immune responses attenuate the development of disease in murine models of EAA. Thus, Treg cells may be a future potential therapeutic target in EAA. Further research is needed to better understand the immunopathogenesis of EAA to target the inflammatory cascade therapeutically.

TREATMENT

Early diagnosis and elimination of antigen exposure are key elements in minimizing morbidity from EAA and treating the disease. Antigen elimination is the most effective approach. For example, maple bark stripper's lung and bagassosis are now rare because of changes in handling organic substrates that minimize growth of microorganisms. Indoor sources of moisture that may lead to microbial contamination, such as humidifiers, leaking pipes, or appliances, and indoor hot tubs should be eliminated. A detailed environmental exposure history is important to identify potential causal antigens and remove the patient from exposure. However, in bird fancier's lung associated with residential exposures, removal of birds from the home may not be sufficient; high levels of bird antigens may persist in the home and require extensive environmental cleanup. Efforts to ensure exposure abatement are often costly and difficult to assess for adequacy. It is therefore important for patients with EAA to receive regular clinical follow-up, PFTs, and imaging to monitor for progression and to direct further efforts at minimizing antigen exposure.

Oral corticosteroids are the first-line pharmacologic agents used at all stages of disease. Corticosteroids can shorten the duration of illness in acute EAA but do not improve long-term prognosis. Generally, patients should be started on high doses of prednisone, followed by gradual tapering once there is clinical improvement. Initiating prednisone at 0.5 mg/kg/day for 1 month, followed by a gradual taper until reaching a maintenance dose of 10 to 15 mg/day, is the recommended empiric regimen. PFTs should be performed within 2 months of therapy initiation, along with a clinical assessment of symptoms and possible steroid side effects. Prednisone should be discontinued when symptoms have resolved or there is no clear clinical or functional response. Inhaled corticosteroids can be useful adjuncts to steroid therapy, along with inhaled β-agonists if airway hyperresponsiveness is prominent. However, no randomized controlled clinical trials (RCTs) support the use of inhaled therapies in EAA. Supplemental oxygen is recommended in patients with hypoxemia.

In EAA patients taking corticosteroids without improvement or with severe steroid side effects, steroid-sparing agents such as azathioprine should be considered because of reported anecdotal success. In patients with progressive fibrotic EAA, early referral for lung transplantation should be considered.

Debate continues as to whether *hot tub lung* represents an infectious or hypersensitivity reaction to nontuberculous mycobacterial (NTM) aerosols and whether treatment with antimycobacterial antibiotics is necessary. The literature suggests that most patients improve with removal from exposure and treatment with corticosteroids. Thus, most immunocompetent patients with hot tub lung do not require prolonged courses of antimycobacterial therapy.

PROGNOSIS

The natural history of EAA is variable and probably depends on the type and duration of antigen exposure and the host immune response. Acute EAA generally resolves within several weeks with corticosteroid therapy and removal from antigen exposure. However, continued symptoms and progressive lung impairment have been reported after recurrent acute attacks and even after a single acute attack. Additionally, persistent airway hyperresponsiveness and emphysema may impact long-term recovery.

Mortality estimates for patients with chronic EAA range from 1% to 10%. Patients with more severe lung fibrosis on biopsy specimens, honeycomb change on imaging, and digital clubbing have a worse prognosis. Moreover, patients with fibrotic EAA can present with acute exacerbations not triggered by recurrent antigen exposure. Unfortunately, they seem to have a similar poor prognosis as those with acute exacerbations of IPF. A recent study has shown that all-cause mortality in patients with EAA is three times higher than in the general population. The reason for this difference is unclear and needs further investigation.

Both prevention of disease and prevention of progression are key areas for intervention. Primary prevention is important in at-risk work environments and begins with informing workers of exposure risks and offering appropriate respiratory protection. Engineering controls and other workplace interventions are essential, such as improving ventilation systems, mechanizing feeding processes on farms, using additives to prevent the growth of mold in hay and silage, preventive maintenance on heating and cooling systems, enclosing selected metalworking fluid machining operations, and regular home cleaning to eliminate microbial colonization. Once EAA has been diagnosed, similar interventions can still be undertaken with a focus on elimination of antigen exposure to prevent disease progression.

CONTROVERSIES AND PITFALLS: A FOCUS ON TREATMENT

Minimal evidence exists to guide treatment decisions for patients with EAA. When to start therapy and choice of pharmacologic agent are often challenging decisions. If, despite antigen elimination, the patient does not improve or even worsens oral corticosteroid therapy should be initiated. The recommended starting dose is 0.5 mg/kg of prednisone (usually 40-60 mg) once daily for 1 month, followed by a gradual taper. PFTs (e.g., DL_{CO}) along with the patient's symptoms should be assessed every 2 to 3 months to determine the clinical response to treatment. Prednisone may be tapered by 5-mg increments every 1 to 2 weeks, with close patient monitoring and adjustment as needed. Corticosteroid therapy should be tapered and discontinued if there is no clear response after 3 months.

Steroid-sparing agents (e.g., azathioprine) have been used with anecdotal success in patients who have failed prednisone or cannot tolerate steroids because of side effects. Some EAA patients require a steroid-sparing immunosuppressive agent for long-term preservation of lung function.

Again, antigen elimination, sometimes with several weeks of tapering oral corticosteroids, is effective for treatment of immunocompetent patients with hot tub lung, with no need for antibiotic therapy.

Long-acting inhaled steroids and β-agonists may be helpful in some EAA patients with airway hyperreactivity. Supplemental oxygen therapy is indicated in patients with hypoxemia. Early referral for lung transplantation should be considered in those with progressive fibrotic EAA.

SUGGESTED READINGS

Camarena A, Aquino-Galvez A, Falfan-Valencia R, et al: PSMB8 (LMP7) but not PSMB9 (LMP2) gene polymorphisms are associated with pigeon breeder's hypersensitivity pneumonitis, *Respir Med* 104:889–894, 2010.

Camarena A, Juarez A, Mejia M, et al: Major histocompatibility complex and tumor necrosis factor-alpha polymorphisms in pigeon breeder's disease, *Am J Respir Crit Care Med* 163:1528–1533, 2001.

Dakhama A, Hegele RG, Laflamme G, et al: Common respiratory viruses in lower airways of patients with acute hypersensitivity pneumonitis, *Am J Respir Crit Care Med* 159:1316–1322, 1999.

Lacasse Y, Assayag E, Cormier Y: Myths and controversies in hypersensitivity pneumonitis, *Semin Respir Crit Care Med* 29:631–642, 2008.

Lacasse Y, Selman M, Costabel U, et al: Clinical diagnosis of hypersensitivity pneumonitis, *Am J Respir Crit Care Med* 168:952–958, 2003.

Lacasse Y, Selman M, Costabel U, et al: Classification of hypersensitivity pneumonitis: a hypothesis, *Int Arch Allergy Immunol* 149:161–166, 2009.

Lynch DA, Rose CS, Way D, et al: Hypersensitivity pneumonitis: sensitivity of high-resolution CT in a population-based study, *AJR Am J Roentgenol* 159:469–472, 1992.

Rose CS, Lara AR: Hypersensitivity pneumonitis. In Mason RJ, et al, editors: *Murray and Nadel's textbook of respiratory medicine*, ed 5, Philadelphia, 2010, Saunders-Elsevier.

Selman M: Hypersensitivity pneumonitis: a multifaceted deceiving disorder, *Clin Chest Med* 25:531–547, 2004.

Selman M: Hypersensitivity pneumonitis. In Schwarz M, King TEJ, editors: *Interstitial lung disease*, Shelton, Conn, 2011, People's Medical Publishing House, pp 597–635.

Chapter **56**
Toxic Inhalational Lung Injury

Lee S. Newman • Kathryn G. Bird

A variety of chemicals, when liberated into the atmosphere as gases, fumes, or mist, can cause irritant lung injury or asphyxiation. As summarized in **Table 56-1**, any level of the respiratory tract can be the target for toxins, which produce a wide range of disorders, from tracheitis and bronchitis to pulmonary edema.

EPIDEMIOLOGY

Smoke inhalation is common among the general population. The use of potentially toxic chemicals in industry continues to rise, and accidental spills, explosions, and fires can result in complex exposures, with little known of the health consequences. The potential health effects produced by inhaled toxins in the United States may be tremendous. More than 500,000 workers risk occupational exposure to ammonia (NH_3) and other gases such as sulfur dioxide (SO_2). More than 100,000 individuals have potential exposure to hydrogen sulfide (H_2S). Tens of thousands risk smoke inhalation from household fires. The number of people environmentally exposed to potentially hazardous levels of air pollutants such as ozone can be estimated in the tens of millions. The threat of biologic and other weaponized agents increases inhalational exposure risks. Also, the World Trade Center collapse showed that firefighters and other rescue workers who respond to emergencies form an additional class of patients at risk from exposures to complex mixtures of dust, fumes, and gas.

ETIOLOGY AND RISK FACTORS

Major risk factors for inhalational exposure and injury are related to the environment and not to the individual. Exposures occur randomly in the general environment, such as when a chemical spill occurs on a highway or railroad, carbon monoxide (CO) leaks in a home, or a person incorrectly mixes household chemicals together and releases a gas or aerosol. Smoke that comprises the pyrolysis products of synthetic materials is a common cause of injury to the respiratory tract, as well as a cause of pulmonary insufficiency and death from fires.

Occupational injuries more often occur when workers handle chemicals, work in areas that are inadequately ventilated, or enter exposed areas with improper protective equipment. **Table 56-2** lists sources of occupational exposure to major chemical causes of irritant lung injury and asphyxiation.

Factors that influence the acute effects of toxic chemicals include solubility, particle size, concentration, duration of exposure, chemical properties, and individual factors such as minute ventilation. The more water-soluble compounds dissolve in the upper respiratory tract and airways, whereas the less water-soluble agents tend to bypass the upper airway and affect peripheral airways and pulmonary parenchyma (**Figure 56-1**).

Pathology

In general, the upper airway can be affected by most inhaled toxins, which result in edema of the nasal passage, posterior oropharynx, and larynx. In severe cases, mucous membrane ulceration and hemorrhage ensue. Toxins of low water solubility may reach the lung parenchyma without necessarily producing upper airway lesions. If breath holding, laryngospasm, and normal "scrubbing" activities of the nasopharynx fail to contain the exposure, lesions develop in the trachea and bronchi (e.g., paralysis of cilia, increased mucus production, goblet cell hyperplasia, injury to airway epithelium, epithelial denudation, exudation, submucosal hemorrhage, edema). Pseudomembranes may form along the trachea and bronchi, causing various degrees of bronchiolitis, bronchiolitis obliterans (**Figure 56-2**), and organizing pneumonia (**Figure 56-3**). Bronchiolitis has been associated with exposures to oxides of nitrogen—nitric oxide (NO), nitrogen dioxide (NO_2), and nitrogen peroxide (N_2O_4)—as well as sulfur dioxide, ammonia, chlorine (Cl_2), phosgene, fly ash that contains trichloroethylene (C_2HCl_3), ozone (O_3), hydrogen sulfide, hydrogen fluoride (HF), metal oxide fumes, dusts (e.g., asbestos, silica, talc, grain dust), freebase cocaine, tobacco smoke, and fire smoke.

Parenchymal injury is less common than airway damage. When alveolar or interstitial injury occurs, both epithelial damage and endothelial damage are observed, resulting in alveolocapillary leak and the pathologic changes of adult respiratory distress syndrome (ARDS). *Diffuse alveolar damage* (DAD) is a common histologic pattern in acute interstitial lung disease caused by inhaled toxins. It is characterized by widespread, diffuse edema, epithelial necrosis and cell sloughing (with exudates that fill the alveolar spaces), and formation of hyaline membranes (**Figure 56-4**). Later, DAD may organize, which leads to proliferation of type II pneumonocytes, resorption of the hyaline membranes and exudates, and fibroblast proliferation. Long-term survivors of such parenchymal injury may fully recover or may have various degrees of permanent interstitial fibrosis.

Pathogenesis

Asphyxiants, such as methane (CH_4) and carbon dioxide (CO_2), displace oxygen (O_2) from the air or, in the case of CO, interfere with normal oxidative metabolism and O_2 transport. Typically, the more soluble gases produce greater injury in the upper airway, whereas less soluble gases injure distal airways and parenchyma. Some of the irritant gases produce direct

Table 56-1 Inhalational Toxins and Range of Toxicity

Toxins	Effects
Ammonia	Mucous membrane irritation and sloughing Bronchiectasis, pulmonary interstitial fibrosis
Ammonia, phosgene, hydrogen sulfide	Laryngeal edema and obstruction
Carbon monoxide, cyanide, hydrogen sulfide	Asphyxiation
Chlorine, phosgene	Acute respiratory distress syndrome
Hydrofluoric acid	Systemic effects, hypocalcemia, hypomagnesemia
Hydrogen chloride, chlorine	Tracheobronchitis
Hydrogen fluoride, mustard gas	Chemical pneumonitis
Hydrogen sulfide	Bacterial pneumonia
Nitric oxide	Systemic effects, methemoglobinemia
Oxides of nitrogen, sulfur oxides	Obliterative bronchiolitis (bronchiolitis obliterans)
Sulfur dioxide, hydrogen chloride, oxides of nitrogen, ozone	Bronchoconstriction, airway edema, asthma

Table 56-2 Inhalational Toxins and Source of Exposure

Toxin	Sources of Exposure
Ammonia	Agriculture, explosives, plastics
Carbon monoxide	Firefighters, smoke inhalation, smelters, miners, transportation, home furnaces
Chlorine	Household cleaners, paper, textiles, sewage treatment, swimming pools
Hydrofluoric acid	Fertilizers, insecticides, glass and ceramic etching, masonry, metalworking, pharmaceuticals, chemical manufacture
Hydrogen chloride	Fertilizers, textiles, dyes, rubber manufacture
Hydrogen cyanide	Metallurgy, electroplating, plastics, polyurethane manufacture
Hydrogen sulfide	Metallurgy, chemical manufacture, wastewater treatment, natural gas and oil drilling, paper mills, coke ovens, rayon manufacture, rubber vulcanization
Mustard gas	Chemical warfare
Oxides of nitrogen	Air pollution, welding, hockey rinks, chemical and dye manufacture, agriculture
Ozone	Welding, air pollution, high altitude, chemical manufacture
Phosgene	Firefighters; paint strippers; chemical, pharmaceutical, and dye manufacturing; chemical warfare
Sulfur dioxide	Air pollution, smelting, power plants, chemical manufacture, paper manufacture, food preparation

cellular injury because they are alkalis (e.g., ammonia) or acids (e.g., phosgene). Others, such as ozone and oxides of nitrogen, form oxygen free radicals that cause respiratory tract injury. These gases may also produce smooth muscle bronchoconstriction and stimulate afferent parasympathetic receptors, which explain some of their ability to induce airway hyperreactivity and bronchoconstriction.

Chronic lower-level exposures to various toxic gases (e.g., SO_2, Cl_2) can induce copious mucus secretion, cough, bronchoconstriction, and bronchitis as a physiologic response to the inhalational exposure. Chronic bronchitis is common among workers exposed to relatively low levels of irritants and may increase their risk for development of chronic airflow obstruction and accelerated longitudinal decline in forced expiratory volume in 1 second (FEV_1). In some cases, nonspecific airway hyperreactivity is induced by persistent, nonspecific irritant exposures.

CLINICAL FEATURES AND DIAGNOSIS

Diagnosis should focus on the nature of the compound inhaled, the magnitude and duration of exposure, and the water solubility of the inhaled agent. Inhalational injury is suspected in those who have facial burns or inflamed nares. Headache and dizziness, along with chest pains and emesis, suggest systemic poisons (e.g., cyanide, H_2S). Unconscious victims found in confined spaces are assumed to have received longer inhalational exposures than conscious ones because of the unprotected airways and concentrated exposures. Evidence of hoarseness, upper airway stridor, wheezing or rales, cough, and sputum production is assessed. Chest radiographs may show pulmonary edema, atelectasis, or infiltrates (**Figure 56-5**), although they are often negative early after exposure. Flow-volume loops are the most sensitive noninvasive indicators of upper and lower airway

obstruction. Hypoxemia in the face of a normal arterial partial pressure of oxygen (PaO_2) suggests CO toxicity. Carboxyhemoglobin levels are obtained for all fire and explosion victims. Metabolic acidosis may indicate cyanide or H_2S intoxication.

In patients who have persistent symptoms months after exposure, bronchial provocation tests with methacholine may help assess whether the patient has *reactive airway dysfunction syndrome*. Computed tomography (CT) may help determine if permanent fibrotic changes have developed.

CHEMICAL IRRITANTS

Ammonia

Ammonia is a colorless, water-soluble, alkaline gas with a pungent odor. Because it is usually transported as a liquid, many accidents occur when it is being transferred from tanks to farm equipment. When it comes in contact with the mucosa, NH_3 reacts with H_2O to form a strong alkali, *ammonium hydroxide* (NH_4OH). Within hours of acute irritation, there may be sloughing of the upper airway mucosa, edema, and obstruction. Laryngeal edema can present without other obvious clinical signs of burns, but if skin burns are present, inhalational injury is likely. Unusual complications include pneumonia and ARDS, which occur within hours to a few days of exposure. Long-term consequences include persistent bronchitis, bronchiectasis, airflow obstruction, interstitial fibrosis, and impaired gas exchange.

Treatment of NH_3 poisoning is supportive: bronchodilators, O_2 therapy, and observation for need for airway protection.

Figure 56-1 Distribution of gases and particulate matter in the respiratory tract influences the site of toxic injury.

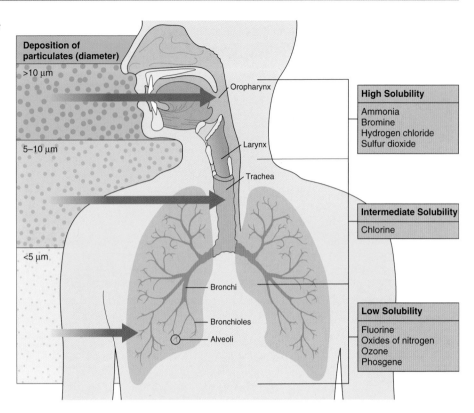

Deposition of particulates (diameter)
>10 μm
5–10 μm
<5 μm

Oropharynx
Larynx
Trachea
Bronchi
Bronchioles
Alveoli

High Solubility
Ammonia
Bromine
Hydrogen chloride
Sulfur dioxide

Intermediate Solubility
Chlorine

Low Solubility
Fluorine
Oxides of nitrogen
Ozone
Phosgene

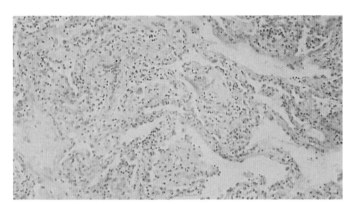

Figure 56-2 Histologic appearance of bronchiolitis obliterans caused by inhalation of oxides of nitrogen in silo filler.

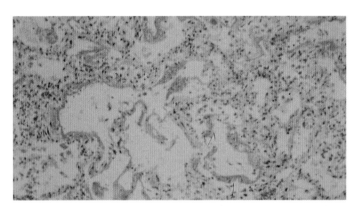

Figure 56-4 Diffuse alveolar damage caused by anhydrous ammonia inhalation. An agricultural worker inhaled the gas when a hose broke during the transfer of this fertilizing agent.

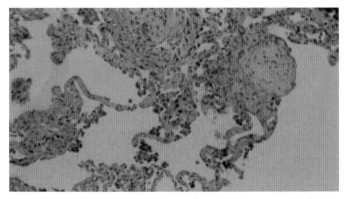

Figure 56-3 Histopathologic features of organizing pneumonia after sulfur dioxide inhalation.

Early intubation may be required to protect the airway from acute laryngeal obstruction.

Hydrogen Chloride

Hydrogen chloride (HCl) is highly water-soluble, and injures the mucosa of the upper airways because of its acidity. Typically encountered in the manufacture of fertilizers, textiles, rubber, and dyes, acute HCl exposure causes mucous membrane irritation of the eyes and airways at levels as low as 5 to 10 parts per million (ppm). Higher levels of exposure can cause acute airflow obstruction and gas exchange abnormalities. Meat wrappers become exposed to HCl when they heat polyvinyl chloride film.

Hydrofluoric Acid

Hydrofluoric acid is a highly corrosive chemical primarily causing dermal injury to the hands. Hydrofluoric acid releases

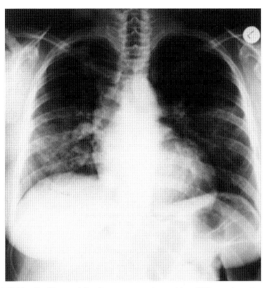

Figure 56-5 Radiographic changes produced by diffuse alveolar damage. Chest radiograph of the same patient as in Figure 56-4 shows acute, diffuse alveolar and interstitial infiltrates.

free hydrogen ions (H^+) that penetrate and corrode the skin, potentially down to bone, producing bone demineralization and necrosis. The respiratory effects parallel those of the skin, except effects in the lungs have a rapid onset and patients present with acute respiratory distress. Hydrofluoric acid is water-soluble and thus predominantly exerts its effects on the upper airways, resulting in rapid onset of tissue damage and bronchoconstriction, in some cases even leading to chemical pneumonitis, delayed-onset pulmonary edema, and death.

Sulfur Dioxide

Sulfur dioxide and sulfuric acid (H_2SO_4) aerosols are produced by fossil fuel combustion. These toxic gases are encountered in power plants and in various industrial processes, such as smelting, chemical manufacture, paper manufacture, food preservation, metal and ore refining, and refrigeration. Past SO_2 air pollution catastrophes have increased mortality rates for patients with chronic lung disease and elderly patients.

As little as 0.5 ppm of SO_2 can be detected in air from its characteristic odor. Levels of 6 to 10 ppm may immediately irritate eyes and the nasopharynx. High exposures ($\geq$50 ppm) injure the larynx, trachea, bronchi, and alveoli. A wide range of individual variability in the response to SO_2 is found, but atopic and asthmatic patients show the most susceptibility. Prior exposure to ozone may potentiate the effect of SO_2 in asthmatic subjects. Classically, patients first experience a burning of the eyes, nose, and throat, with associated cough, chest pain, chest tightness, and dyspnea, along with conjunctivitis, corneal burns, and pharyngeal edema, followed hours later by pulmonary edema. Obliterative bronchiolitis (OB; bronchiolitis obliterans) can develop 2 to 3 weeks after exposure. Persistent airflow obstruction has been observed in smelter workers up to 4 years after SO_2 overexposure, probably because of bronchiolitis obliterans.

Symptomatic treatment for acute SO_2 toxicity may include systemic corticosteroids. Bronchospasm in asthmatic patients may reverse spontaneously after removal from SO_2 exposure, or may require administration of bronchodilators and inhaled corticosteroids.

Chlorine

Chlorine is of intermediate solubility and liberates hydrogen chloride and oxygen free radicals when it contacts water. The result is dose-dependent epithelial cell injury. Low levels of Cl_2 exposure cause irritation of the upper airways and eyes. Increasing levels of exposure injure the nasopharynx and larynx. Higher exposures result in pulmonary edema within 6 to 24 hours. Pulmonary function tests typically show airflow obstruction and air trapping. Long-term consequences include persistent airflow obstruction in some survivors. Clinical management of Cl_2 toxicity is supportive. Even symptomatic patients who have negative physical examinations and laboratory tests must be observed for at least 6 hours because of the potential for a delay in the onset of significant airway toxicity. If symptoms persist, corticosteroids may improve outcome.

Oxides of Nitrogen

The oxides of nitrogen (NO, NO_2, N_2O_4) can produce fatal respiratory injury for some of the millions of workers who come into contact with these gases. Occupations at risk include coal miners after firing of explosives, welders who work with acetylene torches in confined spaces, hockey rink workers, and chemical workers exposed to by-product fumes in the manufacture of dyes, lacquers, and nitric acid (HNO_3). *Silo filler's lung* (silo filler's disease) occurs with inhalation of NO_2 formed from fermented corn or alfalfa in silos. The greatest risk occurs in the first few weeks after filling the silo. Because the oxides of nitrogen have low water solubility, the lower respiratory tract can be exposed to these potent oxidizers. NO_2 reacts with H_2O in the lung to form nitric and nitrous (HNO_2) acids. The oxides dissociate into O_2 free radicals, nitrates, and nitrites, which cause tissue inflammation, lipid peroxidation, and impairment of surfactant activity (among other cellular changes). Notably, nitric oxide has a high affinity for hemoglobin and thus causes methemoglobinemia.

With oxides of nitrogen, exposures of 15 to 25 ppm result in acute mucous membrane irritation of the eyes and throat. At exposure levels of 25 to 100 ppm, toxic pneumonitis and bronchiolitis can develop, often with a smothering sensation and dyspnea. Exposures above 150 ppm are often fatal, associated with OB, chemical pneumonitis, and pulmonary edema. Symptom onset may be delayed, and patients are cautioned that relapses can occur 3 to 6 weeks after initial exposure, with symptoms of cough, chills, fever, and shortness of breath. In some, persistent obstructive lung disease and chronic bronchitis develop. Case reports suggest improvement after corticosteroids in patients exposed to oxides of nitrogen who manifest bronchiolar inflammation.

Phosgene

Also called *carbonyl chloride*, phosgene replaced chlorine as the preferred chemical weapon of World War I and resulted in the majority of "gas attack" fatalities. Phosgene is an intermediate product in the manufacture of isocyanates, pesticides, dyes, and pharmaceuticals. It has a low odor threshold at 1 ppm and produces a characteristic smell of musty hay. As a result of its poor water solubility, phosgene causes only mild upper airway and eye irritant symptoms, and deposits distally in the lung where it hydrolyzes to form hydrochloric acid (aqueous HCl) and CO_2. At high levels of exposure, dyspnea, chest tightness, and cough occur. Acute exposure produces necrosis and sloughing of tracheal, bronchial, and bronchiolar mucosa with associated edema, hemorrhage, and atelectasis. Progressive respiratory failure and ARDS may follow.

Mustard Gas

Sulfur mustard gas (dichlorodiethyl sulfide) was first used as a chemical warfare agent in Europe in 1917. Actually, mustard agents are not gases, but liquids at environmental temperatures. These agents are volatile, enter vapor phase at ambient temperatures, and have low water solubility. Exposure to dichlorodiethyl sulfide produces eye irritation and swelling within 2 to 3 hours. With higher exposure, blurred vision, conjunctival edema, and iritis can occur, with potential for corneal ulceration. The skin becomes pruritic and erythematous, and, 4 to 16 hours later, forms blisters. Acute respiratory damage may be evident within a few hours or, more commonly, several days later. Chemical pneumonitis and pulmonary edema can also occur, with upper airway irritation, sneezing, hoarseness, epistaxis, cough, and dyspnea. Acute injury includes edema, inflammation, and destruction of the airway epithelium, with pseudomembranes developing, similar to those seen with diphtheria. Secondary complications include infection and airway stenosis. The long-term effects of mustard gas include death caused by respiratory infections, chronic bronchitis, and accelerated longitudinal decline in airflow. Additional weaponized agents are discussed later.

Ozone

Ozone is a light blue gas with an acrid "electric" odor. O_3 occurs naturally in the stratosphere, produced by the interaction between O_2 and ultraviolet (UV) light. In the troposphere, O_3 is produced from photochemical reactions between oxides of nitrogen and volatile organic compounds. As a major component of environmental air pollution, O_3 remains a serious pollutant for urban populations worldwide. Its low water solubility causes ozone to principally affect the lower respiratory tract. Healthy individuals exposed to low O_3 concentrations experience acute increases in airway resistance, and decreases in FEV_1 and forced vital capacity, probably through a neural reflex mechanism. With acute exposures to low concentrations, patients can experience chest pain, dyspnea, and cough. Exposure to concentrations as low as 0.08 ppm for 6 hours, with intermittent exercise, may cause lung function and inflammatory changes. Exposure to 0.12 ppm for 1 hour is the U.S. Environmental Protection Agency (EPA) Air Quality Standard.

CHEMICAL ASPHYXIANTS

Nitrous oxide, carbon monoxide, hydrogen cyanide (HCN), and hydrogen sulfide interfere with oxygen delivery, which results in asphyxiation. Others, such as methane, ethane (C_2H_6), argon (Ar), and helium (He_2), are more innocuous at low concentrations, but at high exposure levels can displace oxygen or block the reaction of cytochrome oxidase or hemoglobin, impairing cellular respiratory and O_2 transport. Several important asphyxiants are discussed in the following sections.

Carbon Monoxide

Carbon monoxide is colorless, tasteless, and odorless, and is the major cause of death by poisoning in the United States and most industrialized countries. Exposure results from incomplete combustion of carbon-containing materials such as gasoline, coal, and wood. Home CO exposures occur from furnace gas leaks or fire smoke inhalation. Methylene chloride (CH_2Cl_2), used in paint strippers and household solvents, metabolizes into CO and can be deadly if handled in poorly ventilated areas.

Severe forms of CO poisoning are characterized by unconsciousness, seizures, syncope, coma, neurologic deficits, pulmonary edema, myocardial ischemia, and metabolic acidosis. Lower exposures produce symptoms of headache, nausea, weakness, giddiness, and tinnitus. Confusion typically occurs at carboxyhemoglobin levels greater than 30%, with coma ensuing at 35% to 45%, and death at 50%. Affected individuals are at risk for delayed neuropsychological effects. Carboxyhemoglobin levels correlate poorly with the clinical severity of neurologic sequelae. CO half-life in individuals at rest is approximately 4 hours and can be reduced to 60 to 90 minutes by breathing 100% O_2 by face mask or to less than 60 minutes with O_2 administered by manual bag-assisted ventilation.

Nonrandomized studies show that hyperbaric oxygen reverses the acute effects of CO poisoning and is the most rapid means of reversing acute toxicity. Additional treatments may improve acute neurologic defects. Results of controlled trials are unclear as to the efficacy of hyperbaric oxygen as a treatment for the delayed neuropsychological symptoms. Cardiac monitoring is warranted for patients who have carboxyhemoglobin levels greater than 25% because of the risk of arrhythmias and myocardial infarction.

Hydrogen Cyanide

Individuals exposed to smoke generated by the combustion or pyrolysis of plastics and polyurethanes are at risk of hydrogen cyanide toxicity. The fumes are absorbed through the skin and respiratory tract. By binding to the cytochrome A–cytochrome A_3 subcomplex, hydrogen cyanide blocks oxidative phosphorylation and mitochondrial oxygen utilization, which results in lactic acidosis.

Symptoms produced by exposures to 50 ppm of cyanide gas include headache, tachycardia, tachypnea, and dizziness. Exposures greater than 100 ppm can cause confusion, apnea, and seizures. The patient may emit a bitter almond odor, but this is not a reliable or consistent marker of exposure. Diagnosis rests with the occupational and environmental history. Venous blood appears hyperoxygenated, and the patient may have a distinctive red appearance before respiratory insufficiency, although this also is not a reliable clinical sign. Carboxyhemoglobin levels are measured to differentiate cyanide intoxication from CO poisoning. Treatment focuses on life support measures and detoxification. Early mechanical ventilation, hyperoxygenation, and treatment of metabolic acidosis are critical. Both amyl nitrate and sodium nitrite are recommended.

Hydrogen Sulfide

Hydrogen sulfide is both a respiratory irritant and asphyxiant. As a colorless, naturally occurring gas, H_2S is found in marshes and sulfur springs and as a decay product of organic matter. It is known for its typical "rotten egg" odor. Occupational exposure occurs in the manufacture of chemicals and metals, in petroleum refineries, natural gas plants, coke ovens, paper mills, rubber vulcanization, rayon manufacture, and in tanneries. Heavier than air, H_2S accumulates in low-lying areas; it causes poisoning during oil drilling, wastewater treatment, and natural-gas field leaks. The H_2S reaction with metalloenzymes, such as cytochrome oxidase, accounts for much of its toxicity in humans.

The odor threshold for H_2S is low (0.13 ppm). At concentrations of 50 ppm, H_2S is a mucous membrane irritant. Above 100 ppm, the gas fatigues the sense of olfaction, which makes individuals insensitive to its continued presence. When inhaled, H_2S preferentially affects the lower respiratory tract. At concentrations of 250 ppm, pulmonary edema can occur. At

500 ppm, systemic and neurologic effects develop, with sudden loss of consciousness seen above 700 ppm. Above 1000 ppm, H₂S produces hyperpnea and apnea, which paralyze respiratory drive centers, resulting in death by asphyxia. Prolonged low-level (50 ppm) exposures can cause respiratory tract inflammation and drying; typical symptoms of cough, sore throat, hoarseness, rhinitis, and chest tightness occur between 50 and 250 ppm. At higher acute exposure levels, such symptoms may not manifest because of the rapid absorption of the gas through the lung into the bloodstream.

Management of the patient with H₂S poisoning is generally supportive, with prompt endotracheal intubation and mechanical ventilation for severe cases of intoxication. Oxygen enhances sulfide metabolism and benefits hypoxic tissue. Because the mechanism of H₂S toxicity is similar to that of cyanide, induction of methemoglobinemia with infusion of 3% sodium nitrite or inhalation of amyl nitrate is recommended. Hyperbaric oxygen therapy may be beneficial.

METALS

Arsenic

Arsenic is added to metals as a hardener and is also found in pigments, wood preservatives, herbicides, desiccants, and sheep and cattle dips. This metal has many valences, with As(III), As(V), and arsine gas being the most hazardous. Exposure primarily occurs with smelting and pesticide manufacture and application. Acute inhalational exposure causes abdominal pain, diarrhea, vomiting, peripheral neuropathy, seizures, circulatory collapse, and death. Chronic exposure can cause alopecia, paresthesias, and keratoses on the palms and soles of the feet. More serious symptoms include cardiac failure, renal disease, angiosarcoma of the liver, and lung cancer. Chelation with dimercaprol improves excretion of arsenic.

Beryllium

The light metal beryllium is used as an alloy for its high tensile strength and is found in industries involving nuclear weapons production, aerospace, ceramics, and electronics. Processes that generate beryllium dust and fumes may lead to acute pneumonitis that can largely be avoided through protective measures. *Chronic beryllium disease* (CBD) occurs after seemingly small and short-term exposure to the metal, as a result of a hypersensitivity immune response. Some individuals are genetically predisposed to CBD if exposed. Symptoms include dyspnea, dry cough, and fatigue, with rales (crackles) the most common finding on lung auscultation. The disease is diagnosed through the beryllium lymphocyte proliferation test (BeLPT), which can be performed on blood or bronchoalveolar lavage (BAL). This test distinguishes CBD from sarcoidosis and other similar diseases. Noncaseating granuloma formation and lung fibrosis are pathologic consequences. Immunosuppressant therapy (e.g., corticosteroids) is required as the CBD progresses.

Cadmium

Cadmium is used for electroplating, as a pigment in paint to prevent corrosion, and in batteries. It is also a by-product of smelting and refining. Inhaled cadmium accumulates in the liver and kidneys and can cause headache, myalgia, nausea, fever, cough, dyspnea, and chest tightness. Long-term exposure causes pulmonary fibrosis, emphysema, lung cancer, and prostate cancer. Severe poisoning can be treated with calcium disodium edetate (CaNa₂EDTA) to increase excretion.

Chromium

Chromium provides corrosion resistance for electroplating appliances, automotive parts, machinery, and tools. It may be encountered in mining, welding, and cement workers. Chromium (VI) is the most hazardous of the forms of chromium, known to cause eye and respiratory system irritation, ulceration and erosion of the nasal septum, and lung cancer. Acute exposure can be treated with oxygen and bronchodilators while nasal ulcerations should be treated with 10% CaNa₂EDTA ointment.

Cobalt

Cobalt imparts hardness to alloys and is used as a pigment in glass, paint, and ceramics. Cobalt-related lung disease has been well described in diamond polishers and those working with tungsten carbide grinders. Occupational exposures can cause asthma and several forms of interstitial lung disease, including hard metal disease (cobalt lung, tungsten carbide disease), giant cell pneumonitis, and pulmonary fibrosis, as well as cardiomyopathy and possibly lung cancer. Removal from exposure can help in the management of asthma, hard metal disease, and giant cell pneumonitis.

Nickel

Nickel provides durability and prevents corrosion in alloys. Occupational exposure occurs through mining, milling, and refining. Insoluble nickel accumulates in the respiratory tract and can cause rhinitis, sinusitis, anosmia, asthma, interstitial pneumonitis, and lung cancer. Nonoccupational exposures through skin contact with nickel-containing jewelry are a common cause of nickel allergy and increase the risk for asthma in those occupationally exposed. Exposure can be monitored through excess urine nickel excretion.

INFLAMMATORY AND AUTOIMMUNE AGENTS

Inhalational Fume Fever

A variety of clinically similar conditions are caused by inhalation of metal fumes or dust. Metal fumes of copper, magnesium, and most often zinc are formed during activities such as welding and cause *metal fume fever*. Similarly, the combustion products of polytetrafluoroethylene (PTFE, Teflon) resins may be inhaled and cause *polymer fume fever*. *Organic dust toxic syndrome* occurs through the inhalation of *bioaerosols* (e.g., moldy silage, wood chips, sewage sludge, cotton, grain dust) that are contaminated with bacteria, endotoxins, or fungi.

These inflammatory conditions are characterized by flulike symptoms, including chills, myalgia, headache, fever, malaise, cough, and chest discomfort. On physical examination, crackles may be heard. Diagnosis is made by history and clinical evaluation. Laboratory values may show a leukocytosis with a left shift and elevated serum lactate dehydrogenase. The pathophysiology is not completely understood, but stimulation of the immune system may lead to symptoms, based on studies of cytokine production in BAL fluid and blood of affected individuals.

Treatment is symptomatic, and inhalational fume fever is self-limited, generally peaking at 18 hours and lasting 24 hours. Removal from further exposure is necessary. These conditions share some clinical overlap with *hypersensitivity pneumonitis*, a lung condition caused by bioaerosols and certain chemicals that induce specific cellular and humoral immune responses.

Table 56-3 Categories of Biochemical Poisons and Weapons: Specific Agents, Pulmonary Effects, and Treatment

Toxin	Pulmonary Effect	Treatment
Biotoxins/Poisoning Agents		
Ricin (phytotoxin)	Cough, pulmonary edema	Pulmonary toilet, oxygen, mechanical ventilation, cardiopulmonary resuscitation
Blister Agents/Vesicants		
Lewisite	Respiratory tract irritation, coryza sneezing, hoarseness, epistaxis, dyspnea and cough, pneumonitis, pulmonary edema, respiratory failure	Dimercaprol (antilewisite, British anti-lewisite [BAL])
Lung-Damaging Agents		
Chloropicrin	Coughing, dyspnea, chest tightness, pulmonary edema	β_2-Adrenergic agonists and corticosteroids for bronchospasm
Nerve Agents		
Sarin, Soman, Tabun, VX	Respiratory failure	Atropine, 2-PAM (pralidoxime); benzodiazepines for convulsions
Riot Control/Tearing Agents		
Chloroacetophenone	Rhinorrhea, cough, sneezing, chest tightness, dyspnea, pulmonary edema, bronchospasm	
Vomiting Agents		
Adamsite (diphenylamine chlorarsine)	Rhinorrhea, cough, sneezing	Oxygen; bronchodilators for bronchospasm

Biochemical Toxins and Weaponized Agents

A variety of agents have been developed and used to cause mass injury or disruption. **Table 56-3** provides an overview of pulmonary effects and treatment of these toxicities. With all chemical exposures, individuals should be removed from exposure and given supportive care.

COMPLEX EXPOSURES

In practice, patients with inhalational injuries are frequently exposed to complex mixtures of toxic compounds rather than a single agent. Such admixtures may be poorly characterized, and may contain combustion products, pyrolysis products, metals, particulates, and gas. Recent studies illustrate the ability of such mixtures to produce a range of airway and diffuse interstitial lung lesions.

As a consequence of exposures immediately after the World Trade Center collapse in 2001, pulmonary function decline, reactive airways dysfunction syndrome (RADS), asthma, reactive upper airways dysfunction syndrome (RUDS), sinus complaints, gastroesophageal reflux disease (GERD), and cases of inflammatory pulmonary parenchymal diseases (e.g., sarcoidosis) have been documented among rescue and recovery workers and volunteers. Specifically, in rescue workers with a high level of exposure, 8% experienced new onset of cough, 95% had symptoms of dyspnea, 87% had GERD, 54% had nasal congestion, and 23% of workers were identified as having bronchial hyperreactivity 6 months later. About 16% of rescue workers met the diagnosis criteria for RADS 1 year after the collapse. In a longitudinal study of pulmonary function in rescue workers before and after exposure, the average adjusted FEV_1 decreased 372 mL during the year after September 2001, which translates to an estimated 12 years of aging-related FEV_1 decline.

Factors such as dust alkalinity may have contributed to some of these conditions, although as often the case in acute situations, detailed information about the inhalational exposures in those workers is limited. Detailed qualitative and quantitative analyses of airborne pollutants with their changing composition during initial rescue/recovery and subsequent cleanup have been published, but incomplete air quality monitoring during and early after the structural collapse make full individual assessment of this exposure problematic.

CONTROVERSIES AND PITFALLS

Many of the uncertainties in this arena of pulmonary medicine pertain to the management and treatment of inhalational injury, for which a few general comments apply. In patients with severe inhalational injury, intubation may be required for airway protection. Careful observation, preferably in an intensive care setting, is recommended for suspected cases of significant inhalational injury. Some advocate direct laryngoscopy or fiberoptic bronchoscopy to assess for laryngeal edema. However, no clear guidelines are available to direct clinicians as to when intubation, laryngoscopy, or bronchoscopy is warranted. Although many clinicians may empirically prescribe corticosteroids, such medications have not been proved efficacious for many of the conditions described. Designing randomized controlled trials to treat sporadic acute inhalational injuries is difficult.

A common clinical pitfall is to dismiss prematurely patients who may be at risk for delayed-onset respiratory disorders such as asthma, OB (bronchiolitis obliterans), chemical pneumonitis, or pulmonary edema. Given sufficient dose and solubility, most acutely inhaled substances pose a risk for immediate or delayed-onset pulmonary edema, which warrants careful observation. Even those toxin victims who are thought to be stable and ready for discharge from the emergency department must be given detailed instructions about the warning signs of delayed-onset respiratory tract injury.

Routine spirometry in groups considered at high risk for acute inhalational exposures may be warranted, based on the exposures of New York City firefighter and rescue worker clinics.

SUGGESTED READINGS

Aldrich TK, Gustave J, Hall CB, et al: Lung function in rescue workers at the World Trade Center after 7 years, *N Engl J Med* 362:1263–1272, 2010.

Amshel CE, Fealk MH, Phillips BJ, Caruso DM: Anhydrous ammonia burns: case report and review of the literature, *Burns* 26:493–497, 2000.

Banauch GL, Dhala A, Prezant DJ: Pulmonary disease in rescue workers at the World Trade Center site, *Curr Opin Pulm Med* 11:160–168, 2005.

Das R, Blanc PD: Chlorine gas exposure and the lung: a review, *Toxicol Ind Health* 9:439–455, 1993.

Hnizdo E, Sullivan PA, Moon Bang K, Wagner G: Association between chronic obstructive pulmonary disease and employment by industry and occupation in the US population: a study of data from the Third National Health and Nutrition Examination Survey, *Am J Epidemiol* 156:738–746, 2002.

Mapp CE, Boschetto P, Maestrelli P, Fabbri LM: Occupational asthma, *Am J Respir Crit Care Med* 172:280–305, 2005.

Miller K, Chang A: Acute inhalation injury, *Emerg Med Clin North Am* 21:533–557, 2003.

Newman LS: Current concepts: occupational illness, *N Engl J Med* 333:1128–1134, 1995.

Perkner JJ, Fennelly KP, Balkissoon R, et al: Irritant-associated vocal cord dysfunction, *J Occup Environ Med* 40:136–143, 1998.

US National Institute for Occupational Safety and Health: The emergency response safety and health database, 2008. www.cdc.gov/NIOSH/ershdb/AgentListCategory.html.

Chapter **57**

Pulmonary Embolism

Michael P. Gruber • Todd M. Bull

The philosophies of one age have become the absurdities of the next, and the foolishness of yesterday has become the wisdom of tomorrow.

William Osler

Pulmonary embolism (PE) and *deep vein thrombosis* (DVT) are different manifestations of the same pathologic process best grouped under the designation *venous thromboembolism* (VTE). As a disease entity, VTE is responsible for significant morbidity and mortality while imparting great socioeconomic impact. Appropriately, much attention has been devoted to its diagnosis and treatment. Although the medical literature has at times presented conflicting opinions, increased numbers of better-designed trials are helping to build consensus toward the optimal approach for the management of PE. This is not to say that significant controversies do not still exist. As in all areas of medicine, as one question is answered, others arise. This chapter presents an overview of the most important literature regarding the clinical approach to PE.

EPIDEMIOLOGY, RISK FACTORS, AND PATHOGENESIS

EPIDEMIOLOGY

PE is a common clinical problem. In the United States, hospital-based studies estimate the incidence of PE at 1 case per 1000 persons per year, equating to 200,000 to 300,000 hospital admissions per year. Estimates suggest that as many as 30,000 to 50,000 people die from PE annually in the United States, with an estimated 3-month disease-specific mortality rate of 10%. In nearly 20% of cases, the presenting clinical manifestation is sudden death. Data reported from Europe and other parts of the world are broadly similar.

Significant differences in mortality associated with PE for age, gender, and race have been observed. Age-adjusted PE mortality rates are as much as 50% higher among African Americans than whites. Within and between racial strata, PE mortality rates are 20% to 30% higher in men than in women. African American men have the highest reported mortality from PE, at 6.0 deaths per 100,000 persons, followed by African American women at 4.8 deaths per 100,000 persons. The mortality for PE in white males is 2.4 deaths per 100,000 persons and is the lowest in white females at 2.3 deaths per 100,000 persons. The incidence of PE also is age-dependent, with increasing incidence of death with advancing age. From 1979 to 1998, accounting for both gender and race, age-specific mortality rates doubled for each 10-year age group after 15 to 24 years.

In recent decades, the overall mortality rate from PE has decreased dramatically. From 1998 to 2009, the annual in-hospital mortality decreased by approximately 30%. The decline has been observed across gender and ethnic groups and has been attributed to improved risk factor modification, including improved prophylaxis of DVT, better detection and treatment of DVT, and/or enhanced PE diagnostic techniques, which has led to a decrease in disease misclassification.

RISK FACTORS

The etiopathogenesis of VTE, which includes PE and DVT, is a dynamic process resulting from synergistic interaction between acquired and genetic risk factors. Historically, Rudolph Virchow is credited with describing the classic triad of vascular endothelial injury, hypercoagulability, and venous stasis as the combination of host factors that predispose to VTE. VTE risk factors traditionally are categorized as either genetic (inherited thrombophilia) or acquired.

Inherited Thrombophilia

Inherited thrombophilias may result from qualitative or quantitative defects in coagulation factor inhibitors (antithrombin, protein C, protein S), increased levels or function of coagulation factors (activated protein C resistance, factor V Leiden mutation, prothrombin gene mutation, elevated factor VIII levels), hyperhomocysteinemia, defects in fibrolysis, or altered platelet function. Epidemiologic features of the common inherited thrombophilias are shown in **Table 57-1**.

Antithrombin Deficiency

Formerly termed *antithrombin III*, antithrombin (AT) is a single-chain vitamin K–independent glycoprotein belonging to the serine protease inhibitor superfamily. AT functions as a natural anticoagulant by binding and inactivating thrombin and the activated coagulation factors IXa, Xa, XIa, and XIIa. The AT molecule also has an active heparin-binding site, which, when heparin-bound, has marked affinity and function for binding and inactivating coagulation factors such as thrombin. The augmentation of the inhibitory activity of AT by heparin is the basis for the clinical use of heparin therapy. Mutations in AT lead to decreased ability of the molecule to inhibit the coagulation cascade, thereby leading to increased risk for thrombosis. AT deficiency is inherited as an autosomal dominant trait affecting males and females equally. Most affected persons are heterozygotic for AT deficiency, because homozygotic inheritance typically is fetal-lethal. Heterozygote AT-deficient people have AT levels that are 40% to 70% of normal. Two different types of AT deficiency caused by more

Table 57-1   Inherited Thrombophilias

Disorder/Defect/ Mutation	Prevalence (%)		Inheritance Pattern	Relative Risk	Clinical Feature(s)
	General Population	Patients with VTE			
AT deficiency	0.2	1-3	AD	20	VTE, heparin resistance
Protein C deficiency	0.2-0.4	3-5	AD	10	VTE
Protein S deficiency	0.03-0.1	1-5	AD	10	VTE and ATE
Factor V Leiden	5	10-50	AD	5	VTE and ATE
Prothrombin G20210A	2-5	6-18	AD	3	VTE
Hyperhomocysteinemia	5	10	Not known	3	VTE and premature ASCVD
Elevated factor VIII	11	25	Not known	5	VTE

AD, autosomal dominant; *ASCVD,* atherosclerotic cardiovascular disease; *AT,* antithrombin; *ATE,* arterial thromboembolism; *VTE,* venous thromboembolism.
Data from Franchini M, Veneri D, Salvagno GL, et al: Inherited thrombophilia, *Crit Rev Clin Lab Sci* 43:249–290, 2006.

than 250 mutations have been described: Type I AT deficiency is characterized by a quantitative reduction in normally functioning AT. Type II AT deficiency is characterized by both quantitative and qualitative defects, with three different subtypes classified on the basis of the type of receptor defect: (1) abnormality of active thrombin binding site, (2) abnormality of heparin-binding site, and (3) abnormalities of both thrombin- and heparin-binding sites. These classification categories are clinically relevant in that defects in the active thrombin-binding site confer a higher risk for VTE than defects that involve only the heparin-binding site or that are strictly quantitative.

Despite a low prevalence, AT deficiency is considered the most severe inherited thrombophilia, with increased risk of thrombosis as much as 20-fold over that in the absence of such deficiency. In patients with AT deficiency, VTE typically develops during the latter part of the second or third decade of life. The most common sites of thrombosis include the lower extremity and iliofemoral veins. However, other sites including the upper extremities, mesenteric veins, vena cava, renal veins, and retinal veins have been reported. Thrombotic events in AT-deficient persons often are precipitated by acquired thrombophilic risk factors such as surgery, trauma, pregnancy, drugs, or infection. Approximately 60% of affected persons experience recurrent thrombotic events, and clinical signs of PE are evident in up to 40% of these patients.

The diagnosis of AT deficiency should be determined by a functional assay of heparin cofactor activity, which is able to detect all cases of AT deficiency of clinical relevance. AT levels usually are not influenced by warfarin therapy but can be decreased during the acute phase of a thrombotic event, in disseminated intravascular coagulation, or with the concomitant use of heparin. Heparin therapy can lower AT levels by as much as 30%. Screening for AT deficiency is recommended within at least 2 weeks of an acute thrombotic event or at least 5 days after discontinuation of heparin therapy.

Protein C Deficiency

Protein C is a vitamin K–dependent glycoprotein synthesized in the liver. Protein C is activated by the thrombin-thrombomodulin complex. Protein C circulates as an inactive precursor and exerts its anticoagulant function after activation to the serine protease, activated protein C. Once activated, protein C proteolytically degrades activated coagulation factors Va and VIIIa. More than 160 qualitative or quantitative mutations in protein C have been described. Protein C is inherited as an autosomal dominant trait affecting both males and females

equally. Homozygous persons typically have more severe and earlier-onset thrombophilia.

Two different subtypes of inherited protein C deficiency have been identified. Type I deficiency is a quantitative disorder characterized by parallel reductions in functional and antigenic levels of protein C to 50% of normal levels. Type II deficiency is a qualitative defect with reductions in functional levels of protein C but preserved antigenic function.

The prevalence of protein C deficiency is estimated at 0.2% to 0.4% in the general population and 3% to 5% in people with VTE. Three clinical syndromes are associated with protein C deficiency: (1) VTE in teenagers and adults, (2) neonatal purpura fulminans in homozygous or doubly heterozygous newborns, or (3) warfarin-induced skin necrosis. Acquired protein C deficiency occurs in a variety of clinical settings, including liver disease, infection, septic shock, disseminated intravascular coagulation, acute respiratory distress syndrome, and postoperative states, and in association with chemotherapeutic drugs.

The diagnosis of protein C deficiency should be made by means of functional testing based on activation with thrombin-thrombomodulin or snake venom. Pregnancy and oral contraceptive use can increase plasma protein C levels. Protein C levels are decreased in acute thrombotic events and during therapy with warfarin. In the absence of warfarin therapy and known medical conditions that result in acquired protein C deficiency, patients with a protein C level less than 55% of normal are very likely to have a genetic abnormality, whereas levels from 55% to 65% normal are consistent with either a deficient state or low normal values. Thus, repeat testing and/or genetic testing is recommended in most populations.

Protein S Deficiency

Protein S is a vitamin K–dependent glycoprotein synthesized by hepatocytes, megakaryocytes, and endothelial cells. Protein S functions as a cofactor of activated protein C for the degradation of activated factors Va and VIIIa. Protein S circulates in plasma in equilibrium as a free functionally active form and an inactive form bound to a carrier protein (C4BP). The bioavailability of protein S is closely linked to the concentration of C4BP. C4BP functions as an important regulator in the protein C–protein S inhibitor pathway.

Three subtypes of protein S deficiency have been defined on the basis of total protein S concentrations, free protein S concentrations, and activated protein C cofactor activity. Type I protein S deficiency is associated with approximately 50% of normal protein S levels, more marked decrease in free protein S concentrations, and decreased functional activity. Type II deficiency is characterized by normal total and free protein S levels but decreased functional activity. Type III deficiency, also known as type IIa, is characterized by normal total protein levels but decreased free protein concentrations and decreased functional activity. Conditions that result in reductions in protein C levels, as mentioned in the preceding section, can similarly influence protein S levels. The prevalence of protein S deficiency is estimated to be 0.03% to 0.1% in the general population and 1% to 5% in patients with VTE. The clinical presentation of VTE in patients with protein S deficiency is similar to that in those with protein C deficiency. Warfarin-induced skin necrosis has been reported with protein S deficiency.

Measurement of the free protein S concentration is the preferred screening test for protein S deficiency. As with protein C, acute thrombosis, pregnancy, oral contraceptive use, comorbid disease, or use of warfarin can alter assay results. Heparin does not alter plasma protein S or protein C concentrations and thus is an acceptable antithrombotic agent for use during diagnostic workup. In patients on warfarin therapy, recommendations support waiting at least 2 weeks after discontinuation to investigate for suspected protein S deficiency.

Factor V Leiden and Activated Protein C Resistance

Factor V Leiden is the most common recognized cause of inherited thrombophilia, accounting for 20% to 50% of new VTE cases. Factor V circulates in the plasma as an inactive cofactor. After activation by thrombin, factor Va serves as a cofactor in the conversion of prothrombin to thrombin. In 1993, investigators in Leiden, The Netherlands, identified a single point mutation in the factor V gene in a cohort of patients with unexplained VTE. The molecular defect is a single amino acid change (arginine^{506} to glutamine) at one of the activated protein C (APC) cleavage sites, making the factor V molecule resistant to activated protein C at this site. The result of this genetic defect, termed *factor V Leiden*, is the most common cause of inherited APC resistance, although other mutations have been identified. Factor V Leiden is a common mutation. The prevalence of factor V Leiden in the general population is estimated at 5%. People who are heterozygous for the factor C Leiden mutation have approximately a fivefold increase in VTE risk over that in the general population. People who are homozygous for the mutation are estimated to have an 80-fold increase in VTE risk over that in the general population.

The major clinical manifestation of thrombosis in people with factor V Leiden is venous. Thrombosis in the deep veins of the lower extremities is common, whereas involvement of superficial, portal, and cerebral veins is less common. As might be expected with the high frequency of this mutation in the general population, a synergistic effect with other inherited or acquired VTE risk factors has been observed. In addition to inherited APC resistance, acquired APC resistance has been reported. Users of third-generation oral contraceptives, patients with malignancy, and persons with connective tissue disease—in particular, systemic lupus erythematosus and the antiphospholipid antibody syndrome—have APC resistance.

Activated partial thromboplastin time (aPTT)–based assays serve as the screening test for APC resistance. The aPTT is performed in the presence and then absence of a standardized amount of APC, and the two clotting times are expressed as an APC ratio (aPTT in the presence to aPTT in the absence of APC). APC resistance is associated with a reduced APC ratio.

Results of the standard aPTT screening test may be influenced by a variety of factors, including inflammatory states, pregnancy, oral contraceptives, antiphospholipid antibodies, and anticoagulation. Genetic testing for the factor V Leiden mutation also is available.

Prothrombin Gene Mutation

Prothrombin (factor II), the precursor of thrombin, is a vitamin K–dependent protein synthesized in the liver. In 1996, researchers identified a single nucleotide change (guanine to adenine) at nucleotide position 20210 in the prothrombin gene as a risk factor for thrombosis. The prevalence of this mutation is 6% to 18% in people with VTE and 2% to 5% in the general population. Heterozygote carriers of this mutation have 30% higher plasma prothrombin levels than normal, which corresponds to a three-fold higher risk of thrombosis over that in the general population. In view of the relatively low thrombotic risk, controversy remains as to whether this mutation confers an increased risk for recurrent VTE. Studies have shown that the estimated risk of thrombosis associated with the prothrombin G20210A mutation is significantly increased only in those persons with additional thrombotic risk factors. Moreover, studies have demonstrated that the prothrombin G20210A mutation often is co-inherited with factor V Leiden mutation. Approximately 1% to 10% of symptomatic factor V Leiden carriers also have the prothrombin G20210A gene mutation. Diagnostic evaluation for the prothrombin G20210A gene mutation is best completed by direct genomic DNA analysis.

Elevated Factor VIII Levels

High levels of factor VIII are a strong independent risk factor for VTE. The prevalence of increased factor VIII levels in the general population is approximately 11%. In up to 25% of people presenting with VTE, factor VIII levels are higher than normal. Research has demonstrated that for each 10% increase in factor VIII levels, the risk of single-episode and recurrent VTE increases by 10% and 24%, respectively. Elevation in factor VIII level has been shown to remain an independent risk factor for VTE with institution of appropriate controls for inflammation, blood group antigens, and von Willebrand factor levels.

Hyperhomocysteinemia

Homocysteine is an intermediary amino acid formed by the conversion of methionine to cysteine. Hyperhomocysteinemia may result from either acquired or heritable factors. Homocysteine is metabolized by means of two pathways. The first involves the cystathionine B-synthase (CBS) enzyme and requires vitamin B_6 as a cofactor. The second involves the enzyme methionine synthase and requires both vitamin B_{12} and methyltetrahydrofolate reductase (MTHFR). Acquired forms of hyperhomocysteinemia may result from dietary deficiencies in vitamin B_{12} or B_6 or folate. Inherited forms may result from genetic defects in the CBS or MTHFR enzymes.

Evidence suggests that hyperhomocysteinemia is a risk factor for VTE. In people with homocysteine levels higher than two standard deviations above normal, the odds ratio for VTE is two to three times greater than in the control groups. Elevated homocysteine levels also have been associated with premature coronary artery disease and cerebrovascular disease, although debate regarding the strength of these associations continues.

Screening for hyperhomocysteinemia is suggested in patients with unexplained VTE. Sensitive laboratory assays are available for the quantification of total plasma homocysteine concentrations. If elevated plasma homocysteine levels are identified, additional laboratory evaluation may be warranted. Treatment varies with the underlying cause but typically involves supplementation with folate and vitamins B_{12} and B_6.

Hypercoagulability Testing

Ongoing research continues to identify new and increasingly prevalent inherited thrombophilic defects in patients with VTE. Thus, which patients to screen, which tests to perform, and when to initiate hypercoagulability testing constitute important questions. Despite the high prevalence of inherited defects, only limited evidence or expert opinion indicates that the identification of an inherited thrombophilia influences either the duration of therapy or risk of recurrence. Arguments for screening acknowledge the increasing prevalence of identified inherited thrombophilias and, with the increase in the discovery of new mutations, the identification of persons with multiple prothrombotic defects. Multiple defects are now found in 1% to 2% of patients with initial-episode idiopathic VTE. Thus, the identification of patients with multiple defects may affect the risk of VTE recurrence, duration of anticoagulation therapy, and/or alteration of management when additional risk factors for the acquired form of VTE are present, such as surgery, pregnancy, or hormonal therapy. Arguments against screening cite the lack of available evidence supporting alteration in anticoagulation management in the presence of hereditary thrombophilia. The 2008 American College of Chest Physicians (ACCP) Antithrombotic and Thrombolytic Therapy Evidence-Based Clinical Practice Guidelines state that "the presence of hereditary thrombophilia has not been used as a major factor to guide duration of anticoagulation in VTE in these guidelines because evidence from prospective studies suggests that these factors are not major determinates of risk of recurrence." A 2009 Cochrane database study failed to identify a single randomized controlled trial evaluating the benefit of testing for inherited thrombophilia after VTE in relation to risk of recurrent VTE.

Given the lack of available evidence that testing and identifying inherited thrombophilia influences the duration of therapy, VTE outcomes from screening of asymptomatic relatives, or risk of recurrent VTE, current recommendations for screening are based primarily on clinical judgment and expert opinion. Key points to recognize regarding first-episode VTE are that (1) the strongest risk factor for recurrent VTE is a history of VTE—of particular importance if the first VTE event was idiopathic—and (2) all patients with VTE are at increased risk for recurrence for several years after the initial event. In view of current limitations in medical evidence regarding the impact of inherited thrombophilia with respect to duration of therapy and risk of recurrence, consultation with a hematologic expert is recommended regarding individual patient management decisions.

Screening for Inherited Thrombophilia

In general, the following patient groups may be considered for screening: (1) those with a first VTE before the age of 50 years without an identifiable risk factor such as recent surgery, (2) those with a history of recurrent VTE, and (3) those with a first-degree relative with recurrent VTE. All such patients should be considered "strongly thrombophilic" on the basis of thrombotic history and are appropriate candidates for hereditary thrombophilia testing. The standard testing approach to screening for inherited thrombophilias includes appropriate

studies to detect activated protein C resistance/factor V Leiden mutation, prothrombin gene mutation, antiphospholipid antibodies, antithrombin deficiency, protein C deficiency, and protein S deficiency.

Several factors must be considered in decisions regarding screening for inherited thrombophilia in patients presenting with VTE. First, acute VTE can transiently reduce plasma levels of antithrombin, protein C, and protein S, resulting in erroneously low levels. Second, treatment with heparin can result in up to a 30% decrease in antithrombin levels over the first several days of therapy. Third, warfarin reduces the functional activity of protein C and protein S and can rarely elevate levels of antithrombin, potentially resulting in falsely normal levels of antithrombin in deficient patients. To sidestep the effects of therapy on measured levels, it is recommended to test for these defects at least 2 weeks after cessation of anticoagulation therapy. If levels are obtained at time of presentation and are within normal limits, then a deficiency generally is excluded. If levels are low at time of presentation, then repeat testing is recommended on cessation of initial therapy. Screening tests for factor V Leiden mutation, prothrombin gene mutation, anticardiolipin antibodies, or antiphospholipid antibodies are not affected by concurrent use of heparin or warfarin therapy. If an inherited thrombophilia is identified, it is recommended to screen all first-degree relatives of the patient.

Management of Inherited Thrombophilia

The initial management of VTE in patients with inherited thrombophilia does not differ from that in other patients. The long-term management of patients with VTE and inherited thrombophilia remains an area of question. Because no randomized controlled trials have evaluated the optimal duration of anticoagulation therapy in inherited thrombophilia, therapy must be tailored to the individual patient. General guidelines suggest indefinite anticoagulation in patients with a history of (1) a single episode of idiopathic VTE in the presence of more than one allelic abnormality (e.g., homozygosity for factor V Leiden, heterozygosity for factor V Leiden and prothrombin mutation), (2) one spontaneous life-threatening thrombosis such as near-fatal PE or cerebral, mesenteric, or portal vein thrombosis associated with a heritable risk factor, or (3) one episode of spontaneous thrombosis in association with antiphospholipid antibody syndrome or antithrombin deficiency. In patients with heterozygosity for inherited thrombophilia and a single episode of idiopathic VTE, the recommended duration of anticoagulation therapy remains in question. Expert consultation is advised to determine the optimum duration of anticoagulation.

Acquired Risk Factors

Acquired risk factors for VTE are far more prevalent than inherited thrombophilias. **Box 57-1** lists common risk factors for acquired VTE.

Surgery and Trauma

The risk of VTE among surgical patients can be stratified by patient age, type of surgery, and comorbid conditions. The incidence of VTE in surgical patients is highest for those aged 65 years or older. High-risk procedures include orthopedic surgery; neurosurgery; thoracic, abdominal, or pelvic surgery for malignancy; renal transplantation; and cardiovascular surgery. The risks from surgery may be less with neuraxial anesthesia than with general anesthesia.

Box 57-1 Acquired Risk Factors for Venous Thromboembolism

Age >40 years
Smoking
Obesity (body weight >120 kg)
Malignancy
    Chemotherapy
Oral contraceptive use or hormone replacement therapy
Prolonged immobilization
    Hospitalization
    Prolonged air travel
Surgery/trauma
Acute inflammatory states
    Acute infection
    Inflammatory bowel disease
    Connective tissuedisease
Intravascular devices
    Pacemaker or implantable cardioverter-defibrillator leads
    Indwelling venous catheters
Pregnancy/postpartum period
Atherosclerotic cardiovascular disease
Congestive heart failure
Cerebrovascular accident
Previous venous thromboembolism
Varicose veins/venous stasis
Acquired hypercoagulability
    Nephrotic syndrome
    Lupus anticoagulant
    Antiphospholipid antibody syndrome
    Hyperhomocysteinemia
    Heparin-induced thrombocytopenia

The association between trauma and VTE has long been recognized. As with surgical risks, the risk of VTE after trauma is related to predisposing host factors; the location, nature, and extent of injuries; and the use of prophylaxis. The risk of VTE in trauma victims is highest with advancing age. Injuries involving the lower extremities or pelvis confer the highest VTE risk. Other VTE risk factors associated with trauma include spinal cord injuries with paralysis, head injuries, vascular injuries, circulatory shock on hospital admission, requirement for mechanical ventilation for longer than 3 days, and the need for a major surgical procedure.

Age

The incidence of VTE increases significantly with advancing age for both idiopathic and secondary forms of the condition, suggesting that the biology of aging and not simply an increased accumulation of VTE risk factors may be involved. In one study, the annual incidence rates for VTE increased from 17 per 100,000 persons for patients 40 to 49 years of age to 232 per 100,000 persons for patients 70 to 79 years of age.

Pregnancy

Pregnancy is associated with increased risk for VTE as a consequence of the hypercoagulability associated with this condition, as well as the increased resistance to venous return by compression from the gravid uterus. VTE will develop in approximately 1 in 2000 women during pregnancy. Age-adjusted estimates of the risk of VTE range from 5 to 50 times higher in pregnant than in nonpregnant women. The risk in the postpartum period is approximately five times higher than during pregnancy. Previous superficial vein thrombosis is an independent risk factor for the occurrence of venous thrombosis during pregnancy and in the postpartum period.

Hormone Replacement Therapy

Hormone therapy is associated with a two- to four-fold increased risk of VTE. The risk of thrombosis increases within 4 months of the initiation of therapy and is unaffected by the duration of use. The VTE risk decreases to baseline levels within 3 months of discontinuation of hormone therapy. First- and third-generation oral contraceptives carry a higher risk for VTE than that reported with second-generation agents. Therapy with selective estrogen receptor modulators, including tamoxifen and raloxifene, has been associated with increased rates of VTE.

Cancer

Malignancy accounts for approximately 20% of cases of incident VTE in the community. Many primary malignancies are associated with VTE. Risk for VTE in patients with cancer seems highest among those with pancreatic cancer, lymphoma, malignant brain tumors, hepatocellular carcinoma, leukemia, colorectalcarcinoma, and other digestive cancers. Furthermore, the use of certain chemotherapy regimens in patients with cancer, including thalidomide, tamoxifen, and L-asparaginase, is associated with higher VTE risk.

Obesity

Emerging evidence supports obesity as an independent risk factor for VTE. The relative risk of VTE for obese people is greater in women than in men, with the greatest effect being noted before the age of 40 years. In addition to its role as an independent risk factor in the context of VTE, obesity is a common contributing factor for VTE occurring in people undergoing long-duration air travel and in women concomitantly taking oral contraceptives or hormone replacement agents.

Previous Venous Thromboembolism

Previous VTE is a major risk factor for recurrence. The magnitude of the risk depends on host factors. Persons with reversible risk factors such as immobility or surgery exhibit a lower rate of recurrence than that noted for those with nonmodifiable risk factors, such as malignancy or inherited thrombophilia.

Heparin-Induced Thrombocytopenia

Heparin-induced thrombocytopenia (HIT) is a life-threatening disorder that follows exposure to unfractionated (UF) or, less commonly, low-molecular-weight heparin (LMWH). HIT classically manifests with a low platelet count (less than $150,000/\mu L$) or a relative decrease in platelet count by 50% from baseline typically within 5 to 10 days of the initiation of heparin or LMWH therapy. The incidence of HIT among patients treated with UF heparin is 10 times higher than among those receiving LMWH. In patients with HIT, the risk of thrombosis is more than 30 times that in the control population. The risk of thrombosis remains high for days to weeks after discontinuation of heparin, even after the platelet counts return to normal.

HIT is caused by antibodies against complexes of platelet factor 4 (PF4) and heparin. The heparin-PF4–antibody complex binds to the platelet surface, where it is recognized by circulating IgA, IgG, and IgM antibodies. Immunoglobulin recognition leads to further platelet activation and release of PF4, thus creating a positive feedback loop. The activated platelets aggregate, resulting in thrombocytopenia and thrombosis. Early-onset HIT, defined as that with onset within hours after initiation of heparin therapy, may be seen in approximately 30% of patients with persistent antibodies to heparin if such therapy is given within the previous 3 months. Diagnosis of HIT is based on recognition of the clinical syndrome and specific serologic testing. Serologic assays can detect circulating IgG, IgA, and IgM heparin-dependent antibodies with high sensitivity (97%) but modest specificity (74% to 86%). Therefore, positive results on serologic assays must be confirmed by more specific tests, including serotonin release assays, heparin-induced platelet aggregation assays, or solid phase immunoassays.

The first intervention in a patient with suspected HIT is immediate cessation of all exposure to heparin, including heparin-bonded catheters and heparin flushes. LMWH should be avoided, because it may cross-react with heparin-induced antibodies. In addition to heparin cessation, patients with suspected HIT should be started on alternative anticoagulation because of high risk of thrombosis. In patients with suspected HIT and/or the need for alternative anticoagulation, direct thrombin inhibitors such as lepirudin or argatroban may be used. The duration of alternative anticoagulant therapy and the subsequent use of oral anticoagulants will depend on whether the patient has had a thrombotic event or requires continued anticoagulation. For patients with HIT without evidence of thrombus, therapeutic doses of alternative anticoagulation should be continued until the platelet counts return to normal. Consideration should be given to continuing anticoagulation therapy with alternative anticoagulation or warfarin for 2 to 4 weeks after the diagnosis of HIT, because of persistent high risks of thrombosis over this period. For a patient with HIT and thrombosis, therapeutic doses of alternative anticoagulation should be continued until the platelet count has normalized; then the patient should be transferred to warfarin therapy with at least a 5-day overlap until the international normalized ratio (INR) is in the therapeutic range for at least 48 hours. Skin necrosis and warfarin-induced venous gangrene of the limbs have been reported during shorter periods of overlap or shorter duration of therapeutic INR.

PATHOGENESIS

Between 60% and 90% of pulmonary emboli arise from the deep veins of the lower extremity and pelvis. Other sources of thrombi include the renal veins, upper extremities, or right side of the heart. Iliofemoral thrombi are the most frequently clinically recognized causes of PE. Thrombi dislodge and embolize to the pulmonary arteries, where they cause hemodynamic abnormalities and impair gas exchange. The hemodynamic response to PE is determined by the embolic burden in association with the host's hemodynamic reserve and compensatory adaptive response. After traveling through the right heart, large thrombi may lodge and obstruct the main pulmonary arteries or travel distally within the pulmonary vascular tree, leading to hemodynamic alterations. In addition to the physical obstruction to flow, acute PE triggers the release of vasoactive substances, resulting in further increase in pulmonary vascular resistance and right ventricular afterload. Because right ventricular afterload increases, increased right ventricular wall tension may lead to right ventricular dilatation and hypokinesis with further right ventricular dysfunction, tricuspid regurgitation, and right ventricular failure. Right ventricular pressure overload can lead to flattening or bowing of the interventricular septum toward the left ventricle with resulting impairment of left ventricular filling, systemic arterial hypotension, and cardiac arrest. Increased right ventricular wall stress caused by right ventricular pressure overload may also lead to right-sided stress-induced ischemia.

Impaired gas exchange may result from impaired ventilation-perfusion matching, increased alveolar dead space, or right-to-left shunting through a patent foramen ovale. Stimulation of pulmonary irritant receptors results in hyperventilation, contributing to the observed hypocapnia and respiratory alkalosis. The presence of hypercapnia in acute PE suggests a large amount of physiologic dead space and impaired minute ventilation, which can result from massive PE.

CLINICAL FEATURES

The clinical consequences of PE range from incidental and clinically unimportant to circulatory collapse and sudden death. Equally challenging, the clinical signs and symptoms related to PE are diverse and nonspecific. Therefore, clinicians use a combination of history and examination findings in association with clinical prediction tools to determine appropriate diagnostic tests and the need for therapeutic interventions. Considerations in the differential diagnosis for acute PE are listed in **Box 57-2**.

MEDICAL HISTORY

Patients with PE often have one or more identifiable risk factors for the development of VTE at the time of clinical presentation (see earlier, under "Risk Factors"). Details should be sought regarding the patient's personal and family history of prior VTE, coexisting medical conditions, functional status, travel history, and current medications. Major risk factors for VTE include surgery or trauma within the preceding 30 days, prolonged immobility, advanced age, malignancy, previous VTE, known thrombophilia, recent myocardial infarction or stroke (cerebrovascular accident), or indwelling venous catheter. Moderate risk factors include obesity, use of estrogen or hormone replacement therapy, and family history of VTE. Scoring systems such as the Wells score and the Geneva score have been devised to help assess the patient's probability of being diagnosed with a PE (see under "Diagnosis" later in the chapter).

SYMPTOMS AND SIGNS

Acute PE embolism may manifest with a wide spectrum of signs and symptoms. The most common symptom in angiographically confirmed acute PE is dyspnea (**Table 57-2**). Less frequently, patients with acute PE present with hemoptysis, wheezing, or chest pain. Frequent findings on physical examination include tachypnea (respiratory rate greater than 20 breaths/minute), tachycardia (heart rate greater than 100

Box 57-2 Differential Diagnosis for Acute Pulmonary Embolism

Pneumonia or bronchitis	Rib fracture
Asthma or exacerbation of chronic obstructive lung disease	Pulmonary edema/congestive heart failure
Pleuritis	Thoracic malignancy
Pericarditis/cardiac tamponade	Pulmonary hypertension
Pneumothorax	Myocardial infarction
Musculoskeletal pain	Aortic dissection
Costochondritis	Anxiety

Table 57-2 Frequency of Signs and Symptoms in Acute Pulmonary Embolism

Manifestation	Frequency (%)
Symptoms	
Dyspnea	73
Pleuritic chest pain	66
Cough	37
Leg swelling	33
Hemoptysis	13
Wheezing	9
Chest pain	4
Signs	
Respiratory rate ≥20 breaths/min	70
Crackles	51
Heart rate ≥100 beats/min	30
Third or fourth heart sound	26
Loud pulmonary component of second heart sound	23
Temperature >38.5° C	7
Pleural rub	3

Data from Stein PD, Terrin ML, Hales CA, et al: Clinical, laboratory, roentgenographic, and electrocardiographic findings in patients with acute pulmonary embolism and no pre-existing cardiac or pulmonary disease, *Chest* 100:598-603, 1991.

beats/minute), and crackles on lung auscultation (see Table 57-2). The presence of syncope, cyanosis, jugular venous distention, pulsatile liver, or parasternal heave or auscultation of an accentuated pulmonic component of the second heart sound, right-sided third heart sound, and/or an audible systolic murmur at the left sternal border may reflect significant right ventricular dysfunction.

LABORATORY TESTS

Standard laboratory tests do not significantly contribute to the evaluation of patients with suspected PE. Routine laboratory findings such as increased erythrocyte sedimentation rate and/or leukocytosis are nonspecific. Common laboratory tests performed as part of the evaluation for PE include arterial blood gas analysis and D-dimer, B-type natriuretic peptide (BNP), and troponin assays. Both troponin and BNP measurements have been suggested as prognostic indicators, differentiating between low risk and intermediate risk for PE-related complications, including hemodynamic collapse and death. Elevated levels of BNP and troponin have yet to become incorporated into formal PE guidelines for risk stratification and treatment, although this change is likely in the future. Normal levels of BNP and troponin have high negative predictive values that identify patients at low risk for adverse outcome related to PE. Alternatively, in hemodynamically stable patients with acute PE and elevated BNP and/or troponin levels, echocardiography is indicated to assess for right ventricular dysfunction, which is likely under these circumstances. Because of the short half-life of these markers and the characteristic delay between the acute event and their release into the circulation, if the duration of symptoms is less than 6 hours, a second laboratory measurement of both BNP and troponin levels is clinically warranted.

Arterial Blood Gas Analysis

Arterial blood gas analysis cannot accurately be used as a diagnostic tool to discriminate between patients with and without PE. Typically, patients with acute PE present with hypocapnia and respiratory alkalosis. The partial pressure of oxygen (Po_2) may be increased, decreased, or normal in patients with PE. The alveolar-arterial oxygen gradient, $Po_2(A–a)$, typically is increased; however, this finding also lacks sufficient discriminatory characteristics to be useful as a screening test. Thus, a normal Po_2 and $Po_2(A–a)$ do not obviate the need for further diagnostic investigation in patients with clinical findings suggestive of disease.

D-Dimer Assay

D-dimer is a plasmin-derived fibrin degradation product most commonly measured by a quantitative enzyme-linked immunosorbent assay (ELISA). D-dimer testing is characterized as highly sensitive with a high negative predictive value useful in the exclusion of VTE, particularly in the outpatient or emergency department setting. With most assays, a level higher than 500 ng/mL is considered abnormal. Used in combination with a low clinical probability of disease, a negative result on D-dimer assay (value lower than 500 ng/mL) has a 99% negative predictive value for PE. D-dimer assays lack specificity (30% to 75%). Elevated D-dimer levels are observed in persons with inflammatory states, infection, acute coronary syndromes, or malignancy or patients who have undergone recent surgery. Current evidence supports that a quantitative D-dimer level lower than 500 ng/mL measured by ELISA can exclude the diagnosis of VTE in patient with low/intermediate pretest probability of disease. At present, D-dimer testing should not be used as the sole modality to rule out VTE in patients with high pretest probability for disease. Clinicians should note that D-dimer assays vary in their sensitivities and specificities. Thus, it is important to be aware of the assay used for appropriate interpretation of results.

B-Type Natriuretic Peptide Assay

BNP is a hormone released by ventricular myocardial cells in response to volume overload and wall stretch. Because of its lack of sensitivity and specificity, BNP is not a useful diagnostic test for PE. In the absence of right ventricular dysfunction, BNP levels are typically normal in the setting of acute PE. However, increased levels of BNP seem to have prognostic significance in people with PE.

Elevation of BNP levels (to greater than 90 pg/mL) obtained within 4 hours of admission have a sensitivity of 85% and specificity of 75% for predicting PE-related clinical outcomes such as death, need for emergent thrombolysis, cardiopulmonary resuscitation, mechanical ventilation, vasopressor therapy, or emergency surgical embolectomy. Normal BNP values in the setting of acute PE have a 97% to 100% negative predictive value for in-hospital death.

Troponin Assay

Cardiac troponins are sensitive and specific markers of myocardial cell damage. Troponin elevation in acute PE is presumed to be related to acute right-sided heart strain with resulting myocyte ischemia and microinfarction. Troponin I and troponin T levels are elevated in 30% to 50% of people with large PE.

However, these elevations are mild and short-lived compared with those observed in acute coronary syndromes. Like BNP, troponin levels correlate with right-sided heart dysfunction in acute PE. Normal troponin T values in the setting of acute PE have a 97% to 100% negative predictive value for in-hospital death.

DIAGNOSIS

The diagnosis of pulmonary embolic disease can present a significant challenge. Typical presenting clinical signs of dyspnea and chest pain are nonspecific and can be confused as manifestations of other serious disease states such as acute myocardial infarction or pneumonia. Many patients with thromboembolic disease present with atypical symptoms, and the diagnosis of PE becomes even more difficult when comorbid conditions such as congestive heart failure (CHF) or chronic obstructive pulmonary disease (COPD) could otherwise explain their presenting complaints. Because of the high prevalence of VTE and the potentially serious consequences of misdiagnosis, it is essential to maintain a high degree of clinical suspicion for the possibility of PE.

CLINICAL ASSESSMENT

Typical clinical features of PE have already been described; here, it is important to stress that clinical judgment is an essential initial step in the evaluation of thromboembolic disease and figures prominently in diagnostic algorithms. The importance of the clinician's assessment of the probability of PE initially was highlighted in the 1990 landmark Prospective Investigation of Pulmonary Embolism Diagnosis (PIOPED) study. Physicians in this study were asked to record their clinical impression (high, intermediate, or low probability) as to the likelihood of PE in patients they were treating before learning the results of the radiographic study (ventilation-perfusion scan or pulmonary arteriogram). The clinical impression was based on an agreed-on set of data but without standardized diagnostic algorithms. One very important finding of the PIOPED study was that diagnosis or exclusion of PE was possible only with clear and concordant clinical and radiographic findings. If the clinical impression did not match the findings on imaging (ventilation-perfusion scan in this study), pulmonary thromboembolic disease could not be confirmed or ruled out by that imaging study, and further investigation was necessary. Since the publication of PIOPED, numerous attempts have been made to standardize the definition of "clinical impression." This has resulted in a variety of scoring systems, assigning points to historical, physical, and laboratory features of an individual patient. Patients receive scores on the basis of inherent risk factors and presenting signs that are then used to predict likelihood of disease. Currently, the two most commonly used scoring systems are the *Wells criteria* and the *Geneva score* (Table 57-3). These two scoring systems and subsequent modifications have been validated in a number of studies. By themselves, scoring systems lack adequate sensitivity or specificity to diagnose or exclude disease. Their true usefulness comes in conjunction with other laboratory or imaging studies, allowing the assessment of disease risk.

Electrocardiograms and Chest Radiographs

Electrocardiograms (ECG) and chest radiographs frequently are used in the evaluation of patients initially seen with dyspnea or chest pain. Although these studies are neither adequately

Table 57-3 Wells and Geneva Scoring Systems Used in Risk Assessment for the Diagnosis of Pulmonary Embolism (PE)*

Wells Score	Points	Geneva Score	Points
Previous VTE	1.5	Previous VTE	2
Heart rate >100 beats/min	1.5	Heart rate >100 beats/min	1
Recent surgery or immobilization	1.5	Recent surgery	3
Clinical signs of DVT	3	Age (years)	
		60-79	1
		≥80	2
Alternative diagnosis less likely	3	Paco₂	
		<36 mm Hg	2
		36-38.9 mm Hg	1
Hemoptysis	1	Pao₂	
		<48.7 mm Hg	4
		48.7-59.9 mm Hg	3
		60-71.2 mm Hg	2
		71.3-82.4 mm Hg	1
Cancer	1	Atelectasis	1
		Elevated hemidiaphragm	1
Clinical Probability		*Clinical Probability*	
Low	0-1	Low	0-4
Intermediate	2-6	Intermediate	5-8
High	>6	High	≥9

*Both scoring systems divide patients into groups with low, intermediate, and high clinical probability for the diagnosis of PE. For the Wells score: total points of <2 indicates a low clinical probability for PE, a score of 2-5 is intermediate, and a score of >6 indicates high probability of PE. For the Geneva score: total score of <0-4 indicates low probability for PE, 5-8 points indicates intermediate probability, and a score of 9 points or more indicates high probability for PE. These scoring systems and their variations have been validated in prospective cohorts of patients. In aggregate, a low clinical probability score indicates a subgroup with a 10% prevalence of PE. Intermediate clinical probability indicates prevalence of approximately 30% and high clinical probability indicates >70% prevalence of PE approximately. *DVT*, deep vein thrombosis; *PE*, pulmonary embolism; *VTE*, venous thromboembolism.

sensitive nor specific to diagnose or exclude PE, they can suggest the diagnosis. ECG findings such as T wave inversions in the anterior leads, in particular V1 to V4, are typical of right ventricular strain and should raise suspicion for pulmonary thromboembolic disease (**Figure 57-1**). Other typical ECG changes include a deep S wave in lead I, a Q wave in lead III, and T wave inversions in lead III. Rhythm and conduction abnormalities such as new-onset atrial fibrillation or right bundle branch block occasionally are noted in association with acute PE.

In the evaluation for PE, chest radiographs predominantly serve to exclude other potential explanations for the patient's symptoms (e.g., a lobar infiltrate consistent with pneumonia). Occasionally, the chest radiograph will demonstrate changes suggestive of PE, such as focal oligemia (Westermark sign), a peripheral wedge-shaped density that indicates infarct

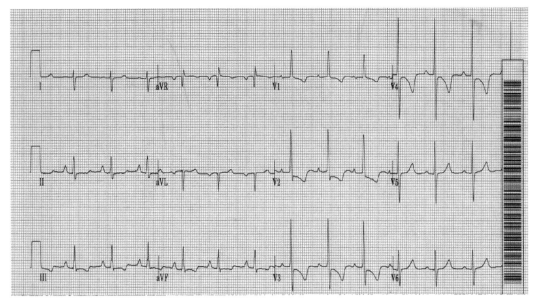

Figure 57-1   Electrocardiogram (ECG) in a patient with right ventricular (RV) strain secondary to thromboembolic disease. Note the right axis deviation, deep S wave in lead I, inverted T wave in lead III, and RV strain pattern in leads V1 to V4. The patient was diagnosed with chronic thromboembolic pulmonary hypertension secondary to multiple pulmonary emboli (PEs).

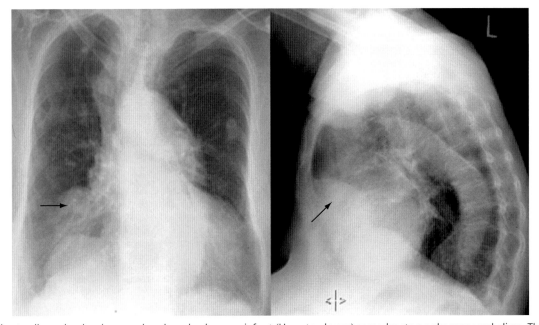

Figure 57-2   Chest radiographs showing a wedge-shaped pulmonary infarct (Hampton hump) secondary to a pulmonary embolism. The infarct is located in the anterior segment of the right middle lobe (*arrows* on both left and right images).

(Hampton hump) (**Figure 57-2**), or an enlarged right descending pulmonary artery (Palla sign).

D-Dimer Assay

Measurement of plasma D-dimer levels in peripheral blood has become an important screening tool to help exclude the presence of VTE. Plasma D-dimer is a degradation product of cross-linked fibrin. After a thrombotic event, endogenous fibrinolysis results in clot dissolution and a measurable increase in plasma D-dimer levels. An elevated D-dimer, however, is not specific for the presence of VTE. Numerous other conditions (e.g., trauma, inflammation, surgery) can raise plasma D-dimer levels; therefore, an abnormal laboratory result has a low positive predictive value for VTE.

Laboratory tests to measure D-dimer levels in peripheral blood have been available since the mid-1980s, but their acceptance as an early screening tool in the evaluation of VTE is relatively recent. Contributing to the initial confusion regarding the usefulness of D-dimer in the assessment of VTE was the presence of significant variability among the various D-dimer assays (ELISA, quantitative latex agglutination, semiquantitative agglutination latex, and whole blood agglutination assays) in both sensitivity and specificity. ELISAs have the highest sensitivity and are therefore superior in their ability to exclude the diagnosis of VTE. Numerous studies have validated the usefulness of D-dimer assays in the evaluation for this entity. A D-dimer ELISA level of less than 500 ng/mL is strong evidence against PE in patients with a low or intermediate clinical probability score. Van Belle and colleagues, reporting for the Christopher Study investigators, demonstrated that the incidence of PE was only 0.5% at 3 months in patients with a low clinical probability score (determined using a modified version of the Wells criteria) and a D-dimer plasma level of 500 ng/mL or less. Other VTE outcome studies have demonstrated similar results, showing the D-dimer assay to have a sensitivity of between 92% and 99% for the diagnosis of VTE. As previously noted, however, the specificity for this study has been reported to be as low as 25%.

Venous Compression Ultrasonography

Ultrasound evaluation of the deep venous system to search for thrombosis frequently is used to assist with the diagnosis of PE. This approach is pragmatic, because the treatments for both DVT and PE are similar, and the first disease process begets the second. Ultrasound imaging frequently is used when the initial tests for PE are nondiagnostic. A positive ultrasound test result confirms the need for anticoagulation and obviates the need for further diagnostic studies. A negative result, however, is more difficult to interpret and requires consideration of certain caveats in considering a treatment plan. In the presence of acute PE, DVT is detectable by compression ultrasound studies in only approximately 50% of cases (50% sensitivity). In patients with nondiagnostic chest imaging studies, compression ultrasound imaging of the proximal vein detects DVT in approximately 5% of cases. Normal findings on bilateral proximal venous ultrasound studies, therefore, do not rule out PE in patients with nondiagnostic lung scans. However, they do imply a reduced probability of this event (negative likelihood ratio of approximately 0.7). Negative results on ultrasound imaging therefore imply a lower short-term risk for development of thromboembolic disease or for a fatal thromboembolic event if anticoagulant therapy is withheld. Some studies have recommended a follow-up serial ultrasound study when anticoagulation therapy is withheld on the basis of initially negative ultrasound findings. These studies, examining a variety of time frames (2 days to 2 weeks), have reported that approximately 2% of patients with an initially negative venous ultrasound will be diagnosed with a DVT by serial testing. If ultrasound imaging continues to yield negative findings during serial examinations, the risk of subsequent symptomatic VTE is low, similar to that observed after a normal-appearing pulmonary angiogram (1% incidence at 6 months).

Contrast Venography

Venography was for many years the only reliable technique to confirm or exclude the possibility of a DVT but is now only of historical interest. Compression ultrasonography has all but replaced this more invasive approach for assessment of suspected DVT. Venography has a reported sensitivity ranging from 70% to 100% and specificity of 60% to 88% for the diagnosis of DVT. Potential complications of contrast venography include nephrotoxicity (secondary to contrast dye), bleeding complications from the venous puncture, and postprocedure phlebitis.

Ventilation-Perfusion Lung Scan

For many years, the ventilation-perfusion lung scan was considered the imaging study of choice to evaluate for PE (**Figure 57-3**). Recently, computed tomography angiography (CTA) has replaced the ventilation-perfusion lung scan as the predominant diagnostic test. However, the ventilation-perfusion scan maintains an important place in the evaluation of patients

for thromboembolic disease who have contraindications to CTA such as renal insufficiency or contrast allergy. As mentioned previously, the PIOPED study correlated the clinical probability of a PE (high, intermediate, or low probability as assessed by history and clinical findings) with the interpretation of the ventilation-perfusion scan (high, intermediate, or low probability or normal perfusion). With concordance of the clinical assessment and the interpretation of the V/Q scan in the high or low probability range, PE can be diagnosed or excluded with reasonable certainty. When the clinical assessment and the interpretation of the ventilation-perfusion scan are discordant (i.e., high clinical probability but low-probability ventilation-perfusion scan, or vice versa), the possibility of PE cannot be adequately assessed, and other studies are required. A normal-appearing ventilation-perfusion scan (with a normal perfusion component) essentially excludes the diagnosis of PE.

Echocardiogram

Transthoracic and transesophageal echocardiography have limited use in the diagnosis of PE. The sensitivity and specificity of these tests are inadequate for diagnosis, because the offending emboli are rarely proximal enough to be visualized. Echocardiography can assist in acute care management decisions for those patients too unstable to be moved from a critical care setting for more definitive imaging studies. Although it is rare to visualize a thrombus within the pulmonary arteries by echocardiogram, changes in right ventricular size and function and increases in tricuspid regurgitation imply acute right heart strain. In the appropriate clinical scenario, these changes in the right ventricle can suggest the diagnosis of acute PE (**Figure 57-4**).

A more important role of echocardiography in the evaluation of patients with PE is that of risk stratification. Multiple studies have demonstrated that patients in whom right ventricular dysfunction develops in association with an acute PE have increased mortality compared with those with preserved right ventricular function. This observation is not surprising, because worsening right ventricular function relates directly to the degree the pulmonary vascular bed is affected by the thrombus and, therefore, the size of the embolic event. Some investigators have suggested that more aggressive therapy, such as thrombolysis, is indicated in patients with right ventricular dysfunction. This issue is discussed further in the section on treatment of PE.

Computed Tomography Angiography

CT pulmonary angiography (i.e., CTA) has become a favored study for the evaluation of PE over the past decade (**Figure 57-5, B**). CTA provides a number of potential advantages over other imaging modalities in the diagnosis of PE, including (1) direct visualization of the embolus, (2) the ability to assess for other potential causes for the patient's complaints such as pneumonia, and (3) imaging algorithms that scan through the pelvis and lower extremities, as well as the chest, allowing simultaneous evaluation for PE and for DVT. The ability to evaluate for other thoracic disease is of no small consequence, because up to two thirds of patients initially suspected to have PE eventually receive another diagnosis for their symptoms. Many of these subsequently diagnosed disorders (i.e., pneumonia, thoracic aorta dissection, pneumothorax) are associated with lung changes that can be visualized on CT scan. The interobserver agreement for CT is better than that for ventilation-perfusion scan. The initial hardware used for assessment of PE was

Figure 57-3 Ventilation-perfusion lung scan. Ventilation images are above their respective perfusion images. Significant heterogeneity is observed between the ventilation and perfusion images, with multiple unmatched defects in the perfusion images, consistent with thromboembolic disease.

Ventilation

Perfusion

Ventilation

Perfusion

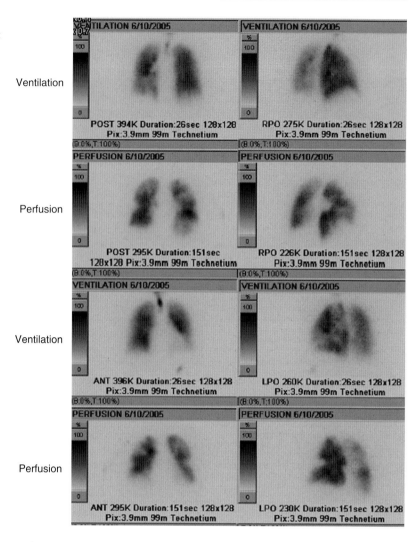

Figure 57-4 Echocardiogram of a patient with markedly dilated right ventricle (RV) and right atrium (RA) secondary to pulmonary thromboembolic disease. The interventricular septum is bowing into and compressing the left ventricle (LV).

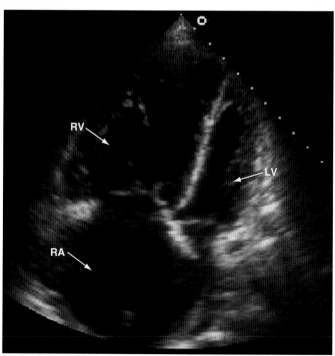

single-detector scanners that provided high specificity for the diagnosis of PE (greater than 90%), but their sensitivity was unacceptable (approximately 72%) for the exclusion of this potentially life-threatening diagnosis. Multidetector (40-, 64-, and 96-slice) scanners in current use, however, have significantly improved the sensitivity and specificity of CTA for the diagnosis of PE. The very high spatial resolution of these studies allows rapid evaluation of pulmonary vessels down to the sixth-order branches during a single breath hold, with consequent increased detection rate for segmental and subsegmental PEs.

A number of outcome studies have demonstrated that a technically adequate negative multidetector CTA study is sufficient to exclude PE (sensitivity and specificity greater than 95%). The Prospective Investigation of Pulmonary Embolism Diagnosis II (PIOPED II) study initially raised some questions regarding the positive and negative predictive power of these studies. The investigators of PIOPED II sought to establish the sensitivity and specificity of multidetector CT scanners in the diagnosis of PE in the same fashion as that used by the original PIOPED for evaluation of ventilation-perfusion scans. These workers undertook a multicenter, prospective study assessing the accuracy of multidetector CTA alone and also of CTA combined with computed tomography venography (CTV) to include venous phase imaging (i.e., CTA-CTV) for the diagnosis of acute PE. However, in contrast with the original PIOPED study, which used pulmonary angiography as the reference test to which ventilation-perfusion lung scan was compared,

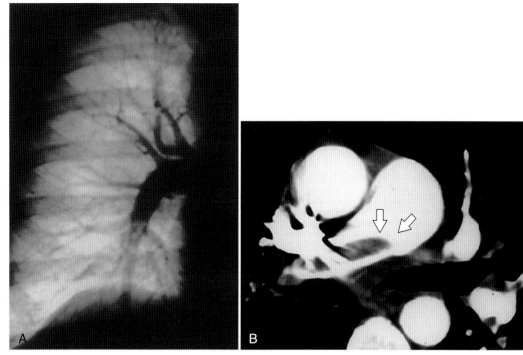

Figure 57-5 Pulmonary imaging for embolism. **A,** Pulmonary angiogram showing a filling defect in the right lower lobe pulmonary artery. **B,** A spiral (helical) computed tomography angiogram, obtained in another case, showing multiple filling defects (*arrows*).

PIOPED II used a composite reference test for VTE that was based on the ventilation-perfusion lung scan, venous compression ultrasound imaging of the lower extremities, and digital subtraction pulmonary angiography (performed in only a minority of cases). They reported the specificity of CTA for the diagnosis of PE to be 96%, but with a sensitivity of only 83%. Venous scanning of the pelvis and lower extremities improved the sensitivity of the study. The sensitivity of CTA-CTV for the diagnosis of PE was 90%, with a specificity of 95%.

PIOPED II also attempted to associate clinical probability with imaging studies to assess positive and negative predictive values. The results were reminiscent of the original PIOPED study in that the positive predictive value of the CT studies was 96% with a concordantly high or low clinical probability, 92% with an intermediate clinical probability, and nondiagnostic with a discordant clinical probability. As discussed earlier, however, a number of large outcome studies demonstrated the efficacy of CTA in the evaluation of PE and the safety of withholding anticoagulation in patients with negative CTA findings. CTA now plays the predominant role in diagnostic algorithms for the evaluation of PE (**Figure 57-6**).

Pulmonary Arteriography

Pulmonary angiography or digital subtraction angiography (DSA) previously had been the "gold standard" modality for the diagnosis of PE (see Figure 57-5, *A*). Because of its invasive nature, it also is associated with the most inherent risk. Arrhythmias, hypotension, bleeding, and nephrotoxicity from contrast dye are potential complications. The mortality rate associated with pulmonary angiography has been estimated at 0.5%, with major nonfatal adverse events occurring with a frequency of 1%. Angiography also is more expensive than the noninvasive means of evaluating for PE and not always immediately available. As other imaging modalities, such as CTA, have gained popularity in the assessment of PE, angiography has become less used, so less experience with its application has been

accrued. Approximately 1% of patients with a normal-appearing pulmonary angiogram will be diagnosed with a VTE at 6 months, implying that the result on angiography was falsely negative. Although large, segmental embolic events are readily appreciated, interobserver variability can be significant in evaluating smaller subsegmental emboli. The main role for DSA at present is for the evaluation of patients with chronic thromboembolic disease being considered for pulmonary endarterectomy (PEA) to assess surgical resectability.

Magnetic Resonance Imaging

Magnetic resonance angiography (MRA) and venography (MRV) were recently evaluated as diagnostic tests for VTE. The multicenter Prospective Investigation of Pulmonary Embolic Disease III (PIOPED III) study evaluated the sensitivity and specificity of MRA and then MRA in combination with MRV (i.e., MRA-MRV) in the assessment of PE. As in PIOPED II, the results were compared with a composite reference standard that included CTA and CTV, ventilation-perfusion scan, venous ultrasonography, D-dimer assay, and clinical assessment. MRA and MRA-MRV fared poorly in the diagnosis of PE. Of interest, the MRA study was technically inadequate in 25% of the 371 patients enrolled. When all enrolled patients were considered, MRA identified only 57% of patients with PE. If only patients with technically adequate studies were considered, the sensitivity of MRA for the diagnosis of PE was 78% and the specificity was 99%. In patients with a technically adequate MRA-MRV study, the sensitivity was 92% and the specificity was 96%; however, in only 52% of patients were both studies technically adequate. These poor results stem from the difficulty of capturing adequate images of the chest vasculature due to motion artifact as well as the difficulty of identifying abrupt termination of contrast in a vessel by MRA. With current MRA technology, the pulmonary vessel without contrast is lost in the background of the lung. In CTA, the same vessel remains visible making a cutoff from PE easier to visualize. The investigators

Figure 57-6 Diagnostic algorithm for evaluation of pulmonary embolism (PE). CTA (or CTA-CTV) is becoming the initial imaging study of choice. Ultrasound imaging and ventilation-perfusion (V/Q) scan can be used in patients in whom CTA is contraindicated (e.g., renal insufficiency) or when additional studies are needed to assist with the diagnosis. *CTA,* computed tomography angiography; *CTV,* computed tomography venography; *ELISA,* enzyme-linked immunosorbent assay; *VTE,* venous thromboembolism.

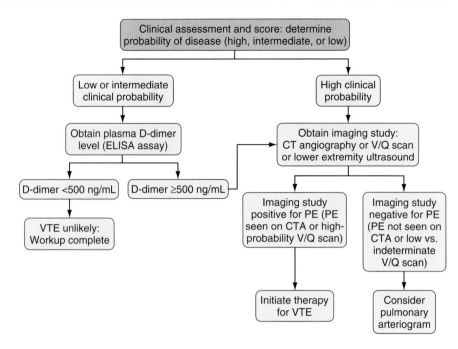

recommended that MRA for evaluation of PE be done only in centers with significant experience in the performance of this study, and only when other tests for the evaluation of PE are contraindicated. Even in with these caveats, however, it is difficult to conceive of many clinical scenarios in which MRA-MRV would be used in the evaluation of PE.

TREATMENT

The basic approach to treatment of PE has not changed appreciably over the past half-century. More recently, however, refinements in recommendations regarding duration of therapy have evolved. In addition, some exciting recent additions of medications for anticoagulation are likely to alter selection and duration of therapy in the near future. The possibility of placement of mechanical barriers to prevent further embolization to the pulmonary vasculature also is now readily available, although data on the appropriate use of these devices are lacking. Thrombolysis remains an option for rapidly dissolving the offending thrombus but is associated with a higher incidence of bleeding complications. The discussion regarding treatment of PE can be divided into two distinct entities: (1) treatment for the acute event and (2) secondary prophylaxis against recurrent VTE.

TREATMENT OF ACUTE PULMONARY EMBOLISM

Anticoagulation

Heparin and Vitamin K Antagonists

The goal of the initial treatment of PE is to obtain adequate, rapid anticoagulation while minimizing bleeding complications. For many years the consensus has been that the initial treatment of acute nonmassive PE should include heparin for a period of at least 5 days overlapping with the initiation of a vitamin K antagonist (VKA). The VKA should be started on the first day of treatment if possible, but recommendations for 5 days of heparin therapy hold even if the desired level of VKA anticoagulation is achieved earlier. This recommendation stems from studies in patients with DVT that demonstrated a higher incidence of recurrence if heparin therapy was truncated.

The goal of therapy with use of UF heparin is an aPTT between 1.5 and 2.0 times the control level. An important development in the use of UF heparin in the treatment of VTE was the implementation of weight-based dosing to rapidly obtain appropriate levels of anticoagulation. This recommendation stemmed from the frequent observation of recurrent thromboembolism in subtherapeutic heparin dosing. UF heparin was the treatment of choice for initial therapy of VTE for decades. More recently, however, LMWH has replaced UF heparin for first-line therapy in most cases. LMWH has better bioavailability and a longer half-life than UF heparin. These features permit once- or twice-daily subcutaneous dosing without the need for coagulation monitoring in appropriate clinical populations (i.e., normal renal function). The ability to obtain a predictable and reliable level of anticoagulation through a subcutaneous route then allows for the possibility of outpatient therapy, significantly decreasing health care costs and increasing patient satisfaction. LMWH was first demonstrated efficacious in the treatment of DVT. In addition, the use of LMWH for at-home therapy of DVT was quickly shown to be both safe and effective. Its use has more recently been studied for initial treatment of acute submassive PE, for which it also was found to be efficacious and safe. These trials showed no difference in morbidity or mortality in patients treated with LMWH versus those treated with UF heparin. A small number of patients in these studies were treated at home or were allowed to go home early receiving subcutaneous LMWH. No difference in outcome was observed in the at-home population. Treatment with LMWH is less commonly associated with HIT than is UF heparin. Although heparin and VKA have played a central role in the treatment of VTE for years, innovations in other medications altering the coagulation cascade are advancing rapidly. Perhaps the most exciting therapeutic advances in the treatment of VTE involve the orally available direct factor Xa inhibitors.

Factor Xa inhibitors

Factor Xa is strategically positioned at the juncture of the intrinsic and extrinsic coagulation pathways proximal to thrombin. The new oral factor Xa inhibitors have excellent bioavailability and induce rapid, predictable systemic anticoagulation.

A recent study comparing 3, 6, or 12 months of the oral Xa inhibitor rivaroxaban against 5 days of subcutaneous enoxaparin followed by 3, 6, or 12 months of an oral vitamin K antagonist demonstrated no significant differences in the primary end point of recurrent VTE (noninferiority). No differences were observed in the incidence of significant bleeding between groups. The investigators simultaneously reported the outcomes of a long-term continuation study in which patients with VTE (DVT or PE) who had already been treated with 6 to 12 months of oral vitamin K antagonists were then randomized to either an additional 6 to 12 months of oral rivaroxaban versus placebo. A significant decrease in the primary end point of recurrent VTE was noted in the patients treated with the oral Xa inhibitor. No statistically significant difference in bleeding events between groups was observed.

These medications have the potential to significantly alter the management of VTE. Their excellent bioavailability, rapid onset, predictable effect, and ease of use will greatly facilitate outpatient therapy. Close monitoring of coagulation levels, as is required with the vitamin K antagonists, is unnecessary, and the risk of over- or underanticoagulation is negligible. In the absence of unforeseen complications, use of these medications may be expected to rapidly become the standard of care in the management of VTE. One potential complicating factor regarding the use of the Xa inhibitors is the lack of a specific antidote for rapid reversal of anticoagulation. Rivaroxaban is cleared both hepatically and through the kidney, and unlike VKAs, it does not interact with food and has few drug-drug interactions. A third study by the same investigators comparing oral rivaroxaban to 5 days of subcutaneous enoxaparin and then 6 to 12 months of an oral vitamin K antagonist in patients with acute PE also demonstrated non-inferiority.

The subcutaneously administered Xa inhibitor fondaparinux also has been demonstrated to be efficacious in the treatment of VTE. Fondaparinux has a relatively long half-life (17 hours) and can be administered once daily. Another factor Xa inhibitor, idraparinux, also is being evaluated in the treatment of VTE. This agent has an even longer half-life (80 hours) than fondaparinux and could thus be administered on a weekly basis. Both fondaparinux and idraparinux are cleared by the kidney and must therefore be used with caution in patients with renal insufficiency.

Direct Thrombin Inhibitors

The direct thrombin inhibitors include hirudin, argatroban, and bivalirudin. Their potential advantage over heparin includes their ability to inactivate clot-bound thrombin and their resistance to circulating inhibitors released by activated platelets including PF4 and heparinase. Of importance, these agents do not cause HIT and are approved for the treatment of this dangerous condition, which is currently their primary role in the treatment of VTE.

Thrombolytics

For many years, significant interest has focused on the use of thrombolytic agents to rapidly dissolve pulmonary emboli in hopes of improving clinical outcomes. These agents have been successfully applied in acute coronary syndromes to help dissolve intracoronary thrombus, so their application to pulmonary vascular thrombus would seem reasonable. Although the use of these agents in the treatment of acute PE has been associated with earlier dissolution of clot, improved physiologic parameters, and resolution of imaging changes, most relevant studies did not show decreased patient mortality. As would be expected, however, an increase in significant bleeding complications was noted in patients receiving thrombolysis compared with those on anticoagulation alone. Attention has since been turned toward identifying subsets of patients with PE who might benefit from this therapy. Jerjes-Sanchez and associates evaluated the efficacy of thrombolytic therapy in patients with massive PE who presented in cardiogenic shock. The study was a small prospective, randomized controlled trial, enrolling a total of only 8 patients before it was terminated early (a total of 40 patients had been planned for enrollment). The 4 patients who received thrombolytics (streptokinase in this study) followed by heparin survived and at 2 years of follow-up demonstrated no evidence of pulmonary hypertension. The 4 who received heparin alone died within 1 to 3 hours of arrival in the emergency department. It is highly unlikely this study will be repeated, and by essentially uniform expert agreement, patients who develop cardiogenic shock related to PE should receive thrombolytics in the absence of major contraindications. A more controversial use of these medications is in patients with PE without hemodynamic compromise but with right ventricular dysfunction. A number of studies have demonstrated that patients with right ventricular dysfunction associated with PE have a significantly increased mortality. It would therefore seem reasonable to treat this group of patients more aggressively.

Two large studies have suggested a potential benefit of thrombolytics in patients with PE and right ventricular dysfunction or pulmonary hypertension, although both of these studies have received criticism regarding their design. The first study, the Management Strategies and Prognosis of Pulmonary Embolism Trial (MAPPET), demonstrated a survival benefit in patients with right ventricular dysfunction who received heparin and a thrombolytic (alteplase, streptokinase, and urokinase were the medications used) compared with heparin alone. The 30-day mortality rate for those who received thrombolysis was 4.7%, versus 11.1% for those receiving heparin alone. In addition, recurrent PE was significantly less frequent in those receiving thrombolytic therapy (7.7% versus 18.7%). This study was not randomized, however, and further inspection of the results reveals that the patients who received heparin alone were significantly older than those who received thrombolysis. This finding is relevant in that older age is a recognized risk factor for mortality in PE. The patients who received thrombolytics plus heparin also had less severe underlying cardiac and pulmonary disease than those receiving heparin alone, which also may have influenced the mortality outcomes.

The second study demonstrating an improvement in outcome for patients receiving thrombolytics was the Management Strategies and Prognosis of Pulmonary Embolism Trial-3 (MAPPET-3). This was a randomized prospective study examining the use of medical thrombolysis in PE associated with right ventricular dysfunction. The primary end point of this study was a combined end point of survival and escalation of therapy. A significant benefit in terms of this combined primary end point was reported in patients who received thrombolytics (alteplase) and heparin versus those who received heparin alone. Close review of this study, however, demonstrates no survival benefit between the two groups. Rather, the difference in the primary end point between groups was due to a difference in escalation of therapy, and in most patients this escalation of therapy related to later thrombolysis for PE. A number of experts have cited this article as evidence of benefit of thrombolytics in patients with PE and right ventricular dysfunction, although other workers are more skeptical of its use in this patient population. An interesting area of current exploration is the potential benefit of thrombolysis for submassive PE with right ventricular dysfunction in terms of long-term exercise tolerance and New York Heart Association (NYHA) functional class.

PROPHYLAXIS AGAINST RECURRENT VENOUS THROMBOEMBOLISM (SECONDARY PREVENTION)

Clear evidence has shown that "early" discontinuation of anticoagulation after an acute VTE results in a substantially increased risk for symptomatic extension of the thrombus, embolization, or recurrence of clot. The difficulty, however, is defining *early*. Most studies examining optimal duration of anticoagulation have found that the longer a person receives anticoagulation after a DVT or PE, the less likely they are to have a repeat VTE. Furthermore, when anticoagulation is discontinued, the risk of VTE increases substantially and is significantly above that in persons without a history of VTE. This elevation in risk is reflected in the clinical scoring systems (Wells score, Geneva score) discussed earlier. Of note, however, chronic anticoagulation presents its own inherent risks, cost, and requirements for lifestyle modification. The challenge then becomes balancing the inherent risk of anticoagulation with the individual patient's risk of recurrent disease. The ACCP has published consensus statement recommendations regarding the duration of chronic anticoagulation to prevent recurrent VTE by considering patient risk factors and presentation (**Table 57-4**). These recommendations by necessity are directed at broad categories of patients. When applying these standards, therefore, clinicians must consider the individual patient's risk of adverse outcomes with anticoagulation. As discussed earlier, however, the recent availability of the oral Xa inhibitors may change the risk-benefit ratio, resulting in longer periods of anticoagulation after VTE. The EINSTEIN investigators demonstrated that continuation of the oral Xa inhibitor rivaroxaban for an additional 6 to 12 months after completion of 6 to 12 months of anticoagulation resulted in significantly fewer episodes of recurrent VTE (1.3% versus 7.1%). Only a slight increase in nonfatal major bleeding (0.7%) was observed in the treatment cohort compared with the placebo cohort (0%).

TREATING PULMONARY EMBOLISM ASSOCIATED WITH MALIGNANCY

The pathophysiology of venous thrombosis in patients with cancer is complex and is influenced by a number of variables, including tumor type, stage, and overall tumor burden. Malignancies such as renal cell carcinoma are associated with a 43% incidence of VTE. Patients with DVT or PE related to cancer have increased 6-month mortality over patients with cancer not complicated by VTE. The CLOT (Randomized Comparison of Low-Molecular-Weight Heparin versus Oral Anticoagulant Therapy for the Prevention of VTE in Patients with Cancer) study demonstrated that LMWH (dalteparin) was more efficacious in the prevention of recurrent VTE in patients with malignancy than warfarin. Patients with cancer complicated by acute DVT, PE, or both were randomly assigned to receive 6 months of either warfarin or the LMWH dalteparin. Patients receiving dalteparin had less recurrent VTE than those receiving warfarin (9% versus 17%).

TREATMENT OF PULMONARY EMBOLISM IN PREGNANCY

Treatment of PE in pregnancy is complicated by risk to both the mother and the fetus. Warfarin is contraindicated in pregnancy because of its ability to cross the placenta and its association with both fetal hemorrhage and teratogenic effects such as central nervous system and neural developmental defects and nasal hypoplasia. Both UF heparin and LMWH can be used in the treatment of VTE in pregnancy, because neither crosses the placenta. Long-term use of UF heparin is associated with an increased risk for osteoporosis, but the risk is lower in patients treated with LMWH. Current recommendations for the treatment of VTE in pregnancy advocate the use of LMWH because of its favorable dosing and monitoring characteristics and its lower toxicity compared with other agents. An important consideration in this context, however, is that the maternal volume of distribution increases significantly during pregnancy, so the LMWH dose must be adjusted accordingly. Full-dose anticoagulation significantly increases the risk of hemorrhage at the time of delivery; therefore, LMWH and UF heparin should be discontinued 24 hours before planned induction of labor.

If spontaneous labor occurs, consideration should be given to reversal of anticoagulation with protamine. Anticoagulation can be restarted within 12 to 24 hours of delivery in the absence of ongoing bleeding. Warfarin, UF heparin, and LWMH are not excreted in breast milk, so these medications can be administered to breast-feeding women.

Pulmonary Embolectomy

Surgical resection of acute PE is a consideration in some patients. The operation is plagued by a high reported mortality (with rates as high as 30% in some series), in part because it typically is undertaken in already critically ill, hemodynamically unstable patients. Patients selected to undergo emergency embolectomy for this indication frequently have been found to have a large PE with resulting right ventricular dysfunction (a marker of increased mortality in itself). In such patients, anticoagulation or therapeutic thrombolysis often has failed to effect improvement or is contraindicated.

Table 57-4 Recommendations for Duration of Anticoagulation in Patients Diagnosed With Venous Thromboembolism (VTE)

Indication for Anticoagulation	Duration of Therapy
First VTE with reversible or transient risk factor	Minimum of 3 months
First episode of idiopathic VTE	Minimum of 6-12 months; consider use for indefinite period
VTE associated with malignancy	LMWH for the first 3-6 months; then indefinitely or until the malignancy resolves
First episode of VTE associated with hypercoagulable state	12 months; suggest indefinitely
Two or more documented episodes of VTE	Indefinite

LMWH, low-molecular-weight heparin.

TREATMENT OF CHRONIC THROMBOEMBOLIC DISEASE

In most patients, the usual histopathologic and clinical course of PE eventuates in complete resolution of the thrombus and restoration of normal pulmonary artery pressures, usually within 30 days of the event. On the basis of a prospective incidence study, however, Pengo and colleagues reported that up to 4% of patients who survive a symptomatic PE may develop a condition termed *chronic thromboembolic pulmonary hypertension* (CTEPH). Most of these patients are seen late in the clinical course after significant pulmonary artery hypertension (PAH) develops; therefore, little is known about the natural history of this disease. In the currently accepted model for the pathogenesis of CTEPH, acute PE, either symptomatic or asymptomatic, serves as the initiating event, followed by disease progression. For reasons that are unknown, these emboli do not resolve but rather become coated by endothelial cells, a process referred to as *endothelialization*, making them inaccessible to endogenous or exogenous thrombolysis. This process eventually results in remodeling and obstruction of the pulmonary vascular bed and PAH.

What predisposes patients to CTEPH is unclear. Increased factor VIII levels have been detected in the peripheral blood of some of these patients, and an increased incidence of anticardiolipin antibodies also has been reported. The predicted 5-year survival rate for untreated severe CTEPH (i.e., mean pulmonary artery pressure greater than 50 mm Hg) is poor, with some estimates as low as 10%.

The treatment for CTEPH differs significantly from that for acute PE. Although these patients require anticoagulation to prevent further embolic events, the endothelialized clot is not accessible to these medications. Therapy, therefore, revolves around either removing the thrombus surgically or treating the elevation in pulmonary artery pressures medically. Surgical resection, termed *pulmonary endarterectomy* (PEA), is the treatment of choice in eligible patients (**Figure 57-7**). It is performed by dissecting away the endothelialized thrombus through careful separation of the thrombus from the pulmonary artery wall. This procedure is associated with significant operative and postoperative risk (as reflected by reported 5% to 10% mortality rates) and should be performed only in experienced centers. When PEA is successful, outcomes include significant improvement in pulmonary artery pressure, right-sided heart function, cardiac output, and functional class. A substantial number of patients (10% to 50%) with CTEPH referred for PEA, however, are deemed to be ineligible because of inaccessible distal thrombus or other serious comorbid conditions. Furthermore, persistent PH after successful PEA is frequent, with substantial

small-vessel occlusion or arteriopathy. For these reasons, medical therapy for CTEPH has been applied. These treatments include nonspecific therapies such as administration of diuretics to improve fluid status, long-term oxygen therapy for hypoxemia, and digoxin to improve right ventricular contractility. More recently, however, novel therapies more specific for the treatment of PAH and approved for the treatment of idiopathic pulmonary artery hypertension (IPAH) have garnered attention as potentially useful in the medical management of CTEPH. Such therapies include use of the prostacyclin analogues (epoprostenol, treprostinil, and iloprost), endothelin receptor antagonists (bosentan), and the phosphodiesterase-5 (PDE-5) inhibitors (sildenafil). Evidence for the success of these medications, however, is limited to case series, retrospective studies, and prospective cohort studies. The only randomized controlled clinical trial to date that has included patients with CTEPH, as well as patients with other causes of PAH, is the Aerosolized Iloprost Randomized (AIR) study. Iloprost is an inhaled prostacyclin analogue approved for the treatment of PAH. This study did not demonstrate significant beneficial effects of inhaled iloprost in the CTEPH population, however.

PREVENTION OF PULMONARY EMBOLISM

General Approach to Prophylaxis

VTE is a major cause of morbidity and mortality. Approximately 10% of in-hospital deaths are attributed to PE. Recognition of the prevalence and consequences associated with VTE has led to recommendations regarding primary prevention or thromboprophylaxis. Thromboprophylaxis has been demonstrated to be highly efficacious in a variety of patient populations and is associated with minimal risk. Recommendations for VTE prophylaxis advocate assessing the individual patient's risk for thrombosis and adjusting the aggressiveness of the approach on the basis of that risk. Although means of assessing patient-specific risk have been described, these systems are cumbersome, have not been adequately validated, and are unlikely to be used routinely in clinical practice. An easier, more applicable method involves a "group-specific" approach applied routinely to all patients falling within a specific target group. A full discussion of these recommendations is reviewed in detail in the Seventh ACCP Conference consensus statement on the prevention of VTE. The statement divides patients into medical and surgical groups. The surgical patients are classified on the basis of individual risk factors, such as age, preexisting conditions, and the type of surgery planned. Recommendations are then made regarding the most appropriate type of thromboprophylaxis. A similar approach is used for medical patients. Of note, most medically managed patients admitted to the hospital in the current era will have at least one and probably multiple risk factors for VTE. Therefore, thromboprophylaxis is indicated in most hospitalized patients and is considered to be an essential component of optimal clinical care.

In most cases, the agents recommended for prophylaxis are anticoagulants. These anticoagulants include subcutaneous UF heparin or LMWH, with occasional recommendations for agents such as Xa inhibitors (fondaparinux) or oral vitamin K antagonists in high-risk groups such as postoperative patients recovering from hip or knee surgery. In a developing consensus, the use of mechanical compressive devices as the sole means of thromboprophylaxis against VTE is discouraged. The ACCP currently recommends that mechanical methods of thromboprophylaxis be used primarily in patients at high risk for bleeding or as an adjunct to anticoagulant-based prophylaxis.

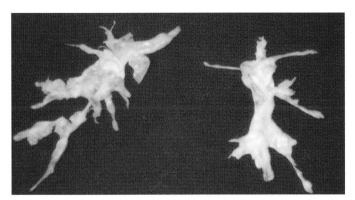

Figure 57-7 Thrombus removed from right and left pulmonary arteries in a patient with chronic thromboembolic pulmonary artery hypertension.

Currently, however, data supporting a role for such methods as adjunctive therapy are limited.

Inferior Vena Cava Filters

The concept of mechanically obstructing the vena cava to prevent embolization to the pulmonary vasculature is not new, being originally conceived by Trousseau in 1868. Techniques to insert this protective barrier have been refined substantially over the years, however, and now the placement of inferior vena cava (IVC) filters can be achieved safely and reliably. More recently, the development of retrievable IVC filters has expanded the number of patients considered for this procedure. The two most common scenarios in which IVC filters are used are (1) inability to anticoagulate and (2) failure of adequate anticoagulation in patients with known VTE. Other scenarios meriting consideration of IVC filter placement include high risk for PE despite use of recommended thromboprophylaxis, such as in trauma victims with lower extremity or pelvic fractures, high risk of death from pulmonary embolic disease in some patients, and/or those with severe pulmonary hypertension and a known DVT.

Only one randomized trial of IVC filters for the treatment of VTE has been published. This study demonstrated a decrease in the incidence of PE in the first 12 days after placement of the device (1.1% versus 4.8%) but an increase in the incidence of DVT at 2 years after placement (11.6% versus 20%). The incidence of PE at 2 years after filter placement was only slightly decreased (3.4% versus 6.2%). An 8-year follow-up study in the same cohort demonstrated a decrease in the recurrence of PE in the patients with IVC filters (6.2% versus 15.1%), but a significantly increased occurrence of DVTs was noted in the patients who received filters (35.7% versus 27.5%). No difference was found in the incidence of the postthrombotic syndrome or mortality between the cohorts. All patients in this study received anticoagulation for a minimum of 3 months, and many remained on anticoagulation indefinitely.

No randomized trials have been conducted to examine the incidence of PE in patients who received an IVC filter but did not receive anticoagulation. Retrievable filters are a potential option in patients who have only a transiently increased risk for VTE (**Figure 57-8**). The filters should be removed before endothelization of the struts occurs, which usually is within 7 to 21 days of placement. An increasing number of case reports and case series, however, have demonstrated the ability to remove retrievable filters months after their placement. The risk of complications rises with delayed removal. Randomized controlled trials demonstrating the efficacy of retrievable filters in terms of outcomes have yet to be performed.

NONTHROMBOTIC PULMONARY EMBOLI

Although most pulmonary emboli arise from DVT, other clinically significant forms of emboli may have an impact on the lung vasculature, as summarized in **Box 57-3**.

Box 57-3 Causes of Nonthrombotic Pulmonary Emboli
Fat embolism
Air embolism
Venous
Arterial
Amniotic fluid embolism
Tumor embolism
Septic pulmonary embolism

Fat Embolism Syndrome

Fat embolism syndrome (FES) is a poorly understood complication of skeletal trauma. Although rare, FES most often occurs after fractures of long bones or other conditions resulting in bone marrow disruption. FES is characterized by the appearance of free fat and fatty acids in the blood, lungs, brain, kidneys, and other organs. The classic triad of respiratory insufficiency, neurologic abnormalities, and petechial rash occurs in 0.5% to 2.0% of solitary long bone fractures. The incidence increases to 5% to 10% in multiple fractures with pelvic involvement.

FES is a clinical diagnosis that typically manifests within 12 to 72 hours of initial injury. Respiratory impairment leads to hypoxemia in up to 30% of patients and, on occasion, to respiratory failure and the need for mechanical ventilation. The chest radiograph often shows diffuse infiltrates but can appear normal. Cerebral symptoms may occur in 60% of patients and tend to follow the pulmonary symptoms. Neurologic findings may range from restlessness, confusion, and altered sensorium to focal deficits, seizures, and coma. The characteristic petechial rash is observed in 50% of patients and usually is found on the neck, in the axillary region, or on the trunk, or petechiae may appear on the conjunctiva. The rash often is the last of the triad to develop and resolves within a range of hours to days.

Treatment of FES includes aggressive supportive care and early ventilatory support. Steroids have been demonstrated to be efficacious as prophylaxis for FES, although experience with steroids as specific treatment remains anecdotal.

Air Embolism

Air embolism is a consequence of entry of air into the vascular system, resulting in mechanical obstruction, end-organ ischemia, and/or hemodynamic compromise. Air can enter the venous system under two simultaneous conditions: (1) presence of a direct communication between the source of air and the venous system and (2) development of a pressure gradient favoring the passage of air into the venous system. Under high pressure, gas may be forced into the venous system such as with laparoscopic procedures, pressurized infusion sets, or mechanical ventilation. Conversely, generating high negative intrathoracic pressures (as in hyperventilation, exacerbation of underlying lung disease, hypovolemia, or upright positioning) may predispose patients to *venous air embolism* by increasing the pressure gradient between the atmosphere and the thorax.

In most instances, venous air embolism occurs in relation to placement of central venous catheters (zero to 2% incidence). The mortality rate for this entity associated with central venous catheters has been reported to be as high as 32%. In humans, the lethal volume of air is estimated to be 300 to 500 mL. With a pressure gradient of only 5 cm H_2O (as with normal tidal breathing), air can pass through a 14 gauge catheter at a rate of 100 mL/second. The clinical symptoms of venous air embolism are nonspecific. Care providers must maintain a high index of suspicion to consider this diagnosis in patients who exhibit sudden cardiopulmonary and/or neurologic decompensation in the appropriate clinical setting. Patients may experience a gasping reflex, light-headedness, dizziness, chest pain, or sudden-onset dyspnea. If venous gas reaches the arterial circulation, myocardial or central nervous system injury may occur. Physical examination may reveal tachycardia, tachypnea, and elevated jugular venous pressure. A mill-wheel murmur, produced by movement of air bubbles in the right ventricle, is considered the only specific sign, but it is a rare, transient, and

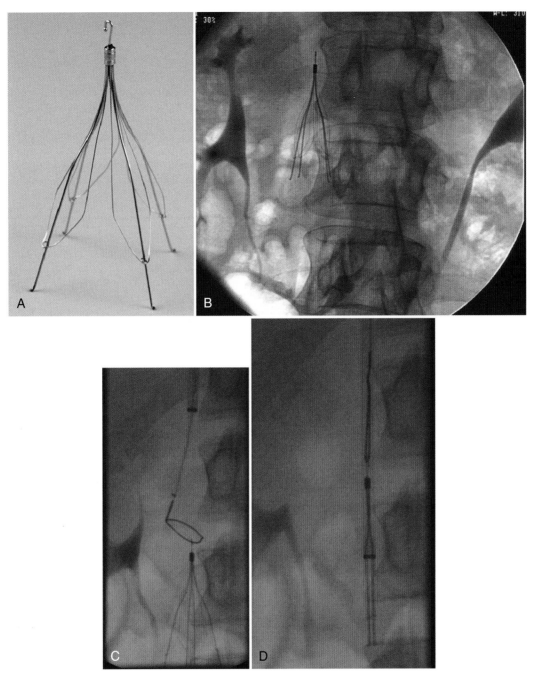

Figure 57-8 Inferior vena cava (IVC) retrievable filter. **A,** Gunter Tulip IVC filter. **B,** Filter is seen after deployment in the IVC. **C,** Preparation for retrieval of the filter. A snare is inserted percutaneously, which is used to engage the end of the filter. **D,** The filter is retracted and drawn into a sheath for percutaneous extraction.

late finding. Wheezing or rales may occur secondary to induced bronchospasm.

Transthoracic or transesophageal echocardiography is the most sensitive method for detection of venous air and may show evidence of both acute right ventricular dilatation and pulmonary hypertension. Indwelling pulmonary artery catheters will show an acute increase in pulmonary artery pressure. Although this finding has a sensitivity of only 45%, the presence of a pulmonary artery catheter at the time of onset of venous air embolism can result in early therapeutic intervention. If venous air embolism is suspected, the patient should be placed left side down in Trendelenburg position, allowing air to migrate toward the right apex of the heart, thereby diminishing pulmonary outflow obstruction. Manual removal of air from an indwelling central line or pulmonary artery catheter may be

attempted and is most effective at or above the right atrial junction, not in the right ventricular or pulmonary artery outflow tract. Closed-chest cardiac massage improves survival to the same extent as that achieved by proper positioning, presumably by mechanically forcing air out of the right ventricle and pulmonary outflow tract. Patients should be administered 100% inspired oxygen (FiO_2) to increase the rate of bubble absorption. For patients with persistence of cardiopulmonary or cerebrovascular deficits despite application of these modalities, hyperbaric oxygen therapy should be initiated.

Amniotic Fluid Embolism Syndrome

Amniotic fluid embolism syndrome (AFES) is a rare complication of pregnancy with variable manifestations and high morbidity and mortality. The reported incidence of this catastrophic syndrome ranges from 1 in 8000 to 1 in 80,000 pregnancies. Amniotic fluid is a complex mixture of both maternal and fetal components, including particulate matter such as fetal squamous cells, lanugo hairs, and variably meconium. Amniotic fluid is postulated to enter the maternal circulation through endocervical veins, through the site of placental insertion, or through uterine trauma. Once in the circulation, amniotic fluid triggers an immunologically mediated systemic inflammatory response leading to cardiovascular compromise, respiratory failure, coagulopathy, and disseminated intravascular coagulation. AFES occurs during labor but before delivery in 70% of cases, after vaginal delivery in 11%, and during cesarean section in 19%. Of the patients in whom AFES developed after delivery, 69% experienced clinical onset within the first 5 minutes post partum. AFES also has been reported to occur as early as the second trimester and as late as 36 hours post partum. AFES may occur during therapeutic abortion, amniocentesis, and labor and delivery and in the setting of abdominal trauma. Factors historically associated with increased risk for AFES include advanced maternal age, multiparity, large fetal size, premature placental separation, fetal death, fetal male sex, meconium staining, and a history of allergy or atopy in the mother.

The clinical presentation of AFES often is dramatic, with sudden-onset respiratory distress, cyanosis, convulsions, and cardiovascular collapse classically occurring during labor and delivery. Rapid progression to asystole or pulseless electrical activity has been described. Among patients who survive the initial event, a major coagulopathy develops later on in 40% of the cases.

The diagnosis of AFES is clinical. Early aggressive support is imperative, because most maternal deaths occur within 1 hour of symptom onset. AFES is a life-threatening condition that necessitates prompt resuscitation, including airway and hemodynamic support in an intensive care setting. The maternal mortality rate for AFES ranges from 30% to 90%. The fetal survival rate is 40% when the fetus is in utero at the time of AFES onset. Furthermore, AFES is associated with significant morbidity, with neurologically intact survival observed in only 15% of maternal survivors in some reports.

Tumor Embolism

Pulmonary tumor embolism occurs when solid tumors seed the systemic circulation with individual cells, clusters of cells, or large tumor fragments. Emboli travel to the pulmonary vasculature, causing microvasculature obstruction. Furthermore, tumor emboli may activate the coagulation system, resulting in concomitant thrombotic obstruction. The pathologic spectrum of tumor embolism ranges from large tumor masses that may mimic PE, on one end, to the more common microvessel embolism in small arterioles and capillaries that cause a subacute clinical syndrome, on the other. The incidence of tumor embolism is estimated by autopsy series to be 3% to 26% in patients with solid tumors. Tumor embolism seems to be more common in patients with mucin-producing adenocarcinomas such as breast, gastric, and lung carcinoma; however, this observation may be explained by the higher prevalence of these tumors within the general population.

CONTROVERSIES AND PITFALLS

Although great progress has been made in expansion of the current understanding and approach to the clinical entity of PE, new developments frequently bring with them new questions and controversies. Some of these dilemmas are discussed next.

ISOLATED SUBSEGMENTAL PULMONARY EMBOLI

The development of faster, multidetector scanners has improved the clinician's ability to see the subsegments of the pulmonary vasculature on CTA. This ability, however, has raised an interesting conundrum: Are isolated small, subsegmental pulmonary emboli clinically meaningful? On one side of this argument are researchers who believe that any thrombus in the pulmonary vasculature is pathologic, and that even if a subsegmental thrombus does not have immediate clinical effects, it implies a risk for subsequent PE that therefore merits anticoagulation. The converse argument is that very small thrombi may intermittently occur in normal people, and that perhaps it is the lungs' role to serve as a filter for these "microclots," thereby preventing them from migrating into the arterial circulation. This possibility, although interesting to consider, has never been substantiated. At present, no consensus has been reached on the appropriate clinical approach toward an isolated subsegmental PE detected by multidetector CTA, and very little expert opinion on this topic has been published.

OUTPATIENT TREATMENT OF PULMONARY EMBOLISM

As discussed earlier in this chapter, LMWH has been demonstrated to be safe and effective in the treatment of submassive PE. The oral Xa inhibitor rivaroxaban currently is being studied in the management of PE and was found to be effective for the treatment of DVT. Initial reports of success with these agents raise the possibility of treating patients with PE at home, thereby avoiding a hospital stay. This paradigm is well accepted in the treatment of DVT, for which it has been demonstrated to be safe and cost-effective, as well as popular from a patient perspective. Some of the studies examining the use of LMWH for the treatment of PE have permitted small percentages of the patients enrolled either to be treated entirely on an outpatient basis or to be discharged early from the hospital to complete home therapy. No increases in adverse events were found in patients managed as outpatients. This possibility of home therapy raises concern, however, because patients with PE have an increased mortality compared with patients with DVT. It is possible that treating them in a less monitored environment will carry an increased risk of death. Also, studies examining the use of LMWH in the treatment of PE have excluded patients with hemodynamically significant thromboembolic disease, a subgroup recognized to have even higher mortality. Realistically, however, more and more patients with PE are being treated as outpatients. This approach merits caution in patients known to have adverse hemodynamic changes or right ventricular dilatation or strain related to the thromboembolic event. This group of patients probably should be observed in an inpatient setting, at least initially in their treatment course.

THROMBOLYTIC THERAPY IN PATIENTS WITH PULMONARY EMBOLISM WITHOUT HEMODYNAMIC INSTABILITY

Convincing evidence is lacking for a survival advantage in hemodynamically stable patients with pulmonary emboli who are treated with thrombolytics plus anticoagulation over that in those treated with anticoagulation alone. Two studies have suggested that thrombolytics improve outcomes in patients with pulmonary emboli and right ventricular dysfunction; however, both have been criticized for suboptimal design. Although it is currently agreed that patients with hemodynamic collapse secondary to PE should receive thrombolysis if possible, controversy exists regarding the use of this therapy in less severely affected patients. However, the use of thrombolytics in hemodynamically stable patients with evidence of right ventricular dysfunction is gaining support in a number of expert societies.

SUGGESTED READINGS

Bauer KA: The thrombophilias: well-defined risk factors with uncertain therapeutic implications, *Ann Intern Med* 135:367–373, 2001.

Buller HR, Agnelli G, Hull RD, et al: Antithrombotic therapy for venous thromboembolic disease: the Seventh ACCP Conference on Antithrombotic and Thrombolytic Therapy, *Chest* 126:401–428, 2004.

Cohn D, Vansenne F, de Borgie C, Middeldorp S: Thrombophilia testing for prevention of recurrent venous thromboembolism, *Cochrane Database Syst Rev* 1:CD007069, 2009.

Decousus H, Leizorovicz A, Parent F, et al: A clinical trial of vena caval filters in the prevention of pulmonary embolism in patients with proximal deep-vein thrombosis. Prevention du Risque d'Embolie Pulmonaire par Interruption Cave Study Group, *N Engl J Med* 338:409–415, 1998.

EINSTEIN Investigators, Bauersachs R, Berkowitz SD, et al: Oral rivaroxaban for symptomatic venous thromboembolism, *N Engl J Med* 363:2499–2510, 2010.

Geerts WH, Pineo GF, Heit JA, et al: Prevention of venous thromboembolism: the Seventh ACCP Conference on Antithrombotic and Thrombolytic Therapy, *Chest* 126:338S-400S, 2004.

Goldhaber SZ: Pulmonary embolism, *Lancet* 363:1295–1305, 2004.

Goldhaber SZ: Thrombolysis in pulmonary embolism: a debatable indication, *Thromb Haemost* 86:444–451, 2001.

Jerjes-Sanchez C, Ramirez-Rivera A, de Lourdes GM, et al: Streptokinase and heparin versus heparin alone in massive pulmonary embolism: a randomized controlled trial, *J Thromb Thrombolysis* 2:227–229, 1995.

Konstantinides S, Geibel A, Heusel G, et al: Heparin plus alteplase compared with heparin alone in patients with submassive pulmonary embolism, *N Engl J Med* 347:1143–1150, 2002.

Park B, Messina L, Dargon P, et al: Recent trends in clinical outcomes and resource utilization for pulmonary embolism in the United States: findings from the nationwide inpatient sample, *Chest* 136:983–990, 2009.

Pengo V, Lensing AW, Prins MH, et al: Incidence of chronic thromboembolic pulmonary hypertension after pulmonary embolism, *N Engl J Med* 350:2257–2264, 2004.

PREPIC Study Group: Eight year follow-up of patients with permanent vena cava filters in the prevention of pulmonary embolism: the PREPIC (Prevention du Risque d'Embolie Pulmonaire par Interruption Cave) randomized study, *Circulation* 112:416–422, 2005.

Stein PD, Chenevert TL, Fowler SE, et al: Gadolinium-enhanced magnetic resonance angiography for pulmonary embolism: a multicenter prospective study (PIOPED III), *Ann Intern Med* 152:434–443, 2010.

Stein PD, Woodard PK, Weg JG, et al: Diagnostic pathways in acute pulmonary embolism: recommendations of the PIOPED II investigators, *Am J Med* 119:1048–1055, 2006.

Value of the ventilation/perfusion scan in acute pulmonary embolism. Results of the prospective investigation of pulmonary embolism diagnosis (PIOPED). The PIOPED Investigators, *JAMA* 263:2753–2759, 1990.

Van Belle A, Buller HR, Huisman MV, et al: Effectiveness of managing suspected pulmonary embolism by use of an algorithm combining clinical probability, D-dimer testing, and computed tomography, *JAMA* 295:172–179, 2006.

Chapter **58**
Pulmonary Hypertension
Kristin B. Highland • Andre Holmes

Pulmonary arterial hypertension (PAH) is a rare, pathologically complex disease characterized by a progressive increase in pulmonary arterial pressure associated with variable degrees of pulmonary vascular remodeling, vasoconstriction, and in situ thrombosis. These changes lead in turn to increased pulmonary vascular resistance (PVR) and eventual right-sided heart failure and death. PAH has a nonspecific clinical expression; therefore, the diagnosis often is established late in the disease course, making treatment problematic. Without treatment, the median survival after diagnosis of idiopathic pulmonary arterial hypertension (IPAH) is only 2.8 years.

DEFINITION

The current definition of *pulmonary hypertension* (PH) is a mean pulmonary artery pressure (mPAP) greater than 25 mm Hg measured with the patient at rest. A systolic pulmonary artery pressure (sPAP) greater than 35 to 40 mm Hg on echocardiogram should prompt further workup for PH, but determination of sPAP is not adequate as a stand-alone test.

In an exhaustive systematic review of the literature that included data from 1887 healthy people enrolled in 47 studies from 13 countries, mPAP measured with the subject at rest was 14.0 ± 3.3 mm Hg; this finding was independent of sex and ethnicity and only slightly influenced by age (in subjects younger than 30 years, 12 ± 3.1 mm Hg; in those older than 50 years, 14.7 ± 4.0 mm Hg). Therefore, if the upper limit of normal is defined by the mean plus two times the standard deviation, the upper limit for mPAP determined at rest in a healthy person is 20.6 mm Hg; this value is considerably lower than the established definition for PH of greater than 25 mm Hg. This same systematic review showed that mPAP measured during exercise was dependent on age, exercise type, and exercise intensity, making it difficult to establish a threshold value that would accurately define exercise-induced PH. As a result, the former exercise criterion of greater than 30 mm Hg was abandoned during the Fourth World Symposium on Pulmonary Hypertension held in 2008 in Dana Point, California.

Although modestly elevated mPAP in the setting of chronic lung disease often is associated with a poor prognosis, the significance of a "borderline" mPAP (20 to 25 mm Hg) in subjects who are otherwise healthy remains unclear. This uncertainty highlights the importance of the clinical assessment and the need for early biomarkers, rather than a focus on hemodynamics alone, especially because these data suggest that the prevalence of mPAP values greater than 25 mm Hg will be substantially higher than that indicated by the known prevalence of PAH.

CLASSIFICATION

Pulmonary hypertension was previously classified as either primary or secondary, depending on the absence or the presence, respectively, of identifiable causes or risk factors. The diagnosis of *primary pulmonary hypertension* was one of exclusion after ruling out all other causes for PH. Subsequent classification schemes have attempted to create categories of PH that share pathologic and clinical features, as well as similar therapeutic options. These classification schemes have allowed investigators to conduct clinical trials in well-defined patient groups with a shared underlying pathogenesis for their PH, resulting in the development of new targeted drug therapies; consequently, improvements in both quality of life and survival can now be expected in this otherwise deadly disease. This more inclusive category of PAH also has afforded increased opportunities for treatment of some less common forms of the disorder that were previously too rare for individual treatment studies. The most recent classification scheme was the product of the aforementioned Fourth World Symposium on Pulmonary Hypertension (**Box 58-1**).

GROUP 1: PULMONARY ARTERIAL HYPERTENSION

PAH is a subset of PH defined as a mPAP greater than 25 mm Hg determined with the patient at rest and a normal pulmonary capillary wedge pressure (PCWP) and/or left ventricular end-diastolic pressure (LVEDP) and a lesion localized to the pulmonary arteriole (**Figure 58-1,** *A* to *C*). Unfortunately, a limitation of these classification schemes is the fact that many of these patients have "multifactorial pulmonary hypertension." The clinician is thus faced with treating PH in a variety of clinical scenarios that often include features from more than one of the World Health Organization (WHO) classification categories (i.e., groups 1 to 5, with an additional 1' grouping as described later on). For example, the clinical presentation may include somewhat elevated pulmonary venous pressures, mild to moderate obstructive or restrictive lung disease, or a form of valvular heart disease that typically would not account for pulmonary hypertension severity. Patients with such "out of proportion" PH are not included in clinical trials; therefore, data pertaining to the safety and efficacy of conventional PAH therapies in this population are extremely limited.

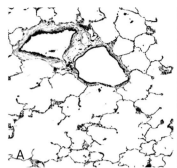
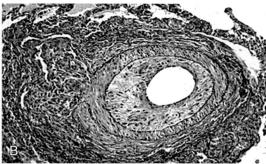
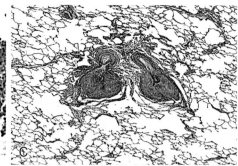

Figure 58-1 Histologic preparations (Von Giesen elastic stain) of normal lung and of specimens from patients with pulmonary arterial hypertension (PAH). **A,** Normal pulmonary arteriole flanked by a normal bronchiole (the latter at the 11 o'clock position). **B,** Concentric obliterative lesion characteristic of PAH. Intimal proliferation with encroachment on the lumen can be seen. A plexiform lesion is present to the left of the artery (at the 9 o'clock position). 40× objective. **C,** Plexiform lesions characteristic of PAH. 10× objective.

Box 58-1	**Updated Clinical Classification of Pulmonary Hypertension**

1 Pulmonary arterial hypertension (PAH)
  1.1 Idiopathic PAH
  1.2 Heritable:
    1.2.1 BMPR2
    1.2.2 ALK-1, endoglin
    1.2.3 Unknown
  1.3 Drug- or toxin-induced
  1.4 Associated with:
    1.4.1 Connective tissue diseases
    1.4.2 Human immunodeficiency virus (HIV) infection
    1.4.3 Portal hypertension
    1.4.4 Congenital heart diseases
    1.4.5 Schistosomiasis
    1.4.6 Chronic hemolytic anemia
  1.5 Persistent pulmonary hypertension of the newborn
1′ Pulmonary venoocclusive disease and/or pulmonary capillary hemangiomatosis
2 Pulmonary hypertension due to left-sided heart disease
3 Pulmonary hypertension due to lung disease and/or hypoxia
4 Chronic thromboembolic pulmonary hypertension (CTEPH)
5 Pulmonary hypertension with multifactorial mechanisms

Idiopathic Pulmonary Arterial Hypertension

IPAH is a rare disease and remains a diagnosis of exclusion. Patients with this sporadic form of PAH do not have a family history of PAH or any identifiable risk factors. A female preponderance, with a gender ratio of 1.7:1, has been recognized, and the mean age at diagnosis is 37 years. The incidence of IPAH is approximately 1 to 2 cases per 1 million population, with a prevalence of approximately 6 per 1 million. Although IPAH originally was believed to be a disease of child-bearing women, cases of IPAH recently have been reported in a number of patients older than 70 years of age.

Heritable Pulmonary Arterial Hypertension

Several germline mutations have been associated with heritable PAH. These include mutations in the genes encoding bone morphogenetic protein receptor type II (i.e., *BMPR2*), active-like kinase type 1 (ALK-1), and endoglin.

Sporadic mutations in *BMPR2* have been identified in approximately 11% to 40% of patients with presumably the idiopathic form of PAH and are seen in 70% to 80% of patients with familial PAH but are relatively uncommon in patients

with so-called associated PAH (i.e., category 1.4 in Box 58-1). Although penetrance is low and only approximately 25% of carriers will go on to develop PAH, genetic anticipation also has been demonstrated (i.e., in affected families, each successive generation has more severe PAH developing at an earlier age). *BMPR2* has been localized to chromosomal region 2q31-32, and inheritance occurs in an autosomal dominant fashion. Recently, it has been suggested that patients with PAH associated with *BMPR2* mutations may represent a subgroup with more severe disease who are less likely to demonstrate vasoreactivity than those with IPAH. Because this mutation can occur sporadically in as many as 25% of patients with PAH and does not occur in all patients with so-called familial PAH, the term *heritable* is now favored over the designation *familial*.

Like BMPR-II, ALK-1 and endoglin also are members of the transforming growth factor-β (TGF-β) superfamily and are located on endothelial cells, and mutations can result in heritable PAH. Mutations in the ALK-1 gene and/or the endoglin gene also are associated with the autosomal dominant disorder hereditary hemorrhagic telangiectasia.

Drug- and Toxin-Induced Pulmonary Arterial Hypertension

A number of risk factors for the development of PAH have been identified (**Box 58-2**). Risk factors for PAH include "any factor or condition that is suspected to play a predisposing or facilitating role in the development of the disease." Such risk factors have been categorized as "definite, very likely, possible, or unlikely, based on the strength of their association with [pulmonary hypertension] and their probable causal role." As a result of the Dana Point symposium, methamphetamine use was reclassified as a very likely risk factor for the development of PAH.

Pulmonary Arterial Hypertension Associated with Connective Tissue Diseases

PAH can occur in any of the connective tissue diseases but most commonly is seen in systemic sclerosis (scleroderma), mixed connective tissue disease, and systemic lupus erythematosus (SLE). The prevalence of PAH among patients with scleroderma is estimated to be between 7% and 12%. Although less well characterized, the prevalence among persons with SLE is thought to be between 1% and 4%. Of note, PAH is not the only cause of pulmonary hypertension in patients with connective tissue disease; these patients frequently have lung fibrosis and cardiac involvement. Experts recommend that all patients with systemic scleroderma have a yearly screening

Box 58-2 Risk Factors for Pulmonary Arterial Hypertension

Definite
Aminorex
Fenfluramine
Dexfenfluramine
Toxic rapeseed oil

Likely
Amphetamines
L-Tryptophan
Methamphetamines

Possible
Cocaine
Phenylpropanolamine
St. John's wort
Chemotherapeutic agents
Selective serotonin reuptake inhibitors

Unlikely
Oral contraceptives
Estrogen
Cigarette smoking

echocardiogram, because untreated PAH in patients with connective tissue disease is associated with a particularly poor prognosis.

Human Immunodeficiency Virus Infection

The prevalence of PAH in the human immunodeficiency virus (HIV)-infected population is approximately 1 per 200 persons. The mechanism for the development of PH remains unclear; it is thought to be a result of the indirect action of the virus through secondary messengers such as cytokines, growth factors, endothelin, or viral proteins. The occurrence of PAH is independent of the $CD4^+$ count, but it seems to be related to the duration of HIV infection. PAH also is more common in those patients infected through intravenous drug abuse. PAH is an independent predictor of mortality in these patients; in a substantial number of cases, however, normalization of pulmonary vascular hemodynamics can be obtained with specific therapy for PAH.

Portal Hypertension

The development of PAH in association with elevated pressure in the portal circulation is known as *portopulmonary hypertension* (POPH). Portal hypertension, rather than the presence of underlying liver disease, is the main determining risk factor for the development of POPH. Approximately 2% to 6% of patients with portal hypertension will also have PH. The diagnosis of POPH usually is made within 4 to 7 years after the diagnosis of portal hypertension. Female sex and autoimmune hepatitis are risk factors for the development of POPH; as a point of interest, hepatitis C infection is associated with a decreased risk. The presence of PAH is a contraindication to liver transplantation, so all patients being referred for transplantation require a screening echocardiogram. Right-sided heart catheterization is absolutely mandatory for the definitive diagnosis of POPH, because several factors may increase PAP in the setting of advanced liver disease. For example, high flow and an elevated cardiac output are associated with the hyperdynamic circulatory state seen in advanced liver disease, and an

increased PCWP secondary to fluid overload and/or diastolic dysfunction also will increase PAP. These conditions generally are associated with a normal PVR.

Congenital Heart Disease

Persistent exposure of the pulmonary vasculature to increased blood flow and pressure results in vascular remodeling, leading to an increased PVR and eventual shunt reversal. Eisenmenger syndrome is defined as congenital heart disease with an initial large and nonrestrictive systemic-to-pulmonary shunt that induces progressive pulmonary vascular disease and PAH, with resultant reversal of flow and cyanosis. This clinical entity represents the most advanced form of PAH associated with congenital heart disease. Although Eisenmenger syndrome occurs more frequently when blood flow is extremely high and the shunt exposes the pulmonary vasculature to systemic-level pressures, such as occurs with a ventricular septal defect, patent ductus arteriosus, or truncus arteriosis, PAH also may occur with low-pressure–high-flow abnormalities such as those seen with atrial septal defects.

Schistosomiasis

Previously, schistosomiasis was categorized in group 4 as PH due to chronic thrombotic and/or embolic disease secondary to embolic obstruction of pulmonary arteries by *Schistosoma* eggs. More recent publications, however, indicate that PH can be similar in presentation to IPAH, with similar histopathologic changes. The mechanism probably is multifactorial and related to POPH, a frequent complication of this disease, and to local vascular inflammation occurring as a result of impacted *Schistosoma* eggs. This is a common cause of PH worldwide: It is estimated that more than 200 million people are infected with schistosomiasis, and anywhere from 4% to 8% of these patients will develop hepatosplenic disease; 4.6% of these will then go on to develop PAH. Schistosomiasis also may cause postcapillary hypertension, reinforcing the need for diagnosis with right-sided heart catheterization.

Chronic Hemolytic Anemia

Increasing evidence suggests that PAH is a complication of chronic hereditary and acquired hemolytic anemias, including sickle cell disease, thalassemia, hereditary spherocytosis, stomatocytosis, and microangiopathic hemolytic anemia. The mechanism of PAH in hemolysis is uncertain but may involve high rates of nitric oxide consumption by free hemoglobin, resulting in a state of resistance to nitric oxide bioactivity.

GROUP 1′: PULMONARY ARTERIAL HYPERTENSION ASSOCIATED WITH PULMONARY VENOUS OR CAPILLARY ABNORMALITIES

Rarely, the typical findings in PAH also are associated with an occlusive venopathy—*pulmonary venoocclusive disease* (PVOD)—or a microvasculopathy—*pulmonary capillary hemangiomatosis* (PCH). Patients with these diseases exhibit features of both PAH and pulmonary venous hypertension, including pulmonary hemosiderosis, interstitial edema, and lymphatic dilatation. PVOD and PCH share similar risk factors including the scleroderma spectrum of disease, HIV infection, and the use of anorexigens. These entities should be suspected in the clinical setting of PAH associated with crackles on auscultation, digital clubbing, and pulmonary edema. Ground glass opacities, septal thickening, and mediastinal adenopathy may be seen on chest computed tomography scans. PVOD and PCH are set aside from the other members of group 1 because the management, response to medical therapy (patients with PVOD and PCH tend to develop pulmonary edema after the administration of PAH-specific therapies), and prognosis are quite different from that of PAH.

GROUP 2: PULMONARY HYPERTENSION DUE TO LEFT-SIDED HEART DISEASE

Pulmonary hypertension due to left-sided heart disease is defined as a mPAP greater than 25 mm Hg measured with the subject at rest with an elevated PCWP and/or LVEDP. It represents the most frequent cause of PH (accounting for more than 90% of the cases). Causes include systolic and diastolic heart failure as well as left-sided valvular disease. Guidelines have defined a PCWP and/or LVEDP less than 15 mm Hg as abnormal. In these patients, the PVR is normal or near normal (less than 3.0 Wood units), and no gradient significant is present between mPAP and pulmonary wedge pressure (i.e., the trans-pulmonary gradient is less than 12 mm Hg). In some patients with left-sided heart disease, the elevation of PAP is out of proportion to that expected from the elevation of the left atrial pressure, resulting in an increased PVR. This is due to either the increase in pulmonary artery vasomotor tone or pulmonary vascular remodeling, or both. No studies using medications approved for PAH have been performed in this patient population, and the efficacy and safety of PAH treatment medications remain unknown.

GROUP 3: PULMONARY HYPERTENSION DUE TO LUNG DISEASE AND/OR HYPOXIA

Pulmonary hypertension associated with disorders of the respiratory system or hypoxemia is a category of PH that is caused mainly by inadequate oxygenation of pulmonary arterial blood as a result of either parenchymal lung disease (e.g., emphysema, interstitial lung disease), impaired control of breathing (e.g., obesity hypoventilation, obstructive sleep apnea), or residence at high altitude. As a rule, mPAP generally is modest (less than 35 mm Hg), and survival depends on the severity of the pulmonary disease, rather than on the severity of the associated hypertension. As with the category of PH out of proportion to left-sided heart disease, large randomized, controlled studies of medications approved for PAH are not available for PH out of proportion to parenchymal lung disease.

GROUP 4: CHRONIC THROMBOEMBOLIC PULMONARY HYPERTENSION

Chronic thromboembolic pulmonary hypertension (CTEPH) is an important category of PH to exclude, because a proximal organized clot in the major pulmonary arteries may be surgically correctable by pulmonary endarterectomy. In all cases, life-long anticoagulation is indicated. The cumulative incidence of CTEPH after a first episode of pulmonary embolism approaches 4% at the 2-year follow-up examination.

GROUP 5: PULMONARY HYPERTENSION OF UNCLEAR OR MULTIFACTORIAL ETIOLOGY

Group 5 consists of several forms of PH for which the etiology is unclear or multifactorial. Potential etiopathogenic disorders include chronic myeloproliferative disorders (polycythemia vera, essential thrombocythemia, chronic myeloid leukemia), systemic disorders (sarcoidosis, pulmonary Langerhans cell histiocytosis, lymphangioleiomyomatosis, neurofibromatosis type 1, antineutrophil cytoplasmic antibody [ANCA]-associated vasculitis), metabolic disorders (type Ia glycogen storage disease, Gaucher disease, thyroid disease), and miscellaneous conditions (tumor obstruction, mediastinal fibrosis, end-stage renal disease).

PATHOBIOLOGY

Normal pulmonary arteries have a thin medial layer of circular muscle whose thickness is less than 5% of the diameter of the vessel (see Figure 58-1, A). Consequently, under physiologic conditions, the pulmonary circulation is characterized by high flow, low pressure, and low vascular resistance. The histopathologic findings in PAH are characterized by variable intimal hyperplasia, medial hypertrophy, adventitial proliferation, and fibrosis culminating in concentric obliterative lesions (see Figure 58-1, B) that occur in close proximity to plexiform lesions (see Figure 58-1, C). The plexiform lesion results from neointimal proliferation and progresses from a cellular to a fibrotic lesion with advancing disease. It is made up of a predominance of endothelial cells in different stages of vascular organization, suggesting an abnormal form of angiogenesis. Pulmonary vascular remodeling also has been associated with in situ thrombosis and infiltration by inflammatory and progenitor cells.

As the vascular pathology progresses, the PVR increases and PAP rises in concert, in order to maintain cardiac output. So long as the right ventricle is able to compensate for the resistance, the pressure continues to increase as the PVR increases. When the contractile reserve of the right ventricle is exhausted, right ventricular systolic failure ensues. A varying degree of right ventricular diastolic dysfunction also is present in PH and is related to right ventricular muscle mass and afterload and correlates with parameters of disease severity. The combination of reduced right ventricular output and diastolic dysfunction enhances diastolic interdependence, severely impairing left ventricular filling and ultimately resulting in hemodynamic deterioration.

Unfortunately, what is known about the pathobiology of PAH largely stems from research in patients with IPAH or from animal models that are meant to represent IPAH. Nevertheless, the pathobiologic features of PAH are thought to result from a multiple-hit hypothesis involving the interaction of a predisposing state with an inciting stimulus (**Figure 58-2**). Consequently, the resulting imbalance favors vasoconstriction, thrombosis, and mitogenesis. Restoration of this balance by inhibition of endothelin and thromboxane or augmentation of nitric oxide and prostacyclin forms the basis of today's current therapies.

Prostacyclin (i.e., prostaglandin I_2 [PGI_2]) is a product of endothelial cells generated by the action of prostacyclin synthase on arachidonic acid. Prostacyclin relaxes smooth muscle by increasing intracellular cyclic adenosine monophosphate (cAMP). It also is an inhibitor of platelet aggregation and smooth muscle cell proliferation. Patients with PAH exhibit increased excretion of urinary metabolites of thromboxane and decreased excretion of urinary metabolites of prostacyclin in comparison with normal control subjects. Likewise, prostacyclin synthase activity is reduced in patients with PAH.

Endothelin-1 is synthesized and secreted by endothelial cells and is metabolized in the normal lung. It is a potent acute

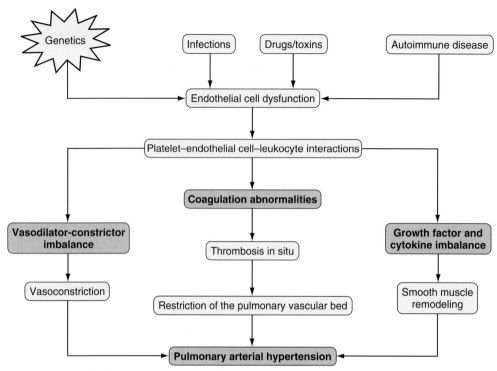

Figure 58-2 Proposed pathogenesis of pulmonary arterial hypertension (PAH). *(From Reed AK, Evans TW, Wort SJ: Pulmonary hypertension. In Albert RK, Spiro SG, Jett JR, editors:* Clinical respiratory medicine, *ed 3, Philadelphia, Mosby, 2008.)*

vasodilator and chronically stimulates cellular proliferation and fibrosis. Patients with PAH exhibit increased plasma levels of endothelin-1 and decreased clearance in comparison with normal control subjects.

Nitric oxide is a potent vasodilator that is produced by endothelial cells from arginine by nitric oxide synthase and acts on the vascular smooth muscle cells via cyclic guanosine monophosphate (cGMP). Phosphodiesterase-5 degrades cGMP, thus counteracting this vasodilatory pathway. Patients with PAH have decreased plasma levels of nitric oxide metabolites; likewise, endothelial nitric oxide synthase (eNOS) expression is reduced in the pulmonary arteries.

Ongoing research on other mediators and pathways (**Table 58-1**) promises new targets for novel therapies.

DIAGNOSTIC APPROACH

The diagnosis of PH is complex and should involve early referral to a provider with expertise in the diagnosis and treatment of the condition. Patients may present because they are concerned about symptoms, because they require further investigation of an incidental finding during previous testing, or because they belong to a high-risk population (e.g., systemic sclerosis, congenital heart disease, liver transplantation evaluation).

SIGNS AND SYMPTOMS

There are no early signs or symptoms of PH. Therefore, annual screening should be performed in high-risk populations (**Table 58-2**). A diagnosis of PH should be considered in any patient who presents with breathlessness in the absence of specific cardiac or pulmonary disease, or in patients who have underlying cardiac or pulmonary disease and present with increasing breathlessness that is not explained by the underlying disease itself. The initial symptoms and signs are nonspecific and may

Table 58-1 Mediators and Pathways in Pulmonary Arterial Hypertension

Increased Activity	Decreased Activity
Endothelin-1	Prostacyclin synthase
Serotonin	Nitric oxide
Thromboxane A_2	Nitric oxide synthase
Angiopoietin-1	Vasoactive intestinal peptide
Plasminogen activator inhibitor-1	Voltage-gated potassium
Growth factors	channels
Oxidant stress	Fibrinolysis
Inflammation	

Table 58-2 Recommendation for Screening for Pulmonary Arterial Hypertension

Risk Factor	Recommendation
Family history of PAH	Yes
Connective tissue disease	
Scleroderma	Yes
Other	No
Congenital heart disease	
Large ASD, nonoperated	Yes
Large VSD, nonoperated	Yes
HIV infection	No
Portal hypertension	No
Consideration for liver transplantation	Yes
Use of appetite-suppressant drugs	No
Previous pulmonary embolism	No
Increasing dyspnea	Yes
Massive/submassive PE	Yes

ASD, atrial septal defect; *HIV,* human immunodeficiency virus; *PE,* pulmonary embolism; *VSD,* ventricular septal defect.

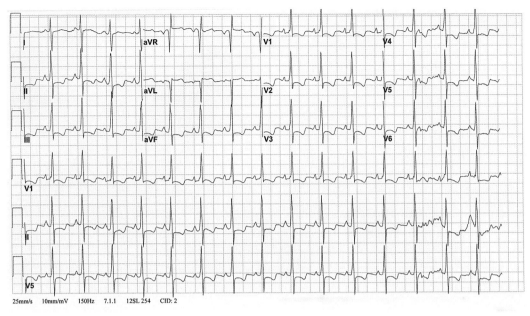

Figure 58-3 Electrocardiogram (ECG) demonstrating right atrial enlargement and right ventricular enlargement with strain in a patient with pulmonary arterial hypertension (PAH).

include fatigue, progressive dyspnea on exertion, palpitations, chest pain, dizziness, and cough. Unfortunately, the mean duration of symptoms before diagnosis reported in most registries approaches 2 years. Exertional dizziness and syncope are suggestive of an inadequate cardiac output and should raise clinical suspicion for PH. As PH progresses, patients go on to develop symptoms and signs of right-sided heart failure including jugular venous distention, right ventricular heave, tricuspid regurgitation, right ventricular gallops, ascites, and edema. Establishing an accurate diagnosis has important implications for therapy.

ELECTROCARDIOGRAM

The electrocardiogram shows abnormalities in 85% of patients with established PH but is not adequately sensitive as a screen for PH. Typical changes include right axis deviation with evidence of right ventricular or right atrial hypertrophy and right ventricular strain (**Figure 58-3**). The degree of these changes does not always reflect the severity of disease, and a normal ECG appearance does not eliminate the diagnosis of PH. Nevertheless, the following ECG findings have negative prognostic implications: (1) right axis deviation, (2) a tall R wave and small S wave with R/S ratio greater than 1 in lead V_1, (3) qR complex in lead V_1, (4) rSR′ pattern in lead V_1, (5) a large S wave and small R wave with R/S ratio less than 1 in lead V_5 or V_6, or (6) S_1-S_2-S_3 pattern (see Figure 58-3).

CHEST RADIOGRAPH

The chest radiograph also is not particularly sensitive for detecting PH. However, incidental findings of enlarged main and hilar pulmonary arterial shadows (right descending greater than 1.6 cm, left greater than 1.8 cm), with concomitant attenuation of peripheral pulmonary vascular markings ("pruning"), and right ventricular hypertrophy as evidenced by a reduced retrosternal clear space on the lateral projection should prompt a workup for PH. Chest radiographic findings

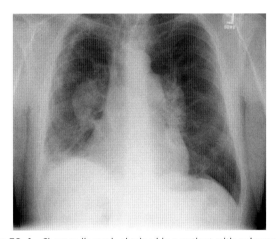

Figure 58-4 Chest radiograph obtained in a patient with pulmonary arterial hypertension (PAH). Note the massively enlarged pulmonary arteries and peripheral "pruning."

also may lead to the diagnosis of an underlying pulmonary process (**Figure 58-4**).

PULMONARY FUNCTION TESTING

Pulmonary function testing is a necessary part of the initial evaluation of all patients with PH, to exclude or characterize the contribution of underlying airway or parenchymal lung disease. On such testing, patients with IPAH and CTEPH typically exhibit a mild to moderate restrictive ventilatory defect and evidence of small airways dysfunction with a reduction in diffusion capacity. No correlation has been observed between the severity of PH and the reduction in diffusion; however, an isolated reduction in diffusion should alert the physician to the possibility of underlying PH. Arterial blood gas analysis typically shows hypoxemia, hypocapnia secondary to alveolar hyperventilation, and an increased alveolar-arterial oxygen gradient. Severe hypoxemia usually is the result of intracardiac shunting.

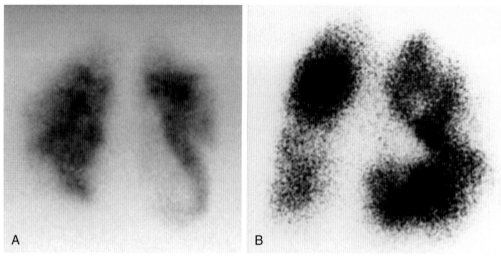

Figure 58-5 **A,** Patchy subsegmental defects on perfusion scan obtained in a patient with pulmonary arterial hypertension (PAH). **B,** Multiple segmental (or larger) defects on perfusion scan obtained in a patient with chronic thromboembolic pulmonary hypertension (CTEPH). *(From Reed AK, Evans TW, Wort SJ: Pulmonary hypertension. In Albert RK, Spiro SG, Jett JR, editors: Clinical respiratory medicine, ed 3, Philadelphia, Mosby, 2008.)*

OVERNIGHT OXIMETRY/POLYSOMNOGRAPHY

Nocturnal desaturation in PH is related primarily to gas exchange abnormalities. Although the clinical consequence of nocturnal desaturation is not well understood, it is likely that hypoxia-induced pulmonary vasoconstriction exacerbates the preexistent pulmonary hypertensive state. Nocturnal desaturation cannot be predicted by exercise desaturation; therefore, overnight oximetry is recommended in all patients with PH. Use of standard oxygen-prescribing guidelines, such as those derived from the Nocturnal Oxygen Treatment Trial, are recommended for hypoxemic patients with PH to maintain an oxygen saturation greater than 90% in adults.

The literature examining the relationship between obstructive sleep apnea and PH is difficult to interpret. In general, pulmonary hypertension associated with obstructive sleep apnea is mild with an average mPAP less than 30 mm Hg. It is recommended that all patients with PH be assessed for sleep-disordered breathing, and polysomnography should be performed if the clinical presentation is highly suggestive of obstructive sleep apnea. Although these patients are at higher risk for other cardiovascular morbidity, routine screening for PH with echocardiography is not recommended in patients with obstructive sleep apnea. In patients with concomitant obstructive sleep apnea and PH, treatment of the sleep apnea with positive-pressure therapy should be provided, with the expectation that pulmonary pressures will decrease, although they may not normalize, particularly when PH is more severe.

VENTILATION-PERFUSION SCAN

PH caused by chronic thromboembolic disease is a potentially surgically curable condition that should be considered in all patients with unexplained PH. A ventilation-perfusion scan is essential to rule out chronic thromboembolic disease in all patients with unexplained pulmonary hypertension; a normal scan effectively excludes a diagnosis of chronic thromboembolic disease. In patients with PAH, the ventilation-perfusion scan typically is normal or displays only minor, patchy perfusion defects, whereas in patients with CTEPH, at least one but often several major segmental or subsegmental mismatches in

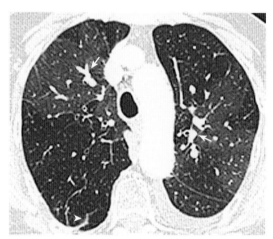

Figure 58-6 Computed tomography angiogram obtained in a patient with chronic thromboembolic pulmonary hypertension (CTEPH). Note the mosaic pattern of perfusion.

ventilation and perfusion will be evident (**Figure 58-5,** *A* and *B*). Unmatched perfusion defects also may be seen in PVOD. The "gold standard" diagnostic modality remains contrast angiography performed at the time of catheterization, which is able to characterize the nature and extent of any thromboembolic disease.

CHEST COMPUTED TOMOGRAPHY

A wide spectrum of abnormalities on computed tomography (CT) scanning has been described in patients with chronic thromboembolic disease. Such abnormalities may include right ventricular enlargement, dilated central pulmonary arteries, presence of persistent thromboembolic material within central pulmonary arteries, increased bronchial artery collateral flow, variability in the size and distribution of pulmonary arteries, parenchymal abnormalities consistent with previous infarcts, or mosaic attenuation of the pulmonary parenchyma (**Figure 58-6**). These are nonspecific findings, however, and their absence does not exclude the presence of surgically accessible disease, because only sixth- or seventh-generation pulmonary arteries

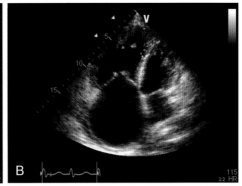

Figure 58-7 **A**, Echocardiogram, four-chamber view, obtained in a normal subject. **B**, Echocardiogram, four-chamber view, obtained in a patient with pulmonary arterial hypertension (PAH). Note the enlarged right atrium, right ventricle with intraventricular septal flattening, and small dimension of the left ventricle.

can be visualized with confidence. Therefore, contrast-enhanced CT should not be used to exclude the diagnosis of chronic thromboembolic disease.

High-resolution CT (HRCT) scanning, however, is required to exclude parenchymal lung disease as the cause of PH and may be particularly useful in helping to make the diagnosis of PVOD.

ECHOCARDIOGRAM

In patients in whom the clinical picture is suggestive of PH or in asymptomatic patients at high risk for the condition, Doppler echocardiography should be performed as a noninvasive screening test to detect elevated sPAP. It provides a noninvasive estimation of right ventricular function and sPAP and can reveal other underlying cardiac abnormalities.

Signs indicative of PH on echocardiogram include increased sPAP or tricuspid regurgitant jet, right atrial and ventricular hypertrophy, flattening of the intraventricular septum, small left ventricular dimension, and a dilated pulmonary artery (**Figure 58-7**, *A* and *B*). A pericardial effusion in the setting of PH carries a poor prognosis. Although echocardiography has been found to correlate with right-sided heart catheterization, Doppler echocardiography generally underestimates systolic PAP in patients with severe PH and overestimates systolic PAP in populations consisting mostly of subjects with normal pressures. Furthermore, the systolic PAP may fall in decompensated right ventricular heart failure (**Figure 58-8**). Echocardiography also is particularly inaccurate in persons with advanced lung disease and both underestimates and overestimates the degree of PH in these patients. With echocardiographic evidence of significant PH, a right-sided heart catheterization should always be undertaken at least once to provide an accurate baseline assessment of the pulmonary hemodynamics and to permit reversibility studies. Echocardiography is, however, useful in following disease progression, removing the need for repeated pulmonary artery catheterizations.

Contrast echocardiography can be useful to assess for intracardiac shunting suggesting the possibility of a congenital heart defect or patent foramen ovale. Agitated saline contrast or commercially available encapsulated microbubble contrast agents also can be used to enhance the spectral tricuspid regurgitant signal. As a general rule, a right ventricular systolic pressure greater than 40 mm Hg generally warrants further evaluation in the patient with unexplained dyspnea. An abnormal right-sided morphology or function also should trigger further evaluation.

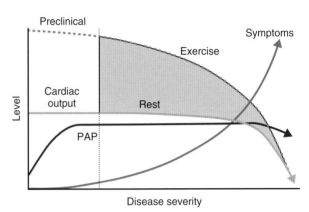

Figure 58-8 Pathophysiology of pulmonary arterial hypertension. In the early stages, cardiac output remains normal at rest but fails to increase appropriately with exercise. With disease progression, cardiac output falls and is subnormal even when the patient is at rest. *PAP*, pulmonary artery pressure. *(From Reed AK, Evans TW, Wort SJ: Pulmonary hypertension. In Albert RK, Spiro SG, Jett JR, editors:* Clinical respiratory medicine, *ed 3, Philadelphia, Mosby, 2008.)*

Exercise echocardiography is challenging both to perform and to interpret and may not be able to discern the extent to which elevated left-sided heart filling pressure may contribute to "exercise-induced pulmonary hypertension." Therefore, no treatment decisions can be made on the basis of exercise-induced pulmonary hypertension alone.

RIGHT-SIDED HEART CATHETERIZATION

In patients with suspected PH, right-sided heart catheterization is required to confirm the presence of PH, to establish the specific diagnosis, and to determine the severity and prognosis of PH. In particular, an elevated right atrial pressure and a depressed cardiac output are associated with worse prognosis and decreased survival. The PCWP is, by definition, normal in PAH. An elevated PCWP in the absence of left-sided heart disease should raise clinical suspicion for PVOD, although the PCWP also is commonly normal, in keeping with the patchy nature of this disease. The transpulmonary gradient (i.e., mPAP – PCWP) is significantly elevated in patients with PAH, but not in patients whose PH is due to increased cardiac output or left-sided heart myocardial or valvular disease. In other words, by definition, both PAP *and* PVR are elevated in patients with PAH.

Right-sided heart catheterization also can be used to evaluate for vasoreactivity and to guide therapy; a favorable acute response to a vasodilator (intravenous epoprostenol, adenosine, or inhaled nitric oxide) is defined as a fall in mPAP of at least 10 mm Hg to 40 mm Hg or less, with an increased or unchanged cardiac output. These "responders" have an improved survival when treated with calcium channel blockers (a 95% 5-year survival rate has been reported). Of note, patients with suspected PVOD should not be subjected to vasoreactivity studies, because such testing may precipitate life-threatening pulmonary edema.

FUNCTIONAL ASSESSMENT

In patients with PAH, serial determinations of functional class and exercise capacity assessed by the 6-minute walk test provide benchmarks for disease severity, response to therapy, progression, and survival. WHO functional classification of patients with PAH is based on a modification of the New York Heart Association (NYHA) system for heart failure and takes syncope into account as a marker of functional status.

The 6-minute walk test is simple and reproducible and has been used as the primary end point in a number of clinical trials for PAH. The 6-minute walk distance correlates inversely with functional class and PVR and directly with baseline cardiac output, peak exercise oxygen consumption, and survival. This test, however, gives no indication of the source of exercise impairment and is less discriminatory for walk distances greater than 450 m ("plateau effect"). Consequently, it is less useful for patients with systemic disease and those assigned to functional class I or II.

Although CPET is used less frequently in PAH clinical trials, owing to a lack of methodologic consistency among different centers, maximal oxygen consumption (peak $\dot{V}o_2$) determined by progressive exercise testing with cycle ergometry was found to be an independent predictor of survival in a study in patients with IPAH. In this study, a peak $\dot{V}o_2$ greater than 10.4 mL/kg/minute was associated with significantly better 1-year survival than lower peak $\dot{V}o_2$ values. Patients with a peak systemic blood pressure higher than 120 mm Hg also enjoyed a better 1-year survival than those patients who did not achieve this systemic blood pressure.

BIOMARKERS

Brain natriuretic peptide (BNP) is released from cardiac myocytes in response to increased ventricular wall tension. ProBNP (the prohormone) is cleaved into active BNP and the more stable amino-terminal (N-terminal) fragment (NT) proBNP. Studies in patients with PAH have demonstrated that plasma BNP and/or proBNP levels are raised in proportion to the extent of right ventricular dysfunction. Growing evidence suggests that BNP may be a potential biomarker for PAH in screening for occult disease, diagnostic evaluation, gauging prognosis, and predicting response to therapy. Baseline and serial changes in BNP correlate well with mortality and other markers such as pulmonary hemodynamics, WHO functional class, and 6-minute walk test. Of note, however, because plasma BNP levels rise in a variety of cardiopulmonary conditions and are affected by several physiologic factors, interpretation of BNP assay results requires experience and good clinical judgment; NT proBNP may have an advantage over BNP, because it is less affected by renal function and age.

Other biomarkers of interest include uric acid and troponin levels. In IPAH, uric acid levels may reflect impaired oxidative metabolism and have been shown to be increased with worsening severity of functional class and hemodynamics and correlated with mortality. Detectable cardiac troponin T also confers a poor prognosis, potentially as a consequence of the effect of right ventricular ischemia.

CARDIAC MAGNETIC RESONANCE IMAGING

Cardiac magnetic resonance imaging (MRI) is now the most accurate means for examination of the structure and function of the right ventricle and is able to accurately assess the size and function of the right ventricle with a high degree of reproducibility. Right ventricular function is an important prognostic indicator in PAH and cardiac MRI of poor right ventricular function, including stroke volume of 25 mL/m^2 or less, right ventricular end-diastolic volume of 84 mL/m^2 or greater, and left ventricular end-diastolic volume of 40 mL/m^2 or less, were found to be independent predictors of mortality and treatment failure, and pulmonary artery stiffness, as measured by relative cross-sectional area change, was predictive of survival in a cohort of 86 patients with PAH studied with MRI. Those with a relative cross-sectional area change of less than 16% had a greater mortality than those with values greater than 16%. The use of noninvasive imaging, such as cardiac MRI, to monitor disease-targeted therapy currently is being evaluated.

OTHER BLOOD TESTS

All patients should have routine hematology, biochemistry, and thyroid function tests. Antinuclear antibody testing frequently gives a positive result in patients with PAH despite absence of connective tissue disease (29% in the National Institutes of Health [NIH] registry) despite the absence of connective tissue disease. These usually are of a nonspecific pattern and are present in low titers. Strongly positive results on serologic testing should lead to further, more specific investigations to exclude PAH related to connective tissue disease. HIV testing should be considered in all patients presenting with apparent PAH.

APPROACH TO THERAPY

Treatment goals for patients with PAH include reduction in clinical signs and symptoms and improvement in exercise tolerance, functional class, hemodynamics, and quality of life, along with decreased need for hospitalization or lung transplantation (or both) and longer survival. The recommended approach to treatment can be divided into two categories: general care and PAH-specific therapy.

GENERAL THERAPY

It is expert opinion that all patients with PAH and documented hypoxemia should be on supplemental oxygen to maintain oxygen saturation above 90%. A sodium-restricted diet also is indicated in patients with PH to help maintain volume status and is particularly important in patients with right ventricular failure. Careful diuresis is indicated in patients with evidence of right ventricular failure. Caution must be exercised to avoid overdiuresis, however, because right ventricular performance is highly dependent on preload for maintenance of adequate cardiac output and systemic blood pressure.

Digoxin may produce a modest increase in cardiac output in patients with PH and right ventricular failure, along with a significant reduction in circulating norepinephrine, although the use of cardiac glycosides in treating right-sided heart dysfunction is controversial owing to the lack of prospective randomized, double-blind, placebo-controlled trials.

Improved survival has been reported with oral anticoagulation in patients with idiopathic PAH, and anticoagulation is recommended for all patients with PAH after analysis of the risk-benefit ratio for bleeding complications.

Arrhythmias, particularly atrial flutter and other tachyarrhythmias, are very poorly tolerated and often result in worsening right ventricular function. Prognosis is improved if sinus rhythm is restored. Cardioversion may be performed electrically or chemically with amiodarone, but ablation therapy may be a better option. Right ventricular failure may worsen with the addition of therapeutic agents that are strong negative inotropes.

Pregnancy and the postpartum period are associated with greater than 50% mortality in patients with PH. Therefore, the WHO recommends adequate birth control and advises discussion of termination of any pregnancy.

Patients should be immunized annually against influenza and pneumococcal pneumonia. They also should be instructed to seek the advice of their PAH treatment center for appropriate management before undergoing any form of elective surgery.

Exposure to high altitudes may contribute to hypoxic pulmonary vasoconstriction. Therefore, patients with an oxygen saturation of less than 92% should receive supplemental oxygen during air travel and when participating in sports and other activities at higher altitudes.

Calcium Channel Blockers

Calcium channel blockers may precipitate right-sided heart failure because of the negative inotropic properties of these agents and should be used only in the rare patient who has a documented vasoreactive response during right-sided heart catheterization. If the functional status of a patient who meets the definition of an acute responder does not improve to class I or II, an alternative or additional PAH therapy should be instituted. Owing to its potential negative inotropic effects, verapamil should be avoided. The main limitations to therapy in responders are systemic hypotension, peripheral edema, and hypoxia caused by increased ventilation-perfusion mismatch. More severe adverse reactions, including arrhythmias, cardiogenic shock, and death, have been reported.

DISEASE-TARGETED THERAPIES

In general, oral therapies are considered first-line treatment for PAH in patients of functional classes II and III, whereas parenteral therapy should be considered in patients of functional class IV. Clinical trials using combination therapy currently are under way. Although currently no consensus has been reached on how to monitor patients for PAH, a clear survival benefit has been recognized for goal-directed therapy. Most experts reevaluate patients every 3 to 4 months by functional class, 6-minute walk testing, and BNP assay. Follow-up echocardiography and right-sided heart catheterization also are done on a routine basis.

Phosphodiesterase Type-5 Inhibitors

The pulmonary vasodilating effects of nitric oxide are mediated through cGMP. Nitric oxide activates guanylate cyclase, which increases cGMP production. Cyclic GMP causes vasorelaxation, but its effects are attenuated by the rapid degradation of cGMP by phosphodiesterase. Sildenafil and tadalafil inhibit phosphodiesterase type 5, thus enhancing relaxation and growth inhibition of vascular smooth muscle cells. Both have demonstrated improvement in exercise capacity and functional class. In its pivotal trial, sildenafil also effected improvement in hemodynamics but did not meet the end point "time to clinical worsening," which was met in the pivotal trail for tadalafil. Side effects include headache, flushing, dyspepsia, and epistaxis. These drugs are contraindicated in patients on nitrates because of the potential for an unsafe drop in blood pressure.

Endothelin Receptor Antagonists

Endothelin-1 is a potent vasoconstrictor and smooth muscle mitogen that is overexpressed in the plasma and lung tissue of patients with PAH. Bosentan is an oral nonselective endothelin receptor antagonist, whereas ambrisentan is an oral selective endothelin type A receptor antagonist. Both of these agents have been shown to improve exercise capacity, functional class, and time to clinical worsening. In one of its pivotal trials, bosentan also was shown to improve hemodynamics. Abnormal hepatic function, defined as elevation of hepatic transaminases to three times the upper limit of normal or higher, is seen in approximately 10% of patients on bosentan and approximately 2% of patients on ambrisentan. Consequently, the U.S. Food and Drug Administration (FDA) mandates monthly liver function testing in those patients on bosentan.

In addition to potential hepatotoxicity, other side effects include anemia and the development of edema. The endothelin receptor antagonists (ERAs) are classified as pregnancy category X, so monthly pregnancy tests are required in women of child-bearing potential.

Prostanoids

Prostacyclin is a potent vasodilator and inhibitor of platelet activation and smooth muscle proliferation. Three prostanoids that have been shown to improve exercise capacity, quality of life, functional class, and hemodynamics are epoprostenol, treprostinil, and iloprost. Regimens proven effective include continuous intravenous epoprostenol therapy; inhaled, subcutaneous, and intravenous treprostinil therapy; and inhaled iloprost. Epoprostenol also has been shown to improve survival. Their respective delivery systems are complex and require collaboration with a clinical center with appropriate expertise.

Expert consensus recommends intravenous epoprostenol therapy as first-line treatment for patients with WHO class IV disease and those with class III disease in whom treatment with other disease-targeting therapies has failed to effect improvement. The main drawbacks to intravenous therapy with epoprostenol are its short half-life (approximately 2 to 5 minutes), invasive mode of delivery, expense, and side effects, which include jaw pain, flushing, diarrhea, headache, backache, leg pain, and hypotension. Catheter-related adverse effects include infection, thrombosis, pump failure, and rebound PAH.

Compared with epoprostenol, treprostinil has a longer half-life (approximately 4 hours), so it can be administered by continuous subcutaneous infusion or intravenously. Treprostinil has a side effect profile similar to that for epoprostenol, with two notable differences: The subcutaneous route is associated with significant pain at the infusion site, often resulting in discontinuation of therapy, and the intravenous route is associated with an increased risk of bloodstream infections, particularly gram-negative infections.

Iloprost is a stable prostacyclin analogue that can be given by inhalation but has a relatively short duration of action and must be inhaled between six and nine times per day, whereas treprostinil can be inhaled four times daily. Both inhaled prostanoids require unique devices for drug delivery and are associated with cough.

Rehabilitation

Data on which to base recommendations regarding exercise are limited; nevertheless, experts recommend low-level aerobic exercise and supervised pulmonary rehabilitation. Patients should be advised to avoid heavy physical exertion or isometric exercise, because such effort may evoke exertional syncope.

Surgical Options

Atrial Septostomy

The use of atrial septostomy should be limited to patients who have signs of right-sided heart failure and syncope and who are on maximal medical therapy. It often is viewed as a bridge to transplantation. Atrial septostomy creates a left-to-right intracardiac shunt that decompresses the right side of the heart, increases left ventricular preload, and augments systemic cardiac output. Thus, despite significant arterial oxygen desaturation, oxygen delivery to the tissues can be improved. The procedure is associated with significant mortality and should be performed only in specialized centers.

Lung Transplantation

Lung transplantation should be considered for patients who fail to improve on prostanoid therapy and those who remain in functional class III or IV. Little difference in efficacy between single lung, bilateral sequential lung, and heart-lung transplantation has been noted, with survival rates of 70% to 80% at 1 year and 50% to 60% at 4 years regardless of the procedure performed. Single-lung transplantation is more complicated in the immediate postoperative period because of reperfusion edema in the transplanted lung. Because of the limited availability of organ transplants, heart-lung blocks are reserved for patients with left-sided heart disease or congenital heart disease coexistent with Eisenmenger syndrome.

Pulmonary Thromboendarterectomy

Pulmonary thromboendarterectomy (PTE) is the treatment of choice for patients with proximal CTEPH and offers a potential cure in carefully selected patients. This procedure is performed in just a few specialized centers. During PTE, organized thromboembolic material is carefully removed from the affected pulmonary arteries under hypothermic circulatory arrest, attempting to restore pulmonary hemodynamics to normal or near normal levels. Those patients with a disproportionately higher PVR than would be expected from the segmental obstruction seen on imaging have a higher mortality and benefit less from PTE. With advances in both surgical technique and postoperative intensive care, the procedure-associated mortality rate has progressively diminished to approximately 6% to 8%. More than 90% of survivors return to functional class I or II. Patients with CTEPH caused by distal disease are not amenable to such treatment, and evidence is emerging for PAH-specific mediations in this group.

SURVIVAL AND OUTLOOK

The natural history of IPAH has been well characterized, with an estimated mean survival period of 2.8 years and 1-, 3-, and 5-year survival rates of 68%, 48%, and 34%. Prognostic indicators generally are related to right ventricular function and

include clinical and echocardiographic evidence of right ventricular failure or dysfunction, poor exercise tolerance, advanced functional class, elevated serum concentrations of BNP, and poor hemodynamics (elevated right atrial pressure, decreased cardiac index). Patients with these risk factors should be considered for early initiation of prostanoid therapy.

Different survival curves have emerged for the different types of PAH. For example, survival typically is better in patients with congenital heart disease than in patients with IPAH, but worse in patients with connective tissue disease (reported rate of 40% at 2 years). This difference highlights another limitation of the classification scheme: Although the different types of PAH share similar pathobiologic features, key differences are recognized: different responses of the right ventricle (congenital heart disease), differences in the pathologic lesions (absence or reduced presence of the plexiform lesion seen in the connective tissue diseases), presence or absence of concomitant left ventricular diastolic dysfunction and/or pulmonary fibrosis (commonly seen in scleroderma), and differing responses to vasodilatation, hyperdynamic or high-flow states (congenital heart disease, portopulmonary hypertension, and chronic hemolysis), and other comorbid conditions seen in all of the "associated" forms of PAH. Fortunately, data suggest that mortality is decreasing in today's era of expanding PAH therapy.

The past decade has brought a more thorough understanding of the pathogenesis of PAH, improved methods of detection, and better treatment options, which together have resulted in improved exercise tolerance and quality of life along with increased time to clinical worsening and survival.

CONTROVERSIES AND PITFALLS

- *Combination therapy*: Combination therapy that uses drugs with different therapeutic mechanisms is an attractive option for patients who fail to improve or deteriorate with first-line treatment (monotherapy), but trials to confirm the value of this approach are ongoing and may be limited by the expense of these therapies. Many experts are interested in the concept of induction therapy followed by tailoring to a maintenance regimen.

- *Out-of-proportion magnitude of pulmonary hypertension*: Most patients present with features of more than one WHO group. Unfortunately, clinical trials are lacking in patients with PH that is out of proportion to their parenchymal lung disease or left heart dysfunction. Decisions on how to treat these patients are limited to anecdotal reports and the clinician's own experience.

- *Peripheral/nonoperable CTEPH*: Data on use of PAH therapies for patients with peripheral or nonoperable CTEPH are evolving, but large clinical trials showing a benefit in this population also are lacking

- *Exercise-induced pulmonary hypertension*: Convincing data show that patients should be treated early for their PH; however the exercise definition (greater than 30 mm Hg) for PH was removed at the most recent symposium in Dana Point. Further studies regarding exercise hemodynamics are sorely needed to allow for earlier detection and treatment, with consequent better prognosis.

- *Associated PAH*: Most of what is known about PAH comes from IPAH; likewise, clinical trials largely comprise patients with IPAH, with a minority of patients with scleroderma spectrum of disease and occasionally diet drugs–related PAH or congenital heart disease. Caution should be taken before applying these data to all forms of PAH.

WEB RESOURCE

Pulmonary Hypertension Association: www.phassociation.org

SUGGESTED READINGS

Badesch DB, Champion HC, Sanchez MA, et al: Diagnosis and assessment of pulmonary arterial hypertension, *J Am Coll Cardiol* 54:S56–S66, 2009.

Barst RJ, Gibbs JS, Ghofrani HA, et al: Updated evidence-based treatment algorithm in pulmonary arterial hypertension, *J Am Coll Cardiol* 54(1 Suppl):S78–S84, 2009.

Hoeper MM, Barberà JA, Channick RN, et al: Diagnosis, assessment, and treatment of non-pulmonary arterial hypertension pulmonary hypertension, *J Am Coll Cardiol* 54(1 Suppl):S85–S96, 2009.

Kovacs G, Berghold A, Scheidl S, Olschewski H: Pulmonary arterial pressure during rest and exercise in healthy subjects: a systematic review, *Eur Respir J* 34:888–894, 2009.

McLaughlin VV, Archer SL, Badesh DB, et al: ACCF/AHA 2009 expert consensus document on pulmonary hypertension, *J Am Coll Cardiol* 53:1573–1619, 2009.

McLaughlin VV, McGoon MD: Pulmonary arterial hypertension, *Circulation* 114:1417–1431, 2006.

McLaughlin VV, Presberg KW, Doyle RL, et al: Prognosis of pulmonary arterial hypertension: ACCP evidence-based clinical practice guidelines, *Chest* 126(1 Suppl):78S–92S, 2004.

Simonneau G, Robbins IM, Beghetti M, et al: Updated clinical classification of pulmonary hypertension, *J Am Coll Cardiol* 54:S43–S54, 2009.

Tuder RM: Pathology of pulmonary arterial hypertension, *Semin Respir Crit Care Med* 30:376–385, 2009.

Tuder RM, Abman SH, Braun T, et al: Development and pathology of pulmonary hypertension, *J Am Coll Cardiol* 54:S3–S9, 2009.

Chapter **59**

Pulmonary Vasculitis and Hemorrhage

Ulrich Specks

PULMONARY VASCULITIS

Pulmonary vasculitis is defined as inflammation of vessels in the lung of different sizes—pulmonary arteries, veins, and capillaries, as well as bronchial arteries. It usually is only one manifestation of a systemic disorder caused by any of a variety of immunologic mechanisms. Moreover, not all respiratory symptoms occurring in patients with vasculitis are caused by inflammation of pulmonary vessels.

Primary vasculitis is separated from secondary vasculitis. The primary systemic vasculitides are a heterogeneous group of syndromes, of unknown etiology, that share a clinical response to immunosuppressive therapy. Their wide spectrum of frequently overlapping clinical manifestations is defined by the size and location of the affected vessels as well as by the nature of the inflammatory infiltrate. Secondary vasculitis may occur in the context of a well-defined underlying disorder or may be attributable to a specific cause such as collagen vascular disease, infection, or therapeutic or illicit drug use.

Most classification schemes and definitions of the vasculitides are based on the size of the most prominently affected vessels. Definitions, nomenclature, and classification schemes have been and remain subject to change. The terms used in this chapter adhere to the nomenclature and definitions put forth by the Chapel Hill consensus conference in 1992.

SMALL VESSEL VASCULITIS

Antineutrophil Cytoplasmic Autoantibody-Associated Vasculitis

The primary systemic small vessel vasculitides are granulomatosis with polyangiitis (GPA) (i.e., Wegener granulomatosis), microscopic polyangiitis (MPA), and eosinophilic granulomatosis with polyangiitis (EGPA) (i.e., Churg-Strauss syndrome). In contrast with the other forms of systemic vasculitis with a predilection for larger vessels, most patients with active GPA and MPA and more than half of the patients with active EGPA have antineutrophil cytoplasmic autoantibodies (ANCA). Of all systemic vasculitides, the ANCA-associated vasculitides are most likely to cause respiratory manifestations. GPA and MPA are discussed together here, because the same diagnostic and therapeutic principles apply; EGPA is considered separately.

Granulomatosis with Polyangiitis and Microscopic Polyangiitis

Definitions and Nomenclature
GPA is characterized by necrotizing granulomatous inflammation involving the respiratory tract and necrotizing vasculitis affecting small to medium-sized vessels. The most commonly affected vessels are capillaries, venules, arterioles, and arteries, but the wall of the aorta also may rarely be affected by necrotizing granulomatous inflammation—hence the term *polyangiitis*. Histopathologic documentation of granulomatous involvement of the respiratory tract is not explicitly required. Radiologic evidence or clinical examination findings highly predictive of granulomatous pathology are sufficient. Consequently, the diagnosis of GPA depends on a correlation of clinical, histopathologic, and serologic features. MPA is defined as necrotizing vasculitis with few or no immune deposits, affecting small vessels including capillaries, venules, or arterioles (polyangiitis). Necrotizing arteritis involving small and medium-sized arteries may be present. Necrotizing glomerulonephritis is very common; pulmonary capillaritis resulting in alveolar hemorrhage occurs frequently. The vasculitis of MPA is indistinguishable from that of GPA, and substantial clinical overlap has been observed. For these reasons, the therapeutic approach to patients with GPA and to those with MPA is governed by the same principles, and most clinical studies and therapeutic trials have combined both diseases.

Histopathologic features that define GPA and separate it from MPA include discrete or confluent necrotizing granulomatous inflammation with vasculitis. Fibrinoid necrosis, microabscesses, focal vasculitis, thrombosis, and fibrous obliteration of the vascular lumen also may be seen. Giant cells are a hallmark of the necrotizing granulomatous inflammation of GPA. Atypical and rare histopathologic features of GPA include organizing pneumonia, bronchocentric inflammation, and a marked number of eosinophils in the inflammatory infiltrates.

For treatment stratification, clinical disease activity is categorized as "limited disease" or "severe disease." *Severe disease* is either life-threatening or associated with involvement of an organ with potentially irreversible loss of function. Consequently, patients with any of the following disease manifestations should be labeled as having severe disease: alveolar hemorrhage, glomerulonephritis, eye involvement (except mere episcleritis), or nervous system involvement including sensorineural hearing loss. *Limited disease* includes essentially all patients who have nonsevere disease. The designation limited disease as used in the United States comprises what European investigators have referred to as "early-systemic disease" and "localized disease." Even though this separation is not based on well-defined biologic distinctions, most disease manifestations leading to the categorization as severe disease are caused by capillaritis. By contrast, most symptoms leading to the classification as limited disease are the result of necrotizing granulomatous inflammation. Patients with limited GPA have a more protracted disease course, a greater likelihood of experiencing a disease relapse after a period of remission, and a higher prevalence of destructive upper respiratory tract disorders (e.g., saddle nose deformity). Tracheobronchial disease involvement also is a feature of GPA not shared with MPA; it may present unique treatment challenges (as discussed later on).

Etiology and Pathogenesis

The etiology of ANCA-associated vasculitis remains unknown. Occupational exposures have been suggested as possible etiologic factors, including inhalation of silica-containing compounds, grain dust, and heavy metals. Infection has been linked to the onset of the disease as well as to relapses. A multifactorial genetic predisposition also may contribute to the development of ANCA-associated vasculitis. Last but not least, ANCA seem to play a pathogenic role for the development of vasculitis.

Clinical Presentation

The median age of patients at diagnosis is 45 years, but children as well as octogenarians may be affected. The average age at onset of GPA is about 10 years younger than for MPA. Men and women are affected equally. More than 90% of patients with GPA are white. The clinical presentation of GPA varies, ranging from subacute nonspecific respiratory illness to rapidly progressive alveolar hemorrhage syndrome. The characteristic disease manifestations of GPA affecting the respiratory tract are caused by necrotizing granulomatous inflammation. Ear, nose, and throat symptoms, initially noted by more than 85% of patients, may include rhinorrhea, purulent or bloody nasal discharge, nasal mucosal drying and crust formation, epistaxis, and otitis media. Paranasal sinus involvement manifesting as deep facial pain, nasal septal perforation, and ulceration of the vomer are important clinical signs. *Staphylococcus aureus* frequently is detected in the nose and sinuses and has been linked to relapses of the disease. Other signs include aphthous lesions of the nasal and oral mucosa and inflammation and destruction of the nasal cartilage leading to the so-called saddle nose deformity. Ulcerated lesions of the larynx and trachea are present in 30% of untreated cases and may cause hemoptysis.

Diagnostic Evaluation

The diagnostic evaluation of patients suspected of having GPA or MPA should include imaging of the chest, pulmonary function testing if the patient has any respiratory symptoms or abnormalities on the chest radiograph, measurements of erythrocyte sedimentation rate, C-reactive protein, complete blood count, serum chemistry panel, urine analysis and microscopy, and testing for ANCA.

Respiratory symptoms usually are associated with unilateral or bilateral radiographic abnormalities including infiltrates, nodules, or mass lesions, which may or may not cavitate. The nodules range in size from a few millimeters to several centimeters across. Solitary nodules also may occur. Unusual manifestations include lymphadenopathy, lobar consolidation, and large pleural effusions.

Tracheobronchial lesions are common and may be asymptomatic or mistaken for evidence of asthma. Pulmonary function testing including inspiratory and expiratory flow-volume loops may provide important clues to the presence of airway narrowing and should be part of the initial evaluation. Bronchoscopic inspection of the tracheobronchial tree is recommended for patients with unexplained respiratory symptoms, abnormalities on pulmonary function tests, or radiographic abnormalities.

Patients with GPA or MPA exhibit variable degrees of elevation of erythrocyte sedimentation rate or C-reactive protein levels. If GPA or MPA is suspected, urine analysis and microscopy and serum creatinine determination are crucial, because early renal involvement may be clinically silent yet can progress rapidly.

In GPA and MPA, ANCA that cause a cytoplasmic immunofluorescence pattern (c-ANCA) on ethanol-fixed neutrophils are caused by the reaction of antibodies with proteinase 3 (PR3) (i.e., PR3-ANCA). By contrast, a variety of antibodies can cause a perinuclear immunofluorescence pattern (p-ANCA) on ethanol-fixed neutrophils. Only those that also react with myeloperoxidase (MPO) are of interest in the context of ANCA-associated vasculitis. Maximal diagnostic accuracy of ANCA testing requires corroboration of a positive target antigen–specific test result (PR3-ANCA or MPO-ANCA) by immunofluorescence assay, or vice versa. Only the PR3-ANCA with c-ANCA combination and the MPO-ANCA with p-ANCA combination are sensitive and specific for ANCA-associated vasculitis.

The clinical utility—as reflected in positive and negative predictive values—of ANCA testing for GPA and MPA is critically dependent on the pretest probability of the disease in the patient tested, as well as on the analytic accuracy of the test method. If applied in patients with clinical features indicating a high pretest probability of GPA or MPA, ANCA testing has a very high positive predictive value. However, occasional false-positive ANCA test results have been reported in a variety of infections. Particularly, subacute bacterial endocarditis may represent a diagnostic dilemma as it may mimic small-vessel vasculitis clinically and has been reported with c-ANCA/PR3-ANCA. With other infections reported with ANCA, either the right pairing of immunofluorescence test results with its corresponding antigen specificity is lacking or their clinical features are distinct from those of GPA or MPA. In patients undergoing evaluation for necrotizing glomerulonephritis with or without alveolar hemorrhage, ANCA may occur in conjunction with anti–glomerular basement membrane (anti-GBM) antibodies. These ANCA usually are of the MPO-ANCA variety. The presence of anti-GBM antibodies seems to determine the prognosis in such double-positive patients.

Most patients with severe GPA or MPA demonstrate a positive result on ANCA testing (for a sensitivity greater than 95%), but up to 30% of patients with limited GPA may not have detectable ANCA. Despite the recognized association between ANCA titers and disease activity, changes in ANCA levels do not reliably predict the disease activity in individual patients. Therefore, serial titers of ANCA should not be used to plan long-term therapy.

Therapy

Standard therapy for GPA and MPA currently follows the same basic principles. Methotrexate (MTX) at a dose of up to 25 mg once a week in combination with oral prednisone is considered the standard of care for patients with limited GPA. However, only one prospective randomized trial has compared MTX and cyclophosphamide (CYC) for remission induction in such patients (Table 59-1). The trial, conducted by the European Vasculitis Study Group (EUVAS), showed that MTX is noninferior to CYC for remission induction, but the side effects were less frequent and less severe. The trial also documented that early discontinuation of immunosuppression in patients with ANCA-associated vasculitis is fraught with a high relapse rate. The largest reported group of patients with limited Wegener's

Table 59-1	Randomized Controlled Trials Informing the Standard of Care in ANCA-Associated Vasculitis			
Treatment Investigated	**Trial Design**	**No. of Patients**	**Main Conclusion**	**Published Study/Name of Trial**
TMP-SMX for remission maintenance in GPA	Randomized (1:1), placebo-controlled	81	TMP-SMX reduces incidence of relapses in WG.	Stegeman et al, 1996/(N/A)
AZA versus CYC for remission maintenance in severe GPA and MPA	Randomized (1:1), controlled, open-label	144	AZA is as effective for remission maintenance as continuation of CYC in severe AAV.	Jayne et al, 2003/ CYCAZAREM
MTX versus CYC for remission induction in early-systemic GPA and MPA	Randomized (1:1), controlled, open-label	100	MTX is not inferior to CYC in early-systemic AAV.	De Groot et al, 2005/ NORAM
PLEX versus intravenous methylprednisolone for GPA and MPA with severe renal disease	Randomized (1:1), controlled, open-label	137	PLEX improves renal survival of methylprednisolone in patients with AAV with severe renal disease.	Jayne et al, 2007/ MEPEX
AZA versus MTX for remission maintenance in severe GPA and MPA	Randomized (1:1), controlled, open-label	126	There is no difference in efficacy (relapse rate) or adverse events rate between AZA and MTX.	Pagnoux et al, 2008/ WEGENT
Etanercept versus placebo added to standard therapy for limited and severe GPA	Randomized (1:1), placebo-controlled, double-blind	180	Etanercept has no benefit in addition to standard therapy.	Wegener's Granulomatosis Etanercept Trial (WGET) Research Group, 2005/WGET
Pulse CYC versus oral daily CYC	Randomized, controlled, open-label	149	Pulse CYC is as effective as oral daily CYC for severe AAV.	De Groot et al, 2009/ CYCLOPS
AZA versus MMF for remission maintenance in GPA and MPA	Randomized, controlled, open-label	156	MMF is inferior to AZA for remission maintenance in GPA and MPA.	Hiemstra et al, 2010/ IMPROVE
RTX versus daily oral CYC, followed by AZA, for remission induction in severe newly diagnosed or relapsing GPA and MPA	Randomized (1:1), double dummy-controlled, double blind	197	RTX is noninferior to CYC for remission induction in severe GPA and MPA. For severe relapses, RTX is superior to CYC. Trial results led to FDA approval of RTX for this indication.	Stone et al, 2010/RAVE
RTX plus 2 pulses of CYC versus intravenous pulse CYC, followed by AZA, for remission induction in severe newly diagnosed GPA and MPA	Randomized (3:1), controlled, open-label	44	RTX is noninferior to CYC followed by AZA for induction of sustained remission (>6 months) in severe GPA and MPA.	Jones et al, 2010/RITUXVAS

AAV, ANCA-associated vasculitis; *ANCA*, antineutrophil cytoplasmic antibodies; *AZA*, azathioprine; *CYC*, cyclophosphamide; *FDA*, U.S. Food and Drug Administration; *GPA*, granulomatosis with polyangiitis; *MMF*, mycophenolate mofetil; *MPA*, microscopic polyangiitis; *MTX*, methotrexate; *PLEX*, plasma exchange; *RTX*, rituximab; *TMP-SMX*, trimethoprim-sulfamethoxazole; *WG*, Wegener granulomatosis.
Data from de Groot K, Harper L, Jayne DR, et al: Pulse versus daily oral cyclophosphamide for induction of remission in antineutrophil cytoplasmic antibody-associated vasculitis: a randomized trial, *Ann Intern Med* 150:670, 2009; de Groot K, Rasmussen N, Bacon PA, et al: Randomized trial of cyclophosphamide versus methotrexate for induction of remission in early systemic antineutrophil cytoplasmic antibody-associated vasculitis, *Arthritis Rheum* 52:2461, 2005; Hiemstra TF, Walsh MW, Mahr A, et al: Mycophenolate mofetil versus azathioprine for remission maintenance in antineutrophil cytoplasmic antibody-associated vasculitis (IMPROVE), *JAMA* 304:2381, 2010; Jayne D, Rasmussen N, Andrassy K, et al: A randomized trial of maintenance therapy for vasculitis associated with antineutrophil cytoplasmic autoantibodies, *N Engl J Med* 349:36, 2003; Jayne DR, Gaskin G, Rasmussen N, et al: Randomized trial of plasma exchange or high-dosage methylprednisolone as adjunctive therapy for severe renal vasculitis, *J Am Soc Nephrol* 18:2180, 2007; Jones RB, Tervaert JW, Hauser T, et al: Rituximab versus cyclophosphamide in ANCA-associated renal vasculitis, *N Engl J Med* 363:211, 2010; Pagnoux C, Mahr A, Hamidou MA, et al: Azathioprine or methotrexate maintenance for ANCA-associated vasculitis, *N Engl J Med* 359:2790, 2008; Stegeman CA, Tervaert JW, de Jong PE, Kallenberg CG: Trimethoprim-sulfamethoxazole (co-trimoxazole) for the prevention of relapses of Wegener's granulomatosis. Dutch Co-Trimoxazole Wegener Study Group, *N Engl J Med* 335:16, 1996; Stone JH, Merkel PA, Spiera R, et al: Rituximab versus cyclophosphamide for ANCA-associated vasculitis, *N Engl J Med* 363:221, 2010; Wegener's Granulomatosis Etanercept Trial (WGET) Research Group: Etanercept plus standard therapy for Wegener's granulomatosis, *N Engl J Med* 352:351, 2005.

granulomatosis (WG) was treated with MTX for remission induction in the context of the Wegener's Granulomatosis Trial (WGET). More than 90% of patients achieved remission with this regimen, and more than 70% achieved a sustained remission (lasting longer than 6 months). These rates are equivalent to those achieved with CYC in severe disease, as discussed next.

CYC at a dose of 2 mg/kg/day in combination with prednisone has been the standard of care for patients with severe GPA or MPA until recently. In contrast with the original regimen introduced by Fauci 40 years ago, the current consensus is to limit the duration of CYC therapy to the first 3 to 6 months of remission induction.

Once remission has been induced and the prednisone taper is well under way, CYC should be switched to either azathioprine (AZA), preferred in patients with renal involvement and any degree of renal insufficiency, or MTX. The first option is supported by the results of a randomized trial showing that AZA is as good as CYC for remission maintenance to 18 months. Another randomized controlled trial has shown that MTX and AZA are equivalent for remission maintenance. By contrast, a recent randomized controlled trial that compared mycophenolate mofetil (MMF) with AZA for remission maintenance has shown that MMF is inferior to AZA for this purpose. Thus, the use of MMF for remission maintenance can be supported only for patients who have failed MTX and AZA, or who have contraindications to both agents. The WGET study, in which MTX was used for remission maintenance, confirmed that long-term remission remains an elusive goal for many patients, because remission was maintained in less than half of the patients.

Whenever CYC is used for remission induction, consideration should be given to the patient's fertility. Young men should be offered sperm banking before therapy is initiated. If time allows, ovarian protection should be offered to young women, in addition to minimizing the cumulative exposure as much as possible.

One randomized controlled trial has evaluated a regimen of intravenous pulse application of CYC compared with daily oral use. The pulse regimen was noninferior to the oral application of CYC for remission, and the frequency of leukopenia, but not infection, was lower. Even though the trial was not powered to detect a difference in relapses, however, the relapse rate was higher after remission induction with the intermittent pulse regimen than with the oral application of CYC.

A metaanalysis of earlier cohort studies had also indicated that intravenous pulse CYC therapy may be safer because of a lower cumulative dose, but a higher relapse rate also was observed after discontinuation. In my own experience, intravenous CYC is best avoided in the intensive care unit setting. However, its use is preferred over oral CYC in patients with questionable compliance, in young women with fertility issues, and in patients who have gastrointestinal problems with oral CYC application.

The four-decade-old standard use of CYC for remission induction in patients with severe GPA and MPA recently has been challenged by the results of two randomized controlled trials. The RAVE (rituximab for ANCA-associated vasculitis) trial was a randomized double-blind, double-placebo-controlled, multicenter trial that compared oral CYC (2 mg/kg/day) to rituximab (RTX) (375 mg/m^2 body surface area/week for 4 weeks) for remission induction in severe GPA or MPA in 197 patients. Once remission was achieved between 3 and 6 months, patients randomized to receive CYC were switched to AZA for remission maintenance for 18 months, whereas patients in the original RTX group then received placebo. No difference was observed in rates of achieving remission at the end of 6 months and maintaining remission at 18 months between the two treatment arms. Among the 101 patients who entered the trial with severe relapsing disease, however, RTX proved superior to CYC. The results of the RAVE trial led to approval by the U.S. Food and Drug Administration (FDA) of RTX for remission induction in severe GPA and MPA.

Another randomized controlled open-label trial conducted in 44 patients with newly diagnosed severe ANCA-associated vasculitis with active renal disease, RITUXVAS (Rituximab versus Cyclophosphamide for ANCA-Associated Renal Vasculitis), showed results complementary to those of the RAVE trial. In the RITUXVAS trial, patients were randomized 3 : 1 to receive RTX (together with two pulses of CYC) compared with standard intravenous pulse CYC therapy followed by oral AZA. The primary outcome was sustained remission (of more than 6 months' duration) at month 12. No difference between the treatment groups was found (RTX 76% versus CYC 82%).

Mycophenolate mofetil (MMF) may represent an alternative to CYC (and RTX) for patients with MPA who have MPO-ANCA and mild renal disease (as defined by creatinine levels less than 3.5 mg/day) and no other life- or organ-threatening disease manifestation. This claim is supported by data from a randomized controlled trial in 35 patients from China comparing oral MMF (1.5 to 2 g/day) with intravenous CYC (0.75 to 1.0 g/m^2 once monthly). In addition, all patients received intravenous methylprednisolone bolus therapy (0.5 g/day for 3 days) followed by oral prednisone (0.6 to 0.8 mg/kg for 4 weeks tapered by 5 mg every week to reach 10 mg/day). These regimens demonstrated equivalent efficacy, but MMF was better tolerated than CYC. A prospective pilot trial in 17 patients conducted at the Mayo Clinic achieved similar results.

For some patients with Wegener granulomatosis (WG) and MPA, the combination of glucocorticoids and cyclophosphamide may not be sufficient to induce a remission quickly. Plasma exchange should be considered early in patients who present with rapidly progressive glomerulonephritis and renal failure, as well as in patients who present with diffuse alveolar hemorrhage (DAH). The use of plasma exchange currently is supported by two studies: The MEPEX (Methylprednisolone Versus Plasma Exchange) trial in 156 patients who presented with a serum creatinine level of 5.5 mg/dL or greater was conducted to compare three pulses of intravenous methylprednisolone with 2 weeks of plasma exchange (seven exchanges at rate of 60 mL/kg) in addition to standard therapy for severe disease (oral prednisone and CYC). Plasma exchange was superior to methylprednisolone with respect to renal recovery. A single-center cohort study of 20 patients presenting with alveolar hemorrhage described 100% survival when plasma exchange was added to standard immunosuppressive therapy. If alveolar hemorrhage is uncontrolled despite aggressive immunosuppressive therapy and plasma exchange, the use of recombinant activated factor VII may be considered.

The term *refractory disease* commonly is used to describe persistent disease activity in patients on the maximal tolerated dose of CYC or in those with contraindications to the use of CYC. A variety of agents have been proposed for use in addition to or instead of the failing regimen in such patients. Over the past decade, RTX has emerged as the agent of choice for treatment of refractory disease, based on over 20 case series and cohort studies comprising more than 200 patients.

Infliximab also has been used in small case series and uncontrolled trials. Of note, however, infliximab therapy was associated with a high frequency of infections with bad outcomes. The WGET showed that etanercept had no effect on remission induction or maintenance when used in addition to standard therapy. Moreover, significantly more malignancies were observed among patients who had received CYC in the etanercept treatment group. Accordingly, the use of etanercept in patients who have received or are receiving CYC is contraindicated. Consequently, no convincing rationale has emerged for the use of antitumor necrosis factor-α (anti-TNF) therapy in patients with GPA.

Several reports have described the use of other agents in patients with refractory disease. Antithymoglobulin has some efficacy but significant side effects. Dispergualine is an agent available in Japan and Europe but not in the United States.

The management of large airway involvement in GPA may present unique challenges. Subglottic stenosis may necessitate dilation procedures paired with local injection of long-acting glucocorticoids with or without mitomycin C, and stenosis of the large airways may warrant bronchoscopic interventions, including dilation by rigid bronchoscopy, yttrium-aluminum-garnet (YAG) laser treatment, and placement of silicone airway stents.

In patients with GPA and MPA, significant morbidity and mortality related to organ damage is not only caused by the disease itself but also attributable to treatment toxicities. Permanent complications have been reported to occur in 86% of patients from GPA itself, including end-stage renal disease, chronic pulmonary dysfunction, diminished hearing, destructive sinus disease, saddle nose deformities, proptosis, and blindness. Among the treated patients, 42% experienced permanent treatment-related problems including chemical (drug-induced) cystitis, osteoporotic fracture, bladder cancer, myelodysplasia, and avascular necrosis. In the 180 patients in the WGET, which reflects more recent standard practice, damage that occurred despite (or because of) therapy included visual impairment, hearing loss, nasal blockage, pulmonary fibrosis, hypertension, renal insufficiency, peripheral neuropathy, gonadal failure, and diabetes mellitus. Only 11% of the enrolled patients did not exhibit a single point on the vascular damage index (which was developed from 61 various items) after 1 year of study enrollment. The WGET investigators also concluded that patients with limited GPA are at a higher risk for GPA-related damage than are those with severe disease.

In the same cohort of 180 patients with GPA, the incidence rate of venous thromboembolism was found to be high in comparison with reported rates in the general population, patients with lupus, and patients with rheumatoid arthritis. This increased risk for thromboembolic disease also has been documented for the other ANCA-associated vasculitides. A high frequency of echocardiographic abnormalities attributable to GPA and associated with an increased mortality was observed in a study of 85 patients with confirmed GPA. Lesions directly related to GPA included regional wall motion abnormalities not matching coronary distributions, left ventricular systolic dysfunction with decreased ejection fraction, pericardial effusions, valvulitis, left ventricular aneurysm, and a large intracardiac mass. Evaluation of unexplained dyspnea in patients with GPA should therefore include echocardiography.

Eosinophilic Granulomatosis With Polyangiitis (Churg-Strauss Syndrome)

The Chapel Hill Consensus definition for EGPA is "eosinophil-rich and granulomatous inflammation involving the respiratory tract, and necrotizing vasculitis affecting small to medium-sized vessels, and associated with asthma and eosinophilia." EGPA is included among the ANCA-associated vasculitides, but only 40% to 70% of patients with active EGPA have detectable ANCA. EGPA is distinguished from GPA and MPA primarily by a high prevalence of asthma and peripheral blood and tissue eosinophilia.

Three distinct phases of the disease have been described: The first is a *prodromal allergic phase* with asthma. This phase may last for a number of years. Second is an *eosinophilic phase* with prominent peripheral and tissue eosinophilia. This phase also may last a number of years, and the manifestations may remit and recur over this period. The differential diagnosis in this phase of the disease includes parasitic infection and chronic eosinophilic pneumonia. The third *vasculitic phase* consists of systemic vasculitis and may be life-threatening. The three phases are not seen in all patients, do not necessarily occur in this order, and may even be concurrent. However, asthma usually predates vasculitic symptoms by a mean of 7 years (range, 0 to 61 years). "Formes frustes" of EGPA also have been described with eosinophilic vasculitis and/or eosinophilic granulomas in isolated organs without evidence of systemic disease.

Pulmonary parenchymal involvement occurs in 38% of patients. Transient alveolar-type infiltrates are most common. These have a predominantly peripheral distribution and are indistinguishable from infiltrates seen in chronic eosinophilic pneumonia. Occasionally, nodular lesions may be seen in EGPA. In contrast with GPA and MPA, alveolar hemorrhage is exceedingly rare in EGPA. Renal involvement is less prominent than in GPA or MPA and does not generally lead to renal failure. By contrast, peripheral nerve involvement, typically in the form of mononeuritis multiplex, is more frequent. Skin, heart, central nervous system, and abdominal viscera also may be involved.

The classic histopathologic picture consists of necrotizing vasculitis, eosinophilic tissue infiltration, and extravascular granulomas. Not all features are found in every case, however, and they are not pathognomonic for the condition. In particular, the finding of a "Churg-Strauss granuloma" on skin biopsy should not lead to confusion with the diagnosis of EGPA. This type of necrotizing extravascular granuloma may be seen in EGPA as well as in other systemic autoimmune diseases including GPA and rheumatoid arthritis.

If ANCA are present, they usually are p-ANCA reacting with MPO. The ANCA status appears to correlate with disease activity. Recent evidence points to a more vasculitic disease phenotype in the presence of ANCA, but this association was not confirmed by all studies. Substantial overlap of organ manifestations between patients with EGPA who are ANCA-positive and those who are ANCA-negative is characteristic.

In recent years, significant attention has been devoted to EGPA detected in patients taking leukotriene receptor antagonists. Available case studies and limited population-based incidence estimates suggest that these agents may lead to unmasking of vasculitic symptoms in asthmatic persons by allowing dose reductions or discontinuation of oral glucocorticoid therapy. There is no evidence suggesting that these agents directly cause the disease.

The prognosis with EGPA is better than that with GPA or MPA, because the overall mortality is lower and not significantly different from that for the normal population. Most deaths are secondary to cardiac involvement.

Systemic glucocorticoids remain the mainstay of therapy. No clinical trials have been conducted to provide clear guidance for therapy for EGPA. It seems most appropriate to treat EGPA according to the principles applied to the management of ANCA-associated vasculitis. Accordingly, CYC should be added to glucocorticoids for remission induction in all patients with disease manifestations that threaten either life or function of a vital organ—particularly those with central or peripheral nerve involvement, glomerulonephritis, heart involvement, or alveolar hemorrhage. MTX, AZA, and MMF have been used as glucocorticoid-sparing agents in less severe disease and for remission maintenance. Refractory disease and that dominated by difficult-to-control eosinophilic inflammation have been reported to respond to interferon-α therapy. Of note, however, continued long-term interferon-α therapy may be necessary, and this treatment carries the risk of substantial toxicity. RTX also has been used successfully in EGPA, particularly ANCA-positive patients with renal disease, but the data are still limited, and use of RTX instead of CYC for patients with severe EGPA cannot be recommended. Anti-interleukin 5 (IL-5) also has recently been reported as a promising agent for treatment of EGPA. The glucocorticoid-sparing effect of anti-IL5 in EGPA has been documented in two separate prospective pilot studies.

Idiopathic Pauciimmune Pulmonary Capillaritis

Occasionally patients present with isolated DAH caused by capillaritis. Despite extensive searching, no evidence of other organ involvement or specific autoantibodies can be detected.

Direct immunofluorescence studies of the lung tissue reveal no immune deposits. This clinicopathologic presentation has been referred to as *idiopathic pauciimmune pulmonary capillaritis* and represents a diagnosis of exclusion. This form of isolated pulmonary capillaritis is histopathologically indistinguishable from that of ANCA-associated vasculitis. Affected patients are best treated with an immunosuppressive regimen selected according to the guidelines for severe GPA and MPA.

MEDIUM-SIZE VESSEL VASCULITIS

Classic Polyarteritis Nodosa

Polyarteritis nodosa (PAN) is not associated with ANCA and does not affect capillaries. Therefore, it does not cause glomerulonephritis or alveolar hemorrhage. However, classic PAN can on rare occasion affect the bronchial or bronchiolar arteries, causing lung hemorrhage by that mechanism. Most cases of classic PAN diagnosed today are associated with viral infections, specifically, hepatitis B and C. Consequently, antiviral therapy plays a prominent role in the management of such cases, in addition to immunosuppression. With classic PAN, relapse is far less likely than with MPA, so PAN generally can be treated with an immunosuppressive regimen of shorter duration.

LARGE VESSEL VASCULITIS

Giant Cell Arteritis

Giant cell arteritis (GCA), also known as *temporal arteritis, cranial arteritis,* and *granulomatous arteritis,* is a generalized inflammatory disorder involving large and medium-sized arteries. It is the most common form of vasculitis in the Northern Hemisphere and affects predominantly elderly patients. The typical features of the disease include new-onset headache, a palpably tender or nodular temporal artery with decreased pulsation, and elevated erythrocyte sedimentation rate (ESR). The clinical illness emerges gradually, with the development of nonspecific systemic signs and symptoms such as low-grade fever, malaise, and weight loss. Headache, variable but often severe, is the most common symptom in GCA. Amaurosis fugax is observed in 20% of patients, and visual loss in 10%. Granulomatous inflammation of the vessel wall is found in 60% of temporal artery biopsy specimens. The aorta also may be affected by the disease, and GCA should be considered as the cause of thoracic aortic aneurysm occurring in elderly patients.

Respiratory symptoms have been reported in up to 25% of patients but rarely require management by a respiratory physician. However, respiratory symptoms may be the initial presentation of giant cell arteritis. Therefore, GCA should be considered in any elderly patient with new-onset cough, hoarseness, or throat pain without other identifiable cause, and the ESR should be measured in such patients. Cough, hoarseness, and throat pain usually resolve promptly with glucocorticoid therapy. Isolated cases of GCA with pleural effusion or multinodular pulmonary lesions also have been reported. Such findings are difficult to interpret in this setting, and GPA should be considered in the differential diagnosis, because it also may involve the temporal artery. Therapy of GCA continues to be based on the use of glucocorticoids without proven alternative. The glucocorticoid-sparing role of MTX for GCA remains controversial.

Takayasu Arteritis

Takayasu arteritis is a large vessel vasculitis affecting predominantly the aorta and its major branches in young patients.

Takayasu arteritis also has been called *pulseless disease, aortic arch syndrome,* or *reverse coarctation.* The disease affects mostly young adult women. It is not limited to patients of Asian descent. Early disease manifestations include constitutional symptoms, low-grade fever, and arthralgias. Variable pulses of the extremities and claudication of affected vascular territories are typical. Renovascular hypertension, pulmonary hypertension, and ischemia of affected organs may be the more disabling complications of this chronically relapsing disease.

Pulmonary complications are the result of a unique arteriopathy predominantly involving the large and medium-size pulmonary vessels. Progressive defects in the outer media of the arteries and ingrowth of granulation tissue–like capillaries associated with thickened intima and subendothelial smooth muscle proliferation lead to pulmonary artery stenoses and occlusion, as well as pulmonary hypertension, in up to half of all patients. The inflammatory infiltrate of the vessel wall is predominantly lymphoplasmocytic, with variable amounts of giant cells. The involvement of pulmonary arteries is common but often asymptomatic. It is detectable by conventional angiography, perfusion scan, or magnetic resonance angiography (MRA). Chest radiographs often are normal in appearance, but computed tomography (CT) may show areas of low attenuation as a result of regional hypoperfusion, subpleural reticulolinear changes, and pleural thickening. Fistula formation between pulmonary artery branches and bronchial arteries, as well as nonspecific inflammatory interstitial lung disease, also has been reported.

Therapy for Takayasu arteritis consists primarily of immunosuppression with glucocorticoids. Other immunosuppressive agents including MTX are used in conjunction with glucocorticoids for remission induction and as glucocorticoid-sparing agents for remission maintenance. Unfortunately, many patients relapse when the glucocorticoid dose is reduced below 15 mg daily. The use of antitumor necrosis factor-α agents may be beneficial for patients with disease refractory to standard therapy. Vascular bypass procedures may restore perfusion to areas affected by severe arterial stenoses, but the improvement is only temporary.

OTHER VASCULITIS SYNDROMES

Behçet Disease

Behçet disease is a rare, chronically relapsing systemic inflammatory disorder characterized by aphthous oral ulcers and at least two or more of the following: aphthous genital ulcers, uveitis, cutaneous nodules or pustules, and meningoencephalitis. Reported prevalence of the disease is 1:16,000 in Japan and 1:20,000 in the United States. A strong association with the major histocompatibility complex antigen HLA-B51 has been recognized. The mean age of patients at the onset of Behçet disease is 35 years. Most studies have reported a predominance of men with the disease over women. Respiratory manifestations are common in Behçet disease and include cough, hemoptysis, chest pain, and dyspnea. Hemoptysis often is massive and fatal. The vasculitis of Behçet disease is immune complex–mediated and may involve vessels of all sizes. Secondary thrombosis with major venous occlusion can occur. Thrombosis may not be preventable in Behçet disease by anticoagulation, but aspirin 80 mg/day has been advocated. Destruction of the elastic lamina of pulmonary arteries causing aneurysm formation, secondary erosion of bronchi, and arterial-bronchial fistulas may result in massive hemoptysis. CT or MRA can be used to detect pulmonary artery aneurysms. Recurrent pneumonia as well as bronchial obstruction secondary to mucosal inflammation also has been described.

Therapy of the underlying disease consists of immunosuppression. Prednisone alone may not be sufficient to control the vasculitis. The addition of other drugs, such as colchicine, chlorambucil, MTX, cyclosporine, or AZA, is recommended. The use of biologic agents, in particular anti-TNF agents, also has been reported recently. The addition of AZA or CYC to glucocorticoids may result in resolution of pulmonary aneurysms. Once pulmonary arteritis has been identified, anticoagulation should be avoided. The prognosis of pulmonary involvement is poor. About one third of patients die within 2 years of developing pulmonary involvement, most from fatal pulmonary hemorrhage. Embolization therapy may be used for treatment and prevention of hemorrhage from pulmonary artery aneurysms.

Henoch-Schönlein Purpura

Henoch-Schönlein purpura (HSP), also known as *anaphylactoid purpura*, *allergic purpura*, or, as more recently proposed, *IgA-associated disease*, is a syndrome characterized by acute-onset purpura, arthritis, colicky abdominal pain, and nephritis. Histopathologic findings include acute arteriolitis and venulitis in the superficial dermis and the bowel. Proliferative and necrotizing glomerulonephritis usually is mild. A similar type of renal lesion is seen in patients with infective subacute bacterial endocarditis, GPA, MPA, systemic lupus erythematosus (SLE), and anti-GBM disease.

Immunofluorescence microscopy shows large deposits of IgA in the skin and kidney. Although HSP is more common in children (mean age of patients, 17 years), adults also may be affected. Palpable purpuric lesions, which usually are distributed over the buttocks and lower extremities, and fever are generally the first clinical manifestations. The purpura may precede, accompany, or follow onset of arthralgias and abdominal colic. The triad of purpura, arthritis, and abdominal pain is present in approximately 80% of patients. Joint involvement typically is monoarticular and transient, involves the large joints, and causes pain that is out of proportion to the objective evidence of synovitis. Peritonitis and melena are common.

Pulmonary manifestations of HSP are rare. Only 26 cases have been reported to date, and capillaritis has been documented histopathologically only in a minority of them. IgA deposits along the pulmonary capillary walls, analogous to those found in vessels of the skin and glomeruli of affected kidneys, are pathognomonic for HSP.

Secondary Vasculitis

Many of the rheumatologic diseases exhibit a secondary vasculitic process in the organs involved. Infectious processes, particularly those secondary to infection with *Aspergillus* and *Mucor* spp., invade vascular structures and produce secondary vasculitis. Certain drugs and chemicals can induce vasculitis. Other uncommon secondary vasculitic entities include benign lymphocytic angiitis and granulomatosis, bronchocentric granulomatosis, and necrotizing sarcoid angiitis.

ALVEOLAR HEMORRHAGE SYNDROMES

Diffuse hemorrhage into the alveolar spaces often is referred to as *diffuse alveolar hemorrhage (DAH) syndrome*. The clinical course of DAH is unpredictable: It may progress rapidly to respiratory failure, and it is always potentially life-threatening. Consequently, this entity should be considered in the differential diagnostic evaluation of any patient with alveolar infiltrates on chest radiograph. The symptoms of DAH are nonspecific.

Patients usually seek care because of dyspnea and cough, possibly associated with fever. Diffuse alveolar infiltrates on the chest radiograph constitute the initial diagnostic hallmark. Depending on the severity of the disease process at the time of evaluation, anemia and hypoxemia may be prominent. Hemoptysis is a common presenting manifestation of DAH but may be absent in up to one third of patients with DAH.

DAH can result from a variety of underlying or associated conditions that cause a disruption of the alveolar-capillary basement membrane integrity. Mechanisms leading to DAH include immunologic inflammatory conditions or agents causing immune complex deposition or capillaritis (e.g., anti-GBM disease or Goodpasture syndrome, SLE, ANCA-associated vasculitis), direct chemical or toxic injury (e.g., from toxic or chemical inhalation, abciximab use, all-*trans*-retinoic acid, trimellitic anhydride, or smoked crack cocaine), physical trauma (e.g., pulmonary contusion), and increased vascular pressure within the capillaries (e.g., mitral stenosis or severe left ventricular failure).

DAH is best confirmed by bronchoalveolar lavage (BAL). Progressively more bloody return fluid indicates alveolar origin of the blood; the presence of greater than 20% hemosiderin-laden macrophages among the total number of alveolar macrophages recovered by BAL is reported to indicate alveolar hemorrhage, even in the absence of ongoing active bleeding. Pulmonary alveolar hemorrhage is significantly associated with the following: thrombocytopenia (less than 50,000 cells/µL), other abnormal coagulation variables, renal failure (creatinine concentration of 2.5 mg/dL or greater), and a history of heavy smoking. The clinical approach to the patient presenting with DAH is aimed at rapid identification of the underlying cause and prompt implementation of appropriate therapy.

Exposure to inhalational toxins such as trimellitic anhydride or pyromellitic dianhydrate, drug abuse including crack cocaine abuse, and tobacco smoke should be identified. The past medical history also will uncover preexisting comorbid conditions, factors, and agents that can cause DAH, including mitral stenosis, coagulation disorders, recent bone marrow or hematopoetic stem cell transplantation, preexisting autoimmune disorders, and various therapeutic drugs. Similarly, the initial physical examination should include a careful search for signs of comorbidity and possible systemic autoimmune disorders.

Initial blood and urine testing should screen for other organ involvement, particularly kidney involvement (complete blood count, blood chemistry profile, urine analysis and microscopy), and determine the current coagulation status (activated partial prothrombin time [aPTT], international normalized ratio [INR]). Baseline markers of inflammation (erythrocyte sedimentation rate and C-reactive protein) are helpful to monitor subsequent responses to therapy. At the same time, specific serologic testing for potential underlying systemic disease processes should be initiated. This includes testing for ANCA, anti-GBM antibodies, antinuclear antibodies, anti–double-stranded DNA antibodies, rheumatoid factor, and antiphospholipid antibodies, as well as determination of complement and creatine kinase levels.

The decision to obtain a biopsy specimen needs to be considered carefully, weighing the risks of the biopsy procedure, the likelihood of obtaining a diagnostic piece of tissue, the likelihood of the biopsy findings to alter the therapeutic approach, and the risks associated with the chosen therapy.

The DAH syndromes can be broadly separated into those in which DAH is caused by or associated with pulmonary capillaritis and those in which pulmonary capillaritis is lacking (bland histologic pattern). Pulmonary capillaritis refers to the specific histopathologic finding of alveolar wall infiltration with inflammatory cells centered on capillary walls and small veins. The inflammatory cells are predominantly neutrophils, but eosinophils or monocytes also may be encountered. Capillaritis usually causes fibrinoid necrosis of alveolar and vessel walls and may culminate in the destruction of the underlying lung architecture. The interstitial infiltration by neutrophils seen in the context of capillaritis needs to be distinguished from the predominant intraalveolar neutrophilic infiltration commonly associated with active infections. Another hallmark of capillaritis is the presence of pyknotic cells and nuclear fragments from neutrophils undergoing apoptosis. This feature, referred to as leukocytoclasis, allows the distinction of true capillaritis from neutrophil margination related to surgical trauma, which can simulate capillaritis.

Most of the syndromes associated with pulmonary capillaritis leading to DAH have been discussed earlier in the chapter. A few unique syndromes or conditions that also may be associated with DAH are described next.

ANTI–GLOMERULAR BASEMENT MEMBRANE ANTIBODY DISEASE (GOODPASTURE SYNDROME)

Anti–glomerular basement membrane antibody (anti-GBM) disease, or Goodpasture syndrome, is a rare autoimmune disease characterized by the presence of autoantibodies directed against the NC1-domain of the alpha-3 chain of basement membrane collagen type IV. This epitope is accessible only to autoantibodies in the basement membranes of kidneys and lungs. DAH occurs in about half of the patients with anti-GBM disease. An additional inhalational injury, particularly smoking, is thought to be required for development of the pulmonary manifestation of this disease. Isolated alveolar hemorrhage in the absence of renal disease is rare in anti-GBM disease. Circulating autoantibodies to basement membrane are detectable in the serum, but the diagnosis of anti-GBM disease hinges on the histopathologic documentation of linear immunoglobulin G (IgG) deposits along the basement membranes in lung or kidney.

Anti-GBM disease is arguably not a vasculitis. Bland pulmonary hemorrhage is the most frequently described histopathologic pattern in DAH associated with anti-GBM disease. Capillaritis occurring as a secondary histopathologic feature, however, has been encountered in some patients. Early implementation of immunosuppressive therapy in conjunction with plasma exchange is the key to a favorable outcome in patients with anti-GBM disease. The pulmonary outcome with anti-GBM disease generally is favorable, but chronic renal failure is common.

VASCULITIDES CAUSING DIFFUSE ALVEOLAR HEMORRHAGE

The various primary vasculitis syndromes that may cause DAH have already been discussed in detail. Worth reiterating here is that the most common cause of the pulmonary-renal syndrome defined as DAH with glomerulonephritis is ANCA-associated vasculitis, either GPA or MPA. By contrast, DAH is rare in the context of EGPA.

SYSTEMIC LUPUS ERYTHEMATOSUS AND OTHER COLLAGEN VASCULAR DISORDERS

The disease manifestations of SLE are highly variable. Pulmonary capillaritis leading to diffuse DAH is rare in SLE, but usually a severe complication of the disease. Direct immunofluorescence microscopy reveals prominent immune complex deposits in the affected tissue of patients with SLE including the lungs. Hence, the development of pulmonary capillaritis in SLE is thought to be immune complex–mediated.

The onset of DAH in patients with SLE usually is abrupt, and it is seldom the first sign of the disease. In the overwhelming majority of patients, the rapid development of pulmonary infiltrates is associated with fever. Hemoptysis may be absent in up to half of the patients. Consequently, the differentiation of DAH from infection may be difficult in SLE and may require diagnostic BAL. Mechanical ventilation, infection, and CYC therapy were identified by univariate analysis as negative prognostic factors in one cohort of patients. The reported mortality rate for DAH in patients with SLE ranges from zero to 90%.

Treatment consists of glucocorticoids and CYC. The use of plasma exchange has been suggested, but its benefit remains unproved.

In all other types of collagen vascular disease or connective tissue disorders, respiratory complications are very common. Pulmonary capillaritis manifesting as DAH is rare, however. Isolated cases have been reported with polymyositis, rheumatoid arthritis, and mixed connective tissue disease. Consequently, serologic testing performed as part of an evaluation of DAH should include studies aimed at the identification of these potential underlying disease entities.

ANTIPHOSPHOLIPID SYNDROME

Antiphospholipid syndrome (APS) is defined by arterial and venous thromboses, or recurrent miscarriages occurring in patients with antiphospholipid antibodies (anticardiolipin antibodies, lupus anticoagulant, or both). If APS occurs in the context of another autoimmune disease, malignancy, or drug exposure, it is labeled *secondary* APS. In the absence of other coexisting disorders, it is considered *primary*. Hypercoagulability can cause pulmonary embolism and infarction, pulmonary microthrombosis, and pulmonary arterial thrombosis with secondary pulmonary hypertension as a consequence. Of note, however, primary pulmonary hypertension and acute respiratory distress syndrome (ARDS) also have been reported as complications of APS.

Diffuse DAH is rare in APS. The clinical presentation is nonspecific and consists of cough, dyspnea, fever, and bilateral pulmonary infiltrates. DAH also can occur in the context of ARDS, and hemoptysis is absent in more than half of the reported patients with APS and DAH. Therefore, early BAL may help in the differential diagnosis. Tissue necrosis from microthrombosis as well as pulmonary capillaritis has been implicated as a cause of DAH in APS. As in SLE, the capillaritis of APS is immune complex–mediated. Most patients respond to glucocorticoids. Yet the coexistence of thrombosis and capillaritis with DAH represents a therapeutic dilemma, in that anticoagulation may need to be interrupted to control the hemorrhage. Early plasma exchange in addition to immunosuppressive therapy should be considered in patients with APS and DAH.

MITRAL VALVE DISEASE

DAH is a well-known feature of mitral stenosis, even though the possibility is rarely considered in clinical practice. Severe mitral insufficiency also can produce alveolar hemorrhage. Hemoptysis can be the presenting feature. It may be caused by the rupture of dilated and varicose bronchial veins early in the course of mitral stenosis or may be a result of the stress failure of pulmonary capillaries. In patients in whom the valvular problem is not corrected surgically, recurrent episodes of DAH may lead to chronic hemosiderosis of the lungs, fibrosis, and punctate calcification or ossification of the lung parenchyma.

IDIOPATHIC PULMONARY HEMOSIDEROSIS

Idiopathic pulmonary hemosiderosis (IPH) is a rare disorder of unknown cause. It is a diagnosis of exclusion. Many such cases reported before the discovery of ANCA probably represented ANCA-associated vasculitis. Most cases of IPH diagnosed today probably are associated with gluten-sensitive sprue (celiac disease). The combination of alveolar hemorrhage and celiac disease also has been called *Lane-Hamilton syndrome.*

In contrast with DAH of other etiology, the DAH of IPH may be subtle and not necessarily associated with hemoptysis. Iron deficiency anemia is a clinical hallmark of IPH. It is thought to be caused by malabsorption of iron in the gastrointestinal tract, rather than recurrent lung hemorrhage. IPH can occur in children or young adults. Patients suspected of having IPH should be tested for antigliadin antibodies, especially because gastrointestinal symptoms may be absent or very subtle. Most patients with IPH attributable to celiac disease respond to a gluten-free diet and do not need immunosuppressive therapy. Repeated DAH in IPH has been reported to progress to lung fibrosis; early appropriate therapy may prevent this outcome.

TOXIC ALVEOLAR HEMORRHAGE

DAH can result from toxic fume inhalation or from blood-borne toxins. Fumes or dust of trimellitic anhydride (a component of certain plastics, paints, and epoxy resins) cause acute rhinitis and asthmatic symptoms if exposure is minor; with greater exposure, alveolar hemorrhage occurs. The trimellitic anhydride–associated hemoptysis-anemia syndrome occurs after "high-dose exposure" to fumes. Isocyanates have caused lung hemorrhage. Illicit drug use, particularly crack cocaine inhalation has also been linked to DAH.

Many medications have been associated with the development of DAH. These include drugs with antiplatelet or anticoagulant effects, including abciximab; immunosuppressive and chemotherapeutic agents, including D-penicillamine, sirolimus, and all-*trans*-retinoic acid; antithyroid drugs such as propylthiouracil; and epoprostenol given by continuous intravenous infusion for primary pulmonary hypertension.

ALVEOLAR HEMORRHAGE AFTER BONE MARROW TRANSPLANTATION

DAH occurs in both allogeneic and autologous hematopoietic stem cell transplantation recipients—specifically those undergoing bone marrow transplantation (BMT)—usually during the first 30 days, with most episodes occurring around day 12 after BMT. Recipients of autologous marrow transplants are at higher risk than recipients of allogeneic marrow transplants. DAH and

diffuse alveolar damage are the two major complications after BMT. The overall incidence of diffuse alveolar damage is 5% to 7%. An autopsy series has found DAH in 24% of recipients of bone marrow transplants. Risk factors for the development of DAH include intensive conditioning chemotherapy and older age (older than 40 years).

Post-BMT alveolar hemorrhage is a form of noninfectious pneumonitis characterized by sudden onset of dyspnea, non-productive cough, fever, and hypoxemia. Hemoptysis is rare, and its absence may lead to incorrect diagnosis. Many cases are identified only at autopsy. The clinical presentation is nonspecific. Chest imaging shows diffuse but patchy alveolar densities with central predominance of distribution. Lung biopsy is rarely indicated. BAL is important to detect DAH and to exclude infections. DAH is a potentially fatal respiratory complication, with a reported mortality rate in excess of 50%. Data that support use of high-dose parenteral glucocorticoids for BMT-associated DAH as beneficial therapy are not convincing, yet it remains standard practice in this setting.

MISCELLANEOUS CAUSES OF ALVEOLAR HEMORRHAGE

The following rare disease entities also can occasionally manifest with alveolar hemorrhage and therefore should be considered in the differential diagnosis: pulmonary lymphangioleiomyomatosis, pulmonary venoocclusive disease, pulmonary capillary hemangiomatosis, and tumor emboli.

SUGGESTED READINGS

Cartin-Ceba R, Fervenza FC, Specks U: Treatment of antineutrophil cytoplasmic antibody-associated vasculitis with rituximab, *Curr Opin Rheumatol* 24:15–23, 2012.

De Groot K, Harper L, Jayne DR, et al: Pulse versus daily oral cyclophosphamide for induction of remission in antineutrophil cytoplasmic antibody–associated vasculitis: a randomized trial, *Ann Intern Med* 150:670, 2009.

Jayne D, Rasmussen N, Andrassy K, et al: A randomized trial of maintenance therapy for vasculitis associated with antineutrophil cytoplasmic autoantibodies, *N Engl J Med* 349:36, 2003.

Jayne DR, Gaskin G, Rasmussen N, et al: Randomized trial of plasma exchange or high-dosage methylprednisolone as adjunctive therapy for severe renal vasculitis, *J Am Soc Nephrol* 18:2180, 2007.

Keogh KA, Specks U: Churg-Strauss syndrome. Clinical presentation, antineutrophil cytoplasmic antibodies, and leukotriene receptor antagonists, *Am J Med* 115:284, 2003.

Lee AS, Specks U: Pulmonary capillaritis, *Semin Respir Crit Care Med* 25:547, 2004.

Polychronopoulos VS, Prakash UB, Golbin JM, et al: Airway involvement in Wegener's granulomatosis, *Rheum Dis Clin North Am* 33:755, 2007.

Sinico RA, Di Toma L, Maggiore U, et al: Prevalence and clinical significance of antineutrophil cytoplasmic antibodies in Churg-Strauss syndrome, *Arthritis Rheum* 52:2926, 2005.

Specks U: Methotrexate for Wegener's granulomatosis: what is the evidence? *Arthritis Rheum* 52:2237, 2005.

Stone JH, Merkel PA, Spiera R, et al: Rituximab versus cyclophosphamide for ANCA-associated vasculitis, *N Engl J Med* 363:221, 2010.

Chapter **60**
Obstructive Sleep Apnea: Epidemiology, Risk Factors, and Pathophysiology

Ferrán Barbé Illa • Miguel Ángel Martínez-García

Obstructive sleep apnea (OSA) is a disorder characterized by repetitive collapse of the upper airway during sleep, resulting in changes in ventilation and intermittent hypoxemia and arousals, which may result in diurnal sleepiness and may lead to cognitive impairment and cardiovascular morbidity. The OSA syndrome is defined on the basis of recognition of symptoms (especially daytime sleepiness) and the objective measurement of disordered breathing during sleep.

EPIDEMIOLOGY

Although obstructive sleep apnea clearly is a common disorder within the general population, its incidence is hard to establish, because methodologic differences among the various epidemiologic studies have made comparisons difficult. First, different tests have been used to diagnose OSA. Overnight polysomnography (PSG) is considered the "gold standard" diagnostic modality, but assessments have been made using other tests instead, such as unattended in-home PSG or respiratory polygraphy, pulse oximetry, and even clinical questionnaires (see Chapter 61). Second, variability in the definitions of different respiratory events (especially hypopnea) and the apnea-hypopnea index (AHI) cutoff value that defines OSA, or clinically significant OSA, is well recognized. In this sense, the chosen oxyhemoglobin desaturation threshold, typically 3% or 4%, used to define hypopnea can lead to different AHI scores; accordingly, estimates of disease severity will vary. Third, differences in sampling of populations (for example, the percentages of elderly and female subjects included) have been noted. Fourth, disparities in signal processing and a lack of standardization in the quantification of airflow (including thermistor, inductance plethysmography, and nasal cannula–pressure transduction) are common. Finally, the quality of validation of equipment and the conclusions of some studies have been questioned because of methodologic limitations such as small sample sizes or inadequate controls for potential confounding variables.

Apart from these differences, epidemiologic studies have focused on two levels of abnormal sleep quantification: OSA, when defined physiologically as increased obstructive breathing events (apneas or hypopneas) during sleep, usually with an AHI of 5 or more events/hour; and the clinical syndrome (the combination of an AHI of 5 or more events/hour and significant self-reported symptoms, especially daytime sleepiness). The real prevalence of OSA probably is underestimated, because a majority of studies used subjective sleepiness as the sole self-reported symptom for definition, although OSA is well known to be associated with other negative outcomes, such as sleep disruption, deterioration of quality of life, cognitive impairment, or cardiovascular disease, which also should be included in the definition of the syndrome.

MIDDLE-AGED POPULATION

It is estimated that 24% of men and 9% of women have OSA, as defined by an AHI of 5 or greater, and that 15% of men and 5% of women between 30 and 60 years have an AHI of 10 or higher. With use of daytime sleepiness as a clinical syndrome, the prevalence ranges between 3% and 7% in men and 2% and 5% in women in the general population (**Box 60-1**). Until recently, population-based epidemiologic studies of OSA were available only for North America, Europe, and Australia. However, more recent studies undertaken in other countries, including China, India, and Korea, report similar prevalence rates. The overall incidence of moderate to severe OSA (defined by an AHI of 15 or higher) occurring over a 5-year period is 11% and 5% in men and in women, respectively, which persists even after adjustment for confounding variables. This means that, even in the absence of any weight change, approximately 20% of men and 10% of women will develop moderate to severe OSA in that period of time.

Most population-based studies have found a two- to threefold higher prevalence of OSA in males than in females. The ratio is even higher for men treated in sleep centers, with reported ratios between 4 : 1 and 8 : 1 or higher. This higher ratio may be the result of multiple factors: Women do not show the "classic" OSA symptomatology—they typically have more comorbid illnesses, use more psychoactive drugs in the absence of a correct diagnosis, and often present with vague, nonspecific symptoms, which widens the differential diagnosis and leads to a higher level of underdiagnosis or misdiagnosis of OSA. An important finding from epidemiologic studies is that gender disparities in prevalence seem to decrease with age, and when women reach postmenopausal status (and are not receiving hormonal replacement treatment), incidence rates for men and women become similar. **Table 60-1** summarizes the most important sleep apnea prevalence studies in middle-aged populations.

ELDERLY POPULATION

The prevalence of OSA in adults increases with age as a result of greater collapsibility of the upper airway and probably reaches a plateau after the age of 65. It is estimated that 65%

Table 60-1 Summary of Middle-Aged Population-Based Studies on Prevalence of Obstructive Sleep Apnea (OSA) and OSA Syndrome (OSAS) in Adults

Study	Country	Age Range (yr)	Sample Size (Gender)	Ethnicity	Diagnostic Method	Criteria	OSA Prevalence	OSAS Prevalence (AHI Cutoff)
Bearpark et al, 1995	Australia	40-65	485 (M)	White	RP	IAH ≥5 IAH ≥10	26% M 10% M	3.1% M (AHI ≥5)
Bixler et al, 2001	United States	20-100	1741 (M+F)	White	PSG	IAH ≥5 IAH ≥10 IAH ≥15	17.7% M, 5% F 10.5% M 7% M, 2% F	3.3% M, 1.2% F (AHI ≥10)
Ip et al, 2001	China	30-60	258 (M+F)	Chinese	PSG	IAH ≥5 IAH ≥15	18.8% M, 3.7% F 5.3% M, 1.2% F	4.1% M, 2.1% F
Durán et al, 2001	Spain	30-70	997 (M+F)	White	PSG (N = 555) RP (N = 442)	IAH ≥5 IAH ≥10 IAH ≥15 IAH ≥20 IAH ≥30	26.2% M, 28% F 19% M, 14.9% F 14.2% M, 8.6% F 9.6% M, 6% F 6.8% M, 4.3% F	3.4% M, 3% F (AHI ≥10)
Kim et al, 2004	Korea	40-69	457 (M+F)	Korean	PSG	IAH ≥5 IAH ≥10 IAH ≥15	27.1% M, 16.8% F 18.9% M, 6.7% F 10.1% M, 4.7% F	4.5% M, 3.2% F (AHI ≥5)
Udwadia et al, 2004	India	35-65	250 (M)	Indian	PSG	IAH ≥5 IAH ≥10 IAH ≥15	19.5% M 11.1% M 8.4% M	7.5%M (AHI ≥5)
Nakayama-Ashida et al, 2008	Japan	23-59	332 (M)	Japanese	RP	IAH ≥5 IAH ≥15	37.4% M 15.7% M	17.6% (AHI ≥5)

AHI, Apnea-hypopnea index; *F*, female; *M*, male; *OSAS*, obstructive sleep apnea syndrome (apnea-hypopnea index cutoff plus symptoms); *PSG*, polysomnography; *RP*, respiratory polygraphy.

Data from Bearpark H, Elliott L, Grunstein R, et al: Snoring and sleep apnea. A population study in Australian men, *Am Respir J Crit Care Med* 1995; 151:1459-1465, 1995; Bixler EO, Vgontzas AN, Lin HM, et al: Prevalence of sleep-disordered breathing in women: effects of gender, *Am Respir J Crit Care Med* 163:608-613, 2001; Ip MS, Lam B, Lauder IJ, et al: A community study of sleep-disordered breathing in middle-aged Chinese men in Hong Kong, *Chest* 119:62-69, 2001; Durán J, Esnaola S, Rubio R, et al: Obstructive sleep apnea-hypopnea and related clinical features in a population-based sample of subjects aged 30 to 70 yr, *Am Respir J Crit Care Med* 163:685-689, 2001; Kim J, In K, Kim J, et al: Prevalence of sleep-disordered breathing in middle-aged Korean men and women, *Am Respir J Crit Care Med* 170:1108-1113, 2004; Udwadia ZF, Doshi V, Lonkar SG, et al: Prevalence of sleep-disordered breathing and sleep apnea in middle-aged urban Indian men, *Am Respir J Crit Care Med* 169:168-173, 2004; Nakayama-Ashida Y, Takegami M, Chin K, et al: Sleep-disordered breathing in the usual lifestyle setting as detected with home monitoring in a population of working men in Japan, *Sleep* 31:419-425, 2008.

Box 60-1 Epidemiologic Features of Obstructive Sleep Apnea (OSA)

- 24% of men and 9% of women have OSA.
- 3% to 7% men and 2% to 5% women have OSA syndrome.
- 65% of older men and 56% of older women have OSA.
- 20% of older men and 15% of older women have OSA syndrome.
- In postmenopausal status, women reach similar incidence rates of OSA than men.
- The overall 5-year incidence of moderate to severe OSA ranges between 5% and 11%.
- Referral to sleep centers for further investigation is four- to eight times more frequent in men than in women.

of older men and 56% of older women between 65 and 95 have OSA as defined by AHI of 10 or greater, and 26% of men and 21% of women between 71 and 100 years have an AHI of 30 or greater. Finally, 20% of older men and 15% of older women have the OSA syndrome (AHI of 10 or higher plus daytime hypersomnia). With age comes an increase in the frequency of both obstructive and central respiratory events. The main problem is to identify the AHI cutoff point that marks the limit of a physiologic and abnormal increase, in order to determine the real prevalence of clinically relevant OSA in the elderly population. In this sense, some investigators state that OSA represents different and distinct clinical entities in middle-aged

adults and in older adults, based on morbidity and mortality data, although this position is controversial. Perhaps there is a more complex model of OSA that varies with the patient's age.

In any case, the two proposed types of OSA consist of (1) a pathologic form of OSA that appears in middle age in those patients who usually are diagnosed in sleep laboratories and (2) OSA that appears after the age of 60 years, with some overlap between the two, mainly caused by physiologic changes (increase in pharyngeal collapsibility) associated with aging, and of less clinical importance. Data also suggest that the interaction between body weight and OSA in elderly persons may be different from that in younger adults. Because of the population-wide increase in longevity, the proportion of elderly persons being treated at sleep units also is increasing; currently one in four sleep studies are performed in patients older than 65 years of age. This scenario will present a scientific challenge in the future, in view of the lack of scientific evidence available on OSA in the elderly. **Table 60-2** summarizes the most important epidemiologic studies describing the prevalence of OSA in older people.

RISK FACTORS FOR OBSTRUCTIVE SLEEP APNEA

Obesity, aging, and male gender are the main risk factors for the development of OSA. It has been estimated that approximately 30% to 40% of AHI variance can be explained by genetic factors. Other risk factors have been proposed,

Table 60-2 Summary of Important Studies on Prevalence of Obstructive Sleep Apnea in Older People

Study	No. of Subjects	Age Range or Mean (SD)	Population	AHI ≥5	AHI ≥10	AHI ≥20
Ancoli-Israel et al, 1991	385	65-95	Community	81%	70% M, 56% F	51% M, 39% F
Bixler et al, 1998	75	65-100	Community	24.8%	23.9%	13.3%
Durán et al, 2001	428	71-100	Community	81% M, 79% F	67% M, 62% F	44% M, 37% F
Young et al, 2002	3448	60-99	Community	54%	20%	
Haas et al, 2005	3643	70.2 (6.9)	Community	46%	36%	

F, female; M, male; SD, standard deviation.
Data from Ancoli-Israel S, Kripke DF, Klauber MR, et al: Sleep-disordered breathing in community-dwelling elderly, *Sleep* 14:486-495, 1991; Bixler EO, Vgontzas AN, Ten Have T, et al: Effects of age on sleep apnea in men: I. Prevalence and severity, *Am Respir J Crit Care Med* 157:144-148, 1998; Durán J, et al. WFSRS. World Conference Sleep Odyssey 2001. Punta del Este. Uruguay, 2001; Young T, Shahar E, Nieto FJ, et al: Predictors of sleep-disordered breathing in community-dwelling adults: the Sleep Heart Health Study, *Arch Intern Med* 162:893-900, 2002; Haas DC, Foster GL, Nieto FJ, et al: Age-dependent associations between sleep-disordered breathing and hypertension: importance of discriminating between systolic/diastolic hypertension and isolated systolic hypertension in the Sleep Heart Health Study, *Circulation* 111:614-621, 2005.

related to increased anatomic or physiologic upper airway collapsibility.

OBESITY

According to recent estimates, 60% of adults in industrialized nations are overweight (body mass index [BMI] of 25 kg/m^2 or higher) and at least 15% are obese (BMI of 30 kg/m^2 or higher). Obesity is a common clinical finding and is present in more than 60% of patients referred for diagnostic sleep evaluations. Twin studies have shown that up to 70% of the variance in obesity within a population may be attributable to genetic factors. Although candidate genes for obesity are numerous, only a few single-gene mutations causally related to obesity have been convincingly detected, including the leptin receptor gene, the leptin gene, the pro-opiomelanocortin gene, the pro-hormone convertase 1 gene, and the melanocortin MC4 receptor gene, but very few studies on candidate genes associated with weight loss or weight gain have been performed, and no work in this area has been carried out specifically in the OSA population.

The prevalence of OSA in obese subjects is as high as 45%. Obesity explains 30% to 50% of the variance in AHI and is the only variable that can be modified. Several researchers have speculated that obesity and OSA may share a common genotype, and linkage analysis identified candidate regions at least on chromosomal arms 2p and 19p, but further studies are needed to confirm these results. Some major epidemiologic studies from around the world have consistently identified body weight as the strongest risk factor for OSA and have demonstrated a positive correlation between changes in OSA incidence and changes in weight over time. The Wisconsin Sleep Cohort showed that an increase of one standard deviation in BMI was associated with a four-fold increase in the prevalence of OSA. The longitudinal analysis component of the same study demonstrated that OSA severity changed approximately 3% for every 1% change in weight over a 4-year period. The Sleep Heart Health Study found that the change in AHI with weight changes over a 5-year period was more pronounced in men, and that the change was greater when associated with a weight increase than with a weight decrease. Corroborating this strong association, some studies have shown that dietary or surgical weight loss leads to reduced OSA severity in many patients and that OSA can even be completely cured in some cases. In other words, patients with mild OSA who gain 10%

of their baseline weight are at a six-fold increased risk for progression of OSA, and an equivalent weight loss can result in a more than 20% improvement with respect to OSA severity.

Whether OSA predisposes affected persons to the preferential accumulation of visceral fat remains to be determined. More evidence is necessary to determine which specific measure of peripheral or central fat distribution is less compromising for OSA. Some investigators have shown that neck circumference, waist circumference, and BMI are independently associated with OSA severity at all ages, although it seems that neck size is the strongest predictor of sleep-disordered breathing, indicating that upper body obesity (fat deposition around the upper airway or fat deposited in the parapharyngeal fat pads), rather than a more generalized distribution of body fat, is important for the development of OSA. In any case, it is advisable to obtain information from all three measures in clinical practice.

The fundamental mechanisms by which obesity leads to an increase in the number of respiratory events during sleep, and weight loss decreases them, are unknown. It has been postulated that fat deposits surrounding the airway play a role in increasing the critical closing pressure. Other potential contributing factors include the reduction of functional residual capacity, ventilatory control system instability, alterations in neural compensatory mechanisms that maintain airway patency, and functional impairment of the upper airway muscles. Obesity also reduces chest wall compliance and increases whole-body oxygen demand, again predisposing affected persons to development of OSA. The degree to which common conditions associated with obesity, such as diabetes, may cause vascular or neuropathic damage to the dilator pharyngeal muscles and reduced upper airway sensation remains to be fully elucidated.

AGING

Aging in itself is associated with numerous physiologic changes, one of them being an increase in upper airway collapsibility, leading to a higher prevalence of OSA. The critical closing pressure of the upper airway in older people is −8.3 ± 2.3 cm H$_2$O, whereas in middle-aged people it is −16 ± 6.9 cm H$_2$O, independent of BMI. This difference may be due to various factors: an age-related decrease in the genioglossus response, an increase in airflow resistance, a decrease in upper airway dilation reflex mechanisms, reduced response to the stimulus of hypoxia, changes in the bony structure surrounding the pharynx, descent of the hyoid bone, increase in soft palate length, or an increase in pharyngeal fat pads. All of these changes lead to a generalized age-related decrease in the size of the upper airway lumen, specifically in men, and a consequent increase in airflow resistance. Age also is associated with an increased incidence of comorbid conditions, postmenopausal hormone status in women, dental disorders, decreased quality of sleep, and intake of psychoactive drugs. All of these factors may increase upper airway collapsibility. Finally, an additional factor that may predispose older persons to development of OSA is the aging-related increase in arousal frequency. Arousals from sleep lead to hyperventilation and relative hypocapnia, which in turn can promote respiratory instability and periodic breathing during subsequent periods of sleep onset.

MALE GENDER

It is not known which mechanisms explain the finding that OSA risk is twice as high in men as in women. Some studies have implicated several factors. First, men have increased fat deposition around the upper airways walls. Although data suggest that, in percentage terms, more women (33.4%) than men (27.5%) have a BMI ≥30 kg/m², magnetic resonance imaging (MRI) studies have shown a decreased proportion of pharyngeal fat and soft tissue volume in the neck of obese women in comparison with obese men. Women in general have lower Mallampati scores, suggesting that the fat does not play as large a role in the female tongue as it does in the male tongue. Second, the upper airway in men is more prone to collapse as a result of its greater overall length with a longer vulnerable segment. Third, PSG characteristics of sleep and breathing patterns differ between women and men. Women tend to have a lower AHI in non–rapid eye movement (REM) sleep but have a similar AHI in REM sleep. Moreover, disordered-breathing events in women are of shorter duration and are associated with less oxyhemoglobin desaturation than in men. Finally, several mechanisms have been proposed to explain how male- or female-specific hormones would affect the propensity to develop OSA. One hypothesis is that the different hormones affect the distribution of body fat. Android body fat distribution (in the upper body and trunk) increases with both age and years after onset of menopause, which is a risk factor for the development of OSA. Hormone levels also have been hypothesized to affect central and neural respiratory control mechanisms. In this sense, progesterone has been shown to be a respiratory stimulant, which might protect premenopausal women from OSA; moreover, combined estrogen-progesterone treatment leads to a decrease in the number of apneic and hypopneic episodes during sleep. On the other hand, lower levels of testosterone may be protective against the development of OSA in women. Some researchers have shown that exogenous androgen therapy in men and women can aggravate OSA severity. It is possible that differing levels of hormones, starting from puberty and further modified by later maturational changes, can affect the development of OSA.

GENETIC PREDISPOSITION

Several studies have confirmed the role of inheritance and familial factors in the genesis of OSA. First-degree relatives of persons with the disorder are more likely to be at risk than first-degree relatives of unaffected persons. Genetic factors explain more than 30% to 40% of the variance in disease

severity, although confounding factors must be taken into account. Some OSA risk factors have a demonstrated genetic basis, such as craniofacial morphology, the volume of the lateral parapharyngeal walls, tongue form, total volume of soft tissue structures, abnormalities in breathing control, and finally, genetic determinants of obesity.

Recently, Larkin and associates conducted the first candidate gene study of OSA. More than 1500 single-nucleotide polymorphisms (SNPs) were genotyped, covering 53 genes representing intermediate disease pathways implicated in the disorder. These workers identified significant associations between sleep-disordered breathing and genetic variants of C-reactive protein, glial cell–derived growth factor, and serotonin 2A receptor genes independently of BMI. These results highlight the potential role of genetic analysis to better describe the different phenotypes of OSA, the risk of inheritance of each type, and its relationship with other diseases.

OTHER PREDISPOSING FACTORS

Box 60-2 shows other predisposing factors that have been associated with increased risk for OSA. Their mechanisms of action are multiple: anatomic variability (e.g., craniofacial malformations), increased airway inflammation (smoking or infections), physiologic factors (sleep position, REM sleep, pregnancy, or ethnicity-related predilection), and depression of dilator pharyngeal muscle function (alcohol consumption, benzodiazepine or sedative use, stroke, and other comorbid conditions).

Although Asians are less obese than whites, disease prevalence in the East is not less than in the West. For a given age, sex, and BMI, however, Asians demonstrate greater disease severity than whites, which can be explained by differences in craniofacial features (persons of Asian ethnicity have a shorter

---

Box 60-2 **Common Risk or Predisposing Factors for Obstructive Sleep Apnea**

Major Factors
Obesity
Male gender
Elderly

Other Factors
Craniofacial abnormalities
    Retrognathia/micrognathia
    Tonsillar hypertrophy (infants)
    Enlarged tongue or soft palate
    Short neck
    Nasal obstruction
Race
Genetic predisposition
Smoking habit
Upper airway inflammation or infection
Alcohol consumption
Medical comorbid conditions
    Stroke
    Hypothyroidism
    Chronic renal insufficiency
    Polycystic ovary syndrome
Pregnancy
Menopausal status
REM phase of sleep
Benzodiazepine use or other psychoactive drug intake
Sleep position

REM, rapid eye movement.

cranial base and a more acute cranial base flexure). On the other hand, also in comparison with whites, African Americans show a greater role for soft tissue factors in susceptibility to OSA. The epidemiologic studies related to racial predisposition to OSA have to be interpreted carefully. Confounding variables, such as comorbid conditions, differing socioeconomic status, and health care disadvantages, could explain the differences in OSA prevalence between races, indicating that race may be a surrogate variable for other predisposing factors.

On the other hand, some epidemiologic studies show that both active smoking and second-hand smoke exposure have been independently associated with habitual snoring and even with an increase in OSA prevalence in some subjects, especially in active smokers. It seems that the inflammation and alteration of some mechanical and neural protective properties of the airway due to cigarette smoke increase the collapsibility of the upper airway. Alcohol intake also can promote pharyngeal collapse, even in normal persons, inducing apneic activity and prolonging apnea duration, probably by reducing respiratory motor output to the upper airway, resulting in hypotonia of the pharyngeal muscles.

The frequency and duration of OSA events and the extent of associated desaturation may increase in the supine compared with the side-lying sleep position. Positional OSA is defined as a supine-measured AHI at least double that measured in the lateral position. The prevalence of positional OSA varies in relation to OSA severity. It was recently identified in 50% of mild, 19% of moderate, and 6.5% of severe OSA cases. The main mechanism has been suggested to involve the effects of gravity on the upper airway size through displacement of the soft tissues, by mandibular retropulsion, and indirectly, by upward displacement of abdominal contents, thereby reducing lung volume and compromising airway cross-sectional area or length. Other studies have shown that one of the main mechanisms is change in the shape of the airway from a transversely oriented ellipse when the subject is supine to a more circular shape with assumption of the side-lying position.

Pregnancy also is associated with a higher prevalence of OSA, particularly in the third trimester. Many changes occur in the respiratory system during pregnancy. Factors recognized to contribute to this phenomenon include elevation of the diaphragm secondary to an enlarged uterus, leading to alterations in pulmonary mechanics including reduced functional residual capacity; an increase in Mallampati score secondary to fluid retention and edema; enlargement of neck circumference; reduced nasal patency; changes in hormonal concentrations (estrogen and progesterone); and weight gain. OSA is an important diagnosis to consider in symptomatic pregnant women, especially in view of possible adverse side effects including pregnancy-induced hypertension and intrauterine growth retardation.

PATHOPHYSIOLOGY

OSA is characterized by repetitive collapse of the upper airway during sleep. The most frequent mechanism of collapse is that in which gravity pulls the tongue toward the back wall of the pharynx in a person who has assumed the supine position. Airway resistance increases during collapse, resulting in increased ventilatory effort, intrathoracic pressure swings, and disruption of sleep (arousals). The activation of the upper airway dilator muscles during arousals causes reopening of the airway and restores ventilation (**Figure 60-1**).

UPPER AIRWAY IN NORMAL SUBJECTS

It has long been recognized that, for what on casual consideration may appear to be a simple tube, the human upper airway is deceptively and enigmatically complex, performing functional tasks such as swallowing and the passage of air for breathing and speech, governed by anatomy and neural controls. Under normal physiologic conditions, the pharynx remains open at all times, except during short closures associated with swallowing, regurgitation, and speech. It is separated into three regions: the *nasopharynx*, extending from the nasal turbinates to the hard palate; the *oropharynx*, composed of the retropalatal region (from the hard palate to the caudal margin of the soft palate) and the retroglossal region (from the caudal margin of the soft palate to the base of the epiglottis); and the *hypopharynx*, extending from the base of the tongue to the larynx. It is composed of more than 20 muscles and soft tissues without rigid or bony support. Pharyngeal muscles can be divided into

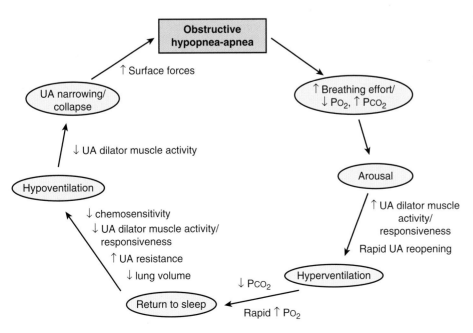

Figure 60-1 Typical pathophysiologic sequence in obstructive sleep apnea. *(From Eckert DJ, Malhotra A: Pathophysiology of adult obstructive sleep apnea, Proc Am Thorac Soc 5:144-153, 2008.)*

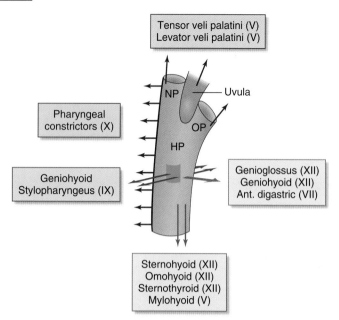

Figure 60-2 Action of upper airway muscles. *Ant.*, anterior, *HP*, hypopharynx; *NP*, nasopharynx; *OP*, oropharynx.

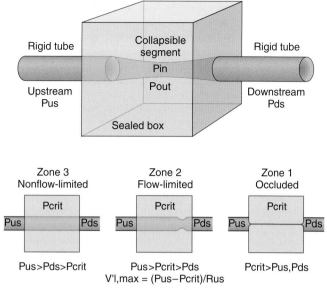

Figure 60-3 Starling resistor model of obstructive sleep apnea. *Pus*, upstream (nasal) segment intraluminal pressure; *Pds*, downstream (tracheal) segment intraluminal pressure; *Pin*, intraluminal pressure in the collapsible segment (pharynx); *Pout*, pressure surrounding collapsible segment; *Rus*, upstream (nasal) airflow resistance. *(From Dempsey JA, Veasey SC, Morgan BJ, O'Donnell CP: Pathophysiology of sleep apnea, Physiol Rev 90:47-112, 2010.)*

three groups: muscles controlling the position of the hyoid bone (geniohyoid and sternohyoid), muscles of the tongue (genioglossus), and palatal muscles (palatopharyngeus, tensor palatini, and levator palatini). The largest of the dilator pharyngeal muscles is the genioglossus, the muscle that forms the major portion of the body of the tongue (**Figure 60-2**).

Human speech requires pharyngeal mobility, such that the hyoid bone, which is a key anchoring site for pharyngeal muscles, is not firmly attached to the skeleton. Thus, the upper airway has rigid support in its proximal and distal segments but has a collapsible portion extending from the hard palate to the larynx, with the size of its lumen being subject to the influence of surrounding pressures and the activity of dilator muscles. Other well-known biologic examples of mobility in respiratory physiology include intrathoracic airway collapse on forced exhalation, collapse of pulmonary capillaries in the lung apex, and collapse of the alae nasi under high inspiratory flow rates.

One mechanistic physiologic representation of this collapsible model is the Starling resistor (**Figure 60-3**). According to this model, when air pressure is applied to the upper airway, the collapsible portion of the upper airway is bound by an upstream segment (nasal segment) and a downstream segment (tracheal segment). Nasal and tracheal segments have their corresponding intraluminal pressures and resistances. The nasal segment has atmospheric pressure at the airway opening. In the surrounding collapsible segment, pressure is generated by soft tissues and structures surrounding the pharynx. Occlusion of the collapsible portions occurs when the surrounding pressure (Pout) becomes greater than the intraluminal pressure (Pin) (transmural pressure [Pout – Pin] above 0).

The oropharynx represents the collapsible segment, the critical closing pressure (Pcrit) of which is defined as the pressure inside the airway at which airway collapse occurs. Flow is partially limited when nasal pressure is higher than Pcrit, Pcrit being higher than tracheal pressure, and total occlusion occurs when Pcrit is greater even than nasal pressure. Pcrit in the human upper airway is determined by lowering the nasal pressure until inspiratory airflow ceases. Its measurements have been shown to define a spectrum of upper airway obstruction ranging from normal breathing to total collapse (apnea),

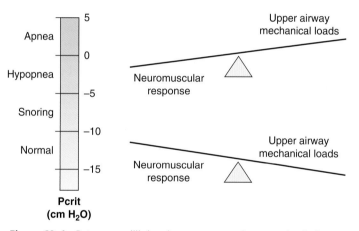

Figure 60-4 Patency equilibrium between upper airway mechanical load and neuromuscular response. *Pcrit*, critical closing pressure of collapsible segment of upper airways. *(Modified from Patil SP, Schneider H, Schwartz AR, Smith PL: Adult obstructive sleep apnea: pathophysiology and diagnosis, Chest 132:325-337, 2007.)*

depending on the equilibrium between mechanical upper airway loads that provoke collapse and neuromuscular dilator functions that maintain upper airway patency. In general, these measures when applied in sleeping or paralyzed humans have shown that passive Pcrit is below –10 cm H_2O in normal subjects with lower airway resistance and minimal CO_2 retention during non-REM sleep. In sleep-disordered breathing, however, it varies, with reported values of –10 to –5 cm H_2O in snorers, –5 to 0 cm H_2O in those with sufficiently high airway resistance to induce airflow limitation and transient hypopneas, and above 0 cm H_2O in patients with apneas associated with complete airway obstruction (**Figure 60-4**). Increases in airway resistance or hypercapnia provoke the activation of the muscle through neural control pathways composed of pressure receptors, sleep-wake brain centers, chemoreceptors, and respiratory centers.

Box 60-3	Factors Contributing to Upper Airway Collapse in Obstructive Sleep Apnea

- Reduction in upper airway caliber by anatomic factors
- Reduction in upper airway dilator muscle activity
- Ventilatory control instability
- Decrease in lung volume during sleep
- Premature arousals during a respiratory event
- Edema and rostral fluid shifts
- Increased surface tension
- Upper airway inflammation
- Increase in respiratory events during REM sleep
- Reduction in intraluminal pressure due to Bernoulli effect

REM, rapid eye movement.

UPPER AIRWAY IN PATIENTS WITH OBSTRUCTIVE SLEEP APNEA

During sleep, the ventilatory system is under automatic control. Even in normal subjects, airway resistance increases during sleep as a consequence of body position, decreased pharyngeal tone, depression of the respiratory drive, and depression of protective reflexes, leading to an increased probability of upper airway collapse. A number of factors contribute to the pathogenesis of OSA, including the activity of the dilated pharyngeal muscles during sleep, upper airway anatomy, lung volume, ventilatory control stability, sleep state stability, rostral fluid shifts, and others; all of these factors probably are mediated, at least in part, by genetic factors.

The primary site of collapse is in the retropalatal and oropharyngeal area in a majority of patients (up to 75%), with frequent caudal extension to the base of the tongue (25% to 44%) and, less often, to the hypopharynx (0 to 33%). The site of collapse depends on the equilibrium of functions exercised by the skeletal structure, soft tissue, and pharyngeal muscles. In obese patients, the most frequent area of collapse evidently is the velopharynx, whereas in nonobese patients, both the velopharynx and the oropharynx constitute the primary site of collapse. The extent of collapse varies by sleep stage, with caudal collapse being more extensive in REM sleep owing to changes in neuromuscular activation (**Box 60-3**).

PATHOGENESIS

ANATOMIC FACTORS

Anatomic factors include increased airway length, lateral wall thickness, tongue volume (macroglossia), skeletal structure (retrognathia or micrognathia), and nasal or pharyngeal abnormalities (nasal obstruction, polyps, or enlarged tonsils, adenoids, or uvula) and probably constitute the most important heritable determinants of OSA. Studies of cephalometric and computed tomography scans have demonstrated differences in the craniofacial structure of patients with OSA in comparison with that of normal subjects, including lower facial weight, reposition of both the maxilla and the mandible, and shorter and medially displaced mandibular rami, all of them correlated with decreased pharyngeal size. The role of enlarged soft tissues has been demonstrated using MRI (**Figure 60-5**). In patients with OSA, pharyngeal lumen is smaller than normal and tissues are narrowed laterally, rather than in the anteroposterior dimension, especially at the retropalatal level, mainly owing to increased thickness of the muscular pharyngeal wall as well as an increase in tongue and total soft tissue volume. The interaction between the bony and soft tissue structures determines upper airway collapsibility. Nevertheless, increased airway length has been observed in subjects with OSA and has been shown to correlate with severity, especially in men. Usually, the longer the upper airway, the greater the risk of collapse.

Data from early physiologic studies suggest that upper airway narrowing and consequent snoring and apnea can be induced by subatmospheric nasal pressure. In theory, inspiratory nasal obstruction would not provoke continuing collapse of the pharynx: With cessation of flow, upstream resistance becomes irrelevant, intrapharyngeal pressure returns to atmospheric, and the pharynx reopens—a cycle generating snoring but not apneas. It is unlikely, however, that the pharynx does behave as a perfect Starling resistor, partly because of hysteresis and partly as a result of surface tension forces from mucus, which will tend to hold the pharynx closed once collapsed. Various observational and cross-sectional studies have documented a relationship among chronic nasal obstruction, snoring, and OSA.

PHARYNGEAL MUSCLE ACTIVITY

Despite compromised anatomic dimensions of the upper airway, subjects with OSA show upper airway collapse only during sleep, because the upper airway musculature can maintain patency during the awake state but has a reduced ability to do so during sleep. This phenomenon is thought to be related to a reduction in upper airway dilator muscle activity, especially in the transition from wakefulness to sleep. Paradoxically, some studies have shown that during the awake state, genioglossus activity is increased in patients with OSA compared with normal subjects, probably because the drive of the upper airway muscles is increased to compensate for anatomic compromise. During sleep, however, the relative decrease in genioglossus activity is greater in patients with OSA than in control subjects. Various mechanisms may explain the reduction in dilator muscle activity seen in patients with OSA: alterations in the mechanoreceptor reflex related to negative intraluminal pressure; changes in the 5-hydroxytryptamine 2A receptor, which has been shown to be the predominant receptor subtype in hypoglossal motor neurons; altered upper airway neuromechanical function; or even an upper airway denervation neuropathy or muscle denervation. In OSA, upper airway neuromuscular compensatory mechanisms during sleep are attenuated compared with those in control subjects in studies using electromyograms and often fail to restore airway patency in the absence of arousals. Furthermore, impaired upper airway afferent neural function has been described, which could attenuate the transmission of information related to intraluminal pressure. This impairment has been observed in the mechanosensitivity receptor of the oropharynx and thermal sensitivity receptors and sensory receptors in the velopharynx and larynx in persons with OSA. Some of these afferent impairments have been associated with OSA severity.

All of these findings point to the presence of an upper airway neuropathy in OSA, probably due to mechanical trauma associated with snoring and apneas, oxidative stress related to hypoxia-reoxygenation, and inflammation resulting from both of these insults. One of these forms of neuropathies appears in the form of muscle denervation, including fiber type grouping, grouped atrophy, and increased fiber size variability. This airway muscle denervation presumably also may result from damage to brain stem motor neurons, as has been reported in a murine model of intermittent hypoxia.

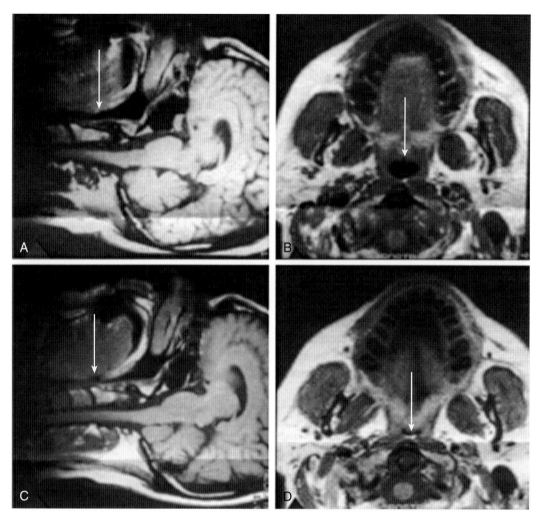

Figure 60-5 Magnetic resonance imaging study of cross-sectional and longitudinal upper airway lumen in a normal subject (*white arrows* in **A** and **B**) and in a patient with obstructive sleep apnea (*white arrows* in **C** and **D**). *(Courtesy J.L. Fernandez, MD.)*

On the other hand, another potential mechanism contributing to altered upper airway muscle function in OSA could be impaired contractile function. In patients with OSA , the upper airway muscle works under considerable load in adverse hypoxic conditions, which could generate some injuries and morphologic changes, increasing force but making the muscle more prone to fatigue. Histologic and biochemical studies have shown an increased proportion of fast-twitch type IIa fibers in the uvula and genioglossus and increased levels of enzymes associated with anaerobic metabolism in patients with OSA, leading to the maintenance of increased muscle contractility at the cost of increased fatigability. Moreover, other factors such as increased airway inflammation and secondary tissue changes could compromise contractile function and alter mechanical coupling of upper airway muscles.

Finally, considerable interest has emerged in the role of some neural pathways and neurotransmitters in the modulation of upper airway muscle activity. Animal studies have shown that the withdrawal of serotoninergic excitation reduces hypoglossal motor output (which drives the major upper airway dilator muscle, i.e., the genioglossus), although human studies using selective serotonin reuptake inhibitors showed only modest effects on OSA severity. Noradrenergic inputs to the hypoglossal motor pool contribute to both the tonic and the phasic components of genioglossus muscle activity in the awake state, and withdrawal of noradrenergic input accounts for some of the reduction in hypoglossal motor activity during non-REM sleep. Glutamatergic inputs seem to play a similar role. The two main inhibitory neurotransmitters in the central nervous system are glycine and gamma-aminobutyric acid (GABA). Stimulation of GABA or glycine receptors suppresses respiration-related genioglossus muscle activity, whereas antagonism of those receptors increases it.

VENTILATORY CONTROL STABILITY

Ventilatory control stability is believed to be an important contributor to OSA pathogenesis, because obstructive events tend to occur during periods of low respiratory drive. One of the most important mechanisms that control the ventilatory system is the hypoxic or hypercapnic ventilatory response ($PaCO_2$ is maintained at a stable level by negative feedback control). This mechanism has a high degree of heritability. During non-REM sleep, reductions in CO_2 below eupneic levels will produce apnea, although this phenomenon does not occur during wakefulness. The CO_2 level at which this occurs (apneic threshold) typically is 1 to 2 mm Hg below waking eupneic levels. Thus, the sudden increase in ventilation occurring in association with arousal, which typically is seen at the termination of apneic and hypopneic episodes, will lead to hypocapnia, so that on returning to sleep, CO_2 is below the apneic threshold, and another apnea ensues. In this manner, postventilatory overshoot and loss of drive to the upper airway may lead to airway collapse with initiation of a subsequent obstructive event.

Other factors may contribute to reduced drive after postapneic hyperpnea, such as vagal stimuli generated during large inspired volumes and baroreceptor-mediated ventilatory inhibition due to postapneic blood pressure surges. Another important concept is *loop gain*, a term used to describe the stability of the respiratory system as a whole and how responsive the system is to a perturbation in breathing during sleep. The higher the loop gain, the lower the ventilatory stability. Patients with OSA have greater ventilatory control instability and higher loop gain when compared with control subjects. The two principal components of loop gain are *controller gain*, representing chemoreceptor responsiveness to hypoxia and hypercapnia (high controller gain is due to increased hypercapnic responsiveness), and *plant gain*, reflecting the effectiveness of a given level of ventilation to eliminate CO_2. In the context of high plant gain, a small change in ventilation would produce a large change in $PaCO_2$. Because upper airway muscles receive input from respiratory control centers, an unstable ventilatory drive will cause greater fluctuation in the activity of these muscles and promote upper airway collapse when ventilatory drive is at its nadir.

LUNG VOLUME AND PHARYNGEAL PATENCY

The interaction between pharyngeal patency and lung volume is believed to be an important contributor to the pathogenesis of OSA. Across the range from residual volume to total lung capacity, there is a lung volume dependence on upper airway diameter that appears to be more pronounced in subjects with OSA. During sleep, airway resistance increases as lung volume decreases. This combination leads to upward displacement of the diaphragm and thorax, with loss of caudal traction on the upper airway, yielding a more collapsible airway. Central obesity is believed to result in a reduction in lung volume during sleep, promoting pharyngeal collapse.

STABILITY OF SLEEP AND UPPER AIRWAY PATENCY

Arousal from sleep is believed to be an important if not essential mechanism for reestablishing airway patency in OSA. The preeminence of arousal is based on a temporal association between arousal and upper airway opening. Arousal mechanisms and upper airway motor neuron pools receive excitatory input from mechanoreceptors and probably also from chemoreceptors. The amount of excitation required to cause arousal is, on average, the same as that required to activate the upper airway motor neuron pool enough to open independently. Because the two systems are subject to different influences, however, the opportunity exists for either event to occur before the other. If arousal occurs prematurely in the context of a respiratory event during sleep, it may abort compensatory mechanisms such as increased pharyngeal dilator muscle activity, engendering ventilatory instability by stimulating hyperventilation. This can in turn promote upper airway collapse and worsening of OSA. These early arousals also have been associated with prolongation of respiratory events and worsened hypoxemia.

EDEMA AND ROSTRAL FLUID SHIFTS

Fluid shifts from the legs to the neck, caused by lower body positive pressure, have been shown to reduce upper airway size and increase collapsibility and appear to play a role in the pathogenesis of OSA. This mechanism is especially important in patients in whom the upper airway lumen is relatively small, because even a small amount of fluid could further compromise its patency. Some studies in patients with heart failure or superior vena cava syndrome corroborate this finding. In these patients, intensive diuresis was associated with an increase in oropharyngeal caliber and a significant reduction in AHI. Finally, vascular tone also may play a role in pharyngeal collapsibility. Animal studies have shown that vasodilatation increases and vasoconstriction decreases upper airway closing and opening pressures.

SURFACE TENSION OF UPPER AIRWAY FLUID

Upper airway collapsibility is affected by the surface tension of the liquid lining the airway, increasing both reopening and closing pressures. Increased surface tension has been reported in patients with OSA over that in normal subjects, as a consequence of mucosal trauma during apneas and use of the oral breathing route. Instillation of a surfactant has been shown to reduce AHI in persons with OSA as a consequence of improvement of airway collapsibility (reduced Pcrit).

UPPER AIRWAY INFLAMMATION

Substantial evidence has shown that inflammation is increased in the upper airway in OSA based on nasal lavage, induced sputum, exhaled breath condensate, and airway mucosal tissue biopsy specimens and that the level of inflammation is related to the severity of OSA. Factors associated with increased inflammation include mechanical trauma associated with snoring, suction collapse and traction during apneas, intense activation of dilator muscles at airway opening, increases in oxidative stress related to hypoxia-reoxygenation and other external factors such as gastroesophageal reflux, alcohol intake, smoking, allergic inflammation, the effect of systemic inflammation, and upper airway infections. Negative consequences appear in the context of repeated intense inflammation, because this could contribute to tissue injury and fibrosis, disorganization of the elastic tissue fibrillar network in uvular tissue, and changes in the connective tissue content, altering airway dimensions and compliance.

RAPID EYE MOVEMENT SLEEP

Hypopneas and apneas increase in duration and are associated with more pronounced hypoxemia during REM sleep in patients with OSA, because REM sleep is associated with decreased upper airway muscle tone, impaired genioglossus reflex responsiveness to negative pressure, and reduced chemosensitivity. Some patients experience OSA only during REM sleep. Certain protective mechanisms, however, tend to reduce event duration: The arousal threshold seems to be higher during REM sleep than during non-REM sleep in patients with OSA, and Pcrit does not change during REM sleep.

BERNOULLI EFFECT

Two physical phenomena cause a reduction in intraluminal pressure as air flows though the upper airway: loss of energy and the Bernoulli effect. The first phenomenon occurs when air flows through a segment (nasal segment) with high resistance, and potential energy is dissipated in overcoming friction, leading to a decrease in intraluminal pharyngeal pressure. The

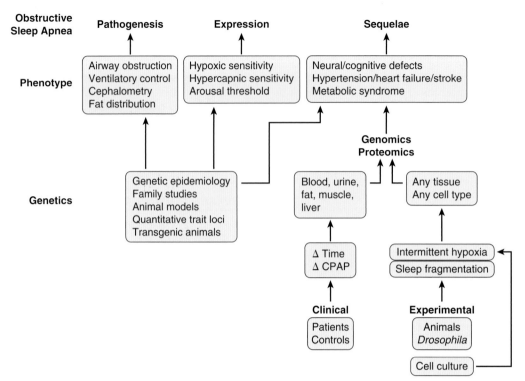

Figure 60-6 Schematic diagram of the relationship among obstructive sleep apnea, phenotype, and genomic-proteomic outcomes. *(From Polotsky VY, O'Donnell CP: Genomics of sleep-disordered breathing,* Proc Am Thorac Soc *4:121-126, 2007.)*

Bernoulli effect is related to the acceleration of the air as it flows through a narrowed segment of the tube, contributing to a decrease in intraluminal pharyngeal pressure.

CONTROVERSIES AND PITFALLS

One of the most controversial issues in the epidemiologic approach to OSA is the difficulty of comparing the results of different studies, because they may use various methodologies and different definitions for the syndrome. Agreement is required on the definition of OSA and the type and applications of diagnostic devices, as well as a global consensus on the definition of hypopnea and what symptoms define OSA, not only in middle-aged men but also in women and elderly persons. More research should be dedicated to specific issues in these two populations: distinguishing between physiologic and pathologic situations in the number and type of respiratory events during sleep in the elderly and, in addition, the clinical presentation of OSA in women, which usually is different from the classical form. On the other hand, although general risk factors for OSA are fairly well known, an additional aspect merits further attention: the analysis of the genomic, proteomic, and metabolomic (metabolite-associated) aspects of the disease. Obstructive events during sleep result in changes in molecular processes that can be assessed, providing a potential molecular signature for the presence and consequences of OSA. Heterogeneity in biologic responses and their changes over time probably explain why some patients with OSA develop hypertension or experience more sleepiness than others, or why some affected persons suffer marked sleep fragmentation and others exhibit more intermittent hypoxia and its consequences. It is possible

that developing and validating genetic and molecular signatures for OSA will provide not only diagnostic but also prognostic information, making the goal of personalized sleep medicine a reality in the near future (**Figure 60-6**).

SUGGESTED READINGS

Amardottir ES, Mackiewicz M, Gislason T, et al: Molecular signatures of obstructive sleep apnea in adults. A review and perspective, *Sleep* 32:447–470, 2009.

Dempsey JA, Veasey SC, Morgan BJ, et al: Pathophysiology of sleep apnea, *Physiol Rev* 90:47–112, 2010.

Eckert DJ, Malhotra A: Pathophysiology of adult obstructive sleep apnea, *Proc Am Thorac Soc* 5:144–153, 2008.

Gaudette E, Kimoff RJ: Pathophysiology of OSA, *Eur Respir Mon* 50:31–50, 2010.

Larkin EK, Patel SR, Goodloe RJ, et al: A candidate gene study of obstructive sleep apnea in European Americans and African Americans, *Am J Respir Crit Care Med* 182:947–953, 2010.

Launois SH, Pepin JL, Levy P: Sleep apnea in the elderly: a specific entity? *Sleep Med Rev* 11:87–97, 2007.

Lin CM, Davidson TM, Ancoli-Israel S: Gender differences in obstructive sleep apnea and treatment implications, *Sleep Med Rev* 12:481–496, 2008.

Lindberg E: Epidemiology of OSA, *Eur Respir Mon* 50:51–68, 2010.

Patil SP, Schneider H, Schwartz AR, et al: Adult obstructive sleep apnea: pathophysiology and diagnosis, *Chest* 132:325–337, 2007.

Polotsky VY, O'Donnell CP: Genomics of sleep-disordered breathing, *Proc Am Thorac Soc* 4:121–126, 2007.

Punjabi NM: The epidemiology of adult obstructive sleep apnea, *Proc Am Thorac Soc* 5:136–143, 2008.

Chapter **61**

Obstructive Sleep Apnea: Clinical Features, Diagnosis, and Treatment*

José M. Marin

CLINICAL FEATURES

The clinical presentations of obstructive sleep apnea (OSA) are legion. Common clinical features can be divided into major and minor categories, as summarized in **Box 61-1**. Patients may present with daytime and/or nocturnal complaints, but commonly, spouses and living companions are the first to push for medical attention.

SNORING

Snoring is the most frequent nocturnal symptom of OSA, occurring in up to 95% of patients with the condition. Snoring has poor predictive value owing to a high prevalence in the general population. In population surveys, the prevalence of snoring increases progressively with age, yet snoring is a hallmark of OSA, and in its absence, the diagnosis of OSA is unlikely. Snoring occurs after sleep onset, although in some patients with OSA it is present even during drowsiness. Its intensity increases with nighttime alcohol consumption and use of sedative drugs. In general, snoring is loudest in the supine position (dorsal recumbency) and decreases in volume in the side-lying position. Periods of silence interrupting loud snoring may reflect occurrence of pathologic apneas.

OTHER NOCTURNAL SIGNS AND SYMPTOMS

Patients with OSA usually fall asleep quickly, although many of them report insomnia and frequent nocturnal awakenings. Insomnia is most likely to reflect the perception of recurrent arousals from sleep and its nonrestorative pattern. Repetitive episodes of airway obstruction can be associated with snoring, gasping, diaphoresis, and restlessness that lead to sleep fragmentation. In severe OSA, choking is reported by more than 30% of patients. Nocturnal awakenings raise a differential diagnosis that should include nocturnal asthma, cardiac failure, and gastroesophageal reflux. Pathologic nocturia (2 episodes or more per night) has a prevalence of 50% among patients with OSA. It is thought to be secondary to hypoxia and atrial stretch, leading to increased atrial natriuretic peptide secretion and subsequent increment in intravascular volume. Effective therapy with continuous positive airway pressure (CPAP) reduces occurrence of these symptoms, thus suggesting a causal relationship between them and OSA.

Bed partners often volunteer witnessing breathing pauses followed by snorting or gasping during sleep, and this is a common reason for referral of the patient to a sleep clinic. Witnessed apneas are considered a good diagnostic predictor of OSA; nevertheless, this finding does not correlate with objective measurements and hence does not predict the severity of the disorder.

EXCESSIVE DAYTIME SLEEPINESS

Sleepiness is difficult to define and is a subjective feeling of impairment of concentration and increased craving for sleep. Excessive daytime sleepiness (EDS) is a nonphysiologic complaint that is not satisfied by a restorative sleep. Sleepiness is reported by 30% to 50% of the general population, so EDS alone is a poor predictor of OSA and requires a differential diagnosis to exclude many other medical conditions associated with this daytime symptom, such as depression, fibromyalgia, chronic insomnia, or hypothyroidism. Patients with OSA sometimes refer to EDS as abnormal daytime tiredness or lack of energy and convey the impression that they must make stringent efforts to remain alert and awake. It is believed that the loss of the restorative function of sleep due to repetitive arousals is the main mechanism to explain the presence of EDS in OSA. The Epworth Sleepiness Scale (**Box 61-2**) is the most popular tool for subjective evaluation (self-assessment) of EDS. A score above 10 of 24 is considered to be clinically relevant. The relationship between the Epworth score and the apnea-hypopnea index (AHI) (as a surrogate index of OSA severity) is relatively poor. In fact, 35% patients with severe OSA identified within sleep clinics do not complain of EDS. This discrepancy is partly due to underestimation or intentional underreporting the severity of sleepiness for personal gain, such as to avoid job loss. On the other hand, patients scoring high in the Epworth scale could have just mild to moderate OSA. EDS is the most disabling symptom among patients with OSA. One example is drowsiness while driving, which is associated with a three-fold increase in risk of accidents in patients with OSA. Poor school or job performance also is frequently reported.

OTHER DAYTIME SIGNS AND SYMPTOMS

On wakening in the morning, half of sufferers report headaches. Morning headache usually is generalized and lessens as the patient begins the usual activities of the day. This symptom may be due to hypercapnia and associated cerebral vasodilation with resultant increase in intracranial pressure. Often,

---

*Additional content for this chapter is available on Expert Consult.

Box 61-1 Common Clinical Features in Obstructive Sleep Apnea

Major Features
Snoring
Excessive daytime sleepiness
Witnessed apneas

Minor Features
Gasping/choking at night
Insomnia
Nocturia
Impotence/decreased libido
Morning headache
Morning dry mouth
Irritability/mood changes
Memory loss
Chronic fatigue

Box 61-2 Epworth Sleepiness Scale: Patient Questionnaire

How often are you likely to doze off or fall asleep in the following situations, in contrast with feeling just tired? This refers to your usual way of life in recent times. Even if you have not done some of these things recently, try to work out how they would have affected you. Use the following scale to choose the *most appropriate number* for each situation:

   0 = would *never* doze
   1 = *slight* chance of dozing
   2 = *moderate* chance of dozing
   3 = *high* chance of dozing
Sitting and reading _____
Watching TV _____
Sitting, inactive in a public place (e.g., a theater or a meeting)
_____As a passenger in a car for an hour without a break _____
Lying down to rest in the afternoon when circumstances permit

_____
Sitting and talking to someone _____
Sitting quietly after lunch without alcohol _____
In a car, while stopped for a few minutes in traffic _____
   TOTAL (example: 24) _____

From Johns MW: A new method for measuring daytime sleepiness: the Epworth Sleepiness Scale, *Sleep* 14:540–545, 1991.

Box 61-3 Physical Findings in Patients with Obstructive Sleep Apnea

General
Obesity
Increased neck circumference

Craniofacial
Retrognathia
Abnormal palate position

Oropharyngeal and Dental
Enlargement of tonsils
Enlargement of peritonsillar tissue
Hypertrophy of uvula
Retrognathia
Micrognathia
Cross-bite
Orthodontia

Nasal
Septal deviation
Turbinate hypertrophy
Nasal polyps

morning headaches disappear after effective treatment of OSA. Symptoms related to cognitive impairment such as memory loss, irritability, personality changes, and depression are frequent but nonspecific. Both sleep fragmentation and nocturnal hypoxemia have been advocated to explain decreased vigilance and psychomotor impairment, respectively. One concern is the observation that OSA treated with CPAP causes only partial resolution of those deficits, suggesting a potentially irreversible anoxic brain damage. In men with OSA, sexual dysfunction including impotence and decreased libido have been reported in 30% to 50% of the cases and appears to be fully reversible with effective treatment of the OSA. Past medical history should be obtained, particularly for those conditions that may occur as a result of OSA, such as hypertension, cardiac failure, myocardial infarction, and motor vehicle crashes.

PHYSICAL EXAMINATION

After a complete history has been obtained, a systematic examination should be performed. In nonobese patients (body mass index [BMI] less than 30 kg/m^2), common physical findings can be observed in the craniofacial, nasal, pharyngeal, and dental areas (**Box 61-3**). Radiographic cephalometry is indicated if craniofacial abnormalities are suspected or if upper airway surgery is planned to treat the patient. The oropharynx must be examined, and the degree of oropharyngeal crowding can be scored using the Friedman Tongue Position, formerly called the modified Mallampati score. For this assessment, the patient is asked to open the mouth widely without protruding the tongue. The observer can assign scores as indicated in **Figure 61-1**. Higher scores suggest the presence of OSA.

Obesity frequently is associated with OSA, in both men and women, but up to 30% of newly diagnosed patients are not obese or overweight. Neck circumference greater than 40 cm is considered a reliable clinical predictor of OSA, and the size of the neck correlates with the severity of disease. Peripheral edema should be sought as a sign of possible coexisting heart failure. Careful assessment for the presence of hypertension, thyroid abnormality, and acromegaly is indicated. Blood samples should be obtained routinely for testing thyroid function and to check for any other hormonal abnormality. In children, the clinical assessment should include evaluation for evidence of Down syndrome, craniofacial disorders, and enlarged tonsils.

DIAGNOSIS

Once the diagnosis of OSA is suspected from the clinical or laboratory features, the presence and severity of the sleep-disordered breathing are confirmed and assessed by a sleep study. Patients should be referred for a sleep study as soon as possible if they have problems with work or driving because of daytime sleepiness. The American Academy of Sleep Medicine (AASM) classified four different levels of sleep testing, as summarized in **Table 61-1**). Inpatient sleep laboratory polysomnography (PSG) remains the "gold standard" modality for the diagnosis of OSA and the initiation of CPAP treatment. Nevertheless, the American Medicare Service recently has turned from full-night attended PSG to portable polygraphy to establish the need for CPAP as a reimbursable therapy for OSA.

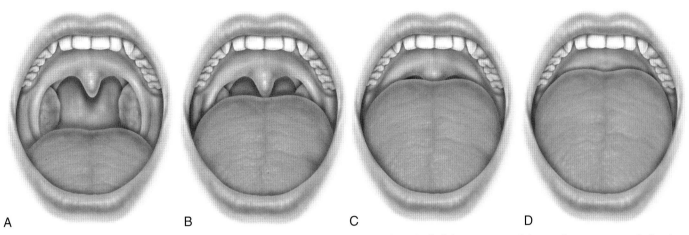

A   B   C   D

Figure 61-1   Friedman tongue position index for visualization of oral structures. **A,** Score I: all of the structures of the oropharynx are seen (soft palate, uvula, lateral pharyngeal pillars, and tonsils). **B,** Score II: allows visualization of the uvula but not the tonsils. **C,** Score III: allows visualization of the soft palate but not the uvula. **D,** Score IV: only the hard palate is seen.   *(From Friedman M, Tanyeri H, La Rosa M, et al: Clinical predictors of obstructive sleep apnea,* Laryngoscope *109:1901–1907, 1999.)*

Table 61-1	AASM Classification of Different Types of Sleep Studies		
Sleep Test	**Description**	**Personnel**	**Minimum Signals Required**
Type 1	In-laboratory PSG	Attended	*At least*: EEG, EOG, EMG, ECG, airflow, respiratory effort, and oxygen saturation
Type 2	Portable PSG	Unattended	Same as for type 1
Type 3	Portable monitor	Attended or unattended	*At least*: respiratory movement, airflow, ECG or pulse rate and oxygen saturation
Type 4	Mono-channel	Unattended	Airflow or pulse oximetry

AASM, American Academy of Sleep Medicine; *ECG*, electrocardiogram; *EEG*, electroencephalogram; *EMG*, electromyogram; *EOG*, electrooculogram; *PSG*, polysomnography.

POLYSOMNOGRAPHY

Polysomnography records neurophysiologic and cardiorespiratory signals, to assess sleep stage. Monitoring includes electroencephalography (EEG), electromyography (EMG) of the anterior tibialis, electrocardiography (ECG), oronasal airflow, snoring, thoracic, and abdominal movements, pulse oximetry, and body position (**Figure 61-2**). The PSG study must be performed in sleep laboratories by trained technicians and is therefore costly and time-consuming but provides the physician with information on both breathing- and non–breathing-related sleep disorders. PSG should be the preferred diagnostic sleep test for snorers with a lower likelihood of OSA, patients with EDS that could be caused by other non–breathing-related disorders during sleep (e.g., narcolepsy, restless legs syndrome), and patients with other medical comorbid conditions (e.g., neuromuscular, cardiac, and respiratory disorders). Apneas and hypopneas are identified, and the number of events per hour of sleep—the apnea-hypopnea index (AHI)—is determined. An AHI of less than 5 is normal. The severity of OSA is classified according to the AHI as mild (5 to 15 events/hour), moderate (15 to 30 events/hour), or severe (more than 30 events/hour). This disease severity classification is correlated with fatal and nonfatal cardiovascular outcomes.

Patients with OSA who are considered candidates for CPAP treatment (see further on) need to have a second attended PSG to determine the optimal level of CPAP to abolish the occurrence of all respiratory events. The so-called split night study combines a diagnostic PSG followed by CPAP titration during the same night. It is an accepted alternative to full-night PSG if the AHI is greater than 40 events/hour during the first two hours of recording.

UNATTENDED SLEEP STUDIES

For hospitalized patients or for persons unable to attend a sleep laboratory, PSG can be performed as an unattended study (type 2 study of the AASM classification). Indications and technical requirements are the same as for type 1 (in-laboratory PSG). Type 3 patient monitors are increasingly used owing to the limited number and capacity of sleep laboratories, as well as the increasing number of persons suspected of having OSA. These devices do not monitor EEG and sleep stages but should record the minimum airflow, respiratory effort, and O_2 saturation (**Figure 61-3**). They cannot evaluate sleep time or detect respiratory event-related arousals. As a result, they tend to underestimate the AHI. On the other hand, for most patients, home sleep studies offer greater convenience, and the study conditions allow close replication of the usual nighttime sleep pattern. The diagnosis of OSA is confirmed and severity determined using the same criteria as for PSG. Type 4 home monitors record continuous single or dual signals during sleep, including O_2 saturation and/or airflow (**Figure 61-4**). Baseline values for SaO_2, mean SaO_2, nadir SaO_2, and O_2 desaturation index (number of episodes of desaturation greater than 3% as divided by recording time) can be collected very easily using home oximetry. Airflow recorders also assess the frequency of apneas and hypopneas, but differentiation between obstructive and central or mixed apneas cannot be achieved.

The utility of type 3 and type 4 studies is greater for diagnosis of OSA in patients with high pretest probability of moderate to severe OSA and not combined sleep or major medical disorders. In most sleep units, however, use of a home monitor recording oxygen saturations, pulse rate, and airflow, calculating the number and severity of apneas, is a perfectly adequate screening test. If done before the patient sees the clinician, it may suffice or may indicate that a more sophisticated sleep

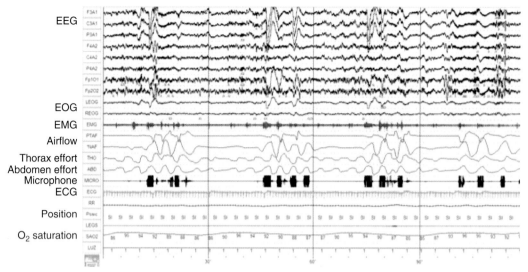

Figure 61-2 Polysomnography tracings showing repetitive obstructive apneic episodes. *ECG*, electrocardiogram; *EEG*, electroencephalogram; *EMG*, electromyogram; *EOG*, electrooculogram.

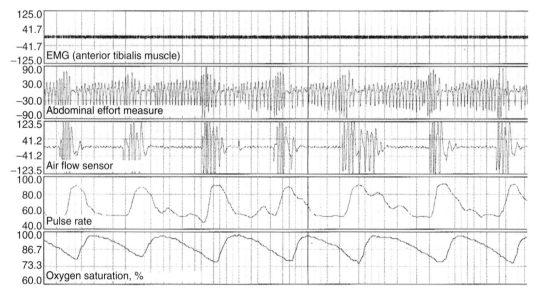

Figure 61-3 Type 3 portable monitor: Recorder tracings showing typical obstructive apneas. Channels included are (*top to bottom*) body movement, abdominal motion, oronasal airflow, pulse rate, and oxygen saturation. *EMG*, electromyogram.

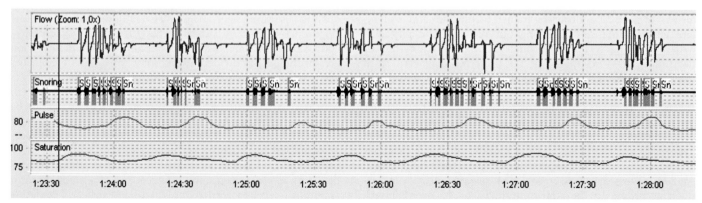

Figure 61-4 Type 4 portable monitor: Example of apneic events recording obtained with a dual sensor using a nasal cannula and a pulse oximeter applied at the patient's home. Channels are (*top to bottom*) airflow, snoring, pulse rate, and oxygen saturation.

Table 61-2   **Common Causes of Excessive Daytime Sleepiness Not Attributable to Obstructive Sleep Apnea**

Feature	Narcolepsy	Restless Legs Syndrome	Insufficient Sleep	Chronic Insomnia
Family history	+	++	−	±
Age at onset (years)	10-20	20-40	20-30	30-50
Predisposing factors	HLA-DQB1*0602 serotype	Iron deficiency	Stress	Psychiatric conditions
Night symptoms	Sleep paralysis	Difficulty falling asleep Leg cramps	Sleep <6 hours/night	Sleep arousals
Daytime symptoms	Cataplexy Hypnagogic hallucinations	Urge to move limbs Worse at evening	Performance impairment	Performance impairment
Other consequences	Depression Social isolation	Anxiety Social isolation	Risk for obesity and diabetes	Higher cardiac risk

HLA, human leukocyte antigen.

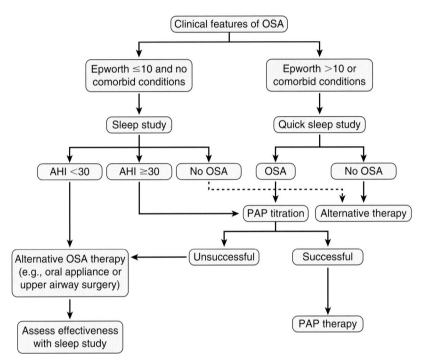

Figure 61-5   Treatment algorithm for obstructive sleep apnea (OSA). This flow diagram shows a general approach to the management of patients with suspected OSA. See Box 61-2 for the Epworth Sleepiness Scale. *AHI*, apnea-hypopnea index; *PAP*, positive airway pressure.

study is needed. A negative result with a portable monitor in patients with symptoms or clinical features highly consistent with OSA also warrants in-laboratory PSG.

OTHER EVALUATIONS

Once the diagnosis of OSA is made, collaboration with an ear, nose, and throat (ENT) specialist may be valuable to search for anatomic obstruction and to formulate a personalized therapy for each patient. Further blood sample analysis or imaging techniques may not be necessary if additional medical conditions are not suspected, although thyroid function abnormalities can still be present without clinical symptoms. In addition, the patient's drug history should be reviewed carefully, because many medicines such as opioids, hypnotics, antidepressants, or antihistamines can cause or aggravate sleep apneas.

DIAGNOSIS

After snoring, EDS is the most common presenting complaint in persons with OSA. Bed partners should be asked about the usual pattern of the patient's sleep, and the physician must

consider other causes of EDS in the differential diagnosis (**Table 61-2**). Apart from OSA, sleep can be interrupted by many other medical conditions, all causing EDS. In particular, patients with asthma and COPD frequently wake up owing to increased nocturnal respiratory symptoms. Heart failure and gastroesophageal reflux must be ruled out as potential causes of poor sleep quality and EDS. As noted, a drug history to identify medications that can cause EDS (e.g., psychiatric drugs, antihistamines, beta blockers) also should be part of a complete evaluation of all patients reporting EDS.

TREATMENT

GENERAL MEASURES

Treatment options should be offered in the context of the severity of the patient's OSA, risk factors, associated comorbid conditions, and personal wishes. A flow diagram outlining a treatment algorithm is shown in **Figure 61-5**. All affected patients should avoid alcohol and sedatives, because these agents reduce upper airway muscle tone and increase severity of OSA.

Weight loss reduces the collapsibility of the upper airway. It has been shown that a 1% reduction in weight is associated with a 3% decrease in AHI in severe OSA. Currently, weight loss is not a primary treatment for OSA but is recommended as an adjunct to other primary therapies and measures such as CPAP. For patients with mild OSA in whom apneas occur only in the supine position and without daytime sleepiness, positional therapy (e.g., with appropriate use of pillows or placement of a tennis ball at the back) may be of benefit. A type 3 or 4 home monitor can evaluate the efficacy of weight loss or positioning measures. No other medical therapies are recommended as primary treatment for OSA of any severity.

SURGICAL TREATMENT

The goal of upper airway surgical procedures is to increase upper airway patency. Surgery remains controversial for the treatment of OSA and is not widely used. A recent Cochrane review concluded that the available evidence does not support the use of surgery for patients with OSA. Nevertheless, it could be indicated if a specific airway abnormality is found. The AASM has identified three potential conditions for the application of upper airway surgery:

1. As a primary therapy for patients with mild OSA who have severe obstructive anatomy that is surgically correctible
2. As secondary treatment for OSA when CPAP or use of an oral appliance (OA) is poorly tolerated or contraindicated or provides inadequate correction or benefit
3. As an adjunctive therapy when obstructive anatomy or functional deficiency compromises other therapies, or to improve tolerance of other OSA treatment

Tonsillectomy or adenoidectomy (or in combination) is the primary treatment for children but does not improve OSA in adults. In patients with craniofacial abnormalities, procedures such as mandibular or genioglossus advancement with tongue and hyoid suspension can be effective when performed by expert surgeons. Uvulopalatopharyngoplasty (UPPP) reduces soft palate redundancy and can be used in patients with mild OSA with retropalatal obstruction. Even in these patients, UPPP reduces AHI to less than 50% of baseline. In patients with hypopharyngeal obstruction or severe OSA, UPPP is not effective at all. Hypopharyngeal procedures such as tongue reduction and tongue advancement or stabilization can be considered in patients with macroglossia or hypopharyngeal obstruction, but again these procedures should be performed by experienced surgeons. Nasal surgery—septoplasty, nasal polypectomy, turbinate reduction, and others—should be considered as adjunctive therapy to increase tolerance to CPAP.

Postsurgical follow-up evaluation should include a sleep study to objectively assess the procedure's success. Further surgical specific outcomes to be evaluated include side effects, complications, anatomic results, patient and spousal satisfaction, and resolution of sleepiness.

ORAL APPLIANCES

The aim with use of OAs is to increase upper airway patency and reduce its collapsibility by improving muscle tone. Most OA devices cover upper and lower teeth and hold the mandible in an advanced position with respect to the resting position. This positioning, in turn, pulls the tongue forward, making pharyngeal collapse with consequent obstruction much less likely to happen. An OA ideally should be custom-made for

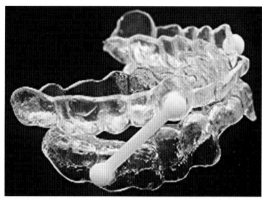

Figure 61-6 Oral appliance. *(From Douglas NJ: Obstructive sleep apnea. In Albert RK, Spiro SG, Jett JR, editors:* Clinical respiratory medicine, *ed 3, Philadelphia, 2008, Mosby.)*

the patient after a dental consultation (**Figure 61-6**); when created using this approach, the device is much more likely to be beneficial.

In clinical trials, OAs are less efficacious at reducing AHI but are associated with better compliance than that typical for CPAP. Available data regarding long-term outcomes with use of these appliances in persons with OSA are limited. No variables predictive of success have been identified, although OAs work better in persons with mild to moderate OSA, but not so well in those with big heavy jaws and masseters, which can generate forces sufficient to destroy the appliance. Also many persons with OSA grind their teeth during sleep; this bruxism also can destroy the appliance. Thus, sleep studies (e.g., with a home monitor) after treatment are recommended to document the efficacy of these devices. Currently, OAs are indicated for persons with simple snoring, patients with mild to moderate OSA, and those unable or unwilling to use CPAP.

POSITIVE AIRWAY PRESSURE

Positive airway pressure (PAP) currently is the management modality of choice for patients with OSA. PAP works by providing pneumatic splinting of the upper airway (**Figure 61-7**). In randomized trials, PAP delivered in continuous mode (i.e., CPAP) has been shown to improve quality of sleep, relieve daytime sleepiness, support maintenance and recovery of neurocognitive and driving abilities, decrease arterial hypertension, and help maximize quality of life in patients with OSA. It also reduces the frequency of cardiovascular events as long-term outcomes in prospective observational studies (**Figure 61-8**).

To determine optimal PAP level, a full-night attended PSG study is the preferred approach for titration. A split-night sleep study, however, may be indicated when AHI higher than 40 is recorded during the initial two hours of PSG. Auto-CPAP (aCPAP) machines continually adjust the applied pressure depending on the patency of the upper airway. Such devices may be used in an unattended setting to determine a fixed CPAP pressure, but this option is valid only for patients without significant comorbid conditions or other non-OSA sleep disorders. When high PAP pressure is required to avoid obstruction, the patient receiving CPAP or aCPAP therapy may experience difficulty with exhaling or can develop hypoventilation. In such cases, a switch to a bilevel system (BiPAP) will allow independent adjustment of inspiratory and expiratory pressures, potentially improving tolerance to the therapy.

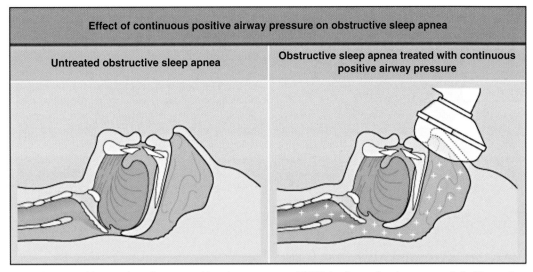

Figure 61-7 Anatomic changes with use of continuous positive airway pressure (CPAP) in obstructive sleep apnea. *Left*, Obstruction of the upper airway at the retrolingual level. *Right*, CPAP works by splinting and dilating the obstructed pharyngeal segment.

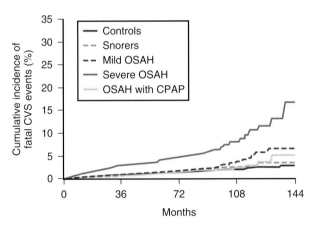

Figure 61-8 Effect of continuous positive airway pressure (CPAP) on mortality. Cumulative incidence of fatal cardiovascular events in patients with untreated obstructive sleep apnea-hypopnea (OSAH) and treated OSAH with CPAP. *(From Marin JM, Carrizo SJ, Vicente E, et al: Long-term cardiovascular outcomes in men with obstructive sleep apnoea/hypopnoea with or without treatment with continuous positive airway pressure: an observational study, Lancet 365:1046–1053, 2005.)*

PAP usually is delivered by nasal mask. Other interfaces such as nasal pillows or full face masks are alternatives to increase patient comfort, ensure a good seal, and avoid leaks. Long-term adherence is predicted by patient sleepiness, average nightly use within the first weeks of therapy, and the reporting of problems during the titration night. PAP is safe, and adverse events are minor and reversible. The most common side effect of PAP is nasal irritation and dryness, which can be treated with an integral heated humidifier. After initial PAP setup, follow-up evaluation is recommended at least once a year and whenever needed to troubleshoot device problems and to assess the cause of any change in clinical features.

ADJUNCTIVE THERAPIES

In obese patients, bariatric surgery may be an acceptable adjunctive therapy in the management of OSA. This surgical procedure is indicated for subjects with a body mass index (BMI) of 40 kg/m² or greater or those with a BMI of 35 kg/m²

or greater with important comorbid conditions. Data from cohort studies show that AHI decreases with weight loss after surgery. If previously initiated, PAP should be maintained after surgery as long as it is indicated (see further on).

Oxygen therapy alone is not recommended for patients with OSA. Such therapy provided during sleep could be added to PAP treatment if, during PAP titration, O_2 was needed to correct hypoxemia in patients with cardiopulmonary comorbidity. No effective drugs are available for treatment of OSA. Use of topical nasal steroids may be beneficial adjunctive therapy in patients with rhinitis and frequently improves nasal suffusion, which many patients complain of during CPAP therapy. Modafinil can be used to relieve residual sleepiness in patients who remain sleepy despite effective PAP treatment.

EFFECTS OF TREATMENT ON MAJOR OUTCOMES

In patients with moderate to severe OSA, maxillofacial surgery is the only surgical procedure for which the degree of improvement in sleepiness achieved was similar to that obtained with CPAP in a randomized trial. No effect on other major clinical outcomes such as motor vehicle crashes or incident cardiovascular events in patients with sleep apnea has been evaluated after surgical procedures or with the use of OAs.

In short-term randomized studies, CPAP reduced blood pressure in patients with severe OSA. This effect was evident only in patients who used the machine for more than 5 hours per night. In specific hypertensive populations such as patients with OSA plus resistant hypertension, CPAP also is effective, but again, the treatment must be used for more than 5 hours per night. The long-term effect of therapy to reduce new-onset hypertension in previously normotensive patients with OSA has not yet been determined. In population and clinic-based long-term observational studies, treatment with CPAP in patients with severe OSA is associated with reduced risk for development of fatal and nonfatal cardiovascular events (i.e., myocardial infarction, stroke). A reduction in frequency of motor vehicle crashes among persons with severe OSA treated with CPAP also has been noted. Today, however, with respect to assessment and validation of the effect of treatment, good long-term randomized controlled trials with strong end points such as cardiovascular events, traffic accidents, or all-cause mortality are lacking. Attempting these kinds of studies poses ethical problems in patients with significant daytime sleepiness: Because CPAP is very effective in alleviating this symptom, it cannot be denied for a long time in a control group.

WHOM TO TREAT AND HOW

Untreated patients with moderate to severe OSA have an increased risk for involvement in motor vehicle crashes and cardiovascular events. Current evidence indicates that persons with excessive daytime sleepiness (e.g., with an Epworth Sleepiness Scale score higher than 10), or who fall asleep while driving to or at work, should be treated no matter what the AHI is. For these patients, PAP is the primary treatment. For patients with AHI greater than 30, CPAP also is indicated as primary treatment regardless of the degree of sleepiness. For those with mild to moderate OSA (AHI between 5 and 30), therapy with CPAP is effective, but OAs and upper airway surgery should be offered and the risks and expected benefits discussed with the patient. Use of OAs is more suitable for thinner and younger patients with mild OSA. Surgery should be limited to patients with mild to moderate OSA who refuse other forms of therapy or as adjunctive treatment for those with upper airway obstruction to improve tolerance to PAP.

CONTROVERSIES AND PITFALLS

OBSTRUCTIVE SLEEP APNEA IN WOMEN

As in chronic obstructive pulmonary disease (COPD), OSA remains underdiagnosed in women. Physicians have a lower suspicion of OSA in females. On the other hand, they are more reluctant than males to complain of snoring. Finally, women reported more sleep and medical comorbidities such as depression, fibromyalgia, hypothyroidism, or chronic fatigue syndrome that ultimately can be attributed as responsible for daytime sleepiness. Hence, the clinicians need to include OSA in their differential diagnosis when evaluating female patients.

OBSTRUCTIVE SLEEP APNEA AND CHRONIC OBSTRUCTIVE PULMONARY DISEASE

The coincidence of OSA and COPD is termed *overlap syndrome*, and it is present in 1% of adults older than 40 years of age. In patients with OSA alone, daytime hypoxemia is rare, but in patients with COPD, the coexistence of OSA is associated with more profound nocturnal hypoxemia than in patients who have only one disorder. Consequently, patients with the overlap syndrome are at high risk for development of pulmonary hypertension. Recently, these patients have been reported to be at increased risk for severe exacerbations of COPD and all-cause mortality compared with patients with COPD and no coexistent OSA. Moreover, treatment of the OSA component of the overlap syndrome with CPAP decreases COPD exacerbations and improves survival. Accordingly, it is paramount in patients with COPD and daytime sleepiness to evaluate the potential coexistence of OSA.

SLEEP LABORATORY VERSUS OUT-OF-LABORATORY DIAGNOSIS

Full overnight polysomnography remains the "gold standard" modality for the diagnosis of sleep-disordered breathing performed in a staffed laboratory setting. Out-of-laboratory diagnosis is rapidly growing in respiratory medicine. The utility of these studies is greatest among patients with high pretest probability of severe disease, who may benefit from expedited diagnosis and treatment. Nevertheless, uncertainty remains regarding the quality of most devices, and pitfalls in automatic scoring have been recognized. Currently, portable systems for the diagnosis of OSA should be applied only by trained physicians, and their use should be limited to patients with suspected OSA not associated with comorbid conditions or other sleep disorders unlikely to be a cause of symptoms.

NON-CONTINUOUS POSITIVE AIRWAY PRESSURE THERAPY

Despite the efficacy of CPAP for relieving symptoms of OSA, many patients experience discomfort with this therapy and look for a curative option. Evidence supports the use of OAs in persons with mild to moderate OSA and weight loss in obese patients. Nevertheless, most surgical therapies lack robust scientific evidence and cannot be recommended as treatment for severe OSA. Controversies exist on when and what procedure to perform on an individual basis. Success depends mainly on the experience of the surgeon.

SUGGESTED READINGS

Centers for Medicare and Medicaid Services: Continuous positive airway pressure (CPAP) therapy for obstructive sleep apnea (OSA). Updated August 28, 2008 (online article): www.cms.gov; accessed on March 28, 2012.

Colten HR, Altevogt BM, editors: *Sleep disorders and sleep deprivation: an unmet public health problem*, Washington, DC, 2006, National Academy Press.

Cross M, Vennelle M, Engleman HM, et al: Comparison of CPAP titration at home or the sleep laboratory in the sleep apnea hypopnea syndrome, *Sleep* 29:1451–1455, 2006.

Deegan PC, McNicholas WT: Predictive value of clinical features for the obstructive sleep apnea syndrome, *Eur Respir J* 9:117–124, 1996.

Douglas NJ: Home diagnosis of the obstructive sleep apnoea/hypopnoea syndrome, *Sleep Med Rev* 7:53–59, 2003.

Epstein LJ, Kristo D, Strollo P, et al: Clinical guideline for the evaluation, management and long-term care of obstructive sleep apnea in adults, *J Clin Sleep Med* 5:263–276, 2009.

Marin JM, Carrizo SJ, Vicente E, et al: Long-term cardiovascular outcomes in men with obstructive sleep apnoea/hypopnoea with or without treatment with continuous positive airway pressure: an observational study, *Lancet* 365:1046–1053, 2005.

Pack AI, Platt AB, Pien GW: Does untreated obstructive sleep apnea lead to death? *Sleep* 31:1067–1068, 2008.

Sundaram S, Bridgman SA, Lim J, Lasserson TJ: Surgery for obstructive sleep apnea, *Cochrane Database Syst Rev* 4:CD001004, 2005.

Yaggi HK, Concato J, Kernan WN, et al: Obstructive sleep apnea as a risk factor for stroke and death, *N Engl J Med* 353:2034–2041, 2005.

Chapter **62**
Obesity Hypoventilation Syndrome

Gimbada B. Mwenge • Daniel Rodenstein

Obesity hypoventilation syndrome is a disorder characterized by the presence of daytime compensated respiratory acidosis (i.e., hypercapnia with normal pH and increased serum bicarbonate), in patients in whom no cause of ventilatory failure can be identified. These patients cannot ensure a normal minute ventilation even in the resting state, although clinical evaluation will rule out disorders associated with decreased muscle force (neuromuscular diseases), abnormal muscle geometry (e.g., kyphoscoliosis), severe airway obstruction and abnormal ventilation-perfusion relationships (e.g., chronic obstructive pulmonary disease [COPD], emphysema), or parenchymal abnormalities (e.g., interstitial lung diseases). In these patients, with performance of a respiratory maneuver consisting of serial deep inspirations, subsequently the arterial carbon dioxide tension ($PaCO_2$) normalizes, and in those in whom hypoxia is present, oxygen saturation (SaO_2) rises by 4% to 6% in less than 2 minutes. Of note, however, they do not sustain adequate minute ventilation and remain hypercapnic, with the kidneys compensating to maintain a normal pH. Another clinical element quite evident is that such persons are obese, frequently morbidly obese, with body mass index (BMI) values in excess of 35 kg/m². It is the association of pathologic obesity and daytime hypercapnia that defines the obesity hypoventilation syndrome.

When these patients are studied in a sleep laboratory, it becomes clear that they are afflicted with some form of sleep-disordered breathing pattern. The vast majority of patients have a moderate to severe form of obstructive sleep apnea (OSA), with a minority showing no obstructed breathing but simply sleep-related hypoxia and hypercapnia (long periods of SaO_2 below 90% and an increase in $PaCO_2$ of about 10 mm Hg developing overnight). The diagnosis of obesity hypoventilation syndrome can be reached with certainty only when other causes of daytime hypercapnia have been excluded.

EPIDEMIOLOGY

The prevalence of obesity hypoventilation syndrome in the general population remains unknown. In the United States, it has been estimated to be between 0.15% and 0.3%. A study conducted in obese hospitalized patients with a BMI greater than 35 kg/m² found a prevalence of 31%. Among patients with OSA, previous European studies (France, Italy, Greece, and Spain) found occurrence rates for obesity hypoventilation syndrome of 9% to 17%. Studies from the United States found a prevalence of greater than 20% in this patient group.

The gender ratio for obesity hypoventilation syndrome remains uncertain: Even if the prevalence seems to be higher in men, some studies found a higher proportion of the cases in women. All reported data come from selected cohorts of hospitalized patients or from sleep laboratories.

RISK FACTORS

Several conditions seem to predispose an obese person to development of the obesity hypoventilation syndrome. Undisputedly, in comparison with patients with OSA, patients diagnosed with this syndrome seem to be more obese, and they have more severe OSA. The main cause of obesity is well recognized to be an excess of food intake in relation to the energy expenditure requirements of the organism, resulting in the constitution of an energy stock essentially in the form of fat deposits. According to worldwide epidemiologic data, the prevalence of obesity is increasing everywhere, and this trend seems to be related essentially to a rapid change in eating habits, themselves influenced by technologic changes and food industry policies. Whether this reflects an improvement in the standard of living is a matter of debate.

The health consequences of obesity should prompt implementation of educational strategies to promote adequate behavioral changes in eating habits. Nevertheless, at the individual level, genetic factors may have an influence on the development of obesity, depending on the balance between what can be termed "catabolic" and "anabolic" genes. More than 250 genes have been identified that have a more or less important influence on the final handling of the energetic balance. The clinical importance of each genetic variant, however, is not yet well appreciated. Only a few monogenetic causes of obesity have been described in humans, the best example being mutations in the gene coding for the melanocortin 4 receptor. It has to be stressed, however, that obesity will not develop if access to food is compromised, or if energy expenditure exceeds energy absorption.

An apnea-hypopnea index (AHI) greater than 50, as measured by the number of apneic or hypopneic episodes per hour of sleep, also seems to be a risk factor for obesity hypoventilation syndrome, because 25% of patients with such AHIs in several studies had the syndrome. Oxygen saturation nadir levels below 60% during polysomnography and moderate to severe restriction found on pulmonary function testing also are predictors for the syndrome, with odds ratios of 4 and 10, respectively. Finally, some studies found that patients with obesity hypoventilation syndrome had greater neck, waist, and hip circumferences and a larger waist-to-hip ratio than their counterparts with OSA.

PATHOPHYSIOLOGY

Obese patients, both eucapnic and hypercapnic, have significant reductions in functional residual capacity and expiratory reserve volume with preservation of inspiratory capacity and often normal or slightly reduced total lung capacity. But obesity is not, however, the only determinant of hypoventilation, because only a third of morbidly obese persons develop hypercapnia. Some differences between eucapnic obese and hypercapnic subjects have been recognized and are summarized next.

Reduced Muscle Strength

The maximal inspiratory and expiratory pressures are normal in eucapnic morbidly obese patients but may be reduced in patients with obesity hypoventilation syndrome, although this is not a universal finding.

Central Respiratory Drive

Many studies found that patients with obesity hypoventilation syndrome do not hyperventilate to the same degree as morbidly obese patients without the syndrome when rebreathing CO_2. This deficit corrects in most patients after normalization of $PaCO_2$. In patients with severe OSA but without hypercapnia, the hypercapnic ventilatory response does not change with continuous positive airway therapy (CPAP). The reversibility of the blunted central drive suggests that this is a secondary phenomenon of the syndrome (and necessary for its persistence), but not the origin of it.

Obstructive Sleep Apnea

OSA may play a role in the pathogenesis of chronic hypercapnia in those patients, because in most cases, treatment of OSA corrects the hypercapnia. Indeed, to compensate for the effect of intermittent periodic breathing and resultant acute hypercapnia, normal subjects as well as patients with OSA will increase their tidal volume in the first breath after an apnea (hyperventilation). With physiologic differences in ventilatory responses between subjects, however, an overload in CO_2 could result. The duration of the apneas also could contribute: When apneic episode duration becomes three times longer than the breathing interval, CO_2 tends to accumulate despite maximal tidal volume, because there is insufficient time for adequate hyperventilation events (**Figure 62-1**). In addition, hypercapnia could blunt the ventilatory responses: The initial ventilation after an apneic episode is directly related to the volume of CO_2 loaded during the preceding respiratory event and thus represents an index of CO_2 ventilatory response. Hypercapnic patients demonstrated depression of this index of ventilatory compensation compared with that in eucapnic patients. It has been shown that the apnea-to-interapnea duration ratio is greater in hypercapnic patients than in eucapnic patients.

One study also has shown impaired CO_2 homeostasis after respiratory events may be mediated by opioids or opioid receptors, because endorphin blockade changed this pattern. Increased cerebrospinal fluid beta-endorphin activity with return to normal values has been reported in subjects with OSA. This finding could explain hypercapnia on awakening after a night full of apneic episodes. To understand why in a period of wakefulness free of apnea the $PaCO_2$ does not normalize, the role of the renal system has to be considered. Hypercapnia leads to respiratory acidosis, which activates the process of renal compensation.

To elucidate the mechanisms that are involved in the development of hypercapnia in patients with OSA, Norman and co-workers have proposed, using a computer model, some hints for prediction of the transition from acute hypercapnia during sleep-disordered breathing (apnea, hypopnea, and hypoventilation) to chronic daytime hypercapnia. In their model, when the ventilatory CO_2 response and renal HCO_3^- excretion were normal, increases in $PaCO_2$ and HCO_3^- did not develop. The bicarbonate excretion during the day compensated for that retained during the night. When CO_2 ventilatory response was very low, however, the model demonstrated a modest rise in $PaCO_2$ and HCO_3^- measured during the awake state over multiple days. Similarly, when renal HCO_3^- excretion rate was lowered to simulate chloride deficiency, the model

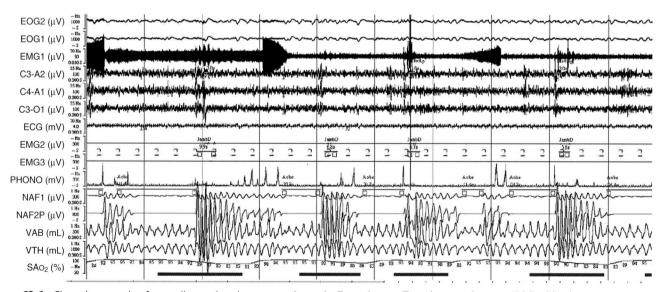

Figure 62-1 Five-minute tracing from a diagnostic polysomnography study. *Top to bottom:* Two electrooculograms (*EOG*); chin electromyogram (*EMG1*); three electroencephalograms (*C3-A2, C4-A1, C3-O1*); electrocardiogram (*ECG*); leg movement electromyograms (*EMG2, EMG3*); snoring recordings (*PHONO*); oronasal flow with a thermocouple (*NAF1*); nasal flow (*NAF2P*); abdominal and thoracic movement from inductive plethysmographic bands (*VAB, VTH*); and oxygen saturation measurement with pulse oximetry (*Sao₂*). The subject is in stage 2 non-REM sleep. Note the absence of nasal flow and persistent abdominal and thoracic movements with falls in oxygen saturation, with successive obstructive apneas ending with loud snoring and leg movements (with one exception). *REM*, rapid eye movement.

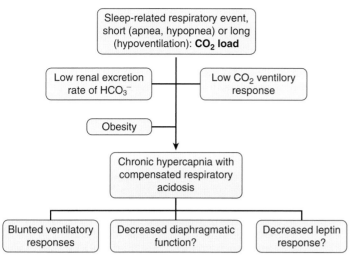

Figure 62-2 Schematic representations of the physiopathology of obesity hypoventilation syndrome. Respiratory events with the combination of low CO_2 ventilatory response and low renal HCO_3^- excretion rate produce a synergistic effect on the degree of elevation of daytime $PaCO_2$. Chronic hypercapnia will then lead to blunted ventilatory responses, possibly decreased diaphragmatic function, and decreased leptin response.

demonstrated a modest rise in daytime $PaCO_2$ and HCO_3^-. The combination of low CO_2 response and low renal HCO_3^- excretion rate produced a synergistic effect on the degree of elevation of daytime $PaCO_2$. These workers suggested that hypercapnia results from an imbalance between the period of CO_2 loading (short = apnea or hypopnea; long = hypoventilation) and inadequate compensation both during sleep and during the awake state. This pulmonary-renal interaction may contribute to the development and perpetuation of chronic daytime hypercapnia, which will lead to a blunted respiratory drive for the next sleep cycle (**Figure 62-2**).

There is clearly a link between the pathogenesis of OSA and pure hypoventilation in patients with obesity hypoventilation syndrome. In their study, De Miguel Díez and colleagues provided ventilatory support to 12 patients with pure obesity hypoventilation syndrome (without sleep apnea), using noninvasive ventilation (NIV), for a minimum period of 1 year. After 3 months subsequent to discontinuation of NIV and disappearance of hypercapnia, 7 patients had developed obstructive sleep apnea syndrome. These data suggest that impairment of the ventilatory drive caused by compensated respiratory acidosis may potentially lead the switch from apnea-hypopnea syndrome to pure obesity hypoventilation syndrome.

Neurohormonal Response (Leptin Resistance)

Leptin is a protein released by adipose tissue. Its functions are to reduce appetite and increase energy expenditure. In obesity, some studies have found high blood levels of leptin but without the expected physiologic effects, suggesting the presence of so-called leptin resistance. Animal studies have shown that this protein is a potent stimulus of ventilation, and absence of or reduction in its action may result in hypoventilation. Serum levels of leptin are decreased or normal after CPAP treatment in patients with OSA. A hypothesis for this association is that the apnea and hypopnea could be the *cause* of the elevation of leptin, rather than the result. Leptin levels are twice as high in patients with obesity hypoventilation syndrome as in patients with similar degrees of obesity and similar AHI values. Leptin levels can be reduced with NIV or weight loss. All of these

observations have led to the idea that resistance to leptin may be the cause of obesity hypoventilation syndrome. A recent study, however, found opposite results: Those patients with the syndrome not associated with a significant number of apneic and hypopneic episodes have lower leptin levels than those obese patients with the same number of obstructive events without daytime hypercapnia and obesity, and leptin levels increased with treatment with NIV. More studies have to be performed to clarify those findings. Clearly, as yet, no comprehensive picture of the neurohumoral interactions in obesity hypoventilation syndrome has emerged.

CLINICAL FEATURES

The following clinical features have been found in a systematic review of the literature including a significant number of patients. Patients typically are diagnosed in the sixth decade of life and prevalence is slightly higher in men (60%). Compared with patients with OSA, patients with obesity hypoventilation syndrome are severely obese (mean, 44 kg/m²; range, 35 to 56 kg/m²). Up to 90% of these patients have OSA, with an AHI in the severe range (mean, 66; range, 20 to 100). Subjects with obesity hypoventilation syndrome are sleepier than those with OSA (on the Epworth sleepiness scale, a score of 14.6 ± 4.9, versus 12.5 ± 4.6). The impact of this excessive sleepiness has the same consequences, with decrements in work performance, concentration lapses, inattention, and increased reaction time. Nocturnal and daytime hypoxemia also characterize obesity hypoventilation syndrome. Depending on the studies, the mean reported daytime PaO_2 is 53 mm Hg (47 to 74 mm Hg). Finally, the nadir of oximetry-measured oxygen saturation (SpO_2) during sleep often is below 60%.

DIAGNOSIS

HISTORY

Most patients with obesity hypoventilation syndrome will have some daytime respiratory complaints (dyspnea) and some degree of excessive daytime sleepiness. They often have comorbid illnesses at the time of diagnosis, such as diabetes and hypertension. All other complaints also are seen in typical eucapnic patients with OSA, including loud snoring, nocturnal choking episodes with witnessed apneas, and excessive daytime sleepiness, nycturia, mood disturbance, and morning headaches. The diagnosis usually is made by a sleep specialist or a respiratory physician. Alternatively, in patients previously treated for OSA successfully, recurrence of symptoms can suggest a shift toward obesity hypoventilation syndrome. Frequently, patients are diagnosed after an episode of acute respiratory failure with admission to intensive care unit.

PHYSICAL EXAMINATION

Physical examination in both eucapnic and hypercapnic patients with obesity hypoventilation syndrome usually reveals a BMI higher than 40 kg/m² and a neck circumference greater than 42 cm in men and 40 in women. The oral examination shows a large tongue with a crowded oropharynx (Mallampati score IV; Friedman tongue position index of 3 or 4). Few specific findings have been recognized to distinguish obesity hypoventilation syndrome from OSA: Abnormal oxygen saturation (SpO_2) detected by finger pulse oximetry during the awake state also should lead clinicians to exclude the syndrome in patients with OSA, because hypoxemia during the awake state is not common in these patients.

Patients with obesity hypoventilation syndrome may present with signs of cor pulmonale: a prominent pulmonic component of the second heart sound on cardiac auscultation, lower extremity edema, injected sclera (thought to be related to elevated $PaCO_2$ and cerebral vasodilatation), hepatomegaly, and prominent jugular veins.

BLOOD GAS ANALYSIS AND SERUM BLOOD CHEMISTRY

Elevated serum venous bicarbonate level has been suggested as an effective screening tool. Of patients with serum bicarbonate levels greater than 27 mmol/L and clinical obesity (BMI higher than 30 kg/m^2), 38% had obesity hypoventilation syndrome in one study. If obesity was severe and lung function showed restriction and severe OSA, the prevalence of obesity hypoventilation syndrome jumped to 56%.

Hypothyroidism is a rare occurrence, but it may be worth excluding with a thyroid-stimulating hormone (TSH) challenge test.

"Awake" (daytime) hypercapnia ($PaCO_2$ greater than 45 mm Hg) in arterial blood is a defining criterion for the diagnosis and frequently is accompanied by daytime hypoxia.

SLEEP LABORATORY DIAGNOSIS

Sleep-disordered breathing can take either of two forms; the most common type is OSA, and the second one is central hypoventilation. Polysomnographic evaluation shows either a typical OSA pattern or periods of fall in SaO_2 in REM stages alone (**Figure 62-3**) or throughout the entire sleep period (**Figure 62-4**). In many cases, sleep-disordered breathing is seen throughout sleep, with steep falls in saturation in non-REM sleep and much steeper falls in the REM stage (see Figure 62-4).

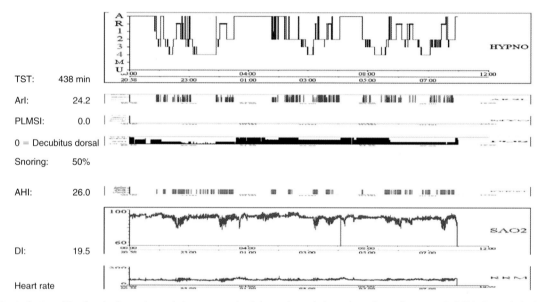

Figure 62-3 *Top to bottom:* The first horizontal panel shows a graph of the wake and sleep data: *A*, awake state; *R*, REM sleep; *1, 2, 3, 4*, non-REM sleep stages; *U*, unknown stage; *M*, movement. The next panels show arousal index (*Arl*), index of periodic leg movements (*PLMSI*), body position (with the supine position indicated as 0), snoring as a percentage of sleep time, apnea-hypopnea index (*AHI*), desaturation index (*DI*) (defined as the number of 4% or greater falls in oxygen saturation [SaO_2] per hour of sleep), and heart rate. Of note, apneas and hypopneas lead to falls in oxygen saturation, but these falls are much steeper during REM sleep. *REM*, rapid eye movement; *TST*, total sleep time.

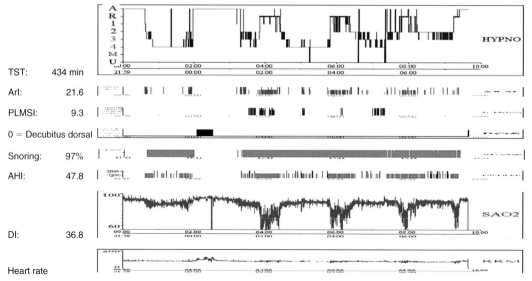

Figure 62-4 Note low SaO_2 throughout the night and deeper falls in SaO_2 related to the period of REM sleep. For abbreviations, see Figure 62-3.

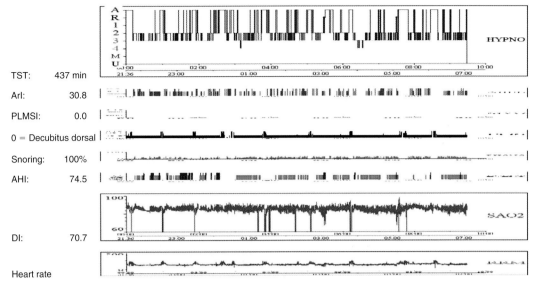

Figure 62-5 Note low SaO₂ throughout the night, with cyclic falls and recoveries, and the almost complete absence of REM sleep. For abbreviations, see Figure 62-3.

In some patients, REM sleep may even be completely absent (**Figure 62-5**).

SPIROMETRY

The most predictable and pronounced effects of obesity on lung function are decrease in functional residual capacity (FRC) and in expiratory reserve volume (ERV) associated with the closure of peripheral lung units and ventilation-to-perfusion ratio abnormalities that appear when the subject is lying down. When obese persons achieve significant weight loss, FRC increases. In patients with obesity hypoventilation syndrome, total lung capacity (TLC) is normal or mildly decreased, whereas ERV and FRC are reduced, compared with values in eucapnic patients, and these changes are more evident in patients with obesity hypoventilation syndrome than in eucapnic patients, even at similar BMI.

CHEST RADIOGRAPHY

Plain chest radiography shows no special features. Nevertheless, this imaging study is recommended to exclude interstitial lung disease and chest wall deformities (severe kyphoscoliosis), or diaphragmatic paralysis.

CARDIAC ECHOGRAPHY

In cases of cor pulmonale, echocardiography may confirm the diagnosis and is useful for follow-up evaluation.

CLINICAL COURSE: MORBIDITY AND MORTALITY

Obesity in itself does not result in a higher rate of morbidity and mortality in intensive care units (ICUs). This has been demonstrated in a matched-patient study that found that BMI did not have a significant impact on mortality in this sample.

Patients with obesity hypoventilation syndrome are heavy users of health care resources for several years before the evaluation and treatment of their sleep-related breathing disorder, and a substantial reduction in days hospitalized is achieved once treatment is instituted. Nowbar and associates showed a clear increase in mortality after hospital discharge in the follow-up evaluation for obesity hypoventilation syndrome compared with simple obesity.

The most common consequences in obesity hypoventilation syndrome include polycythemia, hypothyroidism, pulmonary hypertension, right-sided heart failure, and acute respiratory failure.

MacGregor and associates reported a high level of mortality, including sudden death, in patients with obesity hypoventilation syndrome and a subsequent reduction in mortality with the institution of mechanical ventilation. These findings were reinforced by the study by Budweiser and colleagues that demonstrated improvement of gas exchange and lung function in obesity hypoventilation syndrome after initiation of NIV. These workers also underlined the relationship between a poor survival and the presence of hypoxemia, low pH and elevated inflammation markers.

TREATMENT

WEIGHT REDUCTION

The ideal treatment is weight loss. Restoration of a normal weight reverses respiratory failure, pulmonary hypertension, and sleep-related disordered breathing. The problem is that it is difficult to achieve and maintain significant weight loss in these patients. Bariatric surgery appears to be the most effective means to achieve long-term reduction in body weight. This is a treatment reserved for a minority of subjects, however, owing to increased surgical morbidity and mortality of patients with obesity hypoventilation syndrome. The perioperative mortality rate for this procedure is between 0.5% and 1.5%. The independent risk factors associated with mortality are intestinal leaks and pulmonary embolism. Ideally, patients with obesity hypoventilation syndrome should be supported with CPAP therapy or NIV before undergoing surgical intervention, in order to decrease perioperative morbidity and mortality. Moreover, CPAP or NIV therapy should be reinitiated immediately after extubation, to avoid postoperative respiratory failure.

REVERSAL OF SLEEP-DISORDERED BREATHING

Noninvasive Ventilation

The efficiency of NIV has been extensively studied. It can be expected to produce a successful clinical response, as has been shown in many diseases and conditions associated with hypercapnia (kyphoscoliosis, central alveolar hypoventilation). NIV provides significant long-term improvement in PaO_2 and $PaCO_2$ and relief of subjective sleepiness and dyspnea.

NIV often is used as second-line treatment after a trial with CPAP, which may be warranted owing to lack of adherence to CPAP therapy, lack of improvement in hypercapnia, or the persistence of hypoxemia despite CPAP. It also should be considered in patients with obesity hypoventilation syndrome who experience an episode of acute-on-chronic respiratory failure and in patients who have obesity hypoventilation syndrome without OSA.

Continuous Positive Airway Pressure

CPAP treatment improves AHI, REM duration, arousal indices, and nocturnal oxygen saturation. In some subjects, however, nocturnal desaturation continues despite the treatment. When evaluated in various cohorts of selected patients without severe hypoxia, CPAP alone produced a satisfactory response in 80% of patients, the others needing NIV. Although CPAP and NIV are widely used for treatment of obesity hypoventilation syndrome, no randomized controlled trial has been conducted in unselected patients, to determine if one of these treatments is more effective or efficient, or for any comparison with weight loss. Also lacking are studies systematically evaluating longer-term response (6 months) of patients with obesity hypoventilation syndrome placed on CPAP, so it is unclear what impact this therapy has on outcomes such as hospitalization and survival.

Thus far, no study has yielded a valid method for predicting success or failure with CPAP, thereby predicting the need for NIV. Until good data allow a reasoned choice, the best option appears to be a trial of CPAP. If sleep-disordered breathing and respiratory acidosis are not corrected, a change to NIV is warranted.

Tracheostomy

Performance of a tracheostomy bypasses the upper airway, with consequent reduction in risk for obstructive events. In patients with OSA, tracheostomy was shown to be an effective treatment alternative despite the presence of hypercapnia. For various reasons, however, it is not recommended in most patients with obesity hypoventilation syndrome. Tracheostomy is challenging in the morbidly obese. Complications have occurred with use of both the surgical and percutaneous approaches. Complications most frequently reported with percutaneous tracheostomy are need to abort the procedure, accidental extubation, need for conversion to surgical tracheostomy, paratracheal placement, development of pneumothorax, major bleeding (requiring blood product transfusion or surgical intervention), hypoxia, minor bleeding (requiring pressure dressing or suturing), subcutaneous emphysema, transient hypotension, tube obstruction, malpositioning of the tracheostomy tube after being dislodged, and death. Because CPAP and NIV are effective in most cases, tracheostomy is certainly not a first choice for management of obesity hypoventilation syndrome.

PHARMACOTHERAPY

Very few drug trials have been conducted in patients with obesity hypoventilation syndrome. A recent study by Raurich and co-workers in Spain, performed in 25 patients with obesity hypoventilation syndrome, investigated the relationship between CO_2 response, BMI, and plasma bicarbonate concentration and the effect of acetazolamide on bicarbonate concentration and CO_2 response in ventilated patients with acute respiratory failure. These workers found that the addition of acetazolamide decreased bicarbonate concentration and increased CO_2 response. They suggest that this treatment could be used as a complement in ventilation.

CONCLUSIONS

Obesity hypoventilation syndrome seems to develop only in the presence of massive obesity and represents one of the most serious respiratory complications of obesity. This syndrome is both preventable and treatable, and the treatment apparently is independent of the maintenance or the loss of the excessive weight. If left undiagnosed and untreated, obesity hypoventilation syndrome leads to severe health consequences. Unfortunately, this clinical entity is underdiagnosed—it remains primarily a subject of interest to a small number of physicians puzzled by the interrelation between sleep and breathing, whereas it remains hidden behind obesity for the vast majority of physicians. The increase in the worldwide prevalence of obesity will require a dedicated educational effort by health care professionals to make this disease better known. Otherwise, patients will continue being diagnosed in the ICU setting, once a first episode or several episodes of acute respiratory failure have precipitated a life-threatening crisis necessitating emergency care.

CONTROVERSIES AND PITFALLS

Although considerable advances have added to the current understanding of how the obesity hypoventilation syndrome develops and becomes established, a vast amount of uncertainty remains regarding its clinical presentation and consequences. Some of the unresolved issues are as follows:

- Is the obesity hypoventilation syndrome just a particular form of obesity, so that losing weight would be enough to cure it?
- Does the obesity hypoventilation syndrome prevent weight loss via excessive daytime sleepiness, decrease in energy consumption, and exacerbated hunger sensation?
- What is the simpler and best screening method to identify patients at risk and to prompt an adequate diagnostic process?
- Is polysomnography necessary to manage patients with obesity hypoventilation syndrome?
- Is the respiratory treatment of the sleep-related causes of obesity hypoventilation syndrome (i.e., CPAP for the apnea-hypopnea syndrome or NIV for sleep-related hypoventilation) enough to protect the patient's health, or is weight loss still a mandatory component of management?
- CPAP is an efficient therapy in many patients. A sizable number, however, do not respond to this intervention. What are the predictive factors that could rapidly identify such nonresponders?
- In patients needing NIV, how many can revert to a simpler CPAP treatment?

- In patients needing NIV, when is a shift to CPAP advisable?
- What is the cost-utility ratio of CPAP and NIV in OHS?
- CPAP or NIV treatment seems to decrease mortality, but this has been assessed in a limited number of patients. Long-term follow-up studies in larger cohorts are needed to confirm this major outcome and to determine the confounding effect of persistent obesity on survival.

SUGGESTED READINGS

Banerjee D, Yee BJ, Piper AJ, et al: Obesity hypoventilation syndrome: hypoxemia during continuous positive airway pressure, *Chest* 131:1678–1684, 2007.

Berg G, Delaive K, Manfreda J, et al: The use of health-care resources in obesity-hypoventilation syndrome, *Chest* 120:377–383, 2001.

Budweiser S, Riedl SG, Jorres RA, et al: Mortality and prognostic factors in patients with obesity-hypoventilation syndrome undergoing noninvasive ventilation, *J Intern Med* 261:375–383, 2007.

Chouri-Pontarollo N, Borel JC, Tamisier R, et al: Impaired objective daytime vigilance in obesity-hypoventilation syndrome: impact of noninvasive ventilation, *Chest* 131:148–155, 2007.

De Miguel Díez J, De Lucas Ramos P, Pérez Parra JJ, et al: [Analysis of withdrawal from noninvasive mechanical ventilation in patients with obesity-hypoventilation syndrome. Medium term results.], *Arch Bronconeumol* 39:292–297, 2003.

Lumachi F, Marzano B, Fanti G, et al: Hypoxemia and hypoventilation syndrome improvement after laparoscopic bariatric surgery in patients with morbid obesity, *In Vivo* 24:329–331, 2010.

MacGregor MI, Block AJ, Ball WC Jr: Topics in clinical medicine: serious complications and sudden death in the Pickwickian syndrome, *Johns Hopkins Med J* 126:279–295, 1970.

Marien H, Rodenstein D: Morbid obesity and sleep apnea. Is weight loss the answer? *Clin Sleep Med* 4:339–340, 2008.

Masa JF, Celli BR, Riesco JA, et al: The obesity hypoventilation syndrome can be treated with noninvasive mechanical ventilation, *Chest* 119:1102–1107, 2001.

Norman RG, Goldring RM, Clain JM, et al: Transition from acute to chronic hypercapnia in patients with periodic breathing: predictions from a computer model, *J Appl Physiol* 100:1733–1741, 2006.

Nowbar S, Burkart KM, Gonzales R, et al: Obesity-associated hypoventilation in hospitalized patients: prevalence, effects, and outcome, *Am J Med* 116:1–7, 2004.

Pérez de Llano LA, Golpe R, Ortiz Piquer M, et al: Short-term and long-term effects of nasal intermittent positive pressure ventilation in patients with obesity-hypoventilation syndrome, *Chest* 128:587–594, 2005.

Raurich JM, Rialp G, Ibáñez J, et al: Hypercapnic respiratory failure in obesity-hypoventilation syndrome: CO_2 response and acetazolamide treatment effects, *Respir Care* 55:1442–1448, 2010.

Trakada GP, Steiropoulos P, Nena E, et al: Prevalence and clinical characteristics of obesity hypoventilation syndrome among individuals reporting sleep-related breathing symptoms in northern Greece, *Sleep Breath* 14:381–386, 2010.

Chapter **63**
Scoliosis and Kyphoscoliosis
Anita K. Simonds

Scoliosis refers to lateral curvature of the spine (**Figure 63-1**), a well-recognized clinical entity that was described by Hippocrates as early as 500 BCE. *Kyphosis* indicates backward and *lordosis* forward curvature in an anteroposterior (medial) plane. Many patients who have a thoracic scoliosis are mistakenly described as having a kyphoscoliosis, because the rib angle prominence is misinterpreted as a kyphotic component. In fact, most instances of idiopathic thoracic scoliosis incorporate a lordotic and a rotatory element. The degree of lateral curvature is expressed by the *Cobb angle*, which is calculated from radiograph-based measurements, as shown in **Figure 63-2**.

EPIDEMIOLOGY, RISK FACTORS, AND PATHOPHYSIOLOGY

Spinal curvature is the most common cause of chest wall deformity. The causes of chest wall deformity are shown in **Box 63-1**. By far, the most frequently found scoliosis is the idiopathic variety, which accounts for approximately 80% of cases. *Idiopathic* scoliosis is defined as lateral curvature for which no cause can be identified; *congenital* forms of scoliosis are related to a developmental abnormality of the spine, as in failure of segmentation (e.g., fused vertebrae), failure of formation (e.g., hemivertebrae), or genetic syndromes (e.g., spondylocostal dysostosis or Klippel-Feil or Goldenhar syndrome).

Scoliotic curves of more than 35 degrees are present in 1 in 1000 population, and those that exceed 70 degrees are estimated to occur at a rate of 0.1 in 1000. A gender predilection for more pronounced deformity has been recognized: Females are at greater risk for severe curvature. It has been estimated that approximately 500,000 persons with a scoliotic curve of greater than 30 degrees are living in the United States. Approximately 3 or 4 children per 1000 will require specialist supervision for their spinal curvature, and a third of these will require intervention (e.g., corrective surgery or bracing). Idiopathic scoliosis occurs more often with increasing maternal age and in higher socioeconomic groups, but no association has been found between the incidence of scoliosis and birth order or season of birth. A subclassification of idiopathic scoliosis is based on age at onset of the spinal changes resulting in curvature—infantile (birth to age 3 years), juvenile (3 to 11 years), and adolescent (11 years and older).

Scoliosis is associated with a variety of congenital syndromes. Marfan syndrome affects 1 in 5000 of the population, and approximately 70% of these patients develop a spinal deformity. Diagnosis can be confirmed by linkage to the Marfan syndrome gene *MFS1*, the protein product of which produces fibrillin. Marfan genotype-phenotype correlations

show association with severe mutations in 25% of persons with the syndrome, with 50% of those in the latter half of the exon (exons 33 to 63). Related syndromes may result from mutations in microfibrils that interact with fibrillin in the extracellular matrix. Congenital contractual arachnodactyly (Beals syndrome), in which scoliosis is common, also has been shown to be caused by fibrillin deficiency.

Neurofibromatosis type 1 (NF) is a multisystem disease, with scoliosis being the most common bone manifestation, occurring in 10% to 30% of patients. Genome-wide scans have identified the likely chromosomal locus on 17q11.

GENETICS OF IDIOPATHIC SCOLIOSIS

The genetic basis of idiopathic scoliosis remains unclear, and causation may be multifactorial in that particular growth patterns may exacerbate a genetic predisposition. Support for an underlying genetic cause comes from data showing an incidence of idiopathic scoliosis in 6.94%, 3.69%, and 1.55% in first-, second-, and third-degree relatives, respectively, of 114 affected persons. These findings are consistent with either an autosomal dominant or a multifactorial mode of inheritance. A large kindred with autosomal dominant idiopathic scoliosis has been identified with a chromosomal locus on 17p11. By contrast, congenital scoliosis is relatively common among congenital malformations and is associated with congenital heart and renal tract anomalies. An autosomal recessive form of congenital scoliosis has been found in male and female sibships with consanguineous parents, associated with lack of vertebral segmentation and fused ribs. Mouse models for idiopathic scoliosis have been developed, and the list of candidate genes continues to grow, indicating the underlying etiologic complexity and probable interaction of genetic, environmental, and developmental factors.

Spinal curvature is acquired in neuromuscular disorders (**Figure 63-3**) that involve the chest wall and thoracic musculature before skeletal maturity occurs. Scoliosis develops in more than 50% of boys with Duchenne muscular dystrophy (DMD), and spinal curvature is common in many of the other congenital muscular dystrophies, myopathies, and conditions such as type I and type II spinal muscular atrophy. The introduction of steroid therapy in childhood in DMD may lessen the severity of scoliosis by reducing the rate of loss of muscle strength, such that wheelchair dependency occurs later in adolescence and peak vital capacity is increased, although the number of prospective randomized controlled trials has been limited.

A scoliotic deformity often develops as a sequela of thoracotomy carried out in childhood or young adulthood.

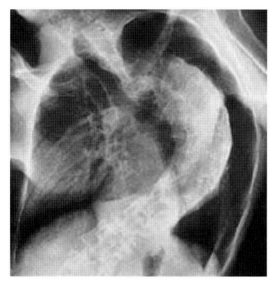

Figure 63-1 Radiograph showing lateral curvature of the spine in a patient with congenital idiopathic scoliosis.

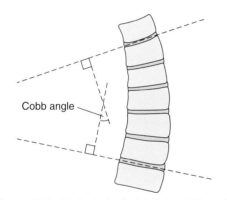

Figure 63-2 Method of calculating the Cobb angle.

Cobb angle

KYPHOSIS

Idiopathic kyphosis is rare. An increase in thoracic kyphosis occurs with age and is exacerbated by factors that increase a tendency to osteoporosis, such as oral corticosteroid therapy. Pott's disease, or tuberculosis (TB) of the spine, is still a common cause of acquired kyphosis in TB-endemic geographic regions.

EFFECTS OF CHEST WALL DEFORMITY ON RESPIRATORY AND CARDIAC FUNCTION

Chest wall disorders affect respiratory function and cause a restrictive ventilatory defect. Any significant scoliosis or kyphosis results in a loss of height, so arm span can be used to predict normal lung volumes. As a general rule, patients who have a thoracic curve of greater than 70 degrees are subject to significant ventilatory limitation.

Lung Volumes

Although both scoliosis and kyphosis diminish lung volumes, which results in a restrictive ventilatory defect, lateral curvature has a more profound effect on chest wall mechanics. Total lung capacity is reduced in all chest wall disorders. In a pure scoliosis, both vital capacity (VC) and expiratory reserve volume are decreased, with relative preservation of residual

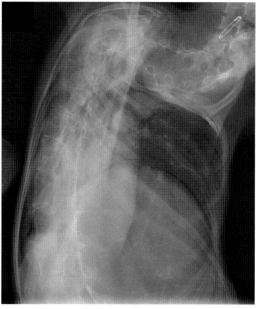

Figure 63-3 Radiograph showing extensive severe neuromuscular scoliosis in a patient with type II spinal muscular atrophy.

Box 63-1 | Classification of Spinal Deformity

Idiopathic Deformities	**Deformity Associated With Neuromuscular Disease**
Idiopathic scoliosis	Cerebral palsy
Idiopathic kyphosis	Poliomyelitis
	Muscular dystrophies
Congenital Deformities	Myopathies
Bone	Hereditary sensory motor
Scoliosis	neuropathies
Kyphosis	Friedreich ataxia
	Syringomyelia
Cord	
Myelodysplasia	**Acquired Deformity**
	Secondary to Insult or Disease
Syndromes in Which	Surgery/trauma
Scoliosis Is Common	Infection
Neurofibromatosis	Pyogenic
Marfan syndrome	Tuberculosis (Pott kyphosis)
Osteogenesis imperfecta	Radiotherapy
Klippel-Feil syndrome	Tumor
Mucopolysaccharidoses	Neuroblastoma
Treacher Collins syndrome	Osteoma
Goldenhar syndrome	Hemangioma
Apert syndrome	Chordoma
Ehlers-Danlos syndrome	Eosinophilic granuloma
Vertebral and epiphyseal	
dysplasias	
Arthrogryposis	

volume (**Table 63-1**). An obstructive ventilatory defect is rare in scoliosis and kyphosis, unless the individual is a smoker, has coexistent asthma, or the scoliosis results in bronchial torsion.

The relationship between pulmonary impairment and the deformity is complex and cannot be predicted accurately from the Cobb angle alone. The four major determinants of a reduced VC are the number of vertebrae involved in the curve, position of the curve closer to the head, Cobb angle, and the degree of loss of normal thoracic kyphosis.

Table 63-1 Typical Results on Pulmonary Function Testing in Patients With Idiopathic Thoracic Scoliosis

Parameter	Effect
Forced expiratory volume in 1 second (FEV$_1$)	Reduced
Forced vital capacity (FVC)	Reduced
FEV$_1$/FVC	Normal
Residual volume	Normal
Total lung capacity	Reduced
Transfer factor for carbon monoxide—diffusion capacity (DL$_{CO}$)	Reduced
Transfer coefficient (K_{CO})—DL$_{CO}$/accessible alveolar volume	Supranormal*

*Transfer coefficient usually is supranormal, but it is reduced in the presence of pulmonary hypertension.

In paralytic scoliosis, lung volumes are reduced not only by chest wall restriction but also by inspiratory muscle weakness.

Chest Wall Mechanics

Chest wall compliance (CCW) is an important determinant of lung volumes and the work of breathing. Patients with a Cobb angle of less than 50 degrees experience a minimal reduction in CCW, whereas CCW is likely to be significantly reduced if the Cobb angle is greater than 100 degrees. A direct relationship between Cobb angle and CCW is not seen in patients with neuromuscular disorders, because respiratory muscle weakness contributes independently to chest wall stiffness. Alteration in chest wall properties cannot be attributed solely to the mechanical deformity of scoliosis, because a decrease in CCW has been found in patients affected by chronic respiratory muscle weakness in the absence of a scoliosis.

Lung Compliance

Although lung expansion is compromised by chest wall properties, primary pulmonary pathology is unusual in patients who have idiopathic scoliosis. Lung compliance is reduced, however, because of a shift in the pressure-volume curve to the right. These changes in pulmonary characteristics arise largely from an alteration in alveolar forces caused by chronic hypoventilation. In patients with neuromuscular disease, microatelectasis and macroatelectasis may complicate the picture. Microatelectasis seems relatively rare, however, because fine-section (thinslice) CT scans have shown areas of atelectasis in only a minority of patients affected by respiratory muscle weakness. Patients with neuromuscular disease who exhibit bulbar weakness or an ineffectual cough are at increased risk for recurrent pneumonia. Severe lateral curvature of the spine in a minority of patients can produce bronchial torsion, and obstruction of the bronchus by this mechanism may lead to recurrent distal infection. Pulmonary fibrosis also is a histopathologic feature in patients who have "old" TB, in whom areas of bronchiectasis may be seen. Cystic lung changes may be noted in some patients with neurofibromatosis.

Gas transfer coefficient tends to be raised in patients with scoliosis in the presence of a low transfer factor (see Table 63-1), because extrathoracic compression squeezes more air than blood out of the lungs, thereby decreasing accessible alveolar volume.

Respiratory Muscles/Thoracic Pump During Sleep

Impaired respiratory muscle function might be expected in idiopathic scoliosis, because the respiratory muscles work at a mechanical disadvantage when chest wall shape is altered. A reduction in transdiaphragmatic pressure and static respiratory mouth pressures have been demonstrated in patients who have scoliosis or a thoracoplasty. These findings tend to support the contention that the efficiency of the respiratory muscles may be affected by relatively small degrees of chest wall deformity. Respiratory muscle action is further reduced by the loss of intercostal muscle tone during rapid eye movement (REM) sleep and a reduced ability to compensate for added respiratory load. The effect of these changes explains why early features of ventilatory failure during sleep predate the development of daytime ventilatory failure.

Control of Breathing

Impaired hypercapnic ventilatory drive usually is secondary to chronic CO$_2$ retention in patients with scoliosis. However, primary drive disorders may complicate some neuromuscular conditions (e.g., myotonic dystrophy) and may be acquired in patients in whom poliomyelitis has compromised brain stem control mechanisms. Generally, however, ventilatory drive is increased in patients with neuromuscular disease, to compensate for respiratory muscle insufficiency.

Pulmonary and Cardiac Hemodynamics

Cor pulmonale is the end-stage result of severe, untreated chest wall deformity. Pulmonary artery pressure becomes elevated at rest with an inverse correlation between pulmonary artery pressure and arterial oxygen tension. In some patients with severe scoliosis, a disproportionate rise in pulmonary artery pressure on exercise can be seen in the absence of hypoxemia, because the restricted thorax is unable to accommodate the increase in cardiac output on exertion.

An additional stress on hemodynamics is the effect of nocturnal hypoventilation on pulmonary artery pressure. The exact level of nocturnal hypoxemia that generates pulmonary hypertension is unknown, but if it is severe, nocturnal arterial blood gas disturbances inevitably lead to daytime problems if the condition is left untreated.

Impact of Adolescent Idiopathic Scoliosis on Exercise Capacity

In a recent case-control study, the relationship among pulmonary function, muscle strength, and exercise ability was explored in 60 patients with adolescent-onset scoliosis (AIS) and Cobb angles greater than 40 degrees, and the findings were compared with data for 25 control subjects. The patients with AIS had mild to moderate ventilatory limitation (FVC of 86% predicted), but both respiratory muscle and limb muscle strength together with exercise capacity were reduced in comparison with those in control subjects. In the AIS group exercise capacity was 58% predicted with a maximum oxygen uptake of 60% predicted. Arterial oxygen saturation values on exercise remained normal. Of note, no relationship was found between the Cobb angle and lung function, muscle function, or exercise capacity. Exercise ability, however, was correlated with inspiratory, expiratory, and limb muscle function, with the main contributor on multiple regression analysis found to be limb muscle function. This finding suggests that generalized muscle dysfunction is key to explaining exercise limitation *in the absence of severe ventilatory impairment* and underscores the point that AIS may be a systemic disease process.

CLINICAL FEATURES

Spinal abnormalities are best evaluated by ascertaining the age at onset, etiology, and location of the curve (e.g., adolescent onset, idiopathic thoracic scoliosis). During physical examination, accompanying features should be sought, such as café-au-lait spots and neurofibromas. Marfan syndrome is a clinical diagnosis that requires the involvement of two of three main systems—ocular, cardiac, and skeletal. A careful search for cardiac lesions is mandatory in patients with early-onset scoliosis, which is associated with an increased incidence of congenital heart disease. Skeletal lesions demonstrated radiologically, such as hemivertebrae and rib fusion, suggest the presence of a congenital scoliosis.

Patients are observed in the standing position and then viewed bending forward, to obtain an indication of the degree of lateral rib hump deformity. Assessment of shoulder and pelvic symmetry, leg length, and gait is helpful. The lower back should be examined for hairy tufts and other cutaneous stigmata of spinal dysraphism, and a full neurologic examination should be performed.

PROGRESSION OF CURVATURE

Detailed studies of the natural history of untreated idiopathic scoliosis are rare, but the younger the age at presentation, the greater the potential for progression, because more of the growth spurt needs to be accommodated, and spinal growth continues until at least the age of 25 years. High and low thoracic curves, together with thoracolumbar curves, seem to be more unstable than lumbar deformities. Curves most likely to progress include those caused by congenital failure of segmentation, infantile idiopathic scoliosis, the angular curve of neurofibromatosis, pronounced paralytic curves, and scoliosis associated with progressive childhood neuromuscular conditions.

In AIS, key determinants of progression are the growth potential of the child at presentation and the magnitude of the curve. On evaluation using standard indices of skeletal maturity, skeletally immature children with a more pronounced curve (20 to 29 degrees) at initial diagnosis had a 68% risk of curve progression, whereas more mature teenagers with similar curves showed a 23% risk of curve progression. Conversely, immature children with lesser curves (5 to 19 degrees) had a 22% chance of curve progression, whereas mature children had only a 1.6% chance of progression. It also has been shown that children with curves of less than 30 degrees at skeletal maturity did not experience curve progression in adulthood, whereas a majority of curves greater than 50 degrees progressed at a rate of approximately 1 degree per year.

DIAGNOSIS

CARDIOPULMONARY DECOMPENSATION: IDENTIFICATION OF HIGH-RISK CASES

Most patients who have a thoracic spinal curvature do not develop cardiorespiratory problems and therefore do not require long-term respiratory follow-up evaluations. It is important to identify the minority at risk for such problems, however, so that appropriate monitoring and therapeutic intervention can be carried out.

Cor pulmonale was the primary cause of death in a series of 102 untreated patients with idiopathic thoracic scoliosis. Age at onset of the scoliosis is crucial to ascertain. Branthwaite showed that in patients in whom cardiorespiratory problems attributable to their scoliosis developed, 90% had an early-onset curvature (i.e., onset before the age of 5 years).

A VC of 50% predicted is an important cutoff value, because respiratory decompensation is much more likely to develop in patients with a VC of less than 50% predicted at presentation than in those with initially larger lung volumes.

In a study by Braithwaite, the mean age of patients in respiratory failure who presented for ventilatory support was 49 years for those with idiopathic scoliosis, 51 years for those with previous poliomyelitis, and 62 years for those who had sequelae of pulmonary TB. Pehrsson and co-workers followed lung function over a period of 20 years in patients with idiopathic scoliosis. Respiratory failure occurred in 25%, all of whom had a VC of less than 45% predicted and a thoracic Cobb angle greater than 110 degrees.

MONITORING HIGH-RISK PATIENTS

Monitoring high-risk patients should include the following:

- Assessment for breathlessness, exercise intolerance and associated limiting factors, frequency of chest infections, and symptoms of nocturnal hypoventilation
- Clinical examination
- Pulmonary function testing
- Arterial blood gas analysis
- Measurement of respiratory muscle strength (e.g., mouth pressures, sniff inspiratory pressure)
- Spinal and chest radiology

Additional investigations may be indicated:

- MRI scanning may be required to delineate spinal cord and vertebral anomalies, and computed tomography may be needed to investigate abnormalities such as pulmonary hypoplasia or bronchial torsion.
- Echocardiography (ECG) is mandatory in all patients with congenital or early-onset scoliosis.

A fall in VC of more than 15% predicted on assuming the supine position indicates significant diaphragm weakness. Daytime hypercapnia is associated with an inspiratory mouth pressure of less than 30% predicted.

As noted, in addition to detecting breathlessness and exercise tolerance, the assessment should identify any symptoms of nocturnal hypoventilation (morning headache, poor sleep quality, frequent arousals, nocturnal confusion, and morning anorexia); if any of these is present, the patient should undergo monitoring of respiration during sleep. A characteristic picture of nocturnal hypoventilation, with episodes of desaturation and CO_2 retention most pronounced in REM sleep, usually is revealed (**Figure 63-4**).

TREATMENT

MANAGEMENT OF SPINAL DEFORMITY

Conservative Management

The success of a conservative approach depends on the age of the patient, the severity of the curvature at presentation, and its propensity to progression. For example, an infantile idiopathic scoliosis may spontaneously regress, whereas a juvenile-onset scoliosis is more likely to progress.

NOCTURNAL HYPOVENTILATION

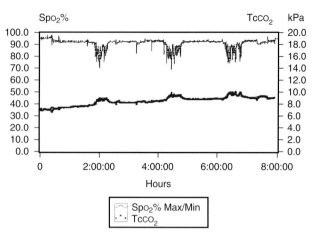

Figure 63-4 Overnight recording of oximetry-determined oxygen saturation (SpO₂) and transcutaneous carbon dioxide tension (TcCO₂) in a patient with early-onset scoliosis. The initial clinical presentation was one of sleep disturbance and morning headaches. The tracings show three periods of dips in SpO₂ and peaks of TcCO₂ in rapid eye movement sleep.

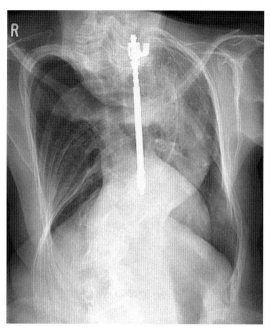

Figure 63-5 Radiograph showing instrumentation in place in a patient with scoliosis treated with a Harrington rod.

Bracing

Devices such as the Milwaukee and Cotrell braces have been used extensively, and these continue to evolve. The mechanical aim of the brace is to re-create a normal thoracic kyphosis, hyperextend the spine, and limit forward flexion, all of which will act to derotate the scoliosis. Bracing probably works more effectively with a kyphosis than with a scoliosis. In paralytic disorders, a circumferential brace can support the trunk, thereby making sitting more comfortable. Vital capacity should always be measured with and without the brace in place.

Surgery for Scoliosis

In general, surgery is performed to correct unacceptable deformity and to prevent progression. It is not carried out to improve ventilatory function.

Thoracic scolioses with curves of more than 45 degrees usually are judged to be unacceptable. A lesser curve associated with a greater degree of rotation, however, may create a rib hump, which is just as concerning to the patient. It is a surgical maxim that even the best operative technique does not completely straighten a spine. An approximately 50% correction of the Cobb angle in smaller curves can be expected from an instrumentation procedure. The best guide to a successful result is the initial amount of spinal flexibility. Also, the greater the degree of rotation, the greater the inflexibility of the curve.

Spinal fusion followed by casting has now been superseded in many situations by rod instrumentation (**Figure 63-5**). The system provides distraction to the concave side of the spine and compression to the convex side, which enhances stabilization and reduces any rotational tendency. Instrumentation is used to stabilize the curve and spinal fusion to prevent growth. A posterior approach is used, but with a severe deformity or very rigid curvature, an anterior approach may be required to release the disk space. The combined anterior and posterior approach carries greater anesthetic and surgical risk. In patients with AIS, surgical complication rates are around 5% to 6%, with wound infections being more common after posterior fusion and pulmonary complications more frequent with use of an anterior approach. Weiss and colleagues have recently debated the pros and cons of surgical correction in AIS.

Preoperative assessment should include the investigations listed previously. In persons with a VC less than 50% predicted, a sleep study should be considered. If there is evidence of nocturnal hypoventilation, use of noninvasive ventilation (NIV) in the perioperative period may be helpful.

A recent consensus conference of scoliosis surgery in patients with Duchenne muscular dystrophy (DMD) highlighted the fact that scoliosis surgery should be carried out in centers with full access to multidisciplinary respiratory and cardiac input. The key aim of scoliosis surgery in these neuromuscular conditions is *not* to improve lung function, because most studies show no major impact on postoperative lung volumes, but to prevent further progression of the curve and to improve comfort and sitting position in a wheelchair. Surgery should optimally be performed in DMD and other neuromuscular conditions when pulmonary function is not too compromised (as reflected in an FVC greater than 30% predicted) but has been carried out safely in patients with VC between 20% and 30% predicted as supportive care such as NIV in the postoperative period and cough assistance with a mechanical insufflator-exsufflator has become available. All patients with DMD are at risk for development of cardiomyopathy, and left ventricular function and ECG should be monitored closely. Surgery-associated risks are likely to increase if left ventricular fractional shortening is less than 25%, and these risks should be carefully balanced against the overall prognosis.

MANAGEMENT OF VENTILATORY IMPAIRMENT

Optimization of Respiratory Function

Individuals should be advised of the adverse effects of smoking and obesity and encouraged to enroll in appropriate intervention programs. The influenza and pneumococcal vaccines are recommended for persons who have ventilatory limitations.

Bisphosphonate therapy reduces the risk of osteoporosis in postmenopausal women and also in men. Care should be taken not to miss the reactivation of TB in patients with a thoracoplasty. Patients who have Marfan syndrome may require β-adrenergic blocker therapy to reduce the risk of aortic dissection.

Exercise should be encouraged, other than for persons with pulmonary hypertension and patients with Marfan syndrome. Pulmonary rehabilitation programs suggest that exercise and a reduction in deconditioning is just as valuable in restrictive disorders as in chronic obstructive pulmonary disease.

Ventilatory Failure

The evidence now clearly shows that ventilatory failure in patients who have chest wall disease can be successfully treated by use of NIV at night. Negative-pressure devices are effective but have been supplanted by noninvasive positive-pressure ventilation systems. In patients with scoliosis who receive NIV, the 5-year survival rate is approximately 80%, with rates of 100% in patients with previous poliomyelitis and greater than 90% in those with post-TB conditions. It seems increasingly likely that persons who have nonprogressive disorders may live a normal or near-normal life span, provided that NIV is introduced before the development of intractable pulmonary hypertension. Patients report good quality of life with use of NIV, and many are able to return to work.

Of note, NIV produces a more favorable outcome than that achieved with long-term oxygen therapy (LTOT) in patients with scoliosis. In a retrospective analysis of consecutive patients with kyphoscoliosis who started LTOT alone or NIV in Belgium, 1-year survival was higher in the NIV treatment group (100% versus 66%), and NIV-managed patients demonstrated a greater improvement in PaO_2 and $PaCO_2$. More recently, these results have been confirmed in a larger Swedish cohort, for which the reported survival rate was three times higher in NIV users than in those receiving LTOT alone, and this was unrelated to baseline arterial blood gas tensions, gender, or respiratory comorbidity. In general, oxygen usually is combined with NIV at night if mean SaO_2 on NIV alone is not above 90%, despite adequate control of $PaCO_2$. Evidence that any one type of ventilator is superior in patients with scoliosis is lacking, although some patients with congenital or idiopathic scoliosis may require relatively high inflation pressures.

NIV also can be used to palliate symptoms of breathlessness and cor pulmonale in patients who have progressive disorders and will alter the natural history of these conditions. A 5-year survival as high as 73% can be achieved in DMD, and many patients with DMD are now surviving into their 30s and early 40s.

CONTROVERSIES AND PITFALLS

CLINICAL SIGNS IN SCOLIOSIS

In patients with severe scoliosis in whom asthma subsequently develops, an important consideration is that a characteristic wheeze may not be heard because of low airflow. Measurement of spirometry and home peak flow monitoring are useful in these cases.

An isolated unifocal wheeze may indicate bronchial torsion or kinking, which can occur in patients with severe scoliosis and may be associated with bronchiectasis or hyperinflation in the distal lung lobe. Bronchial stenting has been successfully used in this situation. In the case shown in **Figure 63-6**, the right bronchus intermedius was partially obstructed by torsion and compression against the spine. The clinical consequence

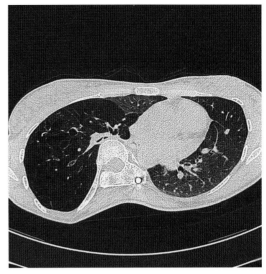

Figure 63-6 Computed tomography scan showing compression of right bronchial tree and hyperinflated right lower lobe with cystic change. The patient had a staphylococcal pneumonia that resulted from the ventilatory obstruction. *(Courtesy P. Rafferty.)*

was development of a staphylococcal pneumonia with cystic changes affecting the right lower lobe.

PREGNANCY AND SCOLIOSIS

A successful outcome from pregnancy is usual in most patients who have adolescent-onset idiopathic scoliosis. In a survey of 118 pregnancies in 64 women who had thoracic scoliosis, no serious medical problems were encountered, with a cesarean rate of 17% for obstetric reasons. More recently, in a study of 142 pregnancies in women who had been treated with Harrington rod surgery, the proportion of cases requiring cesarean section was slightly higher than in the general population, but the rates of complications in pregnancy and delivery did not exceed those in the general population, and the offspring were healthy. About 40% of mothers developed low back pain during pregnancy, but this had resolved by 3 months after delivery in a majority. Likewise, a 2010 survey of cases of mostly idiopathic scoliosis in India shows a higher cesarean rate than for women without scoliosis, and no major problems with maternal health were reported.

However, cardiorespiratory complications can be expected in women with a VC less than 1.0 L. Stable curves are unlikely to progress during pregnancy. Prepregnancy counseling and assessment are sensible in patients with scoliosis, particularly those with congenital or early-onset curves or a VC less than 50% predicted. Assessment should include full pulmonary and cardiologic evaluation and genetic counselling. Pregnancy is contraindicated in the presence of pulmonary hypertension and hypoxemia. If ventilatory problems arise in pregnancy, the situation may be successfully managed by use of NIV.

SUGGESTED READINGS

Bergofsky EH: Thoracic deformities. In Roussos C, editor: *The thorax; part C: disease*, New York, 1995, Marcel Dekker, pp 1915–1949.

Branthwaite MA: Cardiorespiratory consequences of unfused idiopathic scoliosis, *Br J Dis Chest* 80:360–369, 1986.

Buyse B, Meersseman W, Demedts M: Treatment of chronic respiratory failure in kyphoscoliosis: oxygen or ventilation? *Eur Respir J* 22:525–528, 2003.

Chopra S, Adhikari K, Agarwal N, et al: Kyphoscoliosis complicating pregnancy: maternal and neonatal outcome, *Arch Gynecol Obstet* 284:295–297, 2011.

Giampietro PF, Blank RD, Raggio CL, et al: Congenital and idiopathic scoliosis: clinical and genetic aspects, *Clin Med Res* 1:125–136, 2003.

Gustafson T, Franklin KA, Midgren B, et al: Survival of patients with kyphoscoliosis receiving mechanical ventilation or oxygen at home, *Chest* 130:1828–1833, 2006.

Lowe TG, Edgar M, Margulies JY, et al: Etiology of idiopathic scoliosis: current trends in research, *J Bone Joint Surg Am* 82-A:1157–1168, 2000.

Martinez-Llorens J, Ramirez M, Colomina MJ, et al: Muscle dysfunction and exercise limitation in adolescent idiopathic scoliosis, *Eur Respir J* 36:393–400, 2010.

Orvoman E, Hiilesmaa V, Poussa M, et al: Pregnancy and delivery in patients operated by Harrington method for idiopathic scoliosis, *Eur Spine J* 6:304–307, 1997.

Pehrsson K, Bake B, Larsson S, Nachemson A: Lung function in adult idiopathic scoliosis: a 20 year follow up, *Thorax* 46:474–478, 1991.

Simonds AK: Home non-invasive ventilation in restrictive disorders and stable neuromuscular disease. In Simonds AK, editor: *Non-invasive respiratory support: a practical handbook*, ed 3, London, 2007, Arnold, pp 184–188.

Weiss HR, Bess S, Wong MS, et al: Adolescent idiopathic scoliosis—to operate or not? A debate article, *Patient Saf Surg* 2:25, 2008.

Chapter **64**

Diseases of the Thoracic Cage and Respiratory Muscles

Michelle Ramsay • Michael I. Polkey • Nicholas Hart

Dyspnea and alveolar hypoventilation occur in patients with restrictive lung disease as a consequence of an imbalance between the respiratory muscle load and respiratory muscle capacity. Subsequent modification of the neural respiratory drive occurs, which directly reflects this imbalance. This chapter begins with an overview of the anatomy of the respiratory muscle pump and includes a detailed explanation of the pathophysiology of chronic respiratory failure. It provides a comprehensive guide to the physician of how best to assess and investigate a patient with suspected respiratory compromise from respiratory muscle weakness, chest wall disease, or obesity. The second part of the chapter focuses on specific neurologic/neuromuscular and chest wall diseases associated with respiratory impairment.

RESPIRATORY MUSCLE PUMP

The respiratory system is made up of two main components: the respiratory muscle pump, which facilitates airflow, thereby enabling ventilation, and the lungs, which support pulmonary gas exchange (see Chapter 6 for more detailed explanations and for respiratory muscle testing). The respiratory muscle pump itself is made up of the inspiratory muscles, the diaphragm and extradiaphragmatic accessory muscles, and the expiratory muscles, principally the abdominal wall muscles. Inspiration is an active process in which contraction of the diaphragm forces the abdominal contents in an anterocaudal direction to allow the volume of the chest cavity to increase. This expansion, in turn, generates a negative subatmospheric pressure to form a pressure gradient that drives air into the lungs. At rest, expiration is a passive process with the elastic properties of the chest wall and lungs providing the recoil forces that allow the lung volume to return to the functional residual capacity. During exercise and forced expiratory maneuvers (e.g., coughing), however, contraction of the abdominal muscles occurs, pushing the diaphragm upward in the absence of flow limitation.

CLINICAL CONSEQUENCES OF RESPIRATORY MUSCLE PUMP IMBALANCE

Breathlessness, alveolar hypoventilation and hypercapnic respiratory failure result from an imbalance between the respiratory muscle load, capacity, and neural respiratory drive (**Figure 64-1**). By using this model the physician can develop a simple clinical tool to assess the breathless patient and the patient in chronic respiratory failure. More commonly, in patients with

restrictive lung disease, the reduction in capacity occurs as a consequence of intrinsic muscle weakness. On occasion, however, capacity may be relatively preserved, but in the context of a significant respiratory muscle load or poor orientation of the inspiratory muscles (e.g., kyphoscoliosis), this may limit the pressure-generating capacity, so that dyspnea and alveolar hypoventilation can develop subsequently. In critically ill patients, the respiratory muscle weakness may be transient and reversible, such as occurs in respiratory acidosis, hypokalemia, and hypophosphatemia (**Box 64-1**).

An increase in respiratory muscle load occurs in patients with increased airway resistance, chest wall deformity, or obesity. Any of these conditions will accelerate the onset of dyspnea and alveolar hypoventilation in patients with respiratory muscle weakness (**Figure 64-2**).

In healthy subjects, a significant reduction in neural respiratory drive to skeletal muscle, including the respiratory muscles, occurs during sleep. Despite the complete loss of skeletal muscle activity during rapid eye movement (REM) sleep, in normal subjects significant nocturnal hypoxia and hypercapnia are avoided because the activation of the diaphragm to maintain ventilation is preserved. By contrast, in patients with respiratory muscle weakness, especially diaphragmatic weakness and paralysis, hypoventilation during REM sleep often is the first sign of declining respiratory function. Of interest, in patients with idiopathic diaphragmatic paralysis, hypoventilation is prevented by a neuroadaptive mechanism with cyclic activation of the sternocleidomastoid muscle during REM sleep, which maintains ventilation. Also, there is substantial reserve in the respiratory muscle pump such that inspiratory muscle strength must fall to one third of normal before the onset of respiratory failure. Furthermore, clinical deterioration is observed at an earlier stage if an increased load is applied to the system, such as in pneumonia, or if the neural respiratory drive is modified with drugs such as benzodiazepines, opiates, and other anesthetic agents used during routine anesthesia.

ASSESSMENT OF THE RESPIRATORY MUSCLE PUMP

The respiratory muscle pump is essential for effective ventilation and to maintain gas exchange. In addition to a directed clinical history and examination, the physician can use simple bedside tests as well as more advanced measurements of respiratory muscle function to perform a detailed assessment of the patient with restrictive respiratory muscle and chest wall disease.

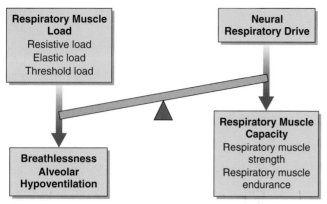

Figure 64-1 The respiratory muscle pump.

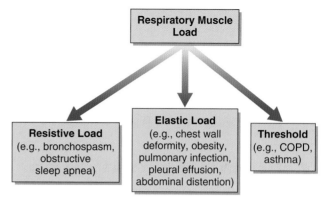

Figure 64-2 Types of respiratory muscle load. *COPD,* chronic obstructive pulmonary disease.

Box 64-1 Causes of Respiratory Muscle Weakness

Neurogenic
Motor neuron disease
Polyneuropathy (e.g., Guillain-Barré syndrome)
Critical illness neuromyopathy
Neuralgic amyotrophy
Poliomyelitis
Spinal cord injury
Trauma of phrenic nerves (e.g., from radiotherapy or coronary artery bypass grafting)

Neuromuscular Junction
Myasthenia gravis
Eaton-Lambert syndrome

Muscular
Muscular dystrophies
Inflammatory myopathies (e.g., polymyositis, dermatomyositis)
Acid maltase deficiency
Thyroid myopathy
Biochemical abnormalities (e.g., acidosis, hypophosphatemia, hypokalemia)
Malnutrition myopathy

Table 64-1 Important Clinical Features in Diseases of the Thoracic Cage and Respiratory Muscles

Disorder	Clinical Manifestations
Sleep-disordered breathing	Morning headache, daytime sleepiness, disrupted sleep pattern, impaired intellectual function, generalized fatigue, loss of appetite and weight
Respiratory muscle weakness	Orthopnea, breathlessness on immersion in water, breathlessness on leaning forward, breathlessness on exertion, poor cough, poor chest expansion, paradoxical abdominal motion during inspiration (inward motion of the anterior abdominal wall due to diaphragm weakness), abdominal muscle recruitment in expiration
Bulbar dysfunction	Low volume voice, difficulty swallowing, drooling, difficulty clearing secretions, poor cough, staccato/slurred speech, coughing on swallowing

Clinical Features

As always, a detailed history will facilitate making a correct diagnosis (Table 64-1). Of particular importance is the rate of onset of symptoms. Acute respiratory muscle weakness tends to progress rapidly, culminating in a medical emergency requiring intubation and mechanical ventilation. Some causes of acute respiratory muscle weakness, such as an acute myasthenic crisis or Guillain-Barré disease, may be reversible, and it is important to facilitate invasive respiratory support in the acute setting until a diagnosis can be made and appropriate therapies initiated. In chronic respiratory failure, the onset may not be clear, but clues to the course of events can be gained from the history. Often patients will describe dyspnea on exertion, but if peripheral muscle weakness precedes respiratory muscle weakness, the consequent loss of significant locomotor function will not permit exertion of sufficient degree to produce dyspnea. Classic features of diaphragm weakness are not always present in patients with generalized neuromuscular disease but may include dyspnea on lying supine, on bending forward, or on immersion in water above the midchest level. If respiratory weakness is severe, patients also may describe symptoms of nocturnal hypoventilation, such as extensive daytime somnolence, reduced concentration, and morning headaches that typically resolve within 30 minutes of waking. Specifically, in the pediatric and adolescent populations, clinicians should be alerted to more subtle clinical features such as failing school performance, recurrent episodes of chest sepsis, reduction in appetite, and weight loss.

In all cases of respiratory muscle weakness, an important aspect of the evaluation is to identify any symptoms that may suggest generalized neuromuscular weakness—in particular, decrements in the patient's speech and swallowing function, as well as weakness of the arms and legs. Weakness of the abdominal muscles may result in difficulty achieving an effective cough to clear secretions and debris from the airways. This impairment leads to issues with sputum retention and increases the risk of chest infection. In the case of chest wall disease, the common causes kyphoscoliosis and obesity usually are self-evident. As highlighted earlier, certain drugs have effects that can accelerate respiratory decline, so attention should be given to the common offenders, such as benzodiazepines, opiates, and corticosteroids. More recently, in particular, in the Duchenne muscular dystrophy (DMD) population, corticosteroids are increasingly being used to maintain locomotor muscle function, and these agents are associated with substantial weight gain and consequent upper airway obstruction. Clinicians must be aware of this potential problem in this younger patient population.

Physical examination requires a careful and considered approach, which must include a thorough neurologic examination to observe for signs of tongue and peripheral muscle fasciculation, peripheral muscle wasting and weakness, and peripheral sensory loss. Other signs, such as pseudohypertrophy of the calf muscles, are observed in patients with muscular dystrophies. Scars of previous operations may indicate possible trauma to underlying neuromuscular structures or an imposed restrictive chest wall deformity, such as from a phrenic nerve crush, thoracoplasty, coronary artery bypass grafting, thyroidectomy, or thymoma resection. With severe diaphragm weakness, abdominal inspiratory paradox is observed: The anterior abdominal wall moves inward as a result of the failure of a weak or paralyzed diaphragm to descend against the force exerted by the abdominal contents. With more generalized weakness, global loss of thoracic expansion on inspiration is observed.

Arterial Blood Gas Analysis

Although arterial blood gas analysis is one of the most common first-line investigations to diagnose chronic respiratory failure, limitations associated with this technique have been recognized. In particular, the daytime partial pressure of carbon dioxide ($PaCO_2$) may be normal despite the presence of substantial inspiratory muscle weakness, nocturnal hypoventilation, and nocturnal hypercapnia. Measurement of arterial blood gas partial pressures is essential, however, to define the severity of respiratory failure. Most commonly, hypoventilation caused by neuromuscular respiratory weakness and chest wall disease manifests with a mild hypoxia, with a partial pressure of oxygen (PaO_2) less than 60 mm Hg, and hypercapnia, with a $PaCO_2$ greater than 45 mm Hg.

The respiratory failure associated with many neurologic and chest wall conditions frequently manifests insidiously, with hypercapnia triggering metabolic compensation and renal retention of bicarbonate to maintain the hydrogen ions and, consequently, arterial pH within the normal range.

In the event of rapid onset of neurologic symptoms, such as in Guillain-Barré syndrome and myasthenic syndrome, or with acute deterioration of chronic respiratory failure, there is less time for renal buffering, so hypercapnic respiratory acidosis will occur.

Pulmonary Function Tests

Patients with respiratory neuromuscular weakness and those with chest wall disease both are characterized by a reduced ability to expand the thoracic rib cage. In turn, this failure to expand the rib cage results in a lack of generation of sufficient negative intrathoracic pressure to facilitate adequate inspiratory airflow. As a result, these patients present with clinical features of a restrictive lung function pattern characterized by a reduced forced vital capacity (FVC) and an elevated ratio of forced expiratory volume in 1 second (FEV_1) to FVC (FEV_1/FVC greater than 80%). Although vital capacity (VC) is in widespread use and is relatively simple to determine, its utility is limited because it has low sensitivity. In particular, significant inspiratory muscle weakness is required before a significant fall in VC is observed. A fall in VC on adoption of the supine position is specific for respiratory muscle weakness, and a fall in VC of more than 20% suggests bilateral diaphragmatic weakness. Of importance, the VC can be preserved in persons with a moderate degree of global respiratory muscle weakness or hemidiaphragm weakness.

The pattern of respiratory muscle weakness must be considered in interpreting results of pulmonary function tests in

Table 64-2 Pulmonary Function Tests for Patients with Predominantly Inspiratory Muscle Weakness and Combined Inspiratory/Expiratory Muscle Weakness

Inspiratory Muscle Weakness	Combined Inspiratory/ Expiratory Muscle Weakness
Reduced VC	Reduced VC
Fall in supine VC >20%	N/A
FEV_1/FVC ratio >80%	FEV_1/FVC ratio >80%
Reduced TLC	Reduced TLC
Normal RV	Increased RV
Reduced FRC	Increased FRC
Reduced TLco	Reduced TLco
"Supranormal" Kco	Reduced Kco

FEV_1, forced expiratory volume in 1 second FRC, functional residual capacity; FVC, forced vital capacity; Kco, gas transfer coefficient corrected for alveolar volume; N/A, not available; RV, residual volume; TLC, total lung capacity; TLco, overall gas transfer; VC, vital capacity.

patients with chest wall disease and respiratory muscle weakness. Although total lung capacity (TLC) and VC are reduced in patients with predominantly inspiratory muscle weakness and combined inspiratory and expiratory muscle weakness, the pattern of weakness influences functional residual capacity (FRC), residual volume (RV), overall gas transfer (DLco), and gas transfer corrected for alveolar volume (**Table 64-2**).

Tests of Respiratory Muscle Function

Because respiratory muscle contraction generates tension, the consequent pressure change that occurs can serve as an in vivo measure for the quantification of respiratory muscle strength. In addition, recent developments have expanded the current understanding of the mechanical actions and interactions of the respiratory muscles. A greater emphasis has been placed on assessing and quantifying respiratory muscle strength and pulmonary mechanics in a variety of patient groups, including children, adolescents, and adults (see Chapter 6 for a more detailed discussion).

Maximal Inspiratory and Expiratory Pressures

Maximal inspiratory and expiratory pressure measurements are clinically useful noninvasive tests with established reference ranges. As with any volitional test, however, results will be dependent on subject motivation and maximal effort, which explains in part the wide range of normal values. Furthermore, the observed pressure depends on mouthpiece design and patient posture, and it often is difficult to distinguish between mild weakness and normal strength on an individual basis. Nevertheless, maximum inspiratory mouth pressure (PImax) can provide a simple rapid estimation of global inspiratory muscle strength (in men, below −80 cm H_2O; in women, below −70 cm H_2O), but it does not allow specific conclusions to be drawn about the function of the diaphragm. If the maneuver is performed from FRC, PImax reflects the strength of the inspiratory muscles, whereas with performance from RV, the test will be influenced by the elastic recoil of the chest wall. In clinical practice, patients find it easier to perform the test from FRC rather than RV, and previous data have shown little difference between the peak or plateau values measured from either RV or FRC.

The strength of the expiratory muscles, principally the abdominal muscles, is assessed by measuring the static expiratory pressure generated at the mouth (PEmax). As with the PImax, the range of the normal values is wide (in men, above +130 cm H_2O; in women, above +100 cm H_2O) and some patients can find this maneuver difficult to perform, particularly those patients with weakness of the orofacial muscles. Thus, as with PImax, although a high value of PEmax excludes expiratory muscle weakness, a low value can be difficult to interpret. PEmax are can be measured from either TLC or FRC. PImax and PEmax measurements are reduced in females and decline with age.

Sniff Inspiratory Pressure

The rapid inspiratory effort of a sniff maneuver (see Chapter 6) is accompanied by momentary equilibration of intrathoracic and upper airway pressures. This equilibration occurs above a pressure of 10 to 12 cm H_2O, so employing sniff nasal pressure (Pn_{sn}) allows noninvasive measurement of inspiratory muscle strength. Pn_{sn} is a particularly useful additional investigation in patients with a low or equivocal PImax to confirm or exclude the presence of inspiratory muscle weakness.

A study of 241 patients with moderate to severe neuromuscular disorders showed a positive correlation between Pn_{sn} and PImax, but with a relatively poor agreement observed between Pn_{sn} and PImax. However, the findings of this study differ from those in earlier studies in that the value of PImax was at least the same as or even greater than Pn_{sn}, particularly in those patients with severe ventilatory restriction, which highlights the potential limitation of Pn_{sn} in this particular patient population. These findings add support to the idea that Pn_{sn} can underestimate inspiratory muscle strength in patients with moderate to severe neuromuscular disease (VC less than 40% of predicted), as demonstrated previously in smaller studies of patients with chronic stable inspiratory muscle weakness and acute respiratory failure. Specifically, as VC falls, a greater decrease occurs in Pn_{sn} than in PImax. Strictly speaking, PImax and Pn_{sn} are not interchangeable measurements but are complementary tests, and they should be used in combination with VC for a complete sequential assessment of inspiratory muscle strength in patients with neuromuscular and chest wall disease. In clinical practice, Pn_{sn} is usually measured through occlusion of one of the nasal passages with a nasal bung fitted with a small piece of tubing that connects to a handheld pressure transducer. Normal Pn_{sn} values are below −70 cm H_2O in men and below −60 cm H_2O in women with the measurement made from FRC.

Cough Gastric Pressure

As with sniffing, patients find coughing a natural maneuver. Although assessment of the cough gastric pressure ($Pgas_{cough}$) requires the insertion of a gastric balloon, the measurement is easy to learn and more reproducible than with PEmax. Although normal values for $Pgas_{cough}$ have been reported, previous studies using $Pgas_{cough}$ as a marker for expiratory muscle strength are described in the literature. Normal $Pgas_{cough}$ values are above +215 cm H_2O in men and above +165 cm H_2O in women.

Cough Peak Flow

Cough peak flow is a simple noninvasive measure of expiratory muscle function, which is considered to be a useful marker of cough function and a reflection of the patient's ability to clear respiratory secretions. Values of less than 160 L/min are reported to be the cutoff level for increased risk of developing

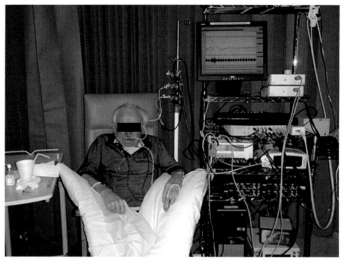

Figure 64-3 Equipment required to measure transdiaphragmatic pressure. *(Courtesy of the patient.)*

chest sepsis. A cough peak flow less than 160 L/min can be augmented by the mechanical insufflator-exsufflator device used with a face mask.

Maximum Transdiaphragmatic Pressure Measurements

The previously described tests provide data only on global respiratory muscle function, rather than on diaphragm function itself. To specifically assess diaphragm function, transdiaphragmatic pressure (Pdi) is measured by placement of a pressure-monitoring catheter in both the esophagus and stomach, to provide measurement of the esophageal and gastric pressures (**Figure 64-3**).

Although transdiaphragmatic pressure during a maximal static maneuver (Pdi_{max}) has been reported, this maneuver gives a wide normal range in naive (i.e., previously untested) subjects. An alternative is to obtain maximal sniff transdiaphragmatic pressure (Pdi_{sn}), which has gained recognition in clinical practice not only because it is a familiar maneuver but because it measures both Pes_{sn} and Pdi_{sn}, providing data on global inspiratory muscle and diaphragm strength (**Figure 64-4**).

Twitch Transdiaphragmatic Pressure

Faraday's law states that in a conducting material, a changing magnetic field will induce an electric current. Magnetic stimulation stores electrical energy in a capacitor and then discharges this energy by way of a coil to generate a rapidly changing magnetic field. This magnetic field has advantages over the electrical stimulus in that it is less attenuated by distance and therefore can more easily penetrate the deep structures in the neck and stimulate the phrenic nerve. This stimulation produces a single "twitch" of the diaphragm that is well tolerated by patients.

Clinical magnetic stimulation to allow bilateral stimulation of the roots supplying the phrenic nerves was first reported in 1989. Subsequent work has demonstrated its clinical usefulness, and this technique provides a nonvolitional assessment of diaphragm strength in a number of patient groups, including children and adolescents, as well as critically ill patients in intensive care in whom motivation and cooperation to perform maximal volitional maneuvers are difficult to achieve. In addition to improved tolerability, magnetic stimulation has advantages over electrical stimulation in that it is easier to stimulate

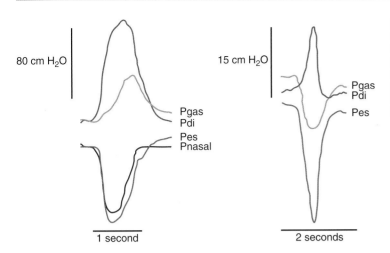

80 cm H$_2$O

15 cm H$_2$O

Pgas
Pdi

Pes
Pnasal

Pgas
Pdi

Pes

1 second

2 seconds

Figure 64-4   Transdiaphragmatic pressure measurements during a sniff maneuver in a healthy subject (*left*) and a patient with diaphragm weakness (*right*). Note the negative deflection of the gastric pressure curve in the patient with diaphragm weakness. *Pdi,* transdiaphragmatic pressure; *Pes,* esophageal pressure; *Pgas,* gastric pressure; *Pnasal,* nasal pressure.   *(From Mustfa N, Moxham J: Respiratory muscle assessment in motor neurone disease,* Q J Med *94:497–502, 2001.)*

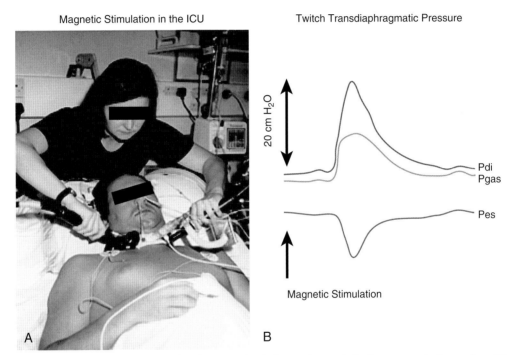

Magnetic Stimulation in the ICU

Twitch Transdiaphragmatic Pressure

20 cm H$_2$O

Pdi
Pgas

Pes

Magnetic Stimulation

A

B

Figure 64-5   An example of bilateral anterior magnetic phrenic nerve stimulation weakness. **A,** Equipment required to perform bilateral anterior magnetic phrenic nerve stimulation. **B,** Example of transdiaphragmatic pressure change generated after a phrenic nerve magnetic twitch stimulus. *ICU,* intensive care unit; *Pdi,* transdiaphragmatic pressure; *Pes,* esophageal pressure; *Pgas,* gastric pressure.   *(From Harris ML, Moxham J: Measuring respiratory and limb muscle strength using magnetic stimulation,* Br J Intensive Care *8:21–28, 1998.)*

the phrenic nerves and reduces the technical difficulties involved in isolation of the nerve (**Figure 64-5**). Further details can be found in the recommended reading section.

Pulmonary Mechanics

The measurement of lung and chest wall compliance can be assessed in restrictive lung disease but requires the placement of an esophageal pressure catheter balloon. Moreover, static compliance requires the patient to be able to relax the respiratory musculature against a closed airway, which most patients with respiratory neuromuscular and chest wall disease find difficult. On the other hand, if an esophageal catheter has been passed to accurately measure global inspiratory muscle strength, dynamic lung compliance (measured as the ratio of change in volume to change in pressure between points of zero flow) is easily measured, providing a useful clinical evaluation of the load on the respiratory system.

Role of Imaging in Respiratory Muscle Weakness and Chest Wall Disease

An elevated hemidiaphragm on a plain chest radiograph often is considered to indicate diaphragmatic weakness or paralysis, but in fact this finding is confirmed by diaphragmatic testing in only approximately 24% of cases. The most recent data indicate that hemidiaphragm elevation on the chest radiograph has a 93% sensitivity but only a 44% specificity for predicting diaphragmatic weakness. Thus, elevation of the hemidiaphragm on the chest radiograph is likely to represent hemidiaphragmatic weakness; however, a normally positioned hemidiaphragm does not exclude weakness on that side.

The contraction of the diaphragm can be directly visualized by other techniques such as fluoroscopic screening, ultrasonography, and dynamic magnetic resonance imaging. Of these, ultrasonography has the advantage of being cheap and radiation-free; however, false positives may occur in approximately 6%

of subjects, and even when correctly identifying weakness, this technique gives no functional information with regard to diaphragm strength. Accordingly, ultrasound imaging should not routinely be used in the assessment of patients with suspected hemidiaphragm or bilateral diaphragm weakness. For these purposes, unilateral and bilateral magnetic phrenic nerve stimulation should be used. Although computed tomography (CT) cross-sectional imaging may have particular value in the assessment of pleural causes of lung restriction, it is relatively unhelpful in obese patients, except to exclude coexisting thromboembolic disease and parenchymal lung disease.

Sleep Studies

Overnight oximetry and capnometry constitute an essential part of the assessment for the early detection of nocturnal hypoventilation. These are recommended investigations in patients with neuromuscular and chest wall disease who report symptoms of sleep-disordered breathing (see Table 64-1). Although some investigators advocate the use of polysomnography, including an electroencephalogram, to confirm and quantify arousals during respiratory events, this study is not necessary in the routine clinical management of these patients. Nocturnal hypoventilation can be managed simply with overnight titration of ventilatory support to a defined level of hypercapnia, irrespective of the sleep stage of the patient.

RESPIRATORY PRESENTATIONS OF NEUROLOGIC AND CHEST WALL DISEASE

The remainder of this chapter describes specific neurologic/neuromuscular disorders and chest wall diseases, as well as obesity, recognized to be associated with restrictive lung disease. These conditions are divided into acute and chronic presentations (Table 64-3), and the neuromuscular conditions are discussed in the context of the disease and grouped according to their impact on the relevant portion of the anatomic pathway from the central cortex to the peripheral muscle (Figure 64-6).

ACUTE DISORDERS AFFECTING THE CENTRAL NERVOUS SYSTEM

Stroke

Stroke (cerebrovascular accident) is one of the most common causes of acute neurologic deterioration. It is the third leading cause of death in both the United Kingdom and the United States affecting 150,000 and 795,000 patients, respectively, each year. The diaphragm has bilateral cortical representation, whereas the expiratory muscles have contralateral representation, similar to that in the limb muscles. Although hypercapnic respiratory failure is uncommon in stroke patients, chest infection is relatively frequent, and it is likely that impaired voluntary cough coupled with poor glottic coordination as well as swallowing difficulties contribute to the episodes of chest sepsis.

Cheyne-Stokes respiration breathing pattern often is observed as a feature associated with many different types of stroke. This pattern consists of a regular crescendo and decrescendo in breathing interspersed with periods of total apnea that cycles approximately every 30 seconds to 2 minutes. It commonly is observed in chronic heart failure and as a preterminal breathing pattern but also may be seen in healthy subjects at altitude.

Certain classic breathing patterns (**Figure 64-7**) are considered to reflect aspects of central nervous system pathology, though these are relatively rare in mainstream respiratory clinical practice. These include (1) *central neurogenic hyperventilation* resulting from a pontine lesion with hyperventilation present throughout both sleep and wakefulness; (2) *cluster breathing* caused by a mid–brain stem lesion, with periods of hyperventilation alternating with distinct periods of apnea; (3) *apneustic breathing* as a consequence of damage to the caudal pons with prolonged pauses after each inspiratory breath resulting in hypoventilation; and (4) *ataxic breathing* observed in patients with cortical lesions of the medulla, which is characterized by an erratic breathing pattern, which differs from the other breathing patterns in having no clear-cut cyclic nature.

Table 64-3   Acute and Chronic Presentations of Neuromuscular Disorders From Central Cortex to Peripheral Muscle

Central Nervous System	Anterior Horn Cell	Peripheral Nerve Disease	Neuromuscular Junction	Muscle
Acute				
Stroke	Rabies	Guillain-Barré syndrome	Botulism	Corticosteroid myopathy
Spinal injury	Poliomyelitis	Critical illness	Shellfish poison	Hypo/hyperkalemia
Tetanus		neuromyopathy	Drugs with neuromuscular	Hypo/hyperthyroidism
		Phrenic nerve injury	blocking effects (e.g.,	Vitamin deficiency (e.g., vitamins
			aminoglycosides)	D and E)
Chronic				
Multiple sclerosis	Motor neuron	Neuralgic amyotrophy	Myasthenia gravis	Duchenne/Becker muscular dystrophy
Arnold-Chiari	disease	Hereditary sensorimotor	Lambert-Eaton syndrome	Myotonic dystrophy
malformation	Spinal muscular	neuropathy		Congenital myopathies
Parkinson disease	atrophy	Chronic inflammatory		Metabolic myopathies (e.g., glycogen
		demyelinating		storage diseases, acid maltase
		polyneuropathy		deficiency)
		Toxins (lead)		Inflammatory myopathy (e.g.,
		Vasculitis		polymyositis, dermatomyositis)
		Porphyria		

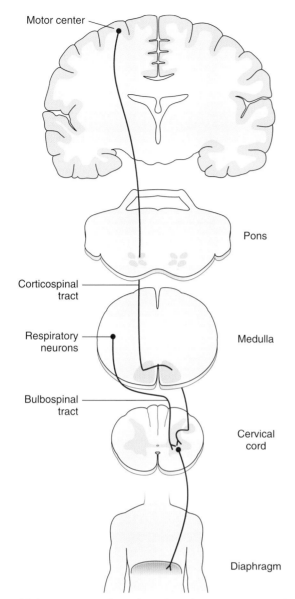

Figure 64-6 Neuromuscular pathway from the motor cortex to the diaphragm.

Labels in figure: Motor center, Pons, Corticospinal tract, Respiratory neurons, Medulla, Bulbospinal tract, Cervical cord, Diaphragm

Spinal Cord Injury

Spinal cord injury (SCI) commonly is a complication of trauma occurring predominantly in young adults, but it also may result from spinal artery infarction or tumor compression. The average age at insult is 34 years, and males are four times more likely to be affected. The extent of any neuromuscular weakness will be dependent on the site of injury, with higher cervical injuries resulting in more profound impairment. SCI at the level of C1 to C3 results in profound respiratory failure secondary to respiratory muscle denervation. Both voluntary and involuntary muscle control are lost. Unless neurologic recovery occurs, the patient will remain tracheostomy ventilator–dependent. SCI at the level of C3 to C6 results in a variable degree of diaphragmatic weakness, with more caudal lesions conferring a better prognosis. Patients may not have long-term ventilator dependence, and some improvement in respiratory muscle function often occurs over time as a consequence of reduction in inflammation and recruitment of other accessory muscles. SCI affecting the lower cervical and upper thoracic spinal cord carries a significantly better prognosis. The intercostal muscles

and the abdominal muscles are affected, but the diaphragm is spared. Patients therefore rarely require long-term mechanical ventilation.

Custom-made corsets that are designed to provide both truncal stability and abdominal support are helpful in such patients. These garments reduce the sensation of respiratory effort by optimizing the operating lung volumes and decreasing abdominal compliance, which in turn enhances diaphragm performance. These patients are susceptible to respiratory tract infections, however, as with other neuromuscular disease, due to the impairment of cough function.

Bilateral diaphragmatic pacing can be considered as an alternative method of ventilatory support in a select group of patients who have high SCI and preserved function of the phrenic nerve–diaphragm unit. The most suitable candidates for pacing are considered to be those patients with a preserved response to peripheral phrenic nerve stimulation but lacking a response to transcranial stimulation of the diaphragm motor area.

Tetanus

Tetanus toxin is produced by the anaerobic bacillus *Clostridium tetani*, which commonly resides in soil. The bacillus enters the human through a wound in the skin, and the toxin travels along peripheral nerves to the central nervous system. Hypertonicity and generalized severe muscular spasms develop when the tetanus toxin blocks the release of inhibitory neurotransmitters at the neuromuscular junction. These spasms often are protracted and can cause death by means of severe resistant laryngospasm and respiratory muscle failure. Potential treatments include wound débridement, penicillin, tetanus antitoxin, neuromuscular blocking agents, sedatives, tracheostomy, intubation, and mechanical ventilation. Preventive vaccination is now common, so this has become a rare condition for which the astute physician needs to maintain an awareness.

Drugs

Opiates, benzodiazepines, and anesthetic agents affect neural drive to the respiratory muscle and, consequently, the tone and coordination of the upper airway, diaphragm, and chest wall muscular contraction. These drugs should be used with caution in patients with underlying respiratory muscle weakness to avoid precipitating life-threatening respiratory failure.

CHRONIC DISORDERS AFFECTING THE CENTRAL NERVOUS SYSTEM

Multiple Sclerosis

Multiple sclerosis is an inflammatory demyelinating condition that can affect any part of the central nervous system. Respiratory manifestations of this condition vary with the anatomic location of the demyelinating lesions. The most common finding is a difficulty performing voluntary tests, but because the central control of breathing depends on connections from the brain stem, respiratory failure is uncommon. More usual practical problems include difficulty with voluntary cough secondary to lesions causing paraplegia and complications such as obstructive sleep apnea arising from the weight gain that results from enforced reduction in physical activity and steroid therapy.

Arnold-Chiari Malformation

Arnold-Chiari malformation is a congenital condition characterized by caudal herniation of the cerebellum and medulla

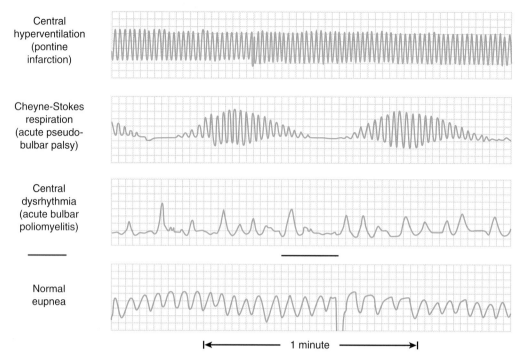

Central hyperventilation (pontine infarction)

Cheyne-Stokes respiration (acute pseudo-bulbar palsy)

Central dysrhythmia (acute bulbar poliomyelitis)

Normal eupnea

|← 1 minute →|

Figure 64-7 Breathing patterns in central nervous system diseases. *(Modified from Plum F, Swanson AG: Central neurogenic hyperventilation in man, AMA Arch Neurol Psychiatry 81:535–549, 1959.)*

through the foramen magnum. The malformation commonly blocks the flow of cerebrospinal fluid out of the posterior fossa, leading to hydrocephalus. It also may be associated with a syringomyelia where it can often interrupt ventilatory control to cause both apnea and apneustic breathing patterns. Whether deterioration can be prevented to some extent by surgical decompression has not yet been established.

Parkinson Disease

Parkinson disease is the most common movement disorder observed in developed countries and frequently is associated with fatal respiratory complications related to infection. Inspiratory muscle weakness occurs late in the progression of the disease, when maximal inspiratory pressures can fall to approximately 30% predicted. Expiratory muscle weakness also is seen; patients are unable to generate a rapid rise in peak expiratory flow. This impairment is akin to the generalized hypokinesia that is a common feature in Parkinson disease and has a deleterious effect on cough function.

Patients with this disease have significant difficulty in coordinating succinct respiratory muscle recruitment, which may partly explain the breathlessness associated with many of the dystonias. Of interest, early in the course of the disease, when no respiratory muscle weakness is evident from objective lung function parameters, the patients are still less able to perform repetitive respiratory muscle contractions than healthy age-matched control subjects. L-Dopa and apomorphine therapy have been shown to reverse these phenomena, suggesting that the defect is one of a central control and coordination of the respiratory muscles.

Patients with Parkinson disease commonly exhibit involuntary movements affecting the upper airways. A saw-tooth flutter wave often is present on the flow-volume loop trace (**Figure 64-8**); this aberration results from repetitive adduction of the vocal cords, occurring at the same frequency as a tremor of 4 to 8 Hz. It can cause significant difficulties if tracheal intubation is required. Obstructive sleep apnea is observed

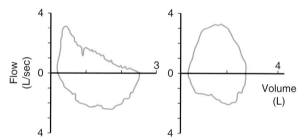

Figure 64-8 Characteristic flow-volume loop in Parkinson disease (*left*) compared with a normal flow-volume loop (*right*). *(From Laghi F, Tobin MJ: Disorders of the respiratory muscles, Am J Respir Crit Care Med 168:10–48, 2003.)*

more frequently in patients with Parkinson disease, although patients also may experience sleep fragmentation because of pain or dystonias. Finally, the related condition of multisystem atrophy is characterized by features of Parkinson disease and autonomic failure. It has been associated with irregular breathing patterns and life-threatening upper airway obstruction related to glottis and vocal cord dysfunction narrowing during sleep.

ACUTE DISORDERS AFFECTING THE ANTERIOR HORN CELLS

Rabies

Rabies is a ribonucleic acid viral disease that has one of the highest fatality rates worldwide. It is transmitted through an infected mammalian bite, primarily from dogs. When the spinal cord is involved an ascending paralysis with clinical features similar to those of Guillain-Barré syndrome is seen, which can ultimately paralyze the respiratory muscles. The condition is now preventable with the rabies vaccination, and rarely seen in industrialized nations.

Poliomyelitis

Poliomyelitis is a rare condition in the Western world consequent to the introduction of the "polio vaccine," which is routinely administered during childhood, although the disease occasionally can occur as a result of the live attenuated vaccine itself. For this reason, since 2000 only the inactive polio vaccine has been used in the United States. In the epidemics in the early 20th century, however, it was the commonest neuromuscular cause of respiratory failure. In fact, the high incidence of acute neuromuscular respiratory failure was directly responsible for the development of and advances in invasive mechanical ventilation and critical care as a specialty. In developed countries, physicians continue to encounter a diminishing number of patients who present with late respiratory failure after having suffered poliomyelitis in youth. This phenomenon is more common in those who received mechanical ventilation, usually in an "iron lung," at the time of the acute illness and in those in whom scoliosis developed subsequently. These so-called postpolio patients respond well to treatment of their chronic respiratory failure with home noninvasive ventilation.

CHRONIC DISORDERS AFFECTING THE ANTERIOR HORN CELLS

Motor Neuron Disease

Motor neuron disease (MND), also known as amyotrophic lateral sclerosis (ALS), has a European annual incidence of approximately 2 to 3 cases per 100,000 population. Only 1% to 3% of MND cases manifest with respiratory muscle weakness and acute respiratory failure. It is uncommon for patients to describe the classical signs of respiratory muscle weakness (see Table 64-1) as a presenting complaint, but respiratory physicians should consider this diagnosis in patients with coexisting muscle wasting and weakness. A more common presentation is one of exertional and positional dyspnea, ineffective cough, and low speech volume in a patient who has already received the diagnosis. Bulbar features, notably aspiration, are common in advanced disease. When muscle weakness is severe, the patient may report disrupted sleep and excessive fatigue, morning headaches and confusion. Physical findings may include tachypnea at rest, inability to complete full sentences, use of accessory muscles, and abdominal inspiratory paradox.

Respiratory muscle weakness may be present in the context of other generalized muscle involvement without chronic respiratory failure. Early detection of respiratory muscle involvement may facilitate appropriate timing of ventilatory support to prevent respiratory crises. Studies have shown that Pn_{sn} is easier to obtain in patients with MND and can be used to predict prognosis. Routine monitoring of Pn_{sn} has been recommended; if the Pn_{sn} is less than 40 cm H_2O, referral for home noninvasive ventilation should be considered. The median survival is 3 to 5 years from onset of symptoms; home noninvasive ventilation has been shown to prolong survival in non-bulbar MND and to enhance health-related quality of life in bulbar MND.

Spinal Muscular Atrophy

Spinal muscular atrophy (SMA) includes a group of genetic autosomal recessive disorders. These disorders are characterized by degeneration of the anterior horn cells and the motor nuclei in the brain stem. Patients with SMA exhibit a progressive symmetric proximal muscular weakness.

The SMAs are classified clinically as types 1 to 4, depending on the age at onset and the progression of symptoms. SMA type 1 is the most aggressive form with rapidly progressive muscular weakness; infants usually develop severe respiratory failure and do not survive longer than a year. SMA type 4 is more indolent and may manifest in the second to third decades of life. The mainstay of treatment is supportive therapy, with a focus on nutritional needs and ventilatory support as symptoms arise.

ACUTE DISORDERS AFFECTING THE PERIPHERAL NERVES

Guillain-Barré Syndrome

Guillain-Barré syndrome is an acute inflammatory demyelinating motor polyneuropathy. Patients characteristically present with a symmetric ascending motor weakness with associated depressed reflexes. Symptoms usually progress over a 2-week period, with 90% of patients reaching the peak of the disease course within 4 weeks. Severe respiratory weakness is a common associated feature, and ventilatory support is required at some point in approximately 10% to 30% of cases. Despite many effective immunomodulatory treatments, the mortality rate for Guillain-Barré syndrome requiring intubation is around 5%.

Inflammatory demyelination starts at the nerve root and progresses in a patchy fashion along the nerve sheath, resulting in weakness and paralysis of the distal muscles. This is confirmed by nerve conduction tests whereby conduction velocity of the signal is slowed or absent. A reduction in the amplitude of the action potential obtained through diaphragm needle electromyelography in response to phrenic nerve stimulation has been correlated with the requirement for invasive ventilation. In view of the risk of respiratory failure, it is essential that respiratory muscle strength is monitored in patients with confirmed or suspected Guillain-Barré syndrome. Predictive indicators for requirement of invasive ventilation are cranial nerve involvement, infection in the preceding 8 days, time from onset of weakness to admission less than 7 days, inability to stand, inability to lift elbow above head, inability to lift head off the pillow, and ineffective cough. Respiratory muscle strength commonly is assessed by serial VC and mouth pressure measurements, for which a declining trend is indicative of impending ventilator failure.

The "20-30-40" rule often is applied in clinical practice, with the combination of a VC less than 20 mL/kg, a maximum inspiratory pressure above −30 cm H_2O, and maximum expiratory pressure below +40 cm H_2O indicating the onset of respiratory failure. A clinical challenge is in maintaining an adequate mouth seal in patients with bulbar involvement, and a full face mask can be attached to the spirometer or pressure monitor to ensure optimal delivery of ventilatory support. A minority of patients, mainly those in their seventh and eighth decade of life with significant bulbar involvement, fail to wean from invasive mechanical ventilation, and these patients will require long-term tracheostomy ventilation.

IATROGENIC DISEASE

Critical Illness Neuromyopathy

Diaphragm weakness is observed in animals exposed to prolonged mechanical ventilation with concomitant use of neuromuscular blocking agents, and a similar observation has been reported in humans, albeit with complete denervation as a result of brain stem death. The importance of ventilator-induced diaphragm dysfunction more generally in critically ill patients remains unclear, although most studies have observed that the nonvolitional twitch transdiaphragmatic pressures are low compared with those obtained in healthy normal subjects.

Although no direct correlation has been found between twitch transdiaphragmatic pressure and duration of mechanical ventilation, previous studies have shown that weaning failure was observed in patients who undergo changes in pulmonary mechanics during a weaning trial such that the respiratory muscle load exceeds the capacity.

Peripheral skeletal muscle weakness associated with critical illness, or intensive care unit–acquired weakness, is beyond the scope of this chapter, but an increasingly abundant literature is accumulating in this important clinical area.

Phrenic Nerve Injury

Anatomically, the phrenic nerve is a long nerve measuring 30 to 40 cm and follows a tortuous path from the cervical spine to the diaphragm, predisposing the nerve to injury. In clinical practice, the most common cause of injury is cardiac surgery, particularly when iced slush has been used for cardioplegia. Other causes of phrenic nerve injury must be considered in patients who have undergone anterior cervical surgery (e.g., thymectomy), internal jugular line central venous access cannulation, and cervical radiotherapy.

CHRONIC DISORDERS AFFECTING THE PERIPHERAL NERVES

Neuralgic Amyotrophy

Neuralgic amyotrophy is a syndrome that classically manifests with a relatively sudden onset of muscle weakness and wasting, which may involve the upper limbs or the diaphragm, or both. In addition to the symptoms of dyspnea on exertion, dyspnea on leaning forward, dyspnea on immersion in water, and orthopnea, there can be associated pain in the appropriate dermatome —in particular, shoulder tip or shoulder blade pain. Previous data have shown that one third of patients with diaphragm paralysis will recover completely, one third will have a partial recovery, and one third will have no recovery at all. This recovery can take between 2 and 5 years. A rare familial syndrome exists, and the clinician should consider this as a cause as well as the rare presentation of a more generalized neurologic condition, such as motor neuron disease, or phrenic nerve palsy due to mediastinal compression from some other cause, such as lymphadenopathy.

Hereditary Motor and Sensory Neuropathy (Charcot-Marie-Tooth Disease)

Hereditary motor and sensory neuropathy (i.e., Charcot-Marie-Tooth disease) is a spectrum of disorders resulting from a genetic mutation in one of many myelin genes. The condition is inherited in an autosomal dominant or recessive pattern, depending on the disorder. It is a chronic degenerative process of the peripheral nerves that results in distal weakness. Phrenic nerve involvement with consequent respiratory failure is a recognized complication but is relatively infrequent.

ACUTE NEUROMUSCULAR JUNCTION DISORDERS

Botulism

Botulism is caused by the neurotoxin produced by the gram-positive anaerobic bacteria, *Clostridium botulinum*. The toxin is absorbed after ingestion, through infantile colonization of the gastrointestinal tract, or through a skin wound, commonly in association with intravenous or subcutaneous drug abuse. The toxin results in an acute presynaptic blockade of the cholinergic neuromuscular junction, leading to a life-threatening generalized paralysis. Mortality is reduced with rapid initiation of invasive ventilatory support, which may be prolonged over many months. Most patients achieve a full recovery, but the respiratory muscles can be slow to recover, and mild respiratory muscle weakness may persist indefinitely.

CHRONIC NEUROMUSCULAR JUNCTION DISORDERS

Myasthenia Gravis

Myasthenia gravis is the most common condition associated with interruption of neuromuscular signaling, but the disorder remains rare, with a prevalence of approximate 15 to 20 cases per 100,000 population. It is caused by antibodies against the acetylcholine receptor in the post synaptic nerve terminal. Patients typically present with a fluctuating muscular weakness that progresses with fatigue of the muscles, which classically is described as most pronounced toward the end of the day. Ocular and bulbar symptoms are the most common manifestations, but respiratory weakness also can occur and occasionally may be a presenting symptom of the condition. Acute respiratory failure can occur in a myasthenic crisis that may be precipitated by factors such as infection and surgery.

The mainstay of treatment is immunosuppression and use of cholinesterase inhibitors, although care must be taken to achieve an optimal balance, because excessive cholinergic blockade can result in issues with increased bronchial secretions or frank cholinergic block of the respiratory muscles. Despite appropriate treatment, a proportion of patients exhibit nocturnal hypoventilation, which will be exacerbated by steroid-induced weight gain.

Thymoma commonly is associated with the myasthenic syndrome, and clinicians must be aware that after thymectomy, acute respiratory failure may occur. Diagnostic considerations in this setting include both postoperative myasthenic syndrome, although risk for this syndrome should be much less after surgery, and phrenic nerve damage incurred during the procedure, because the nerve can be embedded in the tumor, with consequent intentional or unintentional resection.

Lambert-Eaton Myasthenic Syndrome

Lambert-Eaton myasthenic syndrome is a rare condition that affects the release of acetylcholine and reduces neuromuscular signaling at the neuromuscular junction. The disease is caused by antibodies directed against voltage-gated calcium channels. These channels regulate the flow of calcium required for the release of acetylcholine in the presynaptic nerve terminals. The condition is suggested by the presence of proximal muscular weakness, reduced or absent reflexes, and autonomic signs and symptoms such as a dry mouth. A unique feature is the recovery of reflexes and muscle strength with maximal isometric muscular activity and an increase in muscle action potential amplitude observed on repetitive nerve stimulation. Respiratory muscle weakness is uncommon as a presenting feature; more frequently, it occurs late in the disease process. The condition has a strong association with malignancy—in particular, small cell lung cancer, which coexists in up to 50% of cases.

ACUTE MUSCLE DISORDERS

Corticosteroid-Induced Respiratory Myopathy

Corticosteroid-induced myopathy involving the quadriceps is relatively commonly encountered as a consequence of extensive use of corticosteroid treatment for any of various inflammatory and autoimmune conditions. Current available evidence, however, suggests that this is rarely a problem with the respiratory muscles.

Rarer Causes of Acute Myopathy

Myopathy may be associated with many different endocrine and biochemical abnormalities. Commonly, severe hypokalemia causes a rapidly progressive myopathy predominantly affecting proximal muscles. Malabsorption of essential vitamins, such as vitamin D and vitamin E, also may result in a milder generalized myopathy. Hypothyroidism and hyperthyroidism, adrenal insufficiency, and Cushing disease also are associated with myopathy. This can occur at any point in the disease course but occasionally are the presenting manifestation, although such disorders generally are identified in the context of other systemic features. These myopathies rarely involve the respiratory muscles, but if ventilatory failure does occur, their management is supportive while the underlying abnormality is corrected.

CHRONIC MUSCLE DISORDERS

Duchenne Muscular Dystrophy

DMD is an X-linked inherited condition arising from a mutation in the dystrophin gene. It affects males from early childhood, with an incidence of 1 in 3000 births. The decline in function in DMD manifests as a proximal to distal limb muscle weakness, leading to wheelchair dependency by the early teenage years and to respiratory muscle weakness with progression. Respiratory failure is the major cause of death in this group of patients, although mortality also may be associated with the dilated cardiomyopathy that can occur in the absence of respiratory muscle weakness.

As with other progressive neuromuscular conditions, respiratory muscle weakness progresses gradually. The deterioration in respiratory function within these groups manifests initially as nocturnal hypoventilation in REM sleep and progresses to hypoventilation in REM and non-REM sleep and finally to daytime hypercapnia and chronic respiratory failure. This progression in chronic respiratory failure is associated with increasing sleep disturbance, frequency of chest infections, hospital admissions, and deteriorating quality of life. The monitoring of respiratory muscle strength and VC in these patients is a key clinical assessment. VC decreases from the age of 10 years, and a VC of less than 1 L confers a poor prognosis, with mean survival of approximately 2 years without ventilatory support. The presence of scoliosis in these patients may accelerate this process. Mean survival with the onset of chronic respiratory failure is 9.7 months if home nocturnal noninvasive ventilation is not initiated. Although the prophylactic use of home nocturnal noninvasive ventilation before the onset of chronic respiratory failure is controversial, most authorities support the view that noninvasive ventilation brings improvements in gas exchange, normalization of sleep patterns, enhanced quality of life, and prolonged survival. A more recent study indicates that nocturnal ventilatory support should be considered when patients develop nocturnal hypoventilation, and without home noninvasive ventilation, progression to chronic diurnal hypercapnic respiratory failure occurs within 18 months.

Respiratory support also will include secretion clearance, specifically during any episode of pneumonia, with the introduction of a mechanical insufflation-exsufflation device to enhance cough function and secretion management (see earlier under "Cough Peak Flow"). As bulbar function declines, in addition to a reduction in effective cough, patients will be at increased risk for aspiration, and these swallowing problems reduce nutritional intake, resulting in weight loss. Early gastrostomy feeding tube insertion, accomplished with endoscopic or radiologic guidance, is recommended, although evidence supporting this practice is limited. It is possible, with appropriate expertise, to do such procedures with sedation using noninvasive ventilation alone in patients with established respiratory failure.

Other Muscular Dystrophies

Becker muscular dystrophy follows a clinical course similar to that for DMD but typically is of much later onset, with much milder clinical effects. Patients remain ambulatory until the late teenage years, and the degree of respiratory muscle involvement is less. Toward the later stages of the disease, in the fourth decade of life, respiratory failure can develop, and noninvasive ventilation may be required. Facioscapulohumeral muscular dystrophy also is a slowly progressive condition of autosomal dominant inheritance that affects muscles of the face, arms, and shoulders. In approximately 20% of the patients, chest wall and diaphragm involvement may result in respiratory decline necessitating ventilatory support.

Myotonic Dystrophy

Myotonic dystrophy is inherited as an autosomal dominant trait that exhibits generational anticipation. It is a multisystem disorder characterized by features of myotonia (delayed muscle relaxation), progressive skeletal muscle weakness, cardiac conduction deficits and cardiomyopathy, cataracts, frontal baldness, ptosis, testicular failure, hypogammaglobulinemia, and diabetes mellitus. Sleep-disordered breathing is common, with nocturnal hypoventilation and progressive hypercapnia resulting from respiratory muscle weakness and impaired neural respiratory drive. Central and obstructive sleep apnea also may occur as a consequence of upper airway muscular weakness and myotonia. Ventilatory support should be offered on the basis of patient symptoms and arterial carbon dioxide levels. Unfortunately, patients frequently find it difficult to use nocturnal ventilatory support, in part because only a limited symptomatic response is obtained, with persisting daytime somnolence as a consequence of the primary hypersomnolence that accompanies this condition.

Other Rarer Myopathies

Congenital myopathies are a group of inherited disorders of muscle that typically manifest with generalized muscle weakness in infancy. A muscle biopsy is required to characterize the type of myopathy. All patients present with hypotonia and a predominant proximal muscular weakness. The severity of the muscle impairment depends on the individual genetic mutation. A majority of the patients require mechanical ventilation from early life and do not survive childhood.

Metabolic myopathies constitute a heterogenous group of disorders that are related to a deficit in the metabolic pathways of the muscle. Among such disorders, the most common are the glycogen storage diseases. From a respiratory perspective, the most important metabolic myopathy is acid maltase deficiency, because respiratory muscle weakness can be the primary presentation of the condition in the adult-onset form. Treatment is supportive, as with the other myopathic conditions, although enzyme replacement therapy may have a role in slowing the onset of chronic respiratory failure.

Mitochondrial myopathies result from dysfunction of mitochondrial ability to release energy form adenosine triphosphate

(ATP). The clinical manifestations are highly variable but can include respiratory failure.

Idiopathic inflammatory myopathies, including dermatomyositis and polymyositis, manifest with muscular weakness due to inflammatory destructive processes directly affecting the muscle fibers and their blood supply. Dermatomyositis is characterized by typical skin manifestations such as Gottron's papules on the hands and feet and a heliotropic rash over the eyelids and can be associated with malignancy. The muscular weakness may rarely result in respiratory failure. These inflammatory myopathies are associated with interstitial parenchymal lung disease in approximately 20% of cases. Such disease can be rapidly progressive and frequently is fatal.

THORACIC DISORDERS

Chest wall deformities, such as kyphosis, scoliosis, and kyphoscoliosis, and obesity hypoventilation syndrome are described in detail in Chapters 63 and 62, respectively. Obesity itself also has clinical consequences for pulmonary function, and an overview of this issue is presented next, with specific emphasis on pulmonary function tests, pulmonary mechanics, hypercapnic ventilatory response, and respiratory muscle strength.

OBESITY

Clinical Consequences of Obesity

Within the Western world, a well-recognized major public health problem is the growing epidemic of obesity. Although the definition of obesity includes a requirement for a body mass index (BMI) greater than 30 kg/m^2, clinicians are now encountering increasing numbers of patients who are *morbidly obese* (i.e., with a BMI greater than 40 kg/m^2), and more recently, the term *superobese* (BMI greater than 50 kg/m^2) has been adopted to further characterize this patient group. In the United Kingdom, an estimated 25% of the population is obese, with superobesity increasing dramatically over the past decade. By current estimates, superobesity affects 1 in 230 adults in the United States.

With this obesity epidemic, patients are presenting more frequently to respiratory medicine departments and chest clinics with exercise-induced dyspnea, obstructive sleep apnea, and nocturnal hypoventilation necessitating ventilatory support. Observational data on hospitalized obese patients indicate that up to one third of those with a BMI greater than 35 kg/m^2 have hypercapnic respiratory failure.

Respiratory Muscle Pump in Obese Patients

It is hypothesized that breathlessness and alveolar hypoventilation in obese patients result from an imbalance between respiratory muscle load and/or capacity and neural respiratory drive, although the exact pathophysiologic details are yet to be determined. Respiratory muscle capacity, albeit estimated using volitional P_{Imax} and P_{Emax} measurements, was found to be reduced in hypercapnic obese patients compared with eucapnic obese patients. However, direct measurement of diaphragm strength, using Pdi_{max}, demonstrated no difference between eucapnic and hypercapnic obese patients, indicating that diaphragm weakness does not contribute to the development of ventilatory failure in obese patients. By contrast, a difference is seen in respiratory muscle load between hypercapnic obese patients and eucapnic obese subjects with greater upper airway resistance in both sitting and supine positions and reduced respiratory system compliance. This increasing load on the

respiratory muscles results in a reduction in lung volumes, with a reduction in FEV_1 and FVC and an elevated FEV_1/FVC ratio confirming a restrictive defect. In addition, TLC, expiratory reserve volume (ERV), and FRC are all reduced. Of interest, these reductions are more marked in obese patients with hypercapnic respiratory failure than in eucapnic obese subjects with a matched BMI. It is appreciated that in addition to absolute fat load, the distribution of the fat is important in determining the severity of lung restriction.

The obese patient breathes at a lower lung volume, which reduces chest wall and lung compliance. Breathing at a lower lung volume also results in closure of the small airways during early expiration, causing expiratory airflow limitation and development of intrinsic positive end-expiratory pressure (PEEPi). This phenomenon is exacerbated by adoption of a supine position, such as occurs during sleep. It has been shown that in obese patients, moving from a sitting to supine posture is associated with an increase in neural respiratory drive, as measured by the diaphragm electromyogram, with a corresponding increase in diaphragm pressure generation, as measured from transdiaphragmatic pressure swings, but without a corresponding increase in tidal volume. Furthermore, these patients develop PEEPi on change in position, indicating expiratory flow limitation, although it is difficult to separate whether this is a consequence of early airway closure during expiration or upper airway obstruction, or a combination of both mechanisms. More studies in this area are required to confirm the previous data demonstrating changes in hypercapnic ventilatory response in obese hypercapnic patients. These previous studies have shown that obese hypercapnic patients, compared with eucapnic obese subjects, have reduced hypercapnic ventilatory response as a consequence of an inadequate ability to increase tidal volume, resulting in dead space ventilation. Such research will allow investigators to define the pathophysiologic cause of alveolar hypoventilation in obese patients.

CONTROVERSIES AND PITFALLS

Respiratory muscle weakness is a common complication in many neuromuscular and chest wall conditions, and although it may occasionally be a presenting feature of the underlying disorder, it generally is a complication of an already established diagnosis. In view of the impact of chronic respiratory failure on health-related quality of life and the potential life-threatening consequences of respiratory muscle weakness, respiratory muscle function should be monitored at regular intervals with noninvasive respiratory muscle tests in patients with progressive neuromuscular disease. Furthermore, patients with neuromuscular disease or chest wall disease, or both, who present with unexplained dyspnea should be referred for formal respiratory assessment. This evaluation will include a detailed history and clinical examination with a focus on symptoms suggestive of significant muscle weakness, sleep-disordered breathing, and associated complications such as bulbar symptoms. Other components of the evaluation will include a basic lung volume measurement, noninvasive respiratory muscle testing, and, in special circumstances, invasive respiratory muscle testing. It is well to be mindful, however, of the limitations of performing a single measure of respiratory muscle strength in attempting to diagnose respiratory muscle weakness. Previous data have demonstrated that isolated sniff inspiratory nasal pressure often overdiagnosed the severity of weakness in patients with severe restrictive ventilator deficits from neuromuscular disease. Accordingly, for an accurate assessment of respiratory muscle strength, performing an array of noninvasive tests of respiratory muscle function, such as Pn$_{sn}$, PImax, and PEmax, is recommended.

With these clinical data, the timing of initiation of noninvasive ventilation can be planned. In patients with neuromuscular and chest wall disease, recent data suggest that chronic respiratory failure will occur 18 to 24 months after the onset of nocturnal hypoventilation. This will be the time to consider the introduction of noninvasive ventilation, and for those patients who are relatively asymptomatic at this stage and are reluctant to pursue noninvasive ventilation, close monitoring of clinical status is indicated. In addition to ventilatory strategies, clinicians must consider other respiratory adjunctive measures, such as physiotherapy techniques and the use of devices including mechanical insufflation-exsufflation devices for patients with neuromuscular disease in whom poor cough function has been documented.

Finally, clinicians need to be cognizant of the rising trend in obesity and of its negative effects on respiratory function. Thus far, no prospective randomized controlled trials have been conducted to determine an optimal ventilation strategy for treating obesity hypoventilation syndrome. A single-center randomized controlled trial of selected patients with obesity hypoventilation showed equivalence between continuous positive airway pressure and noninvasive ventilation, leading consensus opinion to advocate noninvasive ventilation in patients for whom continuous positive airway pressure has not achieved symptom control. With the increasing incidence of superobesity, it is clear that further research in this area is urgently required.

SUGGESTED READINGS

American Thoracic Society/European Respiratory Society: ATS/ERS statement on respiratory muscle testing, *Am J Respir Crit Care Med* 166:518–624, 2002.

Bassetti CL, Gugger M: Sleep disordered breathing in neurologic diseases, *Swiss Med Wkly* 132:109–115, 2002.

Hart N: Respiratory failure, *Clin Med* 36:242–245, 2008.

Hart N, Polkey MI: Investigation of respiratory muscle function, *Clin Pulm Med* 8:180–187, 2001.

Laghi F, Tobin MJ: Disorders of the respiratory muscles, *Am J Respir Crit Care Med* 168:10–48, 2003.

Luo YM, Moxham J, Polkey MI: Diaphragm electromyelography using an oesophageal catheter: current concepts, *Clin Sci (Lond)* 115:233–244, 2008.

Murphy P, Polkey MI, Hart N: Diagnostic tests in the assessment of patients for home mechanical ventilation. In Elliott MW, Nava S, Schönhofer B, editors: *Principles and practices of non-invasive ventilation and weaning*, London, 2010, Hodder Arnold, pp 151–166.

Mustfa N, Moxham J: Respiratory muscle assessment in motor neurone disease, *Q J Med* 94:497–502, 2001.

Polkey MI, Lyall RA, Davidson AC, et al: Ethical and clinical issues in the use of home non-invasive mechanical ventilation for the palliation of breathlessness in motor neurone disease, *Thorax* 54:367–371, 1999.

Polkey MI, Lyall RA, Moxham J, Leigh PN: Respiratory aspects of neurological disease, *J Neurol Neurosurg Psychiatry* 66:5–15, 1999.

Polkey MI, Moxham J: Clinical aspects of respiratory muscle dysfunction in the critically ill, *Chest* 119:926–939, 2001.

Tobin M: *Principles and practices of mechanical ventilation*, ed 2, New York, 2006, McGraw-Hill.

Chapter **65**

Lung Cancer: Epidemiology, Surgical Pathology, and Molecular Biology

Arnold M. Schwartz • M. Katayoon Rezaei

EPIDEMIOLOGY

INCIDENCE AND SURVIVAL

Lung cancer currently is the highest cause of cancer mortality in the United States and even surpasses the sum of the next four cancer types in both men and women. In terms of incidence, (the number of new cases of cancer in a given year), lung cancer is second only to breast cancer in women and prostate cancer in men. In the United States, estimates of new cases of lung cancer for 2010 were approximately 116,000 in men and 105,000 in women, with approximately 160,000 deaths. Lung cancer deaths accounted for 31% and 27% of overall cancer deaths in men and women, respectively, and are more numerous than deaths due to breast, prostate, and colon cancers combined. In terms of overall causes of death in men, lung cancer is the second most common cause of death, after vascular disease, with deaths due to heart attacks and stroke. The overall 5-year lung cancer survival rate is between 15% and 20% as a consequence of its late stage at onset of symptoms and relatively aggressive clinical behavior. Like other malignancies, lung cancer is a disease of aging, with increasing rates in persons older than 50 years of age, and rarely is diagnosed in those younger than 40 years. Graphing lung cancer incidence according to chronologic age of diagnosis on a logarithmic scale demonstrates a straight line for both men and women, indicating that the carcinogenic pathways probably are similar for both genders and that steroid hormones (estrogen and androgens) do not play a major role in carcinogenesis.

Lung cancer more typically is present in men than in women, and in African Americans than in white Americans; these disparities in incidence probably are due to smoking patterns. The disparity extends to younger persons as well; young African American men and women have significantly higher lung cancer rates than their white counterparts. The incidence of lung cancer in adult African American and in white American male adults in 2008 was 101 and 69 per 100,000, respectively. Both African American and white American women had similar cancer incidences of approximately 55 cases per 100,000. Other ethnic and racial groups, such as Hispanic persons, Native Americans, and Asian or South Pacific Americans have a lower incidence than that for white Americans.

Lung cancer incidence is highest in the developed nations of North America (United States and Canada), the European Union, and countries of the former Soviet Union, where cigarette availability and smoking rates are highest. In 2008, lung cancer was diagnosed worldwide in approximately 1.6 million

people and led to cancer deaths in 1.4 million, and a majority of new cases are reported from China and less developed countries. Since the 1970s, lung cancer incidence has been decreasing in the United States, Canada, United Kingdom, and Australia but has been increasing in Japan and India. Unfortunately, during this same time, lung cancer incidence has been increasing among women in the United States, Canada, Denmark, Norway, and Sweden. Worldwide, lung cancer incidence is more than double for men relative to women, and the relative risk is even higher in Western Asia, Central and Southern America, and Southern Africa.

Although lung cancer is increasing in large developing nations, such as China and India, the socioeconomic demographic features are important in appreciating lung cancer incidence. The risk of lung cancer is inversely associated with education and income and appears to be more closely linked to smoking than risk of disease from occupational or environmental exposures. Data from developing nations are not as robust and accurate as those from Western countries, and analysis of the socioeconomic setting of smoking also involves confounding variables, such as local diet and environmental carcinogens and inhalant exposures.

When the mortality rates (deaths due to disease within a calendar year) for lung cancer in women and men are plotted against the calendar years for the last 50 years, one notes a marked difference in the pattern of the curves (**Figure 65-1**). The incidence rates for men show a marked rise from the early 1950s to the beginning of the 1990s, whereas rates for women lag by about a quarter of a century and then show an identical rise, essentially parallel to those for men, and continuing into the 21st century. By the 1950s, death due to lung cancer far exceeded prostate and colon cancer deaths among men, and by 1990, lung cancer deaths among women exceeded breast and gynecologic cancer deaths. Usually cancer mortality follows cancer incidence; however, in the case of lung cancer, owing to the very high cancer fatality rate (mortality from cancer for persons given a diagnosis of cancer), lung cancer mortality exceeds the most common cancers in both men and women. As a result of the Surgeon General's 1964 report on smoking, men began to stop smoking in the succeeding 20 to 30 years; the incidence and mortality of lung cancer began to decline from a peak in the early 1990s to a level that approximates the mortality rate of the 1970s. The phenomenon of social smoking among women lagged behind that for men; subsequently, both the incidence of lung cancer in women and its associated mortality continue to rise into the present day.

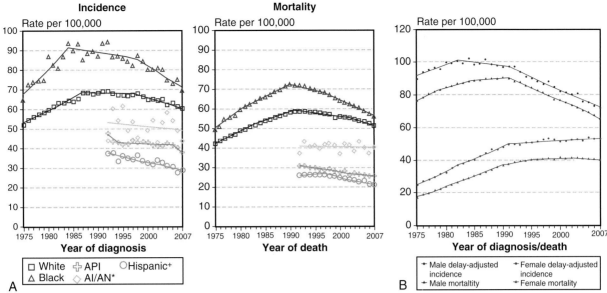

Figure 65-1   A, SEER incidence and U.S. death rates for cancer of the lung and bronchus (men and women). Joinpoint Regression analyses for whites and blacks from 1975 to 2007 and for Asian/Pacific Islanders, American Indians/Alaska Natives, and Hispanics from 1992 to 2007. *API,* Asian Pacific Islander; *AI/AN,* American Indian/Alaska Native. **B,** SEER-delay adjusted rates for cancer of the lung and bronchus mortality differences among men and women of all races in the United States (1975-2007). *SEER,* Surveillance, Epidemiology, and End Results [Program].   *(A, Incidence data for whites and blacks are from the SEER nine areas—San Francisco, Connecticut, Detroit, Hawaii, Iowa, New Mexico, Seattle, Utah, Atlanta. Incidence data for Asian/Pacific Islanders, American Indians/Alaska Natives, and Hispanics are from the SEER thirteen areas—the SEER nine areas plus San Jose-Monterey, Los Angeles, Alaska/ Native Registry, and Rural Georgia. Mortality data are from U.S. mortality files, National Center for Health Statistics, Centers for Disease Control and Prevention [CDC]. Rates are age-adjusted to the 2000 U.S. standard population [19 age groups, Census P25-1103]. Regression lines are calculated using the Joinpoint Regression program Version 3.4.3, April 2010, National Cancer Institute. Joinpoint analyses for whites and blacks during the 1975-2007 period allow a maximum of 4 joinpoints. Analyses for other ethnic groups during the period 1992 to 2007 allow a maximum of 2 joinpoints. *Rates for American Indians/ Alaska Natives are based on the contract health service delivery area [CHSDA] counties. †Hispanic is not mutually exclusive of whites, blacks, Asians/Pacific Islanders, and American Indians/Alaska Natives. Incidence data for Hispanics are based on the NHIA [North American Association of Central Cancer Registries/ NAACCR Hispanic Identification Algorithm] and exclude cases from the Alaska Native Registry. Mortality data for Hispanics exclude cases from Connecticut, the District of Columbia, Maine, Maryland, Minnesota, New Hampshire, New York, North Dakota, Oklahoma, and Vermont. B, Data from SEER nine areas and U.S. mortality files [National Center for Health Statistics, CDC]. Rates are age-adjusted to the 2000 U.S. standard population [19 age groups, Census P25-1103]. Regression lines are calculated using the Joinpoint Regression Program Version 3.4.3, April 2010, National Cancer Institute [http://seer.cancer.gov/statfacts/ html/lungb.html].*

Although *lung cancer* typically refers to the malignant bronchogenic epithelial tumors of the lung, namely, squamous cell carcinoma, adenocarcinoma, large cell carcinoma, and small cell (neuroendocrine) carcinoma, the relative incidence, distribution, and frequency of these tumors over time are characterized by marked differences. In the 1970s, squamous cell carcinoma predominated in incidence over the other bronchogenic carcinomas. Of interest, the age-adjusted incidence rate of adenocarcinoma, among both men and women, continued to rise, so that beginning in the late 1990s and continuing into the early 2000s, adenocarcinomas have become the most frequently encountered lung cancers. The two histologic subgroups of lung cancer most strongly associated with smoking, squamous cell carcinoma and small cell carcinoma, have shown a decrease in their overall incidence, reflecting the trend of decreased cigarette smoking among men. The relative percentages of the major lung cancer histologic types are adenocarcinoma 38%, squamous cell carcinoma 20%, small cell (neuroendocrine) carcinoma 13%, and large cell carcinoma 5%. The remainder are composed of variant carcinomas, sarcomatoid (spindle cell) carcinomas, salivary-type carcinomas, neuroendocrine-carcinoid carcinomas, and others.

The histologic sequence eventuating in squamous cell carcinoma begins with smoking-induced replacement of respiratory epithelium with bronchial squamous metaplasia. Additional cellular and molecular events lead to squamous dysplasia, in situ carcinoma, and ultimately, invasive squamous cell carcinoma. Small cell carcinoma does not have a clearly defined precursor lesion, although it is presumed to be the Kulchitsky cell; however, small cell carcinomas often arise in a setting of squamous metaplasia and dysplasia, indicative of the effects of the smoking environment. Adenocarcinoma, a histologic subtype characterized by formation of malignant-appearing glands, papillae, and intracytoplasmic mucin, also arises in the context of cigarette smoking, yet approximately 25% of lung cancer cases are not attributable to direct smoking. These tumors typically are located peripherally and may be associated with scars that in some cases may be preexisting but also may represent a host desmoplastic response to the tumor. As a histologic subtype, adenocarcinomas of the lung continue to increase in incidence among both men and women.

ETIOLOGY AND RISK FACTORS

The major risk factor associated with lung cancer in a majority of cases is cigarette smoking. The probability that a diagnosis of lung cancer will be made in a nonsmoker is less than 15%. The case for cigarette smoking as a major cause of lung cancer is made by strong epidemiologic evidence and by significant results of animal studies. Both case-control and cohort studies have demonstrated the strong association of smoking with lung cancer and have shown that the association is dose-dependent and linked to current versus past smoking behavior. Initial case-control studies investigating retrospective reviews of smoking behavior in groups with and without lung cancer calculated odds ratios of approximately 10:1 for smoking associated lung cancers. Later, longitudinal cohort studies demonstrated mortality ratios averaging 10:1 for lung cancer deaths in the group of smokers relative to nonsmokers. Moreover, the annual incidence of lung cancer showed a logarithmic relationship with age and duration of smoking. Mortality ratios also demonstrated a dose-response relationship with the number of cigarettes smoked per day. In general, smokers have a 70% increase in mortality relative to nonsmokers.

Cigarette smoking is associated with all the histologic types of bronchogenic carcinoma, however, as discussed above, adenocarcinoma, a smoking related cancer, is also the most common type among nonsmokers. Although a history of many pack-years of cigarette smoking is strongly linked to lung cancer, only a minority of smokers develop lung cancer, suggesting that host biologic and genetic factors may modulate carcinogenic pathways in the development of lung cancer. The clinical history of current or past cigarette smoking also affects the probability of developing lung cancer, with the incidence of lung cancer in heavy smokers more than twice that in light smokers, and more than five-fold that in ex-smokers. Not only is cigarette smoking a risk factor for the development of lung cancer; it is also a predictor of disease recurrence after lung cancer resection in early stage disease. The 5-year overall survival rate for smokers relative to nonsmokers with stage I lung cancer is, respectively, 76% and 92%. There is a modest but real effect of lung cancer attributable to passive or environmental tobacco smoke, based on an update of the Surgeon General's report. Nonsmokers married to smokers incur an approximate 25% relative increase over nonexposed nonsmokers for the induction of lung cancer but of course significantly less than that for active smokers.

In addition to the dominant effect of cigarette smoking, other occupational and environmental conditions are associated with an increased risk of lung cancer. The most well-accepted industrial agents associated with lung cancer are asbestos, hexavalent chromium(VI), arsenic, nickel, and polycyclic aromatic hydrocarbons. Ionizing radiation exposure, as experienced after the atom bomb explosion in Japan (1945), in uranium mining, and with radon encountered in industrial and home settings, also shows hazard rates for lung cancer similar to those for environmental or second-hand cigarette smoke. In persons exposed to industrial chemicals and who also smoke, a synergistic effect may be operative in the development of lung cancer.

Asbestos manufacturing, more so than asbestos mining, is associated with pulmonary fibrosis and lung cancer and also the development of malignant pleural mesothelioma. Asbestos workers who also smoke have a synergistic or multiplicative risk of lung cancer over those who do not smoke. Lung cancer in asbestos-exposed persons usually manifests in a setting of pulmonary asbestosis (interstitial fibrosis). It is believed by some investigators that the fibroinflammatory scarring process of pulmonary asbestosis creates a microenvironment in which cancers develop. On the other hand, other researchers propose that the fibrogenic sequence of interstitial fibrosis due to high asbestos fiber burden may not be the same as the carcinogenic pathway of asbestos-induced malignancies. Both pulmonary fibrosis and asbestos-related bronchogenic carcinomas are dose-dependent on the lung fiber burden. Although pulmonary asbestosis tends to predominate in the lower lobes, the asbestos-induced cancers are found in all lobes of the lung. In the case of pleural diffuse malignant mesothelioma, the tumor may be attributable to asbestos exposure even in the absence of pulmonary fibrosis or smoking.

SURGICAL PATHOLOGY AND CYTOPATHOLOGY

The malignant epithelial tumors of the lung consist of the most common bronchogenic carcinomas: adenocarcinoma, squamous cell carcinoma, small cell carcinoma, and large cell carcinoma, and their subgroups. Less common malignant epithelial tumors include the sarcomatoid carcinomas, neuroendocrine-carcinoid tumors, and salivary gland tumors. Most tumors of the lung are advanced at presentation and tend to be higher-stage cancers. Cancers of the central airways are commonly diagnosed and may occur as an endobronchial mass or as a parenchymal mass with endobronchial extension or extrinsic bronchial compression and a possible resultant obstructive pneumonia. Clinically, affected patients present with cough, hemoptysis, and/or shortness of breath. The central tumors may be approached by interventional bronchoscopy for diagnosis and management. Those tumors that manifest as peripheral scars or solitary pulmonary nodules may be histopathologically assessed by needle core or aspiration biopsy.

Cytologic evaluation of sputum, bronchial washings or brushings, and fine needle aspiration (FNA) biopsy specimens (transbronchial, transesophageal, or percutaneous) has long been utilized in the diagnostic workup of lung masses and as a staging procedure by sampling hilar or mediastinal nodes. The diagnostic accuracy is highly dependent on the sampling method. Cytologic approaches in the right clinical setting can provide valuable information without the need for an invasive procedure such as mediastinoscopy. More recently, it has been shown that the addition of ultrasound guidance to the bronchoscopy or endoscopy procedure improves diagnostic accuracy, with sensitivity of more than 85% and specificity of 100%.

Traditionally, the role of cytologic analysis was to first establish the diagnosis of malignancy and then to further stratify the carcinoma into two main categories of small cell carcinoma and non–small cell carcinoma, for appropriate management. With the advent of targeted therapy, however, this approach no longer provides the necessary information, because major changes have evolved in the treatment of squamous cell carcinoma and adenocarcinoma that may involve approaches dependent on the presence or absence of genetic mutations. Several studies have addressed the feasibility and accuracy of cytologic studies in this respect, especially when immunohistochemical methods are used in conjunction with cytomorphologic examination. Furthermore, it has been shown that molecular studies for *EGFR/KRAS* mutation analysis can be successfully carried out on cytologic preparations.

Adenocarcinoma

Adenocarcinomas are tumors that produce malignant-appearing glands with tubular, acinar, or papillary differentiation and whose cells may demonstrate mucin production and secretion (**Box 65-1**). On gross examination, the tumors may manifest peripherally with pleural retraction (puckering), as central or endobronchial masses, as diffuse pleural involvement resembling a malignant mesothelioma, arising or associated with a scar, or as a diffuse parenchymal pneumonic-like tumor. The histologic pattern and organization may show a well-differentiated acinar pattern with intracytoplasmic vacuoles or more poorly differentiated features with solid malignant growth

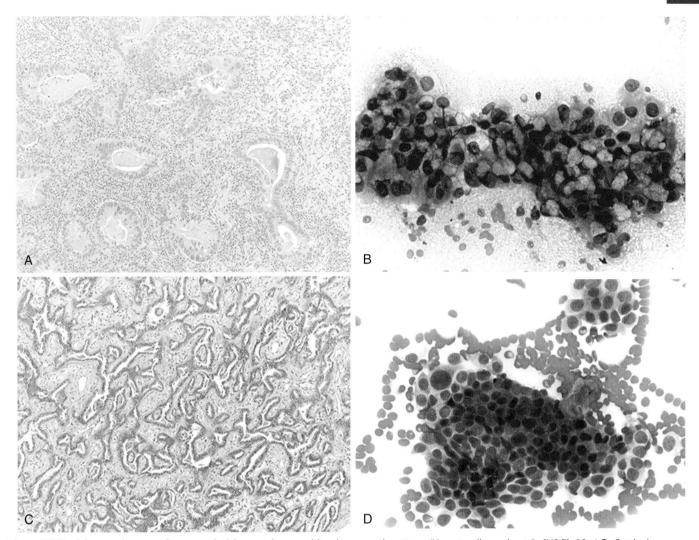

Figure 65-2 Adenocarcinoma, acinar type. **A,** Adenocarcinoma with acinar growth pattern. (Hematoxylin-eosin stain [H&E], 10×.) **B,** Cytologic preparation showing intracytoplasmic vacuoles. (Diff-Quik stain, 40×.) **C,** Adenocarcinoma with tubuloacinar growth pattern. (H&E, 10×.) **D,** Cytologic preparation showing sheetlike growth and intracytoplasmic vacuoles. (Diff-Quik stain, 40×.)

Box 65-1 **Classification of Adenocarcinoma in Resected Specimens**
Preinvasive Lesions Atypical adenomatous hyperplasia (AAH) Adenocarcinoma in situ (AIS) Nonmucinous, mucinous, or mixed types **Minimally Invasive Adenocarcinoma (MIA)** Nonmucinous, mucinous, or mixed types **Invasive Adenocarcinomas** Predominant types: lepidic, acinar, papillary, micropapillary, solid Adenocarcinoma, variants: invasive mucinous, colloid, fetal, enteric

Modified from Travis WD, Brambilla E, Noguchi M, et al: International Association for the Study of Lung Cancer/American Thoracic Society/European Respiratory Society international multidisciplinary classification of lung adenocarcinoma, *J Thorac Oncol* 6:244-285, 2011.

various levels of the airway with malignant changes in respiratory, bronchiolar, and alveolar epithelium. Malignant transformation of these various epithelia may be associated with protean histologic and cytologic characteristics and growth patterns of invasion.

The nature of tumor growth and progression depends on whether the cell of origin is a bronchial gland, ciliated columnar cell, goblet cell, nonciliated bronchiolar cell, or type II pneumocyte. The histologic growth pattern may show a mixture of various types including acinar, papillary, solid, and lepidic (growth along alveolar interstitium), and the cytologic features may include mucinous and nonmucinous differentiation (**Figures 65-2** and **65-3**). The grading of adenocarcinomas is based on the histopathologic assessment of the extent of glandular differentiation and architectural pattern, cytologic expression and pleomorphism, nuclear characteristics and stratification, and mitotic activity and tumor necrosis. Most adenocarcinomas tend to be of mixed pattern, are intermediate in differentiation or moderately differentiated, and show a predominant acinar-type glandular arrangement. As expected, predominantly solid adenocarcinomas tend to demonstrate high-grade, poorly differentiated cytologic features with prominent mitotic activity and tumor necrosis. Adenocarcinomas may have clear cell features resulting from the accumulation

pattern and minimal mucin expression, as demonstrated by histochemical and/or immunohistochemical staining assays. In some cases, the intracytoplasmic vacuole distends the cytoplasm and compressively deforms the nucleus to the cell margin, forming a "signet-ring" cell. The tumors may arise at

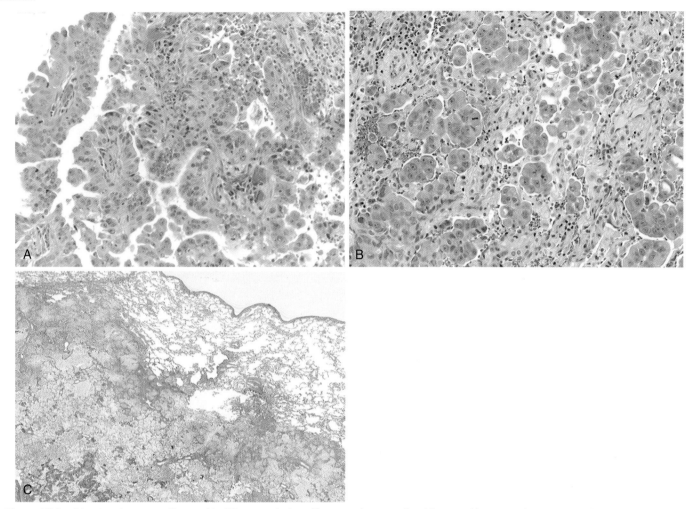

Figure 65-3 Adenocarcinoma, papillary and lepidic types. **A,** A papillary growth pattern is evident on this preparation. (Hematoxylin-eosin stain [H&E], 20×.) **B,** A micropapillary pattern can be seen. (H&E, 20×.) **C,** Mucinous adenocarcinoma with lepidic growth pattern. (H&E, 4×.)

of intracellular glycogen or mucins, and such tumors must be differentiated from metastatic clear cell renal carcinomas; the presence of intracytoplasmic lipid and glycogen is diagnostic of renal tumors of the clear cell type.

Histopathologic characteristics that correlate with a relatively poor prognosis in adenocarcinomas of the lung include a predominant solid pattern and high-grade cytologic features with mitotic figures and tumor necrosis, a micropapillary relative to a papillary histologic pattern, extension to and involvement of the visceral pleura, extensive lymphovascular tumor embolic spread, involvement of bronchial and hilar lymph nodes, and tumor-associated secondary obstructive lobar pneumonia. In addition, resection specimens that show intralobar satellite (metastatic) nodules and involvement of the surgical resection margins are associated with disease recurrence.

The histologic subtypes of adenocarcinoma appear to correlate with a history of cigarette smoking. Relative to nonsmokers, smokers more often have adenocarcinoma of the solid histologic type, and the extent of the solid component within the adenocarcinoma shows a dose-response relationship with pack-years of smoking. The solid subtype of adenocarcinoma also demonstrates a higher frequency of lymphovascular invasion and pleural involvement, and these histopathologic features are predictive for recurrence in stage I adenocarcinoma.

Historically, the most common cases of pulmonary adenocarcinoma were of the mixed type, with several histologic subtypes, and often the tumor had a so-called bronchioloalveolar carcinoma (BAC) growth margin. As originally defined, BAC is characterized by a lepidic growth pattern with atypical tumor cells (nonmucinous serous cells or mucinous cells) proliferating along the interstitial framework and not demonstrating stromal invasion or lymphovascular invasion. Tumors that manifest a BAC pattern often exhibit "ground glass" features on radiographs, and mixed-type invasive adenocarcinomas have central solid density with parenchymal distortion.

As a result of improper utilization and ambiguity of these pathologic terms, a group of international societies proposed a new classification that incorporated the histopathologic pattern, the radiographic features, and the clinical presentation and outcome. On the basis of the accumulated clinical experience with cases in which tumors 3 cm or less in diameter, with a pure lepidic growth pattern, were completely excised, followed by excellent survival, the term *adenocarcinoma in situ* (AIS) was adopted. These preinvasive lesions were judged to be extensions of a precursor lesion, termed *atypical adenomatous hyperplasia* (AAH), which also showed a lepidic growth pattern but were smaller in size (up to 5 mm in diameter). Those tumors that demonstrated an overall AIS pattern but also contained central minimal stromal invasion (less or equal to 5 mm) were

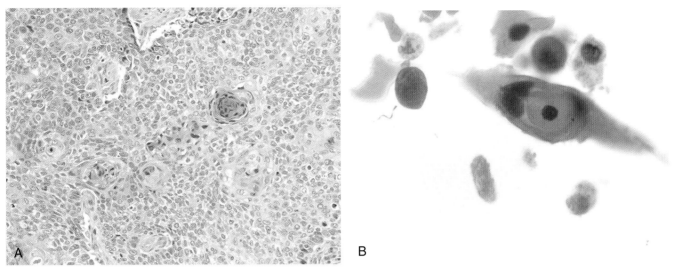

Figure 65-4   Squamous cell carcinoma. **A,** In this preparation, note the keratin pearl. (Hematoxylin-eosin stain, 20×.) **B,** Cytologic preparation showing cytoplasmic keratinization. (Papanicolaou smear, 100×.)

designated *minimally invasive adenocarcinoma* (MIA). These latter cancers usually are nonmucinous and are associated with an excellent clinical outcome. In order to render a diagnosis of AIS or MIA, the entire lesion must be excised and processed for microscopic evaluation. These tumor types are excluded when histologic features of lymphovascular invasion, pleural involvement, and tumor necrosis are identified. It is recommended that the designation BAC be abandoned and that in its place, the proper histologic classification be applied, which may be AIS, MIA, adenocarcinoma with a predominant or mixed lepidic pattern, or mucinous adenocarcinoma. Tumors that were historically diagnosed as "nonmucinous BAC" may now occur as AIS, MIA, or lepidic-dominant adenocarcinomas. Many of these cases tend to be found in women, with immunohistochemical profiles of CK7 and thyroid transcription factor-1 (TTF-1) immunoreactivity and frequent epidermal growth factor receptor (EGFR) mutational status. By contrast, the historical designation of "mucinous BAC" is recommended to be changed to *invasive mucinous adenocarcinoma*, with immunohistochemical profiles of CK20 immunoreactivity and nonreactivity for TTF-1. These tumors frequently are associated with *KRAS* mutation and no *EGFR* mutation.

Invasive adenocarcinomas, representing a considerable majority (greater than 75% of cases), are those that exhibit significant stromal invasion and possible lymphovascular invasion and infiltration of the visceral pleura. These cancers need to be measured, because the size of the invasive component governs the tumor-node-metastasis (TNM) staging and the potential for tumor dissemination. The classification also recommends that the predominant pattern of the adenocarcinoma be designated and that the term "mixed pattern" be abandoned. The assessment of the components of the adenocarcinoma not only is important for the proper classification but also is useful for the correct identification of multiple pulmonary nodules as either multiple primary tumors or T3 or T4 tumors. Obviously, tumors that differ in histologic pattern and those that have an in situ component represent multiple primary tumors. It also is possible to differentiate whether the separate nodules are multiple T1 tumors by determining the relative distribution of the adenocarcinoma subtypes. For example, two nodules of adenocarcinoma may be regarded as separate T1 tumors if one is predominantly of the acinar subtype while the other nodule lacks the acinar pattern and is composed of predominant solid variant.

The consensus classification also addressed the recommended approach with small biopsy specimens (a common problem with fiberoptic biopsy samples) and cytologic preparations. The pathologist must make every attempt to avoid the diagnosis of "lung cancer not otherwise specified," because the identification of a characteristic histologic pattern is important for tumor management. In a majority of cases, the distinction between adenocarcinoma and squamous cell carcinomas may be made using routine hematoxylin-eosin–stained (H&E) sections. In those cases of poorly differentiated carcinomas, mucin histochemical methods and a limited panel of immunohistochemical stains may achieve a more definitive result. Adenocarcinomas will show luminal or intracytoplasmic mucin positivity and TTF-1 immunoreactivity. Squamous cell carcinomas will lack mucin staining and will demonstrate reactivity for p63 or CK5/6 but not TTF-1.

Squamous Cell Carcinoma

Squamous cell carcinoma is a malignant tumor arising from bronchial epithelium with a strong etiologic association with cigarette smoking, in contrast with adenocarcinoma. It most commonly is central in location and arises from the main, lobar, or segmental bronchi. Squamous cell carcinomas usually appear as white or gray masses with a variable degree of fibrosis, frequently associated with central necrosis and cavitations. Histologic hallmarks of squamous origin, namely keratinization and intercellular bridges, are seen in relation to the degree of the differentiation; although readily appreciated in well-differentiated tumors, they may be only focally present or even absent in poorly differentiated ones (**Figure 65-4**). In selected cases, when squamous nature cannot be ascertained by routine light microscopy, immunohistochemistry studies are invaluable. Squamous cell carcinomas usually are immunoreactive for high-molecular-weight keratin, CK5/6, and p63 and generally are nonreactive for TTF-1, CK7, and neuroendocrine markers (CD56, synaptophysin, chromogranin). Although not widely used, electron microscopy also can highlight features of squamous differentiation, such as prominent desmosomes and cytoplasmic aggregates of intermediate keratin filaments.

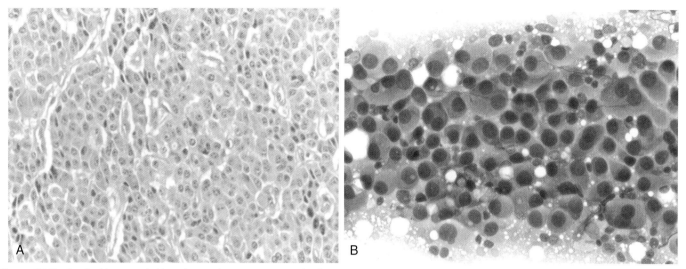

Figure 65-5 Carcinoid tumor. **A,** Note the nesting arrangement of cells. (Hematoxylin-eosin stain, 40×.) **B,** Cytologic preparation showing a uniform cellular pattern. (Diff-Quik stain, 40×.)

Recognizing histologic variants of squamous cell carcinoma, including papillary, clear cell, small cell, and basaloid types, is useful mainly in excluding the various differential diagnostic considerations. Their behavior is primarily a reflection of the degree of differentiation, with basaloid and small cell variants portending a worse outcome.

Pattern of spread is somewhat different depending on the anatomic location. Central tumors either grow along the epithelium, with or without invasion into subepithelial tissue, or expand as an endobronchial polypoid growth. In advanced cases, these tumors may directly involve hilar mediastinal tissue, including lymph nodes. Peripheral tumors, on the other hand, form a solid nodule and may directly break through the pleura into the chest wall or diaphragm.

Staging is governed by the TNM system. Regardless of the location, squamous cell carcinomas are more likely to be locally aggressive and invade adjacent structures. Distant metastasis, albeit far less common than with other subtypes of lung cancer, has a predilection for brain, liver, adrenals, lower gastrointestinal tract, and distant lymph nodes. In general, squamous cell carcinomas are associated with better prognosis and survival rate, as compared with stage-matched adenocarcinomas.

Small Cell Carcinoma and Neuroendocrine (Carcinoid) Tumors

Neuroendocrine tumors, those that contain dense core neurosecretory granules composed of serotonin, histamine, and other bioactive amines, include small cell and large cell neuroendocrine carcinomas and typical and atypical carcinoid tumors. As a group, these tumors represent about one fifth of primary lung neoplasms, with small cell carcinoma being the most common in this category. These tumor types share a histologic pattern of uniform to pleomorphic cells in an organoid arrangement of tumor nests and trabecula (**Figure 65-5**). Carcinoid tumors may be considered as well-differentiated neuroendocrine carcinomas with little to no mitotic activity (less than 2 mitotic figures per 2-mm² microscopic field) or tumor necrosis. Carcinoid tumors may occur in nonsmokers, in whom they manifest as a vascular rich endobronchial mass, although some carcinoid tumors may have a peripheral localization and have spindle cellular features. The tumors are low-grade malignancies with approximately 15% nodal metastases at diagnosis; nevertheless,

affected patients have a greater than 90% 5-year survival. The atypical carcinoid tumors are neuroendocrine carcinomas of intermediate grade that have an organoid arrangement with more irregular and atypical cytologic pattern, identifiable tumor necrosis, and countable mitotic activity (2 to 10 mitoses per 2-mm² microscopic field). In contrast with typical carcinoid tumors, atypical carcinoid may have nearly 50% lymph node metastases on presentation and a lower 5-year survival rate.

The high-grade poorly differentiated neuroendocrine tumors consist of the small cell (neuroendocrine) carcinoma and the large cell neuroendocrine carcinoma. The latter two have, respectively, smaller and larger cells with considerable cytologic atypia, prominent mitotic activity (more than 10 mitotic figures per 2-mm² microscopic field), and abundant tumor necrosis. All of the neuroendocrine tumors will be immunohistochemically reactive with broad-spectrum cytokeratins, CD56, and, specifically, immunoreactive for neuroendocrine markers, such as chromogranin and synaptophysin. The high-grade neuroendocrine carcinomas are immunoreactive for TTF-1, more so than are the intermediate-grade and well-differentiated types.

Close attention to the morphologic details in conjunction with ancillary studies is important to differentiate small cell carcinoma not only from non–small cell carcinoma but also from other neuroendocrine tumors of lung, because they differ substantially in their demographics, clinical presentation, and behavior. Small cell carcinoma of lung generally is a disease of elderly men (mean age, 65 years) who are almost always current or former heavy smokers. These demographic findings are in sharp contrast with those in patients with typical carcinoid, who present at a younger age (mean, 45 to 50 years), with no difference in regard to gender or smoking history. The disparity also extends to associated prognosis and clinical behavior. Whereas typical carcinoid tumors are known for their indolent behavior and excellent survival rates, small cell carcinomas, at the other end of the spectrum, are fatal, with many patients presenting with distant metastasis at the time of diagnosis. Small cell carcinomas typically are central in location and frequently appear radiographically as hilar or perihilar masses with mediastinal lymphadenopathy and lobar collapse. Extensive necrosis is almost always present.

The key histopathologic features in the diagnosis of small cell carcinoma are nuclear morphologic features, such as finely

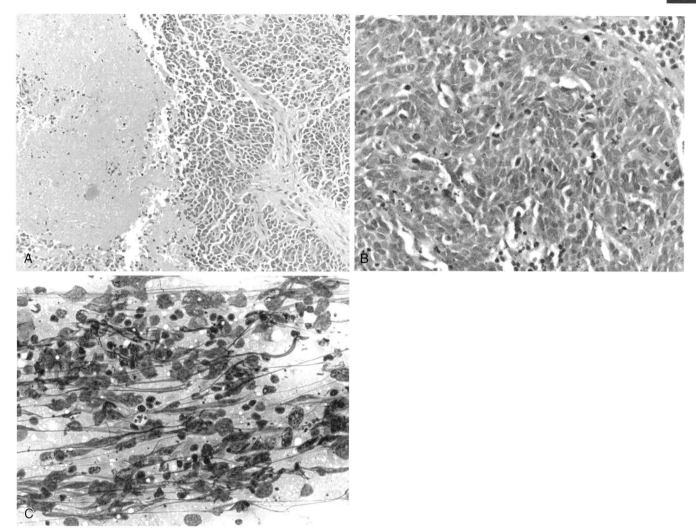

Figure 65-6   Small cell carcinoma. **A,** In this preparation, note the partial nesting pattern and tumor necrosis. (Hematoxylin-eosin stain [H&E], 20×.) **B,** Nuclear molding and mitotic activity are evident in this preparation. (H&E, 40×.) **C,** Cytologic preparation showing inconspicuous cytoplasm and nuclear fragmentation. (Diff-Quik stain, 20×.)

granular chromatin, absence of prominent nucleoli, fragility, molding, and extensive crush artifact, as well as indistinct cytoplasmic borders and high mitotic figure count (more than 10 per 10 high-power fields) (**Figure 65-6**). Large zones of geographic necrosis also are common. Classically, a great deal of emphasis was placed on the small cell size or nuclear size, as suggested by the nomenclature. The usefulness of this criterion is questionable, however, in view of the wide variability in size, with frequent overlap with large cell neuroendocrine carcinomas. Large cell neuroendocrine carcinomas show a low-power neuroendocrine architecture, as seen in carcinoid tumors; however, the cell morphology closely resembles that of non–small cell carcinomas, with vesicular chromatin, prominent nucleoli, and abundant cytoplasm—features completely different from those of small cell carcinoma (**Figure 65-7**). Additionally, these tumors are highly mitotic (more than 10 mitotic figures per 10 high-power fields) and often show extensive necrosis, similar to that in small cell carcinomas, and in keeping with their high-grade nature.

Positive immunoreactivity with at least one neuroendocrine marker (synaptophysin, chromogranin) is required for the diagnosis of small cell carcinoma. By contrast, the main role of immunohistochemistry studies in small cell carcinoma is to exclude a wide range of other high-grade round blue cell tumors in the differential diagnosis. Cytokeratin immunoreactivity, especially the characteristic dotlike positivity, aids in excluding a lymphoid process, reactive or neoplastic, in instances of considerable morphologic overlap, particularly in small and poorly preserved samples. However, strong membranous staining with cytokeratins and diffuse staining with 34βE12 are characteristic of non–small cell carcinomas and generally are not seen in small cell carcinoma. The neuroendocrine markers synaptophysin and chromogranin, although strongly expressed in carcinoid, may be very focal in location or entirely absent in small cell carcinoma, and in such cases, CD56 is a more sensitive indicator of neuroendocrine differentiation. TTF-1, a very useful marker in establishing lung origin in adenocarcinoma, is seen in an overwhelming majority of small cell lung carcinomas, but it also may be expressed by extrapulmonary small cell carcinomas such as bladder and prostate cancers and therefore cannot be used to establish the site of origin. Although Ki-67 (MIB1) proliferation index is not an integral part of the current WHO classification of lung neuroendocrine tumors, it is of value, especially in the evaluation of small biopsy samples and cytologic specimens, when tissue is limited and poor preservation or extensive crush artifact during procurement may be inevitable. It has been suggested that Ki-67 (MIB1) percent positivity may be used as a diagnostic adjunct to morphologic

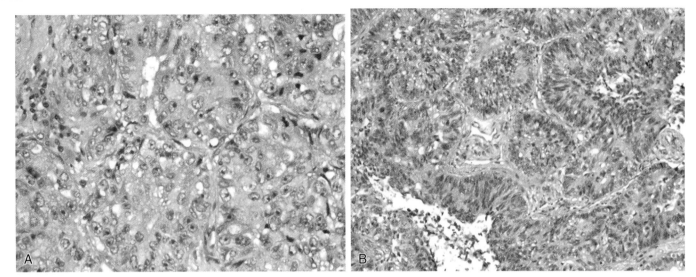

Figure 65-7 Large cell carcinoma. **A,** In this preparation, a high-grade pattern with prominent nucleoli is evident. (Hematoxylin-eosin stain, 40×.) **B,** On this specimen from a large cell neuroendocrine carcinoma, note the trabecular and nesting pattern of a neuroendocrine tumor. (Hematoxylin-eosin stain, 20×.)

examination: for typical carcinoid, less than 2%; for atypical carcinoid, less than 20%; and significantly, greater than 20% for small cell and large cell neuroendocrine carcinomas.

Traditionally, small cell carcinomas have been divided into limited-stage disease (treatable within a single radiation portal) and extensive-stage disease (contralateral or distant metastasis) with regard to prognosis. Recent large-scale analyses have shown the value of TNM staging for all neuroendocrine tumors of the lung, including carcinoid tumors.

Large Cell Carcinoma

By definition, *large cell carcinoma* of lung is an undifferentiated carcinoma lacking morphologic evidence of small cell carcinoma, squamous cell carcinoma, or adenocarcinoma. In other words, it represents a diagnosis of exclusion. These tumors typically are composed of sheets and nests of large polygonal cells with moderate amount of cytoplasm, vesicular chromatin and prominent nucleoli (**Figure 65-7**). Although the classification is purely based on morphologic grounds, judicious use of ancillary studies (as discussed previously), especially with small biopsy specimens, is of significant value in separating the poorly differentiated squamous cell carcinomas and adenocarcinomas from the truly undifferentiated large cell carcinoma. These tumors share similar demographic and clinical features with other non–small cell carcinomas of the lung, because they commonly are seen in elderly men with smoking history.

Large cell carcinomas are preferentially seen at the periphery of the lung. Several histologic subtypes are recognized: basaloid, clear cell, and lymphoepithelioma-like carcinomas. Although grouped under large cell carcinomas in the 2004 WHO classification, large cell neuroendocrine carcinoma, as strictly defined in the previous section, is best categorized as a neuroendocrine tumor, closely resembling small cell carcinoma. Nevertheless, the mere focal expression of neuroendocrine markers as detected on immunohistochemistry studies, seen in some large cell carcinomas, should not be interpreted as diagnostic for large cell neuroendocrine carcinoma. In general, large cell carcinomas are high-grade tumors that are similar in prognosis and pattern of spread to stage-matched non–small cell carcinomas, with performance status at the time of diagnosis and disease extension considered to be the most important

clinical prognostic parameters. Metastases arise most commonly in the hilar and mediastinal nodes, followed by pleura, liver, bone, brain, abdominal nodes, and pericardium. The basaloid subtype carries a worse prognosis, even in the lower stages, with more common metastasis to the brain. On the other hand, lymphoepithelioma-like carcinomas generally are diagnosed at a later stage of disease but are associated with a better prognosis.

Pleural Malignancies

Diffuse malignant mesothelioma is a pleura-based cancer that may be histopathologically composed of a biphasic growth pattern of combined epithelial and sarcomatoid components. The tumor also may manifest in a monophasic form of either epithelioid cancer resembling a pleural adenocarcinoma or a spindle sarcomatoid form resembling a mesenchymal sarcoma. The diagnosis is usually but not exclusively rendered with a history of asbestos exposure, similar to that for pleural asbestosis or asbestos-related diseases and malignancies, but with a lower threshold of lung asbestos burden. Other proposed causes of diffuse malignant mesothelioma are chest radiation therapy and exposure to other mineral silicates, such as vermiculite and erionite. Erionite originally was identified in Turkey but is now appreciated to have widespread deposits in the western United States (i.e., Dakotas, Nevada, Arizona, and California). The diagnosis is based on appropriate clinical, radiographic, and histopathologic findings of a painful pleura-based tumor with scattered multiple nodules or a coalescent tumor encasing the lung. Malignant mesothelioma may obliterate the pleural cavity or be associated with an exudative pleural effusion. The tumor may invade the underlying lung and typically infiltrates through the diaphragm.

Malignant mesothelioma exhibits characteristic surgical pathology features that must be distinguished from reactive mesothelial proliferation and chronic fibrosing pleuritis. Reactive mesothelial hyperplasia frequently is present in the setting of collagen vascular diseases, drug or inflammatory reactions, and trauma or surgery. Of importance, reactive mesothelial hyperplasia lacks invasion of the stromal connective tissue and fat, does not undergo necrosis, and typically is not immunoreactive for EMA (epithelial membrane antigen) and p53 (tumor suppressor gene product). In the setting of exposure to asbestos, collagenous pleural plaques may be identified and associated with either reactive mesothelial hyperplasia or an incipient diffuse malignant mesothelioma. Separation of chronic pleuritis from malignant mesothelioma also is based on the lack of mesothelial invasion in pleuritis and the presence of an organizing zonal layered fibroinflammatory process. Desmoplastic malignant mesothelioma will, on the other hand, show stromal invasion, haphazard growth pattern, and metastatic spread. Reactive mesothelial cells and those of malignant mesothelioma are immunoreactive for cytokeratin. The histopathologic appearance of reactive mesothelial conditions is organized and layered, in contrast to the haphazard cellularity and invasion in malignant mesothelioma.

The histologic pattern of the epithelioid type of diffuse malignant mesothelioma appears as an invasive tubular and papillary malignancy that mimics a pleura-based adenocarcinoma or a metastatic adenocarcinoma. The monophasic sarcomatoid mesotheliomas resemble spindle cell sarcomas, which may manifest as primary or metastatic cancers. The most common form of malignant mesothelioma is the epithelioid variant and may show a variety of histologic features, such as tubulopapillary, glandular, or solid patterns. Cytologic examination of malignant pleural effusions shows irregular clusters of atypical mesothelial-like cells in pools of hyaluronic acid. Malignant mesotheliomas also may present in the peritoneal cavity and mimic ovarian cancers in women. Biphasic mesotheliomas are less common in the abdomen than in the pleura, and abdominal sarcomatoid mesotheliomas are rare. The distinction between malignant mesothelioma and adenocarcinoma in the pleura and peritoneal cavity is based on histologic features and supported by histochemical and immunohistochemical staining and ultrastructural findings. Mesotheliomas will be positive for Alcian blue, a stain that disappears with pretreatment with hyaluronidase. Most adenocarcinomas are histochemically positive for mucicarmine stains, although a few mesotheliomas also may stain positive. On immunohistochemical assays, malignant mesotheliomas will be immunoreactive for calretinin, keratin 5/6, WT-1 protein, and podoplanin (D2-40), in contrast with adenocarcinomas, which are immunoreactive for CEA (carcinoembryonic antigen), MOC-31, B72.3, Ber-EP4, and TTF-1. Both mesotheliomas and adenocarcinomas will be positive on assay for pancytokeratins, which will demonstrate the viability of the tissue for immunohistochemical assessments. Historically, the best diagnostic discriminator for distinguishing malignant mesothelioma from adenocarcinoma has been electron microscopic examination of the tumor. The ultrastructural appearance of malignant mesothelioma on transmission electron microscopy shows long slender microvillous processes with frequent branching and lacking a glycocalyx, in contrast with short blunt straight microvilli of adenocarcinoma, containing a glycocalyx.

MOLECULAR BIOLOGY

The study of cellular and molecular mechanisms of lung cancer has provided insight into lung cancer biology in terms of epidemiology and predisposition to lung cancer, lung cancer carcinogenesis, and cancer progression and resistance to chemotherapy and radiation therapy. Epidemiologic investigations have demonstrated higher levels of lung cancer in patients whose family history included a diagnosis of lung cancer in a first-degree relative. In a case-control study of lung cancer in women, never-smokers with positive family history had an odds

ratio of 5.7 relative to nonsmokers without a family history. Smokers without a family history of lung cancer and smokers with a family history had odds ratios of approximately 15 and 30, respectively, for the development of lung cancer relative to non-smokers without a family history of lung cancer. Among persons who are carriers of a mutated retinoblastoma (*RB*) gene, the mortality rate for lung cancer is 15-fold that in the general population.

The cellular predisposition to lung cancer among cigarette smokers has included protean metabolic phenotypic pathways among smokers at risk for lung cancer. It appears clear that individual metabolism must play a role in carcinogenesis: The overwhelming majority of cancers are found in smokers, but among smokers, only a minority develop lung cancer. The host factors acting on environmental smoke metabolites include the pleiotropic expressions of the cytochrome p450 oxidative enzymes. Polycyclic aromatic hydrocarbons and nitrosamines, components of cigarette smoke and carcinogenic agents, induce the expression of P450 enzymes. In turn, cytochrome P450 metabolism produces reactive oxygenated intermediates that have the capacity for DNA binding and alterations, leading to mutations and cellular dysplasia. Aryl hydrocarbon hydroxylases, as members of the mixed-function oxidases, are induced by and active on cigarette smoke chemicals, and their metabolites are capable of causing DNA mutations and malignant transformation of cells.

One of the fundamental precepts of cancer development is multistep carcinogenesis involving basic steps of initiation (transmissible DNA damage leading to cellular dysplasia with altered regulatory controls), promotion (proliferation of abnormal cellular clones to form a mass), and progression (invasion and metastases). Cellular and molecular events that drive the conversion of preneoplastic conditions to malignant tumors are activations of cellular oncogenes, deletion or inactivation of tumor suppressor genes, enhancement of survival relative to apoptotic pathways, and alterations of DNA repair mechanisms. Early studies found chromosomal 3p deletions in lung cancers, more commonly in small cell carcinomas. *KRAS* activation and the expression of p21, involved in activation of cellular signal transduction pathways, have been identified in lung cancers. Mutations in *KRAS* were identified in adenocarcinomas, especially pronounced in smokers, and were associated with relatively poor survival. Genetic amplification and mutation of the *EGFR* gene, associated with increased or altered protein expression, have been identified predominantly in non–small cell carcinomas. Examples of inactivation of tumor suppressor genes are loss of Rb expression in some small cell carcinomas and inactivation of p53 in non–small cell carcinomas.

Molecular biology studies have provided insight into the initiation and progression of lung cancer. Additional investigations have revealed cellular and molecular changes that modulate the tumor's response to chemotherapy and provide acquired resistance to therapeutic management. Chemotherapeutic agents that act in the folate pathway of pyrimidine and DNA synthesis, such as pemetrexed, may demonstrate reduced efficacy when the functional level of thymidylate synthesis is overexpressed. Similarly, the overexpression of ERCC-1 (excision repair cross-complementation group 1), a repair enzymatic pathway for DNA strand breaks, modifies the therapeutic outcome with platinum drugs that intercalate in the DNA.

Tumors that appear to be markedly governed by a single or small set of pathway gene products are said to show "oncogene addiction." Despite the complexity of genetic and epigenetic tumor cell abnormalities, these "oncogene addiction" pathway genes dominate the progressive and invasive nature of the malignancy, and interruption of their function will lead to tumor regression, thereby promoting a prolonged disease-free interval or overall survival. This molecular condition provides the pharmacologic rationale for targeted therapy. The three genes discussed next appear to be in the "driver's seat" for tumor progression, and blocking their altered function will provide for tumor regression.

Epidermal Growth Factor Receptor Gene

EGFR is a transmembrane signaling protein that transduces extracellular signals, due to binding of EGFR ligands, into intracellular changes mediated by activating tyrosine kinase phosphorylations. EGFR, also called HER1 (human epidermal growth factor receptor 1), is in the same family as HER2, another membrane receptor that is amplified in approximately 20% of breast cancers. In breast cancer, HER2 is biologically associated with a relatively aggressive type of breast cancer, but it also is a therapeutic target for directed antibodies or small molecule tyrosine kinase inhibitors (TKIs). When EGFR is mutated, predominantly in nonsmokers, it adopts an activated state, as if constantly bound to activating ligands or growth factors. EGFR activation induces downstream signals that inhibit apoptosis and stimulate cell proliferation and migration and motility. Targeted TKIs are effective for tumor regression when non–small cell carcinomas have activating EGFR mutations, as opposed to tumors with wild-type EGFR. EGFR-activating mutations tend to be present in a minority of lung cancers (10% to 20%) and appear most commonly in nonmucinous adenocarcinomas exhibiting a well-differentiated acinar or papillary growth pattern with a lepidic growth margin and presenting demographically in younger Asian women who were never-smokers or light smokers. In this last demographic subgroup, the incidence of EGFR mutation may rise to 40% to 50%. Large cell carcinomas also have shown EGFR mutation; however, the rate of such mutations in squamous cell carcinoma is only a few percent, and this low frequency is not sufficient for routine analysis. Immunohistochemical identification of EGFR in tumor tissue has no correlation with clinical tumor response to TKIs. The EGFR mutation is the molecular marker, more significant than EGFR amplification, for targeted therapy and is a predictive factor for a therapeutic response. Fluorescence in situ hybridization (FISH) assays have been attempted to identify EGFR amplification and show some concordance with therapeutic response, because EGFR mutations correlate with amplification. Adenocarcinomas with nonmutated but amplified EGFR gene have been recognized, and these tumors show a partial response to tyrosine kinase inhibition.

The standard tests for EGFR mutations may be performed on formalin-fixed paraffin-embedded tissue and consist of direct DNA sequencing or mutation-specific assays investigating mutations that usually are found in exons 19 and 21. In instances of tumor recurrence due to resistance to TKIs, the sequencing analysis should be expanded to include exons 18 and 20. The acquired resistance tends to occur in about a year after TKI therapy is started and may be related to a new mutation in the active site; other causes for TKI resistance are due to MET gene amplification in 10% to 15% of cases. EGFR genetic testing shows concordant results with the presence of an activating mutation between the primary tumor and its metastasis in a majority of cases; however, an average discordance of 25%, as a result of tumor heterogeneity and progression, has been noted.

KRAS Oncogene

KRAS is an oncogene found on the short arm of chromosome 12 (12p) and shows mutations in approximately 20% of non–small cell lung cancers and amplification of the gene in a smaller set of cancers. The p21 protein (i.e., K-RAS), encoded by KRAS, couples with a cytoplasmic GTPase to convert guanosine triphosphate (GTP) to guanosine diphosphate (GDP) in order to modify transductive signals from the cytoplasm to the nucleus, thereby controlling cellular growth and survival pathways. When KRAS is mutated, GTP is maintained, and the signal is persistently in the "active" state. Activating mutations of KRAS are present in a variety of epithelial tumors, including colon and pancreatic cancers, and lead to activating phosphorylation of mitogen-activated protein kinase (MAPK), inducing nuclear signals of cellular proliferation and tumor progression. KRAS mutations and amplifications demonstrate clinicopathologic correlations with older age combined with male gender, history of heavy cigarette smoking, and advanced disease at presentation, with relatively aggressive tumors and poor clinical outcome. Histologically, KRAS mutations tend to be identified in poorly differentiated adenocarcinomas with solid growth pattern and lacking a lepidic growth pattern. Of interest, the mucinous lepidic pattern is associated with KRAS mutations. These high-grade adenocarcinomas also show lymphovascular invasion, mitotic activity, and tumor necrosis. K-RAS is downstream from EGFR effects and when activated is independent of EGFR status, thereby conveying resistance to tyrosine kinase inhibitors of EGFR function.

EML4/ALK

A new addition to molecular markers that predict a clinically favorable response to targeted therapy is the EML4-ALK translocation. The proper name of the fusion gene product is echinoderm microtubule-associated protein-like 4–anaplastic lymphoma kinase. The short arm of chromosome 2 (2p) may contain multiple small inversions and or translocations whose permutations generate in-frame fusions of the 5′ portion of the EML4 gene with the 3′ end of the ALK gene, creating a chimeric tyrosine kinase with an intracellular kinase domain. Breakpoints of the EML4 gene occur at several possible exon sites, although the breakpoint of the ALK gene tends to be specific for the kinase domain at exon 20. This fusion activation of the ALK gene is infrequent (occurring in less than 10% of non–small cell lung cancers), but the incidence may be enriched in lung cancers present in younger persons without significant smoking history in whom EGFR mutations and KRAS mutations are lacking. EML4-ALK translocations are histologically correlated with high-grade adenocarcinomas exhibiting acinar and solid growth patterns that contain mucinous and signet ring differentiation. From early studies, it appears that tyrosine kinase–targeted therapy for EGFR mutations is not effective treatment for EML4-ALK mutations. EML4-ALK fusion also appears to be selective for adenocarcinomas, because it is lacking in the other types of bronchogenic carcinomas.

The test for the translocation is based on reverse transcriptase–polymerase chain reaction (RT-PCR) assay of tumor tissue RNA, which amplifies and detects certain of the fusion constructs. The assay limitation is due to the identification of only the translocations of EML4 exons 6 and 13 with ALK exon 20. The fusion gene also may be assayed by FISH techniques, and recent studies suggest that immunohistochemical methods also may yield accurate results.

SUGGESTED READINGS

Alberg AJ, Samet JM: Epidemiology of lung cancer, *Chest* 123:21S–49S, 2003.

American Cancer Society: *2010 Cancer facts & figures*, Atlanta, 2010, American Cancer Society.

Brambilla E, Gazdar A: Pathogenesis of lung cancer signalling pathways: roadmap for therapies, *Eur Respir J* 33:1485–1497, 2009.

Cadranel J, Zalcman G, Sequist L: Genetic profiling and epidermal growth factor receptor directed therapy in non-small cell lung cancer, *Eur Respir J* 37:183–193, 2011.

Camidge DR, Hirsch FR, Varella-Garcia M, Franklin WA: Finding ALK-positive lung cancer: what are we really looking for? *J Thorac Oncol* 6:411–413, 2011.

Han SW, Kim TY, Hwang PG, et al: Predictive and prognostic impact of epidermal growth factor receptor mutation in non-small cell cancer patients treated with gefitinib, *J Clin Oncol* 23:2493–2402, 2005.

Haura EB, Camidge DR, Reckamp K, et al: Molecular origins of lung cancer: prospects for personalized prevention and therapy, *J Thorac Oncol* 5:S207–S213, 2010.

Husain AN, Colby TV, Ordonez NG, et al: Guidelines for pathologic diagnosis of malignant mesothelioma, *Arch Pathol Lab Med* 133:1317–1331, 2009.

Idowu M, Powers CN: Lung cancer cytology: potential pitfalls and mimics—a review, *J Clin Exp Pathol* 3:367–385, 2010.

Inamura K, Takeuchi K, Togashi Y, et al: EML4-ALK fusion is linked to histologic characteristics in a subset of lung cancers, *J Thorac Oncol* 3:13–17, 2008.

Mitsudomi T, Kosaka T, Endoh H, et al: Mutations of the epidermal growth factor receptor gene predict prolong survival after gefitinib treatment in patients with non-small-cell lung cancer with post-operative recurrence, *J Clin Oncol* 23:2513–2520, 2005.

Mok TS, Wu YL, Thongprasert S, et al: Gefitinib or carboplatin-paclitaxel in pulmonary adenocarcinoma, *N Engl J Med* 361:947–957, 2009.

Osann KE: Lung cancer in women: the importance of smoking, family history of lung cancer, and medical history of respiratory disease, *Cancer Res* 51:4893–4897, 1991.

Rekhtman N: Neuroendocrine tumors of the lung, *Arch Pathol Lab Med* 134:1628–1638, 2010.

Rekhtman N, Brandt SM, Sigel CS, et al: Suitability of thoracic cytology for new therapeutic paradigms in non-small cell lung carcinoma, *J Thorac Oncol* 6:451–458, 2011.

Samet J, Humble C, Pathak D: Personal and family history of respiratory disease and lung cancer risk, *Am Rev Respir Dis* 134:466–470, 1986.

Schwartz AM, Henson DE: Diagnostic surgical pathology in lung cancer: ACCP evidence-based clinical practice guidelines, ed 2, *Chest* 132:78–91, 2007.

Shaw AT, Yeap BY, Mino-Kenudson M, et al: Clinical features and outcome of patients with non-small cell lung cancer who harbor EML4-ALK, *J Clin Oncol* 27:4247–4251, 2009.

Soda M, Choi YL, Enomoto M, et al: Identification of the transforming EML4-ALK fusion gene in non-small cell lung cancer, *Nature* 448:561–566, 2007.

Takano T, Ohe Y, Sakamoto H, et al: Epidermal growth factor receptor gene mutations and increase copy numbers predict gefitinib sensitivity in patients with recurrent non-small cell lung cancer, *J Clin Oncol* 23:6829–6837, 2005.

Travis WD, Brambilla E, Muller-Hermelink HK, et al: *Pathology and genetics. Tumors of the lung, pleura, thymus, and heart*, Lyon, France, IARC Press, 2004.

Travis WD, Brambilla E, Noguchi M, et al: International Association for the Study of Lung Cancer/American Thoracic Society/European Respiratory Society international multidisciplinary classification of lung adenocarcinoma, *J Thorac Oncol* 6:244–285, 2011.

U.S. Department of Health and Human Services: *How tobacco smoke causes disease: the biology and behavioral basis for smoking attributable disease: a report of the Surgeon General*, Atlanta, 2010, Centers for Disease Control and Prevention, National Center for Chronic Disease Prevention and Health Promotion, Office of Smoking and Health.

U.S. Public Health Service: *Smoking and health. Report of the Advisory Committee to the Surgeon General*, PHS publication no. 1103, Washington, DC, 1964, U.S. Department of Health, Education, and Welfare, Public Health Service, CDC.

Chapter **66**

Lung Cancer: Clinical Evaluation and Staging

Lynn Tanoue

Every patient with lung cancer should undergo a timely and thorough clinical evaluation, starting with a comprehensive history and physical examination. The presence or absence of symptoms will influence subsequent imaging and invasive assessment, and decisions relating to future evaluation and treatment will be guided by the patient's overall health status, including comorbid medical conditions. This general assessment, ultimately leading to the determination of clinical stage, typically will inform further evaluation and will influence the choice of therapy. It is therefore critically important that this process be approached efficiently and comprehensively.

SYMPTOMATIC PRESENTATION

SYMPTOMS AND SIGNS RELATED TO THE PRIMARY TUMOR

Currently, most patients with lung cancer have advanced disease at the time of presentation and are likely to present with symptoms, particularly if local extension, metastasis to distant sites, or a paraneoplastic syndrome is present. Obtaining a thorough history and a review of systems in patients suspected of having lung cancer constitute an important part of the initial evaluation, because the symptom history will influence the choice of imaging studies, the interpretation of those studies, and the institution of early palliative interventions. Symptoms and signs related to the primary tumor most commonly include cough, dyspnea, chest pain, and hemoptysis. Cough is present in up to 75% of patients with lung cancer and may be related to airway involvement, postobstructive pneumonitis, or bronchorrhea. Dyspnea may be associated with primary site–related problems, such as endobronchial or extrinsic airway obstruction, postobstructive atelectasis, infection, or increased airway secretions, or may be related to metastatic disease, with potential manifestations including pleural effusion, lymphangitic tumor spread, pericardial effusion with tamponade, and pulmonary thromboemboli in the setting of hypercoagulability. Hemoptysis with lung cancer usually manifests as intermittent or persistent bloody streaking of the sputum and rarely can be massive. In up to 9% of patients with hemoptysis and lung cancer, the chest radiograph will be normal in appearance, underscoring the need to include endobronchial tumor as a major consideration in the differential diagnosis in patients presenting with hemoptysis and lung cancer risk factors (**Figure 66-1**). With the exception of hemoptysis, these pulmonary symptoms may not necessarily prompt a patient with a history of cigarette use, chronic obstructive pulmonary disease, or interstitial lung disease to seek specific medical attention or, conversely, for the clinician to consider an alternative diagnosis. These may be contributing factors to the consistent observation of a delay of several months between the onset of symptoms and a definitive diagnosis of lung cancer.

SYMPTOMS RELATED TO INTRATHORACIC SPREAD

Intrathoracic spread of lung cancer may occur by direct extension of the primary tumor or by involvement of lymph nodes and other thoracic structures. Chest pain is reported by up to 50% of patients at presentation and often indicates extension of tumor to the mediastinum, chest wall, or pleura. Hoarseness typically heralds involvement of the left recurrent laryngeal nerve, which in its circuitous course into the chest and under the aortic arch is particularly subject to compromise from left-sided cancers spreading to the ipsilateral mediastinal lymph nodes. Recurrent (inferior) laryngeal nerve palsy also may cause aspiration and coughing related to inadequate apposition of the vocal cords. Superior vena cava syndrome occurs more commonly with lung cancer than any other tumor, with small cell carcinoma the most commonly associated histologic subtype. Patients may present with a sensation of facial fullness, dyspnea, dysphagia, and headache or with actual swelling of the face, neck, and upper chest, and typically exhibit distended neck veins as well as a dilated venous pattern over the upper chest and shoulders. Superior sulcus (Pancoast) tumors are associated with a constellation of symptoms, primarily pain from compression or invasion of the brachial plexus (which, because it typically localizes to the shoulder and scapula, may not immediately prompt a pulmonary evaluation per se), Horner syndrome (ptosis, miosis, anhidrosis) due to involvement of the sympathetic chain and stellate ganglion, and upper extremity muscle wasting and pain related to tumor involvement of the eighth cervical and first and second thoracic nerve roots. Extension of tumor to the pericardium can result in pericardial effusion with or without tamponade, as well as arrhythmias. Bulky mediastinal adenopathy itself causes symptoms uncommonly, although dysphagia may result if the esophagus is compressed.

SYMPTOMS RELATED TO METASTATIC SPREAD

Lung cancer can spread distantly to any organ. The presence of constitutional symptoms, particularly weight loss but also fatigue, weakness, or poor appetite, and new symptoms

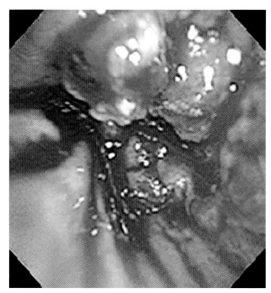

Figure 66-1 Endobronchial tumor in the left main bronchus, which manifested clinically as intermittent hemoptysis accelerating over the course of 2 months. *(Courtesy Jonathan Puchalski, MD.)*

Table 66-1	Paraneoplastic Syndromes Associated with Lung Cancer
Endocrine	Syndrome of inappropriate secretion of antidiuretic hormone (SIADH)/hyponatremia; hypercalcemia; ectopic adrenocorticotropic hormone (ACTH) syndrome; Cushing syndrome; hyperglycemia; hypoglycemia; hyperthyroidism; carcinoid syndrome; gynecomastia; elevated growth hormone; elevated follicle-stimulating hormone (FSH); galactorrhea
Musculoskeletal	Hypertrophic osteoarthropathy (HOP); clubbing, myopathy; dermatomyositis; polymyositis
Neurologic	Lambert-Eaton myasthenic syndrome (LEMS); encephalomyelitis/subacute sensory neuropathy; cerebellar degeneration; opsoclonus-myoclonus; autonomic neuropathy; retinopathy; mononeuritis multiplex; peripheral neuropathy; myopathy
Skin	Acanthosis nigricans; pruritus and urticaria, erythema multiforme; erythroderma; exfoliative dermatitis; hyperpigmentation
Hematologic	Anemia, thrombocytosis, leukocytosis, hypercoagulable state

related to any organ, including musculoskeletal pain, neurologic changes, hoarseness, and abdominal discomfort, should heighten the clinical suspicion for metastatic disease. Laboratory abnormalities, including anemia, abnormalities on liver function tests, and hypercalcemia, also should prompt a search for disease beyond the primary site. Conversely, the absence of any of these symptoms or signs on a thorough initial clinical assessment argues strongly against the presence of metastatic spread. The most common sites of distant spread are lymph glands, liver, bones, adrenal glands, brain and spinal cord, and pleura.

Lymph node metastases typically are seen first in the thorax, in either the ipsilateral hilar area or the mediastinum, and rarely cause symptoms. The supraclavicular fossa should be examined carefully in patients with known or suspected lung cancer, because this is the most common location for palpable malignant adenopathy and offers an easily accessible site for cytologic needle aspiration to establish diagnosis and stage of disease.

Liver metastases may be associated with constitutional symptoms including fever but usually are asymptomatic and often are not associated with any abnormalities on liver function tests. By contrast, bone metastases tend to manifest with pain and may be associated with elevations of alkaline phosphatase or serum calcium levels.

Adrenal metastases typically are unilateral but may be bilateral. Because most adrenal masses actually represent benign adenomas or hyperplasia, a more definitive noninvasive evaluation or biopsy is warranted. Adrenal metastases usually are asymptomatic; adrenal insufficiency related to metastatic invasion of the adrenal glands is rare.

The brain is a common site of spread in patients with lung cancer; conversely, a majority of brain metastases are related to primary sites located in the lung. Overall, intracranial metastasis is present in approximately 10% of all patients with lung cancer at initial diagnosis, with signs and symptoms ranging from headache and confusion to seizures or focal neurologic deficits.

Pleural involvement with tumor may take the form of pleural nodules, direct tumor extension, or malignant pleural effusion. Malignant effusions usually are exudative and may be either serous or bloody. Under the current staging system, the presence of a malignant effusion places the patient in a group with the most advanced stage of clinical disease (stage IV) and establishes nonresectability.

Paraneoplastic Syndromes

Paraneoplastic syndromes occur in approximately 10% of patients with lung cancer (**Table 66-1**). Such syndromes may be the initial presenting complaint triggering an evaluation but also can develop late in the course of disease. Paraneoplastic syndromes are unrelated to direct invasion or distant spread of tumor and in and of themselves do not preclude curative-intent therapy. Endocrine syndromes associated with lung cancers often are characterized by tumor production of biologically active hormones. Lung cancer is the most common cause of cancer-associated hypercalcemia, hyponatremia, and syndromes involving ectopic production of adrenal corticotropic hormone (ACTH).

Hypercalcemia of malignancy is the most frequent of these syndromes and is seen most commonly in patients with squamous cell carcinoma. Hypercalcemia in lung cancer patients usually is related to the ectopic production of parathyroid hormone–related peptide (PTHrP), rather than to the osteolytic effects of bone metastases. Early symptoms—thirst, polyuria, fatigue, constipation, nausea—are nonspecific. Mental status changes, lethargy, and even coma may accompany more severe hypercalcemia. The syndrome of inappropriate secretion of antidiuretic hormone (SIADH) most commonly occurs in patients with small cell lung cancer (SCLC). In some SCLC series, hyponatremia related to SIADH is present in up to 10% to 15% of patients. As with hypercalcemia, the symptoms—weakness, nausea, headache—often are nonspecific; more severe hyponatremia may have serious consequences, including confusion, seizures, and coma. Ectopic ACTH syndrome is seen most commonly with SCLC. The classic features of Cushing syndrome—truncal obesity, myopathy and muscle weakness, diabetes, hypertension, hirsutism—often are absent. In most cases, tumor cells express a precursor hormone that is cleaved to ACTH. A minority of patients produce corticotropin-releasing hormone, which stimulates ACTH production in the pituitary. The distinction between these two processes can be determined by a dexamethasone suppression test.

Nonendocrinologic extrapulmonary syndromes include musculoskeletal abnormalities, most commonly asymptomatic digital clubbing, which can be seen in isolation or in the setting of hypertrophic pulmonary osteoarthropathy (HPO). The pathogenesis of HPO is unknown, but the disorder consists of a proliferative periostitis characterized by symmetric, painful arthropathy that typically involves the ankles, shins, knees, wrists, and elbows. The diagnosis usually is confirmed by the identification of new periosteal bone formation on plain radiographs of the long bones, or by demonstration of diffuse long bone uptake of radionuclide on bone scan or positron emission tomography (PET) imaging. HPO is more commonly seen with adenocarcinoma. Hematologic dyscrasias commonly occurring in patients with lung cancer include anemia, which may compound fatigue and dyspnea; thrombocytosis; and leukocytosis. Eosinophilia is seen only rarely. Lung cancer is the most common cause of hypercoagulability associated with malignancy, which usually declares itself as deep venous thrombosis or thromboembolism, or with classic Trousseau syndrome (migratory superficial thrombophlebitis). Lung cancer, and specifically SCLC, also is the most common cause of a clinically diverse group of paraneoplastic neurologic syndromes (see Table 66-1).

The commonality with several of these syndromes is that they appear to be driven by autoimmune mechanisms. The most common of these is the Lambert-Eaton myasthenic syndrome (LEMS), which occurs in approximately 2% to 4% of patients with SCLC. LEMS is characterized by proximal muscle weakness, hyporeflexia, dysarthria, blurred vision, and autonomic dysfunction. In contrast with myasthenia gravis, muscle strength typically does not improve with the administration of anticholinesterases, but some recovery of strength may be obtained with treatment of the underlying malignancy. LEMS is associated with an antibody that inhibits acetylcholine release by binding to calcium channels in peripheral cholinergic nerve terminals. The diagnosis usually is based on electromyography demonstrating small amplitude of the resting muscle action potential, which increases with repeated nerve stimulation or exercise. The syndrome of encephalomyelitis–subacute sensory neuropathy is associated with antineuronal nuclear-antibody types 1 and 2 (ANNA-1 and ANNA-2), also called anti-Hu and anti-Ri antibodies, respectively, which react with SCLC tumor cell surface proteins and with neuronal nuclear antigens. Anti-Hu antibodies also are seen in patients with SCLC and cerebellar degeneration as well as opsoclonus-myoclonus. Other paraneoplastic neuropathic syndromes include encephalomyelitis, autonomic neuropathy, and cancer-associated retinopathy.

ASYMPTOMATIC PRESENTATION

Approximately 25% of patients with lung cancer present at an early stage of their disease, so only a minority are asymptomatic at the time of diagnosis. The poor overall 5-year survival for patients with lung cancer reflects the disproportionate number of patients who are diagnosed at an advanced stage. Interest in establishing screening for early disease detection in asymptomatic patients has understandably been the focus of many studies. The reasons to develop a reliable lung cancer screening tool are quite evident. Most lung cancers are discovered because of symptom-driven evaluation; a diagnosis of advanced-stage disease unfortunately portends a limited prognosis. By contrast, asymptomatic patients with early-stage cancers are more likely to experience long-term survival with treatment.

Large studies performed since the 1970s evaluating chest radiography, sputum cytologic analysis, and low-radiation-dose chest computed tomography (CT) scanning for lung cancer screening have consistently demonstrated an increase in the number of lung cancers diagnosed and a shift toward identifying earlier-stage disease accompanied by an improvement in survival, but notably without a decrease in lung cancer mortality rates. The National Lung Screening Trial (NLST) is the first large-scale clinical trial to demonstrate a benefit in lung cancer mortality related to screening with low-dose chest CT scanning. The NLST enrolled 53,000 subjects aged 55 to 74 years who were current or former smokers with at least a 30 pack-year history, and who had no previous history of lung cancer. The study compared low-dose chest CT scanning and chest radiography as screening tools, with participants randomized to receiving three annual screens with one or the other modality, with follow-up over another 5 years. The trial was closed in late 2010 when initial results demonstrated that subjects assigned to the CT screening group had 20% less lung cancer deaths than those assigned to chest radiography screening. The disadvantages of screening include a high rate of false-positive findings, which incur additional diagnostic evaluation with the potential for risk or harm related to such evaluation; the anticipated high cost of screening and subsequent evaluation; and the potential consequences of cumulative exposure to radiation from multiple scans. The optimal approach to lung cancer screening inevitably will need to evolve over the coming years, as the results of the NLST are applied to clinical practice, and outcomes related to both benefit and disadvantages can be longitudinally examined.

THE SOLITARY PULMONARY NODULE

The typical presentation of an asymptomatic early stage lung cancer is as a solitary pulmonary nodule (SPN), defined as a solitary lesion 3 cm or less in diameter, surrounded by normal lung and not associated with other thoracic abnormalities such as hilar or mediastinal adenopathy, atelectasis, or pleural effusion. SPNs are common radiographic lesions, frequently identified as incidental findings on chest imaging studies done for issues unrelated to lung cancer. Typical scenarios include routine preoperative evaluation in which a lung nodule or mass is found on the plain chest radiograph, or is identified on a chest CT scan performed for screening purposes or for other reasons unrelated to any chest symptoms, and investigation featuring a CT scan of the abdomen, heart, or spine, in which a portion of the lungs is almost inevitably included.

In evaluating SPNs, it is useful to distinguish small (8 mm or less in diameter) from larger nodules. Small SPNs are very common findings in patients who have participated in CT screening studies for lung cancer, as well as in those undergoing CT scanning for non-lung-related reasons, as noted earlier. In the feasibility study for the NLST performed within the Prostate, Lung, Colorectal, and Ovarian (PLCO) Cancer Screening Trial, 21% of subjects had abnormalities identified on the baseline screening CT scan, most of which were small SPNs. Similarly, in the Mayo Clinic lung cancer screening study, 51% of subjects had abnormalities found on the baseline screening study, with an increase to 69% by the second annual screen, the vast majority of which were small SPNs. The enormous

Table 66-2 Fleischner Society Guidelines for Management of Small Pulmonary Nodules Detected on Computed Tomography (CT) Scans

Nodule Size*	Low-Risk Patient†	High-Risk Patient‡
≤4 mm	No follow-up needed§	Follow-up CT at 12 months; if unchanged, no further follow-up¶
>4-6 mm	Follow-up CT at 12 months; if unchanged, no further follow-up¶	Initial follow-up CT at 6-12 months, then at 18-24 months if no change¶
>6-8 mm	Initial follow-up CT at 6-12 months, then at 18-24 months if no change	Initial follow-up CT at 3-6 months, then at 9-12 months and 24 months if no change
>8 mm	Follow-up CT at around 3, 9, and 24 months, then dynamic contrast-enhanced CT, PET, and/or biopsy	Same as for low-risk patient

NOTE: Guidelines refer to newly detected indeterminate nodules in persons 35 years of age or older.
*Average of length and width.
†Minimal or absent history of smoking and of other known risk factors.
‡History of smoking or of other known risk factors.
§The risk of malignancy in this category (<1%) is substantially less than that determined with a baseline CT scan in an asymptomatic smoker.
¶Nonsolid (ground glass) or partly solid nodules may require longer follow-up period to exclude indolent adenocarcinoma.
PET, positron emission tomography.
Modified from MacMahon H, Austin JH, Gamsu G, et al: Guidelines for management of small pulmonary nodules detected on CT scans: a statement from the Fleischner Society, *Radiology* 237:395-400, 2005.

number of small SPNs generated by an increased volume of CT scanning prompted a position statement from the Fleischner Society proposing guidelines for the management of small (8 mm or less) SPNs detected on CT scans. The recommendations are outlined in **Table 66-2**. Appropriately applied, the guidelines outline algorithms for patients based on their risk of lung cancer, providing timelines for follow-up of incidentally discovered nodules that minimize the number of CT scans necessary in the course of evaluation. These practical recommendations will become even more relevant if CT screening for lung cancer becomes the standard of practice. Of note, these recommendations apply only to patients in whom SPNs are discovered incidentally, unrelated to any known underlying disease, and only for solid SPNs 8 mm or less in diameter. Specifically, the guidelines are not intended to apply to patients known to have or suspected of having malignant disease, patients younger than 35 years of age, or patients with unexplained fever. Furthermore, the recommendations are not fully applicable to persons with nonsolid (ground glass appearance) or partially solid nodules, who may require longer follow-up to permit exclusion of biologically indolent cancers with greater confidence.

Larger SPNs (8 to 30 mm) require further investigation. A review of any previous imaging studies should be the first step, because an established baseline can provide information important to the evaluation. A nodule that is identified as new or growing warrants clinical concern, whereas radiographic stability of a solid SPN over a 2-year period generally is considered to constitute reasonable evidence of benignity. The exception to this general rule is that it is increasingly evident that a 2-year

period of stability is insufficient to allow confident designation of benignity for nodules that are purely of ground glass density. Other CT features also may reliably exclude malignancy, including the presence of fat identifying a hamartoma, complete or laminated calcification of the nodule, the presence of a feeding artery and a draining vein identifying a pulmonary arteriovenous malformation, the "comet tail" sign of swirling bronchovascular structures pointing to the hilum characteristic of rounded atelectasis, and the movement of a nodule within a cavity with positional changes characteristic of a mycetoma.

The larger the nodule, the more likely it is to be a cancer. A majority of asymptomatic pulmonary masses greater than 30 mm in diameter are malignant. **Figure 66-2** outlines a management strategy for SPNs 8 to 30 mm in diameter recommended by the American College of Chest Physicians evidence-based clinical practice guidelines for lung cancer. The algorithm is appealing in its simplicity. The key step is the clinical definition of a pretest probability of malignancy for every patient with an SPN, because this will inform decisions about the extent of evaluation. SPN factors associated with malignancy include larger size, positive smoking history, older age, a previous history of cancer, the location within the lung (higher risk with upper lobe location), and nodule edge characteristics (higher risk with spiculated than with smooth borders) (**Figure 66-3**). Mathematical prediction models incorporating these factors typically perform similarly to the clinical acumen of experienced physicians. Patients with a low probability (less than 5%) of malignancy can be monitored by serial CT imaging. Patients with a high probability (more than 60%) of malignancy should proceed to definitive surgical biopsy or resection. For the large group of patients with an intermediate probability (5% to 60%) of malignancy, the use of a variety of noninvasive and invasive modalities should be considered in deciding whether the SPN should be observed, biopsied, or removed.

Noninvasive imaging modalities commonly used to evaluate SPNs include CT and PET imaging. As already described, certain CT features may establish a benign diagnosis or support the rationale for a period of watchful waiting. By contrast, other findings may more strongly suggest malignancy, including spiculated nodule borders, a dilated bronchus leading into the nodule, and cavitation associated with a thick and irregular wall. CT with dynamic contrast enhancement, in which the demonstration of an increase in Hounsfield units with the administration of contrast is associated with a higher likelihood of malignancy, may be useful in institutions with proficiency in this technique. PET scanning with 18-fluorodeoxyglucose (FDG) is increasingly utilized in the characterization of SPNs. Increased glycolysis is a well-described metabolic characteristic of malignant cells, resulting in enhanced uptake of glucose and FDG. FDG accumulates in these cells because it cannot be completely metabolized.

In SPNs greater than 10 mm in diameter, the sensitivity of PET for identifying malignancy is high (80% to 100%), although specificity is less robust. PET is less sensitive for nodules measuring less than 10 mm in diameter, and its use for evaluating the likelihood of malignancy in small nodules should be discouraged. This modality may yield false-positive results in the setting of inflammation or infection, including tuberculosis, fungal infections, rheumatoid nodules, and sarcoidosis, all of which may mimic lung cancer radiographically. False-negative findings typically are described for patients with well-differentiated tumors, including adenocarcinoma in situ (bronchioloalveolar carcinoma) and carcinoid tumors, for which the tumor metabolic rate presumably is low. PET may be most useful in a situation in

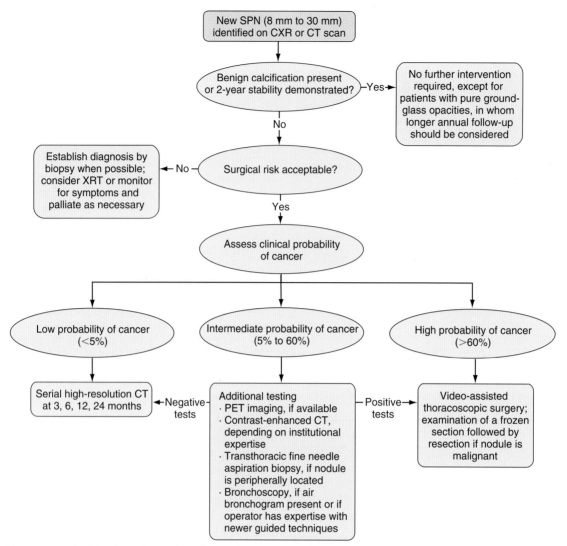

Figure 66-2 Management algorithm for patients with solitary pulmonary nodules (SPNs) 8 to 30 mm in diameter. *CT,* computed tomography; *CXR,* chest radiograph; *PET,* positron emission tomography; *XRT,* radiotherapy. *(From Gould MK, Fletcher J, Iannettoni MD, et al: Evaluation of patients with pulmonary nodules: when is it lung cancer?* Chest *132:108S–130S, 2007.)*

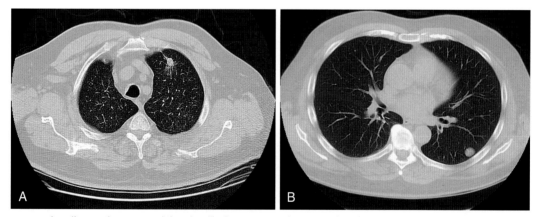

Figure 66-3 Asymptomatic solitary pulmonary nodules visualized on computed tomography. **A,** A 12-mm left upper lobe nodule with spiculated borders in a 74-year-old man with a 50 pack-year smoking history. Surgical resection revealed adenocarcinoma, pT1aN0M0, stage Ia. **B,** A 14-mm left lower lobe nodule with smooth border in a 64-year-old man who was a lifelong nonsmoker. Histopathologic/cytologic evaluation revealed a hamartoma.

which the clinical suspicion for malignancy is low despite suggestive CT findings; in this case, a positive result on PET scanning would lower the threshold to pursue some type of invasive evaluation, whereas a negative result would add reassurance regarding a period of observation.

Invasive modalities of assessing SPNs include surgical removal, bronchoscopic biopsy or aspiration, and percutaneous transthoracic needle aspiration (TTNA). For asymptomatic patients in whom the clinical pretest probability of malignancy is very high and for whom the risk of surgery is acceptable, a strong argument can be made to proceed directly to surgical resection, because this strategy would offer the most efficient, albeit most invasive, approach to establishing a diagnosis and stage, while also potentially providing definitive therapy. In many situations, however, a limited nonsurgical biopsy may be warranted—for example, in patients in whom a benign diagnosis is a strong consideration and a nonsurgical biopsy may potentially be definitive (e.g., tuberculosis or hamartoma), patients in whom surgical resection carries a high risk for complications, and patients who are unwilling to accept a surgical approach without at least an initial attempt to establish a definitive diagnosis. Before bronchoscopy or TTNA is undertaken, a discussion should be held with the patient regarding the possible outcomes, and in particular to consider the approach to be taken should the biopsy be nondiagnostic. This discussion is of particular importance, because a definitive benign diagnosis often is difficult to establish with these procedures, which frequently provide limited biopsy material. Bronchoscopic biopsy has a reasonable diagnostic yield (55%) in nodules greater than 20 mm in diameter, with the yield increasing as nodule size increases and if radiographic evidence of a bronchus leading into the nodule ("bronchus sign") is present. For peripheral nodules less than 20 mm, the diagnostic yield with bronchoscopy is considerably lower, in the range of 10% to 50%, which may be increased by incorporating radial ultrasound or electromagnetic navigational technology to enhance accurate localization.

Percutaneous TTNA commonly is performed under CT or fluoroscopic guidance, with improved diagnostic capability when a core needle biopsy is done in addition to aspiration. TTNA typically is considered for SPN evaluation when bronchoscopy is unlikely to render a diagnosis, usually for SPNs that are relatively small (less than 20 mm) and peripherally located. The diagnostic yield of TTNA for malignant lesions is higher (up to 85%) in studies in which the prevalence of malignancy is high and nodule size is 20 to 40 mm. For smaller nodules, the yield falls, with nondiagnostic biopsy samples obtained in up to 41% of patients with SPNs less than 40 mm in diameter, and in particular when the lesion is benign. The major drawback of TTNA is a high rate of pneumothorax (10% to 35%). Approximately 5% of procedures are complicated by pneumothorax of enough clinical significance to warrant placement of a chest tube. TTNA may pose a higher risk in situations in which the lung traversed by the needle en route to the lesion is emphysematous or bullous, or in patients who are unable to hold their breath as directed during the procedure.

LUNG CANCER STAGING

Staging is an essential and critical part of the management of every patient suspected of having or diagnosed with lung cancer. The staging classifications of the American Joint Committee on Cancer for non–small cell lung cancer (NSCLC) and SCLC now both follow the tumor-node-metastasis (TNM) system. The current seventh edition, published in 2010, was developed by the International Association for the Study of Lung Cancer (IASLC) using an international database of over 80,000 lung cancer cases. The distribution of database cases informing the staging classification spanned four continents: Europe 58%, North America 21%, Asia 14%, and Australia 7%. Although the database still included a majority of white patients and thus may be limited in application to nonwhite patient populations, the magnitude and diversity of the IASLC database constituted a remarkable improvement over the previous

Table 66-3 Designations for Types of Staging Assessments

Prefix	Name	Definition
c	Clinical	Before initiation of any treatment, using any and all information available (e.g., including mediastinoscopy)
p	Pathologic	After resection, based on pathologic assessment
y	Restaging	After part or all of the treatment has been given
r	Recurrence	Stage at time of a recurrence
a	Autopsy	Stage as determined at autopsy

From Detterbeck FC, Boffa DJ, Tanoue LT: The new lung cancer staging system, *Chest* 136:260–271, 2009.

Table 66-4 Staging Designation for Completeness of Surgical Resection

Symbol	Name	Definition
R0	No residual	No identifiable tumor remaining; negative surgical margins
R1	Microscopic residual	Microscopically positive margins but no visible tumor remaining
R2	Gross residual	Gross (visible or palpable) tumor remaining

From Detterbeck FC, Boffa DJ, Tanoue LT: The new lung cancer staging system, *Chest* 136:260–271, 2009.

lung cancer staging system, which had been developed in a largely single-institution North American patient cohort.

SCLC previously was staged according to the Veterans Administration Lung Cancer Study Group (VALSG) two-stage system. In this system, "limited-stage" disease refers to cancer confined to one hemithorax, which may include the ipsilateral lymph nodes. From a practical perspective, a limited-stage SCLC is confined to an area that can be encompassed in a single radiation treatment field. "Extensive-stage" SCLC includes any tumor extending beyond the confines of limited-stage disease, including tumor confined to one hemithorax but involving the pleura. Although this two-stage system is no longer the official staging system for SCLC, it is still clinically appealing in its relatively easy application to treatment planning.

Different types of staging may be used to describe a malignancy during a course of evaluation (**Table 66-3**). The most common staging assessments are the *clinical stage* (indicated by the prefix c), defined as the stage before treatment as determined by all available imaging and biopsy data, and the *pathologic stage* (indicated by the prefix p), defined as the stage determined on the basis of the available imaging and biopsy data, as well as analysis of tissue samples obtained after a surgical resection performed with intent to cure. The completeness of resection is determined histopathologically after surgery (**Table 66-4**). Clinical staging typically is associated with poorer outcomes than those achieved with pathologic staging, the latter being inherently more accurate. All patients will undergo clinical staging; only in a select number will their disease be able to be staged pathologically. Restaging may take place after treatment, at the time of a recurrence, or at autopsy, identified by the prefix y, r, or a, respectively, as outlined in Table 66-3.

Table 66-5 Definitions for Tumor-Node-Metastasis Descriptors

Descriptor			Definition	Subgroups*
T			**Primary tumor**	
	T0		No primary tumor	
	T1		Tumor ≤3 cm,[†] surrounded by lung or visceral pleura, not more proximal than the lobar bronchus	
		T1a	Tumor ≤2 cm[†]	T1a
		T1b	Tumor >2 but ≤3 cm[†]	T1b
	T2		Tumor >3 but ≤7 cm[†] or tumor with any of the following[‡]: invades visceral pleura, involves main bronchus ≥2 cm distal to the carina, atelectasis/obstructive pneumonia extending to hilum but not involving the entire lung	
		T2a	Tumor >3 but ≤5 cm[†]	T2a
		T2b	Tumor >5 but ≤7 cm[†]	T2b
	T3		Tumor >7 cm;	T3$_{>7}$
			or directly invading chest wall, diaphragm, phrenic nerve, mediastinal pleura, or parietal pericardium;	T3$_{Inv}$
			or tumor in the main bronchus <2 cm distal to the carina[§];	T3$_{Centr}$
			or atelectasis/obstructive pneumonitis of entire lung;	T3$_{Centr}$
			or separate tumor nodules in the same lobe	T3$_{Satell}$
	T4		Tumor of any size with invasion of heart, great vessels, trachea, recurrent laryngeal nerve, esophagus, vertebral body, or carina;	T4$_{Inv}$
			or separate tumor nodules in a different ipsilateral lobe	T4$_{IpsiNod}$
N			**Regional lymph nodes**	
	N0		No regional node metastasis	
	N1		Metastasis in ipsilateral peribronchial and/or perihilar lymph nodes and intrapulmonary nodes, including involvement by direct extension	
	N2		Metastasis in ipsilateral mediastinal and/or subcarinal lymph nodes	
	N3		Metastasis in contralateral mediastinal, contralateral hilar, ipsilateral or contralateral scalene, or supraclavicular lymph nodes	
M			**Distant metastasis**	
	M0		No distant metastasis	
	M1a		Separate tumor nodules in a contralateral lobe;	M1a$_{ContrNod}$
			or tumor with pleural nodules or malignant pleural dissemination[‖]	M1a$_{PlDissem}$
	M1b		Distant metastasis	M1b
Special Situations				
TX, NX, MX			T, N, or M status not able to be assessed	
Tis			Focus of in situ cancer	Tis
T1[§]			Superficial spreading tumor of any size but confined to the wall of the trachea or main bronchus	T1$_{SS}$

*These subgroup labels are not defined in the IASLC publications but are added here to facilitate a clear discussion.
[†]In the greatest dimension.
[‡]T2 tumors with these features are classified as T2a if diameter is 5 cm or less.
[§]The uncommon superficial spreading tumor in central airways is classified as T1.
[‖]Pleural effusions are excluded that are cytologically negative, nonbloody, transudative, and clinically judged not to be due to cancer.
From Detterbeck FC, Boffa DJ, Tanoue LT: The new lung cancer staging system, *Chest* 136:260–271, 2009.

The TNM paradigm is based solely on anatomy (**Table 66-5**). The T descriptor characterizes the primary tumor, the N descriptor, involvement of the regional lymph nodes; and the M descriptor, the presence or absence of distant metastases. Combinations of these descriptors are grouped into stages. Even though limitations to the generalized application of the TNM system are increasingly appreciated, it serves as a consistent structure to describe extent of disease and to provide prognosis. Furthermore, staging provides a platform for comparisons between reasonably homogeneous populations in therapeutic clinical trials. It may be tempting to use the clinical stage as the major determinant of therapy, but it is important to recognize that the staging classification system is not intended to be an algorithm for assigning treatment. The designation of stage inherently portends prognosis, because the separation of TNM combinations into stages is fundamentally determined by survival. Two of the limitations of the TNM system become immediately evident. First, the anatomic descriptors yield no

Table 66-6 | **Lung Cancer Stage Groupings by Tumor-Node-Metastasis (TNM) Descriptors***

Stage	TNM Grouping
0	TisN0M0
IA	T1aN0M0
	T1bN0M0
IB	T2aN0M0
IIA	T1aN1M0
	T1bN1M0
	T2aN1M0
	T2bN0M0
IIB	T2bN1M0
	T3N0M0
IIIA	T1N2M0
	T2N2M0
	T3N1M0
	T3N2M0
	T4N0M0
	T4N0M0
	T4N1M0
IIIB	T4N2M0
	Any T N3M0
IV	Any T any N M1a
	Any T any N M1b

*As defined in the seventh edition of the American Joint Commission on Cancer and the Union Internationale Contre le Cancer classification.
From Edge SB, editor: *The American Joint Commission on Cancer cancer staging manual*, ed 7. Chicago, Springer, 2010.

information relating to biologic behavior of the cancer. With a burgeoning recognition that the molecular characteristics of an individual tumor may drive outcomes and more specifically render some tumors very responsive to targeted treatments, the prognostic ability of the TNM system becomes less reliable. Second, patients who share similar survival outcomes may have clinically dissimilar cancers; this divergence becomes clear on examining the stage groupings outlined in **Table 66-6**. Within a given stage of disease, the patients often are not clinically homogeneous, even though they may have similar survival rates. Despite the large size of the IASLC database, outcomes for specific TNM groups with small numbers of patients could not be adequately evaluated, with an inevitable "lumping" rather than "splitting" of these groups. Other issues remain unresolved with use of the current system, including how to incorporate specific radiographic features such as the density of pulmonary nodules, or how to properly prognosticate in clinical situations that fall out of the staging paradigm, for example, the presence of multiple synchronous primary tumors, but the most important limitation is the absence of components reflecting tumor biology. As current understanding of molecular pathways important to neoplasia expands, it seems inevitable that the staging system must incorporate such information in the future.

Ultimately, even with its limitations, the current staging classification represents a major advance in lung cancer care, providing a reliable language to facilitate consistent description and communication, and to give patients, their families, and their physicians insight regarding prognosis. The tools and strategies applied most commonly in the process of clinical evaluation are discussed in the following sections within the context of their use in defining the separate clinical stages.

STAGE I

In the IASLC database, 28% of patients with NSCLC presented with stage I disease. Patients with stage IA lung cancer (T1aN0M0, T1bN0M0) are those with malignant solitary pulmonary nodules 3 cm or less in diameter. These patients typically are asymptomatic. In general, the smaller the SPN, the less likely spread will have occurred beyond the primary site. CT scan should be performed in all patients with known or suspected lung cancer, with inclusion of the upper abdomen for evaluation of the liver and adrenal glands, because these are common sites of metastasis. By definition, CT scanning in stage I disease will not demonstrate enlarged hilar or mediastinal nodes.

In a systematic review of the medical literature performed to inform the American College of Chest Physicians evidence-based guidelines for the diagnosis and management of lung cancer (5111 total evaluable patients with a median prevalence of mediastinal metastasis of 28%), the pooled sensitivity and specificity of CT scanning for identifying mediastinal lymph node metastasis were 51% and 86%, respectively. In the specific clinical situation combining an SPN 3 cm or less and a normal-appearing mediastinum on chest CT, the likelihood of finding malignant mediastinal lymph node involvement by surgical lymph node sampling is low, approximately 6%. Whether this small percentage justifies further noninvasive staging beyond CT scanning is controversial. Overall, PET gives false-negative results in approximately 20% of patients with lung cancer associated with normal-sized but malignant mediastinal nodes. The decision of whether or not to pursue PET imaging must take this into consideration, as well as the possibility that identifying a false-positive abnormality may trigger unnecessary evaluation. Similarly, brain magnetic resonance imaging (MRI) and CT scanning are of low yield in general in patients with lung cancer in whom findings on clinical examination are normal (0 to 10%), and particularly so in patients with clinical stage I NSCLC. Conversely, patients with symptoms suggesting distant disease should undergo further noninvasive imaging, even though the primary tumor may be small.

Patients with stage IB lung cancer have larger solitary tumors (ranging from less than 3 cm to more than 5 cm in diameter). In such cases, the primary tumor may be surrounded by normal lung but also may invade the visceral pleura, involve the main bronchus 2 cm or more distal to the carina, or be associated with atelectasis or obstructive pneumonia not involving the entire lung. The likelihood of finding regional nodal or distant metastasis in the setting of a larger primary lesion is higher than in stage IA, so these patients should undergo PET scanning and brain imaging (MRI or CT with contrast) as part of their staging evaluation (**Figure 66-4**). With the recognition that false-positive results on PET are frequent with nonmalignant inflammation or infection, tissue confirmation should be obtained whenever possible to establish the presence or absence of regional or distant metastasis, because patients should not be denied potentially curative treatments on the basis of imaging alone. Conversely, controversy continues regarding whether a negative result on PET scan in a patient with a T2 or T3 solitary pulmonary lesion and normal mediastinal nodes on CT scan should be followed by tissue biopsy to prove that the mediastinum is truly free of disease. In a metaanalysis evaluating this question, the probability of finding malignant lymph node involvement when both CT and PET findings were negative was approximately 9% (of note, the pretest probability of mediastinal lymph node metastasis was estimated at 35%, and

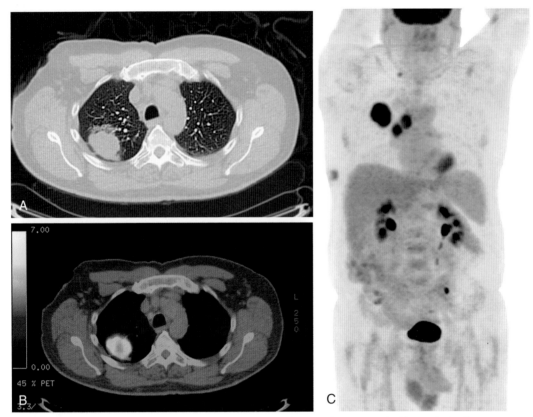

Figure 66-4 The patient was a 69-year-old man with a 45 pack-year smoking history who presented with cough. **A,** Chest computed tomography (CT) scan demonstrates a 4.8-cm right upper lobe mass. The hila and mediastinum appeared normal. **B,** Fused transaxial positron emission tomography (PET) image at the same level as in **A** demonstrates intense fluorodeoxyglucose (FDG) uptake in the right upper lobe mass. **C,** Coronal PET image demonstrates intense FDG uptake in the right upper lobe mass as well as in the right hilum and the mediastinum. Brain magnetic resonance imaging (MRI) was negative. Mediastinoscopy demonstrated adenocarcinoma. Clinical stage was T2aN2M0, stage IIIa.

patients were not differentiated by the size of the primary tumor). Clinicians ultimately must decide whether the overall 9% probability of mediastinal lymph node metastasis in patients with clinical stage IB disease and negative results on CT and PET imaging of the mediastinum warrants further invasive evaluation. This decision may be influenced by the recognition that certain subgroups, including patients with central or larger tumors, have an increased likelihood of mediastinal nodal involvement.

STAGE II

Stage II encompasses a variety of TNM groupings, including those comprising patients who have large lung masses that may invade local structures, patients with small primary tumors and hilar nodal involvement, and patients whose tumors have an endobronchial component within 2 cm of but not involving the main carina. The range of T descriptors in stage II emphasizes that the stage designations are defined by survival outcome, not by anatomy alone. Clinical staging for patients with stage II disease parallels that for stage IB, because the evaluative process typically must include a decision about whether to pursue an invasive mediastinal examination in the setting of negative results of mediastinal imaging on chest CT. Patients with stage II disease are more likely to have occult mediastinal lymph node (N2) involvement, so PET scanning should be routinely included in their staging assessment. The hilar (N1) nodes are difficult to biopsy, except perhaps by a bronchoscopic approach under endobronchial ultrasound (EBUS) guidance. If the ipsilateral N1 nodes are enlarged on CT scan or demonstrate FDG uptake on PET imaging, it usually is not necessary to sample

them before surgery, because they will be removed at the time of resection. However, N1 involvement increases the likelihood that N2 nodes also are involved, even if CT and PET results are negative, and in such cases, invasive evaluation of the mediastinum should be performed to evaluate for the possibility of higher-stage disease. Because by definition the mediastinal nodes in this case are not enlarged, a focused evaluation will not be possible. Accordingly, the most complete mediastinal evaluation possible should be pursued, which may vary institutionally, with preferential use of mediastinoscopy, EBUS, or EBUS with endoscopic ultrasound (EUS).

MRI is not frequently indicated in the evaluation of patients with lung cancer, with the notable exception of patients in whom a more accurate evaluation relating to the bones of the chest cage, the soft tissues and vasculature, or the brachial plexus (in the setting of a superior sulcus [Pancoast] tumor) is necessary. Patients with stage II lung cancer defined by large primary tumors invading adjacent structures often fall into these categories. In these challenging clinical situations, MRI may be superior to CT scanning in distinguishing neoplastic from normal tissues.

STAGE III

Approximately one third of patients with lung cancer present with clinical stage III disease. All patients with evidence of stage III disease on chest CT scan should be evaluated for the presence of distant disease; this may be accomplished by a combination of (1) brain MRI or head CT and (2) PET imaging or abdominal CT scanning with bone scan. The presence of metastatic disease immediately changes the clinical stage to IV. As

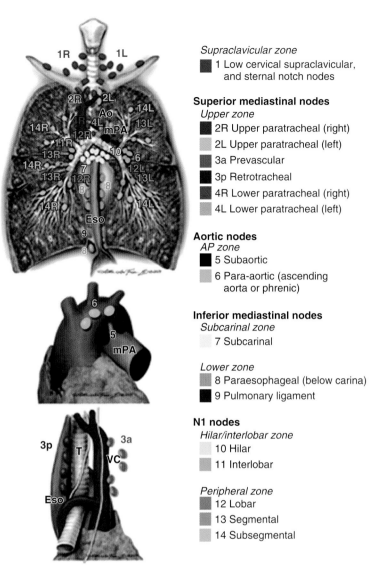

Figure 66-5 The International Association for the Study of Lung Cancer lymph node map. *(From Rusch VW, Asamura H, Watanabe H, et al: The IASLC Lung Cancer Staging Project: a proposal for a new international lymph node map in the forthcoming 7th edition of the TNM classification for lung cancer, J Thorac Oncol 4:568-577, 2009.)*

Supraclavicular zone
■ 1 Low cervical supraclavicular, and sternal notch nodes

Superior mediastinal nodes
Upper zone
■ 2R Upper paratracheal (right)
■ 2L Upper paratracheal (left)
■ 3a Prevascular
■ 3p Retrotracheal
■ 4R Lower paratracheal (right)
■ 4L Lower paratracheal (left)

Aortic nodes
AP zone
■ 5 Subaortic
■ 6 Para-aortic (ascending aorta or phrenic)

Inferior mediastinal nodes
Subcarinal zone
■ 7 Subcarinal

Lower zone
■ 8 Paraesophageal (below carina)
■ 9 Pulmonary ligament

N1 nodes
Hilar/interlobar zone
■ 10 Hilar
■ 11 Interlobar

Peripheral zone
■ 12 Lobar
■ 13 Segmental
■ 14 Subsegmental

with stage II, stage III comprises a wide variety of TNM groupings (see Table 66-6). However, a majority and perhaps the most clinically challenging of these patients with such disease will be defined by involvement of the N2 nodes; careful evaluation of the mediastinum is thus vitally important. The IASLC lymph node map defining the lymph node stations is shown in **Figure 66-5**.

Mediastinal Evaluation: Noninvasive Modalities

Chest CT remains the most accurate anatomic modality for evaluation of the mediastinum. Pathologic enlargement of the mediastinal nodes is defined as a short-axis diameter of 1 cm or greater. CT in the setting of lung cancer is a relatively inaccurate tool for identification of malignant involvement in the mediastinum. Many studies evaluating CT accuracy in this setting have demonstrated that approximately 20% of mediastinal nodes that are not enlarged are actually malignant; conversely, approximately 40% of enlarged mediastinal nodes are actually benign. For all patients with enlarged discrete mediastinal lymph nodes on CT, further evaluation of the mediastinum should be performed before a definitive treatment decision is reached, in view of the high false-positive rate. The exception to this approach would be in patients with bulky mediastinal disease, with lymph node infiltration around vessels and airways so extensive that discrete lymph node measurements are meaningless (**Figure 66-6**). In such cases, malignant involvement of the nodes would be assumed, and the establishment of cell type could be pursued by sampling the most accessible site, either the mediastinal nodes or the primary tumor.

PET scanning is recommended for further evaluation of all patients with clinical stage III lung cancer because of the high likelihood of distant disease. PET scanning is now widely available, with utilization of this modality markedly increasing over the past decade. Abdominal CT with bone scan is a reasonable substitute if PET is unavailable. PET is superior to CT with respect to evaluation of the mediastinum. In a large systematic review including 2865 evaluable patients with lung cancer, the pooled sensitivity and specificity of PET for identifying mediastinal lymph node metastasis were 74% and 85%, respectively. In a separate metaanalysis of patients with enlarged mediastinal lymph nodes, the median sensitivity and specificity of PET were reported at 100% and 78%, respectively. Thus, PET is superior to CT in identifying malignant mediastinal lymph nodes, but approximately 20% of nodes identified as abnormal by PET imaging are actually benign, reflecting the fact that tissues other than cancer can exhibit increased cellular glucose uptake. Because malignant N2 nodal involvement may be the critical factor determining whether a patient is surgically resectable, it is important that tissue confirmation be obtained whenever possible before making a final determination of clinical stage.

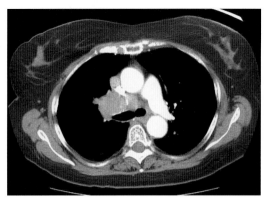

Figure 66-6 The patient was a 62-year-old woman with a 30 pack-year smoking history who presented with cough. Chest computed tomography (CT) reveals a right upper lobe mass with extension of tumor into the mediastinum and precarinal mediastinal adenopathy. Bronchoscopy with endobronchial ultrasound imaging demonstrated endobronchial invasion of tumor at the level of the main carina; biopsy specimens confirmed adenocarcinoma. There was no evidence of distant metastasis. Clinical stage was T4N2M0, stage IIIb.

Table 66-7	**Mediastinal Lymph Node Stations: Accessibility to Minimally Invasive Modalities**

Procedure	Accessible Mediastinal Lymph Node Stations
Mediastinoscopy	Stations 2, 3, 4, 7 (anterior only)
Extended cervical mediastinoscopy	Station 6
Video-assisted thoracoscopic surgery (VATS)	Ipsilateral stations 2, 3, 4, 7; station 6 with left-sided procedure
Parasternal mediastinotomy (Chamberlain procedure)	Station 5 (aortopulmonary window)
Endobronchial ultrasound (EBUS)	Stations 2, 3, 4, 7
Endoscopic ultrasound (EUS)	Stations 4, 5, 7, 8, 9
Transthoracic needle aspiration (TTNA)	All stations

Mediastinal Evaluation: Invasive Modalities

A variety of minimally invasive modalities are available for the evaluation of the mediastinal lymph nodes (**Table 66-7**). TTNA, EUS, extended cervical mediastinoscopy, and EBUS typically are utilized for the purpose of directed biopsy in patients with discrete abnormalities on CT or PET scanning. The choice between these procedures will be decided by the anatomic location of the abnormal nodes and by institutional expertise. The sensitivities of all of the directed minimally invasive techniques are very high, in part because they typically are done in situations in which the prevalence of malignancy in the abnormal nodes also is very high. In theory, all mediastinal lymph nodes are amenable to TTNA, although the individual anatomy will determine whether biopsy is feasible. Ultrasound-guided biopsy techniques using endoscopy or bronchoscopy are increasingly available and have high diagnostic yield.

The specific advantage of EUS is the capability of sampling station 8 and station 9 nodes in the inferior mediastinum, the potential to gain access to subdiaphragmatic structures including the celiac nodes and the adrenal glands, and in some cases the ability to sample the aortopulmonary window (station 5) nodes. Anterior mediastinotomy (Chamberlain procedure) is perhaps the most reliable method for reaching station 5 nodes. EUS is limited in that it cannot reach nodes anterior to the trachea. EBUS allows bronchoscopic access to the pulmonary parenchyma, to nodes in both hila, and to nodes anterior to the trachea as well as in the subcarinal space, affording the opportunity to sample the primary tumor as well as N1 and N2 nodes in a single procedure.

For patients who have no evidence of mediastinal adenopathy on noninvasive imaging, a more comprehensive examination of the mediastinal lymph nodes can be accomplished by mediastinoscopy, EBUS with or without EUS, or video-assisted thoracoscopic surgery (VATS), with the choice between these procedures largely decided by institutional expertise. Mediastinoscopy has long been considered the "gold standard," although it is imperfect. The superior mediastinal nodes (stations 1 to 4) and the anterior portion of the subcarinal space (station 7) are typically accessible to mediastinoscopy, but the posterior subcarinal space, the aortopulmonary window (station 5), and paraaortic nodes (station 6) are not. The station 6 nodes are

the hardest to sample by any means other than surgery (VATS or open thoracotomy). In centers with focused expertise, EBUS performs as well as mediastinoscopy for evaluation of the radiographically negative mediastinum, particularly if combined with EUS. EBUS allows sampling of all nodal stations accessible to standard mediastinoscopy, with the advantage of the ability to access the posterior subcarinal space, inspect the airway for endobronchial lesions, and potentially sample the primary site as well. The addition of EUS to EBUS affords the potential for the most extensive examination of the mediastinum, while providing the opportunity to also sample structures below the diaphragm.

The most invasive approach to mediastinal evaluation is surgical lymphadenectomy. The aortopulmonary window and the paraaortic nodes (stations 5 and 6) may be particularly difficult to access with minimally invasive techniques, and in such cases a surgical approach may be necessary. Both VATS and open thoracotomy offer the opportunity to extensively sample the mediastinum but usually are limited to the ipsilateral nodes. These procedures uncommonly are performed for the sole purpose of examining the mediastinum, with lymph node sampling more typically pursued as an adjunct to resection of the primary tumor. VATS may have the additional benefit of the opportunity to visualize the pleural space, which may be important in a patient with pleural effusion and negative findings on pleural fluid cytologic examination, or to evaluate other abnormalities seen on imaging studies, such as separate pulmonary or pleural nodules or pleural thickening.

STAGE IV

Stage IV lung cancer is defined by the presence of any distant (M1) site of disease. The initial evaluation of any patient with suspected lung cancer should include a thorough history and physical examination and a basic laboratory evaluation. The presence of abnormalities on this initial evaluation is associated with a high likelihood of finding metastatic disease. Constitutional symptoms (e.g., unintentional weight loss, unexplained fevers), focal symptoms (e.g., localized pain, bone pain, unexplained headaches, focal neurologic symptoms) or signs (e.g., hoarseness, hepatomegaly, soft tissue masses), or laboratory abnormalities (e.g., unexplained anemia, hypercalcemia, liver

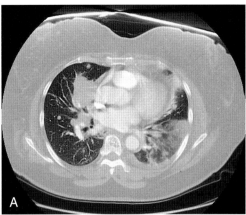
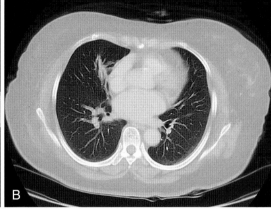

Figure 66-7 The patient was a 66-year-old Asian woman, a lifelong nonsmoker who presented with progressive dyspnea over the course of several weeks. **A,** Chest computed tomography (CT) scan demonstrates a 4-cm mass in the right middle lobe with right hilar adenopathy and multiple bilateral pulmonary nodules. Also evident is mediastinal adenopathy. A palpable right supraclavicular lymph node was biopsied, demonstrating adenocarcinoma. Mutational analysis revealed a deletion in exon 19 of the *EGFR* gene. Clinical stage was T2aN3M1, stage IV. **B,** Chest CT scan obtained in the same patient after 6 weeks of treatment with erlotinib. Marked decrease in the size of the right middle lobe mass with resolution of satellite nodules is evident.

function test abnormalities) should trigger an investigation directed by the specific finding. In such cases, comprehensive imaging is indicated regardless of the size of the primary tumor. All patients with known or suspected lung cancer should undergo chest CT scanning, preferably inclusive of the upper abdomen. Asymptomatic patients whose CT abnormalities indicate a higher likelihood of metastases (e.g., N1 or N2 nodal enlargement, pleural effusion, nodule in a separate ipsilateral or contralateral lobe) should also undergo further noninvasive evaluation. As noted for patients with stage III disease, a complete noninvasive evaluation may consist of (1) brain MRI or head CT plus (2) PET imaging or abdominal CT scan with bone scan. Arguably, all patients suspected of harboring M1 disease should undergo these imaging studies, because prophylactic palliation of asymptomatic sites in organs such as brain or bone may preserve quality of life. However, patients with obvious metastases, such as palpable soft tissue masses, bulky adenopathy outside the thorax, or obvious tumor infiltration in the liver, may not necessarily require further imaging, because spread of disease is clear. In patients in whom the clinical picture is highly suggestive of M1 disease, tissue confirmation at the metastatic site, if feasible, would provide the most efficient means of establishing both diagnosis and stage.

The most common sites of lung cancer metastasis are the brain, adrenal glands, bones, and liver, although any site may be involved. Brain MRI and head CT with contrast are equally sensitive in identifying patients with brain metastases, although MRI is more likely to detect multiple lesions. PET scanning or abdominal CT with contrast in combination with radionuclide bone scan (plus the original chest CT) are suitable for examination of the rest of the body. PET imaging has the advantage of being a single whole-body study; abnormalities seen on the original chest CT study also can be reevaluated for the presence of abnormal metabolic activity.

Two metastatic situations warrant specific mention. The adrenal glands are a common site of lung cancer spread; they also are common sites for benign adenomas, which are found in approximately 3% to 9% of the general population. MRI may be helpful in distinguishing a benign adrenal adenoma from adrenal metastasis. Tissue confirmation of a questionable adrenal nodule may be warranted, particularly if it is the sole potential metastatic site, because resection of an isolated oligometastasis in the adrenal gland (or brain) in a patient with

surgically approachable primary disease can be associated with improved long-term survival. Management of pleural disease also can be challenging in a patient with otherwise resectable lung cancer. One of the major differences between the current and previous editions of the lung cancer staging system is in the designation of pleural dissemination, and particularly malignant pleural effusion, as M1a. Pleural effusions in lung cancer patients can arise for many reasons other than malignant involvement, including parapneumonic effusion in the setting of postobstructive pneumonia and effusions associated with congestive heart failure and pulmonary embolism. Up to 14% of ipsilateral pleural effusions in patients with lung cancer are found to be benign. The sensitivity of pleural fluid cytologic testing for detection of malignancy is approximately 60%, increasing to 85% with three thoracenteses. This approach is not sufficiently sensitive to be reliable when clinical suspicion for pleural dissemination is high but the cytologic findings, even with repeated thoracenteses, are negative. In such cases, pleuroscopy or thoracoscopy should be performed for direct visual inspection of the pleural surfaces, to exclude malignant pleural involvement as definitively as possible before curative-intent surgery is performed for the primary lesion.

FUTURE DIRECTIONS

Even with the many advances accomplished in its newest edition, the current staging system is imperfect. Its most obvious deficiencies are a lack of incorporation of information related to tumor cell type and the absence of any indicators of biologic behavior. It is increasingly evident that distinguishing between cell types within the NSCLC classification is important in identifying populations of patients for the purposes of comparing clinical outcomes, for defining homogeneous groups of patients for clinical trials, and ultimately for assigning treatment. It also is clear that molecular profiling of cancers can play an important role in characterizing subgroups of patients who share common gene mutations or translocations that may drive the neoplastic process, particularly in never-smokers or light smokers with lung adenocarcinoma (**Figure 66-7**). In the future, these distinctions are likely to help define new staging classifications incorporating indicators of biologic activity, with the potential for effectively facilitating personalized patient care.

SUGGESTED READINGS

Aberle DR, Berg CD, Black WC, et al: The National Lung Screening Trial: overview and study design, *Radiology* 258:243–253, 2011.

Detterbeck FC, Boffa DJ, Tanoue LT: The new lung cancer staging system, *Chest* 136:260–271, 2009.

Edge SB, editor: *The American Joint Commission on Cancer cancer staging manual*, ed 7, Chicago, 2010, Springer.

Goldstraw P, Crowley J, Chansky K, et al: The IASLC Lung Cancer Staging Project: proposals for revision of the TNM stage groupings in the forthcoming seventh edition of the TNM classification of malignant tumours, *J Thorac Oncol* 2:706–714, 2007.

Gould MK, Fletcher J, Iannettoni MD, et al: Evaluation of patients with pulmonary nodules: when is it lung cancer? *Chest* 132:108S–130S, 2007.

Gould MK, Kuschner WG, Rydzak CE, et al: Test performance of positron emission tomography and computed tomography for mediastinal staging in patients with non-small cell lung cancer: a meta-analysis, *Ann Intern Med* 139:879–892, 2003.

MacMahon H, Austin JH, Gamsu G, et al: Guidelines for management of small pulmonary nodules detected on CT scans: a statement from the Fleischner Society, *Radiology* 237:395–400, 2005.

Rusch VW, Asamura H, Watanabe H, et al: The IASLC Lung Cancer Staging Project: a proposal for a new international lymph node map in the forthcoming 7th edition of the TNM classification for lung cancer, *J Thorac Oncol* 4:568–577, 2009.

Silvestri G, Littenberg B, Colice G: The clinical evaluation for detecting metastatic lung cancer: a meta-analysis, *Am J Respir Crit Care Med* 152:225–230, 1995.

Silvestri GA, Gould MK, Margolis ML, et al: Noninvasive staging of non-small cell lung cancer, *Chest* 132:178S–201S, 2007.

Toloza E, Harpole L, McCrory DC: Noninvasive staging of non-small cell lung cancer: a review of the current evidence, *Chest* 123:137S–146S, 2003.

Toloza EM, Harpole L, Detterbeck F, et al: Invasive staging of non-small cell lung cancer: a review of the current evidence, *Chest* 123:157S–166S, 2003.

Chapter **67**

Lung Cancer: Treatment

Douglas Arenberg

Lung cancer is one of the most common solid tumors, particularly in industrialized nations, with an incidence similar to breast, colon, and prostate cancer. However, lung cancer accounts for more deaths than all these other cancers combined because of the inherent, often-aggressive biology of lung cancer; the nature of the lung itself, which can readily harbor an advanced tumor in the absence of symptoms; the poor response to treatment; and until recently the lack of an effective screening test.

As with many cancers, therapy for lung cancer includes surgery, chemotherapy, and radiation therapy, either alone or in combination. Definitive treatment increasingly includes combinations of two or all three of these modalities. Improved understanding of the molecular basis of cancer has led to treatments exploiting specific molecular abnormalities (targeted therapy). Lung cancer treatment has become more complex over time, in part because of recognition of tumor-specific and patient-specific traits that predict a greater likelihood of success, or lack of success, with specific drugs. This evolution of "personalized" cancer treatment should not overshadow the following principles of lung cancer treatment, which have remained largely constant over time:

1. Curative therapy should be used whenever feasible.
2. Curative therapy must address all grossly detectable disease, as well as reduce the likelihood of death from occult metastatic disease.
3. Toxicity or risk from treatment can outweigh the benefit when the patient is burdened by significant comorbid illness or when the risk of distant metastasis is extremely low.

Two competing principles are often cited as well: the treatment of lung cancer is strictly dependent on the stage of the disease, but accurate staging is often not possible before treatment (surgery) is rendered. This apparent paradox is resolved by recognizing that the first step in evaluating a patient with suspected lung cancer is the simultaneous determination of (a) whether cancer is the likely diagnosis on clinical grounds, (b) if cancer, whether it appears surgically resectable for cure, and (c) if "yes" to the first two questions, whether the patient can tolerate the required degree of surgical resection (see Chapter 66).

In the subset of patients for whom the answer to all three questions is "yes," surgery is often the next step, and accurate pathologic staging of the disease is determined after complete resection. For patients in whom surgery is not feasible because of locally advanced or metastatic disease, or because of physiologic comorbidity, a biopsy that provides *both* a diagnosis and an accurate staging is necessary. For these patients, the appropriate treatments are chemotherapy and radiotherapy, either alone or in combination, depending on the stage and the likelihood of distant metastasis. However, a significant percentage of patients with advanced disease will be too sick to treat because of a poor performance status or extensive comorbidity.

This chapter divides lung cancer treatment on the basis of tumor anatomy (or staging) and patient physiology (or "performance status"). The following discussion of treatment by *stage* is restricted to non–small cell lung cancer (NSCLC); small cell lung cancer (SCLC) is considered in a separate section.

NON-SMALL CELL LUNG CANCER

STAGE I LUNG CANCER

Stage I disease in NSCLC is completely confined to the lung parenchyma or airway, without nodal spread, and does not arise within 2 cm of the carina. The standard of care for patients with adequate lung function, no other significant comorbid illness (e.g., unstable coronary artery disease, debilitating arthritis), and a nodule with high probability of being lung cancer is surgical resection. Patients with stage I NSCLC who undergo surgery with complete resection of their disease have a high rate of cure with surgery alone (60%-80%).

Based on a randomized trial of NSCLC surgery conducted by the Lung Cancer Study Group, *lobectomy* is the standard surgery for lung cancer. Beginning in 1982, this study compared outcomes of patients who underwent lobectomy versus segmentectomy or wedge resection. The rate of local recurrence was 75% lower in the lobectomy group, and since then, lobectomy has remained the "gold standard" procedure for healthy patients with stage I disease.

Recent data and advances in imaging have led to a reevaluation of this standard. Specifically, several Japanese studies showed that small (≤2 cm) peripheral tumors with a ground-glass appearance on thin-section computed tomography (CT; ≤3 mm) had a low rate of nodal involvement, with 5-year survival of almost 100%, even after limited anatomic resection. Newer studies are re-addressing the appropriate degree of lung resection for patients with small, stage I tumors. One should also bear in mind that the time frame of the Lung Cancer Study Group trial comparing limited resection with lobectomy predated the widespread use of CT and positron emission tomography (PET) scans. Also, the increased use of CT scans to image the chest results in more tumors being detected at smaller sizes. This smaller average size of tumors should not be interpreted to justify abandoning lobectomy as a standard of care, but randomized controlled trials (RCTs) designed to determine the optimum degree of resection in this more modern setting are ongoing.

For now, the standard procedure for stage I NSCLC remains a lobectomy with lymph node dissection. Exceptions to this rule are usually applied for patients with peripheral tumors and limited pulmonary reserve from emphysema. Many surgeons will offer limited pulmonary resection, with or without concomitant *lung volume reduction surgery* (LVRS), to patients with severe emphysema. Published series demonstrating the feasibility of LVRS for patients with severe emphysema universally came from groups participating in RCTs of LVRS. This cannot be overlooked as a contribution to the better-than-expected outcomes in these highly select patients. Patients undergoing evaluation for LVRS who also had lung cancer surgery underwent rigorous pulmonary rehabilitation, with surgery in centers with regimented postoperative pain management, early mobilization, chest physiotherapy, and bronchodilator treatment. Lung cancer surgery for patients with severe emphysema should be done in centers with experience in all these strategies. Preoperative staging of these patients must be thorough, to avoid incomplete resection of tumors with nodal metastases.

The presence or absence of *nodal involvement* is the most important prognostic factor to determine after surgical resection. In addition to lobectomy, mediastinal lymph node dissection is essential to accurate staging of surgically resected lung cancer and must be done as part of any lung cancer resection. Some studies have found a direct correlation between survival and the number of lymph nodes removed at surgery, although this has not been widely validated.

The surgical approach to NSCLC has traditionally employed posterolateral thoracotomy as the standard procedure. The development of video-assisted thoracoscopic surgery (VATS) in the 1990s, followed by its spread through thoracic surgical training programs, has gradually resulted in a greater proportion of NSCLC surgeries being performed by this approach. Various studies show that VATS lobectomy is oncologically equivalent to open lobectomy, such that the tumor-containing lobe is removed intact, and mediastinal lymph node dissection or sampling is completed with equal effectiveness by either approach. VATS lobectomy is associated with less incision pain, reduced length of stay, and faster recovery of preoperative activity levels than open lobectomy. These advantages make VATS the approach of choice for most lobectomies, allowing well-trained thoracic surgeons to offer lobectomy to patients with a broader range of comorbid conditions.

Some patients are not candidates for VATS lobectomy, and occasionally an operation started with the VATS approach is converted to an open procedure at the surgeon's discretion. The open approach is more suited to large (>3 cm) tumors or central tumors located close to the major blood vessels or airway. Patients with these tumors may benefit from the surgeon's greater tactile access in an open chest to ensure resection margins are negative and arteries and airways are removed intact. In addition, patients who have had preoperative chemotherapy or radiation, or who have pleural adhesions or prior chest surgery, may not be candidates for VATS. Tumors with chest wall invasion requiring an en bloc resection usually require an open approach as well. When pneumonectomy is required for complete resection, it is generally performed by thoracotomy. In such situations the size of the specimen requires a large incision to facilitate removal of the specimen, reducing the advantages of VATS.

In general, centers that treat the largest number of patients have the best survival outcomes, for all treatment modalities, but especially for the surgical resection of lung cancer. In the United States, approximately 80% of lung cancer resections between 1996 and 2005 were performed by surgeons for whom lung cancer surgery was not the primary focus of their practice. In this same study, thoracic surgeons (those for whom noncardiac thoracic surgery was the primary focus of their practice) had the lowest operative mortality for patients requiring lobectomy or pneumonectomy. Current evidence-based guidelines from the American College of Chest Physicians (ACCP) advocates that patients being considered for lung cancer surgery should be seen by a "thoracic surgical oncologist with a prominent part of his/her practice focused on NSCLC."

For patients with pathologically confirmed stage I disease, postoperative chemotherapy (adjuvant therapy) is not currently the standard of care. Based on RCT results of postoperative chemotherapy, patients with completely resected, pathologic stage I disease did not have a clear survival benefit with adjuvant chemotherapy. Subgroup analysis of RCTs suggests that patients with the highest risk (based on current understanding of such risk) may benefit from adjuvant therapy. These patients were generally those with large (>4 cm) primary tumors. Many oncologists offer discussions of risks and benefits of adjuvant chemotherapy to patients with large, stage IB tumors (>4 cm) or those with other possible risk factors, such as prominent vascular invasion. On an individualized basis, this practice is reasonable, but adjuvant chemotherapy cannot yet be considered the standard of care for completely resected stage I NSCLC.

For patients with clinical stage I NSCLC who are not candidates for resection because of comorbidity, there are still curative options, and the current standard of care is external beam radiation. An extensive discussion of radiotherapy methods is beyond the scope of this text, but the trend in thoracic oncology for inoperable stage I disease has been toward *stereotactic body radiotherapy* (SBRT) and away from conventionally fractionated *external beam radiotherapy* (EBRT). Conventional radiotherapy is given in doses of 60 to 70 grays (Gy), usually divided into 30 fractions of 2 to 2.5 Gy. SBRT is a form of radiotherapy employing many customized lower-dose beams converging into a volume that encompasses the tumor. These treatments are usually given up to a dose of 50 to 60 Gy over 3 to 5 days of treatment. Tumor motion caused by respiratory excursion can be significant, leading to undertreatment of tumor and overexposure of normal tissue to radiation, if the motion of the tumor is not tracked accurately. SBRT can be delivered more accurately with the use of fiducial markers placed in or near the tumor to track it during the respiratory cycle.

Cure rates with SBRT in stage I NSCLC for patients carefully staged can be excellent; 3-year disease-free survival in a large Phase II trial was close to 50%, with most recurrences being distant disease. Patients with large or centrally located tumors are more likely to be treated with conventionally fractionated EBRT; toxicity was greater in those with central tumors in a Phase II study of SBRT. Some groups treating large numbers of patients with SBRT report late development of chest wall pain or rib fractures. The risk factors for rib fracture include tumors within 2 cm of the chest wall and larger treatment volume. Complications in patients treated with SBRT should be tracked closely because it is a relatively new modality used in this patient population.

Thermal ablation is a minimally invasive therapy that can be used for local control of primary lung tumors. *Radiofrequency ablation* (RFA) uses a radiofrequency probe inserted percutaneously into the tumor, usually under CT guidance, to generate frictional heating that leads to cell death. RFA is the most frequently performed thermal ablation procedure used to treat lung tumors. Although the role of RFA is not clearly defined in lung cancer, small uncontrolled case series support its use for lung metastases. Although RFA is performed more often to treat hepatic and renal tumors, it may be well suited to the lung because of its ability to concentrate thermal energy focally within tumor tissue, with little or no energy spreading to the adjacent aerated normal lung parenchyma. There are no RCTs comparing RFA with radiotherapy in medically inoperable patients.

Based on published data, smaller tumors (<3 cm) may be more effectively treated with RFA than larger tumors. Peripheral tumors surrounded by lung parenchyma and away from hilar structures can be safely treated with RFA. The risk of pneumothorax is significant, as high as 50% in one series. Because this is a newer technology, the role for RFA in treating lung cancer has not been defined by large, well-controlled studies, but centers with experience in this approach can offer this option for inoperable patients, particularly if there is a contraindication to radiotherapy, such as prior irradiation.

A point of emphasis is necessary for defining the term "unresectable" stage I disease. In general, the most qualified person to determine a given patient's suitability for surgery is an experienced thoracic surgeon with lung cancer as a major focus of practice. The benefits of surgery are being extended to more patients with more severe comorbid conditions because of improvements in preoperative care, surgical techniques, and postoperative care. Patients with severe COPD or other comorbid illnesses should not be denied surgery without at least seeing an experienced thoracic surgeon. Furthermore, decisions about any patient's operability should be made in the context of optimum therapy for underlying lung disease.

In some patients a trial of bronchodilators and inhaled or oral corticosteroids might result in improvement in lung function sufficient to reduce surgical risk. The nature of these patients and the increased use of multimodality treatment across all stages of NSCLC make a compelling rationale for a multidisciplinary approach to treating patients with lung cancer.

STAGE II LUNG CANCER

Stage II NSCLC is defined as including mainly (1) tumors with hilar or intralobar nodal metastasis, with tumor confined to one lobe of the lung, or (2) tumors invading the chest wall, without nodal metastasis. Treatment of stage II NSCLC is still primarily surgical resection, and the same principles apply here as in stage I disease. One major difference is that adjuvant chemotherapy has proven survival benefit for patients with stage II disease. If one makes the safe assumption that the risk of systemic chemotherapy is the same whether the patient had stage I or stage II disease, then the favorable risk/benefit data for adjuvant chemotherapy in patients with stage II reflects that occult metastases are more likely to be present in patients with more advanced disease. Therefore, patients with pathologic stage II lung cancer have more to gain with adjuvant chemotherapy than stage I patients. After recovery from surgery, patients who undergo surgical resection of tumors with peribronchial or hilar nodal metastasis (stage II NSCLC) should be referred to a medical oncologist to discuss adjuvant chemotherapy.

Current recommendations suggest all patients with stage II or III disease should receive postoperative chemotherapy. However, metaanalyses of adjuvant trials suggest the number of patients who need to be treated with adjuvant chemotherapy to achieve one additional long-term cure is 24 to 39. To reduce this number, studies looked for additional patient or tumor-specific characteristics that predict benefit (or lack of) from adjuvant treatment. One oft-cited study found tumor biomarkers that may identify patients most likely to benefit from adjuvant chemotherapy. Retrospective examination of tumor specimens from patients enrolled in an adjuvant trial identified *excision repair cross complementation* 1 (ERCC1), an enzyme involved in repairing cisplatin-induced DNA damage, as a possible prognostic and predictive marker. High expression of ERCC1 was associated with a good prognosis, but also identified a patient subgroup who did not benefit from adjuvant (cisplatin-based) chemotherapy. Similarly, high expression of *ribonucleotide reductase* M1 (RRM1, which metabolizes gemcitabine) was identified by immunohistochemistry as predicting better overall survival, but poor response to gemcitabine-containing chemotherapy. Insufficient data are available to recommend the use of biomarker-based selection of any chemotherapy, including adjuvant chemotherapy, but studies are underway to determine whether this improves outcomes relative to empirically chosen chemotherapy and allows fewer patients to be treated while achieving the same survival benefit.

Postoperative radiotherapy for completely resected stage II NSCLC does not have proven survival benefit, may be associated with worse outcomes, and in general should not be used. However, for patients with stage II NSCLC who *cannot tolerate* surgical resection, definitive radiotherapy is the standard of care. Although radiotherapy can provide excellent local control rates, it does not reduce the likelihood of distant metastasis. An unanswered question is whether adjuvant chemotherapy would benefit patients with clinical stage II NSCLC treated with curative radiotherapy. If adjuvant chemotherapy reduces the likelihood of death after surgery for stage II disease, the same approach might benefit patients treated with radiotherapy. No data support this approach, however, and extrapolating surgical data to patients treated with radiotherapy for local control is not appropriate outside of a clinical trial.

STAGE III LUNG CANCER

Stage III NSCLC makes up the largest proportion of any stage and generally includes patients with mediastinal nodal metastasis. Historically, the treatment for stage III lung cancer was thoracic radiotherapy alone, but long-term survival with this approach was poor (<10%), with most patients succumbing to distant metastases. Studies showed that combining systemic chemotherapy with thoracic radiation could improve long-term survival to close to 20%.

The current standard of care for adequately staged patients with stage III NSCLC depends greatly on the patient's comorbid conditions and overall health status. The most commonly used global assessment of these factors in clinical practice is *performance status* (**Box 67-1**). Standard treatments for those with good to excellent Eastern Cooperative Oncology Group performance status (ECOG 0-1) are chemoradiation therapy administered concurrently. For those with less favorable performance status (ECOG 2), sequential chemotherapy followed by radiation therapy is still possible. The rationale for this is that concurrent therapy provides a survival benefit compared with sequential therapy, but at the cost of a greater likelihood of toxicity. Pulmonary toxicity is similar whether treatment is concurrent or sequential, but the occurrence of esophagitis (which can be severe) is more common with concurrent chemoradiation therapy than with sequential therapy. Those with marginal performance status (ECOG 2) may tolerate sequential therapy but are poor candidates for concurrent chemotherapy with thoracic radiation. In general, patients with ECOG performance status 3 or worse are best treated with a palliative approach focused on managing symptoms (i.e., best supportive care). This can include local radiotherapy to minimize complications such as airway obstruction, chest wall pain, or hemoptysis. Patients with poor performance status do not benefit from systemic chemotherapy and are more likely to experience severe toxicity.

The choice of chemotherapy for stage III NSCLC includes a platinum-based drug (cisplatin or carboplatinum) in combination with one other agent with demonstrated activity in NSCLC (**Table 67-1**). *Gemcitabine*, a drug with good single-agent activity often used in adjuvant settings or metastatic disease, is not typically used in combination with radiation because of its tendency to sensitize even normal tissue to the toxic effects of ionizing radiation. The dose of radiation for patients treated concurrently is generally left up to the radiotherapist, but doses used in this setting are lower than those used for primary treatment of early-stage, medically unresectable patients. Most trials delivered radiation doses of about 60 Gy. With better techniques that can limit damage to normal tissues, radiation oncologists are seeking ways to escalate the dose of radiation to increase the rate of cure. PET scans have been used in a course of radiation to adjust the port to a shrinking tumor, permitting a greater dose to metabolically active tumor (and consequently less to healthy tissue), as defined by the PET scan. These ongoing studies are likely to impact on the future treatment of NSCLC.

Given that chemotherapy (typically two cycles) combined with radiation in stage III disease increases local control and

---

Box 67-1 ECOG Performance Status Scale*

0: Asymptomatic (fully active, able to carry on all activity without restriction)

1: Symptomatic but completely ambulatory (restricted in physically strenuous activity but ambulatory and able to carry out work of a light or sedentary nature; e.g., light housework, office work)

2: Symptomatic, <50% time in bed or chair during the day (ambulatory and capable of all self-care but unable to carry out any work activities)

3: Symptomatic, >50% of time spent in bed or chair, but not bedbound (capable of only limited self-care)

4: Bedbound (completely disabled; cannot carry on any self-care; totally confined to bed or chair)

5: Death

From Oken MM et al: Toxicity and response criteria of the Eastern Cooperative Oncology Group, *Am J Clin Oncol* 5:649-655, 1982.
*Eastern Cooperative Oncology Group; also referred to as the World Health Organization (WHO) or Zubrod scale.
Use of performance status scales is central to the oncologist's assessment of both the likelihood of efficacy and the risk of toxicity of systemic chemotherapy.

Table 67-1 Common Chemotherapy Regimens for Non–Small Cell (NSCLC) and Small Cell Lung Cancer

Drug	Most Common Toxicity	Comment
Stage III NSCLC		
Cisplatin *or* Carboplatin *Plus*	Nephrotoxicity Myelosuppression	Two cycles of combination chemotherapy are usually used concurrently with radiation. Patients with marginal performance status usually receive sequential therapy.
Paclitaxel *or*	Neuropathy, allergic reactions, myelosuppression	
Etoposide	Myelosuppression	
Stage IV NSCLC*		
Cisplatin *or* Carboplatin *Plus*	Nephrotoxicity Myelosuppression	Goal: give three or four cycles of two-drug combination. Can be combined with bevacizumab
Any of agents used for stage III disease *or*	Myelosuppression	
Gemcitabine *or*	Myelosuppression	Usually not used in combination with radiotherapy, due to potent radiosensitizing effects and greater incidence of normal tissue toxicity
Pemetrexed	Myelosuppression, mucositis, nausea	Approved only for non–squamous cell lung cancer
Small Cell Lung Cancer		
Cisplatin *or* Carboplatin *Plus*	Nephrotoxicity Myelosuppression	Goal: give four to six cycles of two-drug combination.
Etoposide *or*	Myelosuppression	
Irinotecan	Diarrhea, myelosuppression	
Second-Line Drugs		
Docetaxel	Hepatotoxicity, neutropenia, thrombocytopenia	Usually used as single agent in patients who relapsed after standard therapy
Gefitinib[†] *or* Erlotinib	Skin rash	Response is better in patients with tumors bearing activating-EGFR mutations.

*Patients with activating mutations in epidermal growth factor receptor (EGFR) have better survival when treated with first-line EGFR–tyrosine kinase inhibitors.
[†]Gefitinib is not approved in the United States.

reduces distant metastases, one might conclude that more chemotherapy must be better. However, available studies do not support the role of additional "consolidation" chemotherapy after concurrent chemoradiation. One trial randomized patients to either observation or three cycles of docetaxel after patients had completed standard cisplatin and etoposide (two cycles) with radiation. Subjects receiving docetaxel had more treatment-related toxicity, without improved survival, than the control group. Although trials addressing this question continue, for now there is no role for maintenance or consolidation chemotherapy, even for patients with an apparent complete response.

Another area that remains unsettled is whether there are patients with stage IIIA NSCLC who benefit from some combination of surgery with chemotherapy and radiation therapy. This question has engendered significant debate among experts, but RCTs comparing "definitive" chemoradiation therapy with induction chemoradiation followed by surgery show no differences in survival between the two groups. Does this mean that no patients can benefit from "trimodality" therapy, or that the proper subgroup best suited for this most aggressive approach has yet to be identified? All that can be said with certainty is that the use of neoadjuvant therapy followed by surgical resection cannot yet be considered the standard of care for unselected patients with stage IIIA NSCLC.

One readily identifiable but rare subgroup of patients with stage IIIA NSCLC that most experts would agree should receive surgery is those with T3 tumors (either by chest wall invasion or, in the new staging system, with tumors greater than 7 cm) and hilar nodal metastasis. This group of T3N1, stage IIIA patients are surgical candidates with or without neoadjuvant chemotherapy, as long as they have the physiologic reserve to tolerate complete resection. A consistent finding in trials of neoadjuvant chemotherapy followed by surgery is that patients demonstrating a "complete response" in the mediastinal nodes when restaged before surgery have the best prognosis. Whether this simply identifies a population of patients with a good prognosis (and therefore no need for surgery), or whether surgery itself contributes to favorable long-term survival in this group of patients, cannot currently be answered.

Superior Sulcus Tumors

Tumors in the superior sulcus, sometimes called *Pancoast tumors*, are most often stage IIB (T3N0) or IIIA (T3N1). As for other stage III NSCLCs, chemotherapy with concurrent radiotherapy is the preferred treatment for unresectable patients with acceptable performance status. When potentially resectable (as determined by an experienced thoracic surgeon), Pancoast tumors have been treated with preoperative radiation (30-50 Gy) followed by surgical resection. Studies examining multimodality treatment in patients specifically with superior sulcus tumors show that even with chest wall invasion or nodal involvement, patients with superior sulcus tumors treated with radiation, with or without chemotherapy, followed by surgery have an excellent chance at long-term survival, 30% to 40% at 5 years. In light of these favorable findings in nonrandomized studies, this approach has evolved to be the accepted standard of care.

Given the complexity of these patients, as well as the importance of timing surgery at an appropriate interval after thoracic radiation, patients with superior sulcus tumors offered potentially curative therapy are best served when treated by a multidisciplinary team of NSCLC specialists.

STAGE IV LUNG CANCER

Until the early 1990s, the utility of chemotherapy for metastatic lung cancer was a subject of debate, with a widely held belief being that systemic chemotherapy had no role for patients with stage IV NSCLC. That debate has ended. Studies have demonstrated convincing (but modest) survival benefit with chemotherapy. Metaanalyses show that two-drug chemotherapy regimens are better than single-agent treatment, but the addition of a third agent is associated with greater toxicity, without additional gain in survival. Response to modern combinations of chemotherapy, with more than 50% tumor shrinkage, occurs in 20% to 30% of patients with stage IV NSCLC. Complete clinical remission is rare (<5% of patients), and those who do respond to chemotherapy eventually relapse and die of their disease. Patients with excellent performance status clearly benefit from systemic chemotherapy, but many patients present with ECOG 2 performance status, representing a controversial population regarding the efficacy and risk of systemic chemotherapy for stage IV NSCLC. Subgroup analyses of clinical studies suggest that patients with performance status of 2 can benefit from active treatment, including systemic chemotherapy. Many oncologists treat such patients with a less intense dose schedule.

Despite advances in treatment of advanced NSCLC, therapeutic nihilism has remained prevalent among clinicians, generally more than in other types of solid-organ tumors. A metaanalysis of trials with patients randomly assigned to "best supportive care" versus chemotherapy, including a cisplatin-based regimen, showed a survival benefit in the chemotherapy group. The active chemotherapy group had a reduction in the risk of death of 27% and an absolute improvement in survival of 10% at 1 year. In the 1990s, many promising new chemotherapeutic agents (paclitaxel, docetaxel, irinotecan, vinorelbine, gemcitabine, pemetrexed), each with single-agent activity in advanced disease, were developed for and then used in patients who had stage IV NSCLC. Numerous trials evaluated combinations of one or more of these newer agents with a platinum compound (cisplatin or carboplatinum; see Table 67-1). No one combination of drugs is superior. However, with use of platinum-based combinations, median survival gradually increased to 8 to 9 months, with 1-year survival of 30% to 35%. This compares favorably with untreated patients with stage IV NSCLC, who have median survival of 3 to 4 months, with 1-year survival of approximately 15%. Although no data exist to define the optimum combination of chemotherapeutic agents, newer data are leading to increasingly individualized approaches to care.

Pemetrexed was compared with gemcitabine (both in combination with a platinum compound) in patients with metastatic cancer. The overall population showed no difference between the two drug combinations, but a prespecified subgroup of patients with non–squamous cell histology showed improved outcomes when treated with the platinum-pemetrexed combination. This has resulted in the first histology-based recommendation for systemic chemotherapy in NSCLC.

Erlotinib and *gefitinib*, oral inhibitors of the epidermal growth factor receptor (EGFR) tyrosine kinase, were initially studied and used as second-line or third-line agents for patients with relapsed or metastatic NSCLC. Responses were dramatic in some cases, and larger trials noted common epidemiologic traits in those with excellent responses to these drugs, including nonsmoking (or light smoking) history, female gender, adenocarcinoma histology, and Asian ethnicity. Further studies that sequenced the EGFR gene in tumors of responders and nonresponders found that the drugs were unusually effective in patients' tumors and cell lines bearing a few specific activating mutations affecting the tyrosine kinase domain of the EGFR gene. Further epidemiologic studies confirmed that activating mutations conferring sensitivity to EGFR-TKI drugs were also common in those who shared one or more of the demographic or histologic traits previously noted to confer a high likelihood of response: female, Asian, nonsmoking, or adenocarcinoma. A study in a mostly Asian population, for patients with tumors bearing activating mutations in EGFR, showed that first-line treatment with EGFR-TKI resulted in improved response and overall survival compared with standard chemotherapy among patients with mutant EGFR. In contrast, patients with tumors harboring wild-type EGFR fared better when treated with traditional cytotoxic chemotherapy.

Based on preclinical data demonstrating the importance of angiogenesis in supporting solid-tumor growth, targeted drug development for cancer has included anti-angiogenic agents, particularly drugs targeting vascular endothelial growth factor (VEGF) or its receptors. *Bevacizumab*, a fully human monoclonal antibody against VEGF, is the most advanced antiangiogenic agent in clinical use. In metastatic NSCLC, RCTs have demonstrated a modest but statistically significant survival benefit when bevacizumab was added to standard chemotherapy. In earlier Phase II trials, patients with large central tumors or with squamous cell histology had unacceptably high incidence of serious toxicity, specifically hemoptysis, and were specifically excluded from trials that resulted in the approval of bevacizumab for metastatic NSCLC. Bevacizumab use is also associated with a risk for hypertension and thrombotic complications and is contraindicated in patients with central nervous system (CNS) metastases.

An exciting addition in the field of targeted NSCLC therapy was the report in 2007 of a fusion protein, joining echinoderm microtubule–like 4 (*EML4*) with the anaplastic lymphoma kinase (ALK). EML4-ALK is an activating mutation capable of driving the proliferation of NSCLC cells. Drugs targeting abnormally activated ALK (e.g., crizotinib) were quickly developed and brought to clinical trials, showing great promise in patients bearing ALK mutations. Detecting ALK fusion can be difficult because it is typically formed by a short-segment chromosomal inversion. Fluorescent in situ hybridization (FISH) reagents developed for this purpose, called "break-apart FISH probes," can highlight this chromosomal rearrangement. Similar to mutant EFGR tumors, the prevalence of ALK-mutant NSCLC tumors in most series is small (~5%) and most often found in nonsmokers. Although this finding was relevant to only a small number of cancer patients, the exciting nature of this discovery is that within 2 years after the discovery of ALK's role in transformation of cancer cells, drugs targeting ALK were already in clinical trials, showing dramatic benefit for those with ALK-activating mutations. This pace of progression from discovery to treatment is highly unusual, not just in cancer, but in any field of biomedical research. Additional driving mutations similar to the one that activates ALK will likely be discovered in the future.

In summary, patients with metastatic, stage IV NSCLC and good performance status (ECOG 0-1) are best treated with systemic chemotherapy, with the addition of bevacizumab in those with no contraindication. Patients with ECOG performance status of 2 can also expect to benefit from active treatment, although with a higher risk of toxicity. Diagnoses in all patients should be made with biopsies that yield enough tissue to permit analysis for specific activating mutations in EGFR, or to detect the presence of an activating ALK fusion. Patients with these abnormalities, particularly EGFR mutations, are known (or suspected in the case of ALK) to gain prolonged survival when treated with agents targeted at their specific mutation.

SMALL CELL LUNG CANCER

The rationale for separately discussing SCLC is three-fold. First, the vast majority of patients with small cell lung cancer present with bulky mediastinal lymph node involvement or metastatic disease. Second, SCLC is much more likely to respond to systemic chemotherapy, and therefore patients with borderline performance status may still gain enough benefit from systemic chemotherapy to justify the known risk. Third, the major decision point for SCLC is the distinction between limited-stage and extensive-stage disease. Although small cell lung cancer is considered separately, it is important to recognize that the general principles of oncology for NSCLC still apply for SCLC. For example, the rare patient with SCLC who presents with an isolated pulmonary nodule or mass should be managed just as the patient with NSCLC, with appropriate preoperative staging followed by surgery for patients with acceptable pulmonary reserve. In such patients, postoperative adjuvant chemotherapy may improve long-term survival, but this has not been confirmed in RCTs, because the numbers are so small.

Although the updated (7th edition) staging system for lung cancer (see Chapter 66) has been validated in SCLC as well as NSCLC, the treatment of SCLC has traditionally focused on defining limited-stage versus extensive-stage SCLC. *Limited-stage SCLC*, the purview of the radiation oncologist, is defined by a tumor burden that can be encompassed within a single radiotherapy port with acceptable risk of toxicity. This applies to approximately 30% of patients with SCLC, in whom the addition of thoracic radiotherapy to systemic chemotherapy increases the likelihood of long-term survival. Approximately 20% of patients with limited-stage disease reach 5-year survival. For the remaining 70% of SCLC patients, with *extensive-stage disease*, the recommended treatment is systemic chemotherapy alone, and radiotherapy in these patients is limited to treating CNS metastases or symptomatic skeletal metastases.

As in NSCLC, no data from RCTs can provide the optimum chemotherapy regimen(s) in SCLC. Pooled data from meta-analyses suggest that patients treated with cisplatin-containing regimens have improved survival and acceptable toxicity. The agent most frequently used with cisplatin for SCLC is *etoposide*. RCT data also demonstrate the benefit of etoposide in SCLC, and etoposide in combination with cisplatin has been the standard of care in modern treatment of patients with SCLC. A few generally underpowered studies in SCLC patients have compared cisplatin with carboplatinum, which is generally better tolerated than cisplatin. Results are mixed; some data suggest a slightly better outcome with cisplatin, whereas another study shows equivalence. The number of cycles of chemotherapy varies between four and six. Additional chemotherapy beyond the sixth cycle increases the likelihood of toxicity without any appreciable increase in survival.

PROPHYLACTIC CRANIAL IRRADIATION

In patients treated for stage III or IV NSCLC or for SCLC, systemic chemotherapy is used to treat known or occult metastases. The CNS is a privileged site, and most chemotherapeutic agents are incapable of crossing the blood-brain barrier in sufficient amount to treat CNS metastases. Therefore, many studies address the role of prophylactic cranial irradiation (PCI) to reduce the development of symptomatic metastases. The rationale for this approach is strong, in that many lung cancer deaths result from CNS metastases, particularly with SCLC.

As expected, the strongest data favoring the use of PCI are from studies of patients with SCLC. The patients with the greatest demonstrable benefit are those with limited-stage SCLC in whom chemotherapy and thoracic radiation achieve a complete response. In these patients, PCI reduces the incidence of symptomatic CNS metastases and improves overall survival. PCI has been tested in patients with extensive-stage disease in SCLC as well. The cumulative risk of brain metastases within 1 year was 40.4% in the control group and 14.6% in the group receiving PCI. Median overall survival increased from 5.4 to 6.7 months, and 1-year survival of 27.1% versus 13.3% favored the patients receiving PCI. In NSCLC, the benefits of PCI are less than in SCLC, with one study of patients with mostly stage III NSCLC demonstrating a reduced incidence of symptomatic cranial metastases by more than 50% after PCI, but the difference in survival was statistically too small. This study was ended early because of slow data accrual, leaving the PCI survival benefit uncertain for patients with NSCLC.

PARANEOPLASTIC SYNDROMES AND OTHER COMMON COMPLICATIONS

Paraneoplastic syndromes are defined as systemic or localized effects of tumors unrelated to physical effects of the tumor mass. These syndromes can be divided into those caused by humoral factors produced by the tumor (hormones or other bioactive products) and those caused by immune response to the tumor in the form of autoantibodies. Most of the latter occur in the context of SCLC and result from a variety of antineuronal antibodies. Paraneoplastic syndromes can affect the skin, CNS and peripheral nervous system, vascular system, heart, kidneys, marrow, and muscular or skeletal system (**Table 67-2**).

One common paraneoplastic syndrome involves the inappropriate secretion of ADH by the tumor. The *syndrome of inappropriate antidiuretic hormone* (SIADH) disturbs fluid balance, results in the inability to dilute urine, and causes hyponatremia, which can progress to nausea, vomiting, muscle cramps, confusion, and convulsions. Treatment of SIADH begins with restricted water intake to prevent further hyponatremia (not completely correcting serum sodium level). Salt administration can be used to increase water excretion in the kidney. In extreme cases where sodium correction cannot be achieved using more conservative measures, demeclocycline can be used, and recently, vasopressin receptor antagonists have been tested for use in patients with SIADH.

Compression of the superior vena cava (SVC) and obstruction can occur from direct involvement of the SVC by centrally located tumors. Although this occurs infrequently in lung cancer, patients with lung cancer make up the majority of patients with *superior vena cava syndrome*, with the remainder having lymphoma or fibrotic lymphoid tissue (histoplasmosis or fibrosing mediastinitis). SVC syndrome was once considered a medical emergency, often prompting urgent radiation therapy to relieve the obstruction quickly. However, the principal concern of increased intracranial pressure (ICP) related to impaired venous outflow is rare, because SVC obstruction usually develops gradually and is often accompanied by the development of collateral venous circulation. Emergency treatment is no longer considered necessary for most patients. The importance of accurate histologic diagnosis before starting therapy cannot be overstated, given that the possibilities include

Table 67-2 Paraneoplastic Syndromes: Manifestations of Lung Cancer and Treatment

Syndrome	Manifestations	Treatment
Syndromes Caused by Production of Bioactive Hormones by Tumor		
SIADH	Hyponatremia	Water restriction Demeclocycline
Cushing's syndrome	Hypertension, glucose intolerance, electrolyte abnormalities, muscle weakness, weight loss, hirsutism, osteoporosis	Often improves with treatment of the cancer; can use ketoconazole, metyrapone, or mitotane
Hypercalcemia	Weakness, mental status changes, nausea	Treatment of the cancer Intravenous hydration Bisphosphonates, calcitonin
Syndromes Caused by Humoral Immune Responses to Tumor		
Lambert-Eaton myasthenic syndrome (LEMS)*	Weakness, muscle fatigue, often affects large muscle groups with preserved small muscle function; improvement with repetitive use	Usually improves with treatment of the cancer; can use plasma exchange or agents that increase synaptic depolarization (3,4-diaminopyridine) with or without pyridostigmine
Cerebellar degeneration†	Dizziness, nausea, vertigo, ataxia, and sometimes diplopia; onset can be abrupt	Symptoms often irreversible because of Purkinje cell loss
Limbic encephalitis‡	Cognitive impairment, mood changes, disordered perception, and sleep disturbances	Treatment may result in improvement; immune suppression may help if tumor is also treated.

*Antibody to voltage-gated calcium channel.
†Anti-Yo antibodies, or Purkinje cell antibody type 1 (PCA-1).
‡Anti-Hu antibodies or "antineuronal nuclear antibodies" (ANNA-1).
SIADH, syndrome of inappropriate (secretion of) antidiuretic hormone.

SCLC and NSCLC, as well as lymphoma. Placement of endovascular stents for severely symptomatic patients allows for rapid relief of SVC obstruction and time for proper staging and diagnosis. Important exceptions include patients who present with symptoms of increased ICP (headache, altered consciousness) or central airway obstruction threatening respiratory failure. These situations represent true medical emergencies, and these patients require endovascular stenting and/or emergent radiotherapy to decrease the risk of sudden respiratory failure and death. As always, securing the airway should be the first priority in these patients.

PALLIATIVE CARE

Despite advances in diagnosis, staging, treatment, and even screening, lung cancer will continue to be a major cause of morbidity and mortality. The majority of people diagnosed with lung cancer will die as a result of it, and clinicians must be prepared to manage and palliate acute or chronic, tumor-related symptoms at the end of life, when cancer-specific treatment is no longer indicated.

Principles of *pain management* for cancer patients include (1) recognizing and treating pain promptly; (2) involving the patient and family in pain control; (3) providing multimodal therapy; (4) reassessing and adjusting the management plan, focusing on intensity of pain, functional status, and side effects; and (5) documenting the plan and effectiveness of pain management. Pain control should include not only narcotics but also nonsteroidal antiinflammatory drugs (NSAIDs) and agents to alleviate neuropathic pain. Radiotherapy is an excellent means of rapidly controlling pain related to bony metastasis and should be used aggressively, particularly to reduce the risk of pathologic fracture.

Hemoptysis and large airways obstruction are common, frightening, and potentially life-threatening complications that can be palliated with a variety of approaches. Radiation therapy is a widely available tool to control hemoptysis and should be considered as a first option. Life-threatening hemoptysis can be managed by gaining rapid control of the airway (in patients for whom intubation is not contrary to agreed-on plans, prestated living will, or advance directives), followed by embolization of bronchial circulation. The latter should be attempted only by trained clinicians with significant experience in interventional vascular procedures. Lung, esophageal, or spinal cord infarction are potentially serious complications of bronchial arterial embolization.

Interventional bronchoscopic techniques can be useful for both hemoptysis, if the source of bleeding can be localized to a central airway, and malignant airway obstruction. Airway stents can be used in various ways to debulk the tumor. Balloon dilation, laser therapy, electrocautery, cryotherapy, and argon plasma coagulation can be used to achieve rapid palliation of severe dyspnea. Complex malignant airway obstruction should be managed only in centers with physicians trained and experienced in this procedure. Less rapid means of alleviating airway obstruction include external beam radiotherapy or, for patients who cannot receive EBRT, endobronchial brachytherapy.

Dyspnea occurs frequently in patients with advanced lung cancer, with varied causes. Dyspnea can result from underlying chronic obstructive pulmonary disease, extensive tumor burden, narrowing of a major airway, treatment-related toxicity, cardiovascular disease, or pleural effusion. Whenever possible, treatment of dyspnea should be directed at the underlying cause. When symptoms persist despite maximal treatment of potential contributing causes, however, opiates, oxygen, and bronchodilators can provide relief. Malignant pleural effusions are common and can cause dyspnea. Palliation can be achieved rapidly with therapeutic thoracentesis, but the presence of a pleural effusion does not guarantee that thoracentesis will improve dyspnea. Small to moderate-sized effusions are unlikely to be the root cause of dyspnea, and caution should be exercised before draining effusions ipsilateral to a known or suspected endobronchial obstruction. When a large volume thoracentesis results in lasting relief of dyspnea, placement of an indwelling tunneled pleural catheter can be considered, if the effusion recurs symptomatically.

Pericardial effusions, although less common than pleural effusions, can be life threatening if they produce increased intrapericardial pressure impairing cardiac return and ventricular filling. Pericardial effusions can develop acutely or more slowly, and the rapidity of development is proportional to the likelihood of symptoms. Treatment of the effusion should both relieve intrapericardial pressure from the fluid and prevent reaccumulation. Both goals can be accomplished in a single procedure if fluid drainage is accompanied by placement of an indwelling drain, pericardial window, or catheter-based balloon pericardiostomy.

Palliation and active treatment of cancer were once viewed as "mutually exclusive" approaches, but recent data suggest these may be complementary. In patients with metastatic lung cancer randomized to receive early palliative care or usual care (palliative care consultation only at request of patient, family, or oncologist) in combination with active oncologic treatment, early palliative care not only improved quality of life and lowered rates of depressive symptoms in the intervention group, but also resulted in longer median survival. Palliative care in these patients was delivered by a multidisciplinary team of physicians board-certified in palliative care and advanced-practice nurses. Personnel trained in palliative care should be an integral part of any multidisciplinary lung cancer patient care team. These intriguing findings, although not yet widely validated, suggest that attention to palliation can slow the dying process while providing superior quality of life.

CONCLUSION

Treatment of lung cancer is complex and requires accurate knowledge of both the anatomic stage of the tumor and the patient's overall physiologic condition. Surgical treatment of lung cancer may be an option for patients once thought to be medically unresectable, and patients with borderline physiologic reserve should be seen by a multidisciplinary team. Postoperative adjuvant chemotherapy is now the standard of care for patients with stage II and III non–small cell lung cancer. Therapeutic nihilism for patients who are not candidates for curative surgery should be particularly discouraged; even patients with significant comorbidity can receive curative therapy that preserves quality of life while offering cure or prolonging survival. Patients and clinicians often have an unrealistically pessimistic outlook on the potential benefits of lung cancer treatment. Aggressive multimodality therapy for locally advanced, unresectable (stage III) NSCLC can still offer otherwise healthy patients a significant survival benefit, with 15% to 20% of patients achieving long-term survival. Therefore, patients with clinical stage III NSCLC should be offered realistic but hopeful assessment of their treatment options. Metastatic (stage IV) NSCLC is generally incurable, but also treatable.

Respiratory medicine physicians and other clinicians need to provide cancer patients with the best possible treatment, and in those with metastatic lung cancer and preserved performance status, this includes lung cancer–specific treatment, perhaps alongside early palliative care. Newer treatment options are becoming available at a rapid pace, and the role of novel, targeted therapies is being defined more precisely.

SUGGESTED READINGS

Albain KS, Rusch VW, Crowley JJ, et al: Concurrent cisplatin/etoposide plus chest radiotherapy followed by surgery for stages IIIA (N2) and IIIB non-small-cell lung cancer: mature results of Southwest Oncology Group Phase II study 8805, *J Clin Oncol* 13:1880–1892, 1995.

American College of Chest Physicians: Diagnosis and management of lung cancer: ACCP guidelines (2nd edition), *Chest* 132(suppl 3), 2007. http://chestjournal.chestpubs.org/content/132/3_suppl.toc.

Dillman RO, Seagren SL, Propert KJ, et al: A randomized trial of induction chemotherapy plus high-dose radiation versus radiation alone in stage III non-small-cell lung cancer, *N Engl J Med* 323:940–945, 1990.

Furuse K, Fukuoka M, Kawahara M, et al: Phase III study of concurrent versus sequential thoracic radiotherapy in combination with mitomycin, vindesine, and cisplatin in unresectable stage III non–small-cell lung cancer, *J Clin Oncol* 17:2692–2699, 1999.

Mok TS, Wu YL, Thongprasert S, et al: Gefitinib or carboplatin-paclitaxel in pulmonary adenocarcinoma, *N Engl J Med* 361:947–957, 2009.

Paez JG, Jänne PA, Lee JC, et al: EGFR mutations in lung cancer: correlation with clinical response to gefitinib therapy, *Science* 304:1497–1500, 2004.

Soda M, Choi YL, Enomoto M, et al: Identification of the transforming EML4-ALK fusion gene in non-small-cell lung cancer, *Nature* 448:561–566, 2007.

Temel JS, Greer JA, Muzikansky A, et al: Early palliative care for patients with metastatic non-small-cell lung cancer, *N Engl J Med* 363:733–742, 2010.

Chapter **68**

Benign Lung Tumors*

David E. Midthun

When used together, the words "tumor" and "lung" suggest "malignancy," as expected given the frequency and lethality of lung cancer worldwide. The work of the respiratory medicine physician and the surgeon would be simpler if all focal opacities in the lung were malignant, but in reality, more are benign than malignant, requiring that the two be separated. A *tumor* is defined as abnormal benign or malignant growth, possessing no physiologic function, and arising from uncontrolled cellular proliferation. In a strict sense, "inflammation" is both physiologic and usually controlled, and thus does not fit this definition. However, in everyday practice, physicians know a focal opacity is present on imaging without knowing whether it is "physiologic" or "uncontrolled." This chapter discusses the general approach to benign lung tumors and the most common benign neoplastic and non-neoplastic causes.

DETECTION AND DIAGNOSIS

We tend to use the terms *tumor* and *nodule* (or *mass*) synonymously. Benign tumors may also present primarily in the *airway* versus the lung parenchyma, and certain causes may present in either location or in both locations. Patients presenting with symptoms and found to have tumors on chest x-ray films or computed tomography (CT) imaging studies are more likely to have a lung malignancy.

Incidentally found tumors or nodules in the lung detected at CT screening are more likely to be benign. Studies of CT screening for lung cancer detect one or more nodules in about 25% of participants when CT collimation (slice thickness) is 10 mm and 40% to 60% of participants at 5 mm or less; about 98% of these nodules are benign. Nodule size is generally an excellent guide for determining benign from malignant; less than 1% of nodules 5 mm or less in diameter represent malignancy, even in current or former smokers. This distinction becomes more difficult for larger nodules, with the likelihood of malignancy more than 50% for nodules 2 cm in diameter, and increasing with larger nodule/mass size. A few benign tumors, such as hamartomas and teratomas, may have imaging features such that CT is diagnostic. However, most benign tumors do not have signature characteristics on imaging, and histology is required for diagnosis.

Positron emission tomography (PET) can be helpful in identifying benign from malignant tumors because it is based on the principle that cancer cells have a high rate of *glycolysis* compared with non-neoplastic cells. False-positive PET scans have been reported with infections, sarcoidosis, and other benign conditions. False-negative PET scans may occur with low-grade tumors, carcinoid tumor, and malignancies less than

1 cm in diameter. PET is now most often performed with integrated CT (PET-CT). Avidity on PET-CT is not the same as tissue, and a biopsy should be obtained rather than assuming a diagnosis or a stage.

Once a nodule is 3 cm or larger, and it is not clearly benign by showing evidence of calcification or fat on CT, the likelihood of malignancy is greater than 90%. Therefore, most benign tumors larger than 3 cm are diagnosed at resection because of the high index of suspicion of malignancy. Although most inflammatory lesions show no evidence of growth in follow-up, many benign tumors will grow and prompt concern for malignancy and subsequent removal for diagnosis. Bronchoscopy or transthoracic needle biopsy may be used to diagnose benign tumors, especially when multifocal or complete resection is not feasible.

Obstruction of the trachea and major bronchi is most often caused by squamous cell and small cell carcinoma or carcinoid tumor, but tracheal obstruction may also be caused by benign tumors. Several benign tumors manifest more frequently in the airways rather than the periphery of the lung. The patients may have symptoms of airway obstruction, such as cough, recurrent infection, wheezing, and dyspnea. The endoscopic appearance of a lesion may suggest a diagnosis, but uniformly, histology is required. If the lesion is polypoid and has a low likelihood of malignant behavior, successful treatment may be achieved with endoscopic techniques. Broad-based lesions and those with greater malignant potential are best treated with surgical excision; lung-sparing procedures such as a bronchoplasty or sleeve resection may be appropriate.

CLASSIFICATION

Benign neoplastic tumors are classified histologically according to the World Health Organization (WHO) classification updated in 2004 (**Box 68-1**). These histologic distinctions are more helpful to the pathologist than to the clinician approaching a lung tumor and are more likely to be in the "is it malignant or not" mindset. Although typically benign, many of the benign neoplasms have the potential for malignant transformation.

BENIGN EPITHELIAL NEOPLASMS

Papillomas

Benign epithelial neoplasms are generally rare, although *squamous papilloma* is the most common. Histologically, these are identified as papillary tumors with a squamous cell epithelial surface and delicate connective tissue attachments. They may be solitary or multiple and most often occur in the larynx and trachea, with less than 10% having lower airway involvement

---

*Additional content for this chapter can be found on Expert Consult.

and only 2% within the lung parenchyma (**Figure 68-1**). The squamous type of papilloma has an association with human papillomavirus (HPV types 16, 18, 31, 33, and 35). Obstructive symptoms may develop from airway involvement and are an indication for laryngoscopic or bronchoscopic removal. Recurrent papillomas occur in as many as 20%, and some patients require periodic endoscopic debridement. Malignant transformation to squamous cell carcinoma may occur. Compared with squamous cell papillomas, glandular and mixed-cell papillomas are exceedingly rare.

Adenomas

Alveolar adenomas are rare and typically occur in the lung periphery. They are recognized as solitary tumors with a network of spaces lined by simple cuboidal epithelium and a spindle cell stroma. Although considered neoplasms, adenomas are not recognized as having malignant potential. *Papillary* adenomas also typically occur in the periphery of the lung and also appear to have no malignant potential. *Mucous gland* adenomas more often occur in the central airways and may be difficult to distinguish from low-grade mucoepidermoid carcinomas, although adenomas do not appear to be a malignant precursor. *Pleomorphic* adenomas have features of both epithelial and connective tissue differentiation; they occur in the airway or the lung periphery and may exhibit malignant behavior. *Mucinous cystadenomas* are localized cystic masses filled with mucin and lined by columnar mucinous epithelium; they are usually peripheral and are benign, without malignant progression.

Thymoma

Arising from ectopic thymic tissue, intrapulmonary thymomas are epithelial neoplasms and are otherwise identical to those occurring in the mediastinum. Myasthenia is rarely described with intrapulmonary thymoma, and more common symptoms include cough, fever, chest pain, and dyspnea. Resection is the treatment of choice, and invasion and nodal involvement may occur.

BENIGN MESENCHYMAL NEOPLASMS

Chondroma

Chondromas are benign tumors composed of cartilage and are most often found in the patient with *Carney triad:* pulmonary chondroma, gastric stromal sarcoma, and paraganglioma. Although described as a "triad," most patients will manifest only two different neoplasms. The appearance of chondromas on chest radiograph is usually diagnostic because these are typically multiple, well-circumscribed, calcified nodules occurring in young women (**Figure 68-2**). The main differential of the radiographic appearance of a chondroma is a hamartoma, typically singular. Chondromas are benign, and patients with Carney triad will more likely have symptoms from other, extrapulmonary manifestations.

Inflammatory Myofibroblastic Tumor

Synonyms for inflammatory myofibroblastic tumor (IMT) include inflammatory pseudotumor, plasma cell granuloma, fibrous histiocytoma, and fibroxanthoma. IMT is composed of a mixture of inflammatory cells (with plasma cell predominance), collagen, and spindle cells showing myofibroblastic

---

Box 68-1	Benign Neoplasms

Epithelial
Papilloma
Squamous papilloma*
Glandular papilloma
Mixed papilloma

Adenomas
Alveolar adenoma
Papillary adenoma
Salivary gland–type adenoma
    Mucous gland adenoma
    Pleomorphic adenoma*
Mucinous cystadenoma

Mesenchymal
Thymoma
Chondroma
Inflammatory myofibroblastic tumor*
Nerve sheath tumors*
Solitary fibrous tumor*
Glomus tumor*

Miscellaneous
Hamartoma*
Sclerosing hemangioma
Germ cell tumors
    Teratoma*
Clear cell tumor*
Leiomyoma
Lipoma

Modified from World Health Organization classification, Geneva, 2004, WHO.
*May exhibit malignant behavior.

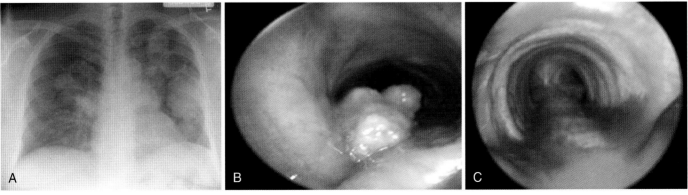

Figure 68-1 **A,** Chest radiograph in 56-year-old man with history of respiratory papillomatosis diagnosed by wedge resection of one of several masses. At bronchoscopy, obstructing papillomas were seen in the trachea (**B**) and distal bronchial tree and were removed with rigid bronchoscopy (**C**).

differentiation. IMTs are the most common benign primary lung tumor in children and usually occur in the airways. In adults these lesions are rare and more often present as solitary parenchymal masses (**Figure 68-3**). Symptoms may include weight loss and fatigue or pain relating to tumor location; chest wall invasion or angioinvasion can occur. Resection is the only proven treatment, and complete excision is usually curative,

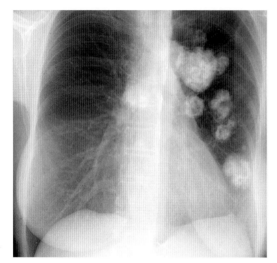

Figure 68-2 Chest radiograph in 25-year-old woman shows multiple calcified pulmonary chondromas. Patient had prior resection of several gastrointestinal stromal tumors (GISTs) and was believed to have Carney triad; she had not demonstrated a paraganglioma.

although recurrence after excision and metastases or progression to sarcoma can occur.

Neurofibromas

The neurofibromatoses (NFs) are autosomal dominant disorders and may be associated with benign peripheral *nerve sheath tumors* in the airway or lung (**Figure 68-4**). A retrospective study of 156 patients with NF found lung nodules or masses present in 5%, not including those with paraspinal or chest wall masses. Neurofibromas and *schwannomas* may also be present in the absence of NF, and there is the potential for malignant change. Clinical signs and symptoms typically relate to airway obstruction (cough, wheezing, dyspnea, hemoptysis).

Solitary Fibrous Tumor of Pleura

Solitary fibrous tumors of the pleura (SFTPs) are spindle cell mesenchymal tumors. They typically arise in the visceral pleura, but also from lung parenchyma or mediastinum, and may become very large (**Figure 68-5**). The terminology of "benign mesothelioma" is no longer used. In one retrospective series of 84 patients, 55% were symptomatic (cough, chest pain, dyspnea); 4% had the paraneoplastic manifestations of hypertrophic pulmonary osteoarthropathy (HPO), 6% had HPO and clubbing, and 1% hypoglycemia. Rarely, SFTP can be malignant.

Glomus Tumor

Glomus tumors are extremely rare, occur more often in males, and are thought to be of glomus cellular origin, having the

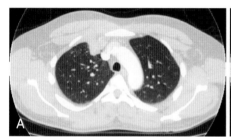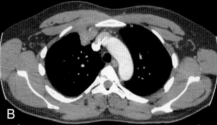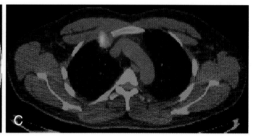

Figure 68-3 Computed tomography (CT) scans in 40-year-old man, never smoker who developed pain in right side of chest, show a mass anteriorly in **A,** right upper lobe of lung, and **B,** mediastinal windows. **C,** Positron emission tomography (PET)–CT shows lesion with moderate activity. Transthoracic needle biopsy was nondiagnostic. Surgical biopsy showed inflammatory myofibroblastic tumor, and patient underwent complete resection.

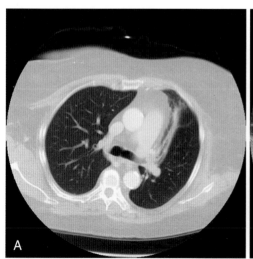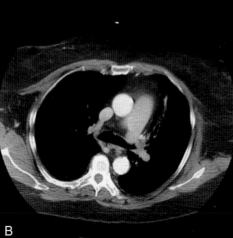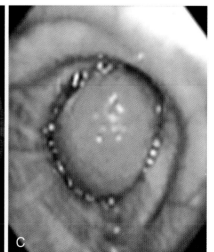

Figure 68-4 **A,** Chest radiograph in 68-year-old woman with history of asthma presenting with worsening cough and dyspnea shows volume loss. **B,** CT scan shows obstruction of left main bronchus. **C,** Bronchoscopy reveals complete obstruction of left main stem by a polypoid tumor. Patient underwent left thoracotomy, with resection of a sleeve of bronchus at takeoff of left upper lobe of lung; pathology revealed a neurofibroma.

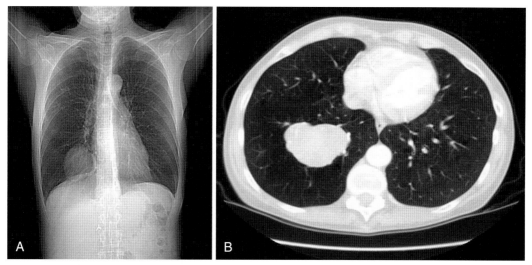

Figure 68-5 **A,** Chest radiograph identifies a mass in an asymptomatic 61-year-old woman, former smoker. **B,** CT scan shows mass without adenopathy, and lobectomy showed this to be a 7-cm solitary fibrous tumor with no involvement of the pleura.

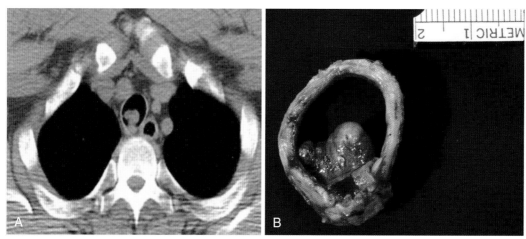

Figure 68-6 **A,** CT chest scan shows a tracheal lesion in 41-year-old man, never smoker, who presented with intermittent hemoptysis for 2 years; chest radiograph was normal. Bronchoscopy showed a broad-based polypoid lesion, and patient underwent tracheal sleeve resection. **B,** Pathology showed glomus tumor.

appearance of smooth muscle. Based on cellular appearance, they are further classified as *classic* glomus tumor, *glomangioma,* and *glomangiomyoma.* Within the chest, glomus tumors are more likely to be in the trachea, but they have been described in the lung and mediastinum (**Figure 68-6**). Successful resection has been reported with surgery or bronchoscopy, and malignant behavior has been observed.

BENIGN NEOPLASMS: MISCELLANEOUS

Hamartoma

Pulmonary hamartomas are the most common benign neoplasms in the lung, comprising cartilage, fat, connective tissue, and smooth muscle. Hamartomas are rare in children; in adults they are usually in the parenchyma, and approximately 10% present endobronchially (**Figure 68-7**). Patients with *parenchymal hamartoma* are usually asymptomatic, and typical features of fat and calcification may be evident on CT images. When lacking classic CT features, parenchymal hamartomas are often diagnosed at resection to exclude malignancy. Rarely, recurrence or sarcomatous transformation has been described.

Sclerosing Hemangioma

Histologic features of sclerosing hemangiomas include papillary, solid, sclerotic, and hemorrhagic structures. Sclerosing hemangiomas usually present as asymptomatic radiographic abnormalities, although cough, hemoptysis, and pain may occur. Sclerosing hemangioma behaves benignly. Although spread to regional lymph nodes is described rarely, when present, it appears to have no negative effect on prognosis, and disease-related death has not been reported.

Benign Teratoma

Teratomas are composed of tissues from more than one germ cell line and have mature and immature forms. Mature pulmonary teratomas are benign and more common in the upper lobes of the lung. Immature teratomas may be malignant. Because teratomas are frequently cystic and contain skin, hair, sweat glands, fat, bone, sebaceous material, or toothlike structures, some of these elements may be visible on CT scans. Patients with teratomas may be asymptomatic or may present with chest pain, hemoptysis, or the unusual symptom of *trichoptysis,* expectorating hair. Surgery is generally recommended, even if the diagnosis is evident from imaging studies (**Figure 68-8**).

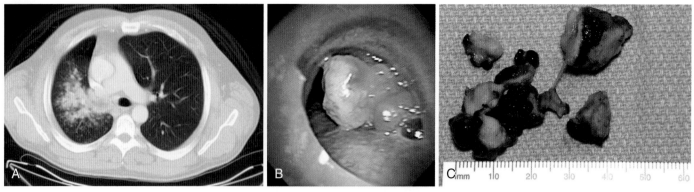

Figure 68-7 **A,** CT chest scan shows complete obstruction of right main bronchus and postobstructive pneumonia in 45-year-old man who presented with fever, sweats, and chills; chest radiograph showed right lung opacity and volume loss. **B,** Bronchoscopy demonstrates a polypoid mass extending into distal trachea. ▣ **C,** Bronchoscopic resection was performed using polypectomy snare, and pathology showed hamartoma. ▣

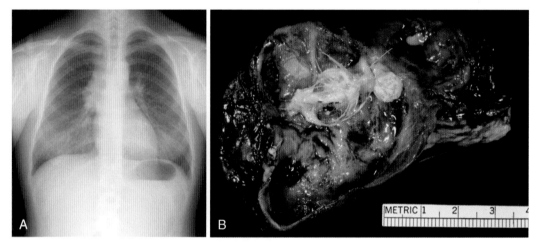

Figure 68-8 **A,** Chest radiograph shows a right hilar mass in 17-year-old girl who had chest discomfort after a basketball game. **B,** Resection shows benign, cystic teratoma.

Clear Cell Tumor

The name "clear cell" tumor comes from presence of cells with abundant clear or eosinophilic cytoplasm containing glycogen; it is also called "sugar tumor." This extremely rare tumor is usually solitary and peripheral, and discovery is incidental. Rarely, malignant features have been described.

Leiomyoma

Leiomyomas are benign smooth muscle tumors occurring in women. When singular, and absent a history of uterine leiomyomas, they most often occur in the airway. Benign leiomyoma may also present in the lung of women with a history of uterine leiomyoma and is termed *benign metastasizing leiomyoma* (BML). BML is characterized by multiple, slow-growing, smooth muscle tumors (**Figure 68-9**). Despite the resemblance to malignancy, the number of mitotic indices is low, and there is no evidence of invasion despite multiple distant lesions. Extrauterine leiomyosarcoma must be excluded. The lung involvement in BML is typically evident 10 to 15 years after the removal of the uterine leiomyoma. BML is usually negative on PET imaging. Treatment includes hormonal therapy, surgical resection, and chemotherapy.

Lipoma

Lipomas are rare, are composed of mature fat cells, and may occur in the airway or less often in the mediastinum. Presenting symptoms depend on the size and location of the lesion, most often dyspnea and cough. CT imaging shows the lesion to be homogeneous and composed of fat (**Figure 68-10**). Local recurrence has been described after resection.

NON-NEOPLASTIC TUMORS

A variety of conditions cause benign lesions in the lung that are not true neoplasms (**Box 68-2**). These conditions need to be considered in the differential diagnosis when evaluating a nodule or mass on imaging studies and include nodular lymphoid hyperplasia, organizing pneumonia, endometriosis, rounded atelectasis, and sequestration, as discussed in earlier chapters.

Amyloid Deposits

As an example of a non-neoplastic tumor, amyloid is composed of a group of fibrillar proteins with beta-pleated-sheet formation, which demonstrates birefringence under polarized light

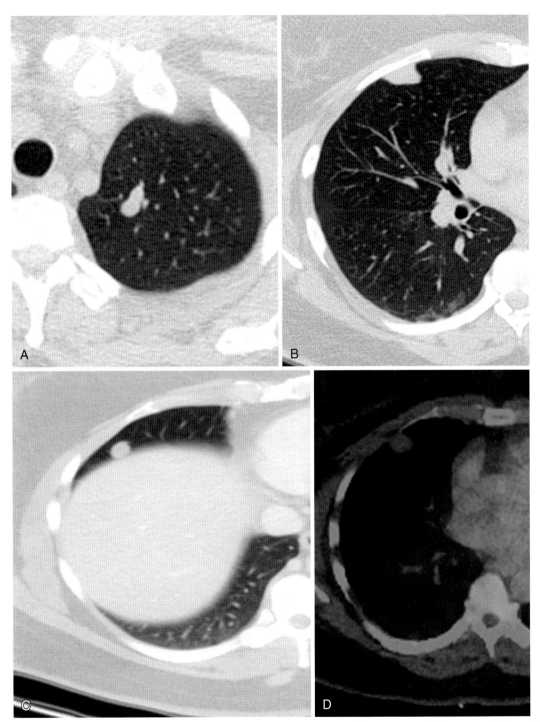

Figure 68-9   A 37-year-old former smoker had an abdominal CT done for pain and a lung nodule was seen. CT chest scans **A**, **B**, and **C** showed multiple lung nodules. **D,** PET-CT scan shows no activity. Patient had no history of malignancy but had a hysterectomy 7 years earlier for fibroid tumors. Needle biopsies of a nodule showed spindle cell neoplasm, consistent with benign metastasizing leiomyoma.

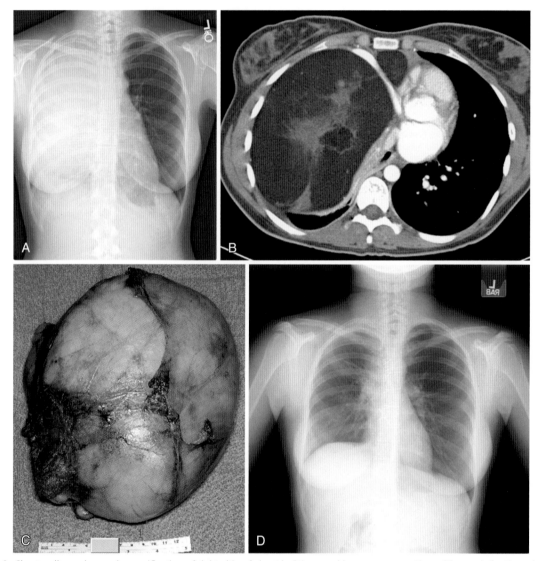

Figure 68-10   A, Chest radiograph reveals opacification of right side of chest in 24-year-old woman presenting with cough for 6 weeks and mild exertional dyspnea. **B,** CT scan shows a large, fat-attenuating mass. **C,** Thoracotomy reveals well-circumscribed benign lipoma (23.0 × 11 cm) with no clonal abnormality. **D,** Radiograph at 8 weeks postoperatively shows reexpansion of right lung.

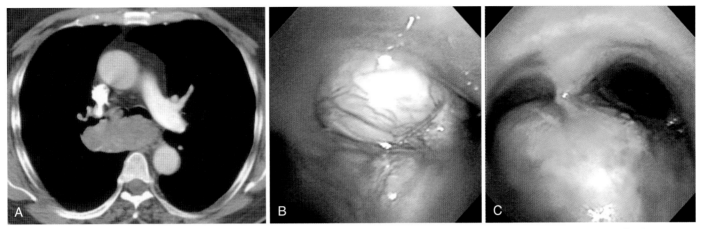

Figure 68-11 **A,** CT scan shows mass obstructing right main stem bronchus in 61-year-old man, never smoker, with 12-year history of asthma, presenting with progressing shortness of breath; chest radiograph showed volume loss in right lung. **B,** Bronchoscopic biopsies show amyloidoma. **C,** Rigid bronchoscopic resection reestablished patency of right main bronchus.

Box 68-2   Non-Neoplastic Tumors

Amyloid deposit (amyloidoma)
Bronchial inflammatory polyp
Endometriosis
Hyalinizing granuloma
Infarct
Micronodular pneumonocyte hyperplasia
Minute meningothelial nodule
Nodular lymphoid hyperplasia
Organizing pneumonia
Rounded atelectasis
Sequestration

---

on Congo red stain. Pulmonary manifestations of amyloidosis include tracheobronchial infiltration, persistent pleural effusions, parenchymal nodules, and amyloidomas **(Figure 68-11)**. Amyloid deposits in the lung may or may not be associated with systemic amyloidosis.

SUGGESTED READINGS

Carney JA: Carney triad: a syndrome featuring paraganglionic, adrenocortical, and possibly other endocrine tumors, *J Clin Endocrinol Metab* 94:3656–3662, 2009.

Gaertner EM, Steinberg DM, Huber M, et al: Pulmonary and mediastinal glomus tumors: report of five cases including a pulmonary glomangiosarcoma—a clinicopathologic study with literature review, *Am J Surg Pathol* 24:1105–1114, 2000.

Gjevre JA, Myers JL, Prakash UB: Pulmonary hamartomas, *Mayo Clin Proc* 71:14–20, 1996.

Harrison-Phipps KM, Nichols FC, Schleck CD, et al: Solitary fibrous tumors of the pleura: results of surgical treatment and long-term prognosis, *J Thorac Cardiovasc Surg* 138:19–25, 2009.

Sakurai H, Hasegawa T, Watanabe S, et al: Inflammatory myofibroblastic tumor of the lung, *Eur J Cardiothorac Surg* 25:155–159, 2004.

Sakurai H, Kaji M, Yamazaki K, et al: Intrathoracic lipomas: their clinicopathological behaviors are not as straightforward as expected, *Ann Thorac Surg* 86:261–265, 2008.

Shah H, Garbe L, Nussbaum E, et al: Benign tumors of the tracheobronchial tree: endoscopic characteristics and role of laser resection, *Chest* 107:1744–1751, 1995.

Travis WD, Brambilla E, Müller-Hermelink HK, et al, editors: *World Health Organization classification of tumors: pathology and genetics of tumors of the lung, pleura, thymus and heart*, ed 4, Geneva, 2004, WHO, pp 78–121.

Utz JP, Swensen SJ, Gertz MA: Pulmonary amyloidosis: the Mayo Clinic experience from 1980 to 1993, *Ann Intern Med* 124:407–413, 1996.

Zamora A, Collard H, Wolters P, et al: Neurofibromatosis-associated lung disease: a case series and literature review, *Eur Respir J* 29:210–214, 2007.

Chapter **69**
Pleural Effusion, Empyema, and Pneumothorax
John M. Wrightson • Helen E. Davies • Y.C. Gary Lee

PLEURAL EFFUSION

Pleural effusion, defined as the accumulation of fluid in the pleural space, is common and affects more than 3000 people per 1 million population each year. Pleural effusions develop when the rate of pleural fluid formation exceeds that of absorption and may be a complication of pleural, pulmonary, and systemic disease or associated with use of certain drugs. A systematic approach is required to determine the underlying cause.

EPIDEMIOLOGY AND PATHOPHYSIOLOGY

EPIDEMIOLOGY

More than 60 causes of pleural effusions have been documented. The relative incidence of different types of effusion varies according to patient demographics and geographic areas. Heart failure is responsible for approximately one third of all pleural effusions (**Table 69-1**), with pleural infection and malignancy accounting for most exudative effusions.

PATHOPHYSIOLOGY

In the healthy person, the pleural cavity contains a small amount of physiologic pleural fluid (less than 10 mL in a 70-kg man), which functions in part to facilitate smooth gliding of the lung over the interior chest wall during respiration. The normal rate of fluid production is approximately 17 mL/day. The fluid is resorbed into lymphatic channels, with an estimated maximal absorptive capacity of 0.2 to 0.3 mL/kg/hour.

With *transudative* effusions, pleural fluid accumulates because of an increase in hydrostatic pressure or a reduction in plasma oncotic pressure; the pleura usually remain normal. By contrast, development of *exudative* effusions normally is the result of various pleural pathologic conditions, resulting in increased vascular permeability and/or impaired fluid resorption (e.g., lymphatic obstruction).

Pleural fluid also can accumulate from extrapleural sources. Transdiaphragmatic migration of peritoneal fluid is well recognized. Abnormal communications between the pleural cavity and the thoracic duct (chylothorax), esophagus, pancreas, renal tract (urinothorax), or dura mater also may lead to development of pleural effusions.

CLINICAL PRESENTATION

Patients may be asymptomatic but often present with dyspnea, chest pain, cough, or other signs or symptoms of underlying disease. Dyspnea is a result of altered diaphragmatic and chest wall mechanics and compression of the lung. Pleuritic chest pain indicates disease involvement of the parietal pleura. Physical examination reveals a stony dull percussion note with decreased fremitus and absence of breath sounds over the effusion. These signs may be difficult to distinguish from those of an elevated hemidiaphragm.

IMAGING

Chest Radiography

Most pleural effusions can be recognized on posteroanterior (greater than 200 mL fluid volume) or lateral (greater than 50 mL fluid volume) chest radiographs. Large effusions may produce contralateral mediastinal shift. Blunting of the costophrenic angle may be the only sign for a small effusion but may also represent pleural thickening.

Thoracic Ultrasound Imaging

The availability of bedside thoracic ultrasound examination by clinicians has had a significant impact on pleural disease management in recent years. The 2010 British Thoracic Society Pleural Disease Guidelines strongly recommended the use of thoracic ultrasound imaging before procedures for pleural fluid. It is particularly useful for the detection (sensitivity approximately 100%), quantification (by depth), and characterization of pleural fluid (**Figures 69-1 to 69-3; Table 69-2**), as well as for guiding intervention. Ultrasonography is invaluable in the differentiation between pleural fluid and collapsed or consolidated lung, thereby avoiding unnecessary pleural procedures and associated complications.

Thoracentesis guided by clinical examination alone could result in organ puncture in 10% of cases. Several large studies have demonstrated improved safety of pleural interventions performed under ultrasound guidance, particularly in reducing iatrogenic pneumothorax or organ puncture. A Mayo Clinic study showed a dramatic reduction (from 8% to 1%) in rate of thoracentesis-related complications since the unit initiated a "pleural safety program" that included pleural ultrasound training and mandated its use before thoracentesis. With adequate

Table 69-1 **Approximate Annual Incidence of Various Types of Pleural Effusions in the United States**

Causative Disorder	Number	Percentage	Percentage of Noncardiac Effusions
Congestive heart failure	500,000	37.4	
Other causes		62.6	
Pneumonia	400,000		48.0
Malignant disease	200,000		24.0
Pulmonary embolism	150,000		18.0
Cirrhosis with ascites	50,000		6.0
Gastrointestinal disease	25,000		3.0
Collagen vascular disease	6000		0.7
Tuberculosis	2500		0.3
Asbestos pleuritis	2000		0.25
Mesothelioma	1500		0.2
TOTAL	1,337,000	100.0	100.0

Modified from Light RW, editor: *Pleural diseases*, ed 4, Philadelphia, Lippincott Williams & Wilkins, 2001.

Table 69-2 **Pleural Fluid Sonographic Appearances**

Sonographic Appearance	Significance
Anechoic (black fluid) (see Figure 69-1)	Transudative or exudative effusion
Septated (multiple lines within fluid) (see Figure 69-2)	Exudative effusion; may suggest possible difficulties inserting chest tube; effusion may drain poorly, although not necessarily
Echogenic (echoes, often swirling, within fluid) (see Figure 69-3)	Exudative effusion; heavily echogenic fluid suggestive of blood or pus

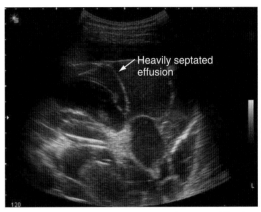

Figure 69-2   A heavily septated effusion is evident on this ultrasound image.

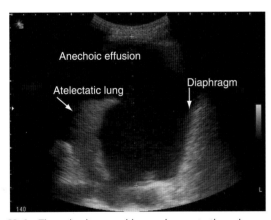

Figure 69-1   Thoracic ultrasound image demonstrating a large anechoic effusion with compressive atelectasis of underlying lung.

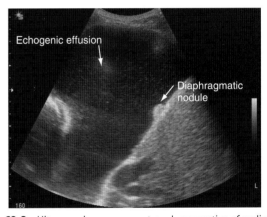

Figure 69-3   Ultrasound appearance strongly suggestive of malignancy, with diaphragmatic nodularity and a large echogenic exudative pleural effusion.

training in this modality, thoracic ultrasound imaging performed by respiratory physicians has been shown to have a safety profile comparable to that when performed by radiologists.

Ultrasound imaging has a high sensitivity (approximately 80%) for detecting pleural malignancy, which can manifest as thickening or nodularity on the visceral, parietal, and diaphragmatic pleural surfaces (see Figure 69-3). Detection of pleural nodularity mandates further investigation (e.g., with chest computed tomography [CT] and pleural biopsy), even if there are no further suspicious features. Ultrasonography also can identify abnormalities beyond the pleural cavity that may provide vital clues to the cause of the effusion, including peripheral lung tumors or abscesses, parenchymal consolidation

and atelectasis, diaphragmatic paralysis or elevation, pericardial effusion, and rib and liver metastases and enables evaluation of supraclavicular and cervical lymphadenopathy (**Figure 69-4**).

Pleural interventions may be guided by site marking or real-time needle visualization; the latter is required to sample small or loculated effusions. The Royal College of Radiologists (in the United Kingdom), the American College of Chest Physicians, the American College of Surgeons, and the American College of Emergency Physicians are among the many agencies that have published ultrasound training guidelines for clinicians. Appropriate training is essential, because potential pitfalls with performance and interpretation of pleural ultrasound studies are recognized.

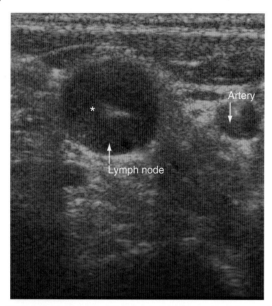

Figure 69-4 Neck ultrasound image showing an enlarged, rounded, hypoechoic lymph node characteristic of malignancy, undergoing fine needle aspiration with a 21-gauge needle (*indicates needle tip).

Computed Tomography and Magnetic Resonance Imaging

CT with pleural phase contrast enhancement highlights pleural abnormalities and aids discrimination of benign from malignant disease (see Chapter 7). Specific "pleural" CT protocols should be adopted for optimal pleural enhancement and abnormality detection; recent data suggest that images should be acquired 60 seconds after injection of 150 mL of an intravenous contrast agent at 2.5 mL/second. The presence of contraction of the hemithorax, mediastinal pleural involvement, and circumferential pleural thickening (especially greater than 1 cm and with nodularity) all are suggestive of pleural malignancy (**Figure 69-5**) but cannot adequately differentiate mesothelioma from metastatic pleural cancers. Magnetic resonance imaging (MRI) can help delineate malignant chest wall involvement and is valuable in selected cases, particularly when (probably benign) pleural abnormalities are to be followed clinically by serial imaging in younger patients.

Positron Emission Tomography

Positron emission tomography (PET)-CT scanning (see Chapter 8) is beginning to emerge as a useful tool in pleural disease management. PET-CT cannot adequately differentiate between benign and malignant effusions, because of the tracer ^{18}F-fluorodeoxyglucose (FDG). FDG-enhanced PET imaging is confounded by avid pleural uptake of FDG in the presence of pleural inflammation (including that due to previous talc pleurodesis and pleural infection). However, FDG-PET may have a role in guiding pleural biopsy in patients with diffuse pleural abnormality to increase sensitivity (**Figure 69-6**). FDG-PET also may identify nonpleural sites that allow tissue sampling to confirm malignancy (e.g., lymphadenopathy or liver metastases). Recent data suggest a role for FDG-PET in monitoring disease response to therapy in malignant mesothelioma, as well as a potential prognostic role.

PET scanning using various novel molecular tracers is in early-phase trials for evaluation of pleural malignancies. For instance, PET scanning using labeled thymidine, essential for deoxyribonucleic acid (DNA) synthesis, can identify sites

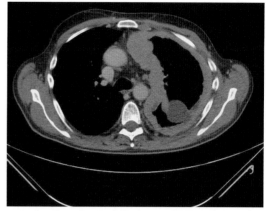

Figure 69-5 Thoracic computed tomography (CT) scan showing circumferential nodular pleural thickening and hemithorax volume loss due to malignant pleural disease.

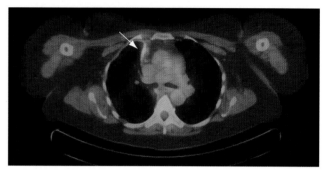

Figure 69-6 Positron emission tomography–computed tomography (PET-CT) image demonstrating localized fluorodeoxyglucose (FDG)-avid mediastinal pleural thickening (*arrow*) in mesothelioma.

of cell proliferation activity and is not confounded by inflammation (**Figure 69-7**). New tracers targeting specific cell biology processes (e.g., annexin, a marker of apoptosis) are likely to provide valuable insight to disease pathobiology.

DIAGNOSTIC APPROACH

Investigation of a pleural effusion should be performed using a systematic approach (**Figure 69-8**), aiming to minimize the number of pleural procedures required to make a diagnosis and thereafter allow definitive treatment.

Thoracentesis, preferably imaging-guided, should be the initial investigation in pleural effusions of uncertain origin. If small (less than 1 cm in depth) effusions require sampling, this procedure should be undertaken using real-time radiologic guidance. Thoracentesis is generally safe and complications are uncommon but include vasovagal syncope (0.6%), pneumothorax, infection, and bleeding. Removal of large amounts of fluid may precipitate reexpansion pulmonary edema, often heralded by cough, chest discomfort (at which point the procedure must be terminated), or acute dyspnea. Pleural manometry has been advocated but is not widely available. If initial pleural fluid analysis is inconclusive, additional investigations are often required, including further imaging, repeat thoracentesis, and thoracoscopic or percutaneous pleural biopsy (see Chapters 13 and 74).

PLEURAL FLUID ANALYSIS

Pleural fluid analysis can help determine the diagnosis or direct further investigations. Recent years have seen a significant

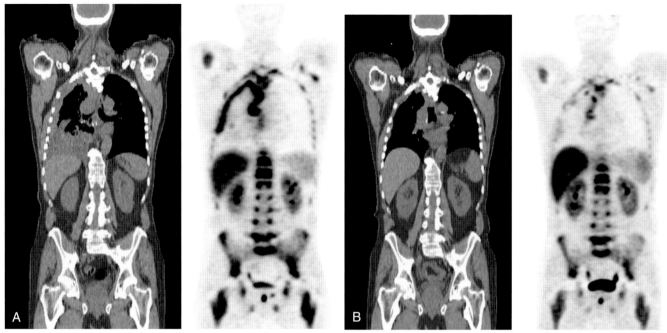

Figure 69-7 Positron emission tomography (PET) imaging using labeled thymidine in a patient with mesothelioma. Images before (**A**) and after (**B**) chemotherapy reveal dramatic improvement in the costal and mediastinal pleural uptake with treatment. *(Courtesy Dr. Roslyn Francis, University of Western Australia, Australia.)*

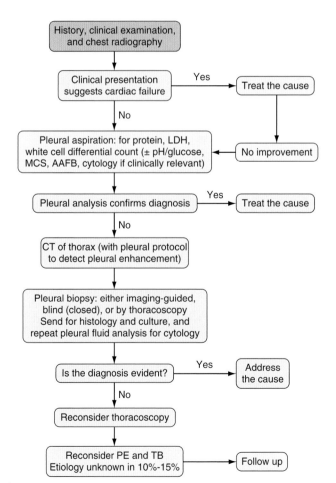

Figure 69-8 Suggested diagnostic approach for a unilateral pleural effusion. (Investigations requested should correlate with suggestive or actual clinical findings.) *AAFB,* acid- and alchohol-fast bacilli; *LDH,* lactate dehydrogenase; *MCS,* microscopy, culture, and sensitivity [testing]; *PE,* pulmonary embolism; *TB,* tuberculosis.

Box 69-1 | **Light's Criteria**

A pleural fluid is an *exudate* if any of the following criteria are met:
1. Pleural fluid-to-serum protein ratio greater than 0.5
2. Pleural fluid-to-serum lactate dehydrogenase (LDH) ratio greater than 0.6
3. Pleural fluid LDH more than two-thirds the upper limit of normal serum LDH

Caveat: False-positive results may occur in patients with cardiac failure on diuretic therapy resulting in a pleural fluid-to-serum protein ratio greater than 0.5. Clinical judgment and measurement of N-terminal pro-BNP will define a true transudate in these circumstances.

---

increase in the tests and biomarkers available for pleural fluid analysis, but the exact role(s) of many of them in the diagnostic algorithm are still to be defined. An understanding of the indications and limitations of the individual tests is essential for clinicians to provide an efficient and cost-effective service.

Bedside Examination of the Fluid

Most pleural fluids are straw-colored (serous), serosanguineous (blood-stained), or hemorrhagic. A genuine hemothorax is characterized by fluid hematocrit greater than 50% of blood hematocrit.

Appearance of the fluid may reveal the diagnosis: presence of pus confirms empyema; food particles in the fluid suggest esophageal perforation; and chylous fluids suggest chylothorax or pseudochylothorax. Pleural fluid that appears milky should be centrifuged: in empyema, a clear supernatant is seen, whereas chyle remains cloudy. The odor of ammonia often is the most important diagnostic clue to the presence of urinothorax.

Separation of Exudates and Transudates

Exudative pleural effusions most commonly are defined by *Light's criteria* (**Box 69-1**), using the fluid-to-serum ratio of

---

Box 69-2 Common Causes of Pleural Effusion for Categories of Pleural Fluid Differential Cell Count

Lymphocytic Effusion (>85% total nucleated cells)
Tuberculosis
Malignancy including lymphoma
Rheumatoid effusion
Sarcoidosis
Yellow nail syndrome
Chylothorax

Eosinophilic Effusion (>10% eosinophils)
Pneumothorax
Hemothorax
Drug-induced pleurisy
Infection (tuberculosis/fungal/parasitic)
Benign asbestos pleural effusion
Churg-Strauss syndrome
Malignancy
Early post-CABG (coronary artery bypass graft)

Neutrophilic Effusion
Acute pleural injury/inflammation
Parapneumonic
Pulmonary embolism

Box 69-3 Conditions Commonly Associated With Low-pH and Low-Glucose Pleural Effusions*

Empyema
Complicated parapneumonic effusion
Malignant effusion
Rheumatoid pleuritis
Tuberculosis
Lupus pleurisy
Esophageal rupture
Urinothorax (transudate)

*Low-pH effusions: pH <7.3; low-glucose effusions: <3.3 mmol/L (60 mg/dL).

---

protein and lactate dehydrogenase, which has an accuracy of 96%. Numerous other markers and criteria have been tested (including measurement of pleural fluid cholesterol values), but none has proved superior. Distinguishing exudates from transudates may narrow the scope of the differential diagnosis and streamline further investigations, although such categorization has limitations: It does not provide the diagnosis and fails to identify concurrent transudative and exudative causes of fluid formation. Research in recent years has focused on disease-specific markers that may provide a definitive diagnosis.

Differential Leukocyte Count

The cellular portion of physiologic pleural fluid consists predominantly of macrophages and monocytes. In disease states, the differential cell count of the pleural fluid may be helpful in determining the cause (**Box 69-2**). Acute pleural inflammation or injury generates chemotaxins, such as interleukin 8, and attracts neutrophils to the pleural space. A neutrophil-predominant effusion is commonly seen with acute bacterial pneumonia or pulmonary infarction. A lymphocyte-rich fluid is more common in disease of insidious onset such as tuberculosis (TB) or malignancy. Tuberculous effusions occasionally (less than 10%) may be neutrophilic. An increased eosinophil count (more than 10% of total leukocytes) is often nonspecific. Most commonly, eosinophil effusions develop secondary to presence of intrapleural air or blood (including pneumothorax or previous interventions) but can also be associated with a range of other diseases, such as Churg-Strauss syndrome or drug-induced pleuritis.

pH and Glucose

Pleural fluid pH (or glucose) measurement can aid disease management. Low glucose levels are associated with a similar spectrum of diseases that give rise to low pH effusions (e.g., infection and connective tissue diseases) (**Box 69-3**) and are equally informative except in patients with hyperglycemia.

Physiologic pleural fluid pH is approximately 7.6 and reflects bicarbonate accumulation within the pleural cavity. Pleural fluid pH should be measured using a blood gas analyzer, and care should be taken to avoid exposure of the fluid to free air or to residual lidocaine, which will potently raise or lower the fluid pH, respectively. pH meters and litmus paper have been shown to give unreliable values. Low pleural fluid pH (e.g., less than 7.3) coexistent with a normal blood pH may result from increased metabolism of leukocytes, bacteria, or tumor cells or hydrogen ion accumulation.

In malignant pleural effusions, a low pH is associated with more extensive tumor involvement of the pleura, a higher chance of positive findings on cytologic examination, a lower success rate for pleurodesis, and a poorer prognosis. In parapneumonic effusion, a low pH (less than 7.2) predicts the need for chest tube drainage, and pH below 7.2 is now often used as a cutoff point to diagnose pleural infection (complicated parapneumonic effusion) in the presence of a compatible clinical history. A recent study of 308 patients confirmed that pleural fluid pH (or glucose) measurements were superior to other biomarkers tested (pleural fluid procalcitonin, C-reactive protein, lipopolysaccharide-binding protein, and triggering receptor expressed on myeloid cells-1 [sTREM-1]) in distinguishing between simple and complicated parapneumonic effusions.

Disease-Specific Tests

The diagnosis of a malignant effusion should be established only by histocytopathologic confirmation of malignant cells in the pleural fluid or tissue. Pleural fluid cytologic examination is the first line of investigation in suspected cases and has a sensitivity up to 60% (dependent on tumor type, extent of disease, and experience of the cytologist). Immunocytochemical analysis plays an invaluable role in cytologic assessment of pleural fluid, improving the differentiation between benign and malignant effusions and between different malignancies (particularly metastatic adenocarcinoma versus mesothelioma). If malignancy is suspected, generally little incremental benefit is obtained from cytologic analysis of pleural fluid on more than two occasions.

Mesothelioma, the most common primary malignant tumor of the pleura, often is challenging to diagnose. Research in recent years has proposed several potential adjunct diagnostic biomarkers. Mesothelin is a U.S. Food and Drug Administration (FDA)-approved diagnostic and prognostic marker for mesothelioma, although it is not recommended as a sole diagnostic marker (having sensitivity of 48% to 84% and specificity of 70% to 100%). False-negative results may occur with sarcomatoid mesothelioma, which often does not express mesothelin. A raised mesothelin level also can be found with other malignancies (most commonly, pancreatic or ovarian carcinoma but also lung adenocarcinoma and lymphoma). Hence, in patients with elevated pleural fluid or blood mesothelin, further investigations should be considered even if cytologic examination demonstrates no malignant cells. Megakaryocyte-potentiating factor (MPF), which originates from the same precursor protein as for mesothelin, has been shown to have a similar diagnostic performance for detection of mesothelioma. After initial interest in the use of osteopontin for mesothelioma identification, subsequent data have shown it to have a lower diagnostic accuracy than mesothelin.

Other tumor markers and pleural fluid cytokine measurements are neither sensitive nor specific enough for clinical use. Cytogenetic evaluation may be a helpful addition to characterize chromosomal markers of hematolymphoid and mesenchymal malignancies. Flow cytometry of the pleural aspirate should be considered if lymphoma is a possibility.

Gram staining and culture of pleural fluid should be performed in an appropriate clinical setting. Direct inoculation of bottled culture media ("blood culture bottles") along with separate microbiologic analysis of pleural fluid in a universal container has been shown to increase microbial yield. In cases characterized by presence of frank pus, the diagnosis of empyema is secured, but Gram staining and culture may help to identify the causative organism(s) and to guide therapy.

Testing for tuberculosis should be conducted if clinically indicated, particularly if the fluid is lymphocyte-predominant (more than 50% of total leukocytes). Direct smears and aspirate cultures have low sensitivities (less than 5% and 10% to 20%, respectively) because tuberculous pleuritis usually develops as a type IV hypersensitivity reaction, with low mycobacterial load in the pleural cavity. Demonstration of caseating granulomas by closed or thoracoscopic pleural biopsy clinches the diagnosis. Debate exists regarding the role of adenosine deaminase (ADA), interferon-γ, interferon-γ release assays (IGRAs), and polymerase chain reaction (PCR) techniques in diagnosing tuberculous pleuritis. ADA, an enzyme present in lymphocytes, commonly is measured in disease-endemic countries, and a high pleural fluid ADA level suggests tuberculous effusions, with a sensitivity of greater than 90%. False-positive results have been reported (especially with empyema, rheumatoid effusions, and lymphoma). In nonendemic areas, a low ADA measurement may help rule out tuberculous pleuritis in some patients. Assays for the isoenzyme ADA_2, which predominates in tuberculous effusions, are not widely available. Unstimulated interferon-γ pleural fluid levels perform about as well as ADA for diagnosis in this setting but are more expensive. Peripheral blood and pleural fluid IGRAs have been shown to be of limited clinical value in the diagnosis of tuberculous pleural effusions.

A raised amylase level (above the serum upper limit of normal or if the pleural fluid–to–serum ratio is more than 1) in an appropriate clinical setting can help confirm effusions from esophageal rupture and pancreatic diseases (acute pancreatitis or pseudocyst). Isoenzyme analysis may further differentiate the source of amylase (salivary or pancreatic) but is rarely needed. A raised amylase is present in some malignant (usually adenocarcinomas) effusions.

In suspected cases of chylothorax, lipoprotein electrophoresis for chylomicrons or a triglyceride concentration greater than 1.24 mmol/L (110 mg/dL) confirms the diagnosis. The presence of cholesterol crystals at microscopy with a pleural fluid cholesterol level more than 5.17 mmol/L (200 mg/dL) is diagnostic of a pseudochylothorax. Chylomicrons are not found in pseudochylothorax fluid.

Pleural fluid levels of rheumatoid factor and antinuclear antibody mirror serum values and add little to clinical management of rheumatoid or systemic lupus erythematosus–related pleuritis. Complement levels can be reduced but are of little clinical value. Very low pleural fluid glucose levels typically are seen in patients with a rheumatoid effusion, and differentiation from empyema fluid may be difficult.

β₂-Transferrin is found in cerebrospinal fluid, and its presence in pleural fluid confirms presence of a duropleural fistula. Raised creatinine values are seen in urinothorax.

PLEURAL BIOPSY

Histologic examination (with or without culture) of pleural tissue can aid in the diagnosis of specific pleural diseases. Tissue can be collected percutaneously (by "blind" or imaging-guided biopsy) or under direct vision (by thoracoscopy or thoracotomy), each with its relative merits (see Chapters 13 and 74).

Percutaneous Biopsy

"Blind" percutaneous pleural biopsy (performed using an Abrams or Cope needle) has been shown to be inferior to imaging-guided biopsy for the diagnosis of malignancy in a randomized controlled trial. Blind biopsy can still be useful in diagnosing diseases with diffuse pleural involvement, especially granulomatous pleuritis (e.g., from TB or rheumatoid arthritis), particularly if thoracoscopic facilities are not readily available. The yield, however, is critically dependent on operator experience and also on the number of passes.

Thoracoscopy

Thoracoscopy is indicated in patients with an undiagnosed exudative pleural effusion after a nondiagnostic thoracentesis. Thoracoscopy can be performed by physicians or surgeons either using local anesthesia and sedation (pleuroscopy) or with the patient under general anesthesia using single-lung ventilation (video-assisted thoracoscopic surgery, [VATS]). Pleuroscopy allows direct visualization of almost the entire pleural surface (**Figure 69-9**), drainage of fluid, parietal pleural biopsy, and pleurodesis by talc poudrage in the same procedure. Diagnostic sensitivity approaches 95% in malignant pleural diseases and almost 100% in tuberculous pleurisy. Complications are few, and mortality rates low (less than 0.5%). VATS has a similarly high diagnostic sensitivity but also allows other invasive interventions during surgery, including lung biopsy. For details of the technique, refer to Chapter 74.

Thoracotomy

Open biopsy with thoracotomy is now seldom indicated. It is a more invasive procedure with significant morbidity, especially postthoracotomy pain.

TREATMENT

Therapeutic objectives in patients with a pleural effusion include treatment of underlying disease, palliation of symptoms, and prevention of fluid recurrence.

MANAGEMENT OF THE UNDERLYING CAUSE

Optimizing the management of the underlying cause (e.g., appropriate diuretic therapy in patients with congestive cardiac failure) is adequate for some effusions. In certain instances (e.g., malignant effusions), however, the underlying cause may not be treatable, and other strategies to prevent reaccumulation of pleural effusions are needed.

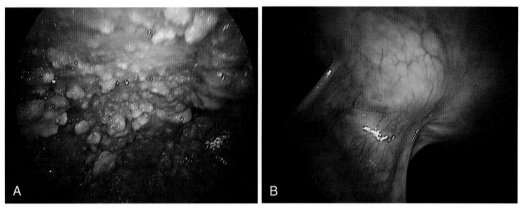

Figure 69-9 **A,** Thoracoscopic view into the right pleural cavity showing multiple tumor nodules covering the parietal pleura. **B,** Thoracoscopy allows identification and biopsy of pleural abnormalities under direct vision while avoiding potentially hazardous structures (e.g., highly vascularized adhesion).

SYMPTOM CONTROL

Thoracentesis

Therapeutic pleural aspiration can be performed at the bedside to relieve breathlessness. For recurrent effusions (e.g., malignant pleural effusions), a definitive procedure to stop fluid reaccumulation, such as pleurodesis, should be considered. If this fails, repeat thoracenteses may be necessary for palliation of breathlessness.

Placement of Indwelling Pleural Catheters

The insertion of a long-term tunneled indwelling pleural catheter (IPC) allows outpatient drainage of refractory malignant pleural effusions. The ambulatory catheters can be inserted as a "day case," avoiding the need for hospital admission. Its presence induces a complete or partial pleurodesis in up to 70% of patients, and the patient (or the caregiver) can drain the effusion as guided by symptoms, averting hospitalization. Implantation of an IPC also is indicated in patients with a symptomatic effusion and underlying trapped lung, as described later. The catheters usually are well tolerated in clinical practice, but reported complications include development of pleural septations, pleural or soft tissue infection, local tumor invasion at the insertion site, and catheter displacement (**Figure 69-10**). A randomized trial is under way to evaluate the use of IPCs as first-line therapy in malignant effusions.

Insertion of a pleuroperitoneal shunt is another alternative if pleurodesis fails. This intervention is contraindicated in the presence of ascites, and potential complications include infection and shunt occlusion (approximately 10%).

Noninvasive Palliation

In terminally ill patients with symptomatic effusions, use of opiates and oxygen therapy to alleviate breathlessness may be appropriate.

PREVENTING FLUID REACCUMULATION

Pleurodesis

The dual aim of pleurodesis is to achieve fusion between the visceral and parietal pleural surfaces and to prevent reaccumulation of pleural fluid (or air). It is indicated in symptomatic malignant pleural effusions and occasionally for recurrent benign effusions when other treatments fail. Dyspnea in patients with malignant effusions often is multifactorial. Only patients with symptomatic improvement consequent to evacuation of the effusion should be considered for pleurodesis.

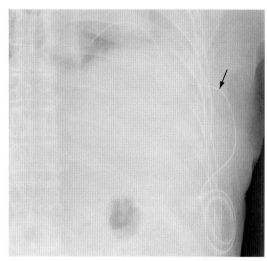

Figure 69-10 Magnified chest radiograph demonstrating a left-sided indwelling pleural catheter (IPC), which has become partly displaced and now has a drainage hole within the subcutaneous tissues (*arrow*).

To achieve successful pleural symphysis, pleural fluid is drained to allow apposition of the pleural layers. Fluid can be drained either at thoracoscopy or using a chest tube. Use of smaller-bore chest tubes (10 to 14F) is associated with less discomfort and allows equal pleurodesis efficacy compared with larger tubes. Pleurodesis, accomplished by mechanical abrasion or using chemical agents, aims to induce damage to the pleura. The resultant acute pleural inflammation, if sufficiently intense, will progress to chronic inflammation with consequent development of pleural adhesions and fibrosis. Pain and fever are common, secondary to the inflammatory process. In animal studies, dampening of this inflammatory process with corticosteroids inhibits pleurodesis. Whether this applies in humans remains unclear.

Pleurodesis is not indicated if close contact of the pleural layers cannot be achieved. The presence of a so-called *trapped lung*, when lung expansion is restricted either by visceral pleura tumor encasement or by endobronchial obstruction, prohibits effective pleurodesis (**Figure 69-11**). With "entrapment" of a significant (greater than 50%) proportion of the lung, insertion of an indwelling pleural catheter should be considered.

Talc is the most commonly used pleurodesis agent worldwide. It can be insufflated as a dry powder (poudrage) during thoracoscopy or instilled through a chest tube as a slurry, with similar efficacy of approximately 75% in a large randomized

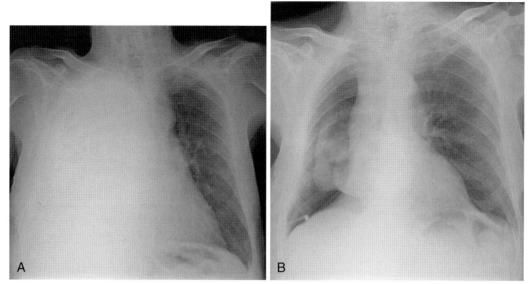

Figure 69-11 Radiographic appearance of trapped lung. The patient had bronchogenic adenocarcinoma and initially was seen with a massive right-sided pleural effusion causing mediastinal shift (**A**). After pleural drainage (with an intercostal tube in situ), his lung failed to reexpand (**B**). Recognizing the presence of trapped lung is important, because pleurodesis not only is unlikely to be successful but may induce visceral fibrosis, causing further restriction of the underlying lung.

study of 482 patients. Adverse effects (e.g., pain, fever) are common after talc pleurodesis and can be serious. The incidence of reported talc-induced acute respiratory distress syndrome (ARDS) ranges from 0 to 9%, and its mechanism remains poorly understood. Particle size, presence of contaminants, and reexpansion pulmonary edema have all been implicated. A randomized controlled trial has confirmed that nongraded talc preparations with "small" particle size (less than 15 µm median diameter) led to more systemic and pulmonary inflammation with resultant hypoxemia. A subsequent study using larger-particle graded talc found no evidence of associated ARDS. In patients with preexisting respiratory compromise, alternative agents (e.g., doxycycline or bleomycin) should be considered. Other agents such as povidone-iodine, silver nitrate, and OK432 are used in some centers.

SPECIFIC ENTITIES ASSOCIATED WITH PLEURAL EFFUSION

CONDITIONS ASSOCIATED WITH TRANSUDATIVE EFFUSIONS

Congestive Cardiac Failure

Effusion secondary to congestive cardiac failure accounts for most transudative effusions worldwide. It is also the most common cause of pleural effusions necessitating acute medical hospital admissions, and as many as 50% to 75% of the hospitalized patients will have pleural effusions, commonly bilateral. Such effusions are thought to arise from transpleural migration of pulmonary interstitial fluid accumulated from elevated pulmonary capillary pressure.

Clinical history and physical examination usually secure the diagnosis. Chest radiography commonly reveals bilateral effusions, cardiomegaly, and venous congestion.

Management is directed at the underlying congestive cardiac failure. Pleurodesis has been performed in refractory cases with variable success. If the patient fails to respond to diuresis or other, atypical features (i.e., unilateral effusion, massive

pleural effusion, or fever) are present, further investigation is warranted.

Occasionally, the pleural fluid may be classified as an exudate using Light's criteria, probably arising because of differential drainage of fluid over protein molecules from the pleural space as a result of diuretic therapy. A plasma-to-effusion protein gradient of more than 3.1 g/dL suggests that the fluid originally formed as a transudate. N-terminal (amino-terminal) pro-brain natriuretic peptide (NT-proBNP) is a sensitive marker of cardiac failure, in both blood and pleural fluid, and can be used to avoid repeated investigations in patients with exudative effusions suspected to be originally caused by cardiac failure. In patients with bilateral transudative pleural effusions with pulmonary hypertension and normal left ventricular function, pulmonary venoocclusive disease (PVOD) should be considered.

Hepatic Hydrothorax

Hepatic hydrothorax occurs in approximately 5% of patients with liver cirrhosis and portal hypertension. Pleural effusions accumulate from transdiaphragmatic migration of ascitic fluid. Fluid also accumulates from the decreased oncotic pressure associated with secondary hypoalbuminemia, and extremely rarely from hemorrhage of congested collateral veins. Most hepatic hydrothoraces are right-sided, and concomitant ascites is frequent but is not a prerequisite. The diagnosis is based on the presence of cirrhotic liver disease, ascites, and transudative fluid on thoracentesis. Spontaneous bacterial empyema may occur and, even with prompt recognition, carries a mortality rate ranging up to 20%.

Management should be directed at treating portal hypertension and reducing the volume of ascitic fluid with diuretic therapy and sodium restriction. This approach frequently fails, and therapeutic thoracenteses may be indicated for symptomatic relief. Loss of electrolytes and protein is a concern. Pleurodesis may be tried in therapy-resistant cases, and repair of any diaphragmatic defects attempted at thoracoscopy. Use of concomitant continuous positive airway pressure (CPAP)

Table 69-3 Characteristics of Simple and Complicated Parapneumonic Effusions and Empyema

Feature	Simple Parapneumonic Effusion	Complicated Parapneumonic Effusion	Empyema
Appearance	Clear/slightly turbid	Often cloudy	Pus
pH	≥7.20	<7.20	Not measured
Glucose*	≥2.2 mmol/L (40 mg/dL)	<2.2 mmol/L (40 mg/dL)	Not measured
Lactate dehydrogenase (LDH)	≤1000 U/L	>1000 U/L	Not measured
Bacteria on Gram stain or culture	No	~25%	~70%

*Glucose threshold advocated in latest British Thoracic Society guidelines, although previous American College of Chest Physicians guidelines suggested 3.3 mmol/L (60 mg/dL).

ventilation at the time of pleurodesis to reverse the peritoneal-pleural gradient has been successful in case reports but remains experimental at present. Transjugular intrahepatic portosystemic shunting (TIPS) can relieve symptomatic hepatic hydrothorax, but liver transplantation, in selected patients, is the only definitive therapy.

Renal Effusions

Pleural effusions may arise in association with nephrotic syndrome, acute glomerulonephritis, or peritoneal dialysis. Transdiaphragmatic migration of peritoneal dialysate often results in a right-sided effusion chemically resembling the dialysis fluid.

Urinothorax is rare but should be considered whenever a low-pH transudative effusion is encountered in clinical practice. It arises secondary to renal obstruction with resultant retroperitoneal urine collection and transfer into the ipsilateral pleural cavity, or a fistula draining into the pleural cavity. An ammonia-like smell is diagnostic, and increased fluid-to-serum creatinine levels are confirmatory.

CONDITIONS ASSOCIATED WITH EXUDATIVE EFFUSIONS

Parapneumonic Effusion and Empyema

Pleural effusions occur in up to 57% of patients with pneumonia and range in size from small subcentimeter effusions to large effusions causing ventilatory embarrassment. A majority of these (approximately 60%) are sterile "simple" parapneumonic effusions reflecting vascular hyperpermeability from pleural inflammation secondary to the underlying pneumonia. "Complicated" parapneumonic effusions are characterized by neutrophilia, low pH and glucose, and often fibrinous septations (caused by fibrin deposition within the procoagulant milieu of the infected pleural space). The current belief is that complicated pleural effusion represents one end of the spectrum of pleural infection and should be treated as such. At the other end of the spectrum is empyema, characterized by frank pleural pus or presence of bacteria in the pleural fluid (**Table 69-3**).

Differentiation between simple and complicated effusions is important, because an infected pleural space requires prompt pleural drainage, being associated with significant morbidity and mortality (15% of patients require surgery, and up to 20% die). Parapneumonic effusion should be suspected in all patients with pneumonia, particularly those in whom clinical improvement fails to occur or laboratory markers of infection remain persistently abnormal. Patients with diabetes mellitus, alcohol or substance abuse, coexisting chronic lung disease, immunosuppression, or rheumatoid arthritis have a higher incidence of pleural infection. Poor dental hygiene is more prevalent in those with anaerobic infection. A low serum albumin less than

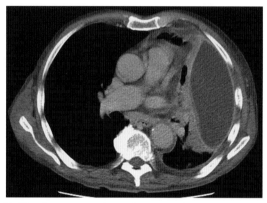

Figure 69-12 A contrast-enhanced computed tomography image of pleural empyema. The "split pleura" sign is demonstrated, with enhancement of both the visceral and the parietal pleural surfaces evident. *(Courtesy Dr. Rachel Benamore, Oxford, United Kingdom.)*

30 g/L, C-reactive protein more than 100 mg/L, platelet count more than 400×10^9/L, serum sodium less than 130 mmol/L, intravenous drug use, and alcohol misuse have been shown to be associated with development of complicated parapneumonic effusion in patients with pneumonia. Recent novel genetic studies also suggest that a variant of the protein tyrosine phosphatase (PTPN22 Trp620) is associated with susceptibility to invasive pneumococcal disease and gram-positive empyema. Primary empyema, in the absence of pneumonia, is responsible for 4% of pleural infection cases.

Chest radiography usually identifies the pleural collection and concomitant pneumonia. In a patient with sepsis, the finding of a new encapsulated effusion in a nonbasal position is strongly suggestive of pleural infection. Ultrasound imaging is of value in the evaluation of pleural infection, allowing fluid characterization and localization (which is particularly important for loculated fluid). In a patient with signs of infection, septations on ultrasound images suggest an infected pleural space with low pH, low glucose, and high lactate dehydrogenase (LDH); heavily echogenic fluid usually represents pus (or blood). Of note, however, the converse does not hold; absence of such sonographic features does not rule out pleural infection. Pleural-phase CT provides detailed information and discriminates between empyema and lung abscess. Empyemas usually are lenticular in shape, with compression of surrounding lung parenchyma. The "split pleura" sign, with enhanced parietal and visceral pleural tissue visible as the surfaces are separated by the pleural collection, is characteristic (**Figure 69-12**). Pleural thickening is seen in 86% to 100% of empyemas and in 56% of parapneumonic effusions. Pleural enhancement and increased attenuation of the extrapleural subcostal fat are suggestive of an infected pleural space.

Frankly purulent or malodorous fluid confirms presence of an empyema. If not purulent on gross examination, the pleural fluid pH should be assessed. A pH less than 7.2, or reduced fluid glucose, indicates a complicated parapneumonic effusion. Positive Gram staining or fluid culture confirms pleural infection and can guide antibiotic choice but is positive in only about 50% to 60% of patients. The use of genetic microbiologic testing to allow organism identification (using PCR and sequencing of the bacterial 16S ribosomal RNA gene) is under investigation. Treatment of complicated parapneumonic effusions or empyema includes appropriate antimicrobial therapy, optimal nutritional support, venothromboembolism prophylaxis, and evacuation of the infected pleural fluid (by chest tube or surgery).

Bacteriology

It is important to differentiate between community- and hospital-acquired pleural infection, because the bacteriology and prognosis differ for the two types. Hospital-acquired cases often are iatrogenic or secondary to hospital-acquired pneumonia and carry a mortality rate several times higher than that for community-acquired cases. The microbiology also varies geographically. In the United Kingdom, gram-positive streptococci account for most community-acquired cases of pleural infection, with the *Streptococcus milleri* group (*Streptococcus constellatus, Streptococcus intermedius, Streptococcus anginosus*) accounting for 24% and *Streptococcus pneumoniae* causing 21%. *Staphylococcus aureus* is isolated in 10% of the cases. Gramnegative organisms, such as *Haemophilus influenzae, Escherichia coli, Pseudomonas* spp., and *Klebsiella* spp. occur in about 10% of cases, particularly in patients with comorbid conditions such as diabetes. Anaerobic pathogens are detected in 12% to 34% of cases, although some studies suggest a much higher incidence. With hospital-acquired infection, methicillin-resistant *Staphylococcus aureus* (MRSA) is responsible for more than a quarter of cases of pleural infection, and gram-negative organisms such as *E. coli, Enterobacter* spp., and *Pseudomonas* spp. are common and particularly associated with critical illness necessitating admission to an intensive care unit.

Antibiotics

All patients should receive antibiotic therapy. Empirical treatment should be initiated while awaiting bacterial culture results and must take into account where the infection was acquired (hospital or community), patient comorbid conditions, and local bacterial resistance patterns. A common antibiotic choice to cover community-acquired pathogens is a beta-lactam antibiotic in conjunction with a beta-lactamase inhibitor (such as amoxicillin and clavulanic acid) or piperacillin-tazobactam. Metronidazole usually is given as well, to ensure adequate anaerobic coverage. Given that hospital-acquired pleural infection is more likely to be caused by resistant pathogens, including gram-negative enteric bacteria and MRSA, a reasonable antibiotic selection in such patients is a carbapenem with vancomycin. Therapy may be modified in the light of positive culture and sensitivity results. Prolonged courses of antibiotics (e.g., 4 to 6 weeks) often are required.

Drainage

Simple parapneumonic effusions generally do not require drainage, but drainage of complicated effusions and empyema is key to their management.

Loculation is common in pleural infection, and imaging-guided insertion of chest drains can ensure optimal placement. Selection of appropriate chest tube size remains contentious, with no randomized trial evidence available, although recent studies have suggested that smaller (less than 15F) Seldinger inserted tubes are less painful, are associated with fewer complications, and perform as well as larger, blunt dissection–inserted tubes. Instillation of intrapleural fibrinolytic agents for complex parapneumonic effusions or empyema has been proposed to disrupt fibrinous septations and potentially improve drainage. However, a large multicenter study, the first Multicenter Intrapleural Sepsis Trial (MIST1), with 454 subjects, failed to demonstrate a benefit on mortality statistics, need for surgery, or duration of hospital stay for patients who received intrapleural streptokinase. A 2008 Cochrane review examining seven fibrinolytic studies concluded that use of fibrinolytics conferred no significant benefit in reducing surgical requirements. The recent MIST2 study examined combination fibrinolytic-plus-DNase therapy in a 2 × 2 factorial randomized controlled trial of tissue-type plasminogen activator (tPA) and deoxyribonuclease (DNase) in 210 patients. This study found that combination tPA and DNase significantly improved pleural fluid drainage (primary outcome) and led to a reduced rate of surgical referral and shorter hospital stay (secondary outcomes), although further studies are needed to define the size of treatment effects.

Prompt referral for surgical drainage is indicated in the 30% of patients who have ongoing sepsis with chronic pleural fluid effusion despite optimal medical treatment. Secondary pleural thickening (fibrothorax) is seen in less than 10%; in this setting, however, residual pleural thickening and lung function impairment always lessen with time and are not indications for surgery. VATS is preferred, but more invasive procedures (e.g., thoracotomy or rib resection with open drainage) are sometimes needed.

Use of VATS as first-line treatment of pleural infection remains contentious, with randomized studies in adults and children failing to show a significant difference in mortality or major morbidity with VATS. Adult studies have shown a shorter hospital stay with VATS (approximately 11 versus 8 days), but a pediatric study showed no difference in length of stay (primary outcome) but a higher cost of VATS.

PLEURAL INFECTION IN CHILDREN

Significant differences exist between pleural infection in children and that in adults in both clinical course and prognosis; the reasons for the differences remain unclear. Pediatric empyema has an incidence of 3.3 per 100,000, and evidence suggests that this rate is rising in many countries. Most cases are secondary to underlying bacterial pneumonia, and *S. pneumoniae* is most commonly isolated. Since the licensing of the 7-valent pneumococcal conjugate vaccine (PCV7) in 2000, active against serotypes 4, 6B, 9V, 14, 18C, 19F, and 23F, the accumulating evidence shows that the nonvaccine serotype 1 is causing increasing numbers of cases of empyema and other invasive pneumococcal disease in some areas.

The diagnosis is based on clinical findings and chest radiography or ultrasonography confirming a pleural collection. Thoracentesis and chest tube drainage may be difficult in babies and young children and usually necessitate use of general anesthesia. Management with adequate fluid therapy, intravenous antibiotics, and antipyretics is sufficient in many cases, and liaison with a tertiary pediatric respiratory care unit is recommended. Advocates of early surgical intervention suggest that if a child is undergoing general anesthesia for chest drain insertion, a definitive procedure such as VATS débridement should be performed; however, no consensus exists. The prognosis in children with empyema is significantly better than that in adults.

TUBERCULOUS PLEURAL EFFUSIONS

Tuberculous pleural effusions represent either primary pleural mycobacterial infection or reactivation of latent infection. Most cases of tuberculous pleuritis develop as a result of a delayed hypersensitivity reaction to the mycobacterial protein, rather than from mycobacterial invasion. The number of organisms within the pleural space often is low.

Acute clinical presentation with pleuritic chest pain and fever is uncommon; more typically, symptoms develop insidiously, with gradual onset of dyspnea and constitutional features. Chest radiographs reveal a pleural effusion with or without parenchymal infiltrates. The pleural fluid is lymphocytic in more than 90% of cases, and fluid glucose and pH may be low. Samples should be sent for staining for acid-fast bacilli and culture for the TB pathogen, although the diagnostic yield usually is low. Obtaining tissue for culture and a histologic diagnosis is important; caseating granulomas frequently are used as a diagnostic surrogate when culture is negative. Because involvement of the pleura in TB commonly is generalized, percutaneous "blind" pleural biopsy is sensitive, although thoracoscopy may further increase yield. The parietal pleura usually have a characteristic appearance of disseminated fine nodules.

Adenosine deaminase (ADA) levels have a high sensitivity and specificity and are routinely used in many countries in which TB is endemic. Low ADA concentrations make tuberculous pleuritis unlikely. High levels also occur in empyema, malignancy (e.g., lymphoma), and collagen vascular diseases.

Spontaneous resolution frequently is seen in tuberculous effusions irrespective of antimycobacterial chemotherapy. Without appropriate treatment, however, approximately 60% of patients will have clinically overt TB develop elsewhere within 5 years. Mycobacterial resistance patterns in cases of tuberculous pleuritis usually are similar to the local resistance patterns of pulmonary TB cases. The treatment of TB is covered in Chapter 31. Thoracentesis may aid symptom relief, and steroids may help to reduce fluid volume, but neither alters the long-term outcome or the incidence of fibrothorax.

PLEURAL EFFUSIONS SECONDARY TO INFECTIONS WITH OTHER ORGANISMS

Viruses, legionnaires disease, *Mycoplasma*, and *Rickettsia* spp. may be associated with pleural effusion in approximately 20% of cases, although they usually are small simple effusions that resolve without needing drainage. The diagnosis is made clinically, with serologic tests, urinary antigen detection (legionnaires disease), or on culture. Pleural fluid commonly is lymphocytic, although neutrophils initially may predominate.

Pulmonary nocardiosis may be complicated by empyema in up to a quarter of cases, and empyema frequently is seen in patients with pulmonary actinomycosis.

Mycotic lung disease accounts for less than 1% of all pleural effusions and usually occurs in immunocompromised hosts. *Candida albicans* is the most common pathogen in fungal empyema and is associated with a high (greater than 70%) mortality rate. Prompt treatment with systemic antifungal

agents and pleural drainage is required. In approximately 4% of patients with (human) blastomycosis and 20% with respiratory coccidioidomycosis, pleural effusions are observed. These generally resolve spontaneously without specific treatment. *Pneumocystis jirovecii* infection is rarely associated with pleural effusion in the immunocompromised host.

Amebic disease can result in empyema, hepatobronchial fistula formation, or a pleural effusion secondary to perforation of an amebic liver abscess. Pleural effusions related to other parasitic infections are extremely rare.

MALIGNANT PLEURAL EFFUSIONS

Malignant pleural effusions (MPEs) are common and affect 660 patients per 1 million population per year. They account for 22% of all pleural effusions and in 20% of patients constitute the presenting manifestation of malignancy. The most common cytologic diagnoses in developed countries are metastatic breast or lung carcinoma, lymphoma, and mesothelioma. Most malignant tumors can metastasize to the pleura. Up to 50% of patients with breast cancer, a quarter of those with bronchogenic carcinoma, and more than 95% of patients with mesothelioma will develop a pleural effusion during their disease course. Symptoms with MPE can be severe, and successful symptom control can contribute to significantly improved quality of life.

Pleural fluid accumulates as a result of increased fluid formation and reduced lymphatic drainage (from malignant involvement of parietal lymphatic channels or mediastinal lymphadenopathy). In some patients with underlying malignancy, a pleural effusion may develop without direct pleural involvement. Such "paramalignant" effusions may be caused by pulmonary embolism, pneumonia, secondary atelectasis, pericardial tumor involvement, hypoproteinemia, or radiotherapy-induced inflammation. Although the distinction is important in cases in which curative resection is considered, some studies have shown that patients with a paramalignant effusion have a prognosis similar to that in persons with frank malignant effusions.

Positive histocytologic confirmation is required for diagnosis. Pleural fluid cytologic examination establishes proof in approximately 60% of the cases, and if findings are negative, thoracoscopy or CT-guided pleural biopsy (if focal pleural abnormality is evident on CT scan) is the logical next step.

Except for a small number of chemotherapy-sensitive tumors (e.g., lymphoma), cure of the underlying malignancy usually is not possible once the cancer has metastasized to the pleura. Management is therefore directed toward controlling symptoms and improving quality of life. Various options are available (as described earlier under "Treatment"); the most appropriate interventions will depend on the patient's symptoms, performance status, and expected survival.

EFFUSIONS SECONDARY TO CONNECTIVE TISSUE DISEASE

Rheumatoid Arthritis

Pleural effusions are the most common thoracic manifestation of rheumatoid arthritis and occur in up to 5% of patients, more frequently men (70%). Often the effusions develop several years after the original diagnosis and in 30% of the cases arise concomitantly with interstitial lung disease or rheumatoid lung nodules. The effusion may persist for years, although spontaneous resorption occasionally is observed. Symptomatic recurrent effusions are rare and may respond to systemic corticosteroid therapy.

Distinguishing rheumatoid effusions from empyema or pseudochylothorax is important but can be difficult. Pleural fluid from a rheumatoid effusion is characterized by leukocytosis, a low glucose, low pH, and increased LDH—features indistinguishable from those of pleural infection. Low complement and elevated pleural fluid rheumatoid factor levels are not diagnostic.

Systemic Lupus Erythematosus

Fifty percent of patients with systemic lupus erythematosus (SLE) will have a pleural effusion, often bilateral and typically exudative (occasionally hemorrhagic), with a lymphocytosis (if the effusion is chronic). Nonsteroidal antiinflammatory medication may relieve pleuritic chest pain, and corticosteroid treatment results in a swift clinical response if the patient remains symptomatic. Pleural effusions arising as a consequence of drug-induced lupus erythematosus are rare.

Other Connective Tissue Disorders

Granulomatosis with polyangiitis (Wegener's) is associated with pleural effusion in approximately 30% of patients and responds to treatment of the underlying condition with immunosuppressant therapy. Pleural effusion may occur in up to 30% of those with Churg-Strauss syndrome; typically, the fluid is rich in eosinophils. The effusions usually are not of any clinical consequence, and most resolve with corticosteroid therapy.

EFFUSION FROM VASCULAR CAUSES

Pleural effusions occur in up to 50% of patients with pulmonary embolism. This diagnosis often is overlooked and should be considered in any patient with an undiagnosed pleural effusion. The pathophysiology remains under debate, and no specific diagnostic features are recognized. Physicians should maintain a high index of clinical suspicion for pulmonary emboli, particularly when other etiologic disorders have been excluded. Effusions normally are exudative, usually are small, and can be blood-stained. Standard treatment of pulmonary emboli should be initiated. The pleural effusion seldom needs drainage and usually will resolve over time.

Effusions after coronary artery bypass graft surgery are common, and in most cases, spontaneous resolution occurs within 6 months. Postcardiac injury syndrome (Dressler syndrome) after myocardial infarction or bypass surgery can result in small bilateral effusions and seldom requires intervention. Sickle cell anemia–related acute chest syndrome results in pleural effusion in 30% to 35% of cases.

DRUG-INDUCED PLEURAL EFFUSIONS

Drug-induced pleural effusions do occur, and a careful drug history may be required to make a diagnosis. Various prescribed medications, including amiodarone, nitrofurantoin, methotrexate, bromocriptine, clozapine, and phenytoin, may result in exudative pleural effusions and eventual pleural fibrosis (see www.pneumotox.com for further causes of drug-induced effusions). Withdrawal of the offending drug, with use of corticosteroids if needed, is sufficient in many cases. Decortication has been attempted but is of no established benefit.

Ovarian hyperstimulation syndrome (OHSS) is an iatrogenic complication occurring in approximately 3% of women undergoing therapeutic ovarian stimulation. It is becoming increasingly recognized as higher numbers of women undergo assisted reproduction procedures, and the exact pathogenesis remains unclear. OHSS is characterized by ovarian enlargement and rapid fluid shifts secondary to increased capillary permeability, which result in intravascular volume depletion. In severe cases, massive ascites with hydrothorax can arise. The treatment is primarily supportive, but fatal cases have been reported.

EFFUSIONS RELATED TO ABDOMINAL DISEASES

Pleural effusions occur in approximately 20% of patients with acute pancreatitis; two thirds are left-sided, and pleural fluid amylase concentrations exceed serum values. Pancreatic pseudocyst, pancreatic-pleural fistula, and abscess formation must be considered if the effusion persists. Effusions also accompany subphrenic abscess in more than 50% of patients. Cholohemothorax secondary to gallstone perforation into the pleural cavity is extremely rare and results in a bilious effusion.

Effusions arising after abdominal surgery are common, and investigation is rarely required, provided secondary infection is excluded.

Meigs syndrome consists of the combination of benign ovarian tumors and coexisting pleural effusion and ascites. These features resolve after tumor resection.

Hemothorax

Hemothorax is characterized by pleural fluid hematocrit values greater than 50% of peripheral blood. The main causes are trauma, iatrogenic (most commonly after thoracic surgery) factors, malignancy, anticoagulation therapy, pulmonary infarction, and aortic rupture. Complications include empyema (1% to 4% of traumatic hemothoraces), trapped lung, and fibrothorax. Treatment is guided by the clinical scenario, but tube thoracostomy to enable evacuation of the blood and assessment of the extent of hemorrhage is advised. Surgical intervention (preferably VATS) is indicated if the bleeding rate is greater than 200 mL/hour. Prophylactic antibiotics usually are administered, although literature evidence to support this practice is scarce.

Chylothorax

Chylothorax develops when disruption of the thoracic duct results in passage of chyle (lymph rich in chylomicrons) into the pleural cavity. The pleural fluid characteristically is milky in appearance (**Figure 69-13**), except in starved patients. Chylothorax must be differentiated from pseudochylothorax and empyema fluid (see under "Pleural Fluid Analysis").

Trauma is the most common cause of chylothorax, which is predominantly iatrogenic secondary to thoracic duct damage during cardiothoracic surgery (e.g., esophagectomy). An important nontraumatic cause is malignancy, especially lymphoma. Congenital chylothorax arises from thoracic duct malformation, and repair of congenital diaphragmatic defects may cause chylothoraces. Lymphangioleiomyomatosis and nonsurgical trauma rarely produce chylothoraces. Chylothorax is idiopathic in 15% of the reported cases. CT scanning should be performed to exclude lymphoma (and other potential causes) in patients without a history of trauma.

Management of chylothorax aims to optimize nutrition, relieve symptoms, and close the thoracic duct defect. Malnourishment secondary to chyle loss can be disabling. Total parenteral nutrition, or a low-fat diet with medium-chain fatty acids, should be adopted to reduce chyle flow. If the patient is symptomatic with dyspnea, fluid can be removed by

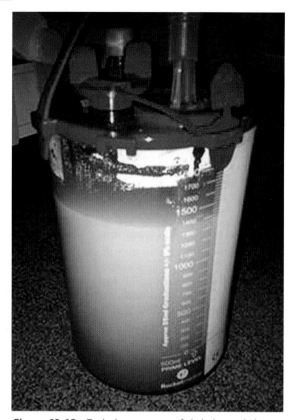

Figure 69-13 Typical appearance of chylothorax drainage.

thoracentesis or chest tube drainage. Pleuroperitoneal shunts have been recommended in the absence of coexisting chyloascites. Pleurodesis has been attempted in refractory cases. With traumatic chylothorax, the defect frequently closes spontaneously. Use of octreotide, a somatostatin analogue, also has been reported, mainly in pediatric-based case series, to enhance thoracic duct closure. Percutaneous thoracic duct embolization performed under radiologic guidance can be attempted before consideration of surgical thoracic duct ligation by VATS or thoracotomy. This approach initially was described in 1998 and offers a minimally invasive treatment strategy for those patients who are unable to tolerate surgical intervention. Catheterization of the thoracic duct is a prerequisite for its use, and anatomic obstruction of the cisterna chyli or retroperitoneal lymphatic chain obviates its use. In patients with underlying lymphoma, radiotherapy or systemic chemotherapy may control the chylothorax.

Pseudochylothorax

Pseudochylothorax, or cholesterol pleurisy, is most commonly associated with tuberculous pleurisy and rheumatoid pleuritis. The pleural fluid has a very high cholesterol content and no chylomicrons. Demonstration of cholesterol crystals is diagnostic. Pseudochylothorax was conventionally thought to result from the accumulation of cholesterol and lecithin-globulin complexes within long-standing pleural effusions enveloped by thickened fibrotic pleura. Recent evidence, however, suggests that such chronicity and pleural fibrosis are not prerequisite in pseudochylothorax from rheumatologic causes. Specific treatment for the condition is seldom indicated. Dyspnea is more likely to be a result of the pleural fibrosis and is seldom relieved by thoracentesis. Respiratory insufficiency, infection, and bronchopleural or pleurocutaneous fistulas are rare complications.

ASBESTOS-RELATED PLEURAL DISEASES

Asbestos fibers have a predisposition to localize to the pleura. Injury to the pleura can result in mesothelioma (see Chapter 70), as well as a range of benign pleural diseases—namely, pleural plaques, diffuse pleural thickening, benign asbestos–related pleural effusions, and round atelectasis.

Circumscribed pleural thickening—pleural plaques—are seen in up to 50% of asbestos-exposed subjects. Plaques occur in the parietal pleura and are of no physiologic consequence. Benign asbestos-related effusions typically are small and unilateral. Their occurrence is dose-dependent on asbestos exposure, with a shorter latency period (within 2 decades of asbestos exposure) than for other asbestos-related pleural disease. The effusion is an exudate, often blood-stained, and may precede the development of diffuse pleural thickening. The diagnosis depends on exclusion of other causes. Prolonged observation is required to exclude mesothelioma. Round atelectasis represents invagination of the visceral pleura and can be diagnosed radiologically by the "comet tail" sign on CT scan. In the absence of classic radiographic features, round atelectasis can mimic lung tumors, and differentiation can be difficult.

Diffuse pleural thickening may occur with asbestos exposure (less than 5%), especially in those with heavy asbestos contact. Significant restrictive lung function changes with resultant dyspnea can occur.

FIBROTHORAX AND PLEURAL THICKENING

Diffuse pleural thickening (fibrothorax) can be secondary to empyema or hemothorax, tuberculous pleurisy, asbestos exposure, collagen vascular disease, and drug-induced pleuritis (e.g., ergot derivatives, such as bromocriptine, pergolide, and methysergide). Pleural fibrosis and thickening also may develop as a result of pleurodesis performed to therapeutically obliterate the pleural space.

Patients with fibrothorax may be asymptomatic or complain of dyspnea. The chest radiograph typically shows concentric pleural thickening, occasionally with evidence of the predisposing cause. Reduction in the size of the hemithorax with an elevated hemidiaphragm suggests chronic fibrosis. Pulmonary function testing usually demonstrates a restrictive pattern. Likewise, long-term survivors of pleurodesis often exhibit radiologic pleural thickening coupled with mild restrictive physiologic changes.

Treatment should be aimed at the underlying cause, with removal of offending agents if possible. Corticosteroids often are administered, and surgical decortication is sometimes attempted; effectiveness of neither approach is established.

OTHER CAUSES OF EXUDATIVE EFFUSIONS

Rarely, exudative effusions may be associated with sarcoidosis, radiotherapy, yellow nail syndrome, familial Mediterranean fever, and amyloidosis.

Approximately 15% of pleural effusions remain undiagnosed despite thorough investigation. Close follow-up may identify those associated with occult malignancy; however, most are benign and resolve spontaneously. It has been postulated, but not proved, that viral infection may be responsible.

CONTROVERSIES AND PITFALLS

Pleural effusions are common. However, pleural effusions often are considered a "side issue" to the underlying systemic or pulmonary disorders causing the effusion. This perspective often results in significant delay in recognition, investigation, and management of the effusion, contributing to morbidity. For example, late recognition of parapneumonic effusions remains commonplace; improved awareness and early intervention would have prevented many cases of empyema.

Advances in imaging will play an increasing role in diagnosis and investigation of pleural disease. High-quality clinical trial data are lacking in pleural disease, and management often is governed by anecdotal experiences.

Several controversies regarding pleural disease management have emerged. The use of some fibrinolytics and other adjunctive therapy (tPA and DNase) in pleural infection has been shown to be beneficial in a randomized controlled trial, but further research is required to define treatment effects. The pros and cons of medical thoracoscopy continue to be debated. The belief that thoracoscopic talc pleurodesis is superior has not been supported by randomized controlled trials. The size of the chest tube and the requisite skills for insertion (i.e., surgical, radiologic, or respiratory medicine) remain controversial.

PNEUMOTHORAX

A pneumothorax exists when air is present within the pleural space and may be classified as spontaneous or traumatic. *Traumatic* pneumothoraces occur as a result of direct or indirect trauma and may be iatrogenic secondary to procedures such as transbronchial or pleural biopsies, thoracentesis, and central venous catheterization.

Spontaneous pneumothoraces are divided into primary and secondary. *Primary* spontaneous pneumothoraces (PSPs) arise in apparently healthy people, whereas *secondary* spontaneous pneumothoraces are associated with underlying pulmonary disease, most commonly chronic obstructive pulmonary disease (COPD). Differentiation between these categories is important, because management and prognosis differ for the two groups (**Box 69-4**).

PRIMARY SPONTANEOUS PNEUMOTHORAX

Primary pneumothorax usually occurs in young male smokers between 20 and 40 years of age. The reported incidence is 18 to 28 per 100,000 for men and 1.2 to 6.0 per 100,000 for women (male-to-female ratio of 5:1). Cigarette smoking is a major risk factor, increasing the lifetime risk of pneumothorax in healthy males from 0.1% in nonsmokers up to 12% in smokers. The risk is dose-related, with relative risk seven times higher in light smokers (1 to 12 cigarettes/day), 21 times higher in moderate smokers, and 102 times higher in those smoking more than 22 cigarettes daily. This trend is less marked in women. The chronic effects of marijuana smoking and its association with bullous lung disease are now recognized as an independent risk factor for pneumothorax.

Mortality rates for primary pneumothorax are extremely low.

PATHOPHYSIOLOGY

Pneumothorax is attributed to the rupture of subpleural blebs and bullae, which represent so-called early emphysematous-like changes (ELCs). Such changes are demonstrated in the lung apices in most patients with primary pneumothorax despite the absence of underlying clinical disease. Pulmonary blebs are air-filled spaces between the lung parenchyma and

| Box 69-4 | Causes of Pneumothorax |

Spontaneous
Primary (most common in young men)
Secondary
    Chronic obstructive pulmonary disease (COPD)
    Asthma
    Cystic fibrosis
    Congenital cysts and bullae
    Pleural malignancy
    Interstitial lung disease
    Bacterial pneumonia
    Pneumocystis jirovecii pneumonia
    Tuberculosis
    Whooping cough
    Langerhans cell histiocytosis (LCH)
    Tuberous sclerosis
    Lymphangioleiomyomatosis (LAM)
    Marfan syndrome
    Esophageal rupture

Traumatic
Penetrating chest wounds
Chest compression injury
    Including external cardiac massage
Iatrogenic
    Pleural aspiration
    Chest tube insertion
    Intercostal nerve block
    Percutaneous lung biopsy
    Radiofrequency ablation of lung lesion
    Transbronchial lung biopsy
    Transbronchial needle aspiration
    Central venous cannulation
    Pacemaker insertion
    Positive-pressure ventilation

the visceral pleura, visible in more than 75% of patients undergoing thoracoscopic treatment for primary pneumothorax. Patients with primary pneumothoraces also tend to be taller and thinner than control subjects, a characteristic associated with an increased pressure gradient from lung base to apex. This feature creates a greater distending pressure on apical alveoli, thereby increasing the likelihood of rupture. However, ELCs are present in up to 25% of control subjects and are not always predictive of pneumothorax.

Fluorescein-enhanced autofluorescence thoracoscopy techniques have identified areas of increased visceral pleural porosity in the absence of other visible abnormality. It is hypothesized that air leakage from these areas may be integral to the formation of primary pneumothoraces. Smoking-induced distal airway inflammation, disturbance of collateral ventilation, congenital anatomic, and morphometric abnormalities may contribute to these changes.

A tendency toward primary pneumothorax is rarely inherited, and the Birt-Hogg-Dube syndrome (inherited as an autosomal dominant trait that has been localized to chromosomal region 17p11.2) is associated with primary pneumothorax, benign skin tumors, and renal tumors. Patients with Marfan syndrome and homocystinuria also have an increased incidence of pneumothorax.

CLINICAL PRESENTATION

Primary pneumothorax may be asymptomatic, but sudden-onset pleuritic chest pain localized to the affected side of the pneumothorax or dyspnea is the most common symptom.

On examination, a hyperresonant percussion note, absence of tactile fremitus, and reduced breath sounds on the affected side may be evident. Tracheal deviation away from the affected side is seen with large, or tension, pneumothoraces. Signs of hemodynamic compromise (hypotension, severe tachycardia, and cyanosis) suggest a tension pneumothorax. Hamman's sign, an audible clicking sound synchronous with the heart sounds, can be heard with a left-sided pneumothorax, and subcutaneous emphysema may be palpable.

DIAGNOSIS

Chest radiographs usually confirm the diagnosis. Expiratory films are no more sensitive than standard films, although lateral decubitus views facilitate the detection of tiny pneumothoraces. In up to 50% of cases, a small ipsilateral pleural effusion also is seen, and mediastinal displacement away from the pneumothorax, subcutaneous emphysema, or pneumomediastinum may coexist. Thoracic ultrasound imaging has a role in ruling out pneumothorax, particularly after interventional procedures, but is hampered by false-positive findings with bullous lung disease (e.g., COPD) or previous pleurodesis and is unable to accurately predict pneumothorax size. CT scanning is rarely necessary acutely in primary pneumothorax and is recommended only if concern exists regarding underlying complex cystic disease or to differentiate between a bulla and pneumothorax.

The "gold standard" for pneumothorax size assessment is CT scanning, but this modality is not used in routine practice. Pneumothorax size may be estimated using chest radiography and *Light's index*: percent pneumothorax = $100 - [100 \times (\text{diameter of deflated lung})^3/(\text{diameter of hemithorax})^3]$. The latest British Thoracic Society guidelines advocate measurement of pneumothorax depth at the level of the hilum, but American College of Chest Physicians guidelines suggest apex-to-cupola depth measurements (**Figure 69-14**). A 2-cm depth is advocated as a sensible cutoff value for intervening in primary pneumothoraces, representing an approximately 50% pneumothorax. For patients with a secondary spontaneous pneumothorax, a 1-cm depth is advocated for intervention.

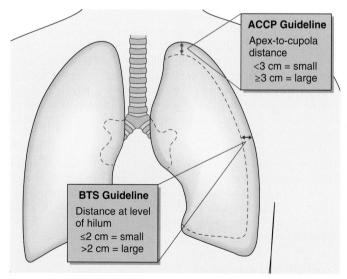

Figure 69-14 Measurement strategies proposed for quantifying pneumothorax size. *ACCP*, American College of Chest Pysicians; *BTS*, British Thoracic Society.

Arterial blood gas measurements may show a reduced PaO_2 and an increase in the alveolar-arterial oxygen gradient, measured as $PO_2(A-a)$.

MANAGEMENT

The management of primary spontaneous pneumothoraces varies widely, with the approach to the patient determined by the clinical presentation. Supplemental high-flow oxygen is advocated by some centers because it can theoretically accelerate pleural air resorption by reducing the partial pressure of nitrogen in the blood. Observation alone may be adequate for patients with small primary pneumothoraces, minimal symptoms, and stable cardiorespiratory status. The rate of spontaneous pleural air resorption is slow (1.25% each 24 hours), and this prolonged course to resolution should be anticipated.

Otherwise, treatment aims to remove air from the pleural space and decrease the risk of recurrence. The former may be achieved by simple aspiration or intercostal tube drainage with or without one-way (e.g., Heimlich) valve insertion. Prevention of recurrence involves removal of risk factors (e.g., smoking cessation) and induction of pleurodesis by means of chemical pleurodesis, thoracoscopy (usually VATS), or rarely, open thoracotomy. The latter two approaches allow identification and resection of abnormal areas (ELC treatment [e.g., bullectomy]) with or without chemical pleurodesis, pleural abrasion, or partial pleurectomy (**Figure 69-15**).

Simple aspiration is the accepted treatment in patients with large or symptomatic small primary pneumothoraces. This technique succeeds in approximately 60% of patients. If complete reexpansion is not achieved but symptoms are relieved, outpatient follow-up is appropriate. Alternatively, a Heimlich flutter valve (thoracic vent) may be inserted and the patient safely discharged with scheduled outpatient review.

Intercostal tube drainage is indicated if pleural aspiration fails to control symptoms. Small (10 to 14F) drains usually are adequate. Once the lung is reexpanded and the drain ceases bubbling for 24 hours, it should be removed. Suction may aid reexpansion but should not be applied before 48 hours to lessen the risk of reexpansion pulmonary edema (RPE). The risk of RPE increases with the length of time the lung has been collapsed. Clamping of the nonbubbling chest tube before removal is a contentious issue. A slow air leak may become apparent only after the drain has been clamped for several hours, so this maneuver may be of value in avoiding premature removal.

SURGICAL TREATMENT

Surgery is indicated in cases of persistent air leak despite adequate tube drainage. Surgery also is indicated in patients with recurrent ipsilateral or first contralateral pneumothorax, synchronous pneumothoraces, or a spontaneous hemothorax, as well as those with job restrictions (e.g., divers, airline pilots).

Minimally invasive VATS allows stapling of blebs and bullae using an Endostapler, laser ablation, or electrocoagulation. Pleurodesis can be induced mechanically with pleural abrasion or partial pleurectomy or chemically (talc poudrage). Recurrence rates after VATS are less than 5%, and this technique is associated with shorter hospital stays and recovery time than with open surgery. The emergence of fluorescein-enhanced autofluorescence thoracoscopy may help identify parenchymal abnormalities not visible on routine thoracoscopy.

Thoracotomy and transaxillary minithoracotomy are indicated only if VATS is unavailable. Recurrence rates are less than

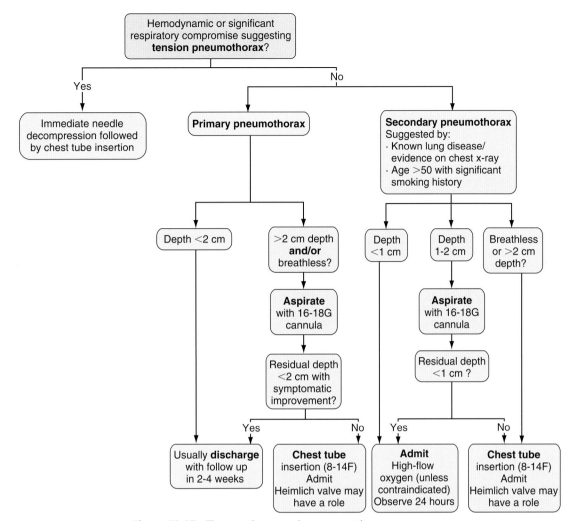

Figure 69-15 Therapeutic approach to pneumothorax management.

1%, but potential morbidity is greater than with minimally invasive procedures.

STRATEGIES FOR AVOIDING RECURRENCE

The risk of recurrence after a primary spontaneous pneumothorax is approximately 30% (16% to 54%) and is greatest in the first few months. Recurrence rates increase with successive pneumothoraces—50% after one recurrence and up to 80% after a third pneumothorax. The risk of contralateral pneumothorax is approximately 15% after a primary event. The recurrence rate is higher in taller patients, smokers, and those with greater number of subpleural blebs or bullae.

Definitive surgical intervention, accomplished by either VATS or open thoracotomy, achieves recurrence rates superior to those after instillation of a pleurodesing agent (usually sterile talc) through the intercostal tube. However, if the patient is unwilling or too frail to undergo surgery, or if thoracoscopy is unavailable, bedside pleurodesis may be appropriate.

SECONDARY SPONTANEOUS PNEUMOTHORAX

Secondary pneumothoraces occur in patients with underlying lung disease, often with impaired respiratory reserve. The reported incidence is similar to that of primary spontaneous pneumothorax, with highest rates (60 cases per 100,000 population per year) in men older than 75 years of age. COPD is a comorbid condition in 60% of patients. *Pneumocystis jirovecii* (i.e., "*Pneumocystis* pneumonia" [PCP]) infection in patients with acquired immunodeficiency syndrome (AIDS) is another risk factor. Other associated conditions are outlined in Box 69-4.

Secondary pneumothorax carries a mortality rate of up to 10%, often indicative of the severity of the underlying lung disease.

CLINICAL PRESENTATION

The symptoms of secondary pneumothorax are similar but often are more severe than those associated with primary pneumothorax. Clinical deterioration may be rapid and of a magnitude disproportionate to the pneumothorax size.

On physical examination, contralateral differences may not be readily apparent in patients with hyperexpanded lungs secondary to COPD.

DIAGNOSIS

Chest radiography confirms the diagnosis in most cases. In patients with underlying lung disease, however, the typical radiographic appearance of a pneumothorax may be altered, and careful distinction between hyperlucent bullae and a pneumothorax must be made. If the diagnosis is in doubt, additional imaging (e.g., CT) should be used before aspiration is attempted.

Arterial blood gas analysis commonly shows hypoxia proportional to the extent of underlying disease and pneumothorax size. Acute hypercapnic respiratory failure may be seen and should resolve after treatment.

MANAGEMENT

Secondary pneumothoraces must be recognized and treated promptly. The evacuation of even a small pneumothorax can rapidly relieve symptoms in these patients.

The initial treatment for most patients is intercostal tube insertion. Observation alone is inappropriate, except in asymptomatic patients with tiny apical pneumothoraces, and aspiration should be considered only in minimally symptomatic patients with small pneumothoraces.

Because air leaks are more common in secondary pneumothoraces, the lung remains unexpanded in approximately 20% of the cases at 7 days. The median time to lung expansion is 5 days, compared with 1 day for primary pneumothoraces. Suction can be applied if the lung fails to spontaneously reinflate.

SURGICAL TREATMENT

Early surgical intervention is recommended in patients with a persistent air leak or failure of reexpansion after 72 hours. VATS is well tolerated by most patients and may supersede more invasive techniques (e.g., open thoracotomy). In persons at high risk for adverse anesthetic events, chemical pleurodesis with delivery of the sclerosing agent through the intercostal tube can be performed.

In other patients in whom tube thoracostomy has failed and surgery is not appropriate, a Heimlich flutter valve can be inserted. Success rates of up to 100% have been reported in patients with advanced AIDS and PCP (see later discussion).

STRATEGIES FOR AVOIDING RECURRENCE

Attempts to prevent recurrence should be considered for all patients after their first secondary pneumothorax, because approximately 45% of this group will have further recurrent episodes.

Open thoracotomy with pleurectomy has the lowest recurrence rate after pneumothorax (approximately 1%), but the less invasive VATS with pleural abrasion or surgical talc pleurodesis usually is preferred and has a recurrence rate of approximately 5%. Many patients, however, will not be suitable candidates for surgical intervention, and chemical pleurodesis performed through a chest tube may be appropriate.

The effect of pleurodesing agents on future lung transplantation must be considered in selected patients. Although not an absolute contraindication, pleurodesis makes transplantation technically more difficult, thereby prolonging the period of donor organ ischemia. Excessive bleeding also is more common. Close liaison with the local transplantation unit is advised for all possible future transplant candidates in whom pleurodesis is contemplated (see Chapter 75).

DISCHARGE AND FOLLOW-UP EVALUATION

Any patient discharged with a residual pneumothorax should have a repeat chest radiograph to ensure complete lung reexpansion. Those who have undergone successful aspiration can be discharged unless an underlying lung abnormality is suspected, when CT imaging may be indicated.

All patients should be cautioned against air travel until 1 week after full lung reexpansion demonstrated on chest radiograph. The risk of recurrence is greatest within the first year, and those with secondary pneumothoraces may wish to avoid flying for a longer period.

Diving should be permanently avoided unless a definitive surgical procedure such as surgical pleurectomy has been performed. Smoking cessation should be strongly encouraged.

SPECIAL SITUATIONS

IATROGENIC PNEUMOTHORAX

Iatrogenic pneumothorax probably is more common than primary and secondary forms of pneumothorax combined, and the incidence is escalating with increasing use of invasive procedures (e.g., transbronchial or percutaneous lung biopsy). Transthoracic needle aspiration accounts for up to one quarter of all cases, especially if the patient has underlying emphysema or aerated lung is traversed during biopsy or radiofrequency ablation of tumor.

A high index of clinical suspicion should be maintained in any patient who becomes breathless after a procedure associated with risk for pneumothorax, and in patients being mechanically ventilated who deteriorate suddenly. The diagnosis is confirmed on a chest radiograph.

In most cases, the patient can be managed with observation and oxygen administration alone. If the patient is more than minimally symptomatic, however, simple aspiration is recommended. Chest tube drainage should be initiated should symptoms persist or if the patient has underlying lung disease. Surgical intervention occasionally is required if the air leak persists (e.g., for longer than 72 hours). Pneumothorax recurrence is not an issue in persons with iatrogenic pneumothoraces unless concomitant lung disease is present.

TENSION PNEUMOTHORAX

Tension pneumothorax constitutes a medical emergency. A defect in the visceral pleural surface acts as a one-way valve, so that air is drawn into the pleural space with inspiration and is unable to leave on expiration. The resulting increase in intrapleural pressure impairs venous return, leading to reduced cardiac output and hypoxemia. Clinically, acute respiratory distress with sweating, tachycardia and hypotension develops; if this disorder goes unrecognized, a pulseless electrical activity (PEA) cardiac arrest may ensue. Tension pneumothorax should be considered when sudden decline occurs in mechanically ventilated patients.

If tension pneumothorax is suspected, treatment should be instituted without delay; awaiting confirmation on the chest radiograph increases the risk of death. The patient should receive high-flow oxygen, and a 16- to 18-gauge cannula should be inserted into the second intercostal space in the midclavicular line. An audible hiss may be noted after insertion. Once enough air has been aspirated to relieve symptoms, an intercostal chest drain should be placed, and a chest radiograph then obtained.

SURGICAL/SUBCUTANEOUS EMPHYSEMA

Surgical emphysema arises as air, under pressure from the pleural space, dissects through the subcutaneous tissue (**Figure 69-16**).

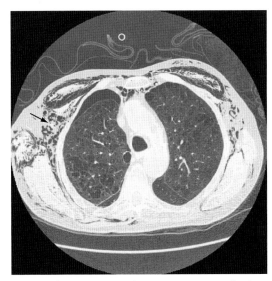

Figure 69-16 Subcutaneous emphysema (*arrow*) complicating secondary pneumothorax related to chronic obstructive pulmonary disease (COPD).

This complication may result from misplacement of a drain with the air holes positioned outside the pleural cavity, from blockage of the drain, or in the presence of a large air leak.

In most cases, no action is required for the surgical emphysema; correction of the drainage problem to prevent further air accumulation in the subcutaneous tissue is adequate. Rarely, acute airway obstruction may develop with secondary respiratory compromise. Tracheostomy may be required to secure the airway and high-flow oxygen applied (in the absence of any contraindications). Skin incision decompression and subcutaneous drains also have been tried.

CATAMENIAL PNEUMOTHORAX

Catamenial pneumothoraces typically develop within 48 hours of onset of menstrual flow and tend to recur. The diagnosis should be considered in women who are seen with recurrent pneumothoraces, with or without a history of endometriosis. This diagnosis often is overlooked, and patients have, on average, five episodes before diagnosis.

The pathogenesis is not fully understood. Most pneumothoraces occur on the right, supporting the hypothesis that air originates from abdominal organs (e.g., endometriotic involvement of the gastrointestinal or uterine tract) and passes into the pleural cavity through diaphragmatic defects. Pleural or diaphragmatic endometriosis may be involved in creating such defects. Alternatively, air may have originated from endometriosis in the lungs.

Treatment of endometriosis with hormonal manipulation is effective in some patients. Alternative therapeutic options include thoracoscopy for pleurodesis and closure of diaphragmatic defects.

PNEUMOTHORAX AND ACQUIRED IMMUNODEFICIENCY SYNDROME

Pneumothorax occurs in 2% to 5% of patients with AIDS. PCP induces a subpleural necrotizing alveolitis responsible for the high frequency and recurrence rate in these patients. Approximately 5% of persons who use prophylactic nebulized pentamidine also will experience spontaneous pneumothoraces.

Management of AIDS-related pneumothorax is notoriously difficult. Early tube thoracostomy and talc pleurodesis or referral for VATS should be considered. Ambulatory drainage with Heimlich valves has been successfully used.

PNEUMOTHORAX IN CYSTIC LUNG DISEASES

Cystic Fibrosis

Development of pneumothorax in patients with cystic fibrosis (CF) carries an important prognostic implication; median survival after pneumothorax is 30 months. The pneumothorax itself is not the cause of demise but is a surrogate marker of end-stage lung disease, because patients with a forced expiratory volume in 1 second (FEV_1) of less than 30% predicted are most at risk. Occurrence of pneumothorax usually is unrelated to acute respiratory illness. Adherence to the standard guidelines for management is recommended, however, with concomitant antibiotic use to avoid secondary infection. Pleurodesis to prevent recurrence of pneumothorax is important, because recurrence rates are approximately 50%. Early liaison with the transplantation team is appropriate if surgical input is required.

Pulmonary Langerhans Cell Histiocytosis

Spontaneous pneumothorax may be the presenting feature in up to 25% of patients with Langerhans cell histiocytosis (LCH). Treatment options are those discussed previously for pneumothorax, together with management of the underlying LCH (see Chapter 54).

Lymphangioleiomyomatosis

In addition to chylothorax, patients with lymphangioleiomyomatosis (LAM) are at risk for development of pneumothorax. This complication is common in this population (affecting up to 80%) and may be the presenting feature of the underlying LAM. Recurrent pneumothoraces occur in two thirds of patients, and early definitive intervention is recommended to reduce recurrence rates. Pleurodesis may increase the rate of perioperative bleeding (occurring as a result of resultant adhesions) but does not preclude successful future lung transplantation (see Chapter 54).

CONTROVERSIES AND PITFALLS

The cause of pneumothorax remains poorly understood. Only a small proportion of subjects with CT evidence of blebs or cystic lung changes actually develop a pneumothorax. Advances in diagnostic technologies (e.g., fluorescein-enhanced autofluorescence thoracoscopy [FEAT]) may shed light on the pathogenesis of pneumothorax. Early evidence casts doubt on whether air leaks truly originate from blebs (as per conventional teachings) or from other abnormal pleural areas identified on FEAT (possibly representing pleura with increased porosity, which may contribute to air leakage). Data from the use of one-way endobronchial valves for persistent air leak demonstrate that a mean of 2.9 valves are required to stop or improve the leak in more than 90% of patients; such data strongly suggest that collateral ventilation between different lung segments and subsegments is important. The concept that pneumothorax can be attributed to one pulmonary (sub) segment and its associated bronchus is overly simplistic.

The optimal management of pneumothoraces remains debatable. The use of suction early in the course of treatment and clamping of the intercostal drain remain controversial topics. Management strategies that use less invasive drainage (e.g., simple aspiration) and early ambulatory drainage with one-way valves are increasingly being adopted by some clinicians. On the other hand, widespread acceptance of minimally invasive thoracoscopic surgery may prompt earlier referral in the future and even first-line thoracoscopic treatment. The best management of pneumothoraces in potential future lung transplant candidates is unclear, and further investigation is needed on optimal timing for air travel in patients with recent pneumothorax.

SUGGESTED READINGS

Havelock T, Teoh R, Laws D, Gleeson F; BTS Pleural Disease Guideline Group: Pleural procedures and thoracic ultrasound: British Thoracic Society Pleural Disease Guideline 2010, *Thorax* 65(Suppl 2):ii61–ii76, 2010.

Light RW, Lee YCG, editors: *Textbook of pleural diseases*, ed 2, London, 2008, Hodder Arnold.

Maskell NA, Davies CW, Nunn AJ, et al: U.K. controlled trial of intrapleural streptokinase for pleural infection (MIST1), *N Engl J Med* 352:865–874, 2005.

Maskell NA, Gleeson FV, Davies RJ: Standard pleural biopsy versus CT-guided cutting-needle biopsy for diagnosis of malignant disease in pleural effusions: a randomised controlled trial, *Lancet* 361:1326–1330, 2003.

Noppen M, Dekeukeleire T, Hanon S, et al: Fluorescein-enhanced autofluorescence thoracoscopy in patients with primary spontaneous pneumothorax and normal subjects, *Am J Respir Crit Care Med* 174:26–30, 2006.

Rahman NM, Maskell NA, West A, et al: Randomized trial of intrapleural tPA and DNase in pleural infection (MIST2), *N Engl J Med* 365:518–526, 2011.

Chapter **70**
Malignant Pleural Mesothelioma
Tarek Meniawy • Bruce W.S. Robinson

Malignant mesothelioma is a neoplasm arising from the mesothelial surface of the pleura, peritoneum, pericardium, and tunica vaginalis, with the majority of cases arising in the pleura. Malignant pleural mesothelioma (MPM) has progressively increased in incidence worldwide, associated with increasing exposure to asbestos in the post–World War II era. The disease is preceded by a long latency period, often more than 30 years. Incidence of MPM is expected to peak in the Western world in the next one or two decades because of regulation of asbestos use and increasing public awareness of its health risks since the 1970s and 1980s. However, MPM will continue to increase in many developing countries, where asbestos remains widely used.

EPIDEMIOLOGY

A relationship between asbestos exposure and development of mesothelioma was first reported in 1960 by Wagner et al., who described a cohort of 33 patients who developed diffuse malignant mesothelioma after exposure to asbestos in the North Western Cape Province of South Africa. Subsequent reports in many countries indicated a rising incidence of mesothelioma. Also, it was reported that the risk of developing mesothelioma was dose dependent, with the rate increasing significantly with time from first exposure, duration of exposure, and cumulative exposure. MPM is often preceded by a prolonged latency period of 20 to 60 years.

A review by Price and Ware of mesothelioma time trends in the United States based on the April 2008 release of the Surveillance Epidemiology and End Result (SEER) data estimated that 2400 cases were diagnosed in 2008, with asbestos likely to be the cause in 58%. They also reported a possible shift in the peak incidence in the United States from a peak between 2000 and 2004 to a peak between 2005 and 2010, and that after 2042, mesothelioma cases diagnosed in the United States will be predominantly caused by "background mesothelioma" rather than asbestos-related MPM.

A similar trend is evident in other Western countries and regions, where several decades of rising incidence of MPM have peaked or will peak in the next 20 to 30 years. The regulatory laws introduced progressively since the 1970s restricted asbestos use in various industries, eventually resulting in a total ban in most developed countries and regions. Again, in many Third World and developing countries where asbestos is still widely used and mesothelioma may also be underreported, incidence will increase for decades.

Mesothelioma has also been linked to nonoccupational and environmental exposure to asbestos in multiple epidemiologic studies. Malignant mesothelioma caused by both occupational and nonoccupational asbestos exposure was notably studied in Wittenoom, Western Australia. In areas of Turkey, exposure to *tremolite* asbestos, commonly used in the white stucco covering walls in houses has been linked to mesothelioma. Another fibrous mineral, *erionite*, has been associated with MPM in three "cancer villages" in the Cappadocia region of Turkey; later reports suggested that this occurs most often in families with genetic predisposition to mineral fiber carcinogenesis.

The *simian virus* 40 (SV40) was proposed to act as a "co-carcinogen" with crocidolite asbestos, resulting in malignant transformation, and was shown to induce mesothelioma in hamsters. The same group subsequently demonstrated SV40 viruslike DNA sequences in patients with malignant mesothelioma. The role of SV40 in mesothelioma remains controversial.

Radiation therapy has been linked to MPM in patients followed up after treatment for non-Hodgkin lymphoma. *Carbon nanotubes*, which are lightweight, strong cylindrical molecules, are increasingly being incorporated into modern manufacturing processes, including electronics, sports equipment, and protective clothing. Initially believed to pose no health risks, they appear to have some similarities to asbestos and were demonstrated to cause mesothelioma when injected into mice. A role for nanotubules in human mesothelioma has not been established, although any long incubation period would make it unlikely that cases would have yet been seen.

Although *smoking* and asbestos exposure can multiplicatively increase the risk of developing lung cancer, smoking has not been demonstrated to have an independent association with mesothelioma.

PATHOGENESIS

Asbestos is a term used to describe a group of mineral fibers of two major types: serpentine and amphibole. *Chrysotile* is the most common *serpentine* asbestos used commercially and has long, curly and pliable fibers. The *amphiboles*, which are short, straight, and stiff, include *crocidolite* (blue asbestos) and *amosite*. Noncommercial amphiboles include tremolite, which is present in the soil in Turkey, Greece, Afghanistan and other regions.

Controversy surrounds the role of different types of asbestos fibers and the exposure threshold for malignant transformation, particularly the role of chrysotile asbestos. The general consensus is that the amphibole crocidolite is the most carcinogenic form of asbestos, and that asbestos fibers of greater length and smaller diameter (high length/width ratio) are more carcinogenic, possibly because they can penetrate farther into the pleura.

Asbestos can affect the pleura by four main processes. First, asbestos fibers can penetrate deeply into the lung and irritate the pleura, eventually leading to either scarring (plaques) or malignant transformation. The fibers may also pierce the mitotic spindle and result in chromosomal damage, with loss of chromosome 22 being the most common gross change. Third, DNA can be damaged through the formation of iron-catalyzed free radicals. Fourth, asbestos can increase expression of proto-oncogenes through phosphorylation of mitogen-activated protein (MAPK) and extracellular signal-regulated kinases (ERK) 1 and 2. In addition, the following six alterations in cell physiology that can dictate malignant growth, as described by Hanahan and Weinberg, also appear to be present in mesothelioma:

1. Mesothelioma cells have increased or *dysregulated growth* through both production of and response to various growth factors.
2. Mesothelioma cells express telomerase and therefore avoid telomere shortening (i.e., become "*immortalized*").
3. Tumor suppressor genes such as p16 and p14, which are important in the Rb and p53 pathways, are absent in mesothelioma, allowing the tumor to *avoid antigrowth signals*.
4. Tumor cells *evade apoptosis* through increased activity of the antiapoptosis molecule Bcl-2.
5. *Increased angiogenesis* occurs through production of angiogenic factors such as vascular endothelial growth factor.
6. Malignant mesothelioma exists in a collagenous environment, and *matrix interactions* and regulation of this environment likely are related to tumor growth.

The SV40 virus may play a role in the pathogenesis of MPM and is a subject of ongoing study to clarify its role. The SV40 large T antigen (SV40Tag) can inhibit p53 and Rb tumor suppressor genes. SV40 infection is also involved in activation of various pathways, including Wnt, ERK, PI3K/Akt, and Notch-1 pathways, and has a co-carcinogenic effect with asbestos.

PATHOLOGY

Gross Pathology

Diffuse MPM is characterized by multiple pleural nodules that progress along the pleural surface, leading to circumferential thickening that encases the lung in a rindlike manner. It may also appear as a single area or multiple areas of thickening or tumor masses. Local invasion of the chest wall, lung, or mediastinum can also occur. *Localized* MPM is a much less common entity involving circumscribed masses that do not show the same diffuse pattern of spread along the pleura.

Histology

A definitive diagnosis of MPM is best made with an adequate biopsy in the context of compatible clinical findings. This often represents a diagnostic challenge because of the relatively low frequency of cases outside large tertiary care centers, the often limited amount of tissue available for examination, the heterogeneity of histologic appearance of the same tumor within a patient, and the differential diagnoses of benign pleural disease or other metastatic malignancies. With the increasing availability of immunohistochemical stains, molecular studies, and electron microscopy, diagnostic accuracy has improved. It remains critical for diagnosis to correlate the pathologic findings with the clinicoradiologic features to reach a definitive diagnosis.

The three main subtypes of diffuse MPM are epithelial (epithelioid), sarcomatous (sarcomatoid), and biphasic mesothelioma, with various histologic patterns within each subtype.

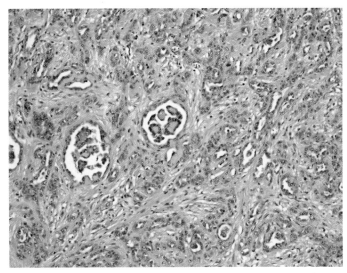

Figure 70-1 Epithelioid mesothelioma with tubulopapillary growth pattern (hematoxylin-eosin stain [H&E]; ×200).

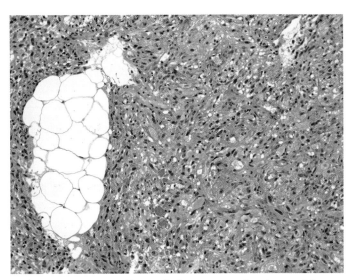

Figure 70-2 Sarcomatoid mesothelioma surrounding chest wall fat (H&E; ×200).

Epithelial Subtype

Epithelioid MPMs are the most common subtype and can be further characterized to a number of patterns. The tubulopapillary pattern contains a mixture of tubules and papillary structures (**Figure 70-1**). Adenomatoid and acinar patterns contain glandlike structures that should be differentiated from adenocarcinomas of other origin (e.g., lung). The solid, well-differentiated pattern has "nests" or sheets of cells that may resemble reactive mesothelium. Differentiating features from *reactive mesothelial hyperplasia* include stromal invasion, presence of necrosis and expansile nodules, as well as immunohistochemical staining patterns. Other types include solid, poorly differentiated, clear cell, and others.

Sarcomatous Subtype

Sarcomatoid MPMs usually show spindle cells, often have more necrosis and atypical cells than epithelioid patterns, may contain anaplastic or giant cells, and include the lymphohistiocytoid and desmoplastic patterns (**Figure 70-2**). The desmoplastic pattern contains dense areas of collagen with small amounts of tumor cells, without significant atypia, and can be difficult to differentiate from nonmalignant pleural conditions such as fibrosing pleuritis; differentiating features include stromal invasion and disorganized growth with uneven thickness.

Biphasic (Mixed) Subtype

Biphasic or mixed MPMs contain elements from both epithelioid and sarcomatoid subtypes, with at least 10% of each required for a diagnosis of "biphasic diffuse MPM."

Cytology

Given that many patients with MPM present with a pleural effusion, cytopathologists and surgical pathologists debate the utility of pleural effusion cytology in the diagnosis. Cell blocks of cytologic samples from pleural effusions used for immunohistochemistry panels similar to those for biopsy specimens have led to more confident diagnosis of MPM when compatible clinicoradiologic findings are present. Morphologic findings alone are not adequate because malignant and reactive epithelial cells share features that make definitive diagnosis difficult. In addition, malignant cells are not usually present in pleural effusions from sarcomatoid effusions, which may contain only reactive mesothelial cells.

The American Thoracic Society, International Mesothelioma Interest Group (IMIG), and European Respiratory Society/European Society of Thoracic Surgeons task force guidelines all acknowledge a role for cytology in the diagnosis of MPM, but favor analysis of a tissue specimen for a definitive diagnosis. In centers with substantial experience in mesothelioma, however, a diagnosis by cytopathology alone is considered possible when combined with immunocytochemical staining.

Immunohisto/Cytochemistry

Immunohistochemistry (IHC) is an important diagnostic tool in MPM. The exact makeup of panels depends on the histologic subtype and type of tumor being considered in the differential diagnosis, as well as the available antibodies. The IMIG consensus statement recommends the use of positive and negative markers with sensitivity or specificity greater than 80% and positivity that considers stain localization and percentage staining (>10%), as follows:

- Reactive mesothelial hyperplasia and epithelioid MPM may be differentiated by a combination of morphologic features and IHC staining; *desmin* is often positive in reactive hyperplasia, and *epithelial membrane antigen* (EMA) and *p53* may be positive in epithelial MPM.
- Malignant mesothelioma (MM) versus metastatic malignancy (often adenocarcinoma) is a common differential diagnosis. Adenocarcinomas often contain intracellular mucin on periodic acid–Schiff stain after digestion, which is only rarely seen in MM. As a general approach, initial IHC workup may include two mesothelial markers and two markers for the malignancy being considered, as well as *pancytokeratin*, which is positive in almost all MPMs, except less common sarcomatoid variants. If the tumor is keratin negative, panels for other cancers (e.g., melanoma, lymphoma) would be considered.
- Positive mesothelioma markers include calretinin, keratin 5/6, WT-1 protein, and podoplanin (D2-40). Markers that favor lung adenocarcinoma include Ber-EP4, which is positive in 95% to 100% of cases, compared to less than 20% of mesotheliomas. Carcinoembryonic antigen (CEA), TTF-1, MOC-31, BG8, B72.3, and CD15 are often positive in adenocarcinoma but only in up to 10% of mesotheliomas.

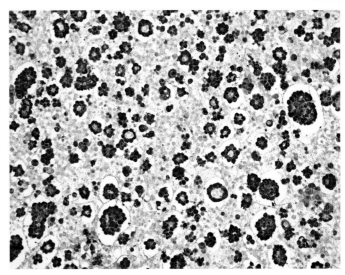

Figure 70-3 Pleural effusion cytology: calretinin stain in malignant mesothelioma (calretinin-immunoperoxidase; ×200).

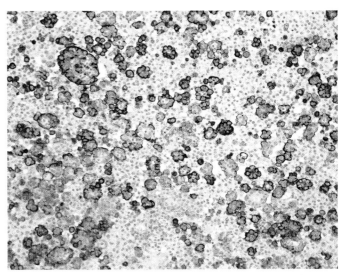

Figure 70-4 Pleural effusion cytology: epithelial membrane antigen (EMA) stain in malignant mesothelioma (EMA-immunoperoxidase; ×200).

- When lung squamous cell carcinoma (SCC) is suspected, keratin 5/6 is not useful, being positive in both mesothelioma and lung SCC, but p63 is useful as it is expressed in almost all SCCs and in 7% of mesotheliomas. MOC-31, BG8, and Ber-EP4 are also often positive in lung SCC.
- If initial IHC panel results are conflicting, these can be expanded to include additional markers.

Immunocytochemistry (ICC) follows the same logic: determine if the cells are of mesothelial origin (e.g., using calretinin; **Figure 70-3**), then determine if they are malignant (e.g., using EMA to determine if there is a dense peripheral staining pattern; **Figure 70-4**). It is essential that the correct anti-EMA antibody is used because some give better results than others, partly contributing to dissent on the role of ICC in diagnosing mesothelioma.

Electron Microscopy

The ultrastructural features of MPM are well described, and electron microscopy (EM) was once the "gold standard" for diagnosing MPM. However, the availability of increasing numbers of suitable antibodies for IHC has largely replaced routine EM, which requires significant expense and expertise and therefore is not widely available outside major centers. MPM diagnosis usually requires a combination of EM features rather than individual features, such as long, thin microvilli, prominent desmosomes, and presence of basal lamina. EM remains useful in well-differentiated to moderately differentiated epithelioid MPM when IHC results are conflicting, especially where differentiation from adenocarcinoma is required.

CLINICAL PRESENTATION

Malignant pleural mesothelioma is most common in men, with age at presentation typically 50 to 70. Presentation at a younger age may also occur in the patient with significant childhood exposure. The insidious onset of symptoms often leads to a delay of 2 to 3 months from initial symptoms to diagnosis, and 25% of patients may not present for evaluation for 6 months or more. Most patients present with a pleural effusion, and the majority develop an effusion at some stage of disease. The most common symptoms at presentation are breathlessness (40%-70%) and chest pain (60%). Constitutional symptoms such as weight loss and fatigue often are not present at diagnosis but develop with progression of disease. Patients may also present with symptoms from local spread causing superior vena cava syndrome, spinal cord compression, pericardial involvement, or chest wall invasion.

The only abnormal physical finding is often of a unilateral pleural effusion, which more frequently (60%) affects the right hemithorax. Tumor spread through the pleural cavity may result in signs of a "fixed" hemithorax. There may be palpable chest wall masses or signs caused by local or distant spread.

There are no specific laboratory features for MPM. Nonspecific findings include anemia, hypergammaglobulinemia, eosinophilia, and thrombocytosis, which is present in 60% to 90% of patients. Pulmonary function tests may show a restrictive pattern, which may result from lung encasement or chest wall involvement.

Distant metastases were present postmortem in 54% to 82% of mesothelioma patients in one large series. However, distant metastases usually are not evident clinically at diagnosis and are not the cause of death. Intracranial metastases may be present infrequently (3%). With the increasing use of positron emission tomography (PET) for diagnostic workup, 5% to 25% of patients may show extrathoracic disease at diagnosis. Miliary spread of mesothelioma has also been described.

DIAGNOSIS

The initial diagnostic workup for patients presenting with an unexplained pleural effusion or pleural thickening is pleural aspiration. Pleural biopsy by sampling an area of the affected pleura with an Abrams needle can be performed, but this blind biopsy is painful and has a yield of only 39% to 60%. In a randomized study, computed tomography (CT) guidance had significantly higher sensitivity than blind biopsy (87% vs. 47%).

Thoracoscopy may be indicated if pleural aspiration is nondiagnostic and for patients who develop recurrent pleural effusions. It has the advantage of a higher sensitivity (98%) and the ability to estimate the extent of involvement of the mediastinum, chest wall and diaphragm, and providing adequate tissue for histologic classification in patients being considered for surgery. If a medical or video-assisted thoracoscopy is not possible, an open biopsy may be necessary. The development of

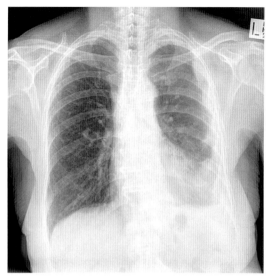

Figure 70-5 Plain chest radiograph of patient with left-sided malignant pleural mesothelioma, demonstrating diffuse pleural thickening and pleural effusion.

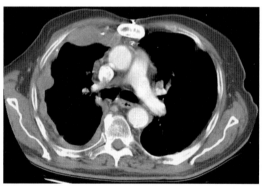

Figure 70-6 Computed tomography scan of patient with right-sided pleural mesothelioma, with diffuse pleural thickening and large focal nodules.

chest wall masses from malignant seeding of biopsy tract sites after thoracocentesis or biopsy is an uncommon complication and may be prevented by radiotherapy to the site after instrumentation, although recent work questions this.

Imaging

The most common finding with MPM on plain chest radiography is a unilateral pleural effusion (**Figure 70-5**). Pleural thickening may also be seen, or in more advanced cases, an encircling "rind" of tumor or lobulated pleural masses. Signs of asbestos exposure, such as pleural plaques, may be present but are not a precursor to mesothelioma.

Computed tomography of the chest may show only a pleural effusion (74%). Pleural-based masses with or without thickening of the interlobular septa are not seen in most patients at presentation but develop later in the disease course (**Figure 70-6**). Lower lobe collapse may result from pleural encasement, pulmonary nodules (60%), or lymphadenopathy affecting the hilar and mediastinal lymph nodes.

Magnetic resonance imaging (MRI), although not commonly used, may be useful in determining the extent of tumor spread, particularly diaphragmatic invasion or assessment of suspected spinal cord metastases.

Positron emission tomography with fluorodeoxyglucose (FDG-PET) may be helpful to distinguish MPM from benign

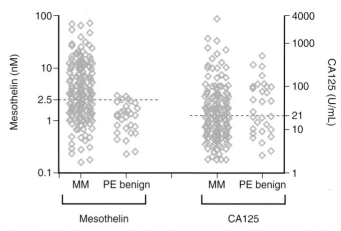

Figure 70-8 Serum mesothelin and cancer antigen 125 *(CA125)* levels in 117 patients with malignant mesothelioma *(MM)* and 30 patients with benign pleural effusions *(PE)* demonstrating similar sensitivity but different specificity levels. At diagnosis, serum mesothelin was elevated in 48% of patients with MM and 3% of patients with benign PE, whereas serum CA125 was elevated in 42% of MM but also in 53% of benign PE.

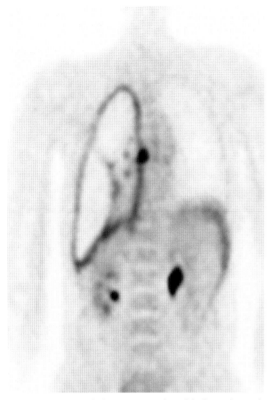

Figure 70-7 Positron emission tomography with fluorodeoxyglucose (PET-FDG) in patient with pleural mesothelioma shows extensive uptake involving right hemithorax with local lymph node involvement.

pleural disease (**Figure 70-7**). PET may also be useful in excluding extrathoracic disease in patients being considered for surgery, but is less accurate for defining locoregional spread to mediastinal lymph nodes. Integrated PET-CT may be more reliable in defining extent of disease than PET, CT, or MRI alone. Changes in PET results may predict response to chemotherapy.

Biomarkers

Two biomarkers, *soluble mesothelin-related peptides* (SMRPs) and osteopontin, have been extensively investigated as potential diagnostic or treatment monitoring markers. *Mesothelin* is a 40-kDa glycoprotein expressed on the surface of mesothelial cells and is overexpressed in mesothelioma. Serum SMRPs were increased in 84% of 44 patients with MPM, and in only three (2%) of 160 control patients. SMRPs measured in pleural effusions have also been investigated. In 192 patients presenting to respiratory clinics, elevated SMRP levels in effusions had a sensitivity of 67% and specificity of 98% for a diagnosis of mesothelioma, often several months before a definitive diagnosis was eventually made (**Figure 70-8**). Their utility has been validated, and SMRPs are now widely available. Of note, the terms *mesothelin* and *SMRP* are often used interchangeably in the literature.

Osteopontin is a glycoprotein that is overexpressed in several cancers. In a report comparing osteopontin levels in MPM patients and in asbestos-exposed patients, a high level of osteopontin had a sensitivity of 77.6% and specificity of 85.5% for mesothelioma, suggesting that it may be useful for distinguishing these two groups. However, osteopontin lacks specificity in other patients with pleural disease compared with SMRPs and thus is not recommended.

STAGING

The current staging system of tumor (T), node (N), metastasis (M) is used by both the International Union against Cancer (UICC) and the American Joint Committee on Cancer (AJCC) and was adopted from the staging system proposed by IMIG in 1995. The AJCC TNM staging system for mesothelioma was published in 2010 (**Table 70-1**). A limitation of staging is that accurate staging, particularly of the T stage, can be determined only by surgical exploration, although initial staging with CT or PET-CT remains valuable.

PROGNOSIS

The median survival of patients with malignant mesothelioma receiving best available treatment is 12 months, or as short as 4 months in patients receiving supportive care alone. The most useful clinical prognostic scoring systems are those derived by the Cancer and Leukaemia Group B (CALGB) and the European Organisation for Research and Treatment of Cancer (EORTC), both validated in subsequent studies. The CALGB index used Cox survival models and regression trees to examine the effects of pretreatment prognostic factors on the survival of 337 patients treated in seven Phase II CALGB clinical trials. Multivariate Cox analysis showed increasing age over 75, pleural involvement, elevated LDH, poor performance status, chest pain, thrombocytosis, and nonepithelial histology to predict a poor prognosis, and six prognostic groups were identified based on these factors. The EORTC identified prognostic factors in 204 patients enrolled in five Phase II trials and reported that a poor performance status, high white blood cell count, male gender, sarcomatous histology, and a probable/possible histologic diagnosis were independent factors of poor prognosis. Patients were classified into a good-prognosis group, with a 40% 1-year survival, and a poor-prognosis group, with a 12% 1-year survival.

An elevated neutrophil/lymphocyte ratio (NLR) at baseline was reported to be an independent prognostic factor in a group of 173 patients undergoing systemic therapy, and normalization of NLR after one cycle of treatment was a predictor of improved survival on subgroup analysis.

Table 70-1	American Joint Committee on Cancer 2010 TNM Staging for Mesothelioma

Primary Tumor (T)

TX	Primary tumor cannot be assessed.
T0	No evidence of primary tumor
T1	Tumor limited to ipsilateral parietal pleura with or without mediastinal pleura and with or without diaphragmatic pleural involvement
T1a	No involvement of visceral pleura
T1b	Tumor also involving visceral pleura

T2	Tumor involving each ipsilateral pleural surface (parietal, mediastinal, diaphragmatic, visceral), with at least one of the following:
	  Involvement of diaphragmatic muscle
	  Extension of tumor from visceral pleura into underlying pulmonary parenchyma

T3	Locally advanced but potentially resectable tumor
	Tumor involving all ipsilateral pleural surfaces (parietal, mediastinal, diaphragmatic, visceral), with at least one of the following:
	  Involvement of endothoracic fascia
	  Extension into mediastinal fat
	  Solitary, completely resectable focus of tumor extending into soft tissues of chest wall
	  Nontransmural involvement of pericardium

T4	Locally advanced, technically unresectable tumor
	Tumor involving all ipsilateral pleural surfaces (parietal, mediastinal, diaphragmatic, visceral) with at least one of the following:
	  Diffuse extension or multifocal masses of tumor in chest wall, with or without associated rib destruction
	  Direct transdiaphragmatic extension of tumor to peritoneum
	  Direct extension of tumor to contralateral pleura
	  Direct extension of tumor to mediastinal organs
	  Direct extension of tumor into the spine
	  Tumor extending through to internal surface of pericardium, with or without a pericardial effusion or tumor involving myocardium

Regional Lymph Nodes (N)

NX	Regional lymph nodes cannot be assessed.
N0	No regional lymph node metastases
N1	Metastases in ipsilateral bronchopulmonary or hilar lymph nodes
N2	Metastases in subcarinal or ipsilateral mediastinal lymph nodes, including ipsilateral internal mammary and peridiaphragmatic nodes
N3	Metastases in contralateral mediastinal, contralateral internal mammary, and ipsilateral or contralateral supraclavicular lymph nodes

Distant metastasis (M)

M0	No distant metastasis
MI	Distant metastasis present

Anatomic Stage/Prognostic Groups

Stage	T	N	M
Stage I	T1	N0	M0
Stage IA	T1a	N0	M0
Stage IB	T1b	N0	M0
Stage II	T2	N0	M0
Stage III	T1, T2	N1	M0
	T1, T2	N2	M0
	T3	N0, N1, N2	M0
Stage IV	T4	Any N	M0
	Any T	N3	M0
	Any T	Any N	M1

From American Joint Committee on Cancer, 2010.

The standardized uptake value (SUV) on PET correlated with survival. Multivariate analysis of 65 patients with MPM demonstrated a longer survival for the group with low-SUV tumors than those with high-SUV lesions.

Gene expression array technology has been investigated as a potential prognostication tool. A molecular predictive test that stratifies patients with good or poor outcomes using relative expression of four genes has been prospectively validated in a group of patients undergoing surgery. Patients with good prognosis had a median survival of 16.8 months, versus 9.5 months for those with poor prognosis. There are no validated tests at present for patients not receiving therapy or for those receiving chemotherapy.

MANAGEMENT

The prognosis of the patient with MPM remains poor, with almost all patients eventually succumbing to their illness. Management options include surgery, chemotherapy, and radiotherapy, with the goal of palliating symptoms or prolongation of survival.

Surgery

The role of surgery in MPM, particularly radical surgery, remains controversial. No randomized controlled trials (RCTs) support radical surgery, and there is considerable difficulty in conducting such trials. Four types of surgery are performed as treatment for mesothelioma: *extrapleural pneumonectomy* (EPP), *pleurectomy/decortication* (P/D), limited pleurectomy, and thoracoscopy with pleurodesis. EPP usually involves an en bloc resection of the lung, pleura, pericardium, and diaphragm, whereas P/D involves resection of the parietal and visceral pleurae, pericardium, and diaphragm but spares the lung.

Although medium-term to long-term survival after multimodality treatment with EPP and radio/chemotherapy has been reported in surgical series from specialized centers, the optimal procedure for patients undergoing resection for early MPM is controversial. Most studies have included exclusively either P/D or EPP as part of multimodality therapy, and selection bias plays a major role in determining the type of surgery, or indeed whether surgery is considered. A retrospective case-control study comparing EPP and P/D for pathologic N2 disease in 57 patients suggested that P/D did not compromise survival for these patients. Retrospectively analyzing outcomes for 663 patients undergoing EPP or P/D at the Memorial Sloan-Kettering Cancer Center, National Cancer Institute, and Karamanos Cancer Institute, Flores et al. reported that patients who underwent P/D had better survival than those undergoing EPP, but acknowledged that the reasons were multifactorial and subject to selection bias, suggesting that therapy should be tailored for individual patients. Operative mortality was 4% for P/D and 7% for EPP.

An important unanswered question is whether radical surgery offers any advantage over nonsurgical therapies. Some patients survived long term after surgery, but these patients might have had slow-growing disease and may have had similar survival without surgery. In most surgical series, the survival benefit could not be specifically attributed to the procedure rather than other components of multimodality therapy. Furthermore, survival analysis for patients who were well enough postoperatively to receive radiotherapy and chemotherapy introduces further selection bias. The Mesothelioma and Radical Surgery (MARS) trial, a feasibility study randomizing patients to trimodality therapy (EPP, chemotherapy, radical

radiotherapy) or identical chemotherapy, followed by appropriate nonsurgical treatment, established that randomization to surgical or nonsurgical resection was feasible, but the study was not powered to address effectiveness and may not provide a definitive answer on the role for surgery. The MARS investigators have proposed a further trial of surgery (MARS-2), that may evaluate P/D as well as respiratory function and quality of life.

For the small proportion of patients presenting with early, potentially resectable MPM, thorough staging with PET-CT, bilateral thoracoscopy, mediastinoscopy, and laparoscopy may avoid major surgery in patients with disease outside the ipsilateral hemithorax. These patients should be counseled on the risks and benefits of radical surgery, including the limitations of available evidence, and referred to a thoracic surgeon with experience in radical surgery, if appropriate.

Limited pleurectomy or thoracoscopy with talc pleurodesis are palliative procedures that can be effective for control of pleural effusions (discussed later).

Radiotherapy

Radiation therapy can be beneficial in mesothelioma but is limited by the need to treat large areas of the hemithorax. Also, the dose is limited by sensitivity of the heart, liver, lung, esophagus, and spinal cord. External beam radiation therapy (EBRT) can palliate symptoms such as painful chest wall metastases in some patients. Radiotherapy has also been used following instrumentation to prevent tumor seeding (discussed above).

Adjuvant radiotherapy is used as a component of multimodality therapy following radical surgery, but there are no RCTs. Intensity-modulated radiation therapy (IMRT) may have reduced toxicity compared with EBRT while improving local control after EPP, but fatal pneumonitis was reported in one smaller series.

Chemotherapy

Systemic platinum-based chemotherapy is the only treatment for the patient with MPM that has a demonstrated survival benefit from RCTs. In 2003 a landmark study of 226 patients with advanced MPM randomized to *cisplatin* and *pemetrexed* combined or cisplatin alone. Median survival improved from 9.3 months for the cisplatin arm to 12.1 months for the cisplatin/pemetrexed group ($p = 0.02$). Radiologic objective response rate, time to progression, and quality of life and symptom distress measures also improved in the two-drug group. In another RCT, the addition of *raltitrexed* to cisplatin showed a similar overall survival benefit: 11.4 months for cisplatin/raltitrexed versus 8.8 months for cisplatin.

Neither of these trials compared chemotherapy to best supportive care, an issue investigated in the MS01study, which compared "active symptoms control" (ASC) to *vinorelbine* or to mitomycin, vinblastine, and cisplatin (MVP). Because of slow accrual, the two chemotherapy arms were combined, and no overall survival benefit was demonstrated over ASC. However, the two chemotherapy arms were significantly different, with vinorelbine demonstrating a 2-month survival advantage that approached significance, suggesting that MVP was not an active regimen in this setting.

The cisplatin/pemetrexed combination has become the standard first-line therapy for patients with MPM in many centers, but *carboplatin* is often substituted for cisplatin for simpler administration and less toxicity, with Phase II evidence of activity and response rates of 20% to 30%. An expanded-access program demonstrated a lower response rate for carboplatin/pemetrexed but similar 1-year survival and time to progression as with cisplatin/pemetrexed. Other regimens with a good response rate include cisplatin and *gemcitabine*, with good response rates in Phase II trials, but this has not been tested in Phase III trials.

There is no second-line therapy with a proven survival advantage that can be considered the standard of care in the MPM patient. It may be reasonable to use pemetrexed in the second-line regimen when not used in first-line therapy, although there is only low-level evidence for this strategy. The timing of initiating chemotherapy (early vs. delayed) in one small randomized study showed an advantage for the early-treatment strategy, but used MVP, not currently considered an active regimen. Other strategies being investigated include the role of maintenance therapy after first-line treatment and the addition of a third cytotoxic agent to initial two-drug chemotherapy.

Targeted Therapies

Several targeted agents have been investigated in mesothelioma, and many more are currently in ongoing trials. A randomized study of cisplatin and gemcitabine with or without the vascular endothelial growth factor (VEGF)–blocking monoclonal antibody (mAb) *bevacizumab* showed disappointing overall efficacy results. Other VEGF–tyrosine kinase (TK) inhibitors have not shown significant activity. Growth factor pathways have also been targeted with selective and multitargeted TK inhibitors, including erlotinib, gefitinib, sorafenib, and sunitinib, but none has a clear role at present in the management of MPM. Other targets and drugs in Phase I and Phase II trials include the proteasome inhibitor *bortezomib* and the mammalian target of rapamycin (mTOR) inhibitor *everolimus*.

Immunotherapy

Mesothelioma appears to be quite sensitive to immunotherapy. MMP expresses self-antigens that include mesothelin and Wilms tumor 1 (WT-1) as well as mutations that represent potential targets for immunotherapies. The recombinant antimesothelin immunotoxin SS1P and the antimesothelin mAb MORAb-009 have shown some activity in Phase I trials in combination with cisplatin and pemetrexed and are the subject of further trials. WT-1 peptide vaccinations, immunogene therapy, systemic and local cytokines, and autologous tumor vaccination are other strategies being investigated.

Response Assessment

The progress of MPM or response to treatment may be assessed by a number of methods. Patients may report an improvement in pain, breathlessness, or functional status. A reduction in size of a chest wall mass or pleural effusion on clinical examination or plain radiography may also indicate a treatment response.

A radiologic response assessment on CT using the Response Evaluation Criteria in Solid Tumors (RECIST) is often required for patients enrolled in clinical trials. However, tumor measurement in mesothelioma is problematic because of the rindlike pattern of growth along the pleural surfaces, which makes bidimensional measurements of discrete tumor masses difficult. A modified version of the RECIST criteria has been developed specifically for mesothelioma and is based on measurement of tumor thickness on multiple levels on CT.

Given its ability to measure tumor metabolic activity rather than size alone, PET scanning has been investigated as a response assessment tool in several cancers. In a prospective study of 20 patients with mesothelioma receiving first-line chemotherapy, the semiquantitative analysis of serial FDG-PET scans performed at baseline and after one cycle of chemotherapy correlated with response to chemotherapy and patient survival. Changes in mesothelin levels are also useful in following progress.

MANAGEMENT OF PLEURAL EFFUSIONS

The management of an initial pleural effusion is thoracocentesis to drain the fluid and initiate the diagnostic workup. Further management of recurrent effusion is guided by rate of reaccumulation, as well as patient symptoms and preferences, and may involve insertion of an indwelling catheter, chemical pleurodesis via catheter or thoracoscopy (most often with talc), or less frequently with partial pleurectomy. Placement of an indwelling (tunneled) catheter is a relatively simple procedure and is the preferred option in many centers because it provides good symptom relief, a low rate of complications, and achieves spontaneous pleurodesis in a significant proportion of patients.

SUPPORTIVE CARE

Pain in patients with MPM may result from involvement of the chest wall or invasion of intercostal nerves or organs. The use of opiates is often helpful, as well as antiinflammatories and agents for management of neuropathic pain, such as pregabalin or valproate sodium. Palliative radiotherapy is also beneficial in some patients. Those with dyspnea may also require opiate analgesia, in addition to addressing any reversible causes such as pleural effusion or anemia.

Psychosocial issues are an important consideration for patients with MPM, who may have feelings of anger or fear compounded by the medicolegal process often associated with this diagnosis.

CONTROVERSIES AND PITFALLS

Patients with MPM often have an insidious onset of symptoms that may lead to a delay in diagnosis. A high index of clinical suspicions and a comprehensive history, including occupational and environmental exposure to asbestos, as well as appropriate investigation may reduce this delay and enable patients to receive potentially beneficial therapies.

Some centers experienced in cytology methods are able to make a definitive diagnosis of MPM on cytologic samples, using specific antibodies, but centers with less experience continue to rely on tissue samples. Definitive diagnosis of MPM may be challenging because of limited available tissue and heterogeneous histologic appearance. Adequate tissue specimens examined by pathologists experienced in diagnosing MPM and using appropriate immunohistochemical panels to differentiate MPM from benign or other malignant disorders, as well as correlation with clinicoradiologic findings, enable a definitive diagnosis in most patients.

Novel biomarkers such as serum or pleural effusion levels of mesothelin may help differentiate benign from malignant causes of pleural effusions that would benefit from further investigation, but these are not in widespread clinical use. Mesothelin has high specificity in blood and pleural fluid and should probably be used more often in the workup of patients suspected of having pleural malignancy.

The role of surgery in the treatment of MPM remains controversial, with improved survival in select patients, who may have had a similar outcome with nonsurgical therapies. For MPM patients considered surgical candidates, comprehensive staging and discussion of available options can avoid a major, potentially futile procedure.

Palliative chemotherapy remains the only treatment modality with a proven survival benefit in patients with advanced MPM able to undergo treatment. Radiotherapy may play a role in palliating symptoms or as a component of multimodality therapy. Because cures are rare, future studies will seek to generate new strategies to circumvent the chemoresistance of MPM.

Malignant pleural mesothelioma research faces many unanswered questions, with limited effective therapies for an aggressive disease with a poor prognosis that will continue to increase in incidence for decades.

CONCLUSION

Controversies surrounding aggressive local therapies will require researchers and mesothelioma patients to accept the critical role for comparative studies and randomization. The many targeted therapies in development should enhance the efficacy of current systemic therapies. Tools and biomarkers for early diagnosis and follow-up continue to be developed, and novel molecular and biologic techniques and therapeutic approaches will ultimately lead to improvements in outcomes. Sequencing the genomes of MPM samples to understand the molecular pathogenesis will uncover new, drug-susceptible targets.

SUGGESTED READING

Cagle PT, Allen TC: Pathology of the pleura: what the pulmonologists need to know, *Respirology* 16:430–438, 2011.

Creaney J, Francis RJ, Dick IM, et al: Serum soluble mesothelin concentrations in malignant pleural mesothelioma: relationship to tumor volume, clinical stage and changes in tumor burden, *Clin Cancer Res* 17:1181–1189, 2011.

Creaney J, Yeoman D, Demelker Y, et al: Comparison of osteopontin, megakaryocyte potentiating factor, and mesothelin proteins as markers in the serum of patients with malignant mesothelioma, *J Thorac Oncol* 3:851–857, 2008.

Edwards JG, Abrams KR, Leverment JN, et al: Prognostic factors for malignant mesothelioma in 142 patients: validation of CALGB and EORTC prognostic scoring systems, *Thorax* 55:731–735, 2000.

Flores RM, Pass HI, Seshan VE, et al: Extrapleural pneumonectomy versus pleurectomy/decortication in the surgical management of malignant pleural mesothelioma: results in 663 patients, *J Thorac Cardiovasc Surg* 135:620–626, e1–e3, 2008.

King J, Thatcher N, Pickering C, et al: Sensitivity and specificity of immunohistochemical antibodies used to distinguish between benign and malignant pleural disease: a systematic review of published reports, *Histopathology* 49:561–568, 2006.

Price B, Ware A: Time trend of mesothelioma incidence in the United States and projection of future cases: an update based on SEER data for 1973 through 2005, *Crit Rev Toxicol* 39:576–588, 2009.

Robinson BW, Lake RA: Advances in malignant mesothelioma, *N Engl J Med* 353:1591–1603, 2005.

Robinson BW, et al: Mesothelin-family proteins and diagnosis of mesothelioma, *Lancet* 362:1612–1616, 2003.

Whitaker D: The cytology of malignant mesothelioma, *Cytopathology* 11:139–151, 2000.

Chapter 71
Disorders of the Mediastinum
Diane C. Strollo • Melissa L. Rosado-de-Christenson

The mediastinum is a central space within the thoracic cavity that is bounded by the sternum anteriorly, the pleura and lungs laterally, the vertebral column posteriorly, the thoracic inlet superiorly, and the diaphragm inferiorly. Although the mediastinum is often arbitrarily divided into compartments, true anatomic planes do not exist, and a mediastinal lesion can occupy more than one compartment. Anatomists and surgeons traditionally divide the mediastinum into four compartments: superior, anterior, middle, and posterior.

The best-known imaging division of the mediastinum is based on the location of a mediastinal mass on the lateral chest radiograph. Because the initial imaging evaluation of mediastinal lesions is typically performed with radiography, localization of a mass in a radiographic mediastinal compartment allows the formulation of a focused differential diagnosis.

This chapter divides the mediastinum into anterior, middle-posterior, and paravertebral compartments (**Figure 71-1**). The *anterior mediastinum* is defined by an imaginary line drawn along the anterior trachea and posterior cardiac border on a lateral chest radiograph. The *paravertebral compartment* is located posterior to an imaginary line drawn to connect the anterior aspects of the thoracic vertebrae. The *middle-posterior mediastinum* is the compartment located between the anterior and paravertebral compartments. Note that the paravertebral regions do not form part of the mediastinum proper.

OVERVIEW OF MEDIASTINAL MASSES

Mediastinal masses are generally described as being predominantly within the anterior, the middle-posterior, or the paravertebral compartment. Cross-sectional imaging allows more accurate localization of mediastinal abnormalities, characterization of the lesions, and visualization of their relationship with and effects on adjacent normal structures.

In adults, approximately 65% of primary mediastinal lesions are located in the anterior mediastinum, 10% in the middle-posterior mediastinum, and 25% in the paravertebral compartment. In contrast, approximately 38% of childhood mediastinal lesions are located in the anterior, 10% in the middle-posterior, and 52% in the paravertebral compartment (**Table 71-1**).

The most common mediastinal masses are intrathoracic hernia, goiter, neurogenic neoplasms, thymic lesions, lymphomas, cysts, and germ cell neoplasms. Thymic and neurogenic neoplasms and foregut cysts are the most frequent primary lesions in adults, and neurogenic neoplasms, foregut cysts, and lymphoma are the predominant lesions in children. Less frequent mediastinal lesions include lymphangioma, pancreatic pseudocyst, extramedullary hematopoiesis, and meningocele. In addition, lung cancer and mediastinal lymph node metastases

may manifest as a mediastinal mass or as extensive mediastinal lymphadenopathy. Non-neoplastic lymphadenopathies, such as sarcoidosis and silicosis, and infectious granulomatous lymphadenopathy may manifest as multiple enlarged mediastinal and hilar lymph nodes and may exhibit calcification.

The nature of mediastinal diseases varies significantly with the patient's age and the clinical presentation. Overall, approximately one third of mediastinal neoplasms are malignant. The mediastinal neoplasms that affect children (40%-50%) are more likely to be malignant than those affecting adults (25%). Most masses (80%-90%) in asymptomatic individuals are benign, whereas approximately 50% of the lesions that produce symptoms are malignant. Conversely, approximately 75% of patients who have malignant neoplasms also have symptoms, compared with less than 50% of patients with benign lesions. Patients with mediastinal masses may experience constitutional symptoms, paraneoplastic syndromes, and symptoms related to compression or invasion of adjacent mediastinal structures. The latter may herald a large, locally invasive or malignant lesion.

The initial evaluation of patients with mediastinal abnormalities includes a detailed history and physical examination to discover specific symptoms and signs of various mediastinal disorders and associated diseases (**Table 71-2**). Posteroanterior (PA) and lateral chest radiography, computed tomography (CT), and occasionally magnetic resonance imaging (MRI) and fluorine 18 (^{18}F) fluorodeoxyglucose (FDG) positron emission tomography (PET) with CT are used for lesion detection and characterization, usually followed by an invasive procedure for tissue diagnosis. However, some mediastinal lesions have a characteristic radiologic appearance, and biopsy may be unwarranted or contraindicated, as in congenital cysts and vascular lesions, respectively. In addition, laboratory evaluation to include a complete blood count, electrolytes, renal and liver function tests, and serologic tests for various autoantibodies and tumor markers may be useful in the initial evaluation and in posttherapy follow-up.

DISEASES OF ANTERIOR MEDIASTINUM

MEDIASTINAL NEOPLASMS

Thymoma

Thymoma is the most common primary mediastinal neoplasm in adults and the most frequent tumor of the anterior mediastinum. It usually affects adults older than 40 years, with no gender predilection. Approximately 30% of patients with thymoma have thoracic symptoms of cough, dyspnea, and/or chest pain; 40% to 70% have symptoms related to one or more of the parathymic syndromes, typically myasthenia gravis

Table 71-1 Compartmental Classification of Mediastinal Disorders

Abnormality/ Source	Disorder/Abnormality
Anterior Mediastinum	
Disorders of thymus gland	Thymomas: thymic carcinoma, thymic carcinoid, thymolipoma, thymic cyst, thymic hyperplasia Lymphoma: Hodgkin disease, non-Hodgkin lymphoma Germ cell neoplasms *Benign:* Mature teratoma *Malignant:* Seminoma, nonseminomatous germ cell neoplasms
Thyroid	Intrathoracic goiter
Parathyroid	Parathyroid adenoma
Pericardial cysts	
Miscellaneous	Mesenchymal neoplasms (lipoma, liposarcoma, angiosarcoma, leiomyoma) Cystic hygroma (mediastinal lymphangioma)
Middle-Posterior Mediastinum	
Lymph node enlargement	Lymphoma Benign mediastinal lymphadenopathy: Granulomatous disease, infectious (tuberculosis, fungal infections) Noninfectious (sarcoidosis, silicosis) *Miscellaneous causes:* Castleman disease Amyloidosis Metastatic mediastinal lymphadenopathy Lung, renal cell, gastrointestinal, and breast carcinoma
Cysts	Foregut cysts Bronchogenic and enteric cysts
Esophageal disorders	Achalasia, benign tumors, esophageal carcinoma, esophageal diverticulum
Vascular lesions	Aneurysms, hemangioma
Miscellaneous	Herniations, pancreatic pseudocyst
Paravertebral Lesions	
Neurogenic neoplasms	*Peripheral nerve neoplasms:* Schwannoma, neurofibroma Malignant peripheral nerve sheath neoplasm *Sympathetic ganglia neoplasms:* Ganglioneuroma, ganglioneuroblastoma, neuroblastoma *Paraganglionic neoplasms:* Pheochromocytoma, paraganglioma
Spinal	Lateral thoracic meningocele Paraspinal abscess (Pott disease)
Miscellaneous	Extramedullary hematopoiesis Thoracic duct cysts

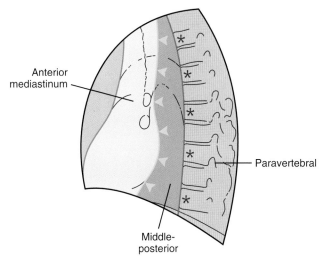

Figure 71-1 Mediastinal compartments on lateral chest radiography. The radiographic anterior mediastinum *(yellow)* is situated anterior to an imaginary line drawn along the anterior tracheal and then continued inferiorly along the posterior heart border. This includes the prevascular space *(blue).* The paravertebral compartment *(gray)* is situated posterior to an imaginary line that joins the anterior thoracic vertebral surfaces. The middle-posterior mediastinum *(pink)* is located between the anterior and the paravertebral compartments. Red asterisks indicate thoracic vertebral bodies.

Table 71-2 Mediastinal Disorders: Constitutional and Paraneoplastic Findings

Diseases	Clinical Findings
Lymphoma	Fever, weight loss, night sweats, pruritus, hypercalcemia
Thymoma	Myasthenia gravis, hypogammaglobulinemia, pure red cell aplasia
Thymic carcinoid secretion	Cushing syndrome, syndrome of inappropriate antidiuretic hormone
Germ cell neoplasm	Gynecomastia, Klinefelter syndrome, hematologic neoplasms
Intrathoracic goiter	Hyper/hypothyroidism
Pheochromocytoma	Hypertension, hypercalcemia, polycythemia, Cushing syndrome
Autonomic ganglia neoplasm	Opsomyoclonus, hypertension, watery diarrhea, Horner syndrome
Sarcoidosis	Hypercalcemia

(MG), but hypogammaglobulinemia, pure red cell aplasia, and nonthymic malignancies may also occur. Some affected patients are asymptomatic and are discovered incidentally because of abnormal chest radiographs. Although the association of thymoma and MG is well recognized, approximately 85% of patients with MG have thymic lymphoid hyperplasia, and only 15% are found to have thymoma. In contrast, 30% to 50% of patients with thymoma may develop MG.

Hypogammaglobulinemia and pure red cell aplasia occur in 10% and 5% of patients who have thymoma, respectively. Non-thymic malignancies occur in 12% to 20% of patients with thymoma and include thyroid carcinoma, lung cancer, and lymphoma.

Thymomas manifest on radiography as rounded, well-circumscribed, unilateral, anterior mediastinal masses (**Figure 71-2**). They are typically located anterior to the aortic root but may be found anywhere from the thoracic inlet to the diaphragm and rarely in the neck. On cross-sectional imaging, thymomas are often homogeneous, soft tissue masses but may exhibit heterogeneity because of cystic change, hemorrhage, or necrosis, especially in large neoplasms. *Drop metastases* to the ipsilateral pleura, pericardium, or upper abdomen through a diaphragmatic hiatus are well documented and represent invasive disease (**Figure 71-3**). Pleural drop metastases may encase

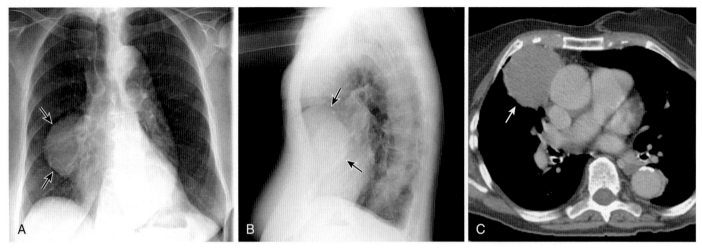

Figure 71-2 Elderly woman with thymoma with microscopic capsular invasion. **A,** Posteroanterior (PA) chest radiograph; **B,** lateral chest radiograph; **C,** contrast-enhanced chest computed tomography (CT) scan (mediastinal window). A 6 × 5 cm discrete homogeneous thymoma *(arrows)* extends inferiorly in the mediastinum without invasion. Thymomas may occur in any location between the thoracic inlet and the diaphragm.

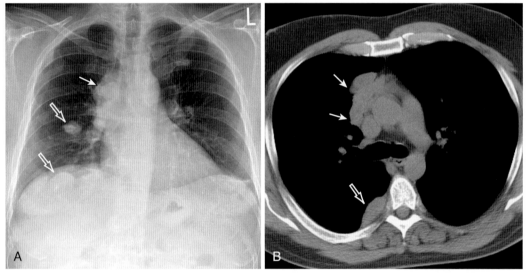

Figure 71-3 Invasive thymoma. **A,** Posteroanterior chest radiograph; **B,** unenhanced chest CT (mediastinal window). Thymoma manifests as a lobular right anterior mediastinal mass *(solid arrows)* with multiple drop metastases to ipsilateral pleura *(open arrows)*.

the lung and mimic diffuse malignant mesothelioma, although associated pleural effusion is infrequent. Lymph node and hematogenous metastases are rare. Mediastinal invasion may be detected with CT and may manifest as an irregular tumoral surface, contralateral extension of thymoma across the midline, and obvious invasion of mediastinal fat and structures. Imaging evidence of local invasion must be correlated with microscopic evidence of capsular transgression and tissue invasion, because encapsulated thymomas may produce fibrous adhesions to adjacent structures. MRI is more sensitive than CT in the detection of vascular invasion. When evaluating a thymic mass, PET-CT may be useful for depicting tumoral invasion, differentiating subgroups of thymic epithelial neoplasms, and staging extent of disease. The maximum standard uptake values (SUVs) of thymoma are typically lower than those of thymic carcinoma. Guided needle biopsy, mediastinotomy, mediastinoscopy, and video-assisted thoracoscopy may establish the diagnosis. However, histologic diagnosis before excisional surgery may not be required in classic cases of thymoma.

Thymomas represent neoplastic proliferation of thymic epithelial cells, intermixed with mature lymphocytes. The histologic typing has been complex and challenging. The Revised

2004 World Health Organization (WHO) classification divides thymic epithelial neoplasms into A, B, and C types on the basis of epithelial cell morphology, the ratio of lymphocytes to epithelial cells, and prognosis. Types A and B correlate with the traditional major histologic cell types of thymoma—epithelial, lymphocytic, mixed lymphoepithelial, and spindle cell. Type C refers to thymic carcinoma. The multidisciplinary International Thymic Malignancy Group (ITMG) assesses diagnostic and therapeutic options of thymoma. Anatomic staging is based on the presence or absence of capsular invasion, determined macroscopically during surgery and confirmed microscopically. Thymomas are now considered malignant neoplasms, and all stages have the potential to metastasize. Most thymomas are completely encapsulated; however, approximately 30% are invasive and grow through the capsule into surrounding adipose tissue, pleura, pericardium, great vessels, and/or heart. Encapsulated and invasive thymomas are microscopically identical, and "invasive" is used to denote capsular invasion.

The treatment of choice for encapsulated and invasive thymomas confined to the mediastinum is surgical resection. Postoperative radiation therapy is included in the treatment of invasive thymoma, but the role of preoperative irradiation is controversial. Chemotherapy with cisplatin-based regimens is generally recommended for metastatic or unresectable recurrent disease, with an overall response rate of 50% to 70% in small studies.

The prognosis of patients with thymoma varies with the stage and extent of surgical resection. Patients with completely resected, encapsulated lesions have the best prognosis. Overall 5-year and 10-year survival rates in patients who have encapsulated thymomas are 75% and 63%, respectively, whereas patients with invasive thymoma have survival rates of 50% and 30%, respectively. Delayed recurrence of thymomas may occur, even in patients with completely resected encapsulated lesions, which emphasizes the importance of long-term follow-up.

The role of thymectomy in the treatment of parathymic syndromes is controversial. Thymectomy is more effective in patients with MG in the absence of a thymoma, with a clinical remission rate of approximately 35% and improvement in another 50%. Neurologic improvement is less likely when MG is associated with thymoma. Thymectomy in patients with pure red cell aplasia results in a 40% to 50% remission rate, in contrast to those with hypogammaglobulinemia, who do not benefit from thymic resection.

Thymic Carcinoma

Thymic carcinomas are a heterogeneous group of aggressive epithelial malignancies with a tendency for early local invasion and distant metastases. Men are more often affected (mean age, 46 years). The Revised 2004 WHO classification of *thymic epithelial neoplasms* describes thymic carcinomas as "nonorganotypic" malignancies (type C) that resemble carcinomas of extrathymic origin, such as lung carcinomas. By traditional histopathologic classification, the two most common cell types are squamous cell and lymphoepithelial-like carcinoma. Unlike thymoma, thymic carcinoma has malignant histologic features and typically manifests as a large, poorly defined, infiltrative, anterior mediastinal mass, frequently with regional lymph node and pulmonary metastases, and pleural and/or pericardial effusions (**Figure 71-4**).

The histologic grade and neoplastic staging determine the therapy and prognosis for the patient with thymic carcinoma. Surgical resection, when feasible, is the preferred treatment. Adjuvant cisplatin-based chemotherapy and concurrent radiotherapy may be used. Response rates are generally poor, with 5-year survival rates of approximately 30%.

Thymic Carcinoid

Thymic carcinoid is a rare, aggressive neuroendocrine neoplasm that typically affects men in the fourth and fifth decades of life. These are large, symptomatic, locally invasive neoplasms with frequent distant metastases. Approximately 35% of affected patients develop endocrine abnormalities caused by ectopic hormone production, most often Cushing syndrome. Multiple endocrine neoplasia syndrome type I (MEN-I) may also occur. However, the syndrome of inappropriate antidiuretic hormone secretion (SIADH) and the carcinoid syndrome are rare. Radiologically, thymic carcinoid is a large, lobular, heterogeneous, and usually invasive anterior mediastinal mass indistinguishable from thymic carcinoma or thymoma (**Figure 71-5**). There may be associated intrathoracic metastatic lymphadenopathy.

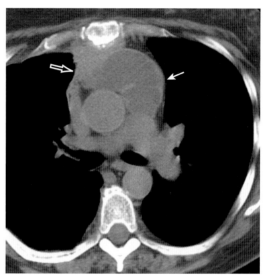

Figure 71-4 Unenhanced chest CT image (mediastinal window) of patient with thymic carcinoma. The heterogeneous left anterior thymic carcinoma extends across the midline of the chest and exhibits multicystic change *(arrow)* and an eccentric mural soft tissue component *(open arrow)*.

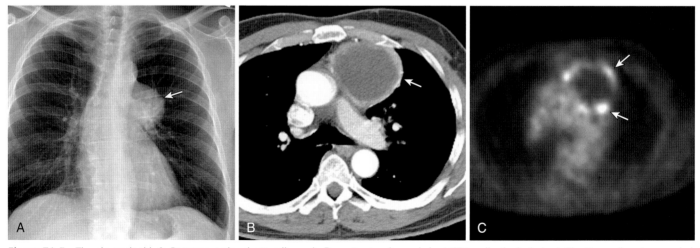

Figure 71-5 Thymic carcinoid. **A,** Posteroanterior chest radiograph; **B,** contrast-enhanced chest CT (mediastinal window). The 6-cm, discrete, rounded left anterior mediastinal thymic carcinoid *(arrow)* exhibits central low attenuation and circumferential mural enhancement. **C,** Fluorodeoxyglucose positron emission tomography (FDG-PET) scan. Multiple FDG-avid foci within the cyst wall *(arrows)* correspond with malignancy.

Surgical resection, when feasible, is the treatment of choice, and response to chemotherapy and radiotherapy is poor.

Mediastinal Lymphoma

Lymphoma represents 10% to 20% of all mediastinal neoplasms in adults. Approximately two thirds of all lymphomas are non-Hodgkin lymphoma (NHL). Mediastinal involvement typically denotes systemic lymphoma but may also represent primary disease. Although both Hodgkin disease (HD) and NHL may affect the mediastinum, mediastinal involvement from systemic lymphoma is much more common in HD than in NHL. *Nodular sclerosis* is the most common subtype of HD to affect the mediastinum. Diffuse, large B-cell lymphoma and lymphoblastic lymphoma represent the most common primary mediastinal subtypes of NHL. Patients affected by NHL have a higher incidence of systemic symptoms and concomitant involvement of extrathoracic and extranodal lymphoid tissue. PET-CT is superior to CT alone in depicting the extent of disease involvement and plays an important role in assessing disease response to therapy and residual viable neoplasm.

Hodgkin Disease

Hodgkin disease is most often seen in adults age 20 to 30 and in those older than 50. Even though the nodular sclerosis subtype is more common in women, HD in general does not exhibit a gender predilection in young patients. Patients who have mediastinal lymphoma tend to be younger. The usual presenting finding is cervical and supraclavicular lymphadenopathy. In less than 25% of patients, HD is limited to the thorax. Approximately one third of patients have systemic symptoms. Patients with mediastinal involvement are generally asymptomatic, although bulky lymphadenopathy may induce symptoms related to mediastinal compression.

Radiologically, most patients with HD have bilateral, asymmetric, mediastinal lymphadenopathy, which frequently involves the prevascular and paratracheal lymph nodes and rarely the posterior mediastinal or juxtacardiac lymph nodes. Nodular sclerosis HD can manifest as a discrete, unilateral anterior mass (**Figure 71-6**) or bilateral mediastinal mass (**Figure 71-7**) or as large, lobular, coalescent lymphadenopathy

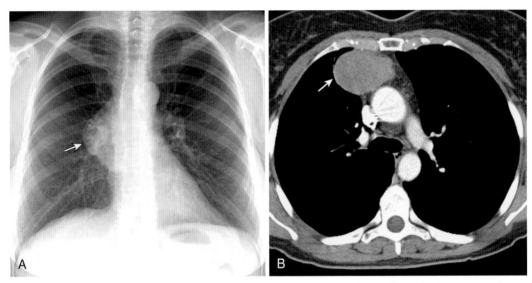

Figure 71-6 Primary mediastinal Hodgkin lymphoma in 45-year-old man. **A,** Posteroanterior chest radiograph; **B,** contrast-enhanced chest CT (mediastinal window). Hodgkin lymphoma manifests as a smooth, homogeneous, right anterior mediastinal mass *(arrow)*, without lymphadenopathy.

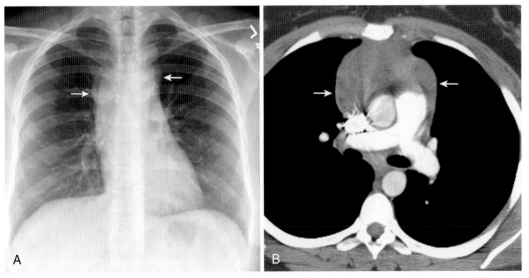

Figure 71-7 Mediastinal mass in Hodgkin disease (HD). **A,** Posteroanterior chest radiograph; **B,** contrast-enhanced chest CT (mediastinal window). Homogeneous central anterior mediastinal mass *(arrows)* extends across the midline bilaterally in woman with HD.

in the anterior mediastinum (**Figure 71-8**). Invasion, compression, and displacement of mediastinal structures, lung, pleura, and chest wall may occur. Affected lymph nodes usually exhibit homogeneous attenuation but may be heterogeneous because of hemorrhage, necrosis, or cystic change. De novo lymph node calcification rarely occurs but may develop 1 to 5 years after radiation therapy. Direct invasion of the lung occurs in 8% to 14% of untreated patients and is usually associated with hilar lymphadenopathy. The diagnosis is established with either core biopsy or surgical excision of affected palpable lymph nodes or masses found on imaging.

Hodgkin disease spreads by means of contiguous nodal chains and is staged anatomically according to the modified Ann Arbor classification, combined with histologic staging: nodular sclerosis, mixed cellularity, lymphocyte predominant, lymphocyte depletion, and unclassified. Stages IA and IIA HD (asymptomatic disease on same side of diaphragm, without bulky lymphadenopathy) have historically been treated with radiation therapy alone. At this time, limited chemotherapy and limited radiotherapy are being evaluated for early-stage disease. More advanced stages are treated with systemic chemotherapy. Bulky mediastinal lymphoma from HD is treated with chemotherapy followed by radiation therapy. Prognosis depends on the stage of the disease, with cure rates of more than 90% achieved in stage IA and IIA disease; even with diffuse or disseminated involvement of one or more extranodal tissues (stage IV), 50% to 60% of patients can be cured with combination chemotherapy. Recurrences may be cured with salvage chemotherapy.

Non-Hodgkin Lymphoma

Non-Hodgkin lymphoma typically affects older patients (compared with those affected by HD) and exhibits a slight male predilection. Diffuse, large B-cell and lymphoblastic lymphomas, the most commonly diagnosed subtype in the mediastinum, occur in younger patients. *Diffuse large B-cell lymphoma* is more common in women, and *lymphoblastic lymphoma* is more common in men and is frequently associated with acute lymphoblastic leukemia (**Figure 71-9**). Both may produce symptoms related to rapid growth and mediastinal invasion, including the superior vena cava syndrome. In addition, diffuse large B-cell lymphoma and lymphoblastic lymphoma may manifest as a primary mediastinal mass without extrathoracic lymphadenopathy. Most patients with NHL are initially seen with advanced disease and systemic symptoms, and approximately half have intrathoracic lymph node enlargement. Thoracic lymphadenopathy is typically isolated or noncontiguous and tends to occur in unusual sites, such as the paravertebral, juxtacardiac, and retrocrural lymph node groups (**Figure 71-10**). Anterior mediastinal involvement is less common than in HD, but imaging features are similar to those of HD.

Non-Hodgkin lymphoma is usually systemic on presentation and spreads unpredictably; thus histologic classification has a better prognostic value than anatomic staging. According to the Revised European-American Classification of Lymphoid Neoplasms, NHL can be classified as indolent, aggressive, or highly aggressive. Indolent NHLs are associated with a more favorable histology and a higher likelihood of nodal disease, but a more advanced clinical stage than the aggressive variety, with a propensity to transform into higher-grade lymphomas. Aggressive NHLs have a less favorable histology, with a tendency for extranodal involvement. Although the prognosis is poor if

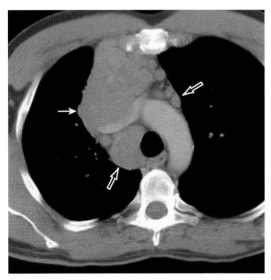

Figure 71-8 Contrast-enhanced chest CT (mediastinal window) of patient with mediastinal Hodgkin disease. A dominant right anterior mediastinal nodal mass *(arrow)* has associated enlarged bilateral contiguous mediastinal nodal groups *(open arrows)*.

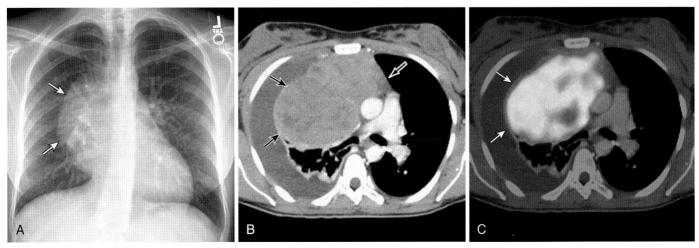

Figure 71-9 Diffuse large B-cell non-Hodgkin lymphoma (NHL). **A,** Posteroanterior chest radiograph; **B** and **C,** contrast-enhanced chest PET-CT images. Heterogeneous right anterior mediastinal NHL *(arrows)* extends across the midline *(open arrow)* and exhibits marked FDG avidity. A moderate right pleural effusion has developed.

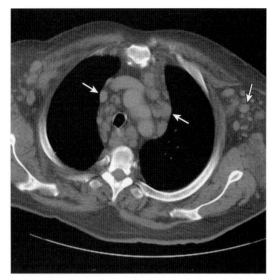

Figure 71-10 Unenhanced chest CT (mediastinal window) of patient with mediastinal non-Hodgkin lymphoma. NHL manifests as multiple enlarged mediastinal and axillary lymph nodes *(arrows)*.

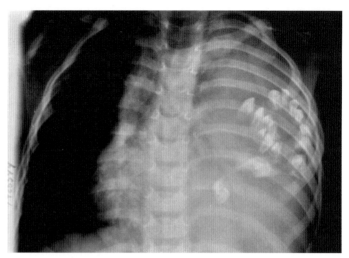

Figure 71-11 Posteroanterior chest radiograph of child with mediastinal mature teratoma. A large mass occupies the entire left hemithorax with mass effect on the mediastinum. Well-formed teeth within the mass, although highly specific for the diagnosis, are an extremely unusual finding.

untreated, aggressive NHLs are potentially more curable than indolent lymphomas. The treatment of indolent NHLs is palliative, and use of radiotherapy or chemotherapy depends on disease stage. PET-CT is an accurate method of assessing remission and prognosis after therapy of aggressive NHL.

Mediastinal Germ Cell Neoplasms

The most common primary extragonadal site of germ cell neoplasms is the anterior mediastinum. These lesions account for 10% to 15% of anterior mediastinal neoplasms in adults. Mediastinal germ cell neoplasms are a diverse group of benign and malignant neoplasms that may originate from ectopic primitive germ cells "misplaced" in the mediastinum during embryogenesis. Most neoplasms that occur in adulthood are benign, but childhood neoplasms are more often malignant. Adults in the third decade of life are most frequently affected. Benign, mature teratomas affect males and females equally, but most malignant mediastinal germ cell neoplasms affect males. Although malignant germ cell neoplasms that manifest as mediastinal masses are typically primary lesions, secondary neoplasia from a primary gonadal germ cell neoplasm should be excluded. Elevation of serum levels of tumor markers, such as alpha fetoprotein (AFP) and beta subunit of human chorionic gonadotropin (β-HCG), in a male with an anterior mediastinal mass strongly suggests the diagnosis of a malignant, nonseminomatous germ cell neoplasm.

Mediastinal Teratomas

Teratomas represent the most common mediastinal germ cell neoplasms, accounting for 60% to 70% of cases, and consist of tissues that may be derived from more than one of the embryonic germ cell layers. Most teratomas are well differentiated and benign, thus the term *mature teratoma*. Uncommon categories include immature teratoma and malignant teratoma or teratocarcinoma. Mature teratoma typically affects children and young adults. Although large tumors may result in symptoms related to local compression, patients with mature teratoma are frequently asymptomatic. Characteristic, but uncommon, symptoms include expectoration of hair (trichoptysis), sebum, or fluid as a result of communication between the tumor and the airways. Radiologically, teratomas are

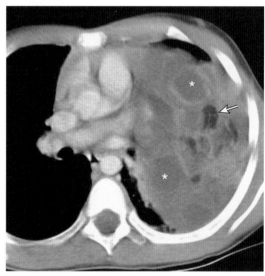

Figure 71-12 Unenhanced chest CT (mediastinal window) of child who has teratoma with immature elements. Teratoma manifests as a large, left anterior mediastinal mass with multicystic *(asterisks)* and fat *(arrow)* components.

spherical, lobular, well-circumscribed, anterior mediastinal masses that may exhibit calcification on radiography (**Figure 71-11**). CT typically demonstrates a multilocular cystic mass, and 75% of lesions contain fat attenuation (**Figure 71-12**). The treatment of choice is surgical excision, and the prognosis is excellent.

Seminomas

Mediastinal seminomas typically affect men in the third and fourth decades of life and represent 40% to 50% of mediastinal malignant germ cell neoplasms of a pure histology. Most patients are symptomatic. β-HCG levels are elevated in 10% of the patients, but AFP level is normal in pure seminomas. The tumor manifests as a large, lobular, well-defined, anterior mediastinal mass. Invasion of mediastinal structures is uncommon, but lymph node, lung, and skeletal metastases may occur. Cisplatin-based chemotherapy for four cycles has largely

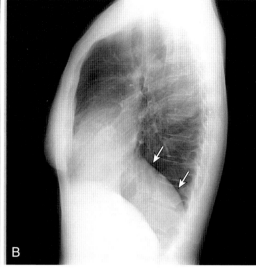

Figure 71-13 **A** and **B,** Posteroanterior and lateral chest radiographs of woman with thymolipoma. Large, soft, left mediastinal thymolipoma *(arrows)* conforms to lower left side of heart and diaphragmatic contours and exhibits multiple punctate calcifications.

replaced previously used radiotherapy alone and results in cure rates of approximately 80%. Radiotherapy is still used in combination with chemotherapy to treat bulky disease and residual neoplasm after chemotherapy.

Nonseminomatous, Malignant Germ-Cell Neoplasms

Nonseminomatous, malignant germ cell neoplasms affect young, symptomatic men and include choriocarcinoma, embryonal carcinoma, endodermal sinus (yolk sac) tumor, and mixed germ-cell neoplasms. Tumor markers (AFP and HCG) are elevated in most patients. A significantly elevated AFP level is usually found in endodermal sinus tumor and embryonal carcinoma, whereas HCG is typically elevated in choriocarcinoma. Nonseminomatous, malignant germ-cell neoplasms may be associated with various hematologic neoplasms, such as acute leukemia or myelodysplastic syndrome, and up to 20% of affected patients have Klinefelter syndrome. These tumors manifest radiologically as large, heterogeneous masses with internal low-attenuation areas corresponding to central necrosis, surrounded by enhancing nodular, irregular soft tissue. Invasion of adjacent structures, pleural and pericardial effusions, and lymph node and distant metastases are common.

Standard treatment involves systemic chemotherapy with cisplatin-containing regimens, followed by surgical resection of residual neoplasm if a positive response is achieved. Patients who respond to therapy are followed with serum tumor markers, which are expected to normalize after treatment. Compared with seminoma, the prognosis is less favorable; however, complete remission rates of 50% to 70% and 5-year survival of approximately 50% can be achieved in patients with nonseminomatous, malignant germ cell neoplasms.

Thymolipoma

Thymolipoma is a rare, benign thymic neoplasm composed of mature adipose and thymic tissues. It usually affects young adults and has no gender predilection. Thymolipomas grow slowly, frequently reaching a large size before diagnosis, and almost half of the patients are asymptomatic. Thymolipomas manifest as large, anterior, inferior mediastinal masses that conform to adjacent thoracic structures and may mimic diaphragmatic elevation and cardiac enlargement on radiography (**Figure 71-13**). These lesions may also exhibit positional changes

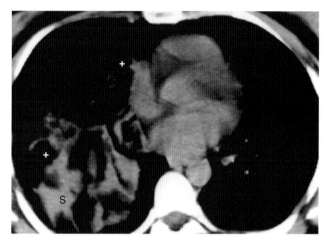

Figure 71-14 Unenhanced chest CT (mediastinal window) of a young woman with thymolipoma. Large anterior mediastinal thymolipoma drapes down into inferior right hemithorax. Note anatomic connection of the thymus and an admixture of fat (+) and soft tissue (S) elements within the lesion.

in shape. CT and MRI demonstrate soft tissue and adipose tissue components and establish an anatomic connection between the lesion and the thymus (**Figure 71-14**). The treatment of choice is surgical resection. The prognosis is excellent.

CYSTS

Thymic Cyst

Thymic cysts are rare anterior mediastinal masses that may be congenital or acquired. Congenital thymic cysts are usually found in the first two decades of life, whereas acquired thymic cysts are seen in association with the acquired immunodeficiency syndrome (AIDS) or thymic inflammation or malignancy (e.g., carcinoma, HD). Radiologically, thymic cysts are well-defined anterior mediastinal masses with cystic unilocular or multilocular appearances on cross-sectional imaging (**Figure 71-15**). Surgical excision is the recommended treatment. The diagnosis of cystic neoplasm should always be considered and excluded, and inflammatory cysts must be carefully examined to exclude associated malignancy.

Pericardial Cyst

Pericardial cysts, also termed *spring water cysts* or *clear water cysts* because of their clear-fluid contents, are uncommon developmental lesions that occur in the radiographic anterior mediastinum. Most are discovered incidentally in asymptomatic middle-aged adults. These cysts are well circumscribed and usually abut the heart, the diaphragm, and the anterior chest wall, typically in the right cardiophrenic angle. CT typically demonstrates a nonenhancing cystic mass of water attenuation and an imperceptible wall (**Figure 71-16**). Unless significant symptoms or atypical imaging features are found, pericardial cysts are followed clinically and radiologically.

GLANDULAR DISORDERS

Thymic Hyperplasia

Thymic hyperplasia most often occurs as a rebound phenomenon in patients who have received chemotherapy for treatment of lymphoma or germ cell neoplasms. Diffuse hyperplasia

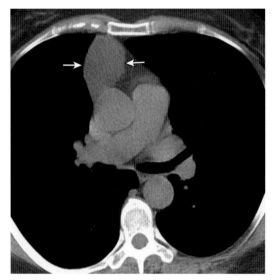

Figure 71-15   Unenhanced chest CT (mediastinal window) of asymptomatic woman with unilocular thymic cyst *(arrows)*, showing water-attenuation contents, an imperceptible wall, and no soft tissue component.

occurs within 2 weeks to 12 months after chemotherapy and may manifest with mediastinal enlargement on radiography or may mimic thymic neoplasia on cross-sectional imaging. On PET-CT, thymic hyperplasia typically exhibits only mild FDG uptake, in contrast to marked uptake by recurrent malignancy. Chemical-shift MRI (in-phase and out-of-phase gradient-echo sequences) may be used successfully to differentiate thymic hyperplasia from thymic neoplasia.

Intrathoracic Goiter

Most intrathoracic goiters result from extension of cervical thyroid goiters into the mediastinum and typically affect women. Although patients are usually asymptomatic, compression of the trachea or esophagus rarely causes symptoms such as dyspnea or dysphagia. The risk of malignant degeneration is small. Most intrathoracic goiters are located in the anterosuperior mediastinum, usually on the right side, but other compartments may be affected. Ectopic intrathoracic goiter without a cervical component rarely occurs. Chest radiography often reveals a cervicothoracic mass that produces mass effect on the trachea. CT demonstrates a lobular, well-defined mass with heterogeneous attenuation resulting from hemorrhage, cystic change, and calcification (**Figure 71-17**). Intense and sustained contrast enhancement is common. In functioning goiters, uptake of radioactive iodine (iodine 123 [^{123}I] or iodine 131 [^{131}I]) and technetium 99 m (^{99m}Tc) pertechnetate is diagnostic. Symptomatic or large goiters may be surgically excised.

Parathyroid Adenoma

Ectopic parathyroid glands in the mediastinum are usually located within or near the thymus gland. Most are encapsulated, functioning, benign adenomas, most often seen in older women who have persistent hyperparathyroidism after surgical parathyroidectomy. Because of their small size, parathyroid adenomas are rarely detected on chest radiography and frequently mimic lymph nodes on CT. Localization may be achieved by ^{99m}Tc sestamibi scintigraphy or dual-isotope digital subtraction imaging with ^{99m}Tc pertechnetate and thallium-201 chloride. Scintigraphic (functional) localization is correlated with CT or MRI (anatomic) identification of a mediastinal soft tissue nodule or mass. Selective venous sampling for parathyroid hormone levels may be necessary. Surgical excision is the treatment of choice.

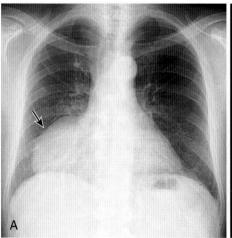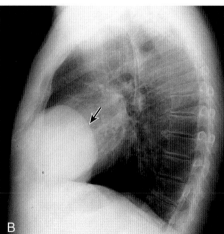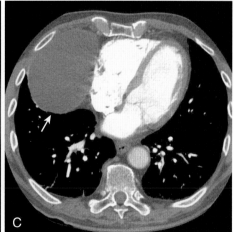

Figure 71-16   Pericardial cyst in asymptomatic man. **A** and **B,** Posteroanterior and lateral chest radiographs; **C,** contrast-enhanced chest CT (mediastinal window). Right cardiophrenic angle pericardial cyst manifests as a unilocular water-attenuation mass *(arrow)* with an imperceptible wall.

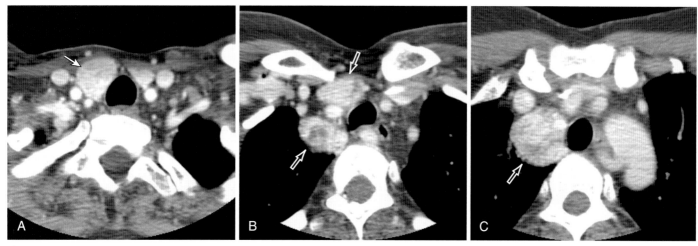

Figure 71-17   A to **C**, Contrast-enhanced chest CT (mediastinal window) in elderly woman with goiter *(arrows)*. The goiter arises from right lobe of thyroid, extends into upper thorax, and exhibits exuberant contrast enhancement.

DISEASES OF MIDDLE-POSTERIOR MEDIASTINUM

LYMPHADENOPATHY

Benign Mediastinal Lymphadenopathy

Infectious and noninfectious granulomatous diseases may involve the mediastinal lymph nodes. Infectious granulomatous diseases include tuberculosis and fungal infections, such as histoplasmosis and coccidioidomycosis. The most important noninfectious granulomatous diseases include *sarcoidosis* and *silicosis.* Lymphadenopathy associated with granulomatous infection is usually unilateral and asymmetric, in contrast to bilateral and symmetric lymph node enlargement with sarcoidosis and silicosis. Many of these disorders cause lymph node calcification, which may exhibit an "eggshell" configuration, characteristic of silicosis and less often sarcoidosis. Although calcified lymph nodes generally represent a benign process, definitive exclusion of malignant lymphadenopathy may be impossible by CT alone, and histologic examination may be required.

Other benign causes of lymph node enlargement include reactive hyperplasia from bacterial or viral lung infections, amyloidosis, drugs such as phenytoin, and Castleman disease (angiofollicular lymphoid hyperplasia or giant lymph node hyperplasia). *Castleman disease* usually manifests in young, asymptomatic adults as incidental, large, well-circumscribed, middle-posterior mediastinal lymph nodes. Nodal hypervascularity results in intense, homogeneous enhancement after intravenous (IV) contrast administration on cross-sectional imaging. The hyaline vascular histologic type accounts for 80% to 90% of cases, whereas the plasma cell and multicentric types represent only 10%. Patients with the *hyaline vascular* type are typically asymptomatic, although symptoms of compression may occur. The *plasma cell* variety may be associated with constitutional symptoms and signs of fever, weight loss, fatigue, anemia, and hypergammaglobulinemia, which may improve after surgical excision. The *multicentric* type is rare and associated with severe systemic symptoms in older patients, generalized lymphadenopathy, and hepatosplenomegaly, with eventual development of NHL.

Metastatic Mediastinal and Hilar Lymphadenopathy

Primary lung, breast, renal cell, gastrointestinal, and prostate carcinomas and malignant melanoma may metastasize to

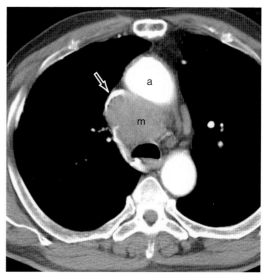

Figure 71-18   Contrast-enhanced chest CT (mediastinal window) in patient with mediastinal squamous cell cancer (SCCA) of lung. SCCA manifests as an anterior mediastinal mass *(m)* that insinuates between the ascending aorta *(a)* and trachea and invades the superior vena cava *(arrow).*

mediastinal or hilar lymph nodes and may manifest as a solitary mass, a dominant mass with lymphadenopathy, or multifocal enlarged lymph nodes (**Figure 71-18**). Ipsilateral mediastinal metastases from lung carcinoma represent N2 disease and may be operable. The diagnosis of metastases is established by a history of a known primary malignancy and confirmed by biopsy. The treatment depends on the underlying neoplasm and its stage.

CYSTS

Foregut Cysts

Congenital foregut cysts represent 20% of mediastinal masses, and 50% to 60% of these are bronchogenic cysts. Enteric cysts, which include esophageal duplication and neurenteric cysts, account for approximately 10% to 15%. Up to 20% of foregut cysts cannot be histologically classified and are termed *nonspecific* or *indeterminate* cysts.

Bronchogenic Cysts

Bronchogenic cysts are thought to originate from abnormal ventral budding of the primitive foregut. Most are located in the mediastinum, most often in subcarinal or paratracheal locations. Up to 15% are reported to arise in the lung; other locations (pleura, diaphragm, pericardium) are rare. These cysts are usually lined by a pseudostratified, columnar, ciliated (respiratory) epithelium; exhibit cartilage and smooth muscle in their walls; and may contain serous fluid, mucus, milk of calcium, blood, or purulent material.

Bronchogenic cysts typically occur in adult men and women but may affect all age groups. Patients are usually asymptomatic, but infection or bleeding eventually produces symptoms in up to two thirds of cases. Radiography usually reveals a well-circumscribed, spherical, middle-posterior mediastinal mass. On CT, these cysts are unilocular homogeneous, nonenhancing masses of variable attenuation, depending on the composition of the fluid (**Figures 71-19** and **71-20**). The cyst wall may contain calcification or enhance after IV administration of contrast. A gas-fluid level within the cyst is exceptionally rare in mediastinal cysts but frequently occurs in pulmonary cysts and indicates communication with the airways or infection. Large cysts in children may compress the airways, with resultant atelectasis, bronchopneumonia, or air trapping.

The treatment of choice is surgical resection (even in the absence of symptoms), although incidental cysts in asymptomatic adults have been followed clinically and radiologically. Bronchoscopic or thoracoscopic needle drainage of cyst fluid typically reveals mucus and bronchial epithelial cells and is reserved for patients with a high risk of surgical complications.

Enteric Cysts

Enteric (esophageal duplication and neurenteric) cysts originate from the dorsal foregut, are usually located in the middle-posterior mediastinum or paravertebral region, and typically manifest in childhood. Enteric cysts are lined by squamous or enteric epithelium and may contain gastric mucosa and/or pancreatic and neural tissue. The cyst walls have two well-defined, smooth muscle layers with a myenteric plexus. *Esophageal duplication cysts* almost always adhere to the esophagus or are located within its wall and can be associated with gastrointestinal (GI) malformations. Similarly, *neurenteric cysts* may be associated with GI and cervical or upper thoracic vertebral anomalies, occasionally with a fibrous attachment to the spine or intraspinal extension.

Most enteric cysts are diagnosed during childhood. Hemorrhage or rupture may occur, especially when gastric epithelium or pancreatic tissue is present. The radiologic features of enteric cysts are similar to those of bronchogenic cysts. Esophageal duplication cysts are usually located close to the distal esophagus on the right side. Most neurenteric cysts are located in the paravertebral region, above the level of the carina on the right side, and approximately one half are associated with scoliosis, anterior spina bifida, vertebral fusion, hemivertebrae, and other vertebral anomalies. MRI is indicated to exclude intraspinal extension. Surgical excision is the treatment of choice. Prognosis after complete resection is excellent.

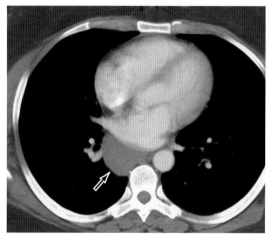

Figure 71-19 Contrast-enhanced chest CT (mediastinal window) of patient with bronchogenic cyst. The cyst *(arrow)* arises in azygoesophageal recess of middle-posterior mediastinum and exhibits water-attenuation contents with an imperceptible wall. Cyst contents do not enhance.

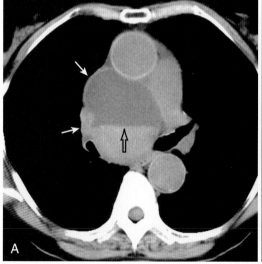
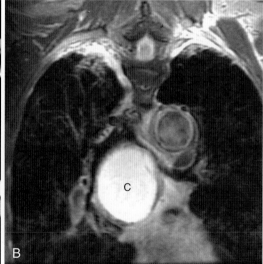

Figure 71-20 Subcarinal bronchogenic cyst. **A,** On contrast-enhanced chest CT (mediastinal window), the cyst *(arrows)* exhibits smooth mural enhancement and "fluid-fluid" level *(open arrow)* from recent hemorrhage. **B,** On T2-weighted coronal magnetic resonance imaging (MRI), the cyst *(c)* splays the main bronchi and exhibits high signal intensity.

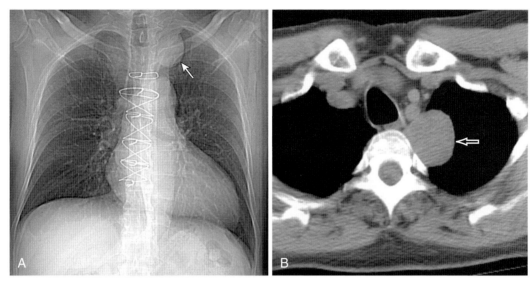

Figure 71-21 Neurofibroma. **A,** Posteroanterior chest radiograph; **B,** unenhanced chest CT (mediastinal window). Rounded, homogeneous left paravertebral neurofibroma *(arrow)* does not exhibit intraspinal extension or skeletal pressure erosion.

OTHER DISORDERS

Vascular Lesions

Vascular lesions constitute approximately 10% of all mediastinal masses and may originate from the arterial or venous portions of the systemic or pulmonary circulation. They may mimic neoplasms on chest radiographs and should be considered in the differential diagnosis before biopsy is performed. The diagnosis is usually established with contrast-enhanced CT, MRI, and angiography.

Herniation

Hiatal hernias are common and result when an abdominal structure, usually the stomach, extends through the esophageal hiatus into the thorax and manifests as a retrocardiac mass. *Morgagni hernias* are congenital defects in the diaphragm that allow herniation of omentum or other abdominal contents into the thorax and typically manifest as right cardiophrenic angle masses. Diagnosis is typically established by identification of abdominal contents in the hernia sac on cross-sectional imaging studies. Treatment of symptomatic cases is surgical.

DISEASES OF PARAVERTEBRAL COMPARTMENT

Neurogenic Neoplasms

Neurogenic neoplasms constitute 15% to 20% of adult and 40% of pediatric mediastinal tumors. Approximately 90% occur in the paravertebral region. Neurogenic neoplasms are the most common cause of a paravertebral mass and account for 75% of primary paravertebral "mediastinal" neoplasms. Approximately 50% of neurogenic neoplasms in children are malignant, whereas in adults most are benign. Approximately half of affected patients are asymptomatic. Neurogenic neoplasms are generally grouped into three categories according to their structure of origin: peripheral nerve, sympathetic ganglia, and paraganglionic neoplasms.

PERIPHERAL NERVE NEOPLASMS

Schwannoma and Neurofibroma

Schwannoma (also termed *neurilemmoma*) and neurofibroma are the most common mediastinal neurogenic neoplasms. More than 90% are benign, and 10% are multiple. They are slow-growing neoplasms and usually arise from a posterior spinal nerve root but can involve any nerve in the thorax. Schwannoma and solitary neurofibroma affect men and women equally in the third and fourth decades. Although these neoplasms may attain large sizes, most patients are asymptomatic. Approximately 30% to 45% of neurofibromas occur in individuals who have *neurofibromatosis* (von Recklinghausen disease). The presence of multiple neurofibromas or a single plexiform neurofibroma is pathognomonic of neurofibromatosis. Malignant transformation of a solitary schwannoma is extremely rare. Patients with neurofibromatosis and neurogenic neoplasms are at increased risk for malignant transformation of one or more lesions. Patients with neurofibromatosis may also have ganglion cell neoplasms develop.

Radiologically, schwannomas and neurofibromas are sharply marginated, spherical, and occasionally lobular paravertebral masses, which usually span one to two rib interspaces but can attain large sizes (**Figure 71-21**). Up to one half of the cases cause splaying and benign pressure erosion of the ribs, vertebral bodies, and neural foramina. Approximately 10% of schwannomas and neurofibromas grow through and widen adjacent neural foramina and expand on either end with a "dumbbell" or hourglass configuration (**Figure 71-22**). Typically, CT reveals a heterogeneous mass that may contain punctate calcification or areas of low attenuation. MRI should always be performed to exclude intraspinal growth of the neoplasm (**Figure 71-23**). The treatment of choice is surgery. Recurrences are uncommon, even when excision is incomplete.

Malignant Peripheral Nerve Sheath Neoplasms

Malignant peripheral nerve sheath neoplasms are a rare group of spindle cell sarcomas thought to represent the malignant counterparts of schwannomas and neurofibromas. These nerve sheath lesions occur equally in men and women in the third to fifth decades, and approximately half occur in patients with neurofibromatosis. The incidence of malignant degeneration of neurogenic neoplasms in patients with neurofibromatosis is approximately 5%. Malignant peripheral nerve sheath neoplasms may also occur sporadically or be induced by radiation. Pain and an enlarging mass are common at presentation. Radiologically, mediastinal malignant peripheral nerve sheath

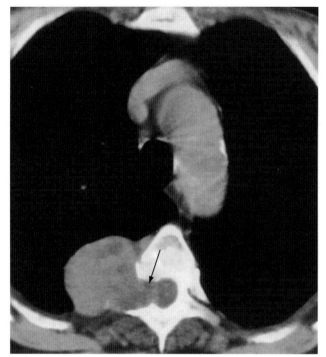

Figure 71-22   Unenhanced chest CT (mediastinal window) of patient with neurofibroma. A spherical mass of heterogeneous attenuation exhibits intraspinal extension *(arrow)* with enlargement and pressure erosion of adjacent neural foramen.

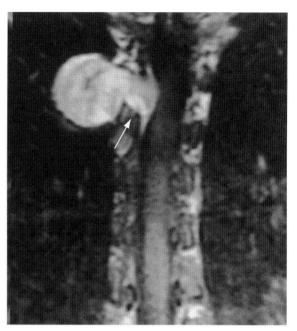

Figure 71-23   Gadolinium-enhanced T1-weighted coronal MR image of patient with neurofibroma. Spherical, heterogeneously enhancing paravertebral neurofibroma exhibits intraspinal extension *(arrow)* and mass effect on spinal cord.

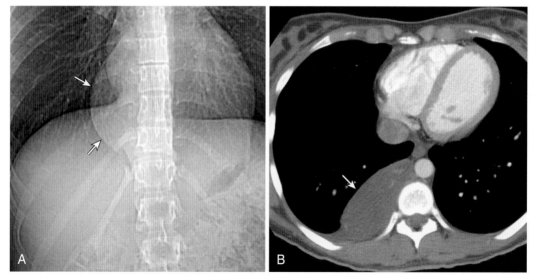

Figure 71-24   Ganglioneuroma in adolescent patient. **A,** Coned-down chest CT scout scan; **B,** contrast-enhanced CT scan (mediastinal window). Oblong, smooth, homogeneous paravertebral ganglioneuroma *(arrow)* does not exhibit intraspinal extension.

neoplasms manifest as sharply marginated, spherical, heterogeneous masses on cross-sectional imaging and may exhibit explosive growth.

SYMPATHETIC GANGLIA NEOPLASMS

Neoplasms of sympathetic ganglia affect both children and young adults, but malignant lesions are most common in children. Ganglioneuroma and ganglioneuroblastoma usually arise in the sympathetic ganglia of the paravertebral region. Approximately one half of neuroblastomas arise from the adrenal glands, and one third are located in the mediastinum, the most common extraabdominal location.

Ganglioneuromas

Ganglioneuromas are benign neoplasms that affect males and females equally. Affected patients are older children (typically >5 years of age) and young adults. One half of patients are symptomatic from local effects of the tumor or intraspinal growth. Radiologically, ganglioneuromas are well-circumscribed, oblong, paravertebral masses that usually span three to five vertebrae and may exhibit skeletal displacement or pressure erosion (**Figure 71-24**). MRI is indicated to exclude intraspinal extension. Surgical excision is the treatment of choice and may necessitate a combined thoracic and neurosurgical approach.

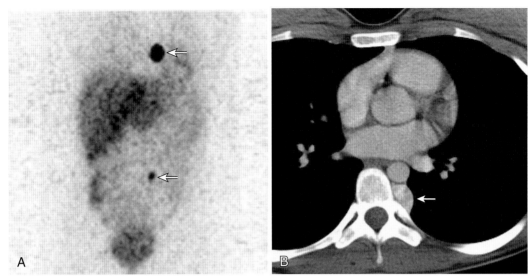

Figure 71-25 **A,** ^{131}I-MIBG scintigraphy of patient with pheochromocytoma. Two foci of pheochromocytoma *(arrows)* in the chest and abdomen exhibit marked uptake of radiotracer. **B,** Contrast-enhanced chest CT (mediastinal window) of left paravertebral pheochromocytoma, manifesting as a smooth nodule *(arrow)* with moderate enhancement.

Ganglioneuroblastomas

Ganglioneuroblastomas are malignant neoplasms that usually affect children younger than 10 years, with no gender predilection. They demonstrate composite histologic, biologic, and radiologic features of ganglioneuromas and neuroblastomas and are not usually distinguishable on imaging. Symptoms, when present, are caused by local mass effect, invasion of adjacent structures, or metastases. Staging and treatment are the same as for neuroblastomas. The prognosis for patients with ganglioneuroblastomas is generally more favorable than in those with neuroblastomas.

Neuroblastomas

Neuroblastomas are highly malignant neoplasms that affect children younger than 5 years, typically boys. Neuroblastomas in children older than 5 have no gender predilection. Two thirds of patients have constitutional symptoms, pain, cough, dyspnea, paraplegia, opsoclonus, and Horner syndrome. Systemic effects, such as hypertension, tachycardia, perspiration, flushing, and severe watery diarrhea, may result from elevation of catecholamine and vasoactive intestinal peptide levels. Radiologically, the masses are paravertebral, occasionally with local invasion, contralateral extension, and skeletal erosion. Approximately 10% exhibit extensive calcification on radiography. On CT, the tumors are heterogeneous because of hemorrhage and necrosis, and calcification may be detected in 80% of cases. MRI should always be used to exclude intraspinal extension and vascular or skeletal involvement. Metaiodobenzylguanidine (MIBG) scintigraphy (^{123}I or ^{131}I) may demonstrate uptake in both primary and metastatic sites.

Neuroblastomas and ganglioneuroblastomas are treated with surgical resection. Adjuvant chemotherapy and irradiation may be used for residual disease or as a primary treatment modality in advanced cases. Radiotherapy in children can lead to delayed complications such as myelitis and scoliosis. The prognosis is generally poor and depends on the age at diagnosis, the size, the degree of histologic differentiation, and the neoplastic stage. Patients with congenital and thoracic lesions have the best prognosis.

PARAGANGLIONIC NEOPLASMS

Pheochromocytoma

Pheochromocytomas are functioning paragangliomas that most often arise from the adrenal glands and occur more frequently in men in the third to fourth decades. Approximately 10% of pheochromocytomas are extraadrenal, and less than 2% are intrathoracic; the latter tend to be more aggressive and multicentric. Symptoms relate to excessive systemic catecholamines or local mass effect. Pheochromocytomas may be part of a multisystem endocrine syndrome (e.g., MEN IIA or IIB). Diagnosis can be established by measurement of urine catecholamines and their metabolites (vanillylmandelic acid, homovanillic acid, metanephrine, normetanephrine). Typically, CT and MRI reveal a well-delineated, enhancing, paravertebral mass. The neoplasm is typically ^{123}I and ^{123}I MIBG avid (**Figure 71-25**). Treatment includes sympathetic α- and β-blockade for 1 to 2 weeks, followed by surgical excision. Chemotherapy and radiotherapy can be used to treat metastatic disease.

Paraganglioma

Paragangliomas are rare neoplasms of paraganglionic tissue. Most are benign, asymptomatic, and nonfunctioning. Radiologically, they typically manifest as sharply marginated, middle-posterior mediastinal nodules or masses, usually located adjacent to the aorta, pulmonary arteries, heart, or costovertebral sulci or within the left atrial wall (**Figure 71-26**). Paragangliomas are hypervascular lesions and demonstrate marked contrast enhancement. The treatment is surgical excision.

SPINAL LESION

Lateral Thoracic Meningocele

Lateral thoracic meningoceles are rare and consist of redundant meninges that protrude through the neural foramen and contain cerebrospinal fluid (CSF). These meningoceles do not exhibit a gender predilection and typically occur in association with neurofibromatosis. Patients are usually asymptomatic adults in the fourth to fifth decades. Radiologic studies demonstrate a

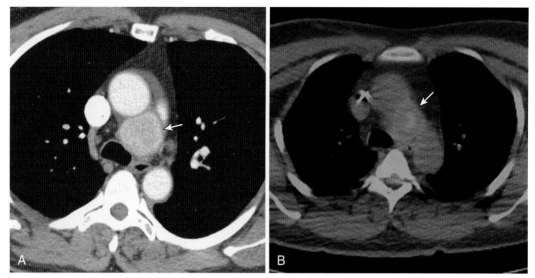

Figure 71-26 **A** and **B,** Contrast-enhanced chest positron emission tomography-computed tomography scan of patient with mediastinal paraganglioma *(arrow)* in the aorticopulmonary region, manifesting as a smooth, rounded mass with moderate homogeneous enhancement and FDG avidity.

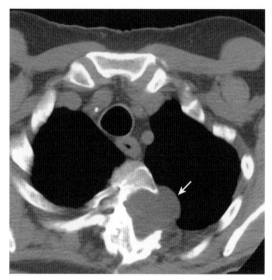

Figure 71-27 Unenhanced contrast CT (mediastinal window) of patient with lateral thoracic meningocele. The rounded meningocele *(arrow)* has attenuation that parallels that of cerebrospinal fluid, an imperceptible wall, and pressure erosion with expansion of neural foramen.

well-circumscribed, paravertebral, cystic lesion, frequently associated with vertebral erosion, kyphoscoliosis, and/or widening of adjacent neural foramina (**Figure 71-27**). Cross-sectional imaging may demonstrate continuity with the thecal sac. CT demonstrates a homogeneous nonenhancing mass of water attenuation, and MRI shows signal intensity equal to that of adjacent CSF. Symptomatic lateral thoracic meningoceles are treated with surgical excision.

MISCELLANEOUS DISORDERS OF THE MEDIASTINUM

Mediastinitis

The term *mediastinitis* is used to refer to a variety of infectious and inflammatory conditions. *Acute mediastinitis* is more common than the chronic form and may be caused by esophageal or tracheobronchial perforation, penetrating chest trauma, postoperative sternal wound infection, extension of an oropharyngeal infection or a paravertebral or vertebral abscess, radiation therapy, malignancy, and rarely anthrax. Patients with acute mediastinitis usually have had sudden onset of high fever, chills, chest pain, dyspnea, and dysphagia. Physical examination may reveal systemic toxicity, respiratory distress, Hamman sign, subcutaneous emphysema, chest wall tenderness, and edema. Chest radiography and CT show mediastinal widening, pneumomediastinum, mediastinal air–fluid levels or fluid collections, and pleural effusions. An esophagram may reveal perforation. Acute mediastinitis is a generally diffuse process but may be localized when secondary to sternal wound infection. The treatment includes surgical drainage, débridement, repair of the traumatic injury, and broad-spectrum antibiotics. The mortality rate is high, especially when the diagnosis is delayed.

Chronic mediastinitis, also termed *fibrosing* or *granulomatous* mediastinitis, is caused by various infectious and inflammatory processes. Histoplasmosis and tuberculosis account for most cases. Noninfectious causes include mediastinal hematoma, radiation therapy, and drugs such as methysergide and hydralazine. Chronic mediastinitis can be associated with various idiopathic and autoimmune diseases, such as retroperitoneal fibrosis, Riedel thyroiditis, pseudotumor of the orbit, sclerosing cholangitis, systemic lupus erythematosus, and rheumatoid arthritis. Dense fibrous tissue, usually located in the paratracheal, carinal, and hilar regions, compresses and obstructs mediastinal structures, such as the superior vena cava, pulmonary vessels, airways, and esophagus. *Superior vena cava syndrome* is the most common clinical manifestation. Chest radiographs, CT, MRI, and perfusion scintigraphy, in addition to endoscopy, help to suggest the diagnosis. The typical CT finding is an infiltrative mediastinal soft tissue mass with calcification and coexistent pulmonary or hepatosplenic calcified granulomas. Noncalcified lesions present a diagnostic dilemma and require exclusion of malignancy. Histologic examination of mediastinal tissue may be necessary to exclude a malignant neoplasm or active infection. Treatment is ineffective and mostly palliative; the benefit of corticosteroids is controversial. In the presence of viable fungal organisms or rising serum antibody titers, antifungal agents can be administered. For patients with superior vena cava syndrome, long-term anticoagulation and vascular stents may be effective.

Pneumomediastinum

Pneumomediastinum is typically caused by overdistention and rupture of alveoli because of increased intrathoracic volume or pressure that results from mechanical ventilation, blunt trauma, asthma, or spontaneous rupture. Air dissects along the pulmonary interstitium into the peribronchovascular tissues and mediastinum and frequently decompresses into the soft tissues of the neck. Less often, pneumomediastinum can be secondary to tracheobronchial or esophageal perforation, a gas-forming infection, traumatic direct entry of air, cervical soft tissue air, or pneumoperitoneum that tracks into the mediastinum.

Mediastinal Hemorrhage

Mediastinal hemorrhage can be spontaneous from rupture of a thoracic or other vascular aneurysm or dissection or can result from blunt or penetrating trauma or invasive medical procedures. Chest radiography typically reveals mediastinal widening. Unenhanced chest CT may show hyperdense areas within the mediastinum or aortic wall, and contrast-enhanced chest CT may reveal an intimal flap or dissection, a contained pseudoaneurysm, or frank extravasation of blood into the mediastinum, pericardium, or pleural space. The treatment depends on the cause and location of the source of bleeding and typically involves surgical repair, especially when the ascending thoracic aorta is involved.

DIFFERENTIAL DIAGNOSIS

Many mediastinal masses are benign and are found incidentally in asymptomatic patients. Large lesions may manifest with symptoms related to compression of adjacent structures. Aggressive or malignant neoplasms may produce constitutional symptoms, paraneoplastic syndromes, invasion of adjacent structures, or metastases. The radiologic evaluation of affected patients begins with chest radiography and is followed by cross-sectional imaging with CT and occasionally MRI. CT is useful in excluding vascular lesions and some benign causes of mediastinal widening, such as lipomatosis. In addition, confident diagnosis can be established for some lesions, including mature teratoma, mediastinal goiter, pericardial cyst, foregut duplication cyst, herniations, and lateral thoracic meningocele. Adjacent structures may also be evaluated for mass effect or invasion. Patients with primary mediastinal masses and cysts usually undergo surgical resection. The presence of lymphadenopathy (in patients with lymphoma and metastatic disease) or certain positive tumor markers may prompt limited biopsy sampling of the lesion, followed by oncologic consultation and chemotherapy with radiation therapy when appropriate. Resection of residual neoplasm will follow in some patients.

The most common *primary anterior mediastinal masses* are thymoma, substernal goiter, and lymphoma. All other lesions are extremely rare. In the correct clinical setting, patients with an anterior mediastinal mass should have serologic evaluation for detection of antibodies to acetylcholine receptors or elevation of AFP and β-HCG to exclude MG and nonseminomatous malignant germ cell neoplasm, respectively. Most primary thymic neoplasms arise in one lobe of the thymus and exhibit unilateral growth; thus an anterior mediastinal mass that extends across the midline is likely an aggressive neoplasm or diffuse malignant lymphadenopathy. Whereas thymoma typically manifests as a homogeneous unilateral thymic mass, *invasive thymoma* may exhibit irregular margins, invasion of mediastinal tissue planes and structures, and drop metastases. Mature teratoma typically manifests as a large, unilateral,

multilocular cystic mass that often exhibits intrinsic fat and calcification. *Intrathoracic goiter* almost always results from contiguous extension of a cervical goiter. *Lymphoma* may affect any mediastinal compartment and classically manifests as lymph node enlargement. The diagnosis is frequently made by biopsy of a palpable peripheral lymph node, and mediastinal involvement is determined by cross-sectional imaging studies. Diagnostic problems may arise when lymphoma manifests with primary mediastinal lymphadenopathy or focal mass. Pericardial cysts are often followed clinically and on imaging.

Middle-posterior mediastinal masses include lesions from many causes. Mediastinal lymphadenopathy is common and may be of benign or malignant etiology to include lymphoma and advanced lung cancer. Mediastinal cysts are typically congenital, classically affect predominantly the middle-posterior mediastinal compartment, and are often surgically excised because of the high incidence of symptoms and complications. Radiologic characteristics can establish the diagnosis of congenital cysts in most cases.

Neurogenic neoplasms are common paravertebral masses. On the basis of morphology, patient age, and presence or absence of symptoms or associated conditions, a prospective diagnosis can usually be established. Lesions of *peripheral nerve* origin typically affect asymptomatic adults, have a spherical morphology, and are cured by excision. Multiple lesions suggest the diagnosis of neurofibromatosis. Neoplasms of *sympathetic ganglia* origin usually affect children and young adults, have an elongate morphology, and have a variable prognosis because of higher frequency of malignant histologic types. Preoperative assessment usually includes MRI to exclude intraspinal extension, with serum and urine catecholamines in some cases to exclude elevated levels and malignancy or clinically active neoplasms. Lateral thoracic meningoceles may mimic neurogenic neoplasms on radiography but are readily diagnosed on cross-sectional imaging.

SUGGESTED READINGS

Boiselle PM, Rosado-de-Christenson ML: Fat attenuation lesions of the mediastinum (pictorial essay), *J Comput Assist Tomogr* 26:881–889, 2001.

Cronin CG, Swords R, Truong MT, et al: Clinical utility of PET/CT in lymphoma, *AJR Am J Roentgenol* 194:W91–W103, 2010.

Henschke CI, Lee IJ, Wu N, et al: CT screening for lung cancer: prevalence and incidence of mediastinal masses, *Radiology* 239:586–590, 2006.

Kim JH, Goo JM, Lee JJ, Chung MJ, et al: Cystic tumors of the anterior mediastinum: radiologic-pathologic correlation, *J Comput Assist Tomogr* 27:714–723, 2003.

Kumar A, Regmi SK, Dutta R, et al: Characterization of thymic masses using (18)F-FDG-PET-CT, *Ann Nucl Med* 23:569–577, 2009.

Rankin S: [(18)F]2-fluoro-2-deoxy-D-glucose PET/CT in mediastinal masses, *Cancer Imaging* 10(spec A):156–160, 2010.

Shepard JO, Maher MM: Imaging of thymoma, *Semin Thorac Cardiovasc Surg* 17:12–19, 2005.

Takahashi K, Al-Janabi NJ: Computed tomography and magnetic resonance imaging of mediastinal tumors, *J Magn Reson Imaging* 32:1325–1339, 2010.

Tanaka O, Kiryu T, Hirose Y, et al: Neurogenic tumors of the mediastinum and chest wall: MR imaging appearance, *J Thorac Imaging* 20:316–320, 2005.

Tateishi U, Muller NL, Johkoh T, et al: Primary mediastinal lymphoma: characteristic features of various histologic subtypes on CT, *J Comput Assist Tomogr* 28:782–789, 2004.

Tian L, Liu LZ, Cui CY, et al: CT findings of primary non-teratomatous germ cell tumors of the mediastinum: a report of 15 cases, *Eur J Radiol* 2011. [Epub ahead of print].

Chapter **72**
Chest Tube Insertion and Management
Stephen D. Cassivi • Claude Deschamps • Nicholas J. Pastis

The pleural cavity can require drainage when, in pathologic states, it contains air (pneumothorax), blood (hemothorax), serum (pleural effusion), lymph (chylothorax), or pus (empyema), or a combination of these. In the presence of these abnormal collections, the pleural cavity pressure may become positive, allowing the lung to collapse partially or fully, leading to hypoxemia. A common procedure used to drain air or fluid collections is the insertion of a chest tube (tube thoracostomy). A properly placed chest tube provides for drainage of air and/or fluid, reestablishes a negative intrapleural pressure, and allows the lung to reexpand within the pleural space. The correct management of a patient who needs a chest tube requires not only the skill to insert it safely, position it well, and minimize discomfort, but also the judgment to know when it is indicated and how to manage it properly after its placement. This requirement implies a sound knowledge of the principles of surgical drains and a working knowledge of the underwater seal drainage system being used.

INDICATIONS AND CONTRAINDICATIONS

Conditions associated with acute or severe respiratory compromise are considered absolute indications for chest tube placement and include tension pneumothorax, large symptomatic pneumothorax, hemothorax, empyema, and previous surgical violation of the pleural space (**Box 72-1**). In addition, under less clear-cut circumstances, appropriate judgment and experience will be required to help determine whether a chest tube is needed or not. Alternatives to chest tube placement, such as observation, thoracentesis, or formal operative drainage, must be considered and the choice individualized according to the clinical situation. Special caution is necessary when the patient's preoperative assessment findings point to an increased possibility of coagulopathy, intrapleural adhesions, or abnormal intrathoracic anatomy. The only contraindications to chest tube placement are a fused pleural space and lack of operative personnel with adequate experience in use of the technique for a safe and effective procedure. In considering placement of a chest tube, either of these circumstances should prompt consultation with a thoracic surgeon.

TECHNIQUE

The technique of chest tube insertion has been described in many publications. A focused yet comprehensive history and physical examination should precede any surgical procedure, even when it is done at the bedside. Chest radiographs and computed tomography (CT) scans, if available, should be thoroughly reviewed before and readily available during the procedure. When possible, a full discussion with the patient, including the specific indication, associated risks, alternatives, and postprocedural care, is indicated before proceeding with insertion of the pleural drain.

SELECTION OF DRAIN TUBE

At present, the most common tube used for chest drainage is a Silastic tube with multiple side holes. It usually has a linear radiopaque stripe running through the most proximal hole (allowing its location to be identified on chest radiographs) and markings to indicate distance in centimeters from the most proximal hole (**Figure 72-1**). These tubes range in size (gauge) up to 40 French (40F). Of note, some tube insertion kits come with a central trochar within the chest tube. Routine use of this trochar is unnecessary, can be dangerous, and is to be discouraged. Smaller chest tubes (14F or smaller) also are available, which can be placed using a Seldinger technique without the need for blunt dissection.

The size of the drain will depend on the indication for insertion and the size of the patient. In general, larger drains are more uncomfortable for the patient and more difficult to insert with use of local anesthesia. Conversely, smaller tubes usually are better tolerated by patients. Traditional consensus among experts has been that smaller chest tubes (14F or smaller) are more likely to clog with thick fluid or particulate matter, as encountered in a hemothorax or empyema, and are more prone to drainage problems from obstruction due to kinking of the tubing. Historically, a general rule has been that most collections are adequately drained with use of a 28F or 32F chest tube. Usually, a simple pneumothorax requires only a small chest tube (14F or smaller), although larger tubes (24F or larger) should be strongly considered for patients on positive-pressure ventilation.

Recently, however, a randomized controlled trial showed that in patients with pleural infection managed with use of smaller chest tubes (14F or smaller), duration of hospital stay, changes on the chest radiograph, and lung function at 3 months were no different from those in patients in whom larger chest tubes were used. In addition, no significant difference was observed in the frequency of either postprocedure death or requirement for thoracic surgery. Pain scores were substantially higher in patients receiving larger tubes. These results suggest that use of smaller-sized tubes may be preferable in the initial treatment of pleural infection.

Placement of long-term indwelling pleural drains also has become a commonly considered technique for the palliation of malignant pleural effusions. The specific technique and indications for use of these drains are discussed later in the chapter.

Box 72-1   Indications for Chest Tube Insertion

Pneumothorax
   Spontaneous
   Traumatic
   Iatrogenic
Pleural effusion (hydrothorax)
   Benign
   Malignant
Hemothorax
   Traumatic
   Iatrogenic
Empyema
Chylothorax
Postoperative (cardiothoracic surgical procedures)

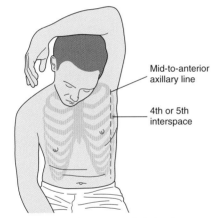

Figure 72-1   Silastic chest tubes. *Top to bottom*: Multiholed straight and angled Silastic chest tubes and Kelly clamp.

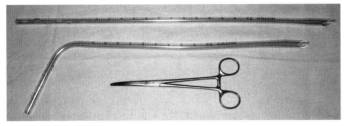

Mid-to-anterior
axillary line

4th or 5th
interspace

Figure 72-2   Preferred site for intercostal drain placement: at a point along the mid-to-anterior axillary line, in the fourth or fifth interspace.

DRAIN INSERTION SITE AND PATIENT POSITIONING

Generally, the optimal site for placement of a chest tube is through the fourth or fifth interspace in the anterior to midaxillary line just beyond the lateral edge of the pectoralis muscle and breast tissue (**Figure 72-2**). This insertion site has the advantage of relatively easy access and avoids the discomfort of a more posteriorly placed tube in patients who often are primarily lying supine in a hospital bed. In addition, it usually is high enough to avoid inadvertent subdiaphragmatic placement yet low enough to adequately drain fluid. Of note, in patients who are primarily lying supine in bed with free-flowing pleural fluid collections, the interspace level of placement of the chest drain is much less important than ensuring the posterior positioning of the tube within the pleural space. Placement of a chest tube in the second or third interspace anteriorly is to be avoided if possible. Such placement does not provide any advantage over the lateral position described previously and is significantly more painful and disfiguring for the patient.

For elective chest drain insertion, the patient should be kept in a relatively comfortable position that facilitates placement of the tube in the location described earlier. Usually, this can be achieved by placing the patient supine or in a semi-Fowler position (with thorax and head elevated 30 to 45 degrees) with the involved side elevated approximately 30 to 45 degrees on wedges or pillows. To improve access to the lateral chest wall, the patient's arm on the involved side is brought above the head (**Figure 72-3**). As with most thoracic procedures, the operator should stand at the patient's back.

PREPARATION, ANESTHESIA, AND INCISION

Before positioning of the patient, all necessary equipment should be made available (**Box 72-2**). A deliberate pause should be taken to verify the patient's identity and to confirm the procedure and correct operative side. When possible, the most recent chest radiograph should be posted in a readily visible location as a separate safety measure to avoid wrong-sided procedures.

The chest wall is cleansed with antiseptic solution and draped in such a way as to provide an operative field approximately 20 cm by 20 cm in size. The skin is infiltrated with 1% lidocaine at the chosen site of insertion with use of a 21-gauge

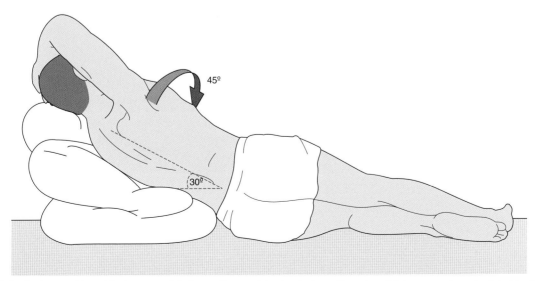

Figure 72-3   Patient positioned for intercostal drainage. The trunk is elevated on pillows to a 30-degree angle and rotated by 45 degrees.

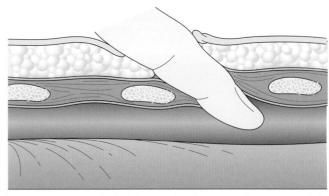

Figure 72-4 For optimal drainage tube placement, the operator's index finger is inserted along the drain tract to exclude adhesions and confirm entry into the chest cavity. Notice that the tract has been created in the interspace over the upper surface of the rib.

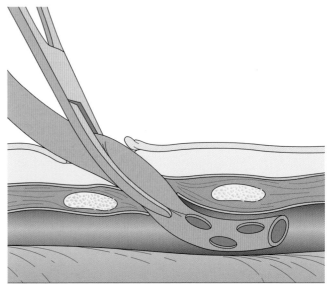

Figure 72-5 Use of a Kelly clamp to guide drain insertion.

needle. Further generous infiltration of the subcutaneous tissues can be done with use of a large-bore needle (18-gauge). Aspirating before injection with this needle will prevent inadvertent vascular injection, as well as indicating the direction and depth of the parietal pleura. The parietal pleura are extremely sensitive and must therefore be thoroughly anesthetized.

A 2-cm transverse incision is made with the scalpel. The incision usually is made one interspace below the interspace planned for insertion, to allow "tunneling" over the superior border of the lower rib. At this stage, one stitch of 0-0 silk suture can be placed at the posterior margin of the incision and tied down, leaving the two ends even and uncut. This suture will be used later to secure the chest tube. Placing the stitch at this point, before initial dissection and entry into the pleural space with its requisite drainage of fluid or air, is much easier. It allows for much more efficient securing of the chest tube once in place within the pleural cavity. In an obese patient, it may be necessary to increase the size of the initial skin incision to permit adequate palpation of the ribs and interspaces.

DRAIN INSERTION

After completion of the initial incision and placement of the securing stitch, a curved Kelly clamp is used to dissect a tract for the chest tube within the subcutaneous and intercostal tissues. "Tunneling" of this tract over the superior border of the lower rib prevents damage to the intercostal neurovascular bundle that lies along the inferior border of each rib. It also reduces the likelihood of air leak at the time of chest tube removal and thereafter while the incision site heals.

Dissecting by use of the Kelly clamp is done with incremental spreading and advancement of the clamp to create a tract for the chest tube. It is important to dissect along only one tract, to avoid subsequent difficulties in finding the dissected path at the moment of tube insertion. This precaution is especially relevant in obese patients. The pleura can be very taut or thickened and can sometimes present significant resistance to entry. Extreme care must be taken on entering the pleural cavity with the Kelly clamp, to control its forward progress and prevent inadvertent entry into underlying structures. Entry into the pleural cavity is signaled by egress of air or fluid and sudden decrease in resistance to forward movement of the clamp. For the patient, breaching of the parietal pleura usually is the most uncomfortable part of the procedure, and it often is useful to provide further local anesthetic to the area before piercing the pleural cavity.

Once the parietal pleura have been breached, the clamp is withdrawn in the open position. The next step is to insert the operator's index finger into the pleural cavity to ensure pleural entry (to exclude subdiaphragmatic placement) and assess for the presence of pleural adhesions and pleural lesions or nodularity (**Figure 72-4**). The chest tube can then be guided into place by use of the Kelly clamp, as illustrated in **Figure 72-5**. Careful placement is an important part of the procedure and, regrettably, often is rushed because of either patient discomfort or ongoing fluid or air leakage. Proper functioning of the tube requires that care be taken at this point to deliberately direct the tube in the desired position. In the most common scenario, in a patient who will for the most part be supine, the tube should be guided posteriorly and then directed cephalad. A tube positioned in this fashion will drain both air and fluid satisfactorily in most cases. To ensure a posterior placement of the drain, the tip of the tube, once in the pleural cavity, must be deliberately directed posteriorly before being advanced. Failure to perform this specific maneuver often will lead to malposition of the tube, either in an anterior direction or within the major fissure, which will then function poorly.

Once the chest tube is positioned correctly, it can be secured in place with the previously placed suture and connected by tubing to the underwater seal chest drainage system

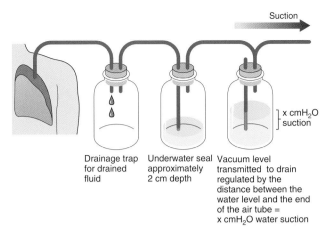

Suction

x cmH$_2$O suction

Drainage trap for drained fluid

Underwater seal approximately 2 cm depth

Vacuum level transmitted to drain regulated by the distance between the water level and the end of the air tube = x cmH$_2$O water suction

Figure 72-6   Underwater seal chest drainage system. Commercially available systems incorporate a multichamber device in one casing that includes (1) a collection chamber to collect fluid and particulate drainage; (2) a waterseal chamber and manometer to ensure one-way egress of air from the pleural space and monitor intrapleural pressures; and (3) suction regulator to control the level of intrapleural suction being applied.

(Figure 72-6). A light dressing is applied to the drain site, and a chest radiograph is obtained to confirm proper tube placement.

CHEST TUBE MANAGEMENT

Specific chest tube management usually is predicated on the condition initially requiring chest drainage. It is nonetheless important to consider the general principles of chest tube management, as well as specific situations that require a particular remedy or response.

GENERAL PRINCIPLES

Once inserted, the chest tube should be closely monitored for the nature (air, fluid, or both) and quantity (slight, moderate, or large air leak or volume of fluid) of pleural drainage. Changes in these parameters, especially if abrupt, should be noted, because they provide important information regarding current pathologic status in the pleural space or drainage system malfunction. The amount of fluid drained hourly should be recorded.

Suction usually is applied to the underwater seal device initially after tube placement, to promote drainage and ensure a negative intrapleural pressure. The amount of suction applied usually is –20 cm of water. It should be emphasized that suction is provided by the underwater seal device and is never directly applied to the chest tube; the former is controlled, whereas the latter may lead to pulmonary or vascular injury. Suction usually can be discontinued and the patient's tube left on "water seal" early in the course of chest tube management if drainage is adequate and the pleural process is resolving. Under certain circumstances, chest tube suction is to be avoided—for example, with placement of a chest tube after a pneumonectomy, or in patients with emphysema and a prominent air leak, such as after lung volume reduction surgery.

A number of observable clues to the functional status of the chest tube and the current status of the pleural space are recognized. Oscillations ("tidaling") of the fluid levels in the water seal or tubing leading to the water seal that are synchronous with the patient's respiratory cycle demonstrate the chest

drain is patent and communicating with the pleural space. It also indicates that the lung has not completely reexpanded to fill the entire pleural space. The situation in which fluid is allowed to pool in dependent portions of tubing connecting the chest drain to the underwater seal device is to be avoided. This condition creates an increased resistance to proper drainage of air and will delay the resolution of the intrapleural process. This problem can be avoided by educating the nursing staff to this potential problem and having them intermittently drain the dependent loop of tubing.

AIR LEAK

When bubbling is observed in the underwater seal device, especially if this is a new or unexpected finding or if the bubbling is continuous (not in cycle with respiration), a thorough survey of the drainage apparatus must be undertaken. An air leak occurring anywhere in the tubing, from the insertion site at the skin to the underwater seal device, as well as any connectors in between, can cause bubbling to appear in the water seal chamber. This can be assessed by placing a clamp on the tubing as near to the insertion site as possible. Bubbling will continue when there is a leak in the tubing. The location of the tubing breach can be found by sequentially moving the clamp toward the underwater seal device and checking at each application for continued bubbling. Air leaks often occur at the connection joint of the chest drain to the underwater seal device's tubing. Once the leak has been located, the damaged tubing or connector should be replaced. The practice of taping the tubing connection joints probably will not prevent or treat occult air leaks but may be useful in reducing the incidence of inadvertent disconnection of the tubing. Unfortunately, a disconnection can still occur, and it may not be as easy to notice underneath a layer of tape. At our hospital, this practice has been replaced with the "banding" of each connection point with a disposable circumferential ratcheted plastic appliance.

CHEST TUBE CLAMPING

In general, chest tube clamping should be avoided. In a few instances, clamping may be necessary or can be a useful adjunct in tube management. Chest drains should be clamped proximally (nearer to the patient) during changing of the tubing or underwater seal device. "Diagnostic" clamping also may be necessary to troubleshoot a continuous air leak when a leak in the tubing system is suspected. Chest tube clamping at the time of drain insertion to prevent reexpansion pulmonary edema is described later in this chapter.

Before removal of a chest tube that has an intermittent or persistent low-grade leak or a wide oscillation of fluid in the tubing, it may be useful to simulate chest tube removal by clamping it for a short period of time (1 to 2 hours). A chest radiograph is then obtained. If the lung remains expanded and there is no evidence of increasing subcutaneous emphysema despite the tube's being clamped, the chest tube can then be removed. If, however, the radiograph shows a pneumothorax or increasing subcutaneous emphysema, or if the patient becomes symptomatic with shortness of breath or pain, the clamp should be promptly removed. Patients in whom the chest tube is clamped for this reason must be closely monitored for symptoms and clinical signs of worsening dyspnea or reaccumulation of the pneumothorax. Routine use of tube clamping before chest tube removal is unnecessary.

CHEST TUBE REMOVAL

Chest tubes are removed when the indication for their placement has resolved: when air leaks have stopped, fluid loss has diminished to a minimal rate (usually less than 300 mL/24 hours), and chest radiography shows the lung to be well expanded. Patients still requiring positive-pressure ventilation with high peak airway pressures are at high risk for new or recurrent air leaks because of barotrauma. In these situations, a chest tube that otherwise would be removed because it has accomplished the drainage for which it was placed should be left in place until the patient has been extubated or the risks of barotrauma have been minimized.

Many techniques are described for chest tube removal, but we recommend the following sequence: After the drain stitch holding the tube in place at the skin has been cut, the patient is asked to take as deep a breath as possible and hold it. Once the patient reaches maximal inspiration, the drain is gently yet swiftly removed. An airtight dressing is then applied to the drain exit site. In our own practice, this method has proved to be the most reliable way to avoid ingress of air into the pleural cavity during chest tube removal. At maximal inspiration, the portion of the respiratory cycle with the most negative intrapleural pressure has been completed. Then, if the patient experiences any discomfort during the removal of the chest drain, the only possible respiratory maneuver at this point will be exhalation, causing increased positive intrapleural pressure and favoring egress of any pleural air.

Some clinicians emphasize the need for a pursestring or mattress stitch to be placed at the time of tube insertion so that this can be tied down at the time of drain removal to ensure wound closure. In our experience, this is not an absolute necessity, and we do not routinely use this adjunctive technique. This technique may potentially be useful in situations in which the chest tube has been in place for several weeks. Although it assists in securing a closure to the drain site, presence of this suture is associated with increased pain after drain removal and requires an early return visit to remove the stitch, 5 to 7 days later.

SPECIAL CONSIDERATIONS

INSERTION DIFFICULTIES

Negative Aspiration

The best opportunity to drain a pleural space is at the time of initial tube insertion. As mentioned previously, needle aspiration at the time of local anesthetic administration allows for confirmation of the presence of air or fluid. If, during needle aspiration, no air or fluid is encountered, further attempts should be made through higher and lower interspaces. If neither air nor fluid (as appropriate) is found, the procedure should be postponed and the situation reevaluated. Further imaging using imaging-guided techniques, for example, or with a more experienced hand, may be required. Failure to follow these precautions may convert a minor difficulty into an emergency, with inadvertent insertion of a drain into the lung or other viscera.

Intrapleural Adhesions

Patients with previous ipsilateral cardiothoracic procedures or a history of a previous pleural process are at increased risk for formation of significant pleural adhesions. These factors should always be taken into consideration in decisions regarding placement of a chest tube. Intrapleural adhesions are detected by palpation. If thin and flimsy, they often can be swept away sufficiently, using the operator's finger, to allow the drain to be inserted safely. If the adhesions are stout, they should be left in place, because further attempts to take these down by finger sweeping may cause tearing and bleeding of the lung or pleural surfaces. The chest tube often can still be inserted and advanced gently to find its own way around various areas of adhesion. If, however, a complete pleural symphysis is encountered, the procedure should be aborted and its indications reconsidered.

Subdiaphragmatic Placement

A chest tube may be incorrectly placed under the diaphragm if the insertion site is chosen too low on the chest or if the diaphragm is elevated higher than expected. This error occurs usually when the operator incorrectly interprets a lower chest opacification as fluid rather than considering the possibility of a raised hemidiaphragm. This mistake usually can be identified when the operator performs finger palpation after breaching the "pleura." If no intraabdominal injuries have occurred, the insertion site can simply be closed, and a higher insertion is then undertaken. Careful monitoring for abdominal injuries is continued after the procedure is properly completed.

This error can be avoided with the recognition that most patients will be for the most part supine during the course of chest drainage after the tube is inserted. Therefore, in free-flowing pleural fluid collections, the positioning of the tube in the pleural space posteriorly is much more important than a low-lying insertion site, which increases the risk of subdiaphragmatic placement.

Impaled Structure

An impaled structure necessitates urgent surgical referral. As with many complications, the optimal management in this situation is to take every measure possible to prevent occurrence of this mishap. As mentioned previously, the use of trocars to assist with chest tube placement may predispose to this type of injury. The use of the technique of blunt finger palpation to guide the drain insertion will avoid this serious injury in most cases.

DIFFICULT MANAGEMENT ISSUES

Subcutaneous Emphysema

Subcutaneous emphysema is a result of leakage of air under sufficient pressure to track into the subcutaneous tissues. As with any gas or fluid, air under pressure will seek the exit path of least resistance. If a chest drain is occluded either by kinking, clamping, or clogging of the tubing with fibrinous material or clot, continued air leak from the pulmonary parenchyma will seek a different path of exit from the pleural space. This also can occur if a volume of "stagnant" fluid remains in a dependent loop of the connecting tubing, as described previously. The increased intrapleural pressure will promote lung collapse and subsequent tracking of air through breaches in the parietal pleura into the subcutaneous tissues.

If subcutaneous emphysema develops, a thorough evaluation of the tubing and collection system is indicated. A chest radiograph is important to assess the lung. Any obstruction within the tubing must be cleared to favor egress of air through the drain over any other pathway. An initial maneuver to consider is to restart suction on the drain by means of the underwater seal device. If the tubing is patent, restarting suction may be all that is needed. Evaluation of the pleural space with computed tomography (CT) may help identify the area

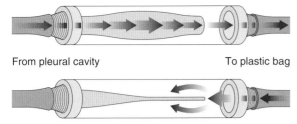

Figure 72-7 Heimlich valve. Air expelled from the pleural cavity opens the flutter valve (*upper*); when pleural pressure falls below atmospheric pressure, the flutter valve is compressed and sealed to prevent inflow of air.

requiring further drainage. The parenchymal air leak may be of such magnitude that a second chest tube is required. On rare occasions, surgical repair of the air leak may be necessary.

Subcutaneous emphysema can be quite disfiguring and thus extremely distressing to affected patients and their families. Appropriate management should therefore include reassurance that although dramatic in appearance, this is rarely a dangerous situation, that the condition usually will require more time to resolve than it took to appear, but that it will ultimately resolve.

Prolonged Air Leak

A prolonged air leak usually is defined as one that persists for more than 1 week. This problem may be secondary to a number of causes. If the air leak is not amenable to surgical repair and is expected to eventually heal spontaneously, a prolonged hospital stay often can be avoided with the use of a Heimlich valve (**Figure 72-7**). As an integral component of a passive drainage system, this one-way flutter valve allows air and fluid to be expelled from the chest cavity while preventing air from entering the pleural space. The patient can be discharged with instructions to return on a weekly basis for a chest radiograph to evaluate the resolution of the air leak.

Special attention must be paid to the attachment of the Heimlich valve to ensure that it is attached in the proper direction. Otherwise, air can be trapped in the pleural space, leading to collapse of the lung and creating the potential for a tension pneumothorax.

Drain Obstruction

Occasionally, a chest drain may become occluded with fibrinous debris or frank clot. If the intrapleural process initially warranting chest tube placement has not resolved, the chest tube occlusion must be cleared. This often can be achieved by "milking" or stripping the tubing. It should be recognized that such stripping of the tubing can create transient negative intrapleural pressures in excess of 400 cm H$_2$O. This maneuver is of questionable benefit and should therefore not be undertaken without the knowledge and consent of the primary surgeon or physician responsible for the chest tube. Another way to clear intraluminal blockage from the chest tube is to pass a Fogarty embolectomy catheter in retrograde fashion up the tube and then draw it back with the balloon inflated, thereby pulling out the debris. This should, of course, be done using meticulous sterile technique. If, after using the appropriate techniques described previously, the drain remains occluded, a new drain may need to be inserted and the occluded drain removed.

Failure of the Lung to Reexpand

After insertion of a chest tube, a frontal (anteroposterior) chest radiograph should be obtained to assess positioning of the tube

and resolution of the intrapleural process that required drain placement. If the lung has not fully reexpanded, an explanation must be sought from among the following scenarios.

First, in the case of a large air leak or initially after lung resection, the lung may not have had enough time to fully reexpand, and no immediate action is necessary. Otherwise, proper intrapleural placement must be confirmed. Definitive confirmation may not be obtainable with the two-dimensional radiograph. It should, however, identify whether all of the chest tube holes are within the pleural space. If this is not the case, the tube may be drawing outside air into the pleural space and tube, thus preventing full reexpansion of the lung. A new sterile tube will then need to be inserted. If the radiograph suggests that all drain holes are appropriately within the pleural space but the lung still is not fully expanded, the explanation may be extrapleural insertion of the tube. Observing a complete lack of any drainage (air or fluid) or oscillation in the tubing can identify this problem. A lateral chest radiograph can help to confirm an intrapleural location of the tube; however, CT is more sensitive.

In cases of hemothorax, chronic pleural effusion, or empyema, the underlying lung may not be able to fully reexpand because of formation of a fibrinous peel or rind overlying the visceral pleura. Drainage of the fluid collection may be complete, yet it leaves an unresolved intrapleural space. If this space does not resolve over the course of a few days of suction applied to the chest drainage tube, surgical decortication may be necessary. Alternatively, bronchoscopy may be indicated to exclude endobronchial blockage preventing reexpansion of the underlying lung parenchyma.

Reexpansion Pulmonary Edema

For drainage of a large intrapleural fluid collection that is compressing underlying lung, consideration should be given to the extremely rare but potentially lethal phenomenon of *reexpansion pulmonary edema*. This pathologic process is due to rapid reexpansion of the previously compressed lung at the time of fluid drainage, leading to a rapid increase in blood flow and pulmonary capillary pressure. Consequent fluid shift across the capillary and alveolar membranes leads in turn to formation of excess extravascular fluid.

The first sign of this process usually is noted at chest tube insertion, when fluid drainage is rapid, at which point the patient begins to cough uncontrollably. Onset of coughing usually occurs when between 800 and 1500 mL of fluid has been acutely drained. When this is observed, the chest tube should be immediately clamped. This maneuver usually will control the patient's urge to cough and prevent further progression of the underlying pathologic process. A controlled drainage is then performed by intermittently unclamping the tube until resolution of the effusion is observed.

Septated Pleural Fluid Infections

In some patients with pleural infections, chest tube drainage may be curtailed or even blocked entirely by the presence of septations, leading to incomplete drainage of fluid through the tube. The breakdown of such septations with the use of fibrinolytic agents may result in improved pleural drainage.

Despite positive results in observational studies, randomized controlled trials of treatment with single fibrinolytic agents have surprisingly not shown a benefit over standard chest tube drainage. However, a randomized controlled trial has demonstrated that the use of combined intrapleural tPA and DNase delivered through chest tubes improved fluid drainage in patients with pleural infections, reduced the frequency of surgical referrals, and shortened hospital stays.

MALIGNANT PLEURAL EFFUSIONS

Malignant pleural effusions require both skill and judgment to effect an optimal palliation for the patient. The important point to recognize in these circumstances is that palliation of dyspnea secondary to fluid compression of the lung is the goal of treatment. In situations in which the patient is close to death, because of progression of the underlying malignancy or other organ dysfunction, it may be appropriate not to proceed with any further invasive maneuvers. If, however, the decision is made to intervene, several therapeutic options are available, including repeated ultrasound-guided thoracenteses, chest tube placement with chemical pleurodesis, and long-term indwelling pleural drain placement. An in-depth discussion of thoracentesis is presented elsewhere in this book.

THERAPEUTIC OPTIONS

Chest Tube With Chemical Pleurodesis

Palliation of a malignant pleural effusion can be achieved by chemical pleurodesis that attempts to obliterate the pleural space, thereby preventing reaccumulation of pleural fluid. This procedure can be accomplished either thoracoscopically with the instillation of a sclerosant on the pleural surfaces or at the bedside by injection of the sclerosant through a chest tube. In most cases, the pleurodesis agent of choice is talc. It produces an inflammatory reaction on the visceral and parietal pleural surfaces that leads to adhesion formation and pleural fusion when these surfaces are in direct apposition. In some instances, an idiosyncratic reaction can occur in which the entire lung becomes inflamed, leading to severe pneumonitis and respiratory distress. For this reason, synchronous bilateral chemical pleurodeses should never be attempted. Recovery after the initial one-sided pleurodesis should be ascertained before embarking on treating the contralateral side, if needed.

Chemical pleurodesis is optimally effective if the lung can completely reexpand, allowing apposition of the visceral and parietal pleural surfaces. Without this contact, as in the case of a "trapped lung," the therapy will be ineffective. Thoracoscopy not only allows evaluation of the ability of the lung to reexpand but also permits complete evacuation of the pleural effusion before instillation of the sclerosant.

Long-Term Indwelling Pleural Drain

With malignant pleural effusions in which the underlying lung is trapped because of tumor or pleural rind, chemical pleurodesis is not the optimal palliative option. If repeated thoracenteses are not wanted, a long-term indwelling pleural drain can be inserted for decompression and consequent relief of dyspnea secondary to recurrent malignant fluid accumulation. This device can be placed by a modified Seldinger technique using local anesthesia or at the time of thoracoscopy. The drain is tunneled under the skin for approximately 7 to 8 cm before entry into the pleural fluid collection. A Teflon cuff built into the drain is positioned just underneath the drain exit site from the skin. The tunneling and use of the Teflon cuff are measures that reduce the likelihood of infection and dislodgment.

These drains are constructed with a one-way valve device at the external end that allows patient self-management of a chronic pleural effusion by drainage on a regular basis, without the risk and inconvenience of repeated thoracenteses. Of interest, in our own experience, even in cases in which the lung has been "trapped" and does not initially fully reexpand, after 8 to 10 weeks of drainage by this method, a functional pleurodesis often can be achieved: The lung seems to gain some degree of reexpansion, along with drawing in of mediastinal, diaphragmatic, and other thoracic soft tissues around the previous fluid-containing cavity, such that no further fluid accumulates in the newly obliterated pleural space. When this occurs, the pleural drain can be removed in an outpatient setting. With use of local anesthesia, the Teflon cuff is freed up just beneath the skin, and the drainage tube is withdrawn.

SUGGESTED READINGS

Baumann MH: What size chest tube? What drainage system is ideal? And other chest tube management questions, *Curr Opin Pulm Med* 9:276–281, 2003.

Cerfolio RJ, Bass CS, Pask AH, Katholi CR: Predictors and treatment of persistent air leaks, *Ann Thorac Surg* 73:1727–1730, 2002.

Davies CW, Gleeson FV, Davies RJ (Pleural Diseases Group, Standards of Care Committee, British Thoracic Society): BTS guidelines for the management of pleural infection, *Thorax* 58(Suppl 2):ii18–ii28, 2003.

Duncan C, Erickson R: Pressures associated with chest tube stripping, *Heart Lung* 11:166–171, 1982.

Gayer G, Rozenman J, Hoffmann C, et al: CT diagnosis of malpositioned chest tubes, *Br J Radiol* 73:786–790, 2000.

Gordon PA, Norton JM, Guerra JM, Perdue ST: Positioning of chest tubes: effects on pressure and drainage, *Am J Crit Care* 6:33–38, 1997.

Heffner JE: Multicenter trials of treatment for empyema—after all these years, *N Engl J Med* 352:926–928, 2005.

Ishikura H, Kimura S: The use of flexible silastic drains after chest surgery: novel thoracic drainage, *Ann Thorac Surg* 81:331–333, 2006.

Light RW: *Parapneumonic effusions and empyema. Pleural diseases*, Philadelphia, 2007, Wolters Kluwer, pp 179–210.

Murthy SC: Air leak and pleural space management, *Thorac Surg Clin* 16:261–265, 2006.

Puntillo K, Ley SJ: Appropriately timed analgesics control pain due to chest tube removal, *Am J Crit Care* 13:292–304, 2004.

Rahman N, Maskell N, Davies C, et al: The relationship between chest tube size and clinical outcomes in pleural infection, *Chest* 137:536–543, 2010.

Rahman N, Maskell N, West A, et al: Intrapleural use of tissue plasminogen activator and DNase in pleural infection, *N Engl J Med* 365:518–526, 2011.

Sewell RW, Fewel JG, Grover FL, Arom KV: Experimental evaluation of reexpansion pulmonary oedema, *Ann Thorac Surg* 26:126–132, 1978.

Tang AT, Velissaris TJ, Weeden DF: An evidence-based approach to drainage of the pleural cavity: evaluation of best practice, *J Eval Clin Pract* 8:333–340, 2002.

Chapter **73**

Preoperative Pulmonary Evaluation

Hilary Petersen • Peter Mazzone

Surgery can influence the patient's pulmonary function. Pulmonary complications of surgery are common, costly, and increase morbidity and mortality in both the near term and the long term. The preoperative assessment of lung function and optimization of the management of preexisting lung conditions can improve outcomes. This chapter discusses surgery-related changes in pulmonary physiology, the impact of common postoperative pulmonary complications, risk factors for these complications, and recommendations for preoperative pulmonary assessment and management, including those related to the evaluation of the lung resection candidate.

PULMONARY PHYSIOLOGY

During and after surgery, ventilation, ventilation-perfusion matching, and airway clearance are altered by many mechanisms. The mechanisms responsible and the degree of impairment are influenced by the type of surgery and the patient's underlying health. The following is a general description of potential physiologic changes related to surgery.

Ventilation   The supine position leads to decreases in all lung volumes, except tidal volume, because of the loss of the mechanical advantage provided by gravity. General anesthesia can worsen the restrictive defect in part through respiratory muscle relaxation and a shift of the balancing recoil forces of the lung and chest wall. Lung and chest wall mechanics are altered by surgery, particularly sternotomy, thoracotomy, and upper abdominal procedures. Diaphragm dysfunction and basal atelectasis may persist long after surgery. The residual effects of anesthesia can impair ventilatory drive in the immediate postoperative period. Shallow breathing related to pain and the effects of opiate use also contribute. In combination, functional residual capacity (FRC) can fall up to 50% for as long as 1 week in high-risk patients undergoing high-risk procedures.

Ventilation-Perfusion Matching   The reduction in FRC can be significant enough to result in atelectatic areas of the lung. Decreases in mucociliary clearance and the cough reflex secondary to anesthetic and opiate use and shallow breathing as a result of pain further contribute to the development of atelectasis. In atelectatic areas of the lung, ideal ventilation-perfusion matching shifts toward shunting where blood flow continues but ventilation is reduced or absent. This effect can be magnified by volatile anesthetic agents that influence hypoxic vasoconstriction. The end result of these changes is postoperative hypoxemia. Anemia and increased oxygen consumption may also contribute to observed oxygenation problems.

Airway Clearance   Many of these mechanisms impair the postoperative patient's ability to clear their airways of mucus. Respiratory muscle dysfunction, atelectasis, pain, and medication use, resulting in a decreased cough reflex or decreased mucociliary clearance, are contributing factors.

POSTOPERATIVE PULMONARY COMPLICATIONS

The frequency of postoperative pulmonary complications (PPCs) varies with type of surgery, the patient's health, and the definition of the complication. Pulmonary complications of surgery are at least as common as cardiac complications and may result in prolonged hospital stays, increased morbidity and mortality, and increased costs (**Table 73-1**).

RISK FACTORS

The many risk factors for PPCs can be classified as patient or surgery related and assigned a simple rating based on the amount and quality of evidence available for support as a risk factor (**Table 73-2**).

Patient-Related Factors

In several studies, chronic obstructive pulmonary disease (COPD) has been found to double the risk of PPCs. The degree of risk is directly related to the severity of obstruction. One study of patients after upper abdominal surgery found that those with decreased breath sounds or other adventitious sounds (e.g., wheezing, rales) had a sixfold increased rate of PPCs.

In contrast, well-controlled *asthma* has not been found to be a risk factor for PPCs. A large retrospective analysis found that rates of bronchospasm, laryngospasm, and respiratory failure in patients with well-controlled asthma were comparable to healthy individuals. Those with poorly controlled asthma (e.g., more frequent albuterol use, recent emergency department visit for asthma) do have an increased risk for PPCs.

Pulmonary hypertension (PH), primary and secondary, may be associated with increased rates of PPCs and in-hospital mortality. In one study, 21% of patients with PH developed respiratory failure versus 3% in matched controls after noncardiac surgery.

A patient's general health may be assessed by using the American Society of Anesthesiologists (ASA) classification system (**Table 73-3**). Studies have shown a direct correlation between a higher ASA class and increased pulmonary complications. Patients with an ASA Class III or higher have a twofold to threefold increase in PPCs compared with those with ASA Class II or lower. Difficulty or inability to perform activities of daily living has also been linked to increased complications.

Table 73-1	Postoperative Pulmonary Complications
Surgery in General	**Lung Resection Surgery**
AECOPD*	Bronchopleural fistulas
Acute lung injury	Empyema
Aspiration events	Nerve injury (phrenic, recurrent laryngeal)
Atelectasis	
Bronchitis and pneumonias	Pleural effusions
Bronchospasm	Pulmonary edema
Pulmonary embolism	Postpneumonectomy syndrome
Respiratory failure	Pulmonary torsion

*Acute exacerbation of chronic obstructive pulmonary disease.

Obesity alone does not seem to increase the risk of PPCs. A wide review of gastric and general surgeries shows that obese and morbidly obese patients have the same risk for PPCs as nonobese patients. However, the presence of a common comorbidity in obese patients, *obstructive sleep apnea* (OSA), does confer increased risk. In a study of patients after hip or knee replacement, those with OSA had longer hospital stays or more frequent transfers to the intensive care unit (ICU). A more recent study found that those with five or more desaturation episodes during the night had greatly increased rates of PPCs. Therefore, patients should be asked about symptoms of OSA preoperatively.

Age is the most significant patient-related predictor for PPCs. Even after adjustment for comorbid conditions, increasing age is an independent risk factor for increased PPCs. Congestive heart failure (CHF) is also an independent risk factor and should be of particular concern in the elderly population.

Cigarette smokers have a moderately increased risk for PPCs, independent of comorbid lung conditions. Smokers have higher rates of wound infections, oxygen desaturation, laryngospasm, and increased coughing with anesthesia, all of which can lead to longer hospital stays and contribute to pulmonary complications. Quitting smoking before surgery lowers the rate of PPCs. Although early data suggested that quitting smoking close to surgery may increase the rate of PPCs, a recent meta-analysis shows this is not true. In general, the sooner a patient can quit smoking, the better it is for the patient, but smoking cessation should be encouraged at any time before surgery.

Surgery-Related Factors

The planned surgery and surgical site have an impact on risk for developing PPCs that is often greater than patient-related factors. Surgical site was the most important predictor for developing postoperative pneumonia and respiratory failure in a cohort of 160,000 U.S. military veterans undergoing major noncardiac surgery. Those undergoing abdominal aortic aneurysm (AAA) repair or thoracic surgery had the highest risk, followed by upper abdominal, neurovascular, and neck surgeries.

Duration of surgery, extent of anesthesia, and invasiveness of the surgery all influence the risk of developing PPCs. Patients undergoing emergency surgeries or surgeries lasting longer than 3 hours are at greater risk for PPCs. Surgeries requiring general anesthesia (GA) carry a greater risk for PPCs than with peripheral nerve blocks. There is questionable evidence about the relative risk of PPCs from surgeries requiring GA versus neuraxial blockade (spinal or epidural anesthesia). A previous large review of various surgeries reported increased rates of pneumonia, respiratory failure, and mortality in patients who received GA compared to those receiving neuraxial blockade. A more

Table 73-2	Selected Risk Factors for Developing Postoperative Pulmonary Complications
Risk Factor	**Level of Prediction**
Systemic Disease	
Asthma (well controlled)	Poor
Congestive heart failure	Good
Chronic obstructive pulmonary disease	Good
Diabetes mellitus	Fair
Human immunodeficiency virus infection	I
Obstructive sleep apnea	Good
Pulmonary hypertension	Fair
Signs and Symptoms	
Abnormal chest auscultation	Good
Arrhythmia	I
Functionally dependent	Good
Impaired mental status	Good
Poor exercise capacity	Fair
Weight loss	Good
Patient Features	
Alcohol user	Good
Cigarette smoker	Good
Corticosteroid use	I
Objective Testing	
Albumin <35 g/L	Good
Blood urea nitrogen >25 mg/dL	Good
Chest radiography, abnormal finding	Good
Spirometry	I
Surgical Site	
Aortic aneurysm	Good
Abdominal	Good
Neurosurgery	Good
Vascular	Good
Hip	Poor
Gynecologic or urologic	Poor
Esophageal	I
Surgical Factors	
Prolonged surgical duration	Good
Emergent surgery	Good
General anesthesia	Fair
Perioperative transfusion	Good

Data from current American Academy of Chest Physicians (AACP) guidelines; Smetana GW et al: *Cleve Clin J Med* 73(Suppl 1):36–41, 2006; and other sources (see Suggested Readings).
Good, ACP "A" or "B" rating or other data to support; *Fair*, ACP "C" rating or other data to support; *Poor*, ACP "D" rating, or is not a risk factor; *I*, indeterminate (insufficient data to support a rating.

Table 73-3 ASA Classification for Surgical Candidates

Class	Patient Status
I	Normal healthy patient
II	Patient with mild systemic disease (e.g., mild asthma)
III	Patient with severe systemic disease, but not incapacitated
IV	Patient with life-threatening illness who is incapacitated
V	Moribund patient
VI	"Brain-dead" patient eligible for organ donation

ASA, American Society of Anesthesiologists.

recent small review of orthopedic surgeries found equal rates of pneumonias in these two groups.

A study of patients undergoing AAA repair found increased rates of PPCs (16%) in open repair compared to endovascular repair (3%). Video-assisted surgeries have reduced PPC rates compared with open approaches. Limited data suggest that patients undergoing cardiothoracic robotic surgery have lower rates of PPCs than those not receiving robotic surgery.

SURGERY IN GENERAL

The most important part of a preoperative pulmonary evaluation is taking a complete history and performing a complete physical examination. For those without pulmonary disease or symptoms, or those with well-controlled chronic lung conditions, routine pulmonary function tests (PFTs) and chest imaging are not indicated.

During the office visit, symptoms or signs of an underlying or undiagnosed pulmonary condition may be discovered. If unexplained dyspnea, coughing, wheezing, other abnormal lung sounds, or chest pain is revealed, testing before an elective surgery may be indicated to identify their cause. Historical clues should aid in distinguishing cardiovascular dyspnea from pulmonary dyspnea and guide which tests should be performed. Pulmonary function testing will help to identify and quantitate physiologic impairment of lung function. If a cardiac etiology is suspected, an electrocardiogram, echocardiogram, brain natriuretic peptide level, and stress test may be performed. Other cardiac risk assessment is beyond the scope of this chapter.

Further testing, such as a chest radiograph, complete blood count, serum chemistries, and thyroid-stimulating hormone (TSH) level can help to determine the cause of cardiopulmonary symptoms and the need for additional testing. If the cause of dyspnea remains unclear, a cardiopulmonary exercise test may help determine its nature and quantify its severity. Additional chest imaging may also be required if a pulmonary cause of a concerning symptom is likely. Screening for PH is not recommended in the preoperative setting, particularly if respiratory symptoms are not present or are otherwise well explained. Since most, if not all, of the conditions causing dyspnea result in increased rates of PPCs, proper diagnosis and treatment optimization of that condition will improve patient outcomes.

During the history and physical examination, patients should be screened for OSA by asking about snoring, witnessed apneas, and daytime somnolence. Neck circumference and obesity should be noted. Validated questionnaires are available for identifying those at risk for OSA (**Box 73-1**). Evidence is

Table 73-4 Risk for Postoperative Respiratory Failure and Pneumonia

Select Preoperative Predictors	Point Value/Score		
	RFRI	PRI	RRI
Age (years)			
Greater than 70	6	13-17	2
60-69	4	9	2
Albumin (<30 g/L)	9	—	1
ASA class			
3	—	—	3
4-5	—	—	5
BUN (>30 mg/dL)	8	3	—
COPD	6	5	2*
Dependent function status	7	6-10	—
Surgery			
AAA	27	15	2
Thoracic	21	14	—
Neurovascular, upper abdomen	14	10,8,3	—
Neck	11	8	—
Emergent	11	3	2
Orofacial	—	—	7

RFRI, respiratory failure risk index (Arozullah AM et al, 2000); *PRI*, pneumonia risk index (Arozullah AM et al, 2001); *RRI*, respiratory risk index (updated; Johnson RG et al, 2007); *ASA*, American Society of Anesthesiologists; *BUN*, blood urea nitrogen; *AAA*, abdominal aortic aneurysm. See Table 73-5.
*Severe chronic obstructive pulmonary disease (COPD).

Box 73-1 Stop-Bang Questionnaire to Screen for Obstructive Sleep Apnea (OSA)

1. Snore: can the patient's snoring be heard through a closed door?
2. Tired: is the patient hypersomnolent during the day?
3. Observed: have there been witnessed apneas?
4. Pressure: does the patient have hypertension?
5. Body mass index: greater than 35?
6. Age: older than 50?
7. Neck circumference: greater than 40 cm?
8. Gender: male?

Modified from Chung F et al: *Anesthesiology* 108:812–821, 2008.
The patient who answers "yes" to three or more of these eight questions is at high risk for OSA.

limited on the usefulness of diagnosing OSA preoperatively with polysomnography, with decisions based on degree of clinical concern and urgency of the surgery.

Validated indices are available for predicting postoperative pneumonia and respiratory failure after major noncardiac surgery. The investigators from three select reviews assigned point values to corresponding risk factors, as summarized in **Tables 73-4** and **73-5**. Clinicians may find these tools helpful in identifying those at risk for postoperative pneumonia and respiratory failure and for selecting perioperative testing and respiratory care for those at high risk.

Table 73-5   Level of Risk Based on Point Value/Score

Risk Level*	Score from RRI	Predicted RF	Class†	Point Total from RFRI	Predicted RF	Point Total from PRI	Predicted Pneumonia
Low	<8	.2%	1	≤10	0.5%	0-15	0.24%
			2	11-19	2.2%	16-25	1.2%
Medium	8-12	1%	3	20-27	5%	26-40	4%
			4	28-40	11.6%	41-5	9.4%
High	>12	6.5%	5	>40	30.5%	>55	15.3%

See Table 73-4 for abbreviations.
RF, respiratory failure.
*Risk level for the RRI, updated respiratory risk index.
†Class indicates level of risk for the PRI and RFRI.

LUNG RESECTION SURGERY

For patients with non–small cell lung cancer (NSCLC), surgical resection with a lobectomy or pneumonectomy offers the best chance at cure. Approximately 20% of lung cancer patients are deemed to be surgical candidates. However, these resections are not without serious risk. The mortality for lobectomy is 2% to 3%, and for pneumonectomy, 4% to 6%. Overall, PPCs range from 20% to 30%. Meticulous patient selection by a multidisciplinary team for these procedures is imperative. The clinician must identify patients who have a poor prognosis without surgery, a low risk of operative mortality, and a high likelihood of tolerating well the reduced lung function after resection. Lung resection surgery is unique in that the reduction in lung function related to surgery does not occur only in the immediate postoperative period but rather persists. Thus, preoperative evaluation must consider not only PPCs but also the long-term effect of the loss of lung function on the patient's quality of life. The following general overview recognizes that decisions about lung resection need to be individualized, considering other treatment options, patient preferences, and comorbidities.

After a complete history and physical examination, the lung resection patient should undergo a thorough pulmonary assessment focusing on pulmonary reserve. All potential lung cancer resection patients should have spirometry performed. Patients with forced expiratory volume in 1 second (FEV_1) measurements above 2 L and 80% of predicted normal values, who are free of cardiopulmonary symptoms, should tolerate resection without the need for additional testing. For all others, a diffusion capacity (DLCO) measurement should be obtained, and *predicted postoperative* (ppo) *lung function* should be calculated.

Estimating postoperative lung function can help determine the risks related to lung resection surgery and identify patients likely to tolerate resection who may not qualify by other measures. An anatomic segment method or radionuclide quantitative perfusion imaging may be used for patients undergoing surgery up to a lobectomy; the latter is preferred for those likely to require a pneumonectomy.

To calculate ppo lung function with the *anatomic segment* method, the fraction of total lung segments that will remain after the resection is multiplied by the preoperative lung function value. The two equations typically used are based on pulmonary segment total (19) or subsegment total (42). Using the former, the predictions correlate well with a lobectomy but less so with a pneumonectomy. Overall, these calculations tend to underestimate actual postoperative lung function, particularly in those with baseline impairment of lung function.

Radionuclide quantitative perfusion studies estimate the relative function of the lung to be resected by quantifying perfusion to the portion of lung to be resected as a fraction of total lung perfusion. Postoperative lung function can be calculated similar to the anatomic segment methods. Radionuclide studies also consistently underestimate FEV_1 values in patients with lower baseline values. Although more accurate than segment methods for postpneumonectomy lung function prediction, the overall predictive value of quantitative perfusion studies is less than ideal.

Pulmonary Function Measures

Although clinicians cannot rely solely on pulmonary function measures to predict the risk of PPCs, perioperative mortality, or unacceptable levels of long-term dyspnea, the FEV_1 value does correlate with these outcomes. As a general rule, a preoperative FEV_1 value of 2 L or greater indicates that a patient without cardiopulmonary symptoms will tolerate a pneumonectomy, and with a value of 1.5 L or greater, a lobectomy. Because absolute values do not consider age, gender, or size, percent of predicted normal values are more useful. Values greater than 80% of predicted normal in those without symptoms support proceeding directly to resection without additional testing. As stated earlier, ppo values as a percentage of normal are also helpful in identifying patients capable of undergoing resection who might have otherwise been rejected based on absolute FEV_1 values.

Guidelines recommend that patients with FEV_1 values below the general parameters just listed and any symptomatic patient should have ppoFEV_1 values calculated. It is difficult and probably inappropriate to apply cutoff values for ppoFEV_1 to an individual patient. As expected, the lower the ppoFEV_1 value, the higher is the rate of complications or unacceptable outcomes. One study noted that no postoperative deaths occurred in patients with ppoFEV_1 greater than 40% after resection, whereas those with ppoFEV_1 less than 40% had a 50% chance of postoperative mortality. Another study found that all patients with a ppoFEV_1 of 30% or lower developed respiratory failure or died after resection.

The DLCO and ppoDLCO are also independent predictors for PPCs and mortality. The majority of patients undergoing lung resection should have DLCO measured. DLCO values may be low despite normal spirometry. As with FEV_1, one cutoff value for resection should not be applied equally to all patients. Lower values correlate with worse outcomes. Those with an absolute DLCO of 60% predicted normal or lower had greater rates of postoperative respiratory failure and death in one study; ppoDLCO values of 40% predicted normal or greater have been used as cutoffs in published guidelines. One study found that patients with ppoFEV$_1$ × ppoDLCO (predicted postoperative product) of less than 1650 have a high mortality rate.

Exercise Testing

When questions remain after standard measures of lung function have been performed and ppo values have been calculated, measures of exercise capacity can be helpful. Cardiopulmonary exercise testing (CPET) with cycle ergometry has been used to assess a patient's fitness for resection. An individual's exercise capacity can be measured as the peak oxygen consumption (VO$_2$ peak). Values greater than 20 ml/kg/min have been used to suggest the ability to tolerate pneumonectomy, 15 ml/kg/min for lobectomy, and less than 10 ml/kg/min for a high-risk group. Many studies have found this value to be an independent predictor for PPCs and mortality. Formal oxygen desaturation studies may be performed as well. A 4% oxygen desaturation is associated with increased PPCs, including respiratory failure, increased ICU stays, and home oxygen requirement. Stair climbing, a 6-minute walk test, and shuttle walking also provide measures of cardiopulmonary capacity that can assist with decisions about resectability.

Box 73-2 summarizes the American College of Chest Physicians (ACCP) recommendations for the preoperative pulmonary evaluation of the lung resection candidate. **Figure 73-1** outlines the ACCP and European Respiratory Society and European Society of Thoracic Surgeons (ERS/ESTS) recommended steps to follow when assessing a patient's pulmonary fitness for lung resection. The differences in these guidelines highlight the lack of consensus in this area and the need to individualize patient decisions.

MANAGEMENT

Most patient-related and surgery-related risk factors are nonmodifiable. The following recommendations should be used in all patients regardless of their risk for PPCs.

Preoperative Measures For patients with airway obstruction (asthma, COPD) the use of inhaled bronchodilators and inhaled and systemic corticosteroids should be based on standard management and optimization of these conditions. It is not necessary to add these treatments in the perioperative setting if the patient's underlying condition is well controlled. There appears to be no risk of increased postoperative infections from a course of corticosteroids lasting less than 1 week. Antibiotics and cough expectorants should only be used in patients who are actively infected or are experiencing an acute exacerbation of COPD. All smokers should be strongly advised to quit smoking as soon as possible before surgery and should be provided with means available to help them quit. Breathing muscle exercises such as incentive spirometry, use of an inspiratory muscle trainer, deep-breathing exercises, or enrollment in a pulmonary rehabilitation program may be advised for those with underlying lung compromise undergoing high-risk surgery. Weight reduction for the obese patient is advised, particularly those with or at risk for OSA.

Patients at high risk for OSA should undergo a sleep study before their scheduled surgery if time permits. If OSA is proven, treatment with continuous positive airway pressure (CPAP)

Box 73-2 Summary of ACCP Guidelines for Lung Cancer Resection

- Patients should not be denied lung resection surgery based on age alone.
- All patients should undergo spirometry.
- An FEV$_1$ of 2 L or greater or 80% predicted in a patient without dyspnea or ILD may proceed to pneumonectomy. FEV$_1$ of 1.5 L or greater in a patient without dyspnea or ILD may proceed to lobectomy.
- If there is undue dyspnea or ILD evident, DLCO is recommended.
- If DLCO or FEV$_1$ is less than 80%, ppo lung function should performed.
- A ppoFEV$_1$ or ppoDLCO less than 40% is consistent with increased PPCs and mortality after resection. Exercise testing is recommended.
- A postoperative predicted product of less than 1650 or a ppoFEV$_1$ of less than 30% indicates an increased risk for PPCs and death. These patients should be counseled on nonsurgical treatment options.
- In patients with a VO$_2$ peak of less than 10 mL/kg/min or a VO$_2$ peak of less than 15, with both ppoFEV$_1$ and ppoDLCO less than 40% predicted, nonsurgical treatment options should be sought.
- Patients who walk less than 25 shuttles on two shuttle walks or less than one flight of stairs should be counseled on nonsurgical options.
- For those with a PaCO$_2$ greater than 45 mm Hg or SaO$_2$ less than 90%, further testing should be performed prior to surgery.
- In lung cancer patients with upper lobe emphysema and FEV$_1$ and DLCO greater than 20%, LVRS combined with resection may be considered.
- Smoking cessation is encouraged for all.

Modified from American College of Chest Physicians recommendations and Colice GL et al: *Chest* 132(3 suppl):161–177, 2007.
ACCP, American College of Chest Physicians; *FEV$_1$*, forced expiratory volume in 1 second; *DLCO*, diffusion capacity; *ILD*, interstitial lung disease; *PPCs*, postoperative pulmonary complications; *VO$_2$ peak*, peak oxygen consumption; *ppo*, predicted postoperative; *LVRS*, lung volume reduction surgery.

should begin as soon as possible. A recent study revealed that patients with newly diagnosed OSA had lower rates of respiratory failure if they had started CPAP therapy before surgery. Currently, data are insufficient to support postponing an elective surgery to optimize sleep apnea therapy.

Surgical Management There is some evidence that the use of regional anesthesia over GA and the choice of a neuromuscular blocker other than pancuronium will reduce PPCs. These choices are rightfully influenced by the anesthesia needs of the procedure. Other operative measures to reduce PPCs include limited anesthesia and thoracotomy times, protective lung ventilation strategies, limited or intermittent hyperinflation to prevent atelectasis, control of secretions, and aspiration prevention measures.

Postoperative Measures After surgery, early ambulation, cough encouragement, mobilization of secretions, and adequate pain control will all help to decrease PPCs. The use of epidural analgesia during and immediately after surgery leads to improved outcomes in patients undergoing lung resection. Selective nasogastric decompression is recommended only for those with nausea or abdominal distention, to prevent

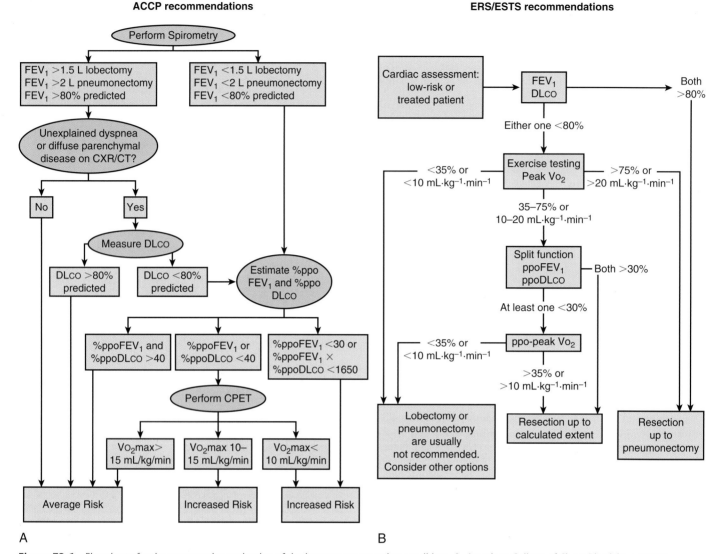

ACCP recommendations

ERS/ESTS recommendations

A

B

Figure 73-1   Flowcharts for the preoperative evaluation of the lung cancer resection candidate. **A,** American College of Chest Physicians (ACCP); **B,** European Respiratory Society and European Society of Thoracic Surgeons (ERS/ESTS). *FEV₁*, forced expiratory volume in 1 second; *CXR*, chest x-ray film (radiograph); *CT*, computed tomography; *DLco*, diffusion capacity; *ppo*, predicted postoperative; *CPET*, cardiopulmonary exercise test.   *(A from Colice GL et al: Chest 132(3 suppl):161–177, 2007; B from Lim E et al: Thorax 65(suppl 3):1–27, 2010.)*

aspiration events. Incentive spirometry and deep-breathing maneuvers are recommended to decrease atelectasis and thereby decrease PPCs. For patients following lung resection surgery, pulmonary rehabilitation has been shown to assist with functional recovery.

CONCLUSION

Postoperative pulmonary complications are common and lend to significant morbidity and mortality as well as increased costs. The preoperative pulmonary evaluation should initially determine the level of risk for complications to provide guidance to the patient and surgeon. Many patient-related and surgery-related risk factors for PPCs are known. Validated clinical tools are available for assessing those at risk for pneumonia and respiratory failure, and evidence-based guidelines assist in assessment of the lung resection candidate. The other goals of the preoperative visit are to optimize the management of underlying diseases, have systems in place to minimize perioperative risks, and educate the patient about the techniques available, to ensure optimal conditions for an uneventful recovery.

SUGGESTED READINGS

Arozullah AM, Khuri SF, Henderson WG, Daley J: Participants in the National Veterans Affairs Surgical Quality Improvement Program: development and validation of a multifactorial risk index for predicting postoperative pneumonia after major noncardiac surgery, *Ann Intern Med* 135:847–857, 2001.

Chung F, Yegneswaran B, Liao P, et al: STOP questionnaire: a tool to screen patients for obstructive sleep apnea, *Anesthesiology* 108:812–821, 2008.

Colice GL, Shafazand S, Griffin JP, et al: Physiologic evaluation of the patient with lung cancer being considered for resectional surgery: American College of Chest Physicians evidenced-based clinical practice guidelines (2nd edition), *Chest* 132(3 suppl):161–177, 2007.

Johnson RG, Arozullah AM, Neumayer L, et al: Multivariable predictors of postoperative respiratory failure after general and vascular surgery: results from the patient safety in surgery study, *J Am Coll Surg* 204:1188–1198, 2007.

Lim E, Baldwin D, Beckles M, et al: Guidelines on the radical management of patients with lung cancer. British Thoracic Society; Society for Cardiothoracic Surgery in Great Britain and Ireland, *Thorax* 65(suppl 3):1–27, 2010.

Mazzone PJ, Arroliga AC: Lung cancer: preoperative pulmonary evaluation of the lung resection candidate, *Am J Med* 118:578–583, 2005.

Myers K, Hajek P, Hinds C, McRobbie H: Stopping smoking shortly before surgery and postoperative complications: a systematic review and meta-analysis, *Arch Intern Med* 171:983–989, 2011.

Poonyagariyagorn H, Mazzone PJ: Lung cancer: preoperative pulmonary evaluation of the lung resection candidate, *Semin Respir Crit Care Med* 29:271–284, 2008.

Smetana GW: Preoperative pulmonary evaluation: identifying and reducing risks for pulmonary complications, *Cleve Clin J Med* 73(suppl 1):36–41, 2006.

Smetana GW, Lawrence VA, Cornell JE: Preoperative pulmonary risk stratification for noncardiothoracic surgery: systematic review for the American College of Physicians, *Ann Intern Med* 144:581–595, 2006.

Sweitzer BJ, Smetana GW: Identification and evaluation of the patient with lung disease, *Med Clin North Am* 93:1017–1030, 2009.

Chapter **74**

Diagnostic Thoracic Surgical Procedures

Chadrick E. Denlinger • Stephen D. Cassivi • Mark S. Allen

Despite the ever-increasing sensitivity of noninvasive diagnostic modalities, especially in diagnostic imaging, diagnostic thoracic surgical procedures add critical information to the diagnostic workup of patients with diverse thoracic diseases. To provide definitive tissue diagnosis and to assess stage and resectability of chest tumors, the general thoracic surgeon is vital in the diagnostic evaluation of patients.

Common thoracic surgical procedures used for diagnosis include, in order of invasiveness, bronchoscopic, cervical, scalene, and supraclavicular lymph node, pleural, mediastinal, and pulmonary biopsy procedures that involve endoscopic, thoracoscopic, or open surgical approaches. There is a spectrum of invasiveness to these procedures, with exploratory thoracotomy representing the most invasive of these diagnostic techniques. The choice of procedure is guided by the particular clinical question to be answered, as well as specific patient characteristics and, at times, the individual surgeon's preference and experience. Overall, these procedures provide a high diagnostic yield, with low morbidity and mortality. Complications, although rare, do occasionally occur, and it is therefore incumbent on referring physicians to understand the nature of these procedures, the level of invasiveness, and the relative risk/benefit ratios.

PREOPERATIVE CONSIDERATIONS

Except for flexible bronchoscopy, which can be performed using topical anesthesia with minimal sedation, most diagnostic surgical interventions require general anesthesia. The physician first determines the appropriateness of the intervention, because some degree of operative risk is always present. A general contraindication to these procedures is excessive risk from comorbid conditions. The referring physician and ultimately the surgeon must assess the patient's overall medical status and ability to withstand the proposed procedure. Furthermore, a diagnostic surgical intervention, no matter how minimally invasive, is unnecessary and unwarranted if the findings of the procedure will not influence the treatment plan for the individual patient.

CLINICAL APPLICATION OF DIAGNOSTIC THORACIC PROCEDURES

The diagnostic thoracic surgical procedures discussed in this chapter have varied applications, with relative advantages and disadvantages (**Table 74-1**) and are typically used in the following three broad areas:

- Assessment of bronchogenic carcinoma
- Diagnosis of interstitial lung disease

- Sampling of indeterminate pleural, pulmonary, and mediastinal lesions

Bronchoscopy

In 1968, Ikeda introduced the first flexible bronchoscope, and over the decades, flexible bronchoscopy has largely supplanted rigid bronchoscopy for diagnostic procedures. Previously, rigid bronchoscopy was the only way to visualize and access the tracheobronchial tree directly. Now, however, the flexible bronchoscope provides access to a greater extent of the airway, can be performed with minimal sedation, and can be routinely performed in the intensive care unit (ICU) as well as the regular patient ward in many hospitals.

Flexible Bronchoscopy

As a diagnostic tool, flexible bronchoscopy offers a relatively noninvasive way to visualize and obtain tissue samples from the airways. The flexible characteristic allows access to subsegmental branches of the tracheobronchial tree. Although flexible bronchoscopy can be done through the endotracheal tube in an anesthetized and intubated patient, this procedure is usually performed with topical anesthesia and conscious sedation. Adjuncts to flexible bronchoscopy continue to evolve, further improving its diagnostic accuracy and utility.

Flexible bronchoscopy not only allows visualization of the tracheobronchial tree, but also provides access for obtaining tissue samples, such as washings, brushings, and bronchoalveolar lavage (BAL) fluid for cytologic and microbiologic analyses. Endobronchial and transbronchial biopsies can be obtained of the airway and lung tissue. In addition, transbronchial needle (Wang) biopsies of mediastinal lymph nodes can be performed through the flexible bronchoscope. This procedure requires a careful evaluation of preoperative images to help blindly pass a needle through the bronchus into the extraluminal lymph node of interest.

Endobronchial Ultrasound

The recent addition of endobronchial ultrasound (EBUS) technology has increased the sensitivity of transbronchial needle biopsies. This special bronchoscope includes the additional feature of a linear ultrasound probe at the end of the scope, which facilitates visualization of lymph nodes outside the airway. Color flow Doppler images also help differentiate lymph nodes from vascular structures. A working channel directs the passage of a transbronchial needle through the region imaged by the ultrasound, to biopsy discrete lymph nodes. EBUS is most frequently used for mediastinal lymph node staging of patients with known or presumed lung cancer. The diagnostic accuracy is similar to that of mediastinoscopy

Table 74-1 Diagnostic Thoracic Surgical Procedures

Procedure	Application	Advantages	Disadvantages
Rigid bronchoscopy	Diagnosis of carcinoma Clear airway obstruction	Removal of secretions/blood Large biopsy specimen may reveal submucosal tumor Opportunity to debulk inoperable tumors or excise benign lesions Assessment of carinal fixation	Poor view of secondary bronchial divisions
Cervical and scalene lymph node biopsy	Diagnosis of enlarged nodes	Safer technique than fine-needle aspiration (FNA) for deeper nodes Large tissue sample	Operative procedure; occasional technical difficulty
Mediastinoscopy	Diagnosis of middle mediastinal pathology (node/mass)	Direct access to mediastinal abnormality Much larger tissue sample than FNA	Operative field restricted to paratracheal and subcarinal areas
Mediastinotomy	Diagnosis of anterior mediastinal pathology (node/mass)	Reaches areas of anterior mediastinum inaccessible to mediastinoscopy Useful for subaortic node sampling May be safer to use than mediastinoscopy in patients who have superior vena cava obstruction Much larger tissue sample than in FNA	Operative field restricted to upper anterior mediastinum More complex operative procedure
Thoracoscopy	Pleural biopsy Biopsy of visceral pleura deposits	Can be effected through single puncture Visually directed biopsy	Limited to small biopsies Dependent on pleural cavity being free of adhesions
Video-assisted thoracoscopic/thoracic surgery (VATS)	Any ipsilateral biopsy or sampling procedure	Complementary to mediastinoscopy and mediastinotomy Excellent view and full operative intervention possible (e.g., wedge excision of pulmonary nodule, dissection of mediastinal mass)	Dependent on pleural cavity being free of adhesions Significant surgical expertise required

for this indication; two recent prospective studies show a similar diagnostic accuracy of EBUS and mediastinoscopy. Clearly, either procedure has great diagnostic value when performed by experienced clinicians.

Navigational Bronchoscopy

Previously, fluoroscopy was used to assist in directing the bronchoscope and biopsy forceps toward indeterminate peripheral lung lesions. The two-dimensional nature of fluoroscopy and the inability directly to "steer" the biopsy forceps were serious drawbacks of this modality. Navigational bronchoscopy using electromagnetic guidance was recently introduced to improve the yield of bronchoscopic lung biopsies. This technology depends on the construction of a virtual three-dimensional airway using CT images. An electromagnetic field created over the patient's chest helps to locate and direct a small endoscopic probe toward the lesion in airways beyond visualization with standard bronchoscopy. This technology can be used in combination with a small, radial ultrasound probe to help determine when the bronchoscope has reached the lesion of interest.

Currently the two most common applications of navigational bronchoscopy are to place fiducial markers or to obtain a tissue diagnosis of small lesions located in airways that are distal to the range of visualization. This technology is most useful for lung lesions within the inner third of the lung parenchyma. Lesions located closer to the periphery of the lung can be biopsied using computed tomography (CT)-guided techniques.

Rigid Bronchoscopy

Rigid bronchoscopy is mostly used for therapeutic airway interventions such as airway dilation, laser debridement, tumor debulking, placement of airway stents, or foreign body retrieval **(Figure 74-1)**. The use of the rigid bronchoscope continues to

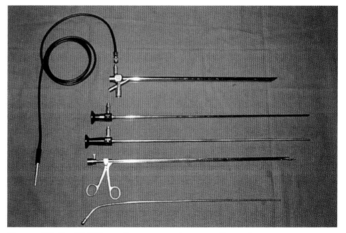

Figure 74-1 Rigid bronchoscopy equipment. *Top to bottom,* Bronchoscope with light cable, straight and right-angled surgical telescopes, biopsy forceps, suction cannula.

be an important diagnostic tool in special circumstances, such as those requiring a better tactile sense when assessing for possible extrinsic tumor invasion of the airway, or when larger biopsies are sought. It is also indispensable when airway control is in question because of hemoptysis or tumor invasion.

Rigid bronchoscopy requires general anesthesia with a muscle relaxant and specific ventilatory strategies. The options most often used include jet ventilation and continuous or intermittent insufflation. In patients with airway control as an overwhelming concern because of an obstructing airway lesion, muscle relaxants are avoided to maintain spontaneous breathing.

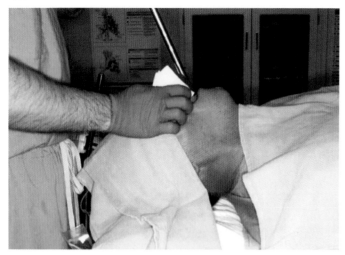

Figure 74-2 Positioning and insertion of rigid bronchoscope. The rigid bronchoscope is inserted with the bevel down while the patient is positioned supine with the neck extended.

Technique

In general, the size of the rigid bronchoscope used for adult men is 8 or 9 mm (outer diameter) and 7 or 8 mm for adult women. Smaller sizes are available for children or smaller adults.

After induction of anesthesia, the patient is positioned supine with the neck extended into the "sniffing" position. Right-handed surgeons use their left thumb to further protect the upper teeth and lips from injury and to serve as the fulcrum in positioning and supporting the bronchoscope throughout the procedure. Protection is also supplemented by use of a rubber tooth guard or saline-soaked gauze sponge. The patient's eyes are also shielded from inadvertent injury with padded covers for the duration of the procedure.

The bronchoscope is inserted through the right side of the patient's mouth with the bevel down (**Figure 74-2**). It is advanced toward the base of the tongue in the posterior oropharynx. The tip of the epiglottis is then identified by carefully elevating the tongue as the scope is brought more into a horizontal position. The scope is then advanced a short distance past the tip of the epiglottis. The protruding superior lip of the bronchoscope is then used to lift gently the tip of the epiglottis, allowing visualization of the vocal cords and laryngeal inlet. The surgeon will then rotate the bronchoscope 90 degrees along its long axis, placing the bevel in the anteroposterior plane to allow easy passage through the vocal cords. The bronchoscope can then be carefully advanced into the trachea under direct vision. To facilitate passage of the bronchoscope into the left or right main stem bronchus, the patient's head is turned to the contralateral side. Visualization of the segmental and subsegmental airways can be facilitated by insertion of a flexible bronchoscope through the lumen of the rigid bronchoscope.

Cervical, Scalene, and Supraclavicular Lymph Node Biopsy

Both bronchogenic and esophageal carcinoma may involve the lymph nodes in the cervical, scalene, and supraclavicular areas. Open biopsy of nonpalpable scalene lymph nodes is no longer a routine preoperative staging, and in fact, this procedure has become rare. Clinically positive or palpable nodes in this area are now accessed by fine-needle aspiration (FNA) directed by either CT or ultrasound imaging, if necessary. Patients who are thought to have lymphoma may require an open surgical biopsy to obtain a sample size adequate to assess for histologic architecture and sufficient tissue quantities for flow cytometry or additional studies required for a complete diagnosis.

A 3 to 4–cm–long skin crease incision is made at the level just above the insertion of the sternocleidomastoid muscle into the medial clavicle. Dissection can proceed between the clavicular and sternal heads of this muscle, or both can be retracted medially. The scalene fat pad lies on the anterior scalene muscle, lateral to the internal jugular vein, and usually receives its blood supply from the transverse cervical artery entering the fat pad inferiorly. This artery should be identified, ligated, and divided. Injury to the phrenic nerve is possible because of its location along the anterior surface of the anterior scalene muscle, deep to the fat pad. Other, rare but significant complications of open surgical lymph node biopsy include pneumothorax and thoracic duct injury with subsequent chylous fistula.

Cervical Mediastinoscopy

Cervical mediastinoscopy is a mainstay of lung cancer staging and was popularized in Europe by Carlens and in North America by Pearson in the 1960s. It is used not only for lung cancer staging but also to assess any lymphadenopathy in the pretracheal, paratracheal, and subcarinal areas. Lymph nodes that are accessible by the standard cervical approach are the highest: the upper and lower paratracheal and subcarinal levels as well as upper lymph nodes of the pulmonary hilum, or stations 1, 2, 4, 7, and 10 in the American Joint Committee on Cancer (AJCC) nomenclature. The "extended" cervical mediastinoscopy, introduced by Ginsberg, allows access to the aortopulmonary window and paraaortic lymph nodes (stations 5 and 6, respectively). More recently, level 5 and 6 lymph node stations are more often biopsied under direct vision by use of left thoracoscopy or anterior mediastinotomy.

Repeat mediastinoscopy, although technically possible, carries a higher risk of complications because of the loss of normal tissue planes to guide the usual dissection. Cervical mediastinoscopy can usually be performed as an outpatient procedure when done as an individual procedure. In many situations, mediastinoscopy is performed as a staged procedure that precedes a pulmonary resection. In experienced hands, mediastinoscopy provides substantial lymph node specimens, which are evaluated immediately by pathologists, who rule out lymph node metastases before the patient proceeds to an anatomic resection of the lung cancer.

Recently in Europe, more extensive procedures, referred to as *transcervical extended mediastinal lymphadenectomy* (TEMLA) and *video-assisted mediastinal lymphadenectomy* (VAMLA), have been proposed as alternatives to conventional cervical mediastinoscopy. These techniques are significantly more involved, with larger lymph node harvests accompanied by significant increases in the length of surgery (2-5 hours). Unfortunately, a recent trial of cervical mediastinoscopy versus TEMLA was prematurely halted before enough cases could be accrued for an adequately powered comparison of morbidity between these two staging procedures. Thus, we cannot accurately assess the risk of morbidity associated with the more invasive staging procedure.

Despite improvements in imaging of the mediastinum with CT imaging and positron emission tomography (PET), cervical mediastinoscopy remains the "gold standard" for preoperative staging of the mediastinum in lung cancer. Of special note is the low positive predictive value (PPV) of PET scans for staging

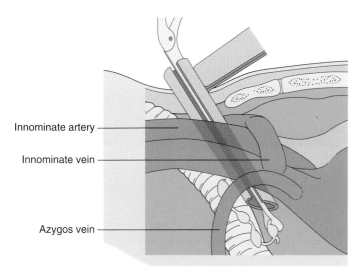

Innominate artery

Innominate vein

Azygos vein

Figure 74-3 Path of cervical mediastinoscope.

the mediastinum in lung cancer. It is therefore imperative that a tissue diagnosis be obtained to document mediastinal metastases before surgical resection is denied. Cervical mediastinoscopy has a diagnostic accuracy of more than 98% in experienced centers and thus remains the mainstay of prethoracotomy mediastinal staging.

Technique

With the patient intubated and under general anesthesia, a bolster is placed under the shoulders to provide adequate neck extension for the procedure. A 2.5-cm transverse incision is made approximately 1 cm above the sternal notch. The pretracheal fascia is exposed by splitting the strap muscles in the midline, with right-angle retractors used to retract the thyroid gland superiorly if necessary. The pretracheal fascia is incised transversely and bluntly dissected off the anterior surface of the trachea with the index finger. This allows direct palpation of the vascular structures, including the aortic arch and innominate vessels, as well as any prominent lymphadenopathy. The mediastinoscope is introduced beneath the pretracheal fascia (**Figure 74-3**). Further blunt dissection can be done under direct vision using the tip of the mediastinoscopy sucker. Systematic dissection and biopsy of the different lymph node levels are then possible.

A spinal needle attached to a syringe can be used to aspirate and thus differentiate in equivocal circumstances between solid masses that can be biopsied and vascular structures that should be avoided. Most small bleeding can be controlled by judicious use of electrocautery or temporary gauze packing. Because of the risk of significant hemorrhage from injury to the many nearby vascular structures, the surgical staff should always be prepared for possible conversion to sternotomy or thoracotomy for definitive control of bleeding. Special care should also be taken when obtaining biopsy samples of lymph nodes in the left paratracheal area, because the left recurrent laryngeal nerve courses nearby and can be injured by aggressive biopsies or injudicious use of electrocautery.

Anterior Mediastinotomy

Anterior mediastinotomy, also known as the *Chamberlain procedure*, is a technique that provides access to the anterior mediastinum. It is typically used to sample lymph nodes in the aortopulmonary window and paraaortic lymph nodes (stations 5 and 6, respectively, in AJCC nomenclature). These nodal stations can also be accessed by extended cervical mediastinoscopy or left thoracoscopy. Although anterior mediastinotomy is somewhat more invasive than cervical mediastinoscopy, patients are usually discharged the day of surgery.

Although this technique is still performed, anterior mediastinotomy is being replaced by video-assisted thoracoscopic surgery (VATS; see next section) in many other centers. The advantage of an anterior mediastinotomy is that if the pleural space is not violated, the patient may go home the day of the procedure. However, the pleural space is often opened, and patient discomfort frequently leads to a brief hospital stay. VATS is becoming increasingly popular as a diagnostic procedure to assess the level 5 and level 6 mediastinal lymph nodes because of the superior visualization this technique provides and the additional ability to visualize the entire thoracic cavity.

Technique

A 3 to 4–cm transverse incision is usually made in the second interspace, just lateral to the lateral sternal border for anterior mediastinotomy. The pectoral muscle can usually be split in the line of its fibers without cutting through muscle. The intercostal muscle is then incised along the upper edge of the second costal cartilage. The internal mammary vessels, located medially, can usually be avoided and preserved. The mediastinal pleura are bluntly pushed laterally to avoid entry into the pleural space. The mediastinoscope is introduced to permit optimal lighting and visualization and obtain appropriate biopsies.

Occasionally, the mediastinal pleura are breached. A chest tube is generally not required if the lung parenchyma has not been damaged. At the end of the procedure, a small catheter can be inserted into the pleural space through the mediastinotomy. The tube is pulled out once the overlying muscular tissues have been almost closed, with the anesthesiologist providing sustained positive-pressure ventilation to evacuate any residual intrapleural air.

Video-Assisted Thoracoscopic Surgery

Minimally invasive access to the lung, pleural space, and mediastinum can be obtained by video-assisted thoracoscopic (thoracic) surgery. VATS is useful in the diagnosis of pleural pathology such as diffuse or focal thickening because of mesothelioma, pleural metastases, asbestos-related plaques, or benign inflammatory pleuritis. Thoracoscopy can also assist in the diagnosis and treatment of pleural fluid collections. In the staging of lung and esophageal cancer, thoracoscopy can provide access, in a minimally invasive way, to the paratracheal, prevascular, aortopulmonary window, paraaortic, subcarinal, paraesophageal, and inferior pulmonary ligament lymph node groups (stations 2 to 9, respectively, in AJCC nomenclature). Tumor invasion of local structures and overall resectability can also be assessed. Thoracoscopy is also used to obtain biopsies of lung tissue to assess discrete nodules or diffuse lung disease.

Thoracoscopy is most effectively done with single-lung ventilation of the contralateral side using a double-lumen endotracheal tube or bronchial blocker. This allows collapse of the lung on the operated side, permitting adequate visualization and maneuverability within the pleural space. Dense pleural adhesions are therefore a contraindication for effective thoracoscopy, as is the inability to tolerate single-lung ventilation.

Although thoracoscopy is a form of minimally invasive surgery, it remains a high-risk procedure when performed in high-risk patients. Of particular note are patients with interstitial lung disease (ILD) requiring lung biopsy to tailor treatment options. These patients usually have severe respiratory compromise before VATS and may already be receiving mechanical ventilation, with a significant proportion having elevated pulmonary artery pressure. Patients with pulmonary hypertension do not tolerate single-lung ventilation well because of their inability to perfuse the ventilated lung preferentially. Therefore, a significant amount of blood is shunted through the nonventilated lung, and the patient experiences significant hypoxemia while attempting single-lung ventilation. In the Mayo Clinic experience, patients with ILD undergoing thoracoscopic lung biopsy had an operative mortality of just under 6%.

Technique

Thoracoscopy is performed by use of single-lung ventilation of the contralateral side. The patient is positioned in the lateral position similar to the positioning used for a posterolateral thoracotomy. When VATS is done for drainage and evaluation of a pleural effusion, a single 1-cm port is usually sufficient. It is placed in the sixth or seventh interspace in the anterior axillary line. Through this port, the camera and a thin suction tip or biopsy forceps can be introduced and maneuvered. For most other applications, one or two additional 1-cm ports are required, usually positioned separately along the fourth or fifth interspace, in the line of a potential posterolateral thoracotomy (**Figure 74-4**). In this way, conversion to thoracotomy simply requires extending the incision between these two upper port sites. The anterior port can be converted to a 5-cm to 7-cm "access" port for removal of a lobectomy specimen, if the procedure requires conversion to a VATS lobectomy, in the case of a biopsied lung nodule found to be an invasive primary lung cancer.

Whereas biopsy for diagnosis of ILD requires only defining several areas of representative pathology, *wedge resection* of an indeterminate pulmonary nodule first necessitates precise localization of the lesion. This is usually done with the surgeon's finger introduced through one of the thoracoscopy incisions (**Figure 74-5**). It is clearly easier to locate larger and peripherally located lesions. Smaller or deeper lesions may not be accessible and may require conversion to open thoracotomy. In general, a pulmonary nodule can be palpated during a VATS exploration if the diameter of the lesion is greater than the depth of lung tissue through which it is felt. Recent experience has been initially promising with radiotracer guidance (technetium 99m) to locate small pulmonary lesions not otherwise discernible thoracoscopically.

Once the area to be biopsied has been located, an endoscopic stapling device can be inserted through a thoracoport and used to perform a wedge resection (**Figure 74-6**). Once the specimen has been resected, it should be removed from the pleural cavity within an endoscopic specimen retrieval bag to avoid port site contamination. A more economical alternative is to use a surgical glove introduced through one of the port sites and held open with two Kelly clamps.

The biopsy specimen should be processed initially on a sterile back table in the operating room. In the case of diffuse lung infiltrates, the staple line can be excised and used for microbiology culture testing, whereas the remainder of the specimen is sent to pathology for histologic evaluation. When an indeterminate lung nodule is excised, a small portion

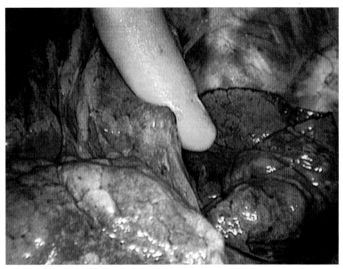

Figure 74-5   Palpation of intrapulmonary nodule during thoracoscopic surgery.

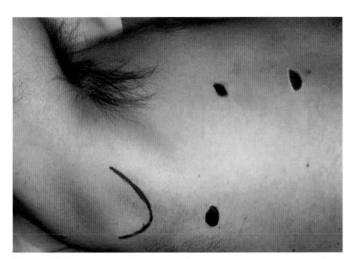

Figure 74-4   Location of thoracoscopic port sites. One port is placed at the seventh interspace in the anterior axillary line. Further ports may be required and are usually placed along the line of a potential posterolateral thoracotomy incision at the level of the fifth interspace.

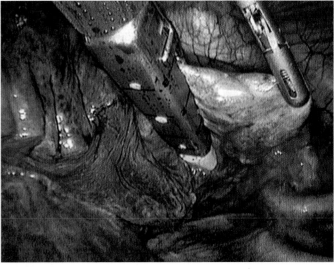

Figure 74-6   Use of endoscopic stapler during video-assisted thoracoscopic surgery (VATS).

should be kept for microbiology cultures, should the evaluation of the rest of the nodule suggest a nonmalignant diagnosis.

After all biopsies have been taken, the pleural cavity should be reassessed for any bleeding or other injury. Special attention should be paid to the staple lines and port sites. Once hemostasis is ascertained, a single, 28-Fr chest tube is introduced through the initial thoracoport in the seventh interspace anteriorly. It is guided posteriorly, with care taken to avoid placement within the fissure. Barring a significant air leak, this tube can usually be removed in 12 to 24 hours and the patient discharged the day after surgery.

Open Thoracotomy

Although a common procedure for thoracic surgeons, open thoracotomy is at the far end of the spectrum of patient morbidity for thoracic surgical procedures performed only for diagnostic purposes and therefore usually the *least* preferred option. However, this procedure is indicated and serves as the best diagnostic modality available in patients who, because of a fused pleural space or the inability to withstand single-lung ventilation, cannot safely undergo thoracoscopy. Frequently, patients referred for open-lung biopsy are critically ill and have significant pulmonary compromise, often requiring mechanical ventilatory assistance. Although open-lung biopsy is generally an accurate diagnostic tool, most studies do not show a survival benefit in critically ill patients with diffuse lung disease, even when a biopsy directs a change in therapy. Special care should be taken to assess the risk of such a procedure and its likely diagnostic yield in the specific patient's situation.

Technique

Usually, the patient undergoing thoracotomy for diagnostic purposes is placed in the lateral position, with both arms flexed forward at the shoulder. The incision is made transversely, one to two fingerbreadths beneath the scapular tip. This provides access to the fourth, fifth, or sixth interspace. Alternately, the patient is positioned supine, and an anterolateral thoracotomy is performed just beneath the mammary fold in the fourth or fifth interspace. As with the thoracoscopic approach, pulmonary resection is usually performed with the assistance of surgical stapling devices. At the end of the procedure, before closing the wound, a single, 28-Fr chest tube is inserted through a separate incision in an interspace beneath the main thoracotomy incision. Guided into the pleural space and positioned posteriorly, this tube will remain until drainage of air or fluid ceases.

CONCLUSION

A spectrum of surgical procedures is available to assist in diagnosis of thoracic diseases. The choice of the optimal diagnostic approach is based on individual patient characteristics, the specific diagnostic dilemma, and the surgeon's preferences and experience. It is essential to have a thorough understanding of the particular clinical situation, the advantages and disadvantages of the procedural alternatives, and the therapeutic implications of each possible diagnostic finding. This will allow the performing clinician to provide the most useful diagnostic answer with the least risk to the patient. Only then will the clinician avoid being more than a mere technician.

SUGGESTED READINGS

Allen MS, Deschamps C, Jones DM, et al: Video-assisted thoracic surgical procedures: the Mayo experience, *Mayo Clinic Proc* 71:351–359, 1996.

Annema JT, van Meerbeeck JP, Rintoul RC, et al: Mediastinoscopy vs. endoscopy for mediastinal nodal staging of lung cancer: a randomized trial, *JAMA* 304:2245–2252, 2010.

Catarino PA, Goldstraw P: The future in diagnosis and staging of lung cancer, *Respiration* 73:717–732, 2006.

Ginsberg RJ, Rice TW, Goldberg M, et al: Extended cervical mediastinoscopy: a single staging procedure for bronchogenic carcinoma of the left upper lobe, *J Thorac Cardiovasc Surg* 94:673–678, 1987.

Hammoud ZT, Anderson RC, Meyers BF, et al: The current role of mediastinoscopy in the evaluation of thoracic disease, *J Thorac Cardiovasc Surg* 118:894–899, 1999.

Kuzdzal J, Zielinski M, Papla B, et al: The transcervical extended mediastinal lymphadenectomy versus cervical mediastinoscopy in non–small cell lung cancer staging, *Eur J Cardiothorac Surg* 31:88–94, 2007.

Leschber G, Holinka G, Linder A: Video-assisted mediastinoscopic lymphadenectomy (VAMLA): a method for systematic mediastinal lymph node dissection, *Eur J Cardiothorac Surg* 24:192–195, 2003.

Nechala P, Graham AJ, McFadden SD, et al: Retrospective analysis of the clinical performance of anterior mediastinotomy, *Ann Thorac Surg* 82:2004–2009, 2006.

Stiles BM, Altes TA, Jones DR, et al: Clinical experience with radiotracer-guided thoracoscopic biopsy of small, indeterminate lung nodules, *Ann Thorac Surg* 82:1191–1197, 2006.

Temes RT, Joste NE, Qualls CR, et al: Lung biopsy: is it necessary? *J Thorac Cardiovasc Surg* 118:1097–1100, 1999.

Yasufuku K, Pierre A, Darling G, et al: A prospective controlled trial of endobronchial ultrasound-guided transbronchial needle aspiration compared with mediastinoscopy for mediastinal lymph node staging of lung cancer, *J Thorac Cardiovasc Surg* 142:1393–1400, 2011.

Chapter **75**
Lung Transplantation

Pamela J. McShane • Luis G. Ruiz • Edward R. Garrity, Jr.

Pulmonary transplantation has become an effective and reliable means to improve survival and quality of life in carefully selected patients with end-stage pulmonary disease. The current success in transplantation is attributed to appropriate referral, early selection, careful evaluation, and improving management of lung allograft donors and recipients. The multidisciplinary approach (**Figure 75-1**), together with meticulous clinical care of each transplant candidate (including understanding of the underlying disease state and optimization of psychosocial status), is of the utmost importance. The concurrent advances in surgical techniques, combined immunosuppressive regimens, surveillance for rejection and institution of prophylaxis, and early treatment of infection have resulted in the excellent survival rates and quality of life witnessed today.

The major challenges of preventing graft rejection and infection continue to impede progress. Lung transplant recipients face higher mortality rates and more frequent loss of graft function than other solid organ transplant recipients. Imbalance between organ supply and demand stresses the allocation system.

HISTORY

The pioneering experiments of numerous researchers who attempted to transplant heart, lung, and combined heart-lung blocks in different animal models laid the foundation for thoracic organ transplantation. In the 1950s, successful canine experiments performed by Demikhov, Metras, Hardin, and Kittle made lung transplantation a reality. In 1963, Dr. James Hardy and his team at the University of Mississippi Medical Center performed the first successful human lung homotransplantation. The recipient was a man with severe emphysema and a nonresectable left-sided lung cancer. His donor had recently died from a massive myocardial infarction. As with most early lung transplant procedures, the allograft was harvested from a non–heart-beating donor, an approach that is currently reemerging as a partial solution for the organ shortage. Immediately after the operation, which lasted less than 3 hours, the patient's oxygen saturation improved, providing the first evidence of adequate allograft function. Unfortunately, the initial success was met with failure, because the recipient died 18 days later from renal failure. Nearly 45 different transplantation attempts followed over the next 20 years. In almost all cases, failure seemed to stem from a lack of adequate bronchial perfusion to the anastomosed airways, which led to necrosis, dehiscence, and infection, in concert with lack of medications adequate to prevent acute rejection.

In the early 1980s, lung transplantation entered a new era. Dr. Bruce Reitz and the Stanford transplant group were able to achieve long-term survival with their series of combined heart-lung transplantations. Part of their success was attributed to the lack of bronchial ischemia as a result of performing the combined heart-lung approach that left the coronary circulation intact to provide collateral blood flow to the main airways after the bronchial artery had been ligated. The concurrent use of cyclosporine, the first effective T cell suppressor drug approved for use in solid organ transplantation in the United States, helped ameliorate acute rejection episodes. Dr. Joel Cooper and the Toronto transplant group also documented success with single-lung transplants and then with en bloc bilateral lung transplants. Improved bronchial healing was achieved with omentopexy (i.e., wrapping omentum around the anastomosis to facilitate neovascularization). Omentopexy has been replaced, first by the telescoping bronchial anastomosis technique first described by Dr. Frank Veith in 1969, and then by the end-to-end technique. In the late 1980s, the bilateral sequential single-lung transplant technique, as developed by the Toronto and San Antonio programs, became the procedure of choice for double-lung transplantation.

Over the next 2 decades, the state of lung transplantation grew sporadically, but quickly, and has now stabilized. The most recent reports from multiple lung transplant centers throughout the world indicate that bilateral and single-lung transplants continue to account for most procedures performed. Heart-lung transplants are now rare and reserved primarily for those patients with the Eisenmenger anomaly or severe primary pulmonary hypertension.

CURRENT TRENDS IN LUNG TRANSPLANTATION

In the United States, the United Network for Organ Sharing (UNOS) has been operating the Organ Procurement and Transplantation Network (OPTN) since 1984. The International Society for Heart and Lung Transplantation (ISHLT), in collaboration with UNOS, created a worldwide registry of all heart and heart-lung transplant procedures in 1982. The Twenty-seventh Report documents that more than 32,000 lung transplant procedures have been performed since that time, with 2769 lung transplant procedures done in 2008 by 158 transplant centers worldwide. Most current transplant procedures involve bilateral sequential or double-lung transplants (**Figure 75-2**). Seventy-three heart-lung transplant procedures were done during that same year.

Although the number of lung transplant procedures has increased substantially in the past 2 decades, the leading indications for lung transplantation remain relatively unchanged: chronic obstructive pulmonary disease (COPD), idiopathic pulmonary fibrosis (IPF), cystic fibrosis (CF), α_1-antitrypsin

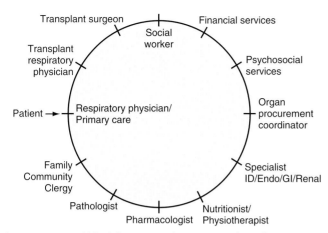

Figure 75-1 Multidisciplinary transplant team. *Endo,* endoscopy; *GI,* gastrointestinal.

(A1A) deficiency with emphysema, and pulmonary arterial hypertension (PAH) (**Figure 75-3**). The type of transplant a patient receives is dictated in part by the recipient's underlying disease: Recipients with COPD and IPF tend to receive single-lung as often as double-lung transplants, whereas those with CF and PAH almost always receive bilateral lung transplants (**Figure 75-4**). Over the past several years, a trend toward performing double-lung transplants and transplanting older people in the 55 to 65 age range has emerged (**Figure 75-5**).

In March 2011, UNOS estimated a total of 1790 patients on the active waiting list in the United States. The median waiting time for those listed in the period 2003 to 2004 was approximately 2 years. The most recent waiting list time is not yet known, but after the implementation of the Lung Allocation Score (LAS), median waiting times seem to have shortened. Twenty-five percent of patients undergo transplantation

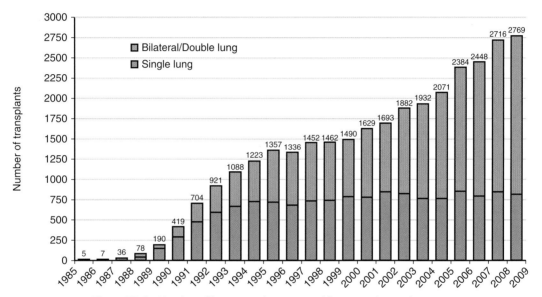

Figure 75-2 Number of lung transplants reported by year and procedure type.

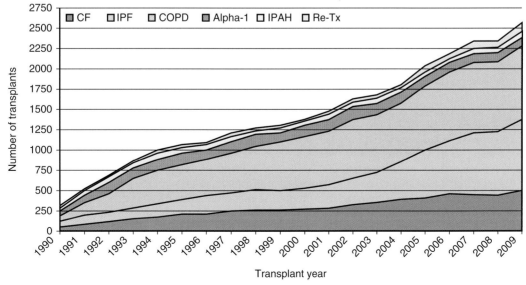

Figure 75-3 Adult lung transplantation major indications by year (%). *Alpha-1,* α_1-antitrypsin deficiency; *CF,* cystic fibrosis; *COPD,* chronic obstructive pulmonary disease; *IPAH,* idiopathic pulmonary arterial hypertension; *IPF,* idiopathic pulmonary fibrosis; *Re-Tx,* repeat transplantation. *(Adapted from Christie JD, Edwards LB, Kucheryavaya AY: The Registry of the International Society for Heart and Lung Transplantation: Twenty-eighth adult lung and heart-lung transplant report—2011,* J Heart Lung Transplant *30:1104-1122, 2011.)*

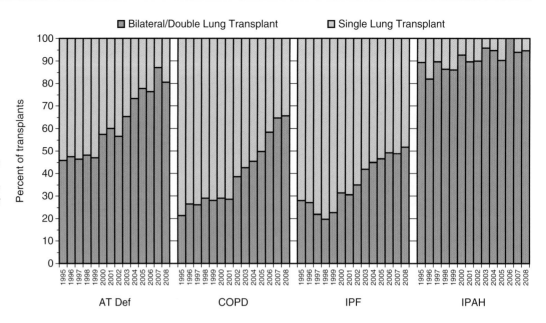

Figure 75-4 Adult lung transplantation procedure types according to indication and year of transplantation. *AT Def,* α1-antitrypsin deficiency emphysema; *COPD,* chronic obstructive pulmonary disease; *IPF,* idiopathic pulmonary fibrosis; *IPAH,* idiopathic pulmonary arterial hypertension. *(Adapted from Christie JD, Edwards LB, Kucheryavaya AY: The Registry of the International Society for Heart and Lung Transplantation: Twenty-eighth adult lung and heart-lung transplant report—2011, J Heart Lung Transplant 30:1104-1122, 2011.)*

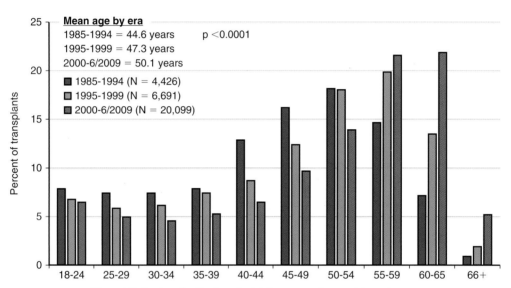

Figure 75-5 Age distribution of adult lung transplant recipients by era.

within 3 months. Today, donors selected for lung donation are older, with a mean age of 38 years, and more donors older than the age of 59 are now accepted.

SURVIVAL

Achieving successful outcomes and maximal survival in the lung transplant population starts with the proper selection of transplant candidates. This entails an understanding of the natural history of the recipient's lung disease and the projected survival with optimal medical and surgical therapy. Identifying potential candidates must be based on their current quality of life and the potential for improvement with and without transplantation. The median survival for lung transplant recipients has improved dramatically over the past several years. Transplant procedures performed from 2000 to 2004 were associated with a median survival of 5 years, significantly higher than for previous years (**Figure 75-6**). The survival curve is not linear, however, because approximately 20% of all recipients die in the first year after transplantation, with most occurring in the

first 90 days. After this rapid decline, survival then stabilizes and follows a more linear trajectory, with an estimated 6% mortality rate per year. First-year mortality is attributable to postoperative graft complications, infection, cardiac failure, rejection, and early toxicity from immunosuppressive medications (**Figure 75-7**).

Several independent factors also seem to affect survival, including older age, higher body mass index (BMI), severe pulmonary hypertension, the type of transplant procedure performed, and the recipient's native pulmonary disease. In recipients older than 65, the expected 5-year median survival is 3.4 years, considerably lower than the overall average 5-year median survival. This is one reason why age older than 65 is considered to be a relative contraindication (**Table 75-1**).

Bilateral lung transplantation (BLTx) is associated with a median survival of 5.6 years, compared with 4.3 years for single lung transplantation (SLTx) (**Figure 75-8**). Although heart-lung transplantation (HLTx) is associated with the lowest median survival rates of approximately 3 years, HLTx procedures also are the least commonly performed. Although it seems that

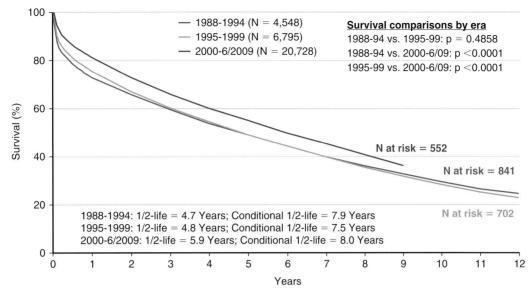

1988-1994: 1/2-life = 4.7 Years; Conditional 1/2-life = 7.9 Years
1995-1999: 1/2-life = 4.8 Years; Conditional 1/2-life = 7.5 Years
2000-6/2009: 1/2-life = 5.9 Years; Conditional 1/2-life = 8.0 Years

Figure 75-6 Kaplan-Meier survival by era for adult lung transplants performed between January 1988 and June 2009. Conditional half-life is the time to 50% survival for the recipients who were alive 1 year after transplantation. *(Adapted from Christie JD, Edwards LB, Kucheryavaya AY: The Registry of the International Society for Heart and Lung Transplantation: Twenty-eighth adult lung and heart-lung transplant report—2011,* J Heart Lung Transplant *30:1104-1122, 2011.)*

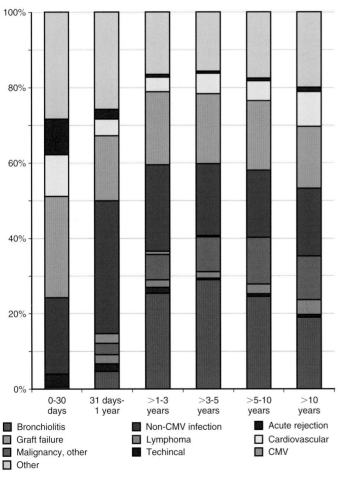

Figure 75-7 Cause of death in time periods after transplantation based on data from transplants performed between January 1997 and June 2009. *(Adapted from Christie JD, Edwards LB, Kucheryavaya AY: The Registry of the International Society for Heart and Lung Transplantation: Twenty-eighth adult lung and heart-lung transplant report—2011,* J Heart Lung Transplant *30:1104-1122, 2011.)*

Table 75-1	**General Contraindications to Lung Transplantation**
Absolute	**Relative**
Malignancy within 5 years (except SCC and BCC)	Age older than 65 years
Untreatable multiorgan dysfunction	Unstable clinical condition
Active hepatitis B and C and HIV infection	Poor rehabilitation potential
Severe spinoskeletal deformity	Pan-resistant colonization (*Burkholderia cepacia* genomovar III)
Current substance addiction	BMI >30 kg/m²
Severe osteoporosis	
Mechanical ventilation	
Poor social support and medical adherence	

BCC, basal cell cancer; *BMI,* body mass index; *HIV,* human immunodeficiency virus; *SCC,* squamous cell cancer.
Modified from Orens JB, Estenne M, Arcasoy SM, et al: International guidelines for the selection of lung transplant candidates: 2006 update—a consensus report from the Pulmonary Scientific Council of the International Society of Heart and Lung Transplantation, *J Heart Lung Transplant* 25:745-755, 2006.

bilateral lung transplant recipients have a better survival, specifically in the COPD group, this finding is controversial, because the observation is retrospective and uncontrolled. One contributing factor may be that older patients tend to receive single-lung transplants, whereas younger patients receive bilateral lung transplants. The highest survival rates are seen in patients with COPD and CF. The lowest survival rates are seen in patients with IPF and PAH, with a relative risk of death exceeding 2.0 in the first year after transplantation (**Figure 75-9**).

GENERAL SELECTION CRITERIA

The International Consensus Guidelines for referral and selection of transplant candidates were published in 1998 as a joint effort from the American Society of Transplant Physicians,

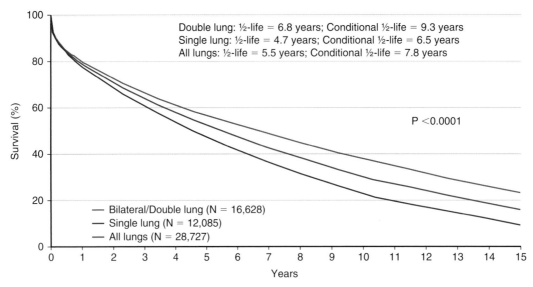

Figure 75-8   Kaplan-Meier survival by procedure type for adult lung transplants performed between January 1994 and June 2009. Conditional half-life is the time to 50% survival for the recipients who were alive 1 year after transplantation.   *(Adapted from Christie JD, Edwards LB, Kucheryavaya AY: The Registry of the International Society for Heart and Lung Transplantation: Twenty-eighth adult lung and heart-lung transplant report—2011, J Heart Lung Transplant 30:1104-1122, 2011.)*

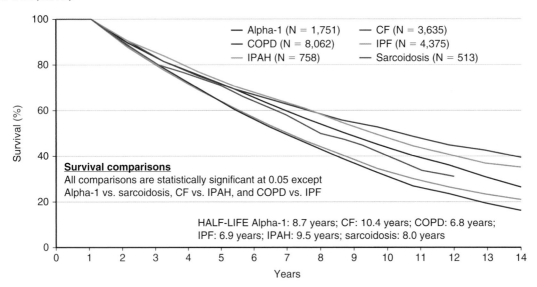

Figure 75-9   Kaplan-Meier survival by diagnosis for adult lung transplants performed between January 1990 and June 2009, conditioned on surviving to one year. *Alpha-1,* α1-antitrypsin–deficiency emphysema; *CF,* cystic fibrosis; *COPD,* chronic obstructive pulmonary disease; *IPAH,* idiopathic pulmonary arterial hypertension; *IPF,* idiopathic pulmonary fibrosis.   *(Adapted from Christie JD, Edwards LB, Kucheryavaya AY: The Registry of the International Society for Heart and Lung Transplantation: Twenty-eighth adult lung and heart-lung transplant report—2011, J Heart Lung Transplant 30:1104-1122, 2011.)*

the American Thoracic Society, the European Respiratory Society, and the International Society for Heart and Lung Transplantation, to facilitate the appropriate timing of referral and proper selection of candidates most likely to benefit from transplantation while ensuring a fair allocation of limited organs. These guidelines were updated in 2006 (**Table 75-2**). In all instances, selected patients with end-stage pulmonary disease should have declining and irreversible lung function despite optimal medical and surgical management. To justify the risk of transplantation, patients should have an estimated survival of less than 2 years.

Two issues regarding this 2-year survival recommendation merit clarification. First, unique to lung transplantation, survival will vary as a function of the recipient's primary disease. Within the first 2 years, survival rates stabilize and allow a more accurate prediction of subsequent survival. Second, the average waiting time for a transplant is close to 2 years. If transplanted

prematurely, patients may lower their survival benefit and keep more terminal candidates from transplantation. Therefore, the most current projected prognosis of lung diseases, the average time on the waiting list, and the median survival after lung transplantation should be considered in determining timing for selection. The new Lung Allocation System in the United States also affects this planning, in that the time to transplantation seems to be shorter, but a median waiting time for patients has not yet been determined. In essence, this is a moving target that will take more time to define.

The typical age for HLTx is younger than 55 years, BLTx younger than 60, and SLTx younger than 65. Medical conditions associated with damage to other organs are considered absolute contraindications. The exception is in rare selected cases with potential for combined heart-lung, lung-kidney, or lung-liver transplantation. For this reason, diagnosis and management of hypertension, diabetes mellitus, gastroesophageal reflux, peptic

Table 75-2 International Guidelines for the Selection of Lung Transplant Candidates: 2006 Update

		Pulmonary Disease		
Guidelines	**COPD**	**CF and Other Causes of Bronchiectasis**	**IPF**	**PPH**
Guidelines for referral	BODE index >5	FEV$_1$ <30% predicted—particularly in young women Exacerbation requiring ICU stay Increasing exacerbations requiring antibiotics Refractory and/or recurrent pneumothorax Recurrent hemoptysis refractory to embolization	Histologic or radiographic evidence of UIP irrespective of FVC Histologic fibrotic NSIP	NYHA class III or IV, irrespective of therapy Rapidly progressive disease
Guidelines for transplantation	BODE index of 7-10 or at least 1 of the following: Hospitalization for exacerbation with acute hypercapnia (Pco$_2$ >50 mm Hg) Pulmonary hypertension or cor pulmonale, or both, despite oxygen therapy FEV$_1$ <20% and either DLco <20% or homogeneous distribution of emphysema	Oxygen-dependent respiratory failure Hypercapnia Pulmonary hypertension	Histologic or radiographic evidence of UIP and any of the following: DLco <39% predicted 10% or greater decline in FVC during 6 months of follow-up Pulse oximetry <88% during a 6-MWT Honeycombing on HRCT (fibrosis score >2) NSIP and DLco <35% NSIP and 10% decline in FVC or 15% decline in DLco during 6 months of follow-up	Persistent NYHA class III or IV on maximal therapy Low (<350 meter) or decline in 6-MWT Failing therapy with intravenous epoprostenol or equivalent CI <2 L/min/m^2 RAP >15 mm Hg

BODE, body mass index, airway obstruction, dyspnea, exercise capacity; *CF,* cystic fibrosis; *CI,* cardiac index; *COPD,* chronic obstructive pulmonary disease; *DLco,* diffusion capacity for carbon monoxide; *FEV$_1$,* forced expiratory volume in 1 second; *FVC,* forced vital capacity; *HRCT,* high-resolution computed tomography; *ICU,* intensive care unit; *IPF,* idiopathic pulmonary fibrosis; *6-MWT,* 6-minute walk test; *NSIP,* Nonspecific interstitial pneumonia; *NYHA,* New York Heart Association; *PPH,* primary pulmonary hypertension; *RAP,* right atrial pressure; *UIP,* usual interstitial pneumonia.
Modified from Orens JB, Estenne M, Arcasoy SM, et al: International guidelines for the selection of lung transplant candidates: 2006 update—a consensus report from the Pulmonary Scientific Council of the International Society of Heart and Lung Transplantation, *J Heart Lung Transplant* 25:745-755, 2006.

ulcer disease, and osteoporosis should be aggressive. Renal impairment is considered an absolute contraindication to transplantation if the creatinine clearance is less than 50 mg/mL/minute.

Cancer screening includes mammography, Papanicolaou smear, PSA assay for prostate, and colonoscopy as medically indicated. A history of cancer is not an absolute contraindication. Eligibility is determined by cancer type and requires documentation of cure without evidence of recurrence or metastasis. In patients with a history of lymphoma, breast, colon, renal, or prostate cancer, a 5-year cancer-free period is required, because these cancers tend to have a longer recurrence period. Less aggressive skin cancers, such as squamous and basal cell, should be in remission for longer than 2 years.

Osteopenia and osteoporosis should be sought with bone densitometry measurements. Bone demineralization should be treated before transplantation by proper nutrition, calcium supplementation, vitamin D, bisphosphonates, and/or hormone replacement. Medications that increase bone resorption should be discontinued. Symptomatic osteoporosis is considered a relative contraindication. The future need for chronic steroid and immunosuppressive therapies will worsen bone loss. This can result in impaired ambulation and suboptimal rehabilitation and limit posttransplantation quality of life.

Nutritional state also affects outcome and postoperative rehabilitation. Candidates should weigh more than 70% but less than 130% of their ideal body weight. Generally speaking, a BMI between 18 and 30 kg/m^2 is acceptable. For patients whose BMI or weight is outside of these limits, a weight gain or weight loss program should be instituted with subsequent reevaluation for candidacy. Percutaneous enteral feeding may be necessary to achieve the desired nutritional goal. Total parenteral nutrition is an option but is not recommended with any enthusiasm because of the attendant risk of infection.

Dependence on tobacco, alcohol, or drugs must be treated, and patients should be substance-free for longer than 6 months. Disabling psychoaffective disorders, noncompliance, and lack of proper social support are relative contraindications. In our institution, social workers assess the support systems to maximize compliance with postoperative interventions and medications. Financial issues, including supplemental aid from hospital programs, insurance companies, and government agencies, as well as family and community support, must be explored preoperatively.

Invasive mechanical ventilation is considered a relative contraindication. Retrospective analyses suggest that acutely ventilated patients have a very high risk of perioperative complications, with a mortality rate surpassing 50%. On the other hand, chronically ventilated patients without other contraindications may have acceptable survival rates if they are otherwise good candidates.

Musculoskeletal disease that limits ambulation and breathing is an absolute contraindication. Less severe disease is acceptable if the recipient can undergo adequate rehabilitation and have a meaningful quality of life after transplantation. Restrictive anatomic deformities of the thorax and skeleton are considered relative contraindications.

Chronic active infection with human immunodeficiency virus (HIV), hepatitis B, and hepatitis C are considered absolute contraindications. Recipients colonized with multidrug-resistant *Burkholderia cepacia* complex (BCC) exhibit an extremely high rate of mortality and graft failure. BCC often is found in patients with CF, and many centers consider this to be an absolute contraindication. Survival in recipients with multidrug-resistant *Pseudomonas aeruginosa* is similar to that in noncolonized patients. Previously treated infection with *Mycobacterium tuberculosis* is not a contraindication. Treatment of various pulmonary infections may be started preoperatively in some patients in an attempt to decrease the pathogen burden. In others, postoperative prophylaxis may be instituted for those who are deemed to be at high risk for infection or reactivation (e.g., with *Aspergillus* colonization). A higher risk of infection still exists in colonized recipients who receive bilateral lung transplants, because many colonizing bacteria and fungi may spill down into the lung from sinuses, nasopharynx, and trachea.

DISEASE-SPECIFIC CONSIDERATIONS FOR REFERRAL AND SELECTION

Chronic Obstructive Pulmonary Disease

Patients with COPD (i.e., emphysema, chronic bronchitis, and obliterative bronchiolitis) have the highest survival rates after transplantation (emphysema related to A1A deficiency is considered a separate condition).

Survival benefit has not been documented in patients with COPD, even though transplantation confers substantial improvement in functional capacity and quality of life. One potential explanation for this discrepancy is that the forced expiratory volume in 1 second (FEV_1) may not be as reliable a referral parameter as, for example, the BODE index (determined by scoring for *body* mass index, airway *obstruction*, *dyspnea*, and *exercise* capacity) (**Table 75-3**). Patients with a BODE index between 7 and 10 should be selected for transplantation. Other criteria for selecting candidates with COPD include severe worsening of pulmonary function, shorter 6-minute walking distance capacity (less than 100 yards), weight loss (BMI less than 20 kg/m²), need for hospital

admission (to the intensive care unit [ICU] in particular), and radiographically homogeneous emphysema. More severely affected patients will show chronic hypoventilation (i.e., $PaCO_2$ greater than 55 mm Hg and evidence of pulmonary hypertension despite oxygen therapy). All patients with COPD should be referred for pulmonary rehabilitation and treated with oxygen therapy, and use of an alternative approach such as lung volume reduction surgery should be either documented as not a viable option or proved to be ineffective.

Pulmonary Fibrosis

IPF is the most progressive of the fibrotic diseases and is defined by the histologic diagnosis of usual interstitial pneumonitis (UIP). No treatment for IPF is known to be effective; accordingly, patients can only be supported with supplemental oxygen, pulmonary rehabilitation, and close clinical surveillance. Prompt referral of appropriate candidates for lung transplantation is essential, because it is the only measure that will prolong survival in those at highest risk for death. IPF has a median survival of 3 years from the time of diagnosis, consistent with the 30% mortality rate documented for patients with IPF awaiting transplantation. Lung function parameters are used to decide when patients should be referred (i.e., a forced vital capacity [FVC] less than 60% to 70% of predicted, a diffusion capacity for carbon monoxide [DLCO] less than 50% to 60% of predicted). Many, however, feel that these cutoffs are too low, because they underestimate mortality. Other variables indicating higher mortality rates include hypoxia developing during a 6-minute walk test (pulse oximetry less than 88%), a resting PaO_2 level less than 50 mm Hg measured in room air, classic radiologic or histologic features of UIP, and a decline in lung function within 6 months of the initial diagnosis.

Other causes of pulmonary fibrosis tend to be associated with a better prognosis. Nonspecific interstitial pneumonia (NSIP), particularly the cellular variant of NSIP, has a 5-year survival rate of 75%. Other fibrotic diseases that may lead to lung transplantation include sarcoidosis, scleroderma, rheumatoid arthritis, mixed connective tissue disorders, asbestosis, histiocytosis X, and lymphangioleiomyomatosis. In general, the same criteria for referral should be used with all of these, because more disease-specific criteria have not yet been developed.

Cystic Fibrosis

Patients with CF frequently have multiorgan involvement and comorbid conditions, including malnutrition, chronic infections of the upper respiratory tract, and colonization with resistant pathogens. Current referral guidelines are inadequate, because good prognostic models for survival in CF do not exist, but patients with an FEV_1 less than 30% predicted or with declining pulmonary function should be referred early. This consideration is most important in female patients younger than 20 years of age, who seem to have a worse prognosis. Severity of disease also may be indicated by an increase in the frequency of hospital admissions, specifically, if ICU care is required. As in COPD, the ability to identify patients with a better prognosis is likely to depend on assessing multiple factors such as the degree of hypoxia and hypercapnia, evidence of cor pulmonale, and limited functional capacity. Colonization with multidrug-resistant *P. aeruginosa*, *Staphylococcus aureus*, *Stenotrophomonas maltophilia*, or *Aspergillus fumigatus* is not a contraindication to transplantation, because these organisms have not been shown to affect posttransplantation survival. The exception is *B. cepacia* genomovar III, which is associated with unacceptably high

	Points			
Variable	**0**	**1**	**2**	**3**
Airflow obstruction (FEV₁ % predicted)	≥65	50-64	36-49	≤35
6-minute walk test (distance in meters)	≥350	250-349	150-249	≤149
MMRC dyspnea scale (range 0-4)	0-1	2	3	4
Body mass index	>21	≤21		

Table 75-3 BODE Index Computation

BODE, body mass index, airway obstruction, dyspnea, exercise capacity; *FEV₁*, forced expiratory volume in 1 second; *MMRC*, Modified Medical Research Council.
Modified from Celli BR, Cote CG, Marin JM, et al: The body-mass index, airflow obstruction, dyspnea, and exercise capacity index in chronic obstructive pulmonary disease, *N Engl J Med* 350:1005–1012, 2004.

posttransplantation mortality. Patients with multidrug-resistant pathogens should undergo frequent evaluation for changes in their colonizing microflora and resistance patterns. This will guide early prophylaxis and treatment in the immediate postoperative period. Complicated pneumothorax and hemoptysis are other indications for early referral.

Patients with CF have excellent survival rates, similar to those in persons with COPD. Although other causes of bronchiectasis also are amenable to transplantation, data on these disorders are insufficient to develop specific guidelines. For the most part, guidelines recommended for patients with CF are used.

Pulmonary Arterial Hypertension

Idiopathic pulmonary hypertension is a progressive and rapidly fatal disease, with an estimated median untreated survival of less than 3 years from the time of diagnosis. Current pulmonary vasodilator therapy (with agents including epoprostenol, treprostinil, sildenafil, and bosentan) has substantially increased survival. Transplantation is, accordingly, reserved for those who do not respond to medical management. Patients in New York Heart Association/World Health Organization (NYHA/WHO) functional class III or IV are at highest risk for death and the most likely to benefit from transplantation. Diminished exercise capacity can be measured by use of a standard 6-minute walk test. Inability to walk a distance of 332 m and degree of right-sided heart failure are important predictors of mortality.

DONOR SELECTION AND MANAGEMENT

The LAS assigns donor lungs to transplant candidates by use of a scoring system determined by medical urgency and net transplant benefit (predicted posttransplantation survival minus predicted wait list survival). Since its implementation in the United States in 2005, median waiting times have shortened markedly. Unfortunately, a scarcity of donated organs remains a limiting problem, leading to use of non–heart-beating donors (Table 75-4), ex vivo donor lung resuscitation, use of "bridges to transplant," and development of different types of lung grafts (Table 75-5).

Currently, the Ideal Donor Selection Criteria are more stringent than those used for selecting other solid organs. In light of the scarcity of available lung grafts, many suggest that donor criteria be made more flexible to expand the existing donor pool. Alternate criteria include donor age older than 55 years, an initial PaO_2/FIO_2 ratio less than 300, the presence of pulmonary infiltrates on chest imaging, purulent secretions, and a positive history of use of tobacco or other inhalant drug (Table 75-6 and Box 75-1). Retrospective studies suggest similar outcomes for ideal and extended lung allograft recipients, specifically with respect to perioperative complications, ICU stay,

requirements for mechanical ventilation, and 1-year survival rate (higher than 80% for both groups). Improved donor management also is under careful investigation, because it may help improve marginal donors and optimize them into ideal candidates. Optimizing donor status with reversal of any limiting physiologic insults is becoming the standard of care in most

Table 75-4 Maastricht Classification for Non–Heart-Beating Donors*

I	Uncontrolled	Brought in dead
II	Uncontrolled	Unsuccessful resuscitation
III	Controlled	Awaiting cardiac arrest
IV	Controlled	Cardiac arrest after brain death
V	Controlled	Cardiac arrest in a hospital inpatient

*Controlled non–heart-beating donors may be eligible for lung donation.

Table 75-5 Types of Lung Grafts

Living donor	Donor donates single lower lobe Recipient receives two lower lobes from two separate donors
Heart-beating donor	Whole brain death May donate one or both lungs, depending on selection criteria
Non–heart-beating donor (NHBD)	Donor has sustained cardiac arrest Resuscitated to unacceptable state and deemed suitable for organ donation
Xenotransplantation	Porcine, bovine, and primate lungs Still under investigation
Artificial lung	Intracorporeal or paracorporeal devices that oxygenate venous blood Still under investigation
Avalon Elite (Wang-Zwische double cannula)	Cannula inserted from the right jugular vein into superior vena cava (SVC) traversing right atrium to inferior vena cava (IVC) Drains venous blood from SVC and IVC and delivers oxygenated blood into the right atrium Achieves minimal to no recirculation and potential total gas exchange

From Wang D, Zhou X, Liu X, et al: Wang-Zwische double-lumen cannula—toward a percutaneous and ambulatory paracorporeal artificial lung, *ASAIO J* 54(6):606-611, 2008.

Table 75-6 Donor Selection Guidelines

Feature	Ideal Donor	Extended Donor
Age (years)	<55	>55
ABO	Identical or compatible	Compatible
Chest radiograph	Clear	Unilateral or focal infiltrate
*PaO$_2$ (mm Hg)	>300	<300 on initial assessment; must be >300 after optimization
Tobacco (smoking) history	<20 pack-years	>20 pack-years
Trauma	Absence of chest trauma	Trauma without significant abnormality
Sputum	No purulent secretions	May be considered, therapeutic suctioning Can be performed
Gram stain	Absence of organisms	Certain organisms may be considered (see Box 75-1)

*Partial pressure of arterial oxygen tension (Pao$_2$) is measured on a fraction of inspired oxygen of 1.0 and a positive end-expiratory pressure of 5 cm H$_2$O.

transplant centers (**Figure 75-10**). Common respiratory insults are caused by aspiration, atelectasis, infection, pulmonary edema, and the hemodynamic instability associated with neurologic dysfunction. Ventilatory strategies to improve alveolar ventilation may be implemented, along with therapeutic bronchoscopy to suction excess secretions and reexpand atelectatic lung. Small-volume bronchoalveolar lavage (BAL) can minimize the amount of alveolar flooding. Adequate tissue perfusion and cardiac function should be aided with vasoactive medications when needed. Repletion of cortisol, vasopressin, and thyroid hormone also may be of benefit (**Figure 75-11**).

DONOR GRAFT MANAGEMENT

Graft ischemic time begins after the lungs have been extracted from the donor. The lungs are flushed with a cold heparinized preservation solution—modified Euro-Collins, low potassium dextran solution (LPD), and University of Wisconsin solutions are the most commonly used—and hypothermic preservation is maintained during transport at 4° C. These solutions have helped reduce the severity of ischemic injury. Additives such as surfactant and platelet and thrombin inhibitors are still under investigation. Donor lungs are matched according to compatibility in size and ABO blood group. A growing trend is for use of prospective lymphocyte and human leukocyte antigen (HLA) cross-matching, especially in sensitized persons. Cytomegalovirus (CMV) and Epstein-Barr virus (EBV) cross-matching is not routine, because such testing often is impractical. Each matching procedure has its supporters for certain situations, however.

LUNG ALLOGRAFT IMPLANTATION

The implantation of a lung allograft (**Figure 75-12**) depends on the planned procedure, surgical experience, and the previous surgical history of the recipient. Before all transplant procedures, the recipient's pulmonary function should be maximized, and management should continue through surgery (e.g., continuing pulmonary vasodilators).

A single-lung transplant often is placed through an anterolateral or posterolateral thoracotomy. Bilateral lung implantation may be performed by means of a transverse sternotomy "clamshell" incision, at the level of the fourth or fifth intercostal spaces, whereas HLTx usually is done through a midsternotomy. Bilateral sequential lung transplantation (BSLT) also can be performed through bilateral anterior thoracotomies; this approach may be preferred because it does not split the sternum and is associated with less chest wall instability. The surgical history of the recipient is important, because previous pleurodesis or cardiothoracic surgery results in fibrous bands and adhesions. This makes resection difficult and may alter the anatomy.

When a single-lung transplant procedure is to be performed, the intact side is preferred.

In most instances, the cold ischemic time for a single-lung transplant is approximately 4 hours and for a bilateral lung transplant is less than 6 hours. Pleural tubes are placed before closure and maintained in place until drainage is less than 200 mL/day. Bronchoscopic evaluation of the airway mucosa, anastomotic sites, and therapeutic suctioning of secretions is performed to document graft viability and optimize function.

Intraoperative and postoperative management of patients with end-stage pulmonary disease is challenging because of poor pulmonary gas exchange, elevated pulmonary vascular resistance, and right ventricular overload. Analgesia is controlled with multiple medications, with avoidance of narcotics if possible because of their effects of decreased respiratory drive and sedative properties. A thoracic epidural often is placed in preparation for surgery to adequately control pain and optimize postoperative lung function. Endotracheal intubation is performed with the largest-diameter dual-lumen tube possible to facilitate clearance of secretions. Mechanical ventilation can increase pulmonary vascular resistance and decrease venous return, leading to systemic hypotension. This potential for such effects is important to consider, because anesthetics used during rapid-sequence induction and surgery should be administered cautiously to avoid a precipitous drop in systemic vascular resistance. In most cases, infusions with propofol and fentanyl are used and combined with a neuromuscular blocker such as pancuronium. A fraction of inspired oxygen at 1.0 is used initially, to reduce hypoxic pulmonary vasoconstriction and limit right-sided heart afterload. Cardiopulmonary bypass is not used routinely and should generally be avoided unless hemodynamic instability arises or simultaneous cardiac surgery is necessary. If bypass is used, aprotinin (which slows fibrinolysis) may be administered to help control the coagulopathic disturbance created by the activation of multiple cytokines from the bypass procedure (although recent studies have suggested aprotinin may be associated with increased thrombotic complications). When single-lung ventilation commences, hypoxia and hypoventilation may ensue. Capnography, along with serial arterial blood gases, can help detect signs of failing single-lung ventilation. This deficit may be corrected with independent dual-lung ventilation and tolerance of moderate respiratory acidosis so long as hemodynamics and oxygenation remain stable.

Pulmonary vasodilators such as inhaled nitric oxide (iNO) are used commonly in the perioperative setting. The effects of iNO at relatively low levels (less than 20 parts per million) are not completely understood, but this agent is preferred because of the selective pulmonary vasodilation occurring at sites receiving adequate alveolar ventilation. iNO also seems to inhibit endothelial dysfunction and capillary leak, suppress oxygen radical formation, and ameliorate ischemia-reperfusion injury to the lung allograft. These benefits could then extend to improvement in early graft function. The adverse effects of iNO at higher concentration levels include methemoglobinemia, pulmonary edema, and cardiac contractile dysfunction. Prostacyclin, in either intravenous or aerosolized form, also is used as a direct pulmonary vasodilator.

The goal of hemodynamic management is to reach a negative fluid balance and limit pulmonary edema. The pulmonary artery occlusion pressure is kept under 10 mm Hg to ensure adequate preload. In most cases, immediate normalization of pulmonary arterial pressures and right ventricular function is expected after transplantation. To prevent alveolar damage, hyperinflation, pulmonary vascular hypertension, and

Collaborative Practice	Phase I Referral	Phase II Declaration of Brain Death and Consent	Phase III Donor Evaluation	Phase IV Donor Management	Phase V Recovery Phase

The following professionals may be involved to enhance the donation process.
 	
Check all that apply.
○ Physician
○ Critical care RN
○ Organ Procurement Organization (OPO)
○ OPO coordinator (OPC)
○ MedicalExaminer (ME)/ Coroner
○ Respiratory
○ Laboratory
○ Pharmacy
○ Radiology
○ Anesthesiology
○ OR/Surgery staff
○ Clergy
○ Social worker
	○ Notify physician regarding OPO referral
	○ Contact OPO ref: Potential donor with severe brain insult
	○ OPC on site and begins evaluation Time _____ Date _____
	○ Ht_____ Wt _____ as documented
	○ ABO as documented _____
	○ Notify house supervisor/ charge nurse of presence of OPC on unit
		○ Brain death documented Time _____ Date _____
		○ Pt accepted as potential donor
		○ MD notifies family of death
		○ Plan family approach with OPC
		○ Offer support services to family (clergy, etc)
		○ OPC/Hospital staff talks to family about donation
		○ Family accepts donation
		○ OPC obtains signed consent & medical/social history Time _____ Date _____
		○ ME/Coroner notified
		○ ME/Coroner releases body for donation
		○ *Family/ME/Coroner denies donation—stop pathway— initiate post-mortem protocol—support family.*
			○ Obtain pre/post transfusion blood for serology testing (HIV, hepatitis, VDRL, CMV)
			○ Obtain lymph nodes and/or blood for tissue typing
			○ Notify OR & anesthesiology of pending donation
			○ Notify house supervisor of pending donation
			○ Chest & abdominal circumference
			○ Lung measurements per CXR by OPC
			○ *Cardiology consult as requested by OPC (see reverse side)*
			○ *Donor organs unsuitable for transplant—stop pathway—initiate post-mortem protocol—support family.*
				○ OPC writes new orders
				○ Organ placement
				○ OPC sets tentative OR time
				○ Insert arterial line/ 2 large-bone IVs
				○ Possibly insert CVP/Pulmonary Artery Catheter
				○ See reverse side
					○ Checklist for OR
					○ Supplies given to OR
					○ Prepare patient for transport to OR
					  ○ IVs ○ Pumps
					  ○ O₂ ○ Ambu
					  ○ Peep valve
					○ Transport to OR
					  Date _____
					  Time _____
					○ OR nurse
					  ○ reviews consent form
					  ○ reviews brain death documentation
					  ○ checks patient's ID band

Labs/Diagnostics		○ Review previous lab results
		○ Review previous hemodynamics
			○ Blood chemistry
			○ CBC + diff
			○ UA ○ C & S
			○ PT, PTT
			○ ABO ○ A Subtype
			○ Liver function tests
			○ Blood culture X 2 / 15 minutes to 1 hour apart
			○ Sputum Gram stain & C & S
			○ Type & Cross Match _____ # units PRBCs
			○ CXR ○ ABGs
			○ EKG ○ Echo
			○ Consider cardiac cath
			○ Consider bronchoscopy
				○ Determine need for additional lab testing
				○ CXR after line placement (if done)
				○ Serum electrolytes
				○ H & H after PRBC Rx
				○ PT, PTT
				○ BUN, serum creatinine after correcting fluid deficit
				○ Notify OPC for
				  ___ PT >14 ___ PTT > 28
				  ___ Urine output
				    ___ < 1 mL/Kg/hr
				    ___ > 3 mL/Kg/hr
				  ___ Hct < 30 / Hgb <10
				  ___ Na >150 mEq/L
					○ Labs drawn in OR as per surgeon or OPC request
					○ Communicate with pathology: Bx liver and/ or kidneys as indicated

Respiratory	○ Pt on ventilator
	○ Suction q 2 hr
	○ Reposition q 2 hr
		○ Prep for apnea testing: set FiO₂ @ 100% and anticipate need to decrease rate if PCO₂ < 45 mm Hg	○ Maximize ventilator settings to achieve SaO₂ 98 - 99%
			○ PEEP = 5cm O₂ challenge for lung placement FiO₂ @ 100%, PEEP @ 5 X 10 min
			○ ABGs as ordered
			○ VS q 1°
				○ Notify OPC for
				  ___ BP < 90 systolic
				  ___ HR < 70 or > 120
				  ___ CVP < 4 or > 11
				  ___ PaO₂ < 90 or
				  ___ SaO₂ < 95%
					○ Portable O₂ @ 100% FiO₂ for transport to OR
					○ Ambu bag and PEEP valve
					○ Move to OR

Treatments/ **Ongoing Care**		○ Use warming/cooling blanket to maintain temperature at 36.5° C - 37.5 °C ○ NG to low intermittent suction	○ Check NG placement & output ○ Obtain actual Ht _____ & Wt _____ if not previously obtained		○ Set OR temp as directed by OPC ○ Post-mortem care at conclusion of case
Medications			○ Medication as requested by OPC	○ Fluid resuscitation—consider crystalloids, colloids, blood products ○ DC meds except pressors & antibiotics ○ Broad-spectrum antibiotic if not previously ordered ○ Vasopressor support to maintain BP > 90 mm Hg systolic ○ Electrolyte imbalance: consider K, Ca, PO₄, Mg replacement ○ Hyperglycemia: consider insulin drip ○ Oliguria: consider diuretics ○ Diabetes insipidus: consider antidiuretics ○ Paralytic as indicated for spinal reflexes	○ DC antidiuretics ○ Diuretics as needed ○ 350 U heparin/kg or as directed by surgeon
Optimal Outcomes	The potential donor is identified & a referral is made to the OPO.	The family is offered the option of donation & their decision is supported.	The donor is evaluated & found to be a suitable candidate for donation.	Optimal organ function is maintained.	All potentially suitable, consented organs are recovered for transplant.

Shaded areas indicate Organ Procurement Coordinator (OPC) Activities.

Figure 75-10 Critical pathway of organ donor management. *(From* Critical pathway for the organ donor, *Richmond, Va, United Network for Organ Sharing, 2006 [poster online]: http://www.Unos.Org/Resources/Pdfs/Criticalpathwayposter.pdf.)*

Figure 75-11 Critical pathway of organ donor management. *CVP*, central venous pressure; *EF*, ejection fraction; *Hgb*, hemoglobin; *PT*, prothrombin time; *PTT*, partial thromboplastin time; *PWCP*, pulmonary capillary wedge pressure; *SVR*, systemic vascular resistance. *(From Critical pathway for the organ donor, Richmond, Va, United Network for Organ Sharing, 2006 [poster online]: http://www.Unos.Org/Resources/Pdfs/Criticalpathwayposter.pdf.)*

Cardio-Thoracic Donor Management

1. Early echocardiogram for all donors—Insert pulmonary artery catheter (PAC) to monitor patient management (placement of the PAC is particularly relevant in patients with an EF < 45% or on high dose inotropes).
   - use aggressive donor resuscitation as outlined below

2. Electrolytes
   - maintain Na < 150 meq/dL
   - maintain K+ > 4.0
   - correct acidosis with Na bicarbonate and mild to moderate hyperventilation (pco_2 30-35 mm Hg)

3. Ventilation — Maintain tidal volume 10-15 mL/kg
   - keep peak airway pressures < 30 mm Hg
   - maintain a mild respiratory alkalosis (pco_2 30-35 mm Hg)

4. Recommend use of hormonal resuscitation as part of a comprehensive donor management protocol — Key elements
   - Tri-iodothyronine (T3): 4 µg bolus; 3 µg/hr continuous infusion
   - Arginine Vasopressin: 1 unit bolus: 0.5-4.0 unit/hour drip (titrate SVR 800-1200 using a PA catheter)
   - Methylprednisolone: 15 mg/kg bolus (repeat q 24° PRN)
   - Insulin: drip at a minimum rate of 1 unit/hour (titrate blood glucose to 120-180 mg/dL)
   - Ventilator: (See above)
   - Volume Resuscitation: Use of colloid and avoidance of anemia are important in preventing pulmonary edema
     - albumin if PT and PTT are normal
     - fresh frozen plasma if PT and PTT abnormal (value ≥ 1.5 × control)
     - packed red blood cells to maintain a PCWP of 8-12 mm Hg and Hgb > 10.0 mg/dL

5. When patient is stabilized/optimized repeat echocardiogram. (An unstable donor has not met 2 or more of the following criteria.)
   - Mean Arterial Pressure ≥ 60
   - CVP ≤ 12 mm Hg
   - PCWP ≤ 12 mm Hg
   - SVR 800-1200 dyne/sec/cm^5
   - Cardiac Index ≥ 2.5 L/min/M^2
   - Left Ventricular Stroke Work Index > 15
   - Dopamine dosage < 10 µg/kg/min

---

anastomotic dehiscence, peak airway pressures are kept under 40 cm H_2O, with a positive end-expiratory pressure close to 5 cm H_2O. Liberation from mechanical ventilation usually is accomplished in the first 1 to 3 days after transplantation.

NONINFECTIOUS COMPLICATIONS

The most common problems in the immediate posttransplantation period are the same as those occurring in most postsurgical patients. Hypoxemia may stem from poor cardiac output, endotracheal tube displacement, or obstruction of uncleared secretions, leading to lobar atelectasis. Additional complications that are unique to lung transplantation include hyperacute rejection, graft dysfunction, and cardiac failure; each may be difficult to differentiate from the others (**Table 75-7**). A suggested reading by Ahya and Kawut has been listed.

HYPERACUTE REJECTION

Hyperacute rejection (HAR) results from a recipient antibody directed against donor endothelial antigens and those in the human leukocyte antigen (HLA) group. This antibody immediately triggers the classic complement cascade with reperfusion of the graft, leading to cell injury and cell death. HAR is extremely rapid in onset, occurring often within

minutes of reperfusion and can be seen intraoperatively as a dusky pallor and swelling of the transplanted lung. Endothelial injury leads to capillary leak, and leukocyte injury leads to microvascular inflammation, thrombosis, and coagulopathy. The capillary injury is manifested as diffuse alveolar infiltrates, low PaO_2/FIO_2 ratio, and increased plateau pressures.

HAR can be avoided by preoperatively performing a leukocyte cross-match test, whereby the recipient's blood is tested against the donor's cells, seeking the presence of leukocyte sensitization and donor cell lysis. The plasma reactivity antibody (PRA) test is another way of checking the recipient's serum against a panel of commonly found HLAs and measuring the degree of sensitization. Patients with a PRA concentration greater than 10% are considered to be at greater risk for rejection and posttransplantation mortality. In our institution, patients with high PRA levels are treated with plasmapheresis followed by intravenous immunoglobulin (IVIG) on the day of transplantation. Prospective cross-matching and/or virtual cross-matching are routinely utilized. This combination treatment seems to provide outcomes comparable to those for recipients without high levels of anti-HLA antibodies. Other methods involve pulse administration of cyclophosphamide or methotrexate along with IVIG to reach a high level of immunosuppression. Desensitization routines vary, and it is as yet unclear how well they work.

Lung transplant techniques				
	Heart-lung	**Bilateral sequential**	**Single lung**	**Live donor lobar**
	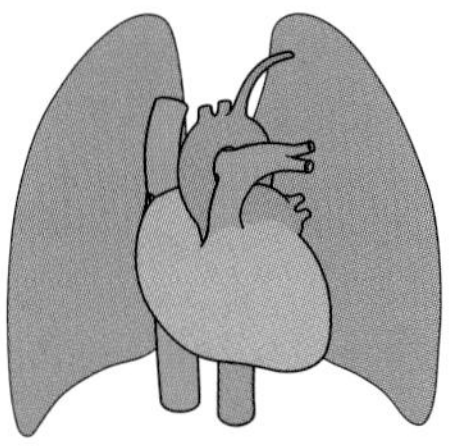	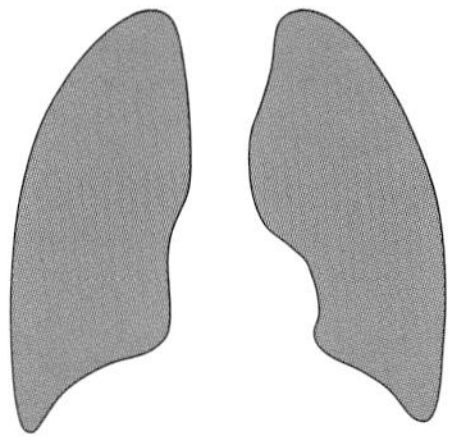	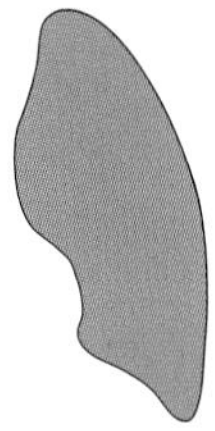	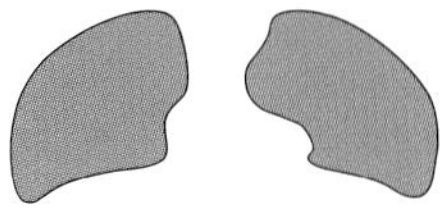
Incision	Midline sternotomy	Horizontal "clam shell" Bilateral anterior thoracotomies preferred Horizontal "clam shell" less frequently used	Lateral thoracotomy	Horizontal "clam shell"
Anastomoses	Tracheal Right atrial Aortic	Left and right bronchial "Double" left atrial Right and left pulmonary artery	Bronchial Left atrial Pulmonary artery	Lobar bronchus to bronchus Lobar vein to superior pulmonary vein Lobar artery to main pulmonary artery
Advantages	Airway vascularity All indications	Access to pleural space No cardiac allograft Less cardiopulmonary bypass	Easiest procedure Increases recipients	Increases donors Can be done "electively"
Disadvantages	Cardiac allograft Organ "consumption"	Airway complications Postoperative pain	Airway complications Poor reserve	Complex undertaking Donor morbidity
Common indications	Congenital heart disease with pulmonary hypertension Heart and lung disease Primary pulmonary hypertension	Cystic fibrosis (CF) Bullous emphysema Primary pulmonary hypertension Bronchiectasis	Emphysema Pulmonary fibrosis Primary pulmonary hypertension	Cystic fibrosis (CF) Pulmonary fibrosis Primary pulmonary hypertension

Figure 75-12 Comparison of the four standard lung replacement techniques, including their common indications.

Table 75-7 **Early Noninfectious Pulmonary Complications**

	Diagnosis			
Feature	**HAR**	**PGD**	**AR**	**HPE**
Onset	Immediate (<2 days)	2-3 days	1 week to 3 months	Immediate (<2 days)
Etiology	Recipient antibodies to donor antigens ABO blood group antigens HLA antigens (DR and B)	Multi-injury: Donor illness, surgical harvest, ischemia preservation hypothermia, reperfusion	Cell-mediated reaction against donor endothelial and epithelial antigens	Pulmonary venous obstruction Cardiogenic shock LV outflow obstruction Fluid overload
Pathology	Alveolar hemorrhage Intravascular fibrin/thrombi Neutrophil interstitial infiltration Capillaritis IgG deposition	DAD Graded by level of hypoxemia	Graded by extent of parenchymal and vascular lymphocytic infiltration T cell infiltration, CD8+ predominant	Alveolar edema
Treatment	Removal of alloantibodies Plasmapheresis IVIG	Negative fluid balance Lung-protective ventilation Nitric oxide Prostaglandins ECMO Retransplantation	Cell-mediated immunosuppression High-dose steroids Antithymocyte globulin Photopheresis Radiation	Negative fluid balance Diuresis Renal replacement therapy Correction/treatment of underlying cause

AR, acute rejection; *DAD*, diffuse alveolar damage; *ECMO*, extracorporeal mechanical oxygenation; *HAR*, hyperacute rejection; *HLA*, human leukocyte antigen; *HPE*; high-pressure pulmonary edema; *IgG*, immunoglobulin G; *IVIG*, intravenous immunoglobulin; *LV*, left ventricle; *PGD*, primary graft dysfunction.

Table 75-8 Recommendations for Grading of Primary Graft Dysfunction Severity

Grade	Pao$_2$/Fio$_2$ Ratio	Radiographic Infiltrates Consistent with Pulmonary Edema
0	>300	Absent
1	>300	Present
2	200-300	Present
3	<200	Present

From Christie JD, Carby M, Bag R, et al: Report of the ISHLT Working Group on Primary Lung Graft Dysfunction. Part II: definition. A consensus statement of the International Society for Heart and Lung Transplantation, *J Heart Lung Transplant* 24(10):1454-1459, 2005.

PRIMARY GRAFT DYSFUNCTION

Primary graft dysfunction (PGD) is the current name for the syndrome of acute lung injury (ALI) after reperfusion of the lung allograft (**Table 75-8**). This entity previously was referred to as ischemia-reperfusion injury, reimplantation edema, or early graft dysfunction. PGD occurs 48 to 72 hours after transplantation and is characterized by development of bilateral diffuse alveolar infiltrates evident on plain chest radiograph coupled with hypoxemia resulting from capillary leak and alveolar flooding and is associated with prolonged ischemic time (i.e., longer than 550 minutes). In approximately 15% of patients, the degree of hypoxemia reaches ALI criteria (Pao$_2$/Fio$_2$ ratio less than 200) with an accompanying mortality rate of more than 60%. Exclusion of other causes of alveolar infiltrates, including high-pressure pulmonary edema, is necessary.

Immediate management is supportive and similar to management of patients with ALI or acute respiratory distress syndrome (ARDS), including generating a negative fluid balance in an attempt to prevent further alveolar flooding by use of open lung plus low tidal volume ventilation (4 to 6 mL/kg of predicted body weight) to limit ventilator-associated lung injury and providing hemodynamic support with vasoactive drugs to maintain adequate perfusion to major organs and the bronchial anastomoses. Renal replacement therapy generally is recommended for oliguric renal injury, because it may facilitate achieving negative fluid balance. Anecdotal evidence suggests that nitric oxide may lower pulmonary arterial pressures, improve ventilation-perfusion mismatch, and protect endothelial cells. Similarly, prostaglandins also may have protective effects in this setting and often are added to the preservation solution as a means of preventing PGD. Extracorporeal membrane oxygenation (ECMO) as a bridge to urgent retransplantation has been used anecdotally with little success.

HIGH-PRESSURE PULMONARY EDEMA

High-pressure pulmonary edema (i.e., a pulmonary artery occlusion pressure greater than 18 mm Hg) can develop as a result of several problems. Fluid overload may occur from blood product transfusion and/or crystalloid infusions. Cardiogenic shock can occur as result of cardiopulmonary bypass or from previously untreated myocardial disease. Pulmonary vascular anastomoses may undergo dehiscence or become thrombosed or stenosed. Diagnosis of pulmonary venous obstruction can be made with transesophageal echocardiography with careful inspection of the pulmonary valve anastomotic sites. Thrombus formation in the pulmonary outflow tract and left atrium can

lead to systemic embolization, necessitating immediate anticoagulation with or without thrombectomy.

ACUTE REJECTION

Acute rejection (AR) is a cell-mediated event activated by donor antigens. It occurs in about 40% of transplant recipients in the first year alone with the highest incidence at 6 months after lung transplantation and is irrespective of specific induction treatment. **Figure 75-13** shows the reported rejection between discharge and 1-year follow-up stratified by immunosuppressive regimen. It manifests with presence of alveolar infiltrates on the chest radiograph, hypoxemia, and fever, but many patients may be asymptomatic. Histologic examination (**Figure 75-14**) is required to diagnose AR, because the clinical presentation mimics that in pulmonary infection, and increasing immunosuppression empirically can lead to toxicity, infection, and malignancy.

AR is associated with an increased risk for development of chronic rejection. For this reason, serial surveillance with fiberoptic bronchoscopy, BAL, and transbronchial biopsy is often routine during the first year after transplantation. Current recommendations are to obtain at least five separate samples that contain both alveolated lung and bronchioles (because both are necessary to grade the level of AR). Treatment centers on increasing the level of immunosuppression by administration of high-dose corticosteroids and optimizing the use of the standard agents. In addition, antithymocyte globulin, photochemotherapy, and lymphoid irradiation may be used.

BRONCHIAL ANASTOMOTIC COMPLICATIONS

Bronchial anastomotic dehiscence may result from ischemic injury, infection, or poor healing. Bronchial artery interruption during the transplant procedure disrupts perfusion to the large airways. High doses of corticosteroids impair wound healing, potentially leading to bronchomalacia and stenosis (**Figure 75-15**). Dehiscence may manifest as pneumomediastinum, pneumopericardium, and/or pneumothorax (**Figure 75-16**). Fiberoptic bronchoscopy is necessary to ensure that all bronchial anastomoses are intact. Correction consists of treating any underlying infection and maintenance of adequate tissue perfusion. Bronchial stent placement, laser ablation, and balloon dilatation often are used in management; rarely is reoperation considered.

PHRENIC NERVE INJURY

Phrenic nerve injury occurs from trauma during intraoperative manipulation of the mediastinum and pericardium. Phrenic nerve dysfunction can occur as a result of hypothermic cardioplegia and stretch injury. Both may complicate weaning. This diagnosis should be suspected in patients who exhibit a paradoxical breathing pattern. An elevated hemidiaphragm may not be obvious on radiography or on fluoroscopic or ultrasound evaluation of diaphragmatic motion if the injury is bilateral. In such instances, a phrenic nerve conduction study would be the definitive diagnostic study of choice.

HYPERINFLATION

Hyperinflation of the native lung may be seen in patients with COPD and unilateral lung transplantation as a result of the higher lung compliance, more severe airway obstruction, and air trapping that occurs in the remaining emphysematous lung.

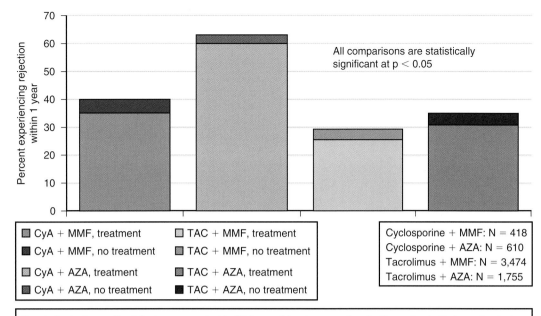

All comparisons are statistically significant at p < 0.05

- ☐ CyA + MMF, treatment
- ■ CyA + MMF, no treatment
- ☐ CyA + AZA, treatment
- ■ CyA + AZA, no treatment

- ☐ TAC + MMF, treatment
- ■ TAC + MMF, no treatment
- ■ TAC + AZA, treatment
- ■ TAC + AZA, no treatment

Cyclosporine + MMF: N = 418
Cyclosporine + AZA: N = 610
Tacrolimus + MMF: N = 3,474
Tacrolimus + AZA: N = 1,755

Treated rejection = Recipient was reported to (1) have at least one acute rejection episode that was treated with an anti-rejection agent; or (2) have been hospitalized for rejection.
No rejection = Recipient had (i) no acute rejection episodes and (ii) was reported either as not hospitalized for rejection or did not recieve anti-rejection agents.

Figure 75-13 Reported rejection between discharge and 1-year follow-up for adult lung transplant follow-ups from July 2004 through June 2010, stratified by maintenance immunosuppressive regimen. Rejection is classified as treated *(lighter color)* or untreated *(darker color)*. AZA, azathioprine; CyA, cyclosporine A; MMF, mycophenolate mofetil; TAC, tacrolimus. Analysis is limited to patients who were alive at the time of the follow-up. *(Adapted from Christie JD, Edwards LB, Kucheryavaya AY: The Registry of the International Society for Heart and Lung Transplantation: Twenty-eighth adult lung and heart-lung transplant report—2011, J Heart Lung Transplant 30:1104-1122, 2011.)*

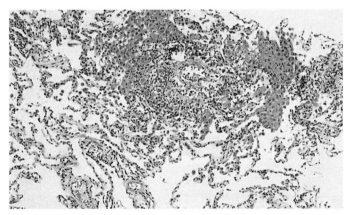

Figure 75-14 Transbronchial lung biopsy specimen showing acute rejection. The lymphocytes surround an arteriole and the infiltrate spreads into surrounding alveolar walls (grade A3).

The hyperinflated lung can compress the transplanted lung and/or the mediastinal structures, causing a substantial reduction in function (**Figure 75-17**).

INFECTIOUS COMPLICATIONS

Infectious complications in the immediate postoperative period are the same as those associated with other major cardiothoracic surgery. Blood-borne infections from indwelling catheters, urinary tract, and wound complications are common. Pneumonia in the acute posttransplantation phase requires careful assessment of the donor's and recipient's microbiologic and clinical histories, including previous bacterial colonization or recent infections. Clinical history is relevant, because it may detect risks for aspiration, nosocomial, and ventilator-associated

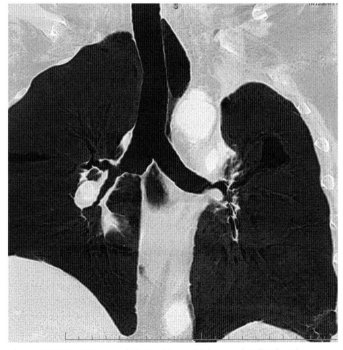

Figure 75-15 CT scan of bilateral bronchial stenosis (distal main bronchi) after bilateral sequential lung transplantation. Poor anastomotic perfusion from septic shock and bacterial pneumonia complicated the immediate postoperative course.

pathogens (**Table 75-9**). Physiologic abnormalities in the transplanted lung also predispose to infection. Impaired mucociliary clearance, denervation of the cough reflex, and disruption of the pulmonary lymphatic and vascular outflow all may act in combination. Infection of the allograft results in inflammation and graft damage. Although prophylaxis seems logical in

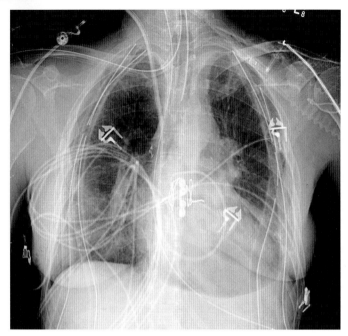

Figure 75-16 Chest radiograph showing pneumopericardium arising as a manifestation of bronchial dehiscence after lung transplantation.

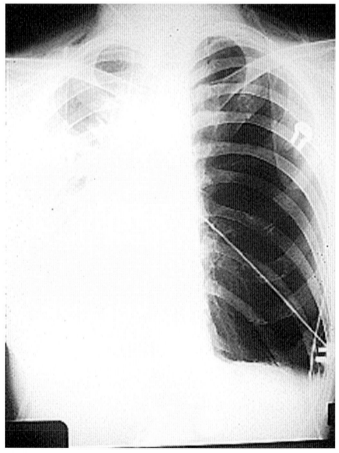

Figure 75-17 Chest radiograph showing right single-lung transplant for emphysema. Severe hyperinflation with mediastinal shift caused by overinflation of the native lung with compression of the transplanted right lung is evident.

preventing future infection, strong clinical evidence to support universal use of prophylaxis is lacking, with variable findings among different transplant centers worldwide.

COMMUNITY-ACQUIRED PNEUMONIA

Pneumonia manifesting in the first month after transplantation usually is bacterial in origin. Community- or hospital-acquired gram-positive and gram-negative bacteria are the most common pathogens. Aspiration is another cause, because donors are at risk of aspiration from emergency intubation, neurologic impairment, and/or critical illness. In donors who have been intubated for more than 48 hours, pneumonia should be considered to be ventilator-associated. Patients with a history of bacterial pneumonia must be treated and guided by the sensitivity and resistance patterns previously documented. With identification of the pathogens responsible for bacterial infection in the donor, appropriate antibiotic coverage should be provided.

Early fiberoptic bronchoscopy with BAL and transbronchial biopsy (TBB) constitutes the standard of care in the early posttransplantation period. Specimens are routinely sent for bacterial, fungal, and viral analysis. Methicillin-resistant *Staphylococcus aureus* (MRSA) and resistant *Pseudomonas aeruginosa* should be suspected in patients at risk for nosocomial infection or colonization, such as in those with CF. Prophylaxis with nebulized antipseudomonal drugs such as tobramycin and colistin may be useful.

OPPORTUNISTIC INFECTIONS

Opportunistic infections are uncommon before the first month after transplantation. They are directly related to the immunosuppressed state that leads to the reactivation of latent infections and an inadequate response to otherwise nonvirulent pathogens. Prophylaxis against *Pneumocystis*, the Herpesviridae family of viruses, and *Aspergillus* will reduce the frequencies of these infections; however, opportunistic infection is a common contributor to posttransplantation morbidity.

Cytomegalovirus (Human Herpesvirus Type 5)

CMV is found in latent stage in nearly 60% of all adults. Routine screening of donor and recipient for CMV IgG allows stratification of patients at highest risk for CMV reactivation and pneumonitis. Primary CMV infection occurs when a CMV-seronegative recipient becomes infected from a CMV-positive graft or blood product. Because primary CMV infection is associated with the highest risk for severe morbidity and mortality, matching CMV-negative recipients to CMV-negative donors is preferred but sometimes is impractical. In cases in which CMV-naive recipients receive a CMV-positive graft, passive immunization with intravenous CMV IgG can be given, followed by inhibition of viral replication with ganciclovir. Other anti-CMV agents include valganciclovir, cidofovir, foscarnet, and leflunomide. These may be used in refractory or resistant cases. Secondary CMV infection and CMV superinfection can cause reactivation pneumonitis in CMV-seropositive recipients; however, these types of infections are not as severe as primary CMV infection. An oral prodrug for cidofovir may be available soon for therapy or prevention.

CMV pneumonitis can be diagnosed by the presence of intranuclear viral inclusion bodies on histologic examination. This condition may be an indirect cause of rejection and the bronchiolitis obliterans syndrome (**Figure 75-18**). CMV

Table 75-9 Infectious Pulmonary Complications

Diagnosis	Community-Acquired	Donor/Recipient-Acquired	Hospital-Acquired	Opportunistic	Reactivation
Onset	<1 month (May occur late as well)	<1 month	<1 month	>1 month	>1 month
Common organisms	*Staphylococcus* *Streptococcus* *Haemophilus* *Chlamydia* *Mycoplasma* *Klebsiella* *Legionella* *Listeria* Community-acquired viruses RSV Adenovirus Parainfluenza virus Influenza virus	Pseudomonas *Stenotrophomonas* *Burkholderia cepacia* genomovar III most virulent MRSA *Aspergillus* MTB Atypical mycobacteria *Toxoplasma*	MRSA *Pseudomonas* *Acinetobacter*	CMV EBV VZV PCP *Nocardia* *Aspergillus* *Candida*	CMV EBV VZV MTB
Late complications	Bronchial anastomosis Rejection	Bronchial anastomosis Rejection	Bronchial anastomosis Rejection	CMV and BOS EBV and PTLD	CMV and BOS EBV and PTLD

BOS, bronchiolitis obliterans syndrome; *CMV*, cytomegalovirus; *EBV*, Epstein-Barr virus; *MRSA*, methicillin-resistant *Staphylococcus aureus*; *MTB*, *Mycobacterium tuberculosis*; *PCP*, *Pneumocystis (jirovecii)* pneumonia; *PTLD*, posttransplant lymphoproliferative disorder; *RSV*, respiratory syncytial virus; *VZV*, varicella-zoster virus.

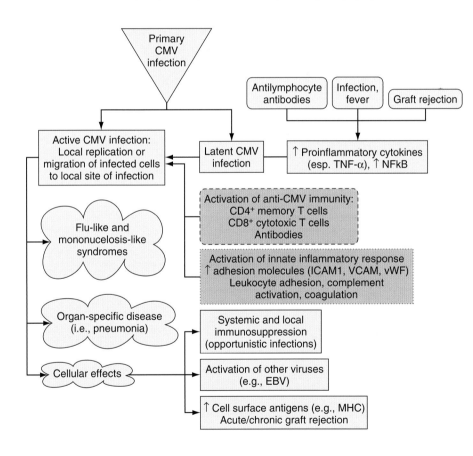

Figure 75-18 The direct and indirect effects of cytomegalovirus infection. The activation of latent cytomegalovirus (CMV) alters many aspects of the innate and adaptive immune response. The indirect effects include predisposition to opportunistic infections, activation of other latent viruses, and graft rejection or graft-versus-host disease. *EBV*, Epstein-Barr virus; *ICAM1*, intercellular adhesion molecule-1; *MHC*, major histocompatibility complex; *TNF-α*, tumor necrosis factor-α; *VCAM*, vascular cell adhesion molecule; *vWF*, von Willebrand factor. *(From Ison MG, Fishman JA: Cytomegalovirus pneumonia in transplant recipients,* Clin Chest Med *26:691–705,viii [Figure 1], 2005.)*

prophylaxis often is given routinely and may delay acute infection (**Table 75-10**). This practice, however, may result in the evolution of resistant strains and predispose the patient to antiviral toxicity, as well as increasing the current cost of care. Alternatively, preemptive monitoring and treatment of infection can be implemented. CMV replication can be detected early by rising serum CMV antigen levels or quantitative CMV polymerase chain reaction (PCR) assay results.

Epstein-Barr Virus

EBV is also routinely screened for in both recipients and donors. Similar to CMV, it carries a high risk for reactivation and can lead to posttransplantation lymphoproliferative disorder (PTLD). PTLD is believed to occur in almost half of the patients who are EBV-seronegative and receive an EBV-seropositive graft. Matching EBV-negative status is therefore extremely important, but often difficult, because few donor agencies screen

Table 75-10 Suggested CMV Prophylaxis After Lung Transplantation

CMV Status	Recipient +	Recipient –

Donor +	• Treatment duration is 3 months
	  1. Days 1-14: Valganciclovir 900 mg PO bid
	  2. Days 15-90: Valganciclovir 900 PO mg daily
		• *Donor +/Recipient – are the highest risk for CMV disease*
		• Prophylaxis may have advantage over preemptive therapy
		• Treatment duration is typically 6 months
		  1. Days 1-14: Valganciclovir 900 mg PO bid
		  2. Days 15-180: Valganciclovir 900 mg PO daily*

Donor –	• Treatment duration is 3 months
	  1. Days 1-14: Valganciclovir 900 mg PO bid
	  2. Days 15-90: Valganciclovir 900 PO mg daily
		• Risk of CMV disease is increased with extensive blood transfusion
		• Leukodepleted and CMV seronegative blood products are recommended
		• If extensive transfusions are necessary, CMV prophylaxis should be considered
		• Monitoring weekly for CMV PCR should be considered
		• We use Acyclovir or Valacyclovir for HSV prophylaxis days 1-90

Additional Considerations:
• Dosing must be adjusted for renal function
• CMV PCR assay is followed routinely if prophylaxis is not given
• Cytogam (CMV immunoglobulin) 150 mg/kg can be added for treatment
• Monitor clinically for signs and symptoms of late onset CMV disease

*When used as prophylaxis, the dose of Valganciclovir is 900 mg daily, versus treatment dose which is 900 mg twice daily.
CMV, cytomegalovirus; *HSV*, herpes simplex virus; *PCR*, polymerase chain reaction.

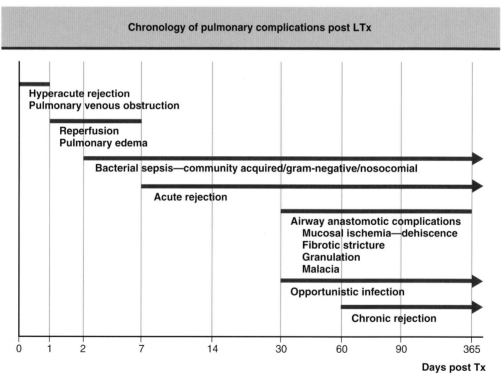

Figure 75-19 The chronology of pulmonary complications in the lung transplant recipient. Some complications occur during a defined time span in the early posttransplantation period, but others occur throughout the follow-up period.

for EBV. PTLD may manifest as a pulmonary nodule, mass, or infiltrate and requires tissue biopsy for diagnosis. Unfortunately, commonly used chemotherapy directed against lymphoproliferative malignancies has not been very successful in treating PTLD. EBV prophylaxis in patients at highest risk is covered by antiviral treatment directed against CMV and herpes simplex virus (HSV). As with all other opportunistic complications, reduction in the level of immunosuppression remains the single most important management strategy, if PTLD occurs.

Aspergillus Spp.

Aspergillus infection is a common infection after solid organ transplantation. It may manifest in a variety of ways, including

a bronchial inflammatory disorder, necrotizing airway infection (with pseudomembrane formation), and invasive pulmonary parenchymal aspergillosis. Invasive fungal infection is difficult to diagnose, because it is angiocentric and not detected on routine BAL or TBB. Surgical biopsy often is necessary to make a definite diagnosis. Prophylaxis with oral amphotericin B, itraconazole, voriconazole, or intravenous liposomal amphotericin may be administered to persons at highest risk for infection. The azoles must be used carefully, because they can interfere with the metabolism of calcineurin inhibitors.

A chronology for the common infectious and noninfectious complications that occur after transplantation over time is presented in **Figure 75-19**.

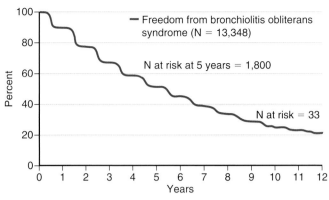

Figure 75-20 Freedom from bronchiolitis obliterans syndrome in adult lung recipients for follow-up assessments between April 1994 and June 2010, conditional on survival to 14 days. *(Adapted from Christie JD, Edwards LB, Kucheryavaya AY: The Registry of the International Society for Heart and Lung Transplantation: Twenty-eighth adult lung and heart-lung transplant report—2011,* J Heart Lung Transplant *30:1104-1122, 2011.)*

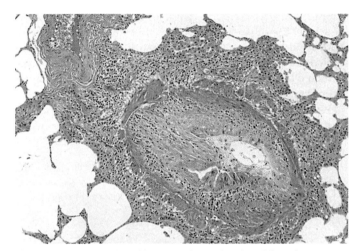

Figure 75-21 Open lung biopsy specimen showing obliterative bronchiolitis. The bronchiolar lumen is obliterated by organizing fibrin, myofibroblasts, and lymphocytes.

CHRONIC REJECTION

Chronic Lung Allograft Dysfunction

Bronchiolitis obliterans syndrome (BOS) is a common clinico-pathologic syndrome of progressive and irreversible airway obstruction with a declining DLCO that occurs as a late complication in graft function with an incidence of almost 50% by the fifth year after transplantation (**Figure 75-20**). On histopathologic examination, BOS is represented by obliterative bronchiolitis (OB)—specifically, fibrosis of the small airways with intimal thickening and sclerosis of its accompanying vessel that lead to near-complete occlusion of the bronchiolar lumen and small airway obstruction (**Figure 75-21**). Chest imaging should yield normal findings in the early stages of BOS, which remains a diagnosis of exclusion at that time. Acute rejection, infection, drug-induced pneumotoxicity, and bronchial anastomotic obstruction must be excluded. Advanced BOS may appear as peripheral bronchiectasis with a loss of vascularity and atelectasis. A staging system has been created to aid in the diagnosis of BOS by the International Society of Heart and Lung Transplantation (**Tables 75-11** and **75-12**). Of importance, not all graft dysfunction is due to OB. A restrictive pattern is present in a significant minority of patients. Imaging may suggest peripheral encroachment of the lung volume and restrictive pulmonary

Table 75-11	**Histologic Classification and Grading of Pulmonary Allograft Rejection**
Acute Rejection	
Grade 0—none	No significant abnormality
Grade 1—minimal	Infrequent perivascular mononuclear cell infiltrates mainly surrounding venules that are 2-3 cells deep
Grade 2—mild	More frequent infiltrates, 5 cells or more deep, involving venules and arterioles
Grade 3—moderate	More exuberant mononuclear cell infiltrate that extends from the perivascular space into the alveolar interstitium
Grade 4—severe	Infiltrate extending into the alveolar space with pneumocyte damage and at times necrosis of vessels and lung parenchyma
Airway inflammation	Lymphocytic bronchitis/bronchiolitis; pathologist may grade
Chronic Rejection	

Chronic airway rejection
  Active
  Inactive	

Chronic vascular rejection-accelerated graft vascular sclerosis	

function tests (PFTs). Therefore, the phraseology "chronic lung allograft dysfunction" (CLAD) is coming into use to account for more than one manifestation of chronic graft failure.

CLAD is believed to be caused by alloimmune tissue injury. Risk factors include a previous history of rejection episodes, viral infections, and the presence of lymphocytic bronchiolitis. Unfortunately, some patients with severe clinical BOS may not show histologic evidence of obliterative bronchiolitis on biopsy, whereas others with significant histologic evidence of BO may be asymptomatic. There is no effective treatment for BOS. Slowing of further progression may be possible with a trial of increased immunosuppression. This may be warranted in patients with an inflammatory-predominant stage of BOS. Retransplantation remains a potential option in a few selected cases. Treatments today do not differ between obstructive and restrictive CLAD.

IMMUNOSUPPRESSION

The goal of immunosuppression in all patients undergoing solid organ transplantation arises from a two-phase host-versus-donor rejection model. In the initial acute posttransplantation period, donor antigen-presenting cells (APCs) activate T cells to react against graft antigens. B cells also are activated by graft antigens and form antibodies directed against them. This first phase, often attenuated, is associated with a high level of immunosuppression and is termed *induction*. Induction is directed against blocking the APC to T cell interaction, preventing T cell proliferation, and B cell alloimmunization. The second phase of immunosuppression is termed *maintenance*. During the maintenance phase, the host apparently adapts to the graft. Doses of immunosuppressants can be lowered to avoid toxicity

Table 75-12 Comparison of Acute Rejection and Bronchiolitis Obliterans Syndrome

Feature	Acute Rejection	Bronchiolitis Obliterans Syndrome
Peak frequency	First 6 months	>3 months
Onset	Abrupt to subacute	Usually subtle
Symptoms/signs	Tightness in chest (immediate postoperative period) Cough (usually not productive) Dyspnea	Dyspnea with heavy exertion Cough (often productive)
Physiologic	Restrictive impairment Desaturation of arterial blood	Obstructive impairment Normoxia until late
Radiologic	Diffuse interstitial infiltrates Pleural effusions	No abnormality until disorder is far advanced Computed tomography evidence of bronchiectasis and mosaic pattern
Hematologic	Leukocytosis	Normal white blood cell count
Histologic	Perivascular mononuclear cell infiltrates Airway inflammation is variable	Obliterative bronchiolitis Atherosclerosis of pulmonary and bronchial arteries Pleural scarring
Response to treatment function	Majority of cases improve rapidly with intravenous corticosteroid	Forced expiratory volume in 1 second at best stabilized Majority of recipients show progressive decline in allograft

and infectious complications while stabilizing the adaptive immune response.

Induction is accomplished with antibodies directed against human lymphoid cells. Antithymocyte globulin and monoclonal antibodies directed against specific CD receptors found on human lymphocytes are used, including muromonab-CD3, alemtuzumab, basiliximab, and daclizumab. Of these, basiliximab and daclizumab have gained favor, because they target activated T cells and have fewer, less severe side effects. Depleting antibodies are used in combination with high-dose methylprednisolone, a calcineurin inhibitor, and an antiproliferative drug such as an antimetabolite or an mTor (mammalian target of rapamycin) inhibitor.

Maintenance therapy is based on a triple-drug regimen that includes a calcineurin inhibitor, an antimetabolite, and a corticosteroid. This triple therapy has been chosen on the basis of studies performed on other solid organ transplants showing improved survival and lower graft rejection episodes over alternate regimens.

CALCINEURIN INHIBITORS

Calcineurin inhibitors block the signal of activation between APCs and T cells. The classic agent in this group is cyclosporine, because it was the first effective immunosuppressant used in transplantation medicine. Tacrolimus is the second most commonly used calcineurin inhibitor and is now preferred in most lung transplant programs. Side effects of these drugs include nephrotoxicity, neurotoxicity, hemolytic uremic syndrome, posttransplantation diabetes mellitus, and hypertension.

ANTIMETABOLITES

The antimetabolites inhibit the proliferation of lymphocytes. They include inhibitors of purine synthesis such as mycophenolate mofetil (MMF) and azathioprine. MMF generally is preferred over azathioprine because of its better side effect profile. Recent studies suggest, however, that the two agents have a similar effectiveness. Accordingly, azathioprine is still preferred at some centers because of its relatively low cost.

MAMMALIAN TARGET OF RAPAMYCIN INHIBITORS

The mTOR inhibitors act by inhibiting the cell cycle and preventing T cell proliferation. Rapamycin, also known as sirolimus, is the classic mTOR inhibitor. Newer mTOR inhibitors include everolimus and temsirolimus. mTOR inhibitors used in conjunction with calcineurin inhibitors increase the incidence of nephrotoxicity and hemolytic uremic syndrome events. The mTOR inhibitors have antineoplastic properties and are used in treatment of several different types of cancers. Accordingly, these agents may have a potential role in treating PTLD. Extreme caution is warranted if mTOR inhibitors are used early after transplantation, because bronchial dehiscence can be a serious complication.

PITFALLS OF IMMUNOSUPPRESSIVE THERAPY

Common complications from the chronic use of immunosuppressive drugs vary, depending on the specific agent and the recipient's predisposing characteristics (Table 75-13). Toxicities may be severe and irreversible, as is evident in cases of posttransplantation malignancy. Frequent checks for metabolic derangements and end-organ toxicity are critical. Unfortunately, serum drug levels do not correlate with the dosage of administered drugs and are not predictive of the potential toxic effects, because these factors vary from person to person.

Reaching and maintaining an adequate level of immunosuppression are difficult, leading some researchers to consider case-by-case analysis for specific genetic polymorphisms that affect drug metabolism to tailor specific treatments to the individual patient. Adjunctive testing of immune activity by the measurement of adenosine triphosphate (ATP) levels may be a more accurate way to adjust dosing. These basic issues warrant further investigation, because they are likely to affect the future of immunosuppressive management.

A current trend is for the use of tacrolimus, MMF, and sirolimus (Figure 75-22). A recent study comparing azathioprine and MMF in lung transplant recipients failed to show a significant difference in prevention of BOS. Although there are multiple reasons why a difference was not observed, there is still

Table 75-13   Maintenance Immunosuppressive Drugs

Agent	Dose	Adverse Effects	Interactions
Cyclosporine (calcineurin inhibitor)	Whole-blood level 250-350 ng/mL	Nephrotoxicity, HUS, neurotoxicity, posttransplantation DM, hirsutism, gingival hyperplasia, gastroparesis, HTN, electrolyte disturbances	Increased by macrolides, azoles, calcium channel blockers, gastric motility agents Decreased by anticonvulsants, rifampin
Tacrolimus (calcineurin inhibitor)	Whole-blood trough level 10-20 ng/mL	Nephrotoxicity, HUS, neurotoxicity, posttransplantation DM, hyperlipidemia, HTN, electrolyte disturbances	Fatty meals decrease absorption Increased by macrolides, azoles, calcium channel blockers, gastric motility agents Decreased by anticonvulsants, rifampin
Azathioprine (antimetabolite)	2-2.5 mg/kg/day Adjust for WBC 4000-6000/mm^3	Leukopenia, anemia, thrombocytopenia, pancreatitis	Allopurinol in combination resulted in higher bone marrow toxicity
Mycophenolate mofetil (antimetabolite)	1000-1500 mg bid	GI symptoms can be improved if given q6h or lower total dose	Antacids, iron, and magnesium decrease absorption Increases levels of acyclovir and ganciclovir
Sirolimus (mTOR inhibitor)	Load 6 mg, then 2 mg/day (goal 10-20 ng/mL level)	Anemia, thrombocytopenia, leucopenia, HTN, electrolyte abnormalities, GI symptoms	Increased by macrolides, azoles, calcium channel blockers, gastric motility agents

DM, diabetes mellitus; *GI,* gastrointestinal; *HTN,* hypertension; *HUS,* hemolytic uremic syndrome; *WBC,* white blood cell count.

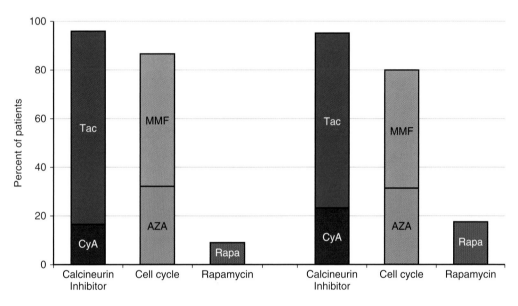

Figure 75-22   Adult lung recipients' maintenance immunosuppression drug combinations at time of follow-up (data for follow-up evaluations performed between January 2002 and June 2005). Conventional combinations analysis was limited to patients receiving prednisone. *AZA,* azathioprine; *Cy,* cyclosporine; *MMF,* mycophenolate mofetil; *Rapa,* rapamycin; *Tac,* tacrolimus.

no definitive evidence to suggest superior outcomes with these newer drugs.

MEDICAL COMPLICATIONS IN LUNG TRANSPLANT SURVIVORS

Lung transplant survivors are at risk for multiple medical complications related to their predisposing illness and toxicities resulting from chronic immunosuppression. The aim of long-term care in the transplant recipient revolves around prevention and early detection of commonly described posttransplantation medical illnesses.

NEUROMUSCULAR

Neuromuscular toxicity is a well-described complication of the calcineurin inhibitors. This complication is thought to be dose-dependent and presents with symptoms ranging from headache

and tremors to seizures and confusion. The posterior leukoencephalopathy syndrome can result in cortical blindness from microvascular injury and encephalopathy. Myopathies are common, especially when the calcineurin inhibitors are used in combination with corticosteroids, presumably caused by direct mitochondrial toxicity. This is an important complication, because the major limiting factor in posttransplantation exercise capacity seems to be related to muscular dysfunction and inadequate mitochondrial activity, rather than to cardiopulmonary deficiency. In patients with seizures, treatment should start with reducing the dose of calcineurin inhibitor and adding an antiepileptic that does not interact with the immunosuppressant regimen.

OSTEOPOROSIS

As discussed earlier, osteoporosis is a relative contraindication to transplantation. Fractures occur commonly after

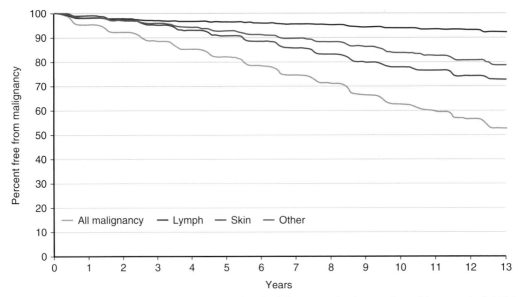

Figure 75-23 Freedom from malignancy for adult lung recipients (data for follow-up evaluations performed between April 1994 and June 2005).

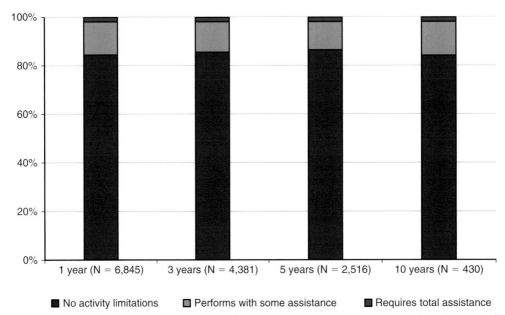

Figure 75-24 Adult lung recipients' functional status of surviving recipients (data for follow-up evaluations performed between April 1994 and June 2005).

transplantation and can be severely debilitating. Advanced age, poor nutrition, immobility, and smoking all contribute to bone demineralization. Corticosteroids and calcineurin inhibitors are known to increase bone resorption and to promote the development of severe osteoporosis. Many centers will treat patients at risk before transplantation with exercise, calcium supplementation, vitamin D, and antiresorptive agents such as the bisphosphonates to reduce the posttransplantation risk.

MALIGNANCY

Posttransplantation malignancy (**Figure 75-23**) frequently is seen after solid organ transplantation. The calcineurin inhibitors and azathioprine have been associated with a higher risk of cancer. Currently, a 10% incidence of tumor development is reported in 5-year survivors, with lymphoid and skin cancers accounting for a majority. Newer immunosuppressive agents, such as the mTOR inhibitors, seem to have antineoplastic properties; evidence that these agents lead to lower cancer risk or decreased mortality is lacking, however.

OTHER MEDICAL COMPLICATIONS AFTER TRANSPLANTATION

Acute and chronic nephrotoxicity is well described with use of the calcineurin inhibitors and is characterized by hyalinosis of afferent arterioles, vacuolization of proximal tubules, and focal areas of interstitial and glomerular fibrosis (**Figure 75-24**). Although renal dysfunction is rather common in 1-year survivors, renal failure requiring dialysis remains rare. Use of calcineurin inhibitors as well as corticosteroids also can lead to diabetes mellitus, hypertension, and dyslipidemia (**Table 75-14**).

Table 75-14 Post-Lung Transplantation Morbidity in Adults

	Follow-ups: April 1994–June 1999		Follow-ups: July 1999–June 2005	
Outcome	Within 1 Year	Total Number with Known Response	Within 1 Year	Total Number with Known Response
Hypertension	48.3%	(N = 3162)	53.2%	(N = 4735)
Renal dysfunction	22.2%	(N = 3088)	27.4%	(N = 4870)
Abnormal creatinine <2.5 mg/dL	12.5%		18.9%	
Creatinine >2.5 mg/dL	8.0%		6.7%	
Chronic dialysis	1.7%		1.8%	
Renal transplantation	0.0%		0.1%	
Hyperlipidemia	11.0%	(N = 3280)	23.9%	(N = 5064)
Diabetes	16.10%	(N = 3129)	26.9%	(N = 4800)
Bronchiolitis obliterans	10.7%	(N = 2817)	7.3%	(N = 4460)

Cumulative prevalence in survivors within 1 year after transplantation (follow-ups: April 1994–June 2005).

SUGGESTED READINGS

Ahya VN, Kawut SM: Noninfectious pulmonary complications after lung transplantation, *Clin Chest Med* 26:613–622, 2005.

Christie JD, Edwards LB, Kucheryavaya AY, et al: Registry of the International Society for Heart and Lung Transplantation: Twenty-Seventh Official Adult Lung and Heart-Lung Transplantation Report, *J Heart Lung Transplant* 29:1104–1118, 2010.

De Soyza A, McDowell A, Archer L, et al: *Burkholderia cepacia* complex genomovars and pulmonary transplantation outcomes in patients with cystic fibrosis, *Lancet* 358:1780–1781, 2001.

Estenne M, Maurer JR, Boehler A, et al: Bronchiolitis obliterans syndrome 2001: an update of the diagnostic criteria, *J Heart Lung Transplant* 21:297–319, 2002.

Kowalski R, Post D, Schneider MC, et al: Immune cell function testing: an adjunct to therapeutic drug monitoring in transplant patient management, *Clin Transplant* 17:77–88, 2003.

McNeil K, Glanville AR, Wahlers T, et al: Comparison of mycophenolate mofetil and azathioprine for prevention of bronchiolitis obliterans syndrome in de novo lung transplant recipients, *Transplantation* 81:998–1003, 2006.

Orens JB, Boehler A, Perot MD, et al: A review of lung transplant donor acceptability criteria, *J Heart Lung Transplant* 22:1183–1200, 2003.

Orens JB, Estenne M, Arcasoy SM, et al: International guidelines for the selection of lung transplant candidates: 2006 update—a consensus report from the Pulmonary Scientific Council of the International Society of Heart and Lung Transplantation, *J Heart Lung Transplant* 25:745–755, 2006.

Shargall Y, Guenther G, Ahya VN, et al: Report of the ISHLT Working Group on Primary Lung Graft Dysfunction part VI: treatment, *J Heart Lung Transplant* 24:1489–1500, 2005.

Steen S, Sjoberg T, Pierre L, et al: Transplantation of lungs from a non-heart beating donor, *Lancet* 357:825–829, 2001.

Woodrow JP, Shlobin OA, Barnett SD, et al: Comparison of bronchiolitis obliterans syndrome to other forms of chronic lung allograft dysfunction after lung transplantation, *J Heart Lung Transplant* 29:1159–1164, 2010.

Chapter **76**
Pregnancy
Stephen E. Lapinsky

The pregnant patient who has pulmonary disease is unique because of altered maternal physiology, the occurrence of diseases specific to pregnancy, and the need to consider two patients in all therapeutic decisions. This chapter focuses on the changes in pulmonary physiology associated with pregnancy, certain pregnancy-specific disorders, and other pulmonary problems encountered in the pregnant patient.

PULMONARY PHYSIOLOGY

PHYSIOLOGIC CHANGES IN PREGNANCY

Hormonal changes in pregnancy affect the upper respiratory tract and cause airway hyperemia and edema resulting in symptoms of rhinitis. Estrogens are likely responsible for many of these effects because they produce capillary congestion and mucous gland hyperplasia. Changes to the thoracic cage result from both the enlarging uterus and the hormonal effects producing ligamentous laxity. The diaphragm is displaced cephalad by up to 4 cm, but the potential loss of lung capacity is partially offset by an increase in the anteroposterior and transverse diameters and by widening of the subcostal angle (**Figure 76-1**). Despite these anatomic changes, diaphragmatic function remains normal, diaphragmatic excursion is not reduced, and the maximum transdiaphragmatic inspiratory pressures that can be generated near term are similar to values generated by patients who are not pregnant. The changes in the chest wall return to normal within 6 months of delivery, although the costal angle may remain widened.

These changes in the thorax produce a progressive decrease in functional residual capacity (FRC) by 10% to 25% by term (**Figure 76-2**). Residual volume decreases slightly, but the major change is in expiratory reserve volume. These alterations are measurable as early as 16 to 24 weeks of gestation and progress to term. The increased diameter of the thoracic cage and the preserved respiratory muscle function allow the vital capacity to remain unchanged, and total lung capacity decreases only minimally. Measurements of airflow and lung compliance are not affected, but chest wall and total respiratory compliance are reduced in the third trimester because of the chest wall changes and increased abdominal pressure. Inconsistencies in results reported for diffusing capacity during pregnancy likely arise from the effects of anemia, variable changes in intravascular volume, and the increase in cardiac output. A small increase may be noted in early pregnancy with a subsequent decrease to normal values by term.

Minute ventilation increases greatly in pregnancy, beginning in the first trimester and reaching 20% to 40% above baseline at term (Figure 76-2), produced mainly by an increase in tidal volume of approximately 30% to 35%. These changes are mediated by the increase in respiratory drive that results from elevated serum progesterone levels. A respiratory alkalosis with compensatory renal excretion of bicarbonate results, with arterial carbon dioxide tension ($PaCO_2$) falling to 28 to 32 mm Hg and plasma bicarbonate falling to 18 to 21 mEq/L. Alveolar-arterial oxygen tension difference ($PO_2[A-a]$) is similar to nonpregnant values, and mean PaO_2 usually exceeds 100 mm Hg at sea level throughout pregnancy. Mild hypoxemia and an increased $PO_2(A-a)$ may develop in the supine position because of airway closure, because FRC diminishes near term. One study suggests that shunt is normally increased in the third trimester to approximately 15% and is not changed significantly by posture. Oxygen consumption increases, beginning in the first trimester, and reaches 20% to 33% above baseline by the third trimester because of fetal demands and maternal metabolic processes. The combination of a reduced FRC and increased oxygen consumption lowers oxygen reserve, which renders the pregnant patient susceptible to the rapid development of hypoxia in response to hypoventilation or apnea.

During labor, hyperventilation increases, and tachypnea (caused by pain or anxiety) may result in marked respiratory alkalosis, augmented in some patients by volume depletion or vomiting. Alkalosis adversely affects fetal oxygenation by reducing uterine blood flow. In some patients, severe pain and anxiety may lead to rapid, shallow breathing with alveolar hypoventilation, atelectasis, and mild hypoxemia. Achieving adequate pain relief with narcotics or epidural analgesia blunts the ventilatory response and can correct the gas exchange abnormalities associated with active labor. The pregnancy-associated changes in lung function reverse significantly in the first 72 hours postpartum and return to baseline within a few weeks.

Changes occur to the pregnant woman's immune system, to facilitate tolerance to paternally derived fetal antigens. Some suppression of cell-mediated immunity occurs; maternal lymphocytes demonstrate a diminished proliferative response to soluble antigens and to allogeneic lymphocytes, and decreased numbers of T-helper cells have been documented. These effects are balanced by an intact or slightly enhanced humoral immune response. These alterations to maternal immunity result in a predisposition to more severe manifestations of some viral and fungal infections.

DYSPNEA IN PREGNANCY

Dyspnea is a common complaint in women who have otherwise normal pregnancies. It may develop in the first or second

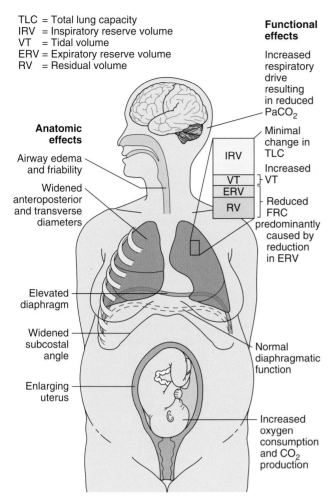

TLC = Total lung capacity
IRV = Inspiratory reserve volume
VT = Tidal volume
ERV = Expiratory reserve volume
RV = Residual volume

Anatomic effects

Airway edema and friability

Widened anteroposterior and transverse diameters

Elevated diaphragm

Widened subcostal angle

Enlarging uterus

Functional effects

Increased respiratory drive resulting in reduced $PaCO_2$

Minimal change in TLC

Increased VT

Reduced FRC predominantly caused by reduction in ERV

Normal diaphragmatic function

Increased oxygen consumption and CO_2 production

Figure 76-1 Pulmonary physiology in pregnancy: anatomic and functional effects of pregnancy that influence pulmonary physiology.

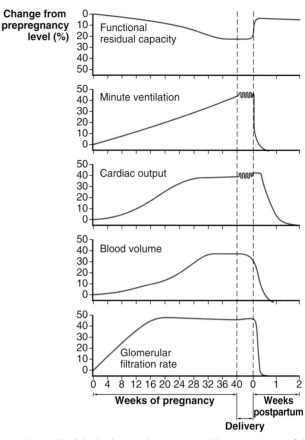

Figure 76-2 Physiologic changes in pregnancy. Shown are some of the physiologic changes that occur during pregnancy and the postpartum period. *(From Lapinsky SE, Kruczynski K, Slutsky AS: Critical care in the pregnant patient,* Am J Respir Crit Care Med *152:427–490, 1995.)*

trimester, and 70% of women complain of dyspnea by the third trimester. The mechanism is not clear but likely represents a normal awareness of increased ventilation; the physiologic increase in minute ventilation results in increased motor cortical stimulation of the respiratory center. The diagnosis of this benign condition is based on the presence of isolated dyspnea not usually affecting daily activities, the absence of associated symptoms, and the exclusion of other, pathologic conditions. Pregnancy also can be associated with increased exercise-induced dyspnea.

COMPLICATIONS AND DISORDERS OF PREGNANCY

PREGNANCY-SPECIFIC DISORDERS

Amniotic Fluid Embolism

Amniotic fluid embolism is a rare obstetric complication (between 1 in 8000 and 1 in 80,000 live births) that carries a mortality rate of 10% to 86% and may account for 10% of maternal deaths. Amniotic fluid embolism is usually associated with labor and delivery, but it may also occur with uterine manipulations or uterine trauma or in the early postpartum period. The mechanism seems to involve amniotic fluid that enters the vascular circulation through endocervical veins or uterine tears. Particulate cellular contents and humoral factors in the amniotic fluid produce acute pulmonary hypertension, predominantly by causing vascular spasm (**Figure 76-3**). Acute

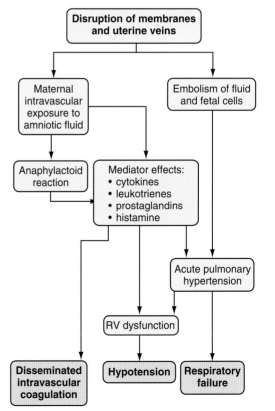

Figure 76-3 Pathophysiology of amniotic fluid embolism: proposed pathophysiologic mechanisms for the development of circulatory shock caused by amniotic fluid embolism. *RV,* right ventricular.

right ventricular dysfunction results from the increased afterload and myocardial dysfunction mediated by humoral factors, associated with secondary left ventricular (LV) failure. The cardiovascular changes of amniotic fluid embolism may resemble those of anaphylaxis, and sensitivity to amniotic fluid contents may be responsible.

The clinical presentation usually involves the sudden onset of severe dyspnea, hypoxemia, and cardiovascular collapse, often accompanied by seizures. Less common presentations include hemorrhage caused by disseminated intravascular coagulation (DIC) and fetal distress. Up to one half of patients may die within the first hour, and cardiac arrest during this period is common.

The diagnosis of amniotic fluid embolism is usually made on the basis of observing the typical clinical picture. Fetal squames in a wedged pulmonary capillary aspirate have been used to confirm the diagnosis, but this is not a specific finding. Less invasive diagnostic tests, such as maternal serum zinc coproporphyrin or sialyl-Tn levels, have been investigated but are not currently in use. The differential diagnosis includes septic shock, pulmonary thromboembolism, abruptio placentae (placental abruption), tension pneumothorax, and myocardial ischemia.

Treatment and Prognosis

Treatment of the pregnant patient with amniotic fluid embolism involves routine resuscitative and supportive measures, with prompt attention to adequate oxygenation, mechanical ventilation, and inotropic support. No specific therapy has been shown to be effective, but some suggest a role for corticosteroids. In view of the inconsistent hemodynamic findings, invasive monitoring may be of value. Survivors of the initial resuscitation are likely to experience the complications of DIC or acute respiratory distress syndrome (ARDS). Neurologic damage caused by hypotension and hypoxemia is common.

Preeclampsia and Pulmonary Edema

Pulmonary edema may rarely occur in association with preeclampsia (i.e., perhaps 3% of preeclamptic patients). The preeclamptic patient is usually volume-depleted, and pulmonary edema usually occurs in the early postpartum period, often associated with aggressive, intrapartum fluid replacement. Other factors that may contribute to the pathogenesis include reduced serum albumin, elevated LV afterload, and systolic and diastolic myocardial dysfunction (**Figure 76-4**). Increased capillary permeability may also occur, aggravated by concomitant conditions such as sepsis, placental abruption, or massive hemorrhage.

Pulmonary edema has been described in chronically hypertensive, obese, pregnant patients in whom preeclampsia develops. Diastolic LV dysfunction results from both the hypertension and the obesity, and pulmonary edema is precipitated by volume overload of pregnancy and hemodynamic stresses of preeclampsia.

Preeclampsia is characterized by hypertension, proteinuria, and peripheral edema, usually in the third trimester. The presentation of pulmonary edema is with acute respiratory distress in the preeclamptic patient, often in the early postpartum period.

Treatment and Prognosis

The standard approach is to restrict fluid, administer diuretics cautiously, and provide ventilatory support if necessary. Invasive monitoring may be useful if inotropic or vasodilator therapy becomes necessary, particularly in the patient with renal dysfunction. Aggressive diuresis must be avoided because filling

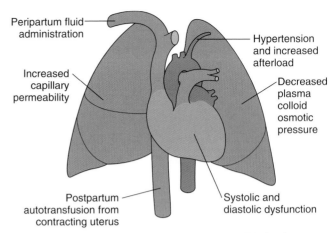

Figure 76-4 Pathophysiologic mechanisms responsible for the development of pulmonary edema in preeclampsia.

pressures should not be reduced to the point of compromising cardiac output and reducing placental perfusion. Volume replacement may be necessary in preeclampsia, particularly if vasodilators are used, because these patients may be extremely volume-depleted. Excessive fluid replacement, however, may precipitate pulmonary or cerebral edema. The ultimate treatment of preeclampsia is delivery of the fetus.

Tocolytic Pulmonary Edema

Beta-adrenergic agonists, as well as several other drugs, including nifedipine, indomethacin, atosiban, and magnesium sulfate, may be used to inhibit uterine contractions in preterm labor. Use of these agents has become less common, however, because a number of studies have demonstrated that tocolysis does not improve neonatal outcome. A complication of these drugs during pregnancy, particularly the β-agonists, is the development of pulmonary edema. The frequency of tocolytic-induced pulmonary edema varies from 0.3% to 9%. Postulated mechanisms include prolonged exposure to catecholamines causing myocardial dysfunction, increased capillary permeability, large volumes of intravenous (IV) fluid administration (often in response to maternal tachycardia), reduced osmotic pressure, and hypotension induced by β-adrenergic stimulation. Glucocorticoids are often administered in preterm labor to enhance fetal lung maturity and may compound fluid retention.

The clinical presentation is of acute respiratory distress with features of pulmonary edema. No specific features characterize tocolytic pulmonary edema. The diagnosis is a clinical one, made in the presence of acute pulmonary edema occurring in the appropriate clinical situation. The differential diagnosis includes cardiogenic pulmonary edema, amniotic fluid embolism, and other conditions (**Table 76-1**). Failure of the pulmonary edema to resolve in 12 to 24 hours requires a search for alternative causes.

Treatment and Prognosis

The tocolytic drug must be discontinued, whereupon pulmonary edema should resolve rapidly; additional treatment is supportive and includes diuresis. Early recognition and management should reduce the need for invasive hemodynamic monitoring and mechanical ventilation.

Peripartum Cardiomyopathy

Cardiac failure may occur in the absence of preexisting heart disease as a result of the hypertension of pregnancy or

Table 76-1	**Acute Respiratory Distress Caused by Complications of Pregnancy and Labor**
Disorder	**Distinguishing Features**
Amniotic fluid embolism	Cardiorespiratory collapse, seizures, disseminated intravascular coagulation
Pulmonary edema caused by preeclampsia	Hypertension, proteinuria
Tocolytic pulmonary edema	Tocolytic administration, rapid improvement with discontinuation
Aspiration pneumonitis	Vomiting, aspiration
Peripartum cardiomyopathy	Gradual onset, signs of heart failure
Venous thromboembolism	Evidence of deep venous thrombosis; radiologic investigations
Pneumomediastinum	Occurs during delivery; subcutaneous emphysema
Air embolism	Related to sexual intercourse or cesarean section; associated hypotension

peripartum cardiomyopathy. This idiopathic dilated cardiomyopathy presents in the last month of pregnancy or in the postpartum period. The diagnosis is made by demonstrating impaired LV function in the absence of other causes of cardiomyopathy. During labor and the early postpartum period, tachycardia and increased cardiac output may precipitate pulmonary edema. Pulmonary thromboembolic events are a common complication of this condition. Management is with diuretics and afterload reduction, bearing in mind that angiotensin-converting enzyme (ACE) inhibitors should not be used during pregnancy because of the development of fetal renal dysfunction. Anticoagulation is recommended in all patients. Other therapeutic interventions that have been used include intravenous immune globulin (IVIG) and bromocriptine. Recovery occurs in approximately half of patients within 6 months, but persistent or progressive cardiac failure develops in a significant proportion. Because mortality is 12% to 18% in the heart failure patients, cardiac transplantation may be considered.

Gestational Trophoblastic Disease

Pulmonary hypertension and pulmonary edema may complicate benign hydatidiform mole, caused by trophoblastic pulmonary embolism. This most often occurs during evacuation of the uterus, and the incidence of pulmonary complications is higher in later gestations. Molar pregnancy may be associated with *choriocarcinoma*, which can produce multiple, discrete pulmonary metastases and occasionally pleural effusions.

Ovarian Hyperstimulation Syndrome

Associated with administration of gonadotropins to stimulate ovulation for in vitro fertilization, the patient with ovarian hyperstimulation syndrome may present with gastrointestinal or respiratory symptoms. Increased capillary permeability results in bilateral pleural effusions and ascites, associated with intravascular volume depletion. Complications include respiratory compromise because of the effusions, shock and renal failure caused by the volume depletion, and pulmonary emboli. Treatment is supportive, with fluid resuscitation and drainage of effusions.

OTHER PULMONARY DISORDERS IN PREGNANCY

Asthma

Asthma affects 5% to 10% of the population and is therefore the most common pulmonary disorder in pregnancy. During pregnancy, the altered hormonal milieu may affect asthma control variably; patients may improve, worsen, or remain unchanged. Although pregnancy does not affect airflow in normal subjects, airway hyperreactivity in asthmatic subjects can be increased. Asthma severity usually returns to prepregnancy levels within 3 months postpartum.

The clinical features of asthma during pregnancy are the same as those in patients who are not pregnant. To differentiate from the dyspnea of pregnancy, objective assessment that uses pulmonary function tests to assess the degree of airflow limitation is essential. Gastroesophageal reflux (GER) is increased in both frequency and severity during pregnancy, and the symptoms of GER should be sought as a contributing factor.

Treatment and Prognosis

Management of the pregnant patient with asthma is similar to that in patients who are not pregnant and includes adequate monitoring, avoidance of precipitating factors, and patient education.

Although physicians may be reluctant to prescribe medications during pregnancy, poorly controlled asthma is potentially more dangerous for the fetus. Inhaled corticosteroids remain the mainstay of therapy, and are considered safe in pregnancy in moderate or low doses (**Table 76-2**). One study suggests a small increased risk of congenital malformation in women using high-dose therapy in the first trimester. The use of a spacer device is encouraged to reduce local side effects and systemic absorption. Although animal data suggest a small risk of cleft palate with systemic corticosteroid use, this has not been demonstrated in humans. Short courses of prednisone should be used to manage poorly controlled asthma when clinically indicated. Inhaled β-agonists seem safe and should be used as required for symptomatic relief. GER, a potentially preventable cause of worsening asthma, is frequently overlooked. Antireflux measures may greatly reduce asthmatic symptoms. Acute attacks are treated by ensuring adequate oxygenation, closely monitoring the fetus, and administering appropriate medications. Concerns over fetal effects of drugs should not cause physicians and patients to avoid use of effective pharmacologic therapy. Updated management algorithms are available through the Working Group on Asthma and Pregnancy of the National Asthma Education and Prevention Program (NAEPP).

Poor asthma control has been reported to increase the incidence of preterm birth, low birth weight, and perinatal mortality. Acute exacerbations may be associated with hypoxemia, which in turn may compromise the fetus.

Pulmonary Thromboembolic Disease

The incidence of venous thromboembolic disease related to pregnancy is 200 per 100,000 woman-years. The incidence is five times greater in the postpartum period than during pregnancy, and it remains an important cause of maternal mortality. Pulmonary embolism results from a hypercoagulable state associated with pregnancy, as well as from hormonally mediated venous stasis and local pressure effects of the uterus on the inferior vena cava (IVC). Pulmonary embolism occurs more frequently in the early postpartum period than during pregnancy, particularly after cesarean section.

Table 76-2 Safety Classification of Asthma Therapy in Pregnancy

Drug	FDA Class
Inhaled bronchodilators	
Albuterol (salbutamol)	C
Terbutaline	B
Ipratropium	B
Salmeterol	C
Formoterol	C
Tiotropium	C
Inhaled corticosteroids	
Beclomethasone	C
Budesonide	B
Fluticasone	C
Leukotriene antagonists	
Zafirlukast	B
Montelukast	B
Other agents	
Theophylline	C
Cromolyn	B
Systemic corticosteroids	C

Data from U.S. Food and Drug Administration (FDA) classification of drug safety in pregnancy; note that the FDA is in the process of revising this approach to labeling. Categories are as follows: *A,* Human studies fail to demonstrate fetal harm. *B,* Animal studies fail to demonstrate harm, but no human studies or animal studies demonstrate risk not shown in human studies. *C,* Animal studies demonstrate risk, or insufficient data available; drugs may be used if benefit outweighs risk. *D,* Human studies demonstrate risk; drugs may be used if benefits justify the risks. *X,* Contraindicated in pregnancy.

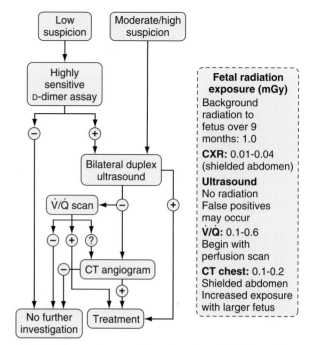

Figure 76-5 Diagnostic approach to thromboembolic disease in pregnancy and radiation exposure of diagnostic tests. +, positive test; −, negative test; ?, nondiagnostic test.

Table 76-3 Management of Thromboembolic Disease in Pregnancy

Therapy	FDA Class*	Comments
Heparin	C	Bone demineralization after prolonged use
Low-molecular-weight heparin	B/C	Good evidence of safety
Warfarin	D/X	Teratogenic, central nervous system abnormalities and bleeding occur, although the risk appears low Sometimes used in second trimester
Alteplase (r-tPA)	C	Consider in acute, life-threatening situations

*See Table 76-2 for U.S. Food and Drug Administration classification of drug safety in pregnancy.

The presentation is similar to that in the patient who is not pregnant. However, the clinical diagnosis of deep venous thrombosis (DVT) and pulmonary embolism is notoriously inaccurate. An overwhelming predilection for DVT in the left leg in the pregnant patient results from anatomic factors.

Investigation of suspected pulmonary embolism follows a similar approach to that in the patient who is not pregnant, and the diagnosis must be pursued aggressively. Duplex ultrasonography is useful for the diagnosis of DVT, although venous Doppler can give false-positive results because of venous obstruction by the gravid uterus. Ventilation-perfusion scanning can be performed with less than 0.5 mGy (<50 mrad) exposure to the fetus and, if necessary, a computed tomography (CT) pulmonary angiogram may be performed with similarly low fetal exposure (**Figure 76-5**). Teratogenicity is generally thought to require exposure greater than 50 to 100 mGy (5-10 rad), but an increased incidence of childhood leukemia may occur with fetal radiation exposures of 20 to 50 mGy (2-5 rad).

The use of radiologic investigations during pregnancy remains a concern for the fetus. However, the risk perceived by pregnant women and their husbands usually far exceeds the actual risk, and it is important to allay these concerns. It is important to establish a diagnosis of pulmonary embolism because of the major implications if such a diagnosis is missed

and the potential effects of unnecessary therapy on the health of mother and fetus.

Treatment and Prognosis

Warfarin therapy during the first trimester has been associated with an embryopathy, and central nervous system abnormalities have been described with second- and third-trimester exposure. Accordingly, warfarin is usually avoided (**Table 76-3**). The anticoagulant of choice is *heparin,* which does not cross the placenta, is not associated with adverse fetal outcome, and can be readily reversed. Low-molecular-weight (LMW) heparins do not seem to cross the placenta and are both safe and effective in pregnancy.

When administered with adequate precautions, streptokinase, urokinase, and tissue plasminogen activator (tPA) have been used successfully without major hemorrhagic complications or significant adverse effects on the fetus or placenta.

Nevertheless, use of these agents should be limited to life-threatening situations. When clinically indicated, an IVC filter can be placed transvenously, although there is some risk of dislodgment because of the dilated venous system and pressure effects during labor.

Women who have a known hypercoagulable state and those with a previous thromboembolism are at increased risk and should receive prophylaxis with anticoagulation throughout pregnancy.

Lower Respiratory Tract Infections

Lower respiratory tract infections are an infrequent occurrence but an important cause of indirect obstetric death. The pregnant patient is susceptible to the usual bacterial pathogens such as *Streptococcus pneumoniae*, *Haemophilus influenzae*, and *Mycoplasma pneumoniae* and is at increased risk of complications such as respiratory failure and empyema. Pregnant women are at increased risk of developing severe respiratory disease related to influenza, particularly the 2009 pandemic H1N1 strain. Less common infections such as varicella pneumonia and coccidioidomycosis may be associated with more severe disease than in nonpregnant patients. These effects are caused by subtle changes in cell-mediated immunity as a result of the pregnant state. *Pneumocystis jirovecii* (previously *P. carinii*) pneumonia may be seen in human immunodeficiency virus (HIV)–positive patients. Pregnancy does not seem to affect the course or incidence of reactivation of tuberculosis.

The clinical features of lower respiratory infection are similar to those in nonpregnant patients. Although dyspnea and increased minute ventilation are common in pregnancy, the respiratory rate is not significantly elevated by the pregnant state.

A chest radiograph is essential for the diagnosis of lower respiratory tract infections and must be considered in any pregnant woman who has a clinical presentation suggestive of pneumonia. Delayed radiography may be partly responsible for the increased morbidity in the pregnant patient population. Further diagnostic investigations include the usual microbiologic cultures, sputum microscopy, and serologic tests as indicated.

Treatment and Prognosis

Usual antibiotic guidelines may be followed, although tetracyclines should be avoided in pregnancy. Quinolones are usually avoided in pregnancy because of an association with arthropathy, but the risk seems to be low. Pregnant women should receive the influenza vaccine, and if disease occurs, treatment with oseltamivir is appropriate. Treatment of varicella pneumonitis is with acyclovir, which decreases mortality and has not been associated with fetal anomalies. Coccidioidomycosis is associated with an extremely high mortality rate, and disseminated disease should be treated with antifungal agents. *P. jirovecii* pneumonia requires treatment with trimethoprim-sulfamethoxazole with folate supplementation, as well as with corticosteroids, if indicated clinically. Although folic acid antagonists and sulfa drugs carry risks for the fetus, pentamidine is associated with higher risks for mother and fetus. Tuberculosis treatment is with isoniazid and rifampin (rifampicin), which have a low risk of adverse fetal effects, as well as ethambutol initially, until sensitivities are available. Pyrazinamide has been used in pregnancy and is recommended by some authorities.

Although pneumonia is associated with an increased risk of mortality, this is probably attributable to underlying diseases rather than to the pneumonia. Fetal complications may occur, as may preterm labor. Transplacental transmission of

Box 76-1	Causes of Acute Respiratory Distress Syndrome in Pregnancy

Pregnancy Specific
Preeclampsia
Amniotic fluid embolism
Chorioamnionitis
Placental abruption
Trophoblastic embolism

Risk Increased by Pregnancy
Gastric acid aspiration
Sepsis, particularly pyelonephritis
Transfusion-related acute lung injury
Air embolism
Pneumonia (e.g., varicella, fungal)

Nonspecific
Trauma
Drugs/toxins
Pancreatitis

varicella-zoster virus (VZV) occurs infrequently (<5%) but can produce limb deformities and neurologic involvement. The nonimmune pregnant woman exposed to VZV should receive prophylaxis with VZV immunoglobulin within 96 hours of exposure, as well as acyclovir if clinical disease develops. Unlike the treatment of active disease, tuberculosis prophylaxis can usually be deferred until after pregnancy, except in the case of recent exposure or skin test conversion.

When investigating and managing lower respiratory tract infections, it is important to consider effects on the fetus (radiation exposure, drug toxicities), but necessary evaluations and interventions should not be avoided inappropriately.

Acute Respiratory Distress Syndrome in Pregnancy

The pregnant patient is at risk for development of ARDS from a number of pregnancy-associated problems (**Box 76-1**). Gastric acid aspiration is a particular risk because of the increased intraabdominal pressure, reduced lower esophageal sphincter tone, and supine position during delivery. Iatrogenic factors such as excessive fluid administration and tocolytic therapy may contribute, as well as reduced albumin level.

The clinical features are similar to those in the nonpregnant patient. The diagnosis is by the usual criteria of hypoxemia in the presence of diffuse pulmonary infiltrates and in the absence of LV failure. A detailed history is critical for identification of the underlying problem.

Treatment and Prognosis

There are no major differences in the management of pregnant patients who have ARDS compared with those who are not pregnant, other than the need for continuous assessment of the fetus. When administering pharmacologic therapy, it is critical to consider the effects on both the fetus and the mother. Ventilatory management includes consideration of the normal physiologic changes of pregnancy. Adequate maternal oxygen saturation is essential for fetal well-being. Alkalosis has an adverse effect on placental perfusion and should be limited. Acidosis seems to be reasonably well tolerated by the fetus. Fetal delivery may benefit both the mother and the fetus, but delivery to improve maternal well-being is not always successful. Epidural anesthesia may reduce the increased oxygen demand produced by uterine contractions.

Survival in the pregnant ARDS patient seems to be similar or better than that in the general population, possibly because of the young age of patients and the reversibility of many predisposing conditions. Specific causes of ARDS that pertain to pregnancy should be sought when assessing patients who have this syndrome. When women of childbearing age are seen with ARDS, they should be checked for pregnancy.

Pleural Disease

Although pleural effusions may accompany obstetric complications such as preeclampsia and choriocarcinoma, small, asymptomatic pleural effusions develop in a substantial proportion of women in the postpartum period. These result from the increased blood volume and reduced colloid osmotic pressure that occur in pregnancy, as well as from impaired lymphatic drainage caused by Valsalva maneuvers that occur during labor. Moderate-size effusions or the presence of symptoms should prompt a full clinical evaluation. Repeated expansion to total lung capacity with or without Valsalva maneuvers of labor may also cause *spontaneous pneumothorax* and *pneumomediastinum*, particularly in patients affected by predisposing conditions such as asthma. This diagnosis should be considered in patients who experience chest discomfort and dyspnea during or immediately after delivery.

Interstitial Lung Disease

Interstitial lung disease (ILD) is uncommon in pregnant women, because most cases occur in women beyond their childbearing years. When ILD is found in pregnant women, certain physiologic effects must be considered. A reduced diffusing capacity may lead to difficulty meeting the increased oxygen consumption requirements of pregnancy. Pulmonary hypertension carries increased risks because cardiac output increases during pregnancy. Minimal data exist on management and outcome of these patients, but restrictive lung disease seems reasonably well tolerated in pregnancy. Patients who have a vital capacity less than 1 L and those who have pulmonary hypertension should consider avoiding pregnancy. Lymphangioleiomyomatosis and systemic lupus erythematosus may worsen as a result of pregnancy.

Management of ILD involves careful assessment and monitoring of the pregnant patient's respiratory and cardiovascular status. Exercise intolerance is common, and patients may require supplemental oxygen early in pregnancy to avoid hypoxemic episodes, because these may be dangerous to the fetus. During labor, maternal effort should be limited and oxygen saturation must be monitored. Invasive hemodynamic monitoring may be indicated in the patient with pulmonary hypertension.

Obstructive Sleep Apnea

Pregnancy may be complicated by obstructive sleep apnea (OSA), with potential adverse effects for mother and fetus. Although upper airway narrowing has been documented in pregnancy, apnea and hypopnea are relatively uncommon because of the respiratory stimulatory effect of progesterone. Usually, OSA is confined to obese patients, perhaps precipitated by pregnancy-associated airway mucosal edema and vascular congestion. OSA may worsen in late pregnancy, coupled with the development of hypertension. The association between OSA and preeclampsia probably results from the generalized edema that occurs. Nocturnal hypoxemia may adversely affect the fetus, and poor fetal growth has been documented in these patients. Treatment with nasal continuous positive airway pressure (CPAP) is safe and effective. Snoring is not associated with fetal risk and is not a good marker for OSA in pregnant women.

Cystic Fibrosis

Advances in the management of patients who have cystic fibrosis (CF) have extended life expectancy into childbearing age. Although fertility is impaired, contraception and planned pregnancy should be considered in the management of these patients. Available data indicate that pregnancy does not increase mortality in patients with stable CF, but poor outcomes can occur in those affected by advanced disease. Those with a forced vital capacity less than 50% predicted and pulmonary hypertension before pregnancy are at greatest risk. Perinatal mortality is increased, related largely to preterm delivery that occurs spontaneously or to maternal CF complications. Management requires a multidisciplinary approach with careful attention to nutrition, glucose monitoring, and genetic counseling. Respiratory exacerbations require early aggressive therapy, with due consideration of the potential fetal toxicity of antibiotics (e.g., aminoglycosides, quinolones) and the altered maternal pharmacokinetics.

Gastric Aspiration

Gastric acid aspiration may occur during labor because of delayed gastric emptying, reduced lower esophageal sphincter tone, and the effects of increased intraabdominal pressure. The presentation is with cough, bronchospasm, and dyspnea, which can progress to ARDS. Prophylaxis with antacids, histamine-2 receptor antagonists, or proton pump inhibitors is often given before cesarean section.

Pulmonary Vascular Disease

Pregnancy in the patient with pulmonary hypertension is associated with an extremely high mortality rate, although this has improved somewhat in the past decade. The increased blood volume and cardiac output during pregnancy may precipitate right ventricular failure. LV filling may also be impaired as a result of ventricular interdependence. Hospitalization is recommended early in the third trimester, with close monitoring, anticoagulation, and oxygen therapy. The cardiovascular effects of labor pose a particular risk, and hemorrhage is poorly tolerated. Invasive hemodynamic monitoring may be of value. Successful pregnancy in these patients requires a multidisciplinary team approach in a referral center.

Pulmonary arteriovenous malformations expand during pregnancy because of the increase in blood volume and venous distensibility, which increases the likelihood of bleeding. Embolization and surgical management have been performed in pregnancy. The "idiopathic hemoptysis" described in pregnancy is related to hyperemia from dilated normal bronchial arteries.

CONTROVERSIES AND PITFALLS

Management of any pregnant patient is complicated by concerns for the fetus, particularly in regard to the effects of radiologic investigations and drug therapy. While not ignoring these effects, the clinician must not avoid investigations and drug treatment essential for maternal well-being. Good evidence exists regarding the risk of radiologic investigations, and most tests for respiratory diseases carry minimal risk to the fetus. Although there is a natural reluctance to prescribe drug therapy in pregnancy, good data and resources exist to identify the actual adverse effects of drug therapy; in many situations the benefit to the mother outweighs any risk to the fetus.

The respiratory medicine physician may be approached by a woman with severe lung disease asking about the risks of pregnancy. The evidence supporting such decisions is minimal, although women with pulmonary hypertension or marked obstructive or restrictive lung disease clearly are at increased risk of potentially fatal complications. Isolated case reports and individual experiences demonstrate the remarkable ability of women with severe disease to tolerate pregnancy, and the desire of a woman to have a baby should not be underestimated. In complex cases, referral to a center with multidisciplinary expertise is advisable.

SUGGESTED READINGS

ANZIC Influenza Investigators and Australasian Maternity Outcomes Surveillance System: Critical illness due to 2009 A/H1N1 influenza in pregnant and postpartum women: population-based cohort study, *BMJ* 340:c1279, 2010.

Bédard E, Dimopoulos K, Gatzoulis MA: Has there been any progress made on pregnancy outcomes among women with pulmonary arterial hypertension? *Eur Heart J* 30:256–265, 2009.

Conde-Agudelo A, Romero R: Amniotic fluid embolism: an evidence-based review, *Am J Obstet Gynecol* 201:445.e1–455.e13, 2009.

Dombrowski MP, Schatz M: ACOG practice bulletin: clinical management guidelines for obstetrician-gynecologists, *Obstet Gynecol* 111(pt 1):457–464, 2008.

Jensen D, Webb KA, Davies GA, O'Donnell DE: Mechanisms of activity-related breathlessness in healthy human pregnancy, *Eur J Appl Physiol* 106:253–265, 2009.

Lapinsky SE: Concise definitive reviews in critical care: cardiopulmonary complications of pregnancy, *Crit Care Med* 33:1616–1622, 2005.

Ratnapalan S, Bentur Y, Koren G: Doctor, will that x-ray harm my unborn child? *CMAJ* 179:1293–1296, 2008.

Scarsbrook AF, Evans AL, Owen AR, et al: Diagnosis of suspected venous thromboembolic disease in pregnancy, *Clin Radiol* 61:1–12, 2006.

Schatz M, Dombrowski MP: Clinical practice: asthma in pregnancy, *N Engl J Med* 360:1862–1869, 2009.

Chapter **77**

Pulmonary Complications of Hematopoietic Stem Cell Transplantation

Rodrigo Cavallazzi • Rodney J. Folz

Hematopoietic stem cell transplantation (HSCT) refers to the transplantation of stem cells from bone marrow, growth factor–stimulated peripheral blood, and umbilical blood for the treatment of malignant and nonmalignant hematologic, autoimmune, and genetic diseases. Transplant recipients are at risk of serious complications as a result of pretransplant cytoreductive conditioning regimens, immunologic sequelae from engraftment of allogeneic lymphoid cells (which mediate graft-versus-host responses), the patient's immunosuppressed status, and infections secondary to immunosuppression. Autopsy studies show that pulmonary complications are responsible for more than 70% of deaths in HSCT recipients.

OVERVIEW OF HEMATOPOIETIC STEM CELL TRANSPLANTATION

TYPES

Hematopoietic stem cell transplantation is classified as autologous, allogeneic, or syngeneic. In *autologous* HSCT, patients receive their own hematopoietic stem cells. In *allogeneic* HSCT, patients receive hematopoietic stem cells from a nonidentical sibling or unrelated matched donor. In *syngeneic* HSCT, patients receive hematopoietic stem cells from a genetically identical twin. The source of the donor hematopoietic stem cells can be bone marrow, peripheral blood, or umbilical cord blood. Because autologous and syngeneic transplants involve stem cells that are immunologically identical to the recipient, reactions between graft and host are avoided. In allogeneic transplants, mismatch between donor and recipient human leukocyte antigens (HLAs) mediate *graft-versus-host disease* (GVHD), which may lead to allograft rejection.

Factors that determine the type of transplant to be performed include the nature and stage of the underlying disease, the availability of a suitable donor, and the medical condition of the recipient. The advantages of allogeneic transplantation over autologous transplantation include a higher likelihood that the stem cell product is free of tumor contamination and graft-versus-host activity.

INDICATIONS

A survey from several countries found that the most common indications for HSCT are lymphoproliferative disorders (55%), leukemias (34%), solid tumors (6%), and nonmalignant disorders (5%). The *lymphoproliferative disorders* included plasma cell disorder, Hodgkin disease, and non-Hodgkin lymphoma. Autologous HSCT was slightly more common than allogeneic HSCT. For allogeneic HSCT, the most frequent malignant disease was acute myeloid leukemia (33%) and the most common nonmalignant disease, bone marrow failure syndrome (6%). For autologous HSCT, the most frequent indication was for a plasma cell disorder (41%); the most common nonmalignant indications included bone marrow failure, hemoglobinopathies, immune deficiencies, inherited diseases of metabolism, and autoimmune disorders.

CONDITIONING REGIMENS

Before undergoing HSCT, patients receive a conditioning regimen with the goals of reducing the tumor burden (with malignancy), ablating the bone marrow, and suppressing the recipient's immune system, thereby allowing engraftment of stem cells. The three regimen types are myeloablative conditioning, reduced-intensity conditioning, and nonmyeloablative conditioning. This classification is based on the duration of cytopenia and the requirement for stem cell support. *Myeloablative* conditioning causes irreversible cytopenia, for which stem cell support is always necessary, whereas *nonmyeloablative* conditioning causes minimal cytopenia, for which stem cell support may not be needed. *Reduced-intensity* conditioning causes cytopenia of variable duration, and stem cell support should be given.

Conventional myeloablative conditioning regimens include cyclophosphamide and total-body irradiation (TBI) or busulfan. The more recent nonmyeloablative or reduced-intensity conditioning regimens have used fludarabine and reduced-dose alkylating agents or TBI. Although these less intensive regimens do not provide a strong cytoreductive effect, they allow engraftment of the donor stem cells with a subsequent potentially beneficial graft-versus-malignancy effect. The nonmyeloablative or reduced-intensity conditioning regimens are associated with reduced transplant-associated morbidity and lower incidence of pulmonary complications after transplantation.

Prophylaxis after allogeneic transplant to prevent GVHD usually involves methotrexate, cyclosporin, corticosteroids, or in vitro T cell depletion of the graft before infusion.

POSTTRANSPLANT PULMONARY COMPLICATIONS

Pulmonary complications after HSCT are common, with an incidence of 40% to 60% and with up to one third of recipients

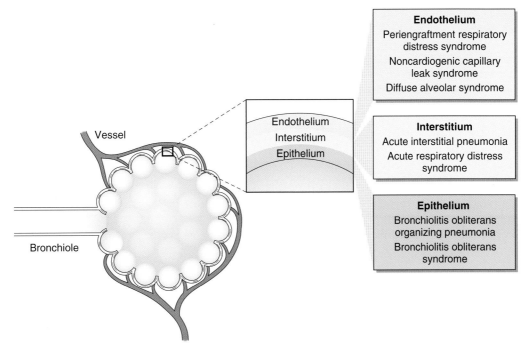

Figure 77-1 Types and location of pulmonary complications after hematopoietic stem cell transplantation (bronchiolitis obliterans organizing pneumonia now called cryptogenic organizing pneumonia).

requiring intensive care after transplantation. Respiratory failure is the most common cause of critical illness, and pneumonia is the leading infectious cause of death after HSCT (**Figure 77-1**). Pulmonary complications can occur early or late in the posttransplant course, can have infectious and noninfectious etiologies, and can present with assorted radiographic findings. The pulmonary complications of HSCT also vary depending on the indication for, type of, and preparative regimen preceding HSCT.

Cellular interactions between graft and host cells are essentially eliminated with autologous transplantation, obviating the need for immunosuppression to prevent or treat GVHD. As such, autologous transplantation is associated with lower incidence of infection, particularly viral pneumonias or cytomegalovirus (CMV) pneumonitis, invasive fungal disease, and other opportunistic infections (e.g., toxoplasmosis), as well as late airflow obstruction defects.

RISK FACTORS FOR PULMONARY DISEASE

Relapse status at transplant and donor-recipient HLA mismatching or nonidentity are risk factors for pulmonary complications and mortality after HSCT (**Box 77-1**). Active phase of malignancy, age over 21 years, and receipt of HLA-nonidentical donor marrow are risk factors for respiratory failure after HSCT.

Abnormalities in pretransplant pulmonary function tests (PFTs) may be predictive of subsequent risk of pulmonary complications and mortality. Reduced diffusing capacity and increased alveolar-arterial oxygen gradient are independent risk factors for interstitial pneumonitis and also independently associated with increased early mortality after HSCT.

Patients with elevated levels of transforming growth factor beta (TGF-β) in plasma, TGF-α in bronchoalveolar lavage (BAL) fluid, and granulocyte-macrophage colony-stimulating factor (GM-CSF) in BAL fluid seem to be at increased risk for

Box 77-1 Risk Factors for Pulmonary Complications After Hematopoietic Stem Cell Transplantation (HSCT)

Donor-recipient human leukocyte antigen mismatch
Relapse status
Active phase of malignancy
Age over 21 years
Pretransplant pulmonary function abnormalities
Reduced diffusion capacity
Increased alveolar-arterial oxygen gradient
Restrictive lung disease
FEV_1 <80% predicted
Elevated pretransplant cytokine levels (TGF-β, TGF-α, GM-CSF)
Allogeneic transplantation
Graft-versus-host disease and type of GVHD prophylaxis
Renal disease

pulmonary complications. One study showed that elevated pretransplant TGF-β levels in patients with breast cancer undergoing autologous HSCT were associated with increased posttransplant risk of pulmonary toxicity and hepatic venoocclusive disease.

Recipients of allogeneic transplantation have more infection complications than recipients of autografts, not only because of chronic immunosuppression, but also because GVHD itself causes an immunodeficient state by affecting the mucosal surfaces, the reticuloendothelial system, and bone marrow. These factors predispose allogeneic recipients to fatal viral pneumonias, multidrug-resistant bacteria, and invasive fungi. Similarly, bronchiolitis obliterans is almost exclusively seen after allogeneic HSCT.

GENETICS AND PULMONARY COMPLICATIONS

Some patients may be genetically predisposed to develop toxicity from the HSCT-related treatments. Indeed, recent studies suggest that certain genetic polymorphisms appear to play a role in the pathogenesis of diverse post-HSCT pulmonary complications. For example, having a polymorphism in the gene for angiotensin-converting enzyme (ACE) increases the likelihood of developing noninfectious pulmonary dysfunction after allogeneic HSCT. Polymorphisms in genes that code for proteins involved in stress-induced oxidant and antioxidant balance may be associated with acute lung injury after HSCT. In some patients, genetic polymorphisms may also be the basis for an increased susceptibility to infection after HSCT. For example, polymorphisms in the mannose-binding lectin gene in both the donor and the recipient are associated with increased risk of major infection.

Although still not routinely used in clinical practice, genetic screening may lead to a more refined prediction of risk for pulmonary complications in future patients undergoing HSCT.

TIME COURSE

Specific pulmonary complications associated with HSCT tend to occur in a relatively well-defined timeline. The timing and intensity of cytoreductive therapies and the resulting pattern of immune reconstitution influence the duration of these intervals.

Preengraftment

The preengraftment phase (0-30 days after transplant) is characterized by prolonged neutropenia and breaks in the mucocutaneous barriers. Accordingly, infectious complications are expected and primarily caused by bacterial and fungal infections. However, most pulmonary complications during this phase are noninfectious and related to regimen-related toxicities.

Early Postengraftment

The early postengraftment period spans days 30 to 100 after transplant and is characterized by persistent impairment in cellular and humoral immunity, in part determined by exogenous immunosuppression, GVHD, deficiency of immunoglobulins, and a loss of protective alveolar macrophages. During this period, neutropenia usually resolves, decreasing the risk of bacterial and fungal infections. The epidemiology of infectious etiologies thus changes to involve predominantly viral infections, especially CMV. With the routine use of antivirals, however, the incidence of posttransplant CMV pneumonia has decreased substantially. Noninfectious etiologies during this time include engraftment syndrome and delayed pulmonary toxicity syndrome.

Late Postengraftment

The late postengraftment period begins at day 100 after transplant. During this time, immune recovery and function are variable and depend on the type of HSCT. Autologous recipients recover more rapidly than allogeneic recipients. T cell responses to alloantigens return to normal, but immunoglobulin levels frequently remain depressed. Viral pathogens cause infections because of poor lymphocyte function, whereas inadequate cellular immunity results in bacterial and fungal pathogens. Noninfectious etiologies are primarily responsible for the pulmonary complications seen during this time, including chronic GVHD, drug-related pulmonary toxicity, bronchiolitis obliterans, restrictive or fibrotic lung disease, and cryptogenic organizing pneumonia (formerly BOOP).

Box 77-2 | **Prevention Strategies for Post-HSCT Opportunistic Infectious**

Infections
Pneumocystis jirovecii (formerly *P. carinii*)
Cytomegalovirus (CMV)
Herpe simplex virus (HSV)
Candida spp.
Aspergillus spp.
Toxoplasma

Prophylaxis
Acyclovir
Ganciclovir
Fluconazole
Posaconazole
Trimethoprim-sulfamethoxazole (TMP-SMX)

HSCT, hematopoietic stem cell transplantation.

INFECTIOUS COMPLICATIONS

The overall risk of pulmonary infection in patients receiving HSCT depends on multiple risk factors, including chemotherapy and radiation-induced neutropenia, lung injury induced by the conditioning regimen, rejection in the form of GVHD, local disruption of host defenses, and intensity of pathogen exposure. In addition, HSCT recipients need to develop a functional immune system from donor-derived cells. Although the production of red blood cells, platelets, and granulocytes occurs soon after HSCT, production of lymphocytes, especially T cells, is considerably delayed. In the first 2 years after transplant, serious infections occur in 50% of otherwise uncomplicated transplants from histocompatible sibling donors and in 80% to 90% of matched unrelated donors or histocompatible recipients with GVHD.

Supportive care in the posttransplant period has changed the microbiology of pneumonia. Prophylactic administration of trimethoprim-sulfamethoxazole (TMP-SMX), antivirals, antifungals, and fluoroquinolones has decreased the incidence of *Pneumocystis jirovecii*, CMV, herpes simplex, and *Candida albicans* infections (**Box 77-2**). Resistant gram-negative and gram-positive bacteria, viruses, and other fungi remain important pathogens.

Bacterial Infections

Bacterial pneumonia is a major cause of morbidity and mortality in patients receiving HSCT. The first month after transplant is notable for pneumonias caused by usual pathogens. Bacterial pneumonia is frequently caused by *Staphylococcus* and *Streptococcus* spp. (24% and 13%, respectively, in one series) and gram-negative organisms, including *Pseudomonas*, *Klebsiella*, *Escherichia*, *Stenotrophomonas*, *Legionella*, *Acinetobacter*, *Serratia*, *Proteus*, *Enterobacter*, and *Citrobacter* spp. Other organisms include *Enterococcus* and rare anaerobes such as *Bacteroides* and *Fusobacterium* spp. Community pathogens emerge after the immediate posttransplant period. *Haemophilus influenzae* is the most common isolate, followed by *Streptococcus pneumoniae* and *Legionella* spp.

Fungal Infections

Fungal disease should be considered in patients with persistent focal radiographic abnormalities that do not respond to empirical antibiotic therapy and in those with nodular opacities on chest imaging, prolonged neutropenia, corticosteroid use, or a history of prior fungal infections.

Invasive aspergillosis is the leading cause of infectious death in HSCT patients, with a mortality of 70% to 90% in allogeneic recipients, despite treatment. The incidence of invasive aspergillosis in allogeneic recipients is 10% to 15%, with a bimodal distribution of cases. During the early preengraftment period that is characterized by profound neutropenia, both allogeneic and autologous recipients are at increased risk for invasive aspergillosis. Allogeneic patients experience a second period of vulnerability, however, during the postengraftment phase, coincident with the development of chronic GVHD, because of the need for augmented immunosuppression. The vulnerability to invasive aspergillosis is higher during the second period than during neutropenia.

Most cases of invasive aspergillosis are limited to the lungs, but sinus and central nervous system involvement can also be seen. Common presenting symptoms include cough and dyspnea, with fever absent in up to two thirds of patients. Concomitant pleuritic chest pain and hemoptysis are clues. Radiographic findings include single or multiple nodules, cavities, and consolidation. The infiltrates are usually focal. The *air crescent sign* describes a central nodule partially or fully surrounded by air, indicating a sequestrum of necrotic lung tissue that has separated from the surrounding parenchyma. The *halo sign* on computed tomography (CT) describes a rim of low attenuation representing edema or hemorrhage that surrounds a pulmonary nodule and is present in more than 90% of patients with neutropenia with invasive pulmonary aspergillosis. The diagnosis of invasive aspergillosis is confirmed by demonstration of fungal elements in diseased tissue and a positive culture result of a specimen from a normally sterile site. In clinical practice, however, biopsy is not usually feasible because of thrombocytopenia or coagulation deficits, and a presumptive diagnosis is often substantiated by high-resolution CT (HRCT) of chest, culture results, or indirect diagnostic tests, such as detection of galactomannan antigen in body fluids.

A randomized clinical trial comparing voriconazole with amphotericin B found that voriconazole led to better survival and improved responses of initial therapy. Therefore, *voriconazole* is recommended as the primary treatment for invasive aspergillosis. The voriconazole loading dosage is 6 mg/kg intravenously (IV) every 12 hours for 1 day, followed by 4 mg/kg IV every 12 hours. Although not the first choice, liposomal *amphotericin B* may be used as an alternative primary therapy. *Posaconazole*, 200 mg every 8 hours, is the first-choice agent for prophylaxis against invasive aspergillosis in high-risk patients, including HSCT recipients with GVHD.

Candida, *Cryptococcus*, and *Zygomycetes* (including *Mucor* and *Rhizopus*) are also important pathogens. The prevalence of invasive zygomycotic infection is 2% and bears a similar clinical course to that of *Aspergillus*. Zygomycetes are angioinvasive, leading to thrombosis, pulmonary infarction, and hemorrhage, with radiographs showing cavitation and halo sign. Mortality rates are high (60%-80%) despite treatment with amphotericin B and surgical resection.

The endemic fungi are encountered less frequently. *Histoplasma* and *Coccidioides* usually occur as reactivation of latent infection. *Blastomyces* usually represents primary disease. Other emerging fungal pathogens reported to cause pulmonary infections include *Fusarium* and *Scedosporium* spp.

Viral Infections

Viral infections, particularly CMV pneumonia, are an important cause of morbidity and mortality in the postengraftment period. *Cytomegalovirus pneumonia* has a nonspecific clinical presentation that includes fever, nonproductive cough, and hypoxia. Chest imaging demonstrates various abnormalities, most frequently bilateral interstitial opacities. A definitive diagnosis relies on demonstrating viral inclusion bodies in lung tissue (which can be difficult on transbronchial biopsy specimens) or detection of virus in BAL fluid by shell vial assay, polymerase chain reaction (PCR), or viral culture (in patients with a compatible clinical presentation). Mortality from CMV pneumonia in posttransplant patients exceeded 90% until the advent of combination therapy with ganciclovir and intravenous immune globulin (IVIG), which improved survival rates to as high as 70%. The use of prophylaxis has not only reduced the incidence but has also delayed the onset of disease, with more CMV infections now occurring 100 days after transplant.

Prophylactic regimens have taken two approaches: (1) universal prophylaxis to all high-risk patients for a defined period after engraftment and (2) preemptive treatment of patients only after detection of subclinical viremia by PCR assay. Both strategies reduce the risk of early CMV disease and are accepted practice guidelines. Seronegative patients who underwent allogeneic transplant from seropositive donors are at highest risk for CMV pneumonia.

The infection pattern of respiratory viruses in HSCT recipients is similar to that in the general population; however, HSCT recipients are more likely to develop lower respiratory tract infection, with mortality of 50% to 70%. Respiratory viruses classically recognized as causing disease in both immunocompetent and immunocompromised individuals include respiratory syncytial virus (RSV), parainfluenza, and influenza. New detection techniques have led to increasing identification of other respiratory viruses, such as human coronavirus, human metapneumovirus, human bocavirus, and human rhinovirus.

In a large prospective study, the 2-year incidence of a first episode of a viral respiratory infection was 29% in recipients of allogeneic HSCT and 15% in recipients of autologous HSCT. The most commonly isolated respiratory viruses were influenza A/B, human RSV, and human metapneumovirus.

Respiratory syncytial virus usually causes an upper respiratory infection, which may progress to fatal pneumonia in the immunocompromised patient. Late airflow obstruction has also been associated with RSV infection. Untreated, RSV pneumonia has a poor prognosis, with mortality approaching 80%. Treatment includes aerosolized *ribavirin;* other agents may be added, although a beneficial effect of concomitant therapy is not well established. Concomitant therapy includes IVIG, RSV-specific immunoglobulin, or palivizumab. Early initiation of treatment appears to be fundamental for the success of antiviral therapy. The role of preemptive therapy in the presence of isolated upper respiratory tract RSV infection is not well defined.

Adenovirus is an uncommon cause of pneumonia and can be isolated in 3% to 5% of patients after HSCT. The incidence is higher in children. It affects the upper and lower respiratory tracts, as well as the gastrointestinal and genitourinary systems. Infection usually develops within the first 3 months of transplantation, with a presentation that might include pharyngitis, tracheitis, bronchitis, pneumonitis, enteritis, hemorrhagic cystitis, or disseminated disease. Mortality with pulmonary involvement may exceed 50%. Cidofovir is used for preemptive (positive viremia despite absence of symptoms) and therapeutic treatment. Some centers have successfully used adenovirus-specific cytotoxic T cells for treatment.

Human metapneumovirus is an RNA paramyxovirus that causes infection in up to 5% of HSCT recipients. Patients usually present with upper respiratory tract symptoms but may also develop pneumonia. The role of antiviral therapy has not been defined in this infection.

Influenza types A and B can cause infection in both immunocompetent and immunocompromised patients, with type A being the most common. The 2009 influenza pandemic was caused by a novel H1N1 influenza A virus, a reassortment of classic swine H1N1, avian Eurasian swine H1N1, and North American human H2N2. Infection by novel H1N1 is characterized by severe disease in patients with specific risk factors, which include immunocompromised status. A cohort study from two medical centers found that HSCT recipients infected with novel H1N1 develop lower respiratory infection in 52% of the cases and have a 30-day mortality of 22%. Zanamivir and oseltamivir are neuraminidase inhibitors used to treat influenza types A and B. Amantadine and rimantadine are adamantanes, which are used only for influenza type A.

Other viral infections include herpes simplex virus (HSV), varicella-zoster virus (VZV), and human herpesvirus (HHV) types 6 and 7. HSV was a common cause of infection in HSCT recipients but incidence has been greatly reduced by acyclovir prophylaxis. HHV-6 has been associated with the idiopathic pneumonia syndrome. Epstein-Barr virus (EBV) infections usually manifest as posttransplant lymphoproliferative disorder.

Pneumocystis Pneumonia

The incidence of *Pneumocystis jirovecii* pneumonia (formerly *P. carinii* pneumonia, PCP) has been greatly reduced by TMP-SMX prophylaxis. Prophylaxis is recommended from time of engraftment to 6 months after transplant in all allogeneic recipients and indefinitely for those on augmented immunosuppressive therapy and those with chronic GVHD. *P. jirovecii* pneumonia presents approximately 60 days after transplantation with cough, dyspnea, fever, and bilateral interstitial and alveolar infiltrates on chest radiography. Diagnostic yield of BAL is almost 90%. Despite TMP-SMX treatment, mortality can be as high as 89% for *P. jirovecii* infections occurring within the first 6 months after transplant versus 40% for late-onset infections.

NONINFECTIOUS COMPLICATIONS

Idiopathic Pneumonia Syndrome

Idiopathic pneumonia syndrome (IPS) refers to a form of severe lung injury in which infectious etiologies, cardiac dysfunction, acute kidney injury, and iatrogenic fluid overload have been excluded. The syndrome encompasses several entities with varying clinical presentation. The heterogeneous clinical manifestations reflect the many lung insults underlying the pathogenesis of IPS, including toxic effects of HSCT conditioning regimens, immunologic cell-mediated injury, and inflammatory cytokines.

The incidence of IPS varies between 2.2% and 15% after allogeneic HSCT; the lower incidence is observed with nonmyeloablative conditioning regimens. The median time of onset for IPS is 22 days after HSCT (range, 4-106 days). There are reports of IPS following autologous HSCT, but it is predominantly seen after allogeneic HSCT. Risk factors for IPS include conventional conditioning regimens, older age, diagnosis of acute leukemia or myelodysplastic syndrome, development of severe acute GVHD, and high-dose TBI.

The insight obtained from animal models has stimulated the classification of the entities under the term *idiopathic pneumonia syndrome* according to the primary anatomic site of cellular damage: interstitial tissue, vascular endothelium, or airway epithelium (see Fig. 77-1). For example, in *interstitial* type of injury, there are increased numbers of cytotoxic T lymphocytes and cells expressing B7 family costimulatory ligands in the alveolar and interstitial spaces. In *vascular endothelium* type of injury, there are injured endothelial cells, and in *airway epithelium* type of injury, injured type II alveolar epithelial cells. This classification reflects complex interactive mechanisms with a pathogenic role attributed to several factors, including increased soluble inflammatory mediators (e.g., tumor necrosis factor alpha), increased host flora–derived lipopolysaccharide, enhanced oxidative stress, depletion of pulmonary surfactant, donor-derived T cell effectors, host antigen-presenting cells, donor accessory cells, and leukocyte recruitment to the lung.

Treatment of the HSCT patient with IPS includes supportive care and, more recently, the combination of corticosteroids. The use of subcutaneous etanercept has been associated with a high clinical response rate in a recent series.

Pulmonary Toxicity

In the immediate posttransplant period, pulmonary toxicity from prior chemo/radiotherapy or the pretransplant conditioning regimen may manifest as fever, dyspnea, cough, hypoxemia, and patchy or diffuse mixed interstitial and alveolar infiltrates on chest radiography. No prospective studies document the efficacy of steroids in these patients, but in clinical practice, prednisone (1-2 mg/kg/day) is used to treat lung toxicity once infection has been excluded.

Pulmonary Edema

Acute pulmonary edema is a complication that tends to occur early, typically in the second week after HSCT. Patients who develop pulmonary edema have fluid retention, as demonstrated by weight gain and a positive fluid balance in the first weeks after HSCT. The fluid retention correlates with left ventricular (LV) end-diastolic diameter measurements by echocardiography. These findings underline the importance of increased LV preload with subsequent elevation in LV end-diastolic pressure and increase in the capillary hydrostatic pressure in the pathophysiology of pulmonary edema after HSCT. Patients may also have underlying cardiac dysfunction secondary to previous treatment with chemotherapeutic agents and chest irradiation.

Noncardiogenic pulmonary edema may result from conditions such as drug-induced pulmonary toxicity, blood product transfusion, and hepatic venooclusive disease.

Diffuse Alveolar Damage

Diffuse alveolar damage is the histologic expression of acute lung injury and acute respiratory distress syndrome. It is therefore the end result of different disease processes, typically sepsis or drug toxicity. The histologic features vary according to the phase: exudative (first week) and organizing. In the exudative phase the histologic analysis reveals intraalveolar edema, interstitial widening, and hyaline membranes. In the organizing phase there is somewhat uniform fibrosis and prominent type 2 pneumocyte hyperplasia.

Diffuse Alveolar Hemorrhage

Diffuse alveolar hemorrhage (DAH) occurs in approximately 5% of autologous and allogeneic recipients. Risk factors include high-dose chemotherapy received before transplant, irradiation, and advanced age. Rapid immune system reconstitution has also been theorized to contribute to DAH. Neutrophil influx into the lung may accentuate the injury and precipitate hemorrhage. The typical symptoms are dyspnea and hemoptysis. Cough and fever may also be present. Although highly suggestive of DAH in the appropriate clinical setting, hemoptysis is not always present. Patients usually are seen during the periengraftment period within the first month after transplantation, but up to 42% of patients with DAH are seen late, after day 30.

Diagnostic criteria proposed to diagnose DAH include alveolar injury, evident as diffuse lung infiltrates or increased alveolar-arterial oxygen gradient; absence of pulmonary infection; BAL fluid with increasingly bloodier return from three separate subsegments; or hemosiderin-laden macrophages at 20% or higher. The radiographic findings of DAH are often nonspecific and include an interstitial or alveolar pattern, usually of bilateral distribution and sparing the peripheral lung areas.

The mainstay of treatment of the HSCT patient with DAH is systemic steroid therapy, which should be instituted promptly. A reported regimen is methylprednisolone, 125 to 250 mg every 6 hours for 5 days, followed by a slow taper over 2 to 4 weeks.

Engraftment Syndrome

Engraftment syndrome is a clinical entity that occurs more often after autologous HSCT but can also follow allogeneic HSCT. A characteristic feature is the development of the syndrome within 96 hours of engraftment. The etiology is unclear but may be attributed to increased cytokine release and neutrophil degranulation during engraftment. The main clinical manifestations of engraftment syndrome include fever, erythrodermal rash, and noncardiogenic pulmonary edema. Patients may also present with hepatic dysfunction, renal insufficiency, weight gain, and transient encephalopathy. Treatment includes supportive care and steroids. For mild cases, steroids may not be warranted.

Delayed Pulmonary Toxicity Syndrome

Delayed pulmonary toxicity syndrome refers to pulmonary toxicity caused by chemotherapy that occurs in patients who undergo autologous HSCT. This syndrome has been associated with regimens containing carmustine and cyclophosphamide. It most often presents between 6 weeks to 3 months after HSCT. It has distinct features that allow the differentiation from idiopathic pneumonia syndrome. For example, delayed pulmonary toxicity syndrome is characterized by high incidence, low mortality, and significant steroid responsiveness. Symptoms include dyspnea, nonproductive cough, and occasional fever. The radiographic abnormalities are nonspecific and do not always correlate with symptoms or worsening pulmonary function. The most common abnormalities on CT scan include ground-glass opacities and mixed linear-nodular opacities. PFTs show decreased diffusion capacity (DL_{CO}), and forced expiratory volume in 1 second (FEV_1), forced vital capacity (FVC), and total lung capacity (TLC) may also be decreased but usually to a lesser extent. Lung biopsy shows alveolar septal thickening, interstitial fibrosis, and type 2 pneumocyte hyperplasia, all consistent with drug toxicity. Treatment consists of steroids.

Interstitial Pneumonitis or Interstitial Lung Disease

Interstitial pneumonitis or interstitial lung disease (ILD) manifests with diminished DL_{CO} and TLC. It can occur at virtually any time after transplantation, with many patients remaining asymptomatic. The pulmonary function changes seen in ILD are usually secondary to treatment with conditioning regimens, particularly those containing carmustine.

Bronchiolitis Obliterans

Bronchiolitis obliterans (obliterative bronchiolitis) is a complication that follows allogeneic HSCT. Rarely, it may also occur after autologous HSCT. The incidence of bronchiolitis obliterans in different reports has ranged from 0% to 48%. Risk factors for obliterative bronchiolitis include chronic GVHD, older age, presence of obstructive disturbance before HSCT, viral infections of the respiratory tract, and busulfan-based conditioning regimens. The close association with GVHD has led some experts to claim that bronchiolitis obliterans may indeed represent the lung manifestation of GVHD.

The activation of donor-derived T lymphocytes plays an important role in the pathogenesis of bronchiolitis obliterans. T cells target the recipient epithelial cells in the bronchioles, leading to an inflammatory reaction. Toll-like receptor–4 signaling in donor-derived hematopoietic cells also appears to be an important factor in causing alloimmunity. Obliterative bronchiolitis tends to occur late, typically more than 100 days after HSCT. The most common symptoms are dry cough, dyspnea, and wheezing. The physical examination may reveal decreased breath sounds, wheezing, and inspiratory squeaks. Furthermore, physical examination often reveals signs of GVHD outside the lung such as skin manifestations. In a minority of patients, there are no respiratory manifestations, and the diagnosis is established by PFTs. The chest radiograph is usually normal, although patients with advanced disease may have signs of hyperinflation, bronchiectasis, and areas of scarring. The HRCT scan is more sensitive for all the previously mentioned abnormalities and valuable in showing air trapping and mosaic attenuation during expiration. PFTs show an obstructive pattern, with FEV_1/FVC ratio less than 0.7 and a decrease in FEV_1 greater than 20% from pretransplant value.

Treatment of the HSCT patient with bronchiolitis obliterans involves corticosteroids, such as prednisone at 1 to 1.5 mg/kg daily, and intensification of immunosuppressive therapy.

Pulmonary Venoocclusive Disease

Pulmonary venoocclusive disease (PVOD) is characterized by *obliterative fibrotic vasculopathy*, which affects mainly the small branches of the pulmonary venous circulation. PVOD may be idiopathic or secondary to another disease. Diseases and risk factors associated with development of PVOD include exposure to chemotherapeutic agents (e.g., carmustine, mitomycin C, bleomycin), autologous and allogeneic HSCT, solid-organ transplantation, radiotherapy, and autoimmune diseases. Patients are seen several months after transplantation with progressive dyspnea on exertion and fatigue. They may also have pleural effusions with right upper quadrant tenderness and ascites. Chest radiography reveals interstitial edema. Abnormalities on HRCT scan include ground-glass opacities with centrolobular distribution, septal thickening, and mediastinal lymphadenopathy.

The diagnosis of PVOD is definitively established by histologic analysis of lung biopsy specimens, but lung biopsy is not indicated because of the high mortality risk. Histologic analysis reveals fibrosis of the venules and small veins in the interlobular septae of the pulmonary circulation, with resultant intraluminal thrombosis. The pulmonary arteries may display medial hypertrophy and eccentric intimal fibrosis. Right-sided cardiac catheterization typically reveals a precapillary pattern of pulmonary hypertension, with an increase in the mean pulmonary artery pressure and normal-range pulmonary capillary wedge pressure. Pulmonary vasodilators can exacerbate the pulmonary edema. Anecdotal reports describe PVOD patient response to high-dose corticosteroids.

Posttransplant Malignancy and Lymphoproliferative Disorder

Posttransplant lymphoproliferative disorder is a term used for different B cell hyperproliferative states that may have benign or malignant behavior. It may follow both solid-organ transplantation and allogeneic HSCT. The lymphoid proliferation is characterized by T cell dysfunction, which results from the conditioning regimen and presence of Epstein-Barr virus. The T cell dysfunction leads to a proliferation of EBV-infected B lymphocytes. Incidence varies from 0.6% to 10%. Risk factors for this disorder include HLA-mismatched donor, T cell depletion of the graft, anti–T cell agents, older age of donor, splenectomy, and mismatch in CMV or EBV status between recipient and donor.

The time from transplantation to development of posttransplant lymphoproliferative disorder is 70 to 90 days. Patients are usually seen within the first 6 months after transplant with lymph node, liver, and spleen involvement, often with relapse with the original malignancy (especially lymphoma) or with secondary lymphomas. Lung involvement is seen in 20% of patients. Treatment consists of reduction in immunosuppressive therapy. Prophylactic administration of rituximab during HSCT has been proposed to prevent posttransplant lymphoproliferative disorder in high-risk patients.

Cryptogenic Organizing Pneumonia (Bronchiolitis Obliterans Organizing Pneumonia)

Cryptogenic organizing pneumonia (COP), formerly bronchiolitis obliterans organizing pneumonia (BOOP), is an inflammatory condition that follows allogeneic and autologous HSCT. The onset of COP varies but usually occurs about 100 days after HSCT. It can be the residue of treated CMV pneumonitis, related to chronic GVHD, or can be idiopathic. Patients present with dry cough, dyspnea, and fever. Physical examination may reveal crackles and inspiratory squeaks. Chest HRCT findings include patchy consolidation, ground-glass attenuation, and randomly distributed nodules. Treatment includes steroid therapy, such as oral prednisone at an initial dose of 1 mg/kg daily, then tapered over 3 to 6 months.

Respiratory Failure

Recipients of HSCT have an overall rate of intensive care unit admission of 15.7%, and the most common cause for ICU admission is respiratory failure followed by shock secondary to sepsis. Independent risk factors for the requirement of assisted mechanical ventilation include older age, active malignancy at transplantation, and donor-recipient HLA mismatch. A review demonstrated that the pooled mortality in HSCT recipients requiring invasive mechanical ventilation is 86.4%. Noninvasive positive-pressure ventilation in select patients with reversible acute respiratory failure is used because observational studies show a survival benefit in HSCT recipients and patients with cancer. In critically ill HSCT recipients, it is also important to comply with the current evidence-based precepts of critical care medicine. For example, in patients with acute respiratory syndrome undergoing mechanical ventilation, a tidal volume of 6 mL/kg of ideal body weight should be targeted.

Other Noninfectious Complications

The term *pulmonary cytolytic thrombi* describes a vasculopathy that occurs in pediatric allogeneic HSCT recipients. It is characterized by an obliterative arteriopathy, occlusive vascular lesions, and hemorrhagic infarcts. This entity can resolve spontaneously without specific therapy. *Pulmonary alveolar proteinosis* has also been reported as a reversible cause of respiratory failure after allogeneic HSCT for acute leukemia.

DIAGNOSTIC EVALUATION

In the diagnostic evaluation of the HSCT patient, information should be obtained on the duration of the pulmonary complication, the radiographic abnormalities, and individual patient factors, such as exposure to toxic drugs, a history of receiving chest radiotherapy, current and previous immunosuppressive regimens and infection prophylaxis, CMV status of donor and recipient, and history of previous opportunistic invasive fungal disease. Useful information may be obtained from PFTs, sputum examination, chest imaging, and serologic studies.

PATTERNS ON IMAGING

The initial imaging evaluation involves a chest radiograph, which can be normal in 15% of symptomatic patients with proven infiltrative lung disease. On the more sensitive chest CT, different patterns may suggest specific disease processes; for example, nodular infiltrates are typical of fungal infections. *Nocardia* and *Cryptococcus* also may present as nodular masses. *Focal infiltrates* usually reflect infectious processes. Noninfectious processes presenting as focal infiltrates include pulmonary emboli, acute radiation pneumonitis, and carcinoma. *Diffuse infiltrates* are nonspecific but often represent pulmonary edema in the preengraftment phase and infections after engraftment. *Pleural effusions* suggest bacterial, mycobacterial, or nocardial infections as well as noninfectious conditions such as pulmonary edema, hepatic venoocclusive disease, pulmonary infarction, and malignancy.

PULMONARY FUNCTION TESTS

Pulmonary function tests should be obtained before HSCT, after transplant in symptomatic patients, and at regularly scheduled intervals in high-risk individuals. Pretransplant abnormalities in DLCO and alveolar-arterial oxygen difference are independent risk factors for interstitial pneumonitis and death. After transplant, typical PFT abnormalities include declining lung volumes, deceasing DLCO, and worsening airflow limitations.

SEROLOGIC STUDIES

The presence of galactomannan, a cell wall component released by *Aspergillus* spp., in serum indicates invasive aspergillosis, as detected by enzyme-linked immunosorbent assay. Using a cutoff optical density of 0.5, the test has a sensitivity of 97.4%, specificity of 90.5%, positive predictive value of 66.1%, and negative predictive value of 99.4%. A galactomannan assay for the diagnosis of invasive aspergillosis has also been evaluated in BAL fluid. Using a cutoff optical density of 0.5, the test showed sensitivity of 86% and specificity of 89%.

An elevated level of $(1,3)$-β-D-glucan in serum is typically associated with invasive aspergillosis and invasive candidiasis but is not specific for a particular fungal infection.

Newer diagnostic techniques have allowed not only a more accurate diagnosis of usual viral respiratory infections but also the detection of emerging viruses that were previously undetected. Nasopharyngeal swab assays employing multiplex PCR can detect up to 20 different respiratory virus types or subtypes in a single rapid test.

Determining CMV serologic status of both recipient and donor is essential in pretransplant screening. The serologic status of the recipient as opposed to the donor is the primary determinant for CMV conversion. A shell vial culture with monoclonal antibody to p72 requires only 48 hours, and tests for antigenemia are rapid, standardized, semiquantitative, and inexpensive. Nucleic acid amplification by PCR on DNA extracted from infected leukocytes also allows rapid diagnosis, detecting infection 2 weeks before viral cultures become positive and 1 week before positive antigenemia, and is highly sensitive.

CONTROVERSIES AND PITFALLS

Bronchoscopy with BAL has the potential to identify the cause of acute respiratory failure in HSCT patients; however, it also carries risks, especially in hypoxemic patients. The role of bronchoscopy was prospectively evaluated in a multicenter observational study in which cancer patients or HSCT recipients with acute respiratory failure received bronchoscopy with BAL, as well as noninvasive diagnostic tests. Noninvasive tests had a diagnostic yield of 66.7%, and BAL bronchoscopy, 50.5%. Although the only investigation that provided a diagnosis in one third of the patients, bronchoscopy with BAL was associated with respiratory deterioration in half the nonintubated patients. Thus, although the routine use of bronchoscopy in HSCT recipients with acute respiratory failure remains controversial, in select patients, bronchoscopy may provide the only means for accurately determining the etiology of lung disease.

Transthoracic needle aspiration under CT or fluoroscopic guidance has a high sensitivity (70%) for detecting pulmonary complications in HSCT patients, with the most common findings being infection and malignancy. However, pneumothorax is also a common complication and may require chest tube placement.

If no diagnosis is made with either bronchoscopy or transthoracic needle aspiration, surgical lung biopsy by either open thoracotomy or a video-assisted thoracoscopic approach may be considered next. Although surgical lung biopsy has a sensitivity of 60% to 80%, the procedure may be associated with worse outcomes and thus should be recommended primarily for hematopoietic stem cell transplant recipients whose test results likely will significantly alter their management.

SUGGESTED READINGS

Afessa B, Azoulay E: Critical care of the hematopoietic stem cell transplant recipient, *Crit Care Clin* 26:133–150, 2010.

Afessa B, Tefferi A, Litzow MR, et al: Diffuse alveolar hemorrhage in hematopoietic stem cell transplant recipients, *Am J Respir Crit Care Med* 166:641–645, 2002.

Azoulay E, Mokart D, Rabbat A, et al: Diagnostic bronchoscopy in hematology and oncology patients with acute respiratory failure: prospective multicenter data, *Crit Care Med* 36:100–107, 2008.

Bacigalupo A, Ballen K, Rizzo D, et al: Defining the intensity of conditioning regimens: working definitions, *Biol Blood Marrow Transplant* 15:1628–1633, 2009.

Boeckh M: The challenge of respiratory virus infections in hematopoietic cell transplant recipients, *Br J Haematol* 143:455–467, 2008.

Dickout WJ, Chan CK, Hyland RH, et al: Prevention of acute pulmonary edema after bone marrow transplantation, *Chest* 92:303–309, 1987.

Espinosa-Aguilar L, Green JS, Forrest GN, et al: Novel H1N1 influenza in hematopoietic stem cell transplantation recipients: two centers' experiences, *Biol Blood Marrow Transplant* 17:566–573, 2010.

Gratwohl A, Baldomero H, Aljurf M, et al: Hematopoietic stem cell transplantation: a global perspective, *JAMA* 303:1617–1624, 2010.

Guo YL, Chen YQ, Wang K, et al: Accuracy of BAL galactomannan in diagnosing invasive aspergillosis: a bivariate metaanalysis and systematic review, *Chest* 138:817–824, 2010.

Herbrecht R, Denning DW, Patterson TF, et al: Voriconazole versus amphotericin B for primary therapy of invasive aspergillosis, *N Engl J Med* 347:408–415, 2002.

Kallianpur AR: Genomic screening and complications of hematopoietic stem cell transplantation: has the time come? *Bone Marrow Transplant* 35:1–16, 2005.

Maertens JA, Klont R, Masson C, et al: Optimization of the cutoff value for the *Aspergillus* double-sandwich enzyme immunoassay, *Clin Infect Dis* 44:1329–1336, 2007.

Mahony J, Chong S, Merante F, et al: Development of a respiratory virus panel test for detection of twenty human respiratory viruses by use of multiplex PCR and a fluid microbead-based assay, *J Clin Microbiol* 45:2965–2970, 2007.

Martino R, Porras RP, Rabella N, et al: Prospective study of the incidence, clinical features, and outcome of symptomatic upper and lower respiratory tract infections by respiratory viruses in adult recipients of hematopoietic stem cell transplants for hematologic malignancies, *Biol Blood Marrow Transplant* 11:781–796, 2005.

Montani D, O'Callaghan DS, Savale L: Pulmonary veno-occlusive disease: recent progress and current challenges, *Respir Med* 104:S23–S32, 2010.

Mullighan CG, Heatley S, Doherty K, et al: Mannose-binding lectin gene polymorphisms are associated with major infection following allogeneic hematopoietic stem cell transplantation, *Blood* 99:3524–3529, 2002.

Onizuka M, Kasai M, Oba T, et al: Increased frequency of the angiotensin-converting enzyme gene D-allele is associated with noninfectious pulmonary dysfunction following allogeneic stem cell transplant, *Bone Marrow Transplant* 36:617–620, 2005.

Pandya CM, Soubani AO: Bronchiolitis obliterans following hematopoietic stem cell transplantation: a clinical update, *Clin Transplant* 24:291–306, 2010.

Soubani AO, Pandya CM: The spectrum of noninfectious pulmonary complications following hematopoietic stem cell transplantation, *Hematol Oncol Stem Cell Ther* 3:143–157, 2010.

Sundin M, Le Blanc K, Ringdén O, et al: The role of HLA mismatch, splenectomy and recipient Epstein-Barr virus seronegativity as risk factors in post-transplant lymphoproliferative disorder following allogeneic hematopoietic stem cell transplantation, *Haematologica* 91:1059–1067, 2006.

Walsh TJ, Anaissie EJ, Denning DW, et al: Treatment of aspergillosis: clinical practice guidelines of the Infectious Diseases Society of America, *Clin Infect Dis* 46:327–360, 2008.

Wilczynski SW, Erasmus JJ, Petros WP, et al: Delayed pulmonary toxicity syndrome following high-dose chemotherapy and bone marrow transplantation for breast cancer, *Am J Respir Crit Care Med* 157:565–573, 1998.

Yanik GA, Ho VT, Levine JE, et al: The impact of soluble tumor necrosis factor receptor etanercept on the treatment of idiopathic pneumonia syndrome after allogeneic hematopoietic stem cell transplantation, *Blood* 112:3073–3081, 2008.

Chapter **78**
Hepatic and Biliary Disease
Aynur Okcay • Michael J. Krowka

The pulmonary consequences of liver disorders can be classified according to whether they predominantly affect the pleural space, the lung parenchyma, or the pulmonary circulation. Unique pulmonary abnormalities occur in patients with severe alpha$_1$-antitrypsin deficiency, primary biliary cirrhosis (PBC), and primary sclerosing cholangitis (PSC). The impact of hepatic dysfunction on the respiratory system during sleep has recently been appreciated (**Table 78-1**).

Hepatopulmonary syndrome (HPS) and *portopulmonary hypertension* (POPH) are the major pulmonary vascular problems that complicate portal hypertension from any cause. HPS, a pulmonary vascular dilation abnormality leading to arterial hypoxemia, occurs in 5% to 15% of patients with portal hypertension. POPH, resulting from pulmonary vascular obstruction or obliteration, has been reported in 4% to 16.5% of patients with advanced liver disease. Pleural effusions related to the formation of ascites develop in 5% to 10% of cirrhotic patients.

Pulmonary function abnormalities can be demonstrated in approximately 50% of patients with advanced liver disease. The most common abnormality is a reduced diffusing capacity for carbon monoxide (DLCO). Abnormal oxygenation measured by increased alveolar-arterial oxygen gradient or reduced arterial oxygen tension (PaO$_2$) is common (40%-50%). Nocturnal oxygenation abnormalities are also common (~50%) and underdiagnosed in patients with advanced liver disease.

RISK FACTORS

Portal hypertension appears to be a prerequisite for the development of either HPS or POPH. Previous portosystemic surgical shunts have been reported in up to 30% of patients with POPH. Conditions leading to abnormal ascites usually precede the development of pleural effusions ("hepatic hydrothorax"). Smoking in the setting of ZZ or SZ α$_1$-antitrypsin deficiency genotypes leads to the greatest risk of emphysema and varying degrees of expiratory airflow obstruction. The Child-Pugh classification for the severity of liver diseases correlates poorly with most pulmonary consequences, with the exception of hepatic hydrothorax. The epidemic of hepatitis C disease does not appear to be related to any unique or common pulmonary abnormality, but the use of interferon-alpha to treat hepatitis C virus (HCV) infection is associated with well-documented drug-induced pulmonary side effects. The clinical presence of ascites or encephalopathy, as well as narcotic and sedative use, appears to predispose to abnormal overnight oximetry and sleep-disordered breathing.

PATHOPHYSIOLOGY

Circulating mediators, associated with the probable genetic predisposition, appear to cause HPS or POPH. Such mediators (causing vasodilation or vasoproliferation, respectively) could arise because of the abnormal metabolism of the dysfunctional liver. However, such specific circulating mediators have yet to be identified in humans.

Hepatopulmonary Syndrome HPS is characterized by arterial hypoxemia caused by precapillary-capillary dilations or direct arteriovenous communications. Excess perfusion for a given area of ventilation, diffusion limitation, and true anatomic shunting contribute to the degree of abnormal arterial oxygenation (**Figure 78-1**). Increased concentrations of exhaled nitric oxide have been demonstrated in HPS. Animal models of HPS have found upregulation of endothelin B receptors causing vasodilation and evidence of angiogenesis.

Portopulmonary Hypertension POPH results from vasoproliferation (endothelium and smooth muscle), along with in situ thrombosis, which causes an increased pulmonary vascular resistance (PVR) to arterial flow. It is important to note the various pulmonary hemodynamic patterns that may exist in the patient with advanced liver disease (**Table 78-2**).

Hepatic Hydrothorax Hepatic hydrothorax is a transudative pleural effusion caused by the formation of ascitic fluid. A combination of negative pleural pressure and positive abdominal pressure forces ascitic fluid into the pleural spaces through diaphragmatic defects and lymphatics. Rarely, the fluid may be chylous; infected pleural fluid may occur in the presence of spontaneous bacterial peritonitis.

Primary Biliary Cirrhosis and Primary Sclerosing Cholangitis PBC has systemic manifestations presumably because of autoimmune phenomena. Pulmonary granulomas, lymphocytic infiltrates, and organizing pneumonia can result. Rarely, both PBC and PSC may be associated with airway inflammation, hilar adenopathy, and mediastinal adenopathy (noncaseating granulomas found at biopsy).

Alpha$_1$-Antitrypsin Deficiency Severe deficiency of the circulating alpha-1 protein is caused by single point mutations in the synthesis of this protein within hepatocytes. Accumulation of polymerized protein within the endoplasmic reticulum of hepatocytes leads to clinically significant deficiency in serum

Table 78-1 Major Pulmonary Consequences of Portal Hypertension (with or Without Cirrhosis)

Area/Disorder	Complications
Pleural space	Hepatic hydrothorax Chylothorax Thoracobiliary fistulas Elevated hemidiaphragms caused by massive ascites
Pulmonary parenchyma	Bronchitis/bronchiectasis Emphysema (ZZ or SZ α_1-antitrypsin deficiency) Organizing pneumonia (PBC) Lymphocytic interstitial pneumonia (PBC) UIP or NSIP (PBC, autoimmune hepatitis/HCV therapy) Hilar/mediastinal lymphadenopathy (PBC, PSC)
Pulmonary circulation	Hepatopulmonary syndrome (HPS) *Pulmonary hypertension* High flow state Excess volume Left ventricular dysfunction Portopulmonary hypertension (POPH)
Sleep-disordered breathing	Frequent and severe nocturnal SaO_2 changes Effects of massive ascites and encephalopathy Obstructive sleep apnea (OSA)

HCV, hepatitis C virus; *NSIP*, nonspecific interstitial pneumonia; *PBC*, primary biliary cirrhosis; *PSC*, primary sclerosing cholangitis; SaO_2, arterial oxygen saturation; *UIP*, usual interstitial pneumonia.

α_1-antitrypsin (especially in ZZ and SZ genotypes). Such deficiency subsequently leaves neutrophil elastase unopposed within the lung, causing lung damage (panacinar emphysema and bronchiectasis).

CLINICAL FEATURES

Exertional dyspnea is the most common, nonspecific presentation of any pulmonary consequence of liver dysfunction.

Hepatopulmonary Syndrome Finger clubbing, cyanosis of the digits, and spider angiomas suggest the arterial hypoxemia of HPS. The chest examination is usually unremarkable; no wheezing or inspiratory crackles are heard. Worsening dyspnea (platypnea) and arterial oxygenation (orthodeoxia) on moving from the supine to the standing position is frequently noted in the HPS patient.

Portopulmonary Hypertension Chest pain, pressure, and palpitations suggest advanced manifestations of POPH. Syncope is especially worrisome for severe POPH. An accentuated second heart sound (increased P_2) is common is POPH. The murmur of tricuspid regurgitation (systolic; over fourth intercostal space to left of sternum) may be heard.

Primary Biliary Cirrhosis and Primary Sclerosing Cholangitis Inspiratory crackles in the lower lung fields heard during auscultation may be associated with the interstitial lung problems that complicate PBC (lymphocytic alveolitis) or chronic aspiration in patients with hepatic encephalopathy. Productive sputum may be related to the airway abnormalities (bronchiectasis) associated with α_1-antitrypsin deficiency or PSC (bronchitis).

Hepatic Hydrothorax Pleural effusion caused by liver dysfunction will be associated with diminished breath sounds depending on the location and extent of the pleural effusion. Egophony (verbalized "e" sounds like "a" to listener) suggests atelectatic lung caused by compressive pleural effusions; affected patients may have significant hypoxemia. Pleural rubs are rare; pleuritic or chest wall pain is not a symptom of hepatic hydrothorax and suggests another diagnosis, such as an autoimmune disorder or pulmonary embolism.

Alpha₁-Antitrypsin Deficiency Signs and symptoms are similar to advanced chronic obstructive lung disease (COPD), especially emphysema (hyperinflation of chest; prolonged expiratory phase with/without wheezing). Chest radiography and computed tomography (CT), however, suggest predominantly lower lung field distribution of emphysematous or bullous abnormality. Such changes are seen only in the severely deficient ZZ or SZ genotypes; MZ genotypes have minimal, if any, lung damage. Approximately 50% of cirrhotic patients with ZZ or SZ phenotypes have abnormal pulmonary function tests (PFTs), such as increased residual volume and reduced forced expiratory volume in 1 second (FEV_1).

Sleep-Disordered Breathing Excess fatigue and daytime hypersomnolence caused by sleep-disordered breathing may be confused with effects of liver disease and anemia. Sleep-related oxygenation abnormalities and effects on liver metabolism, such as insulin resistance resulting from hypoxic liver injury, have been documented. Furthermore, improvement in liver enzyme levels after treatment of obstructive sleep apnea (OSA) with continuous positive airway pressure (CPAP) also supports the diagnosis of hypoxic injury that occurs overnight. Chronic fatigue after liver transplant (LT) has been a major problem regardless of posttransplant duration, greatly impacting the patient's daily functioning and quality of life. A significant relationship was found between severity of post-LT fatigue and sleep quality, as assessed by the Pittsburgh Sleep Quality Index (PSQI).

DIAGNOSIS

Hepatopulmonary Syndrome The HPS diagnosis is established by demonstrating pulmonary vascular dilation as the cause for hypoxemia. Hypoxemia is usually defined as PaO_2 less than 80 mm Hg or alveolar-arterial oxygen gradient greater than 15 to 20 mm Hg. Two noninvasive methods are available to document abnormal pulmonary vascular dilation. Qualitatively, a positive contrast-enhanced transthoracic echocardiogram reflects the passage of microbubbles (usually absorbed during a first pass through normal lungs) through dilated pulmonary vessels, with subsequent detection in the left atrium. Quantitatively, an abnormal brain uptake of technetium-labeled macroaggregated albumin (^{99m}Tc MAA) (uptake > 6%) after lung perfusion reflects the passage of radiolabeled albumin aggregates through the lungs and subsequent uptake in the brain (**Figure 78-2**). Contrast echocardiography is more sensitive than ^{99m}Tc lung scanning to detect pulmonary vascular dilation. A lung biopsy is not necessary. **Figure 78-3** provides a practical clinical algorithm for the evaluation of suspected HPS.

Portopulmonary Hypertension Screening for pulmonary hypertension is accomplished by transthoracic Doppler echocardiography. Increased right ventricular systolic pressure (RVSP) greater than 50 mm Hg suggests but does not prove clinically

Figure 78-1 Mechanisms of arterial hypoxemia in hepatopulmonary syndrome. **A,** Normal ventilation and evenly matched perfusion; no anatomic shunts. **B,** Many capillaries are dilated with blood flow that is not uniform, and ventilation-perfusion excess mismatch occurs. Restricted oxygen diffusion into the center of the dilated capillaries occurs. Anatomic shunts that bypass the alveoli can develop. Hypoxemia evolves from each of these abnormalities. *(From Rodriguez-Roisin R, Krowka MJ: N Engl J Med 358:2378–2387, 2008.)*

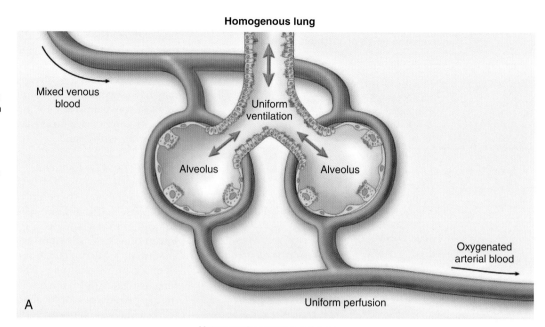

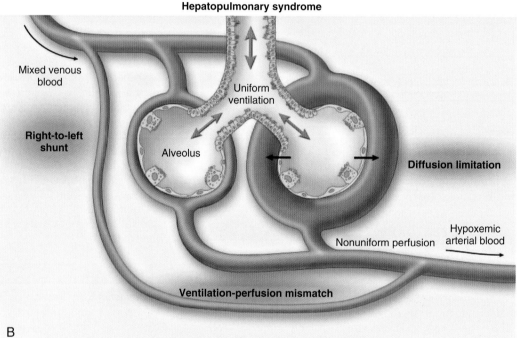

Table 78-2 Pulmonary Hemodynamic Patterns Associated with Advanced Liver Disease

Pattern	MPAP	CO	PAOP	TPG	PVR
High-flow, hyperdynamic circulatory state*	↑	↑↑	↓	↓	↓
Excess volume†	↑	↑	↑	↑↓	↑↓
Portopulmonary hypertension					
Normal volume‡	↑↑↑	↑ → ↓	↓	↑↑↑	↑↑↑
Excess volume	↑↑↑	↑ → ↓	↑	↑↑	↑↑

Specific data associated with these patterns in Okcay A et al: *Hepatology* 44:455, 2009.

CO, cardiac output (normal usually 4-5 L/min); *MPAP,* mean pulmonary artery pressure (normal <25 mm Hg); *PAOP,* pulmonary artery occlusion pressure (same as pulmonary capillary wedge pressure, PCWP); *PVR,* pulmonary vascular resistance (TPG/CO; normal <3 Wood units, or 240 dynes.sec.cm^{-5}); *TPG,* transpulmonary gradient (MPAP − PAOP; normal <12 mm Hg).

*This pattern usually seen in HPS.

†Depending on the duration and reason for excess volume, PVR and TPG may be increased or normal.

‡As POPH worsens, PVR increases, right side of heart fails, and CO declines.

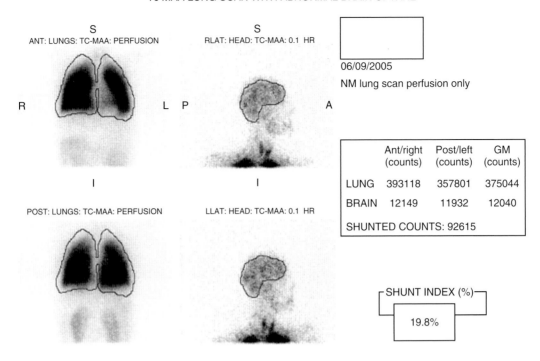

Figure 78-2 Lung perfusion scan with quantified technetium 99 (^{99m}Tc) macroaggregated albumin (MAA) abnormal uptake over the brain. *GM,* geometric mean; *NM,* nuclear medicine.

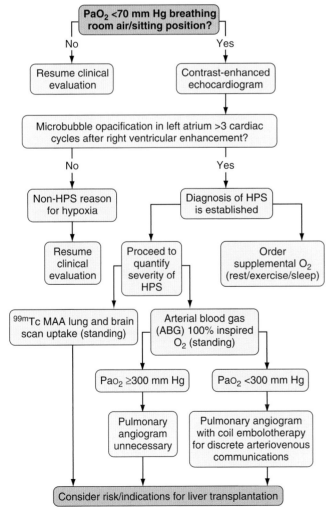

Figure 78-3 Current screening and diagnostic algorithm at the Mayo Clinic for patients with suspected hepatopulmonary syndrome *(HPS).*

significant POPH. A right-sided heart catheterization must be accomplished to establish the diagnosis. **Figure 78-4** provides a screening algorithm used at the Mayo Clinic; clinicians may have other criteria to determine candidates for right-sided heart catheterization. Most centers adhere to the triad of mean pulmonary artery pressure (MPAP) greater than 25 mm Hg, normal pulmonary capillary wedge pressure (PCWP) less than 15 mm Hg, and increased pulmonary vascular resistance (PVR) greater than 240 dynes.sec.cm^{-5}) as definitive criteria for POPH. A lung biopsy is neither necessary nor advised. Chronic pulmonary emboli should be excluded.

Hepatic Hydrothorax   This is a clinical diagnosis based on the chest radiograph showing a pleural effusion that can be right-sided (70%), left-sided (15%), or bilateral (15%). Thoracentesis is usually performed only when dyspnea is extreme, or atypical symptoms (e.g., pain, fever) exist suggesting another process such as empyema or metastatic hepatocellular carcinoma. Hepatic hydrothorax may occur in the absence of clinical ascites.

Alpha$_1$-Antitrypsin Deficiency   Pulmonary dysfunction in the setting of severe α_1-antitrypsin deficiency should be established by standard PFTs, to assess degree of expiratory airflow limitation and hyperinflation, and high-resolution CT (HRCT) of the chest, to assess for subclinical emphysema, bullae, and bronchiectasis. A combination of abnormal serum genotypes (usually ZZ or SZ, with MM normal) and decreased α_1-antitrypsin level confirms the diagnosis.

Sleep-Disordered Breathing   Overnight oximetry (OvOx) using finger pulse monitoring to screen for abnormal nocturnal oxygenation is inexpensive and clinically important. Abnormal OvOx abnormalities include frequent and severe hemoglobin desaturation (**Figure 78-5**). These abnormalities are common

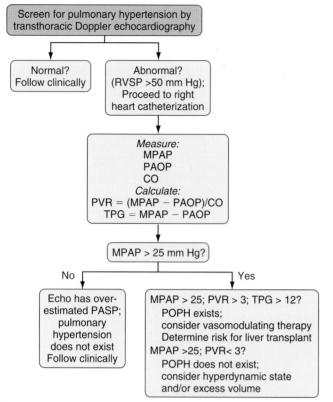

Figure 78-4 Screening, diagnostic, and staging algorithm followed at the Mayo Clinic for patients with portopulmonary hypertension *(POPH)*. *RVSP*, right ventricular systolic pressure; *MPAP*, mean pulmonary artery pressure; *PAOP*, pulmonary artery occlusion pressure (pulmonary capillary wedge pressure); *CO*, cardiac output; *PVR*, pulmonary vascular resistance; *TPG*, transpulmonary gradient; *PASP*, pulmonary artery systolic pressure.

in LT candidates despite a lack of daytime somnolence. Abnormal OvOx is associated with massive ascites, encephalopathy, and increased baseline alveolar-arterial oxygen gradients. If OvOx is abnormal, formal *polysomnography* (PSG; overnight sleep study with multiple variable noninvasive monitoring) should be conducted. PSG is the "gold standard" to diagnose specific sleep-disordered breathing etiologies.

TREATMENT

Hepatopulmonary Syndrome No pharmacologic treatments have proved efficacious in improving arterial hypoxemia caused by HPS. Liver transplantation (LT) is the treatment of choice. Rarely, coil embolization of discrete arteriovenous communications that occur in HPS can improve oxygenation. Supplemental oxygen should be given depending on PaO_2 levels at rest, with exertion, and during sleep.

Portopulmonary Hypertension Significant improvement in pulmonary hemodynamics has been reported with the long-term use of continuous 24-hour intravenous (IV) infusion of the prostacyclins *epoprostenol* and *treprostinil,* as well as with the oral endothelin receptor antagonists *ambrisentan* and *bosentan* and the phosphodiesterase inhibitor *sildenafil.* LT is a high-risk procedure in the patient with POPH and is contraindicated if pulmonary vasomodulating therapy does not result in MPAP less than 50 mm Hg and satisfactory right-sided heart function.

Insp O_2: 0.209 ESS-7 There was 1 drop in
Valid recording time: 6 hrs, 49 mins saturation of at least 4%

Oxygen Saturation (%)		% Time of O_2 Sat	
Beginning	94.9	<90%	0.1
Mean	92.8	<88%	0.0
Maximum	96.0		
Minimum	89.0		

Comments:

Overnight oximetry was performed on room air without any assisted breathing device. Sleep quality was not reported. Baseline oxygen saturation was normal and remained normal through the night. No real abnormality noted.

Impression:

Normal study.

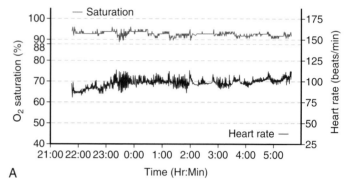

A

Insp O_2: Assume 0.209 ESS-N/A There were 150 drops in
Valid recording time: 8 hrs, 57 mins saturation of at least 4%

Oxygen Saturation (%)		% Time of O_2 Sat	
Beginning	90.9	<90%	41.1
Mean	89.4	<88%	8.8
Maximum	95.0	<85%	3.6
Minimum	72.0	<80%	0.9
		<75%	0.0

Comments:

Overnight oximetry was performed for a total valid sampling time of 8 hours 57 minutes. Baseline saturation was 91% with a mean saturation of 89% and lowest recorded saturation 72%. Overall, 41% of the recorded interval was spent with saturation of less than 90%. There is intermittent oscillatory wave form variability present consistent with disordered breathing in addition to reduced baseline consistent with hypoventilatory or gas exchange abnormality.

Impression:

Consistent with disordered breathing. Reduced baseline saturation consistent with hypoventilatory or gas exchange abnormality.

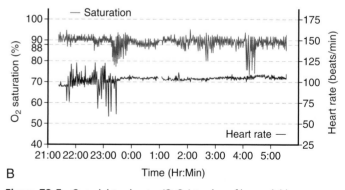

B

Figure 78-5 Overnight oximetry (OvOx) tracing of hemoglobin saturation by oxygen (SaO_2) via finger tip monitoring. **A,** Normal. Minimal variations in SaO_2 and no drops in SaO_2 below 90% saturation. **B,** Desaturator: defined as SaO_2 less than 90% more than 10% of sleep time; and frequent drops in SaO_2 greater than 4%.

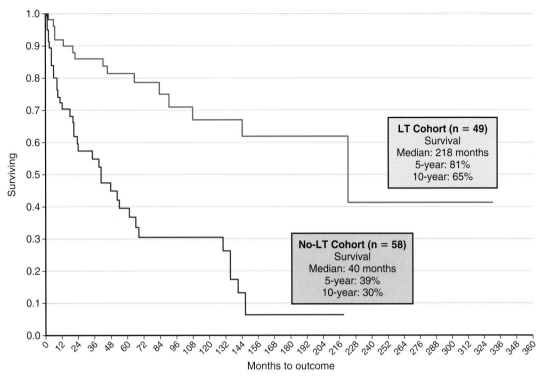

Figure 78-6 Long-term outcome (5-year and 10-year survival) in patients with hepatopulmonary syndrome, lung transplant *(LT)* cohort versus no lung transplant *(no-LT)* cohort. *(From Iyer V et al:* Liver Transpl *17:S130, 2011).*

Hepatic Hydrothorax Salt restriction and aggressive diuresis, as tolerated by renal function, with furosemide and spironolactone are treatment cornerstones. Repetitive thoracentesis is not advised. Chest tube drainage with pleurodesis and video-assisted thoracoscopy rarely provide long-term improvement, by obliterating the pleural space and repairing diaphragmatic defects, respectively. *Transjugular intrahepatic portosystemic shunting* (TIPS) is appropriate treatment for refractory hepatic hydrothorax, as is LT. Outcome of LT is not affected by the presence of hepatic hydrothorax.

Severe α₁-Antitrypsin Deficiency and Abnormal Pulmonary Function In the patient with clinically significant liver disease and severe serum α_1-antitrypsin deficiency (<80 mg/dL), augmentation therapy to replace the protein by weekly or biweekly infusions is appropriate, safe, and may prevent further lung damage. There is no role for treating α_1-antitrypsin liver disease (cirrhosis) with replacement therapy. LT results in the phenotype of the donor liver, normalizes the serum α_1-antitrypsin level, and presumably prevents further lung damage. LT in the patient with serious liver dysfunction caused by ZZ or SZ phenotype may be problematic and must be considered on a case-by-case basis.

Sleep-Disordered Breathing Treatments range from simple supplemental oxygen during sleep by nasal cannula to the use of masks to deliver CPAP or biphasic positive airway pressure (BiPAP). Treating ascites (diuresis) and encephalopathy (oral osmotic laxatives) may be helpful. The effect of LT on sleep-disordered breathing has yet to be studied.

CLINICAL COURSE

Hepatopulmonary Syndrome Few data exist to characterize the clinical course in HPS. In the largest series to date, 5-year

survival associated with LT was 76% versus 23% in non-LT group (**Figure 78-6**). Complete resolution of HPS often follows LT; the time to resolution is directly related to the severity of hypoxemia and may take months. Mortality is rarely a direct consequence of hypoxemia.

Portopulmonary Hypertension The 5-year survival without pulmonary vasodilator treatment is 4% to 14%. Mortality is equally the result of progressive right-sided heart failure and the complications related to liver disease. Long-term survival benefit has been noted with 24-hour continuous IV epoprostenol therapy in POPH versus no treatment. Despite pulmonary vasomodulating therapy, successful outcome during and after LT remains problematic and unpredictable. Despite aggressive therapy, POPH may resolve, remain stable, or progress following LT.

Alpha₁-Antitrypsin Deficiency In patients with the ZZ phenotype, long-term survival is significantly reduced in smokers. No data describe the long-term outcomes in patients with ZZ phenotype, cirrhosis, and pulmonary function abnormalities, with or without LT. The risk of liver cancer increases with age in ZZ patients.

Sleep-Disordered Breathing The effect of arterial hypoxemia (nocturnal or daytime) on hepatic function that may already be impaired is poorly understood. Better nocturnal oxygenation using supplemental oxygen or airway devices may significantly improve quality of life, as well as ameliorate cardiovascular dysfunction (rhythm disturbances, systemic hypertension).

PITFALLS AND CONTROVERSIES

Transjugular intrahepatic portosystemic shunting may or may not have a therapeutic role in the treatment of HPS. TIPS may acutely worsen pulmonary hemodynamics because of increased preload and therefore may be contraindicated in the POPH patient.

The priority for lung transplant in patients with either HPS or POPH is evolving; PaO_2 less than 60 mm Hg from HPS now warrant higher priority for LT. In POPH it is hypothesized that pulmonary hemodynamic improvement with pulmonary vasodilators (goal of MPAP <35 mm Hg and PVR <400 dynes.sec. cm^{-5}, or normalization of PVR with good right ventricular function) may facilitate safe LT and improved long-term survival. The optimal medical therapy (prostacyclins, endothelin receptor antagonists, or phosphodiesterase inhibitors) for POPH has yet to be defined.

The role of hepatitis C infection causing pulmonary dysfunction is debatable. Interferon therapy (standard or pegylated forms) may cause a sarcoidlike reaction within the lungs. Organizing pneumonia has also been reported with such therapy, and discontinuance of therapy and corticosteroids usually resolve the pulmonary process.

Symptoms of fatigue in the patient with advanced liver disease may be caused by treatable sleep-disordered breathing and abnormal nocturnal oxygenation. Therefore, screening overnight oximetry should be a routine diagnostic consideration in such patients.

SUGGESTED READINGS

Cartin-Ceba R, Swanson KL, Wiesner RH, Krowka MJ: Safety and efficacy of ambrisentan in portopulmonary hypertension, *Chest* 139:109–114, 2011.

Gupta S, Castel H, Rao RV, et al: Improved survival after liver transplantation in patients with hepatopulmonary syndrome, *Am J Transplant* 10:354–363, 2010.

Iyer V, Swanson KL, Cartin-Ceba R, Krowka MJ: Liver transplantation in hepatopulmonary syndrome: 5 and 10 year survivals, *Liver Transpl* 17:S130, 2011.

Kelly E, Grenne CM, Carroll TP, et al: Alpha-1 antitrypsin deficiency, *Respir Med* 104:763–772, 2010.

Kiafar C, Gilani N: Hepatic hydrothorax: current concepts of pathophysiology and treatment options, *Ann Hepatol* 7:313–320, 2008.

Krowka MJ, Miller D, Barst R, et al: Portopulmonary hypertension: results from the U.S. REVEAL registry, *Chest* 141:906–915, 2012.

Krowka MJ, Swanson KL, McGoon MD, et al: Portopulmonary hypertension: results of a 10-year screening algorithm, *Hepatology* 44:1140–1152, 2006.

Okcay A, Somers V, Caples S, Krowka MJ: Abnormal screening oximetry in liver transplant candidates (abstract), *Hepatology* 44:455, 2009.

Polito A: Pulmonary reactions to novel chemotherapeutic agents and biomolecules. In Camus P, et al, editors: *Drug-induced and iatrogenic respiratory disease*, London, 2010, Hodder Arnold.

Rodriguez-Roisin R, Krowka MJ: Hepatopulmonary syndrome: a liver-induced lung vascular disorder, *N Engl J Med* 358:2378–2387, 2008.

Singh C, Sager JS: Pulmonary complications of cirrhosis, *Med Clin North Am* 93:871–883, 2009.

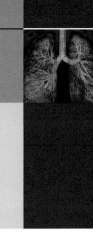

Chapter **79**
Inflammatory Bowel Disease

Frank Schneider • Kristen L. Veraldi

Thoracic involvement by Crohn disease (CD) and ulcerative colitis (UC) is part of the spectrum of extraintestinal manifestations of inflammatory bowel disease (IBD). The distinctive pathologic changes associated with IBD can involve the upper respiratory tract, the large and small airways, the interstitium of the lung, the pleura, and the heart and pericardium. It is often difficult to prove with certainty that a particular lung disease is causally related to an IBD. The presentation is not always temporally related to the bowel disease, and the pathologic findings can overlap with those seen in other inflammatory lung diseases. However, the correlation of pulmonary function with IBD severity and the striking response to corticosteroid therapy by many of the lesions suggests a common mechanism.

Anatomically, the gastrointestinal and respiratory systems have some common features. The cephalad end of the respiratory tract (larynx and trachea) is intimately associated with the foregut until their separation by the mesodermal tracheoesophageal folds. Both epithelia are of endodermal origin, and both mucosal surfaces contain mucosa-associated lymphoid tissue (MALT), columnar epithelium with surface differentiations (villi and cilia), goblet cells, and submucosal glands. The pathogenesis of extraintestinal manifestations is poorly understood. The emerging theme of the proposed mechanisms for bowel damage in IBD is an intricate interplay among innate and acquired immunologic factors, intraluminal microbial flora, and the mucosal barrier separating both. Several studies found a limited repertoire of T cell specificity in IBD patients, suggesting that a cellular immune response is elicited by only a small number of antigens. Autoantibodies, including atypical antinuclear antibodies (ANAs), found in some patients suggest an aberrant B cell functionality. The diapedesis (migration) of inflammatory cells into areas of inflammation suggests abnormalities in the homing of leukocytes. Lastly, increased levels of cytokines (e.g., interferon, tumor necrosis factor) suggest a dysregulation of inflammatory mediators in patients with IBD. Evidence has been found supporting all these mechanisms in sites other than the respiratory tract.

In addition, genetic linkage studies of affected kindred have identified several genes associated with IBD. The first susceptibility gene discovered (IBD1, also known as NOD2) encodes a protein that activates transcription in macrophages on encountering bacterial lipopolysaccharides. Another, more recent, example is the discovery of nonfunctional variants of the interleukin-23 (IL-23) receptor or some of its downstream effectors. IL-23 helps generate Th17 helper cells that play a central role in immune response regulation. Genetic factors are associated not only with the development of IBD but also with its extraintestinal manifestations. A study of more than 250 parent-child and sibling pairs showed concordance of extraintestinal involvement in 70% and over 80% of the pairs, respectively. Other studies more specifically sought associations with certain genes. IBD1 and IL-23 are associated with sacroiliitis and ankylosing spondylitis, respectively. CD patients carrying major histocompatibility complex (MHC) genes *HLA-A2*, *HLA-DR1*, *HLA-DQw5*, *HLA-DRB1*0103* (DR103), or *HLA-B*27* are more likely to develop extraintestinal manifestations. UC patients with *HLA-B*58* have been found to have more joint, skin, and eye manifestations. *HLA-B8* is more common in UC patients with primary sclerosing cholangitis than those without. No specific genetic link has been established between IBD and respiratory tract involvement. However, some genetic alterations may also be involved in other lung diseases; abnormalities of NOD2, for example, have been found in early-onset and advanced pulmonary sarcoidosis.

Thoracic conditions seen in IBD can conceptually be grouped into four categories: (1) nonspecific conditions (e.g., infection), (2) anatomic complications (e.g., fistulas); (3) therapy-related complications (e.g., drug toxicity); and (4) distinctive pathologic changes that statistically show a more-than-incidental association with IBD. This chapter focuses on the fourth category.

EPIDEMIOLOGY

The true incidence of thoracic complications in IBD patients is unknown. There have been no screening tests performed on large populations of IBD patients. The proportion of IBD patients with subjective respiratory symptoms such as cough, sputum production, wheezing, or shortness of breath has been reported to be as high as 50%. One or more pulmonary function tests (PFTs) are abnormal in approximately 40% of IBD patients, with forced expiratory volume in 1 second (FEV_1), inspiratory vital capacity (IVC), or diffusion capacity (DL_{CO}) showing a 10% to 30% reduction. Between 25% and 50% of asymptomatic IBD patients show abnormalities on high-resolution computed tomography (HRCT) scans. Often, the findings are subtle and include ground-glass opacities, mosaicism suggestive of air trapping, peripheral opacities, and cysts. At the other end of the spectrum are case reports and small series of patients with distinctive manifestations of thoracic involvement. These reports, accounting for 155 patients, were recently reviewed (see Suggested Readings). Although nothing is offered to calculate incidence or prevalence, significant symptomatic thoracic involvement by IBD probably is not a common event. However, it is common enough that physicians need to be cognizant of IBD to recognize it and prevent the potentially debilitating consequences of some of its forms.

The temporal relation of the thoracic manifestation to the bowel disease varies. Approximately 80% of patients have an established history of IBD, whereas in about 10% each, the thoracic symptoms precede the bowel disease or develop concomitantly. About one half of patients with airway disease have had a colectomy, and occasionally the onset of airway disease follows the colectomy by days or weeks, suggesting a shift of the inflammatory reaction from the gut to the bronchial tree.

In ulcerative colitis and Crohn disease, the most common anatomic structures involved are the large airways (39%), followed by infiltrative lung disease (23%) and involvement of the serosa (13%). Small airways inflammation (10%), upper airways inflammation (9%), and involvement of the pulmonary vasculature (6%) are slightly less common. In general, respiratory tract involvement is more common in UC than CD patients. In both diseases, however, all compartments of the respiratory tract can be affected, although with slight differences in incidence.

Severity of thoracic involvement in many cases parallels disease activity in the bowel. Patients with active IBD have a greater chance of exhibiting airway obstruction. Inflammation of the bowel also correlates inversely with diffusion capacity. Serosal disease is more common among those with active IBD, while parenchymal disease is often seen in patients with quiescent bowel disease.

Women appear to be more frequently affected (~2:1). When considering only airway disease, this ratio increases up to 4:1. However, pleural involvement is about equally distributed between women and men.

Two thirds of patients with thoracic complications also have other extraintestinal manifestations at the same time, such as involvement of the skin, eyes, joints, or the biliary tract. Smoking does not appear to be a risk factor for developing airway inflammation in IBD, because most patients with this manifestation are nonsmokers.

Interestingly, two recent analyses found that CD patients appear to have a slightly increased risk of lung cancer, whereas the risk appears to be decreased in UC patients (standardized incidence ratios of 1.82 vs. 0.39 and 0.72, respectively).

CLINICAL AND PATHOLOGIC FEATURES

The diagnostic workup should include chest radiograph and CT scan. PFTs should be obtained, if possible, because they can provide a baseline in the course of treatment. Endoscopy complements imaging studies in the detection of upper airway obstruction or stenosis and in obtaining material for microbiology and histologic studies. A complete blood count with differential as well as a metabolic panel should be performed. Erythrocyte sedimentation rate and C-reactive protein may be helpful in following disease activity during treatment. Between 50% and 70% of patients with ulcerative colitis and 10% to 30% of patients with Crohn disease (predominantly those with colonic involvement) show atypical antineutrophil cytoplasmic antibodies (ANCAs), characterized by a fine granular and perinuclear ("snowdrift") pattern. Serologic testing for ANCAs may be helpful in patients with suspected underlying IBD. ANAs can help identify drug-induced lupus syndrome in patients with serositis. Since thromboembolic disease is a known cause of morbidity and mortality in IBD patients, the physician should maintain a low threshold to consider and exclude pulmonary embolism in this population.

This section discusses the different compartments of the respiratory tract involved by IBD, including unique considerations of the particular location, clinical presentation, and its pathologic features (Table 79-1).

AIRWAY DISEASE

Inflammatory bowel disease can affect the entire tracheobronchial tree, including larynx, trachea, and large and small airways, in the form of airway inflammation. Most common is inflammation of the large airways, seen in about 40% of IBD patients. Approximately 10% of patients show involvement of the upper respiratory tract or small airways. Extent and location of involvement are unpredictable; some patients have involvement restricted to a small area, some have patchy disease involving different anatomic levels of the conducting airways, and others show involvement of the entire tracheobronchial tree. The vast majority of patients with airway disease have UC, and only 10% CD. About two thirds of patients are female, with a median age at presentation of 42 years. In about 5% of patients the airway disease predates the diagnosis of IBD, and these patients tend to be much younger (median age, 13 years).

Clinically, laryngeal inflammation affecting the glottis and epiglottis produces narrowing and stenosis. Corresponding symptoms include dry, deep-toned cough with stridor. Severe cases may result in asphyxia, which is why laryngeal inflammation in IBD is one of the three conditions that require emergency treatment. Large airways inflammation in the form of tracheobronchitis manifests with chronic, otherwise unexplained cough that can be dry or productive of copious amounts of mucopurulent sputum. It is this purulent material that led to the historical designation for this condition, "chronic bronchial suppuration." It is also the condition that established the link between IBD and lung disease in 1976. Long-standing chronic inflammation and suppuration lead to bronchiectasis, often with basilar distribution. Small airways disease manifests as airflow obstruction with or without sputum production. Although unlikely to be the dominant feature, microscopic involvement is often found distally from affected large airways.

Radiographically, airway walls appear thickened with a "tram line" pattern. Larger airways show mucus plugging, smaller airways a tree-in-bud appearance. These changes tend to occur in a basilar-predominant distribution, occasionally with associated volume loss. Small airways disease can be associated with a tree-in-bud pattern, diffuse reticular shadows, or mosaic pattern due to air trapping (Figure 79-1). Bronchiectasis after long-standing disease can range from prominent thick-walled bronchi to subtle increases in airway caliber (Figure 79-2).

Bronchoscopically, the large airways show variable, but often severe, inflammation. Scarred bronchial granulomas are sometimes seen in patients with CD.

Histologically, large airways inflammation in IBD is characterized by a mucosal mononuclear inflammatory infiltrate, which is often bandlike and resembles that seen in the bowel mucosa in IBD (Figure 79-3, A). A luminal exudate containing neutrophils is common (Figure 79-3, B). Granulomas are frequently but not always seen in lung biopsies from patients with CD. On the other hand, the presence of a granuloma in a biopsy does not exclude UC as the underlying bowel disease. Small airways inflammation is similarly suppurative, with chronic inflammation of the bronchiolar wall. Occasionally, interstitial foamy macrophages are present in a centrilobular distribution, morphologically resembling diffuse panbronchiolitis. Late-stage small airways involvement may histologically present as constrictive bronchiolitis, which can be patchy throughout the lung and therefore may be missed by the biopsy sampling. An

Table 79-1 Thoracic Involvement in Inflammatory Bowel Disease (IBD)

Pattern of Involvement[a]	UC*	CD*	Symptoms	Imaging	Bronchoscopy/ Pathology[b]	BAL	Treatment	Prognosis/ Outcome
Airway Disease								
Larynx, glottis, epiglottis: Inflammation and narrowing	++	+	Barking cough, noisy breathing, hoarseness, stridor, asphyxia	CT: Normal or narrowing	Glottic/subglottic inflammation (granulomatous in CD), inward bulging, marked stenosis; can show erosion or ulceration	ND	IV CS Laser ablation Emergent tracheostomy	Favorable
Trachea: Inflammation and narrowing	++	+	Dry/productive cough, dyspnea, chronic sputum, hemoptysis	CT: Normal or narrowing	Tracheal inflammation, edema, hemorrhage with consequent stenosis; can be impressive; possible granulomas in CD	ND	IV/oral CS Occasional response to infliximab therapy in CD	Variable
Main bronchi: Simple chronic bronchitis	++	±	Chronic cough, slightly productive, wheeze	Normal	Mild/moderate inflammation and redness of large airways Little or no stenosis	PMN	Inhaled CS with or without short burst of oral CS	Often spectacular effect with CS
Main bronchi: Chronic bronchial suppuration	++	+	Marked chronic cough, wheeze, copious sputum	Thickened bronchial walls "Dirty lungs"	Large airway inflammation, often severe Deep-seated inflammatory cell infiltrate	PMN	Inhaled or oral CS *or* nebulized CS Early treatment recommended	Variable Residual symptoms and physiologic impairment common
Main bronchi: Bronchial distention[c]	+	−	Asymptomatic or cough	CT: Airway distention	ND	ND	CS if patient symptomatic	May recover with CS
Main bronchi: Mucoid impaction	+	−	Asymptomatic	CT: Branched shadows	ND	ND	Watching or CS	Good
Main bronchi: Disseminated endo-bronchial granulomas	−	+	Chronic cough	CT: Normal or narrowing	Spotted granulomas	ND	Oral CS with or without inhaled CS	Unknown
Main bronchi: Bilateral bronchiectasis	++	+	Chronic cough and wheeze Often, abundant sputum Hemoptysis	Thickened and dilated bronchi Mucoid impaction Tree-in-bud pattern distally	Widespread airway inflammation and narrowing Exuberant cellular infiltrate Luminal exudate, metaplastic epithelium	PMN	Inhaled or oral CS Nebulized CS Serial bronchial lavages with CS Rarely resection of affected lobe indicated	Variable residual impairment despite CS treatment is common Refractoriness to all forms of CS unusual
Small airways[d]: Acute purulent bronchiolitis[a]	+	+	Nonproductive cough with or without dyspnea	Small irregular opacities Mosaic on CT	ND	ND	Oral CS (possibly with added inhaled CS)	Variable
Small airways[d]: Granulomatous bronchiolitis[a]	-	+	Nonproductive cough with or without dyspnea	Small irregular opacities Mosaic on CT	ND	Ly	Oral CS	Favorable
Small airways[d]: Diffuse panbronchiolitis pattern	+	−	Dyspnea with or without sputum production	Tree-in-bud pattern Mosaic on CT	Normal/mild inflammation	ND	Oral CS (possibly with added inhaled CS)	May progress to COPD
Small airways[d]: Constrictive bronchiolitis	+	−	Dyspnea	ND	Normal	ND	Inhaled or oral CS	Associated with moderate-to-severe COPD

Continued

Table 79-1 Thoracic Involvement in Inflammatory Bowel Disease (IBD)—cont'd

Pattern of Involvement[a]	UC*	CD*	Symptoms	Imaging	Bronchoscopy/ Pathology[b]	BAL	Treatment	Prognosis/ Outcome
Air Space and Interstitial Disease								
Organizing pneumonia (OP)	+	+	Dry cough, dyspnea, fever, ARF	Bilateral focal or diffuse infiltrates	N	Var	Oral or IV CS, depending on severity	Mostly favorable; this pattern may also be caused by drugs
Eosinophilic pneumonia (EP)[†]	+	±	Dry cough, malaise, dyspnea (and at night); slight fever	Bilateral focal or diffuse infiltrates	N	Eos	Oral or IV CS, depending on severity	Mostly favorable; this pattern may also be caused by drugs
Nonspecific interstitial pneumonia	+	+	Dry cough, dyspnea	Basilar or diffuse opacities	N	Ly	Oral or IV CS, depending on severity	Mostly favorable; this pattern may also be caused by drugs
Infiltrative lung disease, granulomatous	±	++	Dry cough, dyspnea	Diffuse shadowing	N	Ly	Oral or IV CS, depending on severity	Favorable
Infiltrative lung disease, desquamative	+	−	Dyspnea	Disseminated pulmonary opacities	N	ND	Oral or IV CS, depending on severity	Favorable
Sterile necrobiotic nodules	+	−	Dyspnea, sometimes dull chest pain. Can occur with cutaneous pyoderma gangrenosum	Multiple lung nodules, sometimes with cavitation	N	ND	Oral or IV CS, depending on severity	Favorable
Pleural Disease								
Pleural effusion	+	+	Chest discomfort, pleuritic chest pain	Pleural effusion	−	−	Drainage NSAIDs CS	Favorable
Pneumothorax			Stabbing chest pain, dyspnea	Medial pneumothorax to be differentiated from pneumomediastinum	−	−	Exsufflation	Favorable
Pericardial and Cardiac Disease								
Pericarditis Pericardial effusion Myocarditis	+	+	Anterior chest pain, tamponade, arrhythmias, heart block, heart failure	Enlarged heart	−	−	Drainage NSAIDs CS	Favorable; pericardial constriction unusual

*CD, Crohn disease; UC, ulcerative colitis; ++, quite common, suggestive; +, occasional; ±, uncommon; −, not described, does not apply.

[†]In this context, eosinophilic pneumonia is also often referred to as "pulmonary infiltrates with eosinophilia" (PIE).

[a]Location of airway inflammation tends to remain the same with time in a given patient (e.g., in upper airway, trachea, bronchi, or small airway) but may vary depending on the patient and in some cases, time into the disease.

[b]Not all cases reach pathology.

[c]Very few cases/data available for review, or unpublished.

[d]In some patients, pneumothorax or pneumomediastinum occur in association.

Modified from Camus P, Colby TV: *Eur Respir J* 15:5–10, 2000.

ARF, acute respiratory failure; BAL, bronchoalveolar lavage; COPD, chronic obstructive pulmonary disease; CS, corticosteroids or corticosteroid treatment; CT, computed tomography; Eos, eosinophils; IV, intravenous; Ly, lymphocytes; N, normal; ND, no data available; NSAIDs, nonsteroidal antiinflammatory drugs; PMN, polymorphonuclear neutrophil leukocytes; Var, variable.

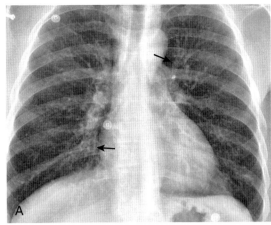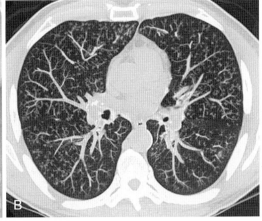

Figure 79-1 Involvement of large and small airways in ulcerative colitis. **A,** Plain chest radiograph of chronic bronchiolitis shows overall increase in nonspecific lung markings ("dirty lung") and occasional "tram tracks" related to bronchial wall thickening *(arrows).* **B,** Chest CT scan of cellular bronchiolitis with tree-in-bud pattern. *(Courtesy Dr. Carl Fuhrman, University of Pittsburgh Medical Center.)*

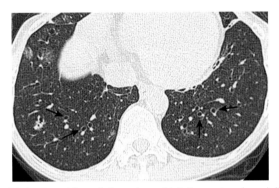

Figure 79-2 Bronchiectasis in patient with inflammatory bowel disease as a result of long-standing chronic bronchitis. The chest CT scan shows increased airway caliber *(arrows)* compared with adjacent pulmonary arteries. *(Courtesy Dr. Carl Fuhrman, University of Pittsburgh Medical Center.)*

expiratory chest CT scan showing air trapping may support a clinical impression of obliterative small airways disease in these patients.

AIR SPACE DISEASE

Inflammatory bowel disease can involve the distal air spaces of the lung in the form of *organizing pneumonia* (OP) or *eosinophilic pneumonia* (EP). The main difficulty with these patterns of involvement is distinguishing them from infection and drug-related lung disease. Clinically, patients present with shortness of breath ranging from moderate dyspnea to acute respiratory failure, sometimes accompanied by fever. Radiographically, OP shows bilateral, ovoid, elongated subpleural opacities, which may contain air bronchograms (**Figure 79-4,** *A* and *B*). EP, similar to non-IBD cases, may assume a masslike appearance or manifest as migratory opacities. Bronchoalveolar lavage (BAL) findings are often nonspecific, but an increase in neutrophils or eosinophils suggests a diagnosis of infection or EP, respectively.

Histologically, OP is characterized by loose, fibroblastic plugs in air spaces (Figure 79-4, *C*), whereas EP shows numerous eosinophils within the interstitium and among fibrinous air space exudates. Both patterns are nonspecific and can also be seen in infections, drug reactions, connective tissue disease, airway obstruction, or cryptogenic (idiopathic) forms of OP

and EP. Biopsies may still be helpful to rule out infection or other causes of air space disease.

INTERSTITIAL LUNG DISEASE

Diffuse interstitial lung diseases described in IBD patients include nonspecific interstitial pneumonia (NSIP) and granulomatous interstitial pneumonia, the latter almost exclusively seen in CD. Rare cases with usual interstitial pneumonia (UIP) or desquamative interstitial pneumonia (DIP) patterns have been reported. In some patients, IBD-related interstitial lung disease has been found to coexist with sarcoidosis. The reason for this association is unknown, but the presence of granulomas and similar T cell subpopulations in both diseases may indicate a pathogenetic connection.

Patients with interstitial lung disease present with shortness of breath and crackles on auscultation. Radiographically, interstitial markings are increased, and often more prominent in the lower lung zones (**Figure 79-5,** *A*). Bronchoscopic examination is normal unless concomitant airway disease is present. Wedge biopsies are necessary for histologic confirmation of diffuse fibrosing lung disease, because transbronchial biopsies are usually too small for assessing the fibrosis pattern. Biopsies show interstitial collagen fibrosis with variable mononuclear inflammatory infiltrates with or without granulomas (Figure 79-5, *B* and *C*). The presence of granulomas should always prompt exclusion of infection with special histochemical stains or preferably by concomitantly submitted tissue culture.

MASSES AND NODULES

Necrobiotic nodules are an uncommon manifestation in ulcerative colitis and Crohn disease. Nodules may occur synchronously with pyoderma gangrenosum lesions in the skin, with common histologic features. One study found that necrobiotic nodules precede the diagnosis of IBD in one third of patients. Patients present with a rapid onset of fever, dyspnea, and chest pain. Imaging studies show multiple rounded lung nodules that may cavitate over time (**Figure 79-6,** *A*). Without intervention, nodules may eventually disappear, leaving a scar. The histologic picture is distinctive, showing aggregates of neutrophils and necrosis without granulomatous features or identifiable infectious organisms (Figure 79-6, *B*). Although drug-induced lung injury can present with lung nodules, these nodules tend

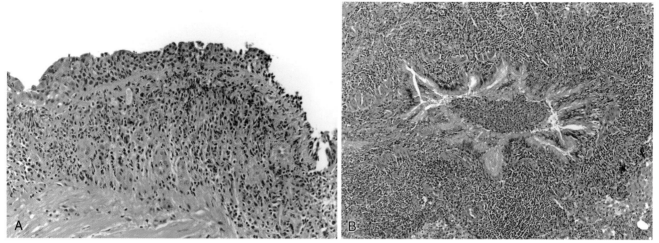

Figure 79-3 **A,** Large airway inflammation in ulcerative colitis. This endobronchial biopsy shows a bandlike mononuclear cell infiltrate underlying metaplastic mucosal epithelium. **B,** Bronchiolitis in ulcerative colitis. A small airway is surrounded by circumferential inflammation and contains a luminal exudate of neutrophils.

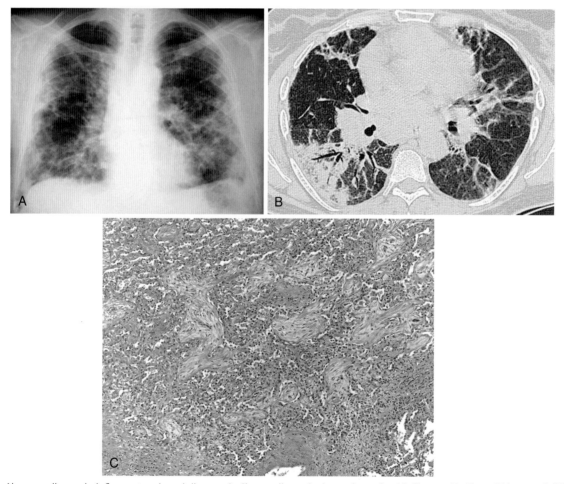

Figure 79-4 Air space disease in inflammatory bowel disease. **A,** Chest radiograph shows dense focal infiltrates. **B,** Chest CT image of different patient shows dense infiltrates with air bronchograms, corresponding histologically to organizing pneumonia **(C).** *(Courtesy Dr. Carl Fuhrman, University of Pittsburgh Medical Center.)*

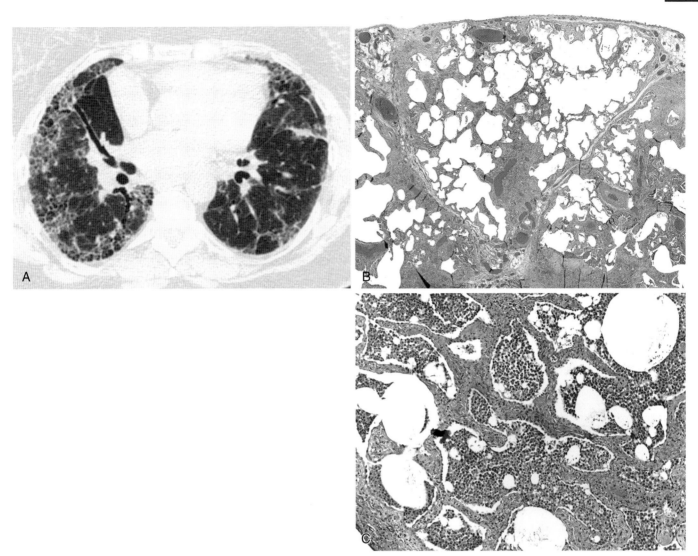

Figure 79-5 Interstitial lung disease in patient with inflammatory bowel disease. **A,** Chest CT image shows prominent interstitial markings with superimposed ground-glass changes. **B,** Corresponding wedge biopsy shows parenchymal remodeling by fibrosis with interstitial inflammation in a usual interstitial pneumonia pattern. Fibroblastic foci are seen at bottom right. **C,** Biopsy of different patient with homogeneous interstitial thickening resembling nonspecific interstitial pneumonia. The air spaces are filled with numerous pigmented macrophages.

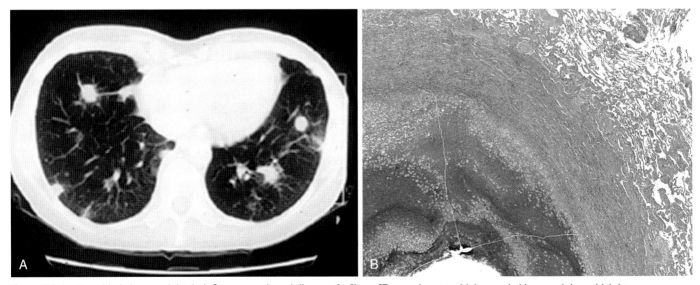

Figure 79-6 Necrobiotic lung nodules in inflammatory bowel disease. **A,** Chest CT scan shows multiple rounded lung nodules, which later may develop cavities. **B,** Corresponding histology reveals a core of blue necrosis with neutrophils *(left)* surrounded by fibrosis and organizing pneumonia.

not to show cavitation radiographically or sterile abscesses histologically.

SEROSAL DISEASE

Serosal membranes may be involved in the form of pleural or pericardial inflammation and thickening or effusions. Patients complain of pleuritic or anterior, sometimes position-dependent, chest pain and sometimes fever. Radiographs or echocardiography may be able to demonstrate an effusion, which if sampled is characteristically exudative and rich in neutrophils. Complications to consider are the possibility of tamponade and associated myocarditis. Electrocardiographic (ECG) changes such as arrhythmias or conduction blocks may indicate myocarditis. Serositis or effusions associated with drug-induced lupus can be identified by the presence of ANAs.

MEDIASTINAL DISEASE

Pneumomediastinum of uncertain pathogenesis has been described in a few UC patients. Because it seems to correlate with disease flares, it could be a result of acute airway obstruction, analogous to the pneumomediastinum seen in asthma attacks. Another possibility is the development of small fistula tracts between colon and mediastinum.

RARE MANIFESTATIONS

Some conditions have only been described in reports of a single or few cases, and the strength of association with IBD is uncertain. These include *eosinophilic pneumonia* (to be distinguished from drug effect), *Langerhans cell histiocytosis* (to be distinguished from reactivation by therapy), and *Wegener granulomatosis* (to be distinguished from primary Wegener granulomatosis which can present with colitis).

DRUG-INDUCED LUNG DISEASE

A major difficulty when encountering patients with apparent lung involvement by IBD is excluding drug-related toxicity. A causal role of drugs in airway inflammation is unlikely for two reasons. First, airway inflammation is common among IBD patients after colectomy and no longer receiving culprit drugs such as sulfasalazine or mesalamine. Second, airway inflammation does not improve on withdrawal of these drugs in patients with no history of colectomy. Infiltrative (air space or interstitial) lung disease, on the other hand, is a pattern associated with several drugs used in IBD patients. Unfortunately, withdrawal of the drug does not always result in stabilization or reversal of the lung disease. Decisions regarding discontinuation of drug therapy must consider the relative severity of the lung disease and the IBD, because drug discontinuation may result in a flare of IBD. **Table 79-2** summarizes toxicity patterns associated with common IBD drugs. An excellent resource for drug-associated pulmonary disease can be found online at Pneumotox.com.

TREATMENT

There are no prospective randomized trials for the treatment of respiratory complications in IBD patients. Before any immunosuppressive therapy is begun, the possibility of superimposed bacterial infection must be considered. Inhaled and systemic corticosteroids are the mainstay of therapy because these agents

Table 79-2 **Biopsy-Proven Lung Changes Related to Drugs Used in Inflammatory Bowel Disease (Other than Infection)**

Drugs	Lung Conditions
Mesalazine Sulfasalazine Balsalazide Olsalazine (5-aminosalicylic acid derivatives)	DAD, EP, OP, HP, chronic interstitial pneumonia
Azathioprine	DAD
6-Mercaptopurine	ND
Methotrexate	DAD, OP, HP, chronic interstitial pneumonia, pulmonary edema, granulomatous inflammation
Infliximab Adalimumab	DAD, EP, OP, chronic interstitial pneumonia
Certolizumab Natalizumab	ND
Cyclosporine	Pulmonary edema
Mycophenolate	Chronic interstitial pneumonia

DAD, diffuse alveolar damage (adult respiratory distress syndrome); *EP*, eosinophilic pneumonia; *HP*, hypersensitivity pneumonitis; *ND*, none documented; *OP*, organizing pneumonia.

rapidly improve symptoms and pulmonary function, as well as imaging, biopsy, and lavage findings. The effectiveness of infliximab and the newer antibodies adalimumab, certolizumab, and natalizumab in thoracic disease remains to be studied. Their use as first-line agents is currently not recommended. *Infliximab* has been found to improve extraintestinal manifestations other than lung disease. Its use may be justified if corticosteroids are insufficient. Mycophenolate mofetil, despite some anecdotal responses, has no proven efficacy and a high incidence of patient intolerance, preventing its use in IBD patients.

EMERGENCIES

The following three thoracic conditions require immediate attention and emergency treatment:

- *Acute upper airway* (glottal and epiglottal) *inflammation* can rapidly lead to airway occlusion and asphyxiation. Treatment should be initiated immediately and should include high-dose corticosteroids and, if needed, securing the airway by intubation, tracheostomy, or laser ablation. Initial corticosteroid administration in this situation should occur intravenously with conversion to oral therapy later. The clinical and visual diagnosis can be confirmed by biopsy of the airway mucosa. A patient with Crohn disease reportedly improved on initiation of infliximab therapy.
- *Diffuse infiltrative lung disease* may result in acute respiratory failure requiring intubation and mechanical ventilation. The two most common differential diagnoses must be ruled out: pulmonary infection, by bronchoscopy with lavage and culture, and drug toxicity, by withdrawal of IBD drug therapy. No evidence shows that surgical lung biopsy improves outcome in these patients; however, it may help guide corticosteroid therapy and rule out infection or other underlying diseases more confidently.

- *Acute pericarditis* with a large pericardial effusion threatening compression or tamponade may require pericardiocentesis or surgical drainage.

AIRWAY INFLAMMATION

Airway inflammation should be treated early and aggressively by administration of inhaled corticosteroids. A high initial dose (e.g., 1500-3000 µg/day of beclomethasone, fluticasone, budesonide, or equivalent in divided doses) is recommended until relief of symptoms or "best" lung function is attained. Effect of treatment can be followed with PFTs, which should be compared to the initial best values attained. Collaboration of the patient is essential, and patients should be instructed to return promptly when symptoms recur or fail to improve. Incomplete response or intermittent flares may be increasingly difficult to control with time.

Inhaled corticosteroids are most effective in large airways inflammation and are less effective in patients with bronchiolitis or bronchiectasis. In some, oral corticosteroids may be necessary and beneficial in addition to inhaled corticosteroids. A common dosing protocol is the administration of prednisone at an initial dose of 0.5 to 1 mg/kg/day, in single or divided dosing, for 4 weeks and then tapered over another 4 to 8 weeks, although the optimal duration of therapy has not been well established. Patients with marked bronchiectasis or abundant suppuration with copious sputum production may respond less well to inhaled corticosteroids and require systemic therapy from the beginning. In most severe cases, 1500 to 2000 µg of nebulized budenoside may increase topical delivery of the medication. Some have even proposed bronchial lavage fluids containing 40 to 80 mg of methylprednisolone, dissolved in 50 to 125 mL of isotonic saline two or three times per week, in addition to inhaled and oral corticosteroids.

Monitoring symptoms, pulmonary function, radiographic changes, and potential adverse effects of corticosteroids (e.g., infection) is essential. No evidence supports antibiotic treatment with macrolides or fluoroquinolones (e.g., erythromycin, azithromycin, ciprofloxacin), although these drugs have shown some efficacy in patients with diffuse panbronchiolitis. In patients receiving high-dose corticosteroids or in those with bronchiectasis, these agents may be useful, and an empirical trial may be justified.

AIR SPACE AND INTERSTITIAL LUNG DISEASE

In patients with infiltrative lung disease and imaging or pathologic findings of OP or EP who are exposed to sulfasalazine, mesalazine, or methotrexate, these medications should be withdrawn. Ensuing clinical improvement supports a drug etiology. Rechallenging the patient with sulfasalazine or mesalazine may induce tolerance and allow continued treatment of the IBD. Despite some reports of successful rechallenge with methotrexate, it is not advised because of its potentially life-threatening adverse effects on the lungs. After infection and drug toxicity are excluded, nonspecific interstitial lung disease, OP, and EP tend to respond well to oral or intravenous corticosteroid therapy. Classification of infiltrative lung disease by histologic diagnosis is preferred over empirical treatment.

SEROSAL DISEASE

Patients with pleuritis or pericarditis usually respond well to nonsteroidal antiinflammatory drugs and corticosteroids.

NSAIDs should be tried first as monotherapy, with subsequent addition of corticosteroids if necessary. High-dose corticosteroid treatment with 1 mg/kg/day of prednisone or equivalent is recommended and can be tapered after 2 to 4 weeks when symptoms have resolved and C-reactive protein has normalized. A slow taper is important because it seems to assist in preventing relapse.

CONTROVERSIES AND PITFALLS

A growing number of case reports and screening studies suggest that both subjective respiratory symptoms and objectively diagnosable disorders of the respiratory system are common in IBD patients. Although pulmonary disease in these patients has been recognized for more than four decades, it is likely underdiagnosed and its true frequency underestimated. Diseases of the large airways, such as bronchiectasis, are relatively common and well-accepted extraintestinal manifestations of IBD. However, the spectrum of respiratory system abnormalities is varied, and it remains a challenge to determine whether findings described in case reports and small studies represent true pulmonary manifestations of IBD versus sequelae of IBD therapies or concomitant but unrelated disease. In particular, diffuse parenchymal lung disease, which is uncommon, has been reported to encompass a range of histopathologic patterns and is confounded by known pulmonary toxicities of common IBD therapies. Current management of these conditions is extrapolated from experience in patients without IBD, which may or may not be applicable in all cases. Prospective studies with appropriately chosen control groups are needed to help define the natural history of pulmonary manifestations and guide the development of longitudinal screening and management recommendations.

CONCLUSION

Latent or mild involvement of the respiratory tract appears to occur in up to 50% of patients with inflammatory bowel disease. The distinctive pathologic changes are much less common but potentially serious and associated with significant long-term morbidity. These changes may precede a diagnosis of IBD, occur during a quiescent phase of the disease, or develop years after colectomy. It is important to diagnose and treat airway disease early in its course to prevent disabling symptoms and the development of bronchiectasis. Infection and drug toxicity are the main differential diagnoses to exclude in infiltrative lung disease.

SUGGESTED READINGS

Adams DH, Eksteen B: Aberrant homing of mucosal T cells and extraintestinal manifestations of inflammatory bowel disease, *Nat Rev Immunol* 6:244, 2006.

Basseri B, Enayati P, Marchevsky A, et al: Pulmonary manifestations of inflammatory bowel disease: case presentations and review, *J Crohns Colitis* 4:390–397, 2010.

Black H, Mendoza M, Murin S: Thoracic manifestations of inflammatory bowel disease, *Chest* 131:524–532, 2007.

Camus P, Colby TV: Respiratory manifestations in ulcerative colitis, *Eur Respir Monogr* 10:168–183, 2006.

Camus P, Colby TV: The lung in inflammatory bowel disease, *Eur Respir J* 15:5–10, 2000.

Camus P, Piard F, Ashcroft T, et al: The lung in inflammatory bowel disease, *Medicine (Baltimore)* 72:151–183, 1993.

Casey MB, Tazelaar HD, Myers JL, et al: Noninfectious lung pathology in patients with Crohn's disease, *Am J Surg Pathol* 27:213–219, 2003.

Chenivesse C, Bautin N, Wallaert B: Pulmonary manifestations in Crohn's disease, *Eur Respir Monogr* 10:151–167, 2006.

Colby TV, Camus P: Pathology of pulmonary involvement in inflammatory bowel disease, *Eur Respir Monogr* 12:199–207, 2007.

Foucher P, Camus P: Pneumotox website, 1997, 2010. www.pneumotox.com.

Hamada S, Ito Y, Imai S, et al: Effect of inhaled corticosteroid therapy on CT scan–estimated airway dimensions in a patient with chronic bronchitis related to ulcerative colitis, *Chest* 139:930–932, 2011.

Higenbottam T, Cochrane GM, Clark TJH, et al: Bronchial disease in ulcerative colitis, *Thorax* 35:581–585, 1980.

Kraft SC, Earle RH, Roesler M, et al: Unexplained bronchopulmonary disease with inflammatory bowel disease, *Arch Intern Med* 136:454–459, 1976.

Mahadeva R, Walsh G, Flower CD, Shneerson JM: Clinical and radiological characteristics of lung disease in inflammatory bowel disease, *Eur Respir J* 15:41–48, 2000.

Marc FJ, André MFJ, Piette JC, et al: A study of 30 patients with or without inflammatory bowel disease and review of the literature, *Medicine (Baltimore)* 86:145–161, 2007.

Pedersen N, Duricova D, Elkjaer M, et al: Risk of extra-intestinal cancer in inflammatory bowel disease: meta-analysis of population-based cohort studies, *Am J Gastroenterol* 105:1480–1487, 2010.

Satsangi J, Grootscholten C, Holt H, et al: Clinical patterns of familial inflammatory bowel disease, *Gut* 38:738–741, 1996.

Chapter **80**
Air Pollution

Seppo T. Rinne • Joel D. Kaufman

Air pollution is a heterogeneous mix of suspended solids, liquids, and gases. Even in the absence of human activity, aerosols are emitted by volcanic activity, windstorms, wildfires, and ocean waves. Traditionally, however, the term *air pollution* refers to the human impact of biomass and fossil fuel combustion, primarily from industry and vehicular traffic. The focus of this chapter is on the air pollutants with the most evidence of ongoing and widespread threat to public health, including both outdoor and indoor pollutants. Specific topics related to air pollution, including environmental tobacco smoke, plant antigens, and windblown agricultural dusts, are primarily addressed in other chapters.

HISTORY

Air pollution has posed a threat to human health since the advent of fire, 500,000 years ago. Evidence of soot in prehistoric caves indicates that early humans were exposed to high levels of indoor air pollution. Outdoor pollution began to rise as populations grew and clustered in cities. During the Industrial Revolution, there was a dramatic increase in coal use by factories and households. The resulting smog caused significant morbidity and mortality, particularly when combined with stagnant atmospheric conditions. During the Great London Smog of 1952, heavy pollution for 5 days caused at least 4000 excess deaths (**Figure 80-1**). This episode highlighted the relationship between air pollution and human health and, together with other episodes, led to clean-air policies in Europe and in the United States. Over the next several decades, with improvements in the regulatory framework, air quality in the developed world steadily improved. Even as energy consumption and greenhouse gas emissions have increased, pollutants that are toxic to humans have been better controlled. Nevertheless, 186 million Americans, or 60% of the population, still live in counties with levels of air pollution higher than U.S. Environmental Protection Agency (EPA) standards (**Figure 80-2**). Air pollution also continues to be a growing problem in cities and households of the developing world.

COMPOSITION OF AIR POLLUTION

Many different substances are considered "air pollutants," which typically exist in combination in the environment; these include *particulate matter* (PM), carbon monoxide (CO), ozone (O_3), nitrogen oxides (NOx), sulfur oxides (SOx), and *volatile organic compounds* (VOCs). The composition varies by season and regions, and the chemistry, state, and size of a pollutant influence the resulting health effects (**Figure 80-3**). Although CO has specific toxicity affecting oxygen transport, many pollutants

appear to cause disease by triggering injury through inflammation and oxidative stress. Physiologic effects can be confirmed by experimental studies, but health impacts of air pollution on populations can be difficult to attribute to a single pollutant because they often share sources and vary together. A multipollutant approach to understanding health effects is becoming more common. Nevertheless, this section discusses some of the physiologic effects of individual pollutants before a description of the health outcomes seen with exposure to air pollution.

Particulate Matter

Among air pollutants, PM is most consistently associated with increased mortality effects at ambient exposure concentrations regularly encountered today. Although PM can be formed by a wide variety of natural and man-made processes, one of the largest sources of PM pollution is through combustion of biomass and fossil fuels. PM is composed of organic and inorganic compounds that vary greatly in size (**Figure 80-4**). *Fine* PM (<2.5 μm) has the most well-recognized health effects, and the *ultrafine* PM fraction (<0.1 μm) may be especially important. Larger PM is filtered and trapped in the proximal respiratory tract, but fine particles can penetrate deep into the lung, where they are efficiently deposited, cause local effects, and may be systemically absorbed.

The composition of PM also influences its health effects. The mechanism of PM toxicity in the lung is still being elucidated but is likely multifactorial and can include impaired ciliary function, damage to epithelial cells, inflammation, and oxidative stress. Neutrophils and macrophages phagocytize the poorly soluble particles and initiate inflammatory cascades. PM also causes oxidative stress by generating reactive oxygen species (ROS) on the surface of particles that may then cause cellular effects. Inflammation and oxidative stress apparently provoke cardiovascular disease through atherosclerosis, thrombogenesis, vasoconstriction, and reduced heart rate variability (**Figure 80-5**).

Epidemiologic studies have associated changes in PM with respiratory symptoms, respiratory tract infections, impaired pulmonary function, asthma exacerbations, chronic obstructive pulmonary disease (COPD), cardiovascular events, cerebrovascular accident (CVA, stroke), lung cancer, and all-cause mortality.

Ozone

The stratospheric ozone layer is a normal part in the Earth's atmosphere that absorbs high-frequency ultraviolet (UV) rays and protects us from their damaging effects. In contrast, ground-level ozone is an air pollutant, which has harmful respiratory and cardiovascular effects. Ground-level O_3 is largely the result

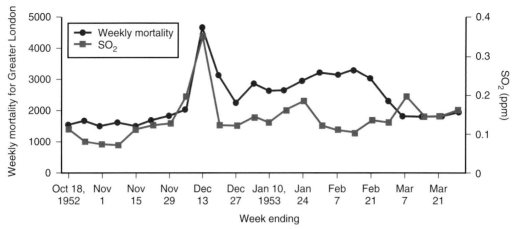

Figure 80-1 Weekly mortality in greater London, October 1952 to March 1953; *S0₂*, oxygen saturation. *(Modified from Bell ML, Davis DL: Reassessment of the lethal London fog of 1952: novel indicators of acute and chronic consequences of acute exposure to air pollution,* Environ Health Perspect *109(suppl 3):389-394, 2001.)*

Figure 80-2 Counties designated as "nonattainment areas" for EPA National Ambient Air Quality Standards (NAAQS) of various pollutants, including particulate matter, ozone, sulfur dioxide, carbon monoxide, and lead. *(From US Environmental Protection Agency Green Book, 2011. www.epa.gov/oaqps001/greenbk/mapnpoll.html.)*

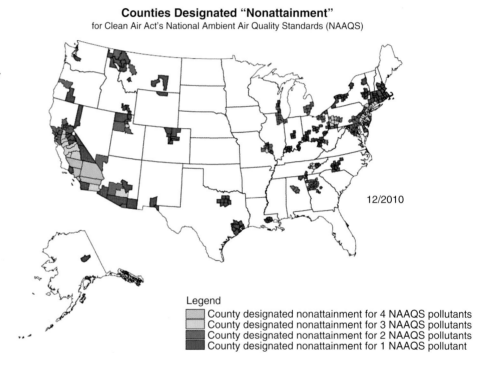

of UV photolysis of NOx and VOCs (products of vehicular and industrial combustion). Inhaled O_3 reacts with biomolecules to form free radicals, which trigger proinflammatory and prooxidative mediators. Increased neutrophils, eosinophils, and inflammatory cytokines have all been noted in bronchoalveolar lavage (BAL) fluid in response to O_3 exposure. Exposure to even very low levels of O_3 leads to airway inflammation and bronchoconstriction. Clinically, exposure to O_3 causes exacerbation of asthma and COPD, impaired pulmonary function, and increased respiratory symptoms, and it has been associated with increased mortality. The effects of O_3 are further potentiated by exposure to PM.

Sulfur Dioxide

Combustion of sulfur-containing fuels, including coal and petroleum, produces sulfur dioxide (SO_2), a highly water-soluble gas that is readily absorbed in the mucosa of the eyes and upper respiratory tract. SO_2 is a strong irritant that leads to local inflammation. SO_2 can also bind to organic PM and affect the distal airways. SO_2 increases vascular distention, mucosal edema, smooth muscle contraction, and intraairway secretions. Lung function in healthy individuals is relatively resistant to the effects of considerable doses of SO_2 (5 ppm), but even lower doses (e.g., <1 ppm) elicit acute and substantial bronchoconstriction in some asthmatic patients. Although SO_2 causes multiple respiratory symptoms, it does not seem to be independently responsible for air pollution–related mortality.

Nitrogen Dioxide

Nitrogen dioxide (NO_2) is formed during the combustion of fossil fuels, predominantly at power plants and in vehicles. Being relatively insoluble, NO_2 is not significantly absorbed by proximal mucosa. Instead, NO_2 travels to the more distal airways, where it reacts with water in the respiratory tree to create nitric acid. HNO_3 causes both local and systemic inflammation. Acutely, this can lead to bronchospasm. NO_2 is

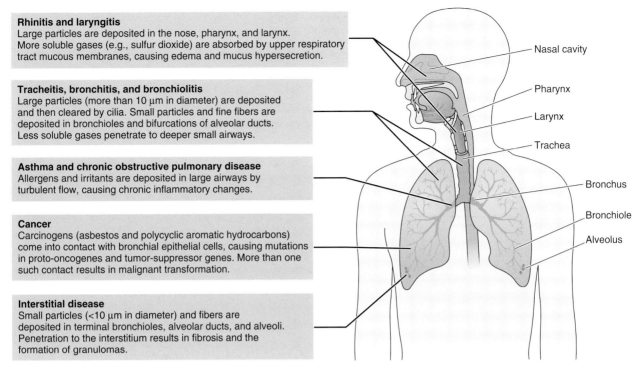

Rhinitis and laryngitis
Large particles are deposited in the nose, pharynx, and larynx.
More soluble gases (e.g., sulfur dioxide) are absorbed by upper respiratory
tract mucous membranes, causing edema and mucus hypersecretion.

Tracheitis, bronchitis, and bronchiolitis
Large particles (more than 10 μm in diameter) are deposited
and then cleared by cilia. Small particles and fine fibers are
deposited in bronchioles and bifurcations of alveolar ducts.
Less soluble gases penetrate to deeper small airways.

Asthma and chronic obstructive pulmonary disease
Allergens and irritants are deposited in large airways by
turbulent flow, causing chronic inflammatory changes.

Cancer
Carcinogens (asbestos and polycyclic aromatic hydrocarbons)
come into contact with bronchial epithelial cells, causing mutations
in proto-oncogenes and tumor-suppressor genes. More than one
such contact results in malignant transformation.

Interstitial disease
Small particles (<10 μm in diameter) and fibers are
deposited in terminal bronchioles, alveolar ducts, and alveoli.
Penetration to the interstitium results in fibrosis and the
formation of granulomas.

Nasal cavity

Pharynx

Larynx

Trachea

Bronchus

Bronchiole

Alveolus

Figure 80-3   Physiologic effects of air pollutants on the respiratory tract.   *(Modified from Beckett WS: Occupational respiratory diseases,* N Engl J Med *342:406-413, 2000.)*

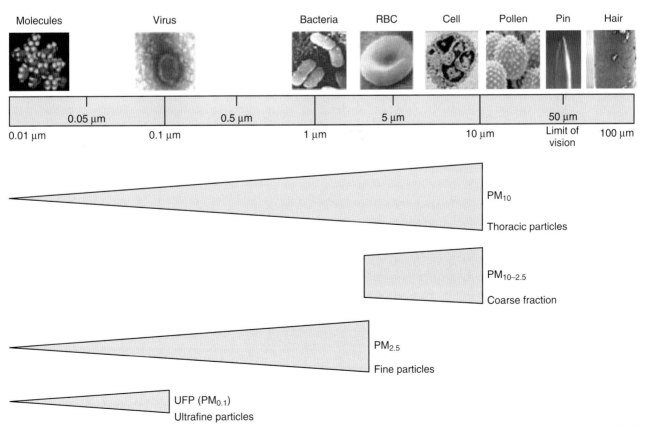

Figure 80-4   Size classification of particulate matter with reference to common structures; *RBC,* red blood cell; *PM,* particulate matter.   *(Modified from Brook RD, Franklin B, Cascio W, et al: Air pollution and cardiovascular disease: a statement for healthcare professionals from the Expert Panel on Population and Prevention Science of the American Heart Association,* Circulation *109:2655-2671, 2004.)*

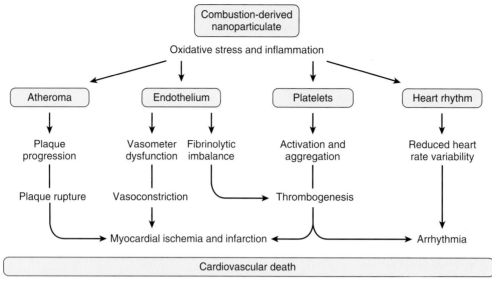

Figure 80-5 Mechanism of cardiovascular disease from exposure to air pollution. *(From Mills NL, Donaldson K, PW Hadoke, et al: Adverse cardiovascular effects of air pollution,* Nat Clin Pract Cardiovasc Med *6:36–44, 2009.)*

generally less potent than other pollutants and is likely to have its most harmful effects by acting in synergy with these other compounds. Although high levels of indoor NO_2 can increase susceptibility to viral infection, this has not been observed with outdoor levels of NO_2 pollution. In epidemiologic research, NO_2 concentrations are often considered a surrogate for exposure to traffic-related air pollution; thus the relationship of NO_2 with disease in these studies is probably caused by other pollutants that share exposure profiles.

Polycyclic Aromatic Hydrocarbons

Polycyclic aromatic hydrocarbons (PAHs) include a number of organic molecules that are found in biomass and fossil fuels or are formed in their combustion. Use of these fuels aerosolizes PAHs along with other VOCs. Although there are many different types of PAH, small and lipophilic PAHs are the most readily absorbed in the respiratory tract. The effects of each PAH species depends on its underlying composition and structure. Many PAHs are irritants to respiratory mucosa. Others, such as benzo[a]pyrene, one of the carcinogens first described, and the dioxins, are mutagenic and carcinogenic, with special concern regarding cancer of the mouth, nasopharynx, larynx, and lung.

OUTDOOR AIR POLLUTION

Outdoor air pollution is influenced by the source of emissions and the surrounding environment. In recent decades, motor vehicles have become a predominant source of pollution, particularly in urban areas. Coal and fossil fuel combustion also continue to be a major source of emissions from industry and power plants. Together, vehicles and power generation make up 90% of outdoor air pollution in the United States. Other sources include biomass combustion from wood fires. During winter months, wood burning is a principal source of pollution in some parts of the United States.

Topography, climate, and local legislation further impact the air quality. In Los Angeles the nearby mountains trap pollutants, largely from local mobile vehicular sources, and intense UV rays act to create high O_3 levels. In Pittsburgh, a major city with some of the highest PM levels in the United States, most

pollution is now largely derived from regional sources, carried by southeasterly winds bringing emissions from more distant power plants and factories. Outside the developed world, there are fewer environmental controls, resulting in higher levels of pollution, especially in areas of rapid industrialization and urbanization. China has many of the most polluted cities in the world, a factor of its heavy coal use and limited environmental protection.

HEALTH EFFECTS OF OUTDOOR AIR POLLUTION

Outdoor air pollution has many diverse health effects, ranging from mild respiratory irritation to hospitalization and death. The World Health Organization estimates that an excess 800,000 deaths occur annually because of exposure to outdoor air pollution. Daily fluctuation in levels of air pollution causes an acute increase in mortality, mostly from cardiovascular causes. Chronic air pollution exposure also contributes to morbidity and mortality through a variety of cardiopulmonary illnesses. Some of the first evidence for mortality of chronic exposure to PM was demonstrated by the Six Cities Study, in which citizens of six U.S. cities (representing a range of air pollution severity) were studied as a prospective cohort. Cities with higher levels of fine PM had an increased risk of all-cause mortality (risk ratio, 1.26 for most polluted vs. least polluted city; **Figure 80-6**). Many other cohort studies confirm this relationship, with improved determination of exposures and health outcomes.

Acute Respiratory Illnesses

Exposure to air pollution produces acute changes in lung function in healthy adults. These changes usually go unnoticed by patients who are not predisposed to bronchospasm. Among patients with asthma and COPD, however, exposure to pollution can lead to serious effects. Asthmatic patients experience increased cough, wheezing, breathlessness, and medication needs on days with high air pollution. Hospitalizations for asthma, COPD, and pneumonia all increase as air pollution rises. There are also more respiratory symptoms and upper respiratory infections in the general population. Even small changes in PM concentration can lead to these effects

(Figure 80-7). For every 10 μg/m³ rise in PM, there is approximately 1% increase in all respiratory diseases. Although this effect size seems small, it has a notable impact when applied to large populations.

Chronic Respiratory Illnesses

Just as acute exposure to air pollution can cause transient changes in pulmonary function, chronic exposure to pollution is associated with structural and functional lung changes. Studies show that children living in more polluted areas have lower forced expiratory volume in 1 second (FEV_1). In patients with cystic fibrosis, exacerbations are more common in communities with higher $PM_{2.5}$ concentrations (PM <2.5 μm in diameter). One study observed that exposure to air pollution in pregnant women led to subsequent impaired lung development in children. There is also evidence that exposure to pollution may contribute to the pathogenesis and incidence of asthma among children. Children living close to motor vehicle

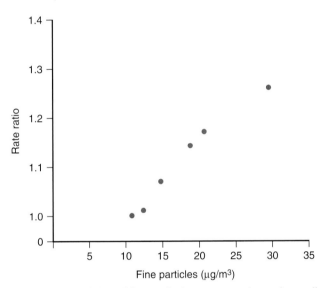

Figure 80-6 Association of fine particulate concentration and mortality from Harvard Six Cities Study. *(Modified from Dockery DW et al: N Engl J Med 329:1753-1759, 1993.)*

traffic have been found to have higher prevalence of asthma and smaller FEV_1 after controlling for potential confounders. European and U.S. cohorts also show that children exposed to higher amounts of air pollution have a higher incidence of asthma.

The association between outdoor air pollution and the development of COPD is less clear, with studies showing inconsistent and inconclusive results. The greatest risk factor for COPD remains tobacco smoke. However, air pollution causes recurrent respiratory symptoms and infections, both of which may contribute to COPD. Similarly, data are limited on the association of outdoor air pollution and lung cancer. Lung cancer is a rare disease with a long latency period, although a few studies found a modest increase in lung cancer with exposure to outdoor air pollution.

Nonrespiratory Illnesses

Some of the most important and well-studied diseases associated with air pollution are cardiovascular illnesses, including ischemic heart disease, arrhythmias, congestive heart failure, and sudden cardiac death. A metaanalysis on air pollution and hospital admissions found that for every 10 μg/m³ increase in PM, there was 0.8% increase in heart failure admissions and 0.7% increase in ischemic heart disease admissions. Driving or otherwise being in traffic has been associated with an acute increase in risk of myocardial infarction (odds ratio, 2.92), although pollution is only one potential culprit. Air pollution has further been associated with ventricular arrhythmias, implantable defibrillator shocks, and atrial fibrillation. The majority of excess deaths associated with air pollution are from cardiovascular causes. There is less conclusive data on the association of air pollution with other nonrespiratory diseases, including stroke, peripheral vascular disease, deep venous thrombosis, and adverse perinatal outcomes.

GENETICS AND AIR POLLUTION

There has been substantial investigation of respiratory gene-environment interactions with special attention to the ambient air pollution. This research may ultimately inform identification of not only especially susceptible populations but also

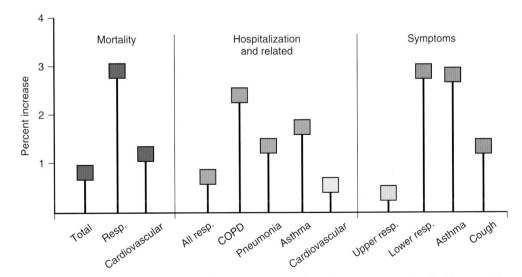

Figure 80-7 Meta-analysis results demonstrating the increase in mortality, morbidity, and symptoms associated with acute, 10 μg/m³ increase in PM_{10}. *COPD*, chronic obstructive pulmonary disease; *resp.*, respiratory. *(Modified from Donaldson K, Mills N, MacNee W, et al: Role of inflammation in cardiopulmonary health effects of PM, Toxicol Appl Pharmacol 207(2 suppl):483-488, 2005.)*

molecular mechanisms involved in the environmental effect. Genes that regulate inflammation and oxidative stress play a significant role in modulating these individual differences. Several studies have identified polymorphisms in oxidative stress genes (*NQO1*, *GSTM1*, and *GSTP1*) and inflammatory genes (*TNF*) that are associated with respiratory symptoms, decreased pulmonary function, and risk of asthma. For example, *NQO1* (NADPH:quinone oxidoreductase 1) is an ROS scavenger. Mutations in this gene have been associated with decreased FEV_1 in healthy individuals exposed to ozone. Polymorphisms of *NQO1* are also correlated with higher rates of asthma among children in Mexico City. Identifying genetic susceptibilities to air pollution not only helps characterize individuals who are at the greatest risk, but also helps target interventions. A clinical trial of children with a mutation in the antioxidant gene *GSTM1* found a protective effect of antioxidants, including vitamins C and E, on pulmonary function. Further studies are needed to characterize these genetic susceptibilities further and focus interventions.

AIR QUALITY INDEX

Governmental agencies worldwide measure and report on the air quality in major cities and suburban areas. The U.S. EPA produces an Air Quality Index (AQI) for more than 100 U.S. cities and regions. The AQI is reported on a scale from 0 to 500, with higher values being more hazardous (**Table 80-1**). An AQI score more than 100 indicates unhealthy air quality, especially when compounded by high-risk weather conditions, such as hot and sunny days. Many newspapers, weather reporters,

and radio stations report this score. On days with high AQI scores, it is recommended that people stay indoors as much as possible. Susceptible individuals should also limit physical activity, which increases ventilation and ultimately leads to five times the amount of PM deposition in lungs.

INDOOR AIR POLLUTION

The vast majority of adverse health effects related to air pollution likely occur in developing countries, where there are higher levels of both outdoor and indoor air pollution. More than half of the world's population depends on solid fuel as the primary source of domestic energy for cooking and heat. Most of this is in rural regions of the developing world where cooking is done over open fires in poorly ventilated homes (**Figure 80-8**). This creates intense exposure to *indoor air pollution* (IAP) with devastating health consequences.

Among households that rely on solid fuels for energy, approximately 95% use *biomass* fuels (wood, charcoal, crop residues, dung) in open indoor fires. Household coal use is less common and is primarily used in parts of China and South Africa. Overall, solid fuels are less efficient and have greater emissions than costlier fuels such as gas and electricity. In fact, although developed countries use several times more energy per household, the fuels used are cleaner with less exposure to pollutants. These differences in domestic energy are referred to as the "energy ladder" (**Figure 80-9**).

Combustion of solid fuels can emit many of the same chemical pollutants as outdoor pollution, including PM, CO, NO_2, SO_2, and PAHs, although the concentrations of these substances tend to be much higher. For example, concentrations of PM in households that rely on solid fuels often reach levels more than 100 times greater than outdoor concentrations. Women and children are disproportionately exposed to this pollution. On average, women in the developing world spend 3 to 7 hours per day near the fire, preparing food. They frequently do so with large children by their side and small children on their backs. As the population with the greatest exposure to IAP, women and children also suffer the most damaging health effects.

Table 80-1	Definitions of Air Quality Index (AQI) Levels by U.S. Environmental Protection Agency	
AQI Levels of Health Concern	**Numeric Value**	**Description**
Good	0-50	Air quality is considered satisfactory, and air pollution poses little or no risk.
Moderate	51-100	Air quality is acceptable; for some pollutants, however, there may be a moderate health concern for a small number of people unusually sensitive to air pollution.
Unhealthy for sensitive groups	101-150	Members of sensitive groups may experience health effects; the general public is not likely to be affected.
Unhealthy	151-200	Everyone may begin to experience health effects; members of sensitive groups may experience more serious health effects.
Very unhealthy	201-300	Health alert; everyone may experience more serious health effects.
Hazardous	301-500	Health warnings of emergency conditions. The entire population is more likely to be affected.

Data from www.airnow.gov. Accessed March 2011.

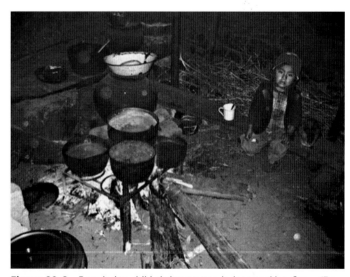

Figure 80-8 Ecuadorian child sitting next to indoor cooking fire. *(From Rinne ST, Rodas EJ, Rinne ML, et al: Use of biomass fuel is associated with infant mortality and child health in trend analysis, Am J Trop Med Hyg 76:585–591, 2007.)*

HEALTH EFFECTS OF INDOOR AIR POLLUTION

The World Health Organization estimates that exposure to solid fuel smoke causes 1.6 million deaths annually, primarily in the developing world (**Figure 80-10**). This includes deaths caused by pneumonia, COPD, and lung cancer (**Table 80-2**). Increasing evidence also is revealing the role of IAP in other infectious and noninfectious diseases. Most diseases associated with outdoor pollution are also linked to IAP exposure. Overall, IAP is responsible for 38.5 million disability-adjusted life years (DALYs), making it the 8th leading cause of DALYs and 11th cause of death worldwide.

Acute Respiratory Illnesses

Worldwide, acute lower respiratory tract infections are the most important cause of mortality in children younger than 5 years. Exposure to IAP more than doubles the risk of developing acute lower respiratory infections. Annually, this leads to 910,000 of the 2 million deaths caused by pneumonia. Several studies also show an association between indoor air pollution and upper respiratory infections, including otitis media and mastoiditis. In addition to infectious diseases, exposure to indoor smoke leads to increased airway reactivity, which can exacerbate asthma and COPD.

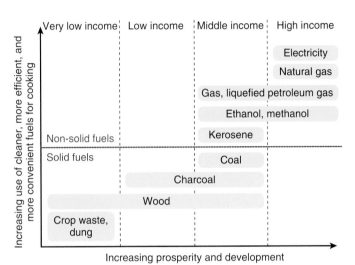

Figure 80-9 "Energy ladder" emphasizing the association of development with household energy. *(Modified from World Health Organization:* Fuel for life: household energy and health, *Geneva, 2006, WHO.)*

Table 80-2 **Results from Metaanalyses on Association of Indoor Air Pollution with Various Health Outcomes**

Health Outcome	Population	Relative Risk	95% CI	Evidence
Pneumonia	Children 0-4 yr	2.3	1.9-2.7	Sufficient
COPD	Women ≥30 yr	3.2	2.3-4.8	Sufficient
	Men ≥30 yr	1.8	1.0-3.2	Sufficient
Lung cancer (coal)	Women ≥30 yr	1.9	1.1-3.5	Sufficient
	Men ≥30 yr	1.5	1.0-2.5	Sufficient
Lung cancer (biomass)	Women ≥30 yr	1.5	1.0-2.1	Insufficient
Asthma	Children 5-14 yr	1.6	1.0-2.5	Insufficient
	Adults ≥15 yr	1.2	1.0-1.5	Insufficient
Cataracts	Adults ≥15 yr	1.3	1.0-1.7	Insufficient

Modified from World Health Organization: *Fuel for life: household energy and health,* Geneva, 2006, WHO.
CI, confidence interval; *COPD,* chronic obstructive pulmonary disease.

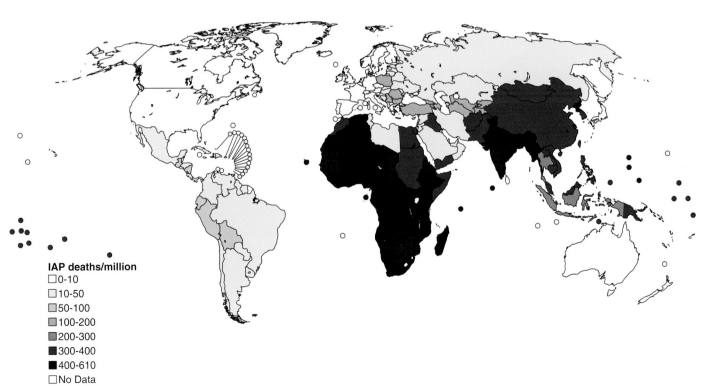

IAP deaths/million
☐ 0-10
☐ 10-50
☐ 50-100
☐ 100-200
☐ 200-300
■ 300-400
■ 400-610
☐ No Data

Figure 80-10 Distribution of mortality from indoor air pollution *(IAP)* throughout the world. *(Modified from World Health Organization:* The World Health Report 2002: reducing risks, promoting healthy life, *Geneva, 2002, WHO.)*

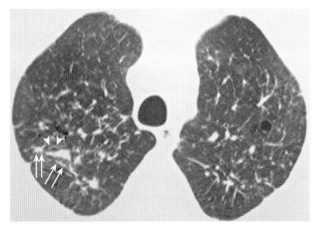

Figure 80-11 Axial high-resolution CT scan of chest demonstrating characteristic findings in domestic acquired particulate lung disease, including nodular interlobular septal thickening *(arrowheads)* and bronchovascular thickening with nodular appearance *(double arrows)*. *(Modified from Diaz JV, Koff J, Gotway MB, et al: Case report: a case of wood-smoke-related pulmonary disease,* Environ Health Perspect *114:759-762, 2006.)*

Chronic Respiratory Illnesses

Chronic exposure to indoor smoke causes a broad range of chronic disorders referred to as *domestic acquired particulate lung disease* (DAPLD) or "hut lung." DAPLD includes noninfectious, nonmalignant diseases such as COPD and pulmonary fibrosis. Women who cook with solid fuels are three times more likely to develop COPD than women who cook with cleaner fuels. Globally, IAP causes 22% of COPD cases. Although most people exposed to chronic indoor smoke develop obstructive pulmonary function, some also have *restrictive* patterns. Bronchoscopy typically reveals anthracotic plaques. Computed tomography (CT) may demonstrate a variety of patterns, including reticulation, peribronchial thickening, nodules, and ground-glass opacities (**Figure 80-11**). Although studies are still few and inconsistent, some reports find a higher incidence of asthma among children exposed to indoor smoke.

Strong evidence links indoor coal smoke to lung cancer, again with most research from China, where coal use is common. Coal smoke has high concentrations of carcinogenic PAHs. Chronic exposure to coal smoke doubles the risk of lung cancer. Few studies have examined the relationship between lung cancer and other solid fuels; but the concern is that exposure to these pollutants also increases risk of malignancy.

Nonrespiratory Illnesses

As discussed previously, exposure to particulate matter from outdoor air pollution has consistently been associated with cardiovascular disease and mortality. Research on similar effects of indoor smoke is minimal, although the same relationships should hold true. If these risks were consistent among households cooking with solid fuels, IAP would represent a major risk factor for morbidity and mortality worldwide.

Unvented cooking with solid fuels has been associated with *poor pregnancy outcomes*, including low birth weight and increased perinatal mortality. This is likely caused by a complex interaction of pollutants in solid-fuel smoke, including PM and CO. PM predisposes to maternal illness affecting fetal growth, whereas CO avidly binds hemoglobin and decreases oxygen delivery to the placenta. On average, babies born to households that cook with biomass fuels weigh 63 g less than those born in households that use cleaner fuels.

Cataracts are common in the developing world and frequently lead to blindness. Large epidemiologic studies in India have shown a 30% increase in cataracts among people living in households dependent on solid fuels after adjusting for confounding factors. The mechanism for this effect remains a matter of speculation.

CONTROVERSIES AND PITFALLS

Environmental influences on respiratory health cannot be interpreted in isolation. Not only are these environmental factors inherently interacting with the genetic predisposition of the individual, but various environmental processes are closely linked. Changes in air pollution are associated with changes in climate, and both are currently driven primarily by fossil fuel combustion. As global warming progresses, it is likely to affect air pollution patterns, although the impact is still uncertain. Global climate change is driven by greenhouse gases, such as carbon dioxide and methane, which are not generally considered to have direct health effects at ambient concentrations. Nevertheless, warmer days are associated with worse air quality, and most scientists believe that climate change will significantly increase the number of summer days that exceed air quality standards. This change in climate will likely increase ground-level ozone as warmer temperatures promote O_3 formation. In contrast, particulate matter levels could conceivably decrease, if global warming leads to increased precipitation or a concerted effort at reducing fossil fuel use.

CONCLUSION

Additional research is needed to define the effects of outdoor air pollution in a multipollutant context. Most published research examines the health effects of individual pollutants, while the interaction between multiple pollutants and the role of particular sources of pollution is likely just as important. Ongoing research should also focus on identifying safe levels of air pollution and effective ways of decreasing exposure to pollution. In the developed world, research into clean energy may provide valuable answers to improving human health as well as the environment. In the developing world, solutions relating to improving indoor air quality and decreasing solid-fuel dependence would also have a widespread and dramatic impact.

SUGGESTED READINGS

Brunekreef B, Holgate ST: Air pollution and health, *Lancet* 360:1233–1242, 2002.

Dockery DW, Pope CA, Xu X, et al: An association between air pollution and mortality in six U.S. cities, *N Engl J Med* 329:1753–1759, 1993.

Fullerton DG, Bruce NN, Gordon SB: Indoor air pollution from biomass fuel smoke is a major health concern in the developing world, *Trans R Soc Trop Med Hyg* 102:843–851, 2008.

Laumbach RJ: Outdoor air pollutants and patient health, *Am Fam Physician* 81:175–180, 2010.

Minelli C, Wei I, Sagoo G, et al: Interactive effects of antioxidant genes and air pollution on respiratory function and airway disease: a HuGE review, *Am J Epidemiol* 173:603–620, 2011.

Perez-Padilla R, Schilmann A, Riojas-Rodriguez H: Respiratory health effects of indoor air pollution, *Int J Tuberc Lung Dis* 14:1079–1086, 2010.

Ren C, Tong S: Health effects of ambient air pollution: recent research development and contemporary methodological challenges, *Environ Health* 7:56, 2008.

Sun Q, Hong X, Wold LE: Cardiovascular effects of ambient particulate air pollution exposure, *Circulation* 121:2755–2765, 2010.

World Health Organization: *Fuel for life: household energy and health,* Geneva, 2006, WHO.

Yang IA, Fong KM, Zimmerman PV, et al: Genetic susceptibility to the respiratory effects of air pollution, *Thorax* 63: 555–563, 2008.

Yang W, Omaye ST: Air pollutants, oxidative stress and human health, *Mutat Res* 674:45–54, 2009.

INDEX

A

Abdominal diseases, pleural effusions related to, 829-830
Abdominal muscles
  action of, 20f
  innervation of, 19
  respiratory, 55
Abscess
  lung, complicating community-acquired pneumonia, 305-306, 306f
  mediastinal, percutaneous sampling of, 187
ACE inhibitor–associated cough, 245-246
Achalasia of cardia, 100f
Acid-base relationships, 45-48
Acidosis, 45
  metabolic
    clinical causes of, 48
    Davenport diagram for, 47f, 48
  respiratory. *See* Respiratory acidosis.
Acinar shadow, in consolidation, 81
Acinus, definition of, 2
Acquired immunodeficiency syndrome (AIDS).
    See also Human immunodeficiency virus
    (HIV) disease.
  definition of, 348t
  indicator diseases for, 348b, 348t
  pneumothorax and, 835
  progression of HIV infection to, 349
ACS. *See* Acute coronary syndrome (ACS).
Actinomyces israelii, in community-acquired pneumonia, 300-301, 301f
Acute coronary syndrome (ACS), dyspnea in, 253-254
Acute coryza, 473
  clinical course and prevention of, 486
  clinical features of, 478
  treatment of, 482
Acute fibrinous organizing pneumonia (AFOP), 635
Acute lung injury-acute respiratory distress syndrome (ALI-ARDS), tidal volumes in management of, 27
Acute lung injury (ALI)
  ARDS from, 454
  mechanical ventilation in, controversy over, 27
Acute respiratory distress syndrome (ARDS), 454-470
  clinical disorders associated with, 455b
  controversies and pitfalls of, 469-470, 470f
  definition of, 455-457, 456b, 457t
  etiology of, 455
  fluid management in, 468-469
  genetics of, 457-458
  histopathology of, 455
  incidence of, 456
  long-term survival with, 469
  mechanical ventilation–induced sepsis and, 460-461

Page numbers followed by *f* indicate figures; *t*, tables; *b*, boxes.

Acute respiratory distress syndrome (ARDS) (*Continued*)
  overview of, 454
  pathophysiology of, 454, 455b
  in pregnancy, 909-910, 909b
  prognosis with, 469
  PEEP in, 462-466, 464f, 464t-465t
  refractory hypoxemia in, rescue strategies for, 466-468
  severity of, 456-457
  supportive treatment for, 468-469
  ventilatory management of, 462
Acyclovir
  for viral lung infections, 339t
  for viral pneumonia, 313-314
Adenocarcinoma
  of lung, 778-781, 779f-780f
    classification of, 779b, 779f-780f
  metastatic, malignant pleural involvement from, 78
Adenoma(s), 811
  parathyroid, 854
Adenovirus infections
  in hematopoietic stem cell transplantation patients, 915
  in non–HIV-infected immunocompromised patients, 340
Adhesions, intrapleural, chest tube insertion with, 866
Adhesive collapse, of lung, 83-84
Adolescent idiopathic scoliosis, impact of, on exercise capacity, 758
Adrenal gland lesions, percutaneous biopsy of, 189-190, 190f
Aeration, loss of, in lobar collapse, 84
Aerobic capacity, assessment of, exercise testing in, 143
Afferent impulses, in dyspnea, 251, 251f
Afferent inputs, to respiratory centers, 50-53, 51f
Age
  community-acquired pneumonia and, 296-297
  postoperative pulmonary complications and, 870
  venous thromboembolism and, 694
AIDS. *See* Acquired immunodeficiency syndrome (AIDS).
Air alveologram, 81
Air bronchogram, in consolidation, 81, 81f
Air embolism, 706-707
  complicating needle biopsy, 185, 185t
Air hunger, in dyspnea, 252
Air pollution, 937-945
  composition of, 937-940
  controversies and pitfalls of, 944
  COPD and, 536
    exacerbations of, 562
  in Great London Smog, 937, 938f
  history of, 937, 938f
  indoor, 942-944, 942f-944f, 943t
  nitrogen dioxide in, 938-940
  outdoor, 940-942, 941f

Air pollution (*Continued*)
  ozone in, 937-938
  particulate matter in, 937, 939f-940f
  physiologic effects of, on respiratory tract, 937, 939f
  polycyclic aromatic hydrocarbons in, 940
  responses to, genetics and, 941-942
  sulfur dioxide in, 938
Air quality index (AQI), 942, 942t
Air space disease
  as emergency, 935
  in inflammatory bowel disease, 931
Airflow
  effort-independent, 25, 26f
  limitation of, in COPD, 542-544
Airflow obstruction
  in COPD, pharmacologic therapy of, 554-556
  measuring, in asthma diagnosis, 506
Airflow resistance, 24-25, 25f-26f
  in obstructive disease, 26, 202, 203f
Airway(s)
  anatomy of, 2-3
  colonization of, community-acquired pneumonia and, 297
  compression of, extrinsic, therapeutic bronchoscopy for, 169
  conducting, 2-3, 3f
  in connective tissue diseases, 654-655
  CT of, 108-110
  in drug-induced respiratory diseases, 237-238
  edema of, in asthma, 493
  generations of, 20, 20f
  inflammation of
    in asthma, 488-491, 501-502
    in COPD, 540
    as emergency, 935
  management of, in ICU, 437-444. *See also* Intensive care unit (ICU), airway management in.
  mucosa of, immune response of, disordered, in asthma, 502
  patency of, in obstructive sleep apnea, sleep stability and, 739
  remodeling of, in asthma, 493, 494f
  responsiveness of, assessment of, in asthma diagnosis, 506, 507t
  smooth muscle of, control of, 202, 203f
    in COPD, 202, 203f
  structural changes in, in asthma, 502
  structural defenses of, 275-277, 277t
  structure of, 19-20
Airway clearance
  in preoperative evaluation, 869
  therapy for, in cystic fibrosis, 574
Airway disease(s)
  asthma as, 487-530. *See also* Asthma.
  bronchiectasis as, 580-587. *See also* Bronchiectasis.
  chronic
    in cystic fibrosis, 571
    in HIV patient, 380-381

Airway disease(s) (*Continued*)
 chronic obstructive pulmonary disease as, 531-567. *See also* Chronic obstructive pulmonary disease (COPD).
 cystic fibrosis as, 568-579. *See also* Cystic fibrosis (CF).
 HRCT in, 119-121
 in inflammatory bowel disease, 928-931, 931f-932f
 in rheumatoid arthritis, 656, 657f
 tracheal narrowing in, 95-96, 95f-96f
 upper airway, 471-486. *See also* Rhinitis; Rhinosinusitis; Upper airway disease.
Airway epithelial cells, 3-4
Airway fluid, surface tension of, obstructive sleep apnea and, 739
Airway hyperresponsiveness
 in asthma, 493, 501, 502f-503f
 COPD and, 537
Airway infections, in cystic fibrosis, treatment of, 574-576, 575t
Airway obstruction
 endoluminal, therapeutic bronchoscopy for, 168-169, 169t
 by mucus, 38
Airway pressure release ventilation, 415, 415f
Airway resistance, lung elastance and, 418, 419f-420f
Airway surface liquid (ASL)
 antimicrobial factors in, 282-283, 282t
 in host defense, 277, 278t
 inadequate, in cystic fibrosis, 568, 570f
Albuterol (Salbutamol)
 formulations, doses and duration of action of, 207t
 with ipratropium for COPD, 556
Alcaligenes xylosoxidans, in cystic fibrosis lung disease, 575
Alcoholism, community-acquired pneumonia and, 297
ALI. *See* Acute lung injury (ALI).
Alkalosis, 45
Allergens
 avoidance of, for asthma, 513
 childhood asthma and, 498
 food, as asthma triggers, 499
 identification and avoidance of, for allergic rhinitis, 480
Allergic bronchopulmonary aspergillosis (ABPA)
 bronchiectasis from, 583
 in cystic fibrosis, 577
 eosinophilic lung disease in, 622-623, 622f, 623b
Allergic rhinitis, 471-472
 clinical course and prevention of, 486
 clinical features of, 478
 global prevalence of, 471, 472f
 pathogenesis of, 471, 473f
 suspected, evaluation for, 479-480
 treatment of, 480-482, 481f
Alveolar-arterial PO$_2$ difference, in gas exchange assessment, 44
Alveolar capillaries, 29, 30f
Alveolar collapse, 38
Alveolar "corner," surface tension and, 30, 31f
Alveolar damage, diffuse. *See* Diffuse alveolar damage (DAD).
Alveolar edema, 34, 34f
Alveolar filling processes, diffuse, 592
Alveolar gas equation, 39f
Alveolar hemorrhage
 after bone marrow transplantation, 730
 in connective tissue diseases, 655

Alveolar hemorrhage (*Continued*)
 diffuse. *See* Diffuse alveolar hemorrhage (DAH).
 toxic, 730
Alveolar hemorrhage syndromes, 728-730. *See also* Diffuse alveolar hemorrhage (DAH).
Alveolar proteinosis, in connective tissue diseases, 655
Alveolar regeneration, in response to retinoic acid, 17
Alveolar ventilation, 39, 39f
Alveolar vessels, lung volumes and, 30, 30f
Alveolitis
 extrinsic allergic, 676-681. *See also* Extrinsic allergic alveolitis (EAA).
 fibrosing
  cryptogenic, classification of, 588
  HRCT in, 71, 115, 115f
Alveologram, air, 81
Alveolus(i), 4-5, 4f
 epithelial cells of, 4-5, 4f-5f
 as functional unit of lung, 37-38
Amantadine
 for viral lung infections, 339t
 for viral pneumonia, 313
Amebiasis, 319
Amebic disease, pleural effusions in, 828
Amikacin, for TB, 392t
Amine precursor uptake and decarboxylation (APUD) cells, 4
Aminolevulinic acid (ALA), in photodynamic therapy, 167
Aminophylline, formulations, doses and duration of action of, 207t
Amiodarone, pulmonary toxicity induced by, 223t
 parenchymal patterns in, 231-232, 231f
Ammonia, as irritant, 683-684, 683t
Amniotic fluid embolism, in pregnancy, 905-906, 905f
Amniotic fluid embolism syndrome, 707-708
Amphotericin B, for invasive aspergillosis, 343t
Amyloid deposits, 814-817, 817f
Amyloidosis, 673
 in connective tissue diseases, 655
Amyotrophy, neuralgic, respiratory presentations of, 772
Anaerobic bacteria, in community-acquired pneumonia, 300
Anatomic dead space, 39
Anemia
 in COPD, 546
 hemolytic, pulmonary arterial hypertension and, 712
Anesthesia
 for bronchoscopy, 162-163
 for chest tube insertion, 863-864
Aneurysm
 aortic, dissecting, chest pain in, 270
 thoracic aortic, 97-98, 99f
Angina, 270
Angiography
 magnetic resonance, 73, 74f
 pulmonary, 74-75, 74f
Angiomyolipoma, lymphangioleiomyomatosis cells in, 667
Angiotensin-converting enzyme (ACE) inhibitor–associated cough, 245-246
Animals, exposure to, childhood asthma and, 498
Ankylosing spondylitis, 661-662
Antacid overdose, metabolic alkalosis from, 48

Anterior horn cells
 acute disorders affecting, 770-771
 chronic disorders affecting, 771
Anterior mediastinal masses, CT evaluation of, 112-113, 112f-113f
Anterior mediastinotomy, diagnostic application of, 877t, 879
Anthrax, pneumonic, 301
Anti-glomerular basement membrane antibody disease, 729
Anti-IgE monoclonal antibody, for asthma, 511
Antibiotics
 for acute rhinosinusitis, 483-484
 childhood asthma and, 497-498
 for COPD, 556
 for COPD exacerbations, 564, 564f
 for cystic fibrosis airway infections, 574-576, 575t
 for exudative effusions, 827
 for nosocomial respiratory infections, 327-328, 327t-328t
 prenatal use of, childhood asthma and, 498
Antibodies, precipitating, in extrinsic allergic alveolitis, 679
Antibody deficiency, in bronchiectasis, 582
Antibody responses, deficiencies in, pathogens associated with, 330, 332t
Anticholinergics. *See* Antimuscarinics.
 for COPD, 555, 555t
 for intrinsic rhinitis, 482
Anticoagulation, for pulmonary embolism, 702-704
Antigen detection, in viral pneumonia diagnosis, 312-313
Antihistamines, for allergic rhinitis, 480-481
Antiinflammatory drugs, 213-220
 for asthma, 510-511
 controversies and pitfalls of, 219-220
 for COPD, 556
 corticosteroids as, 213-216
 investigative, 218-219, 220f
 phosphodiesterase 4 inhibitors as, 216-218
Antileukotrienes, for asthma, 511
Antimetabolites, in lung transplantation, 900, 901t
Antimicrobial molecules, in lung host defense, 282-283, 282t
Antimicrobial peptides, in lung host defense, 283-284
Antimuscarinics
 as bronchodilators, 205-206, 205f
 chemical structures of, 205f
Antineutrophil cytoplasmic autoantibody–associated vasculitis, 722
Antiphospholipid syndrome (APS)
 clinical features of, 660
 diffuse alveolar hemorrhage and, 729
Antiproteinases, in COPD, 541, 542t
Antiretroviral therapy (ART)
 combination (cART), for Kaposi sarcoma, 376
 opportunistic infections and, 372
 with *Pneumocystis* pneumonia, 364
 respiratory symptoms and, 381-382
 with tuberculosis, 365
Antithrombin deficiency, inherited thrombophilia from, 690-691, 691t
α_1-Antitrypsin, for COPD, 556
α_1-Antitrypsin deficiency
 autophagy *versus* endoplasmic reticulum–associated degradation in, 17
 clinical course of, 925
 clinical features of, 921
 in COPD, 537, 537t

α₁-Antitrypsin deficiency *(Continued)*
  in COPD assessment, 550
  diagnosis of, 923
  genetic factors underlying, 8t-9t
  molecular basis of, 7-10, 10f
  pathophysiology of, 920-921
  severe, treatment of, 925
α₁-Antitrypsin polymer, nature of, 17
Antitumor necrosis factor therapy, for
    sarcoidosis, 617t, 618
Antitussive therapies, 248-249
Anxiety, chest pain in, 271
Aorta, thoracic, aneurysm of, 97-98, 99f
Aortic aneurysm, dissecting, chest pain in, 270
Aortic arch, mediastinal anatomy at, 109f
Apnea, sleep, obstructive, 731-748. *See also*
    Obstructive sleep apnea (OSA).
Apneustic breathing, in stroke, 768
Apoptosis, in COPD, 541f, 542
Arachnodactyly, congenital contractual,
    scoliosis in, 756
ARDS. *See* Acute respiratory distress syndrome
    (ARDS).
Arformoterol formulations, doses and duration
    of action of, 207t
Arnold-Chiari malformation, respiratory
    presentations of, 769-770
Arsenic, inhalational injury from, 687
ART. *See* Antiretroviral therapy (ART).
Arterial blood gas(es)
  analysis of
    in diagnosis of HIV-related pneumonia,
      359
    in pulmonary embolism, 696
    in respiratory failure, 765
    in COPD assessment, 549
  measurement of, 140
Arterial cannulation, complications of, 446b
Arterial hypertension, pulmonary. *See*
    Pulmonary arterial hypertension (PAH).
Arterial oxygen assessments, in diagnosis of
    HIV-related pneumonia, 359
Arterial pressure monitoring, in critical illness,
    445-446, 446f
Arterial waveform analysis
  in critical illness, 449-451, 451b, 451f
    transpulmonary lithium indication dilution
      and, 451
    transpulmonary thermodilution with, 451,
      451b, 451f
Arteritis
  giant cell, 727
  Takayasu, 727
Artery(ies)
  bronchial, 5
  pulmonary, 3f, 5
Arthritis
  chest pain in, 270-271
  rheumatoid. *See* Rheumatoid arthritis.
Arthropathy, episodic, in cystic fibrosis, 578
Asbestos
  lung cancer and, 778
  malignant pleural mesothelioma and,
    837-838
  nonmalignant pleural disorders related to,
    646t, 650-651
  pleural diseases related to, 830
Asbestosis, 645-652
  clinical course of, 650
  clinical features of, 648-649
  computed tomography in, 649, 649f
  controversies and pitfalls of, 651-652
  diagnosis of, 649-650
  epidemiology of, 645

Asbestosis *(Continued)*
  etiology of, 645-647
  genetics of, 648
  pathogenesis of, 647-648, 648f
  pathology of, 647, 647f
  pulmonary physiology assessment in, 649
  radiologic findings in, 649, 649f
  risk factors for, 645-647
  treatment of, 650
  uses and sources of exposure in, 646t
Ascariasis, pulmonary, 320
Ascaris lumbricoides, eosinophilia from,
    621-622
Aspergillosis, 315, 316f, 317t
  bronchopulmonary, allergic
    bronchiectasis from, 583
    in cystic fibrosis, 577
    eosinophilic lung disease in, 622-623,
      622f, 623b
  invasive
    in hematopoietic stem cell transplantation
      patients, 915
    in non–HIV-infected
      immunocompromised patients,
      340-343, 341f-342f, 342t-343t
Aspergillus-associated asthma, management of,
    516-517, 517f
Aspergillus infection
  in HIV patient, 355, 356f
  lung transplantation and, 897t, 898, 898f
Aspiration
  fine needle. *See* Fine needle aspiration
    (FNA).
  gastric acid, in pregnancy, 910
  during intubation, prevention of, cricoid
    pressure in, 439, 439f
  risk of
    assessment for, 438, 438b
    drugs reducing, 438t
  of secretions, therapeutic bronchoscopy for,
    171
  tracheal, in pneumonia pathogen
    identification, 293
  transtracheal, in pneumonia pathogen
    identification, 294
Aspiration pneumonia
  complicating community-acquired
    pneumonia, 305, 305f
  in systemic sclerosis, 659
Aspirin-induced asthma, management of, 516
Association study(ies), 10
  genome-wide, 11
Asthma, 487-500
  adult-onset, 498-499
  airway hyperresponsiveness in, 493, 501,
    502f-503f
  airway inflammation in, 488-491, 501-502
  Aspergillus-associated, management of,
    516-517, 517f
  aspirin-induced, management of, 516
  in athletes, management of, 517
  attacks of. *See* Asthma, exacerbations of.
  bronchial thermoplasty for, 172
  bronchodilator use in, 211
  causes of, 487
  in Churg-Strauss syndrome, 626
  clinical subgroups of, 504-505
    management of, 514-519
  controversies and pitfalls of, 519-520
  cough variant, 244-245
    treatment of, 248
  deaths from, world map of, 492f
  definition of, 487, 501-502, 502b
  description of, 487

Asthma *(Continued)*
  diagnosis of, 505-508, 505b, 507t, 508f
  differential diagnosis of, 504b
  difficult-to-treat, 495
  dynamic hyperinflation in, 419-420
  environmental factors in, 496-499
  eosinophilia in, 623-624
  epidemiology of, 487-488, 489t, 490f-492f
  exacerbations of
    acute, 495
    management of, 517-519, 518b, 518t,
      519f
    prevention of, 509
    severity of, guide to, 518t
  genetic factors underlying, 8t-9t, 12
  genetics of, 496, 505
  guided self-management plans for,
    monitoring, 511-512, 512f
  heterogeneity of, 504-505
  history of, 487
  hypereosinophilic, 623-624
  management of, 508-514
    aims of, 508-509, 509b
    recent developments in, 513-514
    stepwise approach to, 509f, 511-512
  natural history of, 493f
  nocturnal, 495
  occupational, 499, 521-530. *See also*
    Occupational asthma (OA).
  pathogenesis of, 488-495
  pathophysiology of, 491-495, 494f, 502-503,
    504b, 504f
  patient education on, 512-513
  pharmacotherapy in, 509-511
  phenotypes of, 496, 515f
  in pregnancy, 500, 907
    management of, 517
    treatment of, 907, 908t
  prevalence of, 492f
  referral to specialist for, 512
  risk factors for, 495-499, 495b
  severe
    factors contributing to, 513b
    management of, 514-516
    recognition and assessment of, in hospital,
      518b
    risk factors for, 513b
  smoking and, 495
  trigger factors for, 495b, 499-500
Asthma Control Questionnaire, 507t
Ataxic breathing, in stroke, 768
Atelectasis
  radiographic signs of, 82-88
  rounded, radiographic signs of, 87-88,
    89f
Athletes, asthma in, management of, 517
Atoll sign, in cryptogenic organizing
    pneumonia, 631-632, 631f
Atopy
  asthma and, 496
  COPD and, 537
Atovaquone
  for bacterial pneumonia, 363
  in *Pneumocystis* pneumonia prophylaxis,
    369-370, 369t
Atrial septostomy, for pulmonary arterial
    hypertension, 720
Atrophic rhinitis, 475
Auto-PEEP, dynamic hyperinflation and, 26,
    419-422, 421f-424f
Autocorrelation, 450
Autofluorescence bronchoscopy (AFB),
    164
Autonomic rhinitis, 474-475

Autophagy
  in α_1-antitrypsin deficiency, endoplasmic
    reticulum–associated degradation *versus*,
    17
  definition of, 17
Azathioprine (AZA)
  for ANCA-associated vasculitis, 724-725,
    724t
  in lung transplantation, 901t
  for sarcoidosis, 617t, 618
Azoospermia, obstructive, in cystic fibrosis,
  571-573
Aztreonam, for *P. aeruginosa* infection in cystic
  fibrosis, 575-576
Azygos vein, dilatation of, 99

B

B-type natriuretic peptide assay, in pulmonary
  embolism, 696
Bacillus anthracis, in community-acquired
  pneumonia, 301
Bacillus Calmette-Guérin (BCG) vaccination,
  for TB, 397
Bacteria
  anaerobic, in community-acquired
    pneumonia, 300
  in cystic fibrosis lung disease, 568-569
  multidrug-resistant, pneumonia patients
    with risk factors for, 327-328
Bacterial infection(s), in HIV patient
  clinical features of, 350-351
  controversies and pitfalls of, 372
  prognosis of, 371
  prophylaxis of, 368-370, 369t
  treatment of, 361, 362t
Bacterial pneumonia
  in hematopoietic stem cell transplantation
    patient, 914
  hemoptysis in, 261-262
  in HIV patient, 350-351, 351f
  in influenza, pathogenesis of, 310-311
  in non–HIV-infected immunocompromised
    patients, 336-337, 336f
Bacteriologic examination, in TB diagnosis,
  389-390
Bacteriologic strategy, for nosocomial
  respiratory infection diagnosis, 325-326,
  326f
Bacteriology, of exudative effusions, 827
Bag mask ventilation, before endotracheal
  intubation in ICU, 438
BAL. *See* Bronchoalveolar lavage (BAL).
Balke protocol, 148
Balloon dilatation, rigid bronchoscopic, 165,
  165f
Bard Biopty biopsy system, 181, 182f
Bartonella henselae infection, in HIV patient,
  351
Base deficit, 48
Bauer Temno biopsy instrument, 181, 182f
Beals syndrome, scoliosis in, 756
Becker muscular dystrophy, respiratory
  presentations of, 773
Behçet disease, 727-728
Behçet syndrome, 662, 662f
Benign lung tumors, 810-817
  classification of, 810, 811b
  detection and diagnosis of, 810
  epithelial, 810-811
  mesenchymal, 811-813
  non-neoplastic, 814-817, 817b, 817f
Bernoulli effect, obstructive sleep apnea and,
  739-740

Beryllium, inhalational injury from, 687
Beryllium disease, chronic, sarcoidosis
  differentiated from, 615
β_2-Agonists
  antiinflammatory effects of, 204-205
  in asthma, 509-510
  bronchodilator action of, 204-205, 205f
  chemical structures of, 205f
  clinical considerations for, 206-208, 207t,
    208f
  for COPD, 555
  side effects of, 207-208, 208t
Bevacizumab, for Stage IV non–small cell lung
  cancer, 806
Bilateral diaphragmatic paralysis, 53, 53f
Bilevel positive airway pressure ventilation,
  415, 416f
Biliary cirrhosis, primary. *See* Primary biliary
  cirrhosis (PBC).
Biliary colic, pain in, 271
Biliary disease, 920-926
Biochemical assays, in diagnosis of HIV-related
  pneumonia, 359-360
Biochemical toxins, 688, 688t
Biomarkers
  of malignant pleural mesothelioma, 841,
    841f
  of pulmonary arterial hypertension, 718
Biomass fuel(s)
  decreased exposure to, for COPD, 554
  indoor air pollution from, 942, 942f
Biopsy(ies)
  common routes for, according to site, 181f
  common sites for, 181f
  lung
    bronchoscopic, 156-157, 156f
      in bronchogenic carcinoma diagnosis,
        160
      in diffuse lung disease diagnosis,
        161-162, 162b
    in connective tissue diseases, 664
    HRCT and, 71-72
    open, in pneumonia pathogen
      identification, 294
  lymph node, diagnostic application of, 877t,
    878
  percutaneous, 180-192. *See also*
    Percutaneous biopsy procedures.
  pleural, 823
    in pneumonia pathogen identification, 293
  surgical, in diffuse lung disease, 595
  transbronchial, in organizing pneumonia
    diagnosis, 634
Biotrauma, in ventilator-induced lung injury,
  420, 458-460
Birt-Hogg-Dube (BHD) syndrome, 670, 670f
  CT appearance and clinical characteristics of,
    671t
Birt-Hogg-Dubé-Rendu syndrome, genetic
  factors underlying, 8t-9t
Blastomycosis, 316-318, 316f, 317t, 318f
  in HIV patient, 357
Blood
  culture of, in pneumonia pathogen
    identification, 293
  flow of, in lungs. *See* Pulmonary blood flow.
Blood buffer line, 46
Blood chemistry, serum, in obesity
  hypoventilation syndrome, 752
Blood gases
  abnormalities of, bronchoscopy and, 162-163
  analysis of, in obesity hypoventilation
    syndrome, 752
  arterial. *See* Arterial blood gas(es).

Blood tests
  in bronchiectasis diagnosis, 582
  in diffuse lung disease diagnosis, 591
BODE index, of COPD severity, 548, 549t
Body cavity–associated lymphoma, in HIV
  patient, 378
Body plethysmography, in lung volume
  measurement, 137, 137f
Bone(s)
  disease of, cystic fibrosis–related, 578
  infections of, nontuberculous mycobacterial
    clinical features of, 400
    treatment of, 403
  lesions of, percutaneous biopsy of, 190-191
Bone and joint tuberculosis, 387
Bone marrow transplantation, alveolar
  hemorrhage after, 730
Borg Scale, Modified, for breathlessness, 547,
  547t
Botulism, respiratory presentations of, 772
Bowel disease, inflammatory, 927-936. *See also*
  Inflammatory bowel disease (IBD).
Brachytherapy, endobronchial, 166-167
Bracing, for scoliosis, 760
Brain natriuretic peptides (BNPs), in acute
  dyspnea, 254
Breastfeeding
  childhood asthma and, 496-497
  tuberculosis treatment during, 394, 397
Breathing
  diaphragmatic, in COPD, 558
  neural control of, 51f, 58-59
  physiology of, 55-56, 55f-56f
  pursed-lip, in COPD, 558
  sleep-disordered. *See* Sleep-disordered
    breathing.
  spontaneous, 34-35
    trial of, initiation of, criteria for, 428b
    ventilation modes delivering assistance to,
      409-415, 410f
  work of, 25-26, 26f
Breathing retraining techniques, for asthma,
  513
Breathing training, for COPD patient, 558
Breathlessness
  in bronchiectasis, 581-582
  in COPD, 546, 547t
Bronchial anastomotic complications, of lung
  transplantation, 894, 896f
Bronchial artery embolization, 75-76, 75f
Bronchial blood supply, 5
Bronchial circulation, 29
Bronchial epithelial cells, 2-3
Bronchial fistula closure, therapeutic
  bronchoscopy for, 171-172
Bronchial signs, of lobar collapse, 84
Bronchial thermoplasty, 172
  for asthma, 514
Bronchiectasis, 580-587
  alternative therapy for, 585-586
  antibiotic therapy for, 584-585, 584f, 585t
  bronchial wall thickening in, 120
  chest radiography in, 97, 97f
  clinical features of, 581-582
  clinical signs of, 582
  complicating community-acquired
    pneumonia, 308
  complications of, 586
  in connective tissue diseases, 655
  controversies and pitfalls of, 587
  CT imaging in, 97, 97f
  cylindrical, 580, 581f
  cystic, 580, 581f
  diagnosis of, 582-583, 582b

Bronchiectasis *(Continued)*
  epidemiology of, 580
  exacerbations of, 583-584, 584b
    antibiotics for, 584-585, 585t
  hemoptysis in, 261, 586
  in HIV patient, 350, 350f
  HRCT identification of, 119-121, 120f-121f,
    121t
  infectious inflammatory cycle of, 581, 581f
  lung transplantation for, 586
  management of, 586
  pathogenesis of, 580-581, 581b
  pathology of, 580, 581f
  physiotherapy for, 586
  prognosis for, 586
  respiratory failure in, 586
  surgery for, 586
  traction, 115, 115f
    in nonspecific interstitial pneumonia,
      592-593, 593f
  underlying causes of, 581b
  vaccinations and, 585
  varicose, 580, 581f
Bronchiectatic disease, nodular, 399, 400f
Bronchiolar stem cell, 16
Bronchiole(s)
  membranous, 3, 3f
  respiratory, 3, 4f
Bronchiolitis
  chronic, in connective tissue diseases, 655
  constrictive, HRCT in, 593
  definition of, 531
  follicular, in connective tissue diseases, 655
  obliterative
    in connective tissue diseases, 655, 655f
    drug-induced, 238
  pathology of, 533, 534f
Bronchiolitis obliterans, in hematopoietic stem
    cell transplantation, 917
Bronchiolitis obliterans organizing pneumonia
    (BOOP)
  after hematopoietic stem cell
    transplantation, 918
  in HIV patient, 380
Bronchitis
  acute, hemoptysis in, 261
  chronic. *See* Chronic bronchitis.
  in connective tissue diseases, 655
  eosinophilic, 245, 246f, 624
    treatment of, 248
  follicular, in connective tissue diseases, 655
  in HIV patient, 350
  industrial, 640
Bronchoalveolar lavage (BAL)
  bronchoscopy and, 157, 157f
  in organizing pneumonia diagnosis, 633-634
  in connective tissue diseases, 663-664, 664f
  in diagnosis of HIV-related pneumonia, 360,
    360f, 360t
  in diffuse lung disease diagnosis, 161-162,
    162t
  in extrinsic allergic alveolitis, 679
Bronchoalveolar stem cells (BASCs), 16
Bronchocentric granulomatosis, 624
Bronchoconstriction, in asthma, 491-493
Bronchodilator(s), 202-212
  actions of
    pharmacologic basis of, 204-206
    physiologic basis for, 202-204
  β₂-agonists as
    clinical considerations for, 206-208, 207t,
      208f
    pharmacologic basis of, 204-205, 205f
    side effects of, 207-208, 208t

Bronchodilator(s) *(Continued)*
  antimuscarinic agents as, pharmacologic basis
    of, 205-206, 205f-206f
  in asthma, 509-510
    vs. COPD, 202-204
  in clinical practice, 211
  controversies and pitfalls with, 211-212
  for COPD, 555-556
  drug delivery for, 210, 210t
  future of, 212
  inhaled, for COPD exacerbations, 564, 564f
  introduction to, 202, 203f
  response to
    assessment of, in asthma diagnosis, 506
    spirometry in assessing, 134-135
  safety of, 212
  synergy of corticosteroids with, 213-214
  synergy of phosphodiesterase 4 inhibitors
    with, 218
  theophylline as, 209-210
Bronchodilator reversibility testing, 204-205,
    211
Bronchogenic carcinoma
  diagnosis of, bronchoscopic, 159-160, 160f
  molecular and immunohistochemical
    assessment of, 161
  staging of, bronchoscopic, 160-161, 161f
Bronchogenic cysts, 856, 856f
  middle mediastinal masses from, 113
Bronchopleural fistula, complicating
    community-acquired pneumonia,
    306-307
Bronchoprovocation testing, 141
Bronchopulmonary aspergillosis, allergic
  bronchiectasis from, 583
  in cystic fibrosis, 577
  eosinophilic lung disease in, 622-623, 622f,
    623b
Bronchopulmonary infection, chronic, COPD
    and, 536
Bronchopulmonary segments, 1-2, 2f, 2t
Bronchoscopy, 154-173
  autofluorescence, 164
  complications of, 162-163
  in diagnosis of HIV-related pneumonia,
    360-361
  diagnostic, indications for, 157-162, 157b
  diagnostic application of, 876
  in diffuse lung disease, 595
  fiberoptic. *See* Fiberoptic bronchoscopy
    (FOB).
  flexible, 154, 155f
    diagnostic application of, 876
  instrumentation for, 154-157, 155f
  monitoring during, 155
  narrow band imaging, 164
  navigational, diagnostic application of,
    877
  navigational systems for, 160
  patient preparation for, 155, 155b
  in pneumonia, in non–HIV-infected
    immunocompromised patients, 336
  in pneumonia pathogen identification, 294
  rigid, 154, 155f
    diagnostic application of, 877-878, 877f,
      877t
  safety factors in, 162
  technique of, 155-157, 156f-157f
  therapeutic
    complications of, 172
    indications for, 157b, 168-172
    techniques of, 165-168, 169t
  types of, 154-157
  ultrathin, 163

Bronchoscopy *(Continued)*
  virtual, 163-164
  white light, 164
Bronchospasm
  acute, drug-induced, 237-238
  catastrophic, drug-induced, 223t
Bronchus(i)
  cartilaginous, 2-3, 3f
  intraparenchymal, structure and function of,
    20
  radiographic anatomy of, 78
Brucella species, in community-acquired
    pneumonia, 301
Brucellosis, 301
Budesonide, nebulized, for COPD
    exacerbations, 564
Buffering, 45
Burkholderia cepacia complex, in cystic fibrosis
    lung disease, 575
Bursitis, chest pain in, 270-271

C

Cadmium, inhalational injury from, 687
Calcification, pleural, radiographic features of,
    106-107, 107f-108f
Calcineurin inhibitors, in lung transplantation,
    900, 901t
Calcium channel blockers, for pulmonary
    arterial hypertension, 719
Calcium metabolism, in sarcoidosis, 615
Canalicular stage, of lung development, 1, 2t
Cancer
  lung, 776-809. *See also* Lung cancer.
    pleural effusions in, 828
    posttransplant, 902, 902f
    pulmonary embolism treatment in, 704
    venous thromboembolism and, 694
Candida species, lung infections from
  in HIV patient, 355
  in non–HIV-infected immunocompromised
    patients, 343-344
Candidate gene approach, to association
    studies, 11
  pitfalls of, 18
CAP. *See* Community-acquired pneumonia
    (CAP).
Capillaries, alveolar, 29, 30f
Capillaritis, pulmonary, pauciimmune,
    idiopathic, 726-727
Capillary stress failure, 38
Caplan syndrome, 640, 640f
Capreomycin, for TB, 392t
Carbon monoxide
  as asphyxiant, 683t, 686
  gas transfer for, in COPD assessment, 549
Carbonyl chloride, as irritant, 685
Carcinoid tumors
  lung, 782-784, 782f
  thymic, 849-850, 849f
Carcinoma, thymic, 849, 849f
Cardia, achalasia of, 100f
Cardiac function, chest wall deformity and,
    757-758, 758t
Cardiac output
  increased, for hypoxemia, 44
  measurement of, using pulmonary artery
    flotation catheter, 448-449, 449b, 449t,
    450f
  thermodilution measurements of, 449, 449b,
    450f
Cardiac sarcoidosis, 614
Cardiac tamponade, echocardiographic features
    of, 199, 200f

Cardiogenic pulmonary edema, noninvasive mechanical ventilation for, 432-433
Cardiomyopathy
  peripartum, 906-907
  restrictive, secondary to chronic respiratory disease, echocardiographic features of, 200-201
Cardiopulmonary decompensation, in scoliosis, 759
Cardiopulmonary exercise testing (CPET), 143-153
  for chronic dyspnea, 259, 259t
  clinical indications for, 143
  clinical protocols for, 147-150
  constant-work rate exercise in laboratory, 149
  exercise intensity in, energy requirements and, 144-145
  incremental, in laboratory, 143, 147-148
  interpretation strategies for, 151, 152f
  patient preparation for, 151
  in preoperative evaluation for lung resection, 873, 874f
  procedures for, 151
  simple, outside laboratory, 149-150, 149f-150f, 150t
Cardiovascular system
  corticosteroid toxicities affecting, 217t
  disorders of
    chest pain in, 270
    in COPD, 546
  examination of, in COPD, 548
  imaging of, MRI in, 73
Cartilaginous bronchi, 2-3, 3f
Caspofungin
  for bacterial pneumonia, 363
  for invasive aspergillosis, 343t
Castleman disease
  mediastinal lymphadenopathy in, 855
  multicentric, in HIV patient, 377
Catamenial pneumothorax, 835
Cataracts, from indoor air pollution, 944
Cathelicidins, in lung host defense, 284
Catheterization
  central venous, in critical illness, 446-447, 447b
  heart, right-sided, in pulmonary arterial hypertension, 717-718
  pulmonary artery, in critical illness, 447-448, 447f, 450f
Catheters, pleural, indwelling, placement of, for pleural effusions, 824, 824f
Cavitating tumors, CT appearance and clinical characteristics of, 671t
Cell biology, 12-17
  intracellular signals in, 12-14
  maintenance of extracellular matrix in, 14-15, 15f
  repair in, 15-17, 16f
Cell-mediated immunity, defects in, pathogens associated with, 330, 332t
Cell senescence, in COPD, 542
Cellular nonspecific interstitial pneumonia, 603-604
Central chemoreceptors, in ventilation, 51f, 52
Central fatigue, respiratory muscle, 57
Central nervous system (CNS)
  acute disorders affecting, 768-769, 770f
  chronic disorders affecting, 769-770
  corticosteroid toxicities affecting, 217t
  depression of, respiratory acidosis from, 47-48
  in dyspnea, 251, 251f
  sarcoidosis involving, 615

Central nervous system tuberculosis, 387-388
Central neurogenic hyperventilation, in stroke, 768, 770f
Central respiratory drive, in obesity hypoventilation syndrome, 750
Central respiratory stimulants, for COPD exacerbations, 565-566
Central venous catheterization, in critical illness, 446-447, 447b
Centrilobular emphysema
  cystic air spaces in, 118, 119f
  pathology of, 533-534
Centrilobular nodules, in extrinsic allergic alveolitis, 678, 678f, 678t
Cerebellar degeneration, in lung cancer, manifestations and treatment of, 807t
Cerebrovascular accident, respiratory presentations of, 768, 770f
Cervical lymph node biopsy, 877t, 878
Cervical mediastinoscopy, diagnostic application of, 877t, 878-879, 879f
CF. See Cystic fibrosis (CF).
Chemical asphyxiants, 683t, 686-687
Chemical irritants, 683-686, 683t
Chemical pleurodesis, chest tube with, for malignant pleural effusions, 868
Chemokines, in lung host defense, 286-287, 287t
Chemoreceptors
  central, in ventilation, 51f, 52
  peripheral, in ventilation, 51f, 52
Chemotherapy
  adjuvant
    for Stage I non–small cell lung cancer, 802
    for Stage II non–small cell lung cancer, 803
  for malignant pleural mesothelioma, 843-844
  restaging lung cancer patients after, 178
  for small cell lung cancer, 806
  for Stage III non–small cell lung cancer, 803-805, 804t
  for Stage IV non–small cell lung cancer, 805
Chemotherapy lung, parenchymal patterns in, 235
Chest drain. See Chest tube.
Chest examination, in COPD, 547-548
Chest pain, 267-274
  causes of, 268b
  clinical presentation of, 269, 270f
  diagnostic tests in, 272-273, 272t
  differential diagnosis of, 267-269
  dysmotility and, 269
  electrocardiographic findings in, 272, 272t
  in esophageal reflux, 269
  history in, 270-271
  musculoskeletal pain and, 268-269, 268f-269f
  in myocardial ischemia, 267
  patient evaluation in, 269-273, 269f
  pericardial, 267
  physical examination in, 272, 272f
  pulmonary, 267
  in pulmonary embolus, 267-268
  treatment of, 273-274
Chest physical therapy, for COPD patient, 558
Chest physiotherapy, in cystic fibrosis, 574
Chest radiography
  in acute dyspnea, 254-255
  in asbestosis, 649, 649f
  in bronchiectasis diagnosis, 582
  in chest pain, 272-273, 272f-273f
  in coal worker's pneumoconiosis, 641-642, 641f-642f

Chest radiography (Continued)
  in connective tissue diseases, 662-663
  in COPD exacerbation, 563, 563f
  in cryptogenic organizing pneumonia, 631f
  in diffuse lung disease diagnosis, 591-592
  in extrinsic allergic alveolitis, 677-678, 678f
  in obesity hypoventilation syndrome, 753
  plain, 63-65
    anatomy on, 76-80
    in COPD assessment, 551
    digital, 64-65
    interpretation of, 80-107
      in airway disease, 95-97, 95f-97f
      in diffuse shadowing, 92-95, 94f
      enhancement characteristics in, 90-92, 92f
      in hilar abnormalities, 101-102, 101f-102f
      in mediastinal abnormalities, 97-101. See also Mediastinal entries; Mediastinum.
      in multiple pulmonary nodules, 92, 93b, 93f-94f
      in pleural disease, 102-107, 102f. See also Pleura; Pleural entries.
      radiographic signs in, 80-90. See also Radiographic signs.
    in latent TB, 396f
    lateral, anatomy of, 78-80, 79f-80f
    in malignant pleural mesothelioma, 840, 840f
    portable, 63-64
    in pulmonary infection classification, 288-289, 289f-290f
    in TB diagnosis, 389, 389f
    technical considerations for, 63-65, 64f-65f
  in pleural effusions, 818
  in pulmonary alveolar microlithiasis, 673-674, 673f
  in pulmonary arterial hypertension, 715, 715f
  in pulmonary embolism, 697-698, 698f
  in sarcoidosis, 610-612, 611f
  of thymoma, 847-848, 848f
Chest tightness, in COPD, 546-547
Chest tube
  with chemical pleurodesis, for malignant pleural effusions, 868
  clamping of, 865
  obstruction of, 867
  removal of, 866
  selection of, 862, 863f
  subdiaphragmatic placement of, 866
  underwater seal chest drainage system and, 864-865, 865f
    air leak in, 865
Chest tube insertion
  anesthesia for, 863-864
  difficulties with, 866
  drain insertion in, 864-865, 864f
  impaled structure during, 866
  incision for, 864
  indications and contraindications for, 862, 863b
  instrument requirements for, 864b
  with intrapleural adhesions, 866
  patient positioning for, 863, 863f
  preparation for, 863-864
  site for, 863, 863f
  special considerations for, 866-868
  subdiaphragmatic placement in, 866
  technique of, 862-865

Chest tube management, 865-866
  air leaks and, 865
    prolonged, 867, 867f
  difficult issues in, 866-868
  lung reexpansion failure and, 867
  reexpansion pulmonary edema and, 867
  subcutaneous emphysema and, 866-867
Chest wall
  defects in. *See also* Chest wall disorder(s).
    hypertransradiancy in, 88, 89f
  disease of, percutaneous sampling of,
      187-188, 188f
  elastic properties of, 22, 22f, 23t
  imaging of, MRI in, 72, 73f
  lungs and, in respiratory system, 22f, 23
  mechanics of, 758
  problems of, chest pain in, 270
  recoil pressures of, transmural pressure
      difference and, 23t
Chest wall disorder(s)
  effects of, on respiratory and cardiac
      function, 757-758, 758t
  imaging in evaluation of, 767-768
  respiratory muscle pump and, 763-768.
      See also Respiratory muscle pump.
  respiratory presentations of, 768-774, 768t
  scoliosis as, 756-762. *See also* Scoliosis.
Cheyne-Stokes respiration, in stroke, 768, 770f
Children
  asthma risks in, 496-498
  pleural infections in, 827-828
  tuberculosis treatment in, 394
Chlamydia species, in community-acquired
    pneumonia, 299
Chlorine, as irritant, 683t, 685
Cholangitis, sclerosing, primary. *See* Primary
    sclerosing cholangitis (PSC).
Chondroma, 811, 812f
Chromium, inhalational injury from, 687
Chronic beryllium disease (CBD), sarcoidosis
    differentiated from, 615
Chronic bronchitis
  cough in, 247
  definition of, 531
  pathology of, 532-533, 533f
Chronic cough
  bronchoscopy in, 157
  causes of, 243, 243t
  definition of, 242
  diagnostic algorithm for, 245f
  management of, common pitfalls in, 249b
  treatment of, 247-249, 248t
  unexplained, 249
Chronic lung disease, restrictive
    cardiomyopathy secondary to,
    echocardiographic features of, 200-201
Chronic obstructive pulmonary disease
    (COPD)
  alternative therapies of, development of, 220
  bronchodilator use in, 211
  cholinergic airway control in, 203f
  clinical features of, 546-547
  clinical signs of, 547
  comorbidities of, 545-546
  defining, 531-532
  diagnostic considerations for, 531-532
  dynamic hyperinflation in, 419-420
  dyspnea in, treatment of, 259
  epidemiology of, 538-539
  etiology of, 534-538
  exacerbations of
    clinical course of, 566
    clinical features of, 562-563
    diagnosis of, 563-564, 563f

Chronic obstructive pulmonary disease
    (COPD) *(Continued)*
    epidemiology of, 562, 563f
    management of, 562-567
    noninvasive mechanical ventilation for, 432
    pathophysiology of, 562, 563b, 563f
    prevention of, 566
    treatment of, 560, 564-566
  exercise in
    hemodynamic response to, 146-147
    lung response to, 145-146
  gene hunting for, 10-12, 11f
  genetic factors underlying, 8t-9t
  hospitalization for, 560-561
  host factors in, 536-538
  lung transplantation for, 888, 888t
  morbidity from, 539
  mortality from, 539
  natural history of, 539-540, 540f
  obstructive sleep apnea and, 748
  pathogenesis of, 540-542, 541f
  pathology of, 532-534, 532b, 533f-535f
  pathophysiology of, 542-545
  patient assessment in, 547-551
  phosphodiesterase 4 inhibitors for, relative
      potency and dosages of, 218t
  prevalence of, 538
  prognosis of, 539-540
  respiratory work in, 26
  risk factors for, 534-536
  severity of
    BODE index of, 548, 549t
    spirometric classification of, 548, 548t
  socioeconomic impact of, 539
  symptoms of, 546-547
  systemic effects of, 545-546
  theophylline for, relative potency and
      dosages of, 218t
  theophylline metabolism in, 210t
  treatability of, 553-554
  treatment of, 553-561
    comprehensive approach to, 554f
    controversies and pitfalls of, 561
    goals of, 553
    in multicomponent disease, 553
    options for, 554b
      for respiratory manifestations, 554-557
      for systemic manifestations, 557-560
  underdiagnosis of, 531
  ventilating patients with, 418-419
Chronic thromboembolic disease, treatment of,
    705, 705f
Chronic thromboembolic pulmonary
    hypertension (CTEPH), 713
  treatment of, 705
Churg-Strauss syndrome (CSS), 626-627, 626f,
    627b, 627t
  management of, 516
  pleural effusions in, 829
Chylothorax, pleural effusions related to,
    829-830, 830f
Cicatrization collapse, of lung, 83
Cidofovir, for viral lung infections, 339t
Cigarette smoking. *See* Smoking/smoke
    exposure.
Ciliary dyskinesia, primary
  bronchiectasis and, 583
  genetic factors underlying, 8t-9t
Ciliated cells, 4
Circulation
  bronchial, 29
  lymphatic, 29
  pulmonary, 29-36. *See also* Pulmonary
      circulation.

Cirrhosis, biliary, primary. *See* Primary biliary
    cirrhosis (PBC).
CL. *See* Compliance, of lungs (CL).
Clara cells, 4
  as progenitor cells, 16
  toxin-resistant variant, 16
Clear cell tumor, 814
Clindamycin-primaquine, for bacterial
    pneumonia, 363
Clinical Pulmonary Infection Score (CPIS),
    323, 325t
Closing volume, 139-140, 139f
Clubbing, digital, in bronchiectasis, 582
Cluster breathing, in stroke, 768
Coagulation, pulmonary circulation and, 33
Coal worker's pneumoconiosis (CWP),
    637-644
  bronchoalveolar lavage in, 643
  chest radiology in, 641-642, 641f
  clinical features of, 640-641
  diagnosis of, 639-643
  epidemiology of, 637
  genetics of, 638
  histopathologic changes in, 638-639, 639f
  lung function in, 642-643
  management of, 643
  nodular pattern on HRCT in, 116
  pathophysiology of, 637-638, 638f
  prevention of, 643
  prognosis of, 643
  serologic and immunologic features of, 643
  sources of exposure in, 637
Cobalt, inhalational injury from, 687
Cobb angle, 756, 757f
Coccidioidomycosis, 316f, 317t, 318, 318f
  in HIV patient, 357
  treatment of, 367, 367t
Cold air challenge, 141
Colistin, for *P. aeruginosa* infection in cystic
    fibrosis, 575-576
Colitis, ulcerative, thoracic involvement in,
    927. *See also* Inflammatory bowel disease
    (IBD).
Collagen vascular disorders, diffuse alveolar
    hemorrhage and, 729
Collectins, in lung host defense, 284
Combination therapy, for COPD, 555t, 556
Common cold, 473
  clinical course and prevention of, 486
  clinical features of, 478
  treatment of, 482
Community-acquired pneumonia (CAP),
    296-308
  Actinomyces israelii in, 300-301, 301f
  age and, 296-297
  airway colonization and, 297
  alcoholism and, 297
  altered immunity and, 297
  anaerobic bacteria in, 300
  Bacillus anthracis in, 301
  Brucella species in, 301
  Chlamydia species in, 299
  clinical presentation of, 296
  clinical stability in, criteria for, 304b
  complications of, 305-308
  controversies and pitfalls for, 308
  Coxiella burnetti in, 300
  environmental factors in, 297
  Francisella tularensis in, 301
  Gram-negative bacilli in, 299-300
  Haemophilus influenzae in, 299
  incidence of, 296
  institutionalization and, 297
  Legionella pneumophila in, 299

Community-acquired pneumonia (CAP) (*Continued*)
in lung transplantation, 896, 897t
microbial etiology prediction in, 292t, 303b
Moraxella catarrhalis in, 301
Mycoplasma pneumoniae in, 299
Nocardia species in, 300
nutrition and, 297
Pasteurella multocida in, 301
pathogens in, 298-301
patient evaluation/diagnostics in, 297-301
risk factors for, 296-297
smoking and, 297
Staphylococcus species in, 298-299
Streptococcus species in, 298
treatment of, 301-305
antimicrobial, 302-303, 303b, 303t-304t
failure to respond to, 304-305, 304f
route and duration of, 303-304, 304t
site of care decision for, 301-302, 302b
vaccine prevention of, recommendations for, 307t, 308
viral, 309
Yersinia pestis in, 301
Compensatory hyperinflation, in lobar collapse, 84
Complement, in host defense system, 283, 283f
Compliance
of lungs (C_L), 22, 22f
in scoliosis, 758
Computed tomography angiography (CTA), in pulmonary embolism, 699-701, 701f
Computed tomography (CT), 65-68, 66f
in acute dyspnea, 255
in asbestosis, 649, 649f
in chest pain, 273, 273f
in COPD assessment, 551
in diagnosis of HIV-related pneumonia, 359, 359f
guiding percutaneous biopsy, 180
in hemoptysis, 263-265, 264f
high-resolution, 68-72. *See also* High-resolution computed tomography (HRCT).
interpretation of, 107-113
intravenous contrast enhancement in, 67-68
in lymphangioleiomyomatosis, 667, 668f
in malignant pleural mesothelioma, 840, 840f
in mediastinal mass evaluation, 111-113, 111f
in nodule growth assessment, 90, 91f
partial volume effect in, 66-67, 67f
in pleural effusions, 820
in pulmonary arterial hypertension, 716-717
in sarcoidosis, 611f-612f
section thickness for, 66-67, 67f
technical considerations for, 66
of thymoma, 847-848, 848f
in upper airway disease diagnosis, 479, 479f
window settings for, 67, 68f
Congenital anomalies, MRA and, 92-95
Congenital contractual arachnodactyly, scoliosis in, 756
Congenital heart disease, pulmonary arterial hypertension and, 712
Congestive heart failure (CHF)
dyspnea in, 253-254
paroxysmal nocturnal dyspnea and orthopnea in, 256
postoperative pulmonary complications and, 870
transudative effusions in, 825

Connective tissue diseases (CTDs), 653-666
activity *versus* severity in, 666
airway pathology in, 654-655
BAL in, 663-664, 664f
chest radiography in, 662-663
clinical course of, 666
clinical features of, 656-662
controversies and pitfalls of, 666
diagnostic flowchart for, 664, 664f
diagnostic testing in, 662-664
epidemiology of, 653
genetics of, 653-654
HRCT in, 663, 663f-664f, 663t
interstitial fibrosis in, 654
lung biopsy in, 664
lung cancer in, 656
lung pathology in, 654-656
mixed, clinical features of, 660
pathogenesis of, 654
pleural effusions secondary to, 828-829
prevention of, 666
pulmonary function tests in, 662
pulmonary hypertension in, 656, 711-712
pulmonary involvement in, 653
treatment of, 664-666
vascular disease and, 654
Conservation of mass equation, 39, 44
Consolidation
causes of, 80t
in diffuse lung disease, 592-593
multifocal, persistent unexplained, 592
in pneumonia, in non–HIV-infected immunocompromised patients, 332-333, 333t, 334f
radiographic signs of, 80-82, 81f-84f
Constrictive bronchiolitis, HRCT in, 593
Continuous positive airway pressure (CPAP), 416-417, 417f
for obesity hypoventilation syndrome, 754
for obstructive sleep apnea, 746-747, 747f
effects on major outcomes, 747-748
Contrast venography, in pulmonary embolism, 699
Cook Quickcore device, 181, 182f
COP. *See* Cryptogenic organizing pneumonia (COP).
COPD. *See* Chronic obstructive pulmonary disease (COPD).
COPD Assessment Test, 550
Cor pulmonale, echocardiographic evaluation of, 199
Coronary artery bypass graft surgery, pleural effusions after, 829
Corticosteroid-induced respiratory myopathy, respiratory presentations of, 772-773
Corticosteroid-sparing agents, for asthma, 511
Corticosteroids
in ARDS management, 469
for Churg-Strauss syndrome, 627
for COPD, 555t, 556
for COPD exacerbations, 564, 564f
for cryptogenic organizing pneumonia, 634-635, 634t
for extrinsic allergic alveolitis, 680
controversies and pitfalls of, 681
for inflammatory diseases, 213-216
inhaled
adult dosing for, 216t
adverse effects of, 217t
for asthma, 510-511
for COPD, 555t, 556
pharmacokinetics of, 215, 215t
receptor affinity of, 215t

Corticosteroids (*Continued*)
for interstitial pneumonias, in connective tissue diseases, 665
molecular mechanisms of, 213, 214f-215f
oral, for asthma, 511
pharmacodynamics of, 213, 214f
pharmacokinetics of, 214-215, 215t-216t
resistance to, 214
for sarcoidosis, 616, 617t
side effects of, 214, 217t
synergy of bronchodilators with, 213-214
systemic
adverse effects of, 217t
pharmacokinetics of, 214-215
tolerability of, 219-220
topical
for acute rhinosinusitis, 484
for allergic rhinitis, 480
for chronic rhinosinusitis, 484-485
for intrinsic rhinitis, 482
toxicity of, prevention and management of, 216
Coryza
acute, 473
clinical course and prevention of, 486
clinical features of, 478
treatment of, 482
diagnosis of, 479
Cough, 242-249
ACE inhibitor–associated, 245-246
acute
common causes of, 243b
definition of, 242-243
antitussive therapies for, 248-249
chronic. *See* Chronic cough.
clinical assessment of, 243-247, 244t
differential diagnosis of, 242-243
in COPD, 546
in defense system, 276, 277t
further investigations of, 247
gastroesophageal reflux–associated, 247
treatment of, 248
reflex, 242, 243f
severity assessment tools for, 246f
solitary, drug-induced, 238
treatment of, 247-249, 248t
in upper airway disease, 246-247
Cough gastric pressure, in respiratory function testing, 766
Cough peak flow, in respiratory function testing, 766
Cough variant asthma, 244-245
treatment of, 248
Coxiella burnetti, in community-acquired pneumonia, 300
CPET. *See* Cardiopulmonary exercise testing (CPET).
Crackles, coarse, in bronchiectasis, 582
Cranial arteritis, 727
Cricoid pressure, in endotracheal intubation in ICU, 439, 439f
Cricothyroidotomy, emergency, 441-443, 444f
Critical illness, hemodynamic monitoring in, 445-453. *See also* Hemodynamic monitoring, in critical illness.
Critical illness neuromyopathy, respiratory presentations of, 771-772
Critical illness polyneuromyopathy (CIPM), 425-426
Critical power, in exercise testing, 144, 144f
Crohn disease, thoracic involvement in, 927. *See also* Inflammatory bowel disease (IBD).
Cryotherapy, endobronchial, 166

Cryptococcosis, 316f, 319
  in HIV patient, treatment of, 366-367, 367t
Cryptococcus, lung infections from
  in HIV patient, 355-356, 356f
  in non–HIV-infected immunocompromised
    patients, 344
Cryptogenic fibrosing alveolitis (CFA),
    classification of, 588
Cryptogenic hemoptysis, 262
Cryptogenic organizing pneumonia (COP)
  after hematopoietic stem cell
    transplantation, 918
  clinical features of, 630-631
  complicating community-acquired
    pneumonia, 307
  HRCT in, 593
  imaging features of, 631-632, 631f-632f,
    632b
  severe, 635
  treatment of, 634-635, 634t
CSS. See Churg-Strauss syndrome (CSS).
CTDs. See Connective tissue diseases (CTDs).
Culture
  blood, in pneumonia pathogen identification,
    293
  mycobacterial, in TB diagnosis, 390
  in viral pneumonia diagnosis, 312
CURB-65 index, 289-290, 291f
Cushing's syndrome, in lung cancer,
    manifestations and treatment of, 807t
Cutaneous sarcoidosis, 612, 613f
Cutis laxa, emphysema secondary to, genetic
    factors underlying, 8t-9t, 14-15, 15f
CWP. See Coal worker's pneumoconiosis
    (CWP).
Cyclophosphamide (CYC)
  for ANCA-associated vasculitis, 723-725,
    724t
  for sarcoidosis, 618
  for scleroderma diffuse lung disease, 665
Cycloserine, for TB, 392t
Cyclosporine, in lung transplantation, 901t
Cylindrical bronchiectasis, 580, 581f
Cyst(s)
  bronchogenic, 856, 856f
  enteric, 856
  foregut, 855
  neuroenteric, posterior mediastinal masses
    from, 113
  pericardial, 854, 854f
  pulmonary, tuberous sclerosis with, genetic
    factors underlying, 8t-9t
  thymic, 853, 854f
Cystic air spaces, 118-119, 118f-119f
Cystic bronchiectasis, 580, 581f
Cystic fibrosis (CF), 568-579
  bone disease related to, 578
  CFTR mutations causing, 14
  clinical course of, 573-574, 573b
  clinical features of, 571, 571b
  complications of, 568-571
  controversies and pitfalls of, 578
  diabetes related to, 577-578
  diagnostic approach to, 571-573, 572f
  gene replacement therapy for, 574
  genetic factors underlying, 7, 8t-9t
  genetics of, 568, 569f
  inflammation in, treatment of, 576
  liver disease in, 577
  lung transplantation for, 888-889
  malignancy in, 578
  pancreatic insufficiency in, 570-571, 576-577
  pathophysiology of, 568-571, 570f
  pharmacotherapy for, 574

Cystic fibrosis (CF) (Continued)
  pneumothorax in, 835
  pregnancy in, 576, 910
  prognosis for, 578
  pulmonary exacerbation in, symptoms and
    signs of, 573b
  therapy of, principles of, 573-574
  treatment of, 574-576
Cystic fibrosis transmembrane regulator
    (CFTR) gene
  in cystic fibrosis, 568, 569f
  mutations of, in bronchiectasis, 580
Cystic hygroma, superior mediastinal masses
    from, 111-112
Cystic lung diseases
  evaluation of patients with, 670-671, 671t
  pneumothorax in, 835
  rare, 667-671
Cystic teratoma, anterior mediastinal masses
    from, 112-113, 113f
Cytokines, in lung host defense, 286, 286t
Cytomegalovirus (CMV) infection
  in hematopoietic stem cell transplantation
    patient, 915
  in HIV patient, 357, 357f
    treatment of, 367-368
  lung transplantation and, 896-897, 897f,
    897t-898t
  in non–HIV-infected immunocompromised
    patient, 337-338, 338f, 339t

D

D-dimer, in acute dyspnea, 254
D-dimer assay, in pulmonary embolism, 696,
    698-699
Dapsone, in Pneumocystis pneumonia
    prophylaxis, 369, 369t
Davenport diagram, 40, 45-46, 46f
  for metabolic acidosis, 47f, 48
  for metabolic alkalosis, 47f, 48
  for respiratory acidosis, 46f, 47
  for respiratory alkalosis, 47f, 48
Daytime sleepiness
  causes of, other than obstructive sleep
    apnea, 745, 745t
  obstructive sleep apnea and, 741, 742b
Dead space, 38
  anatomic, 39
  physiologic, in gas exchange assessment,
    44-45
Deaths, in asthma, beta2-agonists and, 207-208
Debulking, rigid bronchoscopic, 165
Defensins, in lung host defense, 283-284
Demand valve systems, for home oxygen
    therapy in COPD, 560
Dendritic cells, in immune response, 280-281,
    280t
Depression
  central nervous system, respiratory acidosis
    from, 47-48
  chest pain in, 271
  in COPD, 546
Dermatomyositis, 653
  clinical features of, 659-660, 659f
Desensitization, for allergic rhinitis, 481-482
Desquamative interstitial pneumonia (DIP),
    604-605
  characteristics of, 600t
  diagnosis of, 604-605
  histopathologic images of, 601f
  HRCT in, 593, 601f
  physiologic finding in, 604
  prognosis and therapy of, 605

Desquamative interstitial pneumonitis,
    Langerhans cell histiocytosis and, 669
Diabetes
  in COPD, 546
  in cystic fibrosis, 577-578
Diabetic ketoacidosis, metabolic acidosis from,
    48
Diagnostic thoracic surgery, 876-881
  clinical application of, 876-881, 877t
Diaphragm, 51f, 53-54
  actions of, 20f, 53-54, 54f
  dysfunction of, ventilator-induced, 58-59,
    425-426
  fatigue of, 57-58, 58f
  hyperinflation and, 56, 57f
  innervation of, 19
  neuromuscular pathway from motor cortex
    to, 769f
  in normal expiration and inspiration, 53f-54f
  paralysis of, bilateral, 53, 53f
  radiographic anatomy of, 78
  structure and function of, 19
Diaphragmatic breathing, in COPD, 558
Diaphragmatic pacing, bilateral, in spinal cord
    injury, 769
Diet, COPD and, 537
Differential leukocyte count, in pleural fluid,
    822, 822b
Diffuse alveolar damage (DAD)
  in ARDS, 455
  drug-induced, 223t, 235
  in hematopoietic stem cell transplantation
    patients, 916
  in toxic inhalational lung injury, 682, 684f
Diffuse alveolar filling processes, 592
Diffuse alveolar hemorrhage (DAH)
  antiphospholipid syndrome and, 729
  drug-induced, 235-236
  in hematopoietic stem cell transplantation
    patients, 916-917
  idiopathic pulmonary hemosiderosis and, 730
  mitral valve disease and, 729-730
  systemic lupus erythematosus and, 729
  vasculitides causing, 729
Diffuse ground glass infiltration, in pneumonia,
    in non–HIV-infected
    immunocompromised patients, 334, 334f
Diffuse lung disease (DLD)
  bronchoscopic procedures in, 161-162, 162b,
    162t
  classification of, controversies and pitfalls of,
    597-598
  clinical evaluation in, 588-591
  clinical examination in, 591
  clinical history of, 589-591
  diagnostic approach to, 588-598
    blood tests in, 591
    chest radiography in, 591-592
    integrated, 595-597
    pulmonary function tests in, 591
  HRCT in, 70-71, 70f
  incidence and prevalence of, 588, 589t
  infiltrative, as emergency, 934
  longitudinal disease behavior patterns in,
    596, 596t
  optimal diagnosis and regional expertise in,
    controversies and pitfalls of, 598
  rare, 671-674
  smoking-related, 590
  surgical biopsy in, 595
    decision to perform, controversies and
      pitfalls of, 597-598
  treatment of, 597, 665
  underlying causes of, 589, 590t

Diffuse lung shadowing, 92-95, 94f
Diffuse malignant mesothelioma, 784-785
Diffuse panbronchiolitis, cough in, 247
Diffusing capacity (DL) test, 138-139
Diffusion
    in gas exchange, 37
        lung structure and, 37
        mass conservation and, 39-40, 40f
Diffusion limitation, hypoxemia from, 43, 43t
Digital chest radiography, 64-65
Digital clubbing, in bronchiectasis, 582
Digital subtraction pulmonary angiography, 74, 74f
DIP. See Desquamative interstitial pneumonia (DIP).
Dipalmitoyl phosphatidylcholine (DPPC), 24
DIRDs. See Drug-induced respiratory diseases (DIRDs).
Dissecting aortic aneurysm, chest pain in, 270
Disseminated nontuberculous mycobacterial infections
    clinical features of, 400-401
    treatment of, 403-404
Distal intestinal obstruction syndrome, in cystic fibrosis, 577
Distending pressure, 21-22
DLD. See Diffuse lung disease (DLD).
Donor lung
    dysfunction of, primary, 885f, 893t, 894
    management of, 890, 891f-892f
    selection of, 889-890, 889t, 890b
Doppler echocardiography
    in COPD assessment, 550-551
    in peak systolic velocity of lateral tricuspid annulus displacement measurement, 194-196, 195f
    in right ventricular diastolic function assessment, 196, 196f
Doppler monitoring
    transcutaneous, in critical illness, 452-453
    and ultrasound imaging, esophageal, in critical illness, 451-453, 452f
Dorsal respiratory group (DRG) of neurons, 50, 51f
Doxapram, for COPD exacerbations, 565-566
DPPC (dipalmitoyl phosphatidylcholine), 24
Drain tube. See Chest tube; Chest tube entries.
Drainage
    of exudative effusions, 827
    postural, in COPD, 558
Driving pressure, across pulmonary circulation, 29-30, 30f
Drug(s)
    associated with rhinitis, 474b, 475
    as asthma triggers, 499
    causing eosinophilic pneumonia, 623b
    implicated as agents of respiratory injury, 222t
    for inflammatory bowel disease, lung diseases induced by, 934, 934t
    in organizing pneumonia etiology, 632-633, 633b
    pleural effusions induced by, 829
    pulmonary arterial hypertension induced by, 711, 712b
    respiratory presentations of, 769
Drug-induced respiratory diseases (DIRDs), 221-241
    airway involvement in, 237-238
    controversies and pitfalls of, 240
    diagnosis of, 227, 228t, 229b
    drugs/drug families implicated in, 224t-226t
    incidence of, 226-227
    introduction to, 221-223

Drug-induced respiratory diseases (DIRDs) (Continued)
    life-threatening, 231f
    patterns of, 227-240, 230t
        mediastinal, 239-240
        parenchymal, 229-237
        pleural, 238-239, 239f
    risk evaluation for, 226-227
Drug susceptibility testing
    in nontuberculous mycobacterial infections, 402
    in TB diagnosis, 390
Dry powder devices, for bronchodilator delivery, 210
Duchenne muscular dystrophy (DMD)
    respiratory presentations of, 773
    scoliosis in, 756
    surgery for, 760
Dusts, occupational exposure to, COPD and, 536
"Dutch hypothesis," of COPD, 537
Dynamic compression, in respiratory cycle, 25, 25f
Dynamic hyperinflation
    auto-PEEP and, 26, 419-422, 421f-424f
    dyspnea and, 252, 252f
Dysmotility, chest pain in, 269, 271
Dyspnea, 250-260
    acute, 252-256
        biomarkers of, 254
        differential diagnosis of, 252-254, 253t
        initial evaluation of, 252, 252f
        physical examination in, 254
        thoracic imaging in, 254-255
    afferent impulses in, 251, 251f
    central nervous system in, 251, 251f
    chronic, 256-259
        definition of, 256
        diagnostic testing for, 258-259, 258f, 258t-259t
        differential diagnosis of, 256, 257t
        medical history in, 256
        physical examination in, 256-258
        treatment of, 259
    definition of, 250
    language of, 251-252
    in lung cancer, management of, 808
    mechanisms of, 250-251, 251f
    neuromodulation of, by endogenous opioids, 251
    neurophysiologic basis of, 250, 251f
    palliation of, 259
    in pregnancy, 904-905
    sensory receptors in, 250-251, 251f
    treatment of, 255-256, 255t

E

EAA. See Extrinsic allergic alveolitis (EAA).
Echinococcosis, 321
Echocardiography, 193-201
    in acute right-sided heart failure, 198-199, 198f
    in chronic right heart failure, 199
    in critical illness, 453
    Doppler. See Doppler echocardiography.
    in hemodynamic assessment of right heart, 196-197, 197f
    in obesity hypoventilation syndrome, 753
    in peak systolic velocity of lateral tricuspid annulus displacement measurement, 194-196, 195f
    in pericardial constriction, 199-200

Echocardiography (Continued)
    in pericardial effusion and tamponade, 199, 200f
    planes of, right-sided heart structures and, 193, 194t, 195f
    in pulmonary arterial hypertension, 197-198, 717, 717f
    in pulmonary embolism, 699, 700f
    in restrictive cardiomyopathy secondary to chronic respiratory disease, 200-201
    in right ventricular function assessment, 193-196, 195f-196f
    in tricuspid annular plane systolic excursion measurement, 194, 195f
Ectopic ACTH syndrome, in lung cancer, 789-790
Edema
    alveolar, 34, 34f
    high-altitude pulmonary, 34
    hydrostatic, 33
    interstitial, 33-34
    permeability, 33
    pulmonary. See Pulmonary edema.
    rostral fluid shifts and, in obstructive sleep apnea, 739
Effusion
    parapneumonic, complicating community-acquired pneumonia, 306
    pleural, 818-836. See also Pleural effusion(s).
Effusion lymphoma, primary, in HIV patient, 378
Eisenmenger syndrome, 712
Elastase, synthesis and repair of, in COPD, 541-542
Elastic component, of respiratory work, 25-26, 26f
Elastic properties
    of chest wall, 22, 22f, 23t
    of lungs, 22, 22f
    surface tension and, 23-24, 24f
Elastic structures, volumes of, 21-22, 21f
Elderly
    dyspnea in, 250
    obstructive sleep apnea in, 731-734, 733t
Electrocardiography
    in COPD assessment, 550
    in pulmonary arterial hypertension, 715, 715f
    in pulmonary embolism, 697-698, 698f
Electrocautery, endobronchial, 166
Electrophysiologic testing, of respiratory muscle function, 61, 62f
Embolectomy, pulmonary, 704
Embolism
    amniotic fluid, in pregnancy, 905-906, 905f
    pulmonary. See Pulmonary embolism (PE).
Embolization, bronchial artery, 75-76, 75f
Embryonic stage, of lung development, 1, 2t
Emergency respiratory conditions, drug-induced, 223t
EML4/ALK, 786
Emotional extremes, as asthma triggers, 499
Emphysema
    bronchoscopic treatments for, 172
    centrilobular
        cystic air spaces in, 118, 119f
        pathology of, 533-534
    in coal workers, 642, 642f
    CT appearance and clinical characteristics of, 671t
    definition of, 531
    in extrinsic allergic alveolitis, 678t, 679
    in HIV patient, 380-381
    mediastinal, 99-101

Emphysema (Continued)
  oxidative stress in pathogenesis of, 12-13
  panlobular, pathology of, 533-534
  paraseptal, pathology of, 534
  pathology of, 533-534, 535f
  respiratory system pressure-volume curve in, 23
  secondary to cutis laxa, genetic factors underlying, 8t-9t, 14-15, 15f
  secondary to Marfan syndrome, genetic factors underlying, 8t-9t
  secondary to Menkes disease, genetic factors underlying, 8t-9t, 15
  subcutaneous, from chest tube leakage, 866-867
  treatment of, retinoic acid in, controversy over, 17
Empyema, pleural, 826-827, 826f, 826t
Encephalitis, limbic, in lung cancer, manifestations and treatment of, 807t
Encephalomyelitis–subacute sensory neuropathy, in lung cancer, 790
Endobronchial brachytherapy, 166-167
Endobronchial cryotherapy and electrocautery, 166
Endobronchial laser therapy, 165-166
Endobronchial ultrasound (EBUS), diagnostic application of, 876-877
Endobronchial ultrasound (EBUS) techniques, 174-176, 175f
  endoesophageal ultrasound techniques combined with, 177-178, 177f
  for restaging lung cancer patients after chemotherapy, 178
Endoesophageal ultrasound (EUS) techniques, 176-177, 177f
  endobronchial ultrasound techniques combined with, 177-178, 177f
  for restaging lung cancer patients after chemotherapy, 178
Endogenous opioids, in neuromodulation of dyspnea, 251
Endoluminal airway obstruction, therapeutic bronchoscopy for, 168-169, 169t
Endoplasmic reticulum-associated degradation, in α_1-antitrypsin deficiency, autophagy versus, 17
Endoplasmic reticulum overload, as intracellular signal, 13f, 14
Endoplasmic reticulum stress, as intracellular signal, 13-14, 13f
Endothelial cells, in host defense system, 279
Endothelin receptor antagonists, for pulmonary arterial hypertension, 719
Endotracheal intubation, in ICU, 438-441
  awake fiberoptic, 441
  bag mask ventilation in, 438
  confirming, 441
  cricoid pressure in, 439, 439f
  equipment for, 440-441, 440f-441f
  gaseous induction for, 441
  laryngeal anatomy for, 440f-441f, 441
  positioning for, 438, 439f
  preoxygenation in, 439, 439t
  rescue techniques for, 441, 442f
Endotracheal tree, in nosocomial respiratory infections, 322
Endurance training, for ventilatory muscles, in COPD, 558-559
Energy, requirements for, exercise intensity and, 144-145
Energy supply vs. demand, 55, 55f
  load vs. competence and, 56, 56f

Engraftment syndrome, in hematopoietic stem cell transplantation, 917
Enteric cysts, 855
Environmental factors
  in asthma, 496-499
  in community-acquired pneumonia, 297
Eosinophil(s), 620
  in host defense system, 280t, 281, 281f
Eosinophilia
  in Churg-Strauss syndrome, 626
  pulmonary, tropical, 320-321
Eosinophilia syndrome, nonallergic rhinitis with, 474
Eosinophilic bronchitis, 245, 246f
  treatment of, 248
Eosinophilic granulomatosis with polyangiitis, 726. See also Churg-Strauss syndrome (CSS).
Eosinophilic lung disease, 620-628
  clinical classification of, 621b
  controversies and pitfalls of, 628
  parasitic, 621-622
  of unknown origin, 624-628
Eosinophilic pneumonia (EP)
  acute, drug-induced, 223t
  adult, idiopathic, 625-626, 625b, 625f
  chronic, idiopathic, 624-625, 624f, 625b
  in connective tissue diseases, 655
  diagnosis of, 621, 621b
  drug-induced, parenchymal patterns in, 232-233, 232f
  drugs causing, 623b
  histopathologic features of, 620-621
  iatrogenic, 623
  in inflammatory bowel disease, 931
EP. See Eosinophilic pneumonia (EP).
Epidermal growth factor receptor gene (EGFR), 786
Epigenetic regulation, 12
Episodic arthropathy, in cystic fibrosis, 578
Epithelial cells
  airway, 3-4
  alveolar, 4-5, 4f-5f
  bronchial, 2-3
  in host defense system, 278, 278b, 279f
Epithelial neoplasms, benign, 810-811
Epithelial to mesenchyme transition (EMT), from endoplasmic reticulum stress, 14
Epithelium, respiratory, in host defense system, 277, 277t
Epstein-Barr virus (EBV), lung transplantation and, 897-898, 897t
Erdheim-Chester disease, pulmonary manifestations of, 674
Erlotinib, for Stage IV non–small cell lung cancer, 805-806
Erythrocythemia, in COPD assessment, 550
Esophageal reflux, chest pain in, 269, 271
Esophagus
  abnormalities of, imaging in, 98-99, 100f
  carcinoma of, posterior mediastinal masses from, 113
  CT imaging of, 110
  Doppler monitoring and ultrasound imaging of, in critical illness, 451-453, 452f
  rupture of, chest pain in, 271, 271f
Ethambutol, for TB, 391t
Ethionamide, for TB, 392t
Exercise(s)
  as asthma trigger, 499
  capacity for
    impact of adolescent idiopathic scoliosis on, 758
  impaired, 143

Exercise(s) (Continued)
  hemodynamic response to, 146-147
  intensity of, energy requirements and, 144-145
  lower extremity, in COPD, 557
  pulmonary response to
    in healthy humans, 145
    in lung disease, 145-146, 145f
  responses to, in health and disease, 145-147
  upper extremity, in COPD, 557-558
Exercise conditioning, in COPD, 557
Exercise testing, 143-153. See also Cardiopulmonary exercise testing (CPET).
  in COPD assessment, 549-550
Expiration (EXP), 23
Expiratory flow, in COPD assessment, 548-549
Expiratory force, 23, 23f
External intercostal muscles, 53
Extraalveolar vessels, lung volumes and, 30, 30f
Extracellular matrix, maintenance of, 14-15
Extracorporeal membrane oxygenation (ECMO), for refractory hypoxemia in ARDS, 466-467
Extrapulmonary intrathoracic tissues, percutaneous sampling of, 186-188
Extrapulmonary tuberculosis
  clinical features of, 386-387
  treatment of, 394
Extrathoracic lesions, percutaneous biopsy of, 188-191, 189f-190f
Extrinsic allergic alveolitis (EAA), 676-681. See also Hypersensitivity pneumonitis.
  antigens causing, categories of, 677t
  BAL in, 679
  clinical features of, 677
  diagnosis of, clinical prediction rule for, 677t
  diagnostic testing for, 679-680, 680f
  histopathology of, 679-680, 680f
  imaging in, 677-679, 678f, 678t
  immunopathogenesis of, 680
  incidence of, 676
  laboratory studies for, 679
  prognosis for, 680-681
  pulmonary physiology of, 679
  risk factors for, 676
  serum precipitins for, 679
  treatment of, 680
    controversies and pitfalls of, 681
Exudate/transudate separation, in pleural effusions, 821-822
Exudative effusions, 818
  antibiotics for, 827
  bacteriology of, 827
  conditions associated with, 826-827, 826f, 826t
  drainage of, 827
  parapneumonic, 826-827, 826t
Eyes
  corticosteroid toxicities affecting, 217t
  sarcoidosis involving, 612-613, 614f

F

^{18}F-fluorodeoxyglucose (FDG), in PET imaging, 122
Fabry disease, pulmonary manifestations of, 674
Factor V Leiden, inherited thrombophilia from, 691t, 692
Factor VIII elevation, inherited thrombophilia from, 691t, 692
Factor Xa inhibitors, for pulmonary embolism, 702-703

FAM13A, in COPD, 11-12
Familial pneumothorax, genetic factors underlying, 8t-9t
Family structure, childhood asthma and, 497
Farmer's lung, 676. *See also* Extrinsic allergic alveolitis (EAA).
Fascioscapulohumeral muscular dystrophy, respiratory presentations of, 773
Fat embolism syndrome, 706
Fatigue, respiratory muscle, 57-58, 57f-58f
FDG. *See* ¹⁸F-fluorodeoxyglucose (FDG).
Fenoterol
    chemical structure of, 205f
    formulations, doses and duration of action of, 207t
Fever, complicating bronchoscopy, 163
Feyrter cells, 4
Fibered confocal fluorescence microscopy (FCFM), 165
Fiberoptic bronchoscopy (FOB)
    with bronchoalveolar lavage, in organizing pneumonia diagnosis, 633-634
    in hemoptysis, 264-265, 265f
    in sarcoidosis, 615, 616f
Fibroblasts
    in host defense system, 279
    in organizing pneumonia, 629, 630f
Fibrocavitary disease, 399, 399f
Fibromyalgia, chest pain in, 270, 271f
Fibrosing alveolitis
    cryptogenic, classification of, 588
    HRCT in, 71
Fibrothorax, 830
Fibrotic nonspecific interstitial pneumonia, 603-604
Fick principle, 40
Filtering, by pulmonary circulation, 32-33
Fine needle aspiration (FNA)
    with endoesophageal ultrasound, 176-177
    needles for, 181-182, 182f
    percutaneous, in pneumonia pathogen identification, 294
Finger clubbing, in bronchiectasis, 582
Fissures
    interlobar, displacement of, in lobar collapse, 84
    radiographic anatomy of, 78, 78f
Fistulas
    bronchial, therapeutic bronchoscopy for, 171-172
    bronchopleural, complicating community-acquired pneumonia, 306-307
Flexible bronchoscopy, 154, 155f
    diagnostic application of, 876
Flow. *See also* Airflow.
Flow-cycled ventilation, 407, 407f
Flow resistance, 24-25, 25f-26f
Flow-volume curve(s)
    expiratory
        in central airway obstruction, 140, 140f
        in chronic airflow obstruction, 140, 140f
        normal, 133, 134f
    forced vital capacity maneuver and, 25, 26f
Flow-volume loop
    in Parkinson disease, 770, 770f
    in upper airway obstruction, 141, 141f, 258, 258f
Fluid exchange, in pulmonary circulation, 33-34, 33t, 34f
Fluid flux, 33
Fluid management, in ARDS, 468-469
Fluid shifts, rostral, edema and, in obstructive sleep apnea, 739
Fluoroscopy, in bronchoscopy, 156-157

Fluticasone, with salmeterol
    for COPD, 555t, 556
    and tiotropium for COPD, 555t, 556
FOB. *See* Fiberoptic bronchoscopy (FOB).
Follicular bronchiolitis, in connective tissue diseases, 655
Follicular bronchitis, in connective tissue diseases, 655
Food allergens, as asthma triggers, 499
Food-induced rhinitis, 475
Force-frequency curve, of diaphragm, 61, 62f
Forced expiratory flow rate between 25% and 75% (FEF$_{25-75}$), 134
Forced expiratory volume at 1 second (FEV$_1$), cigarette smoking and, 535, 536f
Forced expiratory volume at 1 second to forced vital capacity ratio (FEV$_1$/FVC), in mixed obstruction and restriction, 138
Forced expiratory volume in 6 seconds (FEV$_6$), 134
Forced expiratory volume maneuver, in spirometry, 133, 134f
Forced vital capacity (FVC), maneuver generating, in tests, 25, 26f
Foregut cysts, 855
Foreign body removal, therapeutic bronchoscopy for, 170-171
Formoterol
    chemical structure of, 205f
    formulations, doses and duration of action of, 207t
    with tiotropium, for COPD, 555t, 556
Formoterol fumarate, for COPD, 555, 555t
Foscarnet, for viral lung infections, 339t
Francisella tularensis, in community-acquired pneumonia, 301
FRC. *See* Functional residual capacity (FRC).
Frictional component, of respiratory work, 25-26, 26f
Friedländer's pneumonia, 300
Functional endoscopic sinus surgery (FESS), 482
Functional residual capacity (FRC), 21, 21f
    in obstructive lung disease, 138, 138f
    pressure/force balance and, 22, 22f
    in restrictive lung disease, 138
Fungal infections
    in hematopoietic stem cell transplantation patients, 914-915
    in HIV patient, 355-357
        treatment of, 366-367, 367t
    pleural effusions in, 828
Fungal pneumonias, 315-319, 316f, 317t
    aspergillosis as, 315, 316f, 317t
    blastomycosis as, 316-318, 316f, 317t, 318f
    coccidioidomycosis as, 316f, 317t, 318, 318f
    histoplasmosis as, 315-316, 316f, 317t, 318f
    paracoccidioidomycosis as, 318-319
FVC. *See* Forced vital capacity (FVC).

G

Ganciclovir, for viral lung infections, 339t
Ganglioneuroblastomas, 859
Ganglioneuromas, 858, 858f
Gas distribution, tests of, 139-140, 139f
Gas exchange, 37-49
    acid-base relationships and, 45-48
    basis of, 37-45
    for carbon monoxide, in COPD assessment, 549
    clinical application of, pitfalls in, 48
    clinical assessment of, 44-45
    compensatory mechanisms in, 43-44

Gas exchange *(Continued)*
    in COPD, 544
    in homogeneous lung, 38-40
    pulmonary, in COPD, 544
    ventilation-perfusion inequality and, 42-43, 42f
Gastric acid aspiration, in pregnancy, 910
Gastroesophageal reflux, cough associated with, 247
    treatment of, 248
Gastroesophageal reflux disease (GERD)
    asthma and, 499-500
    in COPD, 546
Gastrointestinal system. *See also* Inflammatory bowel disease (IBD).
    complications of cystic fibrosis involving, 577
    corticosteroid toxicities affecting, 217t
    disorders of
        chest pain in, 271, 271f
        in cystic fibrosis, 571
    sarcoidosis involving, 614
Gastrointestinal tuberculosis, 388
Gaucher disease, pulmonary manifestations of, 674
Gefitinib, for Stage IV non–small cell lung cancer, 805-806
Gender
    asthma and, 496
    dyspnea and, 250
    obstructive sleep apnea and, 734
Genetic diseases, complex, gene hunting for, 10-12
Genetic factors
    in COPD, 537-538, 537b, 537t
    in lung disease, 7, 8t-9t
    in sarcoidosis, 607, 608t
Genetics
    air pollution responses and, 941-942
    of allergic rhinitis, 471
    of ARDS, 457-458
    of asbestosis, 648
    of asthma, 496, 505
    of coal worker's pneumoconiosis, 638
    of cystic fibrosis, 568, 569f
    of extrinsic allergic alveolitis, 676
    of inflammatory bowel disease, 927
    of Kaposi sarcoma, 375
    of nontuberculous mycobacteria, 399
    of obstructive sleep apnea, 734
    pulmonary complications of hematopoietic stem cell transplantation and, 913-914
    of scoliosis, 756
    of tuberculosis, 385
Genitourinary tuberculosis, 387
Genome-wide association studies, 11
Genotyping, in cystic fibrosis diagnosis, 571, 572f
Germ cell neoplasms
    anterior mediastinal masses from, 112-113
    mediastinal, 852
        nonseminomatous, malignant, 853
Gestational trophoblastic disease, 907
Giant cell arteritis, 727
Glomangioma, 812-813
Glomangiomyoma, 812-813
Glomus tumor, 812-813, 813f
Glottis, in pulmonary host defense system, 276-277
(1-3)-β-D-glucan, serum levels of, in diagnosis of HIV-related pneumonia, 360, 360t
Glucocorticoids
    adjuvant, for bacterial pneumonia, 363
    for COPD, 556

Glucose and pH levels, of pleural fluid, 822, 822b
Glycopyrrolate, chemical structure of, 205f
Goblet cells, 2-3
Goiter, intrathoracic, 854, 855f
Goodpasture syndrome, 729
GPA. *See* Granulomatosis with polyangiitis (GPA).
Graft-*versus*-host disease, in hematopoietic stem cell transplantation, 912
Gram-negative bacilli, in community-acquired pneumonia, 299-300
Granuloma(s)
    liver, in sarcoidosis, 614, 614f
    nasal involvement in, 475
    treatment of, 483
Granulomatosis
    bronchocentric, 624
    eosinophilic, with polyangiitis, 726. *See also* Churg-Strauss syndrome (CSS).
    with polyangiitis (GPA), 722-726
        clinical presentation of, 723
        definition and nomenclature of, 722-723
        diagnostic evaluation of, 723
        etiology and pathogenesis of, 723
        large airway involvement in, therapy for, 725
        refractory, therapy for, 725
        therapy for, 723-726, 724t
            complications of, 725-726
        Wegener, with microscopic polyangiitis, therapy for, 725
Granulomatous arteritis, 727
Granulomatous infiltrative lung disease, drug-induced, parenchymal patterns in, 233
Gravitational effect, on blood flow distribution, 30-31
    controversies and pitfalls related to, 35-36
Great vessels
    dilatation of, radiography of, 99, 101f
    in mediastinal anatomy, 107-108, 109f-110f
    mediastinal anatomy at, 78
Ground-glass attenuation, in nonspecific interstitial pneumonia, 592-593, 593f
Ground glass infiltration, diffuse, in pneumonia, in non–HIV-infected immunocompromised patients, 334, 334f
Ground glass opacification, 71, 71f
    causes of, 71b, 117
    and consolidation, 81, 82f
    in extrinsic allergic alveolitis, 678, 678t
    on HRCT, lung density and, 117-118, 117f-118f
Ground glass shadowing, 95
Guillain-Barré syndrome, respiratory presentations of, 771
Gustatory rhinitis, 475

H

Haemophilus influenzae
    in community-acquired pneumonia, 299
    in cystic fibrosis lung disease, 574-575, 575t
Hamartoma, 813, 814f
    mesenchymal, multiple cystic, 670-671
Haplotype, 11
Hay fever. *See also* Allergic rhinitis.
    global prevalence of, 471, 472f
Headache, morning, in obstructive sleep apnea, 741-742
Health status, in COPD assessment, 550

Heart
    catheterization of, right-sided, in pulmonary arterial hypertension, 717-718
    right, hemodynamic assessment of, echocardiographic, 196-197, 197f
    right-sided structures of, 193, 194t, 195f
    sarcoidosis involving, 614
Heart disease
    congenital, pulmonary arterial hypertension and, 712
    left-sided, pulmonary hypertension due to, 713
Heart failure, right-sided
    acute, echocardiographic evaluation of, 198-199, 198f
    chronic, echocardiographic evaluation of, 199
Helium dilution, in lung volume measurement, 136, 136f
Hemangioma, sclerosing, 813
Hematopoietic stem cell transplantation (HSCT)
    bronchiolitis obliterans in, 917
    conditioning regimens for, 912
    cryptogenic organizing pneumonia in, 918
    delayed pulmonary toxicity syndrome in, 917
    diffuse alveolar damage in, 916
    diffuse alveolar hemorrhage in, 916-917
    engraftment syndrome in, 917
    idiopathic pneumonia syndrome in, 916
    indications for, 912
    interstitial lung disease in, 917
    interstitial pneumonitis in, 917
    lymphoproliferative disorder after, 918
    malignancy after, 918
    overview of, 912
    pulmonary alveolar proteinosis after, 918
    pulmonary complications of, 330-331, 912-919
        bacterial pneumonia as, 914
        controversies and pitfalls of, 919
        diagnostic evaluation of, 918-919
        early postengraftment, 914
        fungal, 914-915
        genetics and, 913-914
        imaging patterns in, 918
        infectious, 914-916, 914b
        late postengraftment, 914
        noninfectious, 916-918
        preengraftment, 914
        pulmonary function tests in, 918
        risk factors for, 913, 913b
        serologic studies in, 918-919
        time course of, 914
        viral, 915-916
    pulmonary cytolytic thrombi after, 918
    pulmonary edema in, 916
    pulmonary toxicity in, 916
    pulmonary venoocclusive disease in, 917-918
    respiratory failure after, 918
    types of, 912
Hematoporphyrin derivatives (Photofrin), in photodynamic therapy, 167
Hemidiaphragm elevation, in lobar collapse, 84
Hemodynamic assessment, of right heart, echocardiographic, 196-197, 197f
Hemodynamic monitoring, in critical illness, 445-453
    arterial pressure monitoring in, 445-446, 446b, 446f
    arterial waveform analysis in, 449-451, 451b, 451f

Hemodynamic monitoring, in critical illness *(Continued)*
    central venous catheterization in, 446-447, 447b
    circulation model for, 445
    devices for, 445-449
    esophageal Doppler monitoring and ultrasound imaging in, 451-453, 452f
    pulmonary artery catheterization in, 447-448, 447b, 447f-448f, 449b, 449t, 450f
Hemodynamic response, to exercise, 146-147
Hemodynamics, pulmonary and cardiac, in scoliosis, 758
Hemolytic anemia, pulmonary arterial hypertension and, 712
Hemolytic dyscrasias, in lung cancer, 790
Hemoptysis, 261-266
    bronchial artery embolization for, 75-76, 75f
    in bronchiectasis, 581-582, 586
    bronchoscopy in, 158
    causes of, 261-262, 262b, 262f, 262t
    computed tomography in, 263-265, 264f
    control of, therapeutic bronchoscopy in, 170, 170b, 171f
    cryptogenic, 262
    in cystic fibrosis, 577
    definition of, 261
    diagnostic algorithm for, 265, 265f
    differential diagnosis of, 261-262
    fiberoptic bronchoscopy in, 264-265, 265f
    in lung cancer, management of, 808
    massive, 261, 265-266
    patient evaluation in, 262-265
Hemorrhage
    alveolar, 728-730. *See also* Diffuse alveolar hemorrhage (DAH).
        after bone marrow transplantation, 730
        in connective tissue diseases, 655
        diffuse. *See also* Diffuse alveolar hemorrhage (DAH).
        toxic, 730
    complicating bronchoscopy, 163
    complicating needle biopsy, 185, 185f, 185t
    mediastinal, 861
Hemorrhagic telangiectasia, hereditary, genetic factors underlying, 8t-9t
Hemosiderosis, pulmonary, idiopathic, diffuse alveolar hemorrhage and, 730
Hemothorax
    massive, drug-induced, 223t
    pleural effusions related to, 829
Henderson-Hasselbalch equation, 45-46, 45f-46f
Henoch-Schönlein purpura, 728
Heparin, for pulmonary embolism, 702
Heparin-induced thrombocytopenia, venous thromboembolism and, 694-695
Hepatic hydrothorax
    clinical features of, 921
    diagnosis of, 923
    pathophysiology of, 920
    transudative effusions in, 825-826
    treatment of, 925
Hepatopulmonary syndrome (HPS), 920
    clinical course of, 925, 925f
    clinical features of, 921
    diagnosis of, 921, 923f
    pathophysiology of, 920, 922f
    risk factors for, 920
    treatment of, 924
Hereditary hemorrhagic telangiectasia, genetic factors underlying, 8t-9t

Hereditary motor and sensory neuropathy, respiratory presentations of, 772
Hermansky-Pudlak syndrome, pulmonary manifestations of, 674
Hernia(s)
hiatal, 857
Morgagni, 857
Herpes simplex virus (HSV) infection, in non–HIV-infected immunocompromised patients, 338
Hiatal hernias, 857
High-altitude pulmonary edema (HAPE), 34
High-frequency fatigue, respiratory muscle, 57-58, 57f
High-frequency oscillatory ventilation (HFOV), for refractory hypoxemia in ARDS, 467
High-resolution computed tomography (HRCT), 68-72
in asbestosis, 649, 649f
in bronchiectasis diagnosis, 582
clinical applications of, 64f, 70-72, 70f-71f, 71b
in connective tissue diseases, 663, 663f-664f, 663t
in cryptogenic organizing pneumonia, 631f-632f, 632b
in diffuse lung disease diagnosis, 592-594, 593b, 593f-594f
in extrinsic allergic alveolitis, 678, 678f, 678t
in idiopathic interstitial lung diseases, 601, 601f
indications for, 72b
interpretation of, 114-121
in Langerhans cell histiocytosis, 669, 669f
in sarcoidosis, 611
technical considerations for, 68-70, 69f-70f
Hilar convergence sign, 101
Hilar lymphadenopathy, 592
Hilum
abnormalities of, imaging of, 101-102, 101f-102f
anatomy of
CT, 108
radiographic, 77
displacement of, in lobar collapse, 84
lesions of, percutaneous sampling of, 187
Histatins, in lung host defense, 284
Histiocytosis, Langerhans cell, 668-670
cystic air spaces in, 118f, 119
HRCT in, 593
Histoplasmosis, 315-316, 316f, 317t, 318f
in HIV patient, 356-357, 356f
treatment of, 367, 367t
HIV. See Human immunodeficiency virus (HIV) entries.
HIV-1-associated pulmonary hypertension, 381
Hodgkin disease, 850-851
anterior mediastinal masses from, 113
imaging of, 850f-851f
Home oxygen therapy, in COPD, 559-560
Honeycomb change, in extrinsic allergic alveolitis, 678f, 679
Hormonal rhinitis, 475
Hormone replacement therapy, venous thromboembolism and, 694
Host defenses, 275-287. See also Pulmonary host defense system.
Host factors, in COPD, 536-538
Hot tub lung, 680
HPS. See Hepatopulmonary syndrome (HPS).
HRCT. See High-resolution computed tomography (HRCT).

HSCT. See Hematopoietic stem cell transplantation (HSCT).
Human immunodeficiency virus (HIV) disease. See also Acquired immunodeficiency syndrome (AIDS).
acute primary, 348
aging patient with, pulmonary disease in, 382
antiretroviral therapy in. See Antiretroviral therapy (ART).
background on, 346
bronchoscopy in, 159
CDC classification of, 348t
chronic, 349
chronic rhinosinusitis and, 477
epidemiology of, 346-350, 347f
inflammatory pulmonary disorders in, 379-381, 379f
natural history of, 347-349
neoplasia in, 374-379
noninfectious conditions in, 374-382
predictors of disease in, 372
prognostic markers for, 349
pulmonary function in, 374
pulmonary immune response during, 349-350
pulmonary infections in, 346-373
bacterial, 350-351
controversies and pitfalls of, 372
prognosis of, 371
prophylaxis of, 368-370, 369t
treatment of, 347
clinical course and prevention of, 368-371, 369t
clinical features of, 350-358
diagnosis of, 358-361, 358b
etiologic agents in related infections, 347b
fungal, 355-357, 356f
treatment of, 366-367, 367t
mycobacterial, 351-355
controversies and pitfalls of, 372-373
prognosis of, 371, 371b
prophylaxis of, 370-371
treatment of, 364-366
parasitic, treatment of, 367, 368t
protozoal, 358, 358f
risk factors for, 350
treatment of, 361-368
tuberculosis as, 351-353, 352f-353f, 352t, 394
viral, 357, 357f, 367-368
respiratory symptoms in, 374
virology and immunology of, 346-347
Human metapneumovirus infection
in hematopoietic stem cell transplantation patient, 916
in non–HIV-infected immunocompromised patients, 340
Hunter syndrome, pulmonary manifestations of, 674
Hurler disease, pulmonary manifestations of, 674
Hydrofluoric acid, as irritant, 683t, 684-685
Hydrogen chloride, as irritant, 683t, 684
Hydrogen cyanide, as asphyxiant, 683t, 686
Hydrogen sulfide, as asphyxiant, 683t, 686-687
Hydropneumothorax, radiographic features of, 105f
Hydrostatic edema, 33
Hydrothorax, hepatic. See Hepatic hydrothorax.
transudative effusions in, 825-826
Hydroxychloroquine, for sarcoidosis, 617-618, 617t

Hygiene hypothesis, for asthma, 497, 499
Hyper-IgE, genetic factors underlying, 8t-9t
Hyperacute rejection (HAR), in lung transplantation, 892, 893t
Hypercalcemia
in lung cancer, manifestations and treatment of, 807t
of malignancy, 789-790
Hypercapnic ventilatory response, 52
Hypercoagulability, in lung cancer, 790
Hypercoagulability testing, for inherited thrombophilia, 693
Hypereosinophilic asthma, 623-624
Hypereosinophilic syndromes (HES), idiopathic, 627-628
Hyperhomocysteinemia, inherited thrombophilia from, 691t, 692-693
Hyperinflation
compensatory, in lobar collapse, 84
in COPD, 542-544, 543f
dynamic
auto-PEEP and, 26
dyspnea and, 252, 252f
effect on diaphragm, 56, 57f
in lung transplantation, 894-895, 896f
Hypersensitivity pneumonitis. See also Extrinsic allergic alveolitis (EAA).
causes of, 589-590
subacute, HRCT in, 70-71, 71f, 593, 594f
Hypertension
portal, 712
pulmonary consequences of, 921t
portopulmonary, 712, 920. See also Portopulmonary hypertension (POPH).
pulmonary. See Pulmonary hypertension.
pulmonary arterial, 710. See also Pulmonary arterial hypertension (PAH).
Hypertonic saline, in cystic fibrosis therapy, 574
Hypertransradiancy, 88, 89f-90f
Hypertrophic pulmonary osteoarthropathy (HPO)
in cystic fibrosis, 578
in lung cancer, 790
Hyperventilation
for hypoxemia, 43-44
respiratory alkalosis from, 48
Hypogammaglobulinemia, bronchiectasis from, 582
Hypoventilation
hypoxemia from, 43, 43t
nocturnal, in chest wall disease, 768
Hypoxemia
causes of, 43, 43t
compensatory mechanisms for, 43-44
in COPD exacerbations, 564-565
refractory, in ARDS, rescue strategies for, 466-468
Hypoxia
patients with, noninvasive ventilation in, 433
protein misfolding and, 14
pulmonary hypertension due to, 713
Hypoxic ventilatory response, 52

I

IBD. See Inflammatory bowel disease (IBD).
IC. See Inspiratory capacity (IC).
ICU. See Intensive care unit (ICU).
Idiopathic pneumonia syndrome (IPS), in hematopoietic stem cell transplantation patients, 916

Idiopathic pulmonary fibrosis (IPF), 599-603
  acute exacerbations of, 602
  characteristics of, 600t
  comorbidities of, 602
  diagnosis of, 599
    algorithm for, 602f
    criteria for, 602
  genetic factors underlying, 16
  HRCT in, 593, 593f
  lung transplantation for, 888
  mortality rates for, 602, 602f
  natural history of, 602-603, 603f
  pulmonary hypertension in, 602
  risk factors for, 599
  treatment of, 603
ILDs. See Interstitial lung diseases (ILDs).
Imaging techniques, 63-121
  bronchial artery embolization as, 75-76, 75f
  computed tomography as, 65-68. See also
    Computed tomography (CT).
  in COPD assessment, 551
  magnetic resonance angiography as, 73, 74f
  magnetic resonance imaging as, 72. See also
    Magnetic resonance imaging (MRI).
  in malignant pleural mesothelioma, 840-841,
    840f-841f
  plain chest radiography as, 63-65. See also
    Chest radiography, plain.
  positron emission tomography as, 122-132.
    See also Positron emission tomography
    (PET).
  pulmonary angiography as, 74-75, 74f
  superior vena cava stenting as, 76, 76f
  in upper airway disease diagnosis, 479, 479f
Immune cells, in host defense system, 279-282,
  280t
Immune defects, in chronic rhinosinusitis, 477
Immune receptors, innate, 284-286, 284t,
  285f
Immune reconstitution inflammatory
  syndrome (IRIS), in HIV patient with TB,
  365-366, 366b
Immune response
  adaptive, 275, 276f
  innate, 275, 276f
  pulmonary, during HIV infection, 349-350
Immunity
  airway mucosal, disordered, in asthma, 502
  altered, community-acquired pneumonia
    and, 297
  cell-mediated, defects in, pathogens
    associated with, 330, 332t
Immunocompromise, severe, diseases and
  conditions associated with, 331b
Immunocompromised patients
  non–HIV-infected, pneumonia in, 330-345.
    See also Non–HIV-infected
    immunocompromised patients,
    pneumonia in.
  pulmonary infections in
    bronchoscopy in, 159
    diagnostic approach to, 295f
    microbial etiology prediction in, 293t
    respiratory failure in, noninvasive mechanical
      ventilation for, 433
  viral pneumonia in, 309
Immunodeficiency, degree of, noninfectious
  pulmonary conditions and, 375t
Immunoglobulin A (IgA), absence of, chronic
  rhinosinusitis in, 477
Immunoglobulin E (IgE), immunologic
  occupational asthma mediated by, 523
Immunoglobulins, in bronchiectasis diagnosis,
  582-583

Immunologic system, corticosteroid toxicities
  affecting, 217t
Immunopathogenesis, of extrinsic allergic
  alveolitis, 680
Immunosuppression, for lung transplantation,
  899-900, 901t
  pitfalls of, 900-901
Immunotherapy
  for allergic rhinitis, 481-482
  for malignant pleural mesothelioma, 844
Impaired exercise capacity
  definition of, 143
  identification of, exercise testing in, 143
Indacaterol
  for COPD, 555
  formulations, doses and duration of action
    of, 207t
Industrial bronchitis, 640
Infarction, pulmonary, MRA and, 73
Infection(s). See also Pulmonary infections.
  airway, in cystic fibrosis, treatment of,
    574-576, 575t
  asthma and, 499
  childhood asthma and, 497-498
  complicating bronchoscopy, 154
  COPD exacerbations and, 562, 563b
  lower respiratory tract, in pregnancy, 909
  opportunistic. See Opportunistic
    infection(s).
Infectious agents, associated with organizing
  pneumonia (OP), 632, 633b
Infectious pneumonia, nonbacterial, 315-321
Inferior vena cava filters, in pulmonary
  embolism prevention, 706, 707f
Infertility, in cystic fibrosis, 571-573
  management of, 576
Infiltrative lung disease
  diffuse, as emergency, 934
  granulomatous, drug-induced, parenchymal
    patterns in, 233
Inflammation
  air space, in COPD, 540
  in cystic fibrosis, 570
    treatment of, 576
  drugs for, 213-220. See also
    Antiinflammatory drugs.
  respiratory muscle, 50
  systemic, COPD exacerbations and, 562
  upper airway, obstructive sleep apnea and,
    739
Inflammatory agents, inhalational injury from,
  687-688
Inflammatory bowel disease (IBD), 927-936
  air space disease in, 931, 932f
  airway disease in, 928-931, 931f-932f
  clinical and pathologic features of, 928-934,
    929t-930t
  drug-induced lung disease in, 934, 934t
  epidemiology of, 927-928
  interstitial lung disease in, 931, 933f
  masses and nodules in, 931-934, 933f
  mediastinal disease in, 934
  rare manifestations of, 934
  serosal disease in, 934
  thoracic involvement in, 927, 929t-930t
    controversies and pitfalls of, 935
    emergencies in, 934-935
    treatment of, 934-935
Inflammatory cells, in airway inflammation in
  asthma, 489-490
Inflammatory mediators
  in airway inflammation in asthma, 490-491
  in COPD, 540b
  in lung host defense, 286-287, 286t

Inflammatory myofibroblastic tumor, 811-812,
  812f
Inflammatory pulmonary disorders, in HIV
  patient, 379-381
Inflammometry, for asthma, 513-514, 514f
Infliximab, for ANCA-associated vasculitis, 725
Influenza
  bacterial pneumonia in, pathogenesis of,
    310-311
  pneumonia in, 310
  viral pneumonia related to, primary, 311
Influenza A, in HIV patient, 357, 357f
  prophylaxis of, 370
  treatment of, 368
Influenza virus infection
  in hematopoietic stem cell transplantation
    patients, 916
  in non–HIV-infected immunocompromised
    patients, 340
Inhalational fume fever, 687
Inhalational toxins
  exposure sources for, 682-683
  toxicity range for, 683t
Inherited thrombophilia
  from activated protein C resistance, 692
  from antithrombin deficiency, 690-691, 691t
  from factor V Leiden, 691t, 692
  from factor VIII elevation, 691t, 692
  hypercoagulability testing for, 693
  from hyperhomocysteinemia, 691t, 692-693
  management of, 693
  from protein C deficiency, 691, 691t
  from protein S deficiency, 691-692, 691t
  from prothrombin gene mutation, 691t, 692
  screening for, 693
Injury, respiratory muscle, 50
Innate immune receptors, 284-286, 284t, 285f
Insomnia, obstructive sleep apnea and, 741
Inspiration (INS), 23
Inspiratory capacity (IC), 21, 21f
Inspiratory force, 23, 23f
Inspiratory load, neuromuscular competence
  vs., 55, 55f
  energy supply vs. demand and, 56, 56f
Institutionalization, community-acquired
  pneumonia and, 297
Intensive care unit (ICU)
  airway management in, 437-444
    airway assessment for, 437-438, 438b,
      438f, 438t
    controversies and pitfalls of, 443-444
    drugs used in, 439t
    endotracheal intubation and muscle
      relaxation in, 438-441, 439f-444f,
      439t, 443b. See also Endotracheal
      intubation, in ICU.
    noninvasive ventilation in, 437
  airway support in, indications for, 437
Intercostal muscles, 51f, 53
  action of, 20f
  innervation of, 19
Interferon-γ release assays (IGRAs), 389,
  395-396
Internal intercostal muscles, 53
Interstitial edema, 33-34
Interstitial fibrosis, in connective tissue
  diseases, 654
Interstitial lung diseases (ILDs), 599-606
  acute cellular, drug-induced, 223t
  comparison of, 600t
  controversies and pitfalls of, 605
  diffuse, rare, 667-675
  drug-induced, 222
  as emergency, 935

Interstitial lung diseases (ILDs) (Continued)
exercise in
hemodynamic response to, 146-147
lung response to, 146
genetic factors underlying, 8t-9t
in hematopoietic stem cell transplantation, 917
HRCT and histopathologic images of, 601f
idiopathic pulmonary fibrosis as, 599-603.
See also Idiopathic pulmonary fibrosis (IPF).
in inflammatory bowel disease, 931
in pregnancy, 910
respiratory bronchiolitis, 604. See also Respiratory bronchiolitis interstitial lung disease (RBILD).
Interstitial pneumonia(s)
acute
characteristics of, 600t
diagnosis of, 605
HRCT in, 593
imaging in, 605
prognosis and therapy of, 605
in connective tissue diseases, 655, 656t
desquamative, 604-605. See also Desquamative interstitial pneumonia (DIP).
idiopathic, 596t
lymphoid, 605. See also Lymphoid interstitial pneumonia (LIP).
nonspecific. See Nonspecific interstitial pneumonia (NSIP).
in polymyositis/dermatomyositis, 659-660, 659f
in rheumatoid arthritis, 656-657, 657f-658f
in systemic sclerosis, 653, 658-659, 658f
unusual, histopathologic pattern diagnosis of, 599
Interstitial pneumonitis
desquamative, Langerhans cell histiocytosis and, 669
drug-induced, parenchymal patterns in, 229-231, 230f
in hematopoietic stem cell transplantation, 917
lymphocytic, in HIV patient, 380
nonspecific, in HIV patient, 379-380, 379f
Interstitial pressure, surface tension and, 33
Intraalveolar bud formation, in organizing pneumonia, 629, 630f
Intraparenchymal bronchi, structure and function of, 20
Intrapulmonary lesions, percutaneous biopsy for, 182-186
Intrathoracic goiter, 854, 855f
Intrinsic rhinitis, treatment of, 482
Intubation
difficult, predictors of, 437-438, 438f
endotracheal. See Endotracheal intubation.
Intussusception, in cystic fibrosis, 577
Invasive arterial pressure monitoring, 446
Invasive mechanical ventilation, 406-430
complications of, 422
controversies and pitfalls of, 430
for COPD exacerbations, 565
modes of, 406-407, 407f
combined, 415-416, 415f-416f
delivering assistance to spontaneous breathing, 409-415, 410f-414f
facilitating spontaneous breathing, 416-418, 417f, 417t
targeting volume or pressure, 407-409, 408f-409f
in obstructive airway disease, 418-419

Invasive mechanical ventilation (Continued)
weaning from, 428-429, 429f
failure of, 429-430
Invasive pulmonary aspergillosis (IPA), in non–HIV-infected immunocompromised patients, 340-343, 341f-342f, 342t-343t
Ipatroprium, with albuterol for COPD, 556
IPF. See Idiopathic pulmonary fibrosis (IPF).
Ipratropium, chemical structure of, 205f
Ipratropium bromide
for COPD, 555, 555t
formulations, doses and duration of action of, 207t
IRIS (immune reconstitution inflammatory syndrome), in HIV patient with TB, 365-366, 366b
Irregular emphysema, in coal workers, 642
Irritant receptors, 51f, 52
Isoniazid, for TB, 391t
latent, 396t
Itraconazole, for invasive aspergillosis, 343t
IVIG, for viral lung infections, 339t

J

J receptors, 52
Job's syndrome, genetic factors underlying, 8t-9t
Joint and bone tuberculosis, 387
Joint infections, nontuberculous mycobacterial, treatment of, 403

K

Kanamycin, for TB, 392t
Kaposi sarcoma, in HIV patient, 374-377
clinical course and prevention of, 377
clinical features of, 375, 376f
diagnosis of, 375-376
epidemiology, 374-375
genetics of, 375
pathogenesis of, 374-375
risk factors for, 374-375
treatment of, 376
Kidneys, in acid-base relationships, 45
Kohn, pores of, 4, 4f
KRAS oncogene, 786
Kulchitsky cells, 4
Kyphosis, 757
definition of, 756

L

Lactate dehydrogenase (LDH), in diagnosis of HIV-related pneumonia, 359
Lactate threshold, in exercise testing, 144, 144f
Lactation, tuberculosis treatment during, 394, 397
Lactic acidosis, metabolic acidosis from, 48
Lactoferrin, in airway surface liquid, 282-283, 282t
LAM. See Lymphangioleiomyomatosis (LAM).
Lambert-Eaton myasthenic syndrome (LEMS)
in lung cancer, 790
manifestations and treatment of, 807t
respiratory presentations of, 772
Lamellar bodies, in Type II epithelial cells, 5, 5f, 24
Langerhans cell histiocytosis (LCH), 668-670
CT appearance and clinical characteristics of, 671t
cystic air spaces in, 118f, 119
diagnosis of, 669, 669f

Langerhans cell histiocytosis (LCH) (Continued)
histopathology of, 669, 669f
HRCT in, 593
management of, 669-670
pneumothorax in, 669, 835
Laplace's law, 24
Large cell carcinoma, of lung, 784, 784f
Laryngeal amyloid, 673
Laryngeal mask airway (LMA), in difficult intubation in ICU, 441, 443f
Larynx
anatomy of, for endotracheal intubation in ICU, 440f-441f, 441
structure and function of, 19-20
Laser therapy, endobronchial, 165-166
LCH. See Langerhans cell histiocytosis (LCH).
Legionella pneumophila, in community-acquired pneumonia, 299
Leiomyoma, 814, 815f
Leishmaniasis, in HIV patient, 358
treatment of, 367, 368t
LEMS. See Lambert-Eaton myasthenic syndrome (LEMS).
Leptin resistance, in obesity hypoventilation syndrome, 751
Leukocytes
eosinophil, 620
in host defense system, 279-282, 280t, 281f
Levalbuterol, formulations, doses and duration of action of, 207t
Levofloxacin, for TB, 392t
Light chain deposition disease, CT appearance and clinical characteristics of, 671t
Light's criteria, for pleural effusions, 821-822, 821b
Limbic encephalitis, in lung cancer, manifestations and treatment of, 807t
Lingula, 1-2, 2f, 2t
collapse of, radiographic signs of, 88
Linkage disequilibrium, in association studies, 11
LIP. See Lymphoid interstitial pneumonia (LIP).
Lipoma, 814, 816f
pleural, radiographic features of, 108f
Liver
disease of, 920-926
controversies and pitfalls of, 925-926
in cystic fibrosis, 577
sleep-disordered breathing and, 921.
See also Sleep-disordered breathing.
lesions of, percutaneous biopsy of, 189, 189f
sarcoidosis involving, 614, 614f
LMA (laryngeal mask airway), in difficult intubation in ICU, 441, 443f
Load, respiratory muscle responses to, 57-59, 57f-59f
Load-capacity balance, in breathing, 55-56, 55f-56f
Lobe collapse
left lower, radiographic signs of, 85, 86f
left upper, radiographic signs of, 87, 87f
middle, radiographic signs of, 85, 86f
radiographic signs of, 84
right lower
and middle, radiographic signs of, 87-88, 88f
radiographic signs of, 85, 86f
right upper
and middle, radiographic signs of, 87, 88f
radiographic signs of, 84-85, 85f
Lobectomy, for Stage I non–small cell lung cancer, 801-802

Low-frequency fatigue, of diaphragm, 58, 58f
Lower extremity exercise, in COPD, 557
Lower respiratory tract
    bronchoscopic examination of, 156
    infections of, in pregnancy, 909
Lung(s)
    abscess of, complicating community-acquired
        pneumonia, 305-306, 306f
    in acid-base relationships, 45-48
    anatomy of, 1-6, 2f, 2t
        HRCT, 114-119, 114f
    biopsy of. *See* Biopsy(ies), lung.
    chest wall and, in respiratory system, 22f,
        23
    collapse of, radiographic signs of, 82-88,
        85f-90f
    compliance of, 22, 22f
        in restrictive disease, 26
        in scoliosis, 758
    complications of cystic fibrosis involving,
        576-577
    in connective tissue diseases, 654-656
    density of, increased, HRCT and, 117-118
    development of, 1, 2t
    elastance of, airway resistance and, 418,
        419f-420f
    elastic properties of, 22, 22f
        surface tension and, 23-24, 24f
    function of
        challenges to, caused by structure, 38
        childhood asthma and, 497
        in coal worker's pneumoconiosis, 642-643
        in HIV patient, 374
        in Langerhans cell histiocytosis, 669
        measures of, in preoperative evaluation for
            lung resection, 872-873
        predicted postoperative, 872
        testing of, in diagnosis of HIV-related
            pneumonia, 359
    growth of, COPD and, 536
    hyperexpansion of, hypertransradiancy in,
        68f, 88
    imaging of, 63-121. *See also* Imaging
        techniques.
    infections of. *See* Pulmonary infections.
    injury to
        acute. *See* Acute lung injury (ALI).
        associated with ARDS, 454, 455b
        toxic inhalational, 682-689. *See also* Toxic
            inhalational lung injury.
        ventilator-induced, 422-428, 426f-427f.
            See also Ventilator-induced lung
            injury (VILI).
    interdependence in, 20
    lobes of, 1-2, 2f, 2t
    lymphatic system of, 5-6
    malarial, 319-320
    mass in. *See* Pulmonary mass.
    mechanics of, in respiratory function testing,
        767
    nodules in. *See* Pulmonary nodule(s).
    recoil pressures of, transmural pressure
        difference and, 23t
    recruitment of, 426
        alternative approaches to, 426-428, 428f
        for refractory hypoxemia in ARDS, 466
    regeneration of, 14
        stem cells in, 17
    resection of
        ACCP guidelines for, 873b
        preoperative evaluation for, 872-873,
            874f
        for Stage I non–small cell lung cancer,
            801-802

Lung(s) (*Continued*)
    response to exercise
        in healthy humans, 145
        in lung disease, 145-146, 145f
    segments of, 2t
    structure of, function related to, 37-38
    tumors of
        benign, 810-817. *See also* Benign lung
            tumors.
        malignant, 776-809. *See also* Lung cancer.
    vascular system of, 5
Lung allograft dysfunction
    chronic, 899, 899f, 899t-900t
    primary, 893t-894t, 894
Lung allograft syndromes, respiratory viruses
    and, 340
Lung cancer, 776-809
    adenocarcinoma, 778-781
    asymptomatic presentation of, 790-793
    in connective tissue diseases, 656
    in COPD, 546
    cytologic analysis of, 778-785
    epidemiology of, 776-778
    epidermal growth factor receptor gene and,
        786
    etiology of, 777-778
    in HIV patient, 378-379
    incidence of, 776-777, 777f
    large cell, 784, 784f
    molecular biology of, 785-786
    neuroendocrine (carcinoid), 782-784, 782f
    non–small cell
        Stage I, treatment of, 801-803
        Stage II, treatment of, 803
        Stage III, treatment of, 803-805, 804b, 804t
        Stage IV, treatment of, 805-806
    palliative care for, 808
    pathology of, 778-785
    risk factors for, 777-778
    silicosis and coal worker's pneumoconiosis
        and, 640-641
    small cell, 782-784, 783f
        treatment of, 806
    squamous cell, 781-782, 781f
    Stage I, 795-796, 796f
    Stage II, 796
    Stage III, 796-798, 797f-798f, 798t
    Stage IV, 798-799
    staging of, 793-799, 793t
        future directions for, 799, 799f
        mediastinal lymph node, endoscopic, 174
        repeat, after chemotherapy, 178
        TNM system for, 794-795, 794t-795t
    survival in, 776-777, 777f
    symptomatic presentation of, 788-790
        related to intrathoracic spread, 788
        related to metastatic spread, 788-790,
            789t
        related to primary tumor, 788, 789f
    treatment of, 801-809
        principles of, 801
Lung-chest wall system, 21
Lung disease
    in aging HIV patient, 382
    cystic, rare, 667-671
    diffuse, 588-598. *See also* Diffuse lung
        disease (DLD).
    drug-induced, in inflammatory bowel
        disease, 934
    genetic basis of, 7, 8t-9t
    interstitial, 599-606. *See also* Interstitial lung
        diseases (ILDs).
    nontuberculous mycobacterial, 399,
        399f-401f

Lung disease (*Continued*)
    parenchymal. *See* Parenchymal lung disease.
    pulmonary hypertension due to, 713
    pulmonary response to exercise in, 145-146,
        145f
    treatment of, stem cell technology in, 16-17
Lung injury scoring system, 456, 456t
Lung parenchyma
    in connective tissue diseases, 655
    diseases of. *See* Parenchymal lung diseases.
    magnetic resonance imaging of, 72
Lung transplantation
    allograft dysfunction in
        chronic, 899, 899f, 899t-900t
        primary, 893t-894t, 894
    allograft implantation in, 890-892, 893f
    antimetabolites in, 900, 901t
    in bronchiectasis, 586
    calcineurin inhibitors in, 900, 901t
    community-acquired pneumonia in, 896,
        897t
    complications of
        bronchial anastomotic, 894, 895f-896f
        infectious, 895-900, 897t
        noninfectious, 892-895
    in connective tissue diseases, 665-666
    contraindications to, 885t
    for COPD, 888, 888t
    current trends in, 882-884, 883f-884f
    for cystic fibrosis, 888-889
    in cystic fibrosis, 576
    disease-specific referral/selection
        considerations, 888-889
    donor selection and management for,
        889-890, 889t, 890b, 891f
    grafts for, types of, 889t
    high-pressure pulmonary edema in, 893t,
        894
    history of, 882
    hyperinflation in, 894-895, 896f
    immunosuppression for, 899-900, 901t
        pitfalls of, 900-901
    malignancy complicating, 901f, 902
    medical complications after, 901-902
    morbidity after, 902, 902f, 903t
    mTOR inhibitors in, 900, 901t
    multidisciplinary approach to, 882, 883f
    neuromuscular complications of, 901
    osteoporosis complicating, 901-902
    phrenic nerve injury in, 894
    for pulmonary arterial hypertension, 720,
        889
    for pulmonary fibrosis, 888
    rejection in
        acute, 893t, 894, 895f
        chronic, 899, 899f, 899t-900t
        histologic classification and grading of, 890
        hyperacute, 892, 893t
    in sarcoidosis, 618
    selection criteria for, 885-889, 887t
    survival after, 884-885, 885f-886f
Lung volume(s), 21, 21f
    abnormalities of, interpretation of, 137-138
    alveolar *vs.* extraalveolar vessels and, 30,
        30f
    chest wall deformity and, 757-758, 758t
    in COPD assessment, 549
    measurement of, 136-137, 136f-137f
    pharyngeal patency and, in obstructive sleep
        apnea, 739
    spirometry and, 136
Lung volume reduction surgery (LVRS), for
    Stage I non–small cell lung cancer, 802
Lupus syndrome, drug-induced, 233

Lymph node(s)
  biopsy of, diagnostic application of, 877t,
    878
  CT imaging of, 110-111, 111f
  dissection of, mediastinal, for Stage I
    non–small cell lung cancer, 802
  enlargement of, anterior mediastinal masses
    from, 113
  lesions of, percutaneous biopsy of, 190,
    190f
Lymphadenitis
  cervical
    mycobacterial, clinical features of,
      399-400
    nontuberculous mycobacterial, treatment
      of, 403
    tuberculous, 387
Lymphadenopathy
  hilar, 592
  in lymphangioleiomyomatosis, 667
  mediastinal
    benign, 855
    metastatic, 855, 855f
    radiographic signs of, 97, 98f
Lymphangioleiomyomas, in
    lymphangioleiomyomatosis, 667
Lymphangioleiomyomatosis (LAM), 667-668,
    668f
  CT appearance and clinical characteristics of,
    671t
  cystic air spaces in, 118-119, 119f
  diagnosis of, 667-668
  extrapulmonary manifestations of, 667
  management of, 668
  pneumothorax in, 835
  pulmonary, HRCT in, 593
  tuberous sclerosis with, genetic factors
    underlying, 8t-9t
Lymphatic circulation, 29
Lymphatic malformations, superior mediastinal
    masses and, 111-112
Lymphatic system, of lungs, 5-6
Lymphatics, sarcoidosis involving, 614
Lymphocytic interstitial pneumonitis, in HIV
    patient, 380
Lymphocytic variant of hypereosinophilic
    syndrome, 628
Lymphoid hyperplasia, in rheumatoid arthritis,
    658, 658f
Lymphoid interstitial pneumonia (LIP)
  characteristics of, 600t
  CT appearance and clinical characteristics of,
    671t
  treatment of, 605
Lymphoma. See also specific lymphoma, e.g.
    Non-Hodgkin lymphoma (NHL).
  anterior mediastinal masses from, 113,
    850-852
Lymphoproliferative disorder
  after hematopoietic stem cell
    transplantation, 918
  posttransplantation, FDG-PET imaging in,
    122
Lysosomal storage disorders, pulmonary
    manifestations of, 674
Lysozyme, in airway surface liquid, 282t,
    283

M

Macrophages, in host defense system, 279-280,
    280t
Magnetic resonance angiography (MRA), 73,
    74f

Magnetic resonance imaging (MRI), 72
  cardiac, in pulmonary arterial hypertension,
    718
  in malignant pleural mesothelioma, 840
  in pleural effusions, 820
  in pulmonary embolism, 701-702
Malarial lung, 319-320
Malignancy
  after hematopoietic stem cell
    transplantation, 918
  hypercalcemia of, 789-790
  of lung, 776-809. See also Lung cancer.
  posttransplant, 902, 902f
  pulmonary embolism treatment in, 704
Malignant peripheral nerve sheath neoplasm,
    857-858
Malignant pleural effusions, 828
Malignant pleural mesothelioma (MPM),
    837-845
  biomarkers of, 841, 841f
  biphasic subtype of, 839
  chemotherapy for, 843-844
  clinical presentation of, 840
  controversies and pitfalls of, 844-845
  cytology of, 839
  diagnosis of, 840-841
  electron microscopy of, 839-840
  epidemiology of, 837
  epithelial subtype of, 838, 838f
  histology of, 838-839
  imaging of, 840-841, 840f-841f
  immunohisto/cytochemistry of, 838-840,
    839f
  immunotherapy for, 844
  management of, 843-844
  pathogenesis of, 837-838
  pathology of, 838-840
  pleural effusions in, 844
  prognosis of, 841-843
  radiotherapy for, 843
  response assessment for, 844
  sarcomatous subtype of, 838-839, 838f
  staging of, 841, 842t
  supportive care for, 844
  surgery for, 843
  targeted therapies for, 844
Mallampati test, 437-438, 438f
Malnutrition, in cystic fibrosis, treatment of, 576
Mammalian target of rapamycin (mTOR)
    inhibitors, in lung transplantation, 900,
    901t
Marfan syndrome, 662
  pneumothorax and emphysema secondary
    to, genetic factors underlying, 8t-9t
  scoliosis in, 756
Mask ventilation
  difficult, predictors of, 437
  in difficult intubation in ICU, 441
Mass conservation
  diffusion and, 39-40, 40f
  perfusion and, 40
  ventilation and, 38-39
Mast cells, in immune system, 280, 280t
Maximal exercise (VO_2max), 145
Maximal expiratory pressure, 765-766
Maximal inspiratory pressure, 765-766
Maximal static mouth pressures, in respiratory
    function testing, 59-60, 60f
Maximum voluntary ventilation (MVV), 134
Mechanical ventilation. See also Ventilator
    entries; Ventilator(s).
  diaphragmatic dysfunction from, 58-59
  dynamic hyperinflation and, 419-422,
    421f-424f

Mechanical ventilation (Continued)
  history of, 406
  indications and contraindications for, 406
  invasive, 406-430. See also Invasive
    mechanical ventilation.
  lung injury and, 27
  multiple system organ failure and, 458-459,
    459f
  noninvasive, 431-436. See also Noninvasive
    mechanical ventilation (NIV).
  respiratory system mechanics and, 418,
    419f-420f
  sepsis induced by, 460-461
    multiple system organ dysfunction and,
      461
    ventilator-induced lung injury and,
      461-462
  weaning from, 428-429, 429f
    failure of, 429-430
    noninvasive ventilation and, 434
Mechanotransduction, in ventilator-induced
    lung injury, 460
Mediastinal collections, percutaneous sampling
    of, 187
Mediastinal emphysema, 99-101
Mediastinal hemorrhage, 861
Mediastinal lymph node dissection, for Stage I
    non–small cell lung cancer, 802
Mediastinal lymphadenopathy
  benign, 855
  metastatic, 855, 855f
  radiographic signs of, 97, 98f
Mediastinal lymphoma, 850
  Hodgkin disease as, 850-851. See also
    Hodgkin disease.
  non-Hodgkin, 850-852, 851f-852f. See also
    Non-Hodgkin lymphoma (NHL).
Mediastinal masses
  CT evaluation of, 111-113, 111f
  and nodes, percutaneous sampling of,
    186-187, 187f
  overview of, 846
Mediastinal patterns, drug-induced, 239-240
Mediastinitis, 860
Mediastinoscopy, cervical, diagnostic
    application of, 877t, 878-879, 879f
Mediastinotomy, anterior, diagnostic
    application of, 877t, 879
Mediastinum
  abnormalities of, radiographic signs of,
    97-101, 98f
  anatomy of
    CT, 107-111, 109f-110f
    radiographic, 76-77, 77f
  anterior. See also Thymic entries; Thymus.
    cysts of, 853-854
    definition of, 846, 847f
    diseases of, 846-854
      differential diagnosis of, 861
    glandular disorders of, 854, 855f
    neoplasms of, 846-853
      germ cell, 852
    seminomas of, 852-853
    teratomas of, 852, 852f
  disorders of, 846-861
    compartmental classification of, 846, 847t
    constitutional and paraneoplastic findings
      in, 847t
    differential diagnosis of, 861
    in inflammatory bowel disease, 934
  displacement of, in lobar collapse, 84
  evaluation of, in Stage III lung cancer,
    797-798, 798t
  inflammation of, 860

Mediastinum (Continued)
magnetic resonance imaging of, 72, 73f
middle-posterior
cysts of, 855-856, 856f
definition of, 846, 847f
diseases of, 855-857
differential diagnosis of, 861
herniations in, 857
lymphadenopathy and, 855, 855f
vascular lesions of, 857
paravertebral compartment of
definition of, 846, 847f
diseases of, 857-860
neoplasms of
differential diagnosis of, 861
neurogenic, 857
paraganglionic, 859, 859f-860f
peripheral nerve, 857-858, 857f-858f
sympathetic ganglia, 858-859, 858f
spinal lesions and, 859-860, 860f
Mediator modification, by pulmonary
circulation, 33
Medical Research Council (MRC) Dyspnea
Scale, Modified, for breathlessness, 546,
547t
Medulla, respiratory centers in, 50, 51f
Melioidosis, 300
Membranous bronchioles, 3, 3f
Meningioma, in lymphangioleiomyomatosis,
667
Meningitis, tuberculous, 387-388
Meningocele, thoracic, lateral, 859-860, 860f
Menkes disease, emphysema secondary to,
genetic factors underlying, 8t-9t, 15
Mesenchymal neoplasms, benign, 811-813
Mesothelioma
FDG-PET-CT imaging in assessment of,
129-130, 130f
malignant
diffuse, 784-785
pleural, 837-845. See also Malignant
pleural mesothelioma (MPM).
mesosthelin levels in pleural fluid in,
822-823
Metabolic acidosis
clinical causes of, 48
Davenport diagram for, 47f, 48
Metabolic alkalosis
clinical causes of, 48
Davenport diagram for, 47f, 48
Metals, inhalational injury from, 687
Metapneumovirus, human, infection from, in
non–HIV-infected immunocompromised
patients, 340
Meteorologic changes, as asthma triggers, 499
Metered dose inhalers (MDIs), in obstructive
lung disease, technique for use of, 210,
210t
Methacholine, in bronchoprovocation testing,
141
Methemoglobinemia, drug-induced, 223t, 240
Methotrexate (MTX)
for ANCA-associated vasculitis, 723-725,
724t
for sarcoidosis, 617t, 618
Methylxanthine drugs, for COPD
exacerbations, 565
Microlithiasis, pulmonary alveolar, 673-674,
673f
Microscopic polyangiitis (MPA), 722-726
definition and nomenclature of, 722
diagnostic evaluation of, 723
etiology and pathogenesis of, 723
refractory, therapy for, 725

Microscopic polyangiitis (MPA) (Continued)
therapy for, 723-726, 724t
complications of, 725-726
Wegener granulomatosis with, therapy for,
725
Microscopy, fibered confocal fluorescence, 165
Middle mediastinal masses, CT evaluation of,
113
Migratory superficial thrombophlebitis, in lung
cancer, 790
Miliary tuberculosis, 388, 388f
Miller syndrome, genetic factors underlying, 7
Mini Asthma Quality of Life Questionnaire
(AQLQ), 507t
Mitral valve disease, diffuse alveolar
hemorrhage and, 729-730
Mixed connective tissue disease (MCTD), 653
Molecular assays, in TB diagnosis, 390
Molecular biology, 7-12
Molecular methods, in viral pneumonia
diagnosis, 313
Monoclonal antibody, anti-IgE, for asthma, 511
Monoclonal antibody therapies, for asthma, 514
Monocytes, 279-280
Moraxella catarrhalis, in community-acquired
pneumonia, 301
Morbidity, in COPD, 539
Morgagni hernias, 857
Mortality, from COPD, 539
Mosaicism, in extrinsic allergic alveolitis,
678-679, 678f, 678t
Motor neuron disease, respiratory presentations
of, 771
Moxifloxacin, for TB, 392t
MPA. See Microscopic polyangiitis (MPA).
MPM. See Malignant pleural mesothelioma
(MPM).
MRC Dyspnea Scale, Modified, for
breathlessness, 546, 547t
MRI. See Magnetic resonance imaging (MRI).
Mucin-secreting cells, 3
Mucociliary escalator, in respiratory system
defense, 277, 278t
Mucociliary function, in bronchiectasis
diagnosis, 583
Mucociliary function testing, 479
Mucokinetic agents, for COPD, 556
Mucopolysaccharidoses, pulmonary
manifestations of, 674
Mucosa, airway, immune response of,
disordered, in asthma, 502
Mucus
airway obstruction by, 38
hypersecretion of
in asthma, 493
chronic, COPD and, 536
Mucus clearance defects, chronic rhinosinusitis
and, 477
Multicentric Castleman disease, in HIV
patient, 377
Multiorgan dysfunction syndrome, drug-
induced, 223t
Multiple comparisons, 10
Multiple cystic mesenchymal hamartoma,
670-671
Multiple sclerosis, respiratory presentations of,
769
Multiple system organ failure, mechanical
ventilation and, 458-459, 459f, 461
Muscle(s)
disorders of, respiratory presentations of,
772-774
oxygen utilization by, in health and disease,
147

Muscle(s) (Continued)
paralysis of, in ARDS management, 468
pharyngeal, activity of, in obstructive sleep
apnea, 737-738
respiratory, 50-62. See also Respiratory
muscles.
skeletal, dysfunction/wasting of, in COPD,
545-546
smooth, of airways, control of, 202, 203f
in COPD, 202, 203f
ventilatory, strength and endurance training
for, in COPD, 558-559
Muscular dystrophy
Becker, respiratory presentations of, 773
Duchenne
respiratory presentations of, 773
scoliosis in, 756
surgery for, 760
fascioscapulohumeral, respiratory
presentations of, 773
Musculoskeletal pain, chest pain and, 268-269,
268f-269f
Musculoskeletal system, corticosteroid
toxicities affecting, 217t
Mustard gas, as irritant, 683t, 686
Myasthenia gravis, respiratory presentations of,
772
Mycobacterial infections, 383-405
bronchoscopy in, 159, 159f
in HIV patient, 351-355
controversies and pitfalls of, 372-373
prognosis of, 371
prophylaxis of, 370-371
treatment of, 364-366
in non–HIV-infected immunocompromised
patients, 337
nontuberculous, 397-404. See also
Nontuberculous mycobacteria (NTM).
tuberculosis as, 383-397. See also
Tuberculosis (TB).
Mycobacterium abscessus infection, treatment
of, 402t, 403
Mycobacterium avium complex infection
in HIV patient, 353
treatment of, 366
treatment of, 402-403, 402t
Mycobacterium chelonae infection, treatment of,
403
Mycobacterium fortuitum infection, treatment
of, 403
Mycobacterium kansasii infection
clinical features of, 399, 400f-401f
in HIV patient, 354
treatment of, 366
treatment of, 402t, 403
Mycobacterium malmoense infection, treatment
of, 402t, 403
Mycobacterium tuberculosis, culture and
identification of, in TB diagnosis, 390
Mycobacterium xenopi infection
in HIV patient, 354
treatment of, 402t, 403
Mycophenolate mofetil (MMF)
for ANCA-associated vasculitis, 725
in lung transplantation, 901t
for sarcoidosis, 618
Mycoplasma pneumoniae, in community-
acquired pneumonia, 299
Mycotic lung disease, pleural effusions in, 828
Myeloablative conditioning, for hematopoietic
stem cell transplantation, 912
Myeloproliferative variant of hypereosinophilic
syndrome, 628
Myocardial infarction, chest pain in, 270

Myocardial ischemia
chest pain and, 270
pain in, 267
Myocardial performance index, 194, 195f
Myofibroblastic tumor, inflammatory, 811-812, 812f
Myopathy(ies)
congenital, respiratory presentations of, 773
inflammatory, idiopathic, respiratory presentations of, 774
metabolic, respiratory presentations of, 773
mitochondrial, respiratory presentations of, 773-774
respiratory, corticosteroid-induced, respiratory presentations of, 772-773
Myotonic dystrophy, respiratory presentations of, 773

N

Nares, in defense system, 275-276
Narrow band imaging (NBI), 164
Nasal airways tests, 479
Nasal cannulas, reservoir, for home oxygen therapy in COPD, 560
Nasal cavities, structure and function of, 19
Nasal cytology, 480
Nasal drops, instillation of, 482f
Nasal polyps
chronic rhinosinusitis with, 477-478, 477f, 478b
treatment of, 485-486, 485f
surgical interventions for, 485-486
Nasal potential difference measurement, in cystic fibrosis diagnosis, 571, 572f
Necrobiotic nodules, in inflammatory bowel disease, 931-934, 933f
Needles, for percutaneous biopsy procedures, 181-182
Neoplasms
hemoptysis in, 261
in HIV patient, 374-379
Nerve sheath tumors, 812
Nerves
peripheral
acute disorders affecting, 771
chronic disorders affecting, 772
phrenic, injury to
in lung transplantation, 894
respiratory presentations of, 772
Neuralgic amyotrophy, respiratory presentations of, 772
Neurally adjusted ventilatory assist (NAVA), 413-415, 414f
Neuraminidase inhibitors, for viral pneumonia, 313
Neurilemmoma, 857
Neuroblastomas, 859
Neuroendocrine cells, 4
Neuroendocrine tumors, of lung, 782-784, 782f
Neuroenteric cysts, posterior mediastinal masses from, 113
Neurofibroma(s), 812, 812f, 857, 857f-858f
Neurofibromatosis, 857
Neurofibromatosis type 1, scoliosis in, 756
Neurogenic neoplasms, mediastinal, 857
Neurohormonal response, in obesity hypoventilation syndrome, 751
Neuromuscular competence, inspiratory load vs., 55, 55f
energy supply vs. demand and, 56, 56f

Neuromuscular disorders
from immunosuppressants, 901
respiratory presentations of, 768-774, 768t
Neuromuscular failure, drug-induced, 223t
Neuromuscular junction disorders, 772
Neuromyopathy, critical illness, respiratory presentations of, 771-772
Neuropathy
motor and sensory, hereditary, respiratory presentations of, 772
sensory, encephalomyelitis-subacute, in lung cancer, 798
Neutropenia, pathogens associated with, 330, 332t
Neutrophils, polymorphonuclear, in immune response, 280t, 281-282, 282f
NHL. See Non-Hodgkin lymphoma (NHL).
Nickel, inhalational injury from, 687
Niemann-Pick disease, pulmonary manifestations of, 674
Nitric oxide
exhaled, in asthma assessment, 507t
pulmonary blood flow and, 32
Nitrogen dioxide, in air pollution, 938-940
Nitrogen oxides, as irritants, 683t, 685
Nitrogen washout, in lung volume measurement, 136-137, 137f
NIV. See Noninvasive mechanical ventilation (NIV).
Nocardia asteroides infection, in HIV patient, 351
Nocardia species
in community-acquired pneumonia, 300
infections from, in non–HIV-infected immunocompromised patients, 337
Nocardiosis, pulmonary, pleural effusions in, 828
Nocturnal asthma, 495
Nocturnal hypoventilation, in chest wall disease, 768
Nodular bronchiectatic disease, 399, 400f
Nodular opacities, 94, 94f
Nodular pattern, on HRCT in parenchymal disease, 115-116, 116f
Nodules. See Pulmonary nodule(s).
Non-Hodgkin lymphoma (NHL), 850-852
anterior mediastinal masses from, 113
hilar abnormalities in, 102f
in HIV patient, 377-378, 378f
imaging of, 851f-852f
Nonallergic rhinitis, 473-475
Nonbacterial infectious pneumonia, 315-321
Non–HIV-infected immunocompromised patients
cytomegalovirus infection in, 337-338, 338f, 339t
invasive aspergillosis in, 340-343, 341f-342f, 342t-343t
mycobacterial infections in, 337
nocardial infections in, 337
pneumonia in, 330-345
bacterial, 336-337, 336f
clinical approach to, 330-332, 331t-333t, 333f
clinical assessment of, 332-336
controversies and pitfalls of, 344
diagnostic protocols for, 332-336
overview of, 330
specific clinical entities in, 336-344
Noninvasive arterial blood pressure monitoring, in critical illness, 445-446, 446f

Noninvasive mechanical ventilation (NIV), 431-436
controversies and pitfalls of, 435
for COPD exacerbations, 565, 565b, 565f
equipment for, 431-432
future directions for, 434
indications for, 431
clinical, 432-434
modes of, 431
for obesity hypoventilation syndrome, 754
physiologic effects of, 434
for respiratory muscle resting, in COPD, 559
weaning and, 434
Noninvasive positive-pressure ventilation (NIPPV), for acute dyspnea, 255-256
Nonmyeloablative conditioning, for hematopoietic stem cell transplantation, 912
Nonspecific interstitial pneumonia (NSIP), 603-604
cellular, 603-604
characteristics of, 600t
drug-induced, parenchymal patterns in, 229-231
epidemiology of, 603
fibrotic, 603-604
histopathologic images of, 601f
HRCT in, 593, 593f, 601f
treatment and prognosis of, 604, 604f
Nontuberculous mycobacteria (NTM), 397-404
clinical course of, 404
clinical features of, 399-401, 399f-401f
controversies and pitfalls of, 404
diagnosis of, 401-402, 401b
epidemiology of, 397-398
genetics of, 399
by growth rate, 398t
pathogenesis of, 398-399
prevention of, 404
risk factors for, 398
Nosocomial pneumonia, 322-329
definition of, 322
diagnosis of, 324-326
impact on outcomes, 322
incidence of, 322
prevention of, 323-324, 323b
severe, clinical characteristics of, 290, 290b
Nosocomial respiratory infections, 322-329
definition of, 322
diagnosis of, 324-326
strategies for, 325-326, 326f
epidemiology of, 322
etiologic agents in, 323
pathogenesis of, 322-323
prevention of, 323-324, 323b
treatment of, 327-329, 327f, 327t-328t, 329f
Nosocomial tracheobronchitis
definition of, 322
diagnosis of, 324-325
impact on outcomes, 322
incidence of, 322
pathogenesis of, 322
NSIP. See Nonspecific interstitial pneumonia (NSIP).
NTM. See Nontuberculous mycobacteria (NTM).
Nuclear factor κB, oxidative stress activating, 12
Nucleic acid amplification assays (NAAs), in TB diagnosis, 390

Nutrition
  childhood asthma and, 497
  community-acquired pneumonia and, 297
  evaluation of, in COPD, 559
  prenatal, childhood asthma and, 498

O

OA. See Occupational asthma (OA).
Obesity
  asthma and, 496
  clinical consequences of, 774
  intubation in, positioning for, 439f
  lung volumes in, 138
  obstructive sleep apnea and, 733
  postoperative pulmonary complications and, 870
  respiratory muscle pump and, 774
  venous thromboembolism and, 694
Obesity hypoventilation syndrome, 749-755
  blood gas analysis in, 752
  chest radiography in, 753
  clinical course of, 753
  clinical features of, 751
  continuous positive airway pressure for, 754
  controversies and pitfalls of, 754-755
  diagnosis of, 751-753
  echocardiography in, 753
  epidemiology of, 749
  history in, 751
  morbidity and mortality in, 753
  neurohormonal response in, 751
  noninvasive ventilation for, 754
  obstructive sleep apnea in, 750-751, 750f
  pathophysiology of, 750-751, 750f-751f
  pharmacotherapy of, 754
  physical examination in, 751-752
  reversal of sleep-disordered breathing for, 754
  risk factors for, 749
  serum blood chemistry in, 752
  sleep laboratory diagnosis of, 752-753, 752f-753f
  spirometry in, 753
  tracheostomy for, 754
  treatment of, 753-754
  weight reduction for, 753
Obliterative bronchiolitis
  in connective tissue diseases, 655, 655f
  drug-induced, 238
Obstructive impairment, spirometric abnormalities in, 135
Obstructive lung disease
  lung volume abnormalities in, 138
  metered dose inhaler use in, technique for, 210, 210t
  respiratory work in, 26
  spirometric abnormalities in, 135
  ventilating patients with, 418-419
Obstructive sleep apnea (OSA), 731-748
  anatomic factors in, 737, 738f
  Bernoulli effect and, 739-740
  chronic obstructive pulmonary disease and, 748
  clinical features of, 741-742
  controversies and pitfalls of, 740, 748
  diagnosis of, 742-745
  edema and rostral fluid shifts in, 739
  in elderly population, 731-734, 733t
  epidemiology of, 731-732, 732b
  genetic predisposition to, 734
  lung volume and pharyngeal patency in, 739
  male gender and, 734
  in middle-aged population, 731, 732t

Obstructive sleep apnea (OSA) (Continued)
  obesity and, 733
  in obesity hypoventilation syndrome, 749-751, 750f
  oral appliances for, 746, 746f
  pathogenesis of, 737-740
  pathophysiology of, 735-737, 735f
  pharyngeal muscle activity in, 737-738
  physical examination in, 742, 742b, 743f
  polysomnography in, 743, 744f
  positive airway pressure for, 746-747, 747f
    non-continuous, 748
  postoperative pulmonary complications and, 870
  in pregnancy, 910
  in preoperative pulmonary evaluation, 871, 871b
  in REM sleep, 739
  risk factors for, 732-735, 734b
  stability of sleep and airway patency in, 739
  surface tension of airway fluid in, 739
  treatment of, 745-748
    adjunctive therapies in, 747
    decisions on, 748
    effects of, on major outcomes, 747-748
    surgical, 746
  upper airway collapse in, 737, 737b
  upper airway inflammation and, 739
  ventilatory control stability in, 738-739
  in women, 748
Occupational asthma (OA), 499, 521-530
  causal agents in, 521, 522t
  clinical course of, 528-529, 528f
  clinical features of, 525-526
  controversies and pitfalls of, 530
  diagnosis of, 526-528, 527f-528f, 527t
  epidemiology of, 521, 522t-524t
  immunologic
    IgE-mediated, 523
    non-IgE-mediated, 524-525, 525f
  incidence of, 521, 523t
  management of, 517
  nonimmunologic, 525, 525f-526f
  pathophysiology of, 523-525, 525f-526f
  prevalence of, 521
  prevention of, 529
  risk factors for, 521-523, 524t
  treatment of, 529-530
Occupational exposure
  to dusts, COPD and, 536
  to inhalational toxins, 682, 683t
Occupational rhinitis, 475
Ocular sarcoidosis, 612-613, 614f
Oncogene, KRAS, 786
OP. See Organizing pneumonia (OP).
Opioids, endogenous, in neuromodulation of dyspnea, 251
Opportunistic infection(s)
  antiretroviral therapy and, 372
  drug-induced, 223t
  lung transplantation and, 896-898, 897f-898f, 897t
Optical coherence tomography, 164-165, 164f
Ordered polymer response, 14
Organizing pneumonia (OP), 629-636
  acute fibrinous, 635
  clinical features of, 630-631
  complicating community-acquired pneumonia, 307
  controversies and pitfalls of, 635
  cryptogenic. See Cryptogenic organizing pneumonia (COP).
  HRCT in, 593
  definition of, 629

Organizing pneumonia (OP) (Continued)
  diagnosis of, 633-634
  drug-induced, parenchymal patterns in, 233, 234f
  imaging features of, 631-632, 631f-632f, 632b
  in inflammatory bowel disease, 931
  pathogenesis of, 629, 630f
  secondary, 632-633, 633b
  severe, 635
  treatment of, 634-635, 634t
OSA. See Obstructive sleep apnea (OSA).
Oscillatory ventilation, high-frequency, for refractory hypoxemia in ARDS, 467
Oseltamivir
  for viral lung infections, 339t
  for viral pneumonia, 313
Osler-Weber-Rendu syndrome, genetic factors underlying, 8t-9t
Osteoarthropathy, pulmonary, hypertrophic
  in cystic fibrosis, 578
  in lung cancer, 790
Osteopenia, in cystic fibrosis, 578
Osteopontin, in malignant pleural mesothelioma, 841
Osteoporosis
  in COPD, 545-546
  in cystic fibrosis, 578
  from immunosuppressants, 901-902
Ovarian hyperstimulation syndrome, in pregnancy, 907
Oxidant/antioxidant imbalance, in COPD, 542
Oxidative stress, as intracellular signal, 12-13
Oximetry, overnight, in pulmonary arterial hypertension, 716
Oxitropium bromide, formulations, doses and duration of action of, 207t
Oxygen
  for acute dyspnea, 255
  increased extraction of, from blood, 43
Oxygen therapy
  in COPD exacerbation prevention, 566
  for COPD exacerbations, 564-565
  home, in COPD, 559-560
  for obstructive sleep apnea, 747
Oxygen transport–oxygen utilization pathway, major elements of, 144f
Oxygenation
  extracorporeal membrane, for refractory hypoxemia in ARDS, 466-467
  PEEP and, 464, 464t
Ozone
  in air pollution, 937-938
  as irritant, 683t, 686

P

PAH. See Pulmonary arterial hypertension (PAH).
Pain
  chest, 267-274. See also Chest pain.
  management of, in lung cancer, 808
Palivizumab, for viral lung infections, 339t
Panbronchiolitis, diffuse, cough in, 247
Pancoast tumors, treatment of, 805
Pancreas, complications of cystic fibrosis involving, 577
Pancreatic insufficiency, in cystic fibrosis, 570-571, 577
  treatment of, 576
Pancreatitis, pain in, 271
Panhypogammaglobulinemia, chronic rhinosinusitis in, 477
Panlobular emphysema, pathology of, 533-534

PAP. See Pulmonary alveolar proteinosis (PAP).
Papillomas, 810-811, 811f
Paraaminosalicylic acid (PAS), for TB, 392t
Paracicatricial emphysema, in coal workers, 642
Paracoccidioidomycosis, 318-319
Paragangliomas, 859, 860f
Paraganglionic neoplasms, 859, 859f
Paraganglionoma, posterior mediastinal masses from, 113, 113f
Paragonimiasis, 321
Parainfluenza virus infection, in non–HIV-infected immunocompromised patients, 340
Paralysis
   diaphragmatic, bilateral, 53, 53f
   muscle, in ARDS management, 468
Paraneoplastic syndromes, 789-790, 789t
   manifestations and treatments of, 807-808, 807t
Parapneumonic effusion, 826-827, 826t
   complicating community-acquired pneumonia, 306
Paraseptal emphysema, pathology of, 534
Parasinusitis, in cystic fibrosis, 571
Parasitic infections
   eosinophilic pneumonia in, 621-622
   in HIV patient, treatment of, 367, 368t
Parasitic pneumonias, 319-321
Parathyroid adenoma, 854
Parenchyma. See Lung parenchyma.
Parenchymal lung diseases
   asbestosis as, 645-652. See also Asbestosis.
   coal worker's pneumoconiosis as, 637-644. See also Coal worker's pneumoconiosis (CWP).
   connective tissue diseases as, 653-666. See also Connective tissue diseases (CTDs).
   desquamative interstitial pneumonia as, 604-605
   diffuse, 588-598. See also Diffuse lung disease (DLD).
   eosinophilic, 620-628. See also Eosinophilic lung disease.
   extrinsic allergic alveolitis as, 676-681. See also Extrinsic allergic alveolitis (EAA).
   idiopathic pulmonary fibrosis as, 599-603. See also Idiopathic pulmonary fibrosis (IPF).
   nonspecific interstitial pneumonia as, 603-604. See also Nonspecific interstitial pneumonia (NSIP).
   organizing pneumonia as, 629-636. See also Organizing pneumonia (OP).
   patterns of, on HRCT, 114-119
   rare diffuse interstitial lung diseases as, 667-675
   respiratory bronchiolitis interstitial lung disease as. See also Respiratory bronchiolitis interstitial lung disease (RBILD).
   respiratory bronchiolitis interstitial lung disease as, 604
   sarcoidosis as, 607-619. See also Sarcoidosis.
   silicosis as, 637. See also Silicosis.
   toxic inhalational lung injury as, 682-689. See also Toxic inhalational lung injury.
Parenchymal patterns, of drug-induced respiratory diseases, 229-237
Parietal pleura, 1
Parkinson disease, respiratory presentations of, 770, 770f
Particle deposition, in lungs, 38

Particulate matter (PM), in air pollution, 937, 939f-940f
Passive collapse, of lung, 82
Pasteurella multocida, in community-acquired pneumonia, 301
Pauciimmune pulmonary capillaritis, idiopathic, 726-727
PBC. See Primary biliary cirrhosis (PBC).
PCP. See Pneumocystis jirovecii pneumonia (PCP).
PE. See Pulmonary embolism (PE).
Peak exercise (VO₂peak), 145
Peak expiratory flow (PEF)
   in asthma assessment, 507t
   diurnal variation of, in asthma diagnosis, 506
Peak expiratory flow rate, 134
Peak systolic velocity, of lateral tricuspid annulus displacement, 194-196, 195f
PEEP. See Positive end-expiratory pressure (PEEP).
Pemetrexed, for Stage IV non–small cell lung cancer, 805
Penicillium marneffei infection, in HIV patient, 357
   treatment of, 367, 367t
Pentamidine
   intravenous, for bacterial pneumonia, 363
   in Pneumocystis pneumonia prophylaxis, 369, 369t
Pentoxifylline, for sarcoidosis, 617t, 618
Peptic ulcer disease, pain in, 271
Peptides, antimicrobial, in lung host defense, 283-284
Percutaneous biopsy procedures, 180-192
   common sites for, 181f
   for extrapulmonary intrathoracic tissues, 186-188
   for extrathoracic lesions, 188-191, 189f-190f
   of hilar lesions, 187
   imaging techniques guiding, 180-182
   for intrapulmonary lesions, 182-186
     complications of, 184-185, 185f, 185t
     indications and contraindications for, 182-183, 183f, 183t
     method and procedure for, 183-184, 184f
   for mediastinal collections, 187
   for mediastinal nodes and masses, 186-187, 187f
   pleural, 823
   for pleural and chest wall disease, 187-188, 188f
   ultrasound-guided, 180, 186, 186f
Percutaneous fine needle aspiration, in pneumonia pathogen identification, 294
Percutaneous tracheostomy, 443, 443b
Perfusion
   in gas exchange, 37
   mass conservation and, 40
Pericardial cysts, 854, 854f
Pericardial effusions
   echocardiographic evaluation of, 199, 200f
   in lung cancer, management of, 808
Pericardial pain, 267, 270
Pericardial tuberculosis, 388
Pericarditis, acute, as emergency, 935
Pericardium
   constriction of, echocardiographic detection of, 199-200
   CT imaging of, 111
Perinatal factors, childhood asthma and, 498
Peripartum cardiomyopathy, 906-907
Peripheral chemoreceptors, in ventilation, 51f, 52

Peripheral fatigue, respiratory muscle, 57-58, 57f
Peripheral nerve neoplasms, mediastinal, 857-858, 857f-858f
Peripheral nerves
   acute disorders affecting, 771
   chronic disorders affecting, 772
Permeability edema, 33
Persistent unexplained multifocal consolidation, 592
PET imaging. See Positron emission tomography (PET) imaging.
pH and glucose levels, of pleural fluid, 822, 822b
Pharmacogenetics, future directions for, 18
Pharmacology
   antiinflammatory drugs in, 213-220. See also Antiinflammatory drugs.
   bronchodilators in, 202-212. See also Bronchodilator(s).
   drug-induced respiratory diseases and, 221-241. See also Drug-induced entries; Drug-induced respiratory diseases (DIRDs).
Pharmacotherapy
   in asthma, 509-511
   in COPD, 554-556, 555t
     for exacerbations, 564, 564f
   for cystic fibrosis, 574
   for obesity hypoventilation syndrome, 754
Pharynx
   muscles of, activity of, in obstructive sleep apnea, 737-738
   patency of, lung volumes and, in obstructive sleep apnea, 739
   structure and function of, 19
Pheochromocytomas, 859, 859f
Phosgene, as irritant, 683t, 685
Phosphodiesterase 4 (PDE4) inhibitors
   as antiinflammatories, 216-218
   pharmacodynamics of, 217-218, 218f
   pharmacokinetics of, 218, 219f
   side effects of, 218
Phosphodiesterase inhibitors
   for COPD, 555t, 556
   type-5, for pulmonary arterial hypertension, 719
Photodynamic therapy, bronchoscopy in, 167
Phrenic latency, 61, 62f
Phrenic nerve conduction time, 61, 62f
Phrenic nerve injury
   in lung transplantation, 894
   respiratory presentations of, 772
Physical therapy, chest, for COPD patient, 558
Physiologic assessment
   in COPD, 548-550
   preoperative, 869
Physiologic dead space (Vd/Vt), in gas exchange assessment, 44-45
Physiotherapy, for bronchiectasis, 586
Pirfenidone, for idiopathic pulmonary fibrosis, 603
Plasma exchange, for Wegener granulomatosis with microscopic polyangiitis, 725
Pleura, 1
   biopsy of, 823
     in pneumonia pathogen identification, 293
   calcification of, radiographic features of, 106-107, 107f-108f
   diseases of
     asbestos-related, nonmalignant, 646t, 650-651, 651f
     percutaneous sampling of, 187-188, 188f
     in pregnancy, 910

Pleura (Continued)
  radiographic features of, 102-107
    in rheumatoid arthritis, 656-658
  lipoma of, radiographic features of, 108f
  malignancies of, 784-785
  malignant mesothelioma of, 837-845.
    See also Malignant pleural
    mesothelioma (MPM).
  masses of, radiographic features of, 107,
    108f-109f
  solitary fibrous tumor of, 812, 813f
  thickening of, radiographic features of,
    105-106, 106f-107f
Pleural catheters, indwelling, placement of, for
  pleural effusions, 824, 824f
Pleural diseases, asbestos-related, 830
Pleural drain, indwelling, long-term, for
  malignant pleural effusions, 868
Pleural effusion(s), 818-836. See also Exudative
    effusions; Transudative effusions.
  chest radiography in, 818
  clinical presentation of, 818
  computed tomography in, 820
  controversies and pitfalls of, 830-831
  definition of, 818
  diagnostic approach to, 820-823, 821f
  drug-induced, 238-239, 239f, 829
  entities associated with, 825-830
  epidemiology of, 818, 819t
  imaging of, 818-820
  incidence of, 818, 819t
  magnetic resonance imaging in, 820
  malignant, 828, 868
    therapeutic options for, 868
  in malignant pleural mesothelioma, 844
  massive, drug-induced, 223t
  pathophysiology of, 818
  percutaneous drainage of, 191, 191f
  pleural fluid analysis in, 820-823, 821b-822b
  positron emission tomography in, 820,
    820f-821f
  in pregnancy, 910
  radiography of, 102-103, 102f-103f
  related to abdominal diseases, 829-830
  secondary to connective tissue disease,
    828-829
  secondary to infections with other
    organisms, 828
  thoracic ultrasound imaging in, 818-819,
    819f-820f, 819t
  treatment of, 823-825
    management of underlying cause in, 823
    in preventing fluid reaccumulation,
      824-825
    symptom control in, 824, 824f
  tuberculous, 828
Pleural empyema, 826-827, 826f, 826t
Pleural fibrosis and thickening, 830
Pleural fluid
  analysis of, in pleural effusions, 820-823,
    821b-822b
  bedside examination of, 821
  differential leukocyte count in, 822, 822b
  disease-specific tests on, 822-823
  pH and glucose levels in, 822, 822b
  in pleural disease, 102-103, 102f-103f
  reaccumulation of, in pleural effusions,
    preventing, 824-825, 825f
  sampling of, in pneumonia pathogen
    identification, 293
Pleural infections
  in children, 827-828
  septated, chest tube drainage and, 867-868
Pleural patterns, drug-induced, 238-239, 239f

Pleural pressure, in distribution of ventilation,
  27
Pleural space, structure of, 19
Pleural tuberculosis, 387
Pleurodesis, 824-825, 825f
  chemical, chest tube with, for malignant
    pleural effusions, 868
PMF. See Progressive massive fibrosis (PMF).
Pneumoconiosis(es)
  coal worker's, 637-644. See also Coal
    worker's pneumoconiosis (CWP).
  complicated. See also Progressive massive
    fibrosis (PMF).
    definition of, 641
  definition of, 637
  radiographic classification of, 640t
Pneumocystis, 316f, 317t, 319
Pneumocystis jirovecii pneumonia (PCP)
  in hematopoietic stem cell transplantation
    patients, 916
  in HIV patient, 354-355, 354t, 355f
    controversies and pitfalls of, 373
    deterioration in, 363, 364t
    initiation of antiretroviral therapy in,
      timing of, 364
    prognosis of, 363-364, 371, 371b
    prophylaxis for, 368-370
    treatment of, 361-364, 361t-362t
  in immunocompromised patient, 344, 344f
    bronchoscopy in, 159
  severity of, grading, 361t
Pneumocytes
  type I, 16f
    in gaseous exchange, 15
  type II, 16f
    functions of, 15-16
Pneumomediastinum
  chest pain in, 270, 270f
  imaging of, 99-101, 101f
  in pregnancy, 910
Pneumonectomy, 106f
Pneumonia(s)
  aspiration, complicating community-
    acquired pneumonia, 305, 305f
  bacterial. See Bacterial pneumonia.
  CMV, in hematopoietic stem cell
    transplantation patients, 915
  community-acquired, 296-308. See also
    Community-acquired pneumonia
    (CAP).
  eosinophilic. See Eosinophilic pneumonia
    (EP).
  fungal, 315-319, 316f, 317t. See also Fungal
    pneumonias.
  health care-associated, 308
  infectious, nonbacterial, 315-321
  interstitial. See Interstitial pneumonia(s).
  in non-HIV-infected immunocompromised
    patients, 330-345. See also Non-HIV-
    infected immunocompromised patients,
    pneumonia in.
  nosocomial, 322-329. See also Nosocomial
    pneumonia.
  organizing, 629-636. See also Organizing
    pneumonia (OP).
    complicating community-acquired
      pneumonia, 307
  parasitic, 319-321
  postoperative, risk for, 871, 871t
  ventilator-associated. See Ventilator-
    associated pneumonia (VAP).
  viral, 309-314. See also Viral pneumonia.
Pneumonia Severity Index (PSI), 289-290,
  291f

Pneumonic anthrax, 301
Pneumonitis
  hypersensitivity. See also Extrinsic allergic
    alveolitis (EAA).
    causes of, 589-590
    subacute, HRCT in, 70-71, 71f
  interstitial. See Interstitial pneumonitis.
Pneumothorax, 831-836
  AIDS and, 835
  catamenial, 835
  causes of, 831b
  complicating bronchoscopy, 163, 163f
  complicating needle biopsy, 184-185, 185f,
    185t
  complications of, 105, 105f-106f
  controversies and pitfalls of, 835-836
  in cystic fibrosis, 576-577, 835
  familial, genetic factors underlying, 8t-9t
  iatrogenic, 834
  in Langerhans cell histiocytosis, 669
  in lymphangioleiomyomatosis, 667, 835
  primary spontaneous, 831-833
    clinical presentation of, 831-832
    diagnosis of, 832, 832f
    management of, 832, 833f
    pathophysiology of, 831
    recurrence of, strategies to avoid, 833
    surgical treatment of, 832-833
  in pulmonary Langerhans' cell histiocytosis,
    835
  radiographic features of, 103-105, 104f-105f
  secondary spontaneous, 833-834
    clinical presentation of, 833
    diagnosis of, 833-834
    discharge and follow-up evaluation of, 834
    management of, 834
    recurrence, strategies to avoid, 834
    surgical treatment of, 834
  secondary to Marfan syndrome, genetic
    factors underlying, 8t-9t
  spontaneous
    in coal worker's pneumoconiosis, 640-641
    in pregnancy, 910
  surgical/subcutaneous, 834-835, 835f
  tension, 834
Poliomyelitis, respiratory presentations of, 765
Pollutants, COPD exacerbations and, 562
Pollution, air, 937-945. See also Air pollution.
Polyangiitis
  eosinophilic granulomatosis with, 726.
    See also Churg-Strauss syndrome (CSS).
  granulomatosis with, 722-726. See also
    Granulomatosis with polyangiitis
    (GPA).
  microscopic, 722-726. See also Microscopic
    polyangiitis (MPA).
Polyarteritis nodosa, 727
Polychondritis, relapsing, 661, 661b
Polycyclic aromatic hydrocarbons (PAHs), in
  air pollution, 940
Polycythemia, in COPD assessment, 550
Polymorphonuclear neutrophils, in immune
  response, 280t, 281-282, 282f
Polymyositis, 653
  clinical features of, 659-660, 659f
Polyneuromyopathy, critical illness, 425-426
Polyp(s), nasal
  chronic rhinosinusitis with, 477-478, 477f,
    478b
    treatment of, 485-486, 485f
  surgical interventions for, 485-486
Polysomnography
  in obstructive sleep apnea, 743, 744f
  in pulmonary arterial hypertension, 716

POPH. *See* Portopulmonary hypertension (POPH).
Pores, of Kohn, 4, 4f
Portal hypertension, 712
  pulmonary consequences of, 921t
Portopulmonary hypertension (POPH), 712, 920
  clinical course of, 925
  clinical features of, 921
  diagnosis of, 921-923, 924f
  pathophysiology of, 920, 922t
  risk factors for, 920
  treatment of, 924
Posaconazole, for invasive aspergillosis, 343t
Positioning
  for endotracheal intubation in ICU, 438, 439f
  prone, for refractory hypoxemia in ARDS, 467
Positive airway pressure (PAP)
  non-continuous, for obstructive sleep apnea, 748
  for obstructive sleep apnea, 742, 747f
Positive end-expiratory pressure (PEEP), 417-418, 417f
  in ARDS, 462-466, 464f, 464t-465t
  oxygenation and, 464, 464t
  positive-pressure ventilation and, 35
Positive-pressure ventilation, 35
  noninvasive, 431
    for acute dyspnea, 255-256
Positron emission tomography–computed tomography, integrated, guiding percutaneous biopsy, 180-181, 182f
Positron emission tomography (PET), 122-132
  cameras for, 122-123
  in diagnosis, 124, 125f
  false-negative results with, 124
  false-positive results with, 123-124
  future innovations in, 131-132
  health economics and, 129
  indications for, in respiratory oncology, 127t
  interpretation of, 123-124
  in malignant pleural mesothelioma, 840-841, 841f
  in mesothelioma assessment, 129-130, 130f
  metabolic tracers in, 123
  normal imaging with, 123
  in pleural effusions, 820, 820f-821f
  principles of, 122-123
  in radiotherapy planning, 131
  in sarcoidosis, 611-612
  in small cell lung cancer staging, 129
  in staging, 124-131, 126f, 127t
  survival and, 129
  in therapy assessment, 130-131
  treatment choices and, 127-129, 127f-128f, 128t
Posterior mediastinal masses, CT evaluation of, 113, 113f
Postextubation failure, noninvasive ventilation in, 433-434
Postnatal stage, of lung development, 1, 2t
Postoperative complications, for intrapulmonary lesions, pitfalls and controversies for, 185-186
Posttransplantation lymphoproliferative disorder (PTLD), FDG-PET imaging in, 122
Postural drainage, in COPD, 558
Prednisone
  for ANCA-associated vasculitis, 723-724, 724t
  oral, for COPD exacerbations, 564

Preeclampsia, pulmonary edema and, 906, 906f
Pregnancy, 904-911
  acute respiratory distress causes in, 907t
  amniotic fluid embolism in, 905-906, 905f
  ARDS in, 909-910, 909b
  asthma in, 500, 907
    management of, 517
    treatment of, 905f, 907
  asthma risk factors in, 498
  controversies and pitfalls of, 910-911
  in cystic fibrosis, 576, 910
  dyspnea in, 904-905
  gastric aspiration in, 910
  gestational trophoblastic disease in, 907
  interstitial lung disease in, 910
  lower respiratory tract infections in, 909
  obstructive sleep apnea in, 910
  outcomes of, poor, from indoor air pollution, 944
  ovarian hyperstimulation syndrome in, 907
  peripartum cardiomyopathy in, 906-907
  pleural disease in, 910
  preeclampsia and pulmonary edema in, 906, 906f
  pulmonary embolism treatment in, 704
  pulmonary physiology in, 904-905, 905f
  pulmonary thromboembolic disease in, 907-909, 908f, 908t
  pulmonary vascular disease in, 910
  scoliosis and, 761
  tocolytic pulmonary edema and, 906
  tuberculosis treatment in, 394, 397
  venous thromboembolism and, 694
Preoxygenation, before endotracheal intubation in ICU, 439
Pressure- and volume-limited (PVL) ventilation, for ARDS, 462, 463t
Pressure-cycled ventilation, 407, 407f
Pressure-regulated volume control and volume support, 416
Pressure support ventilation, 410, 411f
Pressure-targeted (-controlled) ventilation, 407-409, 409f
Pressure-volume curve
  of combined thoracic system, 22f
  of lung, 22, 22f
Primary biliary cirrhosis (PBC)
  clinical features of, 921
  pathophysiology of, 920
Primary ciliary dyskinesia, bronchiectasis and, 583
Primary effusion lymphoma, in HIV patient, 378
Primary sclerosing cholangitis (PSC)
  clinical features of, 921
  pathophysiology of, 920
Prinzmetal angina, chest pain and, 270
Prior probability, in association studies, 11
Progressive massive fibrosis, 639
  chest radiology in, 641, 641f-642f
Prone positioning, for refractory hypoxemia in ARDS, 467
Proportional assist ventilation, 413, 414f
Prostanoids, for pulmonary arterial hypertension, 719-720
Protein C deficiency, inherited thrombophilia from, 691, 691t
Protein C resistance, activated, inherited thrombophilia from, 692
Protein S deficiency, inherited thrombophilia from, 691-692, 691t
Proteinase/antiproteinase imbalance, in COPD, 541, 542t

Prothrombin gene mutation, inherited thrombophilia from, 691t, 692
Protozoal infections, in HIV patient, 358, 358f
PSC. *See* Primary sclerosing cholangitis (PSC).
Pseudochylothorax, pleural effusions related to, 830
Pseudoglandular stage, of lung development, 1, 2t
Pseudomediastinum, 861
Pseudomonas aeruginosa, in cystic fibrosis lung disease, 568-569, 571b, 575, 575t
Psittacosis, 299
Psychiatric disorders, chest pain in, 271
Psychiatric nursing practice, etiologic agents in, 323
Psychological support, in COPD, 559
Pulmonary alveolar microlithiasis (PAM), 673-674, 673f
Pulmonary alveolar proteinosis (PAP)
  BAL fluid in, 671-672, 672f
  diagnosis of, 671-672, 672f
  histopathology of, 671-672, 672f
  management of, 672
  opportunistic infections complicating, 672
Pulmonary angiography, 74-75, 74f
Pulmonary arterial hypertension (PAH), 710.
  See also Pulmonary hypertension.
  associated with connective tissue diseases, 711-712
  biomarkers of, 718
  blood tests in, 718
  cardiac magnetic resonance imaging in, 718
  chest computed tomography in, 716-717, 716f
  chest radiograph in, 715, 715f
  chronic hemolytic anemia and, 712
  congenital heart disease and, 712
  controversies and pitfalls of, 720
  definition of, 710
  description of, 710-712, 711f
  diagnostic approach to, 714-718, 714t
  drug and toxin-induced, 711
  echocardiogram in, 717, 717f
  echocardiographic evaluation of, 197-198
  electrocardiograph in, 715, 715f
  functional assessment in, 718
  heritable, 711
  in HIV patients, 712
  idiopathic, 711
  lung transplantation for, 889
  mediators and pathways in, 714t
  overnight oximetry/polysomnography in, 716
  pathophysiology of, 717f
  portal, 712
  pulmonary function testing in, 715
  with pulmonary venous or capillary abnormalities, 712-713
  right-sided heart catheterization in, 717-718
  risk factors for, 712b
  schistosomiasis and, 712
  screening recommendations for, 710-713
  survival and outlook with, 720
  therapy of
    disease-targeted, 719-720
    general, 718-719
  ventilation-perfusion scan in, 716, 716f
Pulmonary arteriography, in pulmonary embolism, 701, 701f
Pulmonary artery(ies), 3f, 5
  radiographic anatomy of, 78, 78f
Pulmonary artery catheterization, in critical illness, 447-449, 447f-448f, 449b, 449t, 450f

Pulmonary artery flotation catheter (PAFC), 447-449, 447b, 447f-448f, 449t, 450f
Pulmonary artery occlusion pressure, measuring, 448, 449t
Pulmonary ascariasis, 320
Pulmonary blood flow
    distribution of, 30-31, 31f
    regulation of, 32, 32f
    ventilation and, inequality of, 38
Pulmonary capillaritis, pauciimmune, idiopathic, 726-727
Pulmonary capillary abnormalities, pulmonary arterial hypertension with, 712-713
Pulmonary capillary hemangiomatosis (PCH), 712-713
Pulmonary circulation, 29-36
    blood flow distribution in, 30-31, 31f
    driving pressure across, 29-30, 30f
    fluid exchange in, 33-34, 33t, 34f
    nonrespiratory functions of, 32-33
    physiology of, 29-30
    respiratory-circulatory interactions and, 34-35
Pulmonary cysts, tuberous sclerosis with, genetic factors underlying, 8t-9t
Pulmonary cytolytic thrombi, after hematopoietic stem cell transplantation, 918
Pulmonary disease. See Lung disease.
Pulmonary edema
    acute, drug-induced, parenchymal patterns in, 234-235, 234f
    cardiogenic, noninvasive mechanical ventilation for, 432-433
    in hematopoietic stem cell transplantation patients, 916
    high-altitude, 34
    high-pressure, in lung transplantation, 893t, 894
    noncardiac, drug-induced, 223t
    preeclampsia and, 906, 906f
    reexpansion, 867
    tocolytic, 906
Pulmonary embolectomy, 704
Pulmonary embolism (PE), 690-709
    acute, treatment of, 702-704
    air, 706-707
    amniotic fluid, 707-708
    arterial blood gas analysis in, 696
    B-type natriuretic peptide assay in, 696
    chest radiographs in, 697-698, 698f
    clinical assessment of, 697-702
    clinical features of, 695-697
    computed tomography angiography in, 699-701, 701f
    contrast venography in, 699
    controversies and pitfalls of, 708-709
    D-dimer assay in, 696, 698-699
    diagnosis of, 697-702, 697t, 702f
    differential diagnosis of, 695b
    echocardiogram in, 699, 700f
    electrocardiograms in, 697-698, 698f
    epidemiology of, 690
    isolated subsegmental, controversies over, 708
    laboratory tests in, 696-697
    magnetic resonance imaging in, 701-702
    medical history in, 695
    MRA and, 73
    nonthrombotic, 706-708, 706b
    pathogenesis of, 695
    pleural effusions in, 829
    prevention of, 705-706
    pulmonary arteriography in, 701, 701f
    risk factors for, 690-695
        acquired, 693-695, 694b

Pulmonary embolism (PE) (Continued)
        inherited, 690-693. See also Inherited thrombophilia.
    symptoms and signs of, 695-696, 696t
    thrombolytic therapy for, without hemodynamic instability, 708-709
    treatment of, 702-708
        with malignancy, 704
        outpatient, controversies over, 708
        in pregnancy, 704
        prophylactic, 704, 704t
    troponin assay in, 696-697
    tumor, 708
    venous compression ultrasonography in, 699
    ventilation-perfusion lung scan in, 699, 700f
Pulmonary embolus, pain in, 267-268
Pulmonary eosinophilia, tropical, 320-321
Pulmonary fibrosis
    drug-induced, 236-237
    idiopathic. See Idiopathic pulmonary fibrosis (IPF).
    lung transplantation for, 888
    reticular pattern on HRCT in, 115, 115f
Pulmonary fissures, radiographic anatomy of, 78, 78f
Pulmonary function testing, 133-142
    bronchoprovocation testing in, 141
    diffusing capacity in, 138-139
    gas distribution tests in, 139-140, 139f
    lung volumes in, 136-138. See also Lung volumes.
    in pulmonary arterial hypertension, 715
    in sarcoidosis, 612
    spirometry in, 133-136. See also Spirogram; Spirometry.
    in upper airway obstruction, 140-141, 140f-141f
Pulmonary function tests
    in connective tissue diseases, 662
    in diffuse lung disease diagnosis, 591
    for pulmonary complications of hematopoietic stem cell transplantation, 918
    in respiratory function weakness, 765, 765t
Pulmonary gas exchange, 37-49. See also Gas exchange.
Pulmonary hemosiderosis, idiopathic, diffuse alveolar hemorrhage and, 730
Pulmonary host defense system, 275, 276f
    antimicrobial molecules in, 282-283, 282t
    antimicrobial peptides in, 283-284
    complement in, 283, 283f
    inflammatory mediators in, 286-287, 286t-287t
    innate immune receptors in, 284-286, 284t, 285f
    specific cell responses in, 277-282
    structural defenses in, 275-277, 277t
Pulmonary hypertension, 710-721. See also Pulmonary arterial hypertension (PAH).
    catastrophic, drug-induced, 223t
    chest pain in, 268
    chronic thromboembolic, 713
    classification of, 710-713, 711b
    in connective tissue diseases, 656
    in COPD, 544-545, 545b
    definition of, 710
    diagnostic approach to, 714-718
    HIV-1-associated, 381
    in idiopathic pulmonary fibrosis, 602
    from left-sided heart disease, 713
    from lung disease and/or hypoxia, 713
    lung structure and, 38
    pathobiology of, 713-714, 714f

Pulmonary hypertension (Continued)
    postoperative pulmonary complications and, 869
    in pregnancy, 910
    primary, genetic factors underlying, 8t-9t
    in sarcoidosis, 609-610
    signs and symptoms of, 714-715
    in systemic sclerosis, 659
    therapy for, 718-720
    thromboembolic, chronic, treatment of, 705
    of unclear or multifactorial etiology, 713
Pulmonary infections
    bronchoscopy in, 158-159
    diagnostic approach to, 288-295
        classification in, 288-289, 289t
        in community acquired pneumonia, 295f
        controversies on, 294
        features in, 288, 289t
        in nosocomial pneumonia, 295f
        pathogen in
            identification of, 292-294
            prediction of, 290-292, 292f, 292t-293t
        pitfalls of, 294-295
        in pneumonia in immunocompromised patient, 295f
        severity in, 289-290, 290b, 291f
    in HIV patients, 346-373
    in immunocompromised patients
        bronchoscopy in, 159
        diagnostic approach to, 295f
        microbial etiology prediction in, 293t
        pneumonia as. See also Pneumonia(s).
        viral, in non–HIV-infected immunocompromised patients, 338-340, 339f, 339t
Pulmonary inflammation, chest pain in, 270
Pulmonary light chain deposition disease (LCDD), 670
Pulmonary lobule, 2, 3f
Pulmonary lymphangioleiomyomatosis, HRCT in, 593
Pulmonary mass, radiographic signs of, 89-90, 90f-91f
Pulmonary mechanics, in respiratory function testing, 767
Pulmonary nodule(s)
    growth of, CT assessment of, 90, 91f
    multiple
        causes of, 93b
        radiographic features of, 92, 93f-94f
    necrobiotic, in inflammatory bowel disease, 931-934, 933f
    in pneumonia, in non–HIV-infected immunocompromised patients, 335-336, 335f
    in rheumatoid arthritis, 658-659
    solitary, in lung cancer, 790-793, 791t, 792f
Pulmonary pain, 267
Pulmonary physiology
    changes in, in pregnancy, 904, 905f
    preoperative evaluation of, 869
Pulmonary physiology assessment
    in asbestosis, 649
    before thoracic surgery, 869
Pulmonary rehabilitation, in COPD, 557
Pulmonary stretch receptors (PSRs), 51f, 52
Pulmonary surfactant
    in alveolus, at air-liquid interface, 24, 24f
    secretion of, type II pneumocytes in, 15-16, 24
Pulmonary thromboembolic disease, in pregnancy, 907-909, 908f, 908t
Pulmonary thromboendarterectomy, for pulmonary arterial hypertension, 720

Pulmonary toxicity
   amiodarone-induced, 223t
   in hematopoietic stem cell transplantation
      patients, 916
Pulmonary toxicity syndrome, delayed, in
   hematopoietic stem cell transplantation,
   917
Pulmonary tuberculosis. *See* Tuberculosis (TB).
Pulmonary vascular disease
   exercise in, lung response to, 146
   in pregnancy, 910
Pulmonary vascular resistance (PVR)
   calculation of, 30
   lung volume and, 30
Pulmonary vasculature. *See also* Pulmonary
   artery(ies); Pulmonary vascular disease;
   Pulmonary vein(s).
   in COPD, 534
Pulmonary vasculitis, 722-728
   antineutrophil cytoplasmic autoantibody–
      associated, 722
   Behçet disease as, 727-728
   definition of, 722
   Henoch-Schönlein purpura as, 728
   large vessel, 727
   medium-size vessel, 727
   secondary, 728
   small vessel, 722-727
Pulmonary vasculopathy, drug-induced, 239
Pulmonary veins, radiographic anatomy of, 78,
   78f
Pulmonary venoocclusive disease (PVOD),
   712-713
   drug-induced, 239
   in hematopoietic stem cell transplantation,
   917-918
Pulmonary venous abnormalities, pulmonary
   arterial hypertension with, 712-713
Pulse contour analysis, in critical illness, 449-450
Pulse power analysis, in critical illness, 450,
   451b, 451f
Purpura, Henoch-Schönlein, 728
Pursed-lip breathing, in COPD, 558
PVOD. *See* Pulmonary venoocclusive disease
   (PVOD).
PVR. *See* Pulmonary vascular resistance (PVR).
Pyrazinamide, for TB, 391t

R

RA. *See* Rheumatoid arthritis (RA).
Rabies, respiratory presentations of, 770
Radiation-induced injury, 237
   of lung, acute drug-induced, 223t
Radiofrequency ablation (RFA), for Stage I
   non–small cell lung cancer, 802-803
Radiography, chest, 63-65. *See also* Chest
   radiography.
Radiotherapy
   cranial, prophylactic, for Stage III or IV lung
      cancer, 806-807
   for malignant pleural mesothelioma, 843
   planning of, PET in, 131
   postoperative, for Stage II non–small cell
      lung cancer, 803
   for small cell lung cancer, 806
   for Stage III non–small cell lung cancer,
      803-805
   stereotactic body, for Stage I non–small cell
      lung cancer, 802
Rapidly adapting pulmonary stretch receptors,
   51f, 52
RBILD. *See* Respiratory bronchiolitis interstitial
   lung disease (RBILD).
Reabsorption collapse, of lung, 84

Reactive airway disease, bronchoprovocation
   testing for, 141
Reactive airways dysfunction syndrome
   (RADS), 521
   pathophysiology of, 525f
Reactive oxygen species (ROS)
   in epigenetic regulation, 12
   genes in protection against, 12
Recoil pressure(s), 21-22, 21f
   transmural pressure difference and, 23t
Recombinant human deoxyribonuclease, in
   cystic fibrosis therapy, 574
Recruitment maneuvers
   for refractory hypoxemia in ARDS, 466
   in ventilator-induced lung injury prevention,
      426
      alternative approaches to, 426-428, 428f
Reduced-intensity conditioning, for
   hematopoietic stem cell transplantation,
   912
Reexpansion pulmonary edema, 867
Rehabilitation
   pulmonary. *See* Pulmonary rehabilitation.
   for pulmonary arterial hypertension, 720
Rejection, in lung transplantation
   acute, 893t, 894, 895f
   chronic, 899, 899f, 899t-900t
   histologic classification and grading of, 899t
   hyperacute, 892, 893t
Relapsing polychondritis, 661, 661b
Renal effusions, 826
Reservoir nasal cannulas, for home oxygen
   therapy in COPD, 560
Residual volume (RV), 21, 21f
   in obstructive lung disease, 138, 138f
   in restrictive lung disease, 138
Respiratory acidosis
   clinical causes of, 47-48
   Davenport diagram for, 46f, 47
   in obesity hypoventilation syndrome, 749
Respiratory alkalosis
   clinical causes of, 48
   Davenport diagram for, 47f, 48
Respiratory bronchioles, 3, 4f, 19-20
Respiratory bronchiolitis interstitial lung
   disease (RBILD)
   characteristics of, 600t
   HRCT in, 593
Respiratory centers, 50
   afferent inputs to, 50-53, 51f
   efferent limb of, 53-56
Respiratory cycle
   distribution of ventilation in, 27
   events of, 23-27
   flow resistance in, 24-25, 25f-26f
   respiratory muscle effort in, 23, 23f
   surface tension in, 23-24, 24f
   work of breathing in, 25-26, 26f
Respiratory disease(s). *See also* Lung disease;
   specific diseases, e.g. Cystic fibrosis (CF).
   acute
      from indoor air pollution, 943
      from outdoor air pollution, 940-941, 941f
   chronic
      from indoor air pollution, 944, 944f
      from outdoor air pollution, 941
   drug-induced, 221-241. *See also* Drug-
      induced *entries;* Drug-induced
      respiratory diseases (DIRDs).
   in HIV patients, risk factors for, 350
   single-gene disorders and, 7-10
Respiratory distress syndrome
   acute, 454-470. *See also* Acute respiratory
      distress syndrome (ARDS).
   genetic factors underlying, 8t-9t, 16

Respiratory epithelium, in host defense system,
   277, 277t
Respiratory failure
   after hematopoietic stem cell
      transplantation, 918
   in bronchiectasis, 586
   in immunocompromised patients,
      noninvasive mechanical ventilation for,
      433
   postoperative, risk for, 871, 871t
Respiratory function
   chest wall deformity and, 757-758, 758t
   in scoliosis, optimization of, 760-761
Respiratory infections. *See also* Pulmonary
   infections.
   as asthma triggers, 499
   bronchoscopy in, 158t
   nosocomial, 322-329. *See also* Nosocomial
      respiratory infections.
Respiratory mechanics, 19-28
   airways in, 19-20, 20f
   application of, controversies and pitfalls in,
      27
   elastic properties of chest wall in, 22, 22f, 23t
   elastic properties of lungs in, 22, 22f
   lung-chest wall system in, 21
   lung interdependence in, 20
   lung volumes in, 21, 21f
   pleural space in, 19
   thoracic structure in, 19, 20f
   volumes of elastic structures in, 21-22, 21f
Respiratory muscle(s), 50-62
   abdominal, 55
   adaptation of, from chronic load increase,
      58, 59f
   diaphragm as, 51f, 53-54, 53f-54f. *See also*
      Diaphragm.
   diseases of, clinical features of, 764-765,
      764t
   effort of, 22f, 23
   fatigue of, 57-58, 57f-58f
   force-frequency relationships in, 57-58, 57f
   function of
      assessment of, 774-775
      tests of, 765-767, 765t, 766f-767f
   function testing of, 59-61
   functional anatomy of, 53-55
   inactivity/unloading of, 58-59
   inflammation and injury of, 58
   intercostals as, 51f, 53
   physiology of, 55-56
   plasticity of, from chronic load increase, 58,
      59f
   responses to load changes, 57-59, 57f-59f
   resting of, in COPD, 559
   scalenes as, 55
   during sleep, in scoliosis, 758
   sternocleidomastoids as, 54
   weak, in COPD, 544
   weakness of
      causes of, 764b
      imaging in evaluation of, 767-768
      in polymyositis/dermatomyositis,
         pulmonary complications of, 659
Respiratory muscle function test, in COPD
   assessment, 550
Respiratory muscle pump, 763-768, 764f
   assessment of, 763-768
   imbalance of, clinical consequences of, 763,
      764b, 764f
   in obese patients, 774
Respiratory muscle-thoracic cage receptors,
   51f, 53
Respiratory myopathy, corticosteroid-induced,
   respiratory presentations of, 772-773

Respiratory oncology, PET imaging in, 127t
Respiratory rhythmogenesis, controversy over, 62
Respiratory stimulants, central, for COPD exacerbations, 565-566
Respiratory syncytial virus (RSV) infection
  in hematopoietic stem cell transplantation patient, 915
  in non–HIV-infected immunocompromised patients, 340
Respiratory system
  imaging of, 63-121. *See also* Imaging techniques.
  lungs and chest wall in, 22f, 23
  recoil pressures of, transmural pressure difference and, 23t
Respiratory viruses
  infections from, in non–HIV-infected immunocompromised patients, 338-340, 339f, 339t
  lung allograft syndromes and, 340
Respiratory work, in dyspnea, 252
Respiratory zone, 19-20
Restrictive cardiomyopathy, secondary to chronic respiratory disease, echocardiographic features of, 200-201
Restrictive impairment, spirometric abnormalities in, 135-136
Restrictive lung disease
  lung volume abnormalities in, 138
  respiratory work in, 26
  spirometric abnormalities in, 135-136
  ventilating patients with, 422
Reticular pattern, on HRCT in parenchymal disease, 114-115, 115f
Reticular shadowing, 93-94, 94f
Reticulonodular shadowing, 94
Retinoic acid
  alveolar regeneration in response to, 17
  in lung regeneration in mice, 16-17
Reverse halo sign, in cryptogenic organizing pneumonia, 631-632, 631f
Reversibility testing, in COPD assessment, 549
Rheumatoid arthritis (RA), 653
  airways disease in, 656, 657f
  clinical features of, 656-658
  interstitial pneumonias in, 656-657, 657f-658f
  lymphoid hyperplasia in, 658, 658f
  pleural disease in, 656
  pleural effusions secondary to, 828-829
  pulmonary nodules in, 657-658
Rheumatoid factor, elevated, in bronchiectasis, 583
Rhinitis, 471-475
  allergic, 471-472. *See also* Allergic rhinitis.
  atrophic, 475
  autonomic, 474-475
  classification of, 472f
    by frequency and severity, 480f
  clinical course and prevention of, 486
  cough due to, treatment of, 248
    cough due to, 246
  definition of, 471
  diagnosis, evaluation, and tests in, 479-480
  differential diagnosis of, 474b, 475
  drug-induced, 475
  drugs associated with, 474b
  food allergen-induced, 475
  food-induced, 475
  gustatory, 475
  hormonal, 475
  idiopathic or intrinsic, 475
    clinical course and prevention of, 486
    treatment of, 482

Rhinitis (Continued)
  infectious, 472-473
  nonallergic, 473-475
    clinical features of, 478
  noninfective, clinical features of, 478
  occupational, 475
Rhinosinusitis, 476-478
  acute, 476-477
    clinical course and prevention of, 486
    clinical features of, 478
    diagnosis of, 479
    treatment of, 483-484, 484f
  chronic, 477-478
    clinical course and prevention of, 486
    clinical features of, 478
    treatment of, 484-485, 485f
Rhodococcus equi infection, in HIV patient, 351
Rhythmogenesis, respiratory, controversy over, 62
Ribavirin
  for viral lung infections, 339t
  for viral pneumonia, 313-314
Ribs
  crowding of, in lobar collapse, 84
  thoracic movement and, 19, 20f
Rifabutin, for TB, 391t
Rifampin, for TB, 391t
  latent, 396t
Rifapentine, for TB, 391t
Right heart, hemodynamic assessment of, echocardiographic, 196-197, 197f
Right ventricular function, echocardiographic assessment of, 193-196, 195f-196f
Rigid bronchoscopic debulking or balloon dilatation, 165, 165f
Rigid bronchoscopy, 154, 155f
  diagnostic application of, 877-878, 877f, 877t
Rimantadine, for viral pneumonia, 313
Rituximab (RTX), for ANCA-associated vasculitis, 725
Roflumilast, for COPD, 556
RV. *See* Residual volume (RV).

S

S-adenosylmethionine (SAM, AdoMet), plasma or serum levels of, in diagnosis of HIV-related pneumonia, 359-360
Saccharin clearance test, 479
Saccular stage, of lung development, 1, 2t
St. George's Respiratory Questionnaire, in COPD, 550
Salbutamol. *See* Albuterol (Salbutamol).
  chemical structure of, 205f
Saline, hypertonic, in cystic fibrosis therapy, 574
Salmeterol
  chemical structure of, 205f
  for COPD, 555, 555t
  with fluticasone, for COPD, 555t, 556
  formulations, doses and duration of action of, 207t
  with theophylline, for COPD, 555t, 556
  with tiotropium
    with COPD, 556
    and fluticasone for COPD, 555t, 556
Sarcoidosis, 607-619
  alternative therapies for, 616-618, 617t
  antitumor necrosis factor therapy for, 617t, 618
  azathioprine for, 617t, 618
  biomarkers of, 616
  bronchoscopy in, 615, 616f

Salmeterol (Continued)
  calcium metabolism in, 615
  chest radiography in, 610-612, 611f
  clinical course of, 618-619
  clinical features of, 609-615, 611f-614f
  CNS in, 615
  controversies and pitfalls of, 619
  corticosteroids for, 616, 617t
  cyclophosphamide for, 618
  diagnosis of, 615, 616f
  epidemiology of, 607
  etiology of, 607
  extrapulmonary, 612-615, 613f
  eyes in, 612-613, 614f
  gastrointestinal in, 614
  genetic factors in, 607, 608t
  heart in, 614
  HRCT in, 71, 593, 594f
  hydroxychloroquine for, 617-618, 617t
  immunosuppressive therapies for, 616-618, 617t
  liver in, 614, 614f
  lung transplantation for, 618
  lymphatics in, 614
  methotrexate for, 617t, 618
  mycophenolate mofetil for, 618
  nodular pattern on HRCT in, 115-116, 116f
  pathophysiology of, 607-609, 609f-610f
  pentoxifylline for, 617t, 618
  pulmonary function testing in, 612
  pulmonary hypertension in, 609-610
  pulmonary manifestations of, 609-612, 611f-612f
  relapse rates for, 616
  risk factors for, 607, 619b
  skin in, 612, 613f
  spleen in, 614
  tetracyclines for, 618
  thalidomide for, 617t, 618
  treatment of, 616-618
  tumor necrosis factor-α blockers for, 618
Sarcoma, Kaposi, 374-377. *See also* Kaposi sarcoma.
Scalene lymph node biopsy, 877t, 878
Scalene muscles, 55
Scar emphysema, in coal workers, 642
Schistosomiasis, 321
  pulmonary arterial hypertension and, 712
Schwannoma, 812, 855
SCLC. *See* Small cell lung cancer (SCLC).
Scleroderma renal crisis, 665
Sclerosing cholangitis, primary. *See* Primary sclerosing cholangitis (PSC).
Sclerosing hemangioma, 813
Scoliosis, 756-762
  adolescent idiopathic, impact of, on exercise capacity, 758
  bracing for, 760
  cardiopulmonary decompensation in, 759
  clinical features of, 759
  clinical signs in, controversies over, 761
  controversies and pitfalls of, 761
  curvature in, progression of, 759
  definition of, 756, 757f
  diagnosis of, 759
  epidemiology of, 756
  genetics of, 756
  monitoring of high-risk patients for, 759
  pathophysiology of, 756
  pregnancy and, 761
  risk factors for, 756
  surgery for, 760, 760f
  treatment of, 759-761
  ventilatory impairment in, management of, 760-761

Scrofula, 387
Secondary lobule of Miller, 2, 3f
Secretions, aspiration of, therapeutic
  bronchoscopy for, 171
Sedation, in ARDS management, 468
Seminomas, mediastinal, 852-853
Senescence, cell, in COPD, 542
Sensory receptors, in dyspnea, 250-251, 251f
Sepsis, mechanical ventilation–induced,
  460-461
  multiple system organ dysfunction and, 461
  ventilator-induced lung injury and, 461-462
Serologic studies, for pulmonary complications
  of hematopoietic stem cell transplantation,
  918-919
Serologic testing
  in pneumonia pathogen identification, 294
  in viral pneumonia diagnosis, 312
Serosal disease
  as emergency, 935
  in inflammatory bowel disease, 934
Sexual dysfunction, obstructive sleep apnea
  and, 741-742
Shunt, 43
  in gas exchange assessment, 44
  hypoxemia from, 43, 43t
Shunt equation, 44, 44f
Signet ring sign, in bronchiectasis, 119-120, 120f
Sildenafil, for idiopathic pulmonary fibrosis, 603
Silhouette sign, in consolidation, 81-82
Silicone embolism syndrome, 236
Silicosis
  accelerated, 641
  acute, 637, 641
  epidemiology of, 637
  histopathologic changes in, 639, 639f
  industries associated with, 638t
  sources of exposure in, 637, 638t
Silo filler's lung, 685. See also Toxic
  inhalational lung injury.
Single-inhaler therapy, for asthma, 514
Single-nucleotide polymorphisms (SNPs)
  disease-associated, in COPD, 11-12
  variation in, in ARDS, 457-458
Sinuses
  drainage pathways of, 476f
  inflammation of lining of. See Rhinosinusitis.
Sirolimus, in lung transplantation, 901t
Sjögren syndrome (SS), 653
  clinical features of, 660, 661b, 661f
  CT appearance and clinical characteristics of,
  671t
Skin
  corticosteroid toxicities affecting, 217t
  infections of, nontuberculous mycobacterial
    clinical features of, 400
    treatment of, 403
  sarcoidosis involving, 612, 613f
Skin tests, for allergic rhinitis, 479-480
Sleep
  REM, obstructive sleep apnea in, 739
  respiratory muscles/thoracic pump during, in
    scoliosis, 758
  stability of, airway patency in obstructive
    sleep apnea and, 739
Sleep apnea, obstructive, 731-748. See also
    Obstructive sleep apnea (OSA).
Sleep-disordered breathing
  clinical course of, 925
  clinical features of, 921
  diagnosis of, 923-924, 924f
  in obesity hypoventilation syndrome,
    749-755. See also Obesity
    hypoventilation syndrome.

Sleep-disordered breathing (Continued)
  obstructive sleep apnea as, 731-748. See also
    Obstructive sleep apnea (OSA).
  treatment of, 925
Sleep studies
  in chest wall disease, 768
  in COPD assessment, 550
  in obesity hypoventilation syndrome,
    752-753, 752f-753f
  in obstructive sleep apnea, 743-745, 743t,
    744f
    in-laboratory vs. out-of-laboratory, 748
Sleepiness, daytime
  causes of, other than obstructive sleep
    apnea, 745, 745t
  obstructive sleep apnea and, 741, 742b
Slowly adapting pulmonary stretch receptors,
  51f, 52
Small airways disease. See also Bronchiolitis.
  definition of, 531
  pathology of, 533, 534f
Small cell lung cancer (SCLC), 782-784, 783f
  staging of, PET imaging in, 129
"Small granular" cells, 4
Smoking/smoke exposure
  asthma and, 495, 499
  cessation of
    for asthma, 513
    for COPD, 554
  community-acquired pneumonia and, 297
  COPD and, 534-536, 536f
  diffuse lung disease related to, 590
  endoplasmic reticulum stress in cells from, 13
  Langerhans cell histiocytosis and, 669
  lung cancer and, 777-778
  oxidative stress from, 12-13
  postoperative pulmonary complications and,
    870
Sneeze, in defense system, 276, 277t
Sniff pressure(s)
  inspiratory, in respiratory function testing, 766
  in respiratory function testing, 60-61, 61f
Snoring, in obstructive sleep apnea, 741
Socioeconomic impact, of COPD, 539
Socioeconomic status, childhood asthma and,
  497
Soft tissues
  corticosteroid toxicities affecting, 217t
  infections of, nontuberculous mycobacterial
    clinical features of, 400
    treatment of, 403
Solitary fibrous tumor of pleura, 812, 813f
Solitary pulmonary nodules (SPNs), in lung
  cancer, 790-793, 791t, 792f
Soluble mesothelin-related peptides (SMRPs),
  in malignant pleural mesothelioma, 841,
  841f
Spinal cord injury (SCI), respiratory
  presentations of, 769
Spinal fusion, for scoliosis, 760, 760f
Spinal muscular atrophy (SMA)
  respiratory presentations of, 771
  scoliosis in, 756, 757f
Spine
  deformity of
    classification of, 757b
    in scoliosis, management of, 759-760
  lesions of, 859-860, 860f
Spiriva (tiotropium). See Tiotropium (Spiriva).
Spirogram
  expiratory, force vital capacity maneuver
    and, 25, 26f
  normal, 21f
  traditional, 133, 134f

Spirometry, 133-136
  in asthma assessment, 507t
  in COPD assessment, 548, 548t-549t
  data from, in upper airway obstruction,
    258f
  expiratory flow measurements in, 133-134
  forced expiratory volume maneuver in, 133,
    134f
  interpretation of abnormalities, 135-136
  limits of normality for, 135
  lung volumes and, 136
  in obesity hypoventilation syndrome, 753
  reference equations for, 135
  reversibility of findings from, 134-135, 211
Spleen, sarcoidosis involving, 614
Spondylitis, ankylosing, 661-662
Spontaneous breathing, 34-35
  trial of, initiation of, criteria for, 428b
  ventilation modes delivering assistance to,
    409-415, 410f
Spontaneous pneumothorax, in pregnancy,
  910
Sputum
  examination of, in pneumonia pathogen
    identification, 292-293, 293f
  induced, in diagnosis of HIV-related
    pneumonia, 360, 360t
  microbiology of, in bronchiectasis diagnosis,
    583, 583t
  microscopy of, in TB diagnosis, 389-390,
    389f
Sputum eosinophil differential count, in
  asthma assessment, 507t
Squamous cell carcinoma, of lung, 781-782,
  781f
Squamous papilloma, 810-811
Staging, PET imaging in, 124-131, 126f, 127t
Staphylococcus aureus, in cystic fibrosis lung
  disease, 574-575, 575t
Staphylococcus species, in community-acquired
  pneumonia, 298-299
Starling equation, modified, 33t
Stem cell(s)
  biology of, 17
  bronchiolar, 16
  bronchoalveolar, 16
  in lung disease treatment, 16-17
Stenotrophomonas maltophilia, in cystic fibrosis
  lung disease, 575
Stenting, tracheobronchial, 167-168, 168f
Stereotactic body radiotherapy, for Stage I
  non–small cell lung cancer, 802
Sternocleidomastoid muscles, 54
Straight back syndrome, 78
Strength training, for ventilatory muscles, in
  COPD, 558-559
Streptococcus species, in community-acquired
  pneumonia, 298
Streptomycin, for TB, 392t
Stress
  endoplasmic reticulum, as intracellular
    signal, 13-14, 13f
  oxidative, as intracellular signal, 12-13
  prenatal, childhood asthma and, 498
Stress ulcer, prophylaxis for, in intubated
  patients, 324
Stretch receptors, 51f, 52
Stridor, 252-253
Stroke, respiratory presentations of, 768, 770f
Strongyloides stercoralis infection, in HIV
  patient, treatment of, 367
Strongyloidiasis, 320
  eosinophilia in, 622
  in HIV patient, 358, 358f

Subaortic fossa, mediastinal anatomy at, 109f
Subcutaneous emphysema, from chest tube leakage, 866-867
Subcutaneous pneumothorax, 834-835, 835f
Subdiaphragmatic placement, of chest tube, 866
Sulfur dioxide
  in air pollution, 938
  as irritant, 683t, 685
Superior mediastinal masses, CT evaluation of, 111-112, 112f
Superior sulcus tumors, treatment of, 805
Superior vena cava
  dilatation of, imaging of, 99, 101f
  obstruction of (SVCO), stenting for, 76
Superior vena cava stenting, 76
Superior vena cava syndrome, in lung cancer, manifestations and treatment of, 807-808
Supraclavicular lymph node biopsy, 877t, 878
Surface tension, 23-24, 24f
  of airway fluid, obstructive sleep apnea and, 739
  interstitial pressure and, 33
Surfactant. See Pulmonary surfactant.
Surgery
  for bronchiectasis, 586
  venous thromboembolism and, 693-694
Sweat testing, in cystic fibrosis diagnosis, 571, 572f
Sympathetic ganglia neoplasms, 858-859, 858f
Synchronized intermittent mandatory ventilation, 415-416, 416f
Syndrome of inappropriate secretion of antidiuretic hormone (SIADH), in lung cancer, 789-790
  manifestations and treatment of, 807, 807t
Systemic diseases, rare, pulmonary manifestations of, 674
Systemic inflammation, COPD exacerbations and, 562
Systemic lupus erythematosus (SLE), 653
  clinical features of, 660, 660f
  diffuse alveolar hemorrhage and, 729
  pleural effusions secondary to, 829
Systemic sclerosis (SSc), 653
  aspiration pneumonia in, 659
  clinical features of, 658-659
  interstitial pneumonia in, 653, 658-659, 658f
  pulmonary hypertension in, 659

T

Tacrolimus, in lung transplantation, 901t
Takayasu arteritis, 727-728
TB. See Tuberculosis (TB).
Telangiectasia, hemorrhagic, hereditary, genetic factors underlying, 8t-9t
Temporal arteritis, 727
Tendinitis, chest pain in, 270-271
Tension pneumothorax, 834
Teratoma(s)
  anterior mediastinal masses from, 112-113, 113f, 852, 852f
  benign, 813, 814f
Terbutaline
  chemical structure of, 205f
  formulations, doses and duration of action of, 207t
Tetanus, respiratory presentations of, 769
Tetracyclines, for sarcoidosis, 618
Tetralogy of Fallot, 100f
Tetraplegic patients, chest wall motion in, 53-54

Thalidomide, for sarcoidosis, 617t, 618
Theophylline
  for asthma, 510
  as bronchodilator, 209-210
    formulations, doses and duration of action of, 207t
  for COPD, 555t, 556
    relative potency and dosages of, 218t
  for COPD exacerbations, 565
  metabolism of, in COPD, 210t
  with salmeterol, for COPD, 555t, 556
Thermal ablation, for Stage I non–small cell lung cancer, 802-803
Thermodilution, transpulmonary, with arterial waveform analysis, 451, 451b, 451f
Thermodilution curves, 450f
Thermoplasty, bronchial, for asthma, 514
Thoracentesis
  in pleural effusion diagnosis, 820
  for pleural effusions, 824
Thoracic aorta
  abnormalities of, imaging of, 97-98, 98f-100f
  aneurysm of, 97-98, 99f
Thoracic cage
  diseases of, clinical features of, 764-765, 764t
  radiographic anatomy of, 78, 79f
Thoracic pump, during sleep, in scoliosis, 758
Thoracoscopy
  for pleural biopsy, 823
  video-assisted, diagnostic application of, 877t, 879-881, 880f
Thoracostomy, tube, 862. See also Chest tube insertion.
Thoracotomy
  open, diagnostic application of, 881
  for pleural biopsy, 823
Thorax
  disorders of, 774
  imaging of, in acute dyspnea, 254-255
  structure of, 19, 20f
  surgery of
    chest tube insertion and management for, 862-868. See also Chest tube insertion.
    diagnostic, 876-881. See also Diagnostic thoracic surgery.
    for lung transplantation, 882-903. See also Lung transplantation.
    postoperative complications of, 869-873, 870t
      risk factors for, 869-871, 870t
    postoperative measures for, 873-874
    preoperative measures for, 873
    pulmonary evaluation before, 869-875
      ASA classification for surgical candidates in, 871t
      for lung resection surgery, 872-873
      for surgery in general, 871, 871b
    surgical management for, 873
Throat swab, in pneumonia pathogen identification, 292
Thrombin inhibitors, direct, for pulmonary embolism, 703
Thrombocytopenia, heparin-induced, venous thromboembolism and, 694-695
Thromboembolic disease
  chronic, treatment of, 705, 705f
  pulmonary, in pregnancy, 907-909, 908f, 908t
Thromboembolic pulmonary hypertension, chronic, 713
Thromboendarterectomy, pulmonary, for pulmonary artery hypertension, 720

Thrombolytics, for pulmonary embolism, 703-704
Thrombophilia, inherited, 690-693, 691t. See also Inherited thrombophilia.
Thrombophlebitis, superficial, migratory, in lung cancer, 790
Thymectomy, 849
Thymolipoma, 853, 853f
Thymoma, 811, 846-849
  clinical findings in, 847t
  imaging of, 847-848, 848f
  treatment of, 848-849
Thymus
  carcinoid of, 849-850, 849f
  carcinoma of, 849, 849f
  CT imaging of, 110
  cysts of, 853, 854f
  hyperplasia of, 854
  neoplasia of, anterior mediastinal masses from, 112, 112f
Thyroid
  CT imaging of, 110
  superior mediastinal masses from, 111, 112f
Tidal volume (VT), 21, 21f
  in acute lung injury–acute respiratory distress syndrome management, 27
  in ARDS management, 461-462
  ventilator-induced lung injury and, 459-460, 459f
Time-cycled ventilation, 407, 407f
Tiotropium (Spiriva)
  chemical structure of, 205f
  for COPD, 555, 555t
  with formoterol, for COPD, 555t, 556
  formulations, doses and duration of action of, 207t
  with salmeterol
    with COPD, 556
    and fluticasone for COPD, 555t, 556
Tissue Doppler imaging (TDI), in peak systolic velocity of lateral tricuspid annulus displacement measurement, 194-196, 195f
Tissue sampling. See Biopsy(ies); Percutaneous biopsy procedures.
TLC. See Total lung capacity (TLC).
TMP-SMX. See Trimethoprim-sulfamethoxazole (TMP-SMX).
Tobacco. See Smoking/smoke exposure.
Tobramycin, for P. aeruginosa infection in cystic fibrosis, 575-576
Tocolytic pulmonary edema, 906
Toll-like receptor-2 (TLR-2), 284t, 285
Toll-like receptor-3 (TLR-3), 284t, 285
Toll-like receptor-4 (TLR-4), 284t, 285
Toll-like receptor-5 (TLR-5), 284t, 285
Toll-like receptor-9 (TLR-9), 284t, 285
Toll-like receptors (TLRs), 284-285, 284t, 285f
Tomography
  computed, 65-68, 66f. See also Computed tomography (CT).
  optical coherence, 164-165, 164f
  positron emission, 122-132. See also Positron emission tomography (PET).
Total lung capacity (TLC), 21, 21f
  in obstructive lung disease, 138, 138f
  in restrictive lung disease, 138
Toxic alveolar hemorrhage, 730
Toxic inhalational lung injury, 682-689
  chemical asphyxiants in, 683t, 686-687
  chemical irritants in, 683-686, 683t
  clinical features of, 683-688
  from complex exposures, 688
  controversies and pitfalls of, 688-689

Toxic inhalational lung injury (Continued)
  diagnosis of, 683-688
  epidemiology of, 682
  etiology of, 682-683, 683t
  pathology of, 682, 684f
  risk factors for, 682-683
Toxins
  biochemical, 688, 688t
  pulmonary arterial hypertension induced by, 711, 712b
Toxocariasis, 320
  blood eosinophilia in, 622
Toxoplasmosis, in HIV patient, 358, 358f
  treatment of, 367, 368t
Trachea, 2-3
  anatomy of, CT, 108-110
  aspiration of, in pneumonia pathogen identification, 293
  narrowing of, 95-96, 95f-96f
  structure and function of, 19-20
  widening of, 96-97, 96f
Tracheal tubes, in nosocomial respiratory infection prophylaxis, 324
Tracheobronchial stenting, 167-168, 168f
Tracheobronchitis, nosocomial. See Nosocomial tracheobronchitis.
Tracheobronchomalacia, therapeutic bronchoscopy for, 169-170, 170f
Tracheostomy, 443, 443b
  for obesity hypoventilation syndrome, 754
Traction bronchiectasis, 115, 115f
  in nonspecific interstitial pneumonia, 592-593, 593f
Transbronchial needle aspiration (TBNA)
  with endobronchial ultrasound, 175, 175f-176f
  in lung cancer staging, 174, 175f
Transbronchoscopic needle aspiration (TBNA)
  bronchoscopy and, 156-157
  in staging, 161
Transbronchoscopic needle biopsy (TBNB), bronchoscopy and, 156-157
Transcervical extended mediastinal lymphadenectomy (TEMLA), 878
Transcutaneous Doppler monitoring, in critical illness, 452-453
Transdiaphragmatic pressure
  in respiratory function testing, 60, 766, 766f-767f
  twitch, in respiratory function testing, 766-767
Transfer factor, 138-139
Transjugular intrahepatic portosystemic shunting (TIPS), for hepatopulmonary syndrome, controversies and pitfalls of, 925-926
Transmural pressure difference, recoil pressures and, 23t
Transplantation
  bone marrow, alveolar hemorrhage after, 730
  lung, 882-903. See also Lung transplantation.
Transpulmonary indicator dilution, in critical illness, 451
Transpulmonary pressure (PL), 418, 420f
Transradiancy, increased, unilateral, 88, 89f-90f
Transtracheal aspiration, in pneumonia pathogen identification, 294
Transtracheal oxygen therapy, for COPD, 560
Transudate/exudate separation, in pleural effusions, 821-822

Transudative effusions, 818
  conditions associated with, 825-826
  congestive cardiac failure and, 825
  hepatic hydrothorax and, 825-826
Trauma, venous thromboembolism and, 693-694
Tree-in-bud changes, in pneumonia, in non–HIV-infected immunocompromised patients, 334-335, 334f-335f
Trichoptysis, in benign teratomas, 813
Tricuspid annular plane systolic excursion (TAPSE), echocardiographic measurement of, 194, 195f
Tricuspid annulus, displacement of, lateral, peak systolic velocity of, 194-196, 195f
Trimethoprim-dapsone, for bacterial pneumonia, 363
Trimethoprim-sulfamethoxazole (TMP-SMX), for Pneumocystis pneumonia, 362-363, 362t
  prophylactic, 368-369, 369t
Trophoblastic disease, gestational, 907
Tropical eosinophilic pneumonia, 621
Tropical pulmonary eosinophilia, 320-321
Troponin assay, in pulmonary embolism (PE), 696-697
Troponin isoforms, in acute dyspnea, 254
Trousseau syndrome, in lung cancer, 790
Tube thoracostomy, 862. See also Chest tube insertion.
Tuberculin skin test, 388-389, 395
Tuberculosis (TB), 383-397
  bone and joint, 387
  in breastfeeding, treatment of, 394
  bronchoscopy in, 159, 159f
  central nervous system, 387-388
  in children, treatment of, 394
  clinical course of, 394
  clinical features of, 385-388, 386f, 388f
  clinical monitoring of, 397
  coal worker's pneumoconiosis and, 640
  diagnosis of, 388-390, 389f
  drug-resistant, 353
    treatment of, 394
  epidemiology of, 383-384, 384f
  extrapulmonary
    clinical features of, 386-387
    treatment of, 394
  gastrointestinal, 388
  genetics of, 385
  genitourinary, 387
  hemoptysis in, 261
  in HIV patient, 351-353, 352f, 352t, 392-394
    controversies and pitfalls of, 372-373
    prognosis of, 371
    prophylaxis of, 370-371
    treatment of, 364-366
  latent
    diagnosis of, 395-396, 396f
    treatment of, 396-397, 396t
  miliary, 388, 388f
  pathogenesis of, 385, 385f-386f
  pericardial, 388
  pleural, 387
  pleural effusions in, 828
  pleural fluid in, 831
  in pregnancy, treatment of, 394
  prevention of, 394-397
  pulmonary, clinical features of, 385-386, 386f
  risk factors for, 384-385, 384t
  treatment of, 390-394, 391t-393t, 393f
  vaccination for, 397

Tuberculous lymphadenitis, 387
Tuberous sclerosis, with pulmonary cysts/lymphangioleiomyomatosis, genetic factors underlying, 8t-9t
Tuberous sclerosis complex, 667-668
Tubular myelin, 15-16
Tularemia, 301
Tumor(s)
  lung
    benign, 810-817. See also Benign lung tumors.
    malignant, 776-809. See also Lung cancer.
    mediastinal. See under Mediastinum.
Tumor embolism, 708
Tumor necrosis factor-α blockers, for sarcoidosis, 618
Tumor-node-metastasis (TNM) status, PET imaging and, 124-127, 126f, 127t
Twitch occlusion test, 57
Twitch Pdi, 61
Twitch transdiaphragmatic pressure, in respiratory function testing, 766-767
Tyrosine kinase inhibitors, for Stage IV non–small cell lung cancer, 805-806

U

Ulcerative colitis, thoracic involvement in, 927. See also Inflammatory bowel disease (IBD).
Ulcers, stress, prophylaxis for, in intubated patients, 324
Ultrasound imaging
  Doppler
    in COPD assessment, 550-551
    esophageal, in critical illness, 451-453, 452f
  endobronchial, 174-176, 175f
    diagnostic application of, 876-877
  endoesophageal, 174-176, 177f
  guiding percutaneous biopsy, 180, 186, 186f
  thoracic, in pleural effusions, 818-819, 819f-820f, 819t
  venous compression, in pulmonary embolism, 699
Ultrathin bronchoscopy, 163
Underwater seal chest drainage system, 864-865, 865f
  air leak in, 865
Unfolded protein response (UPR), 13, 13f
Upper airway
  bronchoscopic examination of, 156
  corticosteroid toxicities affecting, 217t
  description of, 471
  inflammation of
    acute, as emergency, 934
    obstructive sleep apnea and, 739
  normal, 735-736, 736f
  in obstructive sleep apnea patients, 737, 737b
Upper airway disease, 471-486. See also Rhinitis; Rhinosinusitis.
  controversies and pitfalls of, 486
  cough due to, 246-247
Upper airway obstruction
  acute, drug-induced, 223t
  drug-induced, 237
  flow-volume loop in, 258, 258f
  pulmonary function testing in, 140-141
Upper extremity exercise, in COPD, 557-558
Upper respiratory passages, structure and function of, 19
Urine, testing of, in pneumonia pathogen identification, 293

Urinothorax, 826
Usual interstitial pneumonia (UIP)
    histopathologic pattern diagnosis of, 599
    HRCT and histopathologic images of, 601f
    HRCT radiologic pattern diagnosis of, 601

V

Vaccinations
    in bronchiectasis management, 585
    in COPD exacerbation prevention, 566
    in COPD management, 556-557
Valganciclovir, for viral lung infections, 339t
VAP. See Ventilator-associated pneumonia
    (VAP).
Variant angina, chest pain and, 270
Varicella-zoster virus (VZV) infection, in
    non–HIV-infected immunocompromised
    patients, 338
Varicose bronchiectasis, 580, 581f
Vas deferens, congenital bilateral absence of, in
    cystic fibrosis, 572
Vascular disease
    in connective tissue diseases, 654
        treatment of, 665, 665f
    pleural effusions secondary to, 829
Vascular lesions, mediastinal, 857
Vascular malformations, MRA and, 74f, 92-95
Vascular signs, of lobar collapse, 84
Vascular system, of lungs, 5
Vasculitis
    nasal involvement in, 475
    pulmonary, 722-728. See also Pulmonary
        vasculitis.
Vasculogenesis, in lung development, 1
Vasoconstrictors, for allergic rhinitis, 481
Vasodilators, inhaled, for refractory hypoxemia
    in ARDS, 467-468
VC. See Vital capacity (VC).
Veins, bronchial, 5
Venography, contrast, in pulmonary embolism,
    699
Venous compression ultrasonography, in
    pulmonary embolism, 699
Venous thromboembolism (VTE)
    previous, recurrent VTE and, 694
    recurrent, prophylaxis against, 704, 704t
    risk factors for, 699
        acquired, 693-695, 694b
        inherited, 690-693. See also Inherited
            thrombophilia.
Ventilation
    alveolar, 39, 39f
    and blood flow, inequality of, 38
    control of, 50-62
    distribution of, 27
    in gas exchange, 37
    impairment of
        categories of, 136t
        mixed, spirometric abnormalities in, 136
        obstructive, spirometric abnormalities in,
            135
        restrictive, spirometric abnormalities in,
            135-136
    mass conservation and, 38-39
    mechanical. See Mechanical ventilation.
    oscillatory, high-frequency, for refractory
        hypoxemia in ARDS, 467
    positive-pressure, 35
    preoperative evaluation of, 869

Ventilation (Continued)
    pressure- and volume-limited, for ARDS,
        462, 463t
    studies of, MRI in, 72
    wasted, 38
Ventilation-perfusion equation, 41, 41f
Ventilation-perfusion lung scan
    in pulmonary arterial hypertension, 716,
        716f
    in pulmonary embolism, 699, 700f
Ventilation-perfusion (Va/Q) inequality
    alveolar, hypoxemia from, 43
    gas exchange and, 42-43, 42f
Ventilation-perfusion matching, in preoperative
    evaluation, 869
Ventilator(s). See also Mechanical ventilation.
    "hybrid", 432
    ICU, typical, 431-432
    portable home, 432
Ventilator-associated pneumonia (VAP)
    bronchoscopy in, 158-159
    deaths related to, 322
    incidence of, 322
    pathogenesis of, 322
Ventilator-induced diaphragmatic dysfunction
    (VIDD), 58-59, 425-426
Ventilator-induced lung injury (VILI),
    422-428, 426f-427f
    in ARDS, 458-462
    mechanical ventilation–induced sepsis and,
        461-462
    multiple system organ dysfunction and, 461
    pathophysiology of, 459-460, 459f-460f
Ventilator-patient asynchrony, 412-413, 412f
Ventilatory control stability, in obstructive
    sleep apnea, 738-739
Ventilatory failure, in scoliosis, management of,
    761
Ventilatory impairment, in scoliosis,
    management of, 760-761
Ventilatory muscles, strength and endurance
    training for, in COPD, 558-559
Ventilatory therapy, physical modalities of, in
    COPD, 558-559
Ventral respiratory group (VRG) of neurons,
    50, 51f
Ventricle, right, function of, echocardiographic
    assessment of, 193-196, 195f-196f
Video-assisted mediastinal lymphadenectomy
    (VAMLA), 878
Video-assisted thoracoscopic surgery (VATS)
    lobectomy, 802
    diagnostic application of, 877t, 879-881,
        880f
VILI. See Ventilator-induced lung injury
    (VILI).
Viral infections
    childhood asthma and, 497-498
    in hematopoietic stem cell transplantation
        patients, 915-916
    in HIV patient, 357, 357f
        treatment of, 367-368
Viral pneumonia, 309-314
    clinical features of, 312
    clinical studies of, summary of, 310t
    community-acquired, 309
    controversies and pitfalls of, 314
    coronaviruses in, 311
    diagnosis of, 312-313, 313t
    human metapneumovirus in, 311

Viral pneumonia (Continued)
    in immunocompromised patients, 309
    influenza-related, primary, 311
    influenza viruses in, 309-311, 310t
    parainfluenza viruses 1, 2, and 3 in, 311
    pathogens in, 309-312
    respiratory syncytial virus in, 311
    rhinovirus in, 311-312
    treatment of, 313-314
    varicella-zoster virus in, 312
Virtual bronchoscopy, 163-164
Visceral larva migrans, 320
Visceral larva migrans syndrome, blood
    eosinophilia in, 622
Visceral pleura, 1
Vital capacity (VC), 21, 21f
    forced. See Forced vital capacity (FVC).
    in respiratory function testing, 59
    slow, 133-134
Vitamin K antagonists, for pulmonary
    embolism, 702
Volume-cycled ventilation, 406, 407f
Volume-targeted (-controlled) ventilation, 407,
    408f-409f
Vomiting, persistent, metabolic alkalosis from,
    48
von Recklinghausen disease, 857
Voriconazole, for invasive aspergillosis, 343t
VT. See Tidal volume (VT).
VTE. See Venous thromboembolism (VTE).

W

Weaning, from mechanical ventilation,
    428-429, 429f
    failure of, 429-430
    noninvasive ventilation and, 434
Weaponized agents, 688, 688t
Wegener granulomatosis (WG)
    with microscopic polyangiitis, therapy for,
        725
    pleural effusions secondary to, 829
Weight loss
    in COPD, 545
    in obstructive sleep apnea management,
        746-747
Weight reduction, for obesity hypoventilation
    syndrome, 753
Wheezing, in COPD, 546
White light bronchoscopy (WLB), 164
Whole-lung lavage, for pulmonary alveolar
    proteinosis, 672
Work-related asthma, 521. See also
    Occupational asthma (OA).

X

Xpert MTB-RIF, in TB diagnosis, 390

Y

Yersinia pestis, in community-acquired
    pneumonia, 301

Z

Zanamivir
    for viral lung infections, 339t
    for viral pneumonia, 313
Zone of apposition, 19, 53, 54f